HANDBOOK ON INJECTABLE DRUGS

17th EDITION

Lawrence A. Trissel

American Society of Health-System Pharmacists®
Bethesda, Maryland

LAWRENCE A. TRISSEL, F.A.S.H.P., is the author of the *Handbook on Injectable Drugs*.

Any correspondence regarding this publication should be sent to the publisher, American Society of Health-System Pharmacists®, 7272 Wisconsin Avenue, Bethesda, MD 20814, attn: Special Publishing.

The information presented herein reflects the opinions of the author and reviewers. It should not be interpreted as an official policy of ASHP or as an endorsement of any product.

Drug information and its applications are constantly evolving because of on-going research and clinical experience and are often subject to professional judgment and interpretation by the practitioner due to the uniqueness of a clinical situation. The author, reviewers, and ASHP have made every effort to ensure the accuracy and completeness of the information presented in this book. However, the reader is advised that the publisher, author, contributors, editors, and reviewers cannot be responsible for the continued currency of the information, for any errors or omissions, and/or for any consequences arising from the use of the information in the clinical setting.

The reader is cautioned that ASHP makes no representation, guarantee, or warranty, express or implied, that the use of the information contained in this book will prevent problems with insurers and will bear no responsibility or liability for the results or consequences of its use.

Senior Director, eHealth Solutions Division, Publications and Drug Information Systems Office: Jeffery Shick

Director of Product Development and Maintenance, eHealth Solutions Division, Publications and Drug Information Systems Office, and Clinical Informaticist: Edward D. Millikan

Production: Johnna Hershey

ISBN: 978-1-58528-378-1

To those pharmacists who understand that research
is *part of the mission of pharmacy,*
To Cyndi, for keeping the faith, never giving up, and reaching
for her dream,
and, as always,
To Pam, for her love, forbearance, and continuing support

"The end is nothing; the road is all."
Willa Seibert Cather

CONTENTS

ACKNOWLEDGMENTS

I would gratefully like to acknowledge the valuable contributions of the following individuals, who helped in the preparation and review of the seventeenth edition of the *Handbook on Injectable Drugs*:

WILLIAM J. DANA, Pharm.D., FASHP, Quality Assurance Pharmacist, Harris County Hospital District, Houston, Texas

N. PAULINE THOMAS PARKS, M.S., Consultant Pharmacist, Houston, Texas

WENDY D. SMITH, Pharm.D., BCPS, Clinical Pharmacy Specialist in Drug Information and Drug Use Policy, Division of Pharmacy, The University of Texas, M. D. Anderson Cancer Center, Houston, Texas

PREFACE

The *Handbook on Injectable Drugs*, 17th edition, is the most recent contribution in this continuing series. With its publication, all previous editions are considered out of date.

For proper use of this reference work, the reader must review the *How to Use the Handbook* section that immediately follows this preface. This section will acquaint the user of the *Handbook* with its organization, content, structure, summarization strategy, interpretation of the information presented, and limitations of the published literature on which the *Handbook* is based. Without a good working knowledge of these points, the *Handbook* may not be used to its best advantage or even interpreted correctly.

The 17th edition of the *Handbook on Injectable Drugs* brings together information on 332 parenteral drugs commercially available in the United States and in other countries. The information in the 17th edition is accumulated from 2830 references, including 42 new to this edition. As for each previous edition, the monographs have been completely updated. In addition to the updated monographs, two additional monographs on ceftaroline fosamil and telavancin hydrochloride are new to this edition. Also, some monograph reorganization and redundancy pruning has been performed to aid in use of the information, especially in electronic form.

Note of Appreciation

I want to thank a number of individuals who have helped in the creation of the many editions of the *Handbook on Injectable Drugs* over 35 years. Karen Hale, Dan Haas, Mary Baker, Todd Canada, William Dana, N. Pauline Thomas Parks, Wendy Smith, and Quanyun Xu contributed their time and talents to aid me in preparing difficult manuscripts. Their input has helped to make the *Handbook* a better resource for many editions. In addition, Shelly Elliott initially, then Johnna Hershey undertook and conducted the process that makes a book from a difficult manuscript and did so in exemplary form throughout these decades. Thanks to all for your help.

I also want to thank Dr. Roger Anderson who as head of the pharmacy at M. D. Anderson Cancer Center had the vision, foresight, and wisdom to establish the clinical pharmaceutics laboratory that for over 15 years conducted so much of the research, literally hundreds of studies, which contributed so much to our profession's knowledge of the clinical pharmaceutics of parenteral drugs. Unfortunately, those days were ended much too soon because new pharmacy management abruptly stopped our research. Although I am very pleased with what we were able to accomplish, I wish we would have had additional time so that we could have done more.

The individuals who worked so diligently on the numerous drug stability and compatibility research projects that we conducted in our clinical pharmaceutics laboratory in the pharmacy at the University of Texas, M. D. Anderson Cancer Center over those 15 years also deserve special recognition. The hundreds of studies that the following individuals helped to perform created many thousands of research results that are a substantial part of the world's knowledge base on the stabilities and compatibilities of parenteral drugs. Without the outstanding efforts of the individuals acknowledged below, the pharmacy profession in the United States and around the world would have much less of this information that is so valuable in patient care. Thanks to all of you.

Doward Gilbert, Pharm.D.
Delshalonda Ingram, Pharm.D.
Juan Martinez
Abayomi Ogundele, Pharm.D.
Christopher Saenz, Pharm.D.
Kimberly Williams, Pharm.D.
Quanyun Xu, Ph.D.
Yan-Ping Zhang, B.S. Pharm.

And of course my wife, Pam, and daughter, Cyndi, have had to endure the enormous time commitment that the *Handbook* represents 17 times over 35 years, not to mention all of the other manuscripts, books, and databases that have consumed my professional life. I recognize that I have spent much of our lives together with papers, proofs, and publishing deadlines that might have otherwise been spent with them. I have the deepest gratitude for their forbearance, tolerance, and support over many decades that have made my contribution to this work possible.

Final Words

I have spent many decades compiling, writing, revising, and proofing the various editions of *Handbook on Injectable Drugs* and all the other works. To me, the *Handbook* has been a calling, a bedrock professional activity that I have always made paramount, and a true labor of love. From my original conception and design and throughout the tens of thousands of hours spent preparing the many editions of this work, I have always wanted to provide this resource for the benefit of the members of our profession and the patients they serve.

I have thought of the *Handbook* as a principal professional undertaking and contribution that I was here to perform. In *Ecclesiastes IX. 10.* it is written "Whatsoever thy hand findeth to do, do it with thy might." I have tried to conduct all of my professional undertakings, including the *Handbook*, in a manner consistent with this statement. Though much sacrifice of my time and other life goals was required, I have been willing, indeed eager, to continue this difficult and demanding undertaking over all these years in the knowledge that my efforts were providing a useful and valuable informational resource in patient care. For those many individuals, colleagues, and friends who have expressed their gratitude for my efforts, it is I who am grateful. I am grateful for those kind words that have encouraged me throughout the endless procession of late nights and early mornings, weekends, holidays, and vacations, all seemingly countless in number, spent on this undertaking. And to the members of the profession of pharmacy, especially those "in the trenches" of patient care who have found the *Handbook* useful, I am glad I could help. Thank you for this opportunity to serve.

However, the time has come to pass on this cherished work to others who are to continue it in the years to come. Although I will not be a part of the future of the *Handbook*, I will always take pride in my contributions of the past. So thank you again my colleagues and friends. It has been a pleasure.

LAT
December 2011

HOW TO USE THE HANDBOOK

What Is the Handbook?

The *Handbook on Injectable Drugs* is a collection of summaries of information from the published literature on the pharmaceutics of parenteral medications as applied to the clinical setting. The *Handbook* is constructed from information derived from 2830 references with the information presented in the standardized structure described below. The purpose of the *Handbook* is to facilitate the use of this clinical pharmaceutics research by knowledgeable health care professionals for the benefit of patients. The summary information from published research is supplemented with information from the labeling of each product and from other references.

The information base summarized in the *Handbook on Injectable Drugs* is large and highly complex, requiring thoughtful consideration for proper use. The *Handbook* is not, nor should it be considered, elementary in nature or a primer. A single quick glance in a table is not adequate for proper interpretation of this highly complex information base. Proper interpretation includes the obvious need to consider and evaluate all relevant research information and results. Additionally, information on the formulation components, product attributes (especially pH), and the known stability behaviors of each parenteral drug, as well as the clinical situation of the patient, must be included in a thoughtful, reasoned evaluation of clinical pharmaceutics questions.

Who Should Use the Handbook?

The *Handbook on Injectable Drugs* is designed for use as a professional reference and guide to the literature on the clinical pharmaceutics of parenteral medications. The intended audience consists of knowledgeable health care professionals, particularly pharmacists, well versed in the formulation and clinical use of parenteral medications and who have the highly specialized knowledge base, training, and skills set necessary to interpret and apply the information. Practitioners who are not well versed in the formulation, essential properties, and clinical application of parenteral drugs should seek the assistance of more knowledgeable and experienced health care professionals to ensure patient safety.

Users of the *Handbook* must recognize that no reference work, including this one, can substitute for adequate decision-making by health care professionals. Proper clinical decisions must be made considering all aspects of the patient's condition and needs, with particular attention to the special demands imposed by parenteral medications. The *Handbook* cannot make decisions for its users. However, in knowledgeable hands, it is a valuable tool for the proper use of parenteral medications.

Organization of the Handbook

The *Handbook on Injectable Drugs* has been organized as a collection of monographs on each of the drugs. The monographs are arranged alphabetically by nonproprietary name. The names of the drugs follow the style of *USAN and the USP Dictionary of Drug Names*. Also included are some of the trade names and manufacturers of the drug products; this listing is not necessarily comprehensive and should not be considered an endorsement of any product or manufacturer.

All of the information included in the *Handbook* is referenced so that those who wish to study the original sources may find them. In addition, the *American Hospital Formulary Service* Classification System numbers have been included to facilitate the location of therapeutic information on the drugs.

The monographs have been divided into the subheadings described below:

Products—lists many of the sizes, strengths, volumes, and forms in which the drug is supplied, along with other components of the formulation. Instructions for reconstitution (when applicable) are included in this section.

The products cited do not necessarily constitute a comprehensive list of all available products. Rather, some common representative products are described. Furthermore, dosage forms, sizes, and container configurations of parenteral products may undergo significant changes during the lifespan of this edition of the *Handbook*.

Following the product descriptions, the pH of the drug products, the osmotic value(s) of the drug and/or dilutions (when available), and other product information such as the sodium content and definition of units are presented.

Practitioners have not always recognized the value and importance of incorporating product formulation information into the thought process that leads to their decision on handling drug compatibility and stability questions. However, consideration of the product information and formulation components as well as the properties and attributes of the products, especially pH, is essential to proper interpretation of the information presented in the *Handbook*.

Administration—includes route(s) by which the drug can be given, rates of administration (when applicable), and other related administration details.

The administration information is a condensation derived primarily from the product's official labeling and the *American Hospital Formulary Service*. For complete information, including dosage information sufficient for prescribing, the reader should refer to the official labeling and therapeutically comprehensive references such as the *American Hospital Formulary Service*.

Stability—describes the drug's stability and storage requirements. The storage condition terminology of *The United States Pharmacopeia*, 34th ed., is used in the *Handbook on Injectable Drugs*.

The United States Pharmacopeia defines controlled room temperature as "A temperature maintained thermostatically that encompasses the usual and customary working environment of 20 ° to 25 °; that results in a mean kinetic temperature calculated to be not more than 25 °; and that allows for excursions between 15 ° and 30 ° that are experienced in pharmacies, hospitals, and warehouses."[1] (All temperatures are Celsius.)

Protection from excessive heat is often required; excessive heat is defined as any temperature above 40 °C. Similarly, protection from freezing may be required for products that are subject to loss of strength or potency, or destructive alteration of their characteristics in addition to the risk of container breakage.[1]

Some products may require storage at a cool temperature, which is defined as any temperature between 8 and 15 °C, or a cold temperature, which is defined as any temperature not exceeding 8 °C. A refrigerator is defined as a cold place in which the temperature is maintained thermostatically between 2 and 8 °C. Freezer storage refers to a place in which the temperature is maintained thermostatically between −25 and −10 °C.[1]

In addition to storage requirements, aspects of drug stability related to pH, freezing, and exposure to light are presented in this section. Also presented is information on repackaging of the drugs or their dilutions in container/closure systems other than the original package (e.g., prefilling into syringes or in ambulatory pumps). Sorption and filtration

Table 1.
Solution Compatibility

Monograph drug name

Solution	Mfr	Mfr	Conc/L	Remarks	Ref	C/I
(1)	(2)	(3)	(4)	(5)	(6)	(7)

1. Solution in which the test was conducted.
2. Manufacturer of the solution.
3. Manufacturer of the drug about which the monograph is written.
4. Concentration of the drug about which the monograph is written.
5. Description of the results of the test.
6. Reference to the original source of the information.
7. Designation of the compatibility (C) or incompatibility (I) of the test result according to conventional guidelines.

Table 2.
Additive Compatibility

Monograph drug name

Drug	Mfr	Conc/L	Mfr	Conc/L	Test Soln	Remarks	Refs	C/I
(1)	(2)	(3)	(4)	(5)	(6)	(7)	(8)	(9)

1. Test drug.
2. Manufacturer of the test drug.
3. Concentration of the test drug.
4. Manufacturer of the drug about which the monograph is written.
5. Concentration of the drug about which the monograph is written.
6. Infusion solution in which the test was conducted.
7. Description of the results of the test.
8. Reference to the original source of the information.
9. Designation of the compatibility (C) or incompatibility (I) of the test result according to conventional guidelines.

Table 3.
Drugs in Syringe Compatibility

Monograph drug name

Drug (in syringe)	Mfr	Amt	Mfr	Amt	Remarks	Ref	C/I
(1)	(2)	(3)	(4)	(5)	(6)	(7)	(8)

1. Test drug.
2. Manufacturer of the test drug.
3. Actual amount of the test drug.
4. Manufacturer of the drug about which the monograph is written.
5. Actual amount of the drug about which the monograph is written.
6. Description of the results of the test.
7. Reference to the original source of the information.
8. Designation of the compatibility (C) or incompatibility (I) of the test result according to conventional guidelines.

Table 4.
Y-Site Injection Compatibility (1:1 Mixture)

Monograph drug name

Drug	Mfr	Conc	Mfr	Conc	Remarks	Ref	C/I
(1)	(2)	(3)	(4)	(5)	(6)	(7)	(8)

1. Test drug.
2. Manufacturer of the test drug.
3. Concentration of the test drug prior to mixing at the Y-site.
4. Manufacturer of the drug about which the monograph is written.
5. Concentration of the drug about which the monograph is written prior to mixing at the Y-site.
6. Description of the results of the test.
7. Reference to the original source of the information.
8. Designation of the compatibility (C) or incompatibility (I) of the test result according to conventional guidelines.

characteristics of the drugs are provided as well when this information is available. The information is derived principally from the primary published research literature and is supplemented by the product labeling and the *AHFS Drug Information*.

Compatibility Information—tabulates the results of published reports from primary research on the compatibility of the subject drug with infusion solutions and the other drugs. The various citations are listed alphabetically by solution or drug name; the information is completely cross-referenced among the monographs.

Four types of tables are utilized to present the available information, depending on the kind of test being reported. The first type is for information on the compatibility of a drug in various infusion solutions and is depicted in Table 1. The second type of table presents information on two or more drugs in intravenous solutions and is shown in Table 2. The third type of table is used for tests of two or more drugs in syringes and is shown in Table 3. The fourth table format is used for reports of simulated or actual injection into Y-sites and manifolds of administration sets and is shown in Table 4.

Many published articles, especially older ones, do not include all of the information necessary to complete the tables. However, the tables have been completed as fully as possible from the original articles.

Additional Compatibility Information—provides additional information and discussions of compatibility presented largely in narrative form.

Other Information—contains any relevant auxiliary information concerning the drug which does not fall into the previous categories.

The Listing of Concentration

The concentrations of all admixtures in intravenous solutions in the tables have been indicated in terms of concentration per liter to facilitate comparison of the various studies. In some cases, this may result in amounts of the drug that are greater or lesser than those normally administered (as when the recommended dose is tested in 100 mL of vehicle), but the listings do accurately reflect the actual concentrations tested, expressed in standardized terms.

For studies involving syringes, the amounts actually used are indicated. The volumes are also listed if indicated in the original article.

For studies of actual or simulated Y-site injection of drugs, the concentrations are cited in terms of concentration per milliliter of each drug solution prior to mixing at the Y-site. Most published research reports have presented the drug concentrations in this manner, and the *Handbook* follows this convention. For those few published reports that presented the drug concentrations after mixing at the Y-site, the concentrations have been recalculated to be consistent with the more common presentation style to maintain the consistency of presentation in the *Handbook*. Note that the Y-Site Injection Compatibility table is designed with the assumption of a 1:1 mixture of the subject drug and infusion solution or admixture. For citations reporting other than a 1:1 mixture, the actual amounts tested are specifically noted.

Designating Compatibility or Incompatibility

Each summary of a published research report appearing in the Compatibility Information tables bears a compatibility indicator (**C**, **I**, or **?**). A report receives a designation of **C** when the study results indicate that compatibility of the test samples existed under the test conditions. If the study determined an incompatibility existed under the test conditions, then an **I** designation is assigned for the *Handbook* entry for that study result. Specific standardized guidelines are used to assign these compatibility designations. The citation is designated as a report of com-

patibility when results of the original article indicated one or more of the following criteria were met:

1. Physical or visual compatibility of the combination was reported (no visible or electronically detected indication of particulate formation, haze, precipitation, color change, or gas evolution).
2. Stability of the components for at least 24 hours in an admixture under the specified conditions was reported (decomposition of 10% or less).
3. Stability of the components for the entire test period, although in some cases it was less than 24 hours, was reported (time periods less than 24 hours have been noted).

The citation is designated as a report of incompatibility when the results of the original article indicated either or both of the following criteria were met:

1. A physical or visual incompatibility was reported (visible or electronically detected particulate formation, haze, precipitation, color change, or gas evolution).
2. Greater than 10% decomposition of one or more components in 24 hours or less under the specified conditions was reported (time periods of less than 24 hours have been noted in the table).

Reports of test results that do not clearly fit into the compatibility or incompatibility definitions cannot be designated as either. These are indicated with a question mark.

Although these criteria have become the conventional definitions of compatibility and incompatibility, the reader should recognize that the criteria may need to be tempered with professional judgment. Inflexible adherence to the compatibility designations should be avoided. Instead, they should be used as aids in the exercising of professional judgment.

Therapeutic incompatibilities or other drug interactions are not within the scope of the *Handbook* and have not been included.

Interpreting Compatibility Information in the Handbook

As mentioned above, the body of information summarized in the *Handbook* is large and complicated. With the possible exception of a report of immediate gross precipitation, it usually takes some degree of thoughtful consideration and judgment to properly evaluate and appropriately act on the research results that are summarized in this book.

Nowhere is the need for judgment more obvious than when apparently contradictory information appears in two or more published reports. The body of literature in drug–drug and drug–vehicle compatibility is replete with apparently contradictory results. Except for study results that have been documented later to be incorrect, the conflicting information has been included in the *Handbook* to provide practitioners with all of the information for their consideration. The conflicting information will be readily apparent to the reader because of the content of the Remarks section as well as the **C**, **I**, and **?** designations following each citation.

Many or most of the apparently conflicting citations may be the result of differing conditions or materials used in the studies. A variety of factors that can influence the compatibility and stability of drugs must be considered in evaluating such conflicting results, and absolute statements are often difficult or impossible to make. Differences in concentrations, buffering systems, preservatives, vehicles, temperatures, and order of mixing may all play a role. By reviewing a variety of reports, the user of the *Handbook* is better able to exercise professional judgment with regard to compatibility and stability.

The reader must guard against misinterpretation of research results, which may lead to extensions of compatibility and stability that are inappropriate. As an example, a finding of precipitate formation two hours after two drugs are mixed does not imply nor should it be interpreted to mean that the combination is compatible until that time point, when a sudden precipitation occurs. Rather, it should be interpreted to mean that precipitation occurred at some point between mixing and the first observation point at two hours. Such a result would lead to a designation of incompatibility in the *Handbook*.

Precipitation reports can be particularly troublesome for practitioners to deal with because of the variability of the time frames in which they may occur. Apart from combinations that repeatedly result in immediate precipitation, the formation of a precipitate can be unpredictable to some degree. Numerous examples of variable precipitation time frames can be found in the literature, including paclitaxel, etoposide, and sulfamethoxazole–trimethoprim in infusion solutions and calcium and phosphates precipitation in parenteral nutrition mixtures. Differing drug concentrations can also play a role in creating variability in results. A good example of this occurs with co-administered vancomycin hydrochloride and beta-lactam antibiotics. Users of the information in the *Handbook* must always be aware that a marginally incompatible combination might exhibit precipitation earlier or later than that reported in the literature. In many such cases, the precipitation is ultimately going to occur, it is just the timing that is in question. This is of particular importance for precipitate formation because of the potential for serious adverse clinical consequences, including death, which have occurred. Certainly, users of the *Handbook* information should always keep in mind and anticipate the possibility of precipitation and its clinical ramifications. Furthermore, all injections and infusions should be inspected for particulate matter and discoloration. If found, they should be discarded.

In addition, many research reports cite test solutions or concentrations that may not be appropriate for clinical use. An example would be a report of a drug's stability in unsterile water. Although the *Handbook* summary will accurately reflect the test solutions and conditions that existed in a study, it is certainly inappropriate to misinterpret a stability report like this as being an authorization to use the product clinically. In such cases, the researchers may have used the clinically inappropriate diluent to evaluate the drug's stability for extrapolation to a more suitable vehicle that is similar, or they may not have recognized that the diluent is clinically unsuitable. In either event, it is incumbent on the practitioner in the clinical setting to use professional judgment to apply the information in an appropriate manner and recognize what is not acceptable clinically.

Further, it should be noted that many of the citations designated incompatible are not absolute. While a particular admixture may incur more than 10% decomposition within 24 hours, the combination may be useful for a shorter time period. The concept of "utility time" or the time to 10% decomposition may be useful in these cases. Unfortunately, such information is often not available. Included in the Remarks columns of the tables are the amount of decomposition, the time period involved, and the temperature at which the study was conducted when this information is available.

Users of the *Handbook* information should always keep in mind that the information in the *Handbook* must be used as a tool and a guide to the research that has been conducted and published. It is not a replacement for thoughtfully considered professional judgment. It falls to the practitioner to interpret the information in light of the clinical situation, including the patient's needs and status. What is certain is that relying solely on the **C** or **I** designation without the application of professional judgment is inappropriate.

Limitations of the Literature

In addition to conflicting information, many of the published articles have provided only partial evaluations, not looking at all aspects of a drug's stability and compatibility. This is not surprising considering the complexity, difficulty, and costs of conducting such research. There are, in fact, some articles that do provide evaluations of both physical stability/compatibility and chemical stability. But others are devoted only to physical issues, while others examine only chemical stability. Although a finding of precipitation, haze, or other physical effect may constitute an incompatibility (unless transient), the lack of such changes does not rule out chemical deterioration. In some cases, drugs initially designated as compatible because of a lack of visual change were later shown to undergo chemical decomposition. Similarly, the determination of chemical stability does not rule out the presence of unacceptable levels of particulates and/or turbidity in the combination. In a classic case, the drugs leucovorin calcium and fluorouracil were determined to be chemically stable for extended periods by stability-indicating HPLC assays in several studies, but years later, repeated episodes of filter clogging led to the discovery of unacceptable quantities of particulates in combinations of these drugs. The reader must always bear in mind these possibilities when only partial information is available.

And, finally, contemporary practitioners have come to expect that the analytical methods used in reports on the chemical stability of drugs will be validated stability-indicating methods. However, many early studies used methods that were not demonstrated to be stability indicating.

Literature Search for Updating the Handbook

To gather the bulk of the published compatibility and stability information for updating the *Handbook*, a literature search is performed using the *International Pharmaceutical Abstracts* database. By using key terms (e.g., stability), a listing of candidate articles for inclusion in the *Handbook* is generated. From this list, relevant articles are selected. As a supplement to this automated literature searching, a manual search of the references of the articles is also conducted, and any articles not included previously are obtained.

Reference

1. *The United States Pharmacopeia*, 34th ed. Rockville, MD: United States Pharmacopeial Convention; 2011.

Abbreviations

AA	Amino acids (percentage specified)
D	Dextrose solution (percentage unspecified)
D5LR	Dextrose 5% in Ringer's injection, lactated
D5R	Dextrose 5% in Ringer's injection
D–S	Dextrose–saline combinations
D2.5½S	Dextrose 2.5% in sodium chloride 0.45%
D2.5S	Dextrose 2.5% in sodium chloride 0.9%
D5¼S	Dextrose 5% in sodium chloride 0.225%
D5½S	Dextrose 5% in sodium chloride 0.45%
D5S	Dextrose 5% in sodium chloride 0.9%
D10S	Dextrose 10% in sodium chloride 0.9%
D5W	Dextrose 5%
D10W	Dextrose 10%
IM	Isolyte M
IP	Isolyte P
LR	Ringer's injection, lactated
NM	Normosol M
NR	Normosol R
NS	Sodium chloride 0.9%
R	Ringer's injections

REF	Refrigeration		BP	British Pharmacopoeia[a]
RT	Room temperature		BPC	British Pharmaceutical Codex[a]
S	Saline solution (percentage unspecified)		BR	Bristol
½S	Sodium chloride 0.45%		BRD	Bracco Diagnostics
SL	Sodium lactate ⅙ M		BRN	B. Braun
W	Sterile water for injection		BRT	Britianna

BT	Boots
BTK	Biotika
BV	Ben Venue
BW	Burroughs Wellcome
BX	Berlex

Manufacturer and Compendium Abbreviations

AB	Abbott		CA	Calmic
ABX	Abraxis		CAR	Cardinal Health
ACC	American Critical Care		CE	Carlo Erba
AD	Adria		CEN	Centocor
AGT	Aguettant		CER	Cerenex
AH	Allen & Hanburys		CET	Cetus
AHP	Ascot Hospital Pharmaceuticals		CH	Lab. Choay Societe Anonyme
AKN	Akorn		CHI	Chiron
ALP	Alpharma		CI	Ciba
ALT	Altana Pharma		CIS	CIS US
ALZ	Alza		CL	Clintec
AM	ASTA Medica		CN	Connaught
AMG	Amgen		CNF	Centrafarm
AMP	Amphastar		CO	Cole
AMR	American Regent		COR	COR Therapeutics
AMS	Amerisource		CP	Continental Pharma
AND	Andromaco		CPP	CP Pharmaceuticals
ANT	Antigen		CR	Critikon
AP	Asta-Pharma		CSL	CSL Ltd.
APC	Apothecon		CTI	Cell Therapeutics Inc.
APO	Apotex		CU	Cutter
APP	American Pharmaceutical Partners		CUB	Cubist
AQ	American Quinine		CUP	Cura Pharmaceuticals
AR	Armour		CUR	Curomed
ARC	American Red Cross		CY	Cyanamid
AS	Arnar-Stone		DAK	Dakota
ASC	Ascot		DB	David Bull Laboratories
ASP	Astellas Pharma		DCC	Dupont Critical Care
AST	Astra		DI	Dista
ASZ	AstraZeneca		DIA	Diamant
AT	Alpha Therapeutic		DM	Dome
AVE	Aventis		DME	Dupont Merck Pharma
AW	Asta Werke		DMX	Dumex
AY	Ayerst		DRA	Dr. Rentschler Arzneimittel
BA	Baxter		DU	DuPont
BB	B & B Pharmaceuticals		DUR	Dura
BAN	Banyu Pharmaceuticals		DW	Delta West
BAY	Bayer		EA	Eaton
BC	Bencard		EBE	Ebewe
BD	Becton Dickinson		ELN	Elan
BE	Beecham		EN	Endo
BED	Bedford		ENZ	Enzon
BEL	R. Bellon		ES	Elkins-Sinn
BFM	Bieffe Medital		ESL	ESI Lederle
BI	Boehringer Ingelheim		ESP	ESP Pharma
BIO	Bioniche Pharma		EST	Esteve
BK	Berk		EV	Evans
BKN	Baker Norton		EX	Essex
BM	Boehringer Mannheim		FA	Farmitalia
BMS	Bristol-Myers Squibb		FAN	Fandre Laboratories
BN	Breon			

FAU	Faulding		MAR	Marsam
FC	Frosst & Cie		MAY	Mayne Pharma
FED	Federa		MB	May & Baker
FER	Ferring		MDI	Medimmune
FI	Fisons		MDX	Medex
FOR	Forest Laboratories		ME	Merck
FP	Faro Pharma		MG	McGaw
FRE	Fresenius		MGI	MGI Pharma
FRK	Fresenius Kabi		MI	Miles
FUJ	Fujisawa		MJ	Mead Johnson
GEI	Geistich Pharma		MN	McNeil
GEM	Geneva-Marsam		MMD	Marion Merrell Dow
GEN	Genentech		MMT	Meridian Medical Technologies
GG	Geigy		MON	Monarch
GIL	Gilead		MRD	Merrill-Dow
GIU	Giulini		MRN	Merrill-National
GL	Glaxo		MSD	Merck Sharp & Dohme
GNS	Gensia-Sicor		MUN	Mundi Pharma
GO	Goedecke		MY	Maney
GRI	Grifols		MYR	Mayrhofer Pharmazeutika
GRP	Gruppo		NA	National
GRU	Grunenthal		NAB	Nabi
GSK	GlaxoSmithKline		NAP	NAPP Pharmaceuticals
GVA	Geneva		NCI	National Cancer Institute
GW	Glaxo Wellcome		NE	Norwich-Eaton
HAE	Haemonetics		NF	National Formulary[a]
HC	Hillcross		NO	Nordic
HMR	Hoechst Marion Roussel		NOP	Novopharm
HO	Hoechst-Roussel		NOV	Novo Pharm
HOS	Hospira		NVA	Novartis
HR	Horner		NVP	Nova Plus
HY	Hyland		NYC	Nycomed
ICI	ICI Pharmaceuticals		OHM	Ohmeda
ICN	ICN Pharmaceuticals		OM	Omega
IMM	Immunex		OMJ	OMJ Pharmaceuticals
IMS	IMS Ltd.		OMN	Ortho-McNeil
IN	Intra		ON	Orion
INT	Intermune		OR	Organon
IV	Ives		ORC	Orchid
IVX	Ivex		ORP	Orphan Medical
IX	Invenex		ORT	Ortho
JC	Janssen-Cilag		PAD	Paddock
JJ	Johnson & Johnson		PB	Pohl-Boskamp
JN	Janssen		PD	Parke-Davis
JP	Jones Pharma		PE	Pentagone
KA	Kabi		PF	Pfizer
KEY	Key Pharmaceuticals		PFM	Pfrimmer
KN	Knoll		PH	Pharmacia
KP	Kabi Pharmacia		PHC	Pharmachemie
KV	Kabi-Vitrum		PHS	Pharmascience
KY	Kyowa		PHT	Pharma-Tek
LA	Lagap		PHU	Pharmacia & Upjohn
LE	Lederle		PHX	Phoenix
LEM	Lemmon		PO	Poulenc
LEO	Leo Laboratories		PP	Pharmaceutical Partners
LI	Lilly		PR	Pasadena Research
LME	Laboratoire Meram		PRF	Pierre Fabre
LY	Lyphomed		PRK	Parkfields
LZ	Labaz Laboratories		PX	Pharmax
MA	Mallinckrodt		QLM	Qualimed Labs
MAC	Maco Pharma		QU	Quad

RB	Robins
RBP	Ribosepharm
RC	Roche
RI	Riker
RKB	Reckitt & Benckhiser
RKC	Reckitt & Colman
ROR	Rorer
ROX	Roxane
RP	Rhone-Poulenc
RPR	Rhone-Poulenc Rorer
RR	Roerig
RS	Roussel
RU	Rugby
SA	Sankyo
SAA	Sanofi Aventis
SAG	Sageant
SAN	Sanofi
SC	Schering
SCI	Scios
SCN	Schein
SCS	SCS Pharmaceuticals
SE	Searle
SEQ	Sequus
SER	Servier
SGS	SangStat
SHI	Shionogi
SIC	Sicor
SKB	SmithKline Beecham
SKF	Smith Kline & French
SM	Smith
SN	Smith + Nephew
SO	SoloPak
SQ	Squibb
SS	Sanofi-Synthelabo
ST	Sterilab
STP	Sterop
STR	Sterling
STS	Steris
STU	Stuart
SV	Savage
SW	Sanofi Winthrop
SX	Sabex
SY	Syntex

SYN	Synergen
SYO	Synthelabo
SZ	Sandoz
TAK	Takeda
TAP	TAP Holdings
TAY	Taylor
TE	Teva
TEC	Teclapharm
TL	Tillotts
TMC	The Medicines Company
TO	Torigian
TR	Travenol
UP	Upjohn
USB	US Bioscience
USP	United States Pharmacopeiea[a]
USV	USV Pharmaceuticals
UT	United Therapeutics
VHA	VHA Plus
VI	Vitarine
VIC	Vicuron Pharmaceuticals
VT	Vitrum
WAS	Wasserman
WAT	Watson
WAY	Wyeth-Ayerst
WB	Winthrop-Breon
WC	Warner-Chilcott
WED	Weddel
WEL	Wellcome
WI	Winthrop
WL	Warner Lambert
WOC	Wockhardt
WW	Westward
WY	Wyeth
XGN	X-Gen
YAM	Yamanouchi
ZEN	Zeneca
ZLB	ZLB Biopharma
ZNS	Zeneus Pharma

[a]*While reference to a compendium does not indicate the specific manufacturer of a product, it does help to indicate the formulation that was used in the test.*

Commercial Drug Monographs

ABCIXIMAB
AHFS 20:12.18

Products — Abciximab is available as a 2-mg/mL solution, which also contains 0.01 M sodium phosphate, 0.15 M sodium chloride, and 0.001% polysorbate 80 in water for injection. (1)

pH — 7.2. (1)

Trade Name(s) — ReoPro.

Administration — Abciximab is administered by direct intravenous injection or by intravenous infusion using a controlled infusion device after dilution in dextrose 5% or sodium chloride 0.9%. (1; 4)

Stability — The clear, colorless injection in intact vials should be stored under refrigeration and protected from freezing. The vials should not be shaken. No incompatibilities with glass bottles or PVC containers and sets have been observed. (1; 4)

Although refrigerated storage is required, the manufacturer states that the drug may be stored at room temperature for eight days. (2745)

Filtration — The manufacturer recommends filtration through a low protein-binding 0.2- or 5-μm filter during preparation of an intravenous infusion or using a 0.2- or 0.22-μm inline filter during administration. The manufacturer also recommends using a low protein-binding 0.2- or 5-μm syringe filter for bolus doses. (1)

Compatibility Information

Y-Site Injection Compatibility (1:1 Mixture)

Abciximab

Drug	Mfr	Conc	Mfr	Conc	Remarks	Ref	C/I
Adenosine	FUJ	3 mg/mL	LI	36 mcg/mL[a]	Visually compatible for 12 hr at 23 °C	2374	C
Argatroban	GSK	1 mg/mL[a,b,c]	LI	36 mcg/mL[a,b,c]	Physically compatible with no loss of argatroban in 4 hr at 23 °C. Abciximab not tested	2630	C
Atropine sulfate	AMR	0.4 mg/mL	LI	36 mcg/mL[a]	Visually compatible for 12 hr at 23 °C	2374	C
Bivalirudin	TMC	5 mg/mL[a]	CEN	10 mcg/mL[a]	Physically compatible for 4 hr at 23 °C	2373	C
Diphenhydramine HCl	ES	25 mg/mL	LI	36 mcg/mL[a]	Visually compatible for 12 hr at 23 °C	2374	C
Fentanyl citrate	AB	50 mcg/mL	LI	36 mcg/mL[a]	Visually compatible for 12 hr at 23 °C	2374	C
Metoprolol tartrate	AB	1 mg/mL	LI	36 mcg/mL[a]	Visually compatible for 12 hr at 23 °C	2374	C
Midazolam HCl	BED	2 mg/mL	LI	36 mcg/mL[a]	Visually compatible for 12 hr at 23 °C	2374	C

[a]Tested in dextrose 5%.
[b]Tested in sodium chloride 0.9%.
[c]Mixed argatroban:abciximab 1:1 and 4:1.

ACETAZOLAMIDE SODIUM
AHFS 52:40.12

Products — Acetazolamide as the sodium salt is available in 500-mg vials with sodium hydroxide and, if necessary, hydrochloric acid to adjust the pH. Reconstitute the vial with at least 5 mL of sterile water for injection to yield a solution containing not more than 100 mg/mL. (1)

pH — Approximately 9.6. (1)

Osmolality — The osmolality of acetazolamide sodium 500 mg was calculated for the following dilutions (1054):

Diluent	Osmolality (mOsm/kg)	
	50 mL	100 mL
Dextrose 5%	321	291
Sodium chloride 0.9%	348	317

Sodium Content — 2.049 mEq/500 mg (calculated). (846)

Trade Name(s) — Diamox Sodium.

Administration — Administration by direct intravenous injection is preferred. Intramuscular injection is painful due to the alkaline pH and is not recommended. (1; 4)

Stability — Store intact vials at controlled room temperature. (4) The manufacturer states that the reconstituted solution is stable for three days if refrigerated or for 12 hours at room temperature. (1) Other information indicates that the reconstituted solution is stable for one week under refrigeration. However, because the product contains no preservatives, use of the solution within 24 hours after reconstitution is recommended. (4)

pH Effects — The stability of acetazolamide sodium in aqueous solution appears to decrease as the pH increases above 9. At pH 8.8, a 0.25-mg/mL solution retained 96% of the initial amount after three days at 25 °C; at pH 10.8 and 12.7, the remaining drug was 88 and 83%, respectively, after four days. (1230) Acetazolamide exhibits maximum stability at pH 4. (1424)

Sorption — Acetazolamide sodium was shown not to exhibit sorption to PVC bags and tubing, polyethylene tubing, Silastic tubing, and polypropylene syringes. (536; 606)

Compatibility Information

Solution Compatibility

Acetazolamide sodium

Solution	Mfr	Mfr	Conc/L	Remarks	Ref	C/I
Dextrose–Ringer's injection combinations	AB	LE	375 mg	Physically compatible	3	C
Dextrose–Ringer's injection, lactated, combinations	AB	LE	375 mg	Physically compatible	3	C
Dextrose–saline combinations	AB	LE	375 mg	Physically compatible	3	C
Dextrose 2.5%	AB	LE	375 mg	Physically compatible	3	C
Dextrose 5%	AB	LE	375 mg	Physically compatible	3	C
	TR[a]	LE	375 mg	Physically compatible. Losses of 7% in 5 days at 25 °C, 5% in 44 days at 5 °C, and 3% in 44 days at −10 °C	1085	C
Dextrose 10%	AB	LE	375 mg	Physically compatible	3	C
Ionosol products	AB	LE	375 mg	Physically compatible	3	C
Ringer's injection	AB	LE	375 mg	Physically compatible	3	C
Ringer's injection, lactated	AB	LE	375 mg	Physically compatible	3	C
Sodium chloride 0.45%	AB	LE	375 mg	Physically compatible	3	C
Sodium chloride 0.9%	AB	LE	375 mg	Physically compatible	3	C
	TR[a]	LE	375 mg	Physically compatible. Losses of 7% in 5 days at 25 °C, 5% in 44 days at 5 °C, and 3% in 44 days at −10 °C	1085	C
Sodium lactate ⅙ M	AB	LE	375 mg	Physically compatible	3	C

[a]Tested in PVC containers.

Additive Compatibility

Acetazolamide sodium

Drug	Mfr	Conc/L	Mfr	Conc/L	Test Soln	Remarks	Ref	C/I
Ranitidine HCl	GL	50 mg and 2 g		5 g	D5W	Physically compatible. Ranitidine stable for 24 hr at 25 °C. Acetazolamide not tested	1515	C

Drugs in Syringe Compatibility

Acetazolamide sodium

Drug (in syringe)	Mfr	Amt	Mfr	Amt	Remarks	Ref	C/I
Pantoprazole sodium	a	4 mg/1 mL		100 mg/1 mL	Clear solution	2574	C

[a]*Test performed using the formulation WITHOUT edetate disodium.*

Y-Site Injection Compatibility (1:1 Mixture)

Acetazolamide sodium

Drug	Mfr	Conc	Mfr	Conc	Remarks	Ref	C/I
Diltiazem HCl	MMD	5 mg/mL	LE	100 mg/mL	Precipitate forms	1807	I
	MMD	1 mg/mL[b]	LE	100 mg/mL	Visually compatible	1807	C
TPN #203, #204[a]			LE	100 mg/mL	White precipitate forms immediately	1974	I

[a]*Refer to Appendix I for the composition of parenteral nutrition solutions. TPN indicates a 2-in-1 admixture.*
[b]*Tested in sodium chloride 0.9%.*

ACETYLCYSTEINE
AHFS 92:12

Products — Acetylcysteine injection is available in 30-mL single-dose vials as a preservative-free concentrated solution containing 200 mg/mL of drug. Each milliliter also contains sodium hydroxide to adjust pH. This concentrate must be diluted for use. (1)

pH — 6 to 7.5. (1)

Osmolarity — Acetylcysteine injection has an osmolarity of 2600 mOsm/L. (1)

Trade Name(s) — Acetadote.

Administration — Acetylcysteine injection is a concentrate that must be diluted for intravenous infusion. The manufacturer recommends that for patients weighing 40 kg or more a loading dose be added to 200 mL for infusion over 60 minutes. Subsequently, a first maintenance dose should be mixed in 500 mL delivered over 4 hours. The second maintenance dose should be mixed in 1 L delivered over 16 hours. (1)

The total volume must be adjusted for patients under 40 kg and fluid-restricted patients. For patients less than 40 kg but more than 20 kg, the manufacturer recommends a loading dose be added to 100 mL for infusion over 60 minutes. Subsequently, a first maintenance dose should be mixed in 250 mL and delivered over 4 hours. The second maintenance dose should be mixed in 500 mL and delivered over 16 hours. (1)

For patients weighing 20 kg or less, the manufacturer recommends a loading dose be diluted in 3 mL/kg of body weight for infusion over 60 minutes. Subsequently, a first maintenance dose should be mixed in 7 mL/kg of body weight and delivered over 4 hours. The second maintenance dose should be mixed in 14 mL/kg of body weight and delivered over 16 hours. (1)

Acetylcysteine is a reducing agent and is not compatible with oxidizing agents. The drug is incompatible with rubber, and some metals such as iron and copper, liberating hydrogen sulfide gas. Consequently, the use of preparation and administration equipment composed of plastic, glass, and stainless steel or other unreactive metal is recommended. (4)

Stability — Store intact vials of acetylcysteine injection at room temperature. The vials are for single use, and previously opened vials should be discarded and not used. The manufacturer states that the color of acetylcysteine injection may vary from colorless to slight pink or purple after stopper penetration, but this color change does not indicate an adverse effect on drug quality. (1)

Compatibility Information

Solution Compatibility

Acetylcysteine

Solution	Mfr	Mfr	Conc/L	Remarks	Ref	C/I
Dextrose 5%				Compatible for 24 hr at room temperature	1	C
Sodium chloride 0.45%				Compatible for 24 hr at room temperature	1	C

Y-Site Injection Compatibility (1:1 Mixture)

Acetylcysteine

Drug	Mfr	Conc	Mfr	Conc	Remarks	Ref	C/I
Cefepime HCl	BMS	120 mg/mL		100 mg/mL	Over 10% cefepime loss occurs in 1 hr	2513	I
Ceftazidime	GSK	120 mg/mL		100 mg/mL	Over 10% ceftazidime loss occurs in 1 hr	2513	I

ACYCLOVIR SODIUM
AHFS 8:18.32

Products — Acyclovir sodium is available in vials containing 500 mg or 1 g of acyclovir as the sodium salt. Reconstitute the 500-mg vial with 10 mL and the 1-g vial with 20 mL of sterile water for injection; shake well to ensure complete dissolution. Do not use bacteriostatic water for injection containing parabens or benzyl alcohol for reconstitution. The acyclovir concentration in the reconstituted solution is 50 mg/mL; the reconstituted solution must be diluted to a concentration of 7 mg/mL or less for use. (1)

pH — The reconstituted solution has a pH of approximately 11. (1; 4)

Osmolality — The osmolality of acyclovir sodium 500 mg was calculated for the following dilutions (1054):

Diluent	Osmolality (mOsm/kg)	
	50 mL	100 mL
Dextrose 5%	316	289
Sodium chloride 0.9%	342	316

The osmolality of acyclovir sodium 7 mg/mL was determined to be 278 mOsm/kg in dextrose 5% and 299 mOsm/kg in sodium chloride 0.9%. (1375)

Sodium Content — Acyclovir sodium (Glaxo Wellcome) contains 4.2 mEq of sodium per gram of drug. (4)

Administration — Acyclovir sodium is administered by slow intravenous infusion at concentrations of 7 mg/mL or less over a period of one hour. Rapid intravenous administration and administration by other routes must be avoided. (1; 4)

Stability — Intact vials of acyclovir sodium should be stored at controlled room temperature. The reconstituted solution should be used within 12 hours. Refrigeration of the reconstituted solution may cause a precipitate, but this precipitate will dissolve at room temperature, apparently without affecting potency. After dilution for administration, the dose may be stored at room temperature; it should be used within 24 hours. (1; 4) However, storage of acyclovir admixtures at room temperature does not guarantee that no precipitate will form. Precipitation has also been observed in acyclovir sodium infusions in PVC containers after a few days' storage at room temperature. (2190)

If acyclovir sodium is diluted in solutions with dextrose concentrations greater than 10%, a yellow discoloration may appear. This discoloration does not affect the drug's potency. (4)

Acyclovir sodium reconstituted with bacteriostatic water for injection containing benzyl alcohol is as stable as when reconstituted with unpreserved sterile water for injection. However, the manufacturer recommends not using the benzyl alcohol-containing diluent because of concerns about the risks to neonates. The paraben-containing form of bacteriostatic water for injection must not be used for reconstitution because of the potential for precipitate formation. (4)

Precipitation — Short-term refrigerated storage of acyclovir sodium admixtures with concentrations exceeding 1 mg/mL may result in formation of a precipitate that redissolves upon warming to room temperature. However, such solutions should be used immediately after warming to room temperature because of the subsequent appearance of persistent microprecipitates. (2098)

Physical instability is the principal limitation to long-term storage of acyclovir sodium admixtures. Persistent subvisual microprecipitate formation as well as frank persistent precipitation may occur in variable time periods. Such precipitation has been reported to occur after as little as seven days and in varying time periods throughout a 35-day observation period; the appearance of a precipitate is not precisely predictable. (2098)

The formation of large amounts of subvisual particulates has been attributed to an interaction of the highly alkaline acyclovir sodium solution with PVC containers. Some increase in the number of particulates was observed in as little as one day, with substantial increases in seven days. When packaged in ethylene vinyl acetate (EVA) containers, no significant increase in subvisual particulates occurs, even after 28 days of storage. (2190)

Syringes — Acyclovir sodium (American Pharmaceutical Partners) 10 mg/mL in sodium chloride 0.9% and packaged in polypropylene syringes (Becton-Dickinson) was found to be stable for 30 days at room temperature but precipitated in 5 days under refrigeration. (2558)

Sorption — Acyclovir sodium was shown not to exhibit sorption to PVC, polyethylene, and glass containers as well as elastomeric reservoirs. (2014; 2289)

Central Venous Catheter — Acyclovir sodium (GlaxoWellcome) 1 mg/mL in dextrose 5% was found to be compatible with the ARROWg+ard Blue Plus (Arrow International) chlorhexidine-bearing triple-lumen central catheter. Essentially complete delivery of the drug was found with little or no drug loss occurring. Furthermore, chlorhexidine delivered from the catheter remained at trace amounts with no substantial increase due to the delivery of the drug through the catheter. (2335)

Compatibility Information

Solution Compatibility

Acyclovir sodium

Solution	Mfr	Mfr	Conc/L	Remarks	Ref	C/I
Dextrose 5%	TR[a]	BW	5 g	Visually compatible with no loss in 37 days at 25 and 5 °C	1343	C
	BA[a]	BW	1 g	Physically compatible with no loss after 35 days at 23 °C and after 35 days at 4 °C followed by 2 days at 23 °C protected from light	2098	C
	BA[a]	BW	7 g	Physically compatible with 3% or less loss after 28 days at 23 °C protected from light. Subvisible microprecipitate forms by 35 days	2098	C
	BA[a]	BW	7 g	Precipitate forms on refrigeration that redissolves on warming. No loss after 35 days at 4 °C protected from light, but subvisible precipitate forms after 2 more days at 23 °C	2098	C
	BA[a]	BW	10 g	Physically compatible with no loss after 21 days at 23 °C protected from light. Subvisible microprecipitate forms in 28 days, and visible precipitate forms in 35 days	2098	C
	BA[a]	BW	10 g	Precipitate forms on refrigeration that redissolves on warming. No loss after 35 days at 4 °C protected from light, but subvisible precipitate forms after 2 more days at 23 °C	2098	C
	BA[a], BRN[c]	GW	5 g	Visually compatible with little or no loss in 24 hr at 4 and 22 °C	2289	C
Sodium chloride 0.9%	TR[a]	BW	5 g	No loss in 37 days at 25 and 5 °C. Storage at 5 °C resulted in white precipitate that dissolved on warming to 25 °C	1343	C
	BA[a]	BW	1, 7, 10 g	Physically compatible with no loss after 7 days at 23 °C protected from light. Visible precipitate formed within 14 days	2098	C
	BA[a]	BW	1, 7, 10 g	Physically compatible with no loss after 35 days at 4 °C followed by 2 days at 23 °C protected from light	2098	C
	BA[a]	WEL	2.5 and 5 g	No loss in 28 days at 25 °C, but subvisible particulates increase significantly after 7 days due to interaction with PVC containers	2190	C
	BA[b]	WEL	2.5 and 5 g	No loss and little change in subvisible particulates in 28 days at 25 °C	2190	C
	BA[a], BRN[c]	GW	5 g	Visually compatible with little or no loss in 24 hr at 4 and 22 °C	2289	C

[a]Tested in PVC containers.
[b]Tested in ethylene vinyl acetate (EVA) containers.
[c]Tested in polyethylene and glass containers.

Additive Compatibility

Acyclovir sodium

Drug	Mfr	Conc/L	Mfr	Conc/L	Test Soln	Remarks	Ref	C/I
Dobutamine HCl	LI	0.5 g	BW	2.5 g	D5W	Discoloration in 25 min. Cloudiness and brown color in 2 hr due to dobutamine oxidation. No acyclovir loss	1343	I

Additive Compatibility (Cont.)

Acyclovir sodium

Drug	Mfr	Conc/L	Mfr	Conc/L	Test Soln	Remarks	Ref	C/I
Dopamine HCl	SO	0.8 g	BW	2.5 g	D5W	Yellow color developed in 1.5 hr due to dopamine oxidation. No acyclovir loss	1343	I
Fluconazole	PF	1 g	BW	5 g	D5W	Visually compatible with no fluconazole loss in 72 hr at 25 °C under fluorescent light. Acyclovir not tested	1677	C
Meropenem	ZEN	1 g	BW	5 g	NS	Visually compatible for 4 hr at room temperature	1994	C
	ZEN	20 g	BW	5 g	NS	Precipitates immediately	1994	I
Tramadol HCl	GRU	400 mg	WEL	5 g	NS	Precipitation and 20% tramadol loss in 1 hr	2652	I

Drugs in Syringe Compatibility

Acyclovir sodium

Drug (in syringe)	Mfr	Amt	Mfr	Amt	Remarks	Ref	C/I
Caffeine citrate		20 mg/ 1 mL	BW	50 mg/ 1 mL	Precipitates immediately	2440	I
Pantoprazole sodium	[a]	4 mg/ 1 mL		50 mg/ 1 mL	Precipitates within 4 hr	2574	I

[a]Test performed using the formulation WITHOUT edetate disodium.

Y-Site Injection Compatibility (1:1 Mixture)

Acyclovir sodium

Drug	Mfr	Conc	Mfr	Conc	Remarks	Ref	C/I
Allopurinol sodium	BW	3 mg/mL[b]	BW	7 mg/mL[b]	Physically compatible for 4 hr at 22 °C	1686	C
Amifostine	USB	10 mg/mL[a]	BW	7 mg/mL[a]	Subvisible needles form in 1 hr. Visible particles form in 4 hr	1845	I
Amikacin sulfate	BR	5 mg/mL[a]	BW	5 mg/mL[a]	Physically compatible for 4 hr at 25 °C	1157	C
Amphotericin B cholesteryl sulfate complex	SEQ	0.83 mg/mL[a]	GW	7 mg/mL[a]	Physically compatible for 4 hr at 23 °C	2117	C
Ampicillin sodium	WY	20 mg/mL[b]	BW	5 mg/mL[a]	Physically compatible for 4 hr at 25 °C	1157	C
Amsacrine	NCI	1 mg/mL[a]	BW	7 mg/mL[a]	Immediate dark orange turbidity, becoming brownish orange in 1 hr	1381	I
Anidulafungin	VIC	0.5 mg/mL[a]	APP	7 mg/mL[a]	Physically compatible for 4 hr at 23 °C	2617	C
Aztreonam	SQ	40 mg/mL[a]	BW	7 mg/mL[a]	White needles form immediately and become dense precipitate in 4 hr	1758	I
Caspofungin acetate	ME	0.7 mg/mL[b]	BV	7 mg/mL[b]	Physically compatible for 4 hr at room temperature	2758	C
	ME	0.5 mg/mL[b]	BED	5 mg/mL[b]	Fine clear crystals reported	2766	I
Cefazolin sodium	SKF	20 mg/mL[a]	BW	5 mg/mL[a]	Physically compatible for 4 hr at 25 °C	1157	C
Cefotaxime sodium	HO	20 mg/mL[a]	BW	5 mg/mL[a]	Physically compatible for 4 hr at 25 °C	1157	C
Cefoxitin sodium	MSD	20 mg/mL[a]	BW	5 mg/mL[a]	Physically compatible for 4 hr at 25 °C	1157	C

Y-Site Injection Compatibility (1:1 Mixture) (Cont.)

Acyclovir sodium

Drug	Mfr	Conc	Mfr	Conc	Remarks	Ref	C/I
Ceftaroline fosamil	FOR	2.22 mg/mL[a,b,g]	BV	7 mg/mL[a,b,g]	Physically compatible for 4 hr at 23 °C	2826	C
Ceftazidime	SKF	20 mg/mL[a]	BW	5 mg/mL[a]	Physically compatible for 4 hr at 25 °C	1157	C
Ceftriaxone sodium	RC	20 mg/mL[a]	BW	5 mg/mL[a]	Physically compatible for 4 hr at 25 °C	1157	C
Cefuroxime sodium	GL	15 mg/mL[a]	BW	5 mg/mL[a]	Physically compatible for 4 hr at 25 °C	1157	C
Chloramphenicol sodium succinate	ES	20 mg/mL[a]	BW	5 mg/mL[a]	Physically compatible for 4 hr at 25 °C	1157	C
Cisatracurium besylate	GW	0.1 and 2 mg/mL[a]	BW	7 mg/mL[a]	Physically compatible for 4 hr at 23 °C	2074	C
	GW	5 mg/mL[i]	BW	7 mg/mL[a]	White cloudiness forms immediately	2074	I
Clindamycin phosphate	UP	12 mg/mL[a]	BW	5 mg/mL[a]	Physically compatible for 4 hr at 25 °C	1157	C
Cyclosporine	BED	1 mg/mL[a]	BV	5 mg/mL[b]	Crystals form	2794	I
Dexamethasone sodium phosphate	ES	0.2 mg/mL[a]	BW	5 mg/mL[a]	Physically compatible for 4 hr at 25 °C	1157	C
	APP	4 mg/mL	BV	5 mg/mL[b]	Physically compatible	2794	C
Diltiazem HCl	MMD	5 mg/mL	BW	5[a] and 7[b] mg/mL	Cloudiness and precipitate form	1807	I
	MMD	1 mg/mL[b]	BW	5[a] and 7[b] mg/mL	Visually compatible	1807	C
Dimenhydrinate	SE	1 mg/mL[a]	BW	5 mg/mL[a]	Physically compatible for 4 hr at 25 °C	1157	C
Diphenhydramine HCl	ES	1 mg/mL[a]	BW	5 mg/mL[a]	Physically compatible for 4 hr at 25 °C	1157	C
	BA	50 mg/mL	BV	5 mg/mL[b]	Cloudy upon mixing	2794	I
Dobutamine HCl	LI	1 mg/mL[a]	BW	5 mg/mL[a]	Cloudy and brown in 1 hr at 25 °C	1157	I
Docetaxel	RPR	0.9 mg/mL[a]	GW	7 mg/mL[a]	Physically compatible for 4 hr at 23 °C	2224	C
Dopamine HCl	AB	1.6 mg/mL[a]	BW	5 mg/mL[a]	Solution turns dark brown in 2 hr at 25 °C	1157	I
Doripenem	JJ	5 mg/mL[a,b]	BED	7 mg/mL[a,b]	Physically compatible for 4 hr at 23 °C	2743	C
Doxorubicin HCl liposomal	SEQ	0.4 mg/mL[a]	GW	7 mg/mL[a]	Physically compatible for 4 hr at 23 °C	2087	C
Doxycycline hyclate	PF	1 mg/mL[a]	BW	5 mg/mL[a]	Physically compatible for 4 hr at 25 °C	1157	C
Droperidol	MDX	2.5 mg/mL	BV	5 mg/mL[b]	Physically compatible	2794	C
Erythromycin lactobionate	AB	4 mg/mL[a]	BW	5 mg/mL[a]	Physically compatible for 4 hr at 25 °C	1157	C
Etoposide phosphate	BR	5 mg/mL[a]	GW	7 mg/mL[a]	Physically compatible for 4 hr at 23 °C	2218	C
Famotidine	ME	2 mg/mL[b]		7 mg/mL[a]	Visually compatible for 4 hr at 22 °C	1936	C
Fentanyl citrate	HOS	50 mcg/mL	BV	5 mg/mL[b]	Physically compatible	2794	C
Filgrastim	AMG	30 mcg/mL[a]	BW	7 mg/mL[a]	Physically compatible for 4 hr at 22 °C	1687	C
Fluconazole	RR	2 mg/mL	BW	10 mg/mL	Physically compatible for 24 hr at 25 °C	1407	C
Fludarabine phosphate	BX	1 mg/mL[a]	BW	7 mg/mL[a]	Color darkens within 4 hr	1439	I
Foscarnet sodium	AST	24 mg/mL	BW	10 mg/mL	Precipitates immediately	1335	I
	AST	24 mg/mL	BW	7 mg/mL[c]	Acyclovir crystals form immediately	1393	I
Gallium nitrate	FUJ	1 mg/mL[b]	BW	7 mg/mL[b]	Visually compatible for 24 hr at 25 °C	1673	C
Gemcitabine HCl	LI	10 mg/mL[b]	GW	7 mg/mL[b]	Gross precipitation occurs immediately	2226	I
Gentamicin sulfate	TR	1.6 mg/mL[a]	BW	5 mg/mL[a]	Physically compatible for 4 hr at 25 °C	1157	C
	AMS	30 mg/mL[i]	BV	5 mg/mL[b]	White paste-like precipitate	2794	I
Granisetron HCl	SKB	0.05 mg/mL[a]	BW	7 mg/mL[a]	Physically compatible for 4 hr at 23 °C	2000	C
	RC	1 mg/mL	BV	5 mg/mL[b]	Crystals form	2794	I

Y-Site Injection Compatibility (1:1 Mixture) (Cont.)

Acyclovir sodium

Drug	Mfr	Conc	Mfr	Conc	Remarks	Ref	C/I
Heparin sodium	ES	50 units/mL[a]	BW	5 mg/mL[a]	Physically compatible for 4 hr at 25 °C	1157	C
	BD	100 units/mL	BV	5 mg/mL[b]	Physically compatible	2794	C
Hydrocortisone sodium succinate	LY	1 mg/mL[a]	BW	5 mg/mL[a]	Physically compatible for 4 hr at 25 °C	1157	C
Hydromorphone HCl	WB	0.04 mg/mL[a]	BW	5 mg/mL[a]	Physically compatible for 4 hr at 25 °C	1157	C
Idarubicin HCl	AD	1 mg/mL[b]	BW	5 mg/mL[b]	Haze forms and color changes immediately. Precipitate forms in 12 min	1525	I
Imipenem–cilastatin sodium	MSD	5 mg/mL[b]	BW	5 mg/mL[a]	Physically compatible for 4 hr at 25 °C	1157	C
Levofloxacin	OMN	5 mg/mL[a]	BW	50 mg/mL	Cloudy precipitate forms	2233	I
Linezolid	PHU	2 mg/mL[a]	APP	7 mg/mL[a]	Physically compatible for 4 hr at 23 °C	2264	C
Lorazepam	WY	0.04 mg/mL[a]	BW	5 mg/mL[a]	Physically compatible for 4 hr at 25 °C	1157	C
Magnesium sulfate	LY	20 mg/mL[a]	BW	5 mg/mL[a]	Physically compatible for 4 hr at 25 °C	1157	C
Melphalan HCl	BW	0.1 mg/mL[b]	BW	7 mg/mL[b]	Physically compatible for 3 hr at 22 °C	1557	C
Meperidine HCl	WB	1 mg/mL[a]	BW	5 mg/mL[a]	Physically compatible for 4 hr at 25 °C	1157	C
	AB	10 mg/mL	BW	5 mg/mL[a]	White crystalline precipitate forms within 1 hr at 25 °C	1397	I
	WY	100 mg/mL	BW	5 mg/mL[c]	Visually compatible for 24 hr at room temperature in test tubes. No precipitate found on filter from Y-site delivery	2063	C
Meropenem	ZEN	1 mg/mL[b]	BW	5 mg/mL[d]	Visually compatible for 4 hr at room temperature	1994	C
	ZEN	50 mg/mL[b]	BW	5 mg/mL[d]	Precipitate forms	2068	I
Methylprednisolone sodium succinate	LY	0.8 mg/mL[a]	BW	5 mg/mL[a]	Physically compatible for 4 hr at 25 °C	1157	C
Metoclopramide HCl	ES	0.2 mg/mL[a]	BW	5 mg/mL[a]	Physically compatible for 4 hr at 25 °C	1157	C
	SIC	5 mg/mL	BV	5 mg/mL[b]	Crystals form	2794	I
Metronidazole	SE	5 mg/mL	BW	5 mg/mL[a]	Physically compatible for 4 hr at 25 °C	1157	C
Milrinone lactate	SS	0.2 mg/mL[a]	APP	7 mg/mL[a]	Visually compatible for 4 hr at 25 °C	2381	C
Morphine sulfate	WB	0.08 mg/mL[a]	BW	5 mg/mL[a]	Physically compatible for 4 hr at 25 °C	1157	C
	AB	1 mg/mL	BW	5 mg/mL[a]	Precipitate forms in 2 hr at 25 °C	1397	I
Multivitamins	LY	0.01 mL/mL[a]	BW	5 mg/mL[a]	Physically compatible for 4 hr at 25 °C	1157	C
Nafcillin sodium	WY	20 mg/mL[a]	BW	5 mg/mL[a]	Physically compatible for 4 hr at 25 °C	1157	C
Nalbuphine HCl	HOS	10 mg/mL	BV	5 mg/mL[b]	Physically compatible	2794	C
Ondansetron HCl	GL	1 mg/mL[b]	BW	7 mg/mL[a]	Precipitates immediately	1365	I
Oxacillin sodium	BE	20 mg/mL[a]	BW	5 mg/mL[a]	Physically compatible for 4 hr at 25 °C	1157	C
Paclitaxel	NCI	1.2 mg/mL[a]	BW	7 mg/mL[a]	Physically compatible for 4 hr at 22 °C	1556	C
Pemetrexed disodium	LI	20 mg/mL[b]	APP	7 mg/mL[a]	Physically compatible for 4 hr at 23 °C	2564	C
Penicillin G potassium	PF	40,000 units/mL[a]	BW	5 mg/mL[a]	Physically compatible for 4 hr at 25 °C	1157	C
Pentobarbital sodium	WY	2 mg/mL[a]	BW	5 mg/mL[a]	Physically compatible for 4 hr at 25 °C	1157	C
Piperacillin sodium–tazobactam sodium	LE[h]	40 + 5 mg/mL[a]	BW	7 mg/mL[a]	Particles form in 1 hr	1688	I
Potassium chloride	IX	0.04 mEq/mL[a]	BW	5 mg/mL[a]	Physically compatible for 4 hr at 25 °C	1157	C
Propofol	ZEN	10 mg/mL	BW	7 mg/mL[a]	Physically compatible for 1 hr at 23 °C	2066	C

Y-Site Injection Compatibility (1:1 Mixture) (Cont.)

Acyclovir sodium

Drug	Mfr	Conc	Mfr	Conc	Remarks	Ref	C/I
Ranitidine HCl	GL	1 mg/mL[a]	BW	5 mg/mL[a]	Physically compatible for 4 hr at 25 °C	1157	C
Remifentanil HCl	GW	0.025 and 0.25 mg/mL[b]	BW	7 mg/mL[a]	Physically compatible for 4 hr at 23 °C	2075	C
Sargramostim	IMM	10 mcg/mL[b]	BW	7 mg/mL[b]	Few small white particles form in 4 hr	1436	I
Sodium bicarbonate	IX	0.5 mEq/mL[a]	BW	5 mg/mL[a]	Physically compatible for 4 hr at 25 °C	1157	C
Tacrolimus	FUJ				Significant tacrolimus loss within 15 min	191	I
Teniposide	BR	0.1 mg/mL[a]	BW	7 mg/mL[a]	Physically compatible for 4 hr at 23 °C	1725	C
Theophylline	TR	1.6 mg/mL[a]	BW	5 mg/mL[a]	Physically compatible for 4 hr at 25 °C	1157	C
Thiotepa	IMM[e]	1 mg/mL[a]	BW	7 mg/mL[a]	Physically compatible for 4 hr at 23 °C	1861	C
TNA #218 to #226[f]			GW	7 mg/mL[a]	White precipitate forms immediately	2215	I
Tobramycin sulfate	DI	1.6 mg/mL[a]	BW	5 mg/mL[a]	Physically compatible for 4 hr at 25 °C	1157	C
TPN #203, #204[f]			BW	7 mg/mL	White precipitate forms immediately	1974	I
TPN #212 to #215[f]			BW	7 mg/mL[a]	Crystalline needles form immediately, becoming a gross precipitate in 1 hr	2109	I
Trimethoprim–sulfamethoxazole	RC	0.8 + 4 mg/mL[a]	BW	5 mg/mL[a]	Physically compatible for 4 hr at 25 °C	1157	C
Vancomycin HCl	LI	5 mg/mL[a]	BW	5 mg/mL[a]	Physically compatible for 4 hr at 25 °C	1157	C
Vinorelbine tartrate	BW	1 mg/mL[b]	BW	7 mg/mL[b]	Immediate white precipitate	1558	I
Zidovudine	BW	4 mg/mL[a]	BW	7 mg/mL[a]	Physically compatible for 4 hr at 25 °C	1193	C

[a]Tested in dextrose 5%.
[b]Tested in sodium chloride 0.9%.
[c]Tested in both dextrose 5% and sodium chloride 0.9%.
[d]Tested in sterile water for injection.
[e]Lyophilized formulation tested.
[f]Refer to Appendix I for the composition of parenteral nutrition solutions. TNA indicates a 3-in-1 admixture, and TPN indicates a 2-in-1 admixture.
[g]Tested in Ringer's injection, lactated.
[h]Test performed using the formulation WITHOUT edetate disodium.
[i]Tested in sodium chloride 0.45%.

ADENOSINE
AHFS 24:04.04.24

Products — Adenosine is available under the name Adenocard IV as a 3-mg/mL solution with sodium chloride 9 mg/mL in 2- and 4-mL disposable syringes for intravenous bolus injection. Adenosine is also available under the name Adenoscan as a 3-mg/mL solution with sodium chloride 9 mg/mL in 20- and 30-mL vials for intravenous infusion only. (1)

pH — Adenocard IV: from 4.5 to 7.5. Adenoscan: from 4.5 to 7.5. (1)

Trade Name(s) — Adenocard IV, Adenoscan.

Administration — Adenosine injections are administered intravenously. Adenocard IV is given as a rapid bolus injection by the peripheral intravenous route directly into a vein or into an intravenous line close to the patient and is followed by a rapid sodium chloride 0.9% flush. Adenoscan is given by continuous peripheral intravenous infusion only. (1)

Stability — Intact containers of adenosine injections should be stored at controlled room temperature. They should not be refrigerated, because of possible crystal formation. If crystallization occurs, let the solution warm to room temperature to dissolve the crystals. The solution must be clear prior to administration. (1-7/05; 1-1/06)

Adenosine 6 mcg/mL in sodium chloride 0.9% was packaged in 5-mL glass ampuls. Based on analysis of high-temperature-accelerated decomposition, it was projected that the drug solution would be stable for at least five years at 4 and 25 °C. (2115)

Adenosine 2 mg/mL in sodium chloride 0.9% was packaged in glass vials and stored for six months at temperatures ranging from 4 to 72 °C. Analysis found no loss of adenosine in samples stored at 4, 22, and 37 °C. (2277)

Adenosine 80 mg/L and 330 mg/L in cardioplegia solutions having high (100 mmol/L) and low (30 mmol/L) concentrations of potassium was stored at 4 and 23 °C. The solutions also contained THAM 12 mmol/L, magnesium sulfate 9 mmol/L, dextrose 250 mmol/L, and citrate-phosphate-dextrose-adenine solution 20 mL/L. No adenosine loss occurred after 14 days of storage in either solution. (2402)

Syringes — Undiluted adenosine (Fujisawa) 3 mg/mL was packaged as 25 mL in 60-mL polypropylene syringes (Becton Dickinson) and sealed with polyolefin tip caps (Sherwood Medical). The syringes were stored at 25, 5, and −15 °C. The solutions remained visually clear, and analysis showed no loss of adenosine in 7 days at 25 °C, 14 days at 5 °C, and 28 days at −15 °C. The drug's stability in glass vials was essentially identical under the same conditions. (2114)

Adenosine (Fujisawa) diluted to 0.75 mg/mL with several infusion solutions was packaged as 25 mL in 60-mL polypropylene syringes (Becton Dickinson) and sealed with polyolefin tip caps (Sherwood Medical). The syringes were stored at 25, 5, and −15 °C. The solutions remained visually clear, and analysis showed no loss of adenosine in 14 days for dextrose 5% in lactated Ringer's and lactated Ringer's injection and 16 days for dextrose 5% and sodium chloride 0.9%. (2114)

Compatibility Information

Solution Compatibility

Adenosine

Solution	Mfr	Mfr	Conc/L	Remarks	Ref	C/I
Dextrose 5% in Ringer's injection, lactated	BA[a]	FUJ	750 mg	Visually compatible with no loss in 14 days at 25, 5, and −15 °C	2114	C
Dextrose 5%	BA[a]	FUJ	750 mg	Visually compatible with no loss in 16 days at 25, 5, and −15 °C	2114	C
Ringer's injection, lactated	BA[a]	FUJ	750 mg	Visually compatible with no loss in 14 days at 25, 5, and −15 °C	2114	C
Sodium chloride 0.9%	BA[a]	FUJ	750 mg	Visually compatible with no loss in 16 days at 25, 5, and −15 °C	2114	C

[a]*Tested in PVC containers.*

Y-Site Injection Compatibility (1:1 Mixture)

Adenosine

Drug	Mfr	Conc	Mfr	Conc	Remarks	Ref	C/I
Abciximab	LI	36 mcg/mL[a]	FUJ	3 mg/mL	Visually compatible for 12 hr at 23 °C	2374	C

[a]*Tested in PVC containers.*

ALBUMIN HUMAN
AHFS 16:00

Products — Albumin human is available in 20-, 50-, and 100-mL vials as a 25% aqueous solution. Each 100 mL of solution contains 25 g of serum albumin. Albumin human is also available as a 5% aqueous solution in 50-, 250-, 500-, and 1000-mL sizes. The products also contain sodium carbonate, sodium bicarbonate, sodium hydroxide, and/or acetic acid to adjust the pH. (1; 4) The products are heat-treated for inactivation of hepatitis viruses. Sodium caprylate and sodium *N*-acetyltryptophanate are added to the products as stabilizers to prevent denaturation during the heat treatment. Low aluminum-containing albumin human products contain less than 200 mcg/L of aluminum. (1)

pH — From 6.4 to 7.4. (1; 4)

Sodium Content — From 130 to 160 mEq/L. (1; 4)

Trade Name(s) — Albuminar, Albutein, Albumarc, Buminate, Plasbumin.

Administration — Albumin human is administered intravenously either undiluted or diluted in an intravenous infusion solution having sufficient osmolality to be safely administered. (1; 4)

CAUTION—Substantial reduction in tonicity, creating the potential for fatal hemolysis and acute renal failure, may result from the use of sterile water as a diluent. The hemolysis and acute renal failure that result from the use of a sufficient volume of sterile water as a diluent may be life-threatening. (4; 1942; 2072; 2073)

Stability — Albumin human has been variously described as clear amber to deep orange-brown and as a transparent or slightly opalescent pale straw to dark brown solution. The solution should not be used if it is turbid or contains a deposit. Since it contains no preservative, the manufacturer recommends use within four hours after opening the vial. The expiration date is five years after issue from the manufacturer if the labeling recommends storage between 2 and 8 or 10 °C, or not more than three years after issue from the manufacturer if the labeling recommends storage at temperatures not greater than 30 or 37 °C. (4)

The addition of albumin human to parenteral nutrition solutions has resulted in occlusion of filters at concentrations ranging from over 25 g/L to 10.8 g/L. (854; 1634)

Freezing Solutions — Freezing the albumin human solutions may damage the container and result in contamination. (4)

Compatibility Information

Solution Compatibility

Albumin human

Solution	Mfr	Mfr	Conc/L	Remarks	Ref	C/I
Dextrose–Ringer's injection combinations	AB		5 g	Physically compatible	3	**C**
Dextrose–Ringer's injection, lactated, combinations	AB		5 g	Physically compatible	3	**C**
Dextrose–saline combinations	AB		5 g	Physically compatible	3	**C**
Dextrose 2.5%	AB		5 g	Physically compatible	3	**C**
Dextrose 5%	AB		5 g	Physically compatible	3	**C**
Dextrose 10%	AB		5 g	Physically compatible	3	**C**
Ionosol products	AB		5 g	Physically compatible	3	**C**
Ringer's injection	AB		5 g	Physically compatible	3	**C**
Ringer's injection, lactated	AB		5 g	Physically compatible	3	**C**
Sodium chloride 0.45%	AB		5 g	Physically compatible	3	**C**
Sodium chloride 0.9%	AB		5 g	Physically compatible	3	**C**
Sodium lactate ⅙ M	AB		5 g	Physically compatible	3	**C**
TNA #232[a]			9.5 g	Microscopically observed emulsion disruption found with increased fat globule size in 48 hr at room temperature	2267	**?**
TNA #233[a]			9.5 g	Visually apparent emulsion disruption with creaming in 4 hr at room temperature. Increased disruption attributed to the added effect of calcium and magnesium ions	2267	**I**
TNA #234[a]			18.2 g	Creaming and free oil formation visually observed in 24 hr at room temperature	2267	**I**
TNA #235[a]			18.2 g	Visually apparent emulsion disruption with creaming and free oil formation in 4 hr at room temperature. Increased disruption attributed to the added effect of calcium and magnesium ions	2267	**I**

[a]Refer to Appendix I for the composition of parenteral nutrition solutions. TNA indicates a 3-in-1 admixture.

Additive Compatibility

Albumin human

Drug	Mfr	Conc/L	Mfr	Conc/L	Test Soln	Remarks	Ref	C/I
Verapamil HCl	KN	80 mg	ARC	25 g	D5W, NS	Cloudiness develops within 8 hr	764	**I**

Y-Site Injection Compatibility (1:1 Mixture)

Albumin human

Drug	Mfr	Conc	Mfr	Conc	Remarks	Ref	C/I
Diltiazem HCl	MMD	5 mg/mL	AR, AT	5 and 25%	Visually compatible	1807	C
Fat emulsion, intravenous		20%		20%	Immediate emulsion destabilization	2267	I
Lorazepam	WY	0.33 mg/mL[b]		200 mg/mL	Visually compatible for 24 hr at 22 °C	1855	C
Micafungin sodium	ASP	1.5 mg/mL[b]	ZLB	25%	Immediate increase in measured haze	2683	I
Midazolam HCl	RC	5 mg/mL		200 mg/mL	White precipitate forms immediately	1855	I
Vancomycin HCl		20 mg/mL[a]		0.1 and 1%[b]	Heavy turbidity forms immediately and precipitate develops subsequently	1701	I
Verapamil HCl	LY	0.2 mg/mL[a]	HY	250 mg/mL[a]	Slight haze in 1 hr	1316	I
	LY	0.2 mg/mL[b]	HY	250 mg/mL[b]	Slight haze in 3 hr	1316	I

[a]*Tested in dextrose 5%.*
[b]*Tested in sodium chloride 0.9%.*

ALDESLEUKIN
(INTERLEUKIN-2; IL-2)
AHFS 10:00

Products — Aldesleukin is available in single-use vials containing 22 million I.U. (1.3 mg of protein). When reconstituted with 1.2 mL of sterile water for injection, each milliliter contains aldesleukin 18 million I.U. (1.1 mg) along with mannitol 50 mg, sodium dodecyl sulfate 0.18 mg, monobasic sodium phosphate 0.17 mg, and dibasic sodium phosphate 0.89 mg. During reconstitution, the sterile water for injection should be directed at the vial's sides. Swirl the contents gently to cause dissolution and avoid excess foaming. Do not shake the vial. Do not use bacteriostatic water for injection. (1)

Units — The biological potency of aldesleukin is determined by the lymphocyte proliferation bioassay and is expressed in International Units (I.U.). Aldesleukin 18 million I.U. equals 1.1 mg of protein. (1) During the development of aldesleukin, various unit systems were employed. However, the International Unit is now the standard measure of its activity.

pH — The reconstituted product has a pH of 7.2 to 7.8. (1)

Trade Name(s) — Proleukin.

Administration — Aldesleukin is administered intravenously; the reconstituted solution should be diluted in 50 mL of dextrose 5% and infused over 15 minutes. Inline filters should not be used. (1; 4) The drug should be diluted within the concentration range of 30 to 70 mcg/mL for administration. Concentrations of aldesleukin below 30 mcg/mL and above 70 mcg/mL have shown increased variability in drug delivery. Dilution and drug delivery outside this concentration range should be avoided. (1)

If aldesleukin concentrations less than 30 mcg/mL are necessary for short-term intravenous infusion of 15 minutes, the manufacturer recommends diluting the dose in dextrose 5% that contains albumin human 0.1% to prevent variability in the stability and bioactivity of the drug. (4; 1890)

Stability — Aldesleukin is a white to off-white powder; it becomes a colorless to slightly yellow liquid when reconstituted. (1)

Intact vials should be stored under refrigeration and protected from light. (1) However, aldesleukin in intact vials is stable for at least two months at controlled room temperature. (1890) The reconstituted solution, as well as dilutions in infusion solutions for intravenous administration, should also be stored under refrigeration and protected from freezing. Intravenous infusions should be brought to room temperature before administration. (1)

The manufacturer indicates that reconstituted and diluted aldesleukin is stable for 48 hours when stored at room temperature or under refrigeration. Refrigeration is recommended because the product contains no antibacterial preservative. (1)

Syringes — Aldesleukin (Cetus), reconstituted according to label directions, was evaluated for stability when stored in 1-mL plastic syringes (Becton Dickinson). One- and 0.5-mL aliquots were drawn into these syringes and refrigerated for five days. The product was physically stable and retained activity by biological analysis (cell proliferation assay) throughout the study period. (1821)

Reconstituted aldesleukin diluted to a concentration of 220 mcg/mL with dextrose 5% was repackaged aseptically as 1 mL drawn into tuberculin syringes and stored under refrigeration at 2 to 8 °C. The drug was found to be stable for the 14-day study period. (1890)

Ambulatory Pumps — For continuous intravenous infusion of aldesleukin in concentrations of 70 mcg/mL or less via an ambulatory pump at the accompanying higher temperature of near 32 °C, the dose should be diluted in dextrose 5% to which albumin human at a concentration of 0.1% has been added to maintain aldesleukin stability. (1890) The albumin human helps keep aldesleukin in its microaggregate state and helps decrease sorption to surfaces, especially at concentrations below 10 mcg/mL. (4) In the absence of albumin human, visually observed precipitation and loss of aldesleukin activity has been found. At concentrations greater than 70 and less than 100 mcg/mL at 32 °C, aldesleukin is unstable whether albumin human is present or not. (1890)

Aldesleukin (Cetus) 5 to 500 mcg/mL in dextrose 5% was evaluated for stability in PVC containers during simulated administration from pumps (CADD-1, Pharmacia Deltec). At 100 to 500 mcg/mL, aldesleukin was stable for six days at 32 °C and remained visually clear throughout the study period. At concentrations of 5 and 40 mcg/mL, however, albumin human 0.1% was necessary to maintain physical stability. The aldesleukin solutions with albumin human remained clear and remained active for six days at 32 °C. Without albumin human, precipitation occurred within a few hours. (1821)

Sorption — Aldesleukin in low concentrations, particularly less than 10 mcg/mL, undergoes sorption to surfaces such as plastic bags, tubing, and administration devices. Addition of 0.1% albumin human to the solution decreases the extent of sorption. (4) Both glass and PVC containers have been used to infuse aldesleukin with comparable clinical results. However, drug delivery may be more consistent with PVC containers. (1; 4)

Filtration — Inline filters should not be used for aldesleukin. (1; 4)

Compatibility Information

Solution Compatibility

Aldesleukin

Solution	Mfr	Mfr	Conc/L	Remarks	Ref	C/I
Dextrose 5%				Recommended for dilution of aldesleukin	1	C
Sodium chloride 0.9%				Increased aggregation occurs	1	I

Y-Site Injection Compatibility (1:1 Mixture)

Aldesleukin

Drug	Mfr	Conc	Mfr	Conc	Remarks	Ref	C/I
Amphotericin B	SQ	1.6 mg/mL[a]	CHI	33,800 I.U./mL[a]	Visually compatible for 2 hr	1857	C
Calcium gluconate	LY	100 mg/mL	CHI	33,800 I.U./mL[a]	Visually compatible with little or no loss of aldesleukin activity	1857	C
Diphenhydramine HCl	SCN	50 mg/mL	CHI	33,800 I.U./mL[a]	Visually compatible for 2 hr	1857	C
Dopamine HCl	ES	1.6 mg/mL[a]	CHI	33,800 I.U./mL[a]	Visually compatible with little or no loss of aldesleukin activity	1857	C
			CHI	[c]	Unacceptable loss of aldesleukin activity	1890	I
Fluconazole	RR	2 mg/mL[a]	CHI	33,800 I.U./mL[a]	Visually compatible with little or no loss of aldesleukin activity	1857	C
Fluorouracil			CHI	[c]	Unacceptable loss of aldesleukin activity	1890	I
Foscarnet sodium	AST	24 mg/mL	CHI	33,800 I.U./mL[a]	Visually compatible with little or no loss of aldesleukin activity	1857	C
Ganciclovir sodium	SY	10 mg/mL[a]	CHI	33,800 I.U./mL[a]	Aldesleukin bioactivity inhibited	1857	I
Heparin sodium	BA	100 units/mL	CHI	33,800 I.U./mL[a]	Visually compatible with little or no loss of aldesleukin activity	1857	C
			CHI	[c]	Visually compatible but aldesleukin activity was variable depending on rate of delivery. Heparin not tested	1890	?
Lorazepam	WY	2 mg/mL	CHI	33,800 I.U./mL[a]	Globules form immediately	1857	I

Y-Site Injection Compatibility (1:1 Mixture) (Cont.)

Aldesleukin

Drug	Mfr	Conc	Mfr	Conc	Remarks	Ref	C/I
Magnesium sulfate	LY	20 mg/mL[a]	CHI	33,800 I.U./ mL[a]	Visually compatible with little or no loss of aldesleukin activity	1857	C
Metoclopramide HCl	DU	5 mg/mL	CHI	33,800 I.U./ mL[a]	Visually compatible with little or no loss of aldesleukin activity	1857	C
Ondansetron HCl	GL	0.7 mg/mL[a]	CHI	33,800 I.U./ mL[a]	Visually compatible with little or no loss of aldesleukin activity	1857	C
	GL		CHI	5 to 40 mcg/ mL[c]	Visually compatible. Aldesleukin activity retained if each drug infused at a similar rate. Ondansetron not tested	1890	C
Pentamidine isethionate	FUJ	6 mg/mL[a]	CHI	33,800 I.U./ mL[a]	Aldesleukin bioactivity inhibited	1857	I
Potassium chloride	AB	0.2 mEq/mL	CHI	33,800 I.U./ mL[a]	Visually compatible with little or no loss of aldesleukin activity	1857	C
			CHI	c	Loss of aldesleukin activity	1890	I
Prochlorperazine edisylate	SKB	5 mg/mL	CHI	33,800 I.U./ mL[a]	Aldesleukin bioactivity inhibited	1857	I
Promethazine HCl	ES	25 mg/mL	CHI	33,800 I.U./ mL[a]	Aldesleukin bioactivity inhibited	1857	I
Ranitidine HCl	AB	1 mg/mL[b]	CHI	33,800 I.U./ mL[a]	Visually compatible with little or no loss of aldesleukin activity	1857	C
Trimethoprim–sulfamethoxazole	BW	1.6 + 8 mg/ mL[a]	CHI	33,800 I.U./ mL[a]	Visually compatible with little or no loss of aldesleukin activity	1857	C
Vancomycin HCl			CHI	c	Visually compatible. Aldesleukin activity retained. Vancomycin not tested	1890	C

[a]*Tested in dextrose 5%.*
[b]*Tested in sodium chloride 0.45%.*
[c]*Tested in D5W with 0.1% human serum albumin.*

ALFENTANIL HYDROCHLORIDE
AHFS 28:08.08

Products — Alfentanil hydrochloride is available at a concentration equivalent to alfentanil base 500 mcg/mL with sodium chloride for isotonicity in 2-, 5-, 10-, and 20-mL ampuls. (1)

pH — From 4 to 6. (1)

Osmolality — Alfentanil hydrochloride injection is isotonic. (1)

Trade Name(s) — Alfenta.

Administration — Alfentanil hydrochloride is administered by intravenous injection or infusion. For infusion, dilution to 25 to 80 mcg/ mL in a compatible solution has been utilized. (1)

Stability — Alfentanil hydrochloride injection is stable at controlled room temperature when protected from light. (1)

Syringes — Alfentanil hydrochloride (Janssen) 0.5 mg/mL in dextrose 5% was packaged in 20-mL polypropylene syringes (Becton Dickinson) and stored at 20 °C exposed to light and at 8 °C for 16 weeks. The solutions were visually clear and colorless throughout the study. No loss of alfentanil hydrochloride occurred and no leached substances from the plastic syringes appeared. (2191)

Alfentanil hydrochloride (Janssen) 0.167 mg/mL in sodium chloride 0.9% in polypropylene syringes (Sherwood) was physically stable and exhibited little loss in 24 hours stored at 4 and 23 °C. (2191)

Sorption — Alfentanil hydrochloride (Janssen) (concentration unspecified) was found to be compatible with polyethylene, polypropylene, and PVC. (2468)

Compatibility Information

Solution Compatibility

Alfentanil HCl

Solution	Mfr	Mfr	Conc/L	Remarks	Ref	C/I
Dextrose 5% in sodium chloride 0.9%			25 to 80 mg	Physically and chemically stable	1	C
Dextrose 5%			25 to 80 mg	Physically and chemically stable	1	C
Ringer's injection, lactated			25 to 80 mg	Physically and chemically stable	1	C
Sodium chloride 0.9%			25 to 80 mg	Physically and chemically stable	1	C

Drugs in Syringe Compatibility

Alfentanil HCl

Drug (in syringe)	Mfr	Amt	Mfr	Amt	Remarks	Ref	C/I
Atracurium besylate	BW	10 mg/mL		0.5 mg/mL	Physically compatible and atracurium stable for 24 hr at 5 and 30 °C	1694	C
Midazolam HCl	RC	0.2 mg/mL[a]	JN	0.5 mg/mL	Visually compatible. 8% midazolam and 2% alfentanil loss in 3 weeks at 20 °C in light. No alfentanil loss and 7% midazolam loss in 4 weeks at 6 °C in dark	2133	C
Morphine sulfate	DB	0.8 mg/mL[a]	ASZ	55 mcg/mL[a]	No loss of either drug in 182 days at room temperature or refrigerated	2527	C
Ondansetron HCl	GW	1.33 mg/mL[a]	JN	0.167 mg/mL[a]	Physically compatible. Little loss of either drug in 24 hr at 4 or 23 °C	2199	C

[a]Diluted with sodium chloride 0.9%.

Y-Site Injection Compatibility (1:1 Mixture)

Alfentanil HCl

Drug	Mfr	Conc	Mfr	Conc	Remarks	Ref	C/I
Amphotericin B cholesteryl sulfate complex	SEQ	0.83 mg/mL[a]	JN	0.5 mg/mL	Gross precipitate forms	2117	I
Bivalirudin	TMC	5 mg/mL[a]	TAY	0.125 mg/mL[a]	Physically compatible for 4 hr at 23 °C	2373	C
Cisatracurium besylate	GW	0.1, 2, 5 mg/mL[a]	JN	0.125 mg/mL[a]	Physically compatible for 4 hr at 23 °C	2074	C
Dexmedetomidine HCl	AB	4 mcg/mL[b]	TAY	0.5 mg/mL	Physically compatible for 4 hr at 23 °C	2383	C
Etomidate	AB	2 mg/mL	JN	0.5 mg/mL	Visually compatible for 7 days at 25 °C	1801	C
Fenoldopam mesylate	AB	80 mcg/mL[b]	TAY	0.5 mg/mL	Physically compatible for 4 hr at 23 °C	2467	C
Hetastarch in lactated electrolyte	AB	6%	TAY	0.125 mg/mL[a]	Physically compatible for 4 hr at 23 °C	2339	C
Linezolid	PHU	2 mg/mL	TAY	0.5 mg/mL	Physically compatible for 4 hr at 23 °C	2264	C
Propofol	ZEN	10 mg/mL	JN	0.5 mg/mL	Physically compatible for 1 hr at 23 °C	2066	C

Y-Site Injection Compatibility (1:1 Mixture) (Cont.)

Alfentanil HCl

Drug	Mfr	Conc	Mfr	Conc	Remarks	Ref	C/I
Remifentanil HCl	GW	0.025 and 0.25 mg/mL[b]	JN	0.125 mg/mL[a]	Physically compatible for 4 hr at 23 °C	2075	C

[a]Tested in dextrose 5%.
[b]Tested in sodium chloride 0.9%.

ALLOPURINOL SODIUM
AHFS 92:16

Products — Allopurinol sodium is available in single-use vials containing the equivalent of 500 mg of allopurinol in lyophilized form. Reconstitute with 25 mL of sterile water for injection to yield an almost colorless concentrated solution that is clear to slightly opalescent. (1)

pH — 11.1 to 11.8. (4)

Trade Name(s) — Aloprim.

Administration — The reconstituted solution must be diluted for use in sodium chloride 0.9% or dextrose 5% to a final concentration of no greater than 6 mg/mL. The diluted infusion is given as a single infusion daily or in equally divided infusions at 6-, 8-, or 12-hour intervals. The rate of infusion depends on the volume to be infused. (1)

Stability — Allopurinol sodium is supplied as a white lyophilized powder. The intact vials should be stored at controlled room temperature. Administration should begin within 10 hours of reconstitution. The reconstituted solution and diluted infusion solution should not be refrigerated. (1)

Compatibility Information

Y-Site Injection Compatibility (1:1 Mixture)

Allopurinol sodium

Drug	Mfr	Conc	Mfr	Conc	Remarks	Ref	C/I
Acyclovir sodium	BW	7 mg/mL[b]	BW	3 mg/mL[b]	Physically compatible for 4 hr at 22 °C	1686	C
Amikacin sulfate	BR	5 mg/mL[b]	BW	3 mg/mL[b]	Crystals and flakes form within 1 hr	1686	I
Aminophylline	AB	2.5 mg/mL[b]	BW	3 mg/mL[b]	Physically compatible for 4 hr at 22 °C	1686	C
Amphotericin B	SQ	0.6 mg/mL[a,b]	BW	3 mg/mL[b]	Amphotericin B haze lost immediately	1686	I
Aztreonam	SQ	40 mg/mL[b]	BW	3 mg/mL[b]	Physically compatible for 4 hr at 22 °C	1686	C
Bleomycin sulfate	BR	1 unit/mL[b]	BW	3 mg/mL[b]	Physically compatible for 4 hr at 22 °C	1686	C
Bumetanide	RC	0.04 mg/mL[b]	BW	3 mg/mL[b]	Physically compatible for 4 hr at 22 °C	1686	C
Buprenorphine HCl	RKC	0.04 mg/mL[b]	BW	3 mg/mL[b]	Physically compatible for 4 hr at 22 °C	1686	C
Butorphanol tartrate	BR	0.04 mg/mL[b]	BW	3 mg/mL[b]	Physically compatible for 4 hr at 22 °C	1686	C
Calcium gluconate	AMR	40 mg/mL[b]	BW	3 mg/mL[b]	Physically compatible for 4 hr at 22 °C	1686	C
Carboplatin	BR	5 mg/mL[b]	BW	3 mg/mL[b]	Physically compatible for 4 hr at 22 °C	1686	C
Carmustine	BR	1.5 mg/mL[b]	BW	3 mg/mL[b]	Gas evolves immediately	1686	I
Cefazolin sodium	GEM	20 mg/mL[b]	BW	3 mg/mL[b]	Physically compatible for 4 hr at 22 °C	1686	C
Cefotaxime sodium	HO	20 mg/mL[b]	BW	3 mg/mL[b]	Tiny particles form immediately	1686	I
Cefotetan disodium	STU	20 mg/mL[b]	BW	3 mg/mL[b]	Physically compatible for 4 hr at 22 °C	1686	C
Ceftazidime	LI	40 mg/mL[b]	BW	3 mg/mL[b]	Physically compatible for 4 hr at 22 °C	1686	C
Ceftriaxone sodium	RC	20 mg/mL[b]	BW	3 mg/mL[b]	Physically compatible for 4 hr at 22 °C	1686	C

Y-Site Injection Compatibility (1:1 Mixture) (Cont.)

Allopurinol sodium

Drug	Mfr	Conc	Mfr	Conc	Remarks	Ref	C/I
Cefuroxime sodium	GL	20 mg/mL[b]	BW	3 mg/mL[b]	Physically compatible for 4 hr at 22 °C	1686	**C**
Chlorpromazine HCl	RU	2 mg/mL[b]	BW	3 mg/mL[b]	White precipitate forms immediately	1686	**I**
Cisplatin	BR	1 mg/mL	BW	3 mg/mL[b]	Physically compatible for 4 hr at 22 °C	1686	**C**
Clindamycin phosphate	AB	10 mg/mL[b]	BW	3 mg/mL[b]	Tiny particles form immediately and become more numerous over 4 hr	1686	**I**
Cyclophosphamide	MJ	10 mg/mL[b]	BW	3 mg/mL[b]	Physically compatible for 4 hr at 22 °C	1686	**C**
Cytarabine	SCN	50 mg/mL	BW	3 mg/mL[b]	Tiny particles form within 4 hr	1686	**I**
Dacarbazine	MI	4 mg/mL[b]	BW	3 mg/mL[b]	Small particles form within 1 hr and become large pink pellets in 24 hr	1686	**I**
Dactinomycin	MSD	0.01 mg/mL[b]	BW	3 mg/mL[b]	Physically compatible for 4 hr at 22 °C	1686	**C**
Daunorubicin HCl	WY	1 mg/mL[b]	BW	3 mg/mL[b]	Reddish-purple color and haze form immediately. Reddish-brown particles form within 1 hr	1686	**I**
Dexamethasone sodium phosphate	LY	1 mg/mL[b]	BW	3 mg/mL[b]	Physically compatible for 4 hr at 22 °C	1686	**C**
Diphenhydramine HCl	PD	2 mg/mL[b]	BW	3 mg/mL[b]	White precipitate forms immediately	1686	**I**
Doxorubicin HCl	CET	2 mg/mL	BW	3 mg/mL[b]	Immediate dark red color and haze. Reddish-brown particles within 1 hr	1686	**I**
Doxorubicin HCl liposomal	SEQ	0.4 mg/mL[a]	BW	3 mg/mL	Physically compatible for 4 hr at 23 °C	2087	**C**
Doxycycline hyclate	ES	1 mg/mL[b]	BW	3 mg/mL[b]	Immediate brown particles. Hazy brown solution with precipitate in 4 hr	1686	**I**
Droperidol	JN	0.4 mg/mL[b]	BW	3 mg/mL[b]	Immediate turbidity with particles	1686	**I**
Enalaprilat	MSD	0.1 mg/mL[b]	BW	3 mg/mL[b]	Physically compatible for 4 hr at 22 °C	1686	**C**
Etoposide	BR	0.4 mg/mL[b]	BW	3 mg/mL[b]	Physically compatible for 4 hr at 22 °C	1686	**C**
Famotidine	MSD	2 mg/mL[b]	BW	3 mg/mL[b]	Physically compatible for 4 hr at 22 °C	1686	**C**
Filgrastim	AMG	30 mcg/mL[a]	BW	3 mg/mL[a]	Physically compatible for 4 hr at 22 °C	1687	**C**
Floxuridine	RC	3 mg/mL[b]	BW	3 mg/mL[b]	Tiny particles form in 1 to 4 hr	1686	**I**
Fluconazole	RR	2 mg/mL	BW	3 mg/mL[b]	Physically compatible for 4 hr at 22 °C	1686	**C**
Fludarabine phosphate	BX	1 mg/mL[b]	BW	3 mg/mL[b]	Physically compatible for 4 hr at 22 °C	1686	**C**
Fluorouracil	RC	16 mg/mL[b]	BW	3 mg/mL[b]	Physically compatible for 4 hr at 22 °C	1686	**C**
Furosemide	ES	3 mg/mL[b]	BW	3 mg/mL[b]	Physically compatible for 4 hr at 22 °C	1686	**C**
Gallium nitrate	FUJ	0.4 mg/mL[b]	BW	3 mg/mL[b]	Physically compatible for 4 hr at 22 °C	1686	**C**
Ganciclovir sodium	SY	20 mg/mL[b]	BW	3 mg/mL[b]	Physically compatible for 4 hr at 22 °C	1686	**C**
Gentamicin sulfate	ES	5 mg/mL[b]	BW	3 mg/mL[b]	Hazy solution with crystals forms in 1 hr	1686	**I**
Granisetron HCl	SKB	0.05 mg/mL[a]	BW	3 mg/mL[a]	Physically compatible for 4 hr at 23 °C	2000	**C**
Haloperidol lactate	MN	0.2 mg/mL[b]	BW	3 mg/mL[b]	Immediate turbidity. Crystals in 1 hr	1686	**I**
Heparin sodium	ES	100 units/mL[b]	BW	3 mg/mL[b]	Physically compatible for 4 hr at 22 °C	1686	**C**
Hydrocortisone sodium succinate	UP	1 mg/mL[b]	BW	3 mg/mL[b]	Physically compatible for 4 hr at 22 °C	1686	**C**
Hydromorphone HCl	KN	0.5 mg/mL[b]	BW	3 mg/mL[b]	Physically compatible for 4 hr at 22 °C	1686	**C**
Hydroxyzine HCl	ES	4 mg/mL[b]	BW	3 mg/mL[b]	Immediate turbidity and precipitate	1686	**I**

Y-Site Injection Compatibility (1:1 Mixture) (Cont.)

Allopurinol sodium

Drug	Mfr	Conc	Mfr	Conc	Remarks	Ref	C/I
Idarubicin HCl	AD	0.5 mg/mL[b]	BW	3 mg/mL[b]	Immediate reddish-purple color. Particles in 1 hr. Total color loss in 24 hr	1686	**I**
Ifosfamide	MJ	25 mg/mL[b]	BW	3 mg/mL[b]	Physically compatible for 4 hr at 22 °C	1686	**C**
Imipenem–cilastatin sodium	MSD	10 mg/mL[b]	BW	3 mg/mL[b]	Haze and particles form in 1 hr	1686	**I**
Lorazepam	WY	0.1 mg/mL[b]	BW	3 mg/mL[b]	Physically compatible for 4 hr at 22 °C	1686	**C**
Mannitol	BA	15%	BW	3 mg/mL[b]	Physically compatible for 4 hr at 22 °C	1686	**C**
Mechlorethamine HCl	MSD	1 mg/mL	BW	3 mg/mL[b]	Haze and small particles form immediately. Numerous large particles in 4 hr	1686	**I**
Meperidine HCl	WY	4 mg/mL[b]	BW	3 mg/mL[b]	Tiny particles form immediately and increase in number over 4 hr	1686	**I**
Mesna	MJ	10 mg/mL[b]	BW	3 mg/mL[b]	Physically compatible for 4 hr at 22 °C	1686	**C**
Methotrexate sodium	LE	15 mg/mL[b]	BW	3 mg/mL[b]	Physically compatible for 4 hr at 22 °C	1686	**C**
Methylprednisolone sodium succinate	AB	5 mg/mL[b]	BW	3 mg/mL[b]	Haze forms in 1 hr with white precipitate in 24 hr	1686	**I**
Metoclopramide HCl	DU	5 mg/mL	BW	3 mg/mL[b]	Heavy white precipitate forms immediately	1686	**I**
Metronidazole	BA	5 mg/mL	BW	3 mg/mL[b]	Physically compatible for 4 hr at 22 °C	1686	**C**
Mitoxantrone HCl	LE	0.5 mg/mL[b]	BW	3 mg/mL[b]	Physically compatible for 4 hr at 22 °C	1686	**C**
Morphine sulfate	WI	1 mg/mL[b]	BW	3 mg/mL[b]	Physically compatible for 4 hr at 22 °C	1686	**C**
Nalbuphine HCl	DU	10 mg/mL	BW	3 mg/mL[b]	Particles in 1 hr. Crystals in 4 hr	1686	**I**
Ondansetron HCl	GL	1 mg/mL[b]	BW	3 mg/mL[b]	Immediate turbidity becoming precipitate	1686	**I**
Potassium chloride	AB	0.1 mEq/mL[b]	BW	3 mg/mL[b]	Physically compatible for 4 hr at 22 °C	1686	**C**
Prochlorperazine edisylate	SKB	0.5 mg/mL[b]	BW	3 mg/mL[b]	Heavy turbidity forms immediately	1686	**I**
Promethazine HCl	WY	2 mg/mL[b]	BW	3 mg/mL[b]	Immediate turbidity. Particles in 4 hr	1686	**I**
Ranitidine HCl	GL	2 mg/mL[b]	BW	3 mg/mL[b]	Physically compatible for 4 hr at 22 °C	1686	**C**
Sodium bicarbonate	AB	1 mEq/mL	BW	3 mg/mL[b]	Small and large crystals form in 1 hr	1686	**I**
Streptozocin	UP	40 mg/mL[b]	BW	3 mg/mL[b]	Haze and small particles in 1 hr	1686	**I**
Teniposide	BR	0.1 mg/mL[a]	BW	3 mg/mL[a]	Physically compatible for 4 hr at 23 °C	1725	**C**
Thiotepa	LE[c]	1 mg/mL[b]	BW	3 mg/mL[b]	Physically compatible for 4 hr at 22 °C	1686	**C**
Ticarcillin disodium–clavulanate potassium	SKB	31 mg/mL[b]	BW	3 mg/mL[b]	Physically compatible for 4 hr at 22 °C	1686	**C**
Tobramycin sulfate	LI	5 mg/mL[b]	BW	3 mg/mL[b]	Haze and crystals form in 1 hr	1686	**I**
Trimethoprim–sulfamethoxazole	ES	0.8 + 4 mg/mL[b]	BW	3 mg/mL[b]	Physically compatible for 4 hr at 22 °C	1686	**C**
Vancomycin HCl	LY	10 mg/mL[b]	BW	3 mg/mL[b]	Physically compatible for 4 hr at 22 °C	1686	**C**
Vinblastine sulfate	LI	0.12 mg/mL[b]	BW	3 mg/mL[b]	Physically compatible for 4 hr at 22 °C	1686	**C**
Vincristine sulfate	LI	0.05 mg/mL[b]	BW	3 mg/mL[b]	Physically compatible for 4 hr at 22 °C	1686	**C**
Vinorelbine tartrate	BW	1 mg/mL[b]	BW	3 mg/mL[b]	Immediate white precipitate	1686	**I**
Zidovudine	BW	4 mg/mL[b]	BW	3 mg/mL[b]	Physically compatible for 4 hr at 22 °C	1686	**C**

[a]Tested in dextrose 5%.
[b]Tested in sodium chloride 0.9%.
[c]Powder fill formulation tested.

ALPROSTADIL
AHFS 24:12.92

Products — Alprostadil for intravenous use is available as a 500-mcg/mL concentrate in dehydrated alcohol packaged in ampuls and vials. The concentrate must be diluted in a compatible infusion solution for use. (1)

Administration — For continuous intravenous or intra-arterial infusion in neonates, alprostadil concentrate is diluted by adding 500 mcg (one vial of concentrate) to 25, 50, 100, or 250 mL of dextrose 5% or sodium chloride 0.9% to yield 20, 10, 5, or 2 mcg/mL, respectively. The diluted solution is administered using a controlled infusion device. (1)

Stability — Intact containers of alprostadil concentrate should be stored under refrigeration. Alprostadil concentrate diluted for infusion is stable for up to 24 hours in the infusion solution. (1) Alprostadil is reported not to be subjected to increased degradation due to ambient light exposure. (2639)

Undiluted alprostadil concentrate may interact with plastic volumetric infusion chambers changing their appearance and resulting in a hazy solution. Consequently, the infusion solution should be added to the volumetric chamber first with the alprostadil concentrate added into the solution avoiding contact with the chamber walls. (1)

pH Effects — Alprostadil is more stable at acidic pH values compared to neutral and especially alkaline pH. The pH of maximum stability has been reported to be pH 3. (2639)

Syringes — Alprostadil 500 mcg/mL undiluted and also diluted with sodium chloride 0.9% to concentrations near 250 and 125 mcg/mL was packaged in 1-mL polypropylene syringes (Becton Dickinson). After 30 days stored at 4 °C, 5% or less alprostadil loss occurred. (2602)

Compatibility Information

Drugs in Syringe Compatibility

					Alprostadil		
Drug (in syringe)	Mfr	Amt	Mfr	Amt	Remarks	Ref	C/I
Caffeine citrate		20 mg/1 mL	UP	0.5 mg/1 mL	Visually compatible for 4 hr at 25 °C	2440	**C**
Pantoprazole sodium	a	4 mg/1 mL		0.5 mg/1 mL	Clear solution	2574	**C**

[a]Test performed using the formulation WITHOUT edetate disodium.

Y-Site Injection Compatibility (1:1 Mixture)

					Alprostadil		
Drug	Mfr	Conc	Mfr	Conc	Remarks	Ref	C/I
Ampicillin sodium	SQ	100 mg/mL[b]	BED	7.5 mcg/mL[d]	Visually compatible for 1 hr	2746	**C**
Cefazolin sodium	LI	100 mg/mL[b]	BED	7.5 mcg/mL[d,e]	Visually compatible for 1 hr	2746	**C**
Cefotaxime sodium	HO	100 mg/mL[b]	BED	7.5 mcg/mL[d,e]	Visually compatible for 1 hr	2746	**C**
Chlorothiazide sodium	ME	25 mg/mL[b]	BED	7.5 mcg/mL[d]	Visually compatible for 1 hr	2746	**C**
Dobutamine HCl	AB	3 mg/mL[b]	BED	7.5 mcg/mL[d,e]	Visually compatible for 1 hr	2746	**C**
Dopamine HCl	AB	3 mg/mL[b]	BED	7.5 mcg/mL[d,e]	Visually compatible for 1 hr	2746	**C**
Fentanyl citrate	JN	10 mcg/mL[b]	BED	7.5 mcg/mL[d,e]	Visually compatible for 1 hr	2746	**C**
Gentamicin sulfate	ES	1 mg/mL[b]	BED	7.5 mcg/mL[d,e]	Visually compatible for 1 hr	2746	**C**
Levofloxacin	OMN	5 mg/mL[a]	UP	0.5 mg/mL	Precipitate forms	2233	**I**
Methylprednisolone sodium succinate	PH	40 mg/mL[b]	BED	7.5 mcg/mL[d,e]	Visually compatible for 1 hr	2746	**C**

Y-Site Injection Compatibility (1:1 Mixture) (Cont.)

Drug	Mfr	Conc	Mfr	Conc	Remarks	Ref	C/I
				Alprostadil			
Sodium nitroprusside	RC	0.3, 1.2, 3 mg/mL[a]	UP	2 mcg/mL[a]	Visually compatible for 48 hr at 24 °C protected from light	2357	C
	RC	0.3, 1.2, 3 mg/mL[a]	UP	10 mcg/mL[a]	Visually compatible for 48 hr at 24 °C protected from light	2357	C
Tobramycin sulfate	LI	1 mg/mL[b]	BED	7.5 mcg/mL[d,e]	Visually compatible for 1 hr	2746	C
TPN #274[c]			BED	15 mcg/mL[a]	Visually compatible for 1 hr	2746	C
Vancomycin HCl	LI	5 mg/mL[b]	BED	7.5 mcg/mL[d,e]	Visually compatible for 1 hr	2746	C
Vecuronium bromide	OR	1 mg/mL[b]	BED	7.5 mcg/mL[d,e]	Visually compatible for 1 hr	2746	C

[a]Tested in dextrose 5%.
[b]Tested in either dextrose 5% or in sodium chloride 0.9%, but the report did not specify which solution.
[c]Refer to Appendix I for the composition of parenteral nutrition solutions. TPN indicates a 2-in-1 admixture.
[d]Tested in a 1:1 mixture of (1) dextrose 5% and dextrose 5% in sodium chloride 0.45% with and without potassium chloride 20 mEq/L and also in (2) dextrose 10% in sodium chloride 0.45% with and without potassium chloride 20 mEq/L.
[e]Tested in a 1:1 mixture of dextrose 5% and TPN #274 (see Appendix I).

ALTEPLASE
(t-PA)
AHFS 20:12.20

Products — Alteplase is available as a sterile lyophilized powder in 50- and 100-mg vials. The products also contain L-arginine, phosphoric acid, and polysorbate 80. (1)

The pH may have been adjusted with phosphoric acid and/or sodium hydroxide. Intact 50-mg vials contain a vacuum, but the 100-mg vials do not. (1)

The alteplase vials are accompanied by 50- and 100-mL vials of sterile water for injection for the 50- and 100-mg sizes, respectively. Alteplase should be reconstituted with sterile water for injection only; do not use solutions containing preservatives. Use of the accompanying diluent results in a 1-mg/mL concentration. The manufacturer recommends use of a large bore needle to direct the stream into the lyophilized cake of the 50-mg vials. For the 100-mg vials, the special transfer device should be used. The vials should be swirled gently— not shaken—to dissolve the drug. Excessive agitation should be avoided. Although slight foaming may occur, the bubbles will dissipate after standing for several minutes. (1)

Cathflo Activase is available in alteplase 2.2-mg vials with L-arginine 77 mg, polysorbate 80 0.2 mg, and phosphoric acid to adjust pH. Reconstitute with 2.2 mL of sterile water for injection and gently swirl to yield a 1-mg/mL solution; do not shake. If slight foaming occurs, allow the solution to stand for a few minutes until the bubbles dissipate. Do not use bacteriostatic water for injection with a preservative as a diluent. (1)

Specific Activity — Alteplase is a purified glycoprotein with a specific activity of 580,000 I.U./mg. The 50-mg vial contains 29 million I.U., and the 100-mg vial contains 58 million I.U. (1)

pH — Approximately 7.3. (1; 1)

Osmolality — The product has an osmolality of 215 mOsm/kg. (1)

Trade Name(s) — Activase.

Administration — Alteplase is administered by intravenous infusion, directly after reconstitution to a 1-mg/mL concentration or diluted with an equal volume of sodium chloride 0.9% or dextrose 5% to a 0.5-mg/mL concentration. (1; 4) Dilution to a lower concentration may result in precipitation. (4; 1425)

Alteplase has been effective and well tolerated in catheter clearance (1; 2328; 2329; 2330; 2446; 2635).

Stability — Alteplase, an off-white lyophilized powder, becomes a colorless to pale yellow solution on reconstitution. Intact vials should be refrigerated or stored at room temperature with protection from extended exposure to light. The 50-mg vials should not be used unless a vacuum is present. Cathflo Activase should be stored under refrigeration. (1) Although refrigerated storage is required, the manufacturer of Cathflo Activase states that the drug may be stored at room temperature for four months. (2745)

Because alteplase has no bacteriostat, the manufacturer recommends reconstitution immediately before use. However, the solution may be administered within eight hours when stored at room temperature or under refrigeration. (1) Exposure to light does not affect the potency of either reconstituted solutions of alteplase or dilutions in compatible infusion solutions. (1; 4)

Alteplase is stated to be incompatible with the preservatives used in bacteriostatic water for injection because preservatives can interact with the alteplase molecule. (4) Even so, alteplase was reconstituted with sterile water for injection and also bacteriostatic water for injection (benzyl alcohol 0.9%) to yield a 1-mg/mL solution. The test solutions were stored at 37 °C and remained clear and colorless. In vitro clot lysis testing found activity was retained for at least seven days. The USP antimicrobial effectiveness test was performed as well. The samples reconstituted with sterile water failed the test while the samples reconstituted with bacteriostatic water for injection passed. (2668)

pH Effects — Alteplase in solution is stable at pH 5 to 7.5. (4)

Freezing Solutions — A 50-mg vial of alteplase (Genentech), reconstituted with sterile water for injection to a concentration of 1 mg/mL, was diluted with balanced saline solution to a final concentration of 250 mcg/mL. Then 0.3-mL (75 mcg) portions of the diluted solution were drawn into 1-mL tuberculin syringes and frozen at −70 °C. Alteplase activity was retained for at least one year. (2157)

However, others have objected to frozen storage of diluted alteplase solution. It was noted that the alteplase formulation has been designed for optimal stability, and dilution to a concentration lower than 500 mcg/mL might adversely affect the drug's solubility by diluting the formulation's solubilizing components. Furthermore, it was noted that the calcium or magnesium salts contained in some diluents might interact with the phosphates present in the alteplase formulation to form a precipitate. Indeed, precipitated protein has been found in diluted alteplase after room temperature storage for 24 hours. Frozen storage at −20 °C with subsequent thawing has resulted in changed patterns of light scattering as well. It was recommended that dilution with balanced saline solution and storage of dilutions for any length of time at room temperature or frozen should be avoided. (2158)

Use of a diluent containing polysorbate 80, L-arginine, and phosphoric acid to reconstitute and dilute alteplase to 50 mcg/mL is reported to permit frozen storage. Although the report did not specify the exact concentrations of the diluent components, it may have duplicated the alteplase vehicle after reconstitution. Use of this diluent for dilution prevented precipitation of the protein upon frozen storage at −20 °C. In addition, the activity in ophthalmic use was found to be unchanged after storage for six months in the frozen state. (2159)

Alteplase (Genentech) concentrations of 0.5, 1, and 2 mg/mL in sterile water for injection were packaged as 1 mL of solution in 5-mL polypropylene syringes and sealed with rubber tip caps. Sample syringes were stored frozen at −70 and −25 °C for up to 14 days as well as refrigerated at 2 °C. Frozen samples were thawed at room temperature and stored under refrigeration for determination of fibrinolytic activity. Fibrinolytic activity after frozen storage at both −70 and −25 °C remained near nominal initial concentrations for at least 14 days. Furthermore, the activity remained greater than 90% for up to 48 hours in all thawed samples subsequently stored at 2 °C and was comparable to the activity of refrigerated solutions that had never been frozen. However, substantial and unacceptable losses of activity occurred after 72 hours under refrigeration whether previously frozen or not. (2327)

Genentech evaluated the activity of alteplase 1 mg/mL when reconstituted with sterile water for injection, packaged in glass vials, and stored frozen at −20 °C for 32 days, followed by thawing at room temperature. The frozen alteplase solution remained physically and chemically comparable to newly reconstituted alteplase for at least eight hours at room temperature after thawing. (2328)

Alteplase (Genentech) 1 mg/mL in sterile water for injection packaged in polypropylene syringes was frozen at −20 °C for six months. Similar solutions in glass vials were frozen at −70 °C for two weeks, thawed and kept at 23 °C for 24 hours, and then refrozen at −70 °C for 19 days. Little or no loss of alteplase bioactivity was found. (2400)

Compatibility Information

Solution Compatibility

Alteplase

Solution	Mfr	Mfr	Conc/L	Remarks	Ref	C/I
Dextrose 5%	a	GEN	0.5 g	Stable for up to 8 hr at room temperature	1	C
	MG	GEN	160 mg	Precipitates immediately	1425	I
	MG	GEN	90 mg	Precipitate forms in 4 hr	1425	I
Sodium chloride 0.9%	a	GEN	0.5 g	Stable for up to 8 hr at room temperature	1	C
	BA	GEN	10 mg	Physically compatible. Alteplase stable for 24 hr at room temperature	2501	C

*a*Tested in glass and PVC containers.

Additive Compatibility

Alteplase

Drug	Mfr	Conc/L	Mfr	Conc/L	Test Soln	Remarks	Ref	C/I
Dobutamine HCl	LI	5 g	GEN	0.5 g	D5W, NS	Yellow discoloration and precipitate form	1856	I
Dopamine HCl	ACC	5 g	GEN	0.5 g	D5W, NS	About 30% alteplase clot-lysis activity loss in 24 hr at 25 °C	1856	I

Additive Compatibility (Cont.)

Alteplase

Drug	Mfr	Conc/L	Mfr	Conc/L	Test Soln	Remarks	Ref	C/I
Heparin sodium	ES	40,000 units	GEN	0.5 g	NS	Heparin interacts with alteplase. Opalescence forms within 5 min with peak intensity at 4 hr at 25 °C. Alteplase clot-lysis activity reduced slightly	1856	I
Lidocaine HCl	AST	4 g	GEN	0.5 g	D5W	Visually compatible with no alteplase clot-lysis activity loss in 24 hr at 25 °C	1856	C
	AST	4 g	GEN	0.5 g	NS	Visually compatible with 7% alteplase clot-lysis activity loss in 24 hr at 25 °C	1856	C
Morphine sulfate	WY	1 g	GEN	0.5 g	NS	Visually compatible with 5 to 8% alteplase clot-lysis activity loss in 24 hr at 25 °C	1856	C
Nitroglycerin	ACC	400 mg	GEN	0.5 g	D5W, NS	Visually compatible with 2% or less clot-lysis activity loss in 24 hr at 25 °C	1856	C

Y-Site Injection Compatibility (1:1 Mixture)

Alteplase

Drug	Mfr	Conc	Mfr	Conc	Remarks	Ref	C/I
Bivalirudin	TMC	5 mg/mL[a]	GEN	1 mg/mL	Small aggregates form immediately	2373	I
Dobutamine HCl	LI	2 mg/mL[a]	GEN	1 mg/mL	Haze in 20 min spectrophotometrically and in 2 hr visually	1340	I
Dopamine HCl	DU	8 mg/mL[a]	GEN	1 mg/mL	Haze noted in 4 hr	1340	I
Heparin sodium	ES	100 units/mL[a]	GEN	1 mg/mL	Haze noted in 24 hr	1340	I
Lidocaine HCl	AB	8 mg/mL[a]	GEN	1 mg/mL	Physically compatible for 6 days	1340	C
Metoprolol tartrate	CI	1 mg/mL	GEN	1 mg/mL	Visually compatible with no alteplase clot-lysis activity loss in 24 hr at 25 °C	1856	C
Nitroglycerin	DU	0.2 mg/mL[a]	GEN	1 mg/mL	Haze noted in 24 hr	1340	I
Propranolol HCl	AY	1 mg/mL	GEN	1 mg/mL	Visually compatible. 2% clot-lysis activity loss in 24 hr at 25 °C	1856	C

[a]Tested in dextrose 5%.

AMIFOSTINE
AHFS 92:56

Products — Amifostine is available in vials containing, in lyophilized form, 500 mg of amifostine on the anhydrous basis. The vial contents are reconstituted with 9.7 mL of sodium chloride 0.9% to yield a solution containing amifostine 50 mg/mL. (1)

pH — Approximately 7. (234)

Trade Name(s) — Ethyol.

Administration — When used as a chemoprotectant in adults, amifostine is administered once daily as a 15-minute intravenous infusion. The infusion is started 30 minutes before chemotherapy. When used as a radioprotectant in adults, amifostine is administered once daily as a three-minute intravenous infusion started 15 to 30 minutes prior to radiation therapy. Patients should be well hydrated prior to intravenous infusion of amifostine and should maintain a supine position during the infusion. Only limited experience in administration to children or elderly patients is available. (1; 4)

Stability — The intact vials may be stored at controlled room temperatures of 20 to 25 °C. The manufacturer states that the reconstituted solution is chemically stable for 24 hours under refrigeration but only five hours at 25 °C. The product should not be used if cloudiness or a precipitate is observed. (1)

Compatibility Information

Solution Compatibility

Amifostine

Solution	Mfr	Mfr	Conc/L	Remarks	Ref	C/I
Sodium chloride 0.9%	a		5 and 40 g	Stable for 24 hr at 4 °C and 5 hr at 25 °C	1	**C**

[a]Tested in PVC containers.

Y-Site Injection Compatibility (1:1 Mixture)

Amifostine

Drug	Mfr	Conc	Mfr	Conc	Remarks	Ref	C/I
Acyclovir sodium	BW	7 mg/mL[a]	USB	10 mg/mL[a]	Subvisible needles form in 1 hr. Visible particles form in 4 hr	1845	**I**
Amikacin sulfate	DU	5 mg/mL[a]	USB	10 mg/mL[a]	Physically compatible for 4 hr at 23 °C	1845	**C**
Aminophylline	AMR	2.5 mg/mL[a]	USB	10 mg/mL[a]	Physically compatible for 4 hr at 23 °C	1845	**C**
Amphotericin B	AD	0.6 mg/mL[a]	USB	10 mg/mL[a]	Turbidity forms immediately	1845	**I**
Ampicillin sodium	WY	20 mg/mL[b]	USB	10 mg/mL[a]	Physically compatible for 4 hr at 23 °C	1845	**C**
Ampicillin sodium–sulbactam sodium	RR	20 + 10 mg/mL[b]	USB	10 mg/mL[a]	Physically compatible for 4 hr at 23 °C	1845	**C**
Aztreonam	SQ	40 mg/mL[a]	USB	10 mg/mL[a]	Physically compatible for 4 hr at 23 °C	1845	**C**
Bleomycin sulfate	MJ	1 unit/mL[b]	USB	10 mg/mL[a]	Physically compatible for 4 hr at 23 °C	1845	**C**
Bumetanide	RC	0.04 mg/mL[a]	USB	10 mg/mL[a]	Physically compatible for 4 hr at 23 °C	1845	**C**
Buprenorphine HCl	RKC	0.04 mg/mL[a]	USB	10 mg/mL[a]	Physically compatible for 4 hr at 23 °C	1845	**C**
Butorphanol tartrate	BR	0.04 mg/mL[a]	USB	10 mg/mL[a]	Physically compatible for 4 hr at 23 °C	1845	**C**
Calcium gluconate	AMR	40 mg/mL[a]	USB	10 mg/mL[a]	Physically compatible for 4 hr at 23 °C	1845	**C**
Carboplatin	BR	5 mg/mL[a]	USB	10 mg/mL[a]	Physically compatible for 4 hr at 23 °C	1845	**C**
Carmustine	BR	1.5 mg/mL[a]	USB	10 mg/mL[a]	Physically compatible for 4 hr at 23 °C	1845	**C**
Cefazolin sodium	MAR	20 mg/mL[a]	USB	10 mg/mL[a]	Physically compatible for 4 hr at 23 °C	1845	**C**
Cefotaxime sodium	HO	20 mg/mL[a]	USB	10 mg/mL[a]	Physically compatible for 4 hr at 23 °C	1845	**C**
Cefotetan disodium	STU	20 mg/mL[a]	USB	10 mg/mL[a]	Physically compatible for 4 hr at 23 °C	1845	**C**
Cefoxitin sodium	MSD	20 mg/mL[a]	USB	10 mg/mL[a]	Physically compatible for 4 hr at 23 °C	1845	**C**
Ceftazidime	LI	40 mg/mL[a]	USB	10 mg/mL[a]	Physically compatible for 4 hr at 23 °C	1845	**C**
Ceftriaxone sodium	RC	20 mg/mL[a]	USB	10 mg/mL[a]	Physically compatible for 4 hr at 23 °C	1845	**C**
Cefuroxime sodium	GL	30 mg/mL[a]	USB	10 mg/mL[a]	Physically compatible for 4 hr at 23 °C	1845	**C**
Chlorpromazine HCl	SCN	2 mg/mL[a]	USB	10 mg/mL[a]	Subvisible haze forms immediately	1845	**I**
Ciprofloxacin	MI	1 mg/mL[a]	USB	10 mg/mL[a]	Physically compatible for 4 hr at 23 °C	1845	**C**
Cisplatin	BR	1 mg/mL	USB	10 mg/mL[a]	Subvisible haze forms in 4 hr	1845	**I**
Clindamycin phosphate	AST	10 mg/mL[a]	USB	10 mg/mL[a]	Physically compatible for 4 hr at 23 °C	1845	**C**
Cyclophosphamide	MJ	10 mg/mL[a]	USB	10 mg/mL[a]	Physically compatible for 4 hr at 23 °C	1845	**C**
Cytarabine	CET	50 mg/mL	USB	10 mg/mL[a]	Physically compatible for 4 hr at 23 °C	1845	**C**
Dacarbazine	MI	4 mg/mL[a]	USB	10 mg/mL[a]	Physically compatible for 4 hr at 23 °C	1845	**C**
Dactinomycin	ME	0.01 mg/mL[a]	USB	10 mg/mL[a]	Physically compatible for 4 hr at 23 °C	1845	**C**
Daunorubicin HCl	WY	1 mg/mL[a]	USB	10 mg/mL[a]	Physically compatible for 4 hr at 23 °C	1845	**C**

Y-Site Injection Compatibility (1:1 Mixture) (Cont.)

Amifostine

Drug	Mfr	Conc	Mfr	Conc	Remarks	Ref	C/I
Dexamethasone sodium phosphate	AMR	1 mg/mL[a]	USB	10 mg/mL[a]	Physically compatible for 4 hr at 23 °C	1845	**C**
Diphenhydramine HCl	PD	2 mg/mL[a]	USB	10 mg/mL[a]	Physically compatible for 4 hr at 23 °C	1845	**C**
Dobutamine HCl	LI	4 mg/mL[a]	USB	10 mg/mL[a]	Physically compatible for 4 hr at 23 °C	1845	**C**
Docetaxel	RPR	0.9 mg/mL[a]	ALZ	10 mg/mL[b]	Physically compatible for 4 hr at 23 °C	2224	**C**
Dopamine HCl	AST	3.2 mg/mL[a]	USB	10 mg/mL[a]	Physically compatible for 4 hr at 23 °C	1845	**C**
Doxorubicin HCl	CET	2 mg/mL	USB	10 mg/mL[a]	Physically compatible for 4 hr at 23 °C	1845	**C**
Doxycycline hyclate	LY	1 mg/mL[a]	USB	10 mg/mL[a]	Physically compatible for 4 hr at 23 °C	1845	**C**
Droperidol	JN	0.4 mg/mL[a]	USB	10 mg/mL[a]	Physically compatible for 4 hr at 23 °C	1845	**C**
Enalaprilat	MSD	0.1 mg/mL[a]	USB	10 mg/mL[a]	Physically compatible for 4 hr at 23 °C	1845	**C**
Etoposide	BR	0.4 mg/mL[a]	USB	10 mg/mL[a]	Physically compatible for 4 hr at 23 °C	1845	**C**
Famotidine	ME	2 mg/mL[a]	USB	10 mg/mL[a]	Physically compatible for 4 hr at 23 °C	1845	**C**
Floxuridine	RC	3 mg/mL[a]	USB	10 mg/mL[a]	Physically compatible for 4 hr at 23 °C	1845	**C**
Fluconazole	RR	2 mg/mL	USB	10 mg/mL[a]	Physically compatible for 4 hr at 23 °C	1845	**C**
Fludarabine phosphate	BX	1 mg/mL[a]	USB	10 mg/mL[a]	Physically compatible for 4 hr at 23 °C	1845	**C**
Fluorouracil	AD	16 mg/mL[a]	USB	10 mg/mL[a]	Physically compatible for 4 hr at 23 °C	1845	**C**
Furosemide	AB	3 mg/mL[a]	USB	10 mg/mL[a]	Physically compatible for 4 hr at 23 °C	1845	**C**
Gallium nitrate	FUJ	0.4 mg/mL[a]	USB	10 mg/mL[a]	Physically compatible for 4 hr at 23 °C	1845	**C**
Ganciclovir sodium	SY	20 mg/mL[a]	USB	10 mg/mL[a]	Crystalline needles form immediately. Dense precipitate in 1 hr	1845	**I**
Gemcitabine HCl	LI	10 mg/mL[b]	USB	10 mg/mL[b]	Physically compatible for 4 hr at 23 °C	2226	**C**
Gentamicin sulfate	ES	5 mg/mL[a]	USB	10 mg/mL[a]	Physically compatible for 4 hr at 23 °C	1845	**C**
Granisetron HCl	SKB	0.05 mg/mL[a]	USB	10 mg/mL[a]	Physically compatible for 4 hr at 23 °C	2000	**C**
Haloperidol lactate	MN	0.2 mg/mL[a]	USB	10 mg/mL[a]	Physically compatible for 4 hr at 23 °C	1845	**C**
Heparin sodium	ES	100 units/ mL[a]	USB	10 mg/mL[a]	Physically compatible for 4 hr at 23 °C	1845	**C**
Hydrocortisone sodium succinate	UP	1 mg/mL[a]	USB	10 mg/mL[a]	Physically compatible for 4 hr at 23 °C	1845	**C**
Hydromorphone HCl	AST	0.5 mg/mL[a]	USB	10 mg/mL[a]	Physically compatible for 4 hr at 23 °C	1845	**C**
Hydroxyzine HCl	WI	4 mg/mL[a]	USB	10 mg/mL[a]	Subvisible haze forms immediately	1845	**I**
Idarubicin HCl	AD	0.5 mg/mL[a]	USB	10 mg/mL[a]	Physically compatible for 4 hr at 23 °C	1845	**C**
Ifosfamide	MJ	25 mg/mL[a]	USB	10 mg/mL[a]	Physically compatible for 4 hr at 23 °C	1845	**C**
Imipenem–cilastatin sodium	MSD	10 mg/mL[a]	USB	10 mg/mL[a]	Physically compatible for 4 hr at 23 °C	1845	**C**
Leucovorin calcium	LE	2 mg/mL[a]	USB	10 mg/mL[a]	Physically compatible for 4 hr at 23 °C	1845	**C**
Lorazepam	WY	0.1 mg/mL[a]	USB	10 mg/mL[a]	Physically compatible for 4 hr at 23 °C	1845	**C**
Magnesium sulfate	AST	100 mg/mL[a]	USB	10 mg/mL[a]	Physically compatible for 4 hr at 23 °C	1845	**C**
Mannitol	BA	15%	USB	10 mg/mL[a]	Physically compatible for 4 hr at 23 °C	1845	**C**
Mechlorethamine HCl	MSD	1 mg/mL	USB	10 mg/mL[a]	Physically compatible for 4 hr at 23 °C	1845	**C**
Meperidine HCl	WY	4 mg/mL[a]	USB	10 mg/mL[a]	Physically compatible for 4 hr at 23 °C	1845	**C**
Mesna	MJ	10 mg/mL[a]	USB	10 mg/mL[a]	Physically compatible for 4 hr at 23 °C	1845	**C**
Methotrexate sodium	LE	15 mg/mL[a]	USB	10 mg/mL[a]	Physically compatible for 4 hr at 23 °C	1845	**C**

Y-Site Injection Compatibility (1:1 Mixture) (Cont.)

Amifostine

Drug	Mfr	Conc	Mfr	Conc	Remarks	Ref	C/I
Methylprednisolone sodium succinate	AB	5 mg/mL[a]	USB	10 mg/mL[a]	Physically compatible for 4 hr at 23 °C	1845	C
Metoclopramide HCl	ES	5 mg/mL	USB	10 mg/mL[a]	Physically compatible for 4 hr at 23 °C	1845	C
Metronidazole	BA	5 mg/mL	USB	10 mg/mL[a]	Physically compatible for 4 hr at 23 °C	1845	C
Mitomycin	BR	0.5 mg/mL	USB	10 mg/mL[a]	Physically compatible for 4 hr at 23 °C	1845	C
Mitoxantrone HCl	LE	0.5 mg/mL[a]	USB	10 mg/mL[a]	Physically compatible for 4 hr at 23 °C	1845	C
Morphine sulfate	AST	1 mg/mL[a]	USB	10 mg/mL[a]	Physically compatible for 4 hr at 23 °C	1845	C
Nalbuphine HCl	AST	10 mg/mL	USB	10 mg/mL[a]	Physically compatible for 4 hr at 23 °C	1845	C
Ondansetron HCl	GL	1 mg/mL[a]	USB	10 mg/mL[a]	Physically compatible for 4 hr at 23 °C	1845	C
Pemetrexed disodium	LI	20 mg/mL[b]	MDI	10 mg/mL[b]	Physically compatible for 4 hr at 23 °C	2564	C
Potassium chloride	AB	0.1 mEq/mL[a]	USB	10 mg/mL[a]	Physically compatible for 4 hr at 23 °C	1845	C
Prochlorperazine edisylate	SN	0.5 mg/mL[a]	USB	10 mg/mL[a]	Immediate increase in measured haze	1845	I
Promethazine HCl	ES	2 mg/mL[a]	USB	10 mg/mL[a]	Physically compatible for 4 hr at 23 °C	1845	C
Ranitidine HCl	GL	2 mg/mL[a]	USB	10 mg/mL[a]	Physically compatible for 4 hr at 23 °C	1845	C
Sodium bicarbonate	AST	1 mEq/mL	USB	10 mg/mL[a]	Physically compatible for 4 hr at 23 °C	1845	C
Streptozocin	UP	40 mg/mL[a]	USB	10 mg/mL[a]	Physically compatible for 4 hr at 23 °C	1845	C
Teniposide	BR	0.1 mg/mL[a]	USB	10 mg/mL[a]	Physically compatible for 4 hr at 23 °C	1845	C
Thiotepa	LE[c]	1 mg/mL[a]	USB	10 mg/mL[a]	Physically compatible for 4 hr at 23 °C	1845	C
Ticarcillin disodium–clavulanate potassium	SKB	31 mg/mL[a]	USB	10 mg/mL[a]	Physically compatible for 4 hr at 23 °C	1845	C
Tobramycin sulfate	LI	5 mg/mL[a]	USB	10 mg/mL[a]	Physically compatible for 4 hr at 23 °C	1845	C
Trimethoprim–sulfamethoxazole	ES	0.8 + 4 mg/mL[a]	USB	10 mg/mL[a]	Physically compatible for 4 hr at 23 °C	1845	C
Vancomycin HCl	AB	10 mg/mL[a]	USB	10 mg/mL[a]	Physically compatible for 4 hr at 23 °C	1845	C
Vinblastine sulfate	LI	0.12 mg/mL[a]	USB	10 mg/mL[a]	Physically compatible for 4 hr at 23 °C	1845	C
Vincristine sulfate	LI	0.05 mg/mL[a]	USB	10 mg/mL[a]	Physically compatible for 4 hr at 23 °C	1845	C
Zidovudine	BW	4 mg/mL[a]	USB	10 mg/mL[a]	Physically compatible for 4 hr at 23 °C	1845	C

[a]*Tested in dextrose 5%.*
[b]*Tested in sodium chloride 0.9%.*
[c]*Powder fill formulation tested.*

AMIKACIN SULFATE
AHFS 8:12.02

Products — Amikacin sulfate is available in a concentration of 250 mg/mL. Also present are sodium metabisulfite, sodium citrate, and sulfuric acid to adjust pH. (1)

pH — 4.5. (291) The range is 3.5 to 5.5. (4)

Osmolality — The osmolality of amikacin sulfate 500 mg was calculated for the following dilutions (1054):

Diluent	Osmolality (mOsm/kg)	
	50 mL	100 mL
Dextrose 5%	353	319
Sodium chloride 0.9%	383	349

Sodium Content — The sodium content of amikacin sulfate 50 mg/mL is 0.064 mEq/mL; for the 250-mg/mL concentration, the sodium content is 0.319 mEq/mL. (291)

Administration — Amikacin sulfate may be administered by intramuscular injection and intravenous infusion; for intravenous infusion 500 mg may be diluted in 100 to 200 mL of compatible infusion solution and administered to adults over 30 to 60 minutes. The diluent volume should be sufficient for drug infusion over one to two hours in infants and over 30 to 60 minutes in older children. (1; 4)

Stability — Amikacin sulfate is supplied as a colorless to pale yellow or light straw-colored solution. (4) It was reported that aqueous solutions of amikacin sulfate in concentrations of 37.5 to 250 mg/mL retained greater than 90% for up to 36 months at 25 °C, 12 months at 37 °C, and three months at 56 °C. (291) Aqueous solutions of amikacin sulfate are subject to color darkening because of air oxidation. However, this change in color has no effect on potency. (291)

Amikacin base (Bristol) 10 and 50 mg/L in peritoneal dialysis concentrate with 50% dextrose (McGaw) retained about 70% of initial activity in seven hours and about 40 to 50% in 24 hours at room temperature. (1044)

Amikacin sulfate (Bristol) 25 mcg/mL combined separately with the cephalosporins cefazolin sodium (Lilly) and cefoxitin (MSD) at

a concentration of 125 mcg/mL in peritoneal dialysis solution (Dianeal 1.5%) exhibited enhanced rates of lethality to *Staphylococcus aureus, Escherichia coli,* and *Pseudomonas aeruginosa* compared to any of the drugs alone. (1623)

Syringes — Amikacin sulfate (Bristol) 750 mg diluted with 1 mL of sodium chloride 0.9% to a final volume of 4 mL was stable, showing about a 2% loss when stored in polypropylene syringes (Becton Dickinson) for 48 hours at 23 °C under fluorescent light. (1159)

Sorption — Amikacin sulfate was shown not to exhibit sorption to PVC bags or sets and multilayer bags composed of polyethylene, polyamide, and polypropylene. (2269)

Central Venous Catheter — Amikacin sulfate (Apothecon) 1 mg/mL in dextrose 5% was found to be compatible with the ARROWg+ard Blue Plus (Arrow International) chlorhexidine-bearing triple-lumen central catheter. Delivery of the amikacin sulfate ranged from 92 to 98% of the initial concentration among the three lumens. Furthermore, chlorhexidine delivered from the catheter remained at trace amounts with no substantial increase due to the delivery of the drug through the catheter. (2335)

Compatibility Information

Solution Compatibility

Amikacin sulfate

Solution	Mfr	Mfr	Conc/L	Remarks	Ref	C/I
Dextrose 5% in Ringer's injection	BA	BR	250 mg and 5 g	Compatible and stable for 24 hr at 25 °C, 60 days at 4 °C, 30 days at −15 °C	292	C
Dextrose 5% in Ringer's injection, lactated	BA	BR	250 mg and 5 g	Compatible and stable for 24 hr at 25 °C, 60 days at 4 °C, 30 days at −15 °C	292	C
Dextrose 2.5% in sodium chloride 0.45%	BA	BR	250 mg and 5 g	Compatible and stable for 24 hr at 25 °C, 60 days at 4 °C, 30 days at −15 °C	292	C
Dextrose 2.5% in sodium chloride 0.9%	BA	BR	250 mg and 5 g	Compatible and stable for 24 hr at 25 °C, 60 days at 4 °C, 30 days at −15 °C	292	C
Dextrose 5% in sodium chloride 0.2%	BA	BR	250 mg and 5 g	Compatible and stable for 24 hr at 25 °C, 60 days at 4 °C, 30 days at −15 °C	292	C
Dextrose 5% in sodium chloride 0.45%	BA	BR	250 mg and 5 g	Compatible and stable for 24 hr at 25 °C, 60 days at 4 °C, 30 days at −15 °C	292	C
Dextrose 5% in sodium chloride 0.9%	BA	BR	250 mg and 5 g	Compatible and stable for 24 hr at 25 °C, 60 days at 4 °C, 30 days at −15 °C	292	C
Dextrose 10% in sodium chloride 0.9%	BA	BR	250 mg and 5 g	Compatible and stable for 24 hr at 25 °C, 60 days at 4 °C, 30 days at −15 °C	292	C
Dextrose 5%	BA	BR	250 mg and 5 g	Compatible and stable for 24 hr at 25 °C, 60 days at 4 °C, 30 days at −15 °C	292	C
	TR[a]	BR	5 g	Physically compatible and potency retained for 24 hr at room temperature	518	C
	TR[a]	BR	20 g	Physically compatible. 4% loss in 24 hr at room temperature and 6% loss frozen for 30 days at −20 °C	555	C
	MG[b]	BR	4 g	Stable for 48 hr at 25 °C in light	981	C

Solution Compatibility (Cont.)

Amikacin sulfate

Solution	Mfr	Mfr	Conc/L	Remarks	Ref	C/I
	AB[a]	BR	5 g	Visually compatible. Stable for 48 hr at 25 °C in light and 4 °C in dark	1541	C
Dextrose 10%	BA	BR	250 mg and 5 g	Compatible and stable for 24 hr at 25 °C, 60 days at 4 °C, 30 days at −15 °C	292	C
	SO	BR	250 mg/ 21 mL[c]	Visually compatible with no loss in 30 days at 5 °C	1731	C
	SO	BR	500 mg/ 22 mL[c]	Visually compatible with no loss in 30 days at 5 °C	1731	C
Dextrose 20%	BA	BR	250 mg and 5 g	Compatible and stable for 24 hr at 25 °C, 60 days at 4 °C, 30 days at −15 °C	292	C
Normosol M in dextrose 5%	AB	BR	250 mg and 5 g	Compatible and stable for 24 hr at 25 °C, 60 days at 4 °C, 30 days at −15 °C	292	C
Normosol R	AB	BR	250 mg and 5 g	Compatible and stable for 24 hr at 25 °C, 60 days at 4 °C, 30 days at −15 °C	292	C
Normosol R in dextrose 5%	AB	BR	250 mg and 5 g	Compatible and stable for 24 hr at 25 °C, 60 days at 4 °C, 30 days at −15 °C	292	C
Ringer's injection	BA	BR	250 mg and 5 g	Compatible and stable for 24 hr at 25 °C, 60 days at 4 °C, 30 days at −15 °C	292	C
Ringer's injection, lactated	BA	BR	250 mg and 5 g	Compatible and stable for 24 hr at 25 °C, 60 days at 4 °C, 30 days at −15 °C	292	C
Sodium chloride 0.25%	BA	BR	250 mg and 5 g	Compatible and stable for 24 hr at 25 °C, 60 days at 4 °C, 30 days at −15 °C	292	C
Sodium chloride 0.45%	BA	BR	250 mg and 5 g	Compatible and stable for 24 hr at 25 °C, 60 days at 4 °C, 30 days at −15 °C	292	C
Sodium chloride 0.9%	BA	BR	250 mg and 5 g	Compatible and stable for 24 hr at 25 °C, 60 days at 4 °C, 30 days at −15 °C	292	C
	TR[a]	BR	5 g	Physically compatible. Stable for 24 hr at room temperature	518	C
	MG[b]	BR	4 g	Stable for 48 hr at 25 °C in light	981	C
	AB[a]	BR	5 g	Visually compatible. Stable for 48 hr at 25 °C in light and 4 °C in dark	1541	C
Sodium lactate ⅙ M	BA	BR	250 mg and 5 g	Compatible and stable for 24 hr at 25 °C, 60 days at 4 °C, 30 days at −15 °C	292	C
TPN #107[d]			150 mg	Activity retained for 24 hr at 21 °C	1326	C

[a]Tested in PVC containers.
[b]Tested in glass containers.
[c]Tested as a concentrate in glass vials.
[d]Refer to Appendix I for the composition of parenteral nutrition solutions. TPN indicates a 2-in-1 admixture.

Additive Compatibility

Amikacin sulfate

Drug	Mfr	Conc/L	Mfr	Conc/L	Test Soln	Remarks	Ref	C/I
Aminophylline	SE	5 g	BR	5 g	LR, NS, R, SL	Physically compatible and amikacin stable for 24 hr at 25 °C. Aminophylline not analyzed	294	C

Additive Compatibility (Cont.)

Amikacin sulfate

Drug	Mfr	Conc/L	Mfr	Conc/L	Test Soln	Remarks	Ref	C/I
	SE	5 g	BR	5 g	D5LR, D5R, D5S, D5W, D10W	Over 10% amikacin loss after 8 hr but within 24 hr at 25 °C. Aminophylline not analyzed	294	I
Amphotericin B	SQ	100 mg	BR	5 g	D5LR, D5R, D5S, D5W, D10W, LR, NS, R, SL	Precipitates immediately	293	I
Ampicillin sodium	BR	30 g	BR	5 g	D5LR, D5R, D5S, D5W, D10W, LR, NS, R, SL	Over 10% ampicillin loss in 4 hr at 25 °C	•293	I
Ascorbic acid	CO[a]	5 g	BR	5 g	D5LR, D5R, D5S, D5W, D10W, LR, NS, R, SL	Physically compatible and both stable for 24 hr at 25 °C	294	C
Bleomycin sulfate	BR	20 and 30 units	BR	1.25 g	NS	Physically compatible. Bleomycin stable for 1 week at 4 °C. Amikacin not tested	763	C
Calcium chloride	UP	1 g	BR	5 g	D5LR, D5R, D5S, D5W, D10W, LR, NS, R, SL	Physically compatible and both stable for 24 hr at 25 °C	294	C
Calcium gluconate	UP	500 mg	BR	5 g	D5LR, D5R, D5S, D5W, D10W, LR, NS, R, SL	Physically compatible and both stable for 24 hr at 25 °C	294	C
Cefazolin sodium	LI	20 g	BR	5 g	D5LR, D5R, D5S, D5W, D10W, LR, NS, R, SL	Both drugs stable for 8 hr at 25 °C. Turbidity observed at 24 hr	293	I
Cefepime HCl	BR	40 g	BR	6 g	D5W, NS	Visually compatible with 6% cefepime loss in 24 hr at room temperature and 4% loss in 7 days at 5 °C. No amikacin loss	1681	C
Cefotaxime sodium	RS	50 mg	BR	25 mg	D5W	33% loss of amikacin in 2 hr at 22 °C	504	I
	RS	50 mg	BR	15 mg	D5W	Under 8% loss of amikacin in 24 hr at 22 °C	504	C

Additive Compatibility (Cont.)

Amikacin sulfate

Drug	Mfr	Conc/L	Mfr	Conc/L	Test Soln	Remarks	Ref	C/I
Cefoxitin sodium	MSD	5 g	BR	5 g	D5S	9% cefoxitin loss at 25 °C and none at 5 °C in 48 hr. No amikacin loss at 25 °C and 1% at 5 °C in 48 hr	308	C
Ceftazidime	GL	50 mg	BR	25 mg	D5W	28% loss of amikacin in 2 hr at 22 °C	504	I
	GL	50 mg	BR	15 mg	D5W	17% loss of amikacin in 24 hr at 22 °C	504	I
Ceftriaxone sodium	RC	100 mg	BR	15 and 25 mg	D5W	6% loss of amikacin in 24 hr at 22 °C	504	C
Chloramphenicol sodium succinate	PD	10 g	BR	5 g	D5LR, D5R, D5S, D5W, D10W, LR, NS, R, SL	Physically compatible and both stable for 24 hr at 25 °C	293	C
Chlorothiazide sodium	MSD	10 mg	BR	5 g	D5LR, D5R, D5S, D5W, D10W, LR, NS, R, SL	Precipitate forms within 4 hr at 25 °C	294	I
Ciprofloxacin	MI	1.6 g	BR	4.1 g	D5W, NS	Visually compatible and both stable for 48 hr at 25 °C under fluorescent light	1541	C
	BAY	2 g	APC	4.9 g	D5W	Visually compatible with no loss of ciprofloxacin in 24 hr at 22 °C under fluorescent light. Amikacin not tested	2413	C
Clindamycin phosphate	UP	6 g	BR	5 g	D5LR, D5R, D5S, D5W, D10W, LR, NS, R, SL	Physically compatible and amikacin stable for 24 hr at 25 °C. Clindamycin not analyzed	293	C
	UP	9 g	BR	4 g	D5W, NS[b]	Both stable for 48 hr at 25 °C under fluorescent light	981	C
Cloxacillin sodium	BR	10 g	BR	5 g	D5LR, D5R, D5S, D5W, D10W, LR, NS, R, SL	Physically compatible and both stable for 24 hr at 25 °C	293	C
Colistimethate sodium	WC	500 mg	BR	5 g	D5LR, D5R, D5S, D5W, D10W, LR, NS, R, SL	Physically compatible and amikacin stable for 24 hr at 25 °C. Colistimethate not analyzed	293	C
Dexamethasone sodium phosphate	MSD	40 mg	BR	5 g	D5LR, D5R, D5S, D5W, D10W, LR, NS, R, SL	Physically compatible and both stable for 24 hr at 25 °C	294	C
	MSD	40 mg	BR	5 g	D2.5S	16% dexamethasone loss in 4 hr at 25 °C	294	I

Additive Compatibility (Cont.)

Amikacin sulfate

Drug	Mfr	Conc/L	Mfr	Conc/L	Test Soln	Remarks	Ref	C/I
Dimenhydrinate	SE	100 mg	BR	5 g	D5LR, D5R, D5S, D5W, D10W, LR, NS, R, SL	Physically compatible and both stable for 24 hr at 25 °C	294	**C**
Diphenhydramine HCl	PD	100 mg	BR	5 g	D5LR, D5R, D5S, D5W, D10W, LR, NS, R, SL	Physically compatible and both stable for 24 hr at 25 °C	294	**C**
Epinephrine HCl	PD	2.5 mg	BR	5 g	D5LR, D5R, D5S, D5W, D10W, LR, NS, R, SL	Physically compatible and both stable for 24 hr at 25 °C	294	**C**
Fluconazole	PF	1 g	BR	2.5 g	D5W	Visually compatible with no fluconazole loss in 72 hr at 25 °C under fluorescent light. Amikacin not tested	1677	**C**
Furosemide	HO	160 mg	BR	2 g	D5W, NS	Transient cloudiness, then visually compatible for 24 hr at 21 °C	876	**?**
Heparin sodium	AB	30,000 units	BR	5 g	D5LR, D5R, D5S, D5W, D10W, LR, NS, R, SL	Precipitates immediately	294	**I**
Hyaluronidase	SE	150 units	BR	5 g	D5LR, D5R, D5S, D5W, D10W, LR, NS, R, SL	Physically compatible and amikacin stable for 24 hr at 25 °C. Hyaluronidase not analyzed	294	**C**
Hydrocortisone sodium succinate	UP	200 mg	BR	5 g	D5LR, D5R, D5S, D5W, D10W, LR, NS, R, SL	Physically compatible and both stable for 24 hr at 25 °C	294	**C**
Lincomycin HCl	UP	10 g	BR	5 g	D5LR, D5R, D5S, D5W, D10W, LR, NS, R, SL	Physically compatible and both stable for 24 hr at 25 °C	293	**C**
Mannitol	BA	20%	BR	250 mg and 5 g		Compatible and stable for 24 hr at 25 °C, 60 days at 4 °C, 30 days at −15 °C	292	**C**

Additive Compatibility (Cont.)

Amikacin sulfate

Drug	Mfr	Conc/L	Mfr	Conc/L	Test Soln	Remarks	Ref	C/I
Norepinephrine bitartrate	WI	8 mg	BR	5 g	D5LR, D5R, D5S, D5W, D10W, LR, NS, R, SL	Physically compatible and both stable for 24 hr at 25 °C	294	C
Oxacillin sodium	BR	2 g	BR	5 g	D5LR, D5R, D5S, D5W, D10W, LR, NS, R	Physically compatible and both stable for 24 hr at 25 °C	293	C
	BR	2 g	BR	5 g	NR, SL	Oxacillin stable for 8 hr at 25 °C. Over 10% loss in 24 hr	293	I
Penicillin G potassium	LI	20 million units	BR	5 g	D5LR, D5R, D5S, D5W, D10W, LR, NS, R, SL	Physically compatible and both stable for 24 hr at 25 °C	293	C
Pentobarbital sodium	AB	100 mg	BR	5 g	D5LR, D5R, D5S, D5W, D10W, LR, NS, R, SL	Physically compatible and both stable for 24 hr at 25 °C	294	C
Phenobarbital sodium	LI	300 mg	BR	5 g	D5LR, D5R, D5S, D5W, D10W, LR, NS, R, SL	Physically compatible and both stable for 24 hr at 25 °C	294	C
Phenytoin sodium	PD	250 mg	BR	5 g	D5LR, D5R, D5S, D5W, D10W, LR, NS, R, SL	Precipitates immediately	294	I
Phytonadione	MSD	200 mg	BR	5 g	D5LR, D5R, D5S, D5W, D10W, LR, NS, R, SL	Physically compatible and amikacin stable for 24 hr at 25 °C. Phytonadione not analyzed	294	C
Polymyxin B sulfate	BW	200 mg	BR	5 g	D5LR, D5R, D5S, D5W, D10W, LR, NS, R, SL	Physically compatible and amikacin stable for 24 hr at 25 °C. Polymyxin not analyzed	293	C

Additive Compatibility (Cont.)

Amikacin sulfate

Drug	Mfr	Conc/L	Mfr	Conc/L	Test Soln	Remarks	Ref	C/I
Potassium chloride	LI	3 g	BR	5 g	D5LR, D5R, D5S, D5W, D10W, LR, NS, R, SL	Physically compatible and both stable for 24 hr at 25 °C	294	C
Prochlorperazine edisylate	SKF	20 mg	BR	5 g	D5LR, D5R, D5S, D5W, D10W, LR, NS, R, SL	Physically compatible and both stable for 24 hr at 25 °C	294	C
Promethazine HCl	WY	100 mg	BR	5 g	D5LR, D5R, D5S, D5W, D10W, LR, NS, R, SL	Physically compatible and both stable for 24 hr at 25 °C	294	C
Ranitidine HCl	GL	100 mg	BR	1 g	D5W	Physically compatible for 24 hr at ambient temperature in light	1151	C
	GL	50 mg and 2 g		2.5 g	D5W	Physically compatible. Ranitidine stable for 24 hr at 25 °C. Amikacin not tested	1515	C
Sodium bicarbonate	BR	15 g	BR	5 g	D5LR, D5R, D5S, D5W, D10W, LR, NS, R, SL	Physically compatible and both stable for 24 hr at 25 °C	294	C
Succinylcholine chloride	SQ	2 g	BR	5 g	D5LR, D5R, D5S, D5W, D10W, LR, NS, R, SL	Physically compatible and both stable for 24 hr at 25 °C	294	C
Vancomycin HCl	LI	2 g	BR	5 g	D5LR, D5R, D5S, D5W, D10W, LR, NS, R, SL	Physically compatible and amikacin stable for 24 hr at 25 °C. Vancomycin not tested	293	C
Verapamil HCl	KN	80 mg	BR	2 g	D5W, NS	Physically compatible for 24 hr	764	C

[a]*Present as calcium ascorbate.*
[b]*Tested in glass containers.*

Drugs in Syringe Compatibility

Amikacin sulfate

Drug (in syringe)	Mfr	Amt	Mfr	Amt	Remarks	Ref	C/I
Caffeine citrate		20 mg/ 1 mL	BED	250 mg/ 1 mL	Visually compatible for 4 hr at 25 °C	2440	C

Drugs in Syringe Compatibility (Cont.)

Amikacin sulfate

Drug (in syringe)	Mfr	Amt	Mfr	Amt	Remarks	Ref	C/I
Clindamycin phosphate	UP	900 mg/ 6 mL	BR	750 mg/ 4 mL[a]	Physically compatible with little loss of either drug in 48 hr at 25 °C	1159	**C**
Doxapram HCl	RB	400 mg/ 20 mL		100 mg/ 2 mL	Physically compatible with no doxapram loss in 24 hr	1177	**C**
Heparin sodium		2500 units/ 1 mL		100 mg	Turbidity or precipitate forms within 5 min	1053	**I**
Pantoprazole sodium	[b]	4 mg/ 1 mL		250 mg/ 1 mL	Precipitates	2574	**I**

[a]Diluted to 4 mL with 1 mL of sodium chloride 0.9%.
[b]Test performed using the formulation WITHOUT edetate disodium.

Y-Site Injection Compatibility (1:1 Mixture)

Amikacin sulfate

Drug	Mfr	Conc	Mfr	Conc	Remarks	Ref	C/I
Acyclovir sodium	BW	5 mg/mL[a]	BR	5 mg/mL[a]	Physically compatible for 4 hr at 25 °C	1157	**C**
Allopurinol sodium	BW	3 mg/mL[b]	BR	5 mg/mL[b]	Crystals and flakes form within 1 hr	1686	**I**
Amifostine	USB	10 mg/mL[a]	DU	5 mg/mL[a]	Physically compatible for 4 hr at 23 °C	1845	**C**
Amiodarone HCl	LZ	4 mg/mL[c]	BR	5 mg/mL[c]	Physically compatible for 4 hr at room temperature	1444	**C**
Amphotericin B cholesteryl sulfate complex	SEQ	0.83 mg/mL[a]	AB	5 mg/mL[a]	Gross precipitate forms	2117	**I**
Amsacrine	NCI	1 mg/mL[a]	BR	5 mg/mL[a]	Visually compatible for 4 hr at 22 °C	1381	**C**
Anidulafungin	VIC	0.5 mg/mL[a]	APC	5 mg/mL[a]	Physically compatible for 4 hr at 23 °C	2617	**C**
Azithromycin	PF	2 mg/mL[e]	VHA	100 mg/mL[e,o]	Whitish-yellow microcrystals found	2368	**I**
Aztreonam	SQ	40 mg/mL[a]	BMS	5 mg/mL[a]	Physically compatible for 4 hr at 23 °C	1758	**C**
Bivalirudin	TMC	5 mg/mL[a]	APO	5 mg/mL[a]	Physically compatible for 4 hr at 23 °C	2373	**C**
Caspofungin acetate	ME	0.7 mg/mL[b]	HOS	5 mg/mL[b]	Physically compatible for 4 hr at room temperature	2758	**C**
Cefepime HCl	BMS	120 mg/mL[n]		15 mg/mL	Physically compatible with less than 10% cefepime loss. Amikacin not tested	2513	**C**
Ceftaroline fosamil	FOR	2.22 mg/ mL[a,b,d]	HOS	5 mg/mL[a,b,d]	Physically compatible for 4 hr at 23 °C	2826	**C**
Ceftazidime	SKB	125 mg/mL		1.5 mg/mL	Visually compatible with less than 10% loss of both drugs in 1 hr	2434	**C**
	GSK	120 mg/mL[n]		15 mg/mL	Physically compatible with less than 10% ceftazidime loss. Amikacin not tested	2513	**C**
Cisatracurium besylate	GW	0.1, 2, 5 mg/ mL[a]	AB	5 mg/mL[a]	Physically compatible for 4 hr at 23 °C	2074	**C**
Cyclophosphamide	MJ	20 mg/mL[a]	BR	5 mg/mL[a]	Physically compatible for 4 hr at 25 °C	1194	**C**
Dexamethasone sodium phosphate	AMR	4 mg/mL	SQ	50 mg/mL[e]	Visually compatible for 24 hr at room temperature in test tubes. No precipitate found on filter from Y-site delivery	2063	**C**
Dexmedetomidine HCl	AB	4 mcg/mL[b]	APO	5 mg/mL[b]	Physically compatible for 4 hr at 23 °C	2383	**C**

Y-Site Injection Compatibility (1:1 Mixture) (Cont.)

Amikacin sulfate

Drug	Mfr	Conc	Mfr	Conc	Remarks	Ref	C/I
Diltiazem HCl	MMD	5 mg/mL	BR	5[b] and 250 mg/mL	Visually compatible	1807	C
Docetaxel	RPR	0.9 mg/mL[a]	AB	5 mg/mL[a]	Physically compatible for 4 hr at 23 °C	2224	C
Doripenem	JJ	5 mg/mL[a,b]	BED	5 mg/mL[a,b]	Physically compatible for 4 hr at 23 °C	2743	C
Enalaprilat	MSD	0.05 mg/mL[b]	BR	2 mg/mL[a]	Physically compatible for 24 hr at room temperature under fluorescent light	1355	C
Esmolol HCl	DCC	10 mg/mL[a]	BR	5 mg/mL[a]	Physically compatible for 24 hr at 22 °C	1169	C
Etoposide phosphate	BR	5 mg/mL[a]	APC	5 mg/mL[a]	Physically compatible for 4 hr at 23 °C	2218	C
Fenoldopam mesylate	AB	80 mcg/mL[b]	APO	5 mg/mL[b]	Physically compatible for 4 hr at 23 °C	2467	C
Filgrastim	AMG	30 mcg/mL[a]	ES	5 mg/mL[a]	Physically compatible for 4 hr at 22 °C	1687	C
	AMG	10[f] and 40[a] mcg/mL	BMS	5 mg/mL[a]	Visually compatible. Little loss of filgrastim and fluconazole in 4 hr at 25 °C	2060	C
Fluconazole	RR	2 mg/mL	BR	20 mg/mL	Physically compatible for 24 hr at 25 °C	1407	C
Fludarabine phosphate	BX	1 mg/mL[a]	BR	5 mg/mL[a]	Visually compatible for 4 hr at 22 °C	1439	C
Foscarnet sodium	AST	24 mg/mL	BR	20 mg/mL	Physically compatible for 24 hr at room temperature under fluorescent light	1335	C
Furosemide	HO	10 mg/mL	BR	2 mg/mL[c]	Physically compatible for 24 hr at 21 °C	876	C
Gemcitabine HCl	LI	10 mg/mL[b]	APC	5 mg/mL[b]	Physically compatible for 4 hr at 23 °C	2226	C
Granisetron HCl	SKB	0.05 mg/mL[a]	AB	5 mg/mL[a]	Physically compatible for 4 hr at 23 °C	2000	C
Hetastarch in lactated electrolyte	AB	6%	APC	5 mg/mL[a]	Physically compatible for 4 hr at 23 °C	2339	C
Hetastarch in sodium chloride 0.9%	DCC	6%	BR	5 mg/mL[a]	Small crystals form immediately after mixing and persist for 4 hr	1313	I
Hydromorphone HCl	WY	0.2 mg/mL[a]	BR	5 mg/mL[a]	Physically compatible for 4 hr at 25 °C	987	C
Idarubicin HCl	AD	1 mg/mL[b]	BR	5 mg/mL[a]	Visually compatible for 24 hr at 25 °C	1525	C
Labetalol HCl	SC	1 mg/mL[a]	BR	5 mg/mL[a]	Physically compatible for 24 hr at 18 °C	1171	C
Levofloxacin	OMN	5 mg/mL	BED	50 mg/mL	Visually compatible for 4 hr at 24 °C	2233	C
Linezolid	PHU	2 mg/mL	AB	5 mg/mL[a]	Physically compatible for 4 hr at 23 °C	2264	C
Lorazepam	WY	0.33 mg/mL[b]	BMS	5 mg/mL	Visually compatible for 24 hr at 22 °C	1855	C
Magnesium sulfate	IX	16.7, 33.3, 66.7, 100 mg/mL[a]	BR	5 mg/mL[a]	Physically compatible for at least 4 hr at 32 °C	813	C
Melphalan HCl	BW	0.1 mg/mL[b]	BR	5 mg/mL[b]	Physically compatible for 3 hr at 22 °C	1557	C
Meperidine HCl	WY	10 mg/mL[a]	BR	5 mg/mL[a]	Physically compatible for 4 hr at 25 °C	987	C
Midazolam HCl	RC	5 mg/mL	BMS	5 mg/mL	Visually compatible for 24 hr at 22 °C	1855	C
Milrinone lactate	SS	0.2 mg/mL[a]	AB	5 mg/mL[a]	Visually compatible for 4 hr at 25 °C	2381	C
Morphine sulfate	WI	1 mg/mL[a]	BR	5 mg/mL[a]	Physically compatible for 4 hr at 25 °C	987	C
Nicardipine HCl	DCC	0.1 mg/mL[a]	BR	2 mg/mL[a]	Visually compatible for 24 hr at room temperature	235	C
Ondansetron HCl	GL	1 mg/mL[b]	BR	5 mg/mL[a]	Visually compatible for 4 hr at 22 °C	1365	C
Paclitaxel	NCI	1.2 mg/mL[a]	BR	5 mg/mL[a]	Physically compatible for 4 hr at 22 °C	1556	C
Pemetrexed disodium	LI	20 mg/mL[b]	APC	5 mg/mL[a]	Physically compatible for 4 hr at 23 °C	2564	C
Propofol	ZEN	10 mg/mL	DU	5 mg/mL[a]	Immediate precipitate and yellow color	2066	I

Y-Site Injection Compatibility (1:1 Mixture) (Cont.)

Amikacin sulfate

Drug	Mfr	Conc	Mfr	Conc	Remarks	Ref	C/I
Remifentanil HCl	GW	0.025 and 0.25 mg/mL[b]	AB	5 mg/mL[a]	Physically compatible for 4 hr at 23 °C	2075	C
Sargramostim	IMM	10 mcg/mL[b]	BR	5 mg/mL[b]	Visually compatible for 4 hr at 22 °C	1436	C
Teniposide	BR	0.1 mg/mL[a]	BR	5 mg/mL[a]	Physically compatible for 4 hr at 23 °C	1725	C
Thiotepa	IMM[g]	1 mg/mL[a]	DU	5 mg/mL[a]	Physically compatible for 4 hr at 23 °C	1861	C
Tigecycline	WY	1 mg/mL[b]		5 mg/mL[b]	Physically compatible for 4 hr	2714	C
TNA #97 to #104[h]			BR	250 mg/mL	Broken fat emulsion with floating oil	1324	I
TNA #218 to #226[h]			AB	5 mg/mL[a]	Visually compatible for 4 hr at 23 °C	2215	C
TPN #54[h]				250 mg/mL	Physically compatible and activity retained over 6 hr at 22 °C	1045	C
TPN #61[h]		[i]	BR	37.5 mg/ 0.15 mL[j]	Physically compatible	1012	C
		[k]	BR	225 mg/ 0.9 mL[j]	Physically compatible	1012	C
TPN #91[h]		[l]		15 mg[m]	Physically compatible	1170	C
TPN #203, #204[h]			APC	5 mg/mL	Visually compatible for 2 hr at 23 °C	1974	C
TPN #212 to #215[h]			AB	5 mg/mL[a]	Physically compatible for 4 hr at 23 °C	2109	C
Vinorelbine tartrate	BW	1 mg/mL[b]	BR	5 mg/mL[b]	Physically compatible for 4 hr at 22 °C	1558	C
Warfarin sodium	DU	0.1[c] and 2 mg/mL[n]	AB	5 mg/mL[c]	Physically compatible for 24 hr at 23 °C	2011	C
Zidovudine	BW	4 mg/mL[a]	BR	4 mg/mL[a]	Physically compatible for 4 hr at 25 °C	1193	C

[a]*Tested in dextrose 5%.*
[b]*Tested in sodium chloride 0.9%.*
[c]*Tested in both dextrose 5% and sodium chloride 0.9%.*
[d]*Tested in Ringer's injection, lactated.*
[e]*Tested in sodium chloride 0.45%.*
[f]*Tested in dextrose 5% with albumin human 2 mg/mL.*
[g]*Lyophilized formulation tested.*
[h]*Refer to Appendix I for the composition of parenteral nutrition solutions. TNA indicates a 3-in-1 admixture, and TPN indicates a 2-in-1 admixture.*
[i]*Run at 21 mL/hr.*
[j]*Given over 30 minutes by syringe pump.*
[k]*Run at 94 mL/hr.*
[l]*Run at 10 mL/hr.*
[m]*Given over one hour by syringe pump.*
[n]*Tested in sterile water for injection.*
[o]*Injected via Y-site into an administration set running azithromycin.*

Additional Compatibility Information

β-Lactam Antibiotics — In common with other aminoglycoside antibiotics, amikacin activity may be impaired by β-lactam antibiotics. This inactivation is dependent on concentration, temperature, and time of exposure. However, amikacin appears to be less affected by the β-lactam antibiotics than other aminoglycosides such as gentamicin and tobramycin. (68; 574; 575; 654; 740; 816; 824; 973; 1052)

The clinical significance of these interactions appears to be primarily confined to patients with renal failure. (218; 334; 361; 364; 616; 816; 847) Literature reports of greatly reduced aminoglycoside levels in such patients have appeared frequently. (363; 365; 366; 367; 614; 615; 962) In addition, the interaction may be clinically important if assays for aminoglycoside levels in serum are sufficiently delayed. (576; 618; 814; 824; 847; 1052)

Most authors believe that in vitro mixing of penicillins with aminoglycoside antibiotics should be avoided but that clinical use of the drugs in combination can be of great value. It is generally recommended that the drugs be given separately in such combined therapy. (157; 218; 222; 224; 361; 364; 368; 369; 370)

AMINO ACIDS
AHFS 40:20

Products — Amino acids are supplied in a variety of concentrations and sizes, both alone and in kits with dextrose 50% injection. For components, concentrations, and characteristics, see the labeling for the individual products.

Administration — Parenteral nutrition solutions composed of amino acids and high-concentration dextrose, which are strongly hypertonic, may be safely administered only through an indwelling intravenous catheter with the tip in the superior vena cava; they are used for severely depleted patients or those requiring long-term therapy. For moderately depleted patients, parenteral nutrition solutions with dextrose concentrations of 5 to 10%, which are substantially less hypertonic, may be administered peripherally. (4)

It has been recommended that administration sets used to administer lipid emulsions be changed within 24 hours of initiating fusion because of the potential for bacterial and fungal contamination. (2342)

The routine use of appropriate inline filters for the administration of parenteral nutrition has been recommended for patients requiring intensive or prolonged therapy, immunocompromised patients, neonates, children, and patients receiving home parenteral nutrition. Filtration is recommended to reduce intrinsic particulate burdens, protect patients from calcium phosphate or other precipitation, and reduce the risk from potential inadvertent microbial contamination. Inline filters should be positioned as close to the patient as possible. For non-lipid-containing (TPN, 2-in-1) parenteral nutrition, 0.2-μm filters, preferably endotoxin retaining, have been recommended. For lipid-containing (TNA, 3-in-1, AIO) parenteral nutrition, 1.2-μm filters have been recommended. (2346)

Stability — Solution containers should be visually inspected for cloudiness, haze, discoloration, precipitates, and bottle cracks and checked for the presence of vacuum before mixing and prior to administration. Only clear solutions should be administered. It is also recommended that the containers be protected from light until ready for use and from extremes of temperature such as freezing or over 40 °C. Because of the risk of microbiological contamination, manufacturers recommend storing mixed parenteral nutrition solutions for as little time as possible after preparation. Administration of a single bottle should not exceed 24 hours.

A study of the original FreAmine showed that the mixed solution was stable at 4 °C for 12 weeks. Increased temperature enhanced degradation. Decomposition due to the Maillard reaction is visible as a color change from the clear, light, pale yellow of the freshly prepared solution to yellow to red to dark brown. It was noted that the possibility of microbiological contamination limits the desirable storage time. It was recommended that solutions be stored under refrigeration and used as soon as possible after mixing. (186)

The previous study did not report on the stability of tryptophan because of variable and nonreproducible results. (186) In another study, it was shown that the tryptophan content of the original FreAmine was reduced approximately 20% by the presence of the sodium bisulfite 0.1% antioxidant. (187)

An evaluation of amino acid 4.25% injection with dextrose 25% (prepared from FreAmine II 8.5%), without additional additives, stored at 4 °C for two weeks showed little or no change in the concentrations of amino acids, including tryptophan, as well as pH. Particle counts were also normal over the period. When stored at 25 °C, approximately 6% tryptophan loss occurred, but no other changes were observed. (581)

In contrast, parenteral nutrition solutions composed of amino acids solution with ethanol and vitamins (Aminofusin, Pfrimmer) along with dextrose and a variety of electrolytes exhibited a darkening of color on storage at 37, 25, and 5 °C for 60 days. The rate of color change was less at the lowest temperature. A loss of ascorbic acid in the mixture was also demonstrated and was shown to be associated with the color changes. The rate of ascorbic acid decomposition was dependent on air space in the container and storage temperature. In addition, fine white crystals of calcium phosphate precipitated on day 12 at 25 and 37 °C and on day 25 at 5 °C. (580)

A photoreaction of the L-tryptophan in Nephramine essential amino acid injection was reported. The L-tryptophan in combination with bisulfite stabilizer, oxygen, and light yielded an indigo blue color. Although no toxicity was associated with the L-tryptophan degradation and blue color formation, it was recommended that Nephramine remain in its original carton until ready to be mixed with dextrose and that Nephramine mixtures be covered with amber, UV-light-resistant bags to retard the formation of the blue color. It was further noted that a slightly blue solution need not be changed for a colorless one, nor is it necessary to change a slightly blue filter for a white one. (579) However, it has been emphasized that the clinical importance of this reaction is largely undetermined and may not be entirely benign. (1055)

The effects of photoirradiation on a FreAmine II–dextrose 10% parenteral nutrition solution containing 1 mL/500 mL of multivitamins (USV) were evaluated. During simulated continuous administration to an infant at 0.156 mL/min, the amino acids did not change when the bottle, infusion tubing, and collection bottle were shielded with foil. Only 20 cm of tubing in the incubator was exposed to light. However, if the flow was stopped, a marked reduction in methionine (40%), tryptophan (44%), and histidine (22%) occurred in the solution exposed to light for 24 hours. In a similar solution without vitamins, only the tryptophan concentration decreased. The difference was attributed to the presence of riboflavin, a photosensitizer. The authors recommended administering the multivitamin separately and shielding from light. (833)

The stability of amino acids in a parenteral nutrition solution composed of amino acids 3.5%, dextrose 25%, and electrolytes in PVC bags was assessed at 4 and 25 °C over 30 days. No significant decreases of the amino acids occurred in the refrigerated samples. However, the sample stored at room temperature showed significant losses of methionine (10.2%) and arginine (8.2%) in 30 days. (1057)

The long-term stability of the components of a parenteral nutrition solution composed of amino acids, dextrose, electrolytes, and trace metals in PVC bags was determined over a six-month period of storage at 4 °C. None of the amino acids decomposed more than 10% during the first two months. However, at six months, all of the amino acids except tyrosine, lysine, and histidine had degraded by more than 10%; some losses exceeded 25%. The dextrose, electrolytes, and trace elements remained constant for the six-month period. Water loss through the PVC bag was only 0.2%. Visually the color remained unchanged. (1058)

The long-term stability of the components of six parenteral nutrition solutions containing variable amounts of amino acids, dextrose, electrolytes, trace elements, and vitamins, stored in PVC bags at 4 and 25 °C, was evaluated. No significant changes to the amino acids, dextrose, electrolytes, or trace elements were noted during 28 days. (1063)

Peroxide Formation — Potentially toxic peroxide is generated in parenteral nutrition admixtures as a reaction between oxygen and various components catalyzed by riboflavin in the presence of light. This is particularly true in neonatal formulations. (1650; 1653; 1947; 2306; 2309; 2316) Exposure of a neonatal parenteral nutrition admixture to ambient light resulted in the formation of peroxide concentrations up to 300 μm. Light protection from compounding through administration has been recommended as a more achievable approach to reduce the formation of peroxide than avoiding contact with oxygen. (2316)

Exposure of parenteral nutrition admixtures to light during phototherapy has been shown to generate substantially larger amounts of hydrogen peroxide. (2310) In a study of the rate of hydrogen peroxide formation in a TrophAmine 1%-based parenteral nutrition admixture exposed to light, levels of peroxide increased linearly for about eight hours and then reached a plateau at about 940 μm. A similar solution kept in the dark did not generate any detectable peroxide. A hydrogen peroxide concentration of as little as 25 μm has been shown to be lethal to 90% of human cells in culture. The authors speculated that additive hepatic oxidant injury over time might increase hepatic dysfunction as the duration of exposure to parenteral nutrition increases. The presence of sulfite antioxidants in the amino acids helps to reduce the formation of hydrogen peroxide, but the antioxidants are present in insufficient quantities to offer adequate protection. Shielding parenteral nutrition admixtures from light was recommended for neonatal administration. (2309)

The formation of toxic peroxides due to exposure of parenteral nutrition admixtures to light was reduced substantially by using colored administration sets. Both 2-in-1 and 3-in-1 parenteral nutrition admixtures exhibited little protection from peroxide formation when only the bag was shielded from light. Peroxide formation was two to three times higher using light-protected bags with clear tubing when compared to colored tubing. Shielding the parenteral nutrition bags from light and using black, yellow, or orange tubing would reduce peroxide loads down to about 100 μm. (2306)

Freezing Solutions — The acceptability of frozen storage of some parenteral nutrition solutions has been determined. Parenteral nutrition solutions composed of equal parts of Travasol 8.5% with electrolytes and dextrose 70% injection (final concentrations of amino acids and dextrose were 4.25 and 35%, respectively), in PVC containers were stored frozen at −20 °C for 60 days. Both overnight room temperature thawing and 30-minute microwave thawing were utilized. The results indicated that, with either thawing technique, the amino acids, electrolytes, and dextrose were unchanged after 60 days of frozen storage and subsequent thawing. (578)

Plasticizer Leaching — A parenteral nutrition solution containing an amino acid solution, dextrose, and electrolytes in a PVC bag did not leach measurable quantities of diethylhexyl phthalate (DEHP) plasticizer during 21 days of storage at 4 and 25 °C. However, addition of fat emulsion 10 or 20% to the formula caused detectable leaching of DEHP from the PVC containers stored for 48 hours. Higher DEHP levels were found in the 25 °C samples than in the 4 °C samples. The authors recommended limiting the use of lipid-containing parenteral nutrition admixtures to 24 to 36 hours. Use of non-PVC containers and tubing is another option to eliminate the problem of plasticizer leaching. (1430)

Compatibility Information

Solution Compatibility

Amino acids

Solution	Mfr	Mfr	Conc/L	Remarks	Ref	C/I
Fat emulsion 10%, intravenous	VT	MG	AA 8.5%	Mixed in equal parts. Physically compatible for 48 hr at 4 °C and room temperature	32	C
	CU	MG AB TR	8.5% 7% 8.5%	Mixed in equal parts. Physically compatible for 72 hr at room temperature	656	C
	VT		AA 10%	Mixed in equal parts. Changes in 20 min. Coalescence and creaming in 8 hr at 8 and 25 °C	825	I

Additive Compatibility

Amino acids

Drug	Mfr	Conc/L	Mfr	Test Soln	Remarks	Ref	C/I
Albumin human		9.5 g		TNA #232[a,i]	Microscopically observed emulsion disruption found with increased fat globule size in 48 hr at room temperature	2267	?
		9.5 g		TNA #233[a,i]	Visually apparent emulsion disruption with creaming in 4 hr at room temperature. Increased disruption attributed to the added effect of calcium and magnesium ions	2267	I

Additive Compatibility (Cont.)

Amino acids

Drug	Mfr	Conc/L	Mfr	Test Soln	Remarks	Ref	C/I
		18.2 g		TNA #234[a,i]	Creaming and free oil formation visually observed in 24 hours at room temperature	2267	**I**
		18.2 g		TNA #235[a,i]	Visually apparent emulsion disruption with creaming and free oil formation in 4 hr at room temperature. Increased disruption attributed to the added effect of calcium and magnesium ions	2267	**I**
Amikacin sulfate		150 mg		TPN #107[a]	Activity retained for 24 hr at 21 °C	1326	**C**
Aminophylline	SE	500 mg	MG	AA 4.25%, D 25%	No increase in particulate matter in 24 hr at 4 °C	349	**C**
	SE	250 mg to 1.5 g		TPN #25 to #27[a]	Physically compatible and aminophylline stable for at least 24 hr at 25 °C	755	**C**
	SE	1 g		TPN #25 to #27[a]	Physically compatible and aminophylline stable for at least 24 hr at 4 °C	755	**C**
	SE	1 g		TPN #28 to #30[a]	Physically compatible and aminophylline stable for at least 24 hr at 25 °C	755	**C**
		29.3 mg		[b]	No significant change in aminophylline content over 24 hr at 24 to 26 °C	852	**C**
		284 and 638 mg		TNA #180[a]	No theophylline loss and no increase in fat particle size in 24 hr at room temperature	1617	**C**
Amphotericin B	SQ	100 mg	MG	AA 4.25%, D 25%	Turbidity and fine yellow particles form	349	**I**
Ampicillin sodium	BR	1 g	MG	TPN #21[a]	Activity retained for 24 hr at 4 °C	87	**C**
	BR	1 g	MG	TPN #21[a]	12 to 25% ampicillin loss in 24 hr at 25 °C	87	**I**
	BR	1 g	MG	AA 4.25%, D 25%	Increase in microscopic particles noted over 24 hr at 5 °C	349	**I**
	AST	1.5 g		TPN #52[a]	69% ampicillin loss in 24 hr at 29 °C	440	**I**
	AST	1.5 g		TPN #53[a]	22% ampicillin loss in 24 hr at 29 °C	440	**I**
		1 and 3 g		TPN #107[a]	Activity retained for 24 hr at 21 °C	1326	**C**
Aztreonam		2 g		TPN #107[a]	Activity retained for 24 hr at 21 °C	1326	**C**
Cefazolin sodium	LI	1 g	MG	AA 4.25%, D 25%	No increase in particulate matter in 24 hr at 4 °C	349	**C**
	SKF	10 g	TR	TPN #22[a]	Physically compatible with no loss of activity in 24 hr at 22 °C in the dark	837	**C**
		1 g		TPN #107[a]	9% cefazolin loss in 24 hr at 21 °C	1326	**C**
Cefepime HCl	BR	1 and 4 g	AB	AA 4.25%, D 25%, electrolytes	5 to 6% cefepime loss in 8 hr at room temperature and 3 days at 5 °C	1682	**C**
Cefotaxime sodium		1 g		TPN #107[a]	Activity retained for 24 hr at 21 °C	1326	**C**
Cefoxitin sodium		1 g		TPN #107[a]	Activity retained for 24 hr at 21 °C	1326	**C**
Ceftazidime		1 g		TPN #107[a]	Activity retained for 24 hr at 21 °C	1326	**C**
	GL	6 g	AB	AA 5%, D 25%	No substantial amino acid degradation in 48 hr at 22 °C and 10 days at 4 °C. Ceftazidime stability the determining factor	1535	**C**
	GL	1 g		TPN #141 to #143[a]	Visually compatible with 8% ceftazidime loss in 6 hr and 10% loss in 24 hr at 22 °C. 8% ceftazidime loss in 3 days at 4 °C	1535	**C**

Additive Compatibility (Cont.)

Amino acids

Drug	Mfr	Conc/L	Mfr	Test Soln	Remarks	Ref	C/I
	GL	6 g		TPN #141 to #143[a]	Visually compatible with 6% ceftazidime loss in 12 hr and 11 to 13% loss in 24 hr at 22 °C. 7 to 9% ceftazidime loss in 3 days at 4 °C	1535	C
Cefuroxime sodium		1 g		TPN #107[a]	Activity retained for 24 hr at 21 °C	1326	C
Clindamycin phosphate	UP	250 mg	MG	TPN #21[a]	Stable for 24 hr at 4 and 25 °C	87	C
	UP	600 mg	MG	AA 4.25%, D 25%	No increase in particulate matter in 24 hr at 4 °C	349	C
	UP	3 g	TR	TPN #22[a]	Physically compatible with no loss in 24 hr at 22 °C in the dark	837	C
		400 mg[c]		TPN #107[a]	Stable for 24 hr at 21 °C	1326	C
Cyclophosphamide	MJ	500 mg	MG	AA 4.25%, D 25%	No increase in particulate matter in 24 hr at 4 °C	349	C
Cyclosporine	SZ	150 mg	MG	AA 5%, D 25%	Visually compatible with no cyclosporine loss in 72 hr at 21 °C	1616	C
Cytarabine	UP	100 mg	MG	AA 4.25%, D 25%	No increase in particulate matter in 24 hr at 4 °C	349	C
	UP	50 mg		TPN #57[a]	Physically compatible with no cytarabine loss in 48 hr at 25 or 8 °C	996	C
Dopamine HCl	AS	400 mg	MG	AA 4.25%, D 25%	No increase in particulate matter in 24 hr at 4 °C	349	C
Epoetin alfa	ORT	100 units		[d]	96% of the epoetin alfa delivered[e] over 24 hr	1878	C
Famotidine	MSD	20 and 40 mg		TPN #109, #110[a]	Physically compatible with no famotidine loss and little change in amino acids in 48 hr at 21 °C and in 7 days at 4 °C	1331	C
	MSD	20 and 50 mg		TNA #111, #112[a]	Physically compatible. Little loss and no change in fat particle size in 48 hr at 4 and 21 °C	1332	C
	MSD	20 mg		TPN #113[a]	Physically compatible. Little loss in 35 days at 4 °C in light	1334	C
	MSD	20 and 40 mg		TNA #114[a]	Physically compatible. No loss and no change in fat particle size in 72 hr at 21 °C in light	1333	C
	MSD	20 mg		[f]	0 to 5% loss in 48 hr at 25 °C in light or dark and at 5 °C	1344	C
	MSD	16.7 and 33.3 mg		TPN #115, #116[a]	No famotidine loss in 7 days at 23 and 4 °C	1352	C
	MSD	20 mg		TNA #182[a]	Visually compatible. No loss in 24 hr at 24 °C in light	1576	C
	MSD	20 mg		TNA #197 to #200[a]	Physically compatible. No loss in 48 hr at 22 °C in light	1921	C
	MSD	20 mg		TPN #196[a]	Physically compatible. No loss in 48 hr at 22 °C in light	1921	C
Fluorouracil	RC	500 mg	MG	AA 4.25%, D 25%	No increase in particulate matter in 24 hr at 4 °C	349	C
	RC	1 and 4 g		TPN #23[a]	Physically compatible for 42 hr at room temperature in light. Erratic assay results	562	?
	RC	1 g		TPN #23[a]	Physically compatible and fluorouracil stable for 48 hr at room temperature in ambient light	826	C

Additive Compatibility (Cont.)

Amino acids

Drug	Mfr	Conc/L	Mfr	Test Soln	Remarks	Ref	C/I
Folic acid		1 mg		TPN #74[a]	Folic acid stable over 8 hr at room temperature in fluorescent or sunlight	842	C
	USP	0.2 and 10 mg	MG	AA 4.25%, D 25%	Physically compatible. Stable for 7 days at 4 °C and room temperature in dark	895	C
	USP	0.4 mg		TPN #69[a]	Physically compatible and folic acid stable for at least 7 days at 4 and 25 °C protected from light	895	C
	LE	0.25 to 1 mg		TPN #70[a]	Folic acid stable for at least 48 hr at 6 and 21 °C in light or dark conditions	896	C
Furosemide	HO	40 mg	MG	AA 4.25%, D 25%	No increase in particulate matter in 24 hr at 4 °C	349	C
Ganciclovir sodium	SY	3 and 5 g		TPN #183 to #185[a]	Precipitate forms	1744	I
	SY	2 g		TPN #183[a]	Precipitate forms	1744	I
Gentamicin sulfate	SC	80 mg	MG	AA 4.25%, D 25%	No increase in particulate matter in 24 hr at 4 °C	349	C
	SC	800 mg	TR	TPN #22[a]	Physically compatible. No loss in 24 hr at 22 °C in the dark	837	C
	SC	50 mg		TPN #52 and TPN #53[a]	Physically compatible. No loss in 24 hr at 29 °C	440	C
		75 mg		TPN #107[a]	Physically compatible and stable for 24 hr at 21 °C	1326	C
Heparin sodium	RI	20,000 units	MG	AA 4.25%, D 25%	No increase in particulate matter in 24 hr at 4 °C	349	C
		35,000 units		TPN #48 to #51[a]	Heparin activity retained for 24 hr at 25 °C but fell significantly after 24 hr	900	C
	LY	3000 to 20,000 units		TPN #205[a]	Heparin activity retained for 28 days at 4 °C	2025	C
Hydrochloric acid		40, 60, 100 mEq	MG	TPN #24[a]	Physically compatible and changes in amino acid concentrations considered negligible over 24 hr at 25 °C. Hydrochloric acid available from solution	582	C
Imipenem–cilastatin sodium		500 mg		TPN #107[a]	57% imipenem loss in 24 hr at 21 °C	1326	I
	MSD	5 g		TPN #241, #242[a]	8 to 10% imipenem loss within 30 min at 25 °C under fluorescent light	493	I
Insulin, regular	NOV	10 units	[a,i]	TNA #267[a,i]	40 to 60% loss likely due to sorption	2599	I
Iron dextran	FI	100 mg	TR	TPN #31 to #33[a]	Physically compatible with minimal changes to iron dextran and amino acids for 18 hr at room temperature	692	C
	FI	50 mg		TNA #122[a]	Lipid oiling out in 18 to 19 hr with formation of yellow-brown layer	1383	I
	FI			TNA #159 to #166[a]	Physically compatible with no change in particle size distribution in 48 hr at 4 and 25 °C	1648	C
	SCN	10 mg		TPN #207, #208[a]	Rust-colored precipitate forms in 12 hr at 19 °C protected from sunlight	2103	I
	SCN	10 mg		TPN #209[a]	Rust-colored precipitate forms in some samples in 18 to 24 hr at 19 °C protected from sunlight	2103	I
	SCN	10 mg		TPN #210[a]	Visually compatible for 48 hr at 19 °C protected from sunlight. Trace iron precipitation found after 48 hr	2103	?

Additive Compatibility (Cont.)

Amino acids

Drug	Mfr	Conc/L	Mfr	Test Soln	Remarks	Ref	C/I
	SCN	10 mg		TPN #211[a]	Visually compatible for 48 hr at 19 °C protected from sunlight. No iron precipitation found after 48 hr	2103	C
Isoproterenol HCl	WI	2 mg	MG	AA 4.25%, D 25%	No increase in particulate matter in 24 hr at 4 °C	349	C
Lidocaine HCl	AST	1 g	MG	AA 4.25%, D 25%	No increase in particulate matter in 24 hr at 4 °C	349	C
Meperidine HCl	WI	100 mg		TPN #71[a,g]	Physically compatible with no meperidine loss in 36 hr at 22 °C	1000	C
Methotrexate sodium	LE	50 mg	MG	AA 4.25%, D 25%	No increase in particulate matter in 24 hr at 4 °C	349	C
Methyldopate HCl	MSD	500 mg	MG	AA 4.25%, D 25%	No increase in particulate matter in 24 hr at 4 °C	349	C
Methylprednisolone sodium succinate	UP	250 mg	MG	AA 4.25%, D 25%	No increase in particulate matter in 24 hr at 4 °C	349	C
	PHU	25, 63, 125 mg		TNA #237[a,i]	Physically compatible with no substantial change in lipid particle size. Variable assay results, but less than 10% change in drug concentration and less than 8% change in TNA components after 7 days at 4 °C, followed by 24 hr at ambient temperature and light	2347	C
	PHU	25, 63, 125 mg		TPN #236[a,i]	Variable assay results, but less than 10% change in drug concentration and less than 12% change in TPN components after 7 days at 4 °C, followed by 24 hr at ambient temperature and light	2347	C
Metoclopramide HCl	RB	5 and 20 mg	TR	AA 2.75%, D 25%, electrolytes	Metoclopramide chemically stable for 72 hr at room temperature	854	C
	RB	5 mg		TPN #89[a]	Physically compatible with no metoclopramide loss in 24 hr and 10% loss in 48 hr at 25 °C	1167	C
	RB	20 mg		TPN #89[a]	Physically compatible with no metoclopramide loss in 72 hr at 25 °C	1167	C
	RB	5 mg		TPN #90[a]	Physically compatible with no metoclopramide loss in 72 hr at 25 °C	1167	C
	RB	20 mg		TPN #90[a]	Physically compatible with 3% metoclopramide loss in 72 hr at 25 °C	1167	C
Midazolam HCl	RC	600 mg to 1 g		TPN #174 to #176[a]	Precipitates immediately	1624	I
	RC	100 and 500 mg		TPN #174 to #176[a]	Visually compatible with no midazolam loss and less than 10% loss of any amino acid in 5 hr at 22 °C	1624	C
Morphine sulfate	LI	100 mg		TPN #71[a,g]	Physically compatible with no morphine loss in 36 hr at 22 °C	1000	C
Multivitamins	USV	1 vial	TR	AA 4.25%, D 25%	No loss of thiamine HCl in 22 hr at 30 °C	843	C
(M.V.I. Pediatric)	ROR	5 mL		AA 2%, D 12.5%, electrolytes	7% phytonadione loss in 4 hr and 27% loss in 24 hr under ambient temperature and light	1815	I

Additive Compatibility (Cont.)

Amino acids

Drug	Mfr	Conc/L	Mfr	Test Soln	Remarks	Ref	C/I
Multivitamins	LY	10 mL	AB[g,h,l]	AA 2.5%, D 25%	All vitamins stable for 24 hr at 4 °C	926	C
	LY	10 mL	MG[g,h,l]	AA 4.25%, D 25%	All vitamins stable for 24 hr at 4 °C	926	C
Nafcillin sodium		1 and 2 g		TPN #107[a]	Nafcillin activity retained for 24 hr at 21 °C	1326	C
Norepinephrine bitartrate	WI	4 mg	MG	AA 4.25%, D 25%	No increase in particulate matter in 24 hr at 4 °C	349	C
Octreotide acetate	SZ	1.5 mg		TPN #119, #120[a,h]	Little octreotide loss over 48 hr at room temperature in ambient room light	1373	C
	SZ	450 mcg		TNA #139[a,g,i]	Physically compatible with no change in lipid particle size in 48 hr at 22 °C under fluorescent light and 7 days at 4 °C. Octreotide activity highly variable	1540	?
Ondansetron HCl	GL	0.03 and 0.3 g		TNA #190[a]	Physically compatible with no ondansetron loss in 48 hr at 24 °C in light	1766	C
Oxacillin sodium	BR	500 mg	MG	AA 4.25%, D 25%	No increase in particulate matter in 24 hr at 4 °C	349	C
Pantoprazole sodium	ALT[k]	13.3 mg	TPN #265[a]		Yellow discoloration and drug losses of 12% in 3 hr at room temperature in dark	2789	I
Penicillin G potassium	SQ	5 million units	MG	TPN #21[a]	Activity retained for 24 hr at 4 and 25 °C	87	C
	LI	1 million units	MG	AA 4.25%, D 25%	No increase in particulate matter in 24 hr at 4 °C	349	C
	AY	25 million units	TR	TPN #22[a]	Physically compatible with no loss of activity in 24 hr at 22 °C in dark	837	C
		2 g		TPN #107[a]	Activity retained for 24 hr at 21 °C	1326	C
Penicillin G sodium		2 g		TPN #107[a]	Activity retained for 24 hr at 21 °C	1326	C
Phytonadione	MSD	10 mg	MG	AA 4.25%, D 25%	No increase in particulate matter in 24 hr at 4 °C	349	C
Polymyxin B sulfate	NOV	40 mg		TPN #52, #53[a]	Physically compatible with no polymyxin loss in 24 hr at 29 °C	440	C
Ranitidine HCl	GL	83, 167, 250 mg		TPN #58[a]	10% ranitidine loss in 48 hr at 23 °C	997	C
	GL	50 and 100 mg		TPN #59, #60[a,h]	No color change and 7 to 9% ranitidine loss in 24 hr at 24 °C in light. Amino acids unaffected. Darkened color and 10 to 12% ranitidine loss in 48 hr	1010	C
	GL	50 and 100 mg		TNA #92[a,i]	7 to 10% ranitidine loss in 12 hr and 20 to 28% loss in 24 hr at 23 °C in light	1183	I
	GL	50 and 100 mg		TPN #117[a]	Physically compatible and 5% ranitidine loss in 48 hr refrigerated and at 25 °C	1360	C
	GL	50 and 100 mg		TNA #118[a]	Physically compatible. 6 to 10% ranitidine loss in 36 hr under refrigeration and at 25 °C	1360	C
	GL	75 mg		TNA #197 to #200[a]	Physically compatible with 7% or less ranitidine loss in 24 hr at 22 °C in light. About 15% loss in 48 hr	1921	C
	GL	75 mg		TPN #196[a]	Physically compatible with 7% or less ranitidine loss in 24 hr at 22 °C in light. About 12% loss in 48 hr	1921	C

Additive Compatibility (Cont.)

Amino acids

Drug	Mfr	Conc/L	Mfr	Test Soln	Remarks	Ref	C/I
		200 mg		TNA #245[a]	No ranitidine loss and no lipid change in 24 hr at room temperature	486	C
	GL	72 mg		TNA #246[a]	Less than 7% ranitidine loss and no change in emulsion integrity in 14 days at 4 °C	501	C
	GL	72 mg		TPN #247[a]	2% ranitidine loss in 14 days at 4 °C	501	C
Sodium bicarbonate		50 and 150 mEq		TPN #62 to #65	Physically compatible with 10% or less carbon dioxide loss and unchanged pH in 7 days at 25 °C protected from light	1011	C
		100 mEq		TPN #66 to #68[a]	Physically compatible with 10% or less carbon dioxide loss and unchanged pH in 7 days at 25 °C protected from light	1011	C
Tacrolimus	FUJ	100 mg		TPN #201[a,g]	Visually compatible with no loss in 24 hr at 24 °C	1922	C
Tobramycin sulfate	LI	80 mg	MG	AA 4.25%, D 25%	No increase in particulate matter in 24 hr at 4 °C	349	C
Vancomycin HCl		400 mg		TPN #95, #96[a]	Physically compatible and no vancomycin loss for 8 days at room temperature and refrigerated	1321	C
		1 and 6 g		TPN #105, #106[a]	Physically compatible with little or no vancomycin loss in 4 hr at 22 °C	1325	C
		200 mg		TPN #107[a]	Activity retained for 24 hr at 21 °C	1326	C
	LI	500 mg and 1 g		TPN #202[a,h]	Visually compatible and activity retained for 35 days at 4 °C plus 24 hr at 22 °C	1933	C

[a]*Refer to Appendix I for the composition of parenteral nutrition solutions. TNA indicates a 3-in-1 admixture, and TPN indicates a 2-in-1 admixture.*
[b]*Tested in a pediatric parenteral nutrition solution containing 150 mL of dextrose 5% and 30 mL of Vamin glucose with electrolytes and vitamins.*
[c]*Expressed as clindamycin base.*
[d]*TPN composed of amino acids (TrophAmine) 0.5 or 2.25% with dextrose 12.5%, vitamins, trace elements, magnesium sulfate, calcium gluconate, sodium chloride, potassium acetate, and heparin sodium.*
[e]*Delivered from a syringe through microbore tubing, T-connector, and a Teflon neonatal 24-gauge intravenous catheter.*
[f]*Tested in Vamin 14, Vamin 18, Vamin glucose, and Vamin N.*
[g]*Tested in glass containers.*
[h]*Tested in PVC containers.*
[i]*Tested in ethylene vinyl acetate containers.*
[j]*Concentration expressed in milligrams of phenytoin sodium equivalents (PE) per milliliter.*
[k]*Test performed using the formulation WITH edetate disodium.*
[l]*Tested in polyolefin bags.*

Y-Site Injection Compatibility (1:1 Mixture)

Amino acids

Drug	Mfr	Conc	Mfr	Conc	Remarks	Ref	C/I
Acetazolamide sodium	LE	100 mg/mL		TPN #203, #204[g]	White precipitate forms immediately	1974	I
Acyclovir sodium	BW	7 mg/mL		TPN #203, #204[g]	White precipitate forms immediately	1974	I
	BW	7 mg/mL[a]		TPN #212 to #215[g]	Crystalline needles form immediately, becoming a gross precipitate in 1 hr	2109	I
	GW	7 mg/mL[a]		TNA #218 to #226[g]	White precipitate forms immediately	2215	I
Alprostadil	BED	15 mcg/mL[a]		TPN #274[g]	Visually compatible for 1 hr	2746	C
Amikacin sulfate		250 mg/mL		TPN #54[g]	Physically compatible and activity retained over 6 hr at 22 °C	1045	C

Y-Site Injection Compatibility (1:1 Mixture) (Cont.)

				Amino acids			
Drug	Mfr	Conc	Mfr	Conc	Remarks	Ref	C/I
	BR	37.5 mg/ 0.15 mL[j]		TPN #61[c,g]	Physically compatible	1012	C
	BR	225 mg/ 0.9 mL[j]		TPN #61[d,g]	Physically compatible	1012	C
	BR	15 mg[e]		TPN #91[f,g]	Physically compatible	1170	C
	BR	250 mg/mL		TNA #97 to #104[g]	Broken fat emulsion with floating oil	1324	I
	APC	5 mg/mL		TPN #203, #204[g]	Visually compatible for 2 hr at 23 °C	1974	C
	AB	5 mg/mL[a]		TPN #212 to #215[g]	Physically compatible for 4 hr at 23 °C	2109	C
	AB	5 mg/mL[a]		TNA #218 to #226[g]	Visually compatible for 4 hr at 23 °C	2215	C
Aminophylline	DB	1 mg/mL[b]		TPN #189[g]	Visually compatible for 24 hr at 22 °C	1767	C
	AMR	5 and 25 mg/ mL		TPN #203, #204[g]	White precipitate forms immediately	1974	I
	AB	2.5 mg/mL[a]		TPN #212 to #215[g]	Physically compatible for 4 hr at 23 °C	2109	C
	AB	2.5 mg/mL[a]		TNA #218 to #226[g]	Visually compatible for 4 hr at 23 °C	2215	C
Amoxicillin sodium		50 mg/mL[b]		TPN #189[g]	Visually compatible for 24 hr at 22 °C	1767	C
Amphotericin B	PH	0.6 mg/mL[a]		TPN #212 to #215[g]	Precipitate forms immediately	2109	I
	PH	0.6 mg/mL[a]		TNA #218 to #226[g]	Yellow precipitate forms immediately	2215	I
Ampicillin sodium	BR	40 mg/mL[b]		TNA #73[g,h]	Visually compatible for 4 hr at 25 °C	1008	C
	WY	250 mg/ 1.3 mL[i]		TPN #61[c,g]	Heavy precipitate of calcium phosphate	1012	I
	WY	1.5 g/7.5 mL[i]		TPN #61[d,g]	Heavy precipitate of calcium phosphate	1012	I
				TPN #54[g]	Precipitate forms in 30 min at 22 °C	1045	I
	APC	100 and 250 mg/mL		TPN #203, #204[g]	White precipitate forms immediately	1974	I
	SKB	20 mg/mL[b]		TPN #212 to #215[g]	Physically compatible for 4 hr at 23 °C	2109	C
	SKB	20 mg/mL[b]		TNA #218 to #226[g]	Visually compatible for 4 hr at 23 °C	2215	C
Ampicillin sodium–sulbactam sodium	RR	20 + 10 mg/ mL[b]		TPN #212 to #215[g]	Physically compatible for 4 hr at 23 °C	2109	C
	PF	20 + 10 mg/ mL[b]		TNA #218 to #226[g]	Visually compatible for 4 hr at 23 °C	2215	C
Argatroban	SKB	1 mg/mL[a]		TPN #263[g]	Physically compatible for 24 hr at 23 °C	2572	C
Ascorbic acid	DB	20 mg/mL[b]		TPN #189[g]	Visually compatible for 24 hr at 22 °C	1767	C
Atracurium besylate	WEL	10 mg/mL		TPN #189[g]	Visually compatible for 24 hr at 22 °C	1767	C
Aztreonam	SQ	40 mg/mL[a]		TPN #212 to #215[g]	Physically compatible for 4 hr at 23 °C	2109	C
	SQ	40 mg/mL[a]		TNA #218 to #226[g]	Visually compatible for 4 hr at 23 °C	2215	C
Bumetanide	RC	0.04 mg/mL[a]		TPN #212 to #215[g]	Physically compatible for 4 hr at 23 °C	2109	C

Y-Site Injection Compatibility (1:1 Mixture) (Cont.)

Amino acids

Drug	Mfr	Conc	Mfr	Conc	Remarks	Ref	C/I
	RC, BV	0.04 mg/mL[a]		TNA #218 to #226[g]	Visually compatible for 4 hr at 23 °C	2215	C
Buprenorphine HCl	RKC	0.04 mg/mL[a]		TPN #212 to #215[g]	Physically compatible for 4 hr at 23 °C	2109	C
	RKC	0.04 mg/mL[a]		TNA #218 to #226[g]	Visually compatible for 4 hr at 23 °C	2215	C
Butorphanol tartrate	APC	0.04 mg/mL[a]		TPN #212 to #215[g]	Physically compatible for 4 hr at 23 °C	2109	C
	APC	0.04 mg/mL[a]		TNA #218 to #226[g]	Visually compatible for 4 hr at 23 °C	2215	C
Calcium gluconate	DB	10 mg/mL[b]		TPN #189[g]	Visually compatible for 24 hr at 22 °C	1767	C
	AB	40 mg/mL[a]		TPN #212 to #215[g]	Physically compatible for 4 hr at 23 °C	2109	C
	AB	40 mg/mL[a]		TNA #218 to #226[g]	Visually compatible for 4 hr at 23 °C	2215	C
Carboplatin	BMS	5 mg/mL[a]		TPN #212 to #215[g]	Physically compatible for 4 hr at 23 °C	2109	C
	BMS	5 mg/mL[a]		TNA #218 to #226[g]	Visually compatible for 4 hr at 23 °C	2215	C
Caspofungin acetate	ME	0.7 mg/mL[b]		TPN[w]	Immediate white turbid precipitate forms	2758	I
Cefazolin sodium	SKF	20 mg/mL[a]		TNA #73[g,h]	Visually compatible for 4 hr at 25 °C	1008	C
	SKF	200 mg/ 0.9 mL[i]		TPN #61[c,g]	Physically compatible	1012	C
	SKF	1.2 g/5.3 mL[i]		TPN #61[d,g]	Physically compatible	1012	C
	SKB	20 mg/mL[a]		TPN #212, #213[g]	Physically compatible for 4 hr at 23 °C	2109	C
	SKB	20 mg/mL[a]		TPN #214, #215[g]	Microprecipitate forms immediately	2109	I
	SKB	20 mg/mL[a]		TNA #218 to #226[g]	Visually compatible for 4 hr at 23 °C	2215	C
Cefotaxime sodium	HO	200 mg/ 0.7 mL[i]		TPN #61[c,g]	Physically compatible	1012	C
	HO	1.2 g/4 mL[i]		TPN #61[d,g]	Physically compatible	1012	C
	RS	200 mg/mL[k]		TPN #189[g]	Visually compatible for 24 hr at 22 °C	1767	C
	HO	60 mg/mL		TPN #203, #204[g]	Visually compatible for 2 hr at 23 °C	1974	C
	HO	20 mg/mL[a]		TPN #212 to #215[g]	Physically compatible for 4 hr at 23 °C	2109	C
	HO	20 mg/mL[a]		TNA #218 to #226[g]	Visually compatible for 4 hr at 23 °C	2215	C
Cefotetan disodium	STU	20 mg/mL[a]		TPN #212 to #215[g]	Physically compatible for 4 hr at 23 °C	2109	C
	ZEN	20 mg/mL[a]		TNA #218 to #226[g]	Visually compatible for 4 hr at 23 °C	2215	C
Cefoxitin sodium	MSD	20 mg/mL[a]		TNA #73[g,h]	Visually compatible for 4 hr at 25 °C	1008	C
	MSD	200 mg/ 2.1 mL[i]		TPN #61[c,g]	Physically compatible	1012	C
	MSD	1.2 g/ 12.6 mL[i]		TPN #61[d,g]	Physically compatible	1012	C
	MSD	200 mg/mL[k]		TPN #189[g]	Visually compatible for 24 hr at 22 °C	1767	C
	ME	20 mg/mL[a]		TPN #212 to #215[d]	Physically compatible for 4 hr at 23 °C	2109	C

Y-Site Injection Compatibility (1:1 Mixture) (Cont.)

Drug	Mfr	Conc	Mfr	Conc	Remarks	Ref	C/I
				Amino acids			
	ME	20 mg/mL[a]		TNA #218 to #226[g]	Visually compatible for 4 hr at 23 °C	2215	C
Ceftaroline fosamil	FOR	2.22 mg/mL[a,b,v]		TPN #296[g]	Physically compatible for 4 hr at 23 °C	2826	C
Ceftazidime	GL	40 mg/mL[l]		TPN #141 to #143[g]	Visually compatible with 4% or less ceftazidime loss in 2 hr at 22 °C in 1:1 and 1:3 ratios	1535	C
	GL	200 mg/mL[k]		TPN #189[g]	Visually compatible for 24 hr at 22 °C	1767	C
	LI	60 mg/mL		TPN #203, #204[g]	Visually compatible for 2 hr at 23 °C	1974	C
	SKB	40 mg/mL[a]		TPN #212 to #215[g]	Physically compatible for 4 hr at 23 °C	2109	C
	SKB[v]	40 mg/mL[a]		TNA #218 to #226[g]	Visually compatible for 4 hr at 23 °C	2215	C
Cefuroxime sodium	LI	30 mg/mL[a]		TPN #212 to #215[g]	Physically compatible for 4 hr at 23 °C	2109	C
	GL	30 mg/mL[a]		TNA #218 to #226[g]	Visually compatible for 4 hr at 23 °C	2215	C
Chloramphenicol sodium succinate	PD	125 mg/1.25 mL[i]		TPN #61[c,g]	Physically compatible	1012	C
	PD	750 mg/7.5 mL[i]		TPN #61[d,g]	Physically compatible	1012	C
Chlorothiazide sodium	ME	28 mg/mL		TPN #203, #204[g]	White precipitate forms immediately	1974	I
Chlorpromazine HCl	SCN	2 mg/mL[a]		TPN #212 to #215[g]	Physically compatible for 4 hr at 23 °C	2109	C
	SCN	2 mg/mL[a]		TNA #218 to #226[g]	Visually compatible for 4 hr at 23 °C	2215	C
Ciprofloxacin	MI	2 mg/mL[a]	AB	AA 5%, D 25%	Visually compatible for 2 hr at 25 °C under fluorescent light	1628	C
	MI	1 mg/mL[a]		TPN #212 to #215[g]	Amber discoloration forms in 1 to 4 hr	2109	I
	BAY	1 mg/mL[a]		TNA #218 to #226[g]	Visually compatible for 4 hr at 23 °C	2215	C
Cisplatin	BMS	1 mg/mL		TPN #212 to #215[g]	Amber discoloration forms in 1 to 4 hr	2109	I
	BMS	1 mg/mL		TNA #218 to #226[g]	Visually compatible for 4 hr at 23 °C	2215	C
Clindamycin phosphate	UP	12 mg/mL[a]		TNA #73[g,h]	Visually compatible for 4 hr at 25 °C	1008	C
	UP	50 mg/0.33 mL[m]		TPN #61[c,g]	Physically compatible	1012	C
	UP	300 mg/2 mL[m]		TPN #61[d,g]	Physically compatible	1012	C
	AB	10 mg/mL[a]		TPN #212 to #215[g]	Physically compatible for 4 hr at 23 °C	2109	C
	AST	10 mg/mL[a]		TNA #218 to #226[g]	Visually compatible for 4 hr at 23 °C	2215	C
Clonazepam	RC	1 mg/mL[k]		TPN #189[g]	Visually compatible for 24 hr at 22 °C	1767	C
Cyclophosphamide	MJ	10 mg/mL[a]		TPN #212 to #215[g]	Physically compatible for 4 hr at 23 °C	2109	C

Y-Site Injection Compatibility (1:1 Mixture) (Cont.)

<table>
<tr><th colspan="9" style="text-align:center">Amino acids</th></tr>
<tr><th>Drug</th><th>Mfr</th><th>Conc</th><th>Mfr</th><th>Conc</th><th>Remarks</th><th>· Ref</th><th>C/I</th></tr>
<tr><td></td><td>MJ</td><td>10 mg/mL[a]</td><td></td><td>TNA #218 to #226[g]</td><td>Visually compatible for 4 hr at 23 °C</td><td>2215</td><td>**C**</td></tr>
<tr><td>Cyclosporine</td><td>SZ</td><td>5 mg/mL[a]</td><td></td><td>TPN #212, #213[g]</td><td>Physically compatible for 4 hr at 23 °C</td><td>2109</td><td>**C**</td></tr>
<tr><td></td><td>SZ</td><td>5 mg/mL[a]</td><td></td><td>TPN #214, #215[g]</td><td>Small amount of subvisible precipitate forms in 4 hr</td><td>2109</td><td>**I**</td></tr>
<tr><td></td><td>SZ</td><td>5 mg/mL[a]</td><td></td><td>TNA #220, #223[g]</td><td>Small amount of precipitate forms immediately</td><td>2215</td><td>**I**</td></tr>
<tr><td></td><td>SZ</td><td>5 mg/mL[a]</td><td></td><td>TNA #218, #219, #221, #222, #224 to #226[g]</td><td>Visually compatible for 4 hr at 23 °C</td><td>2215</td><td>**C**</td></tr>
<tr><td>Cytarabine</td><td>CHI</td><td>50 mg/mL</td><td></td><td>TPN #212 to #215[g]</td><td>Substantial loss of natural subvisible turbidity occurs immediately</td><td>2109</td><td>**I**</td></tr>
<tr><td></td><td>BED</td><td>50 mg/mL</td><td></td><td>TNA #218 to #226[g]</td><td>Visually compatible for 4 hr at 23 °C</td><td>2215</td><td>**C**</td></tr>
<tr><td>Dexamethasone sodium phosphate</td><td>AMR</td><td>4 mg/mL</td><td></td><td>TPN #203, #204[g]</td><td>Visually compatible for 2 hr at 23 °C</td><td>1974</td><td>**C**</td></tr>
<tr><td></td><td>AMR</td><td>1 mg/mL[a]</td><td></td><td>TPN #212 to #215[g]</td><td>Physically compatible for 4 hr at 23 °C</td><td>2109</td><td>**C**</td></tr>
<tr><td></td><td>FUJ, ES</td><td>1 mg/mL[a]</td><td></td><td>TNA #218 to #226[g]</td><td>Visually compatible for 4 hr at 23 °C</td><td>2215</td><td>**C**</td></tr>
<tr><td>Digoxin</td><td>BW</td><td>12.5 mcg/mL[l]</td><td></td><td>TNA #73[g]</td><td>Visually compatible for 4 hr</td><td>1009</td><td>**C**</td></tr>
<tr><td></td><td>BW</td><td>0.25 mg/mL</td><td></td><td>TPN #212 to #215[g]</td><td>Physically compatible for 4 hr at 23 °C</td><td>2109</td><td>**C**</td></tr>
<tr><td></td><td>ES, WY</td><td>0.25 mg/mL</td><td></td><td>TNA #218 to #226[g]</td><td>Visually compatible for 4 hr at 23 °C</td><td>2215</td><td>**C**</td></tr>
<tr><td>Diphenhydramine HCl</td><td>SCN</td><td>2[a] and 50 mg/mL</td><td></td><td>TPN #212 to #215[g]</td><td>Physically compatible for 4 hr at 23 °C</td><td>2109</td><td>**C**</td></tr>
<tr><td></td><td>SCN, PD</td><td>2[a] and 50 mg/mL</td><td></td><td>TNA #218 to #226[g]</td><td>Visually compatible for 4 hr at 23 °C</td><td>2215</td><td>**C**</td></tr>
<tr><td>Dobutamine HCl</td><td>LI</td><td>1 mg/mL[n]</td><td></td><td>TPN #91[f,g]</td><td>Physically compatible</td><td>1170</td><td>**C**</td></tr>
<tr><td></td><td>LI</td><td>50 mg/mL[b]</td><td></td><td>TPN #189[g]</td><td>Visually compatible for 24 hr at 22 °C</td><td>1767</td><td>**C**</td></tr>
<tr><td></td><td>LI</td><td>5 mg/mL</td><td></td><td>TPN #203, #204[g]</td><td>Visually compatible for 4 hr at 23 °C</td><td>1974</td><td>**C**</td></tr>
<tr><td></td><td>LI</td><td>4 mg/mL[a]</td><td></td><td>TPN #212 to #215[g]</td><td>Physically compatible for 4 hr at 23 °C</td><td>2109</td><td>**C**</td></tr>
<tr><td></td><td>AST</td><td>4 mg/mL[a]</td><td></td><td>TNA #218 to #226[g]</td><td>Visually compatible for 4 hr at 23 °C</td><td>2215</td><td>**C**</td></tr>
<tr><td>Dopamine HCl</td><td>AB</td><td>1.6 mg/mL[l]</td><td></td><td>TNA #73[g]</td><td>Visually compatible for 4 hr</td><td>1009</td><td>**C**</td></tr>
<tr><td></td><td>DB</td><td>1.6 mg/mL[b]</td><td></td><td>TPN #189[g]</td><td>Visually compatible for 24 hr at 22 °C</td><td>1767</td><td>**C**</td></tr>
<tr><td></td><td>AMR</td><td>3.2 mg/mL</td><td></td><td>TPN #203, #204[g]</td><td>Visually compatible for 4 hr at 23 °C</td><td>1974</td><td>**C**</td></tr>
<tr><td></td><td>AB</td><td>3.2 mg/mL[a]</td><td></td><td>TPN #212 to #215[g]</td><td>Physically compatible for 4 hr at 23 °C</td><td>2109</td><td>**C**</td></tr>
<tr><td></td><td>AB</td><td>3.2 mg/mL[a]</td><td></td><td>TNA #222, #223[g]</td><td>Precipitate forms immediately</td><td>2215</td><td>**I**</td></tr>
<tr><td></td><td>AB</td><td>3.2 mg/mL[a]</td><td></td><td>TNA #218 to #222, #224 to #226[g]</td><td>Visually compatible for 4 hr at 23 °C</td><td>2215</td><td>**C**</td></tr>
<tr><td>Doxorubicin HCl</td><td>PH</td><td>2 mg/mL</td><td></td><td>TPN #212 to #215[g]</td><td>Substantial loss of natural subvisible haze occurs immediately</td><td>2109</td><td>**I**</td></tr>
</table>

Y-Site Injection Compatibility (1:1 Mixture) (Cont.)

Drug	Mfr	Conc	Mfr	Conc	Remarks	Ref	C/I
	PH, GEN	2 mg/mL		TNA #218 to #226[g]	Damage to emulsion occurs immediately with free oil formation possible	2215	I
Doxycycline hyclate	PF	10 mg/1 mL[j]		TPN #61[c,g]	Physically compatible	1012	C
	PF	60 mg/6 mL[j]		TPN #61[d,g]	Physically compatible	1012	C
	LY	1 mg/mL[a]		TPN #212 to #215[g]	Physically compatible for 4 hr at 23 °C	2109	C
	FUJ	1 mg/mL[a]		TNA #218 to #226[g]	Damage to emulsion occurs immediately with free oil formation possible	2215	I
Droperidol	AB	0.4 mg/mL[a]		TPN #212 to #215[g]	Physically compatible for 4 hr at 23 °C	2109	C
	AB	0.4 mg/mL[a]		TNA #218 to #226[g]	Damage to emulsion occurs in 1 to 4 hr with free oil formation possible	2215	I
Enalaprilat	MSD	0.1 mg/mL[a]		TPN #212 to #215[g]	Physically compatible for 4 hr at 23 °C	2109	C
	ME	0.1 mg/mL[a]		TNA #218 to #226[g]	Visually compatible for 4 hr at 23 °C	2215	C
Epinephrine HCl	AST	0.2 mg/mL[b]		TPN #189[g]	Visually compatible for 24 hr at 22 °C	1767	C
Erythromycin lactobionate	AB	20 mg/mL[b]		TNA #73[g,h]	Visually compatible for 4 hr at 25 °C	1008	C
	AB	50 mg/1 mL[j]		TPN #61[c,g]	Physically compatible	1012	C
	AB	300 mg/6 mL[j]		TPN #61[d,g]	Physically compatible	1012	C
	DB	10 mg/mL[b]		TPN #189[g]	Visually compatible for 24 hr at 22 °C	1767	C
Famotidine	ME	2 mg/mL[a]		TPN #212 to #215[g]	Physically compatible for 4 hr at 23 °C	2109	C
	ME	2 mg/mL[a]		TNA #218 to #226[g]	Visually compatible for 4 hr at 23 °C	2215	C
Fentanyl citrate	ES	0.05 mg/mL		TPN #203, #204[g]	Visually compatible for 4 hr at 23 °C	1974	C
	ES	0.01 mg/mL[k]		TPN #216[g]	Mixed 1 mL of fentanyl with 9 mL of TPN. Visually compatible for 24 hr	2104	C
	AB, JN	0.0125[a] and 0.05 mg/mL		TPN #212 to #215[g]	Physically compatible for 4 hr at 23 °C	2109	C
	AB	0.0125[a] and 0.05 mg/mL		TNA #218 to #226[g]	Visually compatible for 4 hr at 23 °C	2215	C
Floxacillin sodium	BE	50 mg/mL[b]		TPN #189[g]	Visually compatible for 24 hr at 22 °C	1767	C
Fluconazole	PF	0.5 and 1.75 mg/mL[o]		TPN #146[g,o]	Visually compatible with no fluconazole loss in 2 hr at 24 °C in fluorescent light. Amino acids greater than 93%	1554	C
	PF	0.5 and 1.75 mg/mL[o]		TPN #147, #148[g,o]	Visually compatible with no fluconazole loss in 2 hr at 24 °C in fluorescent light. Amino acids not analyzed	1554	C
	RR	2 mg/mL		TPN #212 to #215[g]	Physically compatible for 4 hr at 23 °C	2109	C
	PF	2 mg/mL		TNA #218 to #226[g]	Visually compatible for 4 hr at 23 °C	2215	C
Fluorouracil	PH	16 mg/mL[a]		TPN #212, #213[g]	Slight subvisible haze, crystals, and amber discoloration form in 1 to 4 hr	2109	I
	PH	16 mg/mL[a]		TPN #214, #215[g]	Turbidity forms immediately	2109	I
	PH	16 mg/mL[a]		TNA #220, #223[g]	Small amount of white precipitate forms immediately	2215	I

Y-Site Injection Compatibility (1:1 Mixture) (Cont.)

Amino acids

Drug	Mfr	Conc	Mfr	Conc	Remarks	Ref	C/I
	PH	16 mg/mL[a]		TNA #218, #219, #221, #222, #224 to #226[g]	Visually compatible for 4 hr at 23 °C	2215	C
Folic acid	AB	15 mg/mL		TPN #189[g]	Visually compatible for 24 hr at 22 °C	1767	C
Foscarnet sodium	AST	24 mg/mL		TPN #121[g]	Physically compatible for 24 hr at 25 °C	1393	C
Furosemide	ES	3.3 mg/mL[l]		TNA #73[g]	Visually compatible for 4 hr	1009	C
		10 mg/mL[b]		TPN #189[g]	Visually compatible for 24 hr at 22 °C	1767	C
	AMR	10 mg/mL		TPN #203, #204[g]	Visually compatible for 2 hr at 23 °C	1974	C
	AB	3 mg/mL[a]		TPN #212 to #215[g]	Small amount of subvisible precipitate forms immediately	2109	I
	AB	3 mg/mL[a]		TNA #218 to #226[g]	Visually compatible for 4 hr at 23 °C	2215	C
Ganciclovir sodium	SY	1 and 5 mg/mL[a]		TPN #144[g]	Visually compatible for 2 hr at 20 °C	1522	C
	SY	10 mg/mL[a]		TPN #144[g]	Heavy precipitate forms within 30 min	1522	I
	SY	3 and 5 mg/mL		TPN #183 to #185[g]	Precipitate forms	1744	I
	SY	2 mg/mL		TPN #183[g]	Precipitate forms	1744	I
	SY	1 mg/mL[p]		TPN #183[g]	Visually compatible with no ganciclovir loss in 3 hr at 24 °C. Less than 10% amino acids loss in 2 hr	1744	C
	SY	2 mg/mL[q]		TPN #184, #185[g]	Visually compatible with no ganciclovir loss in 3 hr at 24 °C. Less than 10% amino acid loss in 3 hr	1744	C
	SY	20 mg/mL[a]		TPN #212 to #215[g]	Gross white precipitate forms immediately	2109	I
	RC	20 mg/mL[a]		TNA #218 to #226[g]	White precipitate forms immediately	2215	I
Gentamicin sulfate	SC	1.6 mg/mL[a]		TNA #73[g,h]	Visually compatible for 4 hr at 25 °C	1008	C
	IX	12.5 mg/1.25 mL[j]		TPN #61[c,g]	Physically compatible	1012	C
	IX	75 mg/1.9 mL[j]		TPN #61[d,g]	Physically compatible	1012	C
		13 and 20 mg/mL		TPN #54[g]	Physically compatible and gentamicin activity retained over 6 hr at 22 °C	1045	C
	IX	5 mg[e]		TPN #91[f,g]	Physically compatible	1170	C
	ES	40 mg/mL		TNA #97 to #104[g]	Physically compatible and gentamicin content retained for 6 hr at 21 °C	1324	C
	DB	1 mg/mL[b]		TPN #189[g]	Visually compatible for 24 hr at 22 °C	1767	C
	ES	10 mg/mL		TPN #203, #204[g]	Visually compatible for 2 hr at 23 °C	1974	C
	AB	5 mg/mL[a]		TPN #212 to #215[g]	Physically compatible for 4 hr at 23 °C	2109	C
	AB, FUJ	5 mg/mL[a]		TNA #218 to #226[g]	Visually compatible for 4 hr at 23 °C	2215	C
Granisetron HCl	SKB	0.05 mg/mL[a]		TPN #212 to #215[g]	Physically compatible for 4 hr at 23 °C	2109	C
	SKB	0.05 mg/mL[a]		TNA #218 to #226[g]	Visually compatible for 4 hr at 23 °C	2215	C

Y-Site Injection Compatibility (1:1 Mixture) (Cont.)

Amino acids

Drug	Mfr	Conc	Mfr	Conc	Remarks	Ref	C/I
Haloperidol lactate	SE	10 mg/mL		TPN #189[g]	Visually compatible for 24 hr at 22 °C	1767	C
	MN	0.2 mg/mL[a]		TPN #212 to #215[g]	Physically compatible for 4 hr at 23 °C	2109	C
	MN	0.2 mg/mL[a]		TNA #218 to #226[g]	Damage to emulsion occurs immediately with free oil possible	2215	I
Heparin sodium	DB	500 units/mL[b]		TPN #189[g]	Visually compatible for 24 hr at 22 °C	1767	C
	AB	100 units/mL		TPN #212 to #215[g]	Physically compatible for 4 hr at 23 °C	2109	C
	AB	100 units/mL		TNA #218 to #226[g]	Damage to emulsion occurs immediately with free oil possible	2215	I
Hydrocortisone sodium succinate	UP	50 mg/mL[b]		TPN #189[g]	Visually compatible for 24 hr at 22 °C	1767	C
	AB	1 mg/mL[a]		TPN #212 to #215[g]	Physically compatible for 4 hr at 23 °C	2109	C
	AB	1 mg/mL[a]		TNA #218 to #226[g]	Visually compatible for 4 hr at 23 °C	2215	C
Hydromorphone HCl	ES	0.5 mg/mL[a]		TPN #212 to #215[g]	Physically compatible for 4 hr at 23 °C	2109	C
	ES	0.5 mg/mL[a]		TNA #219, #222, #224 to #226[g]	Damage to emulsion occurs immediately with free oil formation possible	2215	I
	ES	0.5 mg/mL[a]		TNA #218, #220, #221, #223[g]	Visually compatible for 4 hr at 23 °C	2215	C
Hydroxyzine HCl	ES	2 mg/mL[a]		TPN #212 to #215[g]	Physically compatible for 4 hr at 23 °C	2109	C
	ES	2 mg/mL[a]		TNA #218 to #226[g]	Visually compatible for 4 hr at 23 °C	2215	C
Idarubicin HCl	AD	1 mg/mL[b]		TPN #140[g]	Visually compatible for 24 hr at 25 °C	1525	C
Ifosfamide	MJ	25 mg/mL[a]		TPN #212 to #215[g]	Physically compatible for 4 hr at 23 °C	2109	C
	MJ	25 mg/mL[a]		TNA #218 to #226[g]	Visually compatible for 4 hr at 23 °C	2215	C
Imipenem–cilastatin sodium	ME	10 mg/mL[b]		TPN #212 to #215[g]	Physically compatible for 4 hr at 23 °C	2109	C
	ME	10 mg/mL[b]		TNA #218 to #226[g]	Visually compatible for 4 hr at 23 °C	2215	C
Indomethacin sodium trihydrate	MSD	1 mg/mL[b]	MG[r]	AA 1 and 2%, D 10%	Haze forms in 2 hr and white precipitate forms in 4 hr	1527	I
	MSD	1 mg/mL[b]	MG[r]	AA 1 and 2%, W	Haze forms in 30 min and white precipitate forms in 1 hr	1527	I
Insulin, regular	NOV	2 units/mL[s]		TPN #189[g]	Visually compatible for 24 hr at 22 °C	1767	C
	NOV	1 unit/mL[a]		TPN #212 to #215[g]	Physically compatible for 4 hr at 23 °C	2109	C
	NOV	1 unit/mL[a]		TNA #218 to #226[g]	Visually compatible for 4 hr at 23 °C	2215	C
Isoproterenol HCl	BR	4 mcg/mL[l]		TNA #73[g]	Visually compatible for 4 hr	1009	C
Leucovorin calcium	IMM	2 mg/mL[a]		TPN #212 to #215[g]	Physically compatible for 4 hr at 23 °C	2109	C
	IMM	2 mg/mL[a]		TNA #218 to #226[g]	Visually compatible for 4 hr at 23 °C	2215	C

Y-Site Injection Compatibility (1:1 Mixture) (Cont.)

Amino acids

Drug	Mfr	Conc	Mfr	Conc	Remarks	Ref	C/I
Lidocaine HCl	ES	4 mg/mL[l]		TNA #73[g]	Visually compatible for 4 hr	1009	**C**
Lorazepam	WY	0.1 mg/mL[a]		TPN #212 to #215[g]	Physically compatible for 4 hr at 23 °C	2109	**C**
	WY	0.1 mg/mL[a]		TNA #218 to #226[g]	Damage to emulsion occurs in 1 hr	2215	**I**
Magnesium sulfate	AB	100 mg/mL[a]		TPN #212 to #215[g]	Physically compatible for 4 hr at 23 °C	2109	**C**
	AB	100 mg/mL[a]		TNA #218 to #226[g]	Visually compatible for 4 hr at 23 °C	2215	**C**
Mannitol	BA	15%		TPN #212 to #215[g]	Physically compatible for 4 hr at 23 °C	2109	**C**
	BA	15%		TNA #218 to #226[g]	Visually compatible for 4 hr at 23 °C	2215	**C**
Meperidine HCl	AB	10 mg/mL		TPN #131, #132[g]	Physically compatible for 4 hr at 25 °C under fluorescent light	1397	**C**
	DB	50 mg/mL		TPN #189[g]	Visually compatible for 24 hr at 22 °C	1767	**C**
	AST	4 mg/mL[a]		TPN #212 to #215[g]	Physically compatible for 4 hr at 23 °C	2109	**C**
	AST	4 mg/mL[a]		TNA #218 to #226[g]	Visually compatible for 4 hr at 23 °C	2215	**C**
Meropenem	ZEN	20 mg/mL[a]		TNA #218 to #226[g]	Visually compatible for 4 hr at 23 °C	2215	**C**
Mesna	MJ	10 mg/mL[a]		TPN #212 to #215[g]	Physically compatible for 4 hr at 23 °C	2109	**C**
	MJ	10 mg/mL[a]		TNA #218 to #226[g]	Visually compatible for 4 hr at 23 °C	2215	**C**
Methotrexate sodium	LE	15 mg/mL[a]		TPN #212 to #215[g]	Substantial loss of natural haze with a microprecipitate	2109	**I**
	IMM	15 mg/mL[a]		TNA #218 to #226[g]	Visually compatible for 4 hr at 23 °C	2215	**C**
Methyldopate HCl	MSD	5 mg/mL[a]		TNA #73[g]	Cracked the lipid emulsion	1009	**I**
	MSD	5 mg/mL[b]		TNA #73[g]	Visually compatible for 4 hr	1009	**C**
Methylprednisolone sodium succinate	AB	5 mg/mL[a]		TPN #212 to #215[g]	Physically compatible for 4 hr at 23 °C	2109	**C**
	AB	5 mg/mL[a]		TNA #218 to #226[g]	Visually compatible for 4 hr at 23 °C	2215	**C**
Metoclopramide HCl	AB	5 mg/mL		TPN #212 to #215[g]	Substantial loss of natural haze occurs immediately	2109	**I**
	AB	5 mg/mL		TNA #218 to #226[g]	Visually compatible for 4 hr at 23 °C	2215	**C**
Metronidazole	DB	5 mg/mL		TPN #189[g]	Visually compatible for 24 hr at 22 °C	1767	**C**
	AB	5 mg/mL		TPN #203, #204[g]	Visually compatible for 2 hr at 23 °C	1974	**C**
	SCS	5 mg/mL		TPN #212 to #215[g]	Physically compatible for 4 hr at 23 °C	2109	**C**
	AB	5 mg/mL		TNA #218 to #226[g]	Visually compatible for 4 hr at 23 °C	2215	**C**
Micafungin sodium	ASP	1.5 mg/mL[b]		TPN #268[g]	Physically compatible for 4 hr at 23 °C	2683	**C**
Midazolam HCl	RC	5 mg/mL		TPN #189[g]	White haze and precipitate form immediately. Crystals form in 24 hr	1767	**I**

Y-Site Injection Compatibility (1:1 Mixture) (Cont.)

Amino acids

Drug	Mfr	Conc	Mfr	Conc	Remarks	Ref	C/I
	RC	2 mg/mL[a]		TPN #212 to #215[g]	White cloudiness forms rapidly	2109	I
	RC	2 mg/mL[a]		TNA #218 to #226[g]	Damage to emulsion occurs immediately with free oil formation possible	2215	I
Milrinone lactate	SW	0.4 mg/mL[a]		TPN #217[g]	Visually compatible with no loss of milrinone in 4 hr at 23 °C	2214	C
	SS	0.2 mg/mL[a]		TPN #243, #244[g]	Visually compatible for 4 hr at 24 °C	2381	C
Mitoxantrone HCl	IMM	0.5 mg/mL[a]		TPN #212 to #215[g]	Substantial loss of natural haze occurs immediately	2109	I
	IMM	0.5 mg/mL[a]		TNA #218 to #226[g]	Visually compatible for 4 hr at 23 °C	2215	C
Morphine sulfate	AB	1 mg/mL		TPN #131, #132[g]	Physically compatible for 4 hr at 25 °C	1397	C
	DB	30 mg/mL		TPN #189[g]	Visually compatible for 24 hr at 22 °C	1767	C
	ES	1 mg/mL		TPN #203, #204[g]	Visually compatible for 2 hr at 23 °C	1974	C
	AST	1 mg/mL[a]		TPN #212 to #215[g]	Physically compatible for 4 hr at 23 °C	2109	C
	ES	1 mg/mL[a]		TNA #218 to #226[g]	Visually compatible for 4 hr at 23 °C	2215	C
	ES	15 mg/mL		TNA #218 to #226[g]	Damage to emulsion occurs immediately with free oil formation possible	2215	I
Multivitamins (M.V.I.-12)	ROR			TPN #189[g]	Visually compatible for 24 hr at 22 °C	1767	C
Nafcillin sodium	WY	250 mg/1 mL[i]		TPN #61[c,g]	Physically compatible	1012	C
	WY	1.5 g/6 mL[i]		TPN #61[d,g]	Physically compatible	1012	C
		250 mg/mL		TPN #54[g]	Physically compatible and nafcillin activity retained over 6 hr at 22 °C	1045	C
	BE	20 mg/mL[a]		TPN #212 to #215[g]	Physically compatible for 4 hr at 23 °C	2109	C
	BE, APC	20 mg/mL[a]		TNA #218 to #226[g]	Visually compatible for 4 hr at 23 °C	2215	C
Nalbuphine HCl	AB	10 mg/mL		TPN #212 to #215[g]	Physically compatible for 4 hr at 23 °C	2109	C
	AB, AST	10 mg/mL		TNA #218 to #226[g]	Damage to emulsion occurs immediately with free oil formation possible	2215	I
Nitroglycerin	DU	0.4 mg/mL[a]		TPN #212 to #215[g]	Physically compatible for 4 hr at 23 °C	2109	C
	DU	0.4 mg/mL[a]		TNA #218 to #226[g]	Visually compatible for 4 hr at 23 °C	2215	C
Norepinephrine bitartrate	BN	8 mcg/mL[l]		TNA #73[g]	Visually compatible for 4 hr	1009	C
	AB	16 mcg/mL[a]		TPN #212 to #215[g]	Physically compatible for 4 hr at 23 °C	2109	C
Octreotide acetate	SZ	0.01 mg/mL[a]		TPN #212 to #215[g]	Physically compatible for 4 hr at 23 °C	2109	C
	SZ	0.01 mg/mL[a]		TNA #218 to #226[g]	Visually compatible for 4 hr at 23 °C	2215	C
Ondansetron HCl	GL	1 mg/mL[a]		TPN #212 to #215[g]	Physically compatible for 4 hr at 23 °C	2109	C
	CER	1 mg/mL[a]		TNA #218 to #226[g]	Damage to emulsion occurs immediately with free oil formation possible	2215	I

Y-Site Injection Compatibility (1:1 Mixture) (Cont.)

Amino acids

Drug	Mfr	Conc	Mfr	Conc	Remarks	Ref	C/I
Oxacillin sodium	BE	20 mg/mL[a]		TNA #73[g,h]	Visually compatible for 4 hr at 25 °C	1008	C
	BE	250 mg/ 1.5 mL[i]		TPN #61[c,g]	Physically compatible	1012	C
	BE	1.5 g/9 mL[i]		TPN #61[d,g]	Physically compatible	1012	C
		100 and 150 mg/mL		TPN #54[g]	Physically compatible and 88 to 94% oxacillin activity retained over 6 hr at 22 °C	1045	C
Paclitaxel	MJ	1.2 mg/mL[a]		TPN #212 to #215[g]	Physically compatible for 4 hr at 23 °C	2109	C
	MJ	1.2 mg/mL[a]		TNA #218 to #226[g]	Visually compatible for 4 hr at 23 °C	2215	C
Penicillin G	PF	200,000 units/2 mL[i]		TPN #61[c,g]	Physically compatible	1012	C
	PF	1.2 million units/12 mL[i]		TPN #61[d,g]	Physically compatible	1012	C
		320,000 and 500,000 units/mL		TPN #54[g]	Physically compatible and 88% penicillin activity retained over 6 hr at 22 °C	1045	C
		300 mg/mL[b]		TPN #189[g]	Visually compatible for 24 hr at 22 °C	1767	C
Penicillin G potassium	SQ	40,000 units/ mL[a]		TNA #73[g,h]	Visually compatible for 4 hr at 25 °C	1008	C
	MAR	500,000 units/mL		TPN #203, #204[g]	Visually compatible for 2 hr at 23 °C	1974	C
Pentobarbital sodium	AB	5 mg/mL[a]		TPN #212 to #215[g]	Physically compatible for 4 hr at 23 °C	2109	C
	AB	5 mg/mL[a]		TNA #218 to #226[g]	Damage to emulsion occurs immediately with free oil formation possible	2215	I
Phenobarbital sodium	WY	5 mg/mL[a]		TPN #212 to #215[g]	Physically compatible for 4 hr at 23 °C	2109	C
	WY	5 mg/mL[a]		TNA #218 to #226[g]	Damage to emulsion occurs immediately with free oil formation possible	2215	I
Phenytoin sodium	PD	50 mg/mL		TPN #189[g]	Heavy white precipitate forms immediately	1767	I
Piperacillin sodium–tazobactam sodium	CY[x]	40 + 5 mg/ mL[a]		TPN #212 to #215[g]	Physically compatible for 4 hr at 23 °C	2109	C
	LE[x]	40 + 5 mg/ mL[a]		TNA #218 to #226[g]	Visually compatible for 4 hr at 23 °C	2215	C
Potassium chloride	AST	30 mg/mL[b]		TPN #189[g]	Visually compatible for 24 hr at 22 °C	1767	C
	AB	0.1 mEq/mL[a]		TPN #212 to #215[g]	Physically compatible for 4 hr at 23 °C	2109	C
	AB	0.1 mEq/mL[a]		TNA #218 to #226[g]	Visually compatible for 4 hr at 23 °C	2215	C
Potassium phosphates	AB	3 mmol/mL		TPN #212 to #215[g]	Increased turbidity forms immediately	2109	I
	AB	3 mmol/mL		TNA #218 to #226[g]	Damage to emulsion occurs immediately with free oil formation possible	2215	I
Prochlorperazine edisylate	SCN	0.5 mg/mL[a]		TPN #212 to #215[g]	Physically compatible for 4 hr at 23 °C	2109	C
	SCN, SO	0.5 mg/mL[a]		TNA #218 to #226[g]	Visually compatible for 4 hr at 23 °C	2215	C
Promethazine HCl	SCN	2 mg/mL[a]		TPN #212, #214[g]	Physically compatible for 4 hr at 23 °C	2109	C

Y-Site Injection Compatibility (1:1 Mixture) (Cont.)

Amino acids

Drug	Mfr	Conc	Mfr	Conc	Remarks	Ref	C/I
	SCN	2 mg/mL[a]		TPN #213, #215[g]	Amber discoloration forms in 4 hr	2109	I
	SCN	2 mg/mL[a]		TNA #218 to #226[g]	Visually compatible for 4 hr at 23 °C	2215	C
Propofol	STU	2 and 3 g		TPN #186 to #188[g]	Physically compatible and 6% or less propofol loss in 5 hr at 22 °C	1805	C
	STU	500 mg		TPN #186[g]	Physically compatible but 28% propofol loss in 5 hr at 22 °C	1805	I
	STU	500 mg		TPN #187, #188[g]	Physically compatible and 6% or less propofol loss in 5 hr at 22 °C	1805	C
Ranitidine HCl	GL	2.5 mg/mL[b]		TPN #189[g]	Visually compatible for 24 hr at 22 °C	1767	C
	GL	25 mg/mL		TPN #203, #204[g]	Visually compatible for 2 hr at 23 °C	1974	C
	GL	2 mg/mL[a]		TPN #212 to #215[g]	Physically compatible for 4 hr at 23 °C	2109	C
	GL	2 mg/mL[a]		TNA #218 to #226[g]	Visually compatible for 4 hr at 23 °C	2215	C
Sargramostim	IMM	10 mcg/mL[b]		TPN #133[g]	Visually compatible for 4 hr at 22 °C	1436	C
	IMM	6[t] and 15 mcg/mL[b]		TPN #181[g]	Visually compatible for 2 hr	1618	C
Sodium bicarbonate	AB	1 mEq/mL		TPN #212, #214[g]	Microprecipitate in 1 hr	2109	I
	AB	1 mEq/mL		TPN #213, #215[g]	Physically compatible for 4 hr at 23 °C	2109	C
	AB	1 mEq/mL		TNA #218 to #226[g]	Visually compatible for 4 hr at 23 °C	2215	C
Sodium nitroprusside	AB	0.4 mg/mL[a]		TPN #212 to #215[g]	Physically compatible for 4 hr at 23 °C protected from light	2109	C
	AB	0.4 mg/mL[a]		TNA #218 to #226[g]	Visually compatible for 4 hr at 23 °C protected from light	2215	C
Sodium phosphates	AB	3 mmol/mL		TPN #212 to #215[g]	Increased turbidity forms immediately	2109	I
	AB	3 mmol/mL		TNA #218 to #226[g]	Damage to emulsion occurs immediately with free oil formation possible	2215	I
Tacrolimus	FUJ	1 mg/mL[a]		TPN #212 to #215[g]	Physically compatible for 4 hr at 23 °C	2109	C
	FUJ	1 mg/mL[a]		TNA #218 to #226[g]	Visually compatible for 4 hr at 23 °C	2215	C
Thiotepa	IMM[u]	1 mg/mL[a]		TPN #193[g]	Physically compatible for 4 hr at 23 °C	1861	C
Ticarcillin disodium–clavulanate potassium	BE	30 mg/mL[b]		TPN #189[g]	Visually compatible for 24 hr at 22 °C	1767	C
	SKB	31 mg/mL[a]		TPN #212 to #215[g]	Physically compatible for 4 hr at 23 °C	2109	C
	SKB	31 mg/mL[a]		TNA #218 to #226[g]	Visually compatible for 4 hr at 23 °C	2215	C
Tobramycin sulfate	LI	1.6 mg/mL[a]		TNA #73[g,h]	Visually compatible for 4 hr at 25 °C	1008	C
	DI	12.5 mg/ 1.25 mL[j]		TPN #61[c,g]	Physically compatible	1012	C
	DI	75 mg/ 1.9 mL[j]		TPN #61[d,g]	Physically compatible	1012	C
		20 mg/mL		TPN #54[g]	Physically compatible and tobramycin activity retained over 6 hr at 22 °C	1045	C

Y-Site Injection Compatibility (1:1 Mixture) (Cont.)

Amino acids

Drug	Mfr	Conc	Mfr	Conc	Remarks	Ref	C/I
	LI	5 mg[e]		TPN #91[f,g]	Physically compatible	1170	C
	LI	40 mg/mL		TNA #97 to #104[g]	Physically compatible and tobramycin content retained for 6 hr at 21 °C	1324	C
	AB	5 mg/mL[a]		TPN #212 to #215[g]	Physically compatible for 4 hr at 23 °C	2109	C
	AB	5 mg/mL[a]		TNA #218 to #226[g]	Visually compatible for 4 hr at 23 °C	2215	C
Trimethoprim–sulfamethoxazole	ES	0.8 + 4 mg/mL[a]		TNA #212 to #215[g]	Physically compatible for 4 hr at 23 °C	2109	C
	ES	0.8 + 4 mg/mL[a]		TNA #218 to #226[g]	Visually compatible for 4 hr at 23 °C	2215	C
Vancomycin HCl	LI	50 mg/1 mL[j]		TPN #61[c,g]	Physically compatible	1012	C
	LI	300 mg/6 mL[j]		TPN #61[d,g]	Physically compatible	1012	C
	LI	30 mg[e]		TPN #91[f,g]	Physically compatible	1170	C
	DB	10 mg/mL[b]		TPN #189[g]	Visually compatible for 24 hr at 22 °C	1767	C
	AB	10 mg/mL[a]		TPN #212 to #215[g]	Physically compatible for 4 hr at 23 °C	2109	C
	AB	10 mg/mL[a]		TNA #218 to #226[g]	Visually compatible for 4 hr at 23 °C	2215	C
Vecuronium bromide	OR	2 mg/mL[k]		TPN #189[g]	Visually compatible for 24 hr at 22 °C	1767	C
Zidovudine	BW	4 mg/mL[a]		TPN #212 to #215[g]	Physically compatible for 4 hr at 23 °C	2109	C
	GW	4 mg/mL[a]		TNA #218 to #226[g]	Visually compatible for 4 hr at 23 °C	2215	C

[a] *Tested in dextrose 5%.*
[b] *Tested in sodium chloride 0.9%.*
[c] *Run at 21 mL/hr.*
[d] *Run at 94 mL/hr.*
[e] *Given over one hour by syringe pump.*
[f] *Run at 10 mL/hr.*
[g] *Refer to Appendix I for the composition of parenteral nutrition solutions. TNA indicates a 3-in-1 admixture, and TPN indicates a 2-in-1 admixture.*
[h] *A 32.5-mL sample of parenteral nutrition solution and 50 mL of antibiotic in a minibottle.*
[i] *Given over five minutes by syringe pump.*
[j] *Given over 30 minutes by syringe pump.*
[k] *Tested in sterile water for injection.*
[l] *Tested in both dextrose 5% and sodium chloride 0.9%.*
[m] *Given over 10 minutes by syringe pump.*
[n] *Tested in dextrose 5% infused at 1.2 mL/hr.*
[o] *Varying volumes to simulate varying administration rates.*
[p] *Ganciclovir sodium concentration after mixing was 0.83 mg/mL.*
[q] *Ganciclovir sodium concentration after mixing was 1.4 mg/mL.*
[r] *TrophAmine.*
[s] *Tested in Haemaccel (Behring).*
[t] *With albumin human 0.1%.*
[u] *Lyophilized formulation tested.*
[v] *Tested in Ringer's injection, lactated.*
[w] *Specific composition of the parenteral nutrition admixture not reported. TPN indicates a 2-in-1 admixture.*
[x] *Test performed using the formulation WITHOUT edetate disodium.*

Additional Compatibility Information

Multicomponent (3-in-1; TNA) Admixtures — Because of the potential benefits in terms of simplicity, efficiency, time, and cost, the concept of mixing amino acids, carbohydrates, electrolytes, fat emulsion, and other nutritional components together in the same container has been explored. Within limits, the feasibility of preparing such 3-in-1 parenteral nutrition admixtures has been demonstrated as long as a careful examination of the emulsion mixtures for signs of instability is performed prior to administration.

However, these 3-in-1 mixtures are very complex and inherently unstable. Emulsion stability is dependent on both zeta potential and van der Waals forces, influenced by the presence of dextrose. (2029) The ultimate stability of each unique mixture depends on numerous complicated factors, making definitive stability predictions impossible. Injury and death have resulted from administration of unrecognized precipitation in 3-in-1 parenteral nutrition admixtures. (1769; 1782; 1783) See the section on Calcium and Phosphate. In addition, the use of 3-in-1 admixtures is associated with a higher rate of catheter occlusion and reduced catheter life compared with giving the fat emulsion separately from the parenteral nutrition solution. (705; 1518; 2194)

The use of a 5-μm inline filter for a 3-in-1 admixture (containing Travasol 8.5%, dextrose, Intralipid 10%, various electrolytes, vitamins, and trace elements) showed that fat, in the form of large globules or aggregates, comprised 99.4% of the filter contents. These authors recommend the use of an appropriate filter (≤ 5 μm) for preventing catheter occlusion with 3-in-1 admixtures. (742)

Using light microscopy, the presence of glass particles, talc, and plastic has been observed in administration line samples drawn from 20 adults receiving 3-in-1 parenteral nutrition admixtures and in 20 children receiving 2-in-1 admixtures with separate fat emulsion infusions. Particles ranged from 3 to 5 μm to greater than 40 μm and were more consistently seen in the pediatric admixtures. The authors suggest the use of inline filters given that particulate contamination is present, has no therapeutic value, and can be harmful. (2458)

Combining an amino acids–glucose parenteral nutrition solution containing various electrolytes with fat emulsion 20%, intravenous (Intralipid, Vitrum), resulted in a mixture which, although apparently stable for a limited time, ultimately exhibited a creaming phenomenon. Within 12 hours, a distinct 2-cm layer separated on the upper surface. Microscopic examination revealed aggregates believed to be clumps of fat droplets. Fewer and smaller aggregates were noted in the lower layer. (560; 561)

Amino acids were reported to have no adverse effect on the emulsion stability of Intralipid 10%. In addition, the amino acids appeared to prevent the adverse impact of dextrose and to slow the flocculation and coalescence resulting from mono- and divalent cations. However, significant coalescence did result after a longer time. Therefore, it was recommended that such cations not be mixed with fat emulsion, intravenous. (656)

Three-in-one TNA admixtures prepared with Intralipid 20% and containing mono- and divalent ions as well as heparin sodium 5 units/ mL were found to undergo changes consistent with instability including fat particle shape and diameter changes as well as creaming and layering. The changes were evident within 48 hours at room temperature but were delayed to between one and two months when refrigerated. (58)

Travenol states that 1:1:1 mixtures of amino acids 5.5, 8.5, or 10% (Travenol), fat emulsion 10 to 20% (Travenol), and dextrose 10 to 70% are physically stable but recommends administration within 24 hours. M.V.I.-12 3.3 mL/L and electrolytes may also be added to the admixtures up to the maximum amounts listed in Table 1 (850).

The stability of mixtures of 1 L of Intralipid 20%, 1.5 L of Vamin glucose (amino acids with dextrose 10%), and 0.5 L of dextrose 10% with various electrolytes and vitamins was evaluated. Initial emulsion particle size was around 1 μm. The mixture containing only monovalent cations was stable for at least nine days at 4 °C, with little change in particle size. The mixtures containing the divalent cations, such as calcium and magnesium, demonstrated much greater particle size increases, with mean diameters of around 3.3 to 3.5 μm after nine days at 4 °C. After 48 hours of storage, however, these increases were more modest, around 1.5 to 1.85 μm. After storage at 4 °C for 48 hours followed by 24 hours at room temperature, few particles exceeded 5 μm. It was found that the effect of particle aggregation caused by electrolytes demonstrates a critical concentration before the effect begins. For calcium and magnesium chlorides, the critical concentrations were 2.4 and 2.6 mmol/L, respectively. Sodium and potassium chloride had critical concentrations of 110 and 150 mmol/L, respectively. The rate of particle aggregation increased linearly with increasing electrolyte concentration. The quantity of emulsion in the mixture had a relatively small influence on stability, but higher concentrations exhibited a somewhat greater coalescence. (892)

Instability of the emulsion systems is manifested by (1) flocculation of oil droplets to form aggregates, producing a cream-like layer on top; or (2) coalescence of oil droplets, leading to an increase in the average droplet size and eventually a separation of free oil. The lowering of pH and the adding of electrolytes can adversely affect the mechanical and electrical properties at the oil–water interface, eventually leading to flocculation and coalescence. Amino acids act as buffering agents and provide a protective effect on emulsion stability. Adding electrolytes, especially the divalent ions Mg^{++} and Ca^{++} in excess of 2.5 mmol/L, to simple fat emulsions will cause flocculation. But in mixed parenteral nutrition solutions, the stability of the emulsion will be enhanced, depending on the quantity and nature of the amino acids present. The authors recommended a careful examination of emulsion mixtures for signs of instability prior to administration. (849)

Good stability was reported for an amino acid 4% (Travenol), dextrose 14%, and fat emulsion 4% (Pharmacia) parenteral nutrition solution. The solution also contained electrolytes, vitamins, and heparin sodium 4000 units/L. The aqueous solution was prepared first, with the fat emulsion added subsequently. This procedure allowed visual inspection of the aqueous phase and reduced the risk of emulsion breakdown by the divalent cations. Sample mixtures were stored at 18 to 25 and 3 to 8 °C for up to five days. They were evaluated

Table 1. Maximum Electrolyte Amounts for Travenol 3-in-1 Admixtures (850)

Calcium	8.3 mEq/L
Magnesium	3.3 mEq/L
Sodium	23.3 mEq/L
Potassium	20.0 mEq/L
Chloride	23.3 mEq/L
Phosphate	20 mEq/L
Zinc	3.33 mg/L
Copper	1.33 mg/L
Manganese	0.33 mg/L
Chromium	13.33 mcg/L

visually and with a Coulter counter for particle size measurements. Both room temperature and refrigerated mixtures were stable for 48 hours. A marked increase in particle size was noted in the room temperature sample after 72 hours, but refrigeration delayed the changes. The authors' experience with over 1400 mixtures for administration to patients resulted in one emulsion creaming and another cracking, but the authors had no explanation for the failure of these particular emulsions. (848)

Six parenteral nutrition solutions having various concentrations of amino acids, dextrose, soybean oil emulsion (Kabi-Vitrum), electrolytes, and multivitamins were evaluated. All of the admixtures were stable for one week under refrigeration followed by 24 hours at room temperature, with no visible changes, changes in pH, or significant changes in particle size. (1013) However, other researchers questioned this interpretation of the results. (1014; 1015)

The stability of 3-in-1 parenteral nutrition solutions prepared with 500 mL of Intralipid 20% compared to Soyacal 20%, along with 500 or 1000 mL of FreAmine III 8.5% and 500 mL of dextrose 70% was reported. Also present were relatively large amounts of electrolytes and other additives. All mixtures were similarly stable for 28 days at 4 °C followed by five days at 21 to 25 °C, with little change in the emulsion. A slight white cream layer appeared after five days at 4 °C but was easily redispersed with gentle agitation. The appearance of this cream layer did not statistically affect particle size distribution. The authors concluded that the emulsion mixture remained suitable for clinical use throughout the study period. The stability of other components was not evaluated. (1019)

The stability of 3-in-1 parenteral nutrition admixtures prepared with Liposyn II 10 and 20%, Aminosyn pH 6, and dextrose along with electrolytes, trace metals, and vitamins was reported. Thirty-one different combinations were evaluated. Samples were stored at: (1) 25 °C for one day, (2) 5 °C for two days followed by 30 °C for one day, and (3) 5 °C for nine days followed by 25 °C for one day. In all cases, there was no visual evidence of creaming, free oil droplets, and other signs of emulsion instability. Furthermore, little or no change in the particle size or zeta potential (electrostatic surface charge of lipid particles) was found, indicating emulsion stability. The dextrose and amino acids remained stable over the 10-day storage period. The greatest change of an amino acid occurred with tryptophan, which lost 6% in 10 days. Vitamin stability was not tested. (1025)

The stability of four parenteral nutrition admixtures, ranging from 1 L each of amino acids 5.5% (Travenol), dextrose 10%, and fat emulsion 10% (Travenol) up to a "worst case" of 1 L each of amino acids 10% with electrolytes (Travenol), dextrose 70%, and fat emulsion 10% (Travenol) was reported. The admixtures were stored for 48 hours at 5 to 9 °C followed by 24 hours at room temperature. There were no visible signs of creaming, flocculation, and free oil. The mean emulsion particle size remained within acceptable limits for all admixtures, and there were no significant changes in glucose, soybean oil, and amino acid concentrations. The authors noted that two factors were predominant in determining the stability of such admixtures: electrolyte concentrations and pH. (1065)

Several parenteral nutrition solutions containing amino acids (Travenol), glucose, and lipid, with and without electrolytes and trace elements, produced no visible flocculation or any significant change in mean emulsion particle size during 24 hours at room temperature. (1066)

The compatibility of 10 parenteral nutrition admixtures, evaluated over 96 hours while stored at 20 to 25 °C in both glass bottles and ethylene vinyl acetate bags was reported. A slight creaming occurred in all admixtures, but the cream layer was easily redispersed with

Table 2. Range of Component Amounts for Compatibility Testing of 3-in-1 Admixtures (1067)

Vamin glucose or Vamin N (amino acids 7%)	1000 to 2000 mL
Dextrose 10 to 30%	100 to 550 mL
Intralipid 10 or 20%	500 to 1000 mL
Electrolyte (mmol/L)	
Sodium	20 to 70
Potassium	20 to 55
Calcium	2.3 to 2.9
Magnesium	1.1 to 3.1
Phosphorus	0 to 9.2
Chloride	27 to 71
Zinc	0.005 to 0.03

gentle shaking. No fat globules were visually apparent. The mean drop size was larger in the cream layer, but no globules were larger than 5 μm. Analyses of the concentrations of amino acids, dextrose, and electrolytes showed no changes over the study period. The authors concluded that such parenteral nutrition admixtures could be safely prepared as long as the component concentrations are within the ranges found in Table 2. (1067)

The stability of eight parenteral nutrition admixtures with various ratios of amino acids, carbohydrates, and fat was reported. FreAmine III 8.5%, dextrose 70%, and Soyacal 10 and 20% (mixed in ratios of 2:1:1, 1:1:1, 1:1:½, and 1:1:¼, where 1 = 500 mL) were evaluated. Additive concentrations were high to stress the admixtures and represent maximum doses likely to be encountered clinically. (See Table 3.)

The admixtures were stored at 4 °C for 14 days followed by four days at 22 to 25 °C. After 24 hours, all admixtures developed a thin white cream layer, which readily redispersed on gentle agitation. No free oil droplets were observed. The mean particle diameter remained near the original size of the Soyacal throughout the study. Few particles were larger than 3 μm. Osmolality and pH also remained relatively unchanged. (1068)

Parenteral nutrition 3-in-1 admixtures with Aminosyn and Liposyn can be a problem. Standard admixtures were prepared using Aminosyn 7% 1000 mL, dextrose 50% 1000 mL, and Liposyn 10% 500 mL. Concentrated admixtures were prepared using Aminosyn 10% 500 mL, dextrose 70% 500 mL, and Liposyn 20% 500 mL. Vitamins and trace elements were added to the admixtures along with the following electrolytes (see Table 4).

Samples of each admixture were: (1) stored at 4 °C, (2) adjusted to pH 6.6 with sodium bicarbonate and stored at 4 °C, or (3) adjusted to

Table 3. Range of Component Amounts for Compatibility Testing of 3-in-1 Admixtures (1068)

Sodium acetate	150 mEq
Sodium chloride	210 mEq
Potassium acetate	45 mEq
Potassium chloride	90 mEq
Potassium phosphate	15 mM
Calcium gluconate	20 mEq
Magnesium sulfate	36 mEq
Trace elements	present
Folic acid	5 mg
M.V.I.-12	10 mL

Table 4. Electrolyte Amounts for Compatibility Testing of 3-in-1 Admixtures (1069)

Electrolyte	Standard Admixture	Concentrated Admixture
Sodium	125 mEq	75 mEq
Potassium	95 mEq	74 mEq
Magnesium	25 mEq	25 mEq
Calcium	28 mEq	28 mEq
Phosphate	37 mM	36 mM
Chloride	83 mEq	50 mEq

pH 6.6 and stored at room temperature. The compatibility was evaluated for three weeks.

Visible signs of emulsion deterioration were evident by 96 hours in the standard admixture and by 48 hours in the concentrated admixture. Clear rings formed at the meniscus, becoming thicker, yellow, and oily over time. Free-floating oil was obvious in three weeks in the standard admixture and one week in the concentrated admixture. The samples adjusted to pH 6.6 developed visible deterioration later than the others. The authors indicated that pH may play a greater role than temperature in emulsion stability. However, precipitation (probably calcium phosphate and possibly carbonate) occurred in 36 hours in the pH 6.6 concentrated admixture but not the unadjusted (pH 5.5) samples. Mean particle counts increased for all samples over time but were greatest in the concentrated admixtures. The authors concluded that the concentrated admixtures were unsatisfactory for clinical use because of the early increase in particles and precipitation. Furthermore, they recommended that the standard admixtures be prepared immediately prior to use. (1069)

The physical stability of 10 parenteral nutrition admixtures with different amino acid sources was studied. The admixtures contained 500 mL each of dextrose 70%, fat emulsion 20% (Alpha Therapeutic), and amino acids in various concentrations from each manufacturer. Also present were standard electrolytes, trace elements, and vitamins. The admixtures were stored for 14 days at 4 °C, followed by four days at 22 to 25 °C. Slight creaming was evident in all admixtures but redispersed easily with agitation. Emulsion particles were uniform in size, showing no tendency to aggregate. No cracked emulsions occurred. (1217)

The stability of parenteral nutrition solutions containing amino acids, dextrose, and fat emulsion along with electrolytes, trace elements, and vitamins has been described. In one study the admixtures were stable for 24 hours at room temperature and for eight days at 4 °C. The visual appearance and particle size of the fat emulsion showed little change over the observation periods. (1218) In another study variable stability periods were found, depending on electrolyte concentrations. Stability ranged from four to 25 days at room temperature. (1219)

The effects of dilution, dextrose concentration, amino acids, and electrolytes on the physical stability of 3-in-1 parenteral nutrition admixtures prepared with Intralipid 10% or Travamulsion 10% was studied. Travamulsion was affected by dilution up to 1:14, exhibiting an increase in mean particle size, while Intralipid remained virtually unchanged for 24 hours at 25 °C and for 72 hours at 4 °C. At dextrose concentrations above 15%, fat droplets larger than 5 mcm formed during storage for 24 hours at either 4 °C or room temperature. The presence of amino acids increased the stability of the fat emulsions in the presence of dextrose. Fat droplets larger than 5 mcm formed at a total electrolyte concentration above approximately 240 mmol/L (monovalent cation equivalent) for Travamulsion 10% and 156 mmol/

L for Intralipid 10% in 24 hours at room temperature, although creaming or breaking of the emulsion was not observed visually. (1221)

The stability of 43 parenteral nutrition admixtures composed of various ratios of amino acid products, dextrose 10 to 70%, and four lipid emulsions 10 and 20% with electrolytes, trace elements, and vitamins was studied. One group of admixtures included Travasol 5.5, 8.5, and 10%, FreAmine III 8.5 and 10%, Novamine 8.5 and 11.4%, Nephramine 5.4%, and RenAmine 6.5% with Liposyn II 10 and 20%. In another group, Aminosyn II 7, 8.5, and 10% was combined with Intralipid, Travamulsion, and Soyacal 10 and 20%. A third group was comprised of Aminosyn II 7, 8.5, and 10% with electrolytes combined with the latter three lipid emulsions. The admixtures were stored for 24 hours at 25 °C and for nine days at 5 °C followed by 24 hours at 25 °C. A few admixtures containing FreAmine III and Novamine with Liposyn II developed faint yellow streaks after 10 days of storage. The streaks readily dispersed with gentle shaking, as did the creaming present in most admixtures. Other properties such as pH, zeta-potential, and osmolality underwent little change in all of the admixtures. Particle size increased fourfold in one admixture (Novamine 8.5%, dextrose 50%, and Liposyn II in a 1:1:1 ratio), which the authors noted signaled the onset of particle coalescence. Nevertheless, the authors concluded that all of the admixtures were stable for the storage conditions and time periods tested. (1222)

The stability of 24 parenteral nutrition admixtures composed of various ratios of Aminosyn II 7, 8.5, or 10%, dextrose, and Liposyn II 10 and 20% with electrolytes, trace elements, and vitamins was also studied. Four admixtures were stored for 24 hours at 25 °C, six admixtures were stored for two days at 5 °C followed by one day at 30 °C, and 14 admixtures were stored for nine days at 5 °C followed by one day at 25 °C. No visible instability was evident. Creaming was present in most admixtures but disappeared with gentle shaking. Other properties such as pH, zeta-potential, particle size, and potency of the amino acids and dextrose showed little or no change during storage. (1223)

The emulsion stability of five parenteral nutrition formulas (TNA #126 through #130 in Appendix I) containing Liposyn II in concentrations ranging from 1.2 to 7.1% were reported. The parenteral nutrition solutions were prepared using simultaneous pumping of the components into empty containers (as with the Nutrimix compounder) and sequential pumping of the components (as with Automix compounders). The solutions were stored for two days at 5 °C followed by 24 hours at 25 °C. Similar results were obtained for both methods of preparation using visual assessment and oil globule size distribution. (1426)

The stability of 24 parenteral nutrition admixtures containing various concentrations of Aminosyn II, dextrose, and Liposyn II with a variety of electrolytes, trace elements, and multivitamins in dual-chamber, flexible, Nutrimix containers was studied as well. No instability was visible in the admixtures stored at 25 °C for 24 hours or in those stored for nine days at 5 °C followed by 24 hours at 25 °C. Creaming was observed, but neither particle coalescence nor free oil was noted. The pH, particle size distribution, and amino acid and dextrose concentrations remained acceptable during the observation period. (1432)

The physical stability of 10 parenteral nutrition formulas (TNA #149 through #158 in Appendix I) containing TrophAmine and Intralipid 20%, Liposyn II 20%, and Nutrilipid 20% in varying concentrations with low and high electrolyte concentrations was studied. All test formulas were prepared with an automatic compounder and protected from light. TNA #149 through #156 were stored for 48 hours at 4 °C followed by 24 hours at 21 °C; TNA #157 and #158 were stored for 24 hours at 4 °C followed by 24 hours at 21 °C. Although some minor creaming occurred in all formulas, it was completely reversible with agitation. No other changes were visible, and particle size analysis indicated little variation during the study period. The addition of cysteine hydrochloride 1 g/25 g of amino acids, alone or with L-carnitine 16 mg/g fat, to TNA #157 and #158 did not adversely affect the physical stability of 3-in-1 admixtures within the study period. (1620)

The physical stability of five 3-in-1 parenteral nutrition admixtures (TNA #167 through #171 in Appendix I) was evaluated by visual observation, pH and osmolality determinations, and particle size distribution analysis. All five admixtures were physically stable for 90 days at 4 °C. However, some irreversible flocculation occurred in all combinations after 180 days. (1651)

The stability of several parenteral nutrition formulas (TNA #159 through #166 in Appendix I), with and without iron dextran 2 mg/L was studied. All formulas were physically compatible both visually and microscopically for 48 hours at 4 and 25 °C, and particle size distribution remained unchanged. The order of mixing and deliberate agitation had no effect on physical compatibility. (1648)

The influence of six factors on the stability of fat emulsion in 45 different 3-in-1 parenteral nutrition mixtures was evaluated. The factors were amino acid concentration (2.5 to 7%); dextrose (5 to 20%); fat emulsion, intravenous (2 to 5%); monovalent cations (0 to 150 mEq/L); divalent cations (4 to 20 mEq/L); and trivalent cations from iron dextran (0 to 10 mg elemental iron/L). Although many formulations were unstable, visual examination could identify instability in only 65% of the samples. Electronic evaluation of particle size identified the remaining unstable mixtures. Furthermore, only the concentration of trivalent ferric ions significantly and consistently affected the emulsion stability during the 30-hour test period. Of the parenteral nutrition mixtures containing iron dextran, 16% were unstable, exhibiting emulsion cracking. The authors suggested that iron dextran should not be incorporated into 3-in-1 mixtures. (1814)

The compatibility of eight parenteral nutrition admixtures, four with and four without electrolytes, comparing Liposyn II and Intralipid (TNA #250 through #257 in Appendix I) was reported. The 3-in-1 admixtures were evaluated over two to nine days at 4 °C and then 24 hours at 25 °C in ethylene vinyl acetate (EVA) bags. No substantial changes were noted in the fat particle sizes and no visual changes of emulsion breakage were observed. All admixtures tested had particle sizes in the 2- to 40-μm range. (2465)

The stability of 3-in-1 parenteral nutrition admixtures prepared with Vamin 14 with electrolytes and containing either Lipofundin MCT/LCT 20% or Intralipid 20% was evaluated. The admixtures contained 66.7 mmol/L of monovalent and 6.7 mmol/L of divalent cations. Stability of the fat emulsion was evaluated after 2, 7, and 21 days at 4 °C in EVA bags followed by 24 hours of room temperature to simulate infusion. Microscopy, Coulter counter, photon correlation spectroscopy, and laser diffractometry techniques were used to determine stability. Droplet size by microscopy was noted to increase to 18 to 20 μm after 21 days in both of the admixtures with the Intralipid-containing admixture showing particles this large as early as day 2 and with Lipofundin MCT/LCT at day 7. The Coulter counter assessed particles greater than 2 μm to be approximately 1300 to 1500 with Lipofundin MCT/LCT and 37,000 in the Intralipid-containing admixtures immediately after their preparation. Heavy creaming with a thick firm layer was noted after 2 days with the Intralipid-containing admixture, making particle assessment difficult. The authors concluded that storage limitation of two days for the Intralipid-containing admixture and not more than seven days for the Lipo-

fundin-containing admixture appeared justified. They also noted that calcium and magnesium behaved identically in destabilizing fat emulsion with greater concentrations of divalent cations. (867)

The drop size of 3-in-1 parenteral nutrition solutions in drip chambers is variable, being altered by the constituents of the mixture. In one study, multivitamins (Multibionta, E. Merck) caused the greatest reductions in drop size, up to 37%. This change may affect the rate of delivery if the flow is estimated from drops per minute. (1016) Similarly, flow rates delivered by infusion controllers dependent on predictable drop size may be inaccurate. Flow rates up to 29% less than expected have been reported. Therefore, variable pressure volumetric pumps, which are independent of drop size, should be used rather than infusion controllers. (1215)

The physical instability of 3-in-1 total nutrient admixtures stored for 24 hours at room temperature was reported. The admixtures intended for use in neonates and infants were compounded with TrophAmine 2 to 3%, dextrose 18 to 24%, Liposyn II (Abbott) 2 to 3%, L-cysteine hydrochloride, and the following electrolytes in Table 5.

The emulsion in the admixtures cracked and developed visible free oil within 24 hours after compounding. The incompatibility was considered to create a clinically significant risk of complications if administered. The authors determined that these 3-in-1 total nutrient admixtures containing these concentrations of electrolytes were unacceptable and should not be used. (2619)

Another evaluation of 3-in-1 total nutrient admixtures reported physical instabilities of several formulations evaluated over seven days. The parenteral nutrition admixtures were prepared with dextrose 15% and Intralipos 4% (Fresenius Kabi) along with FreAmine 4.3%, NephrAmine 2.1%, TrophAmine 2.7%, Topanusol 5%, or HepatAmine 4%. Various electrolytes and other components were also present including sodium, potassium, calcium (salt form unspecified), magnesium, trace elements, vitamin K, and heparin. The admixtures were stored at 4 °C and evaluated at zero, three, and seven days. After removal from refrigeration, the samples were subjected to additional exposure to room temperature and temperatures exceeding 28 °C for 24 to 48 hours. Flocculation was found in the admixtures prepared with FreAmine and with TrophAmine after 24 hours storage at room temperature, and after three days under refrigeration followed by 24 hours at room temperature. All of the admixtures developed coalescence after seven days under refrigeration followed by 24 hours at greater than 28 °C. (2621)

The case of a 26-year-old female with Crohn's disease and enterocutaneous fistulae receiving a 3-in-1 parenteral nutrition admixture composed of Travasol 3.6%, dextrose 13.6%, Intralipid 1.5%, sodium chloride 52.3 mEq/L, sodium acetate 27.4 mEq/L, potassium chloride 27.4 mEq/L, potassium acetate 13.7 mEq/L, magnesium sulfate 4.5 mEq/L, calcium gluconate 3.2 mEq/L, MVI-12, and trace elements but no inorganic phosphates was presented. The patient became febrile, short of breath, and developed a dry cough with diffuse crackles in both lungs. After failing to respond to conventional medical therapy, an open lung biopsy was performed and showed widespread

Table 5. Incompatible Electrolyte Ranges in Neonatal 3-in-1 Admixtures (2619)

Sodium	20 to 50 mEq/L
Potassium	13.3 to 40 mEq/L
Calcium chloride	20 to 26.6 mEq/L
Magnesium	3.4 to 5 mEq/L
Phosphates	6.7 to 15 mmol/L

vascular pulmonary thromboses from irregularly shaped crystals leading to the lung perfusion defects. High levels of calcium, potassium, and carbon were detected in the crystals. Subsequent repeat testing in vitro failed to find crystallization. The patient's fever was postulated to contribute to the in vivo crystallization. (2621)

The physical stability of five highly concentrated 3-in-1 parenteral nutrition admixtures for fluid-restricted adults was evaluated. The admixtures were composed of Aminoplasmal (B. Braun) at concentrations over 7% as the amino acids source, dextrose concentrations of about 20%, and a 50:50 mixture of medium-chain triglycerides and long-chain triglycerides (Lipofundin MCT, B. Braun) at concentrations of about 2.5 to 2.7% as the lipid component with electrolytes and vitamins (TNA #269 through #273 in Appendix I). The parenteral nutrition admixtures were prepared in ethylene vinyl acetate bags and stored at room temperature for 30 hours. Electronic evaluation of mean fat particle sizes and globule size distribution found little change over the 30-hour test period. (2721)

Considerations and Recommendations — When multicomponent, 3-in-1, parenteral nutrition admixtures are used, the following points should be considered (490; 703; 892; 893; 1025; 1064; 1070; 1214; 1406; 1951; 2029; 2030; 2215; 2282; 2308):

1. The order of mixing is important. The amino acid solution should be added to either the fat emulsion or the dextrose before final mixing. This practice ensures the protective effect of the amino acids to emulsion disruption by changes in pH and the presence of electrolytes.
2. Electrolytes should not be added directly to the fat emulsions. Instead, they should be added to the amino acids or dextrose before the final mixing.
3. Such 3-in-1 admixtures containing electrolytes (especially divalent cations) are unstable and will eventually aggregate. The mixed systems should be carefully examined visually before use to ensure that a uniform emulsion still exists.
4. Avoid contact of 3-in-1 parenteral nutrition admixtures with heparin, which destabilizes and damages the fat emulsion upon contact. See Heparin section below.
5. The admixtures should be stored under refrigeration if not used immediately.
6. The ultimate stability of the admixtures will be the result of a complex interaction of pH, component concentrations, electrolyte concentrations, and, probably, storage temperature.

Furthermore, the use of a 1.2-μm filter to remove large lipid particles, electrolyte precipitates, and other solid particulates, aggregates, and *Candida albicans* contaminants has been recommended (1106; 1657; 1769; 2061; 2135; 2346), although others recommend a 5-μm filter to minimize the frequency of occlusion alarms. (569; 1951)

Blood Products — Amino acids injection should not be administered simultaneously with blood through the same infusion set because of possible pseudoagglutination. (341)

Calcium and Phosphate — UNRECOGNIZED CALCIUM PHOSPHATE PRECIPITATION IN A 3-IN-1 PARENTERAL NUTRITION MIXTURE RESULTED IN PATIENT DEATH.

The potential for the formation of a calcium phosphate precipitate in parenteral nutrition solutions is well studied and documented (1771; 1777), but the information is complex and difficult to apply to the clinical situation. (1770; 1772; 1777) The incorporation of fat emulsion in 3-in-1 parenteral nutrition solutions obscures any precip-

itate that may be present, which has led to substantial debate about the dangers associated with 3-in-1 parenteral nutrition mixtures and when or if the danger to the patient is warranted therapeutically. (1770; 1771; 1772; 2031; 2032; 2033; 2034; 2035; 2036) Because such precipitation may be life threatening to patients (2037; 2291), the Food and Drug Administration issued a Safety Alert containing the following recommendations (1769):

1. The amounts of phosphorus and of calcium added to the admixture are critical. The solubility of the added calcium should be calculated from the volume at the time the calcium is added. It should not be based upon the final volume.

   Some amino acid injections for TPN admixtures contain phosphate ions (as a phosphoric acid buffer). These phosphate ions and the volume at the time the phosphate is added should be considered when calculating the concentration of phosphate additives. Also, when adding calcium and phosphate to an admixture, the phosphate should be added first.

   The line should be flushed between the addition of any potentially incompatible components.
2. A lipid emulsion in a three-in-one admixture obscures the presence of a precipitate. Therefore, if a lipid emulsion is needed, either (1) use a two-in-one admixture with the lipid infused separately, or (2) if a three-in-one admixture is medically necessary, then add the calcium before the lipid emulsion and according to the recommendations in number 1 above.

   If the amount of calcium or phosphate which must be added is likely to cause a precipitate, some or all of the calcium should be administered separately. Such separate infusions must be properly diluted and slowly infused to avoid serious adverse events related to the calcium.
3. When using an automated compounding device, the above steps should be considered when programming the device. In addition, automated compounders should be maintained and operated according to the manufacturer's recommendations.

   Any printout should be checked against the programmed admixture and weight of components.
4. During the mixing process, pharmacists who mix parenteral nutrition admixtures should periodically agitate the admixture and check for precipitates. Medical or home care personnel who start and monitor these infusions should carefully inspect for the presence of precipitates both before and during infusion. Patients and care givers should be trained to visually inspect for signs of precipitation. They also should be advised to stop the infusion and seek medical assistance if precipitates are noted.
5. A filter should be used when infusing either central or peripheral parenteral nutrition admixtures. At this time, data have not been submitted to document which size filter is most effective in trapping precipitates.

   Standards of practice vary, but the following is suggested: a 1.2-μm air-eliminating filter for lipid-containing admixtures and a 0.22-μm air-eliminating filter for non-lipid-containing admixtures.
6. Parenteral nutrition admixtures should be administered within the following time frames: if stored at room temperature, the infusion should be started within 24 hours after mixing; if stored at refrigerated temperatures, the infusion should be started within 24 hours of rewarming. Because warming parenteral nutrition admixtures may contribute to the formation of precipitates, once administration begins, care should be taken to avoid excessive warming of the admixture.

Persons administering home care parenteral nutrition admixtures may need to deviate from these time frames. Pharmacists who initially prepare these admixtures should check a reserve sample for precipitates over the duration and under the conditions of storage.

7. If symptoms of acute respiratory distress, pulmonary emboli, or interstitial pneumonitis develop, the infusion should be stopped immediately and thoroughly checked for precipitates. Appropriate medical interventions should be instituted. Home care personnel and patients should immediately seek medical assistance.

Calcium Phosphate Precipitation Fatalities — Fatal cases of paroxysmal respiratory failure in two previously healthy women receiving peripheral vein parenteral nutrition were reported. The patients experienced sudden cardiopulmonary arrest consistent with pulmonary emboli. The authors used in vitro simulations and an animal model to conclude that unrecognized calcium phosphate precipitation in a 3-in-1 total nutrition admixture caused the fatalities. The precipitation resulted during compounding by introducing calcium and phosphate near to one another in the compounding sequence and prior to complete fluid addition. This resulted in a temporarily high concentration of the drugs and precipitation of calcium phosphate. Observation of the precipitate was obscured by the incorporation of 20% fat emulsion, intravenous, into the nutrition mixture. No filter was used during infusion of the fatal nutrition admixtures. (2037)

In a follow-up retrospective review, five patients were identified who had respiratory distress associated with the infusion of the 3-in-1 admixtures at around the same time. Four of these five patients died, although the cause of death could be definitively determined for only two. (2291)

Calcium and Phosphate Conditional Compatibility — Calcium salts are conditionally compatible with phosphate in parenteral nutrition solutions. The incompatibility is dependent on a solubility and concentration phenomenon and is not entirely predictable. Precipitation may occur during compounding or at some time after compounding is completed.

NOTE: Some amino acids solutions inherently contain calcium and phosphate, which must be considered in any projection of compatibility.

A study determined the maximum concentrations of calcium (as chloride and gluconate) and phosphate that can be maintained without precipitation in a parenteral nutrition solution consisting of FreAmine II 4.25% and dextrose 25% for 24 hours at 30 °C. It was noted that the amino acids in parenteral nutrition solutions form soluble complexes with calcium and phosphate, reducing the available free calcium and phosphate that can form insoluble precipitates. The concentration of calcium available for precipitation is greater with the chloride salt compared to the gluconate salt, at least in part because of differences in dissociation characteristics. Consequently, a greater concentration of calcium gluconate than calcium chloride can be mixed with sodium phosphate. (608)

In addition to the concentrations of phosphate and calcium and the salt form of the calcium, the concentration of amino acids and the time and temperature of storage altered the formation of calcium phosphate in parenteral nutrition solutions. As the temperature was increased, the incidence of precipitate formation also increased. This finding was attributed, at least in part, to a greater degree of dissociation of the calcium and phosphate complexes and the decreased solubility of calcium phosphate. Therefore, a solution possibly may

be stored at 4 °C with no precipitation, but on warming to room temperature a precipitate will form over time. (608)

The compatibility of calcium and phosphate in several parenteral nutrition formulas for newborn infants was evaluated. Calcium gluconate 10% (Cutter) and potassium phosphate (Abbott) were used to achieve concentrations of 2.5 to 100 mEq/L of calcium and 2.5 to 100 mmol/L of phosphorus added. The parenteral nutrition solutions evaluated were as shown in Table 6. The results were reported as graphic depictions.

The pH dependence of the phosphate–calcium precipitation has been noted. Dibasic calcium phosphate is very insoluble, while monobasic calcium phosphate is relatively soluble. At low pH, the soluble monobasic form predominates; but as the pH increases, more dibasic phosphate becomes available to bind with calcium and precipitate. Therefore, the lower the pH of the parenteral nutrition solution, the more calcium and phosphate can be solubilized. Once again, the effects of temperature were observed. As the temperature is increased, more calcium ion becomes available and more dibasic calcium phosphate is formed. Therefore, temperature increases will increase the amount of precipitate. (609)

Similar calcium and phosphate solubility curves were reported for neonatal parenteral nutrition solutions using TrophAmine (McGaw) 2, 1.5, and 0.8% as the sources of amino acids. The solutions also contained dextrose 10%, with cysteine and pH adjustment being used in some admixtures. Calcium and phosphate solubility followed the patterns reported previously. (609) A slightly greater concentration of phosphate could be used in some mixtures, but this finding was not consistent. (1024)

Using a similar study design, six neonatal parenteral nutrition solutions based on Aminosyn-PF (Abbott) 2, 1.5, and 0.8%, with and without added cysteine hydrochloride and dextrose 10% were studied. Calcium concentrations ranged from 2.5 to 50 mEq/L, and phosphate concentrations ranged from 2.5 to 50 mmol/L. Solutions sat for 18 hours at 25 °C and then were warmed to 37 °C in a water bath to simulate the clinical situation of warming prior to infusion into a child. Solubility curves were markedly different than those for TrophAmine in the previous study. (1024) Solubilities were reported to decrease by 15 mEq/L for calcium and 15 mmol/L for phosphate. The solutions remained clear during room temperature storage, but crystals often formed on warming to 37 °C. (1211)

However, these data were questioned by Mikrut, who noted the similarities between the Aminosyn-PF and TrophAmine products and found little difference in calcium and phosphate solubilities in a preliminary report. (1212) In the full report (1213), parenteral nutrition solutions containing Aminosyn-PF or TrophAmine 1 or 2.5% with dextrose 10 or 25%, respectively, plus electrolytes and trace metals, with or without cysteine hydrochloride, were evaluated under the same conditions. Calcium concentrations ranged from 2.5 to 50 mEq/L, and phosphate concentrations ranged from 5 to 50 mmol/L. In contrast to the previous results (1024), the solubility curves were very

Table 6. Parenteral Nutrition Solutions Evaluated (609)

| Component | Solution Number | | | |
	#1	#2	#3	#4
FreAmine III	4%	2%	1%	1%
Dextrose	25%	20%	10%	10%
pH	6.3	6.4	6.6	7.0[a]

[a] Adjusted with sodium hydroxide.

similar for the Aminosyn-PF and TrophAmine parenteral nutrition solutions but very different from those of the previous Aminosyn-PF study. (1211) The authors again showed that the solubility of calcium and phosphate is greater in solutions containing higher concentrations of amino acids and dextrose. (1213)

Calcium and phosphate solubility curves for TrophAmine 1 and 2% with dextrose 10% and electrolytes, vitamins, heparin, and trace elements were reported. Calcium concentrations ranged from 10 to 60 mEq/L, and phosphorus concentrations ranged from 10 to 40 mmol/L. Calcium and phosphate solubilities were assessed by analysis of the calcium concentrations and followed patterns similar to those reported previously. (608; 609) The higher percentage of amino acids (TrophAmine 2%) permitted a slightly greater solubility of calcium and phosphate, especially in the 10 to 50-mEq/L and 10 to 35-mmol/L ranges, respectively. (1614)

The maximal product of the amount of calcium (as gluconate) times phosphate (as potassium) that can be added to a parenteral nutrition solution, composed of amino acids 1% (Travenol) and dextrose 10%, for preterm infants was reported. Turbidity was observed on initial mixing when the solubility product was around 115 to 130 $mmol^2$ or greater. After storage at 7 °C for 20 hours, visible precipitates formed at solubility products of 130 $mmol^2$ or greater. If the solution was administered through a barium-impregnated silicone rubber catheter, crystalline precipitates obstructed the catheters in 12 hours at a solubility product of 100 $mmol^2$ and in 10 days at 79 $mmol^2$, much lower than the in vitro results. (1041)

The solubility characteristics of calcium and phosphate in pediatric parenteral nutrition solutions composed of Aminosyn 0.5, 2, and 4% with dextrose 10 to 25% were reported. Also present were electrolytes and vitamins. Sodium phosphate was added sequentially in phosphorus concentrations from 10 to 30 mmol/L. Calcium gluconate was added last in amounts ranging from 1 to 10 g/L. The solutions were stored at 25 °C for 30 hours and examined visually and microscopically for precipitation. The authors found that higher concentrations of Aminosyn increased the solubility of calcium and phosphate. Precipitation occurred at lower calcium and phosphate concentrations in the 0.5% solution compared to the 2 and 4% solutions. For example, at a phosphorus concentration of 30 mmol/L, precipitation occurred at calcium gluconate concentrations of about 1, 2, and 4 g/L in the 0.5, 2, and 4% Aminosyn mixtures, respectively. Similarly, at a calcium gluconate concentration of 8 g/L and above, precipitation occurred at phosphorus concentrations of about 13, 17, and 22 mmol/L in the 0.5, 2, and 4% solutions, respectively. The dextrose concentration did not appear to affect the calcium and phosphate solubility significantly. (1042)

The solubility of calcium and phosphorus in neonatal parenteral nutrition solutions composed of amino acids (Abbott) 1.25 and 2.5% with dextrose 5 and 10%, respectively, was evaluated. Also present were multivitamins and trace elements. The solutions contained calcium (as gluconate) in amounts ranging from 25 to 200 mg/100 mL. The phosphorus (as potassium phosphate) concentrations evaluated ranged from 25 to 150 mg/100 mL. If calcium gluconate was added first, cloudiness occurred immediately. If potassium phosphate was added first, substantial quantities could be added with no precipitate formation in 48 hours at 4 °C (Table 7). However, if stored at 22 °C, the solutions were stable for only 24 hours, and all contained precipitates after 48 hours. (1210)

The physical compatibility of calcium gluconate 10 to 40 mEq/L and potassium phosphates 10 to 40 mmol/L in three neonatal parenteral nutrition solutions (TPN #123 to #125 in Appendix I), alone and with retrograde administration of aminophylline 7.5 mg diluted with

Table 7. Maximum Calcium and Phosphorus Concentrations Physically Compatible for 48 Hours at 4 °C (1210)

Calcium (mg/100 mL)	Phosphorus (mg/100 mL)	
	Amino Acids 1.25% + Dextrose 5%[a]	Amino Acids 2.5% + Dextrose 10%[a]
200[b]	50	75
150	50	100
100	75	100
50	100	125
25	150[b]	150[b]

[a]Plus multivitamins and trace elements.
[b]Maximum concentration tested.

1.5 mL of sterile water for injection was reported. Contact of the alkaline aminophylline solution with the parenteral nutrition solutions resulted in the precipitation of calcium phosphate at much lower concentrations than were compatible in the parenteral nutrition solutions alone. (1404)

Additional calcium and phosphate solubility curves were reported for specialty parenteral nutrition solutions based on NephrAmine and also HepatAmine at concentrations of 0.8, 1.5, and 2% as the sources of amino acids. The solutions also contained dextrose 10%, with cysteine and pH adjustment to simulate addition of fat emulsion used in some admixtures. Calcium and phosphate solubility followed the hyperbolic patterns previously reported. (609) Temperature, time, and pH affected calcium and phosphate solubility, with pH having the greatest effect. (2038)

The maximum sodium phosphate concentrations were reported for given amounts of calcium gluconate that could be admixed in parenteral nutrition solutions containing TrophAmine in varying quantities (with cysteine hydrochloride 40 mg/g of amino acid) and dextrose 10%. The solutions also contained magnesium sulfate 4 mEq/L, potassium acetate 24 mEq/L, sodium chloride 32 mEq/L, pediatric multivitamins, and trace elements. The presence of cysteine hydrochloride reduces the solution pH and increases the amount of calcium and phosphate that can be incorporated before precipitation occurs. The results of this study cannot be safely extrapolated to TPN solutions with compositions other than the ones tested. The admixtures were compounded with the sodium phosphate added last after thorough mixing of all other components. The authors noted that this is not the preferred order of mixing (usually phosphate is added first and thoroughly mixed before adding calcium last); however, they believed this reversed order of mixing would provide a margin of error in cases in which the proper order is not followed. After compounding, the solutions were stored for 24 hours at 40 °C. The maximum calcium and phosphate amounts that could be mixed in the various solutions were reported tabularly and are shown in Table 8. (2039) However, these results are not entirely consistent with another study. See Table 9.

The temperature dependence of the calcium–phosphate precipitation has resulted in the occlusion of a subclavian catheter by a solution apparently free of precipitation. The parenteral nutrition solution consisted of FreAmine III 500 mL, dextrose 70% 500 mL, sodium chloride 50 mEq, sodium phosphate 40 mmol, potassium acetate 10 mEq, potassium phosphate 40 mmol, calcium gluconate 10 mEq, magnesium sulfate 10 mEq, and Shil's trace metals solution 1 mL. Although there was no evidence of precipitation in the bottle, tubing and pump cassette, and filter (all at approximately 26 °C) during administration, the occluded catheter and Vicra Loop Lock (next to the patient's body

Table 8. Maximum Amount of Phosphate (as Sodium) (mmol/L) Not Resulting in Precipitation. (2039) See CAUTION Below.[a]

Calcium (as Gluconate)	Amino Acid (as TrophAmine) plus Cysteine HCl 40 mg/g Amino Acid				
	0%	0.4%	1%	2%	3%
9.8 mEq/L	0	27	42	60	66
14.7 mEq/L	0	15	18	30	36
19.6 mEq/L	0	6	15	27	30
29.4 mEq/L	0	3	6	21	24

[a]*CAUTION: The results cannot be safely extrapolated to solutions with formulas other than the ones tested. See text.*

at 37 °C) had numerous crystals identified as calcium phosphate. In vitro, this parenteral nutrition solution had a precipitate in 12 hours at 37 °C but was clear for 24 hours at 26 °C. (610)

Similarly, a parenteral nutrition solution that was clear and free of particulates after two weeks under refrigeration developed a precipitate in four to six hours when stored at room temperature. When the solution was warmed in a 37 °C water bath, precipitation occurred in one hour. Administration of the solution before the precipitate was noticed led to interstitial pneumonitis due to deposition of calcium phosphate crystals. (1427)

The maximum allowable concentrations of calcium and phosphate in a 3-in-1 parenteral nutrition mixture for children (TNA #192 in Appendix I) were reported. Added calcium was varied from 1.5 to 150 mmol/L, and added phosphate was varied from 21 to 300 mmol/L. These mixtures were stable for 48 hours at 22 and 37 °C as long as the pH was not greater than 5.7, the calcium concentration was below 16 mmol/L, the phosphate concentration was below 52 mmol/L, and the product of the calcium and phosphate concentrations was below 250 mmol^2/L^2. (1773)

Calcium phosphate precipitation phenomena was evaluated in a series of parenteral nutrition admixtures composed of dextrose 22%, amino acids (FreAmine III) 2.7%, and fat emulsion (Abbott) 0, 1, and 3.2%. Incorporation of calcium gluconate 19 to 24 mEq/L and phosphate (as sodium) 22 to 28 mmol/L resulted in visible precipitation in the fat-free admixtures. New precipitate continued to form over 14 days, even after repeated filtrations of the solutions through 0.2-μm filters. The presence of the amino acids increased calcium and phosphate solubility, compared with simple aqueous solutions. However, the incorporation of the fat emulsion did not result in a statistically significant increase in calcium and phosphate solubility. The authors noted that the kinetics of calcium phosphate precipitate formation do not appear to be entirely predictable; both transient and permanent precipitation can occur either during the compounding process or at some time afterward. Because calcium phosphate precipitation can be very dangerous clinically, the use of inline filters was recommended. The authors suggested that the filters should have a porosity appropriate to the parenteral nutrition admixture—1.2 μm for fat-containing and 0.2 or 0.45 μm for fat-free nutrition mixtures. (2061)

Laser particle analysis was used to evaluate the formation of calcium phosphate precipitation in pediatric TPN solutions containing TrophAmine in concentrations ranging from 0.5 to 3% with dextrose 10% and also containing L-cysteine hydrochloride 1 g/L. The solutions also contained in each liter sodium chloride 20 mEq, sodium acetate 20 mEq, magnesium sulfate 3 mEq, trace elements 3 mL, and heparin sodium 500 units. The presence of L-cysteine hydrochloride reduces the solution pH and increases the amount of calcium and

phosphate that can be incorporated before precipitation occurs. The results of this study cannot be safely extrapolated to TPN solutions with compositions other than the ones tested. The maximum amount of phosphate that was incorporated without the appearance of a measurable increase in particulates in 24 hours at 37 °C for each of the amino acids concentrations is shown in Table 9. (2196) These results are not entirely consistent with previous results. (2039) See above. The use of more sensitive electronic particle measurement for the formation of subvisible particulates in this study may contribute to the differences in the results.

Calcium and phosphate compatibility was evaluated in a series of parenteral nutrition admixtures composed of Aminosyn II in concentrations ranging from 2% up to 5% (TPN #227 to #231 in Appendix I). The solutions also contained dextrose ranging from 10% up to 25%. Also present were sodium chloride, potassium chloride, and magnesium sulfate in common amounts. Phosphates as the potassium salt and calcium as the acetate salt were added in variable quantities to determine the maximum amounts of calcium and phosphates that could be added to the representative TPN admixtures. The samples were evaluated at 23 and 37 °C over 48 hours by visual inspection in ambient light and using a Tyndall beam and electronically measured for turbidity and microparticulates. The boundaries between the compatible and incompatible concentrations were presented graphically as hyperbolic curves. (2265)

The solubility of calcium acetate versus calcium gluconate with sodium phosphates was evaluated in pediatric parenteral nutrition solutions following storage for 30 hours at 25 °C followed by 30 minutes at 37 °C. Concentrations of Aminosyn PF studied varied from 1 to 3%, dextrose from 10 to 25%, calcium from 5 to 60 mEq/L, and phosphate from 1 to 60 mmol/L. L-cysteine hydrochloride at a dose of 40 mg/g of Aminosyn PF, magnesium 3.2 mEq/L, and pediatric trace elements-4 at 2.4 mL/L of pediatric parenteral nutrition solution were also added. Calcium acetate was found to be less soluble than calcium gluconate when prepared under these concentrations. The maximum concentrations of the calcium salts and sodium phosphates are shown in Table 10. Polarized light microscopy was used to identify the calcium acetate and sodium phosphate crystals adherent to the container walls because simple visual observation was not able to identify the precipitates. The authors recommended the use of calcium

Table 9. Maximum Amount of Phosphate (as Potassium) (mmol/L) Not Resulting in Precipitation. (2196) See CAUTION Below.[a]

Calcium (as Gluconate) (mEq/L)	Amino Acid (as TrophAmine) plus Cysteine HCl 1 g/L					
	0.5%	1%	1.5%	2%	2.5%	3%
10	22	28	38	38	38	43
14	18	18	18	38	38	43
19	18	18	18	33	33	38
24	12	18	18	22	28	28
28	12	18	18	18	18	18
33	12	12	12	12	12	12
37	12	12	12	12	12	12
41	9	9	9	12	12	12
45	0	9	9	12	12	12
49	0	9	9	9	12	12
53	0	9	9	9	9	9

[a]*CAUTION: The results cannot be safely extrapolated to solutions with formulas other than the ones tested. See text.*

Table 10. Maximum Concentrations of Sodium Phosphates and Calcium as Acetate and as Gluconate Not Resulting in Precipitation (2466)

Aminosyn PF (%)	Sodium Phosphates (mmol/L)	Calcium Acetate (mEq/L)	Calcium Gluconate (mEq/L)
1	10	25	50
1	15	15	25
2	10	30	45
2	25	10	12.5
3	20	10	15
3	25	15	17.5

acetate to reduce the iatrogenic aluminum exposure often seen with calcium gluconate in the neonatal population receiving parenteral nutrition. (2466) However, care must be taken to avoid inadvertent calcium phosphate precipitation at the lower concentrations found with calcium acetate if it is substituted for the gluconate salt to reduce aluminum exposure.

Calcium and phosphate compatibility was evaluated in a series of adult formula parenteral nutrition admixtures composed of FreAmine III, in concentrations ranging from 1 to 5% (TPN #258 through #262). The solutions also contained dextrose ranging from 15% up to 25%. Also present were sodium chloride, potassium chloride, and magnesium sulfate in common amounts. Cysteine hydrochloride was added in an amount of 25 mg/g of amino acids from FreAmine III to reduce the pH by about 0.5 pH unit and thereby increase the amount of calcium and phosphates that can be added to the TPN admixtures as has been done with pediatric parenteral nutrition admixtures. Phosphates as the potassium salts and calcium as the gluconate salt were added in variable quantities to determine the maximum amounts of calcium and phosphates that could be added to the test admixtures. The samples were evaluated at 23 and 37 °C over 48 hours by visual inspection in ambient light and using a Tyndall beam and electronic measurement of turbidity and microparticulates. The addition of the cysteine hydrochloride resulted in an increase of calcium and phosphates solubility of about 30% by lowering the solution pH 0.5 pH unit. The boundaries between the compatible and incompatible concentrations were presented graphically as hyperbolic curves. (2469)

A 2-in-1 parenteral nutrition admixture with final concentrations of TrophAmine 0.5%, dextrose 5%, L-cysteine hydrochloride 40 mg/g of amino acids, calcium gluconate 60 mg/100 mL, and sodium phosphates 46.5 mg/mL was found to result in visible precipitation of calcium phosphate within 30 hours stored at 23 to 27 °C. Despite the presence of the acidifying L-cysteine hydrochloride, precipitation occurred at clinically utilized amounts of calcium and phosphates. (2622)

The presence of magnesium in solutions may also influence the reaction between calcium and phosphate, including the nature and extent of precipitation. (158; 159)

The interaction of calcium and phosphate in parenteral nutrition solutions is a complex phenomenon. Various factors play a role in the solubility or precipitation of a given combination, including (608; 609; 1042; 1063; 1427; 2038; 2039; 2061):

1. Concentration of calcium
2. Salt form of calcium
3. Concentration of phosphate
4. Concentration of amino acids
5. Amino acids composition
6. Concentration of dextrose
7. Temperature of solution
8. pH of solution
9. Presence of other additives
10. Order of mixing

Enhanced precipitate formation would be expected from such factors as high concentrations of calcium and phosphate, increases in solution pH, decreased amino acid concentrations, increases in temperature, addition of calcium prior to the phosphate, lengthy standing times or slow infusion rates, and use of calcium as the chloride salt. (854)

Even if precipitation does not occur in the bottle, it has been reported that crystallization of calcium phosphate may occur in a Silastic infusion pump chamber or tubing if the rate of administration is slow, as for premature infants. Water vapor may be transmitted outward and be replaced by air rapidly enough to produce supersaturation. (202) Several other cases of catheter occlusion also have been reported. (610; 1427; 1428; 1429)

Vitamins — As might be expected, vitamin stability has been found to be better during nighttime when compared to daytime because of the influence of photodecomposition. (2307)

A patient receiving 3000 I.U. of retinol daily in a parenteral nutrition solution, nevertheless, experienced two episodes of night blindness. The pharmacy prepared the parenteral nutrition solution in 1-L PVC bags in weekly batches and stored them at 4 °C in the dark until use. A subsequent in vitro study showed losses of vitamin A of 23 and 77% in three- and 14-day periods, respectively, under these conditions. About 30% of the lost vitamin A could be extracted from the PVC bag. (1038)

Losses of vitamin A from multivitamins (USV) in a neonatal parenteral nutrition solution was reported. The solution was prepared in colorless glass bottles and run through an administration set with a burette (Travenol). The total loss of vitamin A was 75% in 24 hours, with about 16% as decomposition in the glass bottle. The decomposition was not noticeable during the first 12 hours, but then vitamin A levels fell rather precipitously to about one-third of the initial amount. The balance of the loss, averaging about 59%, occurred during transit through the administration set. Removal of the inline filter and treatment of the set with albumin human had no effect on vitamin A delivery. The authors recommended a three- to fourfold increase in the amount of vitamin A to compensate for the losses. (1039)

A parenteral nutrition solution in glass bottles exposed to sunlight was reported. Vitamin A decomposed rapidly, losing more than 50% in three hours. The decomposition could be slowed by covering the bottle with a light-resistant vinyl bag, resulting in about a 25% loss in three hours. (1040)

Vitamin E was stable in the parenteral nutrition solution in glass bottles exposed to sunlight, with no loss occurring during six hours of exposure. (1040)

It was reported that 40% retinol losses occurred in two hours and 60% in five hours from parenteral nutrition solutions pumped at 10 mL/hr through standard infusion sets at room temperature. The retinol concentration in the bottle remained constant while the retinol in the effluent decreased. Antioxidants had no effect. Much of the vitamin A was recoverable from hexane washings of the tubing. (1050)

The delivery of vitamins A, D, and E from a parenteral nutrition solution composed of amino acids 3% solution (Pharmacia) in dextrose 10% with electrolytes, trace elements, vitamin K, folate, and vitamin B_{12} was evaluated. To this solution was added 6 mL of multivitamin infusion (USV). The solution was prepared in PVC bags (Travenol), and administration was simulated through a fluid chamber (Buretrol) and infusion tubing with a 0.5-μm filter at 10 mL/hr. During the first 60 to 90 minutes, minimal delivery of the vitamins occurred. This was followed by a rise and plateau in the delivered vitamins, which were attributed to an increasing saturation of adsorptive binding sites in the tubing. Total amounts delivered over 24 hours were 31% for vitamin A, 68% for vitamin D, and 64% for vitamin E. Sorption of the vitamins was found in the PVC bag, fluid chamber, and tubing. Decomposition was not a factor. (836)

Vitamin A was found to rapidly and significantly decompose when exposed to daylight. The extent and rate of loss were dependent on the degree of exposure to daylight which, in turn, depended on various factors such as the direction of the radiation, time of day, and climatic conditions. Delivery of less than 10% of the expected amount was reported. (1047) In controlled light experiments, the decomposition initially progressed exponentially. Subsequently, the rate of decomposition slowed. This result was attributed to a protective effect of the degradation products on the remaining vitamin A. The presence of amino acids provided greater protection. Compared to degradation rates in dextrose 5%, decomposition was reduced by up to 50% in some amino acid mixtures. (1048)

In a parenteral nutrition solution composed of amino acids, dextrose, electrolytes, trace elements, and multivitamins in PVC bags stored at 4 and 25 °C, vitamin A rapidly deteriorated to 10% of the initial concentration in eight hours at 25 °C while exposed to light. The decomposition was slowed by light protection and refrigeration, with a loss of about 25% in four days. Folic acid concentration dropped 40% initially on admixture and then remained relatively constant for 28 days of storage. About 35% of the ascorbic acid was lost in 39 hours at 25 °C with exposure to light. The loss was reduced to a negligible amount in four days by refrigeration and light protection. Thiamine content dropped by about 50% initially but then remained unchanged over 120 hours of storage. (1063)

A 50% loss of vitamin A from a bottle of parenteral nutrition solution prepared with multivitamin infusion (USV) after 5.5 hours of infusion was noted. The amount delivered through an Ivex-2 filter set was only 6.3% of the added amount. Similar quantities were found after 20 hours of infusion. A reduced light exposure and use of ^{3}H-labeled vitamin A confirmed binding to the infusion bottles and tubing. (704)

Subsequently, solutions containing multivitamins (USV) spiked with ^{3}H-labeled retinol were incubated in intravenous tubing protected from light and agitated to simulate flow for five hours. About half of the vitamin A was lost in 30 minutes, and 88 to 96% was lost in five hours. Spectrophotometric assays correlated closely with the radioisotope assays. Hexane rinses and radioactivity determinations on the tubing accounted for the decrease in radioactivity. (1049)

In another experiment, neonatal parenteral nutrition solutions containing multivitamins prepared in bags were delivered at 10 mL/hr through Buretrol sets (Travenol). The bags and sets were protected from light. Spectrophotometric and radioisotope assays showed that about 26% of the vitamin A was lost before the flow was started. At 10 mL/hr, about 67% was lost from the effluent. More rapid flow reduced the extent of loss. Analysis of clinical samples of parenteral nutrition solutions showed losses of 21 to 57% after 20 hours. Because losses after five hours were of the same magnitude, the authors concluded that the loss occurs fairly rapidly and is not due to gradual decomposition. (1049)

The quantity of retinol delivered from an M.V.I.-containing 2-in-1 parenteral nutrition solution and when M.V.I. was added to Intralip-

id 10% was evaluated during simulated administration through a PVC administration set. The parenteral nutrition solution was composed of amino acids 2.8%, dextrose 10%, and standard electrolytes; M.V.I. was added to yield a nominal retinol concentration of 455 mcg/150 mL. Retinol losses were about 80% of the admixed amount after being delivered through the PVC set. When M.V.I. was added to Intralipid 10% in a retinol concentration of 455 mcg/20 mL, retinol losses were reduced to about 10% of the admixed amount. The fat emulsion provides retinol protection from sorption to the PVC administration set. (2027)

Substantially higher amounts of retinol were found to be delivered using polyolefin administration set tubing when compared with PVC tubing during simulated neonatal intensive care administration. Retinol was added to a 2-in-1 parenteral nutrition solution (TPN #206) in concentrations of 25 and 50 I.U./mL and run at 4 and 10 mL/hr through three meter lengths of polyolefin (MiniMed) and PVC (Baxter) intravenous extension set tubing protected from light and passed through a 37 °C water bath. Delivered quantities of retinol varied from 19 to 74% through the PVC tubing and 47 to 87% through the polyolefin tubing. The authors noted that the loss of retinol to the PVC tubing appeared to be saturable. Even so, the use of polyolefin tubing increases the amount of retinol delivered during simulated neonatal administration. (2028)

Substantial loss of retinol all-*trans* palmitate and phytonadione from both TPN and TNA admixtures due to exposure to sunlight was reported. In three hours of exposure to sunlight, essentially total loss of retinol and 50% loss of phytonadione had occurred. The presence or absence of lipids did not affect stability. In contrast, tocopherol concentrations remained essentially unchanged by exposure to sunlight through 12 hours. The container material used to store the nutrition admixtures affected the concentration of the vitamins as well. Losses were greatest (10 to 25%) in PVC containers and were slightly better in EVA and glass containers. (2049)

The photodegradation of vitamins A and E in a 2-in-1 (Synthamin 9, dextrose 20%) admixture and a 3-in-1 (Synthamin 9, dextrose 20%, Intralipid 20%, electrolytes, vitamins, trace elements) admixture after exposure to six hours of indirect daylight was reported. The compounded admixtures were prepared in multilayer bags protected from light and stored at 5 °C for a minimum of five days. The same admixtures were prepared in EVA bags 24 hours prior to use with vitamins added prior to study. Vitamin A decreased to 60 to 80% of the initial concentrations in two to six hours of exposure to indirect daylight. The type of bag had no influence on the photodegradation of vitamin A. Despite fat emulsion, no significant light protection was noted with the 3-in-1 admixture. Vitamin E losses were 15% in six hours with multilayer bags of both admixtures; however, 100% loss was noted with EVA bags within one hour for the 2-in-1 admixture. The presence of the opaque fat emulsion provided some protection; however, losses greater than 50% were noted by six hours in the EVA bags. The authors concluded that the use of multilayer bags prevents vitamin E losses during daylight exposure as compared to EVA bags but only light protection can minimize vitamin A losses. (2459)

The stability of retinol palmitate and tocopherols (δ, γ, and α) in 3-in-1 admixtures of amino acids 4%, dextrose 10%, fat emulsion 3% (Intralipid, Liposyn, and ClinOleic), various electrolytes, vitamins, and trace elements in EVA bags over three days at 4, 25, and 37 °C was evaluated. Retinol palmitate was found to be unstable at room temperature with 33 and 50% degradation at 24 and 72 hours after compounding, respectively. Refrigeration of the admixture reduced the degradation to 29% at 72 hours. The tocopherols displayed varying stability over the temperature range with 16 to 25% degradation after 72 hours. The variation in the tocopherols was theorized to be from the free conversion between the oxidized and reduced forms over the temperatures tested. (2460)

The stability of vitamin E (alpha-tocopherol acetate from M.V.I.-1000 or Soluzyme) and selenium (from Selepen) in amino acids (Abbott) and dextrose in PVC bags was evaluated. Exposure to fluorescent light and room temperature (23 °C) for 24 hours and simulated infusion at 50 mL/hr for eight hours through a Medlon TPN administration set with a 0.22-μm filter did not affect the concentrations of vitamin E and selenium. (1224)

The stability of numerous vitamins in parenteral nutrition solutions composed of amino acids (Kabi-Vitrum), dextrose 30%, and fat emulsion 20% (Kabi-Vitrum) in a 2:1:1 ratio with electrolytes, trace elements, and both fat- and water-soluble vitamins was reported. The admixtures were stored in darkness at 2 to 8 °C for 96 hours with no significant loss of retinyl palmitate, alpha-tocopherol, thiamine mononitrate, sodium riboflavin-5'-phosphate, pyridoxine hydrochloride, nicotinamide, folic acid, biotin, sodium pantothenate, and cyanocobalamin. Sodium ascorbate and its biologically active degradation product, dehydroascorbic acid, totaled 59 and 42% of the nominal starting concentration at 24 and 96 hours, respectively. However, the actual initial concentration was only 66% of the nominal concentration. (1225)

When the admixture was subjected to simulated infusion over 24 hours at 20 °C, either exposed to room light or light protected, or stored for six days in the dark under refrigeration and then subjected to the same simulated infusion, once again the retinyl palmitate, alpha-tocopherol, and sodium riboflavin-5'-phosphate did not undergo significant loss. However, sodium ascorbate and its degradation product, dehydroascorbic acid, had initial combined concentrations of 51 to 65% of the nominal initial concentration, with further declines during infusion. Light protection did not significantly alter the loss of total ascorbic acid. (1225)

The stability of several vitamins from M.V.I.-12 (Armour) admixed in parenteral nutrition solutions composed of different amino acid products, with or without Intralipid 10%, when stored in glass bottles and PVC bags at 25 and 5 °C for 48 hours was reported. Riboflavin, folic acid, and vitamin E were stable in all samples. No vitamin A was lost in any formula in glass bottles, but samples in PVC containers lost as much as 35 and 60% at 5 and 25 °C, respectively, in 48 hours. Thiamine hydrochloride was stable in the parenteral nutrition solutions prepared with amino acid products without sulfites. However, amino acid products containing sulfites (Travasol and FreAmine III) had a 25% thiamine loss in 12 hours and a 50% loss in 24 hours when the solutions were stored at 25 °C; no loss occurred when the solutions were stored at 5 °C. Ascorbic acid was lost from all samples stored at 25 °C, with the greatest losses occurring in solutions stored in plastic bags. No losses occurred in any sample stored at 5 °C. (1431)

In another study, the stability of vitamins A, E, C, riboflavin, thiamine, and folic acid following admixture (as M.V.I.-12) with four different amino acid products (Novamine, Neopham, FreAmine III, Travasol) with or without Intralipid when stored in glass bottles or PVC bags at 25 °C for 48 hours was reported. They found that high-intensity phototherapy light did not affect folic acid, thiamine, or vitamin E; however, ascorbic acid and riboflavin losses were significant with all amino acid products tested. Furthermore, it was noted that vitamin A losses were reduced with the addition of Intralipid to the admixture. When bisulfite was added to the Neopham admixture, riboflavin, folic acid, and ascorbic acid were not affected; however, at a bisulfite concentration of 3 mEq/L, there was substantial losses

of vitamin A and thiamine. The authors also noted that ascorbic acid losses were increased with a more alkaline pH and that bisulfite addition offered some protection presumably by bisulfite being preferentially oxidized. The authors concluded that intravenous multivitamins should be added to parenteral nutrition admixtures immediately prior to administration to reduce losses since commercially available amino acid products may contain bisulfites and have varying pH values. (487)

The stability of five B vitamins was studied over an eight-hour period in representative parenteral nutrition solutions exposed to fluorescent light, indirect sunlight, and direct sunlight. One 5-mL vial of multivitamin concentrate (Lyphomed) and 1 mg of folic acid (Lederle) were added to a liter of parenteral nutrition solution composed of amino acids 4.25%–dextrose 25% (Travenol) with standard electrolytes and trace elements. All five B vitamins tested were stable for eight hours at room temperature when exposed to fluorescent light. In addition, folic acid and niacinamide were stable over eight hours in direct or indirect sunlight. Exposure to indirect sunlight appeared to have little or no effect on thiamine hydrochloride and pyridoxine hydrochloride in eight hours, but 47% of riboflavin-5'-phosphate was lost in that period. Direct sunlight caused a 26% loss of thiamine hydrochloride and an 86% loss of pyridoxine hydrochloride in eight hours. Four-hour exposures of riboflavin-5'-phosphate to direct sunlight resulted in a 98% loss. (842)

The effects of photoirradiation on a FreAmine II–dextrose 10% parenteral nutrition solution containing 1 mL/500 mL of multivitamins (USV) were evaluated. During simulated continuous administration to an infant at 0.156 mL/min, no changes to the amino acids occurred when the bottle, infusion tubing, and collection bottle were shielded with foil. Only 20 cm of tubing in the incubator was exposed to light. However, if the flow was stopped, a marked reduction in methionine (40%), tryptophan (44%), and histidine (22%) occurred in the solution exposed to light for 24 hours. In a similar solution without vitamins, only the tryptophan concentration decreased. The difference was attributed to the presence of riboflavin, a photosensitizer. The authors recommended administering the multivitamins separately and shielding from light. (833)

In further work, the authors simulated more closely conditions occurring during phototherapy in neonatal intensive care units. Riboflavin 1 mg/100 mL was added to a solution of amino acids 2% (Abbott) with dextrose 10%. Infusion was simulated from glass bottles through PVC tubing with a Buretrol at a rate of 4 mL/hr. In addition to the fluorescent room lights, eight daylight bulbs delivered phototherapy. After a simulated 24-hour infusion, riboflavin decreased to about 50% of its initial level. Also, a 7% reduction in total amino acids was noted, including individual losses of glycine (10%), leucine (14%), methionine (24%), proline (10%), serine (9%), tryptophan (35%), and tyrosine (16%). Although the authors did not believe that these losses of amino acids were nutritionally important, they were concerned about the possibility of toxicity from photo-oxidation products. In the same solution without riboflavin, the individual amino acids decreased only slightly. (974)

The extent and rapidity of ascorbic acid decomposition in parenteral nutrition solutions composed of amino acids, dextrose, electrolytes, multivitamins, and trace elements in 3-L PVC bags stored at 3 to 7 °C was reported. About 30 to 40% was lost in 24 hours. The degradation then slowed as the oxygen supply was reduced to the diffusion through the bag. About a 55 to 65% loss occurred after seven days of storage. The oxidation was catalyzed by metal ions, especially copper. In the absence of copper from the trace elements additive, less than 10% degradation of ascorbic acid occurred in 24 hours. The author estimated that 150 to 200 mg is degraded in two to four hours at ambient temperature in the presence of copper but that only 20 to 30 mg is broken down in 24 hours without copper. To minimize ascorbic acid loss, copper must be excluded. Alternatively, inclusion of excess ascorbic acid was suggested. (1056)

Extensive decomposition of ascorbic acid and folic acid was reported in a parenteral nutrition solution composed of amino acids 3.3%, dextrose 12.5%, electrolytes, trace elements, and M.V.I.-12 (USV) in PVC bags. Half-lives were 1.1, 2.9, and 8.9 hours for ascorbic acid and 2.7, 5.4, and 24 hours for folic acid stored at 24 °C in daylight, 24 °C protected from light, and 4 °C protected from light, respectively. The decomposition was much greater than for solutions not containing catalyzing metal ions. Also, it was greater than for the vitamins singly because of interactions with the other vitamins present. (1059)

The stability of ascorbic acid in parenteral nutrition solutions, with and without fat emulsion, was studied. Both with and without fat emulsion, the total vitamin C content (ascorbic acid plus dehydroascorbic acid) remained above 90% for 12 hours when the solutions were exposed to fluorescent light and for 24 hours when they were protected from light. When stored in a cool dark place, the solutions were stable for seven days. (1227)

The stability of several vitamins from M.V.I.-12 (Armour) admixed in parenteral nutrition solutions composed of different amino acid products, with or without Intralipid 10%, when stored in glass bottles and PVC bags at 25 and 5 °C for 48 hours was reported. Ascorbic acid was lost from all samples stored at 25 °C, with the greatest losses occurring in solutions stored in plastic bags. No losses occurred in any sample stored at 5 °C. (1431)

The stability of ascorbic acid and dehydroascorbic acid in a 3-in-1 admixture containing Vamin 14, dextrose 30%, Intralipid 20%, potassium phosphate, Cernevit, and trace elements in EVA bags over a temperature range of 2 to 22 °C was examined. They observed an 89% loss of ascorbic acid and a 37% loss of dehydroascorbic acid over 7 days. The authors concluded that oxygen, trace elements, temperature, and an underfilled bag were the greatest determinants of ascorbic acid loss. (2462)

The long-term stability of ascorbic acid in 3-in-1 admixtures containing amino acids (Eloamin) 10%, dextrose 20%, dextrose 5%, fat emulsion (Elolipid) 20%, calcium gluconate, M.V.C. 9 + 3, and trace elements mixed in EVA and multilayer (Ultrastab) bags at 5 °C was compared. Ascorbic acid losses were greater than 75% in the first 24 hours and 100% after 48 to 72 hours in the EVA bags. In the multilayer bags, ascorbic acid showed a 20 and 40% loss over the first 24 hours with and without fat emulsion, respectively. The initial rapid fall in ascorbic acid was presumably due to the initial oxygen content of the admixtures despite the use of the less oxygen-permeable multilayer bags. The authors noted the ascorbic acid concentration remained stable for up to 28 days in the multilayer bags after the initial fall and recommended adding additional ascorbic acid to compensate for the losses to facilitate extended shelf-life. (2463)

The influence of several factors on the rate of ascorbic acid oxidation in parenteral nutrition solutions was evaluted. Ascorbic acid is regarded as the least stable component in TPN admixtures. The type of amino acid used in the TPN was important. Some, such as FreAmine III and Vamin 14, contain antioxidant compounds (e.g., sodium metabisulfite or cysteine). Ascorbic acid stability was better in such solutions compared with those amino acid solutions having no antioxidant present. Furthermore, the pH of the solution may play a small role, with greater degradation as the pH rises from about 5 to about 7. Adding air to a compounded TPN container can also accel-

erate ascorbic acid decomposition. The most important factor was the type of plastic container used for the TPN. EVA containers (Mixieva, Miramed) allow more oxygen permeation, which results in substantial losses of ascorbic acid in relatively short time periods. In multilayer TPN bags (Ultrastab, Miramed) designed to reduce gas permeability, the rate of ascorbic acid degradation was greatly reduced. TPNs without antioxidants packaged in EVA bags were found to have an almost total loss of ascorbic acid activity occurring in one or two days at 5 °C. In contrast, in TPNs containing FreAmine III or Vamin 14 packaged in the multilayer bags, most of the ascorbic acid content was retained for 28 days at 5 °C. The authors concluded that TPNs made with antioxidant-containing amino acids and packaged in multilayer bags that reduce gas permeability can safely be given extended expiration dates and still retain most of the ascorbic acid activity. (2163)

The initial degradation product of ascorbic acid (dehydroascorbic acid) in a 2-in-1 admixture containing Synthamin 14, glucose 20%, and trace elements over a temperature range of 5 to 35 °C was evaluated. The presence of trace elements, including copper, had no influence on the degradation of dehydroascorbic acid. At room temperature and 5 °C, there was a greater than 50% loss of dehydroascorbic acid noted within two and 24 hours, respectively. The authors concluded this degradation was temperature dependent. (2461)

The degradation of vitamins A, B₁, C, and E from Cernevit (Roche) multivitamins in NuTRIflex Lipid Plus (B. Braun) admixtures prepared in ethylene vinyl acetate (EVA) bags and in multilayer bags was evaluated. After storage for up to 72 hours at 4, 21, and 40 °C, greater vitamin losses occurred in the EVA bags: vitamin A (retinyl palmitate) losses were 20%, thiamine hydrochloride losses were 25%, alpha-tocopherol losses were 20%, and ascorbic acid losses were approximately 80 to 100%. In the multilayer bags (presumably a better barrier to oxygen transfer), losses were less: vitamin A (retinyl palmitate) losses were 5%, thiamine hydrochloride losses were 10%, alpha-tocopherol losses were 0%, and ascorbic acid losses were approximately 25 to 70%. (2618)

Phytonadione stability in a TPN solution containing amino acids 2%, dextrose 12.5%, "standard" electrolytes, and multivitamins (M.V.I. Pediatric) was evaluated over 24 hours while exposed to light. Vitamin loss, about 7% in four hours and 27% in 24 hours, was attributed partly to the light sensitivity of phytonadione. (1815)

Trace Elements — Because of interactions, recommendations to separate the administration of vitamins and trace elements have been made. (1056; 1060; 1061) Others have termed such recommendations premature based on differing reports (895; 896) and the apparent absence of epidemic vitamin deficiency in parenteral nutrition patients. (1062)

The addition of trace elements to a 3-in-1 parenteral nutrition solution with electrolytes had no adverse effect on the particle size of the fat emulsion after eight days of storage at 4 °C. (1017)

The stability of a 3-in-1 parenteral nutrition mixture (TNA #191 in Appendix I) was compared with trace elements added as gluconate salts or chloride salts. TNA #191 with copper 0.24 mg/L, iron 0.5 mg/L, and zinc 2 mg/L in either salt form was physically stable for seven days at 4 and 25 °C. (1787)

Trace elements additives, especially those containing copper ions, have the potential to be incompatible in TPN solutions, resulting in precipitation. In a TPN admixture containing 5% Synthamin 17, 25% dextrose, 1 g of ascorbic acid injection, 14 mmol of calcium chloride, and trace elements solution (David Bull), storage at 20 to 25 °C and 2 to 8 °C, protected from light, resulted in the formation of a discolored solution in three to seven days and an off-white to yellow precipitate in eight to 12 days, respectively. Electron microscopy revealed the presence of numerous bipyramidal, eight-sided crystals in sizes from 3 to 30 μm. The authors proposed that the crystals were calcium oxalate. They suggested that the ascorbic acid decomposed to oxalic acid; the oxalic acid then interacted with calcium ions to form calcium oxalate. The authors did not verify their supposition. They noted that the crystals were conformationally different from calcium phosphate crystals and that no phosphate had been added to the admixture. In addition, mixing ascorbic acid injection 500 mg/5 mL with trace elements solution 5 mL results in the formation of a transparent gel that becomes an opaque flocculent precipitate after five minutes. The authors recommended adding trace elements well away from injections that can act as ligands and with thorough mixing after each addition. Introduction of air and prolonged storage should be avoided. Incorporating trace elements and ascorbic acid on alternate days was also suggested. (2197)

The chromium and zinc contamination of various components of parenteral nutrition solutions by atomic absorption spectrophotometry was evaluated. They analyzed FreAmine III, Aminosyn, TrophAmine, and dextrose 70% and found chromium concentrations were below the limit of detection but zinc ranged from 0.11 to 4.97 mg/L. Additionally, detectable chromium and zinc concentrations were seen with various lots of L-cysteine, potassium and sodium salts (chloride, acetate, and phosphate), calcium gluconate, and magnesium sulfate. The zinc contamination was thought to be a product of manufacturing procedures as it is present in many rubber stoppers and in the materials to produce glass. The authors suggested that the amount of contamination of chromium and zinc present in most pediatric parenteral nutrition solutions may exceed current recommendations, especially for infants less than 10 kg. (2464)

Heparin — Flocculation of fat emulsion (Kabi-Vitrum) was reported during Y-site administration into a line used to infuse a parenteral nutrition admixture containing both calcium gluconate and heparin sodium. Subsequent evaluation indicated that the combination of calcium gluconate (0.46 and 1.8 mmol/125 mL) and heparin sodium (25 and 100 units/125 mL) in amino acids plus dextrose induced flocculation of the fat emulsion within two to four minutes at concentrations that resulted in no visually apparent flocculation in 30 minutes with either agent alone. (1214)

Calcium chloride quantities of 1 and 20 mmol normally result in slow flocculation of fat emulsion 20% over several hours. When heparin sodium 5 units/mL was added, the flocculation rate was accelerated greatly and a cream layer was observed visually in a few minutes. This effect was not observed when sodium ion was substituted for the divalent calcium. (1406)

Similar results were observed during simulated Y-site administration of heparin sodium into nine 3-in-1 nutrient admixtures having different compositions. Damage to the fat emulsion component was found to occur immediately, with the possible formation of free oil over time. (2215)

The destabilization of fat emulsion (Intralipid 20%) was also observed when administered simultaneously with a TPN admixture and heparin. The damage, detected by viscosity measurement, occurred immediately upon contact at the Y-site. The extent of the destabilization was dependent on the concentration of heparin and the presence of MVI Pediatric with its surfactant content. Additionally, phase separation was observed in two hours. The authors noted that TPN admixtures containing heparin should never be premixed with fat emulsion as a 3-in-1 total nutrient admixture because of this emulsion destabilization. The authors indicated their belief that the damage

could be minimized during Y-site co-administration as long as the heparin was kept at a sufficiently low concentration (no visible separation occurred at a heparin concentration of 0.5 unit/mL) and the length of tubing between the Y-site and the patient was minimized. (2282)

However, because the damage to emulsion integrity has been found to occur immediately upon mixing with heparin in the presence of the calcium ions in TPN admixtures (1214; 2215; 2282) and no evaluation and documentation of the clinical safety of using such destabilized emulsions has been performed, use of such damaged emulsions is suspect.

Ranitidine — The stability of ranitidine hydrochloride has been evaluated in a number of TPN solutions with variable results. See Additive Compatibility table. The major mechanism of ranitidine hydrochloride decomposition is oxidation. A number of factors have been found to contribute to ranitidine hydrochloride instability in TPN solutions, including the presence or absence of antioxidants (such as sodium metabisulfite) in the amino acids, the addition of trace elements (which can catalyze ranitidine oxidation), solution pH, and type of plastic container used. In a study of ranitidine hydrochloride stability in several TPN solutions stored at 5 °C, the drug was most stable in FreAmine III–based (contains sodium metabisulfite) admixtures with additives when packaged in multilayer gas impermeable plastic containers (Ultrastab) with about 8% loss in 28 days. In contrast, in ethylene vinyl acetate (EVA) bags, which are permeable to oxygen, losses of approximately 50% occurred in this time period. If Vamin 14 with no antioxidant present was used as the amino acid source, and the solution was packaged in EVA bags, ranitidine hydrochloride losses of approximately 65% occurred in 28 days. Similarly, the addition of air to the bags during compounding increases the extent of ranitidine hydrochloride oxidation substantially. (2195)

Other Information

Titratable Acidity — The acidity of parenteral nutrition solutions can be a factor in the development of metabolic acidosis by a patient. (577; 851) Titratable acidity is a measure of the hydrogen ion content that must be neutralized to raise the pH to a given endpoint and is often expressed as milliequivalents of titrant per liter of reactant. In a study (577) of five amino acid injections and mixtures, the titratable acidities were determined for pH 7.4 by titrating with 0.1220 N sodium hydroxide and 7.54% (0.898 M) sodium bicarbonate. The results are noted in Table 11.

Corresponding (although somewhat lower) values were also obtained for 1:1 mixtures with dextrose 50%. It was concluded that use of sodium bicarbonate to adjust to pH 7.4 was not usually feasible given the large volumes of fluid and increased sodium ion required. However, smaller amounts could be used for smaller pH adjustments. (577)

Table 11. Titratable Acidity of Several Amino Acids Products (577)

	Titratable Acidity	
	NaOH (mEq/L)	NaHCO₃ (mEq/L)
Aminosyn 7%	37	314
FreAmine II 8.5%	16.8	176
Travasol 8.5%	34.7	354
Travasol 8.5% with electrolytes	45.2	420

AMINOCAPROIC ACID
AHFS 20:28.16

Products — Aminocaproic acid is available as a 250-mg/mL concentration in 20-mL vials containing 5 g of drug with hydrochloric acid for pH adjustment. Aminocaproic acid injection is available with benzyl alcohol 0.9% as a preservative and also in preservative-free form. (1; 4)

pH — The pH is adjusted to approximately 6.8 with a range of 6 to 7.6. (1)

Administration — Aminocaproic acid is administered by continuous intravenous infusion after dilution in a suitable infusion solution. Rapid intravenous injection of the undiluted drug should be avoided. (1; 4)

Stability — Intact containers of aminocaproic acid injection should be stored at controlled room temperature. Freezing should be avoided. (1; 4)

Compatibility Information

Solution Compatibility

Aminocaproic acid

Solution	Mfr	Mfr	Conc/L	Remarks	Ref	C/I
Dextrose 5%	BAª	IMM	10 and 100 g	Physically compatible with little or no loss in 7 days at 4 and 23 °C. Yellow discoloration forms after 24 hr at 23 °C but is not associated with drug loss	2096	C
Sodium chloride 0.9%	BAª	IMM	10 and 100 g	Physically compatible with little or no loss in 7 days at 4 and 23 °C	2096	C

ª*Tested in PVC containers.*

Y-Site Injection Compatibility (1:1 Mixture)

Aminocaproic acid

Drug	Mfr	Conc	Mfr	Conc	Remarks	Ref	C/I
Fenoldopam mesylate	AB	80 mcg/mLª	AMR	50 mg/mLª	Physically compatible for 4 hr at 23 °C	2467	C

ª*Tested in sodium chloride 0.9%.*

AMINOPHYLLINE
AHFS 86:16

Products — Aminophylline is available as a 25-mg/mL solution in 10-mL (250 mg) and 20-mL (500 mg) ampuls and vials for intravenous injection. Aminophylline is a 2:1 complex of theophylline and ethylenediamine. It contains excess ethylenediamine to ensure stability (6) and is approximately 79% theophylline by weight. Aminophylline 25 mg is equivalent to 19.7 mg of theophylline. (1)

pH — From 8.6 to 9. (1)

Osmolality — The calculated osmolarity of the injection is 170 mOsm/L. (1) The osmolality was determined to be 114 mOsm/kg by freezing-point depression. (1071)

The osmolality of aminophylline 250 mg was calculated for the following dilutions (1054):

	Osmolality (mOsm/kg)	
Diluent	50 mL	100 mL
Dextrose 5%	300	291
Sodium chloride 0.9%	327	318

Administration — Aminophylline may be administered by intravenous infusion or slow direct intravenous injection. (1; 4)

Stability — The containers should be stored at controlled room temperature and protected from freezing and light. (1; 4) Containers of aminophylline should be inspected for particulate matter and discoloration prior to use. Do not use if crystals are present. (1; 4)

pH Effects — Reports in the literature of aminophylline precipitating in acidic media do not apply to the dilute solutions found in intravenous infusions. Aminophylline should not be mixed in a syringe with other components of an admixture but should be added separately. (6)

Because of the alkalinity of aminophylline-containing solutions, drugs known to be alkali labile should be avoided in admixtures. (6)

Temperature Effects — Aminophylline under simulated summer conditions in paramedic vehicles was exposed to temperatures ranging from 26 to 38 °C over 4 weeks. Analysis found no loss of the drug under these conditions. (2562)

Light Effects — A study of aminophylline (Squibb) 50 mg/mL found no change in theophylline after eight weeks of storage with exposure to fluorescent light. (1231)

Syringes — Aminophylline (Abbott) 5 mg/mL in bacteriostatic water for injection containing benzyl alcohol 0.9% in plastic syringes (Becton-Dickinson) exhibited 2 and 3% losses at 4 and 22 °C, respectively, after 91 days of storage. (1586)

Sorption — Aminophylline was shown not to exhibit sorption to PVC bags and tubing, polyethylene tubing, Silastic tubing, and polypropylene syringes. (536; 606)

Filtration — Aminophylline 500 mg/L in dextrose 5% was passed through an Ivex-2 inline filter at a rate of 2 mL/min. No decrease in the aminophylline concentration occurred over the eight-hour study period. (556)

Central Venous Catheter — Aminophylline (Abbott) 2.5 mg/mL in dextrose 5% was found to be compatible with the ARROWg+ard Blue Plus (Arrow International) chlorhexidine-bearing triple-lumen central catheter. Essentially complete delivery of the drug was found with little or no drug loss occurring. Furthermore, chlorhexidine delivered from the catheter remained at trace amounts with no substantial increase due to the delivery of the drug through the catheter. (2335)

Compatibility Information

Solution Compatibility

Aminophylline

Solution	Mfr	Mfr	Conc/L	Remarks	Ref	C/I
Amino acids 4.25%, dextrose 25%	MG	SE	500 mg	No increase in particulate matter in 24 hr at 5 °C	349	C
Dextrose–Ringer's injection combinations	AB		500 mg	Physically compatible	3	C
Dextrose–Ringer's injection, lactated, combinations	AB		500 mg	Physically compatible	3	C
Dextrose 5% in Ringer's injection, lactated	BA	SE	10 mg	Physically compatible for 24 hr	315	C
Dextrose–saline combinations	AB		500 mg	Physically compatible	3	C
Dextrose 5% in sodium chloride 0.2%	MG	AQ	750 mg	Physically compatible with no aminophylline decomposition in 48 hr at 25 °C. Yellow tinge at 48 hr due to slight dextrose decomposition	556	C
Dextrose 5% in sodium chloride 0.9%			250 mg	Physically compatible	74	C
	BA	SE	10 g	Physically compatible for 24 hr	315	C
	TR[a]	AQ	750 mg	Physically compatible with no aminophylline decomposition in 48 hr at 25 °C. Yellow tinge at 48 hr due to slight dextrose decomposition	556	C
Dextrose 2.5%	AB		500 mg	Physically compatible	3	C
Dextrose 5%			500 mg to 2.5 g	Stable for 24 hr at room temperature	56	C
			250 mg	Physically compatible	74	C
	AB		500 mg	Physically compatible	3	C
	AB	SE	450 mg	Stable for at least 24 hr at room temperature	6	C
	BA	SE	10 g	Physically compatible for 24 hr	315	C
	AB	ES	5 and 10 g	Physically compatible with little or no decomposition in 96 hr under refrigeration	537	C
	TR[a]	AQ	750 mg	Physically compatible with no aminophylline decomposition in 48 hr at 25 °C and 7 days at 5 °C. Yellow tinge in the 25 °C admixture at 48 hr due to slight dextrose decomposition	556	C
	TR[a]	AQ	250 and 500 mg	Physically compatible with no aminophylline decomposition in 48 hr at 25 °C. Yellow tinge in the admixture at 48 hr due to slight dextrose decomposition	556	C

Solution Compatibility (Cont.)

Aminophylline

Solution	Mfr	Mfr	Conc/L	Remarks	Ref	C/I
			250 mg	Stable for at least 24 hr at 24 to 26 °C	852	C
	TR[a]	IX	500 mg	Physically compatible with little or no loss in 48 hr at room temperature	1186	C
	AB	SE	1 g	Physically compatible with no loss in 24 hr at 24 °C under fluorescent light	1198	C
	TR[a]	LY	1 g	Physically compatible with no loss in 24 hr at room temperature under fluorescent light	1358	C
	TR[a]		1 g	Yellow discoloration in 2 hr but theophylline content retained for at least 24 hr	1571	C
	TR[a]	ES	0.5 and 2 g	Visually compatible with little or no aminophylline loss in 48 hr at room temperature	1802	C
Dextrose 10%	AB		500 mg	Physically compatible	3	C
	BA	SE	10 g	Physically compatible for 24 hr	315	C
			250 mg	Stable for at least 24 hr at 24 to 26 °C. Yellow discoloration at 2 hr and increased with time	852	C
Dextrose 20%	BA	SE	10 g	Physically compatible for 24 hr	315	C
			250 mg	Stable for at least 24 hr at 24 to 26 °C. Yellow discoloration at 2 hr and increased with time	852	C
Ionosol products	AB		500 mg	Physically compatible	3	C
Ringer's injection	AB		500 mg	Physically compatible	3	C
Ringer's injection, lactated			250 mg	Physically compatible	74	C
	AB		500 mg	Physically compatible	3	C
	BA	SE	10 g	Physically compatible for 24 hr	315	C
Sodium chloride 0.45%	AB		500 mg	Physically compatible	3	C
Sodium chloride 0.9%	AB		500 mg	Physically compatible	3	C
			250 mg	Physically compatible	74	C
	TR[a]	SE	500 mg	Stable for 24 hr	45	C
	BA[d]	SE	500 mg	Stable for 24 hr	45	C
	BA	SE	10 g	Physically compatible for 24 hr	315	C
	TR[a]	AQ	750 mg	Physically compatible with no decomposition in 48 hr at 25 °C	556	C
	TR[a]		1 g	Theophylline content retained for 24 hr	1571	C
	TR[a]	ES	0.5 and 2 g	Visually compatible with no aminophylline loss in 48 hr at room temperature	1802	C
Sodium lactate ⅙ M	AB		500 mg	Physically compatible	3	C
	BA	SE	10 g	Physically compatible for 24 hr	315	C
TNA #180[b]			234 and 638 mg	No theophylline loss and no increase in fat particle size in 24 hr at room temperature	1617	C
TPN #25 to #27[b]		SE	250 mg to 1.5 g	Physically compatible and aminophylline stable for at least 24 hr at 25 °C	755	C
		SE	1 g	Physically compatible and aminophylline stable for at least 24 hr at 4 °C	755	C
TPN #28 to #30[b]		SE	1 g	Physically compatible and aminophylline stable for at least 24 hr at 25 °C	755	C
TPN[c]			29.3 mg	No significant change in aminophylline content over 24 hr at 24 to 26 °C	852	C

[a]*Tested in PVC containers.*
[b]*Refer to Appendix I for the composition of parenteral nutrition solutions. TNA indicates a 3-in-1 admixture, and TPN indicates a 2-in-1 admixture.*
[c]*Tested in a pediatric parenteral nutrition solution containing 150 mL of dextrose 5% and 30 mL of Vamin glucose with electrolytes and vitamins.*
[d]*Tested in glass containers.*

Additive Compatibility

Aminophylline

Drug	Mfr	Conc/L	Mfr	Conc/L	Test Soln	Remarks	Ref	C/I
Amikacin sulfate	BR	5 g	SE	5 g	LR, NS, R, SL	Physically compatible and amikacin stable for 24 hr at 25 °C. Aminophylline not analyzed	294	C
	BR	5 g	SE	5 g	D5LR, D5R, D5S, D5W, D10W	Over 10% amikacin loss after 8 hr but within 24 hr at 25 °C. Aminophylline not analyzed	294	I
Ascorbic acid	AB	500 mg	SE	500 mg		Physically compatible	6	C
	UP	500 mg	SE	1 g	D5W	Physically incompatible	15	I
Atracurium besylate	BW	500 mg		1 g	D5W	Atracurium unstable due to high pH	1694	I
Bleomycin sulfate	BR	20 and 30 units	ES	250 mg	NS	50% loss of bleomycin in 1 week at 4 °C	763	I
Calcium gluconate		1 g		250 mg	D5W	Physically compatible	74	C
Cefepime HCl	BR	4 g	LY	1 g	NS	37% cefepime loss in 18 hr at room temperature and 32% loss in 3 days at 5 °C. No aminophylline loss	1681	I
Ceftazidime	GL	2 g	ES	1 g	D5W, NS	20 to 23% ceftazidime loss in 6 hr at room temperature	1937	I
	GL	6 g	ES	1 g	D5W, NS	8 to 10% ceftazidime loss in 6 hr at room temperature	1937	I
	GL	2 g	ES	2 g	D5W, NS	35 to 40% ceftazidime loss in 6 hr at room temperature	1937	I
	GL	6 g	ES	2 g	D5W, NS	22% ceftazidime loss in 6 hr at room temperature	1937	I
Ceftriaxone sodium	RC	20 g	AMR	1 g	D5W, NS[a]	Yellow color forms immediately. 3 to 6% ceftriaxone loss and 8 to 12% aminophylline loss in 24 hr	1727	I
	RC	20 g	AMR	4 g	D5W, NS[a]	Yellow color forms immediately. 15 to 20% ceftriaxone loss and 7 to 9% aminophylline loss in 24 hr	1727	I
	RC	40 g	AMR	1 g	D5W, NS[a]	Yellow color forms immediately. 15 to 18% ceftriaxone loss and 1 to 3% aminophylline loss in 24 hr	1727	I
Chloramphenicol sodium succinate	PD	500 mg		250 mg	D5W	Physically compatible	74	C
	PD	10 g	SE	1 g	D5W	Physically compatible	15	C
Chlorpromazine HCl	BP	200 mg	BP	1 g	D5W, NS	Precipitates immediately	26	I
Ciprofloxacin	MI	1.6 g	LY	2 g	D5W, NS	Precipitate forms in 4 hr at 4 and 25 °C	1541	I
						Physically incompatible with loss of ciprofloxacin reported due to pH over 6.0	1924	I
Clindamycin phosphate	UP	600 mg	SE	600 mg		Physically incompatible	101	I
Dexamethasone sodium phosphate		30 mg		625 mg	D5W	Physically compatible and chemically stable for 24 hr at 4 and 30 °C	521	C
Dimenhydrinate	SE	50 mg		250 mg	D5W	Physically compatible	74	C
	SE	500 mg	SE	1 g	D5W	Physically incompatible	15	I
Diphenhydramine HCl	PD	50 mg	SE	500 mg		Physically compatible	6	C
Dobutamine HCl	LI	1 g	SE	1 g	D5W, NS	Cloudy in 6 hr at 25 °C	789	I
	LI	1 g	ES	2.5 g	D5W, NS	White precipitate in 12 hr at 21 °C	812	I

Additive Compatibility (Cont.)

Aminophylline

Drug	Mfr	Conc/L	Mfr	Conc/L	Test Soln	Remarks	Ref	C/I
Dopamine HCl	ACC	800 mg	SE	500 mg	D5W	Physically compatible. At 25 °C, 10% dopamine decomposition occurs in 111 hr	527	C
Doxorubicin HCl	AD					Discolors from red to purple	524	I
Epinephrine HCl	PD	4 mg	SE	500 mg	D5W	At 25 °C, 10% epinephrine decomposition in 1.2 hr in light and 3 hr in dark	527	I
		4 mg		500 mg	D5W	Pink to brown discoloration in 8 to 24 hr at room temperature	845	I
Erythromycin lactobionate	AB	1 g	SE	500 mg		Physically compatible. Erythromycin stable for 24 hr at 25 °C	20	C
Esmolol HCl	DU	6 g	LY	1 g	D5W	Physically compatible with no loss of either drug in 24 hr at room temperature under fluorescent light	1358	C
Fat emulsion, intravenous	VT	10%	ES	1 g		Physically compatible for 48 hr at 4 °C and room temperature	32	C
	VT	10%	DB	500 mg		Lipid coalescence in 24 hr at 25 and 8 °C	825	I
Floxacillin sodium	BE	20 g	ANT	1 g	NS	Physically compatible for 72 hr at 15 and 30 °C	1479	C
Flumazenil	RC	20 mg	AMR	2 g	D5W[b]	Visually compatible. No flumazenil loss in 24 hr at 23 °C in fluorescent light. Aminophylline not tested	1710	C
Furosemide	HO	1 g	ANT	1 g	NS	Physically compatible for 72 hr at 15 and 30 °C	1479	C
Heparin sodium		12,000 units		250 mg	D5W	Physically compatible	74	C
	UP	4000 units	SE	1 g	D5W	Physically compatible	15	C
Hydralazine HCl	BP	80 mg	BP	1 g	D5W	Yellow color produced	26	I
Hydrocortisone sodium succinate	UP	100 mg		250 mg	D5W	Physically compatible	74	C
	UP	500 mg	SE	1 g	D5W	Physically compatible	15	C
	UP	100 mg	SE	500 mg		Physically compatible	6	C
		250 mg		625 mg	D5W	Physically compatible and aminophylline stable for 24 hr at 4 and 30 °C. Total hydrocortisone content changed little but substantial ester hydrolysis	521	C
Hydroxyzine HCl	RR	250 mg	SE	1 g	D5W	Physically incompatible	15	I
Isoproterenol HCl	BN	2 mg	SE	500 mg	D5W	At 25 °C, 10% isoproterenol decomposition in 2.2 to 2.5 hr in light and dark	527	I
Lidocaine HCl	AST	2 g	SE	500 mg		Physically compatible	24	C
	AST	2 g	AQ	1 g	D5W, LR, NS	Physically compatible for 24 hr at 25 °C	775	C
Meropenem	ZEN	1 and 20 g	AMR	1 g	NS	Visually compatible for 4 hr at room temperature	1994	C
Methyldopate HCl	MSD	1 g	SE	500 mg	D, D–S, S	Physically compatible	23	C
	MSD	1 g	SE	500 mg	D5W	Physically compatible. At 25 °C, 10% methyldopate decomposition in 90 hr	527	C
Methylprednisolone sodium succinate	UP	40 to 250 mg		500 mg	D5W, NS	Clear solution for 24 hr	329	C
	UP	80 mg		1 g	D5W	Clear solution for 24 hr	329	C

Additive Compatibility (Cont.)

Aminophylline

Drug	Mfr	Conc/L	Mfr	Conc/L	Test Soln	Remarks	Ref	C/I
	UP	125 mg	SE	500 mg		Precipitate forms after 6 hr but within 24 hr	6	I
	UP	250 mg to 1 g		1 g	D5W	Precipitate forms	329	I
	UP	10 to 20 g		~400 mg	D5S, D5W, LR	Yellow color forms	329	I
	UP	500 mg and 2 g	SE	1 g	D5W	Physically compatible. No aminophylline or methylprednisolone alcohol loss in 3 hr at room temperature, but 7 to 10% ester hydrolysis	1022	C
	UP	500 mg and 2 g	SE	1 g	NS	Physically compatible. No aminophylline or methylprednisolone alcohol loss in 3 hr at room temperature, but 12 to 18% ester hydrolysis	1022	C
Midazolam HCl	RC	50 mg		720 mg	NS	Visually compatible for 4 hr	355	C
	RC	250 mg		720 mg	NS	Transient precipitate that dissipates	355	?
	RC	400 mg		720 mg	NS	Precipitate forms immediately	355	I
Nafcillin sodium	WY	30 g	SE	500 mg	D5W	Nafcillin retained for 24 hr at 25 °C	27	C
	WY	2 g	SE	500 mg	D5W	14% nafcillin loss in 24 hr at 25 °C	27	I
Nitroglycerin	ACC	400 mg	IX	1 g	D5W[c]	Physically compatible with 4% nitroglycerin loss in 24 hr and 6% loss in 48 hr at 23 °C. Aminophylline not tested	929	C
	ACC	400 mg	IX	1 g	NS[c]	Physically compatible with no nitroglycerin loss in 24 hr and 5% loss in 48 hr at 23 °C. Aminophylline not tested	929	C
Norepinephrine bitartrate	WI	8 mg	SE	500 mg	D5W	10% norepinephrine loss in 3.6 hr at 25 °C	527	I
Penicillin G potassium	SQ	1 million units	SE	500 mg	D5W	44% penicillin loss in 24 hr at 25 °C	47	I
	[d]	900,000 units	SE	500 mg	D5W	22% penicillin loss in 6 hr at 25 °C	48	I
Pentazocine lactate	WI	300 mg	SE	1 g	D5W	Physically incompatible	15	I
Pentobarbital sodium	AB	500 mg		500 mg		Physically compatible	3	C
	AB	1 g	SE	1 g	D5W	Physically compatible	15	C
	AB	500 mg	SE	500 mg		Physically compatible	6	C
Phenobarbital sodium	WI	200 mg	SE	1 g	D5W	Physically compatible	15	C
	AB	100 mg	SE	500 mg		Physically compatible	6	C
Potassium chloride	AB	3 g		250 mg	D5W	Physically compatible	74	C
	AB	40 mEq	SE	500 mg		Physically compatible	6	C
Prochlorperazine edisylate	SKF	100 mg	SE	1 g	D5W	Physically incompatible	15	I
Prochlorperazine mesylate	BP	100 mg	BP	1 g	D5W, NS	Precipitates immediately	26	I
Promethazine HCl	BP	100 mg	BP	1 g	D5W, NS	Precipitates immediately	26	I
	WY	250 mg	SE	1 g	D5W	Physically incompatible	15	I
Ranitidine HCl	GL	50 mg and 2 g	ES	500 mg and 2 g	D5W, NS[b]	Physically compatible. 4% or less ranitidine loss in 24 hr at room temperature in light. Aminophylline not tested	1361	C
	GL	50 mg and 2 g	ES	0.5 and 2 g	D5W, NS[b]	Visually compatible. Little loss of either drug in 48 hr at room temperature	1802	C
Sodium bicarbonate	AB	80 mEq	SE	1 g	D5W	Physically compatible	15	C
	AB	40 mEq	SE	500 mg		Physically compatible	6	C

Additive Compatibility (Cont.)

Aminophylline

Drug	Mfr	Conc/L	Mfr	Conc/L	Test Soln	Remarks	Ref	C/I
Terbutaline sulfate	CI	4 mg	SE	500 mg	D5W	Physically compatible. At 25 °C, 10% terbutaline loss in 44 hr in light	527	C
Vancomycin HCl	LI	1 g		250 mg	D5W	Physically compatible	74	C
	LI	5 g	SE	1 g	D5W	Physically incompatible	15	I
Verapamil HCl	KN	80 mg	SE	1 g	D5W, NS	Transient precipitate clears rapidly, then clear for 48 hr	739	?
	KN	400 mg	SE	1 g	D5W	Visible turbidity forms immediately. Filtration removes all verapamil	1198	I
	KN	100 mg	SE	1 g	D5W	Visually clear, but precipitate found by microscopic examination. Filtration removes all verapamil	1198	I

[a]Tested in polyolefin containers.
[b]Tested in PVC containers.
[c]Tested in glass containers.
[d]A buffered preparation was specified.

Drugs in Syringe Compatibility

Aminophylline

Drug (in syringe)	Mfr	Amt	Mfr	Amt	Remarks	Ref	C/I
Caffeine citrate		20 mg/ 1 mL	AB	25 mg/ 1 mL	Visually compatible for 4 hr at 25 °C	2440	C
Dimenhydrinate		10 mg/ 1 mL		50 mg/ 1 mL	Light cloudiness forms immediately	2569	I
Doxapram HCl	RB	400 mg/ 20 mL		250 mg/ 10 mL	Immediate turbidity and precipitation	1177	I
Heparin sodium		2500 units/ 1 mL		240 mg/ 10 mL	Physically compatible for at least 5 min	1053	C
Metoclopramide HCl	RB	10 mg/ 2 mL	ES	80 mg/ 3.2 mL	Physically compatible for 24 hr at 25 °C	1167	C
	RB	10 mg/ 2 mL	ES	500 mg/ 20 mL	Physically compatible for 24 hr at 25 °C	1167	C
	RB	160 mg/ 32 mL	ES	500 mg/ 20 mL	Physically compatible for 24 hr at 25 °C	1167	C
Pantoprazole sodium	[a]	4 mg/ 1 mL		50 mg/ 1 mL	Clear solution	2574	C
Pentobarbital sodium	AB	500 mg/ 10 mL		500 mg/ 2 mL	Physically compatible	55	C

[a]Test performed using the formulation WITHOUT edetate disodium.

Y-Site Injection Compatibility (1:1 Mixture)

Aminophylline

Drug	Mfr	Conc	Mfr	Conc	Remarks	Ref	C/I
Allopurinol sodium	BW	3 mg/mL[b]	AB	2.5 mg/mL[b]	Physically compatible for 4 hr at 22 °C	1686	C
Amifostine	USB	10 mg/mL[a]	AMR	2.5 mg/mL[a]	Physically compatible for 4 hr at 23 °C	1845	C

Y-Site Injection Compatibility (1:1 Mixture) (Cont.)

Aminophylline

Drug	Mfr	Conc	Mfr	Conc	Remarks	Ref	C/I
Amiodarone HCl	LZ	4 mg/mL[c]	ES	5 mg/mL[c]	Haze forms within 15 min and white precipitate forms within 6 hr at 21 °C	1032	I
Amphotericin B cholesteryl sulfate complex	SEQ	0.83 mg/mL[a]	AB	2.5 mg/mL[a]	Physically compatible for 4 hr at 23 °C	2117	C
Anidulafungin	VIC	0.5 mg/mL[a]	AB	2.5 mg/mL[a]	Physically compatible for 4 hr at 23 °C	2617	C
Aztreonam	SQ	40 mg/mL[a]	AMR	2.5 mg/mL[a]	Physically compatible for 4 hr at 23 °C	1758	C
Bivalirudin	TMC	5 mg/mL[a]	AB	2.5 mg/mL[a]	Physically compatible for 4 hr at 23 °C	2373	C
Ceftaroline fosamil	FOR	2.22 mg/mL[d]	AMR	2.5 mg/mL[d]	Physically compatible for 4 hr at 23 °C	2826	C
Ceftazidime	GL	40 mg/mL[a]	ES	2 mg/mL[a]	Visually compatible with 4% ceftazidime loss and 9% theophylline loss in 2 hr at room temperature	1937	C
	GL	40 mg/mL[b]	ES	2 mg/mL[a]	Visually compatible with 5% ceftazidime loss and 4% theophylline loss in 2 hr at room temperature	1937	C
Ciprofloxacin	MI	2 mg/mL[c]	AB	2 mg/mL[c]	Fine white crystals form in 20 min in D5W and 2 min in NS	1655	I
Cisatracurium besylate	GW	0.1 and 2 mg/mL[a]	AB	2.5 mg/mL[a]	Physically compatible for 4 hr at 23 °C	2074	C
	GW	5 mg/mL[a]	AB	2.5 mg/mL[a]	Gray subvisible haze forms in 1 hr	2074	I
Cladribine	ORT	0.015[b] and 0.5[e] mg/mL	AMR	2.5 mg/mL[b]	Physically compatible for 4 hr at 23 °C	1969	C
Clarithromycin	AB	4 mg/mL[a]	EV	2 mg/mL[a]	Needle-like crystals form in 2 hr at 30 °C and 4 hr at 17 °C	2174	I
Clonidine HCl	BI	18 mcg/mL[b]	NYC	0.9 mg/mL[b]	Visually compatible	2642	C
Dexmedetomidine HCl	AB	4 mcg/mL[b]	AB	2.5 mg/mL[b]	Physically compatible for 4 hr at 23 °C	2383	C
Diltiazem HCl	MMD	5 mg/mL	AMR	25 mg/mL[b]	Cloudiness forms	1807	I
	MMD	1 mg/mL[b]	AMR	25 mg/mL[b]	Visually compatible	1807	C
	MMD	5 mg/mL	AMR	2 mg/mL[c]	Visually compatible	1807	C
Dobutamine HCl	LI	4 mg/mL[c]	ES	4 mg/mL[c]	Slight precipitate and color change in 1 hr	1316	I
Docetaxel	RPR	0.9 mg/mL[a]	AB	2.5 mg/mL[a]	Physically compatible for 4 hr at 23 °C	2224	C
Doripenem	JJ	5 mg/mL[a,b]	AMR	2.5 mg/mL[a,b]	Physically compatible for 4 hr at 23 °C	2743	C
Doxorubicin HCl liposomal	SEQ	0.4 mg/mL[a]	AB	2.5 mg/mL[a]	Physically compatible for 4 hr at 23 °C	2087	C
Enalaprilat	MSD	0.05 mg/mL[b]	ES	1 mg/mL[a]	Physically compatible for 24 hr at room temperature under fluorescent light	1355	C
Esmolol HCl	DCC	10 mg/mL[a]	ES	1 mg/mL[a]	Physically compatible for 24 hr at 22 °C	1169	C
Etoposide phosphate	BR	5 mg/mL[a]	AB	2.5 mg/mL[a]	Physically compatible for 4 hr at 23 °C	2218	C
Famotidine	MSD	0.2 mg/mL[a]	LY	2.5 mg/mL[b]	Physically compatible for 14 hr	1196	C
	ME	2 mg/mL[a]		2.5 mg/mL[a]	Visually compatible for 4 hr at 22 °C	1936	C
Fenoldopam mesylate	AB	80 mcg/mL[b]	AB	2.5 mg/mL[b]	Haze and microparticulates form immediately. Yellow turbidity in 4 hr	2467	I
Filgrastim	AMG	30 mcg/mL[a]	AB	2.5 mg/mL[a]	Physically compatible for 4 hr at 22 °C	1687	C
Fluconazole	RR	2 mg/mL	ES	25 mg/mL	Physically compatible for 24 hr at 25 °C	1407	C
	PF	0.5 and 1.5 mg/mL[c]	AMR	0.8 and 1.5 mg/mL[c]	Visually compatible with no loss of either drug in 3 hr at 24 °C	1626	C
Fludarabine phosphate	BX	1 mg/mL[a]	ES	2.5 mg/mL[a]	Visually compatible for 4 hr at 22 °C	1439	C

Y-Site Injection Compatibility (1:1 Mixture) (Cont.)

Aminophylline

Drug	Mfr	Conc	Mfr	Conc	Remarks	Ref	C/I
Foscarnet sodium	AST	24 mg/mL	LY	25 mg/mL	Physically compatible for 24 hr at room temperature under fluorescent light	1335	C
Gallium nitrate	FUJ	1 mg/mL[b]	AMR	25 mg/mL	Visually compatible for 24 hr at 25 °C	1673	C
Gemcitabine HCl	LI	10 mg/mL[b]	AB	2.5 mg/mL[b]	Physically compatible for 4 hr at 23 °C	2226	C
Granisetron HCl	SKB	0.05 mg/mL[a]	AB	2.5 mg/mL[a]	Physically compatible for 4 hr at 23 °C	2000	C
Heparin sodium[f]	RI	1000 units/L[d]	SE	25 mg/mL	Physically compatible for 4 hr at room temperature	322	C
Hetastarch in lactated electrolyte	AB	6%	AMR	2.5 mg/mL[a]	Physically compatible for 4 hr at 23 °C	2339	C
Hydralazine HCl	SO	1 mg/mL[a]	ES	4 mg/mL[a]	Gross color change in 1 hr	1316	I
	SO	1 mg/mL[b]	ES	4 mg/mL[b]	Color change in 1 hr and haze in 3 hr	1316	I
Hydrocortisone sodium succinate[g]	UP	100 mg/L[d]	SE	25 mg/mL	Physically compatible for 4 hr at room temperature	322	C
Labetalol HCl	SC	1 mg/mL[a]	ES	1 mg/mL[a]	Physically compatible for 24 hr at 18 °C	1171	C
Levofloxacin	OMN	5 mg/mL[a]	AMR	25 mg/mL	Visually compatible for 4 hr at 24 °C	2233	C
Linezolid	PHU	2 mg/mL	AB	2.5 mg/mL[a]	Physically compatible for 4 hr at 23 °C	2264	C
Melphalan HCl	BW	0.1 mg/mL[b]	AB	2.5 mg/mL[b]	Physically compatible for 3 hr at 22 °C	1557	C
Meropenem	ZEN	1 and 50 mg/mL[b]	AMR	25 mg/mL	Visually compatible for 4 hr at room temperature	1994	C
Micafungin sodium	ASP	1.5 mg/mL[b]	AMR	2.5 mg/mL[b]	Physically compatible for 4 hr at 23 °C	2683	C
Morphine sulfate	WY	0.2 mg/mL[c]	ES	4 mg/mL[c]	Physically compatible for 3 hr	1316	C
Nicardipine HCl	DCC	0.1 mg/mL[a]	ES	1 mg/mL[a]	Visually compatible for 24 hr at room temperature	235	C
Ondansetron HCl	GL	1 mg/mL[b]	AMR	2.5 mg/mL[a]	Immediate turbidity and precipitation	1365	I
Paclitaxel	NCI	1.2 mg/mL[a]	AB	2.5 mg/mL[a]	Physically compatible for 4 hr at 22 °C	1556	C
Pancuronium bromide	ES	0.05 mg/mL[a]	AB	1 mg/mL[a]	Physically compatible for 24 hr at 28 °C	1337	C
Pemetrexed disodium	LI	20 mg/mL[b]	AB	2.5 mg/mL[a]	Physically compatible for 4 hr at 23 °C	2564	C
Piperacillin sodium–tazobactam sodium	LE[k]	40 + 5 mg/mL[a]	AB	2.5 mg/mL[a]	Physically compatible for 4 hr at 22 °C	1688	C
Potassium chloride		40 mEq/L[e]	SE	25 mg/mL	Physically compatible for 4 hr at room temperature	322	C
Propofol	ZEN	10 mg/mL	AMR	2.5 mg/mL[a]	Physically compatible for 1 hr at 23 °C	2066	C
Ranitidine HCl	GL	0.5 mg/mL	LY	4 mg/mL[a]	Physically compatible for 24 hr	1323	C
Remifentanil HCl	GW	0.025 and 0.25 mg/mL[b]	AB	2.5 mg/mL[a]	Physically compatible for 4 hr at 23 °C	2075	C
Sargramostim	IMM	10 mcg/mL[b]	ES	2.5 mg/mL[b]	Visually compatible for 4 hr at 22 °C	1436	C
Tacrolimus	FUJ	1 mg/mL[b]	ES	2 mg/mL[a]	Visually compatible for 24 hr at 25 °C	1630	C
Teniposide	BR	0.1 mg/mL[a]	AB	2.5 mg/mL[a]	Physically compatible for 4 hr at 23 °C	1725	C
Thiotepa	IMM[h]	1 mg/mL[b]	AMR	2.5 mg/mL[b]	Physically compatible for 4 hr at 23 °C	1861	C
TNA #218 to #226[i]			AB	2.5 mg/mL[a]	Visually compatible for 4 hr at 23 °C	2215	C
TPN #189[i]			DB	1 mg/mL[b]	Visually compatible for 24 hr at 22 °C	1767	C
TPN #203, #204[i]			AMR	5 and 25 mg/mL	White precipitate forms immediately	1974	I

Y-Site Injection Compatibility (1:1 Mixture) (Cont.)

Aminophylline

Drug	Mfr	Conc	Mfr	Conc	Remarks	Ref	C/I
TPN #212 to #215[i]			AB	2.5 mg/mL[a]	Physically compatible for 4 hr at 23 °C	2109	**C**
Vecuronium bromide	OR	0.1 mg/mL[a]	AB	1 mg/mL[a]	Physically compatible for 24 hr at 28 °C	1337	**C**
Vinorelbine tartrate	BW	1 mg/mL[b]	AB	2.5 mg/mL[b]	Visible haze with large particles in 1 hr	1558	**I**
Warfarin sodium	DME	2 mg/mL[j]	ES	4 mg/mL[a]	Haze forms in 4 hr	2078	**I**

[a]*Tested in dextrose 5%.*
[b]*Tested in sodium chloride 0.9%.*
[c]*Tested in both dextrose 5% and sodium chloride 0.9%.*
[d]*Tested in dextrose 5%, sodium chloride 0.9%, and Ringer's injection, lactated.*
[e]*Tested in bacteriostatic sodium chloride 0.9% preserved with benzyl alcohol 0.9%.*
[f]*Tested in combination with hydrocortisone sodium succinate (Upjohn) 100 mg/L.*
[g]*Tested in combination with heparin sodium (Riker) 1000 units/L.*
[h]*Lyophilized formulation tested.*
[i]*Refer to Appendix I for the composition of parenteral nutrition solutions. TNA indicates a 3-in-1 admixture, and TPN indicates a 2-in-1 admixture.*
[j]*Tested in sterile water for injection.*
[k]*Test performed using the formulation WITHOUT edetate disodium.*

AMIODARONE HYDROCHLORIDE
AHFS 24:04.04.20

Products — Amiodarone hydrochloride 50 mg/mL is available in 3-, 9-, and 18-mL vials. Each milliliter also contains polysorbate 80 100 mg, and benzyl alcohol 20.2 mg in water for injection. (1)

pH — The pH is reported to be 4.08. (1053)

Administration — Amiodarone hydrochloride is a concentrate that is administered by intravenous infusion after dilution in a compatible diluent. Intravenous infusion at concentrations of 1 to 6 mg/mL is performed using a volumetric pump and a dedicated central venous catheter with an inline filter when possible; concentrations greater than 2 mg/mL require a central venous catheter. (1; 4) The injection contains polysorbate 80, a surface active agent that alters drop size. The drop size reduction may lead to substantial underdosage if a drop counter infusion set is used. Consequently, the drug must be delivered with a volumetric infusion pump. (1; 1445)

Stability — Amiodarone hydrochloride should be stored at room temperature and protected from light and excessive heat. Light protection is not necessary during administration (1), but exposure to direct sunlight should be avoided. (2258) It is recommended that amiodarone hydrochloride be added only to dextrose 5%. (1) Information on the drug's compatibility in sodium chloride 0.9% has been conflicting. (1443; 1031) Solutions containing less than 0.6 mg/mL of amiodarone hydrochloride in dextrose 5% are unstable and should not be used. (1442)

Precipitation — Amiodarone hydrochloride may precipitate when diluted. Studies found little or no precipitation when the formulation was diluted to very small or very large concentrations. In the middle range, however, at concentrations between 45 mg/mL (90% amiodarone hydrochloride formulation) and about 0.0025 mg/mL in phosphate buffer (pH 7.4), the drug concentration exceeds the solubility of amiodarone hydrochloride in the mixture. Precipitation may occur immediately or on standing. Such precipitation may occur when the

drug enters the bloodstream, contributing to the phlebitis associated with amiodarone hydrochloride. (1818; 1819)

The aqueous solubility of amiodarone hydrochloride is not substantially altered over the pH range of 1.5 to 7.5 (925), but precipitation may occur in alkaline media. (791; 1032)

Amiodarone hydrochloride (Wyeth-Ayerst) 1.2 mg/mL in 250 mL of dextrose 5% has been reported to develop cloudiness upon standing when prepared in glass evacuated bottles (Abbott). The precipitation was attributed to the acetate buffers present in the small amount of residual fluid left in evacuated bottles from steam sterilization. (1982)

Sorption — At concentrations of 1 to 6 mg/mL in dextrose 5% in polyolefin or glass containers, amiodarone hydrochloride is physically compatible, with no loss in 24 hours. In PVC containers, however, the amiodarone hydrochloride loss due to sorption occurs; acceptable potency (less than 10% loss) exists for two hours. Consequently, the manufacturer recommends that all infusions longer than two hours be made in glass or polyolefin containers only. (1)

Similarly, amiodarone hydrochloride is lost due to sorption to PVC infusion sets. (1; 1443) However, the manufacturer states that these losses are accounted for by the recommended dosage schedule. Consequently, PVC sets should be used with this drug, but the recommended infusion regimen must be followed. (1)

Amiodarone hydrochloride 1 mg/mL in dextrose 5% in VISIV polyolefin bags was tested for 24 hours at room temperature near 23 °C. Little or no loss due to sorption was found within the 24-hour study period. (2660)

Plasticizer Leaching — Amiodarone hydrochloride leaches diethylhexyl phthalate (DEHP) plasticizer from PVC tubing. The degree of plasticizer leaching depends on the concentration and rate of administration. Higher concentrations and slower administration rates leach more plasticizer. (1)

Filtration — Amiodarone hydrochloride (Labaz) 0.6 mg/mL in dextrose 5% and sodium chloride 0.9% was filtered through a 0.22-μm cellulose ester membrane filter (Ivex-HP, Millipore) over six hours. No significant drug loss due to binding to the filter was noted. (1034)

Compatibility Information

Solution Compatibility

Amiodarone HCl

Solution	Mfr	Mfr	Conc/L	Remarks	Ref	C/I
Dextrose 5%	MG[a]	LZ	1.8 g	Physically compatible. Little loss in 24 hr at 24 °C in light	1031	C
	TR[b]	LZ	0.6 g	25% loss in 24 hr at room temperature	1443	I
	TR[c]	LZ	0.6 g	Physically compatible with little drug loss in 5 days at room temperature	1443	C
	BA[d]	WY	2 g	Visually compatible with no loss at 5 °C and 3% loss at 25 °C in 32 days	2110	C
	HOS[e]	BED	1 g	Less than 3% loss in 24 hr	2660	C
Sodium chloride 0.9%	MG[a]	LZ	1.8 g	Physically compatible. Little loss in 24 hr at 24 °C in light	1031	C
	TR[c]	LZ	0.6 g	Incompatible in 24 hr at room temperature	1443	I
	BA[d]	WY	2 g	Visually compatible with no loss at 5 °C and 3% loss at 25 °C in 32 days	2110	C
	MYR[c]	EBE	0.84 g	5% loss in 6 hr at room temperature	2258	?

[a]Tested in polyolefin containers.
[b]Tested in PVC containers.
[c]Tested in glass containers.
[d]Tested in amber glass containers.
[e]Tested in VISIV polyolefin containers.

Additive Compatibility

Amiodarone HCl

Drug	Mfr	Conc/L	Mfr	Conc/L	Test Soln	Remarks	Ref	C/I
Dobutamine HCl	LI	1 g	LZ	2.5 g	D5W, NS	Physically compatible for 24 hr at 21 °C	812	C
Floxacillin sodium	BE	20 g	LZ	4 g	D5W	Precipitates immediately	1479	I
Furosemide	ES	200 mg	LZ	1.8 g	D5W, NS[a]	Physically compatible. 8% or less amiodarone loss in 24 hr at 24 °C in light	1031	C
	HO	1 g	LZ	4 g	D5W	Haze in 5 hr and precipitate in 24 to 72 hr at 30 °C. No changes at 15 °C	1479	I
Lidocaine HCl	AB	4 g	LZ	1.8 g	D5W, NS[a]	Physically compatible. 9% or less amiodarone loss in 24 hr at 24 °C in light	1031	C
Potassium chloride	AB	40 mEq	LZ	1.8 g	D5W, NS[a]	Physically compatible. No amiodarone loss in 24 hr at 24 °C in light	1031	C
Procainamide HCl	SQ	4 g	LZ	1.8 g	D5W, NS[a]	Physically compatible. 5% or less amiodarone loss in 24 hr at 24 °C in light	1031	C
Quinidine gluconate	LI	1 g	LZ	1.8 g	D5W[b]	Milky precipitation. 13% amiodarone loss in 6 hr and 23% in 24 hr at 24 °C in light	1031	I
	LI	1 g	LZ	1.8 g	D5W[c]	Milky precipitation. No amiodarone loss in 24 hr at 24 °C in light	1031	I
	LI	1 g	LZ	1.8 g	NS[b]	Physically compatible. 13% amiodarone loss in 24 hr at 24 °C in light	1031	I
	LI	1 g	LZ	1.8 g	NS[c]	Physically compatible. No amiodarone loss in 24 hr at 24 °C in light	1031	C
Verapamil HCl	KN	50 mg	LZ	1.8 g	D5W, NS[a]	Physically compatible. 8% or less amiodarone loss in 24 hr at 24 °C in light	1031	C

[a]Tested in both polyolefin and PVC containers.
[b]Tested in PVC containers.
[c]Tested in polyolefin containers.

Drugs in Syringe Compatibility

Amiodarone HCl

Drug (in syringe)	Mfr	Amt	Mfr	Amt	Remarks	Ref	C/I
Heparin sodium		2500 units/ 1 mL	LZ	150 mg/ 3 mL	Turbidity or precipitate forms within 5 min	1053	**I**
Pantoprazole sodium	a	4 mg/ 1 mL		50 mg/ 1 mL	Precipitates	2574	**I**

[a]*Test performed using the formulation WITHOUT edetate disodium.*

Y-Site Injection Compatibility (1:1 Mixture)

Amiodarone HCl

Drug	Mfr	Conc	Mfr	Conc	Remarks	Ref	C/I
Amikacin sulfate	BR	5 mg/mL[c]	LZ	4 mg/mL[c]	Physically compatible for 4 hr at room temperature	1444	**C**
Aminophylline	ES	5 mg/mL[c]	LZ	4 mg/mL[c]	Haze forms within 15 min and white precipitate forms within 6 hr at 21 °C	1032	**I**
Amoxicillin sodium–clavulanic acid	GSK	10 + 2 mg/ mL	SAN	12.5 mg/mL	Turbidity appeared immediately	2727	**I**
Amphotericin B	BMS	0.5 mg/mL[a]	WY	6 mg/mL[a]	Visually compatible for 24 hr at 22 °C	2352	**C**
Ampicillin sodium–sulbactam sodium	PF	30 mg/mL[b]	WY	6 mg/mL[a]	Immediate opaque white turbidity	2352	**I**
Argatroban	SKB	1 mg/mL[a]	NVP	1.8 mg/mL[a]	Trace precipitate forms immediately	2572	**I**
Atracurium besylate	BA	5 mg/mL[a]	WY	6 mg/mL[a]	Visually compatible for 24 hr at 22 °C	2352	**C**
Atropine sulfate	AB	0.4 mg/mL	WY	6 mg/mL[a]	Visually compatible for 24 hr at 22 °C	2352	**C**
Bivalirudin	TMC	5 mg/mL[a]	WAY	4 mg/mL[a]	Measured haze increases immediately	2373	**I**
Calcium chloride	APP	10 mg/mL[a]	WY	6 mg/mL[a]	Visually compatible for 24 hr at 22 °C	2352	**C**
	APP	100 mg/mL	WY	6 mg/mL[a]	Visually compatible for 24 hr at 22 °C	2352	**C**
Calcium gluconate	AMR	10 mg/mL[a]	WY	6 mg/mL[a]	Visually compatible for 24 hr at 22 °C	2352	**C**
Caspofungin acetate	ME	0.7 mg/mL[b]	SIC	4 mg/mL[b]	Physically compatible for 4 hr at room temperature	2758	**C**
Cefazolin sodium	LI	20 mg/mL[a]	LZ	4 mg/mL[a]	Precipitate forms	1444	**I**
	LI	20 mg/mL[b]	LZ	4 mg/mL[b]	Physically compatible for 4 hr at room temperature	1444	**C**
Ceftaroline fosamil	FOR	2.22 mg/ mL[a,b,f]	SIC	4 mg/mL[a,b,f]	Physically compatible for 4 hr at 23 °C	2826	**C**
Ceftazidime	GW	40 mg/mL[a]	WY	6 mg/mL[a]	Immediate opaque white turbidity	2352	**I**
Ceftriaxone sodium	RC	20 mg/mL[a]	WY	6 mg/mL[a]	Turned yellow in 24 hr at 22 °C, but considered normal for cephalosporins	2352	**C**
Cefuroxime sodium	BA	30 mg/mL[a]	WY	6 mg/mL[a]	Turned yellow in 24 hr at 22 °C, but considered normal for cephalosporins	2352	**C**
Ciprofloxacin	BAY	2 mg/mL[a]	WY	6 mg/mL[a]	Visually compatible for 24 hr at 22 °C	2352	**C**
Clarithromycin	AB	4 mg/mL[a]	SW	3 mg/mL[a]	Visually compatible for 72 hr at both 30 and 17 °C	2174	**C**
Clindamycin phosphate	UP	6 mg/mL[c]	LZ	4 mg/mL[c]	Physically compatible for 4 hr at room temperature	1444	**C**
Dexmedetomidine HCl	AB	4 mcg/mL[b]	WAY	4 mg/mL[b]	Physically compatible for 4 hr at 23 °C	2383	**C**

Y-Site Injection Compatibility (1:1 Mixture) (Cont.)

Amiodarone HCl

Drug	Mfr	Conc	Mfr	Conc	Remarks	Ref	C/I
Digoxin	ES	0.25 mg/mL	WY	6 mg/mL[a]	Immediate opaque white turbidity	2352	**I**
Dobutamine HCl	LI	2 mg/mL[c]	LZ	4 mg/mL[c]	Physically compatible for 24 hr at 21 °C	1032	**C**
Dopamine HCl	ES	1.6 mg/mL[c]	LZ	4 mg/mL[c]	Physically compatible for 24 hr at 21 °C	1032	**C**
Doripenem	JJ	5 mg/mL[a,b]	BED	4 mg/mL[a,b]	Physically compatible for 4 hr at 23 °C	2743	**C**
Doxycycline hyclate	ACC	0.25 mg/mL[c]	LZ	4 mg/mL[c]	Physically compatible for 4 hr at room temperature	1444	**C**
Epinephrine HCl	AMR	1 mg/mL	WY	6 mg/mL[a]	Visually compatible for 24 hr at 22 °C	2352	**C**
Eptifibatide	KEY	0.75 mg/mL	WY	6 mg/mL[a]	Visually compatible for 24 hr at 22 °C	2352	**C**
	KEY	2 mg/mL	WY	6 mg/mL[a]	Visually compatible for 24 hr at 22 °C	2352	**C**
Erythromycin lactobionate	AB	2 mg/mL[c]	LZ	4 mg/mL[c]	Physically compatible for 4 hr at room temperature	1444	**C**
Esmolol HCl	DU	40 mg/mL[a]	WY	4.8 mg/mL[a]	Visually compatible for 24 hr at 23 °C	1877	**C**
Famotidine	ME	10 mg/mL	WY	6 mg/mL[a]	Visually compatible for 24 hr at 22 °C	2352	**C**
Fenoldopam mesylate	AB	80 mcg/mL[b]	WAY	4 mg/mL[b]	Physically compatible for 4 hr at 23 °C	2467	**C**
Fentanyl citrate	BA	50 mcg/mL	WY	6 mg/mL[a]	Visually compatible for 24 hr at 22 °C	2352	**C**
Fluconazole	PF	2 mg/mL[b]	WY	6 mg/mL[a]	Visually compatible for 24 hr at 22 °C	2352	**C**
Furosemide	AMR	1 mg/mL[a]	WY	6 mg/mL[a]	Visually compatible for 24 hr at 22 °C	2352	**C**
	AMR	10 mg/mL	WY	6 mg/mL[a]	Immediate opaque white turbidity	2352	**I**
Gentamicin sulfate	LY	0.8 mg/mL[c]	LZ	4 mg/mL[c]	Physically compatible for 4 hr at room temperature	1444	**C**
	APP	5 mg/mL[a]	WY	6 mg/mL[a]	Visually compatible for 24 hr at 22 °C	2352	**C**
Heparin sodium		300 units/mL[b]			White precipitate forms upon sequential administration	791	**I**
Hetastarch in lactated electrolyte	AB	6%	WAY	4 mg/mL[a]	Physically compatible for 4 hr at 23 °C	2339	**C**
Imipenem–cilastatin sodium	ME	5 mg/mL[a]	WY	6 mg/mL[a]	Immediate haze. Becomes yellow in 24 hr	2352	**I**
Insulin, regular	LI	1 unit/mL[a]	WY	4.8 mg/mL[a]	Visually compatible for 24 hr at 23 °C	1877	**C**
Isoproterenol HCl	ES	4 mcg/mL[c]	LZ	4 mg/mL[c]	Physically compatible for 24 hr at 21 °C	1032	**C**
Labetalol HCl	GL	5 mg/mL	WY	4.8 mg/mL[a]	Visually compatible for 24 hr at 23 °C	1877	**C**
	BED	5 mg/mL	WY	6 mg/mL[a]	Visually compatible for 24 hr at 22 °C	2352	**C**
Lepirudin	HMR	0.4 mg/mL[a]	WY	6 mg/mL[a]	Visually compatible for 24 hr at 22 °C	2352	**C**
Lidocaine HCl	AST	8 mg/mL[c]	LZ	4 mg/mL[c]	Physically compatible for 24 hr at 21 °C	1032	**C**
Lorazepam	WY	1 mg/mL[a]	WY	6 mg/mL[a]	Visually compatible for 24 hr at 22 °C	2352	**C**
Magnesium sulfate	APP	500 mg/mL	WY	6 mg/mL[a]	Immediate opaque white turbidity becoming thick precipitate in 24 hr at 22 °C	2352	**I**
	APP	20 mg/mL[a]	WY	6 mg/mL[a]	Visually compatible for 24 hr at 22 °C	2352	**C**
Methylprednisolone sodium succinate	PHU	125 mg/mL	WY	6 mg/mL[a]	Visually compatible for 24 hr at 22 °C	2352	**C**
Metoprolol tartrate	BED	1 mg/mL	BIO	1.8 mg/mL[a]	Visually compatible for 24 hr at 19 °C	2795	**C**
Micafungin sodium	ASP	1.5 mg/mL[b]	BA	4 mg/mL[b]	Gross milky white precipitate forms	2683	**I**
Midazolam HCl	RC	1 mg/mL[a]	WY	4.8 mg/mL[a]	Visually compatible for 24 hr at 23 °C	1877	**C**
	RC	1 mg/mL[a]	WY	6 mg/mL[a]	Visually compatible for 24 hr at 22 °C	2352	**C**
Milrinone lactate	SAN	0.4 mg/mL[a]	WY	6 mg/mL[a]	Visually compatible for 24 hr at 22 °C	2352	**C**

Y-Site Injection Compatibility (1:1 Mixture) (Cont.)

Amiodarone HCl

Drug	Mfr	Conc	Mfr	Conc	Remarks	Ref	C/I
Morphine sulfate	SX	1 mg/mL[a]	WY	4.8 mg/mL[a]	Visually compatible for 24 hr at 23 °C	1877	C
	WY	1 mg/mL[a]	WY	6 mg/mL[a]	Visually compatible for 24 hr at 22 °C	2352	C
	WY	10 mg/mL	WY	6 mg/mL[a]	Visually compatible for 24 hr at 22 °C	2352	C
Nesiritide	SCI	50 mcg/mL[a,b]		50 mg/mL	Physically compatible for 4 hr	2625	C
Nitroglycerin	AB	0.24 mg/mL[c]	LZ	4 mg/mL[c]	Physically compatible for 24 hr at 21 °C	1032	C
Norepinephrine bitartrate	BN	64 mcg/mL[c]	LZ	4 mg/mL[c]	Physically compatible for 24 hr at 21 °C	1032	C
Penicillin G potassium	PF	100,000 units/mL[c]	LZ	4 mg/mL[c]	Physically compatible for 4 hr at room temperature	1444	C
Phentolamine mesylate	CI	0.04 mg/mL[c]	LZ	4 mg/mL[c]	Physically compatible for 24 hr at 21 °C under fluorescent light	1032	C
Phenylephrine HCl	WI	0.04 mg/mL[c]	LZ	4 mg/mL[c]	Physically compatible for 24 hr at 21 °C	1032	C
Piperacillin sodium–tazobactam sodium	LE[e]	60 + 7.5 mg/mL[a]	WY	6 mg/mL[a]	White haze in 24 hr at 22 °C	2352	I
Potassium chloride	AB	0.04 mEq/mL[c]	LZ	4 mg/mL[c]	Physically compatible for 24 hr at 21 °C	1032	C
Potassium phosphates	APP	0.12 mmol/mL[a]	WY	6 mg/mL[a]	Immediate white cloudiness	2352	I
Procainamide HCl	AHP	8 mg/mL[c]	LZ	4 mg/mL[c]	Physically compatible for 24 hr at 21 °C	1032	C
Sodium bicarbonate	AB	1 mEq/mL	WY	3 mg/mL[a]	Precipitate forms immediately	1851	I
	AB	1 mEq/mL	WY	6 mg/mL[a]	Translucent haze in 1 hr	2352	I
Sodium nitroprusside	BA	0.4 mg/mL[a]	WY	6 mg/mL[a]	Visually compatible for 24 hr at 22 °C	2352	C
	RC	0.3 mg/mL[a]	WAY	1.5 mg/mL[a]	Cloudy precipitate forms within 4 hr at 24 °C protected from light	2357	I
	RC	1.2 and 3 mg/mL[a]	WAY	1.5 mg/mL[a]	Cloudy precipitate forms immediately	2357	I
	RC	0.3 mg/mL[a]	WAY	6 and 15 mg/mL[a]	Visually compatible for 48 hr at 24 °C protected from light	2357	C
	RC	1.2 and 3 mg/mL[a]	WAY	6 and 15 mg/mL[a]	Cloudy precipitate forms immediately	2357	I
Sodium phosphates	APP	0.12 mmol/mL[a]	WY	6 mg/mL[a]	Immediate white cloudiness	2352	I
Tirofiban HCl	ME	0.25 mg/mL[a]	WY	6 mg/mL[a]	Visually compatible for 24 hr at 22 °C	2352	C
Tobramycin sulfate	LI	0.8 mg/mL[c]	LZ	4 mg/mL[c]	Physically compatible for 4 hr at room temperature	1444	C
	LI	5 mg/mL[a]	WY	6 mg/mL[a]	Visually compatible for 24 hr at 22 °C	2352	C
Vancomycin HCl	LI	5 mg/mL[c]	LZ	4 mg/mL[c]	Physically compatible for 4 hr at room temperature	1444	C
	APP	4 mg/mL[a]	WY	6 mg/mL[a]	Visually compatible for 24 hr at 22 °C	2352	C
	APP	10 mg/mL[a]	WY	6 mg/mL[a]	Visually compatible for 24 hr at 22 °C	2352	C
Vasopressin	AMR	0.2 unit/mL[b]	WY	6 mg/mL[a]	Visually compatible for 24 hr at 22 °C	2352	C
	AMR	2 and 4 units/mL[b]	WY	1.5 mg/mL[a]	Physically compatible with vasopressin pushed through a Y-site over 5 sec	2478	C
Vecuronium bromide	OR	1 mg/mL[a]	WY	6 mg/mL[a]	Visually compatible for 24 hr at 22 °C	2352	C

[a]Tested in dextrose 5%.
[b]Tested in sodium chloride 0.9%.
[c]Tested in both dextrose 5% and sodium chloride 0.9%.
[d]Given over three minutes via a Y-site into a running infusion solution of heparin sodium in sodium chloride 0.9%.
[e]Test performed using the formulation WITHOUT edetate disodium.
[f]Tested in Ringer's injection, lactated.

AMMONIUM CHLORIDE
AHFS 40:04

Products — Ammonium chloride additive solution is available in 20-mL vials containing 5.35 g of ammonium chloride, which provides 100 mEq (5 mEq/mL) of NH_4^+ and Cl^- ions. The solution also contains 2 mg/mL of disodium edetate as a stabilizer and hydrochloric acid to adjust the pH. The additive solution is intended to be used only after further dilution in a larger volume of sodium chloride 0.9% injection. (1)

One gram of ammonium chloride contains 18.7 mEq each of ammonium and chloride ions. (4)

pH — About 4.4 with a range of 4 to 6. (1)

Osmolarity — 10 mOsm/mL (calculated). (1)

Administration — Ammonium chloride injection is a concentrate that is generally administered by slow intravenous infusion after dilution of one or two vials (100 to 200 mEq) in 500 to 1000 mL of sodium chloride 0.9% injection. The infusion rate in adults of the diluted solution should not exceed 5 mL/min. (1)

Stability — Store at controlled room temperature and protect from freezing. Highly concentrated solutions of ammonium chloride may crystallize when exposed to low temperatures. If such crystallization does occur, warming to room temperature in a water bath is recommended. (1; 4)

Ammonium chloride is stated to be incompatible with alkalies and their carbonates. (4)

Compatibility Information

Solution Compatibility

Ammonium chloride

Solution	Mfr	Mfr	Conc/L	Remarks	Ref	C/I
Dextrose–Ringer's injection combinations	AB	AB	400 mEq	Physically compatible	3	C
Dextrose–Ringer's injection, lactated, combinations	AB	AB	400 mEq	Physically compatible	3	C
Dextrose–saline combinations	AB	AB	400 mEq	Physically compatible	3	C
Dextrose 2.5%	AB	AB	400 mEq	Physically compatible	3	C
Dextrose 5%	AB	AB	400 mEq	Physically compatible	3	C
Dextrose 10%	AB	AB	400 mEq	Physically compatible	3	C
Ionosol products	AB	AB	400 mEq	Physically compatible	3	C
Ringer's injection	AB	AB	400 mEq	Physically compatible	3	C
Ringer's injection, lactated	AB	AB	400 mEq	Physically compatible	3	C
Sodium chloride 0.45%	AB	AB	400 mEq	Physically compatible	3	C
Sodium chloride 0.9%	AB	AB	400 mEq	Physically compatible	3	C
Sodium lactate ⅙ M	AB	AB	400 mEq	Physically compatible	3	C

Additive Compatibility

Ammonium chloride

Drug	Mfr	Conc/L	Mfr	Conc/L	Test Soln	Remarks	Ref	C/I
Dimenhydrinate	SE	500 mg	AB	20 g	D5W	Physically compatible	15	C

Y-Site Injection Compatibility (1:1 Mixture)

Ammonium chloride

Drug	Mfr	Conc	Mfr	Conc	Remarks	Ref	C/I
Warfarin sodium	DU	0.1 mg/mL[a]	AB	5 mEq/mL	Subvisible haze forms immediately	2011	I
	DU	0.1 mg/mL[b]	AB	5 mEq/mL	Physically compatible for 24 hr at 23 °C	2011	C
	DU	2 mg/mL[c]	AB	5 mEq/mL	Immediate turbidity becoming a precipitate in 24 hr at 23 °C	2011	I

[a]*Tested in dextrose 5%.*
[b]*Tested in sodium chloride 0.9%.*
[c]*Tested in sterile water for injection.*

AMOXICILLIN SODIUM
AHFS 8:12.16.08

Products — Amoxicillin sodium is available in vials containing the equivalent of amoxicillin 250 mg, 500 mg, and 1 g. (38; 115)

For intramuscular injection, reconstitute the vials with the following volumes of sterile water for injection (38; 115):

Vial Size	Volume of Diluent	Final Volume
250 mg	1.5 mL	1.7 mL
250 mg	2.0 mL	2.2 mL
500 mg	2.0 mL	2.4 mL
500 mg	2.5 mL	2.9 mL
1 g	2.5 mL	3.3 mL
1 g	4.0 mL	4.8 mL

Alternatively, the 1-g vial may be reconstituted with lidocaine hydrochloride 1% or procaine hydrochloride 0.5%. However, a greater volume of local anesthetic is required to dissolve amoxicillin 1 g than sterile water for injection. Dividing a 1-g dose into two 500-mg portions given at different sites has been suggested. (38; 115)

For intravenous injection, reconstitute the vials with the following volumes of sterile water for injection (38):

Vial Size	Volume of Diluent	Final Volume
250 mg	5 mL	5.2 mL
500 mg	10 mL	10.4 mL
1 g	20 mL	20.8 mL

Alternatively, the 250-mg vials may be reconstituted with 4.8 mL of diluent to yield a 50-mg/mL solution. The 500-mg vials may be reconstituted with 4.6 mL of diluent to yield a 100-mg/mL solution. (115)

For intravenous infusion, the reconstituted drug may be added to an intravenous solution in a minibag or burette chamber of an administration set. (38)

Sodium Content — Amoxicillin sodium contains 3.3 mmol of sodium per gram of drug. (38)

Trade Name(s) — Amoxil, Clamoxyl, Ibiamox, many others.

Administration — Amoxicillin sodium may be administered by intramuscular injection, direct intravenous injection over three to four minutes, or intermittent intravenous infusion over 30 to 60 minutes. (38; 115)

Stability — Store amoxicillin sodium vials in a cool, dry place protected from light. (38; 115) After reconstitution with sterile water for injection, a transient pink color or slight opalescence may appear. Reconstituted solutions are normally a pale straw color. The reconstituted solution should be administered or diluted immediately in a suitable infusion solution. (38; 115)

Concentration Effects — Amoxicillin sodium 50 mg/mL is substantially less stable in all infusion solutions than at lower concentrations of 10 or 20 mg/mL. (1469)

Freezing Solutions — Amoxicillin sodium 10 mg/mL in sterile water for injection was unstable when stored frozen at between 0 and −20 °C but was stable for 13 days when stored below −30 °C. Amoxicillin sodium 10 mg/mL in sterile water for injection was stable for only two days at 0 °C in the unfrozen state. (1470)

Amoxicillin sodium 10 mg/mL in sodium chloride 0.9% was stable for 10.5 days at 0 °C (unfrozen) and for 14 hours when frozen at −19 °C; in dextrose 5%, the comparative times were 12.5 and 8.4 hours, respectively. (1471)

The processes of freezing and thawing increase the degradation rate of amoxicillin sodium 10 mg/mL in sodium chloride 0.9% in PVC bags (Travenol). Freezing and thawing (natural or microwave) could account for a 5 to 10% loss of amoxicillin; the losses will be affected by the time to reach the equilibrium frozen temperature. (1472)

Sorption — Acetazolamide sodium was shown not to exhibit sorption to PVC bags and tubing, polyethylene tubing, Silastic tubing, polypropylene syringes, and trilayer bags of polyethylene, polyamide, and polypropylene. (536; 606; 1918)

Filtration — Amoxicillin sodium 1.98 mg/mL in sodium chloride 0.9% did not exhibit significant drug loss due to sorption to a 0.22-μm cellulose ester membrane filter (Ivex-HP, Millipore). (1034)

Compatibility Information

Solution Compatibility

Amoxicillin sodium

Solution	Mfr	Mfr	Conc/L	Remarks	Ref	C/I
Dextrose 5%			1 g	9% loss in 4 hr and 34% loss in 24 hr at room temperature	768	I
			10, 20, 50 g	14 and 18% losses in 3 hr at 10 and 20 g/L, respectively, and 14% loss in 1.5 hr at 50 g/L at 25 °C	1469	I
Sodium chloride 0.9%			1 g	10% loss in 24 hr at room temperature	768	C
			10, 20, 50 g	3 and 7% losses in 6 hr at 10 and 20 g/L, respectively, and 12% loss in 4 hr at 50 g/L at 25 °C	1469	I
	TR		10 g	Less than 3% loss in 24 hr at 0 °C	1472	C
Sodium chloride 0.9% with potassium chloride 0.3%			10, 20, 50 g	4 and 9% losses in 8 hr at 10 and 20 g/L, respectively, and 9% loss in 3 hr at 50 g/L at 25 °C	1469	I
Sodium lactate ⅙ M			10, 20, 50 g	10% loss in 6 hr at 10 and 20 g/L and 14% loss in 4 hr at 50 g/L at 25 °C	1469	I

[a]Tested in PVC containers.

Additive Compatibility

Amoxicillin sodium

Drug	Mfr	Conc/L	Mfr	Conc/L	Test Soln	Remarks	Ref	C/I
Ciprofloxacin		2 g		10 g	[a]	Precipitates immediately	1473	I
Dextran 40		10%		10, 20, 50 g	D5W	9, 12, and 12% amoxicillin loss at 10, 20, and 50 g/L, respectively, in 1 hr at 25 °C	1469	I
		10%		10, 20, 50 g	NS	12, 14, and 20% amoxicillin loss at 10, 20, and 50 g/L, respectively, in 3 hr at 25 °C	1469	I
Imipenem–cilastatin sodium	GSK	4 g	MSD	8 g	NS	Blue discoloration formed in 2 hr. Amoxicillin and imipenem losses of 40 and 72%, respectively, in 12 hr	2800	I
Midazolam HCl	RC	50 and 250 mg	BE	10 g	NS	Transient precipitate	355	?
	RC	400 mg	BE	10 g	NS	Precipitate forms immediately	355	I
Pefloxacin		4 g		10 g	D5W, NS	Precipitate forms within 1 hr	1473	I
Sodium bicarbonate		2.74%		10, 20, 50 g		9% amoxicillin loss in 6 and 4 hr at 10 and 20 g/L, respectively, and 15% loss in 4 hr at 50 g/L at 25 °C	1469	I
		8.4%		10, 20, 50 g		10 and 13% amoxicillin loss in 4 hr at 10 and 20 g/L, respectively, and 17% loss in 3 hr at 50 g/L at 25 °C	1469	I

[a]Amoxicillin sodium added to ciprofloxacin solution.

Y-Site Injection Compatibility (1:1 Mixture)

Amoxicillin sodium

Drug	Mfr	Conc	Mfr	Conc	Remarks	Ref	C/I
Lorazepam	WY	0.33 mg/mL[a]	SKB	50 mg/mL	Visually compatible for 24 hr at 22 °C	1855	C
Midazolam HCl	RC	5 mg/mL	SKB	50 mg/mL	White precipitate forms immediately	1855	I
TPN #189[b]				50 mg/mL[a]	Visually compatible for 24 hr at 22 °C	1767	C

[a]Tested in sodium chloride 0.9%.
[b]Refer to Appendix I for the composition of parenteral nutrition solutions. TPN indicates a 2-in-1 admixture.

AMOXICILLIN SODIUM–CLAVULANATE
(CO-AMOXICLAV)
AHFS 8:12.16.08

Products — Amoxicillin sodium–clavulanic acid is available in 600-mg vials containing amoxicillin sodium 500 mg and clavulanic acid 100 mg as the potassium salt and in 1.2-g vials containing amoxicillin sodium 1 g and clavulanic acid 200 mg as the potassium salt. Reconstitute the 600-mg vials with 10 mL and the 1.2-g vials with 20 mL of sterile water for injection. (38; 115)

Sodium and Potassium Content — Amoxicillin sodium–clavulanic acid contains 3.1 mmol of sodium and 1 mmol of potassium in 1.2 g of drug product. The 600-mg vials contain 1.55 mmol of sodium and 0.5 mmol of potassium. (38)

Trade Name(s) — Augmentin, Clavulin, Flanamox.

Administration — Amoxicillin sodium–clavulanic acid may be administered by intravenous injection or intermittent infusion. It is not suitable for intramuscular administration. When given by intravenous injection directly into a vein or via a drip tube, it should be injected slowly over three to four minutes. For intravenous infusion, add the contents of the 600-mg or 1.2-g vial to 50 or 100 mL, respectively, of sterile water for injection or sodium chloride 0.9% and then infuse over 30 to 40 minutes, completing the administration within four hours of reconstitution. (38; 115)

Stability — Amoxicillin sodium–clavulanic acid in intact vials should be stored at 25 °C or below. The injection should be used within 20 minutes after reconstitution with sterile water for injection. (38; 115)

The manufacturer indicates that infusions of amoxicillin sodium–clavulanic acid in sterile water for injection or sodium chloride 0.9% are stable at 5 °C for up to eight hours. Amoxicillin sodium–clavulanic acid is less stable in dextrose, dextran, or bicarbonate-containing infusion solutions and should not be added to them. However, it may be injected into the tubing of running infusions of these solutions. (38; 115)

Amoxicillin sodium–clavulanic acid should not be added to infusion solutions containing dextrose, dextran, sodium bicarbonate, blood products, proteinaceous fluids, or intravenous fat emulsions. (38; 115)

The stability of amoxicillin sodium–clavulanic acid is governed by the more rapid degradation of clavulanic acid compared with amoxicillin. (1474)

Stability is also concentration dependent; amoxicillin sodium–clavulanic acid is less stable in high concentrations. Therefore, it is suggested that reconstituted solutions be used immediately or diluted without delay. (1474)

Freezing Solutions — Amoxicillin sodium–clavulanic acid 1.2 g reconstituted with 20 mL and diluted in 100 mL of sterile water for injection was frozen at −20 °C for four hours, followed by microwave thawing. Solutions retained only 65% of the initial clavulanic acid content. (1474)

Sorption — Amoxicillin sodium–clavulanic acid did not undergo sorption to PVC containers or administration tubing. (1474)

Compatibility Information

Solution Compatibility

Amoxicillin sodium–clavulanic acid

Solution	Mfr	Mfr	Conc/L	Remarks	Ref	C/I
Dextrose 5%	BT[a]	BE	8.33 + 1.67 g	Physically compatible with 10% loss within 30 min at 25 °C and 1.2 hr at 5 °C	1474	**I**
Ringer's injection	BT[a]	BE	8.33 + 1.67 g	Physically compatible with 10% loss in 4.1 hr at 25 °C	1474	**I**[b]
Ringer's injection, lactated	BT[a]	BE	8.33 + 1.67 g	Physically compatible with 10% loss in 4.1 hr	1474	**I**[b]
Sodium chloride 0.9%	BT[a]	BE	8.33 + 1.67 g	Physically compatible with 10% loss in 4.4 hr at 25 °C and 12.5 hr at 5 °C	1474	**I**[b]
Sodium chloride 0.9% with potassium chloride 0.3%	BT[a]	BE	8.33 + 1.67 g	Physically compatible with 10% loss in 3.9 hr at 25 °C	1474	**I**[b]
Sodium lactate ⅙ M	BT[a]	BE	8.33 + 1.67 g	Physically compatible with 10% loss in 4.3 hr at 25 °C	1474	**I**[b]

[a] Tested in polyethylene containers.
[b] Incompatible by conventional standards; may be used in shorter time periods.

Additive Compatibility

Amoxicillin sodium–clavulanic acid

Drug	Mfr	Conc/L	Mfr	Conc/L	Test Soln	Remarks	Ref	C/I
Ciprofloxacin		2 g		10 + 2 g	[a]	Precipitates immediately	1473	**I**
Metronidazole	BAY	5 g	BE	20 + 2 g		Physically compatible with 8% clavulanate loss in 2 hr and 25% loss in 6 hr at 21 °C. 7 to 8% amoxicillin and no metronidazole loss in 6 hr at 21 °C	1920	**I**
Pefloxacin		4 g		10 + 2 g	D5W, NS	Precipitate forms within 1 hr	1473	**I**

[a] Amoxicillin sodium–clavulanic acid added to ciprofloxacin solution.

Y-Site Injection Compatibility (1:1 Mixture)

Amoxicillin sodium–clavulanic acid

Drug	Mfr	Conc	Mfr	Conc	Remarks	Ref	C/I
Amiodarone HCl	SAN	12.5 mg/mL	GSK	10 + 2 mg/mL	Turbidity appeared immediately	2727	**I**
Clarithromycin	AB	4 mg/mL[a]	BE	20 + 4 mg/mL[a]	Visually compatible for 72 hr at both 30 and 17 °C	2174	**C**
Lorazepam	WY	0.33 mg/mL[b]	SKB	20 + 2 mg/mL	Visually compatible for 24 hr at 22 °C	1855	**C**
Midazolam HCl	RC	5 mg/mL	SKB	20 + 2 mg/mL	White precipitate forms immediately	1855	**I**

[a] Tested in dextrose 5%.
[b] Tested in sodium chloride 0.9%.

AMPHOTERICIN B
AHFS 8:14.28

Products — Amphotericin B is available in vials containing 50 mg of drug with sodium desoxycholate 41 mg and sodium phosphates 20.2 mg. Reconstitute with 10 mL of sterile water for injection without preservatives and shake until a clear colloidal dispersion is obtained. The resultant concentration is 5 mg/mL of amphotericin B. Use only sterile water for injection without preservatives for reconstitution because other diluents, such as sodium chloride 0.9% or solutions containing a bacteriostatic agent such as benzyl alcohol, may result in the precipitation of the antibiotic. For infusion, amphotericin B must be further diluted with dextrose 5% with a pH above 4.2. (1; 4)

Although various lipid complex and liposomal products of amphotericin B exist, they are sufficiently different from conventional amphotericin B formulations that extrapolating information to or from the other forms would be inappropriate.

pH — The pH of amphotericin B (Squibb) 100 mg/L in dextrose 5% has been reported as 5.7. (149)

Osmolality — The osmolality of amphotericin B (Squibb) 0.1 mg/mL in dextrose 5% was determined to be 256 mOsm/kg. (1375)

Administration — Amphotericin B is administered by slow intravenous infusion over approximately two to six hours. The recommended concentration of the infusion is 0.1 mg/mL. (1; 4) The drug has also been given intra-articularly, intrathecally, intrapleurally, and by irrigation. (4)

CAUTION: Care should be taken to ensure that the correct drug product, dose, and administration procedure are used and that no confusion with other products occurs.

Stability — Store intact vials at 2 to 8 °C and protect from light. (1; 4) The manufacturer indicates that a 5 to 10% potency loss occurs in one month at room temperature. (1433)

Amphotericin B reconstituted with sterile water for injection without preservatives and stored in the dark is stable for 24 hours at room temperature and for one week under refrigeration at 2 to 8 °C. (1; 4; 108) One report indicates that aqueous solutions may be stable for over a week at both 5 and 28 °C. (352)

Reconstituted amphotericin B may be added to dextrose 5% with a pH above 4.2. Buffers present in the formulation raise the pH of the admixture. If the dextrose 5% has a pH less than 4.2, additional buffer must be added. (1; 4) One or 2 mL of a buffer solution composed of dibasic sodium phosphate anhydrous 1.59 g and monobasic sodium phosphate anhydrous 0.96 g in water for injection is brought to 100 mL. The buffer solution should be sterilized either by filtration or by autoclaving for 30 minutes at 121 °C at 15 pounds pressure. (1) Failure to sterilize this buffer solution coupled with prolonged storage at room temperature has resulted in severe infection. (328)

Amphotericin B was reported to precipitate when added to some evacuated containers due to a small residual amount of fluid that may have acetic acid and sodium acetate buffer or sodium chloride 0.9% solution. Only evacuated containers with residual sterile water should be used for preparing amphotericin B admixtures. (1232)

In an effort to reduce toxicity, amphotericin B has been admixed in Intralipid instead of the more usual dextrose 5%. (1809; 1810; 1811; 2178) However, amphotericin B 0.75 mg/kg/day administered using this approach in 250 mL of Intralipid 20% has been associated with acute pulmonary toxicities, including sudden onset of coughing, tachypnea, cyanosis, and deterioration of oxygen saturation following administration. The temporal relationship between the drug administration and respiratory symptoms suggested a causal relationship. Furthermore, no reduction in renal toxicity or other side effects was observed. It was concluded amphotericin B should not be administered in Intralipid. (2177)

At a concentration of 0.6 mg/mL in Intralipid 10 or 20%, amphotericin B precipitates immediately or almost immediately. The precipitate is not visible to the unaided eye because of the emulsion's dense opacity. Particle size evaluation found thousands of particles larger than 10 μm per milliliter. In dextrose 5%, very few particles were larger than 10 μm. Centrifuging the Intralipid admixtures resulted in rapid visualization of the precipitate as a mass at the bottom of the test tubes. (1808)

However, amphotericin B precipitation is observed in fat emulsion within two to four hours without centrifuging. In concentrations ranging from 90 mg to 2 g/L in Intralipid 20%, amphotericin B precipitate is easily seen as yellow particulate matter on the bottom of the lipid emulsion containers. (1872; 1988) Damage to the emulsion integrity with creaming has also been reported. (1987)

In other reports, the appearance of problems was observed in as little as 15 minutes, and actual amphotericin B precipitate formed within 20 minutes of mixing. Analysis of the precipitate confirmed its identity as amphotericin B. The authors hypothesized that amphotericin B precipitates as a consequence of the excipient desoxycholic acid, which is an anion, attracting oppositely charged choline groups from the egg yolk components of the fat emulsion. As a consequence, desoxycholic acid and phosphatidylcholine form a precipitate and insufficient surfactant remains to keep the amphotericin B dispersed. (2204; 2205)

pH Effects — The pH range for optimum clarity and stability is 6 to 7. (148) At a pH of less than approximately 6, the colloidal dispersion may become turbid. (40; 148) Colloidal particles tend to coagulate rapidly at a pH of less than 5. (4)

Light Effects — Although the manufacturer recommends light protection for aqueous solutions of amphotericin B (1), several reports indicate that for short-term exposure of eight to 24 hours, little difference in potency is observed between light-protected and light-exposed solutions. (150; 335; 353) Longer exposure periods (150) or higher intensity light exposure (2414) may result in unacceptable potency losses, however.

Elastomeric Reservoir Pumps — Amphotericin B (Lyphomed) 0.25 mg/mL in dextrose 5% was evaluated for binding potential to natural rubber elastomeric reservoirs (Baxter). No binding was found after storage for two weeks at 35 °C with gentle agitation. (2014)

Filtration — Various studies have assessed the effects of filtration on the amphotericin B colloidal dispersion with differing results. The use of a 0.22-μm membrane filter was reported to be unacceptable with colloidal solutions adjusted to pH 4.7, 5.6, and 6.5. The concentration of amphotericin B in the filtrate decreased substantially after several hours. A 0.45-μm filter was satisfactory for infusions with a pH of 6.5, but the results at pH 5.6 were inconclusive. At pH 5.6 and 6.5, 1- and 5-μm filters both proved satisfactory in that they did not reduce the concentration of amphotericin B. For the turbid mixtures resulting at pH 4.7, however, all filters sharply reduced the concentration. (148) A report tended to support this finding for the 0.22-μm filter. At pH 5.7, fine particles of amphotericin B formed and were retained by the 0.22-μm filter. (149) No appreciable reduction in concentration with a 0.45-

μm filter was found; but with a 0.22-μm filter, after one hour the concentration of amphotericin B delivered was about 30% of the initial concentration. (152) When amphotericin B 50 mg/500 mL in dextrose 5% was filtered through a 0.22-μm circular cellulose ester membrane (Swinnex) or a 0.22-μm cylindrical cellulose ester filter (Ivex-2), the flow rate decreased dramatically after passage of as little as 30 mL. Flow ceased altogether after 100 to 200 mL. The last sample filtered contained no drug. With a 0.45-μm circular cellulose ester membrane (Swinnex), no loss of activity was determined after filtration of 200 mL.

However, the flow rate had decreased. (598) On the other hand, no significant difference in the amount or concentration of amphotericin B in dextrose 5% with phosphate buffer was found after filtration with 0.22-, 0.45-, and 5-μm filters. (151)

For amphotericin B infusions, only filters with a pore size not less than 1 μm should be used for filtration. (1; 4; 148) This would allow a margin for error that would compensate for possible variations in particle size. (148) Also, limiting the use of filtration to situations where it is believed to be necessary has been recommended. (598; 599)

Compatibility Information

Solution Compatibility

Amphotericin B

Solution	Mfr	Mfr	Conc/L	Remarks	Ref	C/I
Amino acids 4.25%, dextrose 25%	MG	SQ	100 mg	Turbidity and fine yellow particles form	349	I
Dextrose 5% in Ringer's injection, lactated	MG[a]	SQ	100 mg	Precipitate forms in 30 min. About 50% remains in 30 min	539	I
Dextrose 5% in sodium chloride 0.9%	MG[a]	SQ	100 mg	Precipitate forms within 2 hr. 30 to 70% remains in 2 hr	539	I
Dextrose 5%		SQ	70 and 140 mg	Bioactivity not affected over 24 hr at 25 °C in light or dark	335	C
	MG[a]	SQ	100 mg	Physically compatible. Concentration unchanged in 48 hr	539	C
		SQ	50 and 100 mg	No loss of bioactivity in normal light at 25 °C for 24 hr	540	C
	MG[b]	SQ	0.9, 1.2, 1.4 g	Physically compatible with little loss in 36 hr at 6 and 25 °C	1434	C
	MG[b]	SQ	470, 660, 750 mg	Visually compatible with no loss in 24 hr at 25 °C	1537	C
	BA[c]	SQ	100 mg	Visually compatible with no loss in 24 hr at 15 to 25 °C	1544	C
	BA[c]	SQ	100 and 250 mg	Visually compatible with 4% loss in 35 days at 4 °C in dark	1546	C
	BA[c]	SQ	0.2, 0.5, 1 g	Visually compatible. Little loss in 5 days at 4 and 25 °C. Normal turbidity observed at 1 g/L	1728	C
	AB[c]	BMS	50 mg	Visually compatible. No loss protected from light and 5% loss exposed to fluorescent light in 24 hr at 24 °C	2093	C
	AB[c]	BMS	500 mg	Visually compatible. No loss protected from or exposed to fluorescent light in 24 hr at 24 °C	2093	C
			50, 100, 150 mg	Visually compatible with less than 5% loss in 24 hr at 4 and 25 °C when protected from light	2414	C
Dextrose 10%	BA[c]	SQ	100 mg	Visually compatible with no loss in 24 hr at 15 to 25 °C	1544	C
Dextrose 20%	BA[c]	SQ	100 mg	Visually compatible with no loss in 24 hr at 15 to 25 °C	1544	C
Ringer's injection, lactated	MG[a]	SQ	100 mg	Precipitate forms within 2 hr. 80% remains in 2 hr	539	I
Sodium chloride 0.9%	AB	SQ	100 mg	Physically incompatible	15	I
	MG[a]	SQ	100 mg	Precipitate forms within 2 hr. 43% remains in 2 hr	539	I

[a]Tested in both glass and polyolefin containers.
[b]Tested in polyolefin containers.
[c]Tested in PVC containers.

Additive Compatibility

Amphotericin B

Drug	Mfr	Conc/L	Mfr	Conc/L	Test Soln	Remarks	Ref	C/I
Amikacin sulfate	BR	5 g	SQ	100 mg	D5LR, D5R, D5S, D5W, D10W, LR, NS, R, SL	Precipitates immediately	293	I
Calcium chloride	BP	4 g		200 mg	D5W	Haze develops over 3 hr	26	I
Calcium gluconate	BP	4 g		200 mg	D5W	Haze develops over 3 hr	26	I
Chlorpromazine HCl	BP	200 mg		200 mg	D5W	Precipitates immediately	26	I
Ciprofloxacin	MI	2 g		100 mg	D5W	Physically incompatible	888	I
	BAY	2 g	APC	100 mg	D5W	Precipitates immediately	2413	I
Diphenhydramine HCl	PD	80 mg	SQ	100 mg	D5W	Physically incompatible	15	I
Dopamine HCl	AS	800 mg	SQ	200 mg	D5W	Precipitates immediately	78	I
Edetate calcium disodium	RI	4 g		200 mg	D5W	Haze develops over 3 hr	26	I
Fat emulsion, intravenous	CL	10 and 20%	APC, PHT	0.6 g		Precipitate forms immediately but is concealed by opaque emulsion	1808	I
		20%		90 mg		Yellow precipitate forms in 2 hr. Cumulative delivery of only 56% of total amphotericin B dose	1872	I
	CL	20%	APC	10, 50, 100, 500 mg, 1 and 5 g		Emulsion separation occurred rapidly with visible creaming within 4 hr at 27 and 8 °C	1987	I
	KA	20%	SQ	500 mg, 1 and 2 g		Precipitated amphotericin noted on bottom of containers within 4 hr	1988	I
	CL[b]	20%	BMS	50 and 500 mg		Fat emulsion separates into two phases within 8 hr. Little loss protected from or exposed to fluorescent light in 24 hr at 24 °C	2093	I
	KP	20%	BMS	1 and 3 g		Precipitate forms immediately	2518	I
	KP	20%	BMS	150 mg, 300 mg, 1.5 g	D5W[c]	Precipitate forms immediately	2518	I
Fluconazole	PF	1 g	LY	50 mg	D5W	Visually compatible with no fluconazole loss in 72 hr at 25 °C. Amphotericin B not tested	1677	C
Gentamicin sulfate		320 mg		200 mg	D5W	Haze develops over 3 hr	26	I
Heparin sodium	UP	4000 units	SQ	100 mg	D5W	Physically compatible	15	C
	AB	4000 units	SQ	100 mg	D	Physically compatible	21	C
		2000 units	SQ	70 and 140 mg	D5W	Bioactivity not affected over 24 hr at 25 °C	335	C
Hydrocortisone sodium succinate	UP	500 mg	SQ	100 mg	D5W	Physically compatible	15	C
		50 mg	SQ	70 and 140 mg	D5W	Bioactivity not significantly affected over 24 hr at 25 °C	335	C
Magnesium sulfate	IMS	2 and 4 g	SQ	40 and 80 mg	D5W	Physically incompatible in 3 hr at 24 °C with decreased clarity and development of supernatant	1578	I

Additive Compatibility (Cont.)

Amphotericin B

Drug	Mfr	Conc/L	Mfr	Conc/L	Test Soln	Remarks	Ref	C/I
Meropenem	ZEN	1 and 20 g	SQ	200 mg	NS	Precipitate forms	2068	I
Methyldopate HCl		1 g		200 mg	D5W	Haze develops over 3 hr	26	I
Penicillin G potassium	SQ	20 million units	SQ	100 mg	D5W	Physically incompatible	15	I
	SQ	5 million units	SQ	50 mg		Precipitate forms within 1 hr	47	I
	BP	10 million units		200 mg	D5W	Haze develops over 3 hr	26	I
Penicillin G sodium	UP	20 million units	SQ	100 mg	D5W	Physically incompatible	15	I
	BP	10 million units		200 mg	D5W	Haze develops over 3 hr	26	I
Polymyxin B sulfate	BP	20 mg		200 mg	D5W	Haze develops over 3 hr	26	I
Potassium chloride	AB	100 mEq	SQ	100 mg	D5W	Physically incompatible	15	I
	BP	4 g		200 mg	D5W	Haze develops over 3 hr	26	I
Prochlorperazine mesylate	BP	100 mg		200 mg	D5W	Haze develops over 3 hr	26	I
Ranitidine HCl	GL	100 mg	SQ	200 mg	D5W	Color change and particle formation	1151	I
Sodium bicarbonate	AB	2.4 mEq[a]	SQ	50 mg	D5W	Physically compatible for 24 hr	772	C
Streptomycin sulfate	BP	4 g		200 mg	D5W	Haze develops over 3 hr	26	I
Verapamil HCl	KN	80 mg	SQ	100 mg	D5W	Physically incompatible after 8 hr	764	I
	KN	80 mg	SQ	100 mg	NS	Immediate physical incompatibility	764	I

[a] *One vial of Neut added to a liter of admixture.*
[b] *Tested in glass containers.*
[c] *Diluted in dextrose 5% before adding to the fat emulsion.*

Drugs in Syringe Compatibility

Amphotericin B

Drug (in syringe)	Mfr	Amt	Mfr	Amt	Remarks	Ref	C/I
Heparin sodium		2500 units/ 1 mL		50 mg	Physically compatible for at least 5 min	1053	C
Pantoprazole sodium	a	4 mg/ 1 mL		5 mg/ 1 mL	Opacity within 1 hr	2574	I

[a] *Test performed using the formulation WITHOUT edetate disodium.*

Y-Site Injection Compatibility (1:1 Mixture)

Amphotericin B

Drug	Mfr	Conc	Mfr	Conc	Remarks	Ref	C/I
Aldesleukin	CHI	33,800 I.U./mL[a]	SQ	1.6 mg/mL[a]	Visually compatible for 2 hr	1857	C
Allopurinol sodium	BW	3 mg/mL[a]	SQ	0.6 mg/mL[a]	Amphotericin B haze lost immediately	1686	I
Amifostine	USB	10 mg/mL[a]	AD	0.6 mg/mL[a]	Turbidity forms immediately	1845	I
Amiodarone HCl	WY	6 mg/mL[a]	BMS	0.5 mg/mL[a]	Visually compatible for 24 hr at 22 °C	2352	C
Amsacrine	NCI	1 mg/mL[a]	SQ	0.6 mg/mL[a]	Immediate yellow turbidity, becoming yellow flocculent precipitate in 15 min	1381	I
Anidulafungin	VIC	0.5 mg/mL[a]	PHT	0.6 mg/mL[a]	Measured haze went up immediately	2617	I
Aztreonam	SQ	40 mg/mL[a]	PHT	0.6 mg/mL[a]	Yellow turbidity forms immediately and becomes flocculent precipitate in 4 hr	1758	I
Bivalirudin	TMC	5 mg/mL[a]	APO	0.6 mg/mL[a]	Yellow precipitate forms immediately	2373	I
Caspofungin acetate	ME	0.7 mg/mL[b]	XGN	0.6 mg/mL[a]	Immediate yellow turbid precipitate forms	2758	I
Ceftaroline fosamil	FOR	2.22 mg/mL[a,b,c]	XGN	0.6 mg/mL[a]	Increased haze and microparticulates	2826	I
Cisatracurium besylate	GW	0.1 mg/mL[a]	PH	0.6 mg/mL[a]	Physically compatible for 4 hr at 23 °C	2074	C
	GW	2 mg/mL[a]	PH	0.6 mg/mL[a]	Cloudiness forms immediately; gel-like precipitate forms in 1 hr	2074	I
	GW	5 mg/mL[a]	PH	0.6 mg/mL[a]	Turbidity forms immediately	2074	I
Dexmedetomidine HCl	AB	4 mcg/mL[b]	APO	0.6 mg/mL[a]	Yellow precipitate forms immediately	2383	I
Diltiazem HCl	MMD	5 mg/mL	SQ	0.1 mg/mL[a]	Visually compatible	1807	C
Docetaxel	RPR	0.9 mg/mL[a]	PH	0.6 mg/mL[a]	Visible turbidity forms immediately	2224	I
Doripenem	JJ	5 mg/mL[a]	XGN	0.6 mg/mL[a]	Physically compatible for 4 hr at 23 °C	2743	C
	JJ	5 mg/mL[b]	XGN	0.6 mg/mL[a]	Yellow precipitate forms immediately	2743	I
Doxorubicin HCl liposomal	SEQ	0.4 mg/mL[a]	APC	0.6 mg/mL[a]	Fivefold increase in measured particulates in 4 hr	2087	I
Enalaprilat	MSD	1.25 mg/mL	SQ	0.1 mg/mL[a]	Layered haze develops in 4 hr at 21 °C	1409	I
Etoposide phosphate	BR	5 mg/mL[a]	GNS	0.6 mg/mL[a]	Yellow-orange precipitate forms immediately	2218	I
Fenoldopam mesylate	AB	80 mcg/mL[b]	APO	0.6 mg/mL[b]	Yellow precipitate forms immediately	2467	I
Filgrastim	AMG	30 mcg/mL[a]	SQ	0.6 mg/mL[a]	Yellow turbidity and precipitate form	1687	I
Fluconazole	RR	2 mg/mL	SQ	5 mg/mL	Cloudiness and yellow precipitate	1407	I
Fludarabine phosphate	BX	1 mg/mL[a]	SQ	0.6 mg/mL[a]	Precipitate forms in 4 hr at 22 °C	1439	I
Foscarnet sodium	AST	24 mg/mL	SQ	5 mg/mL	Cloudy yellow precipitate forms	1335	I
	AST	24 mg/mL	SQ	0.6 mg/mL[a]	Dense haze forms immediately	1393	I
Gemcitabine HCl	LI	10 mg/mL[b]	PH	0.6 mg/mL[a]	Gross precipitation occurs immediately	2226	I
Granisetron HCl	SKB	0.05 mg/mL[a]	PH	0.6 mg/mL[a]	Large increase in measured turbidity occurs immediately	2000	I
Heparin sodium	SO	100 units/mL[b]	SQ	0.1 mg/mL[a]	Turbidity forms in 45 min	1435	I
Hetastarch in lactated electrolyte	AB	6%	APC	0.6 mg/mL[a]	Immediate gross precipitation	2339	I
Linezolid	PHU	2 mg/mL	AB	0.6 mg/mL[a]	Yellow precipitate forms within 5 min	2264	I
Melphalan HCl	BW	0.1 mg/mL[b]	SQ	0.6 mg/mL[a]	Immediate increase in measured turbidity	1557	I
	BW	0.1 mg/mL[a]	SQ	0.6 mg/mL[a]	Physically compatible but rapid melphalan loss in D5W precludes use	1557	I

Y-Site Injection Compatibility (1:1 Mixture) (Cont.)

Amphotericin B

Drug	Mfr	Conc	Mfr	Conc	Remarks	Ref	C/I
Meropenem	ZEN	1 and 50 mg/mL[b]	SQ	5 mg/mL	Precipitate forms	2068	I
Ondansetron HCl	GL	1 mg/mL[a]	SQ	0.6 mg/mL[a]	Immediate yellow turbid precipitation	1365	I
Paclitaxel	NCI	1.2 mg/mL[a]	SQ	0.6 mg/mL[a]	Immediate increase in measured turbidity followed by separation into two layers in 24 hr at 22 °C	1556	I
Pemetrexed disodium	LI	20 mg/mL[b]	PHT	0.6 mg/mL[a]	Yellow precipitate forms immediately	2564	I
Piperacillin sodium–tazobactam sodium	LE[h]	40 + 5 mg/mL[a]	SQ	0.6 mg/mL[a]	Yellow precipitate forms immediately	1688	I
Propofol	ZEN	10 mg/mL	APC	0.6 mg/mL[a]	Gel-like precipitate forms immediately	2066	I
Remifentanil HCl	GW	0.025 mg/mL[a]	PHT	0.6 mg/mL[a]	Physically compatible for 4 hr at 23 °C	2075	C
	GW	0.25 mg/mL[a]	PHT	0.6 mg/mL[a]	Yellow precipitate forms immediately	2075	I
Sargramostim	IMM	10 mcg/mL[a]	SQ	0.6 mg/mL[a]	Visually compatible for 4 hr at 22 °C	1436	C
	IMM	10 mcg/mL[b]	SQ	0.6 mg/mL[b]	Yellow precipitate forms immediately	1436	I
Tacrolimus	FUJ	1 mg/mL[d]	LY	5 mg/mL[a]	Visually compatible for 24 hr at 25 °C	1630	C
Telavancin HCl	ASP	7.5 mg/mL[a]	XGN	0.1 mg/mL[a]	Increase in measured turbidity	2830	I
Teniposide	BR	0.1 mg/mL[a]	SQ	0.6 mg/mL[a]	Physically compatible for 4 hr at 23 °C	1725	C
Thiotepa	IMM[e]	1 mg/mL[a]	APC	0.6 mg/mL[a]	Physically compatible for 4 hr at 23 °C	1861	C
Tigecycline	WY	1 mg/mL[b]		2 mg/mL[a]	Immediate cloudiness with particulates in 1 hr	2714	I
TNA #218 to #226[g]			PH	0.6 mg/mL[a]	Yellow precipitate forms immediately	2215	I
TPN #212 to #215[g]			PH	0.6 mg/mL[a]	Precipitate forms immediately	2109	I
Vinorelbine tartrate	BW	1 mg/mL[b]	SQ	0.6 mg/mL[f]	Yellow precipitate forms immediately	1558	I
Zidovudine	BW	4 mg/mL[a]	SQ	600 mcg/mL[a]	Physically compatible for 4 hr at 25 °C	1193	C

[a] Tested in dextrose 5%.
[b] Tested in sodium chloride 0.9%.
[c] Tested in dextrose 5%, Ringer's injection, lactated.
[d] Tested in sterile water.
[e] Lyophilized formulation tested.
[f] Tested in both dextrose 5% and sodium chloride 0.9%.
[g] Refer to Appendix I for the composition of parenteral nutrition solutions. TNA indicates a 3-in-1 admixture, and TPN indicates a 2-in-1 admixture.
[h] Test performed using the formulation WITHOUT edetate disodium.

AMPHOTERICIN B CHOLESTERYL SULFATE COMPLEX
AHFS 8:14.28

Products — Amphotericin B cholesteryl sulfate complex is available as a lyophilized powder in 50- and 100-mg vials. The product consists of a 1:1 molar ratio complex of amphotericin B and cholesteryl sulfate along with tromethamine, disodium edetate dihydrate, lactose monohydrate, and sodium hydroxide to adjust pH. (1)

Amphotericin B cholesteryl sulfate complex should be reconstituted with sterile water for injection to form a colloidal dispersion of microscopic, disc-shaped particles. Add 10 mL to the 50-mg vial and 20 mL to the 100-mg vial. Shake gently and rotate the vial until all of the solid material has dissolved. Reconstitution as directed yields opalescent or clear colloidal dispersions containing amphotericin B 5 mg/mL as the cholesteryl sulfate complex. (1)

Amphotericin B cholesteryl sulfate complex must not be reconstituted with sodium chloride or dextrose solutions or mixed with solutions containing sodium chloride or other electrolytes. Furthermore, solutions containing a bacteriostatic agent such as benzyl alcohol should be avoided. Use of any solution other than those recommended may cause precipitate formation. (1)

Although other lipid complex and liposomal amphotericin B products exist, they are sufficiently different from amphotericin B cholesteryl sulfate complex that extrapolating compatibility data to or from other forms would be inappropriate.

Trade Name(s) — Amphotec.

Administration — Amphotericin B cholesteryl sulfate complex is administered intravenously only after dilution in dextrose 5% to a concentration of approximately 0.6 mg/mL (range 0.16 to 0.83 mg/mL). A test dose of 10 mL of the final admixed solution containing 1.6 to 8.3 mg of drug given over 15 to 30 minutes immediately preceding each new course of treatment is recommended. The patient should be observed for the next 30 minutes. Intravenous infusion of the diluted solution is performed at a rate of 1 mg/kg/hr. The infusion time may be shortened to a minimum of two hours for patients who exhibit no evidence of intolerance or reactions. The infusion time may need to be extended for patients who experience reactions or cannot tolerate the fluid volume. (1)

The manufacturer also recommends separating administration from other drugs given through intravenous lines by using a sufficient flush of the line with dextrose 5% to avoid contact. Flushes both before and after administering amphotericin B cholesteryl sulfate complex would be required to avoid inadvertent mixing with other drugs in line. (1)

The functional properties of a drug incorporated into a lipid complex like this one may differ substantially from the functional properties of the original formulation and alternative formulations, including other lipid complexes or liposome formulations. (1) **CAUTION: Care should be taken to ensure that the correct drug product, dose, and administration procedure are used and that no confusion with other products occurs.**

Stability — Intact vials of amphotericin B cholesteryl sulfate complex should be stored at 15 to 30 °C. After reconstitution, the colloidal dispersion should be stored at 2 to 8 °C, protected from freezing, and used within 24 hours. Partial vials should be discarded. (1)

The reconstituted colloidal dispersion diluted to a concentration of 0.16 to 0.83 mg/mL in dextrose 5% should be stored at 2 to 8 °C and used within 24 hours. (1)

Filtration — Amphotericin B cholesteryl sulfate complex is a colloidal dispersion; filtration, including inline filtration, should not be performed. (1)

Compatibility Information

Solution Compatibility

Amphotericin B cholesteryl sulfate complex

Solution	Mfr	Mfr	Conc/L	Remarks	Ref	C/I
Dextrose 5%	BA	SEQ	415 mg	Physically compatible for 4 hr at 23 °C	2117	C
	BA[a]	SEQ	2 g and 100 mg	Stable for 7 days at 4 and 23 °C protected from light. Visible changes and unacceptable microparticulates form after that time. Drug loss due to precipitation	2237	C
Sodium chloride 0.9%	BA	SEQ	415 mg	Microprecipitation occurs immediately	2117	I

[a]*Tested in PVC containers.*

Y-Site Injection Compatibility (1:1 Mixture)

Amphotericin B cholesteryl sulfate complex

Drug	Mfr	Conc	Mfr	Conc	Remarks	Ref	C/I
Acyclovir sodium	GW	7 mg/mL[a]	SEQ	0.83 mg/mL[a]	Physically compatible for 4 hr at 23 °C	2117	C
Alfentanil HCl	JN	0.5 mg/mL	SEQ	0.83 mg/mL[a]	Gross precipitate forms	2117	I
Amikacin sulfate	AB	5 mg/mL[a]	SEQ	0.83 mg/mL[a]	Gross precipitate forms	2117	I
Aminophylline	AB	2.5 mg/mL[a]	SEQ	0.83 mg/mL[a]	Physically compatible for 4 hr at 23 °C	2117	C
Ampicillin sodium	SKB	20 mg/mL[b]	SEQ	0.83 mg/mL[a]	Gross precipitate forms	2117	I
Ampicillin sodium–sulbactam sodium	RR	20 + 10 mg/mL[b]	SEQ	0.83 mg/mL[a]	Gross precipitate forms	2117	I
Aztreonam	SQ	40 mg/mL[a]	SEQ	0.83 mg/mL[a]	Gross precipitate forms	2117	I
Buprenorphine HCl	RKC	0.04 mg/mL[a]	SEQ	0.83 mg/mL[a]	Microprecipitate forms in 4 hr at 23 °C	2117	I
Butorphanol tartrate	APC	0.04 mg/mL[a]	SEQ	0.83 mg/mL[a]	Decreased natural turbidity occurs	2117	I
Calcium chloride	AST	40 mg/mL[a]	SEQ	0.83 mg/mL[a]	Gross precipitate forms	2117	I

Y-Site Injection Compatibility (1:1 Mixture) (Cont.)

Amphotericin B cholesteryl sulfate complex

Drug	Mfr	Conc	Mfr	Conc	Remarks	Ref	C/I
Calcium gluconate	AB	40 mg/mL[a]	SEQ	0.83 mg/mL[a]	Gross precipitate forms	2117	I
Carboplatin	BR	5 mg/mL[a]	SEQ	0.83 mg/mL[a]	Increased turbidity forms immediately	2117	I
Cefazolin sodium	SKB	20 mg/mL[a]	SEQ	0.83 mg/mL[a]	Increased turbidity forms immediately	2117	I
Cefepime HCl	BMS	20 mg/mL[a]	SEQ	0.83 mg/mL[a]	Gross precipitate forms	2117	I
Cefoxitin sodium	ME	20 mg/mL[a]	SEQ	0.83 mg/mL[a]	Physically compatible for 4 hr at 23 °C	2117	C
Ceftazidime	SKB	40 mg/mL[a]	SEQ	0.83 mg/mL[a]	Increased turbidity forms in 4 hr at 23 °C	2117	I
Ceftriaxone sodium	RC	20 mg/mL[a]	SEQ	0.83 mg/mL[a]	Decreased natural turbidity occurs	2117	I
Chlorpromazine HCl	ES	2 mg/mL[a]	SEQ	0.83 mg/mL[a]	Gross precipitate forms	2117	I
Cisatracurium besylate	GW	2 mg/mL[a]	SEQ	0.83 mg/mL[a]	Gross precipitate forms	2117	I
Cisplatin	BR	1 mg/mL	SEQ	0.83 mg/mL[a]	Gross precipitate forms	2117	I
Clindamycin phosphate	UP	10 mg/mL[a]	SEQ	0.83 mg/mL[a]	Physically compatible for 4 hr at 23 °C	2117	C
Cyclophosphamide	MJ	10 mg/mL[a]	SEQ	0.83 mg/mL[a]	Increased turbidity forms immediately	2117	I
Cyclosporine	SZ	5 mg/mL[a]	SEQ	0.83 mg/mL[a]	Decreased natural turbidity occurs	2117	I
Cytarabine	BED	50 mg/mL	SEQ	0.83 mg/mL[a]	Physically compatible for 4 hr at 23 °C	2117	C
Dexamethasone sodium phosphate	ES	2 mg/mL[a]	SEQ	0.83 mg/mL[a]	Physically compatible for 4 hr at 23 °C	2117	C
Diazepam	SW	5 mg/mL	SEQ	0.83 mg/mL[a]	Gross precipitate forms	2117	I
Digoxin	WY	0.25 mg/mL	SEQ	0.83 mg/mL[a]	Microprecipitate forms in 4 hr at 23 °C	2117	I
Diphenhydramine HCl	SCN	2 mg/mL[a]	SEQ	0.83 mg/mL[a]	Microprecipitate and increased turbidity form immediately	2117	I
Dobutamine HCl	AST	4 mg/mL[a]	SEQ	0.83 mg/mL[a]	Gross precipitate forms	2117	I
Dopamine HCl	AB	3.2 mg/mL[a]	SEQ	0.83 mg/mL[a]	Gross precipitate forms	2117	I
Doripenem	JJ	5 mg/mL[a]	INT	0.83 mg/mL[a]	Physically compatible for 4 hr at 23 °C	2743	C
	JJ	5 mg/mL[b]	INT	0.83 mg/mL[a]	Microprecipitate forms	2743	I
Doxorubicin HCl	CHI	2 mg/mL	SEQ	0.83 mg/mL[a]	Gross precipitate forms	2117	I
Doxorubicin HCl liposomal	SEQ	2 mg/mL	SEQ	0.83 mg/mL[a]	Gross precipitate forms	2117	I
Droperidol	AST	2.5 mg/mL	SEQ	0.83 mg/mL[a]	Gross precipitate forms	2117	I
Enalaprilat	ME	0.1 mg/mL[a]	SEQ	0.83 mg/mL[a]	Decreased natural turbidity occurs	2117	I
Esmolol HCl	OHM	10 mg/mL[a]	SEQ	0.83 mg/mL[a]	Microprecipitate forms in 4 hr at 23 °C	2117	I
Famotidine	ME	2 mg/mL[a]	SEQ	0.83 mg/mL[a]	Microprecipitate and increased turbidity form immediately	2117	I
Fentanyl citrate	AB	0.05 mg/mL	SEQ	0.83 mg/mL[a]	Physically compatible for 4 hr at 23 °C	2117	C
Fluconazole	RR	2 mg/mL	SEQ	0.83 mg/mL[a]	Gross precipitate forms	2117	I
Fluorouracil	PH	16 mg/mL[a]	SEQ	0.83 mg/mL[a]	Microprecipitate forms immediately	2117	I
Furosemide	AMR	3 mg/mL[a]	SEQ	0.83 mg/mL[a]	Physically compatible for 4 hr at 23 °C	2117	C
Ganciclovir sodium	RC	20 mg/mL[a]	SEQ	0.83 mg/mL[a]	Physically compatible for 4 hr at 23 °C	2117	C
Gentamicin sulfate	FUJ	5 mg/mL[a]	SEQ	0.83 mg/mL[a]	Gross precipitate forms	2117	I
Granisetron HCl	SKB	0.05 mg/mL[a]	SEQ	0.83 mg/mL[a]	Physically compatible for 4 hr at 23 °C	2117	C
Haloperidol lactate	MN	0.2 mg/mL[a]	SEQ	0.83 mg/mL[a]	Gross precipitate forms	2117	I
Heparin sodium	WY	1000 units/mL[a]	SEQ	0.83 mg/mL[a]	Gross precipitate forms	2117	I

Y-Site Injection Compatibility (1:1 Mixture) (Cont.)

Amphotericin B cholesteryl sulfate complex

Drug	Mfr	Conc	Mfr	Conc	Remarks	Ref	C/I
Hydrocortisone sodium succinate	AB	1 mg/mL[a]	SEQ	0.83 mg/mL[a]	Physically compatible for 4 hr at 23 °C	2117	C
Hydromorphone HCl	ES	0.5 mg/mL[a]	SEQ	0.83 mg/mL[a]	Decreased natural turbidity occurs	2117	I
Hydroxyzine HCl	ES	2 mg/mL[a]	SEQ	0.83 mg/mL[a]	Gross precipitate forms	2117	I
Ifosfamide	MJ	25 mg/mL[a]	SEQ	0.83 mg/mL[a]	Physically compatible for 4 hr at 23 °C	2117	C
Imipenem–cilastatin sodium	ME	10 mg/mL[b]	SEQ	0.83 mg/mL[a]	Gross precipitate forms	2117	I
Labetalol HCl	AH	5 mg/mL	SEQ	0.83 mg/mL[a]	Gross precipitate forms	2117	I
Leucovorin calcium	IMM	2 mg/mL[a]	SEQ	0.83 mg/mL[a]	Gross precipitate forms	2117	I
Lidocaine HCl	AST	10 mg/mL	SEQ	0.83 mg/mL[a]	Gross precipitate forms	2117	I
Lorazepam	WY	0.1 mg/mL[a]	SEQ	0.83 mg/mL[a]	Physically compatible for 4 hr at 23 °C	2117	C
Magnesium sulfate	AST	100 mg/mL[a]	SEQ	0.83 mg/mL[a]	Gross precipitate forms	2117	I
Mannitol	BA	15%	SEQ	0.83 mg/mL[a]	Physically compatible for 4 hr at 23 °C	2117	C
Meperidine HCl	AST	4 mg/mL[a]	SEQ	0.83 mg/mL[a]	Increased turbidity forms immediately	2117	I
Mesna	MJ	10 mg/mL[a]	SEQ	0.83 mg/mL[a]	Microprecipitate forms immediately	2117	I
Methotrexate sodium	IMM	15 mg/mL[a]	SEQ	0.83 mg/mL[a]	Physically compatible for 4 hr at 23 °C	2117	C
Methylprednisolone sodium succinate	PHU	5 mg/mL[a]	SEQ	0.83 mg/mL[a]	Physically compatible for 4 hr at 23 °C	2117	C
Metoclopramide HCl	FAU	5 mg/mL	SEQ	0.83 mg/mL[a]	Gross precipitate forms	2117	I
Metoprolol tartrate	GEM	1 mg/mL	SEQ	0.83 mg/mL[a]	Gross precipitate forms	2117	I
Metronidazole	AB	5 mg/mL	SEQ	0.83 mg/mL[a]	Gross precipitate forms	2117	I
Midazolam HCl	RC	2 mg/mL[a]	SEQ	0.83 mg/mL[a]	Gross precipitate forms	2117	I
Mitoxantrone HCl	IMM	0.5 mg/mL[a]	SEQ	0.83 mg/mL[a]	Gross precipitate forms	2117	I
Morphine sulfate	ES	1 mg/mL[a]	SEQ	0.83 mg/mL[a]	Increased turbidity forms immediately	2117	I
Nalbuphine HCl	AST	10 mg/mL	SEQ	0.83 mg/mL[a]	Gross precipitate forms	2117	I
Naloxone HCl	AST	0.4 mg/mL	SEQ	0.83 mg/mL[a]	Gross precipitate forms	2117	I
Nitroglycerin	AMR	0.4 mg/mL[a]	SEQ	0.83 mg/mL[a]	Physically compatible for 4 hr at 23 °C	2117	C
Ondansetron HCl	CER	1 mg/mL[a]	SEQ	0.83 mg/mL[a]	Gross precipitate forms	2117	I
Paclitaxel	MJ	0.6 mg/mL[a]	SEQ	0.83 mg/mL[a]	Decreased natural turbidity occurs	2117	I
Pentobarbital sodium	AB	5 mg/mL[a]	SEQ	0.83 mg/mL[a]	Decreased natural turbidity occurs	2117	I
Phenobarbital sodium	WY	5 mg/mL[a]	SEQ	0.83 mg/mL[a]	Increased turbidity forms immediately	2117	I
Phenytoin sodium	ES	50 mg/mL[a]	SEQ	0.83 mg/mL[a]	Gross precipitate forms	2117	I
Piperacillin sodium–tazobactam sodium	CY[c]	40 + 5 mg/mL[a]	SEQ	0.83 mg/mL[a]	Microprecipitate forms immediately	2117	I
Potassium chloride	AB	0.1 mEq/mL[a]	SEQ	0.83 mg/mL[a]	Gross precipitate forms	2117	I
Prochlorperazine edisylate	SKB	0.5 mg/mL[a]	SEQ	0.83 mg/mL[a]	Gross precipitate forms	2117	I
Promethazine HCl	ES	2 mg/mL[a]	SEQ	0.83 mg/mL[a]	Gross precipitate forms	2117	I
Propranolol HCl	WY	1 mg/mL	SEQ	0.83 mg/mL[a]	Gross precipitate forms	2117	I
Ranitidine HCl	GL	2 mg/mL[a]	SEQ	0.83 mg/mL[a]	Microprecipitate and increased turbidity form immediately	2117	I
Remifentanil HCl	GW	0.5 mg/mL[a]	SEQ	0.83 mg/mL[a]	Gross precipitate forms	2117	I
Sodium bicarbonate	AB	1 mEq/mL	SEQ	0.83 mg/mL[a]	Gross precipitate forms	2117	I

Y-Site Injection Compatibility (1:1 Mixture) (Cont.)

Amphotericin B cholesteryl sulfate complex

Drug	Mfr	Conc	Mfr	Conc	Remarks	Ref	C/I
Sufentanil citrate	JN	0.05 mg/mL	SEQ	0.83 mg/mL[a]	Physically compatible for 4 hr at 23 °C	2117	C
Ticarcillin disodium–clavulanate potassium	SKB	31 mg/mL[a]	SEQ	0.83 mg/mL[a]	Gross precipitate forms	2117	I
Tobramycin sulfate	AB	5 mg/mL[a]	SEQ	0.83 mg/mL[a]	Gross precipitate forms	2117	I
Trimethoprim–sulfamethoxazole	ES	0.8 + 4 mg/mL[a]	SEQ	0.83 mg/mL[a]	Physically compatible for 4 hr at 23 °C	2117	C
Vancomycin HCl	AB	10 mg/mL[a]	SEQ	0.83 mg/mL[a]	Gross precipitate forms	2117	I
Vecuronium bromide	MAR	1 mg/mL[a]	SEQ	0.83 mg/mL[a]	Gross precipitate forms	2117	I
Verapamil HCl	AMR	2.5 mg/mL	SEQ	0.83 mg/mL[a]	Gross precipitate forms	2117	I
Vinblastine sulfate	FAU	0.12 mg/mL[a]	SEQ	0.83 mg/mL[a]	Physically compatible for 4 hr at 23 °C	2117	C
Vincristine sulfate	FAU	0.05 mg/mL[a]	SEQ	0.83 mg/mL[a]	Physically compatible for 4 hr at 23 °C	2117	C
Vinorelbine tartrate	BW	1 mg/mL[a]	SEQ	0.83 mg/mL[a]	Gross precipitate forms	2117	I
Zidovudine	BW	4 mg/mL[a]	SEQ	0.83 mg/mL[a]	Physically compatible for 4 hr at 23 °C	2117	C

[a]Tested in dextrose 5%.
[b]Tested in sodium chloride 0.9%.
[c]Test performed using the formulation WITHOUT edetate disodium.

AMPHOTERICIN B LIPID COMPLEX
AHFS 8:14.28

Products — Amphotericin B lipid complex is available in 20-mL vials containing 100 mg of amphotericin B in a yellow opaque suspension with L-α-dimyristoylphosphatidylcholine, L-α-dimyristoylphosphatidylglycerol, and sodium chloride in water for injection. The suspension must be diluted in dextrose 5% for administration. Shake the vial gently so that no sediment remains on the vial bottom. Withdraw the dose using a syringe and needle. Attach the 5-μm filter needle that is supplied with the vial, and add the drug suspension into a bag of dextrose 5%. One filter needle may be used for up to four vials of drug. The final concentration is usually 1 mg/mL, although 2 mg/mL may be used in some cases. (1)

Although other colloidal, liposomal, and complexed amphotericin B products exist, they are sufficiently different from amphotericin B lipid complex that extrapolating information to or from other forms would be inappropriate.

pH — 5 to 7. (1)

Trade Name(s) — Abelcet.

Administration — Amphotericin B lipid complex diluted to a concentration of 1 or 2 mg/mL in dextrose 5% is given by intravenous infusion usually delivered over 2 hours. The bag is shaken just prior to infusion; it should not be used if foreign matter is present. If delivery proceeds over more than 2 hours, the bag should be shaken every 2 hours. Use a separate infusion line or flush an existing line with dextrose 5% prior to administration. (1) **CAUTION: Care should be taken to ensure that the correct drug product, dose, and administration procedure are used and that no confusion with other products occurs.**

Stability — Intact vials of amphotericin B lipid complex are stored under refrigeration. They should be protected from light and from freezing. The manufacturer recommends keeping the vials in their original cartons until use. (1)

The manufacturer also states in the labeling that amphotericin B lipid complex diluted in dextrose 5% for administration may be stored for 48 hours under refrigeration with an additional 6 hours at room temperature. (1) However, elsewhere the manufacturer has stated that amphotericin B lipid complex 1 mg/mL in dextrose 5% is stable for 10 days stored under refrigeration. (31)

Amphotericin B lipid complex is incompatible with normal saline and other electrolyte solutions. (1)

Filtration — The manufacturer states that although amphotericin B lipid complex is to be prepared using the 5-μm filter needle provided, it should not be administered using an inline filter. (1)

Compatibility Information

Solution Compatibility

Amphotericin B lipid complex

Solution	Mfr	Mfr	Conc/L	Remarks	Ref	C/I
Dextrose 5%	MAC	ZNS	400 mg, 800 mg, 2 g	Physically compatible. Analytical results were variable but did not indicate substantial loss	2732	**C**

Y-Site Injection Compatibility (1:1 Mixture)

Amphotericin B lipid complex

Drug	Mfr	Conc	Mfr	Conc	Remarks	Ref	C/I
Anidulafungin	VIC	0.5 mg/mL[a]	ELN	1 mg/mL[a]	Physically compatible for 4 hr at 23 °C	2617	**C**
Caspofungin acetate	ME	0.7 mg/mL[b]	ENZ	1 mg/mL[a]	Immediate yellow turbid precipitate	2758	**I**
Doripenem	JJ	5 mg/mL[a]	ENZ	1 mg/mL[a]	Physically compatible for 4 hr at 23 °C	2743	**C**
	JJ	5 mg/mL[b]	ENZ	1 mg/mL[a]	Measured haze increases immediately	2743	**I**
Telavancin HCl	ASP	7.5 mg/mL[a]	ENZ	1 mg/mL[a]	Physically compatible for 2 hr	2830	**C**
Tigecycline	WY	1 mg/mL[b]	ENZ	2 mg/mL[a]	Incompatible with sodium chloride diluent	2714	**I**

[a] Tested in dextrose 5%.
[b] Tested in sodium chloride 0.9%.

AMPHOTERICIN B LIPOSOMAL
AHFS 8:14.28

Products — Amphotericin B liposomal for injection is available as a lyophilized powder in 50-mg vials with hydrogenated soy phosphatidylcholine 213 mg, cholesterol 52 mg, disteaoylphosphatidylglycerol 84 mg, alpha-tocopherols 0.64 mg, sucrose 900 mg, and disodium succinate hexahydrate 27 mg. Each vial contains amphotericin B intercalated into a liposomal membrane.

Reconstitute the vials with 12 mL of sterile water for injection. No other diluent should be used because of potential drug precipitation from electrolytes and preservatives. After addition of the sterile water for injection, shake vigorously for at least 30 seconds to yield a liposomal suspension concentrate of amphotericin B 4 mg/mL. Visually inspect for particulate matter and continue shaking until completely dispersed. (1)

To prepare for administration, pass the concentrate through the 5-μm filter provided using one filter per vial into an appropriate amount of dextrose 5%. The final concentration generally should be 1 to 2 mg/mL, although lower concentrations of 0.2 to 0.5 mg/mL may be used for children. (1)

Although other colloidal and complexed amphotericin B products exist, they are sufficiently different from amphotericin B liposomal that extrapolating information to or from other forms would be inappropriate.

pH — From 5 to 6. (1)

Trade Name(s) — AmBisome.

Administration — Amphotericin B liposomal is administered by intravenous infusion in dextrose 5% using a controlled infusion device over approximately 120 minutes. The administration may be reduced to 60 minutes for patients who tolerate it well. The line should be flushed with dextrose 5% prior to administration or a separate new line must be used. (1) **CAUTION: Care should be taken to ensure that the correct drug product, dose, and administration procedure are used and that no confusion with other products occurs.**

Stability — Intact vials of amphotericin B liposomal for injection are stored at controlled room temperature up to 25 °C. The manufacturer states in the labeling that the reconstituted concentrate may be stored under refrigeration for up to 24 hours. It should be protected from freezing. The single-use vials contain no preservative, and partial vials should be discarded. (1) However, the manufacturer has also stated elsewhere that a concentration of 4 mg/mL in sterile water for injection in glass vials is stable for 14 days under refrigeration and protected from light. (31)

The manufacturer also states that after dilution of amphotericin B liposomal in dextrose 5%, administration should begin within six hours. (1) However, the manufacturer has also indicated that the drug diluted in dextrose 5% for administration is stable for longer time periods. In concentrations of 0.2 mg/mL, the drug is stated to be stable for 24 hours at room temperature exposed to fluorescent light and for 11 days in the refrigerator. In concentrations of 2 mg/mL, the drug is stated to be stable also for 24 hours at room temperature exposed to fluorescent light and for 14 days in the refrigerator. (2577)

Amphotericin B liposomal is incompatible with normal saline and other electrolyte solutions. (1)

Syringes — The manufacturer states that amphotericin B liposomal 4 mg/mL packaged in plastic syringes is stable for 14 days stored under refrigeration and protected from light. (31)

Filtration — The manufacturer states that amphotericin B liposomal diluted for infusion may be administered through an inline filter as long as the filter porosity is not smaller than 1 μm. (1)

Compatibility Information

Y-Site Injection Compatibility (1:1 Mixture)

Amphotericin B liposomal

Drug	Mfr	Conc	Mfr	Conc	Remarks	Ref	C/I
Anidulafungin	VIC	0.5 mg/mL[a]	FUJ	1 mg/mL[a]	Physically compatible for 4 hr at 23 °C	2617	C
Caspofungin acetate	ME	0.7 mg/mL[b]	AST	1 mg/mL[a]	Immediate yellow turbid precipitate	2758	I
Doripenem	JJ	5 mg/mL[a]	ASP	1 mg/mL[a]	Physically compatible for 4 hr at 23 °C	2743	C
	JJ	5 mg/mL[b]	ASP	1 mg/mL[a]	Measured haze increases immediately	2743	I
Telavancin HCl	ASP	7.5 mg/mL[a]	ASP	1 mg/mL[a]	Increase in measured turbidity	2830	I

[a]Tested in dextrose 5%.
[b]Tested in sodium chloride 0.9%.

AMPICILLIN SODIUM
AHFS 8:12.16.08

Products — Ampicillin sodium is available in vials containing the equivalent of ampicillin 125 mg, 250 mg, 500 mg, 1 g, or 2 g. For intramuscular injection, reconstitute the vials with sterile water for injection or bacteriostatic water for injection in the following amounts (1):

Vial Size	Volume of Diluent	Withdrawable Volume	Concentration
125 mg	1.2 mL	1 mL	125 mg/mL
250 mg	1.0 mL	1 mL	250 mg/mL
500 mg	1.8 mL	2 mL	250 mg/mL
1 g	3.5 mL	4 mL	250 mg/mL
2 g	6.8 mL	8 mL	250 mg/mL

For intravenous injection, reconstitute the 125-, 250-, and 500-mg vials with 5 mL of sterile water for injection or bacteriostatic water for injection. For the 1- or 2-g vials, reconstitute with 7.4 or 14.8 mL, respectively, of sterile water for injection or bacteriostatic water for injection. (1)

pH — Ampicillin sodium 10 mg/mL has a pH of 8 to 10. (4) The pH values of various ampicillin sodium solutions are shown below (213):

Percent Ampicillin Sodium	Diluent	Initial pH
2	Sterile water	8.80
5	Sterile water	8.92
10	Sterile water	9.15
2	Sodium chloride 0.9%	8.7
5	Sodium chloride 0.9%	8.9
10	Sodium chloride 0.9%	9.2
2	Dextrose 5%	8.9
5	Dextrose 5%	9.3
10	Dextrose 5%	9.3

Osmolality — Reconstituted with sterile water for injection, ampicillin sodium (Wyeth) 100 mg/mL has an osmolality of 602 mOsm/kg. (50) At 125 mg/mL, Wyeth's product was 702 mOsm/kg and Bristol's product was 675 mOsm/kg. (1071)

In another study, the osmolality of ampicillin sodium (Bristol) diluted in sodium chloride 0.9% was determined to be 493 mOsm/kg at 50 mg/mL and 664 mOsm/kg at 100 mg/mL. (1375)

The osmolality of ampicillin sodium 1 and 2 g was calculated for the following dilutions (1054):

Diluent	Osmolality (mOsm/kg)	
	50 mL	100 mL
1 g		
Dextrose 5%	341	302
Sodium chloride 0.9%	368	328
2 g		
Dextrose 5%	418	346
Sodium chloride 0.9%	444	372

The following maximum ampicillin sodium concentrations were recommended to achieve osmolalities suitable for peripheral infusion in fluid-restricted patients (1180):

Diluent	Maximum Concentration (mg/mL)	Osmolality (mOsm/kg)
Dextrose 5%	62	583
Sodium chloride 0.9%	56	576
Sterile water for injection	112	588

Sodium Content — Ampicillin sodium contains approximately 2.9 to 3.1 mEq of sodium per gram of drug. (1; 4)

Administration — Ampicillin sodium is administered by intramuscular or direct intravenous injection or intravenous infusion. Direct intravenous injection should be made slowly over 10 to 15 minutes. (4)

Stability — The stability of ampicillin sodium in solution under various conditions has been the subject of much work and numerous articles. Several characteristics of the stability of ampicillin sodium have emerged from these studies:

1. The stability is concentration dependent and decreases as the concentration increases.
2. Sodium chloride 0.9% appears to be a suitable diluent for the intravenous infusion of ampicillin sodium.
3. The stability is greatly decreased in dextrose solutions.
4. Storage temperature and the pH of solution affect the stability.

Storage and Usage Times — Savello and Shangraw offered the recommendations in Table 1 regarding storage conditions for ampicillin sodium solutions.

Table 1. Suggested Storage Conditions for Ampicillin Sodium Solutions (210)

Solution	Temperature (°C)	Maximum Storage
Constituted vial	−20	48 hr
	5	4 hr
	27	1 hr
Ampicillin sodium 1% in sodium chloride 0.9%	5	5 days
	27	24 hr
Ampicillin sodium 1% in dextrose 5%	5	4 hr
	27	2 hr

The manufacturer recommends using only freshly prepared ampicillin sodium solutions within one hour of reconstitution. (1)

Concentration Effects — The effect of concentration on ampicillin sodium stability has been attributed to a self-catalyzing effect. (210) As the concentration increases, so does the rate of decomposition. (170; 210) Savello and Shangraw reported that, even though the initial pH values of various concentrations were 9.2 to 9.3, the higher concentrations of the drug maintained their pH longer because of their greater buffer capacity. (210) (See Table 2.)

This concentration dependence of the stability of ampicillin sodium has been related to the polymerization of penicillins in concentrated solutions. (601; 602) Dimerization is the predominant form of degradation with high ampicillin concentrations. The extent of this effect declines as the concentration drops but still remains significant in a 2% solution. At lower concentrations, hydrolysis becomes the determining factor. (603)

In a 50% concentration, ampicillin sodium formed dimer, trimer, tetramer, and pentamer during 24 hours of storage at 24 °C in the dark. The polymer formed through a chain process by linkage of the amino group on the side chain to another molecule with a cleaved β-lactam ring. (1400)

In a 20% ampicillin sodium aqueous solution adjusted to pH 8.5 and stored at 22 °C, 90% of all decomposition products formed within 72 hours were di- and polymers. In a 5% solution, 70% of the decomposition products were di- and polymers. However, a 1% solution formed α-aminobenzylpenicilloic acid as the predominant decomposition product and a dimer concentration of 1 to 2%. The rate of dimerization was almost independent of pH in the range of 7 to 10 but increased strongly with increases in the initial ampicillin sodium concentration. (858)

However, one study showed that if the pH of the solution was held constant at 8 or 9.15, there was little dependence of the rate of decomposition on concentration in the concentration range of 2 to 10%. (213)

Infusion Diluents — Infusion diluents also affect the stability of ampicillin sodium. Sodium chloride 0.9% appears to be a suitable diluent for the intravenous infusion of ampicillin sodium.

Dextrose is thought to exhibit an immense catalytic effect on the hydrolysis of ampicillin sodium (210), decreasing the stability about one-half when compared to sterile water or sodium chloride 0.9%. (213) This has been well documented and has been regarded as an incompatibility. (210; 213) (See Table 3.) This accelerated decomposition associated with dextrose extends to fructose as well, although it is not as extensive. It occurs in the alkaline pH range. Below pH 6 or 7, the decomposition rate with both dextrose and fructose appears to coincide with simple aqueous solutions. (604)

Table 2. Percent Degradation of Ampicillin Sodium Solutions after Reconstitution with Water for Injection at 5 °C after Eight Hours (210)

Percent Concentration	Percent Degradation
1	0.8
5	3.6
10	5.8
15	10.4
20	12.3
25	13.3

Table 3. Percent Degradation of 1% Ampicillin Sodium in Dextrose 5% in Water According to Temperature and Time (210)

Temperature (°C)	4 hr	8 hr	24 hr
−20	13.6	22.3	45.6
0	6.2	11.6	26.3
5	10.1	15.2	29.7
27	21.3	31.1	46.5

Savello and Shangraw further showed that increasing the concentration of dextrose decreased the stability of ampicillin sodium. (See Table 4.)

The stability of ampicillin sodium (Bristol) 50 mg/L in peritoneal dialysis solutions (Dianeal 137 and PD2) with heparin sodium 500 units/L was evaluated at 25 °C. Approximately 93 ± 10% activity remained after 24 hours. (1228)

However, ampicillin sodium (Bristol) 2.5 g/L in peritoneal dialysis concentrate (Travenol) containing dextrose 30% with and without heparin sodium 2500 units/L underwent substantial reduction in activity within as little as 10 minutes. (273)

pH Effects — The pH of the solution also plays a role in its stability. Hydrolysis has been shown to be catalyzed by hydroxide ions. An increase of 1 pH unit in an ampicillin sodium solution has been shown to increase the rate of decomposition 10-fold. (213)

The optimum pH for ampicillin sodium stability has been variously reported as 5.8 (1072), 5.85 at 35 °C (215), approximately 5.2 at 25 °C (604), and 7.5 at room temperature. (209) The pH of ampicillin sodium solutions, however, is in the alkaline range, with higher pH values having been reported at higher concentrations. (213) (See the pH section above.)

Ampicillin sodium (Bristol) 10 g/L was tested for stability at pH 3.4 to 9.2 in various buffer additives. A 7.6% potency loss was reported in 12 hours at room temperature at pH 7.5. Significantly higher degradation rates occurred as the pH varied from 7.5, with about 70% degradation occurring in 12 hours at room temperature at pH 3.4 and 9.2. (209)

In another evaluation, rate constants for ampicillin degradation at various pH values were calculated for an aqueous solution at 25 °C. The pH providing maximum stability was 5.2. When tested in dextrose 10%, a minimum rate of decomposition was observed at approximately pH 5 to 5.5. The amount of ampicillin degradation was 10% or less in 24 hours at 25 °C within a pH range of about 2.75 to 6.75. At pH 8, the time to 10% decomposition was only about two hours. (604)

The stability of ampicillin sodium (Beecham) 250 mg/50 mL and 1 g/100 mL in sodium chloride 0.9% in PVC bags was compared to the stability of the same solutions buffered with potassium acid phosphate 13.6% injection. The 50- and 100-mL containers were buffered with 1 and 2 mL, respectively, lowering the pH by nearly two pH units. Larger quantities of buffer caused precipitation. When stored

Table 4. Percent Degradation of 1% Ampicillin Sodium at 5 °C According to Dextrose Concentration and Time (210)

Percent Dextrose	3 hr	7 hr
5	7.4	13.9
10	10.3	19.4
20	14.2	27.8

at 5 °C, the 250-mg/50-mL solution had a shelf life (t_{90}) of 12 days while the 1-g/100-mL solution had a shelf life of six days. This finding compares favorably to the shelf life of one to two days for the unbuffered solutions. (1820)

Temperature Effects — The storage temperature of ampicillin sodium solutions may also affect stability. It has been stated that freezing ampicillin sodium solutions at −20 °C increases the rate of decomposition over that at 5 °C. For this reason, it has been recommended that ampicillin sodium solutions not be stored in the frozen state. (123; 213)

Apparent increased ampicillin decomposition was found at −20 °C over that at 5 °C in two of the 1% solutions tested (Tables 3 and 5). In a study of ampicillin sodium 2%, about 4 to 6% greater loss was found at −20 °C than at 5 °C in 24 hours in both dextrose 5% and sodium chloride 0.9%. (208)

An explanation of this phenomenon was proposed by Pincock and Kiovsky. Below the freezing point but above the eutectic temperature, there exists a liquid and solid phase in equilibrium. If it is assumed that −20 °C is above the eutectic temperature, then liquid regions of a saturated solution of ampicillin sodium exist, which result in increased decomposition. (214) Solutions of ampicillin sodium stored at −78 °C showed no decomposition within 24 hours. (210)

In a study of long-term storage, ampicillin sodium (Ayerst) 1 g/50 mL in dextrose 5% and also sodium chloride 0.9% was tested in PVC containers frozen at −20 °C for 30 days. In sodium chloride 0.9%, they reported approximately 10% decomposition in one day and approximately 70% decomposition in 30 days. In dextrose 5%, even greater decomposition occurred. They reported about 50% decomposition in one day and virtually total decomposition in 30 days. (299)

Ampicillin sodium (Wyeth) 1 g/50 mL of dextrose 5% was tested in PVC bags frozen at −20 °C for 30 days and then thawed by exposure to ambient temperature or microwave radiation. The admixtures showed essentially total loss of ampicillin activity determined microbiologically. (554) At −30 °C, only 18% of the ampicillin remained in 30 days. A storage temperature of −70 °C was required to retain at least 90% of the original activity for 30 days. (555)

The same concentration in sodium chloride 0.9% showed a 29% loss of ampicillin activity at −20 °C but only about a 4% loss at −30 and −70 °C after 30 days. Subsequent thawing of the −30 and −70 °C samples by exposure to microwave radiation and storage at room temperature for eight hours resulted in additional losses of activity, with the final concentration totaling about 90% of the initial amount. The authors concluded that ampicillin sodium in sodium chloride 0.9% could be stored for 30 days at −30 °C, which was presumably below the eutectic point for this admixture. However, −30 °C was believed to be above the eutectic point for the dextrose 5% admixture because decomposition continued to occur. (555)

Even within acceptable limits for room temperature, significant differences in the rate of ampicillin decomposition can occur. In one solution at 20 °C, a 10% ampicillin loss resulted in 44 hours. This same solution at 30 °C exhibited a 10% loss in 12 hours. Over the

Table 5. Percent Degradation of 1% Ampicillin Sodium in Water According to Temperature and Time (210)

Temperature (°C)	4 hr	8 hr	24 hr
−20	1.3	1.9	5.2
5	0.4	0.8	2.0

range of 20 to 35 °C, each 5 °C rise approximately doubled the rate of decomposition. (604)

Sorption — Acetazolamide sodium was shown not to exhibit sorption to PVC bags and tubing, polyethylene tubing, Silastic tubing, polypropylene syringes, and trilayer solution bags composed of polyethylene, polyamide, and polypropylene. (536; 606; 1035; 1918)

Filtration — Filtration of ampicillin sodium (Wyeth) is stated to result in no adsorption, yielding solutions that maintain their potency. (829)
Ampicillin sodium (Bristol) 1.97 mg/mL in sodium chloride 0.9% was filtered through a 0.22-μm cellulose ester membrane filter (Ivex-

HP, Millipore) over five hours. No significant drug loss due to binding to the filter was noted. (1034)

Central Venous Catheter — Ampicillin sodium (Apothecon) 5 mg/mL in sodium chloride 0.9% was found to be compatible with the AR-ROWg+ard Blue Plus (Arrow International) chlorhexidine-bearing triple-lumen central catheter. Essentially complete delivery of the drug was found with little or no drug loss occurring. Furthermore, chlorhexidine delivered from the catheter remained at trace amounts with no substantial increase due to the delivery of the drug through the catheter. (2335)

Compatibility Information

Solution Compatibility

Ampicillin sodium

Solution	Mfr	Mfr	Conc/L	Remarks	Ref	C/I
Amino acids 4.25%, dextrose 25%	MG	BR	1 g	Increased microscopic particles in 24 hr at 5 °C	349	I
Dextrose 5% in sodium chloride 0.45%			2 g	Stable for up to 2 hr at 25 °C	1	I
			10 g	Stable for up to 1 hr at 4 °C	1	I
Dextrose 5% in sodium chloride 0.9%	MG	BR	1 g	19% loss in 4 hr at 4 °C and 17% in 2 hr at 25 °C	105	I
Dextrose 5%			2 g	Stable for up to 2 hr at 25 °C	1	I
			20 g	Stable for up to 1 hr at 4 and 25 °C	1	I
		BE	1 g	24% loss in 8 hr at 25 °C	211	I
		AY	2 and 4 g	10% loss in 4 hr at room temperature	99	I
	MG	BR	1 g	11% loss in 24 hr at 4 °C and 21% in 24 hr at 25 °C	105	I
	AB	AY	2 g	10% loss in 24 hr at 5 °C and 20% in 24 hr at 25 °C	88	I
		BR	20 g	19% loss in 4 hr at 25 °C. 40% loss in 24 hr at 25 °C	208	I
		BR	10 g	46% loss in 24 hr at −20 °C. 30% loss in 24 hr at 5 °C. 47% loss in 24 hr at 27 °C	210	I
	BA[a], TR	AY	20 g	40% loss in 24 hr at 22 °C and 30% in 24 hr at 5 °C	298	I
			2 g	5% loss in 2 hr and 38% in 24 hr at 20 to 25 °C	307	I
			4 g	10% loss in 2 hr and 45% in 24 hr at 25 °C	307	I
			10 g	12% loss in 2 hr and 50% in 24 hr at 25 °C	307	I
	TR[b]	WY	20 g	35% loss in 8 hr and 52% in 24 hr at room temperature	554	I
	PH	BAY	2 g	10% loss in 3.5 hr at 25 °C	604	I
	PH	BAY	5 g	10% loss in 2.5 hr at 25 °C	604	I
	PH	BAY	15 g	10% loss in 2 hr at 25 °C	604	I
			4 g	10% loss in 4 hr and 28% in 24 hr at room temperature	768	I
			5 g	7% loss in 2 hr and 15% loss in 4 hr at 29 °C. 8% loss in 8 hr at 4 °C	773	I
	TR[b]	WY	10 and 20 g	60% loss in 48 hr at 25 °C and in 7 days at 4 °C	1001	I
	TR[b]	WY	20 g	50% loss at 24 °C and 28% at 4 °C in 1 day	1035	I
	[b]	BR	20 g	No loss during 2 hr storage and 1-hr simulated infusion	1774	C
Dextrose 10%	MG	BR	1 g	17% loss in 6 hr at 4 °C and 18% in 4 hr at 25 °C	105	I
Isolyte M in dextrose 5%	MG	BR	1 g	Stable for 24 hr at 4 and 25 °C	105	C

Solution Compatibility (Cont.)

Ampicillin sodium

Solution	Mfr	Mfr	Conc/L	Remarks	Ref	C/I
Isolyte P in dextrose 5%	MG	BR	1 g	Stable for 24 hr at 4 and 25 °C	105	C
Ringer's injection		AY	2 and 4 g	10% loss in 24 hr at room temperature	99	C
		BAY	2 g	10% loss in 40 hr at 25 °C	604	C
		BAY	5 g	10% loss in 25 hr at 25 °C	604	C
		BAY	15 g	10% loss in 20 hr at 25 °C	604	I
			5 g	9% loss in 8 hr and 18% loss in 24 hr at 29 °C. 3% loss in 24 hr at 4 °C	773	I
Ringer's injection, lactated			30 g	Stable for 8 hr at 25 °C and 24 hr at 4 °C	1	I
		BE	1 g	17% loss in 4 hr at 25 °C	211	I
		BR	1 g	11% loss in 12 hr at 25 °C	87	I
	MG	BR	1 g	17% loss in 6 hr at 4 °C and 25% in 6 hr at 25 °C	105	I
			5 g	20% loss in 2 hr at 29 °C and 11% in 4 hr at 4 °C	773	I
Sodium chloride 0.9%			20 g	Stable for 48 hr at 4 °C	1	C
			30 g	Stable for 8 hr at 25 °C and 24 hr at 4 °C	1	C
		BAY	2 g	10% loss in over 48 hr at 25 °C	604	C
		BAY	5 g	10% loss in 38 hr at 25 °C	604	C
		BAY	15 g	10% loss in 33 hr at 25 °C	604	C
		BE	10 g	Less than 10% decomposition in 24 hr at 25 °C	113	C
		BR	6 g	9% loss in 24 hr at room temperature. 1% loss in 24 hr under refrigeration	127	C
	MG	BR	1 g	Activity retained for 24 hr at 4 and 25 °C	105	C
		AY	2 to 30 g	10% loss in 24 hr at room temperature	99	C
		BR	20 g	4% loss in 24 hr at 5 °C. 12 to 16% loss in 24 hr at 25 °C	208	C
		BR	10 g	4% loss in 24 hr at −20 °C. 3% loss in 24 hr at 5 °C. 8% loss in 24 hr at 27 °C	210	C
		BR	5, 10, 15, 20 g	6 to 12% loss in 24 hr at 25 °C	212	C
		BR	5, 10, 15, 20, 30, 40 g	1 to 6% loss in 24 hr at 5 °C	212	C
	BA[a], TR	AY	20 g	Activity retained for 24 hr at 5 and 22 °C	298	C
			2, 4, 10 g	10% loss in 24 hr at 20 to 25 °C	307	C
		BE	1 g	12% loss in 12 hr at 25 °C and 28% in 24 hr at 25 °C	211	I
		BR	30 and 40 g	15% loss in 24 hr at 25 °C	212	I
			4 g	10% loss in 8 hr and 19% loss in 24 hr at room temperature	768	I
			5 g	10% loss in 8 hr at 29 °C and 3% loss in 24 hr at 4 °C	773	I
	TR[b]	WY	20 g	15% loss in 1 day and 30% in 4 days at 24 °C. 6% loss in 1 day and 10% in 4 days at 4 °C. 13% loss in 4 days at −7 °C	1035	I
	[b]	BR	20 g	No loss during 2 hr storage and 1-hr simulated infusion	1774	C
	AB[c]	WY	60 g	Stable for 24 hr at 5 °C. 10% loss in 6 hr and 20% loss in 24 hr during administration at 30 °C via portable pump	1779	C
	BA[b]	BE	10 g	Visually compatible with 10% loss in 2 days at 5 °C	1820	C

Solution Compatibility (Cont.)

Ampicillin sodium

Solution	Mfr	Mfr	Conc/L	Remarks	Ref	C/I
	BA[b]	BE	5 g	Visually compatible with 10% loss in 1 day at 5 °C	1820	C
Sodium lactate ⅙ M		BR	1 g	37% loss in 4 hr at 25 °C	211	I
		AY	up to 30 g	10% loss in 6 hr at room temperature	99	I
TPN #21[d]		BR	1 g	Activity retained for 24 hr at 4 °C	87	C
		BR	1 g	12 to 25% ampicillin loss in 24 hr at 25 °C	87	I
TPN #52[d]		AST	1.5 g	69% ampicillin loss in 24 hr at 29 °C	440	I
TPN #53[d]		AST	1.5 g	22% ampicillin loss in 24 hr at 29 °C	440	I
TPN #107[d]			1 and 3 g	Activity retained for 24 hr at 21 °C	1326	C

[a]Tested in both PVC and glass containers.
[b]Tested in PVC containers.
[c]Tested in portable pump reservoirs (Pharmacia Deltec).
[d]Refer to Appendix I for the composition of parenteral nutrition solutions. TPN indicates a 2-in-1 admixture.

Additive Compatibility

Ampicillin sodium

Drug	Mfr	Conc/L	Mfr	Conc/L	Test Soln	Remarks	Ref	C/I
Amikacin sulfate	BR	5 g	BR	30 g	D5LR, D5R, D5S, D5W, D10W, LR, NS, R, SL	Over 10% ampicillin loss in 4 hr at 25 °C	293	I
Aztreonam	SQ	10 g	WY	20 g	D5W[a]	10% ampicillin loss in 2 hr and 10% aztreonam loss in 3 hr at 25 °C. 10% ampicillin loss in 24 hr and 10% aztreonam loss in 8 hr at 4 °C	1001	I
	SQ	10 g	WY	5 g	D5W[a]	10% ampicillin loss in 3 hr and 10% aztreonam loss in 7 hr at 25 °C. 10% loss of both drugs in 48 hr at 4 °C	1001	I
	SQ	20 g	WY	20 g	D5W[a]	10% ampicillin loss in 4 hr and 10% aztreonam loss in 5 hr at 25 °C. 10% loss of both drugs in 24 hr at 4 °C	1001	I
	SQ	20 g	WY	5 g	D5W[a]	10% ampicillin loss in 5 hr and 10% aztreonam loss in 8 hr at 25 °C. 10% ampicillin loss in 48 hr and 10% aztreonam loss in 72 hr at 4 °C	1001	I
	SQ	10 g	WY	20 g	NS[a]	10% ampicillin loss in 24 hr and 2% aztreonam loss in 48 hr at 25 °C. 10% ampicillin loss in 2 days and 9% aztreonam loss in 7 days at 4 °C	1001	C
	SQ	10 g	WY	5 g	NS[a]	10% ampicillin loss and no aztreonam loss in 48 hr at 25 °C. 10% ampicillin loss in 3 days and 8% aztreonam loss in 7 days at 4 °C	1001	C

Additive Compatibility (Cont.)

Ampicillin sodium

Drug	Mfr	Conc/L	Mfr	Conc/L	Test Soln	Remarks	Ref	C/I
	SQ	20 g	WY	20 g	NS[a]	10% ampicillin loss in 24 hr and 5% aztreonam loss in 48 hr at 25 °C. 10% ampicillin loss in 2 days and 7% aztreonam loss in 7 days at 4 °C	1001	C
	SQ	20 g	WY	5 g	NS[a]	10% ampicillin loss and no aztreonam loss in 48 hr at 25 °C. 10% ampicillin loss and 5% aztreonam loss in 7 days at 4 °C	1001	C
Cefepime HCl	BR	40 g	BR	1 g	D5W	4% ampicillin loss in 8 hr at room temperature and 5 °C. 7% cefepime loss in 8 hr at room temperature and no loss in 8 hr at 5 °C	1682	?
	BR	40 g	BR	1 g	NS	No ampicillin loss in 24 hr at room temperature and 9% loss in 48 hr at 5 °C. 5% cefepime loss in 24 hr at room temperature and 2% loss in 72 hr at 5 °C	1682	C
	BR	40 g	BR	10 g	D5W	6% ampicillin loss in 2 hr at room temperature and 2% loss in 8 hr at 5 °C. 7% cefepime loss in 2 hr at room temperature and 8 hr at 5 °C	1682	I
	BR	40 g	BR	10 g	NS	6% ampicillin loss in 8 hr at room temperature and 9% loss in 48 hr at 5 °C. 8% cefepime loss in 8 hr at room temperature and 10% loss in 48 hr at 5 °C	1682	I
	BR	4 g	BR	40 g	D5W	10% ampicillin loss in 1 hr at room temperature and 9% loss in 2 hr at 5 °C. 25% cefepime loss in 1 hr at room temperature and 9% loss in 2 hr at 5 °C	1682	I
	BR	4 g	BR	40 g	NS	5% ampicillin loss in 8 hr at room temperature and 4% loss in 8 hr at 5 °C. 4% cefepime loss in 8 hr at room temperature and 6% loss in 8 hr at 5 °C	1682	?
Chlorpromazine HCl	BP	200 mg	BP	2 g	D5W, NS	Precipitates immediately	26	I
Clindamycin phosphate	UP	24 g	WY	10 and 20 g	NS	Physically compatible	1035	C
	UP	3 g	WY	3.7 g	NS	Physically compatible with 4% ampicillin loss in 1 day at 24 °C	1035	C
Dextran 40		10%		4 g	D5W	46% ampicillin loss in 24 hr at 20 °C	834	I
	PH	10%	AY	8 g	D5W	50% loss in 24 hr at room temperature	99	I
	PH	10%	BAY	15 g	D5W	10% ampicillin loss in 1.5 hr at 25 °C	604	I
	PH	10%	BAY	2 g	D5W	10% ampicillin loss in 3.5 hr at 25 °C	604	I
	PH	10%	BAY	5 g	D5W	10% ampicillin loss in 2.3 hr at 25 °C	604	I
	PH	10%	AY	8 g	NS	25% loss in 24 hr at room temperature	99	I
	PH	10%	BAY	15 g	NS	10% ampicillin loss in 2.3 hr at 25 °C	604	I
	PH	10%	BAY	2 g	NS	10% ampicillin loss in 2.8 hr at 25 °C	604	I
	PH	10%	BAY	5 g	NS	10% ampicillin loss in 2.5 hr at 25 °C	604	I
Dopamine HCl	AS	800 mg	BR	4 g	D5W	Color change. 36% ampicillin loss in 6 hr at 23 to 25 °C. Dopamine loss in 6 hr	78	I
Erythromycin lactobionate	AB	3 g	WY	3.7 g	NS	Physically compatible with 6% ampicillin loss in 1 day at 24 °C	1035	C
Fat emulsion, intravenous		10%		20 g		15% ampicillin loss in 24 hr at 23 °C	37	I
	VT	10%	BE	2 g		Lipid coalescence in 24 hr at 25 and 8 °C	825	I

Additive Compatibility (Cont.)

Ampicillin sodium

Drug	Mfr	Conc/L	Mfr	Conc/L	Test Soln	Remarks	Ref	C/I
Floxacillin sodium	BE	20 g	BE	20 g	NS	Physically compatible for 72 hr at 15 and 30 °C	1479	**C**
Furosemide	HO	1 g	BE	20 g	NS	Physically compatible for 72 hr at 15 and 30 °C	1479	**C**
Gentamicin sulfate	RS	160 mg	BE	8 g	D5¼S, D5W, NS	50% gentamicin loss in 2 hr at room temperature	157	**I**
		100 mg		1 g	TPN #107[b]	42% gentamicin loss and 25% ampicillin loss in 24 hr at 21 °C	1326	**I**
Heparin sodium		32,000 units		2 g	NS	Physically compatible and heparin activity retained for 24 hr	57	**C**
		12,000 units	BR	1 g	D10W, LR, NS	Ampicillin stable for 24 hr at 4 °C	87	**C**
	OR	20,000 units	BE	10 g	NS	Both stable for 24 hr at 25 °C	113	**C**
		12,000 units	BR	1 g	D5S	15% ampicillin decomposition in 24 hr at 4 °C	87	**I**
		12,000 units	BR	1 g	D5S, D10W, LR	20 to 25% ampicillin decomposition in 24 hr at 25 °C	87	**I**
Hetastarch in sodium chloride 0.9%		6%		4 g	NS	18% loss in 6 hr and 35% in 24 hr at 20 °C	834	**I**
Hydralazine HCl	BP	80 mg	BP	2 g	D5W	Yellow color produced	26	**I**
Hydrocortisone sodium succinate		200 and 400 mg	BR	1 g	LR	Ampicillin stable for 24 hr at 25 °C	87	**C**
		50 and 100 mg	BR	1 g	LR	14% ampicillin loss in 12 hr at 25 °C	87	**I**
		200 mg	BE	20 g	D–S	32% ampicillin loss in 6 hr at 25 °C	89	**I**
		200 mg	BE	20 g	D5W	23% ampicillin loss in 6 hr at 25 °C	89	**I**
		200 mg	BE	20 g	NS	18% ampicillin loss in 6 hr at 25 °C	89	**I**
		1.8 g	BR	1 g	D5S, D10W, IM, IP, LR	11 to 28% ampicillin loss in 24 hr at 25 °C	87	**I**
		1.8 g	BR	1 g	D5S, D5W, D10W, IM, IP, LR, NS	Ampicillin stable for 24 hr at 4 °C	87	**C**
Lincomycin HCl						Physically compatible for 24 hr at room temperature	1	**C**
Metronidazole	SE	5 g	BR	20 g		9% ampicillin loss in 22 hr at 25 °C and in 12 days at 5 °C. No metronidazole loss	993	**C**
Prochlorperazine mesylate	BP	100 mg	BP	2 g	D5W, NS	Precipitates immediately	26	**I**
Ranitidine HCl	GL	100 mg		2 g	D5W	Physically compatible for 24 hr at ambient temperature under fluorescent light. Ampicillin instability is determining factor	1151	**?**
	GL	50 mg and 2 g		1 g	NS	Physically compatible. Ranitidine stable for 24 hr at 25 °C. Ampicillin not tested	1515	**C**
Sodium bicarbonate		1.4%	AY	2 and 4 g		10% ampicillin loss in 6 hr at room temperature	99	**I**

Additive Compatibility (Cont.)

Ampicillin sodium

Drug	Mfr	Conc/L	Mfr	Conc/L	Test Soln	Remarks	Ref	C/I
		1.4%	BAY	15 g		10% ampicillin loss in 10 hr at 25 °C	604	I
		1.4%	BAY	2 g		10% ampicillin loss in 17 hr at 25 °C	604	I
		1.4%	BAY	5 g		10% ampicillin loss in 14 hr at 25 °C	604	I
Verapamil HCl	KN	80 mg	BR	4 g	D5W, NS	Physically compatible for 24 hr	764	C
	SE	c	WY	40 g	D5W, NS	Cloudy solution clears with agitation	1166	?

[a]Tested in PVC containers.
[b]Refer to Appendix I for the composition of parenteral nutrition solutions. TPN indicates a 2-in-1 admixture.
[c]Final concentration unspecified.

Drugs in Syringe Compatibility

Ampicillin sodium

Drug (in syringe)	Mfr	Amt	Mfr	Amt	Remarks	Ref	C/I
Chloramphenicol sodium succinate	PD	250 and 400 mg/mL in 1.5 to 2 mL	AY	500 mg	No precipitate or color change within 1 hr at room temperature	99	C
	PD	250 and 400 mg/1 mL	AY	500 mg	Physically compatible for 1 hr at room temperature	300	C
Colistimethate sodium	PX	40 mg/2 mL	AY	500 mg	No precipitate or color change within 1 hr at room temperature	99	C
	PX	500 mg/2 mL	AY	500 mg	Physically compatible for 1 hr at room temperature	300	C
Dimenhydrinate		10 mg/1 mL		50 mg/1 mL	Clear solution	2569	C
Erythromycin lactobionate	AB	300 mg/6 mL	AY	500 mg	Precipitate forms in 1 hr at room temperature	300	I
Gentamicin sulfate		80 mg/2 mL	AY	500 mg	Physically incompatible within 1 hr at room temperature	99	I
Heparin sodium		2500 units/1 mL		2 g	Physically compatible for at least 5 min	1053	C
Hydromorphone HCl	KN	2, 10, 40 mg/1 mL	AY	250 mg/1 mL	Visually compatible but 10% loss of ampicillin in 5 hr at room temperature	2082	I
Iohexol	WI	64.7%, 5 mL	BR	30 mg/1 mL	Physically compatible for at least 2 hr	1438	C
Iopamidol	SQ	61%, 5 mL	BR	30 mg/1 mL	Physically compatible for at least 2 hr	1438	C
Iothalamate meglumine	MA	60%, 5 mL	BR	30 mg/1 mL	Physically compatible for at least 2 hr	1438	C
Ioxaglate meglumine–ioxaglate sodium	MA	5 mL	BR	30 mg/1 mL	Physically compatible for at least 2 hr	1438	C
Lidocaine HCl		0.5 and 2.5% in 1.5 mL	BE	500 mg	Physically compatible	89	C

Drugs in Syringe Compatibility (Cont.)

Ampicillin sodium

Drug (in syringe)	Mfr	Amt	Mfr	Amt	Remarks	Ref	C/I
		0.5 and 2.5% in 1.5 mL	BE	250 mg	Occasional turbidity	89	I
Lincomycin HCl	UP	600 mg/ 2 mL	AY	500 mg	Physically incompatible within 1 hr at room temperature	99	I
	UP	600 mg/ 2 mL	AY	500 mg	Precipitate forms within 1 hr at room temperature	300	I
Metoclopramide HCl	RB	10 mg/ 2 mL	BR	250 mg/ 2.5 mL	Incompatible. If mixed, use immediately	1167	I
	RB	10 mg/ 2 mL	BR	1 g/ 10 mL	Incompatible. If mixed, use immediately	1167	I
	RB	160 mg/ 32 mL	BR	1 g/ 10 mL	Incompatible. If mixed, use immediately	1167	I
Pantoprazole sodium	[a]	4 mg/ 1 mL		250 mg/ 1 mL	Clear solution	2574	C
Polymyxin B sulfate	BW	25 mg/ 1.5 mL	AY	500 mg	Physically compatible for 1 hr at room temperature	300	C
	BW	25 mg/ 1.5 mL	AY	250 mg	Precipitate forms within 1 hr at room temperature	300	I
Streptomycin sulfate		1 g/2 mL	AY	500 mg	No precipitate or color change within 1 hr at room temperature	99	C
	BP	1 g/2 mL	AY	500 mg	Physically compatible for 1 hr at room temperature	300	C
	BP	1 g/ 1.5 mL	AY	500 mg	Syrupy solution forms	300	I

[a]*Test performed using the formulation WITHOUT edetate disodium.*

Y-Site Injection Compatibility (1:1 Mixture)

Ampicillin sodium

Drug	Mfr	Conc	Mfr	Conc	Remarks	Ref	C/I
Acyclovir sodium	BW	5 mg/mL[a]	WY	20 mg/mL[b]	Physically compatible for 4 hr at 25 °C	1157	C
Alprostadil	BED	7.5 mcg/mL[m]	SQ	100 mg/mL[n]	Visually compatible for 1 hr	2746	C
Amifostine	USB	10 mg/mL[a]	WY	20 mg/mL[b]	Physically compatible for 4 hr at 23 °C	1845	C
Amphotericin B cholesteryl sulfate complex	SEQ	0.83 mg/mL[a]	SKB	20 mg/mL[b]	Gross precipitate forms	2117	I
Anidulafungin	VIC	0.5 mg/mL[a]	APC	20 mg/mL[b]	Physically compatible for 4 hr at 23 °C	2617	C
Aztreonam	SQ	40 mg/mL[a]	WY	20 mg/mL[b]	Physically compatible for 4 hr at 23 °C	1758	C
Bivalirudin	TMC	5 mg/mL[a]	APO	20 mg/mL[b]	Physically compatible for 4 hr at 23 °C	2373	C
Calcium gluconate	AST	4 mg/mL[b]	WY	40 mg/mL[b]	Physically compatible for 3 hr	1316	C
	AST	4 mg/mL[a]	WY	40 mg/mL[b]	Slight color change in 1 hr	1316	I
Caspofungin acetate	ME	0.7 mg/mL[b]	APP	20 mg/mL[b]	Immediate white turbid precipitate forms	2758	I
Cisatracurium besylate	GW	0.1 and 2 mg/ mL[a]	SKB	20 mg/mL[b]	Physically compatible for 4 hr at 23 °C	2074	C
	GW	5 mg/mL[a]	SKB	20 mg/mL[b]	Gray subvisible haze forms in 1 hr	2074	I
Clarithromycin	AB	4 mg/mL[a]	BE	40 mg/mL[a]	Visually compatible for 72 hr at both 30 and 17 °C	2174	C

Y-Site Injection Compatibility (1:1 Mixture) (Cont.)

Ampicillin sodium

Drug	Mfr	Conc	Mfr	Conc	Remarks	Ref	C/I
Cyclophosphamide	MJ	20 mg/mL[a]	BR	20 mg/mL[b]	Physically compatible for 4 hr at 25 °C	1194	C
Dexmedetomidine HCl	AB	4 mcg/mL[b]	APO	20 mg/mL[b]	Physically compatible for 4 hr at 23 °C	2383	C
Diltiazem HCl	MMD	5 mg/mL	WY	100 mg/mL[b]	Cloudiness forms	1807	I
	MMD	1 mg/mL[b]	WY	100 mg/mL[b]	Visually compatible	1807	C
	MMD	5 mg/mL	WY	10 and 20 mg/mL[b]	Visually compatible	1807	C
Docetaxel	RPR	0.9 mg/mL[a]	SKB	20 mg/mL[b]	Physically compatible for 4 hr at 23 °C	2224	C
Doxapram HCl	RB	2 mg/mL[a]	APO	50 mg/mL[b]	Visually compatible for 4 hr at 23 °C	2470	C
Doxorubicin HCl liposomal	SEQ	0.4 mg/mL[a]	SKB	20 mg/mL[b]	Physically compatible for 4 hr at 23 °C	2087	C
Enalaprilat	MSD	0.05 mg/mL[b]	BR	10 mg/mL[b]	Physically compatible for 24 hr at room temperature under fluorescent light	1355	C
Epinephrine HCl	ES	32 mcg/mL[c]	WY	40 mg/mL[b]	Slight color change in 3 hr	1316	I
Esmolol HCl	DCC	10 mg/mL[a]	WY	20 mg/mL[b]	Physically compatible for 24 hr at 22 °C	1169	C
Etoposide phosphate	BR	5 mg/mL[a]	APC	20 mg/mL[b]	Physically compatible for 4 hr at 23 °C	2218	C
Famotidine	MSD	0.2 mg/mL[a]	ES	20 mg/mL[b]	Physically compatible for 14 hr	1196	C
	ME	2 mg/mL[b]		20 mg/mL[b]	Visually compatible for 4 hr at 22 °C	1936	C
Fenoldopam mesylate	AB	80 mcg/mL[b]	APO	20 mg/mL[b]	Yellow color forms in 4 hr	2467	I
Filgrastim	AMG	30 mcg/mL[a]	WY	20 mg/mL[a]	Physically compatible for 4 hr at 22 °C	1687	C
Fluconazole	RR	2 mg/mL	WY	20 mg/mL	Cloudiness develops	1407	I
Fludarabine phosphate	BX	1 mg/mL[a]	BR	20 mg/mL[b]	Visually compatible for 4 hr at 22 °C	1439	C
Foscarnet sodium	AST	24 mg/mL	WY	20 mg/mL	Physically compatible for 24 hr at room temperature under fluorescent light	1335	C
Gemcitabine HCl	LI	10 mg/mL[b]	SKB	20 mg/mL[b]	Physically compatible for 4 hr at 23 °C	2226	C
Granisetron HCl	SKB	0.05 mg/mL[a]	MAR	20 mg/mL[b]	Physically compatible for 4 hr at 23 °C	2000	C
Heparin sodium	TR	50 units/mL	WY	20 mg/mL[b]	Visually compatible for 4 hr at 25 °C	1793	C
	LEO	10 and 5000 units/mL[b]	NOP	10 mg/mL[b]	Physically compatible with little change in heparin activity in 14 days at 4 and 37 °C. Antibiotic not tested	2684	C
Heparin sodium[o]	RI	1000 units/L[d]	BR	25, 50, 100, 125 mg/mL	Physically compatible for 4 hr at room temperature	322	C
Hetastarch in lactated electrolyte	AB	6%	APC	20 mg/mL[b]	Physically compatible for 4 hr at 23 °C	2339	C
Hetastarch in sodium chloride 0.9%	DCC	6%	BR	20 mg/mL[a]	Visually compatible for 4 hr at room temperature	1313	C
	DCC	6%	BR	20 mg/mL[a]	One or two particles in one of five vials. Fine white strands appeared immediately during Y-site infusion	1315	I
Hydralazine HCl	SO	1 mg/mL[b]	WY	40 mg/mL[b]	Moderate color change in 3 hr	1316	I
	SO	1 mg/mL[a]	WY	40 mg/mL[b]	Moderate color change in 1 hr	1316	I
Hydrocortisone sodium succinate[p]	UP	100 mg/L[d]	BR	25, 50, 100, 125 mg/mL	Physically compatible for 4 hr at room temperature	322	C
Hydromorphone HCl	WY	0.2 mg/mL[a]	BR	20 mg/mL[b]	Physically compatible for 4 hr at 25 °C	987	C
	KN	2, 10, 40 mg/mL	AY	20[a] and 250 mg/mL	Visually compatible. Hydromorphone stable for 24 hr. 10% ampicillin loss in 5 hr	1532	I

Y-Site Injection Compatibility (1:1 Mixture) (Cont.)

Ampicillin sodium

Drug	Mfr	Conc	Mfr	Conc	Remarks	Ref	C/I
Hydroxyethyl starch 130/0.4 in sodium chloride 0.9%	FRK	6%	NOP	10, 25, 40 mg/mL[a]	Visually compatible for 24 hr at room temperature	2770	C
Insulin, regular	LI	0.2 unit/mL[b]	WY	20 mg/mL[b]	Physically compatible for 2 hr at 25 °C	1395	C
Labetalol HCl	SC	1 mg/mL[a]	WY	10 mg/mL[b]	Physically compatible for 24 hr at 18 °C	1171	C
Levofloxacin	OMN	5 mg/mL[a]	MAR	50 mg/mL	Visually compatible for 4 hr at 24 °C	2233	C
Linezolid	PHU	2 mg/mL	APC	20 mg/mL[b]	Physically compatible for 4 hr at 23 °C	2264	C
Magnesium sulfate	IX	16.7, 33.3, 66.7, 100 mg/ mL[a]	WY	20 mg/mL[b]	Physically compatible for at least 4 hr at 32 °C	813	C
Melphalan HCl	BW	0.1 mg/mL[b]	WY	20 mg/mL[b]	Physically compatible for 3 hr at 22 °C	1557	C
Meperidine HCl	WY	10 mg/mL[a]	BR	20 mg/mL[b]	Physically compatible for 4 hr at 25 °C	987	C
Midazolam HCl	RC	1 mg/mL[a]	WY	20 mg/mL[b]	Haze forms immediately	1847	I
Milrinone lactate	SS	0.2 mg/mL[a]	APO	100 mg/mL[b]	Visually compatible for 4 hr at 25 °C	2381	C
Morphine sulfate	WI	1 mg/mL[a]	BR	20 mg/mL[b]	Physically compatible for 4 hr at 25 °C	987	C
Multivitamins	USV	5 mL/L[a]	AY	1 g/50 mL[c]	Physically compatible for 24 hr at room temperature	323	C
Nicardipine HCl	DCC	0.1 mg/mL[a,b]	BR	10 mg/mL[a,b]	Turbidity forms immediately	235	I
Ondansetron HCl	GL	1 mg/mL[b]	BR	20 mg/mL[b]	Immediate turbidity and precipitation	1365	I
Pantoprazole sodium	ALT[l]	0.16 to 0.8 mg/mL[b]	NVP	10 to 40 mg/ mL[a]	Visually compatible for 12 hr at 23 °C	2603	C
Pemetrexed disodium	LI	20 mg/mL[b]	APC	20 mg/mL[b]	Physically compatible for 4 hr at 23 °C	2564	C
Phytonadione	MSD	0.4 mg/mL[c]	WY	40 mg/mL[b]	Physically compatible for 3 hr	1316	C
Potassium chloride		40 mEq/L[d]	BR	25, 50, 100, 125 mg/mL	Physically compatible for 4 hr at room temperature	322	C
Propofol	ZEN	10 mg/mL	WY	20 mg/mL[b]	Physically compatible for 1 hr at 23 °C	2066	C
Remifentanil HCl	GW	0.025 and 0.25 mg/mL[b]	SKB	20 mg/mL[b]	Physically compatible for 4 hr at 23 °C	2075	C
Sargramostim	IMM	10 mcg/mL[b]	BR	20 mg/mL[b]	Few small particles form in 4 hr	1436	I
Tacrolimus	FUJ	1 mg/mL[b]	WY	20 mg/mL[a]	Visually compatible for 24 hr at 25 °C	1630	C
Teniposide	BR	0.1 mg/mL[a]	WY	20 mg/mL[b]	Physically compatible for 4 hr at 23 °C	1725	C
Theophylline	TR	4 mg/mL	WY	20 mg/mL[b]	Visually compatible for 6 hr at 25 °C	1793	C
Thiotepa	IMM[e]	1 mg/mL[a]	WY	20 mg/mL[b]	Physically compatible for 4 hr at 23 °C	1861	C
TNA #73[f]		32.5 mL[g]	BR	40 mg/mL[b]	Visually compatible for 4 hr at 25 °C	1008	C
TNA #218 to #226[f]			SKB	20 mg/mL[b]	Visually compatible for 4 hr at 23 °C	2215	C
TPN #54[f]					Precipitate forms within 30 min at 22 °C	1045	I
TPN #61[f]		[h]	WY	250 mg/ 1.3 mL[i]	Heavy precipitate of calcium phosphate	1012	I
		[j]	WY	1.5 g/7.5 mL[i]	Heavy precipitate of calcium phosphate	1012	I
TPN #203, #204[f]			APC	100 and 250 mg/mL	White precipitate forms immediately	1974	I
TPN #212 to #215[f]			SKB	20 mg/mL[b]	Visually compatible for 4 hr at 23 °C	2109	C

Y-Site Injection Compatibility (1:1 Mixture) (Cont.)

Ampicillin sodium

Drug	Mfr	Conc	Mfr	Conc	Remarks	Ref	C/I
Vancomycin HCl	AB	20 mg/mL[a]	SKB	250 mg/mL[k]	Transient precipitate forms	2189	?
	AB	20 mg/mL[a]	SKB	1, 10, 50 mg/mL[b]	Physically compatible for 4 hr at 23 °C	2189	C
	AB	2 mg/mL[a]	SKB	1[b], 10[b], 50[b], 250[k] mg/mL	Physically compatible for 4 hr at 23 °C	2189	C
Verapamil HCl	SE	2.5 mg/mL	WY	40 mg/mL[c]	White precipitate forms immediately. 91% of verapamil precipitated	1166	I
Vinorelbine tartrate	BW	1 mg/mL[b]	WY	20 mg/mL[b]	Tiny particles form immediately. White particles in turbidity in 1 hr	1558	I

[a] *Tested in dextrose 5%.*
[b] *Tested in sodium chloride 0.9%.*
[c] *Tested in both dextrose 5% and sodium chloride 0.9%.*
[d] *Tested in dextrose 5%, sodium chloride 0.9%, and Ringer's injection, lactated.*
[e] *Lyophilized formulation tested.*
[f] *Refer to Appendix I for the composition of parenteral nutrition solutions. TNA indicates a 3-in-1 admixture, and TPN indicates a 2-in-1 admixture.*
[g] *A 32.5-mL sample of parenteral nutrition solution mixed with 50 mL of antibiotic solution.*
[h] *Run at 21 mL/hr.*
[i] *Given over five minutes by syringe pump.*
[j] *Run at 94 mL/hr.*
[k] *Tested in sterile water for injection.*
[l] *Test performed using the formulation WITHOUT edetate disodium.*
[m] *Tested in either dextrose 5% or in sodium chloride 0.9%, but the report did not specify which solution.*
[n] *Tested in a 1:1 mixture of (1) dextrose 5% and dextrose 5% in sodium chloride 0.45% with and without potassium chloride 20 mEq/L and also in (2) dextrose 10% in sodium chloride 0.45% with and without potassium chloride 20 mEq/L.*
[o] *Tested in combination with hydrocortisone sodium succinate (Upjohn) 100 mg/L*
[p] *Tested in combination with heparin sodium (Rikers) 1000 units/L*

AMPICILLIN SODIUM–SULBACTAM SODIUM
AHFS 8:12.16.08

Products — Ampicillin sodium–sulbactam sodium is available in vials and piggyback bottles containing 1.5 g (ampicillin 1 g plus sulbactam 0.5 g) or 3 g (ampicillin 2 g plus sulbactam 1 g) as the sodium salts. (1)

For intramuscular injection, reconstitute vials with sterile water for injection or lidocaine hydrochloride 0.5 or 2% in the following amounts (1):

Vial Size	Volume of Diluent	Withdrawable Volume	Concentration
1.5 g	3.2 mL	4 mL[a]	375 mg/mL[b]
3.0 g	6.4 mL	8 mL[a]	375 mg/mL[b]

[a] *Sufficient excess is present to permit withdrawal of the volume noted.*
[b] *Ampicillin 250 mg plus sulbactam 125 mg per milliliter.*

For intravenous use, reconstitute piggyback bottles directly with a compatible diluent to the desired concentration between 3 and 45 mg/mL (ampicillin 2 to 30 mg plus sulbactam 1 to 15 mg per milliliter). Standard vials of 1.5 and 3 g may be reconstituted with 3.2 and 6.4 mL of sterile water for injection, respectively, to yield 375-mg/mL solutions (ampicillin 250 mg plus sulbactam 125 mg per milliliter). The reconstituted solution should be diluted immediately in a compatible infusion solution to yield the desired concentration between 3 and 45 mg/mL. (1)

Allow reconstituted solutions to stand so that any foaming may dissipate before inspecting them visually to ensure complete dissolution. (1)

pH — From 8 to 10. (1)

Sodium Content — Each 1.5 g (ampicillin 1 g plus sulbactam 0.5 g as the sodium salts) contains 5 mEq (115 mg) of sodium. (1)

Trade Name(s) — Unasyn.

Administration — Ampicillin sodium–sulbactam sodium may be administered by deep intramuscular injection or intravenous injection or infusion. By direct intravenous injection, the drug should be given slowly over at least 10 to 15 minutes. By infusion, it may be diluted in 50 to 100 mL of compatible diluent and infused over 15 to 30 minutes. (1; 4)

Stability — Intact vials of the white to off-white powder should be stored at room temperature. Aqueous solutions are pale yellow to yellow. Dilute solutions are pale yellow to colorless. The manufacturer recommends that intramuscular solutions be used within one hour after preparation. The administration of diluted solutions for intravenous infusion should be completed within eight hours of preparation to ensure that the potency is maintained throughout the infusion. (1; 4)

Central Venous Catheter — Ampicillin sodium–sulbactam sodium (Pfizer-Roerig) 5 + 2.5 mg/mL in sodium chloride 0.9% was found to be compatible with the ARROWg+ard Blue Plus (Arrow International) chlorhexidine-bearing triple-lumen central catheter. Essentially complete delivery of the drug was found with little or no drug loss occurring. Furthermore, chlorhexidine delivered from the catheter remained at trace amounts with no substantial increase due to the delivery of the drug through the catheter. (2335)

Compatibility Information

Solution Compatibility

Ampicillin sodium–sulbactam sodium

Solution	Mfr	Mfr	Conc/L	Remarks	Ref	C/I
Dextrose 5% in sodium chloride 0.45%			20 + 10 g, 10 + 5 g	Stable for only 4 hr at 4 and 25 °C	1	I
Dextrose 5%			2 + 1 g	Stable for only 4 hr at 25 °C	1	I
			20 + 10 g	Stable for only 4 hr at 4 °C and 2 hr at 25 °C	1	I
Ringer's injection, lactated			30 + 15 g	Stable for 24 hr at 4 °C but only 8 hr at 25 °C	1	I
Sodium chloride 0.9%			30 + 15 g	Stable for 48 hr at 4 °C and 8 hr at 25 °C	1	C
	[a]	PF	20 + 10 g	Visually compatible with 10% loss in 32 hr at 24 °C and 68 hr at 5 °C	1691	C
Sodium lactate ⅙ M			30 + 15 g	Stable for only 8 hr at 4 and 25 °C	1	I

[a]*Tested in PVC containers.*

Additive Compatibility

Ampicillin sodium–sulbactam sodium

Drug	Mfr	Conc/L	Mfr	Conc/L	Test Soln	Remarks	Ref	C/I
Aztreonam	SQ	10 g	PF	20 + 10 g	NS[a]	Visually compatible with 10% ampicillin loss in 30 hr at 24 °C and 94 hr at 5 °C. Ampicillin loss is determining factor	1691	C
Ciprofloxacin	MI	2 g		20 + 10 g	D5W	Physically incompatible	888	I
	BAY	2 g	RR	20 + 10 g	D5W	Precipitates immediately	2413	I
Tramadol HCl	GRU	400 mg	PF	20 + 10 g	NS	Visually compatible with up to 9% tramadol loss in 24 hr at room temperature	2652	C

[a]*Tested in PVC containers.*

Y-Site Injection Compatibility (1:1 Mixture)

Ampicillin sodium–sulbactam sodium

Drug	Mfr	Conc	Mfr	Conc	Remarks	Ref	C/I
Amifostine	USB	10 mg/mL[a]	RR	20 + 10 mg/mL[b]	Physically compatible for 4 hr at 23 °C	1845	C
Amiodarone HCl	WY	6 mg/mL[a]	PF	30 mg/mL[b]	Immediate opaque white turbidity	2352	I
Amphotericin B cholesteryl sulfate complex	SEQ	0.83 mg/mL[a]	RR	20 + 10 mg/mL[b]	Gross precipitate forms	2117	I
Anidulafungin	VIC	0.5 mg/mL[a]	LE	20 + 10 mg/mL[b]	Physically compatible for 4 hr at 23 °C	2617	C
Aztreonam	SQ	40 mg/mL[a]	RR	20 + 10 mg/mL[b]	Physically compatible for 4 hr at 23 °C	1758	C
Bivalirudin	TMC	5 mg/mL[a]	PF	20 + 10 mg/mL[b]	Physically compatible for 4 hr at 23 °C	2373	C
Ciprofloxacin		400 mg[c]		3 + 1.5 g[c]	White crystals form immediately when administered sequentially through a Y-site into running D5S	1887	I
Cisatracurium besylate	GW	0.1 and 2 mg/mL[a]	RR	20 + 10 mg/mL[b]	Physically compatible for 4 hr at 23 °C	2074	C
	GW	5 mg/mL[a]	RR	20 + 10 mg/mL[b]	Subvisible haze develops in 15 min	2074	I
Dexmedetomidine HCl	AB	4 mcg/mL[b]	PF	20 + 10 mg/mL[b]	Physically compatible for 4 hr at 23 °C	2383	C
Diltiazem HCl	MMD	5 mg/mL	RR	45 + 22.5 mg/mL[b]	Cloudiness forms	1807	I
	MMD	1 mg/mL[b]	RR	45 + 22.5 mg/mL[b]	Visually compatible	1807	C
	MMD	5 mg/mL	RR	2 + 1 and 15 + 7.5 mg/mL[b]	Visually compatible	1807	C
Docetaxel	RPR	0.9 mg/mL[a]	RR	20 + 10 mg/mL[b]	Physically compatible for 4 hr at 23 °C	2224	C
Enalaprilat	MSD	0.05 mg/mL[b]	PF	10 + 5 mg/mL[b]	Physically compatible for 24 hr at room temperature under fluorescent light	1355	C
Etoposide phosphate	BR	5 mg/mL[a]	RR	20 + 10 mg/mL[b]	Physically compatible for 4 hr at 23 °C	2218	C
Famotidine	MSD	0.2 mg/mL[a]	RR	20 + 10 mg/mL[b]	Physically compatible for 14 hr	1196	C
Fenoldopam mesylate	AB	80 mcg/mL[b]	PF	20 + 10 mg/mL[b]	Physically compatible for 4 hr at 23 °C	2467	C
Filgrastim	AMG	30 mcg/mL[a]	RR	20 + 10 mg/mL[a]	Physically compatible for 4 hr at 22 °C	1687	C
Fluconazole	RR	2 mg/mL	PF	40 + 20 mg/mL	Physically compatible for 24 hr at 25 °C	1407	C
Fludarabine phosphate	BX	1 mg/mL[a]	RR	20 + 10 mg/mL[b]	Visually compatible for 4 hr at 22 °C	1439	C
Gallium nitrate	FUJ	1 mg/mL[b]	RR	45 + 22.5 mg/mL[b]	Visually compatible for 24 hr at 25 °C	1673	C
Gemcitabine HCl	LI	10 mg/mL[b]	RR	20 + 10 mg/mL[b]	Physically compatible for 4 hr at 23 °C	2226	C

Y-Site Injection Compatibility (1:1 Mixture) (Cont.)

Ampicillin sodium–sulbactam sodium

Drug	Mfr	Conc	Mfr	Conc	Remarks	Ref	C/I
Granisetron HCl	SKB	0.05 mg/mL[a]	RR	20 + 10 mg/mL[b]	Physically compatible for 4 hr at 23 °C	2000	C
Heparin sodium	TR	50 units/mL	PF	20 + 10 mg/mL[b]	Visually compatible for 4 hr at 25 °C	1793	C
Hetastarch in lactated electrolyte	AB	6%	PF	20 + 10 mg/mL[b]	Physically compatible for 4 hr at 23 °C	2339	C
Idarubicin HCl	AD	1 mg/mL[b]	RR	20 + 10 mg/mL[b]	Haze forms and color changes immediately. Precipitate forms in 20 min	1525	I
Insulin, regular	LI	0.2 unit/mL[b]	RR	20 + 10 mg/mL[b]	Physically compatible for 2 hr at 25 °C	1395	C
Linezolid	PHU	2 mg/mL	PF	20 + 10 mg/mL[b]	Physically compatible for 4 hr at 23 °C	2264	C
Meperidine HCl	WY	10 mg/mL[b]	RR	20 + 10 mg/mL[b]	Physically compatible for 1 hr at 25 °C	1338	C
Morphine sulfate	ES	1 mg/mL[b]	RR	20 + 10 mg/mL[b]	Physically compatible for 1 hr at 25 °C	1338	C
Nicardipine HCl	DCC	0.1 mg/mL[a,b]	PF	10 + 5 mg/mL[a,b]	Turbidity forms immediately	235	I
Ondansetron HCl	GL	1 mg/mL[b]	RR	20 + 10 mg/mL[b]	Immediate turbidity and precipitation	1365	I
Paclitaxel	NCI	1.2 mg/mL[a]	RR	20 + 10 mg/mL[b]	Physically compatible for 4 hr at 22 °C	1556	C
Palonosetron HCl	MGI	50 mcg/mL	RR	20 + 10 mg/mL[b]	Physically compatible and no loss of either drug in 4 hr at room temperature	2749	C
Pemetrexed disodium	LI	20 mg/mL[b]	LE	20 + 10 mg/mL[b]	Physically compatible for 4 hr at 23 °C	2564	C
Remifentanil HCl	GW	0.025 and 0.25 mg/mL[b]	RR	20 + 10 mg/mL[b]	Physically compatible for 4 hr at 23 °C	2075	C
Sargramostim	IMM	10 mcg/mL[b]	RR	20 + 10 mg/mL[b]	Few small particles form in 4 hr	1436	I
Tacrolimus	FUJ	1 mg/mL[b]	RR	33.3 + 16.7 mg/mL[a]	Visually compatible for 24 hr at 25 °C	1630	C
Telavancin HCl	ASP	7.5 mg/mL[a,b,g]	BA	20 + 10 mg/mL[a,b,g]	Physically compatible for 2 hr	2830	C
Teniposide	BR	0.1 mg/mL[a]	RR	20 + 10 mg/mL[b]	Physically compatible for 4 hr at 23 °C	1725	C
Theophylline	TR	4 mg/mL	PF	20 + 10 mg/mL[b]	Visually compatible for 6 hr at 25 °C	1793	C
Thiotepa	IMM[d]	1 mg/mL[a]	RR	20 + 10 mg/mL[b]	Physically compatible for 4 hr at 23 °C	1861	C
TNA #218 to #226[e]			PF	20 + 10 mg/mL[b]	Visually compatible for 4 hr at 23 °C	2215	C
TPN #212 to #215[e]			RR	20 + 10 mg/mL[b]	Physically compatible for 4 hr at 23 °C	2109	C
Vancomycin HCl	AB	20 mg/mL[a]	PF	250 + 125 mg/mL[f]	Transient precipitate forms	2189	?

Y-Site Injection Compatibility (1:1 Mixture) (Cont.)

Ampicillin sodium–sulbactam sodium

Drug	Mfr	Conc	Mfr	Conc	Remarks	Ref	C/I
	AB	20 mg/mL[a]	PF	1 + 0.5, 10 + 5, 50 + 25 mg/mL[b]	Physically compatible for 4 hr at 23 °C	2189	C
	AB	2 mg/mL[a]	PF	1 + 0.5[b], 10 + 5[b], 50 + 25[b], 250 + 125[f] mg/mL	Physically compatible for 4 hr at 23 °C	2189	C

[a]*Tested in dextrose 5%.*
[b]*Tested in sodium chloride 0.9%.*
[c]*Concentration and volume not specified.*
[d]*Lyophilized formulation tested.*
[e]*Refer to Appendix I for the composition of parenteral nutrition solutions. TNA indicates a 3-in-1 admixture, and TPN indicates a 2-in-1 admixture.*
[f]*Tested in sterile water for injection.*
[g]*Tested in Ringer's injection, lactated.*

AMSACRINE
(ACRIDINYL ANISIDIDE; m-AMSA)
AHFS 10:00

Products — Amsacrine is available in ampuls containing 1.5 mL of a 50-mg/mL solution (75 mg total) in anhydrous *N,N*-dimethylacetamide (DMA). It is packaged with a vial containing 13.5 mL of 0.0353 M L-lactic acid diluent. (1)

To prepare the drug for use, aseptically add 1.5 mL of the amsacrine solution to the vial of L-lactic acid diluent. The resulting orange-red solution contains amsacrine 5 mg/mL in 10% (v/v) *N,N*-dimethylacetamide and 0.0318 M L-lactic acid. This concentrated solution must be diluted in dextrose 5% for infusion; do not use chloride-containing solutions. (1)

Direct contact of amsacrine solutions with skin or mucous membranes may result in skin sensitization and should be avoided. (234)

Trade Name(s) — Amsidine, Amsidyl.

Administration — Amsacrine is administered by central vein infusion over 60 to 90 minutes after the dose is diluted in 500 mL of dextrose 5%. (1)

Stability — Amsacrine in intact ampuls should be stored at room temperature. (1) When mixed with the L-lactic acid diluent, the amsacrine solution is physically and chemically stable for at least 48 hours at room temperature under ambient light. (234)

Light Effects — The effect of diffuse daylight and fluorescent light on amsacrine 150 mcg/mL in dextrose 5% was studied for 48 hours at 19 to 21 °C; no loss due to light exposure occurred. (1308)

Syringes — Glass syringes are recommended for the transfer of amsacrine concentrate to the L-lactic acid diluent. (115) The DMA solvent may extract UV-absorbing species from plastics and rubber. (967)

The compatibility of amsacrine (Gödecke) concentrated solution in DMA with rubber-free plastic syringes (Injekt, B. Braun) was evaluated at 37 °C and ambient temperature. Storage of the DMA diluent in the plastic syringes resulted in no visible changes to the drug or syringes and did not adversely affect the performance of the syringes. Analysis found a trace amount of oleic acid amide lubricant, about 50 mcg in the 2-mL syringe content, after storage for 24 hours at 37 °C. Storage at ambient temperature resulted in substantially lower amounts of oleic acid amide. The authors concluded the rubber-free Injekt plastic syringes were acceptable alternatives to glass syringes to transfer the amsacrine concentrate. Other plastic syringes incorporating rubber components are not recommended because of the extraction of materials into the drug solution. (2284)

Sorption — Amsacrine 150 mcg/mL in dextrose 5% did not undergo sorption to cellulose propionate and methacrylate butadiene styrene burette chambers and PVC and polybutadiene tubing. (1308)

Compatibility Information

Solution Compatibility

Amsacrine

Solution	Mfr	Mfr	Conc/L	Remarks	Ref	C/I
Dextrose 5%		PD	150 mg[a]	Physically compatible with little or no loss in 48 hr at 20 °C exposed to light	1308	C
		NCI	150 mg	Physically and chemically stable for 48 hours at room temperature in light	234	C
Sodium chloride 0.9%				Amsacrine is incompatible with chloride-containing solutions	1	I

[a]Tested in burette chambers composed of cellulose propionate or methacrylate butadiene styrene.

Additive Compatibility

Amsacrine

Drug	Mfr	Conc/L	Mfr	Conc/L	Test Soln	Remarks	Ref	C/I
Sodium bicarbonate		2 mEq	NCI	[a]	D5W	Amsacrine chemically stable for 96 hr at room temperature	234	C

[a]Concentration unspecified.

Y-Site Injection Compatibility (1:1 Mixture)

Amsacrine

Drug	Mfr	Conc	Mfr	Conc	Remarks	Ref	C/I
Acyclovir sodium	BW	7 mg/mL[a]	NCI	1 mg/mL[a]	Immediate dark orange turbidity, becoming brownish orange in 1 hr	1381	I
Amikacin sulfate	BR	5 mg/mL[a]	NCI	1 mg/mL[a]	Visually compatible for 4 hr at 22 °C	1381	C
Amphotericin B	SQ	0.6 mg/mL[a]	NCI	1 mg/mL[a]	Immediate yellow turbidity, becoming yellow flocculent precipitate in 15 min	1381	I
Aztreonam	SQ	40 mg/mL[a]	NCI	1 mg/mL[a]	Immediate yellow-orange turbidity, becoming a precipitate in 4 hr	1381	I
Ceftazidime	GL	40 mg/mL[a]	NCI	1 mg/mL[a]	Immediate orange precipitate	1381	I
Ceftriaxone sodium	RC	40 mg/mL[a]	NCI	1 mg/mL[a]	Immediate orange turbidity, developing into flocculent precipitate in 4 hr	1381	I
Chlorpromazine HCl	ES	2 mg/mL[a]	NCI	1 mg/mL[a]	Visually compatible for 4 hr at 22 °C	1381	C
Clindamycin phosphate	UP	10 mg/mL[a]	NCI	1 mg/mL[a]	Visually compatible for 4 hr at 22 °C	1381	C
Cytarabine	QU	50 mg/mL	NCI	1 mg/mL[a]	Visually compatible for 4 hr at 22 °C	1381	C
Dexamethasone sodium phosphate	QU	1 mg/mL[a]	NCI	1 mg/mL[a]	Visually compatible for 4 hr at 22 °C	1381	C
Diphenhydramine HCl	PD	2 mg/mL[a]	NCI	1 mg/mL[a]	Visually compatible for 4 hr at 22 °C	1381	C
Famotidine	MSD	2 mg/mL[a]	NCI	1 mg/mL[a]	Visually compatible for 4 hr at 22 °C	1381	C
Fludarabine phosphate	BX	1 mg/mL[a]	NCI	1 mg/mL[a]	Visually compatible for 4 hr at 22 °C	1439	C
Furosemide	ES	3 mg/mL[a]	NCI	1 mg/mL[a]	Yellow turbidity becoming colorless liquid with yellow precipitate	1381	I
Ganciclovir sodium	SY	20 mg/mL[a]	NCI	1 mg/mL[a]	Immediate dark orange turbidity	1381	I
Gentamicin sulfate	SO	5 mg/mL[a]	NCI	1 mg/mL[a]	Visually compatible for 4 hr at 22 °C	1381	C

Y-Site Injection Compatibility (1:1 Mixture) (Cont.)

Amsacrine

Drug	Mfr	Conc	Mfr	Conc	Remarks	Ref	C/I
Granisetron HCl	SKB	0.05 mg/mL[a]	NCI	1 mg/mL[a]	Physically compatible for 4 hr at 23 °C. Precipitate forms in 24 hr	2000	C
Haloperidol lactate	MN	0.2 mg/mL[a]	NCI	1 mg/mL[a]	Visually compatible for 4 hr at 22 °C	1381	C
Heparin sodium	SO	40 units/mL[a]	NCI	1 mg/mL[a]	Orange precipitate forms immediately	1381	I
Hydrocortisone sodium succinate	UP	1 mg/mL[a]	NCI	1 mg/mL[a]	Visually compatible for 4 hr at 22 °C	1381	C
Hydromorphone HCl	AST	0.5 mg/mL[a]	NCI	1 mg/mL[a]	Visually compatible for 4 hr at 22 °C	1381	C
Lorazepam	WY	0.1 mg/mL[a]	NCI	1 mg/mL[a]	Visually compatible for 4 hr at 22 °C	1381	C
Methylprednisolone sodium succinate	UP	5 mg/mL[a]	NCI	1 mg/mL[a]	Immediate orange turbidity and precipitate in 4 hr	1381	I
Metoclopramide HCl	RB	2.5 mg/mL[a]	NCI	1 mg/mL[a]	Orange turbidity becomes orange precipitate in 1 hr	1381	I
Morphine sulfate	ES	1 mg/mL[a]	NCI	1 mg/mL[a]	Visually compatible for 4 hr at 22 °C	1381	C
Ondansetron HCl	GL	1 mg/mL[a]	NCI	1 mg/mL[a]	Orange precipitate forms within 30 min	1365	I
Prochlorperazine edisylate	SKF	0.5 mg/mL[a]	NCI	1 mg/mL[a]	Visually compatible for 4 hr at 22 °C	1381	C
Promethazine HCl	ES	2 mg/mL[a]	NCI	1 mg/mL[a]	Visually compatible for 4 hr at 22 °C	1381	C
Ranitidine HCl	GL	2 mg/mL[a]	NCI	1 mg/mL[a]	Visually compatible for 4 hr at 22 °C	1381	C
Sargramostim	IMM	10 mcg/mL[a]	NCI	1 mg/mL[a]	Visually compatible for 4 hr at 22 °C	1436	C
	IMM	10 mcg/mL[b]	NCI	1 mg/mL[a]	Haze and yellow precipitate form	1436	I
Tobramycin sulfate	LI	5 mg/mL[a]	NCI	1 mg/mL[a]	Visually compatible for 4 hr at 22 °C	1381	C
Vancomycin HCl	LI	10 mg/mL[a]	NCI	1 mg/mL[a]	Visually compatible for 4 hr at 22 °C	1381	C

[a]Tested in dextrose 5%.
[b]Tested in sodium chloride 0.9%.

ANAKINRA
AHFS 92:20

Products — Anakinra is available in prefilled glass syringes containing 100 mg of drug in 0.67 mL of solution. The prefilled syringes have 27-gauge needles protected with latex rubber covers. Each syringe containing 0.67 mL of solution also contains sodium citrate 1.29 mg, sodium chloride 5.48 mg, disodium EDTA 0.12 mg, and 0.7 mg of polysorbate 80 in water for injection. (1)

pH — 6.5. (1)

Trade Name(s) — Kineret.

Administration — Anakinra is administered subcutaneously. (1)

Stability — Anakinra should be stored under refrigeration. Do not shake and protect from freezing and light. It contains no preservative and is for single use. Discard any unused portions. Visually inspect the syringes prior to use for discoloration or particulate matter and discard if either is found. (1)

Compatibility Information

Y-Site Injection Compatibility (1:1 Mixture)

Anakinra

Drug	Mfr	Conc	Mfr	Conc	Remarks	Ref	C/I
Aztreonam	BMS	20 mg/mL[b]	SYN	4 and 36 mg/mL[b]	Physically compatible. No aztreonam loss in 4 hr at 25 °C. Anakinra uncertain	2508	?

Y-Site Injection Compatibility (1:1 Mixture) (Cont.)

Anakinra

Drug	Mfr	Conc	Mfr	Conc	Remarks	Ref	C/I
Cefazolin sodium	GVA	15 mg/mL[b]	SYN	4 and 36 mg/mL[b]	Physically compatible. No cefazolin loss in 4 hr at 25 °C. Anakinra uncertain	2508	?
Cefotaxime sodium	HO	10 mg/mL[b]	SYN	4 and 36 mg/mL[b]	Physically compatible. No cefotaxime loss in 4 hr at 25 °C. Anakinra uncertain	2508	?
Cefoxitin sodium	ME	20 mg/mL[b]	SYN	4 and 36 mg/mL[b]	Physically compatible. No cefoxitin loss in 4 hr at 25 °C. Anakinra uncertain	2508	?
Ceftriaxone sodium	RC	20 mg/mL[a]	SYN	4 and 36 mg/mL[a]	Ceftriaxone stable. 10% anakinra loss in 30 min and 20% in 4 hr at 22 °C	2509	I
	RC	20 mg/mL[b]	SYN	4 and 36 mg/mL[b]	Physically compatible with no loss of either drug in 4 hr at 22 °C	2509	C
Clindamycin phosphate	AST	12 mg/mL[b]	SYN	4 and 36 mg/mL[b]	Physically compatible with little or no loss of either drug in 4 hr at 22 °C	2510	C
Famotidine		1 mg/mL[b]	SYN	4 and 36 mg/mL[b]	Physically compatible with little or no loss of either drug in 4 hr at 22 °C	2511	C
Fluconazole	PF	2 mg/mL[b]	SYN	4 and 36 mg/mL[b]	Physically compatible. No fluconazole loss in 4 hr at 25 °C. Anakinra uncertain	2508	?
Lorazepam	WY	0.1 mg/mL[b]	SYN	4 and 36 mg/mL[b]	Physically compatible with no loss of either drug in 4 hr at 22 °C	2512	C

[a]*Tested in dextrose 5%.*
[b]*Tested in sodium chloride 0.9%.*

ANIDULAFUNGIN
AHFS 8:14.16

Products — Anidulafungin is available in 50-mg vials with 50 mg of fructose, 250 mg of mannitol, 125 mg of polysorbate 80, 5.6 mg of tartaric acid, and sodium hydroxide and/or hydrochloric acid to adjust pH. Anidulafungin is also available in 100-mg vials with 100 mg of fructose, 500 mg of mannitol, 250 mg of polysorbate 80, 11.2 mg of tartaric acid, and sodium hydroxide and/or hydrochloric acid to adjust pH. The 50- and 100-mg vials of drug are accompanied by 15- and 30-mL vials, respectively, of a special diluent composed of 20% (w/w) dehydrated alcohol in water for use in reconstitution. (1)

Reconstitute the 50- and 100-mg vials with 15 and 30 mL, respectively, of the accompanying special diluent to yield a concentrated solution containing anidulafungin 3.33 mg/mL. This concentrate must be diluted in dextrose 5% or sodium chloride 0.9% for administration. The manufacturer recommends diluting 50-, 100-, and 200-mg quantities of anidulafungin in 50, 100, and 200 mL, respectively. (1)

Trade Name(s) — Eraxis.

Administration — Anidulafungin is administered by intravenous infusion at a rate not exceeding 1.1 mg/min after dilution in dextrose 5% or sodium chloride 0.9%. No other solution should be used. (1)

Stability — Intact vials of anidulafungin should be stored refrigerated and protected from freezing. (1)

The reconstituted anidulafungin solution should be stored at controlled room temperature and used within one hour after reconstitution. Anidulafungin diluted in dextrose 5% or sodium chloride 0.9% for infusion should also be stored refrigerated and used within 24 hours. The reconstituted and diluted solutions of anidulafungin should be protected from freezing. (1)

Compatibility Information

Y-Site Injection Compatibility (1:1 Mixture)

Anidulafungin

Drug	Mfr	Conc	Mfr	Conc	Remarks	Ref	C/I
Acyclovir sodium	APP	7 mg/mL[a]	VIC	0.5 mg/mL[a]	Physically compatible for 4 hr at 23 °C	2617	C
Amikacin sulfate	APC	5 mg/mL[a]	VIC	0.5 mg/mL[a]	Physically compatible for 4 hr at 23 °C	2617	C

Y-Site Injection Compatibility (1:1 Mixture) (Cont.)

Anidulafungin

Drug	Mfr	Conc	Mfr	Conc	Remarks	Ref	C/I
Aminophylline	AB	2.5 mg/mL[a]	VIC	0.5 mg/mL[a]	Physically compatible for 4 hr at 23 °C	2617	C
Amphotericin B	PHT	0.6 mg/mL[a]	VIC	0.5 mg/mL[a]	Measured haze went up immediately	2617	I
Amphotericin B lipid complex	ELN	1 mg/mL[a]	VIC	0.5 mg/mL[a]	Physically compatible for 4 hr at 23 °C	2617	C
Amphotericin B liposomal	FUJ	1 mg/mL[a]	VIC	0.5 mg/mL[a]	Physically compatible for 4 hr at 23 °C	2617	C
Ampicillin sodium	APC	20 mg/mL[b]	VIC	0.5 mg/mL[a]	Physically compatible for 4 hr at 23 °C	2617	C
Ampicillin sodium–sulbactam sodium	LE	20 + 10 mg/mL[b]	VIC	0.5 mg/mL[a]	Physically compatible for 4 hr at 23 °C	2617	C
Carboplatin	BMS	5 mg/mL[a]	VIC	0.5 mg/mL[a]	Physically compatible for 4 hr at 23 °C	2617	C
Cefazolin sodium	APC	20 mg/mL[a]	VIC	0.5 mg/mL[a]	Physically compatible for 4 hr at 23 °C	2617	C
Cefepime HCl	DUR	20 mg/mL[a]	VIC	0.5 mg/mL[a]	Physically compatible for 4 hr at 23 °C	2617	C
Cefoxitin sodium	APP	20 mg/mL[a]	VIC	0.5 mg/mL[a]	Physically compatible for 4 hr at 23 °C	2617	C
Ceftazidime	GSK	40 mg/mL[a]	VIC	0.5 mg/mL[a]	Physically compatible for 4 hr at 23 °C	2617	C
Ceftriaxone sodium	RC	20 mg/mL[a]	VIC	0.5 mg/mL[a]	Physically compatible for 4 hr at 23 °C	2617	C
Cefuroxime sodium	GSK	30 mg/mL[a]	VIC	0.5 mg/mL[a]	Physically compatible for 4 hr at 23 °C	2617	C
Ciprofloxacin	AB	2 mg/mL[a]	VIC	0.5 mg/mL[a]	Physically compatible for 4 hr at 23 °C	2617	C
Cisplatin	SIC	1 mg/mL[b]	VIC	0.5 mg/mL[a]	Physically compatible for 4 hr at 23 °C	2617	C
Clindamycin phosphate	AB	10 mg/mL[a]	VIC	0.5 mg/mL[a]	Physically compatible for 4 hr at 23 °C	2617	C
Cyclophosphamide	MJ	10 mg/mL[a]	VIC	0.5 mg/mL[a]	Physically compatible for 4 hr at 23 °C	2617	C
Cyclosporine	NOV	5 mg/mL[a]	VIC	0.5 mg/mL[a]	Physically compatible for 4 hr at 23 °C	2617	C
Cytarabine	BED	50 mg/mL	VIC	0.5 mg/mL[a]	Physically compatible for 4 hr at 23 °C	2617	C
Daunorubicin HCl	BED	1 mg/mL[a]	VIC	0.5 mg/mL[a]	Physically compatible for 4 hr at 23 °C	2617	C
Dexamethasone sodium phosphate	AMR	1 mg/mL[a]	VIC	0.5 mg/mL[a]	Physically compatible for 4 hr at 23 °C	2617	C
Digoxin	GW	0.25 mg/mL	VIC	0.5 mg/mL[a]	Physically compatible for 4 hr at 23 °C	2617	C
Dobutamine HCl	AB	4 mg/mL[a]	VIC	0.5 mg/mL[a]	Physically compatible for 4 hr at 23 °C	2617	C
Docetaxel	AVE	2 mg/mL[a]	VIC	0.5 mg/mL[a]	Physically compatible for 4 hr at 23 °C	2617	C
Dopamine HCl	AMR	3.2 mg/mL[a]	VIC	0.5 mg/mL[a]	Physically compatible for 4 hr at 23 °C	2617	C
Doripenem	JJ	5 mg/mL[a,b]	PF	0.5 mg/mL[a,b]	Physically compatible for 4 hr at 23 °C	2743	C
Doxorubicin HCl	GNS	2 mg/mL[a]	VIC	0.5 mg/mL[a]	Physically compatible for 4 hr at 23 °C	2617	C
Epinephrine HCl	AMR	50 mcg/mL	VIC	0.5 mg/mL[a]	Physically compatible for 4 hr at 23 °C	2617	C
Ertapenem sodium	ME	20 mg/mL[b]	VIC	0.5 mg/mL[a]	Microparticulates form immediately	2617	I
Erythromycin lactobionate	AB	5 mg/mL[b]	VIC	0.5 mg/mL[a]	Physically compatible for 4 hr at 23 °C	2617	C
Etoposide phosphate	BMS	5 mg/mL[a]	VIC	0.5 mg/mL[a]	Physically compatible for 4 hr at 23 °C	2617	C
Famotidine	BV	2 mg/mL[a]	VIC	0.5 mg/mL[a]	Physically compatible for 4 hr at 23 °C	2617	C
Fentanyl citrate	AB	50 mcg/mL	VIC	0.5 mg/mL[a]	Physically compatible for 4 hr at 23 °C	2617	C
Fluconazole	PF	2 mg/mL	VIC	0.5 mg/mL[a]	Physically compatible for 4 hr at 23 °C	2617	C
Fluorouracil	APP	16 mg/mL[a]	VIC	0.5 mg/mL[a]	Physically compatible for 4 hr at 23 °C	2617	C
Furosemide	AB	3 mg/mL[a]	VIC	0.5 mg/mL[a]	Physically compatible for 4 hr at 23 °C	2617	C
Ganciclovir sodium	RC	20 mg/mL[a]	VIC	0.5 mg/mL[a]	Physically compatible for 4 hr at 23 °C	2617	C
Gemcitabine HCl	LI	10 mg/mL[a]	VIC	0.5 mg/mL[a]	Physically compatible for 4 hr at 23 °C	2617	C

Y-Site Injection Compatibility (1:1 Mixture) (Cont.)

Anidulafungin

Drug	Mfr	Conc	Mfr	Conc	Remarks	Ref	C/I
Gentamicin sulfate	AB	5 mg/mL[a]	VIC	0.5 mg/mL[a]	Physically compatible for 4 hr at 23 °C	2617	C
Heparin sodium	AB	100 units/mL	VIC	0.5 mg/mL[a]	Physically compatible for 4 hr at 23 °C	2617	C
Hydrocortisone sodium succinate	PHU	1 mg/mL[a]	VIC	0.5 mg/mL[a]	Physically compatible for 4 hr at 23 °C	2617	C
Ifosfamide	BMS	25 mg/mL[a]	VIC	0.5 mg/mL[a]	Physically compatible for 4 hr at 23 °C	2617	C
Imipenem–cilastatin sodium	ME	5 mg/mL[b]	VIC	0.5 mg/mL[b]	Physically compatible for 4 hr at 23 °C	2617	C
Leucovorin calcium	BED	2 mg/mL[a]	VIC	0.5 mg/mL[a]	Physically compatible for 4 hr at 23 °C	2617	C
Levofloxacin	OMN	5 mg/mL[a]	VIC	0.5 mg/mL[a]	Physically compatible for 4 hr at 23 °C	2617	C
Linezolid	PH	2 mg/mL	VIC	0.5 mg/mL[a]	Physically compatible for 4 hr at 23 °C	2617	C
Meperidine HCl	AB	10 mg/mL[a]	VIC	0.5 mg/mL[a]	Physically compatible for 4 hr at 23 °C	2617	C
Meropenem	ASZ	2.5 mg/mL[b]	VIC	0.5 mg/mL[a]	Physically compatible for 4 hr at 23 °C	2617	C
Methylprednisolone sodium succinate	PH	5 mg/mL[a]	VIC	0.5 mg/mL[a]	Physically compatible for 4 hr at 23 °C	2617	C
Metronidazole	BA	5 mg/mL	VIC	0.5 mg/mL[a]	Physically compatible for 4 hr at 23 °C	2617	C
Midazolam HCl	BA	1 mg/mL[a]	VIC	0.5 mg/mL[a]	Physically compatible for 4 hr at 23 °C	2617	C
Morphine sulfate	ES	15 mg/mL	VIC	0.5 mg/mL[a]	Physically compatible for 4 hr at 23 °C	2617	C
Mycophenolate mofetil HCl	RC	6 mg/mL[a]	VIC	0.5 mg/mL[a]	Physically compatible for 4 hr at 23 °C	2617	C
Norepinephrine bitartrate	BED	0.12 mg/mL[a]	VIC	0.5 mg/mL[a]	Physically compatible for 4 hr at 23 °C	2617	C
Paclitaxel	MJ	0.6 mg/mL[a]	VIC	0.5 mg/mL[a]	Physically compatible for 4 hr at 23 °C	2617	C
Pantoprazole sodium	WAY[c]	0.4 mg/mL[a]	VIC	0.5 mg/mL[a]	Physically compatible for 4 hr at 23 °C	2617	C
Phenylephrine HCl	BA	1 mg/mL[a]	VIC	0.5 mg/mL[a]	Physically compatible for 4 hr at 23 °C	2617	C
Piperacillin sodium–tazobactam sodium	LE[c]	40 + 5 mg/mL[a]	VIC	0.5 mg/mL[a]	Physically compatible for 4 hr at 23 °C	2617	C
Potassium chloride	APP	0.1 mEq/mL[a]	VIC	0.5 mg/mL[a]	Physically compatible for 4 hr at 23 °C	2617	C
Quinupristin–dalfopristin	AVE	5 mg/mL[a]	VIC	0.5 mg/mL[a]	Physically compatible for 4 hr at 23 °C	2617	C
Ranitidine HCl	GSK	2 mg/mL[a]	VIC	0.5 mg/mL[a]	Physically compatible for 4 hr at 23 °C	2617	C
Sodium bicarbonate	APP	1 mEq/mL	VIC	0.5 mg/mL[a]	Haze increases immediately and microparticulates occur in 4 hr	2617	I
Tacrolimus	FUJ	20 mcg/mL[a]	VIC	0.5 mg/mL[a]	Physically compatible for 4 hr at 23 °C	2617	C
Ticarcillin disodium–clavulanate potassium	GSK	31 mg/mL[a]	VIC	0.5 mg/mL[a]	Physically compatible for 4 hr at 23 °C	2617	C
Tobramycin sulfate	AB	5 mg/mL[a]	VIC	0.5 mg/mL[a]	Physically compatible for 4 hr at 23 °C	2617	C
Trimethoprim–sulfamethoxazole	ES	0.8 + 4 mg/mL[a]	VIC	0.5 mg/mL[a]	Physically compatible for 4 hr at 23 °C	2617	C
Vancomycin HCl	APP	10 mg/mL[a]	VIC	0.5 mg/mL[a]	Physically compatible for 4 hr at 23 °C	2617	C
Vincristine sulfate	FAU	50 mcg/mL[a]	VIC	0.5 mg/mL[a]	Physically compatible for 4 hr at 23 °C	2617	C
Voriconazole	PF	4 mg/mL[a]	VIC	0.5 mg/mL[a]	Physically compatible for 4 hr at 23 °C	2617	C
Zidovudine	GSK	4 mg/mL[a]	VIC	0.5 mg/mL[a]	Physically compatible for 4 hr at 23 °C	2617	C

[a]Tested in dextrose 5%.
[b]Tested in sodium chloride 0.9%.
[c]Test performed using the formulation WITHOUT edetate disodium.

ANTIHEMOPHILIC FACTOR (RECOMBINANT)
AHFS 20:28.16

Products — Antihemophilic factor (recombinant) is available in forms prepared by differing processes. Helixate FS, Kogenate, and Kogenate FS are prepared using human factor VIII genes in baby hamster kidney cells while Advate, Recombinate, and ReFacto are prepared from human factor VIII genes in Chinese hamster ovary cells. The products are available in sizes of 250, 500, 1000, 2000, and 3000 international units (I.U.) with sterile water for injection diluent. The vials of drug are sealed under vacuum. (1; 4)

After reconstitution, Kogenate contains excipients of glycine 10 to 30 mg/mL, up to 500 mcg/1000 I.U. of imidazole, up to 600 mcg/1000 I.U. of polysorbate 80, calcium chloride 2 to 5 mM, human albumin 1 to 4 mg/mL, and sodium chloride. (1)

Helixate FS and Kogenate FS are formulated with sucrose. After reconstitution, the products contain excipients of sucrose 0.9 to 1.3%, L-histidine 18 to 23 mM, glycine 21 to 25 mg/mL, calcium chloride 2 to 3 mM, up to 35 mcg/mL of polysorbate 80, up to 20 mcg/1000 I.U. of imidazole, up to 5 mcg/1000 I.U. of tri-n-butyl phosphate. (1)

After reconstitution, Recombinate contains excipients of human albumin 12.5 mg/mL, calcium 0.2 mg/mL, polyethylene glycol 3350 1.5 mg/mL, histidine 55 mM, polysorbate 80 1.5 mcg/I.U., and sodium 0.18 mEq/mL. (1)

Reconstituted ReFacto contains excipients of sodium chloride, sucrose, L-histidine, calcium chloride, and polysorbate 80. (1)

To reconstitute, allow the vials to come to room temperature, and use the transfer needle provided or syringe and needle to transfer the diluent into the vial of drug. The vacuum will draw in the diluent. Direct the stream against the vial wall and avoid excessive foaming. Incomplete diluent transfer warrants discarding the vial. Remove the transfer needle and swirl the vial with gentle agitation to dissolve the powder. It should not be vigorously shaken. Do not refrigerate after reconstitution. (1)

Trade Name(s) — Advate, Helixate FS, Kogenate, Kogenate FS, ReFacto.

Administration — Antihemophilic factor (recombinant) is administered intravenously. The drug should be withdrawn from the vial into a syringe using the sterile filter needle provided. The use of plastic syringes has been suggested because proteins tend to adhere more to glass syringes than to plastic ones. (1)

Stability — The products should be stored under refrigeration protected from light; freezing should be avoided because of possible damage to the diluent container. Intact vials of drug may be stored up to three months at room temperature up to 25 °C (Kogenate, ReFacto) or 30 °C (Recombinate). The products do not contain an antimicrobial preservative; use within three hours after reconstitution is recommended. (1; 4)

Antihemophilic factor VIII (ADVATE, Baxter) when reconstituted as directed was found to exhibit about 8% loss of activity within 24 hours when stored at controlled room temperature. (2748)

Sorption — Antihemophilic factor (recombinant) (Bayer) 1 I.U./mL in sodium chloride 0.9% was delivered at a rate of 1 mL/min through administration tubing composed of PVC (Terumo) and polybutadiene (Terumo). No loss of antihemophilic factor (recombinant) occurred with the polybutadiene administration tubing. However, losses of 10 to 16% occurred through the PVC sets. (2448)

Filtration — Antihemophilic factor (recombinant) (Bayer) 1 I.U./mL in sodium chloride 0.9% was delivered at a rate of 1 mL/min through administration tubing composed of PVC with 0.2-μm inline filters composed of degenerated polysulfone (Terumo), polyethersulfone (JMS), and degenerated polyethersulfone (Nipro). No added loss of antihemophilic factor (recombinant) due to sorption to the filter occurred with the polysulfone filter. However, only 50 to 60% of the antihemophilic factor (recombinant) was delivered with the polyethersulfone filters. About 15% of the loss was attributable to the PVC tubing (see Sorption), but the balance resulted from the filters. (2448)

ANTITHYMOCYTE GLOBULIN (RABBIT)
AHFS 92:44

Products — Antithymocyte globulin (rabbit) is available as a lyophilized powder in 25-mg vials with glycine 50 mg, mannitol 50 mg, and sodium chloride 10 mg. The vial of drug is accompanied by a 5-mL vial of sterile water for injection for use as a diluent. (1)

Allow the vials of antithymocyte globulin (rabbit) and diluent to warm to room temperature before reconstitution. Reconstitute the vial of drug with the diluent provided immediately before use. Direct the flow of diluent to the side of the vial. Rotate the vial gently to dissolve the drug, resulting in a 5-mg/mL solution. Inspect for particulate matter before use; the solution should be clear and not opaque. Should some particulate matter remain, continue rotating gently until all particulate matter is dissolved. (1; 4)

pH — From 6.6 to 7.4. (1)

Trade Name(s) — Thymoglobulin.

Administration — Antithymocyte globulin (rabbit) is administered intravenously into a high-flow vein after dilution in dextrose 5% or sodium chloride 0.9% to an approximate concentration of 0.5 mg/mL. The manufacturer recommends that each vial to be administered be diluted in 50 mL of infusion solution. The total volume usually ranges between 50 and 500 mL. Invert the bag gently once or twice to mix the solution before administration. (1; 4)

Antithymocyte globulin (rabbit) diluted for administration is infused through a 0.22-μm filter over a minimum of six hours for the first infusion and over at least four hours subsequently.

Stability — Intact vials of antithymocyte globulin (rabbit) should be stored under refrigeration and protected from light and freezing. After reconstitution, the drug is stable for 24 hours but should be used within four hours because of the absence of preservatives. (1; 4) Mixed in an infusion solution, immediate use is recommended. (1)

Antithymocyte globulin (rabbit) is for single use and contains no preservative. Any unused drug remaining should be discarded. (1)

Sorption — The manufacturer states that no interaction of antithymocyte globulin (rabbit) with glass bottles or PVC bags or administration sets has been found. (4)

Compatibility Information

Additive Compatibility

Antithymocyte globulin (rabbit)

Drug	Mfr	Conc/L	Mfr	Conc/L	Test Soln	Remarks	Ref	C/I
Heparin sodium[a]	ES	2000 units	SGS	200 and 300 mg	D5W	Immediate haze and precipitation	2488	I
	ES	2000 units	SGS	200 and 300 mg	NS	Physically compatible for 24 hr at 23 °C	2488	C
Hydrocortisone sodium succinate[b]	PHU	50 mg	SGS	200 and 300 mg	D5W	Immediate haze and precipitation	2488	I
	PHU	50 mg	SGS	200 and 300 mg	NS	Physically compatible for 24 hr at 23 °C	2488	C

[a]*Hydrocortisone sodium succinate (Pharmacia Upjohn) 50 mg/L was also present.*
[b]*Heparin sodium (Elkins-Sinn) 2000 units/L was also present.*

Y-Site Injection Compatibility (1:1 Mixture)

Antithymocyte globulin (rabbit)

Drug	Mfr	Conc	Mfr	Conc	Remarks	Ref	C/I
Heparin sodium	ES	2 units/mL[a]	SGS	0.2 mg/mL[a]	Haze and precipitate form immediately	2488	I
	ES	2 units/mL[a]	SGS	0.3 mg/mL[a]	Haze and precipitate form immediately	2488	I
	ES	2 units/mL[b]	SGS	0.2 mg/mL[b]	Physically compatible for 4 hr at 23 °C	2488	C
	ES	2 units/mL[b]	SGS	0.3 mg/mL[b]	Physically compatible for 4 hr at 23 °C	2488	C
	ES	100 units/mL[a,b]	SGS	0.2 mg/mL[a,b]	Physically compatible for 4 hr at 23 °C	2488	C
	ES	100 units/mL[a,b]	SGS	0.3 mg/mL[a,b]	Physically compatible for 4 hr at 23 °C	2488	C
Hydrocortisone sodium succinate	PHU	0.5 mg/mL[a,b]	SGS	0.2 and 0.3 mg/mL[a,b]	Physically compatible for 4 hr at 23 °C	2488	C
	PHU	1 mg/mL[a,b]	SGS	0.2 and 0.3 mg/mL[a,b]	Physically compatible for 4 hr at 23 °C	2488	C

[a]*Tested in dextrose 5%.*
[b]*Tested in sodium chloride 0.9%.*

APOMORPHINE HYDROCHLORIDE
AHFS 28:36.20.08

Products — Apomorphine hydrochloride is available as 10-mg/mL injections with sodium metabisulfite 1 mg in 1-, 2-, and 5-mL ampuls and may also contain sodium hydroxide and/or hydrochloric acid to adjust pH during manufacturing. (38; 115)

pH — From 3 to 4. (115)

Trade Name(s) — APO-go, Apokinon, Apomine.

Administration — Apomorphine hydrochloride is administered subcutaneously by intermittent injection or continuous infusion using a controlled infusion device. (38; 115)

Stability — Containers should be stored under refrigeration (115) or at controlled room temperature (38) and protected from freezing and exposure to light. (38; 115) Apomorphine hydrochloride injection should be clear and colorless and should not be used if it has turned green. (38)

Light Effects — Apomorphine hydrochloride is very sensitive to exposure to light. In sodium chloride 0.9%, apomorphine hydrochloride (Teclapharm) 0.01 mg/mL and 0.1 mg/mL lost 44 and 24%, respectively, in one day when stored at room temperature without light protection. (2403)

Compatibility Information

Solution Compatibility

Apomorphine HCl

Solution	Mfr	Mfr	Conc/L	Remarks	Ref	C/I
Sodium chloride 0.9%	FRE[a]	TEC	100 mg	Physically compatible with about 8% loss in 14 days at room temperature and about 7% loss in 28 days at 4 °C plus 7 days at room temperature when protected from light	2403	C
	FRE[a]	TEC	10 mg	Physically compatible with about 7% loss in 24 days at room temperature and about 9% loss in 7 days at 4 °C plus 24 hr at room temperature when protected from light	2403	C

[a]Tested in PVC containers.

ARGATROBAN
AHFS 20:12.04.12

Products — Argatroban is available as a 100-mg/mL solution in 2.5-mL (250-mg) vials. Each vial also contains D-sorbitol 750 mg and dehydrated alcohol 1000 mg. The concentrate must be diluted 100-fold for use. Mix thoroughly after dilution by repeated inversion of the solution container for one minute. Slight haziness may form due to transient microprecipitation, but the solution should clear with adequate mixing. (1)

pH — After dilution for use, the pH is 3.2 to 7.5. (1)

Administration — Argatroban is administered by continuous intravenous infusion after 100-fold dilution in dextrose 5%, sodium chloride 0.9%, or Ringer's injection, lactated, resulting in a final concentration of 1 mg/mL. For a 2.5-mL vial, the contents are mixed with 250 mL of infusion solution. (1)

Stability — Argatroban is a clear, colorless to pale yellow slightly viscous solution. If the injection is cloudy or contains particulates, it should be discarded. Intact vials are stored at room temperature and retained in the original carton to protect from light. Freezing should be avoided. (1)

Argatroban diluted for administration in a suitable infusion solution is stable for 24 hours at room temperature exposed to normal room light and for 96 hours at room temperature or under refrigeration in the dark. The solutions should not be exposed to direct sunlight. (1)

Compatibility Information

Y-Site Injection Compatibility (1:1 Mixture)

Argatroban

Drug	Mfr	Conc	Mfr	Conc	Remarks	Ref	C/I
Abciximab	LI	36 mcg/mL[a,b,d]	GSK	1 mg/mL[a,b,d]	Physically compatible with no loss of argatroban in 4 hr at 23 °C. Abciximab not tested	2630	C
Amiodarone HCl	NVP	1.8 mg/mL[a]	SKB	1 mg/mL[a]	Trace precipitate forms immediately	2572	I
Atropine sulfate	AMR	0.4 mg/mL	GSK	1 mg/mL[b]	Visually compatible for 24 hr at 23 °C	2391	C
Diltiazem HCl	BV	5 mg/mL	GSK	1 mg/mL[b]	Visually compatible for 24 hr at 23 °C	2391	C
Diphenhydramine HCl	ES	50 mg/mL	GSK	1 mg/mL[b]	Visually compatible for 24 hr at 23 °C	2391	C
Dobutamine HCl	LI	12.5 mg/mL	GSK	1 mg/mL[b]	Visually compatible for 24 hr at 23 °C	2391	C
Dopamine HCl	AMR	80 mg/mL	GSK	1 mg/mL[b]	Visually compatible for 24 hr at 23 °C	2391	C
Eptifibatide	COR	2 mg/mL[e]	GSK	1 mg/mL[a,b,e]	Physically compatible with no loss of either drug in 4 hr at 23 °C	2630	C

Y-Site Injection Compatibility (1:1 Mixture) (Cont.)

Argatroban

Drug	Mfr	Conc	Mfr	Conc	Remarks	Ref	C/I
Fenoldopam mesylate	AB	0.1 mg/mL[a]	SKB	1 mg/mL[a]	Physically compatible for 24 hr at 23 °C	2572	C
Fentanyl citrate	ES	50 mcg/mL	GSK	1 mg/mL[b]	Visually compatible for 24 hr at 23 °C	2391	C
Furosemide	AB	10 mg/mL	SKB	1 mg/mL[a]	Physically compatible for 24 hr at 23 °C	2572	C
Hydrocortisone sodium succinate	PHU	50 mg/mL	GSK	1 mg/mL[b]	Visually compatible for 24 hr at 23 °C	2391	C
Lidocaine HCl	BA	8 mg/mL[a]	SKB	1 mg/mL[a]	Physically compatible for 24 hr at 23 °C	2572	C
Metoprolol tartrate	AB	1 mg/mL	GSK	1 mg/mL[b]	Visually compatible for 24 hr at 23 °C	2391	C
Midazolam HCl	AB	2 mg/mL	GSK	1 mg/mL[b]	Visually compatible for 24 hr at 23 °C	2391	C
Milrinone lactate	NVP	0.4 mg/mL[a]	SKB	1 mg/mL[b]	Physically compatible for 24 hr at 23 °C	2572	C
Morphine sulfate	ES	10 mg/mL	GSK	1 mg/mL[b]	Visually compatible for 24 hr at 23 °C	2391	C
Nesiritide	SCI	6 mcg/mL[a]	SKB	1 mg/mL[a]	Physically compatible for 24 hr at 23 °C	2572	C
Nitroglycerin	BA	0.2 mg/mL[a]	SKB	1 mg/mL[a]	Physically compatible for 24 hr at 23 °C	2572	C
Norepinephrine bitartrate	AB	1 mg/mL	GSK	1 mg/mL[b]	Visually compatible for 24 hr at 23 °C	2391	C
Phenylephrine HCl	AMR	10 mg/mL	GSK	1 mg/mL[b]	Visually compatible for 24 hr at 23 °C	2391	C
Sodium nitroprusside	AB	0.2 mg/mL[a]	SKB	1 mg/mL[a]	Physically compatible for 24 hr at 23 °C	2572	C
Tirofiban HCl	ME	0.05 mg/mL[f]	GSK	1 mg/mL[a,b,f]	Physically compatible with no loss of either drug in 4 hr at 23 °C	2630	C
TPN #263[c]			SKB	1 mg/mL[a]	Physically compatible for 24 hr at 23 °C	2572	C
Vasopressin	AMR	0.4 unit/mL[a]	SKB	1 mg/mL[a]	Physically compatible for 24 hr at 23 °C	2572	C
Verapamil HCl	AMR	2.5 mg/mL	GSK	1 mg/mL[b]	Visually compatible for 24 hr at 23 °C	2391	C

[a] *Tested in dextrose 5%.*
[b] *Tested in sodium chloride 0.9%.*
[c] *Refer to Appendix I for the composition of parenteral nutrition solutions. TPN indicates a 2-in-1 admixture.*
[d] *Mixed argatroban:abciximab 1:1 and 4:1.*
[e] *Mixed argatroban:eptifibatide 1:1 and 16:1.*
[f] *Mixed argatroban:tirofiban hydrochloride 1:1 and 8:1.*

ARIPIPRAZOLE
AHFS 28:16.08.04

Products — Aripiprazole is available in 1.3-mL vials containing 9.75 mg (7.5 mg/mL) of drug with sulfobutylether β-cyclodextrin 150 mg/mL, tartaric acid, and sodium hydroxide in water for injection. (1)

Trade Name(s) — Abilify.

Administration — Aripiprazole injection is administered by deep intramuscular injection only. Other routes should not be used. (1)

Stability — Intact vials of aripiprazole should be stored in the original cartons at controlled room temperature. (1)

Compatibility Information

Drugs in Syringe Compatibility

Aripiprazole

Drug (in syringe)	Mfr	Amt	Mfr	Amt	Remarks	Ref	C/I
Lorazepam	HOS	0.2 mg/ 0.1 mL	BMS	6.75 mg/ 0.9 mL	Visually compatible for 30 min	2719	C
	HOS	0.6 mg/ 0.3 mL	BMS	5.25 mg/ 0.7 mL	Visually compatible for 30 min	2719	C
	HOS	1 mg/ 0.5 mL	BMS	3.75 mg/ 0.5 mL	Visually compatible for 30 min	2719	C
	HOS	1.4 mg/ 0.7 mL	BMS	2.25 mg/ 0.3 mL	Visually compatible for 30 min	2719	C
	HOS	1.8 mg/ 0.9 mL	BMS	0.75 mg/ 0.1 mL	Visually compatible for 30 min	2719	C

ARSENIC TRIOXIDE
AHFS 10:00

Products — Arsenic trioxide is available as a 1-mg/mL solution in 10-mL ampuls. Sodium hydroxide and/or hydrochloric acid may have been used during manufacturing to adjust pH to near 8.0. (1)

pH — From 7.5 to 8. (1)

Trade Name(s) — Trisenox.

Administration — Arsenic trioxide must be diluted with 100 to 250 mL of dextrose 5% or sodium chloride 0.9% for use. It is administered by intravenous infusion over one to two hours. (1)

Stability — Arsenic trioxide injection is clear and colorless. Intact ampuls should be stored at room temperature and protected from freezing. Discard unused portions of the drug properly. After dilution for use, arsenic trioxide is stated to be stable for 24 hours at room temperature and 48 hours under refrigeration. (1)

Compatibility Information

Solution Compatibility

Arsenic trioxide

Solution	Mfr	Mfr	Conc/L	Remarks	Ref	C/I
Dextrose 5%	BA[a]	CTI	10 mg and 80 mg	Physically compatible with little change in arsenic concentration in 14 days under refrigeration and at room temperature	2456	C
	BA[a]	CTI	10, 80, 150 mg	Physically compatible with less than 10% change in arsenic concentration in 72 hr under refrigeration and at room temperature	2457	C
Sodium chloride 0.9%	BA[a]	CTI	10 mg and 80 mg	Physically compatible with little change in arsenic concentration in 14 days under refrigeration and at room temperature	2456	C
	BA[a]	CTI	10, 80, 150 mg	Physically compatible with less than 10% change in arsenic concentration in 72 hr under refrigeration and at room temperature	2457	C

[a]*Tested in PVC containers.*

ASCORBIC ACID
AHFS 88:12

Products — Ascorbic acid is provided as a sodium ascorbate solution equivalent to 500 mg/mL of ascorbic acid in 1- and 2-mL containers. The pH may be adjusted with sodium bicarbonate or sodium hydroxide. Edetate disodium and sodium hydrosulfite 0.5% antioxidant may also be present. (1)

Pressure may build up during storage of containers of ascorbic acid. At room temperature, the pressure may become excessive. When opening ascorbic acid, ampuls should be wrapped in a protective covering. (1)

pH — From 5.5 to 7. (1)

Administration — Intramuscular injection of ascorbic acid is preferred, but it may also be given subcutaneously or intravenously. (1; 4) Intravenously, it should be added to a large volume of a compatible diluent and infused slowly. (1)

Stability — To avoid excessive pressure inside the ampuls, they should be stored in the refrigerator and not allowed to stand at room temperature before use. (1)

Although refrigeration is recommended, Lilly has stated that its ascorbic acid had a maximum room temperature stability of 96 hours. (853) Intact ampuls of commercial ascorbic acid (Vitarine) have been reported to be stable for four years at room temperatures not exceeding 25 °C. (60)

Ascorbic acid in solution is rapidly oxidized in air and alkaline media. (4; 2292)

The stability of ascorbic acid from a multiple vitamin product in dextrose 5% and sodium chloride 0.9%, in both PVC and ClearFlex containers, was evaluated. Analysis showed that ascorbic acid was stable at 23 °C when protected from light, exhibiting less than a 10% loss in 24 hours. When exposed to light, however, ascorbic acid had losses of approximately 50 to 65% in 24 hours. (1509)

Ascorbic acid (Abbott) develops a grayish-brown color if left exposed to a stainless steel 5-μm filter needle (Monoject) for as little as one hour. (1645)

pH Effects — Literature reports of incompatibilities between various acid-labile drugs such as penicillin G potassium (47; 165) and erythromycin lactobionate (20) with pure ascorbic acid do not pertain to ascorbic acid injection, USP. The official product has a pH of 5.5 to 7 (4; 17) and exists as a mixture of sodium ascorbate and ascorbic acid, with the sodium salt predominating. Pure ascorbic acid is quite acidic. A solution of ascorbic acid 500 mg in 2 mL of diluent had a pH of 2. The incompatibilities between pure ascorbic acid and penicillin G potassium have been attributed to the pH rather than being a characteristic of the ascorbate ion. (166)

Light Effects — Ascorbic acid gradually darkens on exposure to light. A slight color developed during storage does not impair the therapeutic activity. (4) Protect the intact containers from light by keeping them in the carton until ready for use. (1)

Sorption — Pure ascorbic acid (Merck) did not display significant sorption to a PVC plastic test strip in 24 hours. (12)

Compatibility Information

Solution Compatibility

Ascorbic acid

Solution	Mfr	Mfr	Conc/L	Remarks	Ref	C/I
Dextrose–Ringer's injection combinations	AB	AB	1 g	Physically compatible	3	C
Dextrose–Ringer's injection, lactated, combinations	AB	AB	1 g	Physically compatible	3	C
Dextrose–saline combinations	AB	AB	1 g	Physically compatible	3	C
Dextrose 5% in sodium chloride 0.45%		BTK	1.25 g	5% loss in 24 hr at room temperature	1775	C
Dextrose 2.5%	AB	AB	1 g	Physically compatible	3	C
Dextrose 5%	AB	AB	1 g	Physically compatible	3	C
		BTK	1.25 g	5% loss in 24 hr at room temperature	1775	C
	BRN	AMR	10 g	Physically compatible with no loss in 24 hr at 24 °C in the dark	2629	C
Dextrose 10%	AB	AB	1 g	Physically compatible	3	C
		BTK	1.25 g	4% loss in 24 hr at room temperature	1775	C
Ionosol products	AB	AB	1 g	Physically compatible	3	C
Ringer's injection	AB	AB	1 g	Physically compatible	3	C
		BTK	1.25 g	6% loss in 24 hr at room temperature	1775	C
Ringer's injection, lactated	AB	AB	1 g	Physically compatible	3	C
		BTK	1.25 g	6% loss in 24 hr at room temperature	1775	C
Sodium chloride 0.45%	AB	AB	1 g	Physically compatible	3	C

Solution Compatibility (Cont.)

Ascorbic acid

Solution	Mfr	Mfr	Conc/L	Remarks	Ref	C/I
Sodium chloride 0.9%	AB	AB	1 g	Physically compatible	3	C
		BTK	1.25 g	4% loss in 24 hr at room temperature	1775	C
	BRN	AMR	10 g	Physically compatible with 3% loss in 24 hr at 24 °C in the dark	2629	C
Sodium lactate ⅙ M	AB	AB	1 g	Physically compatible	3	C

Additive Compatibility

Ascorbic acid

Drug	Mfr	Conc/L	Mfr	Conc/L	Test Soln	Remarks	Ref	C/I
Amikacin sulfate	BR	5 g	CO[a]	5 g	D5LR, D5R, D5S, D5W, D10W, LR, NS, R, SL	Physically compatible and both stable for 24 hr at 25 °C	294	C
Aminophylline	SE	500 mg	AB	500 mg		Physically compatible	6	C
	SE	1 g	UP	500 mg	D5W	Physically incompatible	15	I
Bleomycin sulfate	BR	20 and 30 units	PD	2.5 and 5 g	NS	Loss of all bleomycin in 1 week at 4 °C	763	I
Calcium chloride	UP	1 g	UP	500 mg	D5W	Physically compatible	15	C
Calcium gluconate	UP	1 g	UP	500 mg	D5W	Physically compatible	15	C
Chloramphenicol sodium succinate	PD	1 g	AB	1 g		Physically compatible	6	C
	PD		UP			Concentration-dependent incompatibility	15	I
Chlorpromazine HCl	SKF	250 mg	UP	500 mg	D5W	Physically compatible	15	C
Colistimethate sodium	WC	500 mg	UP	500 mg	D5W	Physically compatible	15	C
Cyanocobalamin	AB	1 mg	AB	1 g		Physically compatible	3	C
Diphenhydramine HCl	PD	80 mg	UP	500 mg	D5W	Physically compatible	15	C
Erythromycin lactobionate	AB	1 g	AB	1 g		Physically compatible	3	C
	AB	5 g	UP	500 mg	D5W	Physically incompatible	15	I
Fat emulsion, intravenous	VT	10%	VI	1 g		Physically compatible for 48 hr at 4 °C and room temperature	32	C
	VT	10%	DB	500 mg		Lipid coalescence in 24 hr at 25 and 8 °C	825	I
Heparin sodium	UP	4000 units	UP	500 mg	D5W	Physically compatible	15	C
Hydrocortisone sodium succinate	UP		UP			Concentration-dependent incompatibility	15	I
Methyldopate HCl	MSD	1 g	AB	1 g	D, D–S, S	Physically compatible	23	C
Nafcillin sodium	WY	5 g	UP	500 mg	D5W	Physically incompatible	15	I
Penicillin G potassium		1 million units	AB	1 g		Physically compatible	3	C
	SQ	10 million units	PD	500 mg	D5W	1% penicillin loss in 8 hr	166	C

Additive Compatibility (Cont.)

Ascorbic acid

Drug	Mfr	Conc/L	Mfr	Conc/L	Test Soln	Remarks	Ref	C/I
Polymyxin B sulfate	BW	200 mg	UP	500 mg	D5W	Physically compatible	15	C
Prochlorperazine edisylate	SKF	100 mg	UP	500 mg	D5W	Physically compatible	15	C
Promethazine HCl	WY	250 mg	UP	500 mg	D5W	Physically compatible	15	C
Sodium bicarbonate	AB	80 mEq	UP	500 mg	D5W	Physically incompatible	15	I
Theophylline		2 g		1.9 g	D5W	Yellow discoloration. 8% ascorbic acid loss in 6 hr and 15% in 24 hr. No theophylline loss	1909	I
Verapamil HCl	KN	80 mg	LI	1 g	D5W, NS	Physically compatible for 24 hr	764	C

[a]As calcium ascorbate.

Drugs in Syringe Compatibility

Ascorbic acid

Drug (in syringe)	Mfr	Amt	Mfr	Amt	Remarks	Ref	C/I
Cefazolin sodium	LI	1 g/3 mL	LI	1 mL	Precipitate forms within 3 min at 32 °C	766	I
Doxapram HCl	RB	400 mg/ 20 mL		500 mg/ 2 mL	Immediate turbidity changing to precipitation in 24 hr	1177	I
Metoclopramide HCl	RB	10 mg/ 2 mL	AB	250 mg/ 0.5 mL	Physically compatible for 48 hr at 25 °C	1167	C
	RB	160 mg/ 32 mL	AB	250 mg/ 0.5 mL	Physically compatible for 48 hr at 25 °C	1167	C

Y-Site Injection Compatibility (1:1 Mixture)

Ascorbic acid

Drug	Mfr	Conc	Mfr	Conc	Remarks	Ref	C/I
Etomidate	AB	2 mg/mL	AB	500 mg/mL	Yellow color and precipitate form in 24 hr	1801	I
Propofol	STU	2 mg/mL	AB	500 mg/mL	No visible change in 24 hr at 25 °C. Yellow color forms within 7 days	1801	?
TPN #189[c]			DB	20 mg/mL[b]	Visually compatible for 24 hr at 22 °C	1767	C
Warfarin sodium	DU	0.1[a,b] and 2[d] mg/mL	SCN	0.5 mg/mL[a,b]	Physically compatible for 24 hr at 23 °C	2011	C

[a]Tested in dextrose 5%.

[b]Tested in sodium chloride 0.9%.

[c]Refer to Appendix I for the composition of parenteral nutrition solutions. TPN indicates a 2-in-1 admixture.

[d]Tested in sterile water for injection.

Additional Compatibility Information

Parenteral Nutrition Solutions — A 35% ascorbic acid loss was reported from a parenteral nutrition solution, composed of amino acids, dextrose, electrolytes, trace elements, and multivitamins, in 39 hours at 25 °C with exposure to light. The loss was reduced to a negligible amount in four days by refrigeration and light protection. (1063)

The extent and rapidity of ascorbic acid decomposition in parenteral nutrition solutions composed of amino acids, dextrose, electrolytes, multivitamins, and trace elements in 3-L PVC bags stored at 3 to 7 °C was reported. About 30 to 40% was lost in 24 hours. The degradation then slowed as the oxygen supply was reduced to the diffusion through the bag. About a 55 to 65% loss occurred after seven days of storage. The oxidation was catalyzed by metal ions, especially copper. In the absence of copper from the trace elements additive, less than 10% degradation of ascorbic acid occurred in 24 hours. The author estimated that 150 to 200 mg is degraded in two to four hours at ambient temperature in the presence of copper but that only 20 to 30 mg is broken down in 24 hours without copper. To minimize ascorbic acid loss, copper must be excluded. Alternatively, inclusion of excess ascorbic acid was suggested. (1056)

Extensive decomposition of ascorbic acid and folic acid was reported in a parenteral nutrition solution composed of amino acids 3.3%, dextrose 12.5%, electrolytes, trace elements, and M.V.I.-12 (USV) in PVC bags. Half-lives were 1.1, 2.9, and 8.9 hours for ascorbic acid and 2.7, 5.4, and 24 hours for folic acid stored at 24 °C in daylight, 24 °C protected from light, and 4 °C protected from light, respectively. The decomposition was much greater than for solutions not containing catalyzing metal ions. Also, it was greater than for the vitamins singly because of interactions with the other vitamins present. (1059)

Ascorbic acid decomposition in TPN admixtures has been reported to result in the formation of precipitated calcium oxalate. Oxalic acid forms as one of the decomposition products of ascorbic acid. The oxalic acid reacts with calcium in the TPN admixture to form the precipitate. (1060)

The stability of numerous vitamins in parenteral nutrition solutions composed of amino acids (Kabi-Vitrum), dextrose 30%, and fat emulsion 20% (Kabi-Vitrum) in a 2:1:1 ratio with electrolytes, trace elements, and both fat- and water-soluble vitamins was reported. The admixtures were stored in darkness at 2 to 8 °C for 96 hours. Sodium ascorbate and its biologically active degradation product, dehydroascorbic acid, totaled 59 and 42% of the nominal starting concentration at 24 and 96 hours, respectively. However, the actual initial concentration was only 66% of the nominal concentration. (1225)

When the admixture was subjected to simulated infusion over 24 hours at 20 °C, either exposed to room light or light protected, or stored for six days in the dark under refrigeration and then subjected to the same simulated infusion, once again the retinyl palmitate, alpha-tocopherol, and sodium riboflavin-5′-phosphate did not undergo significant loss. However, sodium ascorbate and its degradation product, dehydroascorbic acid, had initial combined concentrations of 51 to 65% of the nominal initial concentration, with further declines during infusion. Light protection did not significantly alter the loss of total ascorbic acid. (1225)

The stability of ascorbic acid in parenteral nutrition solutions, with and without fat emulsion, was studied. Both with and without fat emulsion, the total vitamin C content (ascorbic acid plus dehydroascorbic acid) remained above 90% for 12 hours when the solutions were exposed to fluorescent light and for 24 hours when they were protected from light. When stored in a cool dark place, the solutions were stable for seven days. (1227)

The stability of several vitamins from M.V.I.-12 (Armour) was reported when admixed in parenteral nutrition solutions composed of different amino acid products, with or without Intralipid 10%, when stored in glass bottles and PVC bags at 25 and 5 °C for 48 hours. Ascorbic acid was lost from all samples stored at 25 °C, with the greatest losses occurring in solutions stored in plastic bags. No losses occurred in any sample stored at 5 °C. (1431)

In another study, the stability of several vitamins (as M.V.I.-12) following admixture with four different amino acid products (Novamine, Neopham, FreAmine III, Travasol) with or without Intralipid was reported when stored in glass bottles or PVC bags at 25 °C for 48 hours. Under high-intensity phototherapy light, ascorbic acid losses were significant with all amino acid products tested. When bisulfite was added to the Neopham admixture, ascorbic acid was

unaffected. Ascorbic acid losses were increased with a more alkaline pH and that bisulfite addition offered some protection presumably by bisulfite being preferentially oxidized. The authors concluded that intravenous multivitamins should be added to parenteral nutrition admixtures immediately prior to administration to reduce losses since commercially available amino acid products may contain bisulfites and have varying pH values. (487)

The stability of ascorbic acid and dehydroascorbic acid was evaluated in a 3-in-1 admixture containing Vamin 14, dextrose 30%, Intralipid 20%, potassium phosphate, Cernevit, and trace elements in ethylene vinyl acetate (EVA) bags over a temperature range of 2 to 22 °C. They observed an 89% loss of ascorbic acid and 37% loss of dehydroascorbic acid over 7 days. Oxygen, trace elements, temperature, and an underfilled bag were the greatest determinants of ascorbic acid loss. (2462)

The long-term stability of ascorbic acid in 3-in-1 admixtures containing amino acids (Eloamin) 10%, dextrose 20%, fat emulsion (Elolipid) 20%, calcium gluconate, M.V.C. 9 + 3, and trace elements mixed in EVA and multilayer (Ultrastab) bags at 5 °C was evaluated. Ascorbic acid losses were greater than 75% in the first 24 hours and 100% after 48 to 72 hours in the EVA bags. In the multilayer bags, ascorbic acid showed a 20 and 40% loss over the first 24 hours with and without fat emulsion, respectively. The initial rapid fall in ascorbic acid was presumably due to the initial oxygen content of the admixtures despite the use of the less oxygen-permeable multilayer bags. The ascorbic acid concentration remained stable for up to 28 days in the multilayer bags after the initial fall. Adding additional ascorbic acid to compensate for the losses was recommended to facilitate extended shelf-life. (2463)

Because of these interactions, recommendations to separate the administration of vitamins and trace elements have been made. (1056; 1060; 1061) Other researchers have termed such recommendations premature based on differing reports (895; 896) and the apparent absence of epidemic vitamin deficiency in parenteral nutrition patients. (1062)

The influence of several factors on the rate of ascorbic acid oxidation in parenteral nutrition solutions was evaluated. Ascorbic acid is regarded as the least stable component in TPN admixtures. The type of amino acid used in the TPN was important. Some, such as FreAmine III and Vamin 14, contain antioxidant compounds (e.g., sodium metabisulfite or cysteine). Ascorbic acid stability was better in such solutions compared with those amino acid solutions having no antioxidant present. Furthermore, the pH of the solution may play a small role, with greater degradation as the pH rises from about 5 to about 7. Adding air to a compounded TPN container can also accelerate ascorbic acid decomposition. The most important factor was the type of plastic container used for the TPN. EVA containers (Mixieva, Miramed) allow more oxygen permeation, which results in substantial losses of ascorbic acid in relatively short time periods. In multilayer TPN bags (Ultrastab, Miramed) designed to reduce gas permeability, the rate of ascorbic acid degradation was greatly reduced. TPNs without antioxidants packaged in EVA bags had an almost total loss of ascorbic acid activity in one or two days at 5 °C. In contrast, in TPNs containing FreAmine III or Vamin 14 and packaged in the multilayer bags, most of the ascorbic acid content was retained for 28 days at 5 °C. The TPNs made with antioxidant-containing amino acids and packaged in multilayer bags that reduce gas permeability can safely be given extended expiration dates and still retain most of the ascorbic acid activity. (2163)

The initial degradation product of ascorbic acid (dehydroascorbic acid) was evaluated in a 2-in-1 admixture containing Synthamin 14, glucose 20%, and trace elements over a temperature range of 5 to 35 °C. The presence of trace elements, including copper, had no influence on the degradation of dehydroascorbic acid. At room temperature and 5 °C, there was a greater than 50% loss of dehydroascorbic acid noted within two and 24 hours, respectively. The authors concluded this degradation was temperature dependent. (2461)

The degradation of vitamins A, B₁, C, and E from Cernevit (Roche) multivitamins was evaluated in NuTRIflex Lipid Plus (B. Braun) admixtures prepared in ethylene vinyl acetate (EVA) bags and in multilayer bags. After storage for up to 72 hours at 4, 21, and 40 °C, greater vitamin losses occurred in the EVA bags: vitamin A (retinyl palmitate) losses were 20%, thiamine hydrochloride losses were 25%, alpha-tocopherol losses were 20%, and ascorbic acid losses were approximately 80 to 100%. In the multilayer bags (presumably a better barrier to oxygen transfer), losses were less: vitamin A (retinyl palmitate) losses were 5%, thiamine hydrochloride losses were 10%, alpha-tocopherol losses were 0%, and ascorbic acid losses were approximately 25 to 70%. (2618)

The vitamins in Cernevit (Baxter) diluted in three 2-in-1 parenteral nutrition admixtures were tested for stability over 48 hours. While all of the vitamins retained their initial concentrations, ascorbic acid exhibited losses of about 5%, 13%, and 17% in TPNs with dextrose concentrations of 10, 15, and 25%, respectively. (2796)

ASPARAGINASE
AHFS 10:00

Products — Asparaginase is available in vials containing 10,000 I.U. of asparaginase and 80 mg of mannitol in lyophilized form. (1)

For intravenous administration, reconstitute with 5 mL of sterile water for injection or sodium chloride 0.9% to yield a solution containing 2000 I.U./mL. For intramuscular injection, reconstitute with 2 mL of sodium chloride 0.9%. (1)

To prepare a skin test solution for intradermal administration, 0.1 mL of the 2000-I.U./mL reconstituted solution (200 I.U.) is added to 9.9 mL of diluent to yield a 20-I.U./mL solution. (1)

pH — Approximately 7.4. (4)

Trade Name(s) — Elspar.

Administration — Asparaginase is administered intravenously, over not less than 30 minutes, through the sidearm of a running intravenous infusion of sodium chloride 0.9% or dextrose 5%. It may also be administered intramuscularly using a volume no greater than 2 mL; larger volumes require two injection sites. (1; 4)

Stability — It is recommended that intact vials of asparaginase be stored under refrigeration. (1)

The manufacturer indicates that the reconstituted solution should be stored under refrigeration and can be used within eight hours as long as the solution is clear. If the solution becomes turbid, it should be discarded. (1)

Ordinary shaking during reconstitution does not result in inactivation. However, one source indicates that vigorous shaking may result in some loss of potency. Vigorous shaking also can cause foaming, making it difficult to withdraw the entire vial contents. (4)

pH Effects — Asparaginase is stable over a wide pH range of 4.5 to 11, but its activity is completely lost outside this pH range. Returning the drug to pH 8.5 restores drug activity lost at extremes of pH. (2538)

Filtration — Reconstituted solutions of asparaginase may occasionally develop small numbers of gelatinous fibers on standing. Filtration through a 5-μm filter will remove the fibers with no loss of potency, but filtration through a 0.2-μm filter may result in some potency loss. (1; 4)

Compatibility Information

Solution Compatibility

Asparaginase

Solution	Mfr	Mfr	Conc/L	Remarks	Ref	C/I
Ringer's injection, lactated	a	MSD		Activity retained for 7 days at 8 °C	2538	C
Sodium chloride 0.9%	a	MSD		Activity retained for 7 days at 8 °C	2538	C

a Tested in polyolefin containers.

Y-Site Injection Compatibility (1:1 Mixture)

				Asparaginase			
Drug	*Mfr*	*Conc*	*Mfr*	*Conc*	*Remarks*	*Ref*	*C/I*
Methotrexate sodium		30 mg/mL	BEL	120 I.U./mL[a]	Visually compatible for 4 hr at room temperature	1788	**C**
Sodium bicarbonate		1.4%	BEL	120 I.U./mL[a]	Visually compatible for 4 hr at room temperature	1788	**C**

[a]*Tested in dextrose 5%.*

ATRACURIUM BESYLATE
AHFS 12:20.20

Products — Atracurium besylate is available as a 10-mg/mL aqueous solution in 5-mL single-use vials and 10-mL multiple-dose vials with benzyl alcohol 0.9% as a preservative. The pH is adjusted with benzenesulfonic acid. (1)

pH — Adjusted to 3.25 to 3.65. (1)

Administration — Atracurium besylate is administered by rapid intravenous injection or by intravenous infusion in concentrations of 0.2 and 0.5 mg/mL. It must not be given by intramuscular injection. Do not administer in the same syringe or through the same needle as an alkaline solution. (1; 4)

Stability — Atracurium besylate injection is a clear, colorless solution; it should be stored under refrigeration and protected from freezing. Nevertheless, the drug undergoes slow decomposition of about 6% per year. (1; 4) The estimated t_{90} at 5 °C is approximately 18 months. (859) At 25 °C, the rate of decomposition is stated to increase to about 5% per month. (1; 4) The manufacturers have indicated that intact vials of atracurium besylate may be used for 14 days when stored at room temperature. (1; 1181) Other research indicates that atracurium besylate injection in intact containers may be stable even longer at room temperature. Intact containers were found to retain 92% of the concentration after three months at 20 °C. (777)

pH Effects — Atracurium besylate is unstable in the presence of both acids and bases. (4) Maximum stability in aqueous solution was observed at about pH 2.5. (859)

Atracurium besylate, which has an acid pH, should not be mixed with alkaline solutions such as barbiturates. The atracurium besylate may be inactivated and precipitation of a free acid of the admixed drug may occur, depending on the resultant pH. (4)

Syringes — Atracurium besylate (Burroughs Wellcome) 10 mg/mL was repackaged as 10 mL of solution in 12-mL plastic syringes (Monoject) and stored at 5, 25, and 40 °C. The samples remained visually clear throughout the study. No loss occurred in the refrigerated samples and about 4% loss occurred in the room temperature samples after 42 days of storage. At 40 °C, 15% was lost in 21 days. Exposure of atracurium to elevated temperatures should be avoided. (2141)

Atracurium 10 mg/mL repackaged in polypropylene syringes exhibited little change in concentration after four weeks of storage at room temperature when not exposed to direct light. (2164)

Compatibility Information

Solution Compatibility

				Atracurium besylate		
Solution	*Mfr*	*Mfr*	*Conc/L*	*Remarks*	*Ref*	*C/I*
Dextrose 5% in sodium chloride 0.9%		BW	200 and 500 mg	Physically compatible and chemically stable for 24 hr at 5 and 25 °C	1694	**C**
Dextrose 5%		BW	200 and 500 mg	Physically compatible and chemically stable for 24 hr at 5 and 30 °C	1694	**C**
		BW	1 and 5 g	Chemically stable for 48 hr	1693	**C**
	BA[a]	BW	0.5 g	About 50% loss in 14 days stored at 5 and 25 °C	2141	**I**
Ringer's injection, lactated		BW	200 and 500 mg	Increased rate of atracurium degradation limits utility time to 8 hr at 25 °C	1694	**I**
	TR	BW	500 mg	About 6% loss in 12 hr at 22 °C	1692	**I**
		BW	1 and 5 g	About 10 to 12% loss in 24 hr at 30 °C	1693	**I**

Solution Compatibility (Cont.)

Atracurium besylate

Solution	Mfr	Mfr	Conc/L	Remarks	Ref	C/I
Sodium chloride 0.9%		BW	200 and 500 mg	Physically compatible and chemically stable for 24 hr at 5 and 25 °C	1694	C
		BW	1 and 5 g	Chemically stable for 24 hr	1693	C
	BAᵃ	BW	0.5 g	About 60% loss in 14 days at 5 and 25 °C	2141	I
	TR	BW	500 mg	About 1% loss in 12 hr at 22 °C	1692	C

ᵃ*Tested in glass containers.*

Additive Compatibility

Atracurium besylate

Drug	Mfr	Conc/L	Mfr	Conc/L	Test Soln	Remarks	Ref	C/I
Aminophylline		1 g	BW	500 mg	D5W	Atracurium unstable due to high pH	1694	I
Cefazolin sodium		10 g	BW	500 mg	D5W	Atracurium unstable and particles form	1694	I
Ciprofloxacin	BAY	1.6 g	GW	2 g	D5W	Visually compatible with no loss of ciprofloxacin in 24 hr at 22 °C under fluorescent light. Atracurium not tested	2413	C
Dobutamine HCl		1 g	BW	500 mg	D5W	Physically compatible and atracurium stable for 24 hr at 5 and 30 °C	1694	C
Dopamine HCl		1.6 g	BW	500 mg	D5W	Physically compatible and atracurium stable for 24 hr at 5 and 30 °C	1694	C
Esmolol HCl		10 g	BW	500 mg	D5W	Physically compatible and atracurium stable for 24 hr at 5 and 30 °C	1694	C
Gentamicin sulfate		2 g	BW	500 mg	D5W	Physically compatible and atracurium stable for 24 hr at 5 and 30 °C	1694	C
Heparin sodium		40,000 units	BW	500 mg	D5W	Particles form at 5 and 30 °C	1694	I
Isoproterenol HCl		4 mg	BW	500 mg	D5W	Physically compatible and atracurium stable for 24 hr at 5 and 30 °C	1694	C
Lidocaine HCl		2 g	BW	500 mg	D5W	Physically compatible and atracurium stable for 24 hr at 5 and 30 °C	1694	C
Morphine sulfate		1 g	BW	500 mg	D5W	Physically compatible and atracurium stable for 24 hr at 5 and 30 °C	1694	C
Potassium chloride		80 mEq	BW	500 mg	D5W	Physically compatible and atracurium stable for 24 hr at 5 and 30 °C	1694	C
Procainamide HCl		4 g	BW	500 mg	D5W	Physically compatible and atracurium stable for 24 hr at 5 and 30 °C	1694	C
Quinidine gluconate		8.3 g	BW	500 mg	D5W	Particles form and atracurium unstable at 5 and 30 °C	1694	I
Ranitidine HCl		500 mg	BW	500 mg	D5W	Atracurium unstable due to high pH	1694	I
Sodium nitroprusside		2 g	BW	500 mg	D5W	Physically incompatible. Haze, particles, and yellow color form	1694	I
Vancomycin HCl		5 g	BW	500 mg	D5W	Physically compatible and atracurium stable for 24 hr at 5 and 30 °C	1694	C

Drugs in Syringe Compatibility

Atracurium besylate

Drug (in syringe)	Mfr	Amt	Mfr	Amt	Remarks	Ref	C/I
Alfentanil HCl		0.5 mg/mL	BW	10 mg/mL	Physically compatible and atracurium stable for 24 hr at 5 and 30 °C	1694	C
Fentanyl citrate		50 mcg/mL	BW	10 mg/mL	Physically compatible and atracurium stable for 24 hr at 5 and 30 °C	1694	C
Midazolam HCl		5 mg/mL	BW	10 mg/mL	Physically compatible and atracurium stable for 24 hr at 5 and 30 °C	1694	C
Sufentanil citrate		50 mcg/mL	BW	10 mg/mL	Physically compatible and atracurium stable for 24 hr at 5 and 30 °C	1694	C

Y-Site Injection Compatibility (1:1 Mixture)

Atracurium besylate

Drug	Mfr	Conc	Mfr	Conc	Remarks	Ref	C/I
Amiodarone HCl	WY	6 mg/mL[a]	BA	5 mg/mL[a]	Visually compatible for 24 hr at 22 °C	2352	C
Cefazolin sodium	LY	10 mg/mL[a]	BW	0.5 mg/mL[a]	Physically compatible for 24 hr at 28 °C	1337	C
Cefuroxime sodium	GL	7.5 mg/mL[a]	BW	0.5 mg/mL[a]	Physically compatible for 24 hr at 28 °C	1337	C
Clarithromycin	AB	4 mg/mL[a]	GW	1 mg/mL[a]	Visually compatible for 72 hr at both 30 and 17 °C	2174	C
Dexmedetomidine HCl	HOS				Stated to be compatible	1	C
Diazepam	ES	5 mg/mL	BW	0.5 mg/mL[a]	Cloudy solution forms immediately	1337	I
Dobutamine HCl	LI	1 mg/mL[a]	BW	0.5 mg/mL[a]	Physically compatible for 24 hr at 28 °C	1337	C
Dopamine HCl	SO	1.6 mg/mL[a]	BW	0.5 mg/mL[a]	Physically compatible for 24 hr at 28 °C	1337	C
Epinephrine HCl	AB	4 mcg/mL[a]	BW	0.5 mg/mL[a]	Physically compatible for 24 hr at 28 °C	1337	C
Esmolol HCl	DCC	10 mg/mL[a]	BW	0.5 mg/mL[a]	Physically compatible for 24 hr at 28 °C	1337	C
Etomidate	AB	2 mg/mL	BW	10 mg/mL	Visually compatible for 7 days at 25 °C	1801	C
Fenoldopam mesylate	AB	80 mcg/mL[b]	BA	0.5 mg/mL[b]	Physically compatible for 4 hr at 23 °C	2467	C
Fentanyl citrate	ES	10 mcg/mL[a]	BW	0.5 mg/mL[a]	Physically compatible for 24 hr at 28 °C	1337	C
Gentamicin sulfate	ES	2 mg/mL[a]	BW	0.5 mg/mL[a]	Physically compatible for 24 hr at 28 °C	1337	C
Heparin sodium	SO	40 units/mL[a]	BW	0.5 mg/mL[a]	Physically compatible for 24 hr at 28 °C	1337	C
Hetastarch in lactated electrolyte	AB	6%	GW	0.5 mg/mL[a]	Physically compatible for 4 hr at 23 °C	2339	C
Hydrocortisone sodium succinate	AB	1 mg/mL[a]	BW	0.5 mg/mL[a]	Physically compatible for 24 hr at 28 °C	1337	C
Isoproterenol HCl	ES	4 mcg/mL[a]	BW	0.5 mg/mL[a]	Physically compatible for 24 hr at 28 °C	1337	C
Lorazepam	WY	0.5 mg/mL[a]	BW	0.5 mg/mL[a]	Physically compatible for 24 hr at 28 °C	1337	C
Midazolam HCl	RC	0.05 mg/mL[a]	BW	0.5 mg/mL[a]	Physically compatible for 24 hr at 28 °C	1337	C
	RC	0.1 mg/mL[a]	GW	1 and 5 mg/mL[a]	Visually compatible with no loss of either drug in 3 hr at 25 °C	2112	C
	RC	0.5 mg/mL[a]	GW	5 mg/mL[a]	Visually compatible with no loss of either drug in 3 hr at 25 °C	2112	C
	RC	0.5 mg/mL[a]	GW	1 mg/mL[a]	Visually compatible with no loss of midazolam and 4% loss of atracurium in 3 hr at 25 °C	2112	C
Milrinone lactate	SW	0.4 mg/mL[a]	BW	1 mg/mL[a]	Visually compatible with little or no loss of either drug in 4 hr at 23 °C	2214	C

Y-Site Injection Compatibility (1:1 Mixture) (Cont.)

Atracurium besylate

Drug	Mfr	Conc	Mfr	Conc	Remarks	Ref	C/I
Morphine sulfate	WY	1 mg/mL[a]	BW	0.5 mg/mL[a]	Physically compatible for 24 hr at 28 °C	1337	C
Nitroglycerin	SO	0.4 mg/mL[a]	BW	0.5 mg/mL[a]	Physically compatible for 24 hr at 28 °C	1337	C
Propofol	STU	2 mg/mL	BW	10 mg/mL	Oil droplets form within 24 hr, followed by phase separation at 25 °C	1801	I
	ZEN	10 mg/mL	BW	10 mg/mL	Emulsion broke and oiled out	2066	I
	ASZ, BA	10 mg/mL		10 mg/mL	Emulsion disruption upon mixing	2336	I
	ASZ, BA	10 mg/mL		5 mg/mL[a]	Emulsion disruption upon mixing	2336	I
	BA	10 mg/mL		0.5 mg/mL[a]	Emulsion disruption upon mixing	2336	I
	ASZ	10 mg/mL		0.5 mg/mL[a]	Physically compatible for at least 1 hr at room temperature	2336	C
Ranitidine HCl	GL	0.5 mg/mL[a]	BW	0.5 mg/mL[a]	Physically compatible for 24 hr at 28 °C	1337	C
Sodium nitroprusside	ES	0.2 mg/mL[a]	BW	0.5 mg/mL[a]	Physically compatible for 24 hr at 28 °C	1337	C
TPN #189[b]			WEL	10 mg/mL	Visually compatible for 24 hr at 22 °C	1767	C
Trimethoprim–sulfamethoxazole	ES	0.64 + 3.2 mg/mL[a]	BW	0.5 mg/mL[a]	Physically compatible for 24 hr at 28 °C	1337	C
Vancomycin HCl	ES	5 mg/mL[a]	BW	0.5 mg/mL[a]	Physically compatible for 24 hr at 28 °C	1337	C

[a]Tested in dextrose 5%.
[b]Refer to Appendix I for the composition of parenteral nutrition solutions. TPN indicates a 2-in-1 admixture.

ATROPINE SULFATE
AHFS 12:08.08

Products — Atropine sulfate injection is available in concentrations of 0.4 mg/0.5 mL, 0.4 mg/1 mL, 0.5 mg/1 mL, and 1 mg/1 mL and 1 mg/mL in 20-mL multiple-dose vials. Sodium chloride may be present for isotonicity and sulfuric acid may have been used to adjust pH during manufacturing.

Atropine sulfate is also available in a concentration of 0.05 mg/mL in 5-mL prefilled syringes and 0.1 mg/mL in 5- and 10-mL prefilled syringes. (1) Multiple-dose vials also contain methylparaben or benzyl alcohol as a preservative. (4)

pH — From 3 to 6.5. (1)

Osmolarity — Atropine sulfate injection has an osmolarity of 308 mOsm/L. (1)

Administration — Atropine sulfate injection may be administered by subcutaneous, intramuscular, or direct (usually rapid) intravenous injection. (1; 4)

Stability — Atropine sulfate injection should be stored at controlled room temperature. Freezing should be avoided. (1; 4) Minimum hydrolysis occurs at pH 3.5. (1072)

Temperature Effects — Atropine sulfate 0.1 mg/mL in auto-injector syringes (Abbott) was evaluated for stability over 45 days under use conditions in paramedic vehicles. Temperatures fluctuated with locations and conditions and ranged from 6.5 °C (43.7 °F) to 52 °C (125.6 °F) in high desert conditions. No visually apparent changes occurred, and little or no loss of atropine sulfate was found. (2548)

In another study, atropine sulfate injection under simulated summer conditions in paramedic vehicles was exposed to temperatures ranging from 26 to 38 °C over 4 weeks. Analysis found no loss of the drug under these conditions. (2562)

Syringes — Atropine 1 mg/mL repackaged in polypropylene syringes exhibited little change in concentration after four weeks of storage at room temperature not exposed to direct light. (2164)

Extemporaneously compounded atropine sulfate 2-mg/mL injection in sodium chloride 0.9% for use in the event of a terrorist nerve gas attack was packaged in polypropylene syringes (Becton Dickinson) with sealed tips. The injection was adjusted to pH 3.5 with sulfuric acid during compounding. No visible changes were reported, and analysis found no loss of the drug over 364 days at 5 °C protected from light, 364 days at 23 °C exposed to light, and 28 days at 35 °C exposed to light. (2781)

Compatibility Information

Solution Compatibility

Atropine sulfate

Solution	Mfr	Mfr	Conc/L	Remarks	Ref	C/I
Sodium chloride 0.9%	BA[a]		1 g	Physically compatible with little or no atropine loss in 72 hr at 6, 23, and 34 °C	2522	C

[a]Tested in PVC containers.

Additive Compatibility

Atropine sulfate

Drug	Mfr	Conc/L	Mfr	Conc/L	Test Soln	Remarks	Ref	C/I
Dobutamine HCl	LI	167 mg	AB	16.7 mg	NS	Physically compatible for 24 hr	552	C
	LI	1 g	ES	50 mg	D5W, NS	Physically compatible for 24 hr at 21 °C	812	C
Floxacillin sodium	BE	20 g	ANT	60 mg	W	Haze forms in 24 hr and precipitate forms in 48 hr at 30 °C. No change at 15 °C	1479	I
Furosemide	HO	1 g	ANT	60 mg	W	Physically compatible for 72 hr at 15 and 30 °C	1479	C
Meropenem	ZEN	1 and 20 g	ES	40 mg	NS	Visually compatible for 4 hr at room temperature	1994	C
Sodium bicarbonate	AB	2.4 mEq[a]		0.4 mg	D5W	Physically compatible for 24 hr	772	C
Verapamil HCl	KN	80 mg	IX	0.8 mg	D5W, NS	Physically compatible for 24 hr	764	C

[a]One vial of Neut added to a liter of admixture.

Drugs in Syringe Compatibility

Atropine sulfate

Drug (in syringe)	Mfr	Amt	Mfr	Amt	Remarks	Ref	C/I
Buprenorphine HCl					Physically and chemically compatible	4	C
Butorphanol tartrate	BR	4 mg/ 2 mL	ST	0.4 mg/ 1 mL	Physically compatible for 30 min at room temperature	566	C
Chlorpromazine HCl	SKF	50 mg/ 2 mL		0.6 mg/ 1.5 mL	Physically compatible for at least 15 min	14	C
	PO	50 mg/ 2 mL	ST	0.4 mg/ 1 mL	Physically compatible for at least 15 min	326	C
Dimenhydrinate	HR	50 mg/ 1 mL	ST	0.4 mg/ 1 mL	Physically compatible for at least 15 min	326	C
Diphenhydramine HCl	PD	50 mg/ 1 mL	ST	0.4 mg/ 1 mL	Physically compatible for at least 15 min	326	C
Droperidol	MN	2.5 mg/ 1 mL	ST	0.4 mg/ 1 mL	Physically compatible for at least 15 min	326	C
Fentanyl citrate	MN	100 mcg/ 1 mL		0.6 mg/ 1.5 mL	Physically compatible for at least 15 min	14	C
	MN	0.05 mg/ 1 mL	ST	0.4 mg/ 1 mL	Physically compatible for at least 15 min	326	C
Glycopyrrolate	RB	0.2 mg/ 1 mL	ES	0.4 mg/ 1 mL	Physically compatible. pH in glycopyrrolate stability range for 48 hr at 25 °C	331	C

Drugs in Syringe Compatibility (Cont.)

Atropine sulfate

Drug (in syringe)	Mfr	Amt	Mfr	Amt	Remarks	Ref	C/I
	RB	0.2 mg/ 1 mL	ES	0.8 mg/ 2 mL	Physically compatible. pH in glycopyrrolate stability range for 48 hr at 25 °C	331	C
	RB	0.4 mg/ 2 mL	ES	0.4 mg/ 1 mL	Physically compatible. pH in glycopyrrolate stability range for 48 hr at 25 °C	331	C
Heparin sodium		2500 units/ 1 mL		0.5 mg/ 1 mL	Physically compatible for at least 5 min	1053	C
Hydromorphone HCl	KN	4 mg/ 2 mL	ES	0.4 mg/ 0.5 mL	Physically compatible for 30 min	517	C
Hydroxyzine HCl	PF	100 mg/ 4 mL		0.6 mg/ 1.5 mL	Physically compatible for at least 15 min	14	C
	NF	50 mg/ 1 mL	USP	0.4 mg/ 0.4 mL	Hydroxyzine stable for at least 10 days at 3 and 25 °C	49	C
	PF	50 mg/ 1 mL	ST	0.4 mg/ 1 mL	Physically compatible for at least 15 min	326	C
	PF	100 mg/ 2 mL		0.4 mg/ 1 mL	Physically compatible	771	C
	PF	50 mg/ 1 mL		0.4 mg/ 1 mL	Physically compatible	771	C
Meperidine HCl	WY	100 mg/ 1 mL		0.6 mg/ 1.5 mL	Physically compatible for at least 15 min	14	C
	WI	50 mg/ 1 mL	ST	0.4 mg/ 1 mL	Physically compatible for at least 15 min	326	C
Metoclopramide HCl	NO	10 mg/ 2 mL	GL	0.4 mg/ 1 mL	Physically compatible for 15 min at room temperature	565	C
Midazolam HCl	RC	5 mg/ 1 mL	IX	0.4 mg/ 1 mL	Physically compatible for 4 hr at 25 °C	1145	C
Milrinone lactate	STR	5.25 mg/ 5.25 mL	IX	2 mg/ 2 mL	Physically compatible. No loss of either drug in 20 min at 23 °C	1410	C
Morphine sulfate	WY	15 mg/ 1 mL		0.6 mg/ 1.5 mL	Physically compatible for at least 15 min	14	C
	ST	15 mg/ 1 mL	ST	0.4 mg/ 1 mL	Physically compatible for at least 15 min	326	C
Nalbuphine HCl	EN	10 mg/ 1 mL	WY	0.2 mg	Physically compatible for 36 hr at 27 °C	762	C
	EN	5 mg/ 0.5 mL	WY	0.2 mg	Physically compatible for 36 hr at 27 °C	762	C
	EN	10 mg/ 1 mL	WY	0.5 mg	Physically compatible for 36 hr at 27 °C	762	C
	EN	5 mg/ 0.5 mL	WY	0.5 mg	Physically compatible for 36 hr at 27 °C	762	C
	DU	10 mg/ 1 mL		0.4 and 1 mg	Physically compatible for 48 hr	128	C
	DU	20 mg/ 1 mL		0.4 and 1 mg	Physically compatible for 48 hr	128	C
Ondansetron HCl	GW	1.33 mg/ mL[b]	GNS	0.133 mg/mL[b]	Physically compatible. Under 6% ondansetron and under 7% atropine losses in 24 hr at 4 or 23 °C	2199	C
Pantoprazole sodium	[a]	4 mg/ 1 mL		0.4 mg/ 1 mL	Incompatible after 4 hr	2574	I

Drugs in Syringe Compatibility (Cont.)

Atropine sulfate

Drug (in syringe)	Mfr	Amt	Mfr	Amt	Remarks	Ref	C/I
Pentazocine lactate	WI	30 mg/ 1 mL		0.6 mg/ 1.5 mL	Physically compatible for at least 15 min	14	C
	WI	30 mg/ 1 mL	ST	0.4 mg/ 1 mL	Physically compatible for at least 15 min	326	C
Pentobarbital sodium	WY	100 mg/ 2 mL		0.6 mg/ 1.5 mL	Physically compatible for at least 15 min	14	C
	AB	50 mg/ 1 mL	ST	0.4 mg/ 1 mL	Physically compatible for at least 15 min	326	C
	AB	100 mg/ 2 mL	LI	0.6 mg/ 1.5 mL	Precipitate forms in 24 hr at room temperature	542	I
Prochlorperazine edisylate	SKF			0.6 mg/ 1.5 mL	Physically compatible for at least 15 min	14	C
	PO	5 mg/ 1 mL	ST	0.4 mg/ 1 mL	Physically compatible for at least 15 min	326	C
Promethazine HCl	WY	50 mg/ 2 mL		0.6 mg/ 1.5 mL	Physically compatible for at least 15 min	14	C
	PO	50 mg/ 2 mL	ST	0.4 mg/ 1 mL	Physically compatible for at least 15 min	326	C
Ranitidine HCl	GL	50 mg/ 2 mL	GL	0.4 mg/ 1 mL	Physically compatible for 1 hr at 25 °C	978	C
Scopolamine HBr	ST	0.4 mg/ 1 mL	ST	0.4 mg/ 1 mL	Physically compatible for at least 15 min	326	C

[a]Test performed using the formulation WITHOUT edetate disodium.
[b]Tested in sodium chloride 0.9%.

Y-Site Injection Compatibility (1:1 Mixture)

Atropine sulfate

Drug	Mfr	Conc	Mfr	Conc	Remarks	Ref	C/I
Abciximab	LI	36 mcg/mL[a]	AMR	0.4 mg/mL	Visually compatible for 12 hr at 23 °C	2374	C
Amiodarone HCl	WY	6 mg/mL[a]	AB	0.4 mg/mL	Visually compatible for 24 hr at 22 °C	2352	C
Argatroban	GSK	1 mg/mL[b]	AMR	0.4 mg/mL	Visually compatible for 24 hr at 23 °C	2391	C
Bivalirudin	TMC	5 mg/mL[a,b]	AMR	0.4 mg/mL	Visually compatible for 6 hr at 23 °C	2680	C
Dexmedetomidine HCl	HOS				Stated to be compatible	1	C
Doripenem	JJ	5 mg/mL[a,b]	BA	0.4 mg/mL	Physically compatible for 4 hr at 23 °C	2743	C
Etomidate	AB	2 mg/mL	GNS	0.4 mg/mL	Visually compatible for 7 days at 25 °C	1801	C
Famotidine	MSD	0.2 mg/mL[a]	AST	0.1 mg/mL[a]	Physically compatible for 4 hr at 25 °C	1188	C
Fenoldopam mesylate	AB	80 mcg/mL[b]	APP	0.1 mg/mL[b]	Physically compatible for 4 hr at 23 °C	2467	C
Fentanyl citrate	JN	25 mcg/mL[a]	LY	0.4 mg/mL	Physically compatible for 48 hr at 22 °C	1706	C
Heparin sodium	UP	1000 units/L[c]	BW	0.5 mg/mL	Physically compatible for 4 hr at room temperature	534	C
Hydrocortisone sodium succinate	UP	10 mg/L[c]	BW	0.5 mg/mL	Physically compatible for 4 hr at room temperature	534	C
Hydromorphone HCl	AST	0.5 mg/mL[a]	LY	0.4 mg/mL	Physically compatible for 48 hr at 22 °C	1706	C
Meropenem	ZEN	1 and 50 mg/ mL[b]	ES	0.4 mg/mL	Visually compatible for 4 hr at room temperature	1994	C

Y-Site Injection Compatibility (1:1 Mixture) (Cont.)

Atropine sulfate

Drug	Mfr	Conc	Mfr	Conc	Remarks	Ref	C/I
Methadone HCl	LI	1 mg/mL[a]	LY	0.4 mg/mL	Physically compatible for 48 hr at 22 °C	1706	C
Morphine sulfate	AST	1 mg/mL[a]	LY	0.4 mg/mL	Physically compatible for 48 hr at 22 °C	1706	C
Nafcillin sodium	WY	33 mg/mL[b]		0.4 mg/mL	No precipitation	547	C
Palonosetron HCl	MGI	50 mcg/mL	AMR	0.4 mg/mL	Physically compatible and no loss of either drug in 4 hr at room temperature	2771	C
Potassium chloride	AB	40 mEq/L[c]	BW	0.5 mg/mL	Physically compatible for 4 hr at room temperature	534	C
Propofol	STU	2 mg/mL	GNS	0.4 mg/mL	Oil droplets form within 7 days at 25 °C. No visible change in 24 hr	1801	?
	ZEN	10 mg/mL	AST	0.1 mg/mL[a]	Physically compatible for 1 hr at 23 °C	2066	C
Tirofiban HCl	ME	50 mcg/mL[a,b]	APP	0.4 mg/mL	Physically compatible with no loss of either drug in 4 hr at 23 °C	2356	C
	ME	50 mcg/mL[a,b]	AMR	1 mg/mL	Physically compatible with no loss of either drug in 4 hr at 23 °C	2356	C

[a]*Tested in dextrose 5%.*
[b]*Tested in sodium chloride 0.9%.*
[c]*Tested in dextrose 5%, dextrose 5% in Ringer's injection, dextrose 5% in Ringer's injection, lactated, Ringer's injection, lactated, and sodium chloride 0.9%.*

AZATHIOPRINE SODIUM
AHFS 92:44

Products — Azathioprine sodium is available in 20-mL vials containing the equivalent of 100 mg of azathioprine with sodium hydroxide to adjust the pH. Reconstitute by adding 10 mL of sterile water for injection and swirling until a clear solution results. (1)

pH — Approximately 9.6. (1)

Trade Name(s) — Imuran.

Administration — Azathioprine sodium is administered intravenously. Infusions are usually administered over 30 to 60 minutes but have been given over five minutes to eight hours. (1; 4)

In the event of spills or leaks, the manufacturer recommends sodium hypochlorite 5% (household bleach) and sodium hydroxide (concentration unspecified) to inactivate azathioprine. (1200)

Stability — Azathioprine sodium, a yellow powder, should be stored at controlled room temperature and protected from light. It is stated to be stable in neutral or acid solutions but is hydrolyzed to mercapto-purine in alkaline solutions (1; 4), especially on warming. (1) Maximum stability occurs at pH 5.5 to 6.5. (1633) Hydrolysis to mercaptopurine also occurs in the presence of sulfhydryl compounds such as cysteine. (1; 4)

Use of azathioprine sodium within 24 hours after reconstitution is recommended because the product contains no preservatives. (1; 4) Azathioprine sodium is stated to be incompatible with methylparaben, propylparaben, and phenol. (108) Chemically, azathioprine sodium 10 mg/mL in aqueous solution is stable for about two weeks at room temperature. (4) After this time, hydrolysis of azathioprine to mercaptopurine increases.

Storage of the reconstituted solution in the original vial and in plastic syringes (Jelco) at 20 to 25 °C under fluorescent light resulted in no decomposition or precipitation in 16 days. At 4 °C in the dark, a visible precipitate formed after four days. (605)

Azathioprine sodium (Burroughs Wellcome) 100 mg/50 mL diluted in dextrose 5%, sodium chloride 0.9%, or sodium chloride 0.45% in PVC bags (Travenol) was stored at 20 to 25 °C under fluorescent light and at 4 °C in the dark. No decomposition occurred in the solutions over 16 days of storage. However, a precipitate formed in the dextrose 5% admixtures by the 16th day. No precipitate was observed after eight days of storage. (605)

Compatibility Information

Solution Compatibility

Azathioprine sodium

Solution	Mfr	Mfr	Conc/L	Remarks	Ref	C/I
Dextrose 5%	TR[a]	BW	2 g	Physically compatible and chemically stable for 8 days at 23 and 4 °C. Precipitate forms in 16 days	605	C
Sodium chloride 0.45%	TR[a]	BW	2 g	Physically compatible and chemically stable for 16 days at 23 and 4 °C	605	C
Sodium chloride 0.9%	TR[a]	BW	2 g	Physically compatible and chemically stable for 16 days at 23 and 4 °C	605	C

[a]*Tested in PVC containers.*

AZITHROMYCIN
AHFS 8:12.12.92

Products — Azithromycin is available as a powder in vials containing the equivalent of 500 mg of azithromycin along with citric acid 413.6 mg and sodium hydroxide. The drug is packaged under vacuum. Reconstitute with 4.8 mL of sterile water for injection and shake until the drug is dissolved yielding a 100-mg/mL solution. Because of the vacuum, a non-automated syringe is recommended to ensure that the correct amount of diluent is added. (1)

pH — From 6.4 to 6.6. (4)

Trade Name(s) — Zithromax.

Administration — Azithromycin is administered only by intravenous infusion over not less than 60 minutes after dilution to a concentration of 1 to 2 mg/mL in a compatible infusion solution. It should not be given by any other routes. (1)

Stability — Intact vials should be stored at room temperature. (4) The clear, colorless reconstituted solution is stable for 24 hours at room temperature. (1)

Compatibility Information

Solution Compatibility

Azithromycin

Solution	Mfr	Mfr	Conc/L	Remarks	Ref	C/I
Dextrose 5% in Ringer's injection, lactated		PF	1 to 2 g	Stable for 24 hr at room temperature and 7 days refrigerated	1	C
Dextrose 5% in sodium chloride 0.45%		PF	1 to 2 g	Stable for 24 hr at room temperature and 7 days refrigerated	1	C
Dextrose 5%		PF	1 to 2 g	Stable for 24 hr at room temperature and 7 days refrigerated	1	C
Normosol M in dextrose 5%		PF	1 to 2 g	Stable for 24 hr at room temperature and 7 days refrigerated	1	C
Normosol R in dextrose 5%		PF	1 to 2 g	Stable for 24 hr at room temperature and 7 days refrigerated	1	C
Ringer's injection, lactated		PF	1 to 2 g	Stable for 24 hr at room temperature and 7 days refrigerated	1	C
Sodium chloride 0.45%		PF	1 to 2 g	Stable for 24 hr at room temperature and 7 days refrigerated	1	C
Sodium chloride 0.9%		PF	1 to 2 g	Stable for 24 hr at room temperature and 7 days refrigerated	1	C

Additive Compatibility

Azithromycin

Drug	Mfr	Conc/L	Mfr	Conc/L	Test Soln	Remarks	Ref	C/I
Ciprofloxacin						Physically incompatible with loss of ciprofloxacin reported due to pH over 6.0	1924	**I**

Y-Site Injection Compatibility (1:1 Mixture)

Azithromycin

Drug	Mfr	Conc	Mfr	Conc	Remarks	Ref	C/I
Amikacin sulfate	VHA	100 mg/mL[c,d]	PF	2 mg/mL[b]	Whitish-yellow microcrystals found	2368	**I**
Aztreonam	BMS	200 mg/mL[c,d]	PF	2 mg/mL[b]	White microcrystals found	2368	**I**
Bivalirudin	TMC	5 mg/mL[a]	PF	2 mg/mL[a]	Physically compatible for 4 hr at 23 °C	2373	**C**
Caspofungin acetate	ME	0.5 mg/mL[b]	NVP	2 mg/mL[b]	Physically compatible over 60 min	2766	**C**
Cefotaxime sodium	HMR	200 mg/mL[c,d]	PF	2 mg/mL[b]	White microcrystals found	2368	**I**
Ceftaroline fosamil	FOR[a,b,g]	2.22 mg/mL	BA	2 mg/mL[a,b,g]	Physically compatible for 4 hr at 23 °C	2826	**C**
Ceftazidime	GW	80 mg/mL[c,d]	PF	2 mg/mL[b]	Amber and white microcrystals found	2368	**I**
Ceftriaxone sodium	RC	66.7 mg/mL[c,d]	PF	2 mg/mL[b]	White and yellow microcrystals found	2368	**I**
Cefuroxime sodium	VHA	100 mg/mL[c,d]	PF	2 mg/mL[b]	White and yellow microcrystals	2368	**I**
Ciprofloxacin	BAY	2 mg/mL[a,d]	PF	2 mg/mL[b]	Amber microcrystals found	2368	**I**
Clindamycin phosphate	PHU	30 mg/mL[c,d]	PF	2 mg/mL[b]	Amber and white microcrystals found	2368	**I**
Dexmedetomidine HCl	AB	4 mcg/mL[b]	PF	2 mg/mL[b]	Physically compatible for 4 hr at 23 °C	2383	**C**
Diphenhydramine HCl	ES	50 mg/mL[d]	PF	2 mg/mL[b]	Visually compatible	2368	**C**
Dolasetron mesylate	HMR	20 mg/mL[d]	PF	2 mg/mL[b]	Visually compatible	2368	**C**
Doripenem	JJ	5 mg/mL[a,b]	BA	2 mg/mL[a,b]	Physically compatible for 4 hr at 23 °C	2743	**C**
Droperidol	AMR	2.5 mg/mL[d]	PF	2 mg/mL[b]	Visually compatible	2368	**C**
Famotidine	ME	2 mg/mL[d]	PF	2 mg/mL[b]	Grayish-white microcrystals found	2368	**I**
Fentanyl citrate	AB	50 mcg/mL[d]	PF	2 mg/mL[b]	Whitish-yellow microcrystals found	2368	**I**
Furosemide	AMR	10 mg/mL[d]	PF	2 mg/mL[b]	White microcrystals found	2368	**I**
Gentamicin sulfate	AMR	21 mg/mL[c,d]	PF	2 mg/mL[b]	Whitish-yellow microcrystals found	2368	**I**
Hetastarch in lactated electrolyte	AB	6%	PF	2 mg/mL[a]	Physically compatible for 4 hr at 23 °C	2339	**C**
Imipenem–cilastatin sodium	ME	5 mg/mL[b,d]	PF	2 mg/mL[b]	Whitish-yellow microcrystals found	2368	**I**
Ketorolac tromethamine	AB	15 mg/mL[d]	PF	2 mg/mL[b]	Amber microcrystals found	2368	**I**
Levofloxacin	ORT	5 mg/mL[d]	PF	2 mg/mL[b]	White and amber microcrystals found	2368	**I**
Morphine sulfate	WY	1 mg/mL[d]	PF	2 mg/mL[b]	White microcrystals found	2368	**I**
Ondansetron HCl	GW	2 mg/mL[d]	PF	2 mg/mL[b]	Visually compatible	2368	**C**
Piperacillin sodium–tazobactam sodium	LE[e]	100 + 12.5 mg/mL[b,d]	PF	2 mg/mL[b]	White microcrystals found	2368	**I**
Potassium chloride	BA	20 mEq/L[f]	PF	2 mg/mL[b]	White microcrystals found	2368	**I**
Telavancin HCl	ASP	7.5 mg/mL[a,b,g]	APP	2 mg/mL[a,b,g]	Physically compatible for 2 hr	2830	**C**

Y-Site Injection Compatibility (1:1 Mixture) (Cont.)

Azithromycin

Drug	Mfr	Conc	Mfr	Conc	Remarks	Ref	C/I
Ticarcillin disodium–clavulanate potassium	SKB	103.3 mg/mL[b,d]	PF	2 mg/mL[b]	Amber microcrystals found	2368	I
Tigecycline	WY	1 mg/mL[b]		2 mg/mL[b]	Physically compatible for 4 hr	2714	C
Tobramycin sulfate		21 mg/mL[d]	PF	2 mg/mL[b]	White microcrystals found	2368	I

[a]*Tested in dextrose 5%.*
[b]*Tested in sodium chloride 0.9%.*
[c]*Tested in sodium chloride 0.45%.*
[d]*Injected via Y-site into an administration set running azithromycin.*
[e]*Test performed using the formulation WITHOUT edetate disodium.*
[f]*Tested in dextrose 5% in sodium chloride 0.45%.*
[g]*Tested in Ringer's injection, lactated.*

AZTREONAM
AHFS 8:12.07.16

Products — Aztreonam is available in vials containing 1 or 2 g of drug. Approximately 780 mg of arginine per gram of drug is also present. Aztreonam is also available in 1- and 2-g sizes as frozen premixed solutions in dextrose 3.4 and 1.4%, respectively, for intravenous infusion. (1; 4)

For intramuscular injection, reconstitute each gram of drug in vials with at least 3 mL of one of the following diluents (1):

Sterile water for injection
Bacteriostatic water for injection (benzyl alcohol or parabens)
Sodium chloride 0.9%
Bacteriostatic sodium chloride 0.9% (benzyl alcohol)

For intravenous bolus injection, use the vials. Reconstitute with 6 to 10 mL of sterile water for injection. (1)

For intravenous infusion, reconstitute a vial of aztreonam with at least 3 mL of sterile water for injection per gram and further dilute with a compatible infusion solution to yield a concentration not exceeding 2% (w/v). (1)

On adding the diluent to the vial or bottle, shake the contents immediately and vigorously. Discard any unused portion of the reconstituted solution. (1)

The frozen premixed solutions may also be used for intravenous infusion after thawing and warming to room temperature. (1; 4)

pH — Aqueous solutions of aztreonam have pH values of 4.5 to 7.5. (1)

Sodium Content — Aztreonam is sodium free. (1)

Trade Name(s) — Azactam.

Administration — Aztreonam may be administered by intravenous injection or infusion or by deep intramuscular injection into a large muscle mass. By intravenous injection, the dose should be given slowly, over three to five minutes, directly into a vein or the tubing of a compatible infusion solution. Intermittent infusion at concentrations not exceeding 1 g/50 mL should be completed within 20 to 60 minutes. (1; 4)

Stability — The intact vials should be stored at controlled room temperature and protected from excessive temperatures. Exposure to strong light may cause yellowing of the powder. (1; 4)

Aztreonam solutions range from colorless to light straw to yellow. They may develop a slight pink tint on standing without potency being affected. (1)

Aztreonam solutions at concentrations of 2% (w/v) or less should be used within 48 hours if stored at room temperature or seven days if refrigerated. Solutions with concentrations exceeding 2% (w/v) should be used immediately after preparation unless sterile water for injection or sodium chloride 0.9% is used. In these two excepted solutions, aztreonam at concentrations exceeding 2% (w/v) may be used up to 48 hours at room temperature or seven days under refrigeration. (1)

Aztreonam with cloxacillin sodium and aztreonam with vancomycin hydrochloride admixtures are stable in Dianeal 137 with dextrose 4.25% for 24 hours at room temperature. (1)

pH Effects — In aqueous solutions, aztreonam undergoes hydrolysis of the β-lactam ring. Specific base catalysis occurs at pH greater than 6. At pH 2 to 5, isomerization of the side chain predominates. The lowest rates of decomposition occur at pH 5 to 7, with maximum stability occurring at pH 6. (1072)

Freezing Solutions — Aztreonam in any compatible infusion solution is stable for up to three months when frozen at −20 °C. Frozen solutions should be thawed at room temperature or by overnight refrigeration and should not be refrozen. Thawed solutions should be used within 24 hours at room temperature or 72 hours under refrigeration. (1; 4)

The commercially available frozen injection should be thawed at room temperature or under refrigeration and should not be refrozen. The manufacturer indicates that thawed solutions are stable for 48 hours at room temperature or 14 days under refrigeration. (4)

Central Venous Catheter — Aztreonam (Squibb) 10 mg/mL in dextrose 5% was found to be compatible with the ARROWg+ard Blue Plus (Arrow International) chlorhexidine-bearing triple-lumen central catheter. Essentially complete delivery of the drug was found with little or no drug loss occurring. Furthermore, chlorhexidine delivered from the catheter remained at trace amounts with no substantial increase due to the delivery of the drug through the catheter. (2335)

Compatibility Information

Solution Compatibility

Aztreonam

Solution	Mfr	Mfr	Conc/L	Remarks	Ref	C/I
Dextrose 5% in Ringer's injection, lactated				Manufacturer recommended solution	1	C
Dextrose–saline combinations				Manufacturer recommended solution	1	C
Dextrose 5%	TR[a]	SQ	10 g	Physically compatible with 6% loss in 48 hr at 25 °C and 3% in 7 days at 4 °C	1001	C
	TR[a]	SQ	20 g	Physically compatible with 2% loss in 48 hr at 25 °C and 3% in 7 days at 4 °C	1001	C
	MG[b]	SQ	20 g	Physically compatible with no loss in 48 hr at 25 °C under fluorescent light	1026	C
Dextrose 5 and 10%				Manufacturer recommended solutions	1	C
Ionosol B in dextrose 5%				Manufacturer recommended solution	1	C
Isolyte E in dextrose 5%				Manufacturer recommended solution	1	C
Isolyte M in dextrose 5%				Manufacturer recommended solution	1	C
Normosol M in dextrose 5%				Manufacturer recommended solution	1	C
Normosol R				Manufacturer recommended solution	1	C
Normosol R in dextrose 5%				Manufacturer recommended solution	1	C
Ringer's injection				Manufacturer recommended solution	1	C
Ringer's injection, lactated				Manufacturer recommended solution	1	C
Sodium chloride 0.9%	TR[a]	SQ	10 and 20 g	Physically compatible with little or no loss in 48 hr at 25 °C and 7 days at 4 °C	1001	C
	MG[b]	SQ	20 g	Physically compatible with no loss in 48 hr at 25 °C under fluorescent light	1026	C
	BA	SQ	20 g	10% loss in 37 days at 25 °C and more than 120 days at 4 °C. No loss in 120 days at −20 °C	1600	C
	[a]	SQ	10 g	Visually compatible with no loss in 96 hr at 5 and 24 °C	1691	C
				Manufacturer recommended solution	1	C
Sodium lactate ⅙ M				Manufacturer recommended solution	1	C
TPN #107[c]			2 g	Activity retained for 24 hr at 21 °C	1326	C

[a]Tested in PVC containers.
[b]Tested in glass containers.
[c]Refer to Appendix I for the composition of parenteral nutrition solutions. TPN indicates a 2-in-1 admixture.

Additive Compatibility

Aztreonam

Drug	Mfr	Conc/L	Mfr	Conc/L	Test Soln	Remarks	Ref	C/I
Ampicillin sodium	WY	20 g	SQ	10 g	D5W[a]	10% ampicillin loss in 2 hr and 10% aztreonam loss in 3 hr at 25 °C. 10% ampicillin loss in 24 hr and 10% aztreonam loss in 8 hr at 4 °C	1001	I
	WY	5 g	SQ	10 g	D5W[a]	10% ampicillin loss in 3 hr and 10% aztreonam loss in 7 hr at 25 °C. 10% loss of both drugs in 48 hr at 4 °C	1001	I

Additive Compatibility (Cont.)

Aztreonam

Drug	Mfr	Conc/L	Mfr	Conc/L	Test Soln	Remarks	Ref	C/I
	WY	20 g	SQ	20 g	D5W[a]	10% ampicillin loss in 4 hr and 10% aztreonam loss in 5 hr at 25 °C. 10% loss of both drugs in 24 hr at 4 °C	1001	I
	WY	5 g	SQ	20 g	D5W[a]	10% ampicillin loss in 5 hr and 10% aztreonam loss in 8 hr at 25 °C. 10% ampicillin loss in 48 hr and 10% aztreonam loss in 72 hr at 4 °C	1001	I
	WY	20 g	SQ	10 g	NS[a]	10% ampicillin loss in 24 hr and 2% aztreonam loss in 48 hr at 25 °C. 10% ampicillin loss in 2 days and 9% aztreonam loss in 7 days at 4 °C	1001	C
	WY	5 g	SQ	10 g	NS[a]	10% ampicillin loss and no aztreonam loss in 48 hr at 25 °C. 10% ampicillin loss in 3 days and 8% aztreonam loss in 7 days at 4 °C	1001	C
	WY	20 g	SQ	20 g	NS[a]	10% ampicillin loss in 24 hr and 5% aztreonam loss in 48 hr at 25 °C. 10% ampicillin loss in 2 days and 7% aztreonam loss in 7 days at 4 °C	1001	C
	WY	5 g	SQ	20 g	NS[a]	10% ampicillin loss and no aztreonam loss in 48 hr at 25 °C. 10% ampicillin loss and 5% aztreonam loss in 7 days at 4 °C	1001	C
Ampicillin sodium–sulbactam sodium	PF	20 + 10 g	SQ	10 g	NS[a]	Visually compatible with 10% ampicillin loss in 30 hr at 24 °C and 94 hr at 5 °C. Ampicillin loss is determining factor	1691	C
Cefazolin sodium	LI	5 and 20 g	SQ	10 and 20 g	D5W, NS[a]	Physically compatible. Little loss of either drug in 48 hr at 25 °C and 7 days at 4 °C in the dark	1020	C
Cefoxitin sodium	MSD	10 and 20 g	SQ	10 and 20 g	NS[a]	3 to 5% aztreonam loss and no cefoxitin loss in 7 days at 4 °C	1023	C
	MSD	10 and 20 g	SQ	10 and 20 g	D5W[a]	3 to 6% cefoxitin loss and no aztreonam loss in 7 days at 4 °C	1023	C
	MSD	10 and 20 g	SQ	10 and 20 g	D5W, NS[a]	Both drugs stable for 12 hr at 25 °C. Yellow color and 6 to 12% aztreonam and 9 to 15% cefoxitin loss in 48 hr at 25 °C	1023	I
Ciprofloxacin	BAY	1.6 g	SQ	39.7 g	D5W	Visually compatible with no loss of ciprofloxacin in 24 hr at 22 °C under fluorescent light. Aztreonam not tested	2413	C
Clindamycin phosphate	UP	3 and 6 g	SQ	10 and 20 g	D5W, NS[a]	Physically compatible with little or no loss of either drug in 48 hr at 25 °C and 7 days at 4 °C	1002	C
	UP	9 g	SQ	20 g	D5W[b]	Physically compatible with 3% clindamycin loss and 5% aztreonam loss in 48 hr at 25 °C under fluorescent light	1026	C
	UP	9 g	SQ	20 g	NS[b]	Physically compatible with 2% clindamycin loss and no aztreonam loss in 48 hr at 25 °C under fluorescent light	1026	C
Gentamicin sulfate	SC	200 and 800 mg	SQ	10 and 20 g	D5W, NS[a]	Little aztreonam loss in 48 hr at 25 °C and 7 days at 4 °C. Gentamicin stable for 12 hr at 25 °C and 24 hr at 4 °C. Up to 10% loss in 48 hr at 25 °C and 7 days at 4 °C	1023	C

Additive Compatibility (Cont.)

Aztreonam

Drug	Mfr	Conc/L	Mfr	Conc/L	Test Soln	Remarks	Ref	C/I
Linezolid	PHU	2 g	SQ	20 g	c	Physically compatible with no linezolid loss in 7 days at 4 and 23 °C protected from light. About 9% aztreonam loss at 23 °C and less than 4% loss at 4 °C in 7 days	2263	**C**
Mannitol		5 and 10%				Manufacturer recommended solution	1	**C**
Metronidazole	MG	5 g	SQ	10 and 20 g		Pink color develops in 12 hr, becoming cherry red in 48 hr at 25 °C. Pink color develops in 3 days at 4 °C. No loss of either drug detected	1023	**I**
Nafcillin sodium	BR	20 g	SQ	20 g	D5W, NS[a]	Cloudiness and precipitate form. 7% aztreonam and 11% nafcillin loss in 24 hr at room temperature	1028	**I**
Tobramycin sulfate	LI	200 and 800 mg	SQ	10 and 20 g	D5W, NS[a]	Little or no loss of either drug in 48 hr at 25 °C and 7 days at 4 °C	1023	**C**
Vancomycin HCl	AB	10 g	SQ	40 g	D5W, NS	Immediate microcrystalline precipitate. Turbidity and precipitate over 24 hr	1848	**I**
	AB	1 g	SQ	4 g	D5W	Physically compatible. Little loss of either drug in 31 days at 4 °C. 10% aztreonam loss in 14 days at 23 °C and 7 days at 32 °C	1848	**C**
	AB	1 g	SQ	4 g	NS	Physically compatible. Little loss of either drug in 31 days at 4 °C. 8% aztreonam loss in 31 days at 23 °C and 7 days at 32 °C	1848	**C**

[a]*Tested in PVC containers.*
[b]*Tested in glass containers.*
[c]*Admixed in the linezolid infusion container.*

Drugs in Syringe Compatibility

Aztreonam

Drug (in syringe)	Mfr	Amt	Mfr	Amt	Remarks	Ref	C/I
Clindamycin phosphate	UP	600 mg/ 4 mL	SQ	2 g	Physically compatible with 2% clindamycin loss and 8% aztreonam loss in 48 hr at 25 °C under fluorescent light	1164	**C**

Y-Site Injection Compatibility (1:1 Mixture)

Aztreonam

Drug	Mfr	Conc	Mfr	Conc	Remarks	Ref	C/I
Acyclovir sodium	BW	7 mg/mL[a]	SQ	40 mg/mL[a]	White needles form immediately and become dense precipitate in 4 hr	1758	**I**
Allopurinol sodium	BW	3 mg/mL[b]	SQ	40 mg/mL[b]	Physically compatible for 4 hr at 22 °C	1686	**C**
Amifostine	USB	10 mg/mL[a]	SQ	40 mg/mL[a]	Physically compatible for 4 hr at 23 °C	1845	**C**
Amikacin sulfate	BMS	5 mg/mL[a]	SQ	40 mg/mL[a]	Physically compatible for 4 hr at 23 °C	1758	**C**

Y-Site Injection Compatibility (1:1 Mixture) (Cont.)

Aztreonam

Drug	Mfr	Conc	Mfr	Conc	Remarks	Ref	C/I
Aminophylline	AMR	2.5 mg/mL[a]	SQ	40 mg/mL[a]	Physically compatible for 4 hr at 23 °C	1758	C
Amphotericin B	PHT	0.6 mg/mL[a]	SQ	40 mg/mL[a]	Yellow turbidity forms immediately and becomes flocculent precipitate in 4 hr	1758	I
Amphotericin B cholesteryl sulfate complex	SEQ	0.83 mg/mL[a]	SQ	40 mg/mL[a]	Gross precipitate forms	2117	I
Ampicillin sodium	WY	20 mg/mL[b]	SQ	40 mg/mL[a]	Physically compatible for 4 hr at 23 °C	1758	C
Ampicillin sodium–sulbactam sodium	RR	20 + 10 mg/mL[b]	SQ	40 mg/mL[a]	Physically compatible for 4 hr at 23 °C	1758	C
Amsacrine	NCI	1 mg/mL[a]	SQ	40 mg/mL[a]	Immediate yellow-orange turbidity, becoming a precipitate in 4 hr	1381	I
Anakinra	SYN	4 and 36 mg/mL[b]	BMS	20 mg/mL[b]	Physically compatible. No aztreonam loss in 4 hr at 25 °C. Anakinra uncertain	2508	?
Azithromycin	PF	2 mg/mL[b]	BMS	200 mg/mL[g,h]	White microcrystals found	2368	I
Bivalirudin	TMC	5 mg/mL[a]	DUR	40 mg/mL[a]	Physically compatible for 4 hr at 23 °C	2373	C
Bleomycin sulfate	MJ	1 unit/mL[b]	SQ	40 mg/mL[a]	Physically compatible for 4 hr at 23 °C	1758	C.
Bumetanide	RC	0.04 mg/mL[a]	SQ	40 mg/mL[a]	Physically compatible for 4 hr at 23 °C	1758	C
Buprenorphine HCl	RKC	0.04 mg/mL[a]	SQ	40 mg/mL[a]	Physically compatible for 4 hr at 23 °C	1758	C
Butorphanol tartrate	BMS	0.04 mg/mL[a]	SQ	40 mg/mL[a]	Physically compatible for 4 hr at 23 °C	1758	C
Calcium gluconate	AMR	40 mg/mL[a]	SQ	40 mg/mL[a]	Physically compatible for 4 hr at 23 °C	1758	C
Carboplatin	BMS	5 mg/mL[a]	SQ	40 mg/mL[a]	Physically compatible for 4 hr at 23 °C	1758	C
Carmustine	BMS	1.5 mg/mL[a]	SQ	40 mg/mL[a]	Physically compatible for 4 hr at 23 °C	1758	C
Caspofungin acetate	ME	0.7 mg/mL[b]	BMS	40 mg/mL[b]	Physically compatible for 4 hr at room temperature	2758	C
	ME	0.5 mg/mL[b]	BMS	20 mg/mL[b]	Physically compatible over 60 min	2766	C
Cefazolin sodium	MAR	20 mg/mL[a]	SQ	40 mg/mL[a]	Physically compatible for 4 hr at 23 °C	1758	C
Cefotaxime sodium	HO	20 mg/mL[a]	SQ	40 mg/mL[a]	Physically compatible for 4 hr at 23 °C	1758	C
Cefotetan disodium	STU	20 mg/mL[a]	SQ	40 mg/mL[a]	Physically compatible for 4 hr at 23 °C	1758	C
Cefoxitin sodium	MSD	20 mg/mL[a]	SQ	40 mg/mL[a]	Physically compatible for 4 hr at 23 °C	1758	C
Ceftazidime	LI	40 mg/mL[a]	SQ	40 mg/mL[a]	Physically compatible for 4 hr at 23 °C	1758	C
Ceftriaxone sodium	RC	20 mg/mL[a]	SQ	40 mg/mL[a]	Physically compatible for 4 hr at 23 °C	1758	C
Cefuroxime sodium	LI	30 mg/mL[a]	SQ	40 mg/mL[a]	Physically compatible for 4 hr at 23 °C	1758	C
Chlorpromazine HCl	SCN	2 mg/mL[a]	SQ	40 mg/mL[a]	Dense white turbidity forms immediately	1758	I
Ciprofloxacin	MI	1 mg/mL[a]	SQ	20 mg/mL[c]	Physically compatible for 24 hr at 22 °C	1189	C
	MI	1 mg/mL[a]	SQ	40 mg/mL[a]	Physically compatible for 4 hr at 23 °C	1758	C
Cisatracurium besylate	GW	0.1, 2, 5 mg/mL[a]	SQ	40 mg/mL[a]	Physically compatible for 4 hr at 23 °C	2074	C
Cisplatin	BMS	1 mg/mL	SQ	40 mg/mL[a]	Physically compatible for 4 hr at 23 °C	1758	C
Clindamycin phosphate	AST	10 mg/mL[a]	SQ	40 mg/mL[a]	Physically compatible for 4 hr at 23 °C	1758	C
Cyclophosphamide	MJ	10 mg/mL[a]	SQ	40 mg/mL[a]	Physically compatible for 4 hr at 23 °C	1758	C
Cytarabine	CET	50 mg/mL	SQ	40 mg/mL[a]	Physically compatible for 4 hr at 23 °C	1758	C
Dacarbazine	MI	4 mg/mL[a]	SQ	40 mg/mL[a]	Physically compatible for 4 hr at 23 °C	1758	C
Dactinomycin	ME	0.01 mg/mL[a]	SQ	40 mg/mL[a]	Physically compatible for 4 hr at 23 °C	1758	C

Y-Site Injection Compatibility (1:1 Mixture) (Cont.)

Aztreonam

Drug	Mfr	Conc	Mfr	Conc	Remarks	Ref	C/I
Daptomycin	CUB	16.7 mg/mL[b,i]	BMS	16.7 mg/mL[b,i]	Physically compatible with little loss of either drug in 2 hr at 25 °C	2553	C
Daunorubicin HCl	WY	1 mg/mL[a]	SQ	40 mg/mL[a]	Haze forms immediately	1758	I
Dexamethasone sodium phosphate	AMR	1 mg/mL[a]	SQ	40 mg/mL[a]	Physically compatible for 4 hr at 23 °C	1758	C
Dexmedetomidine HCl	AB	4 mcg/mL[b]	BMS	40 mg/mL[b]	Physically compatible for 4 hr at 23 °C	2383	C
Diltiazem HCl	MMD	5 mg/mL	SQ	20 and 333 mg/mL[b]	Visually compatible	1807	C
	MMD	1 mg/mL[b]	SQ	333 mg/mL[b]	Visually compatible	1807	C
Diphenhydramine HCl	PD	2 mg/mL[a]	SQ	40 mg/mL[a]	Physically compatible for 4 hr at 23 °C	1758	C
Dobutamine HCl	LI	4 mg/mL[a]	SQ	40 mg/mL[a]	Physically compatible for 4 hr at 23 °C	1758	C
Docetaxel	RPR	0.9 mg/mL[a]	BMS	40 mg/mL[a]	Physically compatible for 4 hr at 23 °C	2224	C
Dopamine HCl	AST	3.2 mg/mL[a]	SQ	40 mg/mL[a]	Physically compatible for 4 hr at 23 °C	1758	C
Doxorubicin HCl	CET	2 mg/mL	SQ	40 mg/mL[a]	Physically compatible for 4 hr at 23 °C	1758	C
Doxorubicin HCl liposomal	SEQ	0.4 mg/mL[a]	SQ	40 mg/mL[a]	Physically compatible for 4 hr at 23 °C	2087	C
Doxycycline hyclate	ES	1 mg/mL[a]	SQ	40 mg/mL[a]	Physically compatible for 4 hr at 23 °C	1758	C
Droperidol	JN	0.4 mg/mL[a]	SQ	40 mg/mL[a]	Physically compatible for 4 hr at 23 °C	1758	C
Enalaprilat	MSD	0.05 mg/mL[b]	SQ	10 mg/mL[a]	Physically compatible for 24 hr at room temperature under fluorescent light	1355	C
	MSD	0.1 mg/mL[a]	SQ	40 mg/mL[a]	Physically compatible for 4 hr at 23 °C	1758	C
Etoposide	BMS	0.4 mg/mL[a]	SQ	40 mg/mL[a]	Physically compatible for 4 hr at 23 °C	1758	C
Etoposide phosphate	BR	5 mg/mL[a]	SQ	40 mg/mL[a]	Physically compatible for 4 hr at 23 °C	2218	C
Famotidine	ME	2 mg/mL[a]	SQ	40 mg/mL[a]	Physically compatible for 4 hr at 23 °C	1758	C
Fenoldopam mesylate	AB	80 mcg/mL[b]	BMS	40 mg/mL[b]	Physically compatible for 4 hr at 23 °C	2467	C
Filgrastim	AMG	30 mcg/mL[a]	SQ	40 mg/mL[a]	Physically compatible for 4 hr at 22 °C	1687	C
	AMG	30 mcg/mL[a]	SQ	40 mg/mL[a]	Physically compatible for 4 hr at 23 °C	1758	C
Floxuridine	RC	3 mg/mL[a]	SQ	40 mg/mL[a]	Physically compatible for 4 hr at 23 °C	1758	C
Fluconazole	RR	2 mg/mL	SQ	40 mg/mL	Visually compatible for 24 hr at 25 °C	1407	C
	RR	2 mg/mL	SQ	40 mg/mL[a]	Physically compatible for 4 hr at 23 °C	1758	C
Fludarabine phosphate	BX	1 mg/mL[a]	SQ	40 mg/mL[a]	Visually compatible for 4 hr at 22 °C	1439	C
	BX	1 mg/mL[a]	SQ	40 mg/mL[a]	Physically compatible for 4 hr at 23 °C	1758	C
Fluorouracil	AD	16 mg/mL[a]	SQ	40 mg/mL[a]	Physically compatible for 4 hr at 23 °C	1758	C
Foscarnet sodium	AST	24 mg/mL	SQ	40 mg/mL	Physically compatible for 24 hr at room temperature under fluorescent light	1335	C
	AST	24 mg/mL	SQ	40 mg/mL[c]	Physically compatible for 24 hr at 25 °C under fluorescent light	1393	C
Furosemide	AB	3 mg/mL[a]	SQ	40 mg/mL[a]	Physically compatible for 4 hr at 23 °C	1758	C
Gallium nitrate	FUJ	0.4 mg/mL[a]	SQ	40 mg/mL[a]	Physically compatible for 4 hr at 23 °C	1758	C
Ganciclovir sodium	SY	20 mg/mL[a]	SQ	40 mg/mL[a]	White needles form immediately. Dense precipitate in 1 hr	1758	I
Gemcitabine HCl	LI	10 mg/mL[b]	SQ	40 mg/mL[b]	Physically compatible for 4 hr at 23 °C	2226	C
Gentamicin sulfate	ES	5 mg/mL[a]	SQ	40 mg/mL[a]	Physically compatible for 4 hr at 23 °C	1758	C
Granisetron HCl	SKB	0.05 mg/mL[a]	SQ	40 mg/mL[a]	Physically compatible for 4 hr at 23 °C	2000	C

Y-Site Injection Compatibility (1:1 Mixture) (Cont.)

Aztreonam

Drug	Mfr	Conc	Mfr	Conc	Remarks	Ref	C/I
Haloperidol lactate	MN	0.2 mg/mL[a]	SQ	40 mg/mL[a]	Physically compatible for 4 hr at 23 °C	1758	C
Heparin sodium	ES	100 units/ mL[a]	SQ	40 mg/mL[a]	Physically compatible for 4 hr at 23 °C	1758	C
	TR	50 units/mL	BV	20 mg/mL[a]	Visually compatible for 4 hr at 25 °C	1793	C
Hetastarch in lactated electrolyte	AB	6%	BMS	40 mg/mL[a]	Physically compatible for 4 hr at 23 °C	2339	C
Hydrocortisone sodium succinate	UP	1 mg/mL[a]	SQ	40 mg/mL[a]	Physically compatible for 4 hr at 23 °C	1758	C
Hydromorphone HCl	KN	0.5 mg/mL[a]	SQ	40 mg/mL[a]	Physically compatible for 4 hr at 23 °C	1758	C
Hydroxyzine HCl	WI	4 mg/mL[a]	SQ	40 mg/mL[a]	Physically compatible for 4 hr at 23 °C	1758	C
Idarubicin HCl	AD	0.5 mg/mL[a]	SQ	40 mg/mL[a]	Physically compatible for 4 hr at 23 °C	1758	C
Ifosfamide	MJ	25 mg/mL[a]	SQ	40 mg/mL[a]	Physically compatible for 4 hr at 23 °C	1758	C
Imipenem–cilastatin sodium	MSD	10 mg/mL[a]	SQ	40 mg/mL[a]	Physically compatible for 4 hr at 23 °C	1758	C
Insulin, regular	LI	0.2 unit/mL[b]	SQ	20 mg/mL	Physically compatible for 2 hr at 25 °C	1395	C
Leucovorin calcium	LE	2 mg/mL[a]	SQ	40 mg/mL[a]	Physically compatible for 4 hr at 23 °C	1758	C
Linezolid	PHU	2 mg/mL	SQ	40 mg/mL[a]	Physically compatible for 4 hr at 23 °C	2264	C
Lorazepam	WY	0.1 mg/mL[a]	SQ	40 mg/mL[a]	Haze forms within 1 hr	1758	I
Magnesium sulfate	AST	100 mg/mL[a]	SQ	40 mg/mL[a]	Physically compatible for 4 hr at 23 °C	1758	C
Mannitol	BA	15%	SQ	40 mg/mL[a]	Physically compatible for 4 hr at 23 °C	1758	C
Mechlorethamine HCl	MSD	1 mg/mL	SQ	40 mg/mL[a]	Physically compatible for 4 hr at 23 °C	1758	C
Melphalan HCl	BW	0.1 mg/mL[b]	SQ	40 mg/mL[b]	Physically compatible for 3 hr at 22 °C	1557	C
Meperidine HCl	AB	10 mg/mL	SQ	20 mg/mL[a]	Physically compatible for 4 hr at 25 °C	1397	C
	WY	4 mg/mL[a]	SQ	40 mg/mL[a]	Physically compatible for 4 hr at 23 °C	1758	C
Mesna	MJ	10 mg/mL[a]	SQ	40 mg/mL[a]	Physically compatible for 4 hr at 23 °C	1758	C
Methotrexate sodium	LE	15 mg/mL[a]	SQ	40 mg/mL[a]	Physically compatible for 4 hr at 23 °C	1758	C
Methylprednisolone sodium succinate	AB	5 mg/mL[a]	SQ	40 mg/mL[a]	Physically compatible for 4 hr at 23 °C	1758	C
Metoclopramide HCl	ES	5 mg/mL	SQ	40 mg/mL[a]	Physically compatible for 4 hr at 23 °C	1758	C
Metronidazole	BA	5 mg/mL	SQ	40 mg/mL[a]	Orange color forms in 4 hr	1758	I
Mitomycin	BMS	0.5 mg/mL	SQ	40 mg/mL[a]	Reddish-purple color forms in 4 hr	1758	I
Mitoxantrone HCl	LE	0.5 mg/mL[a]	SQ	40 mg/mL[a]	Heavy precipitate forms in 1 hr	1758	I
Morphine sulfate	AB	1 mg/mL	SQ	20 mg/mL[a]	Physically compatible for 4 hr at 25 °C	1397	C
	AST	1 mg/mL[a]	SQ	40 mg/mL[a]	Physically compatible for 4 hr at 23 °C	1758	C
Nalbuphine HCl	AST	10 mg/mL	SQ	40 mg/mL[a]	Physically compatible for 4 hr at 23 °C	1758	C
Nicardipine HCl	DCC	0.1 mg/mL[a]	SQ	10 mg/mL[a]	Visually compatible for 24 hr at room temperature	235	C
Ondansetron HCl	GL	1 mg/mL[b]	SQ	40 mg/mL[a]	Visually compatible for 4 hr at 22 °C	1365	C
	GL	0.03 and 0.3 mg/mL[a]	SQ	40 mg/mL[a]	Visually compatible with little loss of either drug in 4 hr at 25 °C	1732	C
	GL	1 mg/mL[a]	SQ	40 mg/mL[a]	Physically compatible for 4 hr at 23 °C	1758	C
Pemetrexed disodium	LI	20 mg/mL[b]	BMS	40 mg/mL[a]	Physically compatible for 4 hr at 23 °C	2564	C
Piperacillin sodium–tazobactam sodium	LE[f]	40 + 5 mg/ mL[a]	SQ	40 mg/mL[a]	Physically compatible for 4 hr at 22 °C	1688	C
Potassium chloride	AB	0.1 mEq/mL[a]	SQ	40 mg/mL[a]	Physically compatible for 4 hr at 23 °C	1758	C

Y-Site Injection Compatibility (1:1 Mixture) (Cont.)

Aztreonam

Drug	Mfr	Conc	Mfr	Conc	Remarks	Ref	C/I
Prochlorperazine edisylate	ES	0.5 mg/mL[a]	SQ	40 mg/mL[a]	Haze and tiny particles form within 4 hr	1758	**I**
Promethazine HCl	SCN	2 mg/mL[a]	SQ	40 mg/mL[a]	Physically compatible for 4 hr at 23 °C	1758	**C**
Propofol	ZEN	10 mg/mL	SQ	40 mg/mL[a]	Physically compatible for 1 hr at 23 °C	2066	**C**
Quinupristin–dalfopristin	AVE	2 mg/mL[a]		20 mg/mL[a]	Physically compatible	1	**C**
Ranitidine HCl	GL	1 mg/mL[b]	SQ	16.7 mg/mL[b]	No loss of either drug in 4 hr at 22 °C	1632	**C**
	GL	2 mg/mL[a]	SQ	40 mg/mL[a]	Physically compatible for 4 hr at 23 °C	1758	**C**
Remifentanil HCl	GW	0.025 and 0.25 mg/mL[b]	SQ	40 mg/mL[a]	Physically compatible for 4 hr at 23 °C	2075	**C**
Sargramostim	IMM	10 mcg/mL[b]	SQ	40 mg/mL[b]	Visually compatible for 4 hr at 22 °C	1436	**C**
	IMM	10 mcg/mL[b]	SQ	40 mg/mL[a]	Physically compatible for 4 hr at 23 °C	1758	**C**
Sodium bicarbonate	AB	1 mEq/mL	SQ	40 mg/mL[a]	Physically compatible for 4 hr at 23 °C	1758	**C**
Streptozocin	UP	40 mg/mL[a]	SQ	40 mg/mL[a]	Red color forms in 1 hr	1758	**I**
Teniposide	BR	0.1 mg/mL[a]	SQ	40 mg/mL[a]	Physically compatible for 4 hr at 23 °C	1725; 1758	**C**
Theophylline	TR	4 mg/mL	BV	20 mg/mL[a]	Visually compatible for 6 hr at 25 °C	1793	**C**
Thiotepa	LE	1 mg/mL[a]	SQ	40 mg/mL[a]	Physically compatible for 4 hr at 23 °C	1758	**C**
	IMM[d]	1 mg/mL[a]	SQ	40 mg/mL[a]	Physically compatible for 4 hr at 23 °C	1861	**C**
Ticarcillin disodium–clavulanate potassium	SKB	31 mg/mL[a]	SQ	40 mg/mL[a]	Physically compatible for 4 hr at 23 °C	1758	**C**
Tigecycline	WY	1 mg/mL[b]		20 mg/mL[b]	Physically compatible for 4 hr	2714	**C**
TNA #218 to #226[e]			SQ	40 mg/mL[a]	Visually compatible for 4 hr at 23 °C	2215	**C**
Tobramycin sulfate	LI	5 mg/mL[a]	SQ	40 mg/mL[a]	Physically compatible for 4 hr at 23 °C	1758	**C**
TPN #212 to #215[e]			SQ	40 mg/mL[a]	Physically compatible for 4 hr at 23 °C	2109	**C**
Trimethoprim–sulfamethoxazole	ES	0.8 + 4 mg/mL[a]	SQ	40 mg/mL[a]	Physically compatible for 4 hr at 23 °C	1758	**C**
Vancomycin HCl	LI	67 mg/mL[b]	SQ	200 mg/mL[b]	White granular precipitate forms immediately in tubing when given sequentially	1364	**I**
	AB	10 mg/mL[a]	SQ	40 mg/mL[a]	Physically compatible for 4 hr at 23 °C	1758	**C**
Vinblastine sulfate	LI	0.12 mg/mL[a]	SQ	40 mg/mL[a]	Physically compatible for 4 hr at 23 °C	1758	**C**
Vincristine sulfate	LI	0.05 mg/mL[a]	SQ	40 mg/mL[a]	Physically compatible for 4 hr at 23 °C	1758	**C**
Vinorelbine tartrate	BW	1 mg/mL[b]	SQ	40 mg/mL[b]	Physically compatible for 4 hr at 23 °C	1558	**C**
Zidovudine	BW	4 mg/mL[a]	SQ	40 mg/mL[a]	Physically compatible for 4 hr at 25 °C	1193	**C**
	BW	4 mg/mL[a]	SQ	40 mg/mL[a]	Physically compatible for 4 hr at 23 °C	1758	**C**

[a]*Tested in dextrose 5%.*
[b]*Tested in sodium chloride 0.9%.*
[c]*Tested in both dextrose 5% and sodium chloride 0.9%.*
[d]*Lyophilized formulation tested.*
[e]*Refer to Appendix I for the composition of parenteral nutrition solutions. TNA indicates a 3-in-1 admixture, and TPN indicates a 2-in-1 admixture.*
[f]*Test performed using the formulation WITHOUT edetate disodium.*
[g]*Tested in sodium chloride 0.45%.*
[h]*Injected via Y-site into an administration set running azithromycin.*
[i]*Final concentration after mixing.*

BACLOFEN
AHFS 12:20.12

Products — Baclofen injection is available as a preservative-free injection in intrathecal refill kits at a concentration of 0.5 mg/mL in 20-mL ampuls and at a concentration of 2 mg/mL in 5-mL ampuls. Each milliliter of solution contains baclofen 0.5 or 2 mg (500 or 2000 mcg, respectively) with sodium chloride 9 mg in water for injection. (1)

Baclofen preservative-free intrathecal injection is also available in intrathecal screening kits at a concentration of 0.05 mg/mL in 1-mL ampuls. Each milliliter of solution contains baclofen 0.05 mg (50 mcg) with sodium chloride 9 mg in water for injection. (1)

pH — From 5 to 7. (1)

Tonicity — Baclofen injection is an isotonic solution. (1; 4)

Sodium Content — Contains 0.15 mEq per milliliter. (4)

Trade Name(s) — Lioresal Intrathecal.

Administration — For screening, baclofen injection must be diluted with sterile, preservative-free sodium chloride 0.9% injection to a concentration of 50 mcg/mL. The dilution is administered by direct intrathecal injection via lumbar puncture or catheter over at least one minute using barbotage. In maintenance treatment, baclofen injection is also given by intrathecal infusion using an implantable infusion control device; concentration and rate of delivery must be carefully titrated to each patient's needs. (1; 4)

Stability — Baclofen injection may be stored at controlled room temperatures not exceeding 30 °C. It should be protected from freezing. (1; 4) The product is stable in implantable infusion pumps at a temperature of 37 °C. (4) It should not be autoclaved. The product contains no preservatives and is intended for single-use only; unused portions must be discarded. (1; 4)

Baclofen injection must be diluted only with sterile, preservative-free sodium chloride 0.9%. It is compatible with cerebrospinal fluid. (1; 4)

Implantable Pumps — Baclofen 0.5 mg/mL was filled into an implantable pump (Fresenius model VIP 30) and associated capillary tubing and stored at 37 °C. No baclofen loss and no contamination from components of pump materials occurred during eight weeks of storage. (1903)

Compatibility Information

Solution Compatibility

Baclofen

Solution	Mfr	Mfr	Conc/L	Remarks	Ref	C/I
Sodium chloride 0.9%	BA		1 g	Visually compatible with no loss in 10 weeks at 37 °C protected from light	2359	C

Additive Compatibility

Baclofen

Drug	Mfr	Conc/L	Mfr	Conc/L	Test Soln	Remarks	Ref	C/I
Clonidine HCl		0.2 g		1 g	NS	Visually compatible with no loss of either drug in 10 weeks at 37 °C in dark	2359	C
Morphine sulfate	DB	1 and 1.5 g	CI	200 mg	NS[a]	Physically compatible. Little loss of either drug in 30 days at 37 °C	1911	C
	DB	1 g	CI	800 mg	NS[a]	Physically compatible. Little baclofen loss and less than 7% morphine loss in 29 days at 37 °C	1911	C
	DB	1.5 g	CI	800 mg	NS[a]	Physically compatible. Little loss of either drug in 30 days at 37 °C	1911	C
	DB	7.5 g	CI	1.5 g	NS[a]	Physically compatible. Little loss of either drug in 30 days at 37 °C	2170	C
	DB	15 g	CI	1 g	NS[a]	Physically compatible. Little loss of either drug in 30 days at 37 °C	2170	C
	DB	21 g	CI	200 mg	NS[a]	Physically compatible. 7% baclofen loss and little morphine loss in 30 days at 37 °C	2170	C

[a] Tested in glass containers.

BENZTROPINE MESYLATE
AHFS 28:36.08

Products — Benztropine mesylate is available in 2-mL ampuls containing 2 mg of drug with sodium chloride in water for injection. (1)

pH — From 5 to 8. (4)

Trade Name(s) — Cogentin.

Administration — Benztropine mesylate may be administered by intramuscular or, rarely, intravenous injection. (1; 4)

Stability — Store the ampuls at controlled room temperature. Avoid freezing and storing at temperatures over 40 °C. (4)

Compatibility Information

Drugs in Syringe Compatibility

Benztropine mesylate

Drug (in syringe)	Mfr	Amt	Mfr	Amt	Remarks	Ref	C/I
Chlorpromazine HCl	STS	50 mg/ 2 mL	MSD	2 mg/ 2 mL	Visually compatible for 60 min	1784	C
Fluphenazine HCl	LY	5 mg/ 2 mL	MSD	2 mg/ 2 mL	Visually compatible for 60 min	1784	C
Haloperidol lactate	MN	0.25, 0.5, 1 mg	MSD	2 mg	Visually compatible for 24 hr at 21 °C	1781	C
	MN	2 mg	MSD	2 mg	Precipitate forms within 4 hr at 21 °C	1781	I
	MN	3, 4, 5 mg	MSD	2 mg	Precipitate forms within 15 min at 21 °C	1781	I
	MN	0.25 and 0.5 mg	MSD	1 mg	Visually compatible for 24 hr at 21 °C	1781	C
	MN	1 to 5 mg	MSD	1 mg	Precipitate forms within 15 min at 21 °C	1781	I
	MN	0.25 to 5 mg	MSD	0.5 mg	Precipitate forms within 15 min at 21 °C	1781	I
	MN	10 mg/ 2 mL	MSD	2 mg/ 2 mL	White precipitate forms within 5 min	1784	I
Metoclopramide HCl	RB	10 mg/ 2 mL	MSD	2 mg/ 2 mL	Physically compatible for 48 hr at 25 °C	1167	C
	RB	160 mg/ 32 mL	MSD	2 mg/ 2 mL	Physically compatible for 48 hr at 25 °C	1167	C

Y-Site Injection Compatibility (1:1 Mixture)

Benztropine mesylate

Drug	Mfr	Conc	Mfr	Conc	Remarks	Ref	C/I
Fluconazole	RR	2 mg/mL	MSD	1 mg/mL	Physically compatible for 24 hr at 25 °C	1407	C
Tacrolimus	FUJ	1 mg/mL[a]	MSD	1 mg/mL	Visually compatible for 24 hr at 25 °C	1630	C

[a]Tested in sodium chloride 0.9%.

BIVALIRUDIN
AHFS 20:12.04.12

Products — Bivalirudin is available as a white lyophilized powder. Each vial contains bivalirudin 250 mg with mannitol 125 mg and sodium hydroxide to adjust pH. Reconstitute with 5 mL of sterile water for injection and swirl to dissolve yielding a 50-mg/mL solution. The reconstituted solution must be diluted for use. (1)

pH — From 5 to 6. (1)

Sodium Content — Approximately 12.5 mg per vial. (1)

Trade Name(s) — Angiomax.

Administration — Bivalirudin is administered by intravenous injection and infusion. It should not be administered by other routes. Reconstituted bivalirudin must be diluted to a concentration of 0.5 or 5 mg/mL for infusion. (1; 4)

Stability — Bivalirudin vials should be stored at room temperature. The drug is a white lyophilized powder that becomes a clear or opalescent colorless to slightly yellow solution upon reconstitution. The reconstituted solution is stable for 24 hours under refrigeration; freezing should be avoided. The drug has no antibacterial preservative and unused portions should be discarded. (1)

Compatibility Information

Solution Compatibility

Bivalirudin

Solution	Mfr	Mfr	Conc/L	Remarks	Ref	C/I
Dextrose 5%			0.5 to 5 mg/mL	Stable for 24 hr at room temperature	1	C
Sodium chloride 0.9%			0.5 to 5 mg/mL	Stable for 24 hr at room temperature	1	C

Y-Site Injection Compatibility (1:1 Mixture)

Bivalirudin

Drug	Mfr	Conc	Mfr	Conc	Remarks	Ref	C/I
Abciximab	CEN	10 mcg/mL[a]	TMC	5 mg/mL[a]	Physically compatible for 4 hr at 23 °C	2373	C
Alfentanil HCl	TAY	0.125 mg/mL[a]	TMC	5 mg/mL[a]	Physically compatible for 4 hr at 23 °C	2373	C
Alteplase	GEN	1 mg/mL	TMC	5 mg/mL[a]	Small aggregates form immediately	2373	I
Amikacin sulfate	APO	5 mg/mL[a]	TMC	5 mg/mL[a]	Physically compatible for 4 hr at 23 °C	2373	C
Aminophylline	AB	2.5 mg/mL[a]	TMC	5 mg/mL[a]	Physically compatible for 4 hr at 23 °C	2373	C
Amiodarone HCl	WAY	4 mg/mL[a]	TMC	5 mg/mL[a]	Measured haze increases immediately	2373	I
Amphotericin B	APO	0.6 mg/mL[a]	TMC	5 mg/mL[a]	Yellow precipitate forms immediately	2373	I
Ampicillin sodium	APO	20 mg/mL[b]	TMC	5 mg/mL[a]	Physically compatible for 4 hr at 23 °C	2373	C
Ampicillin sodium–sulbactam sodium	PF	20 + 10 mg/mL[b]	TMC	5 mg/mL[a]	Physically compatible for 4 hr at 23 °C	2373	C
Atropine sulfate	AMR	0.4 mg/mL	TMC	5 mg/mL[a,b]	Visually compatible for 6 hr at 23 °C	2680	C
Azithromycin	PF	2 mg/mL[a]	TMC	5 mg/mL[a]	Physically compatible for 4 hr at 23 °C	2373	C
Aztreonam	DUR	40 mg/mL[a]	TMC	5 mg/mL[a]	Physically compatible for 4 hr at 23 °C	2373	C
Bumetanide	OHM	40 mcg/mL[a]	TMC	5 mg/mL[a]	Physically compatible for 4 hr at 23 °C	2373	C
Butorphanol tartrate	APO	40 mcg/mL[a]	TMC	5 mg/mL[a]	Physically compatible for 4 hr at 23 °C	2373	C
Calcium gluconate	APP	40 mg/mL[a]	TMC	5 mg/mL[a]	Physically compatible for 4 hr at 23 °C	2373	C
Cefazolin sodium	APO	20 mg/mL[a]	TMC	5 mg/mL[a]	Physically compatible for 4 hr at 23 °C	2373	C
Cefepime HCl	BMS	20 mg/mL[a]	TMC	5 mg/mL[a]	Physically compatible for 4 hr at 23 °C	2373	C

Y-Site Injection Compatibility (1:1 Mixture) (Cont.)

Bivalirudin

Drug	Mfr	Conc	Mfr	Conc	Remarks	Ref	C/I
Cefotaxime sodium	HO	20 mg/mL[a]	TMC	5 mg/mL[a]	Physically compatible for 4 hr at 23 °C	2373	**C**
Cefotetan disodium	ZEN	20 mg/mL[a]	TMC	5 mg/mL[a]	Physically compatible for 4 hr at 23 °C	2373	**C**
Cefoxitin sodium	ME	20 mg/mL[a]	TMC	5 mg/mL[a]	Physically compatible for 4 hr at 23 °C	2373	**C**
Ceftazidime	GW	40 mg/mL[a]	TMC	5 mg/mL[a]	Physically compatible for 4 hr at 23 °C	2373	**C**
Ceftriaxone sodium	RC	20 mg/mL[a]	TMC	5 mg/mL[a]	Physically compatible for 4 hr at 23 °C	2373	**C**
Cefuroxime sodium	GW	30 mg/mL[a]	TMC	5 mg/mL[a]	Physically compatible for 4 hr at 23 °C	2373	**C**
Chlorpromazine HCl	ES	2 mg/mL[a]	TMC	5 mg/mL[a]	Gross white precipitate forms immediately	2373	**I**
Ciprofloxacin	BAY	2 mg/mL[a]	TMC	5 mg/mL[a]	Physically compatible for 4 hr at 23 °C	2373	**C**
Clindamycin phosphate	AB	10 mg/mL[a]	TMC	5 mg/mL[a]	Physically compatible for 4 hr at 23 °C	2373	**C**
Dexamethasone sodium phosphate	APP	1 mg/mL[a]	TMC	5 mg/mL[a]	Physically compatible for 4 hr at 23 °C	2373	**C**
Diazepam	AB	5 mg/mL	TMC	5 mg/mL[a]	Yellowish precipitate forms immediately	2373	**I**
Digoxin	GW	0.25 mg/mL	TMC	5 mg/mL[a]	Physically compatible for 4 hr at 23 °C	2373	**C**
Diltiazem HCl	BA	5 mg/mL	TMC	5 mg/mL[a]	Physically compatible for 4 hr at 23 °C	2373	**C**
	BV	5 mg/mL	TMC	5 mg/mL[a,b]	Visually compatible for 6 hr at 23 °C	2680	**C**
Diphenhydramine HCl	ES	2 mg/mL[a]	TMC	5 mg/mL[a]	Physically compatible for 4 hr at 23 °C	2373	**C**
Dobutamine HCl	AB	4 mg/mL[a]	TMC	5 mg/mL[a]	Physically compatible for 4 hr at 23 °C	2373	**C**
	BV	12.5 mg/mL[d]	TMC	5 mg/mL[a,b]	Cloudiness forms immediately	2680	**I**
Dopamine HCl	AB	3.2 mg/mL[a]	TMC	5 mg/mL[a]	Physically compatible for 4 hr at 23 °C	2373	**C**
	AMR	80 mg/mL	TMC	5 mg/mL[a,b]	Visually compatible for 6 hr at 23 °C	2680	**C**
Doxycycline hyclate	APP	1 mg/mL[a]	TMC	5 mg/mL[a]	Physically compatible for 4 hr at 23 °C	2373	**C**
Droperidol	AMR	2.5 mg/mL	TMC	5 mg/mL[a]	Physically compatible for 4 hr at 23 °C	2373	**C**
Enalaprilat	BED	0.1 mg/mL[a]	TMC	5 mg/mL[a]	Physically compatible for 4 hr at 23 °C	2373	**C**
Ephedrine sulfate	TAY	5 mg/mL[a]	TMC	5 mg/mL[a]	Physically compatible for 4 hr at 23 °C	2373	**C**
Epinephrine HCl	AMR	50 mcg/mL[a]	TMC	5 mg/mL[a]	Physically compatible for 4 hr at 23 °C	2373	**C**
Epoprostenol sodium	GW	10 mcg/mL[a]	TMC	5 mg/mL[a]	Physically compatible for 4 hr at 23 °C	2373	**C**
Eptifibatide	KEY	2 mg/mL	TMC	5 mg/mL[a]	Physically compatible for 4 hr at 23 °C	2373	**C**
Erythromycin lactobionate	AB	5 mg/mL[b]	TMC	5 mg/mL[a]	Physically compatible for 4 hr at 23 °C	2373	**C**
Esmolol HCl	BA	10 mg/mL[a]	TMC	5 mg/mL[a]	Physically compatible for 4 hr at 23 °C	2373	**C**
Famotidine	ME	2 mg/mL[a]	TMC	5 mg/mL[a]	Physically compatible for 4 hr at 23 °C	2373	**C**
Fentanyl citrate	AB	50 mcg/mL	TMC	5 mg/mL[a]	Physically compatible for 4 hr at 23 °C	2373	**C**
	TAY	50 mcg/mL	TMC	5 mg/mL[a,b]	Visually compatible for 6 hr at 23 °C	2680	**C**
Fluconazole	PF	2 mg/mL	TMC	5 mg/mL[a]	Physically compatible for 4 hr at 23 °C	2373	**C**
Furosemide	AMR	3 mg/mL[a]	TMC	5 mg/mL[a]	Physically compatible for 4 hr at 23 °C	2373	**C**
Gentamicin sulfate	AB	5 mg/mL[a]	TMC	5 mg/mL[a]	Physically compatible for 4 hr at 23 °C	2373	**C**
Haloperidol lactate	MN	0.2 mg/mL[a]	TMC	5 mg/mL[a]	Physically compatible for 4 hr at 23 °C	2373	**C**
Heparin sodium	AB	100 units/mL	TMC	5 mg/mL[a]	Physically compatible for 4 hr at 23 °C	2373	**C**
Hydrocortisone sodium succinate	PHU	1 mg/mL[a]	TMC	5 mg/mL[a]	Physically compatible for 4 hr at 23 °C	2373	**C**
	PHU	50 mg/mL	TMC	5 mg/mL[a,b]	Visually compatible for 6 hr at 23 °C	2680	**C**
Hydromorphone HCl	AST	0.5 mg/mL[a]	TMC	5 mg/mL[a]	Physically compatible for 4 hr at 23 °C	2373	**C**
Isoproterenol HCl	AB	20 mcg/mL[a]	TMC	5 mg/mL[a]	Physically compatible for 4 hr at 23 °C	2373	**C**

Y-Site Injection Compatibility (1:1 Mixture) (Cont.)

Bivalirudin

Drug	Mfr	Conc	Mfr	Conc	Remarks	Ref	C/I
Labetalol HCl	FP	2 mg/mL[a]	TMC	5 mg/mL[a]	Physically compatible for 4 hr at 23 °C	2373	C
Levofloxacin	ORT	5 mg/mL[a]	TMC	5 mg/mL[a]	Physically compatible for 4 hr at 23 °C	2373	C
Lidocaine HCl	AST	10 mg/mL[a]	TMC	5 mg/mL[a]	Physically compatible for 4 hr at 23 °C	2373	C
Lorazepam	ESL	0.5 mg/mL[a]	TMC	5 mg/mL[a]	Physically compatible for 4 hr at 23 °C	2373	C
Magnesium sulfate	APP	100 mg/mL[a]	TMC	5 mg/mL[a]	Physically compatible for 4 hr at 23 °C	2373	C
Mannitol	BA	15%	TMC	5 mg/mL[a]	Physically compatible for 4 hr at 23 °C	2373	C
Meperidine HCl	AST	10 mg/mL[a]	TMC	5 mg/mL[a]	Physically compatible for 4 hr at 23 °C	2373	C
Methylprednisolone sodium succinate	PHU	5 mg/mL[a]	TMC	5 mg/mL[a]	Physically compatible for 4 hr at 23 °C	2373	C
Metoclopramide HCl	FAU	5 mg/mL	TMC	5 mg/mL[a]	Physically compatible for 4 hr at 23 °C	2373	C
Metoprolol tartrate	AB	1 mg/mL	TMC	5 mg/mL[a,b]	Visually compatible for 6 hr at 23 °C	2680	C
Metronidazole	BA	5 mg/mL	TMC	5 mg/mL[a]	Physically compatible for 4 hr at 23 °C	2373	C
Midazolam HCl	BA	1 mg/mL[a]	TMC	5 mg/mL[a]	Physically compatible for 4 hr at 23 °C	2373	C
	AB	2 mg/mL	TMC	5 mg/mL[a,b]	Visually compatible for 6 hr at 23 °C	2680	C
Milrinone lactate	SAN	0.2 mg/mL[a]	TMC	5 mg/mL[a]	Physically compatible for 4 hr at 23 °C	2373	C
Morphine sulfate	AST	1 mg/mL[a]	TMC	5 mg/mL[a]	Physically compatible for 4 hr at 23 °C	2373	C
	ES	10 mg/mL	TMC	5 mg/mL[a,b]	Visually compatible for 6 hr at 23 °C	2680	C
Nalbuphine HCl	AST	10 mg/mL	TMC	5 mg/mL[a]	Physically compatible for 4 hr at 23 °C	2373	C
Nitroglycerin	AMR	0.4 mg/mL[a]	TMC	5 mg/mL[a]	Physically compatible for 4 hr at 23 °C	2373	C
Norepinephrine bitartrate	AB	0.12 mg/mL[a]	TMC	5 mg/mL[a]	Physically compatible for 4 hr at 23 °C	2373	C
Phenylephrine HCl	AMR	1 mg/mL[a]	TMC	5 mg/mL[a]	Physically compatible for 4 hr at 23 °C	2373	C
	AMR	10 mg/mL	TMC	5 mg/mL[a,b]	Visually compatible for 6 hr at 23 °C	2680	C
Piperacillin sodium–tazobactam sodium	LE[c]	40 + 5 mg/mL[a]	TMC	5 mg/mL[a]	Physically compatible for 4 hr at 23 °C	2373	C
Potassium chloride	APP	0.1 mEq/mL[a]	TMC	5 mg/mL[a]	Physically compatible for 4 hr at 23 °C	2373	C
Procainamide HCl	ES	10 mg/mL[a]	TMC	5 mg/mL[a]	Physically compatible for 4 hr at 23 °C	2373	C
Prochlorperazine edisylate	SKB	0.5 mg/mL[a]	TMC	5 mg/mL[a]	Gross white precipitate forms immediately	2373	I
Promethazine HCl	ES	2 mg/mL[a]	TMC	5 mg/mL[a]	Physically compatible for 4 hr at 23 °C	2373	C
Ranitidine HCl	GW	2 mg/mL[a]	TMC	5 mg/mL[a]	Physically compatible for 4 hr at 23 °C	2373	C
Reteplase	CEN	1 unit/mL[a]	TMC	5 mg/mL[a]	Small aggregates form immediately	2373	I
Sodium bicarbonate	AMR	1 mEq/mL	TMC	5 mg/mL[a]	Physically compatible for 4 hr at 23 °C	2373	C
Sodium nitroprusside	BA	2 mg/mL[a]	TMC	5 mg/mL[a]	Physically compatible for 4 hr at 23 °C protected from light	2373	C
Sufentanil citrate	ES	50 mcg/mL	TMC	5 mg/mL[a]	Physically compatible for 4 hr at 23 °C	2373	C
Theophylline	BA	4 mg/mL[a]	TMC	5 mg/mL[a]	Physically compatible for 4 hr at 23 °C	2373	C
Ticarcillin disodium–clavulanate potassium	SKB	31 mg/mL[a]	TMC	5 mg/mL[a]	Physically compatible for 4 hr at 23 °C	2373	C
Tirofiban HCl	ME	50 mcg/mL[a]	TMC	5 mg/mL[a]	Physically compatible for 4 hr at 23 °C	2373	C
Tobramycin sulfate	GNS	5 mg/mL[a]	TMC	5 mg/mL[a]	Physically compatible for 4 hr at 23 °C	2373	C
Trimethoprim–sulfamethoxazole	GNS	0.8 + 4 mg/mL[a]	TMC	5 mg/mL[a]	Physically compatible for 4 hr at 23 °C	2373	C
Vancomycin HCl	AB	10 mg/mL[a]	TMC	5 mg/mL[a]	Gross white precipitate forms immediately	2373	I

Y-Site Injection Compatibility (1:1 Mixture) (Cont.)

Bivalirudin

Drug	Mfr	Conc	Mfr	Conc	Remarks	Ref	C/I
Verapamil HCl	AB	1.25 mg/mL[a]	TMC	5 mg/mL[a]	Physically compatible for 4 hr at 23 °C	2373	C
	AMR	2.5 mg/mL	TMC	5 mg/mL[a,b]	Visually compatible for 6 hr at 23 °C	2680	C
Warfarin sodium	DU	2 mg/mL	TMC	5 mg/mL[a]	Physically compatible for 4 hr at 23 °C	2373	C

[a]Tested in dextrose 5%.
[b]Tested in sodium chloride 0.9%.
[c]Test performed using the formulation WITHOUT edetate disodium.
[d]NOTE: Undiluted dobutamine hydrochloride concentrate must be diluted for administration. This concentration is not acceptable for intravenous administration.

BLEOMYCIN SULFATE
AHFS 10:00

Products — Bleomycin sulfate is available in vials containing 15 and 30 units of bleomycin as the sulfate. For intramuscular or subcutaneous administration, reconstitute the 15-unit vial with 1 to 5 mL and the 30-unit vial with 2 to 10 mL of sterile water for injection, sodium chloride 0.9%, or bacteriostatic water for injection, yielding a solution containing 3 to 15 units/mL. For intravenous injection, reconstitute the 15-unit vial with a minimum of 5 mL and the 30-unit vial with a minimum of 10 mL of sodium chloride 0.9%, resulting in a solution of not more than 3 units/mL. For intrapleural administration, 60 units is dissolved in 50 to 100 mL of sodium chloride 0.9%. (1; 4)

Units — Bleomycin sulfate is a mixture of cytotoxic glycopeptide antibiotics. A unit of bleomycin is equal to the term milligram activity, which was formerly used. One unit of bleomycin is equivalent in activity to 1 mg of bleomycin A_2 reference standard. (4)

pH — The pH of the reconstituted solution varies from 4.0 to 6, depending on the diluent. (1)

Administration — Bleomycin sulfate may be administered by intramuscular, subcutaneous, intravenous, or intrapleural injection. Intravenous injections should be given slowly over a 10-minute period. (1; 4)

Stability — Intact vials are stable under refrigeration and bear an expiration date. (1) They are stated to be stable for 28 days at room temperature. (1181; 1433) Bleomycin sulfate solutions reconstituted with sodium chloride 0.9% are reported to be stable for four weeks when stored at 2 to 8 °C (4; 1369), for two weeks (4) or longer (860; 1369) at room temperature, and for 10 days at 37 °C. (1073) However, because of the risk of microbial contamination in products without preservatives, it is recommended that the solutions be used within 24 hours of reconstitution. (1; 4; 860)

Ogawa et al. reported that immersion of a needle with an aluminum component in bleomycin sulfate (Bristol) 3 units/mL resulted in no visually apparent reaction after seven days at 24 °C. (988)

In the event of spills or leaks, the use of sodium hypochlorite 5% (household bleach) or potassium permanganate 1% has been recommended to inactivate bleomycin sulfate. (1200)

pH Effects — Bleomycin sulfate (Bristol) is stable in solution over a pH range of 4 to 10. (763)

Filtration — Bleomycin sulfate was shown not to exhibit substantial sorption to cellulose ester (Ivex-2), cellulose nitrate/cellulose acetate (Millex OR), nylon, or Teflon (Millex FG) filters. (533; 1415; 1416; 1577)

Compatibility Information

Solution Compatibility

Bleomycin sulfate

Solution	Mfr	Mfr	Conc/L	Remarks	Ref	C/I
Dextrose 5%	a		150 units	About 54% loss in 28 days at room temperature in the dark	1369	I
	BA[b]	BR	300 and 3000 units	About 10% loss in 8 to 10 hr and 11 to 16% loss in 24 hr at 23 °C in glass and PVC	1441	I
	c	BEL	15 units	No loss in 24 hr at room temperature in light	1577	C

Solution Compatibility (Cont.)

Bleomycin sulfate

Solution	Mfr	Mfr	Conc/L	Remarks	Ref	C/I
Sodium chloride 0.9%				Stable for 24 hr at room temperature	1	C
	[a]		150 units	About 4% loss in 28 days at room temperature in the dark	1369	C
	BA[b]	BR	300 and 3000 units	Little or no loss in 24 hr at 23 °C in glass and PVC	1441	C
	[c]	BEL	15 units	No loss in 48 hr at room temperature in light	1577	C

[a]Tested in PVC containers.
[b]Tested in both glass and PVC containers.
[c]Tested in glass, PVC, and high-density polyethylene containers.

Additive Compatibility

Bleomycin sulfate

Drug	Mfr	Conc/L	Mfr	Conc/L	Test Soln	Remarks	Ref	C/I
Amikacin sulfate	BR	1.25 g	BR	20 and 30 units	NS	Physically compatible. Bleomycin stable for 1 week at 4 °C. Amikacin not tested	763	C
Aminophylline	ES	250 mg	BR	20 and 30 units	NS	50% loss of bleomycin in 1 week at 4 °C	763	I
Ascorbic acid	PD	2.5 and 5 g	BR	20 and 30 units	NS	Loss of all bleomycin in 1 week at 4 °C	763	I
Cefazolin sodium	LI	1 g	BR	20 and 30 units	NS	43% loss of bleomycin activity in 1 week at 4 °C	763	I
Dexamethasone sodium phosphate	MSD	50 mg	BR	20 and 30 units	NS	Physically compatible and bleomycin activity retained for 1 week at 4 °C. Dexamethasone not tested	763	C
Diazepam	RC	50 and 100 mg	BR	20 and 30 units	NS	Physically incompatible	763	I
Diphenhydramine HCl	PD	100 mg	BR	20 and 30 units	NS	Physically compatible and bleomycin activity retained for 1 week at 4 °C. Diphenhydramine not tested	763	C
Fluorouracil	RC	1 g	BR	20 and 30 units	NS	Physically compatible and bleomycin activity retained for 1 week at 4 °C. Fluorouracil not tested	763	C
Gentamicin sulfate	SC	50, 100, 300, 600 mg	BR	20 and 30 units	NS	Physically compatible and bleomycin activity retained for 1 week at 4 °C. Gentamicin not tested	763	C
Heparin sodium	RI	10,000 to 200,000 units	BR	20 and 30 units	NS	Physically compatible and bleomycin activity retained for 1 week at 4 °C. Heparin not tested	763	C
Hydrocortisone sodium succinate	AB	300 mg, 750 mg, 1 g, 2.5 g	BR	20 and 30 units	NS	60 to 100% loss of bleomycin activity in 1 week at 4 °C	763	I
Methotrexate sodium	LE	250 and 500 mg	BR	20 and 30 units	NS	About 60% loss of bleomycin activity in 1 week at 4 °C	763	I

Additive Compatibility (Cont.)

Bleomycin sulfate

Drug	Mfr	Conc/L	Mfr	Conc/L	Test Soln	Remarks	Ref	C/I
Mitomycin	BR	10 mg	BR	20 and 30 units	NS	20% loss of bleomycin activity in 1 week at 4 °C	763	I
	BR	50 mg	BR	20 and 30 units	NS	52% loss of bleomycin activity in 1 week at 4 °C	763	I
Nafcillin sodium	BR	2.5 g	BR	20 and 30 units	NS	Substantial loss of bleomycin activity in 1 week at 4 °C	763	I
Penicillin G sodium	SQ	2 million units	BR	20 and 30 units	NS	77% loss of bleomycin activity in 1 week at 4 °C	763	I
	SQ	5 million units	BR	20 and 30 units	NS	41% loss of bleomycin activity in 1 week at 4 °C	763	I
Streptomycin sulfate	PF	4 g	BR	20 and 30 units	NS	Physically compatible and bleomycin activity retained for 1 week at 4 °C. Streptomycin not tested	763	C
Terbutaline sulfate	GG	7.5 mg	BR	20 and 30 units	NS	36% loss of bleomycin activity in 1 week at 4 °C	763	I
Tobramycin sulfate	LI	500 mg	BR	20 and 30 units	NS	Physically compatible and bleomycin activity retained for 1 week at 4 °C. Tobramycin not tested	763	C
Vinblastine sulfate	LI	10 and 100 mg	BR	20 and 30 units	NS	Physically compatible and bleomycin activity retained for 1 week at 4 °C. Vinblastine not tested	763	C
Vincristine sulfate	LI	50 and 100 mg	BR	20 and 30 units	NS	Physically compatible and bleomycin activity retained for 1 week at 4 °C. Vincristine not tested	763	C

Drugs in Syringe Compatibility

Bleomycin sulfate

Drug (in syringe)	Mfr	Amt	Mfr	Amt	Remarks	Ref	C/I
Cisplatin		0.5 mg/ 0.5 mL		1.5 units/ 0.5 mL	Physically compatible for 5 min at room temperature followed by 8 min of centrifugation	980	C
Cyclophosphamide		10 mg/ 0.5 mL		1.5 units/ 0.5 mL	Physically compatible for 5 min at room temperature followed by 8 min of centrifugation	980	C
Doxorubicin HCl		1 mg/ 0.5 mL		1.5 units/ 0.5 mL	Physically compatible for 5 min at room temperature followed by 8 min of centrifugation	980	C
Droperidol		1.25 mg/ 0.5 mL		1.5 units/ 0.5 mL	Physically compatible for 5 min at room temperature followed by 8 min of centrifugation	980	C
Fluorouracil		25 mg/ 0.5 mL		1.5 units/ 0.5 mL	Physically compatible for 5 min at room temperature followed by 8 min of centrifugation	980	C
Furosemide		5 mg/ 0.5 mL		1.5 units/ 0.5 mL	Physically compatible for 5 min at room temperature followed by 8 min of centrifugation	980	C
Heparin sodium		500 units/ 0.5 mL		1.5 units/ 0.5 mL	Physically compatible for 5 min at room temperature followed by 8 min of centrifugation	980	C

Drugs in Syringe Compatibility (Cont.)

Bleomycin sulfate

Drug (in syringe)	Mfr	Amt	Mfr	Amt	Remarks	Ref	C/I
Leucovorin calcium		5 mg/ 0.5 mL		1.5 units/ 0.5 mL	Physically compatible for 5 min at room temperature followed by 8 min of centrifugation	980	C
Methotrexate sodium		12.5 mg/ 0.5 mL		1.5 units/ 0.5 mL	Physically compatible for 5 min at room temperature followed by 8 min of centrifugation	980	C
Metoclopramide HCl		2.5 mg/ 0.5 mL		1.5 units/ 0.5 mL	Physically compatible for 5 min at room temperature followed by 8 min of centrifugation	980	C
Mitomycin		0.25 mg/ 0.5 mL		1.5 units/ 0.5 mL	Physically compatible for 5 min at room temperature followed by 8 min of centrifugation	980	C
Vinblastine sulfate		0.5 mg/ 0.5 mL		1.5 units/ 0.5 mL	Physically compatible for 5 min at room temperature followed by 8 min of centrifugation	980	C
Vincristine sulfate		0.5 mg/ 0.5 mL		1.5 units/ 0.5 mL	Physically compatible for 5 min at room temperature followed by 8 min of centrifugation	980	C

Y-Site Injection Compatibility (1:1 Mixture)

Bleomycin sulfate

Drug	Mfr	Conc	Mfr	Conc	Remarks	Ref	C/I
Allopurinol sodium	BW	3 mg/mL[b]	BR	1 unit/mL[b]	Physically compatible for 4 hr at 22 °C	1686	C
Amifostine	USB	10 mg/mL[a]	MJ	1 unit/mL[b]	Physically compatible for 4 hr at 23 °C	1845	C
Aztreonam	SQ	40 mg/mL[a]	MJ	1 unit/mL[b]	Physically compatible for 4 hr at 23 °C	1758	C
Cisplatin		1 mg/mL		3 units/mL	Drugs injected sequentially in Y-site with no flush. No precipitate seen	980	C
Cyclophosphamide		20 mg/mL		3 units/mL	Drugs injected sequentially in Y-site with no flush. No precipitate seen	980	C
Doxorubicin HCl		2 mg/mL		3 units/mL	Drugs injected sequentially in Y-site with no flush. No precipitate seen	980	C
Doxorubicin HCl liposomal	SEQ	0.4 mg/mL[a]	MJ	1 unit/mL[b]	Physically compatible for 4 hr at 23 °C	2087	C
Droperidol		2.5 mg/mL		3 units/mL	Drugs injected sequentially in Y-site with no flush. No precipitate seen	980	C
Etoposide phosphate	BR	5 mg/mL[a]	MJ	1 unit/mL[b]	Physically compatible for 4 hr at 23 °C	2218	C
Filgrastim	AMG	30 mcg/mL[a]	BR	1 unit/mL[a]	Physically compatible for 4 hr at 22 °C	1687	C
Fludarabine phosphate	BX	1 mg/mL[a]	BR	1 unit/mL[b]	Visually compatible for 4 hr at 22 °C	1439	C
Fluorouracil		50 mg/mL		3 units/mL	Drugs injected sequentially in Y-site with no flush. No precipitate seen	980	C
Furosemide		10 mg/mL		3 units/mL	Drugs injected sequentially in Y-site with no flush. No precipitate seen	980	C
Gemcitabine HCl	LI	10 mg/mL[b]	MJ	1 unit/mL[b]	Physically compatible for 4 hr at 23 °C	2226	C
Granisetron HCl	SKB	0.05 mg/mL[a]	MJ	1 unit/mL[b]	Physically compatible for 4 hr at 23 °C	2000	C
Heparin sodium		1000 units/ mL		3 units/mL	Drugs injected sequentially in Y-site with no flush. No precipitate seen	980	C
Leucovorin calcium		10 mg/mL		3 units/mL	Drugs injected sequentially in Y-site with no flush. No precipitate seen	980	C
Melphalan HCl	BW	0.1 mg/mL[b]	BR	1 unit/mL[b]	Physically compatible for 3 hr at 22 °C	1557	C

Y-Site Injection Compatibility (1:1 Mixture) (Cont.)

Bleomycin sulfate

Drug	Mfr	Conc	Mfr	Conc	Remarks	Ref	C/I
Methotrexate sodium		25 mg/mL		3 units/mL	Drugs injected sequentially in Y-site with no flush. No precipitate seen	980	C
Metoclopramide HCl		5 mg/mL		3 units/mL	Drugs injected sequentially in Y-site with no flush. No precipitate seen	980	C
Mitomycin		0.5 mg/mL		3 units/mL	Drugs injected sequentially in Y-site with no flush. No precipitate seen	980	C
Ondansetron HCl	GL	1 mg/mL[b]	BR	1 unit/mL[b]	Visually compatible for 4 hr at 22 °C	1365	C
Paclitaxel	NCI	1.2 mg/mL[a]	MJ	1 unit/mL[a]	Physically compatible for 4 hr at 22 °C	1556	C
Piperacillin sodium–tazobactam sodium	LE[d]	40 + 5 mg/mL[a]	BR	1 unit/mL[b]	Physically compatible for 4 hr at 22 °C	1688	C
Sargramostim	IMM	10 mcg/mL[b]	MJ	1 unit/mL[b]	Visually compatible for 4 hr at 22 °C	1436	C
Teniposide	BR	0.1 mg/mL[a]	BR	1 unit/mL[b]	Physically compatible for 4 hr at 23 °C	1725	C
Thiotepa	IMM[c]	1 mg/mL[a]	MJ	1 unit/mL[b]	Physically compatible for 4 hr at 23 °C	1861	C
Vinblastine sulfate		1 mg/mL		3 units/mL	Drugs injected sequentially in Y-site with no flush. No precipitate seen	980	C
Vincristine sulfate		1 mg/mL		3 units/mL	Drugs injected sequentially in Y-site with no flush. No precipitate seen	980	C
Vinorelbine tartrate	BW	1 mg/mL[b]	BR	1 unit/mL[b]	Physically compatible for 4 hr at 22 °C	1558	C

[a]*Tested in dextrose 5%.*
[b]*Tested in sodium chloride 0.9%.*
[c]*Lyophilized formulation tested.*
[d]*Test performed using the formulation WITHOUT edetate disodium.*

BORTEZOMIB
AHFS 10:00

Products — Bortezomib is available in vials containing 3.5 mg with mannitol 35 mg. Reconstitute the drug with 3.5 mL of sodium chloride 0.9%. (1)

Trade Name(s) — Velcade.

Administration — Bortezomib is administered by intravenous bolus injection. (1)

Stability — Intact vials should be stored at controlled room temperature and left in the original box to protect from light during storage. (1)

The manufacturer states that bortezomib reconstituted as directed with sodium chloride 0.9% in the original vial or in a syringe should be used within eight hours after preparation. (1) However, bortezomib (Janssen-Cilag) reconstituted with sodium chloride 0.9% to a concentration of 1 mg/mL in the original vials was reported to be stable for at least five days under refrigeration protected from light. (2663)

Bortezomib reconstituted with sodium chloride 0.9% to a concentration of 1 mg/mL was found to undergo little or no loss for 42 days stored at 23 °C or refrigerated at 4 °C. (2768)

Bortezomib (Janssen-Cilag) 1 mg/mL in sodium chloride 0.9% did not result in the loss of viability of *Staphylococcus aureus* within 120 hours at room temperature. Diluted solutions should be stored under refrigeration whenever possible, and the potential for microbiological growth should be considered when assigning expiration periods. (2740)

Syringes — Bortezomib (Janssen-Cilag) 1 mg/mL in sodium chloride 0.9% was packaged in 5-mL polypropylene plastic syringes (Becton-Dickinson) and stored at room temperature exposed to neon light and under refrigeration in the dark. The drug solutions remained clear and colorless throughout the study at both temperatures. About 8 to 9% loss occurred in five days at room temperature and in seven days refrigerated and protected from light. (2663)

BUMETANIDE
AHFS 40:28.08

Products — Bumetanide is available as a 0.25-mg/mL solution in 2-, 4-, and 10-mL vials. The solution also contains sodium chloride 0.85%, ammonium acetate 0.4%, disodium edetate 0.01%, and benzyl alcohol 1% with sodium hydroxide to adjust the pH. (1)

pH — Adjusted to approximately 7. (1; 4)

Administration — Bumetanide is administered by intramuscular injection, direct intravenous injection over one to two minutes, and by intravenous infusion. (1; 4)

Stability — Bumetanide discolors when exposed to light. The injection should be stored at controlled room temperature and protected from light. Bumetanide is reported to be stable at pH 4 to 10. (4) Precipitation may occur at pH values less than 4. (1644)

Sorption — Substantial sorption to glass and PVC containers does not occur. (1; 4)

Central Venous Catheter — Bumetanide (Ohmeda) 0.04 mg/mL in dextrose 5% was found to be compatible with the ARROWg+ard Blue Plus (Arrow International) chlorhexidine-bearing triple-lumen central catheter. Essentially complete delivery of the drug was found with little or no drug loss occurring. Furthermore, chlorhexidine delivered from the catheter remained at trace amounts with no substantial increase due to the delivery of the drug through the catheter. (2335)

Compatibility Information

Solution Compatibility

Bumetanide

Solution	Mfr	Mfr	Conc/L	Remarks	Ref	C/I
Dextrose 5%				Compatible and stable for 24 hr	1	C
	AB[a]	RC	20 mg	4 to 5% loss occurs within 3 hr with no further loss throughout 72 hr at 24 °C under fluorescent light	2090	C
	AB[a]	RC	200 mg	Little or no loss occurs within 72 hr at 24 °C under fluorescent light	2090	C
Ringer's injection, lactated				Compatible and stable for 24 hr	1	C
Sodium chloride 0.9%				Compatible and stable for 24 hr	1	C

[a]Tested in PVC containers.

Additive Compatibility

Bumetanide

Drug	Mfr	Conc/L	Mfr	Conc/L	Test Soln	Remarks	Ref	C/I
Dobutamine HCl	LI	1 g	RC	125 mg	D5W, NS	Immediate yellow discoloration with yellow precipitate within 6 hr at 21 °C	812	I
Floxacillin sodium	BE	20 g	LEO	6 mg	NS	Physically compatible for 72 hr at 15 and 30 °C	1479	C
Furosemide	HO	1 g	LEO	6 mg	NS	Physically compatible for 72 hr at 15 and 30 °C	1479	C

Drugs in Syringe Compatibility

Bumetanide

Drug (in syringe)	Mfr	Amt	Mfr	Amt	Remarks	Ref	C/I
Doxapram HCl	RB	400 mg/ 20 mL		0.5 mg/ 1 mL	Physically compatible with 3% doxapram loss in 24 hr	1177	C

Y-Site Injection Compatibility (1:1 Mixture)

Bumetanide

Drug	Mfr	Conc	Mfr	Conc	Remarks	Ref	C/I
Allopurinol sodium	BW	3 mg/mL[b]	RC	0.04 mg/mL[b]	Physically compatible for 4 hr at 22 °C	1686	C
Amifostine	USB	10 mg/mL[a]	RC	0.04 mg/mL[a]	Physically compatible for 4 hr at 23 °C	1845	C
Aztreonam	SQ	40 mg/mL[a]	RC	0.04 mg/mL[a]	Physically compatible for 4 hr at 23 °C	1758	C
Bivalirudin	TMC	5 mg/mL[a]	OHM	40 mcg/mL[a]	Physically compatible for 4 hr at 23 °C	2373	C
Caspofungin acetate	ME	0.7 mg/mL[b]	BED	0.04 mg/mL[b]	Physically compatible for 4 hr at room temperature	2758	C
Ceftaroline fosamil	FOR	2.22 mg/mL[a,b,g]	HOS	40 mcg/mL[a,b,g]	Physically compatible for 4 hr at 23 °C	2826	C
Cisatracurium besylate	GW	0.1, 2, 5 mg/mL[a]	BV	0.04 mg/mL[a]	Physically compatible for 4 hr at 23 °C	2074	C
Cladribine	ORT	0.015[b] and 0.5[c] mg/mL	RC	0.04 mg/mL[b]	Physically compatible for 4 hr at 23 °C	1969	C
Clarithromycin	AB	4 mg/mL[a]	LEO	0.5 mg/mL	Visually compatible for 72 hr at both 30 and 17 °C	2174	C
Dexmedetomidine HCl	AB	4 mcg/mL[b]	BED	40 mcg/mL[b]	Physically compatible for 4 hr at 23 °C	2383	C
Diltiazem HCl	MMD	1[b] and 5 mg/mL	RC	0.25 mg/mL	Visually compatible	1807	C
Docetaxel	RPR	0.9 mg/mL[a]	RC	0.04 mg/mL[a]	Physically compatible for 4 hr at 23 °C	2224	C
Doripenem	JJ	5 mg/mL[a,b]	BED	0.04 mg/mL[a,b]	Physically compatible for 4 hr at 23 °C	2743	C
Etoposide phosphate	BR	5 mg/mL[a]	RC	0.04 mg/mL[a]	Physically compatible for 4 hr at 23 °C	2218	C
Fenoldopam mesylate	AB	80 mcg/mL[b]	BA	40 mcg/mL[b]	Trace haze forms immediately	2467	I
Filgrastim	AMG	30 mcg/mL[a]	RC	0.04 mg/mL[a]	Physically compatible for 4 hr at 22 °C	1687	C
Gemcitabine HCl	LI	10 mg/mL[b]	RC	0.04 mg/mL[b]	Physically compatible for 4 hr at 23 °C	2226	C
Granisetron HCl	SKB	0.05 mg/mL[a]	RC	0.04 mg/mL[a]	Physically compatible for 4 hr at 23 °C	2000	C
Hetastarch in lactated electrolyte	AB	6%	OHM	0.04 mg/mL[a]	Physically compatible for 4 hr at 23 °C	2339	C
Lorazepam	WY	0.33 mg/mL[b]	LEO	0.5 mg/mL	Visually compatible for 24 hr at 22 °C	1855	C
Melphalan HCl	BW	0.1 mg/mL[b]	RC	0.04 mg/mL[b]	Physically compatible for 3 hr at 22 °C	1557	C
Meperidine HCl	AB	10 mg/mL	RC	0.25 mg/mL	Physically compatible for 4 hr at 25 °C	1397	C
Micafungin sodium	ASP	1.5 mg/mL[b]	BED	40 mcg/mL[b]	Physically compatible for 4 hr at 23 °C	2683	C
Midazolam HCl	RC	5 mg/mL	LEO	0.5 mg/mL	White precipitate forms immediately	1855	I
Milrinone lactate	SW	0.4 mg/mL[a]	RC	0.25 mg/mL	Visually compatible with little or no loss of either drug in 4 hr at 23 °C	2214	C
Morphine sulfate	AB	1 mg/mL	RC	0.25 mg/mL	Physically compatible for 4 hr at 25 °C	1397	C
Nesiritide	SCI	50 mcg/mL[a,b]		0.25 mg/mL	Physically incompatible	2625	I
Oxaliplatin	SS	0.5 mg/mL[a]	BA	0.04 mg/mL[a]	Physically compatible for 4 hr at 23 °C	2566	C
Pemetrexed disodium	LI	20 mg/mL[b]	BA	0.04 mg/mL[a]	Physically compatible for 4 hr at 23 °C	2564	C
Piperacillin sodium–tazobactam sodium	LE[f]	40 + 5 mg/mL[a]	RC	0.04 mg/mL[a]	Physically compatible for 4 hr at 22 °C	1688	C
Propofol	ZEN	10 mg/mL	RC	0.04 mg/mL[a]	Physically compatible for 1 hr at 23 °C	2066	C
Remifentanil HCl	GW	0.025 and 0.25 mg/mL[b]	RC	0.04 mg/mL[a]	Physically compatible for 4 hr at 23 °C	2075	C

Y-Site Injection Compatibility (1:1 Mixture) (Cont.)

Bumetanide

Drug	Mfr	Conc	Mfr	Conc	Remarks	Ref	C/I
Teniposide	BR	0.1 mg/mL[a]	RC	0.04 mg/mL[a]	Physically compatible for 4 hr at 23 °C	1725	C
Thiotepa	IMM[d]	1 mg/mL[a]	RC	0.04 mg/mL[a]	Physically compatible for 4 hr at 23 °C	1861	C
TNA #218 to #226[e]			RC, BV	0.04 mg/mL[a]	Visually compatible for 4 hr at 23 °C	2215	C
TPN #212 to #215[e]			RC	0.04 mg/mL[a]	Physically compatible for 4 hr at 23 °C	2109	C
Vinorelbine tartrate	BW	1 mg/mL[b]	RC	0.04 mg/mL[b]	Physically compatible for 4 hr at 22 °C	1558	C

[a]Tested in dextrose 5%.
[b]Tested in sodium chloride 0.9%.
[c]Tested in bacteriostatic sodium chloride 0.9% preserved with benzyl alcohol 0.9%.
[d]Lyophilized formulation tested.
[e]Refer to Appendix I for the composition of parenteral nutrition solutions. TNA indicates a 3-in-1 admixture, and TPN indicates a 2-in-1 admixture.
[f]Test performed using the formulation WITHOUT edetate disodium.
[g]Tested in Ringer's injection, lactated.

BUPIVACAINE HYDROCHLORIDE
AHFS 72:00

Products — Bupivacaine hydrochloride is available in concentrations of 0.25, 0.5, and 0.75% (2.5, 5, and 7.5 mg/mL, respectively) in single-dose containers. The 0.25 and 0.5% concentrations also come in 50-mL multiple-dose vials with methylparaben 1 mg/mL as a preservative. Sodium hydroxide or hydrochloric acid is used to adjust the pH. (1; 4)

Bupivacaine hydrochloride is also available in concentrations of 0.25, 0.5, and 0.75% with epinephrine 1:200,000 as the bitartrate. In addition to bupivacaine hydrochloride, each milliliter contains epinephrine bitartrate 0.005 mg, sodium metabisulfite 0.5 mg, and disodium edetate 0.1 mg. Multiple-dose vials contain methylparaben 1 mg/mL as a preservative while single-dose containers are preservative free. Sodium hydroxide or hydrochloric acid is used to adjust the pH. (1; 4)

A hyperbaric solution of bupivacaine hydrochloride is available in 2-mL ampuls. Each milliliter contains bupivacaine hydrochloride 7.5 mg and dextrose 82.5 mg (8.25%) with sodium hydroxide or hydrochloric acid to adjust the pH. (1; 4)

pH — Bupivacaine hydrochloride injection and the hyperbaric solution have a pH of 4 to 6.5. Bupivacaine hydrochloride with epinephrine 1:200,000 has a pH of 3.3 to 5.5. (4)

Specific Gravity — The hyperbaric solution has a specific gravity of 1.030 to 1.035 at 25 °C and 1.03 at 37 °C. (4)

Trade Name(s) — Marcaine, Sensorcaine, Sensorcaine-MPF.

Administration — Bupivacaine hydrochloride may be administered by infiltration or by epidural, spinal, or peripheral or sympathetic nerve block as a single injection or repeat injections. Injections should be made slowly, with frequent aspirations, to guard against intravascular injection. Products containing preservatives should not be used for epidural or caudal block. (1; 4)

Stability — Bupivacaine hydrochloride injections should be stored at controlled room temperature; freezing should be avoided. (1; 4) Products containing epinephrine should be protected from light during storage. Partially used containers that do not contain antibacterial preservatives should be discarded after entry. (4)

Bupivacaine hydrochloride without epinephrine and the hyperbaric solution may be autoclaved at 121 °C and 15 psi for 15 minutes. Products containing epinephrine should not be autoclaved. (1; 4)

Bupivacaine hydrochloride with epinephrine should not be used if a pinkish color, a color darker than "slightly" yellow, or a precipitate develops. (1; 4)

Syringes — The stability of bupivacaine (salt form unspecified) 5 mg/mL repackaged in polypropylene syringes was evaluated. Little or no change in concentration was found after four weeks of storage at room temperature not exposed to direct light. (2164)

Bupivacaine hydrochloride (Astra) 1 mg/mL in sodium chloride 0.9% was packaged in two types in polypropylene syringes. The Omnifix (B. Braun) syringes had polyisoprene piston tips while the Terumo syringes had no natural or synthetic rubber in the product. Stored at 4, 21, and 35 °C for 30 days, the test solutions exhibited no visible or pH changes. Although the pH remained within the stability range for the drug, this does not demonstrate stability. (2387)

Ambulatory Pumps — Bupivacaine hydrochloride (Astra) 7.5 mg/mL was filled into 50-mL ambulatory pump cassette reservoirs (Pharmacia Deltec) and stored at room temperature protected from light for 90 days. The drug concentration increased 12% during the observation period, possibly because of loss of water from the solutions. (1850)

Implantable Pumps — Bupivacaine hydrochloride 7.5 mg/mL in dextrose 8.25% (Marcaine spinal) stability was evaluated in SynchroMed implantable pumps over 12 weeks at 37 °C. Little or no loss of bupivacaine hydrochloride and no adverse effects on the pumps occurred. (2583)

An admixture of bupivacaine hydrochloride 25 mg/mL, clonidine hydrochloride 2 mg/mL, and morphine sulfate 50 mg/mL in sterile water for injection was reported to be physically and chemically stable for 90 days at 37 °C in SynchroMed implantable pumps. Little or no loss of any of the drugs occurred. (2585)

Compatibility Information

Solution Compatibility

Bupivacaine HCl

Solution	Mfr	Mfr	Conc/L	Remarks	Ref	C/I
Sodium chloride 0.9%	AB[b]	AST	1.25 g	Visually compatible with no loss in 32 days at 3 °C in the dark and 23 °C exposed to light	1718	C
	AB[a]	AB	625 mg and 1.25 g	Visually compatible with no loss in 72 hr at 24 °C under fluorescent light	1870; 2058	C
	GRI[a]		850 mg	No change in concentration in 28 days at 4 °C and room temperature	1910	C

[a]Tested in PVC containers.
[b]Tested in polypropylene syringes.

Additive Compatibility

Bupivacaine HCl

Drug	Mfr	Conc/L	Mfr	Conc/L	Test Soln	Remarks	Ref	C/I
Buprenorphine HCl	RC	180 mg	AST	3 g	a	No loss of either drug in 30 days at 18 °C	1932	C
Clonidine HCl with fentanyl citrate	BI JN	9 mg 35 mg	AST	1 g	NS[a]	Visually compatible with less than 10% change of any drug in 28 days at 4 °C and 24 days at 25 °C in the dark	2437	C
Diamorphine HCl		0.125 g	GL	1.25 g	NS	Visually compatible with 8% diamorphine loss and no bupivacaine loss in 28 days at room temperature	1791	C
	NAP	20 mg	AST	150 mg	NS[c]	5% diamorphine and no bupivacaine loss in 14 days at 7 °C. Both drugs were stable for 6 months at −20 °C	2070	C
Epinephrine bitartrate with fentanyl citrate	AB JN	0.69 mg 1.25 mg	WI	440 mg	d	No bupivacaine and fentanyl loss and 10% epinephrine loss in 30 days at 3 and 23 °C then 48 hr at 30 °C	1627	C
Epinephrine bitartrate with fentanyl citrate	IVX	2 mg 2 mg	IVX	1 g		Visually compatible with less than 10% loss of epinephrine and no loss of other drugs in 182 days at 4 and 22 °C	2613	C
Fentanyl citrate	JN	20 mg	WI	1.25 g	NS[a]	Physically compatible with little or no loss of either drug in 30 days at 3 and 23 °C	1396	C
		2 mg		1.25 g	NS[a]	Physically compatible with no bupivacaine loss and about 6 to 7% fentanyl loss in 30 days at 4 and 23 °C	2305	C
		2 mg		600 mg	NS[a]	Physically compatible with no bupivacaine loss and about 2 to 4% fentanyl loss in 30 days at 4 and 23 °C	2305	C

Additive Compatibility (Cont.)

Bupivacaine HCl

Drug	Mfr	Conc/L	Mfr	Conc/L	Test Soln	Remarks	Ref	C/I
Fentanyl citrate with clonidine HCl	JN BI	35 mg 9 mg	AST	1 g	NS[a]	Visually compatible with less than 10% change of any drug in 28 days at 4 °C and 24 days at 25 °C in the dark	2437	C
Fentanyl citrate with epinephrine bitartrate	JN AB	1.25 mg 0.69 mg	WI	440 mg	[d]	No bupivacaine and fentanyl loss and 10% epinephrine loss in 30 days at 3 and 23 °C then 48 hr at 30 °C	1627	C
Fentanyl citrate with epinephrine bitartrate	IVX	2 mg 2 mg	IVX	1 g		Visually compatible with less than 10% loss of epinephrine and no loss of other drugs in 182 days at 4 and 22 °C	2613	C
Hydromorphone HCl	KN	20 mg	AB	625 mg and 1.25 g	NS[a]	Visually compatible with little or no loss of either drug in 72 hr at 24 °C under fluorescent light	1870	C
	KN	100 mg	AB	625 mg and 1.25 g	NS[a]	Visually compatible with little or no loss of either drug in 72 hr at 24 °C under fluorescent light	1870	C
Morphine sulfate		1 g	AST	3 g	[a]	Little loss of either drug in 30 days at 18 °C	1932	C
	SCN	100 mg	AB	625 mg and 1.25 g	NS[a]	Visually compatible. No loss of either drug in 72 hr at 24 °C in light	2058	C
	SCN	500 mg	AB	625 mg and 1.25 g	NS[a]	Visually compatible. No loss of either drug in 72 hr at 24 °C in light	2058	C
Sufentanil citrate	JN	5 mg	AST	2 g	NS[b]	9% sufentanil loss and 5% bupivacaine loss in 30 days at 32 °C. No loss of either drug in 30 days at 4 °C	1756	C
	JN	20 mg		3 g	NS[b]	5% sufentanil loss and no bupivacaine loss in 10 days at 5, 26, and 37 °C	1751	C
	JN	5 mg	AST	2 g	NS[a]	Buffered with pH 4.6 citrate buffer. Visually compatible with no loss of either drug in 48 hr at 32 °C	2042	C
	JN	12 mg	AST	40 mg	NS[a]	Visually compatible with no loss of either drug in 43 days at 4 and 25 °C	2455	C
Ziconotide acetate	ELN	25 mg[f]	BB	5 g[e]		90% ziconotide retained for 22 days at 37 °C. No bupivacaine loss in 30 days	2751	C

[a]Tested in PVC containers.
[b]Tested in PVC/Kalex 3000 (phthalate ester) CADD pump reservoirs.
[c]Tested in PVC containers.
[d]Tested in portable infusion pump reservoirs (Pharmacia Deltec).
[e]Bupivacaine HCl powder dissolved in ziconotide acetate.
[f]Tested in SynchroMed II implantable pumps.

Drugs in Syringe Compatibility

Bupivacaine HCl

Drug (in syringe)	Mfr	Amt	Mfr	Amt	Remarks	Ref	C/I
Clonidine HCl	FUJ	100 mcg/ 1 mL	SAN	3.75 mg/ 1 mL	Physically and chemically stable for 14 days at room temperature	2069	C
	FUJ	100 mcg/ 1 mL	SAN	60 mg/ 8 mL	Physically and chemically stable for 14 days at room temperature	2069	C
Clonidine HCl with fentanyl citrate	BI JN	0.45 mg 1.75 mg	AST	50 mg	Diluted to 50 mL with NS. Visually compatible with less than 10% loss of any drug in 25 days at 4 and 25 °C in the dark	2437	C
Clonidine HCl with morphine sulfate	BI ES	0.03 mg/ mL 0.2 mg/ mL	SW	1.5 mg/ mL	Diluted to 5 mL with NS. Visually compatible with no new GC/MS peaks in 1 hr at room temperature	1956	C
Diamorphine HCl	EV	1 and 10 mg/ mL	AST	0.5%	10 to 11% diamorphine loss in 5 weeks at 20 °C and 3 to 7% loss in 8 weeks at 6 °C. No bupivacaine loss at 6 or 20 °C in 8 weeks	1952	C
Fentanyl citrate with clonidine HCl	JN BI	1.75 mg 0.45 mg	AST	50 mg	Diluted to 50 mL with NS. Visually compatible with less than 10% loss of any drug in 25 days at 4 and 25 °C in the dark	2437	C
Fentanyl citrate with ketamine HCl	JN PD	0.01 mg/ mL 2 mg/mL	SW	1.5 mg/ mL	Diluted to 5 mL with NS. Visually compatible with no new GC/MS peaks in 1 hr at room temperature	1956	C
Hydromorphone HCl	KN	65 mg/ mL	AST	7.5 mg/ mL	Visually compatible for 30 days at 25 °C	1660	C
Iohexol		1 mL	AST	0.25 and 0.125%[a], 4 mL	Visually compatible with no bupivacaine loss in 24 hr at room temperature. Iohexol not tested	1611	C
Ketamine HCl with fentanyl citrate	PD JN	2 mg/mL 0.01 mg/ mL	SW	1.5 mg/ mL	Diluted to 5 mL with NS. Visually compatible with no new GC/MS peaks in 1 hr at room temperature	1956	C
Morphine sulfate		1 mg/mL	AST	3 mg/mL	Little loss of either drug in 30 days at 18 °C	1932	C
	[d]	5 mg/mL[e]	[d]	2.5 mg/ mL[e]	Physically compatible. Little morphine or bupivacaine loss in 60 days at 23 °C in fluorescent light and at 4 °C	2378	C
	[d]	50 mg/ mL[f]	[d]	25 mg/ mL[f]	Physically compatible. Little morphine or bupivacaine loss in 60 days at 23 °C in fluorescent light and at 4 °C in dark. Slight yellow discoloration at 23 °C not indicative of decomposition	2378	C
Morphine sulfate with clonidine HCl	ES BI	0.2 mg/ mL 0.03 mg/ mL	SW	1.5 mg/ mL	Diluted to 5 mL with NS. Visually compatible with no new GC/MS peaks in 1 hr at room temperature	1956	C

Drugs in Syringe Compatibility (Cont.)

Bupivacaine HCl

Drug (in syringe)	Mfr	Amt	Mfr	Amt	Remarks	Ref	C/I
Sodium bicarbonate	AB	4%, 0.05 to 0.6 mL	AST, WI	0.25, 0.5[b], 0.75%[b], 20 mL	Precipitate forms in 1 to 2 min up to 2 hr at lowest amount of bicarbonate	1724	I
		1.4%, 1.5 mL	BEL	0.5%[c], 20 mL	No epinephrine loss in 7 days at room temperature. Bupivacaine not tested	1743	C
		4.2 and 8.4%, 1.5 mL	BEL	0.5%[c], 20 mL	5 to 7% epinephrine loss in 7 days at room temperature. Bupivacaine not tested	1743	C

[a]*Diluted 1:1 in sodium chloride 0.9%.*
[b]*Tested with and without epinephrine hydrochloride 1:200,000 added.*
[c]*Tested with epinephrine hydrochloride 1:200,000 added.*
[d]*Extemporaneously compounded from morphine sulfate and bupivacaine hydrochloride powder.*
[e]*Tested in sodium chloride 0.9%.*
[f]*Tested in sterile water for injection.*

BUPRENORPHINE HYDROCHLORIDE
AHFS 28:08.12

Products — Buprenorphine hydrochloride is available in 1-mL ampuls. Each milliliter contains buprenorphine 0.3 mg (as the hydrochloride) with anhydrous dextrose 50 mg in water for injection. The pH is adjusted with hydrochloric acid. (1)

pH — From 4.0 to 6.0. (17)

Osmolality — The osmolality was 297 mOsm/kg. (1233)

Trade Name(s) — Buprenex.

Administration — Buprenorphine hydrochloride is administered by deep intramuscular injection or by intravenous injection slowly over at least two minutes. (1; 4) It has also been given by continuous intravenous infusion at a concentration of 15 mcg/mL in sodium chloride 0.9% and by epidural injection at a concentration of 6 to 30 mcg/mL. (4)

Stability — The clear solution should be stored at 15 to 30 °C and protected from prolonged exposure to light and exposure to temperatures in excess of 40 °C and freezing. (1; 4) Buprenorphine hydrochloride may undergo substantial decomposition when autoclaved. (4)

Central Venous Catheter — Buprenorphine hydrochloride (Reckitt & Colman) 0.04 mg/mL in dextrose 5% was found to be compatible with the ARROWg+ard Blue Plus (Arrow International) chlorhexidine-bearing triple-lumen central catheter. Essentially complete delivery of the drug was found with little or no drug loss occurring. Furthermore, chlorhexidine delivered from the catheter remained at trace amounts with no substantial increase due to the delivery of the drug through the catheter. (2335)

Compatibility Information

Solution Compatibility

Buprenorphine HCl

Solution	Mfr	Mfr	Conc/L	Remarks	Ref	C/I
Dextrose 5%			150 mg	Stated to be compatible	4	C
Ringer's injection, lactated			150 mg	Stated to be compatible	4	C
Sodium chloride 0.9%			150 mg	Stated to be compatible	4	C

Additive Compatibility

Buprenorphine HCl

Drug	Mfr	Conc/L	Mfr	Conc/L	Test Soln	Remarks	Ref	C/I
Bupivacaine HCl	AST	3 g	RC	180 mg	[a]	No loss of either drug in 30 days at 18 °C	1932	**C**
Floxacillin sodium	BE	20 g		75 mg	W	Thick haze forms in 24 hr and precipitate forms in 47 hr at 30 °C. No change at 15 °C	1479	**I**
Furosemide	HO	1 g		75 mg	W	Haze for 6 hr at 30 °C. No change at 15 °C	1479	**I**
Glycopyrrolate with haloperidol lactate	ON	25 mg 104 mg	RKC	84 mg	NS[a]	Visually compatible with less than 10% loss of any drug in 30 days at 4 and 25 °C in the dark	2436	**C**
Haloperidol lactate with glycopyrrolate	ON	104 mg 25 mg	RKC	84 mg	NS[a]	Visually compatible with less than 10% loss of any drug in 30 days at 4 and 25 °C in the dark	2436	**C**

[a]*Tested in PVC containers.*

Drugs in Syringe Compatibility

Buprenorphine HCl

Drug (in syringe)	Mfr	Amt	Mfr	Amt	Remarks	Ref	C/I
Atropine sulfate					Physically and chemically compatible	4	**C**
Diazepam					Incompatible	4	**I**
Diphenhydramine HCl					Physically and chemically compatible	4	**C**
Droperidol					Physically and chemically compatible	4	**C**
Glycopyrrolate with haloperidol lactate	ON	1.2 mg 5 mg	RKC	4 mg	Diluted to 48 mL with NS. Visually compatible with less than 10% loss of any drug in 30 days at 4 and 25 °C in the dark	2436	**C**
Haloperidol lactate with glycopyrrolate	ON	5 mg 1.2 mg	RKC	4 mg	Diluted to 48 mL with NS. Visually compatible with less than 10% loss of any drug in 30 days at 4 and 25 °C in the dark	2436	**C**
Heparin sodium		2500 units/ 1 mL	BM	300 mg/ 1 mL	Visually compatible for at least 5 min	1053	**C**
Hydroxyzine HCl					Physically and chemically compatible	4	**C**
Lorazepam					Incompatible	4	**I**
Midazolam HCl	RC	5 mg/ 1 mL	NE	0.3 mg/ 1 mL	Physically compatible for 4 hr at 25 °C	1145	**C**
Promethazine HCl					Physically and chemically compatible	4	**C**
Scopolamine HBr					Physically and chemically compatible	4	**C**

Y-Site Injection Compatibility (1:1 Mixture)

Buprenorphine HCl

Drug	Mfr	Conc	Mfr	Conc	Remarks	Ref	C/I
Allopurinol sodium	BW	3 mg/mL[b]	RKC	0.04 mg/mL[b]	Physically compatible for 4 hr at 22 °C	1686	C
Amifostine	USB	10 mg/mL[a]	RKC	0.04 mg/mL[a]	Physically compatible for 4 hr at 23 °C	1845	C
Amphotericin B cholesteryl sulfate complex	SEQ	0.83 mg/mL[a]	RKC	0.04 mg/mL[a]	Microprecipitate forms in 4 hr at 23 °C	2117	I
Aztreonam	SQ	40 mg/mL[a]	RKC	0.04 mg/mL[a]	Physically compatible for 4 hr at 23 °C	1758	C
Cisatracurium besylate	GW	0.1, 2, 5 mg/mL[a]	RKC	0.04 mg/mL[a]	Physically compatible for 4 hr at 23 °C	2074	C
Cladribine	ORT	0.015[b] and 0.5[c] mg/mL	RKC	0.04 mg/mL[b]	Physically compatible for 4 hr at 23 °C	1969	C
Docetaxel	RPR	0.9 mg/mL[a]	RKC	0.04 mg/mL[a]	Physically compatible for 4 hr at 23 °C	2224	C
Doxorubicin HCl liposomal	SEQ	0.4 mg/mL[a]	RKC	0.04 mg/mL[a]	Partial loss of measured natural turbidity	2087	I
Etoposide phosphate	BR	5 mg/mL[a]	RKC	0.04 mg/mL[a]	Physically compatible for 4 hr at 23 °C	2218	C
Filgrastim	AMG	30 mcg/mL[a]	RKC	0.04 mg/mL[a]	Physically compatible for 4 hr at 22 °C	1687	C
Gemcitabine HCl	LI	10 mg/mL[b]	RKC	0.04 mg/mL[b]	Physically compatible for 4 hr at 23 °C	2226	C
Granisetron HCl	SKB	0.05 mg/mL[a]	RKC	0.04 mg/mL[a]	Physically compatible for 4 hr at 23 °C	2000	C
Linezolid	PHU	2 mg/mL	RKC	0.04 mg/mL[a]	Physically compatible for 4 hr at 23 °C	2264	C
Melphalan HCl	BW	0.1 mg/mL[b]	RKC	0.04 mg/mL[b]	Physically compatible for 3 hr at 22 °C	1557	C
Oxaliplatin	SS	0.5 mg/mL[a]	RKC	0.04 mg/mL[a]	Physically compatible for 4 hr at 23 °C	2566	C
Pemetrexed disodium	LI	20 mg/mL[b]	RKB	0.04 mg/mL[a]	Physically compatible for 4 hr at 23 °C	2564	C
Piperacillin sodium–tazobactam sodium	LE[f]	40 + 5 mg/mL[a]	RKC	0.04 mg/mL[a]	Physically compatible for 4 hr at 22 °C	1688	C
Propofol	ZEN	10 mg/mL	RKC	0.04 mg/mL[a]	Physically compatible for 1 hr at 23 °C	2066	C
Remifentanil HCl	GW	0.025 and 0.25 mg/mL[b]	RKC	0.04 mg/mL[a]	Physically compatible for 4 hr at 23 °C	2075	C
Teniposide	BR	0.1 mg/mL[a]	RKC	0.04 mg/mL[a]	Physically compatible for 4 hr at 23 °C	1725	C
Thiotepa	IMM[d]	1 mg/mL[a]	RKC	0.04 mg/mL[a]	Physically compatible for 4 hr at 23 °C	1861	C
TNA #218 to #226[e]			RKC	0.04 mg/mL[a]	Visually compatible for 4 hr at 23 °C	2215	C
TPN #212 to #215[e]			RKC	0.04 mg/mL[a]	Physically compatible for 4 hr at 23 °C	2109	C
Vinorelbine tartrate	BW	1 mg/mL[b]	RKC	0.04 mg/mL[b]	Physically compatible for 4 hr at 22 °C	1558	C

[a]Tested in dextrose 5%.
[b]Tested in sodium chloride 0.9%.
[c]Tested in bacteriostatic sodium chloride 0.9% preserved with benzyl alcohol 0.9%.
[d]Lyophilized formulation tested.
[e]Refer to Appendix I for the composition of parenteral nutrition solutions. TNA indicates a 3-in-1 admixture, and TPN indicates a 2-in-1 admixture.
[f]Test performed using the formulation WITHOUT edetate disodium.

BUSULFAN
AHFS 10:00

Products — Busulfan is available as a 6-mg/mL concentrated solution dissolved in a vehicle composed of 33% w/w N,N-dimethylacetamide and 67% w/w polyethylene glycol 400. The product is packaged in 10-mL colorless single-use ampuls along with 25-mm 5-μm nylon membrane filters. The concentrated injection must be diluted for administration. (1)

pH — Busulfan diluted for infusion to a concentration greater than 0.5 mg/mL has a pH of 3.4 to 3.9. (1)

Trade Name(s) — Busulfex.

Administration — Busulfan must be diluted for administration. Sodium chloride 0.9% and dextrose 5% are both recommended diluents for busulfan infusion. The quantity of infusion solution should be ten times the volume of the busulfan concentrate dose to ensure that the final concentration is equal to or greater than 0.5 mg/mL. (1)

Appropriate gloves should be worn during preparation; accidental skin exposure may result in skin reactions. To prepare the infusion admixture, break open the ampul top and withdraw the contents through the 5-μm nylon filter. The filter and needle are removed and a new needle is attached. The busulfan is added into an intravenous solution bag that already contains the appropriate amount of sodium chloride 0.9% or dextrose 5%, making sure that the drug flows into and throughout the solution. The drug should always be added to the diluent. The solution should be mixed thoroughly by inverting several times. Other diluents should not be used.

Busulfan admixtures should be administered intravenously through a central venous catheter as a two-hour infusion every six hours for four consecutive days (a total of 16 doses). More rapid infusion has not been tested and is not recommended. An infusion pump should be used to control the flow rate. The central venous catheter should be flushed before and after busulfan administration with about 5 mL of sodium chloride 0.9% or dextrose 5%. (1)

Stability — Busulfan injection in intact ampuls is a clear colorless solution and should be stored under refrigeration at 2 to 8 °C. Busulfan diluted for infusion in sodium chloride 0.9% or dextrose 5% is stable for up to eight hours at 25 °C. Admixed in sodium chloride 0.9%, the drug is stable for up to 12 hours under refrigeration at 2 to 8 °C. (1)

Busulfan concentrate injection (Pierre Fabre Pharma) 6 mg/mL did not support the growth of *Staphylococcus aureus* and *Candida albicans* within two hours at room temperature. Busulfan 0.5 mg/mL in sodium chloride 0.9% did not support the growth of with loss of viability of *Staphylococcus aureus*, *Enterococcus faecium*, and *Pseudomonas aeruginosa* over 24 to 48 hours at room temperature but did not affect the growth of *Candida albicans*. Diluted solutions should be stored under refrigeration whenever possible, and the potential for microbiological growth should be considered when assigning expiration periods. (2740)

Filtration — Busulfan injection is packaged with 25-mm 5-μm nylon filters for use in withdrawing the injection from the opened ampuls. The use of filters other than this type is not recommended. (1)

Compatibility Information

Solution Compatibility

Busulfan

Solution	Mfr	Mfr	Conc/L	Remarks	Ref	C/I
Dextrose 5%	BA[a], MG[b]		0.5 g	Physically compatible. Under 10% loss in 8 hr at 23 °C but over 20% loss in 24 hr	2183	I[c]
	BA[a], MG[b]		0.1 g	Physically compatible. Under 10% loss in 4 hr at 23 °C but 19% loss in 8 hr	2183	I[c]
Sodium chloride 0.9%	BA[a], MG[b]		0.5 g	Physically compatible. Under 10% loss in 8 hr at 23 °C but over 20% loss in 24 hr	2183	I[c]
	BA[a], MG[b]		0.1 g	Physically compatible. Under 10% loss in 4 hr at 23 °C but 13% loss in 8 hr	2183	I[c]
	[d]	ORP	0.5 g	Precipitation in about 19 hr at 4 °C. Substantial busulfan loss from precipitation	2739	I
	[e]	ORP	0.5 g	Precipitation appears when frozen. Precipitation in about 19 hr at 4 °C. Substantial busulfan loss from precipitation	2739	I
	[d,e]	ORP	0.5 g	Physically stable for 19 to 36 hr at 13 to 15 °C. Under 10% loss until precipitation	2739	?
	[b]	PRF	0.24 g	10% loss in 8 hr at 25 °C;12% loss in 24 hr at 4 °C	2785	I[c]
	[b]	PRF	0.12 g	10% loss in 12 hr at 25 °C and 4 °C	2785	I[c]

[a]Tested in PVC containers.
[b]Tested in polyolefin containers.
[c]Incompatible by conventional standards but may be used in shorter periods of time.
[d]Tested in Freeflex polypropylene bags.
[e]Tested in glass containers.

BUTORPHANOL TARTRATE
AHFS 28:08.12

Products — Butorphanol tartrate is available in concentrations of 1 mg/mL in 1-mL vials and also 2 mg/mL in 1- and 2-mL single-use vials. (1)

Each milliliter of solution also contains citric acid 3.3 mg, sodium citrate 7.29 mg, and sodium chloride 6.4 mg. (1)

pH — From 3.0 to 5.5. (1)

Trade Name(s) — Stadol.

Administration — Butorphanol tartrate may be administered by intramuscular or intravenous injection. (1; 4)

Stability — Butorphanol tartrate injection should be stored at controlled room temperature and protected from light. Freezing should be avoided. (1; 4)

Central Venous Catheter — Butorphanol tartrate (Apothecon) 0.04 mg/mL in dextrose 5% was found to be compatible with the ARROWg+ard Blue Plus (Arrow International) chlorhexidine-bearing triple-lumen central catheter. Essentially complete delivery of the drug was found with little or no drug loss occurring. Furthermore, chlorhexidine delivered from the catheter remained at trace amounts with no substantial increase due to the delivery of the drug through the catheter. (2335)

Compatibility Information

Drugs in Syringe Compatibility

Butorphanol tartrate

Drug (in syringe)	Mfr	Amt	Mfr	Amt	Remarks	Ref	C/I
Atropine sulfate	ST	0.4 mg/ 1 mL	BR	4 mg/ 2 mL	Physically compatible for 30 min at room temperature	566	C
Chlorpromazine HCl	MB	25 mg/ 1 mL	BR	4 mg/ 2 mL	Physically compatible for 30 min at room temperature	566	C
Dimenhydrinate	HR	50 mg/ 1 mL	BR	4 mg/ 2 mL	Gas evolves	761	I
Diphenhydramine HCl	PD	50 mg/ 1 mL	BR	4 mg/ 2 mL	Physically compatible for 30 min at room temperature	566	C
Droperidol	MN	5 mg/ 2 mL	BR	4 mg/ 2 mL	Physically compatible for 30 min at room temperature	566	C
Fentanyl citrate	MN	0.1 mg/ 2 mL	BR	4 mg/ 2 mL	Physically compatible for 30 min at room temperature	566	C
Hydroxyzine HCl	PF	50 mg/ 1 mL	BR	2 mg/ 1 mL	Physically compatible	771	C
	PF	100 mg/ 2 mL	BR	1 mg/ 1 mL	Physically compatible	771	C
Meperidine HCl	WI	50 mg/ 1 mL	BR	4 mg/ 2 mL	Physically compatible for 30 min at room temperature	566	C
Methotrimeprazine HCl		25 mg/ 1 mL	BR	4 mg/ 2 mL	Physically compatible for 30 min at room temperature	566	C
Metoclopramide HCl	NO	10 mg/ 2 mL	BR	4 mg/ 2 mL	Physically compatible for 30 min at room temperature	566	C
Midazolam HCl	RC	5 mg/ 1 mL	BR	2 mg/ 1 mL	Physically compatible for 4 hr at 25 °C	1145	C
Morphine sulfate	AH	15 mg/ 1 mL	BR	4 mg/ 2 mL	Physically compatible for 30 min at room temperature	566	C
Pentazocine lactate	WI	30 mg/ 1 mL	BR	4 mg/ 2 mL	Physically compatible for 30 min at room temperature	566	C
Pentobarbital sodium	AB	50 mg/ 1 mL	BR	4 mg/ 2 mL	Precipitates immediately	761	I

Drugs in Syringe Compatibility (Cont.)

Butorphanol tartrate

Drug (in syringe)	Mfr	Amt	Mfr	Amt	Remarks	Ref	C/I
Prochlorperazine edisylate	MB	5 mg/ 1 mL	BR	4 mg/ 2 mL	Physically compatible for 30 min at room temperature	566	C
Promethazine HCl	WY	25 mg/ 1 mL	BR	4 mg/ 2 mL	Physically compatible for 30 min at room temperature	566	C
Scopolamine HBr	ST	0.4 mg/ 1 mL	BR	4 mg/ 2 mL	Physically compatible for 30 min at room temperature	566	C

Y-Site Injection Compatibility (1:1 Mixture)

Butorphanol tartrate

Drug	Mfr	Conc	Mfr	Conc	Remarks	Ref	C/I
Allopurinol sodium	BW	3 mg/mL[b]	BR	0.04 mg/mL[b]	Physically compatible for 4 hr at 22 °C	1686	C
Amifostine	USB	10 mg/mL[a]	BR	0.04 mg/mL[a]	Physically compatible for 4 hr at 23 °C	1845	C
Amphotericin B cholesteryl sulfate complex	SEQ	0.83 mg/mL[a]	APC	0.04 mg/mL[a]	Decreased natural turbidity occurs	2117	I
Aztreonam	SQ	40 mg/mL[a]	BMS	0.04 mg/mL[a]	Physically compatible for 4 hr at 23 °C	1758	C
Bivalirudin	TMC	5 mg/mL[a]	APO	40 mcg/mL[a]	Physically compatible for 4 hr at 23 °C	2373	C
Cisatracurium besylate	GW	0.1, 2, 5 mg/ mL[a]	APC	0.04 mg/mL[a]	Physically compatible for 4 hr at 23 °C	2074	C
Cladribine	ORT	0.015[b] and 0.5[c] mg/mL	APC	0.04 mg/mL[b]	Physically compatible for 4 hr at 23 °C	1969	C
Dexmedetomidine HCl	AB	4 mcg/mL[b]	APO	40 mcg/mL[b]	Physically compatible for 4 hr at 23 °C	2383	C
Docetaxel	RPR	0.9 mg/mL[a]	APC	0.04 mg/mL[a]	Physically compatible for 4 hr at 23 °C	2224	C
Doxorubicin HCl liposomal	SEQ	0.4 mg/mL[a]	APC	0.04 mg/mL[a]	Physically compatible for 4 hr at 23 °C	2087	C
Enalaprilat	MSD	0.05 mg/mL[b]	BR	0.4 mg/mL[a]	Physically compatible for 24 hr at room temperature under fluorescent light	1355	C
Esmolol HCl	DCC	10 mg/mL[a]	BR	0.04 mg/mL[a]	Physically compatible for 24 hr at 22 °C	1169	C
Etoposide phosphate	BR	5 mg/mL[a]	APC	0.04 mg/mL[a]	Physically compatible for 4 hr at 23 °C	2218	C
Fenoldopam mesylate	AB	80 mcg/mL[b]	APO	40 mcg/mL[b]	Physically compatible for 4 hr at 23 °C	2467	C
Filgrastim	AMG	30 mcg/mL[a]	BR	0.04 mg/mL[a]	Physically compatible for 4 hr at 22 °C	1687	C
Fludarabine phosphate	BX	1 mg/mL[a]	BR	0.04 mg/mL[a]	Visually compatible for 4 hr at 22 °C	1439	C
Gemcitabine HCl	LI	10 mg/mL[b]	APC	0.04 mg/mL[b]	Physically compatible for 4 hr at 23 °C	2226	C
Granisetron HCl	SKB	0.05 mg/mL[a]	APC	0.04 mg/mL[a]	Physically compatible for 4 hr at 23 °C	2000	C
Hetastarch in lactated electrolyte	AB	6%	APC	0.04 mg/mL[a]	Physically compatible for 4 hr at 23 °C	2339	C
Labetalol HCl	SC	1 mg/mL[a]	BR	0.04 mg/mL[a]	Physically compatible for 24 hr at 18 °C	1171	C
Linezolid	PHU	2 mg/mL	APC	0.04 mg/mL[a]	Physically compatible for 4 hr at 23 °C	2264	C
Melphalan HCl	BW	0.1 mg/mL[b]	BR	0.04 mg/mL[b]	Physically compatible for 3 hr at 22 °C	1557	C
Midazolam HCl	RC	f	BR	f	Crystalline midazolam precipitate forms	2144	I
Nicardipine HCl	DCC	0.1 mg/mL[a]	BR	0.4 mg/mL[a]	Visually compatible for 24 hr at room temperature	235	C
Oxaliplatin	SS	0.5 mg/mL[a]	APO	0.04 mg/mL[a]	Physically compatible for 4 hr at 23 °C	2566	C
Paclitaxel	NCI	1.2 mg/mL[a]	BR	0.04 mg/mL[a]	Physically compatible for 4 hr at 22 °C	1556	C

Y-Site Injection Compatibility (1:1 Mixture) (Cont.)

Butorphanol tartrate

Drug	Mfr	Conc	Mfr	Conc	Remarks	Ref	C/I
Pemetrexed disodium	LI	20 mg/mL[b]	BMS	0.04 mg/mL[a]	Physically compatible for 4 hr at 23 °C	2564	C
Piperacillin sodium–tazobactam sodium	LE[g]	40 + 5 mg/mL[a]	BR	0.04 mg/mL[a]	Physically compatible for 4 hr at 23 °C	1688	C
Propofol	ZEN	10 mg/mL	APC	0.04 mg/mL[a]	Physically compatible for 1 hr at 23 °C	2066	C
Remifentanil HCl	GW	0.025 and 0.25 mg/mL[b]	APC	0.04 mg/mL[a]	Physically compatible for 4 hr at 23 °C	2075	C
Sargramostim	IMM	10 mcg/mL[b]	BR	0.04 mg/mL[b]	Visually compatible for 4 hr at 22 °C	1436	C
Teniposide	BR	0.1 mg/mL[a]	BR	0.04 mg/mL[a]	Physically compatible for 4 hr at 23 °C	1725	C
Thiotepa	IMM[d]	1 mg/mL[a]	APC	0.04 mg/mL[a]	Physically compatible for 4 hr at 23 °C	1861	C
TNA #218 to #226[e]			APC	0.04 mg/mL[a]	Visually compatible for 4 hr at 23 °C	2215	C
TPN #212 to #215[e]			APC	0.04 mg/mL[a]	Physically compatible for 4 hr at 23 °C	2109	C
Vinorelbine tartrate	BW	1 mg/mL[b]	BR	0.04 mg/mL[b]	Physically compatible for 4 hr at 22 °C	1558	C

[a]Tested in dextrose 5%.
[b]Tested in sodium chloride 0.9%.
[c]Tested in bacteriostatic sodium chloride 0.9% preserved with benzyl alcohol 0.9%.
[d]Lyophilized formulation tested.
[e]Refer to Appendix I for the composition of parenteral nutrition solutions. TNA indicates a 3-in-1 admixture, and TPN indicates a 2-in-1 admixture.
[f]Concentration unspecified.
[g]Test performed using the formulation WITHOUT edetate disodium.

CAFFEINE CITRATE
AHFS 28:20.92

Products — Caffeine citrate is available as a 20-mg/mL solution in 3-mL (60-mg) vials. Each milliliter provides caffeine base 10 mg/mL with citric acid monohydrate 5 mg and sodium citrate dihydrate 8.3 mg/mL in water for injection. (1)

pH — The pH is adjusted to 4.7. (1)

Trade Name(s) — Cafcit.

Administration — Caffeine citrate injection is administered slowly intravenously using a syringe pump over 30 minutes as a loading dose and over 10 minutes as a maintenance dose. (1; 4)

Stability — Intact vials of the clear, colorless injection should be stored at room temperature. The injection contains no antibacterial preservative and unused portions should be discarded. (1)

Syringes — Caffeine citrate 10 mg/mL was repackaged in glass and plastic syringes (Becton Dickinson) and stored at room temperature and at 4 °C. Less than 4% loss occurred over 60 days. (139)

Compatibility Information

Solution Compatibility

Caffeine citrate

Solution	Mfr	Mfr	Conc/L	Remarks	Ref	C/I
Dextrose 5%			10 mg/mL	Physically compatible and chemically stable for 24 hr at room temperature	1	C
Dextrose 5% in sodium chloride 0.2%			5 mg/mL	Physically compatible and chemically stable for 24 hr at room temperature	193; 483	C
Dextrose 5% in sodium chloride 0.2% and potassium chloride 20 mEq/L			5 mg/mL	Physically compatible and chemically stable for 24 hr at room temperature	193; 483	C

Drugs in Syringe Compatibility

Caffeine citrate

Drug (in syringe)	Mfr	Amt	Mfr	Amt	Remarks	Ref	C/I
Acyclovir sodium	BW	50 mg/ 1 mL		20 mg/ 1 mL	Precipitates immediately	2440	**I**
Alprostadil	UP	0.5 mg/ 1 mL		20 mg/ 1 mL	Visually compatible for 4 hr at 25 °C	2440	**C**
Amikacin sulfate	BED	250 mg/ 1 mL		20 mg/ 1 mL	Visually compatible for 4 hr at 25 °C	2440	**C**
Aminophylline	AB	25 mg/ 1 mL		20 mg/ 1 mL	Visually compatible for 4 hr at 25 °C	2440	**C**
Calcium gluconate		100 mg/ 1 mL		20 mg/ 1 mL	Physically compatible and chemically stable for 24 hr at room temperature	1	**C**
Cefotaxime sodium	HO	200 mg/ 1 mL		20 mg/ 1 mL	Visually compatible for 4 hr at 25 °C	2440	**C**
Clindamycin phosphate	UP	150 mg/ 1 mL		20 mg/ 1 mL	Visually compatible for 4 hr at 25 °C	2440	**C**
Dexamethasone sodium phosphate	ES	4 mg/ 1 mL		20 mg/ 1 mL	Visually compatible for 4 hr at 25 °C	2440	**C**
Dimenhydrinate		10 mg/ 1 mL		10 mg/ 1 mL	Clear solution	2569	**C**
Dobutamine HCl	GNS	12.5 mg/ 1 mL		20 mg/ 1 mL	Visually compatible for 4 hr at 25 °C	2440	**C**
Dopamine HCl	SO	80 mg/ 1 mL		20 mg/ 1 mL	Visually compatible for 4 hr at 25 °C	2440	**C**
Epinephrine HCl	IMS	0.1 mg/ 1 mL		20 mg/ 1 mL	Visually compatible for 4 hr at 25 °C	2440	**C**
Fentanyl citrate	ES	50 mcg/ 1 mL		20 mg/ 1 mL	Visually compatible for 4 hr at 25 °C	2440	**C**
Furosemide	AST	10 mg/ 1 mL		20 mg/ 1 mL	Precipitates immediately	2440	**I**
Gentamicin sulfate	ES	10 mg/ 1 mL		20 mg/ 1 mL	Visually compatible for 4 hr at 25 °C	2440	**C**
Heparin sodium	AB	10 units/ 1 mL		20 mg/ 1 mL	Visually compatible for 4 hr at 25 °C	2440	**C**
Isoproterenol HCl	SW	0.2 mg/ 1 mL		20 mg/ 1 mL	Visually compatible for 4 hr at 25 °C	2440	**C**
Lidocaine HCl	AB	1%, 1 mL		20 mg/ 1 mL	Visually compatible for 4 hr at 25 °C	2440	**C**
Lorazepam	SW	2 mg/ 1 mL		20 mg/ 1 mL	Haze forms immediately becoming two layers over time	2440	**I**
Metoclopramide HCl	ES	5 mg/ 1 mL		20 mg/ 1 mL	Visually compatible for 4 hr at 25 °C	2440	**C**
Morphine sulfate	SW	4 mg/ 1 mL		20 mg/ 1 mL	Visually compatible for 4 hr at 25 °C	2440	**C**
Nitroglycerin	SO	5 mg/ 1 mL		20 mg/ 1 mL	White precipitate forms immediately becoming two layers over time	2440	**I**
Oxacillin sodium	APC	50 mg/ 1 mL		20 mg/ 1 mL	White precipitate forms immediately becoming two layers over time	2440	**I**

Drugs in Syringe Compatibility (Cont.)

Caffeine citrate

Drug (in syringe)	Mfr	Amt	Mfr	Amt	Remarks	Ref	C/I
Pancuronium bromide	GNS	1 mg/ 1 mL		20 mg/ 1 mL	Visually compatible for 4 hr at 25 °C	2440	C
Pantoprazole sodium	a	4 mg/ 1 mL		10 mg/ 1 mL	Precipitates	2574	I
Phenobarbital sodium	ES	130 mg/ 1 mL		20 mg/ 1 mL	Visually compatible for 4 hr at 25 °C	2440	C
Phenylephrine HCl	ES	10 mg/ 1 mL		20 mg/ 1 mL	Visually compatible for 4 hr at 25 °C	2440	C
Sodium bicarbonate	AST	4.2%, 1 mL		20 mg/ 1 mL	Visually compatible for 4 hr at 25 °C	2440	C
Sodium nitroprusside	ES	25 mg/ 1 mL		20 mg/ 1 mL	Visually compatible for 4 hr at 25 °C	2440	C
Vancomycin HCl	LI	50 mg/ 1 mL		20 mg/ 1 mL	Visually compatible for 4 hr at 25 °C	2440	C

[a]*Test performed using the formulation WITHOUT edetate disodium.*

Y-Site Injection Compatibility (1:1 Mixture)

Caffeine citrate

Drug	Mfr	Conc	Mfr	Conc	Remarks	Ref	C/I
Dopamine HCl		0.6 mg/mL[a]		20 mg/mL	Compatible and stable for 24 hr at room temperature	1	C
Doxapram HCl	RB	2 mg/mL[a]	BI	20 mg/mL	Visually compatible for 4 hr at 23 °C	2470	C
Fentanyl citrate		10 mcg/mL[a]		20 mg/mL	Compatible and stable for 24 hr at room temperature	1	C
Heparin sodium		1 unit/mL[a]		20 mg/mL	Compatible and stable for 24 hr at room temperature	1	C
Levofloxacin	OMN	5 mg/mL[a]		5 mg/mL	Visually compatible for 4 hr at 24 °C	2233	C

[a]*Tested in dextrose 5%.*

CALCITRIOL
AHFS 88:16

Products — Calcitriol is available as 1 mL of solution in ampuls. Each milliliter of the Calcijex (Abbott) aqueous solution contains calcitriol 1 mcg, polysorbate 20 4 mg, sodium ascorbate 2.5 mg, and hydrochloric acid and/or sodium hydroxide to adjust pH. (1)

Calcitriol injection (American Regent) utilizes a different formulation. Each milliliter of solution contains calcitriol 1 mcg, polysorbate 20 4 mg, sodium ascorbate 10 mg, sodium chloride 1.5 mg, dibasic sodium phosphate anhydrous 7.6 mg, monobasic sodium phosphate monohydrate 1.8 mg, and edetate disodium dihydrate. (1)

pH — The Calcijex (Abbott) injection has a target pH of 6.5 with a range of 5.9 to 7.0. Calcitriol injection (American Regent) has a pH in the range of 6.7 to 7.7. (1)

Tonicity — The injection is an isotonic solution. (1)

Trade Name(s) — Calcijex.

Administration — Calcitriol is given by intravenous injection. For patients undergoing hemodialysis, it may be administered by rapid intravenous injection through the catheter after a period of hemodialysis. (4)

Stability — Calcitriol injection is a clear, colorless to yellow solution. It should be stored at controlled room temperature and protected from light. (1; 4) Freezing and excessive heat should be avoided, although brief exposure to temperatures up to 40 °C does not adversely affect the injection. (4)

The product does not contain a preservative, and the manufacturers recommend discarding any unused solution. (1; 4)

Syringes — Calcitriol (Abbott) 1 and 2 mcg/mL undiluted and 0.5 mcg/mL diluted in dextrose 5%, sodium chloride 0.9%, and water for injection was evaluated for stability. It was stored in 1-mL polypropylene tuberculin syringes (Becton Dickinson) for eight hours at room temperature while exposed to normal room light. Little or no loss occurred during the study period. (1662)

Sorption — The sorption potential of calcitriol (Abbott) to PVC bags and administration sets and to polypropylene syringes was evaluated by determining the apparent calcitriol polymer–water partition coefficients. The mean apparent partition coefficient was 66 times greater for PVC than polypropylene. In this test, 50% of the calcitriol was lost to PVC within two hours while approximately 4% was lost to polypropylene in 20 days. (1662)

Similar results were reported for calcitriol 1.5 mcg in 2000 mL of Dianeal PD-2, Midpeliq 250, and Peritoliq 250 in polyvinyl chloride peritoneal dialysis solution bags. Losses of up to 75% occurred in 72 hours due to sorption to the container material. However, the same combinations in polypropylene and glass containers exhibited only about 10 to 20% loss in 72 hours. (2695)

Peritoneal Dialysis Solutions — Calcitriol (Abbott) in concentrations of 0.5 to 2 mcg/L in Dianeal (Baxter) with dextrose 1.5 and 4.5% and in Inpersol (Abbott) with dextrose 1.5% lost about 50% in two hours and about 75% in 20 hours due to sorption to the plastic bag. (502)

CALCIUM CHLORIDE
AHFS 40:12

Products — Calcium chloride is available in 10-mL single-dose vials and prefilled syringes containing 1 g of calcium chloride (dihydrate), providing 13.6 mEq (270 mg) of calcium and 13.6 mEq of chloride in water for injection. The pH may have been adjusted with hydrochloric acid and/or calcium hydroxide. (1; 4)

pH — From 5.5 to 7.5 diluted in water to a 5% concentration. (1; 4)

Osmolarity — The 10% injection is labeled as having an osmolarity of 2.04 mOsm/mL. (1)

The osmolality of a calcium chloride 10% solution was determined by osmometer to be 1765 mOsm/kg. (1233)

Administration — Calcium chloride is administered by direct intravenous injection or by continuous or intermittent intravenous infusion. Intravenous administration should be performed slowly at a rate not exceeding 0.7 to 1.8 mEq/min. The drug may also be injected into the ventricular cavity in cardiac resuscitation. It must not be injected into the myocardium. Severe necrosis and sloughing may result if calcium chloride is injected intramuscularly or subcutaneously or leaks into the perivascular tissue. (1; 4)

Stability — The injection is clear and colorless. Intact vials should be stored at controlled room temperature. The single-use vials do not contain a preservative; the manufacturer recommends discarding any unused solution. (1)

Calcium chloride injection under simulated summer conditions in paramedic vehicles was exposed to temperatures ranging from 26 to 38 °C over 4 weeks. Analysis found no loss of the drug under these conditions. (2562)

Compatibility Information

Additive Compatibility

Calcium chloride

Drug	Mfr	Conc/L	Mfr	Conc/L	Test Soln	Remarks	Ref	C/I
Amikacin sulfate	BR	5 g	UP	1 g	D5LR, D5R, D5S, D5W, D10W, LR, NS, R, SL	Physically compatible and both stable for 24 hr at 25 °C	294	C
Amphotericin B		200 mg	BP	4 g	D5W	Haze develops over 3 hr	26	I
Ascorbic acid	UP	500 mg	UP	1 g	D5W	Physically compatible	15	C

Additive Compatibility (Cont.)

Calcium chloride

Drug	Mfr	Conc/L	Mfr	Conc/L	Test Soln	Remarks	Ref	C/I
Ceftriaxone sodium						Incompatible. Precipitate may form in calcium-containing solutions	2222; 2731; 2784	I
Chloramphenicol sodium succinate	PD	10 g	UP	1 g	D5W	Physically compatible	15	C
Dobutamine HCl	LI	182 mg	UP	9 g	NS	Physically compatible for 20 hr. Haze forms at 24 hr	552	I
	LI	1 g	ES	2 g	D5W, NS	Deeply pink in 24 hr at 25 °C	789	I
	LI	1 g	ES	50 g	D5W, NS	Physically compatible for 24 hr at 21 °C	812	C
Dopamine HCl	AS	800 mg	UP		D5W	No dopamine loss in 24 hr at 25 °C	312	C
Fat emulsion, intravenous	CU	10%		1 g		Immediate flocculation with visually apparent layer in 2 hr at room temperature	656	I
	CU	10%		500 mg		Flocculation within 4 hr at room temperature	656	I
	VT	10%	DB	1 g		Coalescence and creaming in 8 hr at 8 and 25 °C	825	I
	KV	10%		10 and 20 mEq		Immediate flocculation, aggregation, and creaming	1018	I
Hydrocortisone sodium succinate	UP	500 mg	UP	1 g	D5W	Physically compatible	15	C
Isoproterenol HCl	WI	4 mg	UP	1 g		Physically compatible	59	C
Lidocaine HCl	AST	2 g	UP	1 g		Physically compatible	24	C
Magnesium sulfate	DB	50 to 10 g	DB	20 to 4 g	D5W, NS	Visible precipitate or microprecipitate forms at room temperature	2597	I
	DB	4 g	DB	2 g	D5W, NS	No visible precipitate. Microscopic examination was inconclusive	2597	?
	DB	2.5 g	DB	2 g	TPN #266[a]	No visible precipitate or microprecipitate in 24 hr at room temperature	2597	C
Norepinephrine bitartrate	WI	8 mg	UP	1 g	D, D–S, S	Physically compatible	77	C
Penicillin G potassium	SQ	20 million units	UP	1 g	D5W	Physically compatible	15	C
Penicillin G sodium	UP	20 million units	UP	1 g	D5W	Physically compatible	15	C
Pentobarbital sodium	AB	1 g	UP	1 g	D5W	Physically compatible	15	C
Phenobarbital sodium	WI	200 mg	UP	1 g	D5W	Physically compatible	15	C
Sodium bicarbonate	AB		UP		D5W	Conditionally compatible depending on concentrations	15	?
	AB	2.4 mEq[b]		1 g	D5W	Physically compatible for 24 hr	772	C
Verapamil HCl	KN	80 mg	ES	2 g	D5W, NS	Physically compatible for 24 hr	764	C

[a] Refer to Appendix I for the composition of parenteral nutrition solutions. TPN indicates a 2-in-1 admixture.
[b] One vial of Neut added to a liter of admixture.

Drugs in Syringe Compatibility

Calcium chloride

Drug (in syringe)	Mfr	Amt	Mfr	Amt	Remarks	Ref	C/I
Milrinone lactate	STR	5.25 mg/ 5.25 mL	AB	3 g/ 30 mL	Physically compatible. No milrinone loss in 20 min at 23 °C	1410	**C**
Pantoprazole sodium	[a]	4 mg/ 1 mL		100 mg/ 1 mL	Precipitates	2574	**I**

[a]*Test performed using the formulation WITHOUT edetate disodium.*

Y-Site Injection Compatibility (1:1 Mixture)

Calcium chloride

Drug	Mfr	Conc	Mfr	Conc	Remarks	Ref	C/I
Amiodarone HCl	WY	6 mg/mL[a]	APP	10 mg/mL[a]	Visually compatible for 24 hr at 22 °C	2352	**C**
	WY	6 mg/mL[a]	APP	100 mg/mL	Visually compatible for 24 hr at 22 °C	2352	**C**
Amphotericin B cholesteryl sulfate complex	SEQ	0.83 mg/mL[a]	AST	40 mg/mL[a]	Gross precipitate forms	2117	**I**
Ceftaroline fosamil	FOR	2.22 mg/ mL[a,b,e]	AMR	40 mg/mL[a,b,e]	Physically compatible for 4 hr at 23 °C	2826	**C**
Dobutamine HCl	LI	4 mg/mL[c]	AB	4 mg/mL[c]	Physically compatible for 3 hr	1316	**C**
Doxapram HCl	RB	2 mg/mL[a]	APP	100 mg/mL	Visually compatible for 4 hr at 23 °C	2470	**C**
Epinephrine HCl	ES	0.032 mg/ mL[c]	AB	4 mg/mL[c]	Physically compatible for 3 hr	1316	**C**
Esmolol HCl	DCC	10 mg/mL[a]	AB	20 mg/mL[a]	Physically compatible for 24 hr at 22 °C	1169	**C**
Hydroxyethyl starch 130/0.4 in sodium chloride 0.9%	FRK	6%	HOS	20, 40, 80 mg/mL[a]	Visually compatible for 24 hr at room temperature	2770	**C**
Micafungin sodium	ASP	1.5 mg/mL[b]	AB	40 mg/mL[b]	Physically compatible for 4 hr at 23 °C	2683	**C**
Milrinone lactate	SS	0.2 mg/mL[a]	AMR	20 mg/mL[a]	Visually compatible for 4 hr at 25 °C	2381	**C**
Morphine sulfate	WY	0.2 mg/mL[c]	AB	4 mg/mL[c]	Physically compatible for 3 hr	1316	**C**
Paclitaxel	NCI	1.2 mg/mL[a]	AST	20 mg/mL[a]	Physically compatible for 4 hr at 22 °C	1556	**C**
Propofol	ZEN	10 mg/mL	AST	40 mg/mL[a]	White precipitate forms in 1 hr	2066	**I**
Sodium bicarbonate	AB	1 mEq/mL	AB	4 mg/mL[c]	Slight haze or precipitate in 1 hr	1316	**I**
Sodium nitroprusside	RC	0.3, 1.2, 3 mg/mL[a]	AST	0.4 and 1.36 mEq/ mL[d]	Visually compatible for 48 hr at 24 °C protected from light	2357	**C**
	RC	1.2 and 3 mg/ mL[a]	AST	0.8 mEq/mL[d]	Visually compatible for 48 hr at 24 °C protected from light	2357	**C**

[a]*Tested in dextrose 5%.*
[b]*Tested in sodium chloride 0.9%.*
[c]*Tested in both dextrose 5% and sodium chloride 0.9%.*
[d]*Tested in dextrose 5% in sodium chloride 0.2%.*
[e]*Tested in Ringer's injection, lactated.*

Additional Compatibility Information

Calcium and Phosphate — UNRECOGNIZED CALCIUM PHOSPHATE PRECIPITATION IN A 3-IN-1 PARENTERAL NUTRITION MIXTURE RESULTED IN PATIENT DEATH.

The potential for the formation of a calcium phosphate precipitate in parenteral nutrition solutions is well studied and documented (1771; 1777), but the information is complex and difficult to apply to the clinical situation. (1770; 1772; 1777) The incorporation of fat emulsion in 3-in-1 parenteral nutrition solutions obscures any precipitate that is present, which has led to substantial debate on the dangers associated with 3-in-1 parenteral nutrition mixtures and when or if the danger to the patient is warranted therapeutically. (1770; 1771; 1772; 2031; 2032; 2033; 2034; 2035; 2036) Because such precipitation may be life-threatening to patients (2037; 2291), the Food and Drug Administration issued a Safety Alert containing the following recommendations (1769):

1. "The amounts of phosphorus and of calcium added to the admixture are critical. The solubility of the added calcium should be calculated from the volume at the time the calcium is added. It should not be based upon the final volume.

   Some amino acid injections for TPN admixtures contain phosphate ions (as a phosphoric acid buffer). These phosphate ions and the volume at the time the phosphate is added should be considered when calculating the concentration of phosphate additives. Also, when adding calcium and phosphate to an admixture, the phosphate should be added first.

   The line should be flushed between the addition of any potentially incompatible components.

2. A lipid emulsion in a three-in-one admixture obscures the presence of a precipitate. Therefore, if a lipid emulsion is needed, either (1) use a two-in-one admixture with the lipid infused separately, or (2) if a three-in-one admixture is medically necessary, then add the calcium before the lipid emulsion and according to the recommendations in number 1 above.

   If the amount of calcium or phosphate which must be added is likely to cause a precipitate, some or all of the calcium should be administered separately. Such separate infusions must be properly diluted and slowly infused to avoid serious adverse events related to the calcium.

3. When using an automated compounding device, the above steps should be considered when programming the device. In addition, automated compounders should be maintained and operated according to the manufacturer's recommendations.

   Any printout should be checked against the programmed admixture and weight of components.

4. During the mixing process, pharmacists who mix parenteral nutrition admixtures should periodically agitate the admixture and check for precipitates. Medical or home care personnel who start and monitor these infusions should carefully inspect for the presence of precipitates both before and during infusion. Patients and care givers should be trained to visually inspect for signs of precipitation. They also should be advised to stop the infusion and seek medical assistance if precipitates are noted.

5. A filter should be used when infusing either central or peripheral parenteral nutrition admixtures. At this time, data have not been submitted to document which size filter is most effective in trapping precipitates.

Standards of practice vary, but the following is suggested: a 1.2-μm air-eliminating filter for lipid-containing admixtures and a 0.22-μm air-eliminating filter for non-lipid-containing admixtures.

6. Parenteral nutrition admixtures should be administered within the following time frames: if stored at room temperature, the infusion should be started within 24 hours after mixing; if stored at refrigerated temperatures, the infusion should be started within 24 hours of rewarming. Because warming parenteral nutrition admixtures may contribute to the formation of precipitates, once administration begins, care should be taken to avoid excessive warming of the admixture.

   Persons administering home care parenteral nutrition admixtures may need to deviate from these time frames. Pharmacists who initially prepare these admixtures should check a reserve sample for precipitates over the duration and under the conditions of storage.

7. If symptoms of acute respiratory distress, pulmonary emboli, or interstitial pneumonitis develop, the infusion should be stopped immediately and thoroughly checked for precipitates. Appropriate medical interventions should be instituted. Home care personnel and patients should immediately seek medical assistance."

Calcium Phosphate Precipitation Fatalities — Fatal cases of paroxysmal respiratory failure in two previously healthy women receiving peripheral vein parenteral nutrition were reported. The patients experienced sudden cardiopulmonary arrest consistent with pulmonary emboli. The authors used in vitro simulations and an animal model to conclude that unrecognized calcium phosphate precipitation in a 3-in-1 total nutrition admixture caused the fatalities. The precipitation resulted during compounding by introducing calcium and phosphate near to one another in the compounding sequence and prior to complete fluid addition. This resulted in a temporarily high concentration of the drugs and precipitation of calcium phosphate. Observation of the precipitate was obscured by the incorporation of 20% fat emulsion, intravenous, into the nutrition mixture. No filter was used during infusion of the fatal nutrition admixtures. (2037)

In a follow-up retrospective review, five patients were identified who had respiratory distress associated with the infusion of the 3-in-1 admixtures at around the same time. Four of these five patients died, although the cause of death could be definitively determined for only two. (2291)

Calcium and Phosphate Conditional Compatibility — Calcium salts are conditionally compatible with phosphate in parenteral nutrition solutions. The incompatibility is dependent on a solubility and concentration phenomenon and is not entirely predictable. Precipitation may occur during compounding or at some time after compounding is completed.

NOTE: Some amino acid solutions inherently contain calcium and phosphate, which must be considered in any projection of compatibility.

A study determined the maximum concentrations of calcium (as chloride and gluconate) and phosphate that can be maintained without precipitation in a parenteral nutrition solution consisting of FreAmine II 4.25% and dextrose 25% for 24 hours at 30 °C. It was noted that the amino acids in parenteral nutrition solutions form soluble complexes with calcium and phosphate, reducing the available free calcium and phosphate that can form insoluble precipitates. The concentration of calcium available for precipitation is greater with the chloride salt compared to the gluconate salt, at least in part because of differences in dissociation characteristics. Consequently, a greater concentration of calcium gluconate than calcium chloride can be mixed with sodium phosphate. (608)

In addition to the concentrations of phosphate and calcium and the salt form of the calcium, the concentration of amino acids and the time and temperature of storage altered the formation of calcium phosphate in parenteral nutrition solutions. As the temperature was increased, the incidence of precipitate formation also increased. This finding was attributed, at least in part, to a greater degree of dissociation of the calcium and phosphate complexes and the decreased solubility of calcium phosphate. Therefore, a solution possibly may be stored at 4 °C with no precipitation, but on warming to room temperature a precipitate will form over time. (608)

The maximum allowable concentrations of calcium and phosphate in a 3-in-1 parenteral nutrition mixture for children (TNA #192 in Appendix I) were reported. Added calcium was varied from 1.5 to 150 mmol/L, and added phosphate was varied from 21 to 300 mmol/L. These mixtures were stable for 48 hours at 22 and 37 °C as long as the pH was not greater than 5.7, the calcium concentration was below 16 mmol/L, the phosphate concentration was below 52 mmol/L, and the product of the calcium and phosphate concentrations was below 250 mmol²/L². (1773)

The presence of magnesium in solutions may also influence the reaction between calcium and phosphate, including the nature and extent of precipitation. (158; 159)

The interaction of calcium and phosphate in parenteral nutrition solutions is a complex phenomenon. Various factors play a role in the solubility or precipitation of a given combination, including (608; 609; 1042; 1063; 1210; 1234; 1427; 2778):

1. Concentration of calcium
2. Salt form of calcium
3. Concentration of phosphate
4. Concentration of amino acids
5. Amino acids composition
6. Concentration of dextrose
7. Temperature of solution
8. pH of solution
9. Presence of other additives
10. Order of mixing

Enhanced precipitate formation would be expected from such factors as high concentrations of calcium and phosphate, increases in solution pH, decreases in amino acid concentrations, increases in temperature, addition of calcium before phosphate, lengthy standing times or slow infusion rates, and use of calcium as the chloride salt. (854)

Even if precipitation does not occur in the container, it has been reported that crystallization of calcium phosphate may occur in a Silastic infusion pump chamber or tubing if the rate of administration is slow, as for premature infants. Water vapor may be transmitted outward and be replaced by air rapidly enough to produce supersaturation. (202) Several other cases of catheter occlusion have been reported. (610; 1427; 1428; 1429)

CALCIUM GLUCONATE
AHFS 40:12

Products — Calcium gluconate is available from various manufacturers in 10-, 50-, and 100-mL vials as a 10% solution. Each milliliter contains 94 mg of calcium gluconate with calcium d-saccharate tetrahydrate 4.5 mg in water for injection, providing 9.3 mg (0.465 mEq) of elementary calcium. The pH may be adjusted with sodium hydroxide and/or hydrochloric acid. (1)

pH — From 6 to 8.2. (1; 4)

Osmolarity — The osmolarity is stated to be 0.68 mOsm/mL. (1)

The osmolality of a calcium gluconate 10% solution was determined by osmometer to be 276 mOsm/kg. (1233)

Administration — Calcium gluconate is usually administered intravenously as a 10% solution, slowly by direct intravenous injection, or by continuous or intermittent intravenous infusion. Intravenous administration should be performed slowly at a rate not exceeding 0.7 to 1.8 mEq/min. (1; 4) Calcium gluconate has been given by intramuscular or, rarely, subcutaneous injection to adults (4), but these routes are not recommended because of possible tissue necrosis, sloughing, and abscess formation. (1) Numerous reports indicate that tissue irritation and necrosis may occur from intramuscular or subcutaneous injection or extravasation from intravenous administration, especially in infants and children. (183; 184; 185; 359)

Stability — Calcium gluconate injection is a supersaturated solution that has been stabilized by the addition of calcium d-saccharate. It should be stored at controlled room temperature. Freezing should be avoided. Do not use it if a precipitate is present. (1)

Compatibility Information

Solution Compatibility

Calcium gluconate

Solution	Mfr	Mfr	Conc/L	Remarks	Ref	C/I
Dextrose 5% in Ringer's injection, lactated	BA	PD	2 g	Physically compatible for 24 hr	315	C
Dextrose 5% in sodium chloride 0.9%			1 g	Physically compatible	74	C
	BA	PD	2 g	Physically compatible for 24 hr	315	C
Dextrose 5%			1 g	Physically compatible	74	C
	BA	PD	2 g	Physically compatible for 24 hr	315	C
Dextrose 10%	BA	PD	2 g	Physically compatible for 24 hr	315	C
		BP	18 g	Physically compatible for 30 hr at room temperature under fluorescent light	1347	C
Dextrose 20%	BA	PD	2 g	Physically compatible for 24 hr	315	C
Ringer's injection, lactated			1 g	Physically compatible	74	C
	BA	PD	2 g	Physically compatible for 24 hr	315	C
Sodium chloride 0.9%			1 g	Physically compatible	74	C
	BA	PD	2 g	Physically compatible for 24 hr	315	C
Sodium lactate ⅙ M	BA	PD	2 g	Physically compatible for 24 hr	315	C

Additive Compatibility

Calcium gluconate

Drug	Mfr	Conc/L	Mfr	Conc/L	Test Soln	Remarks	Ref	C/I
Amikacin sulfate	BR	5 g	UP	500 mg	D5LR, D5R, D5S, D5W, D10W, LR, NS, R, SL	Physically compatible and both stable for 24 hr at 25 °C	294	C
Aminophylline		250 mg		1 g	D5W	Physically compatible	74	C
Amphotericin B		200 mg	BP	4 g	D5W	Haze develops over 3 hr	26	I
Ascorbic acid	UP	500 mg	UP	1 g	D5W	Physically compatible	15	C
Ceftriaxone sodium						Incompatible. Precipitate may form in calcium-containing solutions	2222; 2731; 2784	I
Chloramphenicol sodium succinate	PD	500 mg		1 g	D5W	Physically compatible	74	C
	PD	10 g	UP	1 g	D5W	Physically compatible	15	C
	PD	10 g	UP	1 g		Physically compatible	6	C
Dobutamine HCl	LI	182 mg	VI	9 g	NS	Small particles form within 4 hr. White precipitate and haze after 15 hr	552	I
	LI	1 g	ES	2 g	D5W, NS	Deeply pink in 24 hr at 25 °C	789	I
	LI	1 g	IX	50 g	D5W, NS	Small white particles in 24 hr at 21 °C	812	I
Fat emulsion, intravenous	VT	10%	PR	2 g		Produced cracked emulsion	32	I
	KV	10%		7.2 and 9.6 mEq		Immediate flocculation, aggregation, and creaming	1018	I
Floxacillin sodium	BE	20 g	ANT	2 g	NS	White precipitate forms immediately	1479	I

Additive Compatibility (Cont.)

Calcium gluconate

Drug	Mfr	Conc/L	Mfr	Conc/L	Test Soln	Remarks	Ref	C/I
Furosemide	HO	1 g	ANT	2 g	NS	Physically compatible for 72 hr at 15 and 30 °C	1479	C
Heparin sodium		12,000 units		1 g	D5W	Physically compatible	74	C
	UP	4000 units	UP	1 g	D5W	Physically compatible	15	C
	AB	20,000 units	UP	1 g		Physically compatible	21	C
Hydrocortisone sodium succinate	UP	100 mg		1 g	D5W	Physically compatible	74	C
	UP	500 mg	UP	1 g	D5W	Physically compatible	15	C
Lidocaine HCl	AST	2 g	ES	2 g	D5W, LR, NS	Physically compatible for 24 hr at 25 °C	775	C
Magnesium sulfate	DB	50 to 10 g	DB	60 to 12 g	D5W, NS	Visible precipitate or microprecipitate forms at room temperature	2597	I
	DB	5 g	DB	6 g	D5W, NS	No visible precipitate or microprecipitate in 24 hr at room temperature	2597	C
Methylprednisolone sodium succinate	UP	40 mg		1 g	D5S	Physically incompatible	329	I
Norepinephrine bitartrate	WI	8 mg		1 g	D5W	Physically compatible	74	C
Penicillin G potassium		1 million units		1 g	D5W	Physically compatible	74	C
	SQ	20 million units	UP	1 g	D5W	Physically compatible	15	C
Penicillin G sodium	UP	20 million units	UP	1 g	D5W	Physically compatible	15	C
Phenobarbital sodium	WI	200 mg	UP	1 g	D5W	Physically compatible	15	C
Potassium chloride		3 g		1 g	D5W	Physically compatible	74	C
Prochlorperazine edisylate	SKF	100 mg	UP	1 g	D5W	Physically compatible	15	C
Sodium bicarbonate	AB		UP		D5W	Conditionally compatible depending on concentrations	15	?
Tobramycin sulfate	LI	5 g		16 g	D5W	Physically compatible. No tobramycin loss in 60 min at room temperature	984	C
	LI	1 g		33 g	D5W	Physically compatible. No tobramycin loss in 60 min at room temperature	984	C
Vancomycin HCl	LI	1 g		1 g	D5W	Physically compatible	74	C
Verapamil HCl	KN	80 mg	IX	2 g	D5W, NS	Physically compatible for 48 hr	739	C

Drugs in Syringe Compatibility

Calcium gluconate

Drug (in syringe)	Mfr	Amt	Mfr	Amt	Remarks	Ref	C/I
Caffeine citrate		20 mg/ 1 mL		100 mg/ 1 mL	Physically compatible and chemically stable for 24 hr at room temperature	1	C

Drugs in Syringe Compatibility (Cont.)

Calcium gluconate

Drug (in syringe)	Mfr	Amt	Mfr	Amt	Remarks	Ref	C/I
Dimenhydrinate		10 mg/ 1 mL		100 mg/ 1 mL	Clear solution	2569	C
Metoclopramide HCl	RB	10 mg/ 2 mL	ES	1 g/ 10 mL	Possible precipitate formation	924	I
	RB	160 mg/ 32 mL	ES	1 g/ 10 mL	Incompatible. If mixed, use immediately	1167	I
Pantoprazole sodium	a	4 mg/ 1 mL		100 mg/ 1 mL	Precipitates	2574	I

[a]Test performed using the formulation WITHOUT edetate disodium.

Y-Site Injection Compatibility (1:1 Mixture)

Calcium gluconate

Drug	Mfr	Conc	Mfr	Conc	Remarks	Ref	C/I
Aldesleukin	CHI	33,800 I.U./ mL[a]	LY	100 mg/mL	Visually compatible with little or no loss of aldesleukin activity	1857	C
Allopurinol sodium	BW	3 mg/mL[b]	AMR	40 mg/mL[b]	Physically compatible for 4 hr at 22 °C	1686	C
Amifostine	USB	10 mg/mL[a]	AMR	40 mg/mL[a]	Physically compatible for 4 hr at 23 °C	1845	C
Amiodarone HCl	WY	6 mg/mL[a]	AMR	10 mg/mL[a]	Visually compatible for 24 hr at 22 °C	2352	C
Amphotericin B cholesteryl sulfate complex	SEQ	0.83 mg/mL[a]	AB	40 mg/mL[a]	Gross precipitate forms	2117	I
Ampicillin sodium	WY	40 mg/mL[b]	AST	4 mg/mL[b]	Physically compatible for 3 hr	1316	C
	WY	40 mg/mL[b]	AST	4 mg/mL[a]	Slight color change in 1 hr	1316	I
Aztreonam	SQ	40 mg/mL[a]	AMR	40 mg/mL[a]	Physically compatible for 4 hr at 23 °C	1758	C
Bivalirudin	TMC	5 mg/mL[a]	APP	40 mg/mL[a]	Physically compatible for 4 hr at 23 °C	2373	C
Cefazolin sodium	LI	40 mg/mL[c]	AST	4 mg/mL[c]	Physically compatible for 3 hr	1316	C
Ceftaroline fosamil	FOR	2.22 mg/mL[e]	ABX	40 mg/mL[e]	Physically compatible for 4 hr at 23 °C	2826	C
Ciprofloxacin	MI	2 mg/mL[a]	LY	10%	Visually compatible for 2 hr at 25 °C	1628	C
Cisatracurium besylate	GW	0.1, 2, 5 mg/ mL[a]	AB	40 mg/mL[a]	Physically compatible for 4 hr at 23 °C	2074	C
Cladribine	ORT	0.015[b] and 0.5[d] mg/mL	AMR	40 mg/mL[b]	Physically compatible for 4 hr at 23 °C	1969	C
Dexmedetomidine HCl	AB	4 mcg/mL[b]	APP	40 mg/mL[b]	Physically compatible for 4 hr at 23 °C	2383	C
Dobutamine HCl	LI	4 mg/mL[c]	AST	4 mg/mL[c]	Physically compatible for 3 hr	1316	C
Docetaxel	RPR	0.9 mg/mL[a]	FUJ	40 mg/mL[a]	Physically compatible for 4 hr at 23 °C	2224	C
Doripenem	JJ	5 mg/mL[a,b]	AMR	40 mg/mL[a,b]	Physically compatible for 4 hr at 23 °C	2743	C
Doxapram HCl	RB	2 mg/mL[a]	APP	100 mg/mL	Visually compatible for 4 hr at 23 °C	2470	C
Doxorubicin HCl liposomal	SEQ	0.4 mg/mL[a]	AB	40 mg/mL[a]	Physically compatible for 4 hr at 23 °C	2087	C
Enalaprilat	MSD	0.05 mg/mL[b]	ES	0.092 mEq/ mL[a]	Physically compatible for 24 hr at room temperature	1355	C
Epinephrine HCl	ES	0.032 mg/ mL[c]	AST	4 mg/mL[c]	Physically compatible for 3 hr	1316	C
Etoposide phosphate	BR	5 mg/mL[a]	FUJ	40 mg/mL[a]	Physically compatible for 4 hr at 23 °C	2218	C

Y-Site Injection Compatibility (1:1 Mixture) (Cont.)

Calcium gluconate

Drug	Mfr	Conc	Mfr	Conc	Remarks	Ref	C/I
Famotidine	MSD	0.2 mg/mL[a]	LY	0.00465 mEq/mL[b]	Physically compatible for 14 hr	1196	C
Fenoldopam mesylate	AB	80 mcg/mL[b]	APP	40 mg/mL[b]	Physically compatible for 4 hr at 23 °C	2467	C
Filgrastim	AMG	30 mcg/mL[a]	AST	40 mg/mL[a]	Physically compatible for 4 hr at 22 °C	1687	C
Fluconazole	RR	2 mg/mL	ES	100 mg/mL	Cloudiness develops	1407	I
Gemcitabine HCl	LI	10 mg/mL[b]	FUJ	40 mg/mL[b]	Physically compatible for 4 hr at 23 °C	2226	C
Granisetron HCl	SKB	0.05 mg/mL[a]	AB	40 mg/mL[a]	Physically compatible for 4 hr at 23 °C	2000	C
Heparin sodium[k]	RI	1000 units/L[e]	ES	100 mg/mL	Physically compatible for 4 hr at room temperature	322	C
Hetastarch in lactated electrolyte	AB	6%	FUJ	40 mg/mL[a]	Physically compatible for 4 hr at 23 °C	2339	C
Hydrocortisone sodium succinate[l]	UP	100 mg/L[e]	ES	100 mg/mL	Physically compatible for 4 hr at room temperature	322	C
Hydroxyethyl starch 130/0.4 in sodium chloride 0.9%	FRK	6%	PP	20, 30, 40 mg/mL[a]	Visually compatible for 24 hr at room temperature	2770	C
Indomethacin sodium trihydrate	MSD	1 mg/mL[b]	AMR	100 mg/mL	Fine yellow precipitate forms within 1 hr	1527	I
Labetalol HCl	SC	1 mg/mL[a]	AMR	0.23 mEq/mL[a]	Physically compatible for 24 hr at 18 °C	1171	C
Linezolid	PHU	2 mg/mL	AMR	40 mg/mL[a]	Physically compatible for 4 hr at 23 °C	2264	C
Melphalan HCl	BW	0.1 mg/mL[b]	AST	40 mg/mL[b]	Physically compatible for 3 hr at 22 °C	1557	C
Meropenem	ZEN	1 mg/mL[b]	AMR	4 mg/mL[f]	Visually compatible for 4 hr at room temperature	1994	C
	ZEN	50 mg/mL[b]	AMR	4 mg/mL[f]	Yellow discoloration forms in 4 hr at room temperature	1994	I
Micafungin sodium	ASP	1.5 mg/mL[b]	AMR	40 mg/mL[b]	Physically compatible for 4 hr at 23 °C	2683	C
Midazolam HCl	RC	1 mg/mL[a]	FUJ	100 mg/mL	Visually compatible for 24 hr at 23 °C	1847	C
Milrinone lactate	SW	0.4 mg/mL[a]	LY	0.465 mEq/mL	Visually compatible with no loss of milrinone in 4 hr at 23 °C	2214	C
	SS	0.2 mg/mL[a]	AMR	50 mg/mL[a]	Visually compatible for 4 hr at 25 °C	2381	C
Nicardipine HCl	DCC	0.1 mg/mL[a]	ES	0.092 mEq/mL[a]	Visually compatible for 24 hr at room temperature	235	C
Oxaliplatin	SS	0.5 mg/mL[a]	APP	40 mg/mL[a]	Physically compatible for 4 hr at 23 °C	2566	C
Pemetrexed disodium	LI	20 mg/mL[b]	APP	40 mg/mL[a]	White microparticulates form within 4 hr	2564	I
Piperacillin sodium–tazobactam sodium	LE[j]	40 + 5 mg/mL[a]	AMR	40 mg/mL[a]	Physically compatible for 4 hr at 22 °C	1688	C
Potassium chloride		40 mEq/L[e]	ES	100 mg/mL	Physically compatible for 4 hr at room temperature	322	C
Prochlorperazine edisylate	SCN	5 mg/mL	AMR	10 mg/mL[b]	Visually compatible for 24 hr at room temperature	2063	C
Propofol	ZEN	10 mg/mL	AMR	40 mg/mL[a]	Physically compatible for 1 hr at 23 °C	2066	C
Remifentanil HCl	GW	0.025 and 0.25 mg/mL[b]	AB	40 mg/mL[a]	Physically compatible for 4 hr at 23 °C	2075	C
Sargramostim	IMM	10 mcg/mL[b]	AMR	40 mg/mL[b]	Visually compatible for 4 hr at 22 °C	1436	C
Tacrolimus	FUJ	1 mg/mL[b]	ES	100 mg/mL	Visually compatible for 24 hr at 25 °C	1630	C
Telavancin HCl	ASP	7.5 mg/mL[e]	APP	40 mg/mL[e]	Physically compatible for 2 hr	2830	C

Y-Site Injection Compatibility (1:1 Mixture) (Cont.)

Calcium gluconate

Drug	Mfr	Conc	Mfr	Conc	Remarks	Ref	C/I
Teniposide	BR	0.1 mg/mL[a]	AMR	40 mg/mL[a]	Physically compatible for 4 hr at 23 °C	1725	C
Thiotepa	IMM[h]	1 mg/mL[a]	AMR	40 mg/mL[a]	Physically compatible for 4 hr at 23 °C	1861	C
TNA #218 to #226[i]			AB	40 mg/mL[a]	Visually compatible for 4 hr at 23 °C	2215	C
TPN #189[i]			DB	10 mg/mL[b]	Visually compatible for 24 hr at 22 °C	1767	C
TPN #212 to #215[i]			AB	40 mg/mL[a]	Physically compatible for 4 hr at 23 °C	2109	C
Vinorelbine tartrate	BW	1 mg/mL[b]	AMR	40 mg/mL[b]	Physically compatible for 4 hr at 22 °C	1558	C

[a]*Tested in dextrose 5%.*
[b]*Tested in sodium chloride 0.9%.*
[c]*Tested in both dextrose 5% and sodium chloride 0.9%.*
[d]*Tested in bacteriostatic sodium chloride 0.9% preserved with benzyl alcohol 0.9%.*
[e]*Tested in dextrose 5%, Ringer's injection, lactated, and sodium chloride 0.9%.*
[f]*Tested in sterile water for injection.*
[g]*Tested in dextrose 5% in sodium chloride 0.9%.*
[h]*Lyophilized formulation tested.*
[i]*Refer to Appendix I for the composition of parenteral nutrition solutions. TNA indicates a 3-in-1 admixture, and TPN indicates a 2-in-1 admixture.*
[j]*Test performed using the formulation WITHOUT edetate disodium.*
[k]*Tested in combination with hydrocortisone sodium succinate (Upjohn) 100 mg/L.*
[l]*Tested in combination with heparin sodium (Riker) 1000 units/L.*

Additional Compatibility Information

Calcium and Phosphate — UNRECOGNIZED CALCIUM PHOSPHATE PRECIPITATION IN A 3-IN-1 PARENTERAL NUTRITION MIXTURE RESULTED IN PATIENT DEATH.

The potential for the formation of a calcium phosphate precipitate in parenteral nutrition solutions is well studied and documented (1771; 1777), but the information is complex and difficult to apply to the clinical situation. (1770; 1772; 1777) The incorporation of fat emulsion in 3-in-1 parenteral nutrition solutions obscures any precipitate that is present, which has led to substantial debate on the dangers associated with 3-in-1 parenteral nutrition mixtures and when or if the danger to the patient is warranted therapeutically. (1770; 1771; 1772; 2031; 2032; 2033; 2034; 2035; 2036) Because such precipitation may be life-threatening to patients (2037; 2291), the Food and Drug Administration issued a Safety Alert containing the following recommendations (1769):

1. "The amounts of phosphorus and of calcium added to the admixture are critical. The solubility of the added calcium should be calculated from the volume at the time the calcium is added. It should not be based upon the final volume.

   Some amino acid injections for TPN admixtures contain phosphate ions (as a phosphoric acid buffer). These phosphate ions and the volume at the time the phosphate is added should be considered when calculating the concentration of phosphate additives. Also, when adding calcium and phosphate to an admixture, the phosphate should be added first.

   The line should be flushed between the addition of any potentially incompatible components.

2. A lipid emulsion in a three-in-one admixture obscures the presence of a precipitate. Therefore, if a lipid emulsion is needed, either (1) use a two-in-one admixture with the lipid infused separately, or (2) if a three-in-one admixture is medically necessary,

then add the calcium before the lipid emulsion and according to the recommendations in number 1 above.

   If the amount of calcium or phosphate which must be added is likely to cause a precipitate, some or all of the calcium should be administered separately. Such separate infusions must be properly diluted and slowly infused to avoid serious adverse events related to the calcium.

3. When using an automated compounding device, the above steps should be considered when programming the device. In addition, automated compounders should be maintained and operated according to the manufacturer's recommendations.

   Any printout should be checked against the programmed admixture and weight of components.

4. During the mixing process, pharmacists who mix parenteral nutrition admixtures should periodically agitate the admixture and check for precipitates. Medical or home care personnel who start and monitor these infusions should carefully inspect for the presence of precipitates both before and during infusion. Patients and care givers should be trained to visually inspect for signs of precipitation. They also should be advised to stop the infusion and seek medical assistance if precipitates are noted.

5. A filter should be used when infusing either central or peripheral parenteral nutrition admixtures. At this time, data have not been submitted to document which size filter is most effective in trapping precipitates.

   Standards of practice vary, but the following is suggested: a 1.2-μm air-eliminating filter for lipid-containing admixtures and a 0.22-μm air-eliminating filter for non-lipid-containing admixtures.

6. Parenteral nutrition admixtures should be administered within the following time frames: if stored at room temperature, the infusion should be started within 24 hours after mixing; if stored at refrigerated temperatures, the infusion should be started within 24 hours of rewarming. Because warming parenteral nutrition admixtures may contribute to the formation of precipi-

tates, once administration begins, care should be taken to avoid excessive warming of the admixture.

Persons administering home care parenteral nutrition admixtures may need to deviate from these time frames. Pharmacists who initially prepare these admixtures should check a reserve sample for precipitates over the duration and under the conditions of storage.

7. If symptoms of acute respiratory distress, pulmonary emboli, or interstitial pneumonitis develop, the infusion should be stopped immediately and thoroughly checked for precipitates. Appropriate medical interventions should be instituted. Home care personnel and patients should immediately seek medical assistance."

Calcium Phosphate Precipitation Fatalities — Fatal cases of paroxysmal respiratory failure in two previously healthy women receiving peripheral vein parenteral nutrition were reported. The patients experienced sudden cardiopulmonary arrest consistent with pulmonary emboli. The authors used in vitro simulations and an animal model to conclude that unrecognized calcium phosphate precipitation in a 3-in-1 total nutrition admixture caused the fatalities. The precipitation resulted during compounding by introducing calcium and phosphate near to one another in the compounding sequence and prior to complete fluid addition. This resulted in a temporarily high concentration of the drugs and precipitation of calcium phosphate. Observation of the precipitate was obscured by the incorporation of 20% fat emulsion, intravenous, into the nutrition mixture. No filter was used during infusion of the fatal nutrition admixtures. (2037)

In a follow-up retrospective review, five patients were identified who had respiratory distress associated with the infusion of the 3-in-1 admixtures at around the same time. Four of these five patients died, although the cause of death could be definitively determined for only two. (2291)

Calcium and Phosphate Conditional Compatibility — Calcium salts are conditionally compatible with phosphate in parenteral nutrition solutions. The incompatibility is dependent on a solubility and concentration phenomenon and is not entirely predictable. Precipitation may occur during compounding or at some time after compounding is completed.

NOTE: Some amino acid solutions inherently contain both calcium and phosphate, which must be considered in any projection of compatibility.

A study determined the maximum concentrations of calcium (as chloride and gluconate) and phosphate that can be maintained without precipitation in a parenteral nutrition solution consisting of FreAmine II 4.25% and dextrose 25% for 24 hours at 30 °C. It was noted that the amino acids in parenteral nutrition solutions form soluble complexes with calcium and phosphate, reducing the available free calcium and phosphate that can form insoluble precipitates. The concentration of calcium available for precipitation is greater with the chloride salt compared to the gluconate salt, at least in part because of differences in dissociation characteristics. Consequently, a greater concentration of calcium gluconate than calcium chloride can be mixed with sodium phosphate. (608)

In addition to the concentrations of phosphate and calcium and the salt form of the calcium, the concentration of amino acids and the time and temperature of storage altered the formation of calcium phosphate in parenteral nutrition solutions. As the temperature was increased, the incidence of precipitate formation also increased. This finding was attributed, at least in part, to a greater degree of disso-

ciation of the calcium and phosphate complexes and the decreased solubility of calcium phosphate. Therefore, a solution possibly may be stored at 4 °C with no precipitation, but on warming to room temperature a precipitate will form over time. (608)

The compatibility of calcium and phosphate in several parenteral nutrition formulas for newborn infants was evaluated. Calcium gluconate 10% (Cutter) and potassium phosphate (Abbott) were used to achieve concentrations of 2.5 to 100 mEq/L of calcium and 2.5 to 100 mmol/L of phosphorus added. The parenteral nutrition solutions evaluated were as shown in Table 1. The results were reported as graphic depictions.

The pH dependence of the phosphate–calcium precipitation has been noted. Dibasic calcium phosphate is very insoluble, while monobasic calcium phosphate is relatively soluble. At low pH, the soluble monobasic form predominates; but as the pH increases, more dibasic phosphate becomes available to bind with calcium and precipitate. Therefore, the lower the pH of the parenteral nutrition solution, the more calcium and phosphate can be solubilized. Once again, the effects of temperature were observed. As the temperature is increased, more calcium ion becomes available and more dibasic calcium phosphate is formed. Therefore, temperature increases will increase the amount of precipitate. (609)

Similar calcium and phosphate solubility curves were reported for neonatal parenteral nutrition solutions using TrophAmine (McGaw) 2, 1.5, and 0.8% as the sources of amino acids. The solutions also contained dextrose 10%, with cysteine and pH adjustment being used in some admixtures. Calcium and phosphate solubility followed the patterns reported previously. (609) A slightly greater concentration of phosphate could be used in some mixtures, but this finding was not consistent. (1024)

Using a similar study design, six neonatal parenteral nutrition solutions based on Aminosyn-PF (Abbott) 2, 1.5, and 0.8%, with and without added cysteine hydrochloride and dextrose 10% were studied. Calcium concentrations ranged from 2.5 to 50 mEq/L, and phosphate concentrations ranged from 2.5 to 50 mmol/L. Solutions sat for 18 hours at 25 °C and then were warmed to 37 °C in a water bath to simulate the clinical situation of warming prior to infusion into a child. Solubility curves were markedly different than those for TrophAmine in the previous study. (1024) Solubilities were reported to decrease by 15 mEq/L for calcium and 15 mmol/L for phosphate. The solutions remained clear during room temperature storage, but crystals often formed on warming to 37 °C. (1211)

However, these data were questioned by Mikrut, who noted the similarities between the Aminosyn-PF and TrophAmine products and found little difference in calcium and phosphate solubilities in a preliminary report. (1212) In the full report (1213), parenteral nutrition solutions containing Aminosyn-PF or TrophAmine 1 or 2.5% with dextrose 10 or 25%, respectively, plus electrolytes and trace metals, with or without cysteine hydrochloride, were evaluated under the same conditions. Calcium concentrations ranged from 2.5 to 50 mEq/L,

Table 1. Parenteral Nutrition Solutions (609)

Component	Solution Number			
	#1	#2	#3	#4
FreAmine III	4%	2%	1%	1%
Dextrose	25%	20%	10%	10%
pH	6.3	6.4	6.6	7.0[a]

[a] Adjusted with sodium hydroxide.

and phosphate concentrations ranged from 5 to 50 mmol/L. In contrast to the previous results (1024), the solubility curves were very similar for the Aminosyn-PF and TrophAmine parenteral nutrition solutions but very different from those of the previous Aminosyn-PF study. (1211) The authors again showed that the solubility of calcium and phosphate is greater in solutions containing higher concentrations of amino acids and dextrose. (1213)

Calcium and phosphate solubility curves for TrophAmine 1 and 2% with dextrose 10% and electrolytes, vitamins, heparin, and trace elements were reported. Calcium concentrations ranged from 10 to 60 mEq/L, and phosphorus concentrations ranged from 10 to 40 mmol/L. Calcium and phosphate solubilities were assessed by analysis of the calcium concentrations and followed patterns similar to those reported previously. (608; 609) The higher percentage of amino acids (TrophAmine 2%) permitted a slightly greater solubility of calcium and phosphate, especially in the 10 to 50-mEq/L and 10 to 35-mmol/L ranges, respectively. (1614)

The maximal product of the amount of calcium (as gluconate) times phosphate (as potassium) that can be added to a parenteral nutrition solution, composed of amino acids 1% (Travenol) and dextrose 10%, for preterm infants was reported. Turbidity was observed on initial mixing when the solubility product was around 115 to 130 $mmol^2$ or greater. After storage at 7 °C for 20 hours, visible precipitates formed at solubility products of 130 $mmol^2$ or greater. If the solution was administered through a barium-impregnated silicone rubber catheter, crystalline precipitates obstructed the catheters in 12 hours at a solubility product of 100 $mmol^2$ and in 10 days at 79 $mmol^2$, much lower than the in vitro results. (1041)

The solubility characteristics of calcium and phosphate in pediatric parenteral nutrition solutions composed of Aminosyn 0.5, 2, and 4% with dextrose 10 to 25% were reported. Also present were electrolytes and vitamins. Sodium phosphate was added sequentially in phosphorus concentrations from 10 to 30 mmol/L. Calcium gluconate was added last in amounts ranging from 1 to 10 g/L. The solutions were stored at 25 °C for 30 hours and examined visually and microscopically for precipitation. The authors found that higher concentrations of Aminosyn increased the solubility of calcium and phosphate. Precipitation occurred at lower calcium and phosphate concentrations in the 0.5% solution compared to the 2 and 4% solutions. For example, at a phosphorus concentration of 30 mmol/L, precipitation occurred at calcium gluconate concentrations of about 1, 2, and 4 g/L in the 0.5, 2, and 4% Aminosyn mixtures, respectively. Similarly, at a calcium gluconate concentration of 8 g/L and above, precipitation occurred at phosphorus concentrations of about 13, 17, and 22 mmol/L in the 0.5, 2, and 4% solutions, respectively. The dextrose concentration did not appear to affect the calcium and phosphate solubility significantly. (1042)

The solubility of calcium and phosphorus in neonatal parenteral nutrition solutions composed of amino acids (Abbott) 1.25 and 2.5% with dextrose 5 and 10%, respectively, was evaluated. Also present were multivitamins and trace elements. The solutions contained calcium (as gluconate) in amounts ranging from 25 to 200 mg/100 mL. The phosphorus (as potassium phosphate) concentrations evaluated ranged from 25 to 150 mg/100 mL. If calcium gluconate was added first, cloudiness occurred immediately. If potassium phosphate was added first, substantial quantities could be added with no precipitate formation in 48 hours at 4 °C (Table 2). However, if stored at 22 °C, the solutions were stable for only 24 hours, and all contained precipitates after 48 hours. (1210)

The physical compatibility of calcium gluconate 10 to 40 mEq/L and potassium phosphates 10 to 40 mmol/L in three neonatal paren-

Table 2. Maximum Calcium and Phosphorus Concentrations Physically Compatible for 48 Hours at 4 °C (1210)

	Phosphorus (mg/100 mL)	
Calcium (mg/100 mL)	Amino Acids 1.25% + Dextrose 5%[a]	Amino Acids 2.5% + Dextrose 10%[a]
200[b]	50	75
150	50	100
100	75	100
50	100	125
25	150[b]	150[b]

[a] Plus multivitamins and trace elements.
[b] Maximum concentration tested.

teral nutrition solutions (TPN #123 to #125 in Appendix I), alone and with retrograde administration of aminophylline 7.5 mg diluted with 1.5 mL of sterile water for injection was reported. Contact of the alkaline aminophylline solution with the parenteral nutrition solutions resulted in the precipitation of calcium phosphate at much lower concentrations than were compatible in the parenteral nutrition solutions alone. (1404)

The maximum allowable concentrations of calcium and phosphate in a 3-in-1 parenteral nutrition mixture for children (TNA #192 in Appendix I) was reported. Added calcium was varied from 1.5 to 150 mmol/L, while added phosphate was varied from 21 to 300 mmol/L. The mixtures were stable for 48 hours at 22 and 37 °C as long as the pH was not greater than 5.7, the calcium concentration was below 16 mmol/L, the phosphate concentration was below 52 mmol/L, and the product of the calcium and phosphate concentrations was below 250 $mmol^2/L^2$. (1773)

Additional calcium and phosphate solubility curves were reported for specialty parenteral nutrition solutions based on NephrAmine and also HepatAmine at concentrations of 0.8, 1.5, and 2% as the sources of amino acids. The solutions also contained dextrose 10%, with cysteine and pH adjustment to simulate addition of fat emulsion used in some admixtures. Calcium and phosphate solubility followed the hyperbolic patterns previously reported. (609) Temperature, time, and pH affected calcium and phosphate solubility, with pH having the greatest effect. (2038)

The maximum sodium phosphate concentrations were reported for given amounts of calcium gluconate that could be admixed in parenteral nutrition solutions containing TrophAmine in varying quantities (with cysteine hydrochloride 40 mg/g of amino acid) and dextrose 10%. The solutions also contained magnesium sulfate 4 mEq/L, potassium acetate 24 mEq/L, sodium chloride 32 mEq/L, pediatric multivitamins, and trace elements. The presence of cysteine hydrochloride reduces the solution pH and increases the amount of calcium and phosphate that can be incorporated before precipitation occurs. The results of this study cannot be safely extrapolated to TPN solutions with compositions other than the ones tested. The admixtures were compounded with the sodium phosphate added last after thorough mixing of all other components. The authors noted that this is not the preferred order of mixing (usually phosphate is added first and thoroughly mixed before adding calcium last); however, they believed this reversed order of mixing would provide a margin of error in cases in which the proper order is not followed. After compounding, the solutions were stored for 24 hours at 40 °C. The maximum calcium and phosphate amounts that could be mixed in the various solutions were reported tabularly and are shown in Table 3. (2039) However,

Table 3. Maximum Amount of Phosphate (as Sodium) (mmol/L) Not Resulting in Precipitation (2039) See CAUTION Below.[a]

Calcium (as Gluconate)	Amino Acid (as TrophAmine) with Cysteine HCl 40 mg/g of Amino Acid				
	0%	0.4%	1%	2%	3%
9.8 mEq/L	0	27	42	60	66
14.7 mEq/L	0	15	18	30	36
19.6 mEq/L	0	6	15	27	30
29.4 mEq/L	0	3	6	21	24

[a]CAUTION: The results cannot be safely extrapolated to solutions with formulas other than the ones tested. See text.

these results are not entirely consistent with another study. (2196) See below.

The temperature dependence of the calcium–phosphate precipitation has resulted in the occlusion of a subclavian catheter by a solution apparently free of precipitation. The parenteral nutrition solution consisted of FreAmine III 500 mL, dextrose 70% 500 mL, sodium chloride 50 mEq, sodium phosphate 40 mmol, potassium acetate 10 mEq, potassium phosphate 40 mmol, calcium gluconate 10 mEq, magnesium sulfate 10 mEq, and Shil's trace metals solution 1 mL. Although there was no evidence of precipitation in the bottle, tubing and pump cassette, and filter (all at approximately 26 °C) during administration, the occluded catheter and Vicra Loop Lock (next to the patient's body at 37 °C) had numerous crystals identified as calcium phosphate. In vitro, this parenteral nutrition solution had a precipitate in 12 hours at 37 °C but was clear for 24 hours at 26 °C. (610)

Similarly, a parenteral nutrition solution that was clear and free of particulates after two weeks under refrigeration developed a precipitate in four to six hours when stored at room temperature. When the solution was warmed in a 37 °C water bath, precipitation occurred in one hour. Administration of the solution before the precipitate was noticed led to interstitial pneumonitis due to deposition of calcium phosphate crystals. (1427)

A 2-mL fluid barrier of dextrose 5% in a microbore retrograde infusion set failed to prevent precipitation when used between calcium gluconate 200 mg/2 mL and sodium phosphate 0.3 mmol/0.1 mL. (1385)

Calcium phosphate precipitation phenomena was evaluated in a series of parenteral nutrition admixtures composed of dextrose 22%, amino acids (FreAmine III) 2.7%, and fat emulsion (Abbott) 0, 1, and 3.2%. Incorporation of calcium gluconate 19 to 24 mEq/L and phosphate (as sodium) 22 to 28 mmol/L resulted in visible precipitation in the fat-free admixtures. New precipitate continued to form over 14 days, even after repeated filtrations of the solutions through 0.2-μm filters. The presence of the amino acids increased calcium and phosphate solubility, compared with simple aqueous solutions. However, the incorporation of the fat emulsion did not result in a statistically significant increase in calcium and phosphate solubility. The authors noted that the kinetics of calcium phosphate precipitate formation do not appear to be entirely predictable; both transient and permanent precipitation can occur either during the compounding process or at some time afterward. Because calcium phosphate precipitation can be very dangerous clinically, the use of inline filters was recommended. The authors suggested that the filters should have a porosity appropriate to the parenteral nutrition admixture—1.2 μm for fat-containing and 0.2 or 0.45 μm for fat-free nutrition mixtures. (2061)

Laser particle analysis was used to evaluate the formation of calcium phosphate precipitation in pediatric TPN solutions containing TrophAmine in concentrations ranging from 0.5 to 3% with dextrose 10% and also containing L-cysteine hydrochloride 1 g/L. The solutions also contained in each liter sodium chloride 20 mEq, sodium acetate 20 mEq, magnesium sulfate 3 mEq, trace elements 3 mL, and heparin sodium 500 units. The presence of L-cysteine hydrochloride reduces the solution pH and increases the amount of calcium and phosphate that can be incorporated before precipitation occurs. The results of this study cannot be safely extrapolated to TPN solutions with compositions other than the ones tested. The maximum amount of phosphate that was incorporated without the appearance of a measurable increase in particulates in 24 hours at 37 °C for each of the amino acids concentrations is shown in Table 4. (2196) These results are not entirely consistent with previous results. (2039) See above. The use of more sensitive electronic particle measurement for the formation of subvisual particulates in this study may contribute to the differences in the results.

The solubility of calcium acetate versus calcium gluconate with sodium phosphates was evaluated in pediatric parenteral nutrition solutions following storage for 30 hours at 25 °C followed by 30 minutes at 37 °C. Concentrations of Aminosyn PF studied varied from 1 to 3%, dextrose from 10 to 25%, calcium from 5 to 60 mEq/L, and phosphate from 1 to 60 mmol/L. L-cysteine hydrochloride at a dose of 40 mg/g of Aminosyn PF, magnesium 3.2 mEq/L, and pediatric trace elements-4 at 2.4 mL/L of pediatric parenteral nutrition solution were also added. Calcium acetate was found to be less soluble than calcium gluconate when prepared under these concentrations. The maximum concentrations of the calcium salts and sodium phosphates are shown in Table 5. Polarized light microscopy was used to identify the calcium acetate and sodium phosphate crystals adherent to the container walls because simple visual observation was not able to identify the precipitates. The authors recommended the use of calcium acetate to reduce the iatrogenic aluminum exposure often seen with calcium gluconate in the neonatal population receiving parenteral nutrition. (2466) However, care must be taken to avoid inadvertent calcium phosphate precipitation at the lower concentrations found with calcium acetate if it is substituted for the gluconate salt to reduce aluminum exposure.

Calcium and phosphate compatibility was evaluated in a series of adult formula parenteral nutrition admixtures composed of FreAmine III, in concentrations ranging from 1 to 5% (TPN #258 through #262).

Table 4. Maximum Amount of Phosphate (as Potassium) (mmol/L) Not Resulting in Precipitation (2196) See CAUTION Below.[a]

Calcium (as Gluconate) (mEq/L)	Amino Acid (as TrophAmine) plus Cysteine HCl 1 g/L					
	0.5%	1%	1.5%	2%	2.5%	3%
10	22	28	38	38	38	43
14	18	18	18	38	38	43
19	18	18	18	33	33	38
24	12	18	18	22	28	28
28	12	18	18	18	18	18
33	12	12	12	12	12	12
37	12	12	12	12	12	12
41	9	9	9	12	12	12
45	0	9	9	12	12	12
49	0	9	9	9	12	12
53	0	9	9	9	9	9

[a]CAUTION: The results cannot be safely extrapolated to solutions with formulas other than the ones tested. See text.

Table 5. Maximum Concentrations of Sodium Phosphates and Calcium as Acetate and as Gluconate Not Resulting in Precipitation (2466)

Aminosyn PF (%)	Sodium Phosphates (mmol/L)	Calcium Acetate (mEq/L)	Calcium Gluconate (mEq/L)
1	10	25	50
1	15	15	25
2	10	30	45
2	25	10	12.5
3	20	10	15
3	25	15	17.5

The solutions also contained dextrose ranging from 15% up to 25%. Also present were sodium chloride, potassium chloride, and magnesium sulfate in common amounts. Cysteine hydrochloride was added in an amount of 25 mg/g of amino acids from FreAmine III to reduce the pH by about 0.5 pH unit and thereby increase the amount of calcium and phosphates that can be added to the TPN admixtures as has been done with pediatric parenteral nutrition admixtures. Phosphates as the potassium salts and calcium as the gluconate salt were added in variable quantities to determine the maximum amounts of calcium and phosphates that could be added to the test admixtures. The samples were evaluated at 23 and 37 °C over 48 hours by visual inspection in ambient light and using a Tyndall beam and electronic measurement of turbidity and microparticulates. The addition of the cysteine hydrochloride resulted in an increase of calcium and phosphates solubility of about 30% by lowering the solution pH 0.5 pH unit. The boundaries between the compatible and incompatible concentrations were presented graphically as hyperbolic curves. (2469)

A 2-in-1 parenteral nutrition admixture with final concentrations of TrophAmine 0.5%, dextrose 5%, L-cysteine hydrochloride 40 mg/g of amino acids, calcium gluconate 60 mg/100 mL, and sodium phosphates 46.5 mg/mL was found to result in visible precipitation of calcium phosphate within 30 hours stored at 23 to 27 °C. Despite the presence of the acidifying L-cysteine hydrochloride, precipitation occurred at clinically utilized amounts of calcium and phosphates. (2622)

The presence of magnesium in solutions may also influence the reaction between calcium and phosphate, including the nature and extent of precipitation. (158; 159)

The interaction of calcium and phosphate in parenteral nutrition solutions is a complex phenomenon. Various factors play a role in the solubility or precipitation of a given combination, including (608; 609; 1042; 1063; 1210; 1234; 1427; 2778):

1. Concentration of calcium
2. Salt form of calcium
3. Concentration of phosphate
4. Concentration of amino acids
5. Amino acids composition
6. Concentration of dextrose
7. Temperature of solution
8. pH of solution
9. Presence of other additives
10. Order of mixing

Enhanced precipitate formation would be expected from such factors as high concentrations of calcium and phosphate, increases in solution pH, decreases in amino acid concentrations, increases in temperature, addition of calcium before phosphate, lengthy standing times or slow infusion rates, and use of calcium as the chloride salt. (854)

Even if precipitation does not occur in the container, it has been reported that crystallization of calcium phosphate may occur in a Silastic infusion pump chamber or tubing if the rate of administration is slow, as for premature infants. Water vapor may be transmitted outward and be replaced by air rapidly enough to produce supersaturation. (202) Several other cases of catheter occlusion also have been reported. (610; 1427; 1428; 1429)

Aluminum — Calcium gluconate injection in glass vials is a significant source of aluminum, which has been associated with neurological impairment in premature neonates. Aluminum is leached from the glass vial during the autoclaving of the vials for sterilization. The use of calcium gluconate injection in polyethylene plastic vials in countries where it is available has been recommended to reduce the aluminum burden for neonates. (2322)

CARBOPLATIN
AHFS 10:00

Products — Carboplatin is available as a lyophilized powder in vials containing 150 mg with an equal amount of mannitol. Reconstitute the vials with 15 mL of dextrose 5%, sodium chloride 0.9%, or sterile water for injection. The reconstituted solutions have a carboplatin concentration of 10 mg/mL. (1)

Carboplatin is also available as a 10-mg/mL aqueous injection in 5-mL (50-mg) and 60-mL (600-mg) vials. (1)

pH — A 1% solution has a pH of 5 to 7. (1)

Trade Name(s) — Paraplatin.

Administration — Carboplatin is administered by intravenous infusion over a period of at least 15 minutes or longer. It has also been administered as a continuous intravenous infusion over 24 hours. It may be diluted with compatible diluents to a concentration as low as 0.5 mg/mL for administration. (1; 4)

Because of an interaction occurring between carboplatin and the metal aluminum, resulting in precipitate formation and loss of potency, only administration equipment such as needles, syringes, catheters, and sets that contain no aluminum should be used for this drug. (1)

Stability — Intact vials should be stored at controlled room temperature and protected from light. (1; 4)

The manufacturer states that reconstituted solutions are stable for eight hours at a room temperature not exceeding 25 °C. Because no antibacterial preservative is present, the manufacturer recommends that carboplatin solutions should be discarded eight hours after dilution. (1) However, other information indicates that the drug may be stable for a much longer time. At a concentration of 15 mg/mL in sterile water for injection or at concentrations of 2 and 0.5 mg/mL in dextrose 5%, no decomposition occurs in 24 hours at 22 to 25 °C. (234)

Cisplatin formation in carboplatin 1 mg/mL in sodium chloride 0.9% at 25 °C with exposure to fluorescent light was evaluated. Less than 0.1% of the carboplatin had converted to cisplatin in two hours, and 0.7% had converted in 24 hours. (1695)

Carboplatin 1 mg/mL in sterile water for injection was reported to exhibit less than a 10% loss in 14 days at room temperature. (1379)

Carboplatin (Bristol-Myers Oncology) 1 mg/mL in sterile water for injection was stable in PVC reservoirs (Parker Micropump) for 14 days at 4 and 37 °C, exhibiting no loss. (1696)

The manufacturer states that carboplatin 10 mg/mL aqueous injection in multiple-dose vials is stable for up to 14 days at 25 °C even with multiple needle entries. (1)

pH Effects — The pH range of maximum stability has been reported to be pH 4 to 6 (1919) to 6.5. (1369) The degradation rate increases above pH 6.5. (1369)

Syringes — Carboplatin 10-mg/mL aqueous solution prefilled into plastic syringes exhibited no decomposition in five days at 4 °C and only a 3% loss in 24 hours at 37 °C. (1238)

Carboplatin 10 mg/mL (Bristol-Myers Squibb) was repackaged into 30-mL polypropylene syringes for use in the Intelliject portable syringe pump. The carboplatin solution exhibited no visual changes, and no loss of carboplatin content was found when stored at 25 °C for eight days. No evidence of interaction between carboplatin and the syringe plastic was identified, and no impact on the functioning of the syringe pump was observed. (2147)

Sorption — Carboplatin (Ribosepharm) 0.72 mg/mL in dextrose 5% exhibited little or no loss due to sorption in polyethylene and PVC containers compared to glass containers over 72 hours at room and refrigeration temperatures. (2420; 2430) Simulated infusion of carboplatin 10 mg/mL through a Silastic catheter over 24 hours at 37 °C did not affect the delivered drug concentration. (1238)

Compatibility Information

Solution Compatibility

Carboplatin

Solution	Mfr	Mfr	Conc/L	Remarks	Ref	C/I
Dextrose 5% in sodium chloride 0.2%	AB[a]	NCI	1 g	Physically compatible. 2% loss in 24 hr at 25 °C	1087	C
Dextrose 5% in sodium chloride 0.45%	AB[b]	NCI	1 g	Physically compatible. 2% loss in 24 hr at 25 °C	1087	C
Dextrose 5% in sodium chloride 0.9%	AB[a]	NCI	1 g	Physically compatible. 4% loss in 24 hr at 25 °C	1087	C
Dextrose 5%	[a]	NCI	500 mg and 2 g	Physically compatible. No loss for 24 hr at 25 °C	234	C
	AB[a]	NCI	100 mg and 1 g	Physically compatible. 1.5% loss in 6 hr at 25 °C	1087	C
	[c]	BR	2.4 g	No loss in 9 days at 23 °C in the dark	1757	C
	[c]	BR	1 g	Visually compatible. Little loss in 28 days at 4, 22, and 35 °C	1823	C
	[a]	BR	1 g	Visually compatible. 6% loss in 28 days at 4, 22, and 35 °C	1823	C
	[d]	BR	1 g	Visually compatible. No loss in 28 days at 4, 22, and 35 °C	1823	C
	[e]	BR	1 g	Visually compatible. Little loss in 28 days at 4 and 22 °C. Concentration increased by 14% in 28 days at 35 °C due to moisture transfer through container	1823	C
	BA[a]	BMS	500 mg and 4 g	Visually compatible. 5% loss at 25 °C and no loss at 4 °C in the dark in 21 days	2099	C
	BA[a]	BMS	750 mg and 2 g	Visually compatible with no loss at 25 and 4 °C in the dark in 7 days	2099	C
	[f]	BR	6 g	Little loss in 14 days at 37 °C in the dark	2321	C
	FRE,[c] MAC[g]	TE	0.7 and 2.15 g	Physically compatible. Stable for 84 days at 4 °C and 24 hr at 25 °C	2777	C

Solution Compatibility (Cont.)

Carboplatin

Solution	Mfr	Mfr	Conc/L	Remarks	Ref	C/I
Sodium chloride 0.9%				Use within 8 hr	1	C
	AB[a]	NCI	1 g	Physically compatible. 5% loss in 24 hr at 25 °C	1087	C
			7 g	8% loss in 24 hr at 27 °C	1379	C

[a]Tested in glass containers.
[b]Tested in both glass and PVC containers.
[c]Tested in PVC containers.
[d]Tested in ethylene vinyl acetate containers.
[e]Tested in elastomeric balloon reservoirs (Baxter Infusor).
[f]Tested in Pharmacia Deltec medication cassette reservoirs.
[g]Tested in polyolefin containers.

Additive Compatibility

Carboplatin

Drug	Mfr	Conc/L	Mfr	Conc/L	Test Soln	Remarks	Ref	C/I
Cisplatin		200 mg		1 g	NS	Under 10% drug loss in 7 days at 23 °C	1954	C
Etoposide		200 mg		1 g	W	Under 10% drug loss in 7 days at 23 °C	1954	C
Floxuridine		10 g		1 g	W	Under 10% drug loss in 7 days at 23 °C	1954	C
Fluorouracil		10 g		1 g	W	Greater than 20% carboplatin loss in 24 hr at room temperature	1379	I
	DB	1 g	BR	100 mg	D5W	9% carboplatin loss in 5 hr at 25 °C	2415	I
Ifosfamide		1 g		1 g	W	Both drugs stable for 5 days at room temperature	1379	C
Mesna		1 g		1 g	W	More than 10% carboplatin loss in 24 hr at room temperature	1379	I
Paclitaxel	BMS	300 mg and 1.2 g	BMS	2 g	NS	No paclitaxel loss but carboplatin losses of less than 2, 5, and 6 to 7% at 4, 24, and 32 °C, respectively, in 24 hr. Physically compatible for 24 hr but microparticles of paclitaxel form after 3 to 5 days	2094	C
	BMS	300 mg and 1.2 g	BMS	2 g	D5W	No paclitaxel and carboplatin loss at 4, 24, and 32 °C in 24 hr. Physically compatible for 24 hr but microparticles of paclitaxel form after 3 to 5 days	2094	C
Sodium bicarbonate		200 mmol		1 g		13% carboplatin loss in 24 hr at 27 °C	1379	I

Y-Site Injection Compatibility (1:1 Mixture)

Carboplatin

Drug	Mfr	Conc	Mfr	Conc	Remarks	Ref	C/I
Allopurinol sodium	BW	3 mg/mL[b]	BR	5 mg/mL[b]	Physically compatible for 4 hr at 22 °C	1686	C
Amifostine	USB	10 mg/mL[a]	BR	5 mg/mL[a]	Physically compatible for 4 hr at 23 °C	1845	C
Amphotericin B cholesteryl sulfate complex	SEQ	0.83 mg/mL[a]	BR	5 mg/mL[a]	Increased turbidity forms immediately	2117	I
Anidulafungin	VIC	0.5 mg/mL[a]	BMS	5 mg/mL[a]	Physically compatible for 4 hr at 23 °C	2617	C

Y-Site Injection Compatibility (1:1 Mixture) (Cont.)

Carboplatin

Drug	Mfr	Conc	Mfr	Conc	Remarks	Ref	C/I
Aztreonam	SQ	40 mg/mL[a]	BMS	5 mg/mL[a]	Physically compatible for 4 hr at 23 °C	1758	C
Caspofungin acetate	ME	0.7 mg/mL[b]	MAY	5 mg/mL[b]	Physically compatible for 4 hr at room temperature	2758	C
Cladribine	ORT	0.015[b] and 0.5[c] mg/mL	BR	5 mg/mL[b]	Physically compatible for 4 hr at 23 °C	1969	C
Doripenem	JJ	5 mg/mL[a,b]	SIC	5 mg/mL[a,b]	Physically compatible for 4 hr at 23 °C	2743	C
Doxorubicin HCl liposomal	SEQ	0.4 mg/mL[a]	BR	5 mg/mL[a]	Physically compatible for 4 hr at 23 °C	2087	C
Etoposide phosphate	BR	5 mg/mL[a]	BR	5 mg/mL[a]	Physically compatible for 4 hr at 23 °C	2218	C
Filgrastim	AMG	30 mcg/mL[a]	BR	5 mg/mL[a]	Physically compatible for 4 hr at 22 °C	1687	C
Fludarabine phosphate	BX	1 mg/mL[a]	BR	5 mg/mL[a]	Visually compatible for 4 hr at 22 °C	1439	C
Gemcitabine HCl	LI	10 mg/mL[b]	BR	5 mg/mL[b]	Physically compatible for 4 hr at 23 °C	2226	C
Granisetron HCl	SKB	1 mg/mL	BR	1 mg/mL[b]	Physically compatible with little or no loss of either drug in 4 hr at 22 °C	1883	C
Linezolid	PHU	2 mg/mL	BR	5 mg/mL[a]	Physically compatible for 4 hr at 23 °C	2264	C
Melphalan HCl	BW	0.1 mg/mL[b]	BR	5 mg/mL[b]	Physically compatible for 3 hr at 22 °C	1557	C
Micafungin sodium	ASP	1.5 mg/mL[b]	BA	5 mg/mL[b]	Physically compatible for 4 hr at 23 °C	2683	C
Ondansetron HCl	GL	1 mg/mL[b]	BR	5 mg/mL[a]	Visually compatible for 4 hr at 22 °C	1365	C
	GL	16 to 160 mcg/mL		0.18 to 9.9 mg/mL	Physically compatible when carboplatin given over 10 to 60 min via Y-site	1366	C
Oxaliplatin	SS	0.5 mg/mL[a]	BR	5 mg/mL[a]	Physically compatible for 4 hr at 23 °C	2566	C
Paclitaxel	NCI	1.2 mg/mL[a]		5 mg/mL[a]	Physically compatible for 4 hr at 22 °C	1528	C
Palonosetron HCl	MGI	50 mcg/mL	BMS	5 mg/mL[a]	Physically compatible. No palonosetron and 2% carboplatin loss in 4 hr	2579	C
Pemetrexed disodium	LI	20 mg/mL[b]	BMS	5 mg/mL[a]	Physically compatible for 4 hr at 23 °C	2564	C
Piperacillin sodium–tazobactam sodium	LE[f]	40 + 5 mg/mL[a]	BR	5 mg/mL[a]	Physically compatible for 4 hr at 22 °C	1688	C
Propofol	ZEN	10 mg/mL	BR	5 mg/mL[a]	Physically compatible for 1 hr at 23 °C	2066	C
Sargramostim	IMM	10 mcg/mL[b]	BR	5 mg/mL[b]	Visually compatible for 4 hr at 22 °C	1436	C
Teniposide	BR	0.1 mg/mL[a]	BR	5 mg/mL[a]	Physically compatible for 4 hr at 23 °C	1725	C
Thiotepa	IMM[d]	1 mg/mL[a]	BMS	5 mg/mL[a]	Physically compatible for 4 hr at 23 °C	1861	C
TNA #218 to #226[e]			BMS	5 mg/mL[a]	Visually compatible for 4 hr at 23 °C	2215	C
Topotecan HCl	SKB	56 mcg/mL[a,b]	BR	0.9 mg/mL[a,b]	Visually compatible. Little loss of either drug in 4 hr at 22 °C	2245	C
TPN #212 to #215[e]			BMS	5 mg/mL[a]	Physically compatible for 4 hr at 23 °C	2109	C
Vinorelbine tartrate	BW	1 mg/mL[b]	BR	5 mg/mL[b]	Physically compatible for 4 hr at 22 °C	1558	C

[a] Tested in dextrose 5%.
[b] Tested in sodium chloride 0.9%.
[c] Tested in bacteriostatic sodium chloride 0.9% preserved with benzyl alcohol 0.9%.
[d] Lyophilized formulation tested.
[e] Refer to Appendix I for the composition of parenteral nutrition solutions. TNA indicates a 3-in-1 admixture, and TPN indicates a 2-in-1 admixture.
[f] Test performed using the formulation WITHOUT edetate disodium.

CARMUSTINE (BCNU)
AHFS 10:00

Products — Carmustine is available in vials containing 100 mg of drug, packaged with a vial containing 3 mL of dehydrated alcohol injection, USP, for use as a diluent. (1)

Dissolve the contents of the vial of carmustine with 3 mL of dehydrated alcohol injection, USP. Further dilute with 27 mL of sterile water for injection. The resultant solution will contain 3.3 mg/mL of carmustine in 10% ethanol. (1)

Avoid accidental contact of the reconstituted solution with the skin. Transient hyperpigmentation in the affected areas has occurred. (1; 4)

Trade Name(s) — BiCNU.

Administration — Carmustine is administered as an intravenous infusion over one to two hours. Shorter durations may result in pain and burning at the injection site and flushing. (1; 4)

Stability — The product consists of vacuum-dried pale yellow flakes or is a congealed mass. Intact vials are stored under refrigeration and are stable for at least three years. (1) Intact vials are stable for seven days at room temperatures not exceeding 25 °C. (1181; 1236; 1433) Room temperature storage of intact vials results in slow decomposition, with approximately 3% degradation occurring in 36 days. (285)

Reconstitution as directed results in a colorless to pale yellow solution. This solution is stable for eight hours at room temperature protected from light. (4) About a 6% loss occurs in three hours and about an 8% loss occurs in six hours. (285) A loss of 20% in 21 hours was also reported. (484)

Refrigeration of the solution significantly increases its stability. In 24 hours at 2 to 8 °C with protection from light, approximately 4% decomposition occurs. (1; 285)

Carmustine has a melting point of approximately 30.5 to 32 °C. At this temperature, the drug liquifies, becoming an oily film on the bottom of the vial. Should this occur, the manufacturer recommends that the vials be discarded, because the melting is a sign of decomposition. (1) However, one study showed that storage of the vials at 37 °C for 15 minutes followed by storage at 22 to 25 °C resulted in no decomposition in eight days and about an 8% loss in 37 days. Storage of the vials at 37 °C for seven days resulted in about 10% decomposition. (862)

In 95% ethanol, carmustine 2 mg/mL is reported to be stable for at least 24 hours at 22 to 25 and 37 °C. (862) Under refrigeration, carmustine 0.5 to 0.6 mg/mL in 95% ethanol or absolute ethanol is stable at 0 to 5 °C for up to three months. (863)

pH Effects — The degradation rate for carmustine in aqueous solution was reported to be at a minimum between pH 5.2 and 5.5 (619) and 3.3 and 4.8. (1237) Above pH 6, the degradation rate increases greatly. (619) Decomposition of 10% occurred in less than two hours at pH 6.5 but in 5.5 hours at optimum pH. (1237)

Light Effects — Increased decomposition rates were reported when carmustine, in solution, was exposed to increasing intensities of light. (1237) However, in another study, no clear effect on rate of carmustine loss from exposure to light was demonstrated. Some samples seemed to demonstrate increased rate of loss due to light exposure while others did not. (2337)

Sorption — The manufacturer recommends the use of glass containers for carmustine administration. (1; 4) The rate of loss of carmustine from infusion admixtures in dextrose 5% in PVC containers is substantially greater than the rate of loss in glass (519; 1237; 1658; 2430) or polyolefin (1237; 1658) containers.

Substantial loss to PVC, ethylene vinyl acetate, and polyurethane infusion sets was also noted. Only a set lined with polyethylene proved resistant to carmustine sorption, resulting in little loss in two hours. (1237)

Carmustine (Bristol-Myers Squibb) 0.2 mg/mL in dextrose 5% was evaluated for loss of drug content in glass, polyethylene, and PVC containers. At room temperature, about 40% loss of drug occurred in glass containers in 72 hours. In polyethylene containers, a slightly larger loss occurred, about 50% loss in 72 hours. The greatest loss occurred in PVC containers with about 65% loss in 72 hours. Carmustine losses of 5% occurred in 5.5 hours, 2.5 hours, and 45 minutes in glass, polyethylene, and PVC containers, respectively. The increased losses in polyethylene and PVC containers were attributed to sorption. Under refrigeration, glass and polyethylene containers were similar with less than 10% loss in 72 hours. However, in PVC containers about 20% loss due to sorption occurred in that time frame. (2420; 2430)

Compatibility Information

Solution Compatibility

Carmustine

Solution	Mfr	Mfr	Conc/L	Remarks	Ref	C/I
Dextrose 5%	a	BMS	0.2 mg/mL	Stable for 8 hr at room temperature	1	C
	TR[a]	BR	1.25 g	10% loss in 7.7 hr at room temperature	519	I
	TR[b]	BR	1.25 g	18.5% loss in 1 hr at room temperature	519	I
	CU	BR	100 mg	No decomposition over 90-min study period	523	C
	MG, TR[a]		1.25 g	10% loss in 7.7 to 8.3 hr at room temperature exposed to light	1658	I
	MG[c]		1.25 g	10% loss in 7 hr at room temperature exposed to light	1658	I

Solution Compatibility (Cont.)

Solution	Carmustine Mfr	Mfr	Conc/L	Remarks	Ref	C/I
	TR[b]		1.25 g	10% loss in 0.6 hr at room temperature exposed to light	1658	I
	FAN[a]	BMS	100 mg	7% loss in 2 hr and 12% loss in 4 hr at 25 °C in light or dark. 7% loss in 48 hr at 4 °C	2337	I[e]
	MAC[b]	BMS	100 mg	10% loss in 1 hr at 25 °C in light or dark. 5% loss in 12 hr and 12% loss in 24 hr at 4 °C	2337	I
	BFM[d]	BMS	100 mg	5 to 8% loss in 4 hr and 11 to 14% loss in 6 hr at 25 °C in light or dark. 5% loss in 48 hr and 15% loss in 7 days at 4 °C	2337	I[e]
	FAN[a]	BMS	500 mg	9% loss in 4 hr and 17% loss in 6 hr at 25 °C in light or dark. 9% loss in 48 hr at 4 °C	2337	I[e]
	MAC[b]	BMS	500 mg	7% loss in 1 hr and 10 to 13% loss in 2 hr at 25 °C in light or dark. 7% loss in 12 hr and 18% loss in 24 hr at 4 °C	2337	I
	BFM[d]	BMS	500 mg	9% loss in 6 hr and 13 to 15% loss in 8 hr at 25 °C in light or dark. 5% loss in 48 hr and 15% loss in 7 days at 4 °C	2337	I[e]
	FAN[a]	BMS	1 g	4% loss in 4 hr and 9% loss in 6 hr in dark and 9% loss in 4 hr in light at 25 °C. 4% loss in 48 hr and 13% loss in 7 days at 4 °C	2337	I[e]
	MAC[b]	BMS	1 g	4 to 7% loss in 1 hr and 10% loss in 2 hr at 25 °C in light or dark. 7% loss in 6 hr and 12% loss in 24 hr at 4 °C	2337	I
	BFM[d]	BMS	1 g	7 to 10% loss in 6 hr and 10 to 14% loss in 8 hr at 25 °C in light or dark. 9% loss in 48 hr and 14% loss in 7 days at 4 °C	2337	I[e]
	HOS[f]	BMS	1 g	About 7% loss in 6 hr	2660; 2792	I[e]
Sodium chloride 0.9%	CU	BR	100 mg	No decomposition over 90-min study period	523	C

[a]Tested in glass containers.
[b]Tested in PVC containers.
[c]Tested in polyolefin containers.
[d]Polyethylene-lined trilayer containers.
[e]Incompatible by conventional standards but may be used in lesser time periods.
[f]Tested in VISIV polyolefin containers.

Additive Compatibility

Drug	Carmustine Mfr	Conc/L	Mfr	Conc/L	Test Soln	Remarks	Ref	C/I
Sodium bicarbonate	AB	100 mEq	BR	100 mg	D5W, NS	10% carmustine loss in 15 min and 27% in 90 min	523	I

Y-Site Injection Compatibility (1:1 Mixture)

Drug	Carmustine Mfr	Conc	Mfr	Conc	Remarks	Ref	C/I
Allopurinol sodium	BW	3 mg/mL[b]	BR	1.5 mg/mL[b]	Gas evolves immediately	1686	I
Amifostine	USB	10 mg/mL[a]	BR	1.5 mg/mL[a]	Physically compatible for 4 hr at 23 °C	1845	C
Aztreonam	SQ	40 mg/mL[a]	BMS	1.5 mg/mL[a]	Physically compatible for 4 hr at 23 °C	1758	C

Y-Site Injection Compatibility (1:1 Mixture) (Cont.)

Carmustine

Drug	Mfr	Conc	Mfr	Conc	Remarks	Ref	C/I
Etoposide phosphate	BR	5 mg/mL[a]	BR	1.5 mg/mL[a]	Physically compatible for 4 hr at 23 °C	2218	C
Filgrastim	AMG	30 mcg/mL[a]	BR	1.5 mg/mL[a]	Physically compatible for 4 hr at 22 °C	1687	C
Fludarabine phosphate	BX	1 mg/mL[a]	BR	1.5 mg/mL[a]	Visually compatible for 4 hr at 22 °C	1439	C
Gemcitabine HCl	LI	10 mg/mL[b]	BR	1.5 mg/mL[b]	Physically compatible for 4 hr at 23 °C	2226	C
Granisetron HCl	SKB	0.05 mg/mL[a]	BMS	1.5 mg/mL[a]	Physically compatible for 4 hr at 23 °C	2000	C
Melphalan HCl	BW	0.1 mg/mL[b]	BR	1.5 mg/mL[b]	Physically compatible for 3 hr at 22 °C	1557	C
Ondansetron HCl	GL	1 mg/mL[b]	BR	1.5 mg/mL[a]	Visually compatible for 4 hr at 22 °C	1365	C
Piperacillin sodium–tazobactam sodium	LE[d]	40 + 5 mg/ mL[a]	BR	1.5 mg/mL[a]	Physically compatible for 4 hr at 22 °C	1688	C
Sargramostim	IMM	10 mcg/mL[b]	BR	1.5 mg/mL[b]	Visually compatible for 4 hr at 22 °C	1436	C
Teniposide	BR	0.1 mg/mL[a]	BR	1.5 mg/mL[a]	Physically compatible for 4 hr at 23 °C	1725	C
Thiotepa	IMM[c]	1 mg/mL[a]	BMS	1.5 mg/mL[a]	Physically compatible for 4 hr at 23 °C	1861	C
Vinorelbine tartrate	BW	1 mg/mL[b]	BR	1.5 mg/mL[b]	Physically compatible for 4 hr at 22 °C	1558	C

[a]*Tested in dextrose 5%.*
[b]*Tested in sodium chloride 0.9%.*
[c]*Lyophilized formulation tested.*
[d]*Test performed using the formulation WITHOUT edetate disodium.*

CASPOFUNGIN ACETATE
AHFS 8:14.16

Products — Caspofungin acetate (Merck) is available in vials of 50 and 70 mg of drug. The 50-mg vials also contain 39 mg of sucrose and 26 mg of mannitol. The 70-mg vials also contain 54 mg of sucrose and 36 mg of mannitol. The pH is adjusted during manufacturing with glacial acetic acid and sodium hydroxide. (1)

Equilibrate the refrigerated vials to room temperature. Reconstitute both the 50- and 70-mg vials with 10.8 mL of sterile water for injection, sodium chloride 0.9%, or bacteriostatic water for injection and mix gently until dissolved. Do NOT use dextrose-containing solutions. Withdrawing 10 mL of the reconstituted solution will provide the full 50 or 70 mg as a clear solution. Do not use hazy, precipitated, or discolored solutions. The reconstituted solution should be withdrawn within one hour after reconstitution for preparation of the intravenous infusion. (1)

pH — Approximate pH 6.6. (1)

Osmolality — Caspofungin acetate diluted as directed for infusion is near isotonicity. (2722)

Trade Name(s) — Cancidas.

Administration — Caspofungin acetate is administered by intravenous infusion over a period of one hour. Transfer the appropriate volume of reconstituted solution to a 250-mL bag or bottle of sodium chloride 0.9%, 0.45%, or 0.225%, or Ringer's injection, lactated. Alternatively, the reconstituted caspofungin acetate can be added to a smaller volume of these infusion solutions as long as the final concentration does not exceed 0.5 mg/mL. (1)

Stability — Intact vials of caspofungin acetate should be stored between 2 and 8 °C. Intact vials exposed to ambient room temperature for longer than 48 hours should be discarded. (1)

The reconstituted solution may be stored for up to one hour after reconstitution at room temperature up to 25 °C but should be withdrawn within one hour after reconstitution to prepare the intravenous infusion solution. (1)

Caspofungin acetate is unstable in dextrose-containing solutions; such solutions should not be used for reconstitution or dilution of this drug. (1)

Compatibility Information

Solution Compatibility

Caspofungin acetate

Solution	Mfr	Mfr	Conc/L	Remarks	Ref	C/I
Dextrose 5%		ME		Unstable in dextrose-containing solutions	1	I
Ringer's injection, lactated		ME	0.5 g	Stable for 24 hr at 25 °C and 48 hr at 4 °C	1	C
Sodium chloride 0.225%		ME	0.5 g	Stable for 24 hr at 25 °C and 48 hr at 4 °C	1	C
Sodium chloride 0.45%		ME	0.5 g	Stable for 24 hr at 25 °C and 48 hr at 4 °C	1	C
Sodium chloride 0.9%		ME	0.5 g	Stable for 24 hr at 25 °C and 48 hr at 4 °C	1	C
	[a]	ME	0.2, 0.28, 0.5 g	Physically compatible with less than 10% drug loss in 60 hr at 25 °C and 14 days at 5 °C	2828	C

[a]Tested in Intermate and Homepump Eclipse elastomeric pump reservoirs.

Y-Site Injection Compatibility (1:1 Mixture)

Caspofungin acetate

Drug	Mfr	Conc	Mfr	Conc	Remarks	Ref	C/I
Acyclovir sodium	BV	7 mg/mL[b]	ME	0.7 mg/mL[b]	Physically compatible for 4 hr at room temperature	2758	C
	BED	5 mg/mL[b]	ME	0.5 mg/mL[b]	Fine clear crystals reported	2766	I
Amikacin sulfate	HOS	5 mg/mL[b]	ME	0.7 mg/mL[b]	Physically compatible for 4 hr at room temperature	2758	C
Amiodarone HCl	SIC	4 mg/mL[b]	ME	0.7 mg/mL[b]	Physically compatible for 4 hr at room temperature	2758	C
Amphotericin B	XGN	0.6 mg/mL[a]	ME	0.7 mg/mL[b]	Immediate yellow turbid precipitate forms	2758	I
Amphotericin B lipid complex	ENZ	1 mg/mL[a]	ME	0.7 mg/mL[b]	Immediate yellow turbid precipitate	2758	I
Amphotericin B liposomal	AST	1 mg/mL[a]	ME	0.7 mg/mL[b]	Immediate yellow turbid precipitate	2758	I
Ampicillin sodium	APP	20 mg/mL[b]	ME	0.7 mg/mL[b]	Immediate white turbid precipitate forms	2758	I
Azithromycin	NVP	2 mg/mL[b]	ME	0.5 mg/mL[b]	Physically compatible over 60 min	2766	C
Aztreonam	BMS	40 mg/mL[b]	ME	0.7 mg/mL[b]	Physically compatible for 4 hr at room temperature	2758	C
	BMS	20 mg/mL[b]	ME	0.5 mg/mL[b]	Physically compatible over 60 min	2766	C
Bumetanide	BED	0.04 mg/mL[b]	ME	0.7 mg/mL[b]	Physically compatible for 4 hr at room temperature	2758	C
Carboplatin	MAY	5 mg/mL[b]	ME	0.7 mg/mL[b]	Physically compatible for 4 hr at room temperature	2758	C
Cefazolin sodium	CUR	20 mg/mL[b]	ME	0.7 mg/mL[b]	Immediate white turbid precipitate forms	2758	I
	SZ	100 mg/mL[b]	ME	0.5 mg/mL[b]	Fine white crystals reported	2766	I
Cefepime HCl	BMS	20 mg/mL[b]	ME	0.7 mg/mL[b]	Immediate white turbid precipitate forms	2758	I
Ceftaroline fosamil	FOR	2.22 mg/mL[a,b,h]	ME	0.5 mg/mL[b,h]	Increased haze and particulates	2826	I
Ceftazidime	GSK	40 mg/mL[b]	ME	0.7 mg/mL[b]	Immediate white turbid precipitate forms	2758	I
Ceftriaxone sodium	ORC	20 mg/mL[b]	ME	0.7 mg/mL[b]	Immediate white turbid precipitate forms	2758	I
	NVP	20 mg/mL[b]	ME	0.5 mg/mL[b]	Amber crystals and white paste form	2766	I

Y-Site Injection Compatibility (1:1 Mixture) (Cont.)

Caspofungin acetate

Drug	Mfr	Conc	Mfr	Conc	Remarks	Ref	C/I
Ciprofloxacin	HOS	2 mg/mL[b]	ME	0.7 mg/mL[b]	Physically compatible for 4 hr at room temperature	2758	C
	BAY	2 mg/mL[c]	ME	0.5 mg/mL[b]	Physically compatible over 60 min	2766	C
Cisplatin	APP	0.5 mg/mL[b]	ME	0.7 mg/mL[b]	Physically compatible for 4 hr at room temperature	2758	C
Clindamycin phosphate	BED	10 mg/mL[b]	ME	0.7 mg/mL[b]	Immediate white turbid precipitate forms	2758	I
	HOS	60 mg/mL[d]	ME	0.5 mg/mL[b]	Fine white crystals reported	2766	I
Cyclosporine	BED	5 mg/mL[b]	ME	0.7 mg/mL[b]	Physically compatible for 4 hr at room temperature	2758	C
Cytarabine	MAY	50 mg/mL	ME	0.7 mg/mL[b]	Microparticles form within 4 hr	2758	I
Daptomycin	CUB	10 mg/mL[b]	ME	0.7 mg/mL[b]	Physically compatible for 4 hr at room temperature	2758	C
Daunorubicin HCl	BED	1 mg/mL[b]	ME	0.7 mg/mL[b]	Physically compatible for 4 hr at room temperature	2758	C
Diltiazem HCl	HOS	5 mg/mL	ME	0.7 mg/mL[b]	Physically compatible for 4 hr at room temperature	2758	C
Diphenhydramine HCl	BA	50 mg/mL	ME	0.5 mg/mL[b]	Physically compatible with diphenhydramine HCl given i.v. push over 2 to 5 min	2766	C
Dobutamine HCl	HOS	4 mg/mL[b]	ME	0.7 mg/mL[b]	Physically compatible for 4 hr at room temperature	2758	C
	BA	1 mg/mL[c]	ME	0.5 mg/mL[b]	Physically compatible over 60 min	2766	C
Dolasetron mesylate	SAA	20 mg/mL	ME	0.5 mg/mL[b]	Physically compatible with dolasetron mesylate given i.v. push over 2 to 5 min	2766	C
Dopamine HCl	AMR	3.2 mg/mL[b]	ME	0.7 mg/mL[b]	Physically compatible for 4 hr at room temperature	2758	C
	BA	3.2 mg/mL[c]	ME	0.5 mg/mL[b]	Physically compatible over 60 min	2766	C
Doripenem	JJ	5 mg/mL[a,b]	ME	0.5 mg/mL[b]	Physically compatible for 4 hr at 23 °C	2743	C
Doxorubicin HCl	BED	1 mg/mL[b]	ME	0.7 mg/mL[b]	Physically compatible for 4 hr at room temperature	2758	C
Epinephrine HCl	AMP	0.05 mg/mL[b]	ME	0.7 mg/mL[b]	Physically compatible for 4 hr at room temperature	2758	C
Ertapenem sodium	ME	20 mg/mL[b]	ME	0.7 mg/mL[b]	Immediate white turbid precipitate forms	2758	I
Etoposide phosphate	SIC	5 mg/mL[b]	ME	0.7 mg/mL[b]	Physically compatible for 4 hr at room temperature	2758	C
Famotidine	BA	2 mg/mL[b]	ME	0.5 mg/mL[b]	Physically compatible with famotidine i.v. push over 2 to 5 min	2766	C
Fentanyl citrate	HOS	0.05 mg/mL	ME	0.7 mg/mL[b]	Physically compatible for 4 hr at room temperature	2758	C
	HOS	0.05 mg/mL	ME	0.5 mg/mL[b]	Physically compatible with fentanyl citrate i.v. push over 2 to 5 min	2766	C
Fluconazole	HOS	2 mg/mL[c]	ME	0.5 mg/mL[b]	Physically compatible over 60 min	2766	C
Furosemide	AMR	3 mg/mL[b]	ME	0.7 mg/mL[b]	Immediate white turbid precipitate forms	2758	I
	HOS	10 mg/mL	ME	0.5 mg/mL[b]	Gelatinous material reported	2766	I

Y-Site Injection Compatibility (1:1 Mixture) (Cont.)

Caspofungin acetate

Drug	Mfr	Conc	Mfr	Conc	Remarks	Ref	C/I
Ganciclovir sodium	RC	20 mg/mL[b]	ME	0.7 mg/mL[b]	Physically compatible for 4 hr at room temperature	2758	**C**
Gentamicin sulfate	HOS	5 mg/mL[b]	ME	0.7 mg/mL[b]	Physically compatible for 4 hr at room temperature	2758	**C**
Heparin sodium	HOS	100 units/mL	ME	0.7 mg/mL[b]	Immediate white turbid precipitate forms	2758	**I**
	BA	100 units/mL	ME	0.5 mg/mL[b]	Fine white crystalline material reported	2766	**I**
Hydralazine HCl	APP	20 mg/mL	ME	0.5 mg/mL[b]	Physically compatible with hydralazine HCl i.v. push over 2 to 5 min	2766	**C**
Hydrocortisone sodium succinate	HOS	1 mg/mL[b]	ME	0.7 mg/mL[b]	Physically compatible for 4 hr at room temperature	2758	**C**
Hydromorphone HCl	BA	1 mg/mL[b]	ME	0.7 mg/mL[b]	Physically compatible for 4 hr at room temperature	2758	**C**
	HOS	1 mg/mL	ME	0.5 mg/mL[b]	Physically compatible with hydromorphone HCl i.v. push over 2 to 5 min	2766	**C**
Ifosfamide	BA	20 mg/mL[b]	ME	0.7 mg/mL[b]	Physically compatible for 4 hr at room temperature	2758	**C**
Imipenem–cilastatin sodium	ME	5 mg/mL[b]	ME	0.7 mg/mL[b]	Physically compatible for 4 hr at room temperature	2758	**C**
Insulin, regular	NOV	1 unit/mL[b]	ME	0.7 mg/mL[b]	Physically compatible for 4 hr at room temperature	2758	**C**
	NOV	1 unit/mL[b]	ME	0.5 mg/mL[b]	Physically compatible over 60 min	2766	**C**
Levofloxacin	JN	5 mg/mL[b]	ME	0.7 mg/mL[b]	Physically compatible for 4 hr at room temperature	2758	**C**
	HOS	5 mg/mL[a]	ME	0.5 mg/mL[b]	Physically compatible over 60 min	2766	**C**
Linezolid	PHU	2 mg/mL[b]	ME	0.7 mg/mL[b]	Physically compatible for 4 hr at room temperature	2758	**C**
	PF	2 mg/mL	ME	0.5 mg/mL[b]	Physically compatible over 60 min	2766	**C**
Lorazepam	HOS	0.5 mg/mL[b]	ME	0.7 mg/mL[b]	Physically compatible for 4 hr at room temperature	2758	**C**
Magnesium sulfate	AMR	100 mg/mL[b]	ME	0.7 mg/mL[b]	Physically compatible for 4 hr at room temperature	2758	**C**
	HOS	40 mg/mL	ME	0.5 mg/mL[b]	Physically compatible over 60 min	2766	**C**
Melphalan HCl	CAR	1 mg/mL[b]	ME	0.7 mg/mL[b]	Physically compatible for 4 hr at room temperature	2758	**C**
Meperidine HCl	HOS	10 mg/mL[b]	ME	0.7 mg/mL[b]	Physically compatible for 4 hr at room temperature	2758	**C**
Meropenem	ASZ	2.5 mg/mL[b]	ME	0.7 mg/mL[b]	Physically compatible for 4 hr at room temperature	2758	**C**
	ASZ	10 mg/mL[b]	ME	0.5 mg/mL[b]	Physically compatible over 30 min	2766	**C**
Methylprednisolone sodium succinate	PHU	5 mg/mL[b]	ME	0.7 mg/mL[b]	Immediate white turbid precipitate forms	2758	**I**
Metronidazole	BA	5 mg/mL	ME	0.7 mg/mL[b]	Physically compatible for 4 hr at room temperature	2758	**C**
	BA	5 mg/mL	ME	0.5 mg/mL[b]	Physically compatible over 60 min	2766	**C**
Midazolam HCl	APP	2 mg/mL[b]	ME	0.7 mg/mL[b]	Physically compatible for 4 hr at room temperature	2758	**C**

Y-Site Injection Compatibility (1:1 Mixture) (Cont.)

Caspofungin acetate

Drug	Mfr	Conc	Mfr	Conc	Remarks	Ref	C/I
Milrinone lactate	BA	0.2 mg/mL[b]	ME	0.7 mg/mL[b]	Physically compatible for 4 hr at room temperature	2758	C
Mitomycin	BED	0.5 mg/mL[b]	ME	0.7 mg/mL[b]	Physically compatible for 4 hr at room temperature	2758	C
Morphine sulfate	BA	15 mg/mL	ME	0.7 mg/mL[b]	Physically compatible for 4 hr at room temperature	2758	C
	HOS	2 mg/mL	ME	0.5 mg/mL[b]	Physically compatible with morphine sulfate i.v. push over 2 to 5 min	2766	C
Mycophenolate mofetil HCl	RC	6 mg/mL[b]	ME	0.7 mg/mL[b]	Physically compatible for 4 hr at room temperature	2758	C
Nafcillin sodium	SZ	20 mg/mL[b]	ME	0.7 mg/mL[b]	Transient turbidity becomes white precipitate	2758	I
Norepinephrine bitartrate	BED	0.128 mg/mL[b]	ME	0.7 mg/mL[b]	Physically compatible for 4 hr at room temperature	2758	C
Ondansetron HCl	BED	2 mg/mL	ME	0.5 mg/mL[b]	Physically compatible with ondansetron HCl i.v. push over 2 to 5 min	2766	C
Pantoprazole sodium	WY[e]	0.4 mg/mL[b]	ME	0.7 mg/mL[b]	Physically compatible for 4 hr at room temperature	2758	C
	WY[e]	0.4 mg/mL[b]	ME	0.5 mg/mL[b]	White particles reported	2766	I
Phenylephrine HCl	BA	1 mg/mL[b]	ME	0.7 mg/mL[b]	Physically compatible for 4 hr at room temperature	2758	C
Piperacillin sodium–tazobactam sodium	WY[e]	40 + 5 mg/mL[b]	ME	0.7 mg/mL[b]	Immediate white turbid precipitate forms	2758	I
	WY[f]	80 + 10 mg/mL[b]	ME	0.5 mg/mL[b]	Black particles reported	2766	I
Potassium chloride	APP	0.1 mEq/mL[b]	ME	0.7 mg/mL[b]	Physically compatible for 4 hr at room temperature	2758	C
	BA	0.04 mEq/mL[b]	ME	0.5 mg/mL[b]	Physically compatible over 60 min	2766	C
Potassium phosphates	APP	0.5 mmol/mL[b]	ME	0.7 mg/mL[b]	Immediate white turbid precipitate forms	2758	I
Quinupristin–dalfopristin	MON	5 mg/mL[b]	ME	0.7 mg/mL[b]	Physically compatible for 4 hr at room temperature	2758	C
Tacrolimus	AST	0.02 mg/mL[b]	ME	0.7 mg/mL[b]	Physically compatible for 4 hr at room temperature	2758	C
Telavancin HCl	ASP	7.5 mg/mL[b]	ME	0.5 mg/mL[b]	Physically compatible for 2 hr	2830	C
Tobramycin sulfate	SIC	5 mg/mL[b]	ME	0.7 mg/mL[b]	Physically compatible for 4 hr at room temperature	2758	C
TPN[g]			ME	0.7 mg/mL[b]	Immediate white turbid precipitate forms	2758	I
Trimethoprim–sulfamethoxazole	SIC	0.8 + 4 mg/mL[b]	ME	0.7 mg/mL[b]	Immediate white turbid precipitate forms	2758	I
Vancomycin HCl	HOS	10 mg/mL[b]	ME	0.7 mg/mL[b]	Physically compatible for 4 hr at room temperature	2758	C
	HOS	4 mg/mL[b]	ME	0.5 mg/mL[b]	Physically compatible over 60 min	2766	C

Y-Site Injection Compatibility (1:1 Mixture) (Cont.)

Caspofungin acetate

Drug	Mfr	Conc	Mfr	Conc	Remarks	Ref	C/I
Vasopressin	APP	0.2 unit/mL[b]	ME	0.5 mg/mL[b]	Physically compatible	2641	C
Vincristine sulfate	MAY	0.05 mg/mL[b]	ME	0.7 mg/mL[b]	Physically compatible for 4 hr at room temperature	2758	C
Voriconazole	PF	4 mg/mL[b]	ME	0.7 mg/mL[b]	Physically compatible for 4 hr at room temperature	2758	C
	PF	2 mg/mL[b]	ME	0.5 mg/mL[b]	Physically compatible over 60 min	2766	C

[a]*Tested in dextrose 5%.*
[b]*Tested in sodium chloride 0.9%.*
[c]*Tested as the premixed infusion solution.*
[d]*Tested in sodium chloride 0.45%.*
[e]*Test performed using the formulation WITH edetate disodium.*
[f]*Test performed using the formulation WITHOUT edetate disodium.*
[g]*Specific composition of the parenteral nutrition admixture not reported. TPN indicates a 2-in-1 admixture.*
[h]*Tested in Ringer's injection, lactated.*

CEFAZOLIN SODIUM
AHFS 8:12.06.04

Products — Cefazolin as the sodium salt is available in 500-mg and 1-, 10-, and 20-g vials. For intramuscular administration, reconstitute the 500-mg vial with 2 mL and the 1-g vial with 2.5 mL and shake well until dissolved yielding 225 or 330 mg/mL, respectively. Sterile water for injection or bacteriostatic water for injection may be used for either the 500-mg or 1-g vials while 0.9% sodium chloride only may be used for the 500-mg vial. (1; 4)

For direct intravenous injection, further dilute the reconstituted cefazolin sodium with approximately 5 mL of sterile water for injection. (1; 4)

For intermittent intravenous infusion, reconstituted cefazolin sodium should be diluted further in 50 to 100 mL of compatible infusion solution. (1; 4)

The 10-g bulk vials may be reconstituted with sterile water for injection, bacteriostatic water for injection, or sodium chloride 0.9%. The 10-g vial should be reconstituted with 45 or 96 mL to yield concentrations of 1 g/5 mL or 1 g/10 mL, respectively. (1)

Cefazolin sodium (Braun) is available as 1 g in a dual chamber flexible container. The diluent chamber contains dextrose solution for use as a diluent. (1)

Cefazolin sodium is also available frozen in PVC bags in concentrations of 500 mg and 1 g in 50 mL of dextrose 5%. (4)

pH — From 4.5 to 6. The frozen premixed solutions have a pH of 4.5 to 7. (4)

Osmolality — The osmolality of a 225-mg/mL concentration in sterile water for injection was determined to be 636 mOsm/kg by freezing-point depression. (1071)

The osmolality of cefazolin sodium 1 and 2 g was calculated for the following dilutions (1054):

	Osmolality (mOsm/kg)	
Diluent	50 mL	100 mL
1 g		
Dextrose 5%	321	291
Sodium chloride 0.9%	344	317
2 g		
Dextrose 5%	379	324
Sodium chloride 0.9%	406	351

Cefazolin sodium (Braun) 1 g in dual chamber flexible containers has an osmolality of 290 mOsm/kg when activated with the dextrose solution diluent. (1)

The frozen premixed solutions have osmolalities of 260 to 320 mOsm/kg for the 500 mg/50-mL concentration and 310 to 380 mOsm/kg for the 1 g/50-mL concentration. (4)

The following maximum cefazolin sodium concentrations were recommended to achieve osmolalities suitable for peripheral infusion in fluid-restricted patients (1180):

Diluent	Maximum Concentration (mg/mL)	Osmolality (mOsm/kg)
Dextrose 5%	77	507
Sodium chloride 0.9%	69	494
Sterile water for injection	138	404

Sodium Content — Each gram of cefazolin sodium contains 48 mg or approximately 2 mEq of sodium. (1; 4)

Administration — Cefazolin sodium may be administered by deep intramuscular injection or by intravenous injection. By direct intravenous injection, it is given over three to five minutes directly into the vein or tubing of a running infusion solution. It may also be given by intermittent infusion in 50 to 100 mL of compatible diluent or by continuous infusion. (1)

Stability — Intact containers of the sterile powder should be stored at controlled room temperature. Reconstituted solutions of cefazolin sodium are light yellow to yellow. Protection from light is recommended for both the powder and its solutions. (1; 4)

The manufacturer recommends that solutions of cefazolin sodium be discarded after 24 hours at room temperature or 10 days under refrigeration. (1) This recommendation is made to reduce the potential for the growth of microorganisms and to minimize an increase in color and a change in pH. (276) A test of cefazolin sodium 250 mg/mL in water for injection showed that the drug lost less than 3% in 14 days at 5 °C. A loss of 8 to 10% was noted in four days at 25 °C. (276)

Cefazolin sodium (Braun) 1 g in dual chamber flexible plastic containers with dextrose solution diluent should be used within 24 hours after activation if stored at room temperature and in seven days if stored under refrigeration. (1)

Crystallization — Crystal formation has also been observed in reconstituted cefazolin sodium 330 mg/mL stored at room temperature after complete dissolution when sodium chloride 0.9% is the diluent. The crystals formed initially are fine and may be easily overlooked. At 330 mg/mL, cefazolin sodium is near its saturation point, and the room temperature and ionic content of the diluent are important for maintaining the drug in solution. In an evaluation of cefazolin sodium reconstituted with 2.5 mL of either sodium chloride 0.9% or sterile water for injection and stored at 24 or 26 °C, none of the vials reconstituted with sterile water for injection formed crystals within 24 hours. However, when sodium chloride 0.9% was the diluent, all vials had crystals. Consequently, sterile water for injection was recommended as the diluent when possible. (875) The crystals of cefazolin sodium can be redissolved by hand-warming the vials or by immersion in a 35 °C water bath for two minutes. The clear solution will then be suitable for use. (1075)

pH Effects — Cefazolin sodium solutions are relatively stable at pH 4.5 to 8.5. Above pH 8.5, rapid hydrolysis of the drug occurs. Below pH 4.5, precipitation of the insoluble free acid may occur. (4; 284)

Cefazolin sodium in solutions containing dextrose, fructose, sucrose, dextran 40 or 70, mannitol, sorbitol, or glycerol in concentrations up to 15% was most stable at pH 5 to 6.5. At neutral and alkaline pH, the rate of degradation was accelerated by the carbohydrates and alcohols. (820)

Cefazolin sodium 3.33 mg/mL was evaluated in several aqueous buffer solutions. The drug was most stable in pH 4.5 acetate buffer, exhibiting 10% decomposition in three days at 35 °C and in five days at 25 °C. In pH 5.7 acetate buffer, a 13% loss occurred in three days at 35 °C and a 10% loss occurred in five days at 25 °C. No loss occurred in either acetate buffer in seven days at 4 °C. (1147)

In pH 7.5 phosphate buffer, a yellow color and particulate matter developed after three to four days at 35 °C. This change was accompanied by a 6% cefazolin loss in one day and an 18% loss in three days. At 25 and 4 °C, 10 and 5% cefazolin losses occurred, respectively, in five days. (1147)

Freezing Solutions — Solutions of cefazolin sodium 125, 225, and 330 mg/mL frozen in the original containers at −20 °C immediately after reconstitution with sterile water for injection, bacteriostatic water for injection, or sodium chloride 0.9% are stated to be stable for 12 weeks. Thawed solutions are stable for 24 hours at room temperature or 10 days under refrigeration; they should not be refrozen. (4)

When reconstituted with water for injection, dextrose 5%, or sodium chloride 0.9% in concentrations of 1 g/2.5 mL, 500 mg/100 mL, and 10 g/45 mL, cefazolin sodium retained more than 90% potency for up to 26 weeks when frozen within one hour after reconstitution at −10 and −20 °C. In a concentration of 500 mg/100 mL in dextrose 5% in Ringer's injection, lactated, Ionosol B in dextrose 5%, Normosol M in dextrose 5%, Plasma-Lyte in dextrose 5%, or Ringer's injection, lactated, cefazolin sodium was stable for up to four weeks when frozen within one hour after reconstitution at −10 °C. (277)

In another study, cefazolin sodium (SKF) 1 g/50 mL of dextrose 5% and also sodium chloride 0.9% in PVC containers was frozen at −20 °C for 30 days. The results indicate that potency was retained for the duration of the study. (299)

Cefazolin sodium (Lilly) 1 g/100 mL in dextrose 5% in PVC bags was frozen at −20 °C for 30 days and then thawed by exposure to ambient temperature or microwave radiation. The solutions showed no evidence of precipitation or color change and showed no loss of potency as determined microbiologically. Subsequent storage of the admixture at room temperature for 24 hours also yielded a physically compatible solution which exhibited a 3 to 6% loss of potency. (554)

In an additional study, cefazolin sodium (Lilly and SKF) 10 mg/mL in 50, 100, and 250 mL of dextrose 5% and sodium chloride 0.9% in PVC bags was frozen at −20 °C for 48 hours. Thawing was then performed by exposure to microwave radiation carefully applied so that the solution temperature did not exceed 20 °C and so that a small amount of ice remained at the endpoint. This procedure avoids accelerated decomposition due to inadvertent excessive temperature increases. The solutions were stored for four hours at room temperature. Both brands of cefazolin sodium retained at least 90% of the initial activity as determined by microbiological assay. In addition, the solutions did not exhibit color changes or significant pH changes. (627)

An approximate fourfold increase in particles of 2 to 60 μm was produced by freezing and thawing cefazolin sodium (Lilly) 2 g/100 mL of dextrose 5% (Travenol). The reconstituted drug was filtered through a 0.45-μm filter into PVC bags of solution and frozen for seven days at −20 °C. Thawing was performed at room temperature (29 °C) for 12 hours. Although the total number of particles increased significantly, no particles greater than 60 μm were observed; the solution complied with USP standards for particle sizes and numbers in large volume parenteral solutions. (822)

No loss of cefazolin sodium (SKF) was reported from a solution containing 73.2 mg/mL in sterile water for injection in PVC and glass containers after 30 days at −20 °C. Subsequent thawing and storage for four days at 5 °C, followed by 24 hours at 37 °C to simulate the use of a portable infusion pump, also did not result in a cefazolin loss. (1391)

The manufacturer warns against continued heating of a completely thawed solution, which can result in accelerated drug decomposition and possibly dangerous pressure increases in the container. (627)

Cefazolin sodium (Braun) 1 g in dual chamber flexible containers should not be frozen. (1)

Syringes — Cefazolin sodium (SKF) 1 and 2 g/10 mL in sterile water for injection, packaged in plastic syringes (Monoject), exhibited a 10% cefazolin loss in 13 days at 24 °C. At 4 °C, the drug exhibited less than a 10% loss during the 28-day study period. Frozen at −15 °C, less than 10% drug loss occurred in three months. (1178)

Cefazolin sodium (Apothecon) 50 mg/mL in sodium chloride 0.9% was packaged in 5-mL polypropylene syringes (Becton-Dickinson) and stored at 23 and 5 °C. About 10% loss was found after 12 days of storage at 23 °C. About 3% loss was found after 22 days of refrigerated storage. (2474)

Filtration — Cefazolin sodium (SKF) 10 g/L in dextrose 5% and also in sodium chloride 0.9% was filtered through 0.45- and 0.22-μm Millipore membrane filters at time zero and at 4, 8, and 24 hours after mixing. No significant difference in concentration occurred between any of the filtered samples compared to unfiltered solutions at these time intervals. It was concluded that filtration of cefazolin sodium solutions through these membrane filters could be performed without adversely affecting the drug concentration. (375)

Central Venous Catheter — Cefazolin sodium (SmithKline Beecham) 5 mg/mL in dextrose 5% was found to be compatible with the AR-ROWg+ard Blue Plus (Arrow International) chlorhexidine-bearing triple-lumen central catheter. Essentially complete delivery of the drug was found with little or no drug loss occurring. Furthermore, chlorhexidine delivered from the catheter remained at trace amounts with no substantial increase due to the delivery of the drug through the catheter. (2335)

Cefazolin sodium 10 mg/mL with heparin sodium 5000 units/mL as an antibiotic lock in polyurethane central hemodialysis catheters lost about 50% of the antibiotic over 72 hours at 37 °C. The loss was attributed to sorption to the catheters. Nevertheless, the reduced antibiotic concentration (about 5 mg/mL) remained effective against common microorganisms in catheter-related bacteremia in hemodialysis patients. (2515; 2516)

Compatibility Information

Solution Compatibility

Cefazolin sodium

Solution	Mfr	Mfr	Conc/L	Remarks	Ref	C/I
Amino acids 4.25%, dextrose 25%	MG	LI	1 g	No increase in particulate matter in 24 hr at 5 °C	349	C
Dextrose 5% in Ringer's injection, lactated				Manufacturer recommended solution	1	C
		LI	5 g	Stable for 14 days at 5 °C. 8% loss in 4 days at 25 °C	276	C
Dextrose–saline combinations				Manufacturer recommended solution	1	C
Dextrose 5%				Manufacturer recommended solution	1	C
		LI	5 g	4% loss in 14 days at 5 °C, 6% loss in 4 days at 25 °C	276	C
	BA[a], TR	SKF	20 g	Stable for 24 hr at 5 and 22 °C	298	C
	TR[b]	LI	10 g	Physically compatible with 3% loss in 24 hr at room temperature	554	C
	MG[c]	SKF	10 g	Physically compatible with no loss in 48 hr at room temperature under fluorescent light	983	C
	BA[a]	BR	10 g	Visually compatible with 7% loss in 30 days at 4 °C	2142	C
	TR[a]	LI	20 g	7% loss in 5 days at 24 °C and 5% loss in 24 days at 4 °C	336	C
	BA[e]	NOP	5 and 40 g	Less than 10% loss in 7 days at 23 °C and 28 days at 4 °C	2819	C
Dextrose 10%				Manufacturer recommended solution	1	C
Ionosol B in dextrose 5%		LI	5 g	2% loss in 14 days at 5 °C, 1 to 4% loss in 4 days at 25 °C	276	C
Normosol M in dextrose 5%		LI	5 g	3% loss in 14 days at 5 °C, 1 to 4% loss in 4 days at 25 °C	276	C
Ringer's injection				Manufacturer recommended solution	1	C
Ringer's injection, lactated				Manufacturer recommended solution	1	C
		LI	5 g	Stable for 14 days at 5 °C. 9% loss in 7 days at 25 °C	276	C
Sodium chloride 0.9%				Manufacturer recommended solution	1	C
		LI	5 g	4% loss in 7 days at 5 °C, 8% loss in 4 days at 25 °C	276	C
	BA[a], TR	SKF	20 g	Stable for 24 hr at 5 and 22 °C	298	C

Solution Compatibility (Cont.)

Cefazolin sodium

Solution	Mfr	Mfr	Conc/L	Remarks	Ref	C/I
	MG[c]	SKF	10 g	Physically compatible with no loss in 48 hr at room temperature under fluorescent light	983	C
		LI	3.33 g	Physically compatible with 5% loss at 25 °C in 3 days. No loss in 7 days at 4 °C	1147	C
	TR[b]	LI	20 g	9% loss in 7 days at 24 °C and 5% loss in 15 days at 4 °C	336	C
	HOS[e]	NOP	5 and 40 g	Less than 10% loss in 7 days at 23 °C and 28 days at 4 °C	2819	C
TPN #22[d]		SKF	10 g	Physically compatible with no loss of activity in 24 hr at 22 °C in the dark	837	C
TPN #107[d]			1 g	9% cefazolin loss in 24 hr at 21 °C	1326	C

[a]Tested in both glass and PVC containers.
[b]Tested in PVC containers.
[c]Tested in glass containers.
[d]Refer to Appendix I for the composition of parenteral nutrition solutions. TPN indicates a 2-in-1 admixture.
[e]Tested in Accufusor reservoirs.

Additive Compatibility

Cefazolin sodium

Drug	Mfr	Conc/L	Mfr	Conc/L	Test Soln	Remarks	Ref	C/I
Amikacin sulfate	BR	5 g	LI	20 g	D5LR, D5R, D5S, D5W, D10W, LR, NS, R, SL	Both drugs stable for 8 hr at 25 °C. Turbidity observed at 24 hr	293	I
Atracurium besylate	BW	500 mg		10 g	D5W	Atracurium unstable and particles form	1694	I
Aztreonam	SQ	10 and 20 g	LI	5 and 20 g	D5W, NS[a]	Physically compatible. Little loss of either drug in 48 hr at 25 °C and 7 days at 4 °C in the dark	1020	C
Bleomycin sulfate	BR	20 and 30 units	LI	1 g	NS	43% loss of bleomycin activity in 1 week at 4 °C	763	I
Clindamycin phosphate	UP	9 g	SKF	10 g	D5W[b]	Physically compatible with no clindamycin loss and 8% cefazolin loss in 48 hr at room temperature under fluorescent light	983	C
	UP	9 g	SKF	10 g	NS[b]	Physically compatible with no clindamycin loss and 3% cefazolin loss in 48 hr at room temperature under fluorescent light	983	C
Clindamycin phosphate[d]	UP	9 g	SKF	10 g	D5W, NS[b]	10% cefazolin loss in 4 hr in D5W and 12 hr in NS at 25 °C. No clindamycin and gentamicin loss in 24 hr	1328	I
Famotidine	YAM	200 mg	FUJ	10 g	D5W	Visually compatible with 10% cefazolin and 5% famotidine loss in 24 hr at 25 °C. 9% cefazolin and 5% famotidine loss in 48 hr at 4 °C	1763	C
Fluconazole	PF	1 g	SM	10 g	D5W	Visually compatible with no fluconazole loss in 72 hr at 25 °C under fluorescent light. Cefazolin not tested	1677	C

Additive Compatibility (Cont.)

Cefazolin sodium

Drug	Mfr	Conc/L	Mfr	Conc/L	Test Soln	Remarks	Ref	C/I
Gentamicin sulfate[e]	ES	800 mg	SKF	10 g	D5W, NS[b]	10% cefazolin loss in 4 hr in D5W and 12 hr in NS at 25 °C. No clindamycin and gentamicin loss in 24 hr	1328	I
Linezolid	PHU	2 g	APC	10 g	[c]	Physically compatible with 5% or less loss of each drug in 3 days at 23 °C and 7 days at 4 °C protected from light	2262	C
Meperidine HCl		0.5 g	FUJ	10 g	D5W	Visually compatible. 5% loss of each drug in 5 days at 25 °C. 5% cefazolin and 7% meperidine loss in 20 days at 4 °C	1966	C
Metronidazole	SE	5 g	LI	10 g		5% cefazolin loss and no metronidazole loss in 7 days at 25 °C. No loss of either drug in 12 days at 5 °C	993	C
	AB	5 g	LI	10 g		Visually compatible with no loss of either drug in 72 hr at 8 °C	1649	C
Ranitidine HCl	GL	100 mg		2 g	D5W	Color change within 24 hr	1151	?
	GL	50 mg and 2 g		1 g	D5W	Ranitidine stable for only 6 hr at 25 °C. Cefazolin not tested	1515	I
Tenoxicam	RC	200 mg	FUJ	5 g	D5W	Visually compatible with less than 10% loss of both drugs in 48 hr at 25 °C and in 72 hr at 4 °C in the dark	2441	C
Verapamil HCl	KN	80 mg	SKF	2 g	D5W, NS	Physically compatible for 24 hr	764	C

[a]Tested in PVC containers.
[b]Tested in glass containers.
[c]Admixed in the linezolid infusion container.
[d]Tested in combination with gentamicin sulfate 800 mg/L.
[e]Tested in combination with clindamycin phosphate 9 g/L.

Drugs in Syringe Compatibility

Cefazolin sodium

Drug (in syringe)	Mfr	Amt	Mfr	Amt	Remarks	Ref	C/I
Ascorbic acid	LI	1 mL	LI	1 g/3 mL	Precipitate forms within 3 min at 32 °C	766	I
Dimenhydrinate		10 mg/ 1 mL		100 mg/ 1 mL	Clear solution	2569	C
Heparin sodium		2500 units/ 1 mL		2 g	Physically compatible for at least 5 min	1053	C
Hydromorphone HCl	KN	2, 10, 40 mg/ 1 mL	SKF	>200 mg/1 mL	Precipitate forms	2082	I
	KN	2, 10, 40 mg/ 1 mL	SKF	150 mg/ 1 mL	Visually compatible with less than 10% loss of each drug in 24 hr at room temperature	2082	C
Lidocaine HCl	AST	0.5%, 3 mL	SKF	1 g	Precipitate forms within 3 to 4 hr at 4 °C	532	I
Pantoprazole sodium	[a]	4 mg/ 1 mL		100 mg/ 1 mL	Precipitates immediately	2574	I

[a]Test performed using the formulation WITHOUT edetate disodium.

Y-Site Injection Compatibility (1:1 Mixture)

Cefazolin sodium

Drug	Mfr	Conc	Mfr	Conc	Remarks	Ref	C/I
Acyclovir sodium	BW	5 mg/mL[a]	SKF	20 mg/mL[a]	Physically compatible for 4 hr at 25 °C	1157	C
Allopurinol sodium	BW	3 mg/mL[b]	GEM	20 mg/mL[b]	Physically compatible for 4 hr at 22 °C	1686	C
Alprostadil	BED	7.5 mcg/mL[o,p]	LI	100 mg/mL[n]	Visually compatible for 1 hr	2746	C
Amifostine	USB	10 mg/mL[a]	MAR	20 mg/mL[a]	Physically compatible for 4 hr at 23 °C	1845	C
Amiodarone HCl	LZ	4 mg/mL[a]	LI	20 mg/mL[a]	Precipitate forms	1444	I
	LZ	4 mg/mL[b]	LI	20 mg/mL[b]	Physically compatible for 4 hr at room temperature	1444	C
Amphotericin B cholesteryl sulfate complex	SEQ	0.83 mg/mL[a]	SKB	20 mg/mL[a]	Increased turbidity forms immediately	2117	I
Anakinra	SYN	4 and 36 mg/mL[b]	GVA	15 mg/mL[b]	Physically compatible. No cefazolin loss in 4 hr at 25 °C. Anakinra uncertain	2508	?
Anidulafungin	VIC	0.5 mg/mL[a]	APC	20 mg/mL[a]	Physically compatible for 4 hr at 23 °C	2617	C
Atracurium besylate	BW	0.5 mg/mL[a]	LY	10 mg/mL[a]	Physically compatible for 24 hr at 28 °C	1337	C
Aztreonam	SQ	40 mg/mL[a]	MAR	20 mg/mL[a]	Physically compatible for 4 hr at 23 °C	1758	C
Bivalirudin	TMC	5 mg/mL[a]	APO	20 mg/mL[a]	Physically compatible for 4 hr at 23 °C	2373	C
Calcium gluconate	AST	4 mg/mL[c]	LI	40 mg/mL[c]	Physically compatible for 3 hr	1316	C
Caspofungin acetate	ME	0.7 mg/mL[b]	CUR	20 mg/mL[b]	Immediate white turbid precipitate forms	2758	I
	ME	0.5 mg/mL[b]	SZ	100 mg/mL[b]	Fine white crystals reported	2766	I
Cisatracurium besylate	GW	0.1 mg/mL[a]	SKB	20 mg/mL[a]	Physically compatible for 4 hr at 23 °C	2074	C
	GW	2 mg/mL[a]	SKB	20 mg/mL[a]	Gray subvisible haze forms immediately	2074	I
	GW	5 mg/mL[a]	SKB	20 mg/mL[a]	Gray haze forms immediately	2074	I
Cyclophosphamide	MJ	20 mg/mL[a]	SKF	20 mg/mL[a]	Physically compatible for 4 hr at 25 °C	1194	C
Dexmedetomidine HCl	AB	4 mcg/mL[b]	LI	20 mg/mL[b]	Physically compatible for 4 hr at 23 °C	2383	C
Diltiazem HCl	MMD	5 mg/mL	LI	20 and 200 mg/mL[b]	Visually compatible	1807	C
	MMD	1 mg/mL[b]	LI	200 mg/mL[b]	Visually compatible	1807	C
Docetaxel	RPR	0.9 mg/mL[a]	APC	20 mg/mL[a]	Physically compatible for 4 hr at 23 °C	2224	C
Doxapram HCl	RB	2 mg/mL[a]	APO	100 mg/mL[a]	Visually compatible for 4 hr at 23 °C	2470	C
Doxorubicin HCl liposomal	SEQ	0.4 mg/mL[a]	SKB	20 mg/mL[a]	Physically compatible for 4 hr at 23 °C	2087	C
Enalaprilat	MSD	0.05 mg/mL[b]	SKF[e]	20 mg/mL	Physically compatible for 24 hr at room temperature under fluorescent light	1355	C
Esmolol HCl	DCC	10 mg/mL[a]	LI	10 mg/mL[a]	Physically compatible for 24 hr at 22 °C	1169	C
Etoposide phosphate	BR	5 mg/mL[a]	APC	20 mg/mL[a]	Physically compatible for 4 hr at 23 °C	2218	C
Famotidine	MSD	0.2 mg/mL[a]	LY	20 mg/mL[b]	Physically compatible for 14 hr	1196	C
	ME	2 mg/mL[b]		20 mg/mL[a]	Visually compatible for 4 hr at 22 °C	1936	C
Fenoldopam mesylate	AB	80 mcg/mL[b]	APO	20 mg/mL[b]	Physically compatible for 4 hr at 23 °C	2467	C
Filgrastim	AMG	30 mcg/mL[a]	LI	20 mg/mL[a]	Physically compatible for 4 hr at 22 °C	1687	C
Fluconazole	RR	2 mg/mL	LY	40 mg/mL	Physically compatible for 24 hr at 25 °C	1407	C
Fludarabine phosphate	BX	1 mg/mL[a]	LEM	20 mg/mL[a]	Visually compatible for 4 hr at 22 °C	1439	C
Foscarnet sodium	AST	24 mg/mL	SKF	40 mg/mL	Physically compatible for 24 hr at room temperature under fluorescent light	1335	C
Gallium nitrate	FUJ	1 mg/mL[b]	GEM	100 mg/mL[b]	Visually compatible for 24 hr at 25 °C	1673	C

Y-Site Injection Compatibility (1:1 Mixture) (Cont.)

Cefazolin sodium

Drug	Mfr	Conc	Mfr	Conc	Remarks	Ref	C/I
Gemcitabine HCl	LI	10 mg/mL[b]	APC	20 mg/mL[b]	Physically compatible for 4 hr at 23 °C	2226	C
Granisetron HCl	SKB	0.05 mg/mL[a]	SKB	20 mg/mL[a]	Physically compatible for 4 hr at 23 °C	2000	C
Heparin sodium	TR	50 units/mL	SKB	20 mg/mL[a]	Visually compatible for 4 hr at 25 °C	1793	C
	LEO	10 and 5000 units/mL[b]	NOP	10 mg/mL[b]	Physically compatible with little change in heparin activity in 14 days at 4 and 37 °C. Antibiotic not tested	2684	C
Hetastarch in lactated electrolyte	AB	6%	LI	20 mg/mL[a]	Physically compatible for 4 hr at 23 °C	2339	C
Hetastarch in sodium chloride 0.9%	DCC	6%	SKF	20 mg/mL[a]	Visually compatible for 4 hr at room temperature	1313	C
	DCC	6%	SKF	20 mg/mL[a]	Simulation in vials showed no incompatibility, but white precipitate formed in Y-site during infusion	1315	I
Hydromorphone HCl	WY	0.2 mg/mL[a]	SKF	20 mg/mL[a]	Physically compatible for 4 hr at 25 °C	987	C
	KN	2, 10, 40 mg/mL	SKF	20[a] and 150 mg/mL	Visually compatible and both drugs stable for 24 hr	1532	C
	KN	2, 10, 40 mg/mL	SKF	>200 mg/mL	Precipitate forms immediately	1532	I
Hydroxyethyl starch 130/0.4 in sodium chloride 0.9%	FRK	6%	NOP	20, 30, 40 mg/mL[a]	Visually compatible for 24 hr at room temperature	2770	C
Idarubicin HCl	AD	1 mg/mL[b]	LI	20 mg/mL[a]	Precipitate forms in 1 hr	1525	I
Insulin, regular	LI	0.2 unit/mL[b]	LI	20 mg/mL[a]	Physically compatible for 2 hr at 25 °C	1395	C
Labetalol HCl	SC	1 mg/mL[a]	LI	10 mg/mL[a]	Physically compatible for 24 hr at 18 °C	1171	C
Lidocaine HCl	AB	8 mg/mL[c]	LI	40 mg/mL[c]	Physically compatible for 3 hr	1316	C
Linezolid	PHU	2 mg/mL	SKB	20 mg/mL[a]	Physically compatible for 4 hr at 23 °C	2264	C
Magnesium sulfate	IX	16.7, 33.3, 66.7, 100 mg/mL[a]	LI	20 mg/mL[a]	Physically compatible for at least 4 hr at 32 °C	813	C
Melphalan HCl	BW	0.1 mg/mL[b]	GEM	20 mg/mL[b]	Physically compatible for 3 hr at 22 °C	1557	C
Meperidine HCl	WY	10 mg/mL[a]	SKF	20 mg/mL[a]	Physically compatible for 4 hr at 25 °C	987	C
Midazolam HCl	RC	1 mg/mL[a]	MAR	20 mg/mL[a]	Visually compatible for 24 hr at 23 °C	1847	C
Milrinone lactate	SS	0.2 mg/mL[a]	APO	100 mg/mL[a]	Visually compatible for 4 hr at 25 °C	2381	C
Morphine sulfate	WI	1 mg/mL[a]	SKF	20 mg/mL[a]	Physically compatible for 4 hr at 25 °C	987	C
Multivitamins	USV	5 mL/L[a]	SKF	1 g/50 mL[a]	Physically compatible for 24 hr at room temperature	323	C
Nicardipine HCl	DCC	0.1 mg/mL[a]	SKF	20 mg/mL[a]	Visually compatible for 24 hr at room temperature	235	C
Ondansetron HCl	GL	1 mg/mL[b]	LEM	20 mg/mL[a]	Visually compatible for 4 hr at 22 °C	1365	C
	GL	0.03 and 0.3 mg/mL[a]	LI	20 mg/mL[a]	Visually compatible with little loss of either drug in 4 hr at 25 °C	1732	C
Palonosetron HCl	MGI	50 mcg/mL	WAT	20 mg/mL[a]	Physically compatible and no loss of either drug in 4 hr at room temperature	2749	C
Pancuronium bromide	ES	0.05 mg/mL[a]	LY	10 mg/mL[a]	Physically compatible for 24 hr at 28 °C	1337	C
Pantoprazole sodium	ALT[m]	0.16 to 0.8 mg/mL[b]	NOP	20 to 40 mg/mL[a]	Visually compatible for 12 hr at 23 °C	2603	C
Pemetrexed disodium	LI	20 mg/mL[b]	GVA	20 mg/mL[a]	Slight color darkening occurs over 4 hr	2564	I

Y-Site Injection Compatibility (1:1 Mixture) (Cont.)

Cefazolin sodium

Drug	Mfr	Conc	Mfr	Conc	Remarks	Ref	C/I
Pentamidine isethionate	FUJ	3 mg/mL[a]	SKB	20 mg/mL[a]	Cloudy precipitation forms immediately	1880	I
Promethazine HCl	ES	25 mg	LI	10 mg/mL[a]	Cloudiness forms then dissipates	1753	?
Propofol	ZEN	10 mg/mL	MAR	20 mg/mL[a]	Physically compatible for 1 hr at 23 °C	2066	C
Ranitidine HCl	GL	1 mg/mL[b]	FUJ	20 mg/mL[b]	Visually compatible with little loss of either drug in 4 hr at 25 °C	2259	C
	GL	1 mg/mL[b]	FUJ	20 mg/mL[b]	Visually compatible with no cefazolin loss and 3% ranitidine loss in 4 hr	2362	C
Remifentanil HCl	GW	0.025 and 0.25 mg/mL[b]	SKB	20 mg/mL[a]	Physically compatible for 4 hr at 23 °C	2075	C
Sargramostim	IMM	10 mcg/mL[b]	LEM	20 mg/mL[b]	Visually compatible for 4 hr at 22 °C	1436	C
Tacrolimus	FUJ	1 mg/mL[b]	BR	40 mg/mL[a]	Visually compatible for 24 hr at 25 °C	1630	C
Teniposide	BR	0.1 mg/mL[a]	MAR	20 mg/mL[a]	Physically compatible for 4 hr at 23 °C	1725	C
Theophylline	TR	4 mg/mL	SKB	20 mg/mL	Visually compatible for 6 hr at 25 °C	1793	C
Thiotepa	IMM[f]	1 mg/mL[a]	MAR	20 mg/mL[a]	Physically compatible for 4 hr at 23 °C	1861	C
TNA #73[g]		32.5 mL[h]	SKF	20 mg/mL[a]	Visually compatible for 4 hr at 25 °C	1008	C
TNA #218 to #226[g]			SKB	20 mg/mL[a]	Visually compatible for 4 hr at 23 °C	2215	C
TPN #61[g]		[i]	SKF	200 mg/ 0.9 mL[j]	Physically compatible	1012	C
		[k]	SKF	1.2 g/5.3 mL[j]	Physically compatible	1012	C
TPN #212, #213[g]			SKB	20 mg/mL[a]	Physically compatible for 4 hr at 23 °C	2109	C
TPN #214, #215[g]			SKB	20 mg/mL[a]	Microprecipitate forms immediately	2109	I
Vancomycin HCl	AB	20 mg/mL[a]	SKB	200 mg/mL[l]	Transient precipitate forms	2189	?
	AB	20 mg/mL[a]	SKB	10 and 50 mg/mL[a]	Gross white precipitate forms immediately	2189	I
	AB	20 mg/mL[a]	SKB	1 mg/mL[a]	Physically compatible for 4 hr at 23 °C	2189	C
	AB	2 mg/mL[a]	SKB	200 mg/mL[l]	Physically compatible for 4 hr at 23 °C	2189	C
	AB	2 mg/mL[a]	SKB	50 mg/mL[a]	Subvisible haze forms immediately	2189	I
	AB	2 mg/mL[a]	SKB	1 and 10 mg/mL[a]	Physically compatible for 4 hr at 23 °C	2189	C
Vecuronium bromide	OR	0.1 mg/mL[a]	LY	10 mg/mL[a]	Physically compatible for 24 hr at 28 °C	1337	C
Vinorelbine tartrate	BW	1 mg/mL[b]	GEM	20 mg/mL[b]	Measured turbidity increases immediately	1558	I
Warfarin sodium	DU	2 mg/mL[l]	SKB	20 mg/mL[a]	Visually compatible with no warfarin loss in 30 min	2010	C
	DME	2 mg/mL[l]	SKB	20 mg/mL[a]	Visually compatible for 24 hr at 24 °C	2078	C

[a]*Tested in dextrose 5%.*
[b]*Tested in sodium chloride 0.9%.*
[c]*Tested in both dextrose 5% in water and sodium chloride 0.9%.*
[d]*Tested in dextrose 5%, Ringer's injection, lactated, sodium chloride 0.45%, and sodium chloride 0.9%.*
[e]*Tested in premixed infusion solution.*
[f]*Lyophilized formulation tested.*
[g]*Refer to Appendix I for the composition of parenteral nutrition solutions. TNA indicates a 3-in-1 admixture, and TPN indicates a 2-in-1 admixture.*
[h]*A 32.5-mL sample of parenteral nutrition solution combined with 50 mL of antibiotic solution.*
[i]*Run at 21 mL/hr.*
[j]*Given over five minutes by syringe pump.*
[k]*Run at 94 mL/hr.*
[l]*Tested in sterile water for injection.*
[m]*Test performed using the formulation WITHOUT edetate disodium.*
[n]*Tested in either dextrose 5% or in sodium chloride 0.9%, but the report did not specify which solution.*
[o]*Tested in a 1:1 mixture of (1) dextrose 5% and dextrose 5% in sodium chloride 0.45% with and without potassium chloride 20 mEq/L and also in (2) dextrose 10% in sodium chloride 0.45% with and without potassium chloride 20 mEq/L.*
[p]*Tested in a 1:1 mixture of dextrose 5% and TPN #274 (see Appendix I).*

Additional Compatibility Information

Peritoneal Dialysis Solutions — The stability of cefazolin sodium 75 and 150 mg/L, alone and with gentamicin sulfate 8 mg/L, was evaluated in a peritoneal dialysis solution of dextrose 1.5% with heparin sodium 1000 units/L. Cefazolin activity was retained for 48 hours at both 4 and 26 °C at both concentrations, alone and with gentamicin. Gentamicin activity was also retained over the study period. At 37 °C, however, cefazolin losses were greater, with about a 10 to 12% loss occurring in 48 hours. Gentamicin losses ranged from 4 to 8% in this time period. (1029)

Gentamicin 4 mcg/mL in Dianeal PDS with dextrose 1.5 and 4.25% (Travenol) was evaluated with cefazolin sodium 125 mcg/mL, heparin 500 units, and albumin 80 mg in 2-L bags. The gentamicin content was retained for 72 hours. (1413)

The stability of cefazolin sodium (Lilly) 0.5 mg/mL in Dianeal PD-1 with dextrose 1.5 and 4.25% (Travenol) was studied. The drug was stable, exhibiting losses of 10.5% or less in 14 days at 4 °C, eight days at 25 °C, and 24 hours at 37 °C. However, losses of 11.7 and 14.6% occurred in the solutions containing dextrose 1.5% and dextrose 4.25%, respectively, in 11 days at 25 °C. (1480)

Cefazolin sodium (Lilly) 125 mcg/mL combined separately with the aminoglycosides amikacin sulfate (Bristol), gentamicin sulfate (Schering), and tobramycin sulfate (Lilly) at a concentration of 25 mcg/mL in peritoneal dialysis solution (Dianeal 1.5%) exhibited enhanced rates of lethality to *Staphylococcus aureus*, *Escherichia coli*, and *Pseudomonas aeruginosa* compared to any of the drugs alone. (1623)

Cefazolin sodium (Fujisawa) 0.333 mg/mL in PD-2 with dextrose 1.5% (Baxter) peritoneal dialysis solution with and without heparin sodium 1000 units/1.5 L was stored at 4, 25, and 37 °C. No visible changes occurred, and less than 10% loss of cefazolin occurred in 20 days at 4 °C, 11 days at 25 °C, and 24 hours at 37 °C. (2388)

Cefazolin sodium (Fujisawa) 0.5 mg/mL in Extraneal PD (Baxter) containing 7.5% icodextrin was physically compatible and chemically stable for 30 days at 4 °C with about 7% cefazolin loss and for 7 days at room temperature with about 9% loss. At 37 °C, 8% cefazolin loss occurred in 24 hours. (2480)

Cefazolin sodium 125 and 500 mg/mL (Apothecon) was evaluated for stability at 38 °C in Dianeal PD-2 with dextrose 1.5, 2.5, and 4.25% and in Extraneal 7.5% with and without added heparin. Less than 10% loss occurred in 48 hours and 10 to 14% loss in 60 hours. (2655)

CEFEPIME HYDROCHLORIDE
AHFS 8:12.06.16

Products — Cefepime hydrochloride is available as 1 and 2 g of cefepime in vials. The products contain L-arginine in an approximate concentration of 725 mg/g of cefepime. (1)

For intramuscular administration, reconstitute the 1- and 2-g vials with 1.3 or 2.4 mL, respectively, of sterile water for injection, sodium chloride 0.9%, dextrose 5%, lidocaine hydrochloride 0.5 or 1%, or bacteriostatic water for injection preserved with parabens or benzyl alcohol to yield 280 mg/mL. (1)

For intravenous injection, reconstitute the 1- and 2-g vials with 10 mL of compatible diluent yielding 100- or 160-mg/mL solutions, respectively. The reconstituted solutions should be added to compatible intravenous solutions for intermittent infusion. (1)

pH — From 4 to 6. (1)

Trade Name(s) — Maxipime.

Administration — Cefepime hydrochloride is administered by deep intramuscular injection and by intermittent intravenous infusion over approximately 30 minutes. (1; 4)

Stability — The intact vials should be stored between 2 and 25 °C and protected from light. Reconstituted solutions may vary from colorless to amber. Both the powder and reconstituted solutions may darken during storage like other cephalosporins. When stored as recommended, the drug is not adversely affected. Reconstituted solutions of cefepime hydrochloride in compatible diluents are stable for 24 hours at room temperatures of 20 to 25 °C and for seven days under refrigeration. (1)

Cefepime hydrochloride (Bristol-Myers Squibb) 0.125 and 0.25 mg/mL in Inpersol peritoneal dialysis solution with dextrose 4.25% is stable, exhibiting 3% loss in seven days at 5 °C, 2% loss in 24 hours at room temperature, and 8% loss in 24 hours at 37 °C. (1682)

Cefepime hydrochloride (Bristol-Myers Squibb) 0.1 mg/mL in Delflex solution with dextrose 1.5% stored at various temperatures was evaluated for physical and chemical stability. No visible particulates or changes in color or clarity were observed in any sample. Cefepime exhibited no loss in 14 days at 4 °C, 7% loss in seven days at 25 °C, and 4% loss in 24 hours and 9% loss in 48 hours at body temperature. (2283)

Cefepime hydrochloride (Bristol-Myers Squibb) 0.48 mg/mL was found to exhibit less than 10% loss in icodextrin 7.5% peritoneal dialysis solution (Extraneal) after 7 days at refrigerator temperature, 2 days at room temperature, and 4 hours at 37 °C. (2616)

pH Effects — Cefepime hydrochloride is most stable at pH values in the range of 4 to 5. At higher pH values, cefepime hydrochloride is less stable. Cefepime hydrochloride decomposition results in alkaline degradation products, which may increase the rate of loss. (2513; 2514; 2515)

Syringes — Cefepime hydrochloride (Bristol-Myers Squibb) 100 and 200 mg/mL in dextrose 5%, sodium chloride 0.9%, and sterile water for injection was packaged as 10 mL of solution in 10-mL polypropylene syringes and capped (Becton Dickinson). The samples were stored frozen at −20 °C for 90 days and were also tested without having been frozen. The solutions remained stable for up to 14 days refrigerated at 4 °C, losing 10% or less of the cefepime. In samples stored at room temperature of about 23 °C, less than 10% loss occurred in one day in most cases, but losses as high as 13% occurred in two days in some (but not all) samples that were evaluated. (2220; 2221) Samples refrigerated up to five days followed by room temperature storage exhibited similar stability, exhibiting less than 10% loss in one day but higher losses after two days. (2220)

Cefepime hydrochloride (Bristol-Myers Squibb) 20 mg/mL in sodium chloride 0.9% was packaged in 10-mL polypropylene syringes (Becton Dickinson) and stored at 25 and 5 °C. The drug solutions remained clear, but the color deepened to a darker yellow during storage at room temperature. About 5% loss occurred in two days and 11% loss in four days at 25 °C. About 3% loss was found after 21 days at 5 °C. The losses were comparable to the drug solution stored

in a glass flask, indicating sorption to syringe components did not occur. (2341)

Central Venous Catheter — Cefepime hydrochloride (Bristol-Myers Squibb) 5 mg/mL in dextrose 5% was found to be compatible with the ARROWg+ard Blue Plus (Arrow International) chlorhexidine-bearing triple-lumen central catheter. Delivery of the cefepime hydrochloride ranged from 92 to 95% of the initial concentration among the three lumens. Furthermore, chlorhexidine delivered from the catheter remained at trace amounts with no substantial increase due to the delivery of the drug through the catheter. (2335)

Compatibility Information

Solution Compatibility

Cefepime HCl

Solution	Mfr	Mfr	Conc/L	Remarks	Ref	C/I
Amino acids 4.25%, dextrose 25% with electrolytes	AB	BR	1 and 4 g	5 to 6% loss in 8 hr at room temperature and 3 days at 5 °C	1682	C
Dextrose 5% in Ringer's injection, lactated	[a]	BR	1 and 40 g	Visually compatible with 2 to 6% loss in 24 hr at room temperature exposed to light and about 2 to 3% loss in 7 days at 5 °C	1680	C
Dextrose 5% in sodium chloride 0.9%	[a]	BR	1 and 40 g	Visually compatible with 3 to 5% loss in 24 hr at room temperature exposed to light and 1 to 3% loss in 7 days at 5 °C	1680	C
Dextrose 5%	[b]	BR	1 g	Visually compatible with 2 to 4% loss in 24 hr at room temperature exposed to light and 1 to 2% loss in 7 days at 5 °C	1680	C
	[b]	BR	40 g	Visually compatible with 4 to 7% loss in 24 hr at room temperature exposed to light and about 2% loss in 7 days at 5 °C	1680	C
	BA[a]	BMS	20 g	6% loss in 2 days at 25 °C and in 23 days at 5 °C. Increase in yellow color	2102	C
	BFM[c]	BMS	8 g	8 to 9% loss in 48 hr at 24 °C and in 15 days at 4 °C. Amber discoloration	2150	C
	BA[a]	BMS	20 g	Visually compatible and stable for 30 days frozen at −20 °C followed by 11 days at 4 °C	2390	C
Dextrose 10%	[a]	BR	1 and 40 g	Visually compatible with 3 to 5% loss in 24 hr at room temperature exposed to light and 1 to 3% loss in 7 days at 5 °C	1680	C
Normosol M in dextrose 5%	AB[a]	BR	1 and 40 g	Visually compatible with 2 to 5% loss in 24 hr at room temperature exposed to light and 2% loss in 7 days at 5 °C	1680	C
Normosol R	AB[a]	BR	1 and 40 g	Visually compatible with 2 to 5% loss in 24 hr at room temperature exposed to light and 1 to 2% loss in 7 days at 5 °C	1680	C
Normosol R in dextrose 5%	AB[a]	BR	1 g	Visually compatible with 2% loss in 24 hr at room temperature exposed to light	1680	C

Solution Compatibility (Cont.)

Cefepime HCl

Solution	Mfr	Mfr	Conc/L	Remarks	Ref	C/I
Sodium chloride 0.9%	b	BR	1 and 40 g	Visually compatible with 2 to 5% loss in 24 hr at room temperature exposed to light and about 1 to 3% loss in 7 days at 5 °C	1680	**C**
	BA[a]	BMS	20 g	6% loss in 2 days at 25 °C and in 23 days at 5 °C. Increase in yellow color	2102	**C**
	BFM[c]	BMS	8 g	8% loss in 72 hr at 24 °C and in 15 days at 4 °C. Amber discoloration	2150	**C**

[a]Tested in PVC containers.
[b]Tested in both glass and PVC containers.
[c]Tested in polyethylene-lined trilayer (Clear-Flex) containers.

Additive Compatibility

Cefepime HCl

Drug	Mfr	Conc/L	Mfr	Conc/L	Test Soln	Remarks	Ref	C/I
Amikacin sulfate	BR	6 g	BR	40 g	D5W, NS	Visually compatible with 6% cefepime loss in 24 hr at room temperature and 4% loss in 7 days at 5 °C. No amikacin loss	1681	**C**
Aminophylline	LY	1 g	BR	4 g	NS	37% cefepime loss in 18 hr at room temperature and 32% loss in 3 days at 5 °C. No aminophylline loss	1681	**I**
Ampicillin sodium	BR	1 g	BR	40 g	D5W	4% ampicillin loss in 8 hr at room temperature and 5 °C. 7% cefepime loss in 8 hr at room temperature and no loss in 8 hr at 5 °C	1682	**?**
	BR	1 g	BR	40 g	NS	No ampicillin loss in 24 hr at room temperature and 9% loss in 48 hr at 5 °C. 5% cefepime loss in 24 hr at room temperature and 2% loss in 72 hr at 5 °C	1682	**C**
	BR	10 g	BR	40 g	D5W	6% ampicillin loss in 2 hr at room temperature and 2% loss in 8 hr at 5 °C. 7% cefepime loss in 2 hr at room temperature and 8 hr at 5 °C	1682	**I**
	BR	10 g	BR	40 g	NS	6% ampicillin loss in 8 hr at room temperature and 9% loss in 48 hr at 5 °C. 8% cefepime loss in 8 hr at room temperature and 10% loss in 48 hr at 5 °C	1682	**I**
	BR	40 g	BR	4 g	D5W	10% ampicillin loss in 1 hr at room temperature and 9% loss in 2 hr at 5 °C. 25% cefepime loss in 1 hr at room temperature and 9% loss in 2 hr at 5 °C	1682	**I**
	BR	40 g	BR	4 g	NS	5% ampicillin loss in 8 hr at room temperature and 4% loss in 8 hr at 5 °C. 4% cefepime loss in 8 hr at room temperature and 6% loss in 8 hr at 5 °C	1682	**?**
Clindamycin phosphate	UP	0.25 g	BR	40 g	D5W, NS	7% or less cefepime loss in 24 hr at room temperature and 10% or less loss in 7 days at 5 °C. No clindamycin loss in 24 hr at room temperature and 8% or less loss in 7 days at 5 °C	1682	**C**

Additive Compatibility (Cont.)

Cefepime HCl

Drug	Mfr	Conc/L	Mfr	Conc/L	Test Soln	Remarks	Ref	C/I
	UP	6 g	BR	4 g	D5W, NS	7% or less cefepime loss in 24 hr at room temperature and 10% or less loss in 7 days at 5 °C. No clindamycin loss in 24 hr at room temperature and 8% or less loss in 7 days at 5 °C	1682	C
Gentamicin sulfate	ES	1.2 g	BR	40 g	D5W, NS	Cloudy in 18 hr at room temperature	1681	I
Heparin sodium	MG	10,000 and 50,000 units	BR	4 g	D5W, NS	Visually compatible with 4% cefepime loss in 24 hr at room temperature and 3% in 7 days at 5 °C. No heparin loss	1681	C
Metronidazole	AB, ES, SE	5 g	BR	4 and 40 g		4 to 5% cefepime loss in 24 hr at room temperature exposed to light and up to 10% loss in 7 days at 5 °C. No metronidazole loss. Orange color develops in 18 hr at room temperature and 24 hr at 5 °C	1682	?
	SCS	5 g	BMS	2.5, 5, 10, and 20 g	[a]	Visually compatible. 7 to 9% cefepime loss in 48 hr at 23 °C; 2 to 8% cefepime loss in 7 days at 4 °C. 7% or less metronidazole loss in 7 days at 4 and 23 °C	2324	C
	AB	5 g	ELN	3.3, 6.6, 10, 20 g	[a]	Physically compatible and less than 6% metronidazole loss at 4 and 23 °C in 14 days. 2 to 5% cefepime loss in 14 days at 4 °C. At 23 °C, 10 to 12% cefepime loss in 72 hr	2726	C
Potassium chloride	AB	10 and 40 mEq	BR	4 g	D5W, NS	Visually compatible with 2% cefepime loss in 24 hr at room temperature or 7 days at 5 °C	1681	C
Theophylline	BA	800 mg	BR	4 g	D5W	Visually compatible. 3% cefepime loss in 24 hr at room temperature and 7 days at 5 °C. No theophylline loss	1681	C
Tobramycin sulfate	AB	0.4 g	BR	40 g	D5W, NS	Cloudiness forms immediately	1682	I
	AB	2 g	BR	2.5 g	D5W, NS	Cloudiness forms immediately	1682	I
Vancomycin HCl	LI	5 g	BR	4 g	D5W, NS	4% cefepime loss in 24 hr at room temperature in light and 2% loss in 7 days at 5 °C. No vancomycin loss. Cloudiness in 5 days at 5 °C	1682	C
	LI	1 g	BR	40 g	D5W, NS	4% cefepime loss in 24 hr at room temperature in light and 2% loss in 7 days at 5 °C. No vancomycin loss and no cloudiness	1682	C

[a]*Tested in PVC containers.*

Y-Site Injection Compatibility (1:1 Mixture)

Cefepime HCl

Drug	Mfr	Conc	Mfr	Conc	Remarks	Ref	C/I
Acetylcysteine		100 mg/mL	BMS	120 mg/mL[c]	Over 10% cefepime loss occurs in 1 hr	2513	I
Amikacin sulfate		15 mg/mL	BMS	120 mg/mL[c]	Physically compatible with less than 10% cefepime loss. Amikacin not tested	2513	C
Amphotericin B cholesteryl sulfate complex	SEQ	0.83 mg/mL[a]	BMS	20 mg/mL[a]	Gross precipitate forms	2117	I
Anidulafungin	VIC	0.5 mg/mL[a]	DUR	20 mg/mL[a]	Physically compatible for 4 hr at 23 °C	2617	C
Bivalirudin	TMC	5 mg/mL[a]	BMS	20 mg/mL[a]	Physically compatible for 4 hr at 23 °C	2373	C
Caspofungin acetate	ME	0.7 mg/mL[b]	BMS	20 mg/mL[b]	Immediate white turbid precipitate forms	2758	I
Clarithromycin		50 mg/mL	BMS	120 mg/mL[c]	Physically compatible with less than 10% cefepime loss. Clarithromycin not tested	2513	C
Dexmedetomidine HCl	AB	4 mcg/mL[b]	BMS	20 mg/mL[b]	Physically compatible for 4 hr at 23 °C	2383	C
Dobutamine HCl		1 mg/mL	BMS	120 mg/mL[c]	Physically compatible with less than 10% cefepime loss. Dobutamine not tested	2513	C
		250 mg/mL	BMS	120 mg/mL[c]	Precipitates	2513	I
Docetaxel	RPR	0.9 mg/mL[a]	BMS	20 mg/mL[a]	Physically compatible for 4 hr at 23 °C	2224	C
Dopamine HCl		0.4 mg/mL	BMS	120 mg/mL[c]	Physically compatible with less than 10% cefepime loss. Dopamine not tested	2513	C
Doxorubicin HCl liposomal	SEQ	0.4 mg/mL[a]	BMS	20 mg/mL[a]	Physically compatible for 4 hr at 23 °C	2087	C
Erythromycin lactobionate		5 mg/mL	BMS	120 mg/mL[c]	Over 10% cefepime loss occurs in 1 hr	2513	I
Etoposide phosphate	BR	5 mg/mL[a]	BMS	20 mg/mL[a]	Increased haze and particulates form within 1 hr	2218	I
Fenoldopam mesylate	AB	80 mcg/mL[b]	BMS	20 mg/mL[b]	Physically compatible for 4 hr at 23 °C	2467	C
Fluconazole		2 mg/mL	BMS	120 mg/mL[c]	Physically compatible with less than 10% cefepime loss. Fluconazole not tested	2513	C
Furosemide		10 mg/mL	BMS	120 mg/mL[c]	Physically compatible with less than 10% cefepime loss. Furosemide not tested	2513	C
Gentamicin sulfate		6 mg/mL	BMS	120 mg/mL[c]	Physically compatible with less than 10% cefepime loss. Gentamicin not tested	2513	C
Granisetron HCl	SKB	0.05 mg/mL[a]	BMS	20 mg/mL[a]	Physically compatible for 4 hr at 23 °C	2000	C
Hetastarch in lactated electrolyte	AB	6%	BMS	20 mg/mL[a]	Physically compatible for 4 hr at 23 °C	2339	C
Insulin, regular		100 units/mL	BMS	120 mg/mL[c]	Physically compatible with less than 10% cefepime loss. Insulin not tested	2513	C
Isosorbide dinitrate		0.2 mg/mL	BMS	120 mg/mL[c]	Physically compatible with less than 10% cefepime loss. Isosorbide not tested	2513	C
Ketamine HCl		10 mg/mL	BMS	120 mg/mL[c]	Physically compatible with less than 10% cefepime loss. Ketamine not tested	2513	C
Methylprednisolone sodium succinate		50 mg/mL	BMS	120 mg/mL[c]	Physically compatible with less than 10% cefepime loss. Methylprednisolone not tested	2513	C
Midazolam HCl		5 mg/mL	BMS	120 mg/mL[c]	Over 10% cefepime loss occurs in 1 hr	2513	I
Milrinone lactate	SS	0.2 mg/mL[a]	BMS	100 mg/mL	Visually compatible for 4 hr at 25 °C	2381	C
Morphine sulfate		1 mg/mL	BMS	120 mg/mL[c]	Physically compatible with less than 10% cefepime loss. Morphine not tested	2513	C

Y-Site Injection Compatibility (1:1 Mixture) (Cont.)

Cefepime HCl

Drug	Mfr	Conc	Mfr	Conc	Remarks	Ref	C/I
Mycophenolate mofetil HCl	RC	5.9 mg/mL[a]		20 mg/mL[a]	Physically compatible with no mycophenolate mofetil loss in 4 hr	2738	C
Nicardipine HCl		1 mg/mL	BMS	120 mg/mL[c]	Precipitates	2513	I
Phenytoin sodium		50 mg/mL	BMS	120 mg/mL[c]	Precipitates	2513	I
Propofol		1 mg/mL	BMS	120 mg/mL[c]	Precipitates	2513	I
Remifentanil HCl		0.2 mg/mL	BMS	120 mg/mL[c]	Physically compatible with less than 10% cefepime loss. Remifentanil not tested	2513	C
Sufentanil citrate		5 mcg/mL	BMS	120 mg/mL[c]	Physically compatible with less than 10% cefepime loss. Sufentanil not tested	2513	C
Telavancin HCl	ASP	7.5 mg/mL[a,b,d]	SAG	40 mg/mL[a,b,d]	Physically compatible for 2 hr	2830	C
Theophylline		20 mg/mL	BMS	120 mg/mL[c]	Over 25% cefepime loss in 1 hr	2513	I
Tigecycline	WY	1 mg/mL[b]	ELN	40 mg/mL[b]	Physically compatible for 4 hr	2714	C
Tobramycin sulfate		6 mg/mL	BMS	120 mg/mL[c]	Physically compatible with less than 10% cefepime loss. Tobramycin not tested	2513	C
Valproate sodium		100 mg/mL	BMS	120 mg/mL[c]	Physically compatible. Under 10% cefepime loss. Valproate not tested	2513	C
Vancomycin HCl		30 mg/mL	BMS	120 mg/mL[c]	Physically compatible with less than 10% cefepime loss. Vancomycin not tested	2513	C

[a]Tested in dextrose 5%.
[b]Tested in sodium chloride 0.9%.
[c]Tested in sterile water for injection.
[d]Tested in Ringer's injection, lactated.

CEFOTAXIME SODIUM
AHFS 8:12.06.12

Products — Cefotaxime sodium is available in vials containing the equivalent of 500 mg and 1 and 2 g of cefotaxime (as sodium) and in infusion bottles containing the equivalent of 1 g of cefotaxime (as sodium). It is also available in 10- and 20-g pharmacy bulk packages. (1)

For intravenous administration, the contents of any size vial may be reconstituted with 10 mL of sterile water for injection. (See Table 1.) The 1- and 2-g infusion bottles may be reconstituted with 50 or 100 mL of dextrose 5% or sodium chloride 0.9%. For intramuscular injection, reconstitute with sterile water for injection or bacteriostatic water for injection in the amounts shown in Table 1. (1)

The pharmacy bulk packages may be reconstituted according to the manufacturer's directions, and the dose should be diluted appropriately for administration. (1; 4)

After addition of the diluent, shake to dissolve the contents and inspect for particulate matter or discoloration. (1)

For intravenous infusion, the primary solution may be diluted further to 50 to 1000 mL in a compatible diluent. (1) (See Additional Compatibility Information.)

Cefotaxime sodium is also available as a frozen premixed iso-osmotic infusion solution of 1 or 2 g in dextrose 3.4 or 1.4%, respectively, buffered with sodium citrate. Hydrochloric acid and sodium hydroxide, if needed, are used to adjust the pH during manufacturing. (1; 4)

pH — Injectable solutions of the drug have pH values ranging from 5 to 7.5. (1)

Table 1. Reconstitution of Cefotaxime Sodium (1)

Vial Size	Volume of Diluent	Withdrawable Volume	Approximate Concentration
Intravenous			
500 mg	10 mL	10.2 mL	50 mg/mL
1 g	10 mL	10.4 mL	95 mg/mL
2 g	10 mL	11.0 mL	180 mg/mL
Intramuscular			
500 mg	2 mL	2.2 mL	230 mg/mL
1 g	3 mL	3.4 mL	300 mg/mL
2 g	5 mL	6.0 mL	330 mg/mL

Osmolality — A solution of cefotaxime sodium 1 g/14 mL of sterile water for injection is isotonic. (1)

The osmolality of cefotaxime sodium 1, 2, and 3 g was calculated for the following dilutions (1054):

Diluent	Osmolality (mOsm/kg)	
	50 mL	100 mL
1 g		
Dextrose 5%	350	319
Sodium chloride 0.9%	375	344
2 g		
Dextrose 5%	343	327
Sodium chloride 0.9%	406	351
3 g		
Dextrose 5%	433	344
Sodium chloride 0.9%	458	382

The frozen premixed solutions have osmolalities of 340 to 420 mOsm/kg for the 1-g/50 mL concentration and 450 to 540 mOsm/kg for the 2-g/50 mL concentration. (4)

The osmolality of cefotaxime sodium (Hoechst) 50 mg/mL was determined to be 326 mOsm/kg in dextrose 5% and 333 mOsm/kg in sodium chloride 0.9%. (1375)

The following maximum cefotaxime sodium concentrations were recommended to achieve osmolalities suitable for peripheral infusion in fluid-restricted patients (1180):

Diluent	Maximum Concentration (mg/mL)	Osmolality (mOsm/kg)
Dextrose 5%	86	577
Sodium chloride 0.9%	73	555
Sterile water for injection	147	525

Sodium Content — Cefotaxime sodium contains approximately 2.2 mEq (50.5 mg) of sodium per gram of cefotaxime activity. (1)

Trade Name(s) — Claforan.

Administration — Cefotaxime sodium may be administered by deep intramuscular injection; doses of 2 g should be divided between different injection sites. It may also be administered by direct intravenous injection over three to five minutes directly into the vein or into the tubing of a running compatible infusion solution. In addition, cefotaxime sodium may be administered in 50 to 100 mL of compatible diluent over 20 to 30 minutes by intermittent intravenous infusion or by continuous intravenous infusion. (1; 4)

The manufacturer states that cefotaxime sodium should not be admixed with aminoglycosides. (1) However, they may be administered separately to the same patient. (1; 792)

Stability — Intact vials of cefotaxime sodium should be stored below 30 °C. The dry powder is off-white to pale yellow in color. Solutions may range from light yellow to amber, depending on the diluent, concentration, and storage conditions. Both the dry material and solutions may darken and should be protected from elevated temperatures and excessive light. Discoloration of the powder or solution may indicate a loss of potency. (1; 4)

Store the frozen premixed cefotaxime sodium infusions at −20 °C or below. Thaw at room temperature or under refrigeration. Accelerated thawing using water bath immersion or microwave irradiation should not be used. Thawed solutions should not be refrozen. (1; 4)

When reconstituted as described in the Products section, cefotaxime sodium is stable in the original containers as indicated in Table 2. Storage of reconstituted solutions in disposable glass or plastic syringes for five days under refrigeration is also recommended. (1)

Cefotaxime sodium (Hoechst-Roussel) 1 g/10 mL reconstituted with sterile water for injection or 1 g/50 mL in dextrose 5% in PVC bags exhibited no visible changes in 24 hours at 5 and 25 °C. Although increased levels of particulate matter were observed in most solutions, the increases were significant only in solutions stored at 25 °C. (986)

The stability of cefotaxime sodium (Hoechst-Roussel) 125 mg/L in peritoneal dialysis solutions (Dianeal 137 and PD2) with heparin sodium 500 units/L was evaluated at 25 °C by microbiological assay. Approximately 95 ± 6% activity remained after 24 hours. (1228)

The stability of cefotaxime sodium (Hoechst-Roussel) 1 mg/mL in Dianeal PD-1 with dextrose 1.5 and 4.25% (Travenol) was reported. At 25 °C, the drug exhibited an 8% loss in 24 hours and a 16% loss in 48 hours in both solutions. Storage at 37 °C for 12 hours resulted in 11 and 14% losses in the solutions containing dextrose 1.5% and dextrose 4.25%, respectively. (1481)

pH Effects — The primary factor in the stability of cefotaxime sodium is solution pH. (792) Cefotaxime sodium in aqueous solutions is stable at pH 5 to 7 (1) or 4.3 to 6.2. (1077) The theoretical pH of minimum decomposition is 5.13. (793) However, between pH 3 and 7, the hydrolysis rate is virtually independent of pH. (1072) Determination of decomposition kinetics in various aqueous buffer systems at 25 °C showed 10% decomposition occurring in 24 hours or longer over a pH range of 3.9 to 7.6. At pH 2.2 and 8.4, 10% decomposition occurred in about 13 hours. (793)

The manufacturer recommends that cefotaxime sodium not be diluted in solutions with a pH greater than 7.5. (1; 4)

Freezing Solutions — When reconstituted as recommended, cefotaxime sodium may be stored frozen in the vial or in disposable glass or plastic syringes for 13 weeks. Similarly, dilutions of cefotaxime sodium in dextrose 5% or sodium chloride 0.9% in PVC bags may be stored frozen for 13 weeks. Thawing at room temperature is recommended; frozen solutions should not be heated. Once thawed, the solutions are stable for 24 hours at room temperature or five days at less than 5 °C. Thawed solutions should not be refrozen. (1; 4)

Table 2. Manufacturer's Recommended Storage Times of Reconstituted Cefotaxime Sodium (1)

Vial Size	Concentration	Storage Temperature	
		22 °C	5 °C
500 mg	230 mg/mL	12 hr	7 days
	50 mg/mL	24 hr	7 days
1 g	300 mg/mL	12 hr	7 days
	95 mg/mL	24 hr	7 days
(Infusion bottle)	10 to 20 mg/mL	24 hr	10 days
2 g	330 mg/mL	12 hr	7 days
	180 mg/mL	12 hr	7 days
(Infusion bottle)	20 to 40 mg/mL	24 hr	10 days

Syringes — Cefotaxime sodium (Aventis) 50 mg/mL in sodium chloride 0.9% packaged in 5-mL polypropylene plastic syringes is visually compatible and undergoes about 10% loss in 2 days at 25 °C and about 3% loss in 18 days at 5 °C. (2371)

Sorption — Cefotaxime sodium (Aventis) 50 mg/mL in sodium chloride 0.9% packaged in polypropylene plastic syringes exhibited no evidence of sorption when compared to glass containers. (2371)

Central Venous Catheter — Cefotaxime sodium (Hoechst-Roussel) 5 mg/mL in dextrose 5% was found to be compatible with the AR-ROWg+ard Blue Plus (Arrow International) chlorhexidine-bearing triple-lumen central catheter. Delivery of the cefotaxime sodium ranged from 93 to 95% of the initial concentration among the three lumens. Furthermore, chlorhexidine delivered from the catheter remained at trace amounts with no substantial increase due to the delivery of the drug through the catheter. (2335)

Compatibility Information

Solution Compatibility

Cefotaxime sodium

Solution	Mfr	Mfr	Conc/L	Remarks	Ref	C/I
Dextrose–saline combinations				Stable for 24 hr at room temperature and 5 days refrigerated	1	C
Dextrose 5%				Stable for 24 hr at room temperature and 5 days refrigerated	1	C
	TR[a]	HO	10 g	Physically compatible. 3% loss in 24 hr at 24 °C. No loss in 22 days at 4 °C and 63 days at −10 °C	751; 1077	C
	AB[b]	HO	20 g	Physically compatible. Little loss in 24 hr at 25 °C	994	C
Dextrose 10%				Stable for 24 hr at room temperature and 5 days refrigerated	1	C
Ringer's injection, lactated				Stable for 24 hr at room temperature and 5 days refrigerated	1	C
Sodium chloride 0.9%				Stable for 24 hr at room temperature and 5 days refrigerated	1	C
	TR[a]	HO	10 g	Physically compatible with 2% loss in 24 hr at 24 °C. No loss in 22 days at 4 °C and 63 days at −10 °C	751; 1077	C
	AB[b]	HO	20 g	Physically compatible. Little loss in 24 hr at 25 °C	994	C
Sodium lactate ⅙ M				Stable for 24 hr at room temperature and 5 days refrigerated	1	C
TPN #107[c]			1 g	Activity retained for 24 hr at 21 °C	1326	C

[a]Tested in PVC containers.
[b]Tested in both glass bottles and PVC bags.
[c]Refer to Appendix I for the composition of parenteral nutrition solutions. TPN indicates a 2-in-1 admixture.

Additive Compatibility

Cefotaxime sodium

Drug	Mfr	Conc/L	Mfr	Conc/L	Test Soln	Remarks	Ref	C/I
Amikacin sulfate	BR	25 mg	RS	50 mg	D5W	33% loss of amikacin in 2 hr at 22 °C	504	I
	BR	15 mg	RS	50 mg	D5W	Under 8% loss of amikacin in 24 hr at 22 °C	504	C
Clindamycin phosphate	UP	9 g	HO	20 g	D5W, NS[a]	Physically compatible with no clindamycin loss and 3% cefotaxime loss in 24 hr at 25 °C	994	C
Fusidate sodium	LEO	500 mg		2.5 g	D–S	Physically compatible and chemically stable for 48 hr at room temperature	1800	C

Additive Compatibility (Cont.)

Cefotaxime sodium

Drug	Mfr	Conc/L	Mfr	Conc/L	Test Soln	Remarks	Ref	C/I
Gentamicin sulfate	SC	9 mg	RS	50 mg	D5W	30% loss of gentamicin in 2 hr at 22 °C	504	I
	SC	6 mg	RS	50 mg	D5W	4% loss of gentamicin in 24 hr at 22 °C	504	C
Metronidazole	AB	5 g	HO	10 g		Both drugs stable for 72 hr at 8 °C	1547	C
	AB	5 g	HO	10 g		Visually compatible with 10% cefotaxime loss in 19 hr at 28 °C and 8% loss in 96 hr at 5 °C. No metronidazole loss in 96 hr at 5 or 28 °C	1754	C
Verapamil HCl	KN	80 mg	HO	4 g	D5W, NS	Physically compatible for 24 hr	764	C

[a]Tested in both glass and PVC containers.

Drugs in Syringe Compatibility

Cefotaxime sodium

Drug (in syringe)	Mfr	Amt	Mfr	Amt	Remarks	Ref	C/I
Caffeine citrate		20 mg/ 1 mL	HO	200 mg/ 1 mL	Visually compatible for 4 hr at 25 °C	2440	C
Dimenhydrinate		10 mg/ 1 mL		100 mg/ 1 mL	Clear solution	2569	C
Doxapram HCl	RB	400 mg/ 20 mL		500 mg/ 4 mL	Precipitates immediately	1177	I
Heparin sodium		2500 units/ 1 mL	HO	2 g	Physically compatible for at least 5 min	1053	C
	HOS	5000 units/mL	WW	10 mg/ mL	Physically compatible. No cefotaxime loss in 3 days at 4 °C. Losses of 7 and 14% in 1 and 2 days at 27 °C	2820	C
Pantoprazole sodium	[a]	4 mg/ 1 mL		100 mg/ 1 mL	Precipitates immediately	2574	I

[a]Test performed using the formulation WITHOUT edetate disodium.

Y-Site Injection Compatibility (1:1 Mixture)

Cefotaxime sodium

Drug	Mfr	Conc	Mfr	Conc	Remarks	Ref	C/I
Acyclovir sodium	BW	5 mg/mL[a]	HO	20 mg/mL[a]	Physically compatible for 4 hr at 25 °C	1157	C
Allopurinol sodium	BW	3 mg/mL[b]	HO	20 mg/mL[b]	Tiny particles form immediately	1686	I
Alprostadil	BED	7.5 mcg/ mL[l,m]	HO	100 mg/mL[k]	Visually compatible for 1 hr	2746	C
Amifostine	USB	10 mg/mL[a]	HO	20 mg/mL[a]	Physically compatible for 4 hr at 23 °C	1845	C
Anakinra	SYN	4 and 36 mg/ mL[b]	HO	10 mg/mL[b]	Physically compatible. No cefotaxime loss in 4 hr at 25 °C. Anakinra uncertain	2508	?
Azithromycin	PF	2 mg/mL[b]	HMR	200 mg/mL[i,j]	White microcrystals found	2368	I
Aztreonam	SQ	40 mg/mL[a]	HO	20 mg/mL[a]	Physically compatible for 4 hr at 23 °C	1758	C
Bivalirudin	TMC	5 mg/mL[a]	HO	20 mg/mL[a]	Physically compatible for 4 hr at 23 °C	2373	C

Y-Site Injection Compatibility (1:1 Mixture) (Cont.)

Cefotaxime sodium

Drug	Mfr	Conc	Mfr	Conc	Remarks	Ref	C/I
Cisatracurium besylate	GW	0.1 mg/mL[a]	HO	20 mg/mL[a]	Physically compatible for 4 hr at 23 °C	2074	C
	GW	2 mg/mL[a]	HO	20 mg/mL[a]	Subvisible haze forms in 4 hr	2074	I
	GW	5 mg/mL[a]	HO	20 mg/mL[a]	Subvisible haze forms immediately	2074	I
Cyclophosphamide	MJ	20 mg/mL[a]	HO	20 mg/mL[a]	Physically compatible for 4 hr at 25 °C	1194	C
Dexmedetomidine HCl	AB	4 mcg/mL[b]	HO	20 mg/mL[b]	Physically compatible for 4 hr at 23 °C	2383	C
Diltiazem HCl	MMD	5 mg/mL	HO	10 and 180 mg/mL[b]	Visually compatible	1807	C
	MMD	1 mg/mL[b]	HO	180 mg/mL[b]	Visually compatible	1807	C
Docetaxel	RPR	0.9 mg/mL[a]	HO	20 mg/mL[a]	Physically compatible for 4 hr at 23 °C	2224	C
Etoposide phosphate	BR	5 mg/mL[a]	HO	20 mg/mL[a]	Physically compatible for 4 hr at 23 °C	2218	C
Famotidine	MSD	0.2 mg/mL[a]	HO	20 mg/mL[b]	Physically compatible for 14 hr	1196	C
	ME	2 mg/mL[b]		20 mg/mL[a]	Visually compatible for 4 hr at 22 °C	1936	C
Fenoldopam mesylate	AB	80 mcg/mL[b]	HO	20 mg/mL[b]	Physically compatible for 4 hr at 23 °C	2467	C
Filgrastim	AMG	30 mcg/mL[a]	HO	20 mg/mL[a]	Particles form in 4 hr	1687	I
Fluconazole	RR	2 mg/mL	HO	20 mg/mL	Cloudiness and amber color develop	1407	I
Fludarabine phosphate	BX	1 mg/mL[a]	HO	20 mg/mL[a]	Visually compatible for 4 hr at 22 °C	1439	C
Gemcitabine HCl	LI	10 mg/mL[b]	HO	20 mg/mL[b]	Subvisible haze forms in 1 hr. Increased haze and a microprecipitate in 4 hr	2226	I
Granisetron HCl	SKB	0.05 mg/mL[a]	HO	20 mg/mL[a]	Physically compatible for 4 hr at 23 °C	2000	C
Hetastarch in lactated electrolyte	AB	6%	HO	20 mg/mL[a]	Physically compatible for 4 hr at 23 °C	2339	C
Hetastarch in sodium chloride 0.9%	DCC	6%	HO	20 mg/mL[a]	Small crystals form immediately after mixing and persist for 4 hr	1313	I
Hydromorphone HCl	WY	0.2 mg/mL[a]	HO	20 mg/mL[a]	Physically compatible for 4 hr at 25 °C	987	C
Levofloxacin	OMN	5 mg/mL[a]	HO	200 mg/mL	Visually compatible for 4 hr at 24 °C	2233	C
Lorazepam	WY	0.33 mg/mL[b]	RS	10 mg/mL	Visually compatible for 24 hr at 22 °C	1855	C
Magnesium sulfate	IX	16.7, 33.3, 66.7, 100 mg/mL[a]	HO	20 mg/mL[a]	Physically compatible for at least 4 hr at 32 °C	813	C
Melphalan HCl	BW	0.1 mg/mL[b]	HO	20 mg/mL[b]	Physically compatible for 3 hr at 22 °C	1557	C
Meperidine HCl	WY	10 mg/mL[a]	HO	20 mg/mL[a]	Physically compatible for 4 hr at 25 °C	987	C
Midazolam HCl	RC	1 mg/mL[a]	HO	20 mg/mL[a]	Visually compatible for 24 hr at 23 °C	1847	C
	RC	5 mg/mL	RS	10 mg/mL	Visually compatible for 24 hr at 22 °C	1855	C
Milrinone lactate	SS	0.2 mg/mL[a]	HO	150 mg/mL[a]	Visually compatible for 4 hr at 25 °C	2381	C
Morphine sulfate	WI	1 mg/mL[a]	HO	20 mg/mL[a]	Physically compatible for 4 hr at 25 °C	987	C
Ondansetron HCl	GL	1 mg/mL[b]	HO	20 mg/mL[a]	Visually compatible for 4 hr at 22 °C	1365	C
Pemetrexed disodium	LI	20 mg/mL[b]	APP	20 mg/mL[a]	Slight color darkening occurs over 4 hr	2564	I
Pentamidine isethionate	FUJ	3 mg/mL[a]	HO	20 mg/mL[a]	Fine precipitate forms immediately	1880	I
Propofol	ZEN	10 mg/mL	HO	20 mg/mL[a]	Physically compatible for 1 hr at 23 °C	2066	C
Remifentanil HCl	GW	0.025 and 0.25 mg/mL[b]	HO	20 mg/mL[a]	Physically compatible for 4 hr at 23 °C	2075	C
Sargramostim	IMM	10 mcg/mL[b]	HO	20 mg/mL[b]	Visually compatible for 4 hr at 22 °C	1436	C
Teniposide	BR	0.1 mg/mL[a]	HO	20 mg/mL[a]	Physically compatible for 1 hr at 23 °C	1725	C

Y-Site Injection Compatibility (1:1 Mixture) (Cont.)

Cefotaxime sodium

Drug	Mfr	Conc	Mfr	Conc	Remarks	Ref	C/I
Thiotepa	IMM[c]	1 mg/mL[a]	HO	20 mg/mL[a]	Physically compatible for 1 hr at 23 °C	1861	C
Tigecycline	WY	1 mg/mL[b]		40 mg/mL[b]	Physically compatible for 4 hr	2714	C
TNA #218 to #226[d]			HO	20 mg/mL[a]	Visually compatible for 4 hr at 23 °C	2215	C
TPN #61[d]		[e]	HO	200 mg/ 0.7 mL[f]	Physically compatible	1012	C
		[g]	HO	1.2 g/4 mL[f]	Physically compatible	1012	C
TPN #189[d]			RS	200 mg/mL[e]	Visually compatible for 24 hr at 22 °C	1767	C
TPN #203, #204[d]			HO	60 mg/mL	Visually compatible for 2 hr at 23 °C	1974	C
TPN #212 to #215[d]			HO	20 mg/mL[a]	Physically compatible for 4 hr at 23 °C	2109	C
Vancomycin HCl		12.5, 25, 30, 50 mg/mL[h]		100 mg/mL[h]	White precipitate forms immediately	1721	I
		5 mg/mL[h]		100 mg/mL[h]	No precipitate visually observed over 7 days at room temperature, but nonvisible incompatibility cannot be ruled out	1721	?
	AB	20 mg/mL[a]	HO	200 mg/mL[h]	Transient precipitate forms	2189	?
	AB	20 mg/mL[a]	HO	50 mg/mL[a]	White cloudiness forms immediately	2189	I
	AB	20 mg/mL[a]	HO	1 and 10 mg/mL[a]	Physically compatible for 4 hr at 23 °C	2189	C
	AB	2 mg/mL[a]	HO	1[a], 10[a], 50[a], 200[h] mg/mL	Physically compatible for 4 hr at 23 °C	2189	C
Vinorelbine tartrate	BW	1 mg/mL[b]	HO	20 mg/mL[b]	Physically compatible for 4 hr at 22 °C	1558	C

[a]*Tested in dextrose 5%.*
[b]*Tested in sodium chloride 0.9%.*
[c]*Lyophilized formulation tested.*
[d]*Refer to Appendix I for the composition of parenteral nutrition solutions. TNA indicates a 3-in-1 admixture, and TPN indicates a 2-in-1 admixture.*
[e]*Run at 21 mL/hr.*
[f]*Given over five minutes by syringe pump.*
[g]*Run at 94 mL/hr.*
[h]*Tested in sterile water for injection.*
[i]*Tested in sodium chloride 0.45%.*
[j]*Injected via Y-site into an administration set running azithromycin.*
[k]*Tested in either dextrose 5% or in sodium chloride 0.9%, but the report did not specify which solution.*
[l]*Tested in a 1:1 mixture of (1) dextrose 5% and dextrose 5% in sodium chloride 0.45% with and without potassium chloride 20 mEq/L and also in (2) dextrose 10% in sodium chloride 0.45% with and without potassium chloride 20 mEq/L.*
[m]*Tested in a 1:1 mixture of dextrose 5% and TPN #274 (see Appendix I).*

CEFOTETAN DISODIUM
AHFS 8:12.07.12

Products — Cefotetan disodium is available in 1- and 2-g vials and infusion bottles and 10-g pharmacy bulk packages. (1)

For intramuscular injection, reconstitute the vials with sterile water for injection, bacteriostatic water for injection, sodium chloride 0.9%, or lidocaine hydrochloride 0.5 or 1%. Then shake well to dissolve and let stand until clear. Recommended volumes for reconstitution are shown in Table 1. (1)

For intravenous use, reconstitute the vials with sterile water for injection in the amounts noted in Table 1, shake well to dissolve, and let stand until clear. (1)

Reconstitute the 10-g pharmacy bulk package with sterile water for injection, dextrose 5%, or sodium chloride 0.9% according to the instructions on the package label. Then shake it well to dissolve and let stand until clear. (1)

Cefotetan disodium (Braun) is available as 1 and 2 g in a dual chamber flexible container. The diluent chamber contains dextrose solution 3.58% for the 1-g container and 2.08% for the 2-g container for use as a diluent. (1)

pH — Reconstituted solutions have a pH of 4.5 to 6.5. (1)

Osmolarity — Concentrations of 100 to 200 mg/mL in sterile water for injection have osmolarities of 400 to 800 mOsm/L, respectively. In-

Table 1. Recommended Dilutions of Cefotetan Disodium Vials (1; 4)

Vial Size	Volume of Diluent	Withdrawable Volume	Approximate Concentration
Intramuscular			
1 g	2 mL	2.5 mL	400 mg/mL
2 g	3 mL	4.0 mL	500 mg/mL
Intravenous			
1 g	10 mL	10.5 mL	95 mg/mL
2 g	10 to 20 mL	11 to 21 mL	182 to 95 mg/mL

tramuscular concentrations of 375 to 471.5 mg/mL are extremely hypertonic, with osmolarities greater than 1500 mOsm/L. (4)

Cefotetan disodium (Braun) 1 and 2 g in dual chamber flexible containers has an osmolality of 290 mOsm/kg when activated with the dextrose solution diluent. (1)

Sodium Content — Each gram of cefotetan disodium contains approximately 3.5 mEq (80 mg) of sodium. (1)

Administration — Cefotetan disodium may be administered by deep intramuscular injection, direct intravenous injection over three to five minutes, and intermittent intravenous infusion in 50 to 100 mL of dextrose 5% or sodium chloride 0.9% infused over 20 to 60 minutes. The manufacturer recommends temporarily discontinuing other solutions being administered at the same site. (1; 4)

Stability — Intact vials should be stored at 22 °C or less and protected from light. Cefotetan disodium powder is white to pale yellow. So-

lutions may vary from colorless to yellow, depending on the concentration. (1)

When reconstituted as recommended, cefotetan disodium solutions are stable for 24 hours at room temperature (25 °C) and 96 hours under refrigeration (5 °C). In disposable glass or plastic syringes, the drug also is stable for 24 hours at room temperature and 96 hours under refrigeration. (1; 4)

Cefotetan disodium (Braun) 1 and 2 g in dual chamber flexible plastic containers with dextrose solution diluent should be used within 12 hours after activation if stored at room temperature and in five days if stored under refrigeration. (1)

Freezing Solutions — The manufacturer states that solutions reconstituted as recommended are stable for at least one week when frozen at −20 °C. (1) The manufacturer also has stated that cefotetan disodium as the reconstituted solution in vials is stable for one year at −20 °C; in a large volume parenteral solution, it is stable for 30 weeks at −20 °C. (283) Thawing should be performed at room temperature, and thawed solutions should not be refrozen. (1; 4)

Cefotetan disodium (Braun) 1 and 2 g in dual chamber flexible containers should not be frozen. (1)

Central Venous Catheter — Cefotetan disodium (Zeneca) 5 mg/mL in dextrose 5% was found to be compatible with the ARROWg+ard Blue Plus (Arrow International) chlorhexidine-bearing triple-lumen central catheter. Essentially complete delivery of the drug was found with little or no drug loss occurring. Furthermore, chlorhexidine delivered from the catheter remained at trace amounts with no substantial increase due to the delivery of the drug through the catheter. (2335)

Compatibility Information

Solution Compatibility

Cefotetan disodium

Solution	Mfr	Mfr	Conc/L	Remarks	Ref	C/I
Dextrose 5%	TR[a]	STU	2 g	4% loss at 20 °C and 0 to 2% loss at 4 and −20 °C in 14 days	966	**C**
	[a]	AY	20 and 40 g	Visually compatible with 10% loss in 3.5 days at 23 °C and 13 days at 4 °C	1591	**C**
	TR[a]	STU	20 g	8% loss in 2 days and 11% loss in 3 days at 25 °C. 6% loss in 41 days at 5 °C. No loss in 60 days at −10 °C	1598	**C**
Sodium chloride 0.9%	[a]	AY	20 and 40 g	Visually compatible with 10% loss in 3.5 days at 23 °C and 14 days at 4 °C	1591	**C**
	TR[a]	STU	20 g	8% loss in 2 days and 11% loss in 3 days at 25 °C. 5% loss in 41 days at 5 °C. No loss in 60 days at −10 °C	1598	**C**

[a]*Tested in PVC containers.*

Drugs in Syringe Compatibility

Cefotetan disodium

Drug (in syringe)	Mfr	Amt	Mfr	Amt	Remarks	Ref	C/I
Doxapram HCl	RB	400 mg/ 20 mL		1 g/ 10 mL	Immediate turbidity	1177	I
Promethazine HCl	ES	25 mg/ 1 mL	ZEN	10 mg/ mL[a]	White precipitate, resembling cottage cheese, forms immediately	1753	I

[a]Tested in dextrose 5%.

Y-Site Injection Compatibility (1:1 Mixture)

Cefotetan disodium

Drug	Mfr	Conc	Mfr	Conc	Remarks	Ref	C/I
Allopurinol sodium	BW	3 mg/mL[b]	STU	20 mg/mL[b]	Physically compatible for 4 hr at 22 °C	1686	C
Amifostine	USB	10 mg/mL[a]	STU	20 mg/mL[a]	Physically compatible for 4 hr at 23 °C	1845	C
Aztreonam	SQ	40 mg/mL[b]	STU	20 mg/mL[b]	Physically compatible for 4 hr at 23 °C	1758	C
Bivalirudin	TMC	5 mg/mL[a]	ZEN	20 mg/mL[b]	Physically compatible for 4 hr at 23 °C	2373	C
Dexmedetomidine HCl	AB	4 mcg/mL[b]	ZEN	20 mg/mL[b]	Physically compatible for 4 hr at 23 °C	2383	C
Diltiazem HCl	MMD	5 mg/mL	STU	10 and 200 mg/mL[b]	Visually compatible	1807	C
	MMD	1 mg/mL[b]	STU	200 mg/mL[b]	Visually compatible	1807	C
Docetaxel	RPR	0.9 mg/mL[a]	ZEN	20 mg/mL[a]	Physically compatible for 4 hr at 23 °C	2224	C
Etoposide phosphate	BR	5 mg/mL[a]	ZEN	20 mg/mL[a]	Physically compatible for 4 hr at 23 °C	2218	C
Famotidine	MSD	0.2 mg/mL[a]	STU	20 mg/mL[b]	Physically compatible for 14 hr	1196	C
Fenoldopam mesylate	AB	80 mcg/mL[b]	ZEN	20 mg/mL[b]	Physically compatible for 4 hr at 23 °C	2467	C
Filgrastim	AMG	30 mcg/mL[a]	STU	20 mg/mL[a]	Physically compatible for 4 hr at 22 °C	1687	C
Fluconazole	RR	2 mg/mL	STU	40 mg/mL	Physically compatible for 24 hr at 25 °C	1407	C
Fludarabine phosphate	BX	1 mg/mL[a]	STU	20 mg/mL[a]	Visually compatible for 4 hr at 22 °C	1439	C
Gemcitabine HCl	LI	10 mg/mL[b]	ZEN	20 mg/mL[b]	Physically compatible for 4 hr at 23 °C	2226	C
Granisetron HCl	SKB	0.05 mg/mL[a]	STU	20 mg/mL[a]	Physically compatible for 4 hr at 23 °C	2000	C
Heparin sodium	TR	50 units/mL	STU	40 mg/mL[a]	Visually compatible for 4 hr at 25 °C	1793	C
Hetastarch in lactated electrolyte	AB	6%	ZEN	20 mg/mL[a]	Physically compatible for 4 hr at 23 °C	2339	C
Insulin, regular	LI	0.2 unit/mL[b]	STU	20 and 40 mg/mL[a]	Physically compatible for 2 hr at 25 °C	1395	C
Linezolid	PHU	2 mg/mL	ZEN	20 mg/mL[a]	Physically compatible for 4 hr at 23 °C	2264	C
Melphalan HCl	BW	0.1 mg/mL[b]	STU	20 mg/mL[b]	Physically compatible for 3 hr at 22 °C	1557	C
Meperidine HCl	WY	10 mg/mL[b]	STU	20 and 40 mg/mL[a]	Physically compatible for 1 hr at 25 °C	1338	C
Morphine sulfate	ES	1 mg/mL[b]	STU	20 and 40 mg/mL[a]	Physically compatible for 1 hr at 25 °C	1338	C
Paclitaxel	NCI	1.2 mg/mL[a]	STU	20 mg/mL[a]	Physically compatible for 4 hr at 22 °C	1556	C
Palonosetron HCl	MGI	50 mcg/mL	ASZ	20 mg/mL[b]	Physically compatible and no loss of either drug in 4 hr at room temperature	2749	C
Pemetrexed disodium	LI	20 mg/mL[b]	ASZ	20 mg/mL[a]	Color darkening and brownish discoloration occur immediately	2564	I

Y-Site Injection Compatibility (1:1 Mixture) (Cont.)

Cefotetan disodium

Drug	Mfr	Conc	Mfr	Conc	Remarks	Ref	C/I
Promethazine HCl	ES	25 mg	ZEN	10 mg/mL[a]	White precipitate forms immediately	1753	**I**
Propofol	ZEN	10 mg/mL	STU	20 mg/mL[a]	Physically compatible for 1 hr at 23 °C	2066	**C**
Remifentanil HCl	GW	0.025 and 0.25 mg/mL[b]	ZEN	20 mg/mL[a]	Physically compatible for 4 hr at 23 °C	2075	**C**
Sargramostim	IMM	10 mcg/mL[b]	STU	20 mg/mL[b]	Visually compatible for 4 hr at 22 °C	1436	**C**
Tacrolimus	FUJ	1 mg/mL[b]	STU	40 mg/mL[a]	Visually compatible for 24 hr at 25 °C	1630	**C**
Teniposide	BR	0.1 mg/mL[a]	STU	20 mg/mL[a]	Physically compatible for 4 hr at 23 °C	1725	**C**
Theophylline	TR	4 mg/mL	STU	40 mg/mL[a]	Visually compatible for 6 hr at 25 °C	1793	**C**
Thiotepa	IMM[c]	1 mg/mL[a]	STU	20 mg/mL[a]	Physically compatible for 4 hr at 23 °C	1861	**C**
TNA #218 to #226[d]			ZEN	20 mg/mL[a]	Visually compatible for 4 hr at 23 °C	2215	**C**
TPN #212 to #215[d]			STU	20 mg/mL[a]	Physically compatible for 4 hr at 23 °C	2109	**C**
Vancomycin HCl	AB	20 mg/mL[a]	ZEN	200 mg/mL[e]	Transient precipitate forms followed by white precipitate in 4 hr	2189	**I**
	AB	20 mg/mL[a]	ZEN	10 and 50 mg/mL[a]	Gross white precipitate forms immediately	2189	**I**
	AB	20 mg/mL[a]	ZEN	1 mg/mL[a]	Subvisible haze forms immediately. White precipitate in 4 hr	2189	**I**
	AB	2 mg/mL[a]	ZEN	1[a], 10[a], 50[a], 200[e] mg/mL	Physically compatible for 4 hr at 23 °C	2189	**C**
Vinorelbine tartrate	BW	1 mg/mL[b]	STU	20 mg/mL[b]	Tiny particles form immediately. Turbidity in 4 hr	1558	**I**

[a]Tested in dextrose 5%.
[b]Tested in sodium chloride 0.9%.
[c]Lyophilized formulation tested.
[d]Refer to Appendix I for the composition of parenteral nutrition solutions. TNA indicates a 3-in-1 admixture, and TPN indicates a 2-in-1 admixture.
[e]Tested in sterile water for injection.

CEFOXITIN SODIUM
AHFS 8:12.07.12

Products — Cefoxitin sodium is available in vials containing the equivalent of 1 and 2 g of cefoxitin (as sodium). It is also available in 10-g bulk bottles. (1)

For intravenous administration, reconstitute the vial contents with sterile water for injection. The 1-g vials may be reconstituted with 10 mL resulting in a 95-mg/mL concentration. The 2-g vials may be reconstituted with 20 or 10 mL resulting in 95 or 180 mg/mL, respectively. The 10-g bulk bottles may be reconstituted with 93 or 43 mL resulting in 100 or 200 mg/mL, respectively. After addition of the diluent, shake the vial and allow the solution to stand until it becomes clear. (1; 4)

For intravenous infusion, the primary solution may be diluted further in 50 to 1000 mL of compatible diluent. (1)

Cefoxitin sodium (Braun) is available as 1 and 2 g in a dual chamber flexible container. The diluent chamber contains dextrose solution. (1)

pH — Reconstituted solutions have a pH of 4.2 to 7. The frozen premixed infusion and reconstituted drug in dual chamber containers have a pH of about 6.5. (1; 4)

Osmolality — The osmolality of cefoxitin sodium 1 and 2 g was calculated for the following dilutions (1054):

Diluent	Osmolality (mOsm/kg)	
	50 mL	100 mL
1 g		
Dextrose 5%	326	293
Sodium chloride 0.9%	352	319
2 g		
Dextrose 5%	388	329
Sodium chloride 0.9%	415	355

The osmolality of cefoxitin sodium (MSD) 50 mg/mL was determined to be 348 mOsm/kg in dextrose 5% and 361 mOsm/kg in sodium chloride 0.9%. (1375)

Cefoxitin sodium (Braun) 1 and 2 g in dual chamber flexible containers has an osmolality of 290 mOsm/kg when activated with the dextrose solution diluent. (1)

The following maximum cefoxitin sodium concentrations were recommended to achieve osmolalities suitable for peripheral infusion in fluid-restricted patients (1180):

Diluent	Maximum Concentration (mg/mL)	Osmolality (mOsm/kg)
Dextrose 5%	62	531
Sodium chloride 0.9%	56	508
Sterile water for injection	112	437

Sodium Content — Each gram of cefoxitin sodium contains 2.3 mEq (53.8 mg) of sodium. (1)

Administration — Cefoxitin sodium may be administered by direct intravenous injection over three to five minutes directly into the vein or slowly into the tubing of a running compatible infusion solution, or by continuous or intermittent intravenous infusion. The manufacturer recommends temporarily discontinuing other solutions being administered at the site. (1; 4)

The manufacturer recommends that cefoxitin sodium not be mixed with aminoglycoside antibiotics such as amikacin sulfate, gentamicin sulfate, and tobramycin sulfate. (1) However, compatibility studies show that such admixtures may indeed be sufficiently stable to allow combined mixture in the same solution.

Stability — Intact vials of cefoxitin sodium should be stored between 2 and 25 °C. Exposure to temperatures above 50 °C should be avoided. The powder is white to off-white in color. Solutions may range from colorless to light amber. (1) Both the dry material and solutions may darken, depending on storage conditions. Although moisture plays a role in the rate and intensity of the darkening, exposure to oxygen is the most significant factor. However, this discoloration is stated not to affect potency or relate to any significant chemical change. The concern over color is purely aesthetic. (865)

Exposure of cefoxitin sodium (MSD) 40 mg/mL in sterile water for injection to 37 °C for 24 hours, to simulate the use of a portable infusion pump, resulted in about a 3 to 4% cefoxitin loss. (1391)

Cefoxitin sodium solutions reconstituted as indicated in Table 1 are stable for 48 hours at 25 °C and at least seven days and, in some cases, up to one month at 5 °C. (308)

Cefoxitin sodium (MSD) 1 and 2 g/10 mL in sterile water for injection, packaged in plastic syringes (Monoject), exhibited a 10% cefoxitin sodium loss in two days at 24 °C and 23 days at 4 °C. Less than 10% loss occurred in 3 months frozen at −15 °C. (1178)

pH Effects — Cefoxitin sodium at 1 and 10 mg/mL in aqueous solution is stable over pH 4 to 8. The time to 10% decomposition when stored at 25 °C was essentially independent of pH, ranging from 40 to 44 hours at pH 4 to 5 to 33 hours at pH 8. Under refrigeration, a pH 7 (unbuffered) aqueous solution showed 10% decomposition in 26 days. At pH less than 4, precipitation of the free acid may occur. Above pH 8, hydrolysis of the β-lactam group may result. (308)

In another study, cefoxitin sodium in aqueous solution at 25 °C exhibited minimum rates of decomposition at pH 5 to 7. The solutions in this pH range showed 10% decomposition in about two days. At pH 3, about 40 hours elapsed before 10% decomposition occurred. However, at pH 9, only 14 hours was required to incur a 10% loss. (630)

Freezing Solutions — The stability of cefoxitin sodium reconstituted with the diluents as shown in Table 2 was evaluated in the frozen state at −20 °C. The solutions retained adequate potency for at least 30 weeks. (308) Thawed solutions should not be refrozen. (1) Frozen premixed cefoxitin solutions should also not be refrozen after thawing. The manufacturer states that the thawed solution may be stored for 24 hours at room temperature or 21 days under refrigeration. (1)

An approximate twofold increase in particles of 2 to 60 μm produced by freezing and thawing cefoxitin sodium (MSD) 2 g/100 mL of dextrose 5% (Travenol) was reported. The reconstituted drug was filtered through a 0.45-μm filter into PVC bags of solution and frozen for seven days at −20 °C. Thawing was performed at room temperature (29 °C) for 12 hours. Although the total number of particles increased significantly, no particles greater than 60 μm were observed; the solutions complied with USP standards for particle sizes and numbers in large volume parenteral solutions. (822)

A 3% or less cefoxitin sodium (MSD) loss was reported from a solution containing 40 mg/mL in sterile water for injection in PVC and glass containers after 30 days at −20 °C. Subsequent thawing and storage for four days at 5 °C, followed by 24 hours at 37 °C to simulate the use of a portable infusion pump, resulted in an additional 3 to 4% cefoxitin sodium loss. (1391)

Cefoxitin sodium in sodium chloride 0.9%, Ringer's injection, lactated, and dextrose 5% in PVC bags is stable for 26 weeks if kept frozen. (4)

Cefoxitin sodium (Braun) 1 and 2 g in dual chamber flexible containers should not be frozen. (1)

Sorption — Cefoxitin sodium was shown not to exhibit sorption to PVC bags and tubing, polyethylene tubing, Silastic tubing, and polypropylene syringes. (536; 606)

Central Venous Catheter — Cefoxitin sodium (Merck) 5 mg/mL in dextrose 5% was found to be compatible with the ARROWg+ard Blue Plus (Arrow International) chlorhexidine-bearing triple-lumen central catheter. Essentially complete delivery of the drug was found with little or no drug loss occurring. Furthermore, chlorhexidine delivered from the catheter remained at trace amounts with no substantial increase due to the delivery of the drug through the catheter. (2335)

Table 1. Stability of Reconstituted Cefoxitin Sodium 1 g (308)

Diluent	Volume	Remarks
Bacteriostatic water for injection (benzyl alcohol)	2 mL	9% decomposition in 48 hr at 25 °C. 4% in 7 days and 10% in 1 month at 5 °C
Bacteriostatic water for injection (parabens)	2 mL	9% decomposition in 48 hr at 25 °C. 5% in 7 days and 12% in 1 month at 5 °C
Dextrose 5%	10 mL	9% decomposition in 48 hr at 25 °C, 2% in 7 days at 5 °C
Lidocaine HCl 0.5% (with parabens)	2 mL	8% decomposition in 48 hr at 25 °C. 5% in 7 days and 10% in 1 month at 5 °C
Lidocaine HCl 1% (with parabens)	2 mL	7% decomposition in 48 hr at 25 °C. 2% in 7 days and 10% in 1 month at 5 °C
Sodium chloride 0.9%	10 mL	8% decomposition in 48 hr at 25 °C
Water for injection	10 mL	10% decomposition in 48 hr at 25 °C, 1% in 7 days at 5 °C
Water for injection	4 mL	7% decomposition in 48 hr at 25 °C, 2% in 7 days at 5 °C
Water for injection	2 mL	8% decomposition in 48 hr at 25 °C. 2% in 7 days and 10% in 1 month at 5 °C
(In plastic syringe)	10 mL	6% decomposition in 24 hr and 11% in 48 hr at 25 °C

Table 2. Stability of Reconstituted Cefoxitin Sodium 1 g Frozen at −20 °C (308)

Diluent	Volume	Remarks
Bacteriostatic water for injection (benzyl alcohol)	10 mL	2% decomposition in 30 weeks. Thawed solutions showed 6% decomposition in 24 hr at 25 °C and 1% in 7 days at 5 °C
Bacteriostatic water for injection (parabens)	10 mL	2% decomposition in 30 weeks. Thawed solutions showed no decomposition in 24 hr at 25 °C and 1% in 7 days at 5 °C
Dextrose 5%	10 mL	3% decomposition in 30 weeks. Thawed solutions showed 8% decomposition in 24 hr at 25 °C and 6% in 7 days at 5 °C
Lidocaine HCl 0.5%	2 mL	2% cefoxitin decomposition in 26 weeks. Thawed solutions showed 6% decomposition in 24 hr at 25 °C. Lidocaine stable
Sodium chloride 0.9%	10 mL	5% decomposition in 30 weeks. Thawed solutions showed 3% decomposition in 24 hr at 25 °C and 6% in 7 days at 5 °C
Water for injection	10 mL	1% decomposition in 30 weeks. Thawed solutions showed 3% decomposition in 24 hr at 25 °C and 5% in 7 days at 5 °C
Water for injection	4 mL	No decomposition in 13 weeks

Compatibility Information

Solution Compatibility

Cefoxitin sodium

Solution	Mfr	Mfr	Conc/L	Remarks	Ref	C/I
Dextrose 5% in Ringer's injection, lactated	[a]	MSD	1, 2, 10, 20 g	5 to 8% loss in 24 hr and 12 to 13% in 48 hr at 25 °C. 3 to 5% in 7 days at 5 °C	308	C
Dextrose 5% in sodium chloride 0.2%	[a]	MSD	1 g	5% loss in 24 hr and 11% in 48 hr at 25 °C	308	C
Dextrose 5% in sodium chloride 0.45%	[a]	MSD	1 g	4% loss in 24 hr and 10% in 48 hr at 25 °C	308	C
Dextrose 5% in sodium chloride 0.9%	[a]	MSD	1 g	4% loss in 24 hr and 10% in 48 hr at 25 °C	308	C
Dextrose 5%	[a]	MSD	1, 2, 10 g	6 to 7% loss in 24 hr and 11 to 13% in 48 hr at 25 °C. 3 to 6% in 7 days at 5 °C	308	C
	[a]	MSD	20 g	7.5% loss in 24 hr and 13% in 48 hr at 25 °C. 4% in 7 days at 5 °C. No loss noted in 13 weeks at −20 °C	308	C
	TR[b]	MSD	1 g	9% loss in 24 hr and 11% in 48 hr at 25 °C	308	C
	TR[b]	MSD	20 g	No loss noted in 24 hr but 11% loss in 48 hr at 24 °C. 3% loss in 13 days at 5 °C	525	C
	TR[b]	MSD	20 g	Physically compatible with 5% loss in 24 hr at room temperature. No loss in 30 days at −20 °C	554	C
	[b]		10 and 20 g	Visually compatible and 3% loss after storage at −20 °C for 72 hr, thawed, and 6 hr at room temperature	629	C

Solution Compatibility (Cont.)

Cefoxitin sodium

Solution	Mfr	Mfr	Conc/L	Remarks	Ref	C/I
	MG[a]	MSD	20 g	Physically compatible with no loss in 24 hr and 6% loss in 48 hr at room temperature	983	C
Dextrose 10%	[a]	MSD	1 g	6% loss in 24 hr and 11% in 48 hr at 25 °C	308	C
Ionosol B in dextrose 5%	AB[a]	MSD	1, 2, 10 g	6 to 8% loss in 24 hr and 12 to 13% in 48 hr at 25 °C. 3 to 6% in 7 days at 5 °C	308	C
Normosol M in dextrose 5%	AB[a]	MSD	1, 2, 10, 20 g	4 to 6% loss in 24 hr and 11 to 12% in 48 hr at 25 °C. 3 to 5% in 7 days at 5 °C	308	C
Ringer's injection	[a]	MSD	1 g	2% loss in 24 hr and 12% in 48 hr at 25 °C	308	C
Ringer's injection, lactated	[a]	MSD	1, 2, 10, 20 g	5 to 7% loss in 24 hr and 10 to 12% in 48 hr at 25 °C. 3% in 7 days at 5 °C	308	C
	TR[b]	MSD	1 g	7% loss in 24 hr and 9% in 48 hr at 25 °C	308	C
Sodium chloride 0.9%	[a]	MSD	1 g	5% loss in 24 hr and 11% in 48 hr at 25 °C	308	C
	[a]	MSD	10 and 20 g	8 to 10% loss in 24 hr and 13 and 15% in 48 hr at 25 °C. 4 to 5% in 48 hr at 5 °C	308	C
	[b]	MSD	1 g	4 to 7% loss in 24 hr and 8 to 9% loss in 48 hr at 25 °C	308	C
	TR[b]	MSD	20 g	No loss noted in 24 hr but 12% loss in 48 hr at 24 °C. 3% loss in 13 days at 5 °C	525	C
	[b]		10 and 20 g	Visually compatible and 3% loss after storage at −20 °C for 72 hr, thawing, and 6 hr at room temperature	629	C
	MG[a]	MSD	20 g	Physically compatible with no loss in 24 hr and 6% loss in 48 hr at room temperature	983	C
Sodium lactate ⅙ M	[a]	MSD	1 g	5% loss in 24 hr and 8% in 48 hr at 25 °C	308	C
TPN #107[c]			1 g	Activity retained for 24 hr at 21 °C	1326	C

[a]*Tested in glass containers.*
[b]*Tested in PVC containers.*
[c]*Refer to Appendix I for the composition of parenteral nutrition solutions. TPN indicates a 2-in-1 admixture.*

Additive Compatibility

Cefoxitin sodium

Drug	Mfr	Conc/L	Mfr	Conc/L	Test Soln	Remarks	Ref	C/I
Amikacin sulfate	BR	5 g	MSD	5 g	D5S	9% cefoxitin loss at 25 °C and none at 5 °C in 48 hr. No amikacin loss at 25 °C and 1% at 5 °C in 48 hr	308	C
Aztreonam	SQ	10 and 20 g	MSD	10 and 20 g	D5W, NS[a]	Both drugs stable for 12 hr at 25 °C. Yellow color and 6 to 12% aztreonam and 9 to 15% cefoxitin loss in 48 hr at 25 °C	1023	I
	SQ	10 and 20 g	MSD	10 and 20 g	D5W[a]	3 to 6% cefoxitin loss and no aztreonam loss in 7 days at 4 °C	1023	C
	SQ	10 and 20 g	MSD	10 and 20 g	NS[a]	3 to 5% aztreonam loss and no cefoxitin loss in 7 days at 4 °C	1023	C
Clindamycin phosphate	UP	9 g	MSD	20 g	D5W[b]	Physically compatible with no loss of either drug in 48 hr at room temperature	983	C
	UP	9 g	MSD	20 g	NS[b]	Physically compatible with no clindamycin loss and 7% cefoxitin loss in 48 hr at room temperature	983	C

Additive Compatibility (Cont.)

Cefoxitin sodium

Drug	Mfr	Conc/L	Mfr	Conc/L	Test Soln	Remarks	Ref	C/I
Gentamicin sulfate	SC	400 mg	MSD	5 g	D5S	4% cefoxitin loss in 24 hr and 11% in 48 hr at 25 °C. 2% in 48 hr at 5 °C. 9% gentamicin loss in 24 hr and 23% in 48 hr at 25 °C. 2% in 48 hr at 5 °C	308	C
Mannitol		10%	MSD	1, 2, 10, 20 g		4 to 5% cefoxitin loss in 24 hr and 10 to 11% in 48 hr at 25 °C. 2 to 5% cefoxitin loss in 7 days at 5 °C	308	C
Metronidazole	SE	5 g	MSD	30 g		9% cefoxitin loss in 48 hr at 25 °C and 3% in 12 days at 5 °C. No metronidazole loss	993	C
Multivitamins	USV	50 mL	MSD	10 g	W	5% cefoxitin loss in 24 hr and 10% in 48 hr at 25 °C; 3% in 48 hr at 5 °C	308	C
Ranitidine HCl	GL	50 mg and 2 g		10 g	D5W	Ranitidine stable for only 4 hr at 25 °C. Cefoxitin not tested	1515	I
Sodium bicarbonate	AB	200 mg	MSD	1 g	W	5 to 6% cefoxitin loss in 24 hr and 11 to 12% in 48 hr at 25 °C. 2 to 3% loss in 7 days at 5 °C	308	C
Tobramycin sulfate	LI	400 mg	MSD	5 g	D5S	5% cefoxitin loss in 24 hr and 11% in 48 hr at 25 °C. 3% in 48 hr at 5 °C. 8% tobramycin loss in 24 hr and 37% in 48 hr at 25 °C. 3% in 48 hr at 5 °C	308	C
Verapamil HCl	KN	80 mg	MSD	4 g	D5W, NS	Physically compatible for 24 hr	764	C

[a]Tested in PVC containers.
[b]Tested in glass containers.

Drugs in Syringe Compatibility

Cefoxitin sodium

Drug (in syringe)	Mfr	Amt	Mfr	Amt	Remarks	Ref	C/I
Heparin sodium		2500 units/ 1 mL	MSD	2 g	Physically compatible for at least 5 min	1053	C
Pantoprazole sodium	[a]	4 mg/ 1 mL		100 mg/ 1 mL	Precipitates immediately	2574	I

[a]Test performed using the formulation WITHOUT edetate disodium.

Y-Site Injection Compatibility (1:1 Mixture)

Cefoxitin sodium

Drug	Mfr	Conc	Mfr	Conc	Remarks	Ref	C/I
Acyclovir sodium	BW	5 mg/mL[a]	MSD	20 mg/mL[a]	Physically compatible for 4 hr at 25 °C	1157	C
Amifostine	USB	10 mg/mL[a]	MSD	20 mg/mL[a]	Physically compatible for 4 hr at 23 °C	1845	C
Amphotericin B cholesteryl sulfate complex	SEQ	0.83 mg/mL[a]	ME	20 mg/mL[a]	Physically compatible for 4 hr at 23 °C	2117	C

Y-Site Injection Compatibility (1:1 Mixture) (Cont.)

Cefoxitin sodium

Drug	Mfr	Conc	Mfr	Conc	Remarks	Ref	C/I
Anakinra	SYN	4 and 36 mg/mL[b]	ME	20 mg/mL[b]	Physically compatible. No cefoxitin loss in 4 hr at 25 °C. Anakinra uncertain	2508	?
Anidulafungin	VIC	0.5 mg/mL[a]	APP	20 mg/mL[a]	Physically compatible for 4 hr at 23 °C	2617	C
Aztreonam	SQ	40 mg/mL[a]	MSD	20 mg/mL[a]	Physically compatible for 4 hr at 23 °C	1758	C
Bivalirudin	TMC	5 mg/mL[a]	ME	20 mg/mL[a]	Physically compatible for 4 hr at 23 °C	2373	C
Cisatracurium besylate	GW	0.1 mg/mL[a]	ME	20 mg/mL[a]	Physically compatible for 4 hr at 23 °C	2074	C
	GW	2 and 5 mg/mL[a]	ME	20 mg/mL[a]	Subvisible haze forms immediately	2074	I
Cyclophosphamide	MJ	20 mg/mL[a]	MSD	20 mg/mL[a]	Physically compatible for 4 hr at 25 °C	1194	C
Dexmedetomidine HCl	AB	4 mcg/mL[b]	ME	20 mg/mL[b]	Physically compatible for 4 hr at 23 °C	2383	C
Diltiazem HCl	MMD	5 mg/mL	MSD	10 and 200 mg/mL[b]	Visually compatible	1807	C
	MMD	1 mg/mL[b]	MSD	200 mg/mL[b]	Visually compatible	1807	C
Docetaxel	RPR	0.9 mg/mL[a]	ME	20 mg/mL[a]	Physically compatible for 4 hr at 23 °C	2224	C
Doxorubicin HCl liposomal	SEQ	0.4 mg/mL[a]	ME	20 mg/mL[a]	Physically compatible for 4 hr at 23 °C	2087	C
Etoposide phosphate	BR	5 mg/mL[a]	ME	20 mg/mL[a]	Physically compatible for 4 hr at 23 °C	2218	C
Famotidine	MSD	0.2 mg/mL[a]	MSD	20 mg/mL[b]	Physically compatible for 14 hr	1196	C
	ME	2 mg/mL[b]		20 mg/mL[a]	Visually compatible for 4 hr at 22 °C	1936	C
Fenoldopam mesylate	AB	80 mcg/mL[b]	ME	20 mg/mL[b]	Microparticulates form immediately	2467	I
Filgrastim	AMG	30 mcg/mL[a]	MSD	20 mg/mL[a]	Haze, particles, and filaments form immediately	1687	I
Fluconazole	RR	2 mg/mL	MSD	40 mg/mL	Physically compatible for 24 hr at 25 °C	1407	C
Foscarnet sodium	AST	24 mg/mL	MSD	40 mg/mL	Physically compatible for 24 hr at room temperature under fluorescent light	1335	C
Gemcitabine HCl	LI	10 mg/mL[b]	ME	20 mg/mL[b]	Physically compatible for 4 hr at 23 °C	2226	C
Granisetron HCl	SKB	0.05 mg/mL[a]	ME	20 mg/mL[a]	Physically compatible for 4 hr at 23 °C	2000	C
Hetastarch in lactated electrolyte	AB	6%	ME	20 mg/mL[a]	Physically compatible for 4 hr at 23 °C	2339	C
Hetastarch in sodium chloride 0.9%	DCC	6%	MSD	20 mg/mL[a]	Precipitate in 1 hr at room temperature	1313	I
Hydromorphone HCl	WY	0.2 mg/mL[a]	MSD	20 mg/mL[a]	Physically compatible for 4 hr at 25 °C	987	C
Linezolid	PHU	2 mg/mL	ME	20 mg/mL[a]	Physically compatible for 4 hr at 23 °C	2264	C
Magnesium sulfate	IX	16.7, 33.3, 66.7, 100 mg/mL[a]	MSD	20 mg/mL[a]	Physically compatible for at least 4 hr at 32 °C	813	C
Meperidine HCl	WY	10 mg/mL[a]	MSD	20 mg/mL[a]	Physically compatible for 4 hr at 25 °C	987	C
	WY	10 mg/mL[b]	MSD	40 mg/mL[a]	Physically compatible for 1 hr at 25 °C	1338	C
Morphine sulfate	WI	1 mg/mL[a]	MSD	20 mg/mL[a]	Physically compatible for 4 hr at 25 °C	987	C
	ES	1 mg/mL[b]	MSD	40 mg/mL[a]	Physically compatible for 1 hr at 25 °C	1338	C
Ondansetron HCl	GL	1 mg/mL[b]	MSD	20 mg/mL[a]	Visually compatible for 4 hr at 22 °C	1365	C
Pemetrexed disodium	LI	20 mg/mL[b]	APP	20 mg/mL[a]	Immediate brown discoloration	2564	I
Pentamidine isethionate	FUJ	3 mg/mL[a]	ME	20 mg/mL[c]	Immediate cloudy precipitation	1880	I
Propofol	ZEN	10 mg/mL	ME	20 mg/mL[a]	Physically compatible for 1 hr at 23 °C	2066	C

Y-Site Injection Compatibility (1:1 Mixture) (Cont.)

Cefoxitin sodium

Drug	Mfr	Conc	Mfr	Conc	Remarks	Ref	C/I
Ranitidine HCl	GL	1 mg/mL[b]	BAN	20 mg/mL[b]	Visually compatible. No cefoxitin loss. Under 8% ranitidine loss in 4 hr at 25 °C	2259	C
	GL	1 mg/mL[b]	BAN	20 mg/mL[b]	Visually compatible with no cefoxitin loss and 7% ranitidine loss in 4 hr	2362	C
Remifentanil HCl	GW	0.025 and 0.25 mg/mL[b]	ME	20 mg/mL[a]	Physically compatible for 4 hr at 23 °C	2075	C
Teniposide	BR	0.1 mg/mL[a]	MSD	20 mg/mL[a]	Physically compatible for 4 hr at 23 °C	1725	C
Thiotepa	IMM[e]	1 mg/mL[a]	ME	20 mg/mL[a]	Physically compatible for 4 hr at 23 °C	1861	C
TNA #73[f]		32.5 mL[g]	MSD	20 mg/mL[a]	Visually compatible for 4 hr at 25 °C	1008	C
TNA #218 to #226[f]			ME	20 mg/mL[a]	Visually compatible for 4 hr at 23 °C	2215	C
TPN #61[f]		[h]	MSD	200 mg/ 2.1 mL[i]	Physically compatible	1012	C
		[j]	MSD	1.2 g/ 12.6 mL[i]	Physically compatible	1012	C
TPN #189[f]			MSD	200 mg/mL[k]	Visually compatible for 24 hr at 22 °C	1767	C
TPN #212 to #215[f]			ME	20 mg/mL[a]	Physically compatible for 4 hr at 23 °C	2109	C
Vancomycin HCl	AB	20 mg/mL[a]	ME	180 mg/mL[k]	Transient precipitate forms	2189	?
	AB	20 mg/mL[a]	ME	50 mg/mL[a]	Immediate gross white precipitate	2189	I
	AB	20 mg/mL[a]	ME	10 mg/mL[a]	Visible haze forms in 4 hr at 23 °C	2189	I
	AB	20 mg/mL[a]	ME	1 mg/mL[a]	Physically compatible for 4 hr at 23 °C	2189	C
	AB	2 mg/mL[a]	ME	1[a], 10[a], 50[a], 180[k] mg/mL	Physically compatible for 4 hr at 23 °C	2189	C

[a]*Tested in dextrose 5%.*
[b]*Tested in sodium chloride 0.9%.*
[c]*Tested in dextrose 4%.*
[d]*Tested in premixed infusion solution.*
[e]*Lyophilized formulation tested.*
[f]*Refer to Appendix I for the composition of parenteral nutrition solutions. TNA indicates a 3-in-1 admixture, and TPN indicates a 2-in-1 admixture.*
[g]*A 32.5-mL sample of parenteral nutrition solution combined with 50 mL of antibiotic solution.*
[h]*Run at 21 mL/hr.*
[i]*Given over five minutes by syringe pump.*
[j]*Run at 94 mL/hr.*
[k]*Tested in sterile water for injection.*

CEFTAROLINE FOSAMIL
AHFS 8:12.06.20

Products — Ceftaroline fosamil is available in vials containing 400 and 600 mg of anhydrous ceftaroline fosamil with L-arginine. (1)

Reconstitute the 400- and 600-mg vials with 20 mL of sterile water for injection and mix gently, yielding concentrations of 20- and 30-mg/mL, respectively. (1)

pH — From 4.8 to 6.5. (1)

Trade Name(s) — Teflaro.

Administration — Ceftaroline fosamil is administered by intravenous infusion in 250-mL of compatible infusion solution over approximately one hour. (1)

Stability — Ceftaroline fosamil vials should be stored under refrigeration. The intact vials are stable for no longer than seven days at room temperature. The powder is pale yellowish-white to light yellow in color. After reconstitution, ceftaroline fosamil solution is clear and light to dark yellow in color. (1)

Compatibility Information

Solution Compatibility

Ceftaroline fosamil

Solution	Mfr	Mfr	Conc/L	Remarks	Ref	C/I
Dextrose 2.5%		FOR		Stable for 6 hr at 25 °C and 24 hr at 4 °C	1	**C**
Dextrose 5%		FOR		Stable for 6 hr at 25 °C and 24 hr at 4 °C	1	**C**
Ringer's injection, lactated		FOR		Stable for 6 hr at 25 °C and 24 hr at 4 °C	1	**C**
Sodium chloride 0.45%		FOR		Stable for 6 hr at 25 °C and 24 hr at 4 °C	1	**C**
Sodium chloride 0.9%		FOR		Stable for 6 hr at 25 °C and 24 hr at 4 °C	1	**C**

Y-Site Injection Compatibility (1:1 Mixture)

Ceftaroline fosamil

Drug	Mfr	Conc	Mfr	Conc	Remarks	Ref	C/I
Acyclovir sodium	BV	7 mg/mL[a,b,c]	FOR	2.22 mg/mL[a,b,c]	Physically compatible for 4 hr at 23 °C	2826	**C**
Amikacin sulfate	HOS	5 mg/mL[a,b,c]	FOR	2.22 mg/mL[a,b,c]	Physically compatible for 4 hr at 23 °C	2826	**C**
Aminophylline	AMR	2.5 mg/mL[a,b,c]	FOR	2.22 mg/mL[a,b,c]	Physically compatible for 4 hr at 23 °C	2826	**C**
Amiodarone HCl	SIC	4 mg/mL[a,b,c]	FOR	2.22 mg/mL[a,b,c]	Physically compatible for 4 hr at 23 °C	2826	**C**
Amphotericin B	XGN	0.6 mg/mL[a]	FOR	2.22 mg/mL[a,b,c]	Increased haze and microparticulates	2826	**I**
Azithromycin	BA	2 mg/mL[a,b,c]	FOR	2.22 mg/mL[a,b,c]	Physically compatible for 4 hr at 23 °C	2826	**C**
Bumetanide	HOS	40 mcg/mL[a,b,c]	FOR	2.22 mg/mL[a,b,c]	Physically compatible for 4 hr at 23 °C	2826	**C**
Calcium chloride	AMR	40 mg/mL[a,b,c]	FOR	2.22 mg/mL[a,b,c]	Physically compatible for 4 hr at 23 °C	2826	**C**
Calcium gluconate	ABX	40 mg/mL[a,b,c]	FOR	2.22 mg/mL[a,b,c]	Physically compatible for 4 hr at 23 °C	2826	**C**
Caspofungin acetate	ME	0.5 mg/mL[b,c]	FOR	2.22 mg/mL[a,b,c]	Increased haze and particulates	2826	**I**
Ciprofloxacin	BED	2 mg/mL[a,b,c]	FOR	2.22 mg/mL[a,b,c]	Physically compatible for 4 hr at 23 °C	2826	**C**
Cisatracurium besylate	HOS	0.5 mg/mL[a,b,c]	FOR	2.22 mg/mL[a,b,c]	Physically compatible for 4 hr at 23 °C	2826	**C**
Clindamycin phosphate	BED	10 mg/mL[a,b,c]	FOR	2.22 mg/mL[a,b,c]	Physically compatible for 4 hr at 23 °C	2826	**C**
Cyclosporine	BED	5 mg/mL[a,b,c]	FOR	2.22 mg/mL[a,b,c]	Physically compatible for 4 hr at 23 °C	2826	**C**
Dexamethasone sodium phosphate	SIC	1 mg/mL[a,b,c]	FOR	2.22 mg/mL[a,b,c]	Physically compatible for 4 hr at 23 °C	2826	**C**
Diazepam	HOS	5 mg/mL	FOR	2.22 mg/mL[a,b,c]	Turbid precipitation forms	2826	**I**
Digoxin	BA	0.25 mg/mL	FOR	2.22 mg/mL[a,b,c]	Physically compatible for 4 hr at 23 °C	2826	**C**

Y-Site Injection Compatibility (1:1 Mixture) (Cont.)

Ceftaroline fosamil

Drug	Mfr	Conc	Mfr	Conc	Remarks	Ref	C/I
Diltiazem HCl	HOS	5 mg/mL	FOR	2.22 mg/mL[a,b,c]	Physically compatible for 4 hr at 23 °C	2826	C
Diphenhydramine HCl	BA	2 mg/mL[a,b,c]	FOR	2.22 mg/mL[a,b,c]	Physically compatible for 4 hr at 23 °C	2826	C
Dobutamine HCl	HOS	4 mg/mL[a]	FOR	2.22 mg/mL[a]	Haze increases and particulates appear	2826	I
	HOS	4 mg/mL[b,c]	FOR	2.22 mg/mL[b,c]	Physically compatible for 4 hr at 23 °C	2826	C
Dopamine HCl	HOS	3.2 mg/mL[a,b,c]	FOR	2.22 mg/mL[a,b,c]	Physically compatible for 4 hr at 23 °C	2826	C
Doripenem	SHI	5 mg/mL[b]	FOR	2.22 mg/mL[a,b,c]	Physically compatible for 4 hr at 23 °C	2826	C
Enalaprilat	SIC	0.1 mg/mL[a,b,c]	FOR	2.22 mg/mL[a,b,c]	Physically compatible for 4 hr at 23 °C	2826	C
Esomeprazole sodium	ASZ	0.4 mg/mL[a,b,c]	FOR	2.22 mg/mL[a,b,c]	Physically compatible for 4 hr at 23 °C	2826	C
Famotidine	ABX	2 mg/mL[a,b,c]	FOR	2.22 mg/mL[a,b,c]	Physically compatible for 4 hr at 23 °C	2826	C
Fentanyl citrate	HOS	50 mcg/mL	FOR	2.22 mg/mL[a,b,c]	Physically compatible for 4 hr at 23 °C	2826	C
Filgrastim	AMG	30 mcg/mL[a]	FOR	2.22 mg/mL[a,b,c]	Microparticulates formed	2826	I
Fluconazole	BED	2 mg/mL	FOR	2.22 mg/mL[a,b,c]	Physically compatible for 4 hr at 23 °C	2826	C
Furosemide	HOS	3 mg/mL[a,b,c]	FOR	2.22 mg/mL[a,b,c]	Physically compatible for 4 hr at 23 °C	2826	C
Gentamicin sulfate	HOS	5 mg/mL[a,b,c]	FOR	2.22 mg/mL[a,b,c]	Physically compatible for 4 hr at 23 °C	2826	C
Granisetron HCl	CUP	50 mcg/mL[a,b,c]	FOR	2.22 mg/mL[a,b,c]	Physically compatible for 4 hr at 23 °C	2826	C
Haloperidol lactate	BED	0.2 mg/mL[a,b,c]	FOR	2.22 mg/mL[a,b,c]	Physically compatible for 4 hr at 23 °C	2826	C
Heparin sodium	HOS	100 units/mL	FOR	2.22 mg/mL[a,b,c]	Physically compatible for 4 hr at 23 °C	2826	C
Hydrocortisone sodium succinate	PF	1 mg/mL[a,b,c]	FOR	2.22 mg/mL[a,b,c]	Physically compatible for 4 hr at 23 °C	2826	C
Hydromorphone HCl	HOS	0.5 mg/mL[a,b,c]	FOR	2.22 mg/mL[a,b,c]	Physically compatible for 4 hr at 23 °C	2826	C
Hydroxyzine HCl	ABX	2 mg/mL[a,b,c]	FOR	2.22 mg/mL[a,b,c]	Physically compatible for 4 hr at 23 °C	2826	C
Insulin, regular	NOV	1 unit/mL[a,b,c]	FOR	2.22 mg/mL[a,b,c]	Physically compatible for 4 hr at 23 °C	2826	C
Labetalol HCl	HOS	5 mg/mL	FOR	2.22 mg/mL[a]	Increase in measured haze and microparticulates	2826	I
	HOS	5 mg/mL	FOR	2.22 mg/mL[b,c]	Increase in measured haze	2826	I

Y-Site Injection Compatibility (1:1 Mixture) (Cont.)

Drug	Mfr	Conc	Mfr	Conc	Remarks	Ref	C/I
				Ceftaroline fosamil			
Levofloxacin	OMN	5 mg/mL[a,b,c]	FOR	2.22 mg/mL[a,b,c]	Physically compatible for 4 hr at 23 °C	2826	C
Lidocaine HCl	HOS	10 mg/mL	FOR	2.22 mg/mL[a,b,c]	Physically compatible for 4 hr at 23 °C	2826	C
Lorazepam	HOS	0.5 mg/mL[a,b,c]	FOR	2.22 mg/mL[a,b,c]	Physically compatible for 4 hr at 23 °C	2826	C
Magnesium sulfate	AMR	100 mg/mL[a,b]	FOR	2.22 mg/mL[a,b]	Physically compatible for 4 hr at 23 °C	2826	C
	AMR	100 mg/mL[c]	FOR	2.22 mg/mL[c]	Increase in measured haze	2826	I
Mannitol	HOS	15%	FOR	2.22 mg/mL[a,b,c]	Physically compatible for 4 hr at 23 °C	2826	C
Meperidine HCl	HOS	10 mg/mL[a,b,c]	FOR	2.22 mg/mL[a,b,c]	Physically compatible for 4 hr at 23 °C	2826	C
Methylprednisolone sodium succinate	PHU	5 mg/mL[a,b,c]	FOR	2.22 mg/mL[a,b,c]	Physically compatible for 4 hr at 23 °C	2826	C
Metoclopramide HCl	HOS	5 mg/mL	FOR	2.22 mg/mL[a,b,c]	Physically compatible for 4 hr at 23 °C	2826	C
Metoprolol tartrate	HOS	1 mg/mL	FOR	2.22 mg/mL[a,b,c]	Physically compatible for 4 hr at 23 °C	2826	C
Metronidazole	BA	5 mg/mL	FOR	2.22 mg/mL[a,b,c]	Physically compatible for 4 hr at 23 °C	2826	C
Midazolam HCl	BV	2 mg/mL[a,b,c]	FOR	2.22 mg/mL[a,b,c]	Physically compatible for 4 hr at 23 °C	2826	C
Milrinone lactate	BED	0.2 mg/mL[a,b,c]	FOR	2.22 mg/mL[a,b,c]	Physically compatible for 4 hr at 23 °C	2826	C
Morphine sulfate	BA	15 mg/mL	FOR	2.22 mg/mL[a,b,c]	Physically compatible for 4 hr at 23 °C	2826	C
Moxifloxacin HCl	BAY	1.6 mg/mL	FOR	2.22 mg/mL[a,b,c]	Physically compatible for 4 hr at 23 °C	2826	C
Multivitamins	BA	5 mL/L[a,b,c]	FOR	2.22 mg/mL[a,b,c]	Physically compatible for 4 hr at 23 °C	2826	C
Norepinephrine bitartrate	BED	0.128 mg/mL[a,b,c]	FOR	2.22 mg/mL[a,b,c]	Physically compatible for 4 hr at 23 °C	2826	C
Ondansetron HCl	WOC	1 mg/mL[a,b,c]	FOR	2.22 mg/mL[a,b,c]	Physically compatible for 4 hr at 23 °C	2826	C
Pantoprazole sodium	WY[d]	0.4 mg/mL[a,b,c]	FOR	2.22 mg/mL[a,b,c]	Physically compatible for 4 hr at 23 °C	2826	C
Potassium chloride	HOS	0.1 mEq/mL[a,b,c]	FOR	2.22 mg/mL[a,b,c]	Physically compatible for 4 hr at 23 °C	2826	C
Potassium phosphates	HOS	0.5 mmol/mL[a]	FOR	2.22 mg/mL[a]	Increase in measured haze and microparticulates	2826	I
	HOS	0.5 mmol/mL[b,c]	FOR	2.22 mg/mL[b,c]	Increase in measured haze	2826	I
Promethazine HCl	SIC	2 mg/mL[a,b,c]	FOR	2.22 mg/mL[a,b,c]	Physically compatible for 4 hr at 23 °C	2826	C
Propofol	HOS	10 mg/mL	FOR	2.22 mg/mL[a,b,c]	Physically compatible for 4 hr at 23 °C	2826	C

Y-Site Injection Compatibility (1:1 Mixture) (Cont.)

Ceftaroline fosamil

Drug	Mfr	Conc	Mfr	Conc	Remarks	Ref	C/I
Ranitidine HCl	BED	2 mg/mL[a,b,c]	FOR	2.22 mg/mL[a,b,c]	Physically compatible for 4 hr at 23 °C	2826	C
Remifentanil HCl	HOS	0.25 mg/mL[a,b,c]	FOR	2.22 mg/mL[a,b,c]	Physically compatible for 4 hr at 23 °C	2826	C
Sodium bicarbonate	HOS	1 mEq/mL	FOR	2.22 mg/mL[a,b,c]	Physically compatible for 4 hr at 23 °C	2826	C
Sodium phosphates	HOS	0.5 mmol/mL[a,b,c]	FOR	2.22 mg/mL[a,b,c]	Increase in measured haze	2826	I
Tobramycin sulfate	SIC	5 mg/mL[a,b,c]	FOR	2.22 mg/mL[a,b,c]	Physically compatible for 4 hr at 23 °C	2826	C
Trimethoprim–sulfamethoxazole	SIC	0.8 + 4 mg/mL[a,b,c]	FOR	2.22 mg/mL[a,b,c]	Physically compatible for 4 hr at 23 °C	2826	C
TPN #276[e]			FOR	2.22 mg/mL[a,b,c]	Physically compatible for 4 hr at 23 °C	2826	C
Vasopressin	APP	1 unit/mL[a,b,c]	FOR	2.22 mg/mL[a,b,c]	Physically compatible for 4 hr at 23 °C	2826	C
Voriconazole	PF	4 mg/mL[a,b,c]	FOR	2.22 mg/mL[a,b,c]	Physically compatible for 4 hr at 23 °C	2826	C

[a]*Tested in dextrose 5%.*
[b]*Tested in sodium chloride 0.9%.*
[c]*Tested in Ringer's injection, lactated.*
[d]*Test performed using the formulation WITH edetate disodium.*
[e]*Refer to Appendix I for the composition of parenteral nutrition solutions. TPN indicates a 2-in-1 admixture.*

CEFTAZIDIME
AHFS 8:12.06.12

Products — Ceftazidime is supplied in vials containing 500 mg, 1 g, and 2 g of drug (under reduced pressure), infusion packs containing 1 and 2 g of drug, and 6-g pharmacy bulk packages. The dosage forms contain sodium carbonate 118 mg per gram of ceftazidime. The sodium salt of ceftazidime and carbon dioxide are formed during reconstitution. (1; 4) The use of a venting needle has been suggested for ease of use. (1136) Spraying or leaking of the solution after needle withdrawal has been reported, especially with smaller vials. (1137) The use of larger vials reduces the occurrence of such leakage. (1137; 1138) Care must be taken if a multiple-additive set with a two-way valve is used for reconstitution. The negative pressure in the product may cause inaccuracies in the volume of diluent added to the vial. In one test, almost 3 mL extra entered the vial during reconstitution. (1240) Vials have been vented prior to reconstitution but clamping the tubing from the supply bottle prior to adding the diluent to the vial when multiple-additive sets are used is recommended. (1241)

Ceftazidime is also supplied in frozen solutions containing 1 and 2 g/50 mL of dextrose 4.4 and 3.2%, respectively. (1; 4)

For intramuscular injection, ceftazidime should be reconstituted with sterile water for injection, bacteriostatic water for injection, or lidocaine hydrochloride 0.5 or 1% using 1.5 mL for the 500-mg vial and 3 mL for the 1-g vial. Any carbon dioxide bubbles that are withdrawn into the syringe should be expelled prior to injection. (1; 4)

For direct intravenous injection, ceftazidime should be reconstituted with sterile water for injection. Carbon dioxide will form during dissolution, but the solution will clear in about one to two minutes. (1; 4)

For intravenous infusion, the reconstituted solution can be added to a compatible infusion solution (after expelling any carbon dioxide bubbles that have entered the syringe). Alternatively, the 1- or 2-g infusion packs can be reconstituted with 100 mL of compatible infusion solution, yielding a 10- or 20-mg/mL solution, respectively. (1; 4) To reconstitute the infusion packs, add the diluent in two increments. Initially, add 10 mL with shaking to dissolve the drug. To release the carbon dioxide pressure, insert a venting needle through the closure only after the drug has dissolved and become clear (about one to two minutes). Then add the remaining 90 mL and remove the venting needle. Additional pressure may develop, especially during storage, and should be released prior to use. (4)

The 6-g pharmacy bulk package should be reconstituted with 26 mL of a compatible diluent to yield 30 mL of solution containing 200 mg/mL of ceftazidime. The carbon dioxide pressure that develops should be released using a venting needle. The 200-mg/mL concentrated solution must be diluted further for intravenous use. (1)

Table 1. Reconstitution for Intravenous Injection (1)

Product	Volume of Diluent	Withdrawable Volume	Concentration
500 mg	5.3 mL	5.7 mL	100 mg/mL
1 g	10 mL	10.6 mL	100 mg/mL
2 g	10 mL	11.5 mL	170 mg/mL

pH — From 5 to 8. (1; 4)

Osmolality — The osmolality of ceftazidime (Fortaz, Glaxo) 50 mg/mL was determined to be 321 mOsm/kg in dextrose 5% and 330 mOsm/kg in sodium chloride 0.9%. (1375)

The following maximum ceftazidime concentrations were recommended to achieve osmolalities suitable for peripheral infusion in fluid-restricted patients (1180):

Diluent	Maximum Concentration (mg/mL)	Osmolality (mOsm/kg)
Dextrose 5%	70	503
Sodium chloride 0.9%	63	486
Sterile water for injection	126	302

Sodium Content — Each gram of ceftazidime activity provides 2.3 mEq (54 mg) of sodium from the sodium carbonate present in the formulation. (1; 4)

Trade Name(s) — Fortaz, Tazicef.

Administration — Ceftazidime may be administered by deep intramuscular injection, by direct intravenous injection over three to five minutes directly into a vein or through the tubing of a running compatible infusion solution, or by intermittent intravenous infusion over 15 to 30 minutes. The manufacturer recommends temporarily discontinuing other solutions being administered at the same site during ceftazidime infusion. The drug may be instilled intraperitoneally in a concentration of 250 mg/2 L of compatible dialysis solution. (1; 4)

Stability — Intact vials should be stored at controlled room temperature and protected from light. (1) Approximately 2% decomposition has been reported after 12 months of storage at 37 °C with protection from light. (1136)

Reconstituted ceftazidime solutions are light yellow to amber, depending on the diluent and concentration, and may darken on storage. Color changes do not necessarily indicate a potency loss. (1; 4)

Solutions in sterile water for injection at 95 to 280 mg/mL, in lidocaine hydrochloride 0.5 or 1% or bacteriostatic water for injection at 280 mg/mL, and in sodium chloride 0.9% or dextrose 5% at 10 or 20 mg/mL in piggyback infusion packs are stable for 24 hours at room temperature and seven days under refrigeration. Tazicef and Tazidime in sterile water for injection at 95 to 280 mg/mL or in sodium chloride 0.9% at 10 to 20 mg/mL are stable for 24 hours at room temperature and seven days under refrigeration. (1)

One report of ceftazidime in concentrations of 1, 40, and 333 mg/mL in water indicated no loss after 24 hours at 4 °C and six hours at 25 °C. About a 4 to 6% loss was reported after 24 hours at 25 °C. (1136)

Ceftazidime vials reconstituted with sterile water for injection to a concentration of 270 mg/mL were evaluated for stability at four temper-

atures. About 8 to 9% ceftazidime loss occurred in 7 days under refrigeration at 4 °C and in 4 days at 10 °C. At 20 °C about 7 to 8% loss occurred in 24 hours, but at a higher room temperature of 30 °C about 5% loss occurred in six hours and 12% loss occurred in 18 hours. (2285)

Freezing Solutions — Ceftazidime products differ in their reported stabilities, both during frozen storage of their solutions and after thawing. Table 2 summarizes the reported stabilities. (4)

The commercially available frozen ceftazidime solutions (Fortaz, Glaxo) of 1 and 2 g/50 ml of sodium chloride 0.9%, when thawed, are stable for 24 hours at room temperature or seven days under refrigeration. (4)

Ceftazidime (Fortaz, Glaxo) 1 g/50 mL in sodium chloride 0.9% was stored frozen at −20 °C. About 7% loss occurred in 97 days. After thawing at room temperature, subsequent storage refrigerated for 4 days and at room temperature for 24 hours resulted in additional loss with only about 90% of the ceftazidime remaining. (500)

Less than a 2% ceftazidime (Fortaz, Glaxo) loss was reported from a solution containing 36.6 mg/mL in sterile water for injection in PVC and glass containers after 30 days at −20 °C. Subsequent thawing and storage for four days at 5 °C, followed by 24 hours at 37 °C to simulate the use of a portable infusion pump, resulted in little additional ceftazidime loss. (1391)

Ceftazidime (Fortaz, Glaxo) 100 and 200 mg/mL in sterile water for injection in glass vials and polypropylene syringes (Becton Dickinson) was stored frozen at −20 °C for 91 days followed by eight hours at 22 °C. Losses of about 5 and 10% occurred in the 100- and 200-mg/mL concentrations, respectively. Freezing at −20 °C for 91 days followed by refrigeration at 4 °C for four days resulted in losses of about 10 and 6% in the 100- and 200-mg/mL concentrations, respectively. Particle counts remained within USP limits throughout the study. (1580)

Usually, frozen solutions should be thawed at room temperature or under refrigeration. Other techniques are not recommended. Thawed solutions should not be refrozen. (1; 4)

Light Effects — Ceftazidime reconstituted with sterile water for injection to a concentration of 270 mg/mL exhibited no substantial difference in stability when stored protected from light or exposed to daylight. (2285)

Table 2. Reported Stabilities of Frozen and Thawed Solutions of Ceftazidime Products (1; 4)

Concentration	Fortaz	Tazicef
280 mg/mL	3 months[a]	3 months[a]
Thawed/RT[b]	8 hr	8 hr
Thawed/4 °C[c]	4 days	4 days
100 to 180 mg/mL	6 months[a,d]	3 months[e]
Thawed/RT	24 hr	8 hr
Thawed/4 °C	7 days	4 days
10 to 20 mg/mL[f]	9 months[a]	
Thawed/RT	24 hr	
Thawed/4 °C	7 days	

[a] *In sterile water for injection.*
[b] *Thawed and stored at room temperature.*
[c] *Thawed and stored at 4 to 5 °C.*
[d] *In sodium chloride 0.9%.*
[e] *In sodium chloride 0.9% and dextrose 5%.*
[f] *In infusion packs.*

Syringes — Ceftazidime (Fortaz, Glaxo) 100 and 200 mg/mL in sterile water for injection in polypropylene syringes (Becton Dickinson) and glass vials exhibited a 5% or less loss in eight hours at 22 °C and 96 hours at 4 °C. (1580)

Ceftazidime (Hospira) 1 mg/mL in sodium chloride 0.9% in plastic syringes was stored at room temperature, refrigerated, and frozen at −20 °C. About 10% ceftazidime loss occurred in 3 days at room temperature and in 17 days refrigerated. No loss occurred in the frozen samples over 60 days. (2793)

Ambulatory Pumps — Ceftazidime (Fortaz, Glaxo) at a concentration of 60 mg/mL in water for injection was filled into PVC portable infusion pump reservoirs (Pharmacia Deltec). Storage at −20 °C resulted in less than 3% loss in 14 days. The thawed reservoirs were then stored under refrigeration at 6 °C. Losses totaled 10% after five days of refrigerated storage. Under simulated use conditions at 30 °C, ceftazidime decomposes at a rate of about 10% in 18 hours. The authors concluded prefilling of reservoirs with ceftazidime solutions for home use was not advisable. (2008)

Central Venous Catheter — Ceftazidime (Fortaz, Glaxo Wellcome) 10 mg/mL in dextrose 5% was found to be compatible with the ARROWg+ard Blue Plus (Arrow International) chlorhexidine-bearing triple-lumen central catheter. Furthermore, chlorhexidine delivered from the catheter remained at trace amounts with no substantial increase due to the delivery of the drug through the catheter. (2335)

Ceftazidime 10 mg/mL with heparin sodium 5000 units/mL as an antibiotic lock in polyurethane central hemodialysis catheters lost about 50% of the antibiotic over 72 hours at 37 °C. The loss was attributed to sorption to the catheters. Nevertheless, the reduced antibiotic concentration (about 5 mg/mL) remained effective against common microorganisms in catheter-related bacteremia in hemodialysis patients. (2515; 2516)

Compatibility Information

Solution Compatibility

Ceftazidime

Solution	Mfr	Mfr	Conc/L	Remarks	Ref	C/I
Amino acids 5%, dextrose 25%	AB	GL	6 g	No substantial amino acid degradation in 48 hr at 22 °C and 10 days at 4 °C. Ceftazidime stability the determining factor	1535	C
Dextrose–saline combinations			1 to 40 g	Physically and chemically stable for 24 hr at room temperature and 7 days refrigerated	1	C
Dextrose 5% in sodium chloride 0.9%		GL	20 g	5% loss in 24 hr at 25 °C and no loss in 48 hr at 4 °C	1136	C
Dextrose 5%			1 to 40 g	Physically and chemically stable for 24 hr at room temperature and 7 days refrigerated	1	C
	MG[a]	GL	20 g	Physically compatible with 5% drug loss in 24 hr and 9% in 48 hr at 25 °C under fluorescent light	1026	C
		GL	20 g	6% loss in 24 hr at 25 °C. No loss in 24 hr and 3% loss in 48 hr at 4 °C	1136	C
	TR[a]		40 g	Physically compatible with 8% loss in 2 days at 25 °C, 6% loss in 21 days at 5 °C, and 6% loss in 90 days at −10 °C	1341	C
	[b]	GL	40 g	Physically compatible with 7% loss in 1 day and 19% loss in 3 days at 23 °C; 8% loss in 10 days at 4 °C	1353	C
	BA[b]	GL	2 and 6 g	Visually compatible with 7 to 9% loss in 24 hr at room temperature	1937	C
	[b]		4 g	Visually compatible with little or no loss in 24 hr at room temperature and 4 °C	1953	C
	BA[b], BRN[a,c]	GW	10 g	Visually compatible with little or no loss in 24 hr at 4 and 22 °C	2289	C
	BA[d]	GW	40 g	10% loss in about 12 hr at 37 °C in the dark	2421	I
	[f]	GW	40 g	Losses of 5, 8, and 10% in 20 hr at 20 °C, and losses of 9, 17, and 21% in 20 hr at 35 °C in glass, polypropylene, and PVC containers, respectively	2539	C
Dextrose 10%			1 to 40 g	Physically and chemically stable for 24 hr at room temperature and 7 days refrigerated	1	C

Solution Compatibility (Cont.)

Solution	Mfr	Mfr	Conc/L	Remarks	Ref	C/I
Ringer's injection			1 to 40 g	Physically and chemically stable for 24 hr at room temperature and 7 days refrigerated	1	C
Ringer's injection, lactated			1 to 40 g	Physically and chemically stable for 24 hr at room temperature and 7 days refrigerated	1	C
		GL	20 g	6% loss in 24 hr at 25 °C and 1% loss in 48 hr at 4 °C	1136	C
Sodium chloride 0.9%			1 to 40 g	Physically and chemically stable for 24 hr at room temperature and 7 days refrigerated	1	C
	MG[a]	GL	20 g	Physically compatible with 2% drug loss in 24 hr and 5% in 48 hr at 25 °C under fluorescent light	1026	C
		GL	20 g	7% loss in 24 hr at 25 °C and no loss in 48 hr at 4 °C	1136	C
	TR[a]		40 g	Physically compatible with 5% loss in 2 days and 12% loss in 3 days at 25 °C; 7% loss in 28 days at 5 °C and 6% loss in 90 days at −10 °C	1341	C
	[b]	GL	40 g	Physically compatible with 3% loss in 1 day and 14% loss in 3 days at 25 °C; 10% loss in 14 days at 5 °C	1353	C
	BA[b]	GL	2 and 6 g	Visually compatible with 4 to 6% loss in 24 hr at room temperature	1937	C
	[b]		4 g	Visually compatible with little or no loss in 24 hr at room temperature and 4 °C	1953	C
	KA[h]	GL	60 g	Visually compatible with little or no loss of ceftazidime and little formation of pyridine in 14 days frozen at −20 °C	2113	C
	KA[h]	GL	60 g	Visually compatible with 9% loss of ceftazidime but formation of potentially toxic pyridine 0.53 mg/mL in 14 days at 4 °C	2113	?
	BA[b], BRN[a,c]	GW	10 g	Visually compatible with little or no loss in 24 hr at 4 and 22 °C	2289	C
	BA[d]	GW	40 g	10% loss occurred in about 12 to 16 hr at 37 °C in the dark	2421	I
	[f]	GW	40 g	Losses of 1, 3, and 6% in 20 hr at 20 °C, and losses of 6, 11, and 13% in 20 hr at 35 °C in glass, polypropylene, and PVC containers, respectively	2539	C
Sodium lactate ⅙ M			1 to 40 g	Physically and chemically stable for 24 hr at room temperature and 7 days refrigerated	1	C
TPN #107[g]			1 g	Activity retained for 24 hr at 21 °C	1326	C
TPN #141 to #143[g]		GL	1 g	Visually compatible with 8% ceftazidime loss in 6 hr and 10% loss in 24 hr at 22 °C. 8% ceftazidime loss in 3 days at 4 °C	1535	C
		GL	6 g	Visually compatible with 6% ceftazidime loss in 12 hr and 11 to 13% loss in 24 hr at 22 °C. 7 to 9% ceftazidime loss in 3 days at 4 °C	1535	C

[a]Tested in glass containers.
[b]Tested in PVC containers.
[c]Tested in polyethylene plastic containers.
[d]Tested in Infusor LV 10 (elastomeric), Easypump LT 125 (elastomeric), Ultra-Flow (PVC), and Outbound (polyethylene) infusion device reservoirs.
[e]Tested in Singleday Infusors (Baxter).
[f]Tested in glass, polypropylene, and PVC containers.
[g]Refer to Appendix I for the composition of parenteral nutrition solutions. TPN indicates a 2-in-1 admixture.
[h]Tested in elastomeric ambulatory pumps (Homepump, Block Medical).

Additive Compatibility

Ceftazidime

Drug	Mfr	Conc/L	Mfr	Conc/L	Test Soln	Remarks	Ref	C/I
Amikacin sulfate	BR	25 mg	GL	50 mg	D5W	28% loss of amikacin in 2 hr at 22 °C	504	I
	BR	15 mg	GL	50 mg	D5W	17% loss of amikacin in 24 hr at 22 °C	504	I
Aminophylline	ES	1 g	GL	2 g	D5W, NS	20 to 23% ceftazidime loss in 6 hr at room temperature	1937	I
	ES	1 g	GL	6 g	D5W, NS	8 to 10% ceftazidime loss in 6 hr at room temperature	1937	I
	ES	2 g	GL	2 g	D5W, NS	35 to 40% ceftazidime loss in 6 hr at room temperature	1937	I
	ES	2 g	GL	6 g	D5W, NS	22% ceftazidime loss in 6 hr at room temperature	1937	I
Ciprofloxacin	MI	2 g		20 g	D5W	Physically incompatible	888	I
	BAY	2 g	SKB	19.8 g	D5W	Visually compatible but pH changed by more than 1 unit	2413	?
Clindamycin phosphate	UP	9 g	GL	20 g	D5W[b]	Physically compatible with 9% clindamycin loss and 11% ceftazidime loss in 48 hr at 25 °C under fluorescent light	1026	C
	UP	9 g	GL	20 g	NS[b]	Physically compatible with 5% clindamycin loss and 7% ceftazidime loss in 48 hr at 25 °C under fluorescent light	1026	C
Floxacillin sodium	GSK	40 g	GSK	40 g	NS, W	Physically compatible. Under 10% loss in 24 hr at room temperature and 4 °C	2658	C
	GSK	120 g	GSK	60 g	NS, W	Physically compatible. Under 10% loss in 24 hr at room temperature and 4 °C	2658	C
	GSK	240 g	GSK	180 g	NS, W	Physically compatible. Under 10% loss in 24 hr at room temperature and 4 °C	2658	C
Fluconazole	PF	1 g	GL	20 g	D5W	Visually compatible with no fluconazole loss in 72 hr at 25 °C under fluorescent light. Ceftazidime not tested	1677	C
Gentamicin sulfate	SC	6 and 9 mg	GL	50 mg	D5W	10 to 20% gentamicin loss in 2 hr at 22 °C	504	I
Heparin sodium		10,000 and 50,000 units		4 g	D5W, NS	Ceftazidime stable for 24 hr at room temperature and 7 days refrigerated	4	C
Linezolid	PHU	2 g	GW	20 g	[c]	Physically compatible with no linezolid loss in 7 days at 4 and 23 °C protected from light. Ceftazidime losses of 5% in 24 hr and 12% in 3 days at 23 °C and about 3% in 7 days at 4 °C	2262	C
Metronidazole		5 g	GL	20 g		No loss of either drug in 4 hr	1345	C
	AB	5 g	LI	10 g		Visually compatible with little or no loss of either drug in 72 hr at 8 °C	1849	C
Potassium chloride		10 and 40 mEq		4 g	D5W, NS	Ceftazidime stable for 24 hr at room temperature and 7 days refrigerated	4	C
Ranitidine HCl	GL	500 mg	GL	10 g	D2.5½S	8% ranitidine loss in 4 hr and 37% loss in 24 hr at 22 °C	1632	I
Sodium bicarbonate		4.2%	GL	20 g		11% ceftazidime loss in 24 hr at 25 °C. 3% loss in 48 hr at 4 °C	1136	C

Additive Compatibility (Cont.)

Ceftazidime

Drug	Mfr	Conc/L	Mfr	Conc/L	Test Soln	Remarks	Ref	C/I
Tenoxicam	RC	200 mg	LI	5 g	D5W[a]	Visually compatible for up to 72 hr with yellow discoloration. 10% loss of ceftazidime in 96 hr and of tenoxicam in 168 hr at 4 and 25 °C	2557	C
	RC	200 mg	LI	5 g	D5W[b]	Visually compatible with about 10% loss of both drugs in 168 hr at 4 and 25 °C	2557	C

[a]Tested in PVC containers.
[b]Tested in glass containers.
[c]Admixed in the linezolid infusion container.

Drugs in Syringe Compatibility

Ceftazidime

Drug (in syringe)	Mfr	Amt	Mfr	Amt	Remarks	Ref	C/I
Dimenhydrinate		10 mg/ 1 mL		100 mg/ 1 mL	Clear solution	2569	C
Hydromorphone HCl	KN	2, 10, 40 mg/ 1 mL	GL	180 mg/ 1 mL	Visually compatible with less than 10% loss of either drug in 24 hr at room temperature	2082	C
Pantoprazole sodium	[a]	4 mg/ 1 mL		100 mg/ 1 mL	Precipitates immediately	2574	I

[a]Test performed using the formulation WITHOUT edetate disodium.

Y-Site Injection Compatibility (1:1 Mixture)

Ceftazidime

Drug	Mfr	Conc	Mfr	Conc	Remarks	Ref	C/I
Acetylcysteine		100 mg/mL	GSK	120 mg/mL[k]	Over 10% ceftazidime loss occurs in 1 hr	2513	I
Acyclovir sodium	BW	5 mg/mL[a]	SKF	20 mg/mL[a]	Physically compatible for 4 hr at 25 °C	1157	C
Allopurinol sodium	BW	3 mg/mL[b]	LI	40 mg/mL[a]	Physically compatible for 4 hr at 22 °C	1686	C
Amifostine	USB	10 mg/mL[a]	LI	40 mg/mL[a]	Physically compatible for 4 hr at 23 °C	1845	C
Amikacin sulfate		1.5 mg/mL	SKB	125 mg/mL	Visually compatible with less than 10% loss of both drugs in 1 hr	2434	C
		15 mg/mL	GSK	120 mg/mL[k]	Physically compatible with less than 10% ceftazidime loss. Amikacin not tested	2513	C
Aminophylline	ES	2 mg/mL[a]	GL	40 mg/mL[a]	Visually compatible with 4% ceftazidime loss and 9% theophylline loss in 2 hr at room temperature	1937	C
	ES	2 mg/mL[a]	GL	40 mg/mL[b]	Visually compatible with 5% ceftazidime loss and 4% theophylline loss in 2 hr at room temperature	1937	C
Amiodarone HCl	WY	6 mg/mL[a]	GW	40 mg/mL[a]	Immediate opaque white turbidity	2352	I
Amphotericin B cholesteryl sulfate complex	SEQ	0.83 mg/mL[a]	SKB	40 mg/mL[a]	Increased turbidity forms in 4 hr at 23 °C	2117	I
Amsacrine	NCI	1 mg/mL[a]	GL	40 mg/mL[a]	Immediate orange precipitate	1381	I
Anidulafungin	VIC	0.5 mg/mL[a]	GSK	40 mg/mL[a]	Physically compatible for 4 hr at 23 °C	2617	C

Y-Site Injection Compatibility (1:1 Mixture) (Cont.)

Ceftazidime

Drug	Mfr	Conc	Mfr	Conc	Remarks	Ref	C/I
Azithromycin	PF	2 mg/mL[b]	GW	80 mg/mL[c,d]	Amber and white microcrystals found	2368	I
Aztreonam	SQ	40 mg/mL[a]	LI	40 mg/mL[a]	Physically compatible for 4 hr at 23 °C	1758	C
Bivalirudin	TMC	5 mg/mL[a]	GW	40 mg/mL[a]	Physically compatible for 4 hr at 23 °C	2373	C
Caspofungin acetate	ME	0.7 mg/mL[b]	GSK	40 mg/mL[b]	Immediate white turbid precipitate forms	2758	I
Ciprofloxacin	MI	1 mg/mL[a]	SKF	20 mg/mL[f]	Physically compatible for 24 hr at 22 °C	1189	C
Cisatracurium besylate	GW	0.1 and 2 mg/mL[a]	SKB	40 mg/mL[a]	Physically compatible for 4 hr at 23 °C	2074	C
	GW	5 mg/mL[a]	SKB	40 mg/mL[a]	Subvisible haze forms immediately	2074	I
Clarithromycin		50 mg/mL	SKB	125 mg/mL	Precipitates immediately	2434	I
		10 mg/mL	SKB	125 mg/mL	Trace precipitation	2434	I
		50 mg/mL	GSK	120 mg/mL[k]	Precipitates	2513	I
Daptomycin	CUB	16.7 mg/mL[b,e]	GSK	16.7 mg/mL[b,e]	Physically compatible with no loss of either drug in 2 hr at 25 °C	2553	C
Dexmedetomidine HCl	AB	4 mcg/mL[b]	GW	40 mg/mL[b]	Physically compatible for 4 hr at 23 °C	2383	C
Diltiazem HCl	MMD	5 mg/mL	GL	10 and 170 mg/mL[b]	Visually compatible	1807	C
	MMD	1 mg/mL[b]	GL	170 mg/mL[b]	Visually compatible	1807	C
Dobutamine HCl		1 mg/mL	GSK	120 mg/mL[k]	Physically compatible with less than 10% ceftazidime loss. Dobutamine not tested	2513	C
		250 mg/mL	GSK	120 mg/mL[k]	Precipitates	2513	I
Docetaxel	RPR	0.9 mg/mL[a]	SKB	40 mg/mL[a]	Physically compatible for 4 hr at 23 °C	2224	C
Dopamine HCl		0.4 mg/mL	GSK	120 mg/mL[k]	Physically compatible with less than 10% ceftazidime loss. Dopamine not tested	2513	C
Doxapram HCl	RB	2 mg/mL[a]	GW	40 mg/mL[a]	Visually compatible for 4 hr at 23 °C	2470	C
Doxorubicin HCl liposomal	SEQ	0.4 mg/mL[a]	SKB	40 mg/mL[a]	Partial loss of measured natural turbidity	2087	I
Enalaprilat	MSD	0.05 mg/mL[b]	GL	10 mg/mL[a]	Physically compatible for 24 hr at room temperature under fluorescent light	1355	C
Epinephrine HCl		50 mcg/mL	GSK	120 mg/mL[k]	Physically compatible with less than 10% ceftazidime loss. Epinephrine not tested	2513	C
Erythromycin lactobionate		50 mg/mL	SKB	125 mg/mL	Precipitates immediately	2434	I
		10 mg/mL	SKB	125 mg/mL	Trace precipitation	2434	I
		5 mg/mL	GSK	120 mg/mL[k]	Precipitates	2513	I
Esmolol HCl	DCC	10 mg/mL[a]	GL	10 mg/mL[a]	Physically compatible for 24 hr at 22 °C	1169	C
Etoposide phosphate	BR	5 mg/mL[a]	SKB	40 mg/mL[a]	Physically compatible for 4 hr at 23 °C	2218	C
Famotidine	MSD	0.2 mg/mL[a]	GL	20 mg/mL[b]	Physically compatible for 14 hr	1196	C
	ME	2 mg/mL[b]		20 mg/mL[a]	Visually compatible for 4 hr at 22 °C	1936	C
Fenoldopam mesylate	AB	80 mcg/mL[b]	GW	40 mg/mL[b]	Physically compatible for 4 hr at 23 °C	2467	C
Filgrastim	AMG	30 mcg/mL[a]	LI	40 mg/mL[a]	Physically compatible for 4 hr at 22 °C	1687	C
	AMG	10[g] and 40[a] mcg/mL	LI	10 mg/mL[a]	Visually compatible. Little loss of filgrastim and fluconazole in 4 hr at 25 °C	2060	C
Fluconazole	RR	2 mg/mL	GL	20 mg/mL	Precipitates immediately	1407	I
		2 mg/mL	SKB	125 mg/mL	Visually compatible with less than 10% loss of ceftazidime in 30 min. Fluconazole not tested	2434	C
		2 mg/mL	GSK	120 mg/mL[k]	Physically compatible with less than 10% ceftazidime loss. Fluconazole not tested	2513	C

Y-Site Injection Compatibility (1:1 Mixture) (Cont.)

Drug	Mfr	Conc	Mfr	Conc	Remarks	Ref	C/I
				Ceftazidime			
Fludarabine phosphate	BX	1 mg/mL[a]	GL	40 mg/mL[a]	Visually compatible for 4 hr at 22 °C	1439	C
Foscarnet sodium	AST	24 mg/mL	GL	20 mg/mL	Physically compatible for 24 hr at room temperature under fluorescent light	1335	C
	AST	24 mg/mL	GL	20 mg/mL[f]	Physically compatible for 24 hr at 25 °C under fluorescent light	1393	C
Furosemide		10 mg/mL	SKB	125 mg/mL	Visually compatible with less than 10% loss of ceftazidime in 30 min. Furosemide not tested	2434	C
		10 mg/mL	GSK	120 mg/mL[k]	Physically compatible with less than 10% ceftazidime loss. Furosemide not tested	2513	C
Gallium nitrate	FUJ	1 mg/mL[b]	LI	100 mg/mL[b]	Visually compatible for 24 hr at 25 °C	1673	C
Gemcitabine HCl	LI	10 mg/mL[b]	SKB	40 mg/mL[b]	Physically compatible for 4 hr at 23 °C	2226	C
Gentamicin sulfate		0.6 mg/mL	SKB	125 mg/mL	Visually compatible with less than 10% loss of both drugs in 1 hr	2434	C
		6 mg/mL	GSK	120 mg/mL[k]	Physically compatible with less than 10% ceftazidime loss. Gentamicin not tested	2513	C
Granisetron HCl	SKB	1 mg/mL	SKB	16.7 mg/mL[b]	Physically compatible with little or no loss of either drug in 4 hr at 22 °C	1883	C
Heparin sodium	TR	50 units/mL	LI	20 mg/mL	Visually compatible for 4 hr at 25 °C	1793	C
Hetastarch in lactated electrolyte	AB	6%	GW	40 mg/mL[a]	Physically compatible for 4 hr at 23 °C	2339	C
Hydromorphone HCl	KN	2, 10, 40 mg/mL	GL	40[a] and 180 mg/mL	Visually compatible and both drugs stable for 24 hr	1532	C
Idarubicin HCl	AD	1 mg/mL[b]	LI	20 mg/mL[a]	Haze forms in 1 hr	1525	I
Insulin, regular		100 units/mL	GSK	120 mg/mL[k]	Physically compatible with less than 10% ceftazidime loss. Insulin not tested	2513	C
Isosorbide dinitrate		0.2 mg/mL	GSK	120 mg/mL[k]	Physically compatible with less than 10% ceftazidime loss. Isosorbide not tested	2513	C
Ketamine HCl		10 mg/mL	SKB	125 mg/mL	Visually compatible with less than 10% loss of ceftazidime in 24 hr. Ketamine not tested	2434	C
		10 mg/mL	GSK	120 mg/mL[k]	Physically compatible with less than 10% ceftazidime loss. Ketamine not tested	2513	C
Labetalol HCl	SC	1 mg/mL[a]	GL	10 mg/mL[a]	Physically compatible for 24 hr at 18 °C	1171	C
Linezolid	PHU	2 mg/mL	SKB	40 mg/mL[a]	Physically compatible for 4 hr at 23 °C	2264	C
Melphalan HCl	BW	0.1 mg/mL[b]	LI	40 mg/mL[b]	Physically compatible for 3 hr at 22 °C	1557	C
Meperidine HCl	AB	10 mg/mL	LI	20 and 40 mg/mL[a]	Physically compatible for 4 hr at 25 °C	1397	C
Methylprednisolone sodium succinate		50 mg/mL	GSK	120 mg/mL[k]	Physically compatible. Less than 10% ceftazidime loss. Methylprednisolone not tested	2513	C
Midazolam HCl	RC	1 mg/mL[a]	LI	20 mg/mL[a]	Haze forms in 1 hr	1847	I
		5 mg/mL	SKB	125 mg/mL	Precipitates immediately	2434	I
		5 mg/mL	GSK	120 mg/mL[k]	Precipitates	2513	I
Milrinone lactate	SS	0.2 mg/mL[a]	GW	100 mg/mL[a]	Visually compatible for 4 hr at 25 °C	2381	C
Morphine sulfate	AB	1 mg/mL	LI	20 and 40 mg/mL[a]	Physically compatible for 4 hr at 25 °C	1397	C

Y-Site Injection Compatibility (1:1 Mixture) (Cont.)

Ceftazidime

Drug	Mfr	Conc	Mfr	Conc	Remarks	Ref	C/I
		1 mg/mL	GSK	120 mg/mL[k]	Physically compatible with less than 10% ceftazidime loss. Morphine not tested	2513	C
Nicardipine HCl	DCC	0.1 mg/mL[a]	GL	10 mg/mL[a]	Visually compatible for 24 hr at room temperature	235	C
		1 mg/mL	SKB	125 mg/mL	Precipitates immediately	2434	I
		1 mg/mL	GSK	120 mg/mL[k]	Precipitates	2513	I
Ondansetron HCl	GL	1 mg/mL[b]	GL	40 mg/mL[a]	Visually compatible for 4 hr at 22 °C	1365	C
	GL	16 to 160 mcg/mL		100 to 200 mg/mL	Physically compatible when ceftazidime given as 5-min bolus via Y-site	1366	C
	GL	0.03 and 0.3 mg/mL[a]	LI	40 mg/mL[a]	Visually compatible with less than 10% loss of either drug in 4 hr at 25 °C	1732	C
Paclitaxel	NCI	1.2 mg/mL[a]	LI	40 mg/mL[a]	Physically compatible for 4 hr at 22 °C	1556	C
Pemetrexed disodium	LI	20 mg/mL[b]	GW	40 mg/mL[a]	Color darkening and brownish discoloration occur over 4 hr	2564	I
Pentamidine isethionate	FUJ	3 mg/mL[a]	LI	20 mg/mL[a]	Fine precipitate forms immediately	1880	I
Phenytoin sodium		50 mg/mL	GSK	120 mg/mL[k]	Precipitates	2513	I
Propofol	ZEN	10 mg/mL	SKB	40 mg/mL[a]	Physically compatible for 1 hr at 23 °C	2066	C
		1 mg/mL	SKB	125 mg/mL	Physically incompatible	2434	I
		1 mg/mL	GSK	120 mg/mL[k]	Precipitates	2513	I
Ranitidine HCl	GL	1 mg/mL[b]	GL	20 mg/mL[a]	8% ranitidine loss and no ceftazidime loss in 4 hr at 22 °C	1632	C
Remifentanil HCl		0.2 mg/mL	GSK	120 mg/mL[k]	Physically compatible with less than 10% ceftazidime loss. Remifentanil not tested	2513	C
Sargramostim	IMM	10 mcg/mL[b]	GL	40 mg/mL[b]	Particles and filaments form in 4 hr	1436	I
	IMM	6[h] and 15 mcg/mL[b]	LI	40 mg/mL[f]	Visually compatible for 2 hr	1618	C
Sufentanil citrate		50 mcg/mL	SKB	125 mg/mL	Visually compatible with less than 10% loss of ceftazidime in 24 hr. Sufentanil not tested	2434	C
		5 mcg/mL	GSK	120 mg/mL[k]	Physically compatible with less than 10% ceftazidime loss. Sufentanil not tested	2513	C
Tacrolimus	FUJ	1 mg/mL[b]	GL	20 mg/mL[a]	Visually compatible for 24 hr at 25 °C	1630	C
	FUJ	10 and 40 mcg/mL[a]	GW	40 and 200 mg/mL[a]	Visually compatible with no loss of either drug in 4 hr at 24 °C	2216	C
Telavancin HCl	ASP	7.5 mg/mL[a,b,l]	HOS	40 mg/mL	Physically compatible for 2 hr	2830	C
Teniposide	BR	0.1 mg/mL[a]	LI	40 mg/mL[a]	Physically compatible for 4 hr at 23 °C	1725	C
Theophylline	TR	4 mg/mL	LI	20 mg/mL	Visually compatible for 6 hr at 25 °C	1793	C
		20 mg/mL	GSK	120 mg/mL[k]	Over 25% ceftazidime loss in 1 hr	2513	I
Thiotepa	IMM[i]	1 mg/mL[a]	LI	40 mg/mL[a]	Physically compatible for 4 hr at 23 °C	1861	C
Tigecycline	WY	1 mg/mL[b]		40 mg/mL[b]	Physically compatible for 4 hr	2714	C
TNA #218 to #226[j]			SKB	40 mg/mL[a]	Visually compatible for 4 hr at 23 °C	2215	C
Tobramycin sulfate		0.6 mg/mL	SKB	125 mg/mL	Visually compatible with less than 10% loss of both drugs in 1 hr	2434	C
		6 mg/mL	GSK	120 mg/mL[k]	Physically compatible with less than 10% ceftazidime loss. Tobramycin not tested	2513	C

Y-Site Injection Compatibility (1:1 Mixture) (Cont.)

Drug	Mfr	Conc	Mfr	Conc	Remarks	Ref	C/I
				Ceftazidime			
TPN #141 to #143[j]			GL	40 mg/mL[f]	Visually compatible with 4% or less ceftazidime loss in 2 hr at 22 °C in 1:1 and 1:3 ratios	1535	C
TPN #189[j]			GL	200 mg/mL[k]	Visually compatible for 24 hr at 22 °C	1767	C
TPN #203, #204[j]			LI	60 mg/mL	Visually compatible for 2 hr at 23 °C	1974	C
TPN #212 to #215[j]			SKB	40 mg/mL[a]	Physically compatible for 4 hr at 23 °C	2109	C
Valproate sodium		100 mg/mL	SKB	125 mg/mL	Physically compatible. Under 10% ceftazidime loss. Valproate not tested	2434	C
		100 mg/mL	GSK	120 mg/mL[k]	Physically compatible. Under 10% ceftazidime loss. Valproate not tested	2513	C
Vancomycin HCl		10 mg/mL[a]		50 mg/mL[k]	Precipitates immediately	873	I
	AB	20 mg/mL[a]	SKB	10[a], 50[a], 200[k] mg/mL	Gross white precipitate forms immediately	2189	I
	AB	20 mg/mL[a]	SKB	1 mg/mL[a]	Physically compatible for 4 hr at 23 °C	2189	C
	AB	2 mg/mL[a]	SKB	1[a], 10[a], 50[a], 200[k] mg/mL	Physically compatible for 4 hr at 23 °C	2189	C
		30 mg/mL	SKB	125 mg/mL	Precipitates immediately	2434	I
		30 mg/mL	GSK	120 mg/mL[k]	Precipitates	2513	I
Vinorelbine tartrate	BW	1 mg/mL[b]	LI	40 mg/mL[b]	Physically compatible for 4 hr at 22 °C	1558	C
Warfarin sodium	DME	2 mg/mL[k]	SKB	20 mg/mL[a]	Haze forms in 24 hr at 24 °C	2078	I
Zidovudine	BW	4 mg/mL[a]	GL	20 mg/mL[a]	Physically compatible for 4 hr at 25 °C	1193	C

[a]*Tested in dextrose 5%.*
[b]*Tested in sodium chloride 0.9%.*
[c]*Tested in sodium chloride 0.45%.*
[d]*Injected via Y-site into an administration set running azithromycin.*
[e]*Final concentration after mixing.*
[f]*Tested in both dextrose 5% and sodium chloride 0.9%.*
[g]*Tested in dextrose 5% with human albumin 2 mg/mL.*
[h]*With human albumin 0.1%.*
[i]*Lyophilized formulation tested.*
[j]*Refer to Appendix I for the composition of parenteral nutrition solutions. TNA indicates a 3-in-1 admixture, and TPN indicates a 2-in-1 admixture.*
[k]*Tested in sterile water for injection.*
[l]*Tested in Ringer's injection, lactated.*

Additional Compatibility Information

Peritoneal Dialysis Solutions — Ceftazidime 2 mg/mL in Dianeal with dextrose 1.5% is stated to be stable for 10 days under refrigeration, 24 hours at room temperature, and at least four hours at 37 °C. (4)

Ceftazidime (Glaxo) 125 mg/L and tobramycin sulfate (Lilly) 8 mg/L in Dianeal PD-2 with dextrose 2.5% (Baxter) were visually compatible and chemically stable. After 16 hours of storage at 25 °C under fluorescent light, the loss of both drugs was less than 3%. Additional storage for eight hours at 37 °C, to simulate the maximum peritoneal dwell time, showed tobramycin sulfate concentrations of 96% and ceftazidime concentrations of 92 to 96%. (1652)

Ceftazidime (Glaxo) 0.1 mg/mL in Dianeal PD-2 with dextrose 1.5% in PVC containers was physically and chemically stable for 24 hours at 25 °C exposed to light, exhibiting about 9% loss; additional storage for eight hours at 37 °C resulted in additional loss of about 6%. Under refrigeration at 4 °C protected from light, no loss occurred

in seven days. Additional storage for 16 hours at 25 °C followed by eight hours at 37 °C resulted in about 6% loss. (1989)

Ceftazidime (Glaxo) 0.1 mg/mL admixed with teicoplanin (Marion Merrell Dow) 0.025 mg/mL in Dianeal PD-2 with dextrose 1.5% in PVC containers did not result in a stable mixture. Large (but variable) teicoplanin losses generally in the 20% range were noted in as little as two hours at 25 °C exposed to light. Ceftazidime losses of about 9% occurred in 16 hours. Refrigeration and protection from light of the peritoneal dialysis admixture reduced losses of both drugs to negligible levels. Even so, the authors did not recommend admixing these two drugs because of the high levels of teicoplanin loss at room temperature. (1989)

Ceftazidime (Glaxo) 0.1 mg/mL in Dianeal PD-2 with dextrose 1.5% with or without heparin sodium 1 unit/mL in PVC bags was chemically stable for up to six days at 4 °C (about 3 to 4% loss), four days at 25 °C (about 9 to 10% loss), and less than 12 hours at body temperature of 37 °C. (866)

The addition of vancomycin hydrochloride (Lederle) 0.05 mg/mL to this peritoneal dialysis solution demonstrated similar stability with the ceftazidime being the defining component. Ceftazidime was chemically stable for up to six days at 4 °C (about 3% loss), three days at 25 °C (about 9 to 10% loss), and 12 hours at body temperature of 37 °C with the vancomycin exhibiting less loss throughout. (866)

Vancomycin hydrochloride (Lilly) 1 mg/mL admixed with ceftazidime (Lilly) 0.5 mg/mL in Dianeal PD-2 (Baxter) with 1.5% and also 4.25% dextrose were evaluated for compatibility and stability. Samples were stored under fluorescent light at 4 and 24 °C for 24 hours and at 37 °C for 12 hours. No precipitation or other change was observed by visual inspection in any sample. No loss of either drug occurred in the samples stored at 4 °C and no loss of vancomycin hydrochloride and about 4 to 5% ceftazidime loss occurred in the samples stored at 24 °C in 24 hours. Vancomycin hydrochloride losses of 3% or less and ceftazidime loss of about 6% were found in the samples stored at 37 °C for 12 hours. No difference in stability was found between samples at either dextrose concentration. (2217)

Ceftazidime (GlaxoWellcome) 0.125 mg/mL in Delflex peritoneal dialysis solution bags with 2.5% dextrose (Fresenius) was stable with 10% loss occurring in 7 days at refrigerator temperature and 3 days at room temperature. (2573)

CEFTRIAXONE SODIUM
AHFS 8:12.06.12

Products — Ceftriaxone sodium is available in vials containing the equivalent of 250 mg, 500 mg, 1 g, and 2 g of ceftriaxone. It is also available in 1- and 2-g piggyback bottles and 10-g bulk pharmacy containers. (1)

For intramuscular use, reconstitute the vials with a compatible diluent in the amounts indicated (1):

Vial Size	Volume of Diluent for 250 mg/mL	Volume of Diluent for 350 mg/mL
250 mg	0.9 mL	a
500 mg	1.8 mL	1.0 mL
1 g	3.6 mL	2.1 mL
2 g	7.2 mL	4.2 mL

^a*This vial size not recommended for 350-mg/mL concentration because withdrawal of the entire contents may not be possible.*

More dilute solutions for intramuscular injection may be prepared if required. (1)

For intermittent intravenous infusion, reconstitute the vials with a compatible diluent in the amounts indicated to yield a 100-mg/mL solution (1):

Vial Size	Volume of Diluent
250 mg	2.4 mL
500 mg	4.8 mL
1 g	9.6 mL
2 g	19.2 mL

After reconstitution, withdraw the entire vial contents and further dilute in a compatible infusion solution to the desired concentration. Concentrations between 10 and 40 mg/mL are recommended, but lower concentrations may be used. (1)

The piggyback bottles should be reconstituted with 10 or 20 mL of compatible diluent for the 1- or 2-g size, respectively. After reconstitution, further dilution to 50 to 100 mL with a compatible infusion solution is recommended. (1)

The bulk pharmacy container should be reconstituted with 95 mL of a compatible diluent. The solution is not for direct administration and must be diluted further before use. (4)

Ceftriaxone sodium (Braun) is available as 1 or 2 g in a dual chamber flexible container. The diluent chamber contains dextrose solution. (1)

Ceftriaxone sodium is also available as a frozen premixed infusion solution of 1 or 2 g in 50 mL of dextrose 3.8 or 2.4%, respectively, in water. It should be thawed at room temperature. (1; 4)

pH — The pH of the reconstituted drug in dual chamber containers is approximately 6.7. (1), and the frozen premixed infusion solutions have a pH of approximately 6.6 (range 6 to 8). (4)

Osmolality — The frozen premixed infusion solutions have osmolalities of 276 to 324 mOsm/kg. (4)

The osmolality of ceftriaxone sodium (Roche) 50 mg/mL was determined to be 351 mOsm/kg in dextrose 5% and 364 mOsm/kg in sodium chloride 0.9%. (1375)

Ceftriaxone sodium (Braun) 1 or 2 g in dual chamber flexible containers has an osmolality of 290 mOsm/kg when activated with the dextrose diluent. (1)

Sodium Content — Ceftriaxone sodium contains approximately 3.6 mEq (83 mg) of sodium per gram of ceftriaxone activity. (1)

Trade Name(s) — Rocephin.

Administration — Ceftriaxone sodium is administered by deep intramuscular injection or intermittent intravenous infusion over 15 to 30 minutes in adults or over 10 to 30 minutes in pediatric patients. (1; 4)

Stability — Intact vials of ceftriaxone sodium should be stored at room temperature of 25 °C or below and protected from light. After reconstitution, normal exposure to light is permitted. Solutions may vary from light yellow to amber, depending on length of storage, diluent, and concentration. (1)

Reconstituted solutions of ceftriaxone sodium are stable, exhibiting less than a 10% potency loss for the time periods indicated (1):

Diluent	Ceftriaxone Concentration (mg/mL)	25 °C	4 °C
Sterile water for injection	100	2 days	10 days
Sterile water for injection	250, 350	24 hr	3 days
Sodium chloride 0.9%	100	2 days	10 days
Sodium chloride 0.9%	250, 350	24 hr	3 days
Dextrose 5%	100	2 days	10 days
Dextrose 5%	250, 350	24 hr	3 days
Bacteriostatic water for injection (benzyl alcohol 0.9%)	100	24 hr	10 days
Bacteriostatic water for injection (benzyl alcohol 0.9%)	250, 350	24 hr	3 days
Lidocaine HCl 1% (without epinephrine)	100	24 hr	10 days
Lidocaine HCl 1% (without epinephrine)	250, 350	24 hr	3 days

Ceftriaxone sodium (Braun) 1 or 2 g in dual chamber flexible plastic containers with dextrose solution diluent should be used within 24 hours after activation if stored at room temperature and in seven days if stored under refrigeration. (1)

Ceftriaxone sodium (Roche) 1 mg/mL in Dianeal PD-1 with dextrose 1.5 and 4.25% was stable, retaining at least 90% for 14 days at 4 °C, 24 hours at 23 °C, or six hours at 37 °C. (1592)

Ceftriaxone sodium at concentrations of 10 to 40 mg/mL is incompatible with calcium-containing solutions, including Ringer's injection and Ringer's injection, lactated. Precipitation has been observed to form rapidly. (2222) Fatalities in neonates and infants have been reported to the FDA.

The FDA states that ceftriaxone sodium and calcium-containing solutions should not be given concomitantly to neonates less than 28 days of age; ceftriaxone sodium should not be used in these neonates if they are receiving or expected to receive calcium-containing intravenous solutions. (2731; 2784)

For patients over 28 days of age, the FDA states that ceftriaxone sodium and calcium-containing intravenous solutions may be administered sequentially as long as the infusion lines are thoroughly flushed between the separate infusions. The FDA states that ceftriaxone sodium and calcium-containing intravenous solutions should not be given simultaneously via Y-site to any patient regardless of age. (2731; 2784)

pH Effects — The pH of maximum stability for ceftriaxone sodium has been variously reported as 2.5 to 4.5 (1080) and 7.2. (1244)

Freezing Solutions — The manufacturer indicates that ceftriaxone sodium 10 to 40 mg/mL in dextrose 5% or sodium chloride 0.9%, when frozen at −20 °C in PVC or polyolefin containers, is stable for 26 weeks. Thawing should be performed at room temperature; thawed solutions should not be refrozen. (1)

The frozen premixed infusion solutions are stable for at least 90 days at −20 °C. Thawed solutions are stable for 72 hours at room temperature or 21 days at 5 °C. (4)

Ceftriaxone sodium (Roche) 250 and 450 mg/mL in dextrose 5%, 250 mg/mL in bacteriostatic water for injection, and 450 mg/mL in lidocaine hydrochloride 1% (Lyphomed) were evaluated for stability and pharmaceutical integrity during frozen storage at −15 °C. The solutions were packaged in 10-mL polypropylene syringes with attached needles (Becton Dickinson) and frozen for eight weeks. Some syringes were stored further at 4 °C for 10 days for at 20 °C for three days. Ceftriaxone sodium losses of 5% or less were found after eight weeks of frozen storage. However, particulate matter levels were unacceptable in most samples. While additional storage at 4 °C for 10 days did not cause unacceptable drug loss, storage at 20 °C for three days resulted in 12% drug loss. (1824)

Ceftriaxone sodium (Roche) 2 g/100 mL of dextrose 5% in polyolefin containers was found to remain stable for 14 weeks frozen at −20 °C with no loss of drug occurring. Subsequent thawing in a microwave oven and storage at about 4 °C resulted in 10% drug loss in 44 to 56 days, depending on the power level used for thawing. (2724)

Ceftriaxone sodium (Braun) 1 or 2 g in dual chamber flexible containers should not be frozen. (1)

Syringes — Bailey et al. reported the stability of ceftriaxone sodium (Roche) 10 and 40 mg/mL in dextrose 5% and sodium chloride 0.9% packaged in polypropylene syringes. The solutions were visually compatible and lost 5% or less ceftriaxone in 48 hours at 4 and 20 °C and ten days stored frozen at −10 °C. (1720)

Plumridge et al. reported on the stability of ceftriaxone sodium (Roche) 100 mg/mL in sterile water for injection packaged in polypropylene syringes (Terumo). About 9 to 10% loss of ceftriaxone occurred in five days at 20 °C and 40 days at 4 °C. However, the room temperature samples underwent color intensification that the authors found unacceptable after about 72 hours. Little or no loss occurred during 180 days of frozen storage at −20 °C. (1990)

O'Connell et al. evaluated the stability of reconstituted ceftriaxone sodium 100 mg/mL packaged in 10-mL polypropylene syringes. Stored under refrigeration at 8 °C, about 5% loss occurred in 10 days and 8% in 13 days. (1999)

Elastomeric Reservoir Pumps — Ceftriaxone sodium (Roche) 10 mg/mL in both dextrose 5% and sodium chloride 0.9% was evaluated for binding potential to natural rubber elastomeric reservoirs (Baxter). No binding was found after storage for two weeks at 35 °C with gentle agitation. (2014)

Central Venous Catheter — Ceftriaxone sodium (Roche) 5 mg/mL in dextrose 5% was found to be compatible with the ARROWg+ard Blue Plus (Arrow International) chlorhexidine-bearing triple-lumen central catheter. Essentially complete delivery of the drug was found with little or no drug loss occurring. Furthermore, chlorhexidine delivered from the catheter remained at trace amounts with no substantial increase due to the delivery of the drug through the catheter. (2335)

Compatibility Information

Solution Compatibility

Ceftriaxone sodium

Solution	Mfr	Mfr	Conc/L	Remarks	Ref	C/I
Dextrose 5% in sodium chloride 0.45%		RC	10 to 40 g	Less than 10% loss in 2 days at 25 °C. Incompatible if refrigerated	1	C
		RC	10 g	3% loss in 48 hr at 20 °C. 5% loss in 72 hr and 9% in 96 hr at 4 °C	965	C
Dextrose 5% in sodium chloride 0.9%		RC	10 to 40 g	Less than 10% loss in 2 days at 25 °C. Incompatible if refrigerated	1	C
Dextrose 5%		RC	10 to 40 g	Less than 10% loss in 2 days at 25 °C and 10 days at 4 °C	1	C
		RC	10 g	No loss in 48 hr and 8% in 72 hr at 20 °C. 4% loss in 72 hr and 9% in 96 hr at 4 °C	965	C
	TR[b]	RC	2 g	Little or no loss in 14 days at 20, 4, and −20 °C	966	C
	MG[c]	RC	20 g	Physically compatible with 5% drug loss in 24 hr and 9% in 48 hr at 25 °C	1026	C
	[b]	RC	40 g	Physically compatible with 12% loss in 3 days at 23 °C and 10% loss in 14 days at 4 °C	1243	C
	[a]	RC	1 g	10% loss calculated to occur in 48 hr at 20 °C	1244	C
		RC	10 g	Physically compatible with 8% loss in 7 days at room temperature. 5 to 8% loss in 12 weeks at 5 and −20 °C	1245	C
		RC	50 g	Physically compatible with no loss in 24 hr but 12 to 17% loss in 7 days at room temperature. 5 to 7% loss in 12 weeks at 5 and −20 °C	1245	C
	BA[d]	RC	5 and 40 g	Less than 10% loss in 4 days at 23 °C and 21 days at 4 °C	2819	C
			5 and 40 g	Color darkening occurs but only about 3% ceftriaxone loss occurs in 20 days at 4 °C	2598	C
Dextrose 10%		RC	10 to 40 g	Less than 10% loss in 2 days at 25 °C and 10 days at 4 °C	1	C
		RC	10 g	No loss in 48 hr and 8% in 72 hr at 20 °C. 2% loss in 72 hr and 8% in 96 hr at 4 °C	965	C
Ionosol B in dextrose 5%		RC	10 to 40 g	Less than 10% loss in 24 hours at 25 °C	1	C
Normosol M in dextrose 5%	[a]	RC	1 to 40 g	Less than 10% loss in 24 hours at 25 °C	1	C
Ringer's injection, lactated		RC	10 and 13 g	Precipitate forms relatively rapidly	2222	I
Sodium chloride 0.9%		RC	10 to 40 g	Less than 10% loss in 2 days at 25 °C and 10 days at 4 °C	1	C
		RC	10 g	4% loss in 48 hr and 14% in 72 hr at 20 °C. 3% loss in 48 hr and 9% in 72 hr at 4 °C	965	C
	MG[c]	RC	20 g	Physically compatible with 10% drug loss in 24 hr and 16% in 48 hr at 25 °C under fluorescent light	1026	C
	[b]	RC	40 g	Physically compatible with 5% loss in 3 days at 23 °C and 9% loss in 30 days at 4 °C	1243	C
	[a]	RC	1 g	10% loss calculated to occur in 10 days at 20 °C	1244	C
		RC	10 g	Physically compatible with 9% loss in 7 days at room temperature. 11 to 12% loss in 6 weeks at 5 °C	1245	C

Solution Compatibility (Cont.)

Ceftriaxone sodium

Solution	Mfr	Mfr	Conc/L	Remarks	Ref	C/I
		RC	50 g	Physically compatible with 8 to 9% loss in 7 days at room temperature. 5% loss in 5 weeks and 15% in 8 weeks at 5 °C	1245	**C**
			5 and 40 g	Color darkening occurs but only about 3% ceftriaxone loss occurs in 20 days at 4 °C	2598	**C**
	HOS[d]	RC	40 g	Less than 10% loss in 4 days at 23 °C and 14 days at 4 °C	2819	**C**
	HOS[d]	RC	5 g	Less than 10% loss in 7 days at 23 °C and 21 days at 4 °C	2819	**C**
Sodium lactate ⅙ M		RC	10 to 40 g	Less than 10% loss in 24 hr at 25 °C	1	**C**

[a]*Tested in glass, PVC, and polyethylene containers.*
[b]*Tested in PVC containers.*
[c]*Tested in glass containers.*
[d]*Tested in Accufusor reservoirs.*

Additive Compatibility

Ceftriaxone sodium

Drug	Mfr	Conc/L	Mfr	Conc/L	Test Soln	Remarks	Ref	C/I
Amikacin sulfate	BR	15 and 25 mg	RC	100 mg	D5W	6% loss of amikacin in 24 hr at 22 °C	504	**C**
Aminophylline	AMR	1 g	RC	20 g	D5W, NS[a]	Yellow color forms immediately. 3 to 6% ceftriaxone loss and 8 to 12% aminophylline loss in 24 hr	1727	**I**
	AMR	4 g	RC	20 g	D5W, NS[a]	Yellow color forms immediately. 15 to 20% ceftriaxone loss and 7 to 9% aminophylline loss in 24 hr	1727	**I**
	AMR	1 g	RC	40 g	D5W, NS[a]	Yellow color forms immediately. 15 to 18% ceftriaxone loss and 1 to 3% aminophylline loss in 24 hr	1727	**I**
Calcium chloride						Incompatible. Precipitate may form in calcium-containing solutions	2222; 2731; 2784	**I**
Calcium gluconate						Incompatible. Precipitate may form in calcium-containing solutions	2222; 2731; 2784	**I**
Clindamycin phosphate	UP	12 g	RC	20 g	D5W[b]	10% ceftriaxone loss in 4 hr and 17% in 24 hr at 25 °C under fluorescent light. No clindamycin loss in 48 hr	1026	**I**
	UP	12 g	RC	20 g	NS[b]	10% ceftriaxone loss in 1 hr and 12% in 24 hr at 25 °C under fluorescent light. 6% clindamycin loss in 48 hr	1026	**I**
Gentamicin sulfate	SC	9 mg	RC	100 mg	D5W	13% loss of gentamicin in 8 hr at 22 °C	504	**I**
	SC	6 mg	RC	100 mg	D5W	5% loss of gentamicin in 24 hr at 22 °C	504	**C**
Linezolid	PHU	2 g	RC	10 g	[d]	Physically compatible, but up to 37% ceftriaxone loss in 24 hr at 23 °C and 10% loss in 3 days at 4 °C	2262	**I**

Additive Compatibility (Cont.)

Ceftriaxone sodium

Drug	Mfr	Conc/L	Mfr	Conc/L	Test Soln	Remarks	Ref	C/I
Mannitol		5 and 10%	RC	10 to 40 g		Less than 10% loss in 24 hr at 25 °C	1	C
Metronidazole	AB	5 g	RC	10 g		Visually compatible with little or no loss of either drug in 72 hr at 8 °C	1849	C
	BA	5 g	RC	10 g		Visually compatible with no metronidazole loss and with 6% ceftriaxone loss in 3 days and 8% in 4 days at 25 °C	2101	C
Sodium bicarbonate		5%	RC	10 to 40 g		Less than 10% loss in 24 hr at 25 °C	1	C
Theophylline	BA[c]	4 g	RC	40 g		Yellow color forms immediately. 14% ceftriaxone loss and no theophylline loss in 24 hr	1727	I

[a]Tested in polyolefin containers.
[b]Tested in glass containers.
[c]Tested in PVC containers.
[d]Admixed in the linezolid infusion container.

Drugs in Syringe Compatibility

Ceftriaxone sodium

Drug (in syringe)	Mfr	Amt	Mfr	Amt	Remarks	Ref	C/I
Lidocaine HCl	LY	1%	RC	450 mg/mL	5% ceftriaxone loss in 8 weeks at −15 °C but solution failed the particulate matter test	1824	I
	DW	1%	RC	250 and 450 mg/mL	10% ceftriaxone loss in 3 days at 20 °C, 7 to 8% loss in 35 days at 4 °C, and 4 to 6% loss in 168 days at −20 °C. Lidocaine not tested	1991	C

Y-Site Injection Compatibility (1:1 Mixture)

Ceftriaxone sodium

Drug	Mfr	Conc	Mfr	Conc	Remarks	Ref	C/I
Acyclovir sodium	BW	5 mg/mL[a]	RC	20 mg/mL[a]	Physically compatible for 4 hr at 25 °C	1157	C
Allopurinol sodium	BW	3 mg/mL[b]	RC	20 mg/mL[b]	Physically compatible for 4 hr at 22 °C	1686	C
Amifostine	USB	10 mg/mL[a]	RC	20 mg/mL[a]	Physically compatible for 4 hr at 23 °C	1845	C
Amiodarone HCl	WY	6 mg/mL[a]	RC	20 mg/mL[a]	Turned yellow in 24 hr at 22 °C, but considered normal for cephalosporins	2352	C
Amphotericin B cholesteryl sulfate complex	SEQ	0.83 mg/mL[a]	RC	20 mg/mL[a]	Decreased natural turbidity occurs	2117	I
Amsacrine	NCI	1 mg/mL[a]	RC	40 mg/mL[a]	Immediate orange turbidity, developing into flocculent precipitate in 4 hr	1381	I
Anakinra	SYN	4 and 36 mg/mL[a]	RC	20 mg/mL[a]	Ceftriaxone stable. 10% anakinra loss in 30 min and 20% in 4 hr at 22 °C	2509	I
	SYN	4 and 36 mg/mL[b]	RC	20 mg/mL[b]	Physically compatible with no loss of either drug in 4 hr at 22 °C	2509	C
Anidulafungin	VIC	0.5 mg/mL[a]	RC	20 mg/mL[a]	Physically compatible for 4 hr at 23 °C	2617	C
Azithromycin	PF	2 mg/mL[b]	RC	66.7 mg/mL[f,g]	White and yellow microcrystals found	2368	I

Y-Site Injection Compatibility (1:1 Mixture) (Cont.)

Ceftriaxone sodium

Drug	Mfr	Conc	Mfr	Conc	Remarks	Ref	C/I
Aztreonam	SQ	40 mg/mL[a]	RC	20 mg/mL[a]	Physically compatible for 4 hr at 23 °C	1758	C
Bivalirudin	TMC	5 mg/mL[a]	RC	20 mg/mL[a]	Physically compatible for 4 hr at 23 °C	2373	C
Caspofungin acetate	ME	0.7 mg/mL[b]	ORC	20 mg/mL[b]	Immediate white turbid precipitate forms	2758	I
	ME	0.5 mg/mL[b]	NVP	20 mg/mL[b]	Amber crystals and white paste form	2766	I
Cisatracurium besylate	GW	0.1, 2, 5 mg/mL[a]	RC	20 mg/mL[a]	Physically compatible for 4 hr at 23 °C	2074	C
Daptomycin	CUB	16.7 mg/mL[b,h]	RC	16.7 mg/mL[b,h]	Physically compatible with 4 to 5% loss of both drugs in 2 hr at 25 °C	2553	C
Dexmedetomidine HCl	AB	4 mcg/mL[b]	RC	20 mg/mL[b]	Physically compatible for 4 hr at 23 °C	2383	C
Diltiazem HCl	MMD	5 mg/mL	RC	40 mg/mL[b]	Visually compatible	1807	C
Docetaxel	RPR	0.9 mg/mL[a]	RC	20 mg/mL[a]	Physically compatible for 4 hr at 23 °C	2224	C
Doxorubicin HCl liposomal	SEQ	0.4 mg/mL[a]	RC	20 mg/mL[a]	Physically compatible for 4 hr at 23 °C	2087	C
Etoposide phosphate	BR	5 mg/mL[a]	RC	20 mg/mL[a]	Physically compatible for 4 hr at 23 °C	2218	C
Famotidine	ME	2 mg/mL[b]		20 mg/mL[a]	Visually compatible for 4 hr at 22 °C	1936	C
Fenoldopam mesylate	AB	80 mcg/mL[b]	RC	20 mg/mL[b]	Physically compatible for 4 hr at 23 °C	2467	C
Filgrastim	AMG	30 mcg/mL[a]	RC	20 mg/mL[a]	Particles and filaments form in 1 hr	1687	I
Fluconazole	RR	2 mg/mL	RC	40 mg/mL	Precipitates immediately	1407	I
Fludarabine phosphate	BX	1 mg/mL[a]	RC	20 mg/mL[a]	Visually compatible for 4 hr at 22 °C	1439	C
Foscarnet sodium	AST	24 mg/mL	RC	20 mg/mL[c]	Physically compatible for 24 hr at 25 °C under fluorescent light	1393	C
Gallium nitrate	FUJ	1 mg/mL[b]	RC	40 mg/mL[b]	Visually compatible for 24 hr at 25 °C	1673	C
Gemcitabine HCl	LI	10 mg/mL[b]	RC	20 mg/mL[b]	Physically compatible for 4 hr at 23 °C	2226	C
Granisetron HCl	SKB	0.05 mg/mL[a]	RC	20 mg/mL[a]	Physically compatible for 4 hr at 23 °C	2000	C
Heparin sodium	TR	50 units/mL	RC	20 mg/mL	Visually compatible for 4 hr at 25 °C	1793	C
Hydroxyethyl starch 130/0.4 in sodium chloride 0.9%	FRK	6%	RC	20, 30, 40 mg/mL[a]	Visually compatible for 24 hr at room temperature	2770	C
Labetalol HCl	GL	2.5[d] and 5 mg/mL	RC	20[a,b] and 100[d] mg/mL	Fluffy white precipitate forms immediately	1964	I
Linezolid	PHU	2 mg/mL	RC	20 mg/mL[a]	Physically compatible for 4 hr at 23 °C	2264	C
Melphalan HCl	BW	0.1 mg/mL[b]	RC	20 mg/mL[b]	Physically compatible for 3 hr at 22 °C	1557	C
Meperidine HCl	AB	10 mg/mL	RC	20 and 40 mg/mL[a]	Physically compatible for 4 hr at 25 °C	1397	C
Methotrexate sodium		30 mg/mL	RC	100 mg/mL	Visually compatible for 4 hr at room temperature	1788	C
Morphine sulfate	AB	1 mg/mL	RC	20 and 40 mg/mL[a]	Physically compatible for 4 hr at 25 °C	1397	C
Paclitaxel	NCI	1.2 mg/mL[a]	RC	20 mg/mL[a]	Physically compatible for 4 hr at 22 °C	1556	C
Pantoprazole sodium	ALT[i]	0.16 to 0.8 mg/mL[b]	RC	20 to 40 mg/mL[a]	Visually compatible for 12 hr at 23 °C	2603	C
Pemetrexed disodium	LI	20 mg/mL[b]	RC	20 mg/mL[a]	Physically compatible for 4 hr at 23 °C	2564	C
Pentamidine isethionate	FUJ	3 mg/mL[a]	RC	20 mg/mL[a]	Heavy white precipitate forms immediately	1880	I
Propofol	ZEN	10 mg/mL	RC	20 mg/mL[a]	Physically compatible for 1 hr at 23 °C	2066	C

Y-Site Injection Compatibility (1:1 Mixture) (Cont.)

Ceftriaxone sodium

Drug	Mfr	Conc	Mfr	Conc	Remarks	Ref	C/I
Remifentanil HCl	GW	0.025 and 0.25 mg/mL[b]	RC	20 mg/mL[a]	Physically compatible for 4 hr at 23 °C	2075	C
Sargramostim	IMM	10 mcg/mL[b]	RC	20 mg/mL[b]	Visually compatible for 4 hr at 22 °C	1436	C
Sodium bicarbonate		1.4%	RC	100 mg/mL	Visually compatible for 4 hr at room temperature	1788	C
Tacrolimus	FUJ	1 mg/mL[b]	RC	40 mg/mL[a]	Visually compatible for 24 hr at 25 °C	1630	C
Telavancin HCl	ASP	7.5 mg/mL[a,b]	HOS	20 mg/mL[a,b]	Physically compatible for 2 hr	2830	C
Teniposide	BR	0.1 mg/mL[a]	RC	20 mg/mL[a]	Physically compatible for 4 hr at 23 °C	1725	C
Theophylline	TR	4 mg/mL	RC	20 mg/mL	Visually compatible for 6 hr at 25 °C	1793	C
Thiotepa	IMM[e]	1 mg/mL[a]	RC	20 mg/mL[a]	Physically compatible for 4 hr at 23 °C	1861	C
Tigecycline	WY	1 mg/mL[b]		40 mg/mL[b]	Physically compatible for 4 hr	2714	C
Vancomycin HCl	LI	20 mg/mL	RC	100 mg/mL	White precipitate forms immediately	1398	I
	AB	20 mg/mL[a]	RC	250 mg/mL[d]	Transient precipitate forms	2189	?
	AB	20 mg/mL[a]	RC	10 and 50 mg/mL[a]	Gross white precipitate forms immediately	2189	I
	AB	20 mg/mL[a]	RC	1 mg/mL[a]	Subvisible haze forms immediately	2189	I
	AB	2 mg/mL[a]	RC	1[a], 10[a], 50[a], 250[d] mg/mL	Physically compatible for 4 hr at 23 °C	2189	C
Vinorelbine tartrate	BW	1 mg/mL[b]	RC	20 mg/mL[b]	Tiny particles form immediately, becoming more numerous in 4 hr at 22 °C	1558	I
Warfarin sodium	DME	2 mg/mL[d]	RC	20 mg/mL[a]	Visually compatible for 24 hr at 24 °C	2078	C
Zidovudine	BW	4 mg/mL[a]	RC	20 mg/mL[a]	Physically compatible for 4 hr at 25 °C	1193	C

[a]*Tested in dextrose 5%.*
[b]*Tested in sodium chloride 0.9%.*
[c]*Tested in both dextrose 5% and sodium chloride 0.9%.*
[d]*Tested in sterile water for injection.*
[e]*Lyophilized formulation tested.*
[f]*Tested in sodium chloride 0.45%.*
[g]*Injected via Y-site into an administration set running azithromycin.*
[h]*Final concentration after mixing.*
[i]*Test performed using the formulation WITHOUT edetate disodium.*

CEFUROXIME SODIUM
AHFS 8:12.06.08

Products — Cefuroxime sodium is available in vials containing 750 mg and 1.5 g of drug as the sodium salt. The drug is also available in a 7.5-g pharmacy bulk package. (1)

The vials should be reconstituted with sterile water for injection. For intravenous administration, the 750- and 1.5-g vials may be reconstituted with 8.3 and 16 mL, respectively, to yield a 90-mg/mL solution. (1)

For intramuscular administration, reconstitute the 750-mg vial with 3 mL of sterile water for injection yielding a 225-mg/mL intramuscular suspension. The suspension should be dispersed with shaking before the dose is withdrawn. (1)

The 7.5-g pharmacy bulk package should be reconstituted with 77 mL of sterile water for injection to yield a 95-mg/mL concentration. (1)

Cefuroxime sodium is also available as a frozen premixed solution containing 750 mg or 1.5 g in 50-mL PVC bags. Approximately 1.4 g of dextrose hydrous has been added to the 750-mg bags to adjust the osmolality. Both the 750-mg and 1.5-g bags also contain sodium citrate hydrous 300 and 600 mg, respectively. The pH is adjusted with hydrochloric acid and may have been adjusted with sodium hydroxide. (1)

Cefuroxime sodium (Braun) is available as 750 mg and 1.5 g in a dual chamber flexible container. The diluent chamber contains dextrose solution for use as a diluent. (1)

pH — The reconstituted vials have a pH of 6 to 8.5. The frozen premixed solutions have a pH of 5 to 7.5. (1)

Osmolality — The osmolality of the frozen premixed cefuroxime sodium solutions is approximately 300 mOsm/kg. (1)

Cefuroxime sodium (Braun) in 750 mg and 1.5 g in dual chamber flexible containers has an osmolality of 290 mOsm/kg when activated with the dextrose solution diluent. (1)

The osmolality of cefuroxime sodium (Glaxo) 30 mg/mL was determined to be 315 mOsm/kg in dextrose 5% and 314 mOsm/kg in sodium chloride 0.9%. At a concentration of 50 mg/mL, the osmolality was determined to be 329 mOsm/kg in dextrose 5% and 335 mOsm/kg in sodium chloride 0.9%. (1375)

The following maximum cefuroxime sodium concentrations were recommended to achieve osmolalities suitable for peripheral infusion in fluid-restricted patients (1180):

Diluent	Maximum Concentration (mg/mL)	Osmolality (mOsm/kg)
Dextrose 5%	76	568
Sodium chloride 0.9%	68	541
Sterile water for injection	137	489

Sodium Content — Cefuroxime sodium vials contain 2.4 mEq (54.2 mg) per gram of cefuroxime activity. The frozen premixed 750-mg and 1.5-g solutions contain 4.8 mEq (111 mg) and 9.7 mEq (222 mg), respectively. (1)

Trade Name(s) — Zinacef.

Administration — Cefuroxime sodium is administered by deep intramuscular injection, by direct intravenous injection over three to five minutes directly into the vein or into the tubing of a running infusion solution, by intermittent intravenous infusion over 15 to 60 minutes, or by continuous intravenous infusion. The manufacturer recommends temporarily discontinuing the primary solution when giving the drug by Y-site infusion. (1; 4)

Stability — Intact vials should be stored at controlled room temperature and protected from light. The drug is present as a white to off-white powder. Solutions may range in color from light yellow to amber. Both the powder and solutions of cefuroxime sodium darken, depending on storage conditions, without affecting their potency. (1; 4)

The reconstituted suspension for intramuscular injection and the 90 to 100-mg/mL intravenous solution concentrations are stable for 24 hours at room temperature and 48 hours when refrigerated at 5 °C. The bulk pharmacy vial reconstituted to a concentration of 95 mg/mL is stable for 24 hours at room temperature or seven days under refrigeration. Dilution to concentrations of 1 to 30 mg/mL in compatible diluents results in solutions that are stable for 24 hours at room temperature or seven days under refrigeration. (1; 4)

Cefuroxime sodium (Braun) in 750 mg and 1.5 g in dual chamber flexible plastic containers with dextrose solution diluent should be used within 24 hours after activation if stored at room temperature and in seven days if stored under refrigeration. (1)

pH Effects — The pH of maximum stability is in the range of 4.5 to 7.3. (712)

Freezing Solutions — Commercial, frozen, premixed cefuroxime sodium injections are stable for at least 90 days after shipment when stored at −20 °C. Frozen solutions should be thawed at room temperature or under refrigeration. Some solution components may precipitate in the frozen state, but the precipitate redissolves upon thawing and reaching room temperature. Thawed solutions are stable for 24 hours at room temperature or 28 days at 5 °C. (1; 4)

Extemporaneously prepared solutions of cefuroxime sodium 750 mg or 1.5 g added to 50- to 100-mL PVC bags of dextrose 5% or sodium chloride 0.9% are stable for six months at −20 °C. The manufacturer does not recommend the use of water baths or microwaves for thawing. Following thawing at room temperature, the solutions are stable for 24 hours at room temperature or seven days under refrigeration. The thawed solutions should not be refrozen. (1; 4)

Minibags of cefuroxime sodium in dextrose 5% or sodium chloride 0.9%, frozen at −20 °C for up to 35 days, were thawed at room temperature and in a microwave oven, with care taken that the thawed solution temperature never exceeded 25 °C. No significant differences in cefuroxime concentrations occurred between the two thawing methods. (1192)

Cefuroxime sodium (Glaxo) 30 and 60 mg/mL in sterile water for injection in PVC portable infusion pump reservoirs (Pharmacia Deltec) and glass vials exhibited a 4% loss after 30 days at −20 °C. Subsequent storage for four days at 3 °C resulted in about a 10% loss in the PVC bags and a 4% loss in the glass vials. (1581)

Cefuroxime sodium 1.5 g/100 mL in dextrose 5% in polyolefin bags was reported to be physically and chemically stable for 98 days stored at −20 °C. Less than 10% drug loss occurred upon microwave thawing and subsequent refrigerated storage for 18 to 21 days. (2592)

Cefuroxime sodium (Braun) in 750 mg and 1.5 g in dual chamber flexible containers should not be frozen. (1)

Ambulatory Pumps — Cefuroxime sodium (Glaxo) 22.5 and 45 mg/mL in sterile water for injection in PVC portable infusion pump reservoirs (Pharmacia Deltec) exhibited a 4 to 6% loss in eight hours and an 11 to 12% loss in 16 hours at 30 °C. No loss occurred in 7 days at 3 °C. (1581)

Central Venous Catheter — Cefuroxime sodium (Glaxo Wellcome) 10 mg/mL in dextrose 5% was found to be compatible with the ARROWg+ard Blue Plus (Arrow International) chlorhexidine-bearing triple-lumen central catheter. Essentially complete delivery of the drug was found with little or no drug loss occurring. Furthermore, chlorhexidine delivered from the catheter remained at trace amounts with no substantial increase due to the delivery of the drug through the catheter. (2335)

Compatibility Information

Solution Compatibility

Cefuroxime sodium

Solution	Mfr	Mfr	Conc/L	Remarks	Ref	C/I
Dextrose–saline combinations			1 to 30 g	Less than 10% loss in 24 hr at room temperature and 7 days refrigerated	1	C
Dextrose 5%			1 to 30 g	Less than 10% loss in 24 hr at room temperature and 7 days refrigerated	1	C
	MG[a]	GL	15 g	5% loss in 48 hr at 25 °C under fluorescent light	1164	C
	[b]		6 g	Visually compatible with little or no loss in 24 hr at room temperature and 4 °C	1953	C
	BA[a]	GL	15 g	Visually compatible with 7% loss in 11 days at 4 °C	2142	C
	BA[a,b]	GL	5 and 10 g	Physically compatible with about 7% cefuroxime loss in 24 hr and 13% loss in 48 hr at 25 °C. About 4% loss at 5 °C and no loss at −10 °C in 30 days	712	C
	[d]		15 g	Visually compatible with about 6% loss by in 31 days at 4 °C	2661	C
Dextrose 10%			1 to 30 g	Less than 10% loss in 24 hr at room temperature and 7 days refrigerated	1	C
Ringer's injection			1 to 30 g	Less than 10% loss in 24 hr at room temperature and 7 days refrigerated	1	C
Ringer's injection, lactated			1 to 30 g	Less than 10% loss in 24 hr at room temperature and 7 days refrigerated	1	C
Sodium chloride 0.9%			1 to 30 g	Less than 10% loss in 24 hr at room temperature and 7 days refrigerated	1	C
	MG[a]	GL	15 g	5% loss in 48 hr at 25 °C under fluorescent light	1164	C
	[b]		6 g	Visually compatible with little or no loss in 24 hr at room temperature and 4 °C	1953	C
	BA[a,b]	GL	5 and 10 g	Physically compatible with about 7% cefuroxime loss in 24 hr and 13% loss in 48 hr at 25 °C. About 4% loss at 5 °C and no loss at −10 °C in 30 days	712	C
Sodium lactate ⅙ M			1 to 30 g	Less than 10% loss in 24 hr at room temperature and 7 days refrigerated	1	C
TPN #107[c]			1 g	Activity retained for 24 hr at 21 °C	1326	C

[a] Tested in glass containers.
[b] Tested in PVC containers.
[c] Refer to Appendix I for the composition of parenteral nutrition solutions. TPN indicates a 2-in-1 admixture.
[d] Tested in polyolefin containers.

Additive Compatibility

Cefuroxime sodium

Drug	Mfr	Conc/L	Mfr	Conc/L	Test Soln	Remarks	Ref	C/I
Ciprofloxacin	MI	2 g		30 g	D5W	Physically incompatible	888	I
	BAY	2 g	GW	30 g	D5W	Visually compatible for 6 hr, but small particles appeared by 24 hr at about 22 °C	2413	I
Clindamycin phosphate	UP	9 g	GL	15 g	D5W	Physically compatible with 4% clindamycin loss and 6 to 8% cefuroxime loss in 48 hr at 25 °C under fluorescent light	1164	C

Additive Compatibility (Cont.)

Cefuroxime sodium

Drug	Mfr	Conc/L	Mfr	Conc/L	Test Soln	Remarks	Ref	C/I
	UP	9 g	GL	15 g	NS	Physically compatible with 9% clindamycin and cefuroxime losses in 48 hr at 25 °C under fluorescent light	1164	C
Floxacillin sodium	BE	20 g	GL	37.5 g	W	Physically compatible for 72 hr at 15 and 30 °C	1479	C
	BE	10 g	GL	7.5 g	D5W, NS	Physically compatible for 48 hr. Both drugs stable for 1 hr at room temperature	1036	C
Furosemide	HO	1 g	GL	37.5 g	W	Physically compatible for 72 hr at 15 and 30 °C	1479	C
Gentamicin sulfate	EX	800 mg	GL	7.5 g	D5W, NS[b]	Physically compatible with no loss of either drug in 1 hr	1036	C
		100 mg		1 g	TPN #107[c]	32% gentamicin loss in 24 hr at 21 °C	1326	I
Metronidazole		5 g	GL	7.5 g	[b]	Physically compatible with no loss of either drug in 1 hr	1036	C
		5 g	GL	15 g		No loss of either drug in 4 hr at 24 °C	1376	C
		5 g	GL	7.5 g		10% cefuroxime loss in 16 days at 4 °C and 35 hr at 25 °C. No metronidazole loss in 15 days at 4 and 25 °C	1565	C
	IVX	5 g	GL	7.5 and 15 g		Physically compatible. No loss of metronidazole and about 6% cefuroxime loss in 49 days at 5 °C	2192	C
Midazolam HCl	RC	50, 250, 400 mg	GL	7.5 g	NS	Visually compatible for 4 hr	355	C
Ranitidine HCl	GL	100 mg	GL	1.5 g	D5W	Color change in 24 hr at ambient temperature in light	1151	?
	GL	50 mg and 2 g		6 g	D5W	Ranitidine stable for only 6 hr at 25 °C. Cefuroxime not tested	1515	I

[a]Tested in both glass and PVC containers.
[b]Tested in PVC containers.
[c]Refer to Appendix I for the composition of parenteral nutrition solutions. TPN indicates a 2-in-1 admixture.
[d]Tested in glass containers.

Drugs in Syringe Compatibility

Cefuroxime sodium

Drug (in syringe)	Mfr	Amt	Mfr	Amt	Remarks	Ref	C/I
Dimenhydrinate		10 mg/ 1 mL		100 mg/ 1 mL	Clear solution	2569	C
Doxapram HCl	RB	400 mg/ 20 mL	GL	750 mg/ 7 mL	Immediate turbidity	1177	I
Pantoprazole sodium	[a]	4 mg/ 1 mL		100 mg/ 1 mL	Precipitates immediately	2574	I

[a]Test performed using the formulation WITHOUT edetate disodium.

Y-Site Injection Compatibility (1:1 Mixture)

Cefuroxime sodium

Drug	Mfr	Conc	Mfr	Conc	Remarks	Ref	C/I
Acyclovir sodium	BW	5 mg/mL[a]	GL	15 mg/mL[a]	Physically compatible for 4 hr at 25 °C	1157	C
Allopurinol sodium	BW	3 mg/mL[b]	GL	20 mg/mL[b]	Physically compatible for 4 hr at 22 °C	1686	C
Amifostine	USB	10 mg/mL[a]	GL	30 mg/mL[a]	Physically compatible for 4 hr at 23 °C	1845	C
Amiodarone HCl	WY	6 mg/mL[a]	BA	30 mg/mL[a]	Turned yellow in 24 hr at 22 °C, but considered normal for cephalosporins	2352	C
Anidulafungin	VIC	0.5 mg/mL[a]	GSK	30 mg/mL[a]	Physically compatible for 4 hr at 23 °C	2617	C
Atracurium besylate	BW	0.5 mg/mL[a]	GL	7.5 mg/mL[a]	Physically compatible for 24 hr at 28 °C	1337	C
Azithromycin	PF	2 mg/mL[b]	VHA	100 mg/mL[f,g]	White and yellow microcrystals	2368	I
Aztreonam	SQ	40 mg/mL[a]	LI	30 mg/mL[a]	Physically compatible for 4 hr at 23 °C	1758	C
Bivalirudin	TMC	5 mg/mL[a]	GW	30 mg/mL[a]	Physically compatible for 4 hr at 23 °C	2373	C
Cisatracurium besylate	GW	0.1 mg/mL[a]	LI	30 mg/mL[a]	Physically compatible for 4 hr at 23 °C	2074	C
	GW	2 mg/mL[a]	LI	30 mg/mL[a]	White cloudiness forms immediately	2074	I
	GW	5 mg/mL[a]	LI	30 mg/mL[a]	Turbidity forms immediately	2074	I
Clarithromycin	AB	4 mg/mL[a]	GW	60 mg/mL[a]	White precipitate forms in 3 hr at 30 °C and 24 hr at 17 °C	2174	I
Cyclophosphamide	MJ	20 mg/mL[a]	GL	30 mg/mL[a]	Physically compatible for 4 hr at 25 °C	1194	C
Dexmedetomidine HCl	AB	4 mcg/mL[b]	GW	30 mg/mL[b]	Physically compatible for 4 hr at 23 °C	2383	C
Diltiazem HCl	MMD	5 mg/mL	LI	15 and 100 mg/mL[b]	Visually compatible	1807	C
	MMD	1 mg/mL[b]	LI	100 mg/mL[b]	Visually compatible	1807	C
Docetaxel	RPR	0.9 mg/mL[a]	LI	30 mg/mL[a]	Physically compatible for 4 hr at 23 °C	2224	C
Etoposide phosphate	BR	5 mg/mL[a]	GW	30 mg/mL[a]	Physically compatible for 4 hr at 23 °C	2218	C
Famotidine	MSD	0.2 mg/mL[a]	GL	15 mg/mL[b]	Physically compatible for 14 hr	1196	C
	ME	2 mg/mL[b]		20 mg/mL[a]	Visually compatible for 4 hr at 22 °C	1936	C
Fenoldopam mesylate	AB	80 mcg/mL[b]	GW	30 mg/mL[b]	Physically compatible for 4 hr at 23 °C	2467	C
Filgrastim	AMG	30 mcg/mL[a]	GL	20 mg/mL[a]	Haze, particles, and filaments form immediately	1687	I
Fluconazole	RR	2 mg/mL	GL	30 mg/mL	Precipitates immediately	1407	I
Fludarabine phosphate	BX	1 mg/mL[a]	GL	30 mg/mL[a]	Visually compatible for 4 hr at 22 °C	1439	C
Foscarnet sodium	AST	24 mg/mL	GL	30 mg/mL	Physically compatible for 24 hr at room temperature under fluorescent light	1335	C
Gemcitabine HCl	LI	10 mg/mL[b]	GW	30 mg/mL[b]	Physically compatible for 4 hr at 23 °C	2226	C
Granisetron HCl	SKB	0.05 mg/mL[a]	LI	30 mg/mL[a]	Physically compatible for 4 hr at 23 °C	2000	C
Hetastarch in lactated electrolyte	AB	6%	LI	30 mg/mL[a]	Physically compatible for 4 hr at 23 °C	2339	C
Hydromorphone HCl	WY	0.2 mg/mL[a]	GL	30 mg/mL[a]	Physically compatible for 4 hr at 25 °C	987	C
Linezolid	PHU	2 mg/mL	GL	30 mg/mL[a]	Physically compatible for 4 hr at 23 °C	2264	C
Melphalan HCl	BW	0.1 mg/mL[b]	GL	20 mg/mL[b]	Physically compatible for 3 hr at 22 °C	1557	C
Meperidine HCl	WY	10 mg/mL[a]	GL	30 mg/mL[a]	Physically compatible for 4 hr at 25 °C	987	C
Midazolam HCl	RC	1 mg/mL[a]	LI	15 mg/mL[a]	Particles form in 8 hr	1847	I
Milrinone lactate	SS	0.2 mg/mL[a]	LI	100 mg/mL[a]	Visually compatible for 4 hr at 25 °C	2381	C
Morphine sulfate	WI	1 mg/mL[a]	GL	30 mg/mL[a]	Physically compatible for 4 hr at 25 °C	987	C
Ondansetron HCl	GL	1 mg/mL[b]	LI	30 mg/mL[a]	Visually compatible for 4 hr at 22 °C	1365	C

Y-Site Injection Compatibility (1:1 Mixture) (Cont.)

		Cefuroxime sodium					
Drug	*Mfr*	*Conc*	*Mfr*	*Conc*	*Remarks*	*Ref*	*C/I*
Pancuronium bromide	ES	0.05 mg/mL[a]	GL	7.5 mg/mL[a]	Physically compatible for 24 hr at 28 °C	1337	C
Pemetrexed disodium	LI	20 mg/mL[b]	GSK	30 mg/mL[a]	Physically compatible for 4 hr at 23 °C	2564	C
Propofol	ZEN	10 mg/mL	LI	30 mg/mL[a]	Physically compatible for 1 hr at 23 °C	2066	C
Remifentanil HCl	GW	0.025 and 0.25 mg/mL[b]	LI	30 mg/mL[a]	Physically compatible for 4 hr at 23 °C	2075	C
Sargramostim	IMM	10 mcg/mL[b]	GL	30 mg/mL[b]	Visually compatible for 4 hr at 22 °C	1436	C
Tacrolimus	FUJ	1 mg/mL[b]	LI	30 mg/mL[a]	Visually compatible for 24 hr at 25 °C	1630	C
Teniposide	BR	0.1 mg/mL[a]	GL	20 mg/mL[a]	Physically compatible for 4 hr at 23 °C	1725	C
Thiotepa	IMM[c]	1 mg/mL[a]	LI	30 mg/mL[a]	Physically compatible for 4 hr at 23 °C	1861	C
TNA #218 to #226[d]			GL	30 mg/mL[a]	Visually compatible for 4 hr at 23 °C	2215	C
TPN #212 to #215[d]			LI	30 mg/mL[a]	Physically compatible for 4 hr at 23 °C	2109	C
Vancomycin HCl	AB	20 mg/mL[a]	GW	150 mg/mL[e]	Transient precipitate forms followed by a subvisible haze	2189	I
	AB	20 mg/mL[a]	GW	50 mg/mL[a]	Gross white precipitate forms immediately	2189	I
	AB	20 mg/mL[a]	GW	10 mg/mL[a]	Subvisible haze forms immediately	2189	I
	AB	20 mg/mL[a]	GW	1 mg/mL[a]	Physically compatible for 4 hr at 23 °C	2189	C
	AB	2 mg/mL[a]	GW	1[a], 10[a], 50[a], 150[e] mg/mL	Physically compatible for 4 hr at 23 °C	2189	C
Vecuronium bromide	OR	0.1 mg/mL[a]	GL	7.5 mg/mL[a]	Physically compatible for 24 hr at 28 °C	1337	C
Vinorelbine tartrate	BW	1 mg/mL[b]	GL	20 mg/mL[b]	Large increase in measured turbidity occurs immediately	1558	I

[a]*Tested in dextrose 5%.*
[b]*Tested in sodium chloride 0.9%.*
[c]*Lyophilized formulation tested.*
[d]*Refer to Appendix I for the composition of parenteral nutrition solutions. TNA indicates a 3-in-1 admixture, and TPN indicates a 2-in-1 admixture.*
[e]*Tested in sterile water for injection.*
[f]*Tested in sodium chloride 0.45%.*
[g]*Injected via Y-site into an administration set running azithromycin.*

CHLORAMPHENICOL SODIUM SUCCINATE
AHFS 8:12.08

Products — Chloramphenicol sodium succinate is available in vials containing the equivalent of chloramphenicol 1 g as the sodium succinate salt. The manufacturer recommends reconstitution with 10 mL of an aqueous diluent such as water for injection or dextrose 5% to yield a solution containing 100 mg/mL (10%) of chloramphenicol. (1; 4)

pH — From 6.4 to 7. (4; 6)

Osmolality — Chloramphenicol sodium succinate 100 mg/mL in sterile water for injection has an osmolality of 533 mOsm/kg as determined by freezing-point depression. (1071)

The osmolality of chloramphenicol sodium succinate 1 g was calculated for the following dilutions (1054):

	Osmolality (mOsm/kg)	
Diluent	50 mL	100 mL
Dextrose 5%	341	303
Sodium chloride 0.9%	368	330

The osmolality of chloramphenicol sodium succinate (Parke-Davis) 20 mg/mL was determined to be 330 mOsm/kg in dextrose 5% and 344 mOsm/kg in sodium chloride 0.9%. At 50 mg/mL, the osmolality was determined to be 417 and 422 mOsm/kg, respectively. (1375)

The following maximum chloramphenicol sodium succinate concentrations were recommended to achieve osmolalities suitable for peripheral infusion in fluid-restricted patients (1180):

Diluent	Maximum Concentration (mg/mL)	Osmolality (mOsm/kg)
Dextrose 5%	71	554
Sodium chloride 0.9%	64	538
Sterile water for injection	128	473

Sodium Content — Chloramphenicol sodium succinate contains 2.25 mEq (52 mg) of sodium per gram of drug. (1; 4)

Administration — Chloramphenicol sodium succinate injection at a concentration not exceeding 100 mg/mL may be administered by direct intravenous injection over at least one minute. (1; 4)

Stability — Intact vials should be stored at controlled room temperature. The reconstituted solution is stable for 30 days at room temperature. (4; 6) Cloudy solutions should not be used. (4)

pH Effects — Chloramphenicol is stable over a pH range of 2 to 7, with maximum stability at pH 6. (1072) Chloramphenicol activity was retained for 24 hours at pH 3.6 to 7.5 in dextrose 5%. (6)

Sorption — Acetazolamide sodium was shown not to exhibit sorption to PVC bags and tubing, polyethylene tubing, Silastic tubing, and polypropylene syringes. (536; 606)

Compatibility Information

Solution Compatibility

Chloramphenicol sodium succinate

Solution	Mfr	Mfr	Conc/L	Remarks	Ref	C/I
Dextrose–Ringer's injection combinations	AB	PD	1 g	Physically compatible	3	C
Dextrose–Ringer's injection, lactated, combinations	AB	PD	1 g	Physically compatible	3	C
Dextrose 5% in Ringer's injection, lactated	AB			Stable for 24 hr	6	C
Dextrose–saline combinations	AB	PD	1 g	Physically compatible	3	C
Dextrose 5% in sodium chloride 0.9%		PD	500 mg	Physically compatible	74	C
	AB			Stable for 24 hr	6	C
		PD	2 g	Stable for 24 hr	109	C
Dextrose 2.5%	AB	PD	1 g	Physically compatible	3	C
Dextrose 5%	AB	PD	1 g	Physically compatible	3	C
		PD	500 mg	Physically compatible	74	C
	AB			Stable for 24 hr	6	C
		PD	2 g	Stable for 24 hr	109	C
			10 g	4% loss in 24 hr at room temperature	768	C
Dextrose 10%	AB	PD	1 g	Physically compatible	3	C
	AB			Stable for 24 hr	6	C
		PD	2 g	Stable for 24 hr	109	C
Ionosol products	AB	PD	1 g	Physically compatible	3	C
Normosol M in dextrose 5%	AB			Stable for 24 hr	6	C
Normosol R	AB			Stable for 24 hr	6	C
Ringer's injection	AB	PD	1 g	Physically compatible	3	C
	AB			Stable for 24 hr	6	C
Ringer's injection, lactated	AB	PD	1 g	Physically compatible	3	C
		PD	500 mg	Physically compatible	74	C
	AB			Stable for 24 hr	6	C
Sodium chloride 0.45%	AB	PD	1 g	Physically compatible	3	C

Solution Compatibility (Cont.)

Chloramphenicol sodium succinate

Solution	Mfr	Mfr	Conc/L	Remarks	Ref	C/I
Sodium chloride 0.9%	AB	PD	1 g	Physically compatible	3	C
		PD	500 mg	Physically compatible	74	C
	AB			Stable for 24 hr	6	C
		PD	2 g	Stable for 24 hr	109	C
			10 g	4% loss in 24 hr at room temperature	768	C
Sodium lactate ⅙ M	AB	PD	1 g	Physically compatible	3	C

Additive Compatibility

Chloramphenicol sodium succinate

Drug	Mfr	Conc/L	Mfr	Conc/L	Test Soln	Remarks	Ref	C/I
Amikacin sulfate	BR	5 g	PD	10 g	D5LR, D5R, D5S, D5W, D10W, LR, NS, R, SL	Physically compatible and both stable for 24 hr at 25 °C	293	C
Aminophylline	SE	1 g	PD	10 g	D5W	Physically compatible	15	C
		250 mg	PD	500 mg	D5W	Physically compatible	74	C
Ascorbic acid	AB	1 g	PD	1 g		Physically compatible	6	C
	UP		PD			Concentration-dependent incompatibility	15	I
Calcium chloride	UP	1 g	PD	10 g	D5W	Physically compatible	15	C
Calcium gluconate		1 g	PD	500 mg	D5W	Physically compatible	74	C
	UP	1 g	PD	10 g	D5W	Physically compatible	15	C
	UP	1 g	PD	10 g		Physically compatible	6	C
Chlorpromazine HCl	BP	200 mg	BP	4 g	D5W	Precipitates immediately	26	I
	BP	200 mg	BP	4 g	NS	Haze develops over 3 hr	26	I
Colistimethate sodium	WC	500 mg	PD	10 g	D5W	Physically compatible	15	C
	WC	500 mg	PD	10 g		Physically compatible	6	C
Cyanocobalamin	AB	1 mg	PD	1 g		Physically compatible	6	C
Dimenhydrinate	SE	50 mg	PD	500 mg	D5W	Physically compatible	74	C
Dopamine HCl	AS	800 mg	PD	4 g	D5W	Both drugs stable for 24 hr at 25 °C	78	C
Ephedrine sulfate	AB	50 mg	PD	1 g		Physically compatible	6	C
Erythromycin lactobionate	AB		PD		D5W	May precipitate at some concentrations	15	I
Fat emulsion, intravenous	VT	10%	PD	2 g		Physically compatible for 48 hr at 4 °C and room temperature	32	C
	VT	10%	PD	2 g		Physically compatible for 24 hr at 8 and 25 °C	825	C
Heparin sodium	UP	4000 units	PD	10 g	D5W	Physically compatible	15	C
	AB	20,000 units	PD	1 g		Physically compatible	6; 21	C
		12,000 units	PD	500 mg	D5W	Physically compatible	74	C
Hydrocortisone sodium succinate	UP	500 mg	PD	10 g	D5W	Physically compatible	15	C
	UP	500 mg	PD	1 g		Physically compatible	6	C

Additive Compatibility (Cont.)

Chloramphenicol sodium succinate

Drug	Mfr	Conc/L	Mfr	Conc/L	Test Soln	Remarks	Ref	C/I
	UP	100 mg	PD	500 mg	D5W	Physically compatible	74	C
Hydroxyzine HCl	RR	250 mg	PD	10 g	D5W	Physically incompatible	15	I
Lidocaine HCl	AST	2 g	PD	1 g		Physically compatible	24	C
Lincomycin HCl						Physically compatible for 24 hr at room temperature	1	C
Magnesium sulfate	LI	16 mEq	PD	10 g	D5W	Physically compatible	15	C
Methyldopate HCl	MSD	1 g	PD	1 g	D, D–S, S	Physically compatible	23	C
Methylprednisolone sodium succinate	UP	40 mg	PD	1 g	D5W	Clear solution for 20 hr	329	C
	UP	80 mg	PD	2 g	D5W	Clear solution for 20 hr	329	C
Nafcillin sodium	WY	500 mg	PD	1 g		Physically compatible	27	C
Oxacillin sodium	BR	2 g	PD	1 g		Physically compatible	6	C
	BR	500 mg	PD	500 mg	D5S, D5W	Therapeutic availability maintained	110	C
	BR	2 g	PD	1 g	D5S, D5W	Therapeutic availability maintained	110	C
Oxytocin	PD	5 units	PD	1 g		Physically compatible	6	C
Penicillin G potassium		1 million units	PD	1 g		Physically compatible	3	C
	SQ	1 million units	PD	500 mg	D5S, D5W	Therapeutic availability maintained	110	C
	SQ	5 million units	PD	1 g		Physically compatible	47	C
	SQ	10 million units	PD	1 g		Physically compatible	6	C
	SQ	5 and 10 million units	PD	1 g	D5S, D5W	Therapeutic availability maintained	110	C
	SQ	20 million units	PD	10 g	D5W	Physically compatible	15	C
Penicillin G sodium	UP	20 million units	PD	10 g	D5W	Physically compatible	15	C
Pentobarbital sodium	AB	200 mg	PD	1 g		Physically compatible	6	C
Phenylephrine HCl[a]	WI	2.5 g	PD	500 mg	D5W, NS	Phenylephrine stable for 24 hr at 22 °C	132	C
Phytonadione	MSD	50 mg	PD	1 g		Physically compatible	6	C
Polymyxin B sulfate	BW	200 mg	PD	10 g	D5W	Physically incompatible	15	I
	BW	200 mg	PD	10 g		Precipitate forms within 1 hr	6	I
Potassium chloride		20 and 40 mEq	PD	500 mg and 1 g	D2.5½S, D5W	Therapeutic availability maintained	110	C
	AB	40 mEq	PD	1 g		Physically compatible	6	C
		3 g	PD	500 mg	D5W	Physically compatible	74	C

Additive Compatibility (Cont.)

Chloramphenicol sodium succinate

Drug	Mfr	Conc/L	Mfr	Conc/L	Test Soln	Remarks	Ref	C/I
Prochlorperazine edisylate	SKF	100 mg	PD	10 g	D5W	Physically incompatible	15	I
Prochlorperazine mesylate	BP	100 mg	BP	4 g	NS	Haze develops over 3 hr	26	I
Promethazine HCl	WY	250 mg	PD	10 g	D5W	Physically incompatible	15	I
Ranitidine HCl	GL	100 mg		2 g	D5W	Physically compatible for 24 hr at ambient temperature	1151	C
Sodium bicarbonate	AB	80 mEq	PD	1 g		Physically compatible	6	C
	AB	80 mEq	PD	10 g	D5W	Physically compatible	15	C
Vancomycin HCl	LI	5 g	PD	10 g	D5W	Physically incompatible	15	I
Verapamil HCl	KN	80 mg	PD	2 g	D5W, NS	Physically compatible for 24 hr	764	C

aTested both with and without sodium bicarbonate 7.5 g/L.

Drugs in Syringe Compatibility

Chloramphenicol sodium succinate

Drug (in syringe)	Mfr	Amt	Mfr	Amt	Remarks	Ref	C/I
Ampicillin sodium	AY	500 mg	PD	250 and 400 mg/mL in 1.5 to 2 mL	No precipitate or color change within 1 hr at room temperature	99	C
	AY	500 mg	PD	250 and 400 mg/1 mL	Physically compatible for 1 hr at room temperature	300	C
Cloxacillin sodium	BE	250 mg	PD	250 and 400 mg/1.5 to 2 mL	No precipitate or color change within 1 hr at room temperature	99	C
	AY	250 mg	PD	250 and 400 mg/mL	Physically compatible for 1 hr at room temperature	300	C
Glycopyrrolate	RB	0.2 mg/1 mL	PD	100 mg/1 mL	Gas evolves	331	I
	RB	0.2 mg/1 mL	PD	200 mg/2 mL	Gas evolves	331	I
	RB	0.4 mg/2 mL	PD	100 mg/1 mL	Gas evolves	331	I
Heparin sodium	AB	20,000 units/1 mL	PD	1 g	Physically compatible for at least 30 min	21	C
		2500 units/1 mL		1 g	Physically compatible for at least 5 min	1053	C
Iohexol	WI	64.7%, 5 mL	PD	33 mg/1 mL	Physically compatible for at least 2 hr	1438	C
Iopamidol	SQ	61%, 5 mL	PD	33 mg/1 mL	Physically compatible for at least 2 hr	1438	C

Drugs in Syringe Compatibility (Cont.)

Chloramphenicol sodium succinate

Drug (in syringe)	Mfr	Amt	Mfr	Amt	Remarks	Ref	C/I
Iothalamate meglumine	MA	60%, 5 mL	PD	33 mg/ 1 mL	Physically compatible for at least 2 hr	1438	C
Ioxaglate meglumine–ioxaglate sodium	MA	5 mL	PD	33 mg/ 1 mL	Physically compatible for at least 2 hr	1438	C
Metoclopramide HCl	RB	10 mg/ 2 mL	PD	250 mg/ 2.5 mL	White precipitate forms immediately at 25 °C	1167	I
	RB	10 mg/ 2 mL	PD	2 g/ 20 mL	White precipitate forms immediately at 25 °C	1167	I
	RB	160 mg/ 32 mL	PD	2 g/ 20 mL	White precipitate forms immediately at 25 °C	1167	I
Penicillin G sodium		1 million units	PD	250 and 400 mg in 1.5 to 2 mL	No precipitate or color change within 1 hr at room temperature	99	C

Y-Site Injection Compatibility (1:1 Mixture)

Chloramphenicol sodium succinate

Drug	Mfr	Conc	Mfr	Conc	Remarks	Ref	C/I
Acyclovir sodium	BW	5 mg/mL[a]	ES	20 mg/mL[a]	Physically compatible for 4 hr at 25 °C	1157	C
Cyclophosphamide	MJ	20 mg/mL[a]	ES	20 mg/mL[a]	Physically compatible for 4 hr at 25 °C	1194	C
Enalaprilat	MSD	0.05 mg/mL[b]	PD	10 mg/mL[a]	Physically compatible for 24 hr at room temperature under fluorescent light	1355	C
Esmolol HCl	DCC	10 mg/mL[a]	PD	10 mg/mL[a]	Physically compatible for 24 hr at 22 °C	1169	C
Fluconazole	RR	2 mg/mL	PD	20 mg/mL	Gas production	1407	I
Foscarnet sodium	AST	24 mg/mL	PD	20 mg/mL	Physically compatible for 24 hr at room temperature under fluorescent light	1335	C
Hydromorphone HCl	WY	0.2 mg/mL[a]	LY	20 mg/mL[a]	Physically compatible for 4 hr at 25 °C	987	C
Labetalol HCl	SC	1 mg/mL[a]	PD	10 mg/mL[a]	Physically compatible for 24 hr at 18 °C	1171	C
Magnesium sulfate	IX	16.7, 33.3, 66.7, 100 mg/ mL[a]	PD	20 mg/mL[a]	Physically compatible for at least 4 hr at 32 °C	813	C
Meperidine HCl	WY	10 mg/mL[a]	LY	20 mg/mL[a]	Physically compatible for 4 hr at 25 °C	987	C
Morphine sulfate	WI	1 mg/mL[a]	LY	20 mg/mL[a]	Physically compatible for 4 hr at 25 °C	987	C
Nicardipine HCl	DCC	0.1 mg/mL[a]	PD	10 mg/mL[a]	Visually compatible for 24 hr at room temperature	235	C
Tacrolimus	FUJ	1 mg/mL[b]	PD	20 mg/mL[a]	Visually compatible for 24 hr at 25 °C	1630	C
TPN #61[c]		[d]	PD	125 mg/ 1.25 mL[e]	Physically compatible	1012	C
		[f]	PD	750 mg/ 7.5 mL[e]	Physically compatible	1012	C

[a]Tested in dextrose 5%.
[b]Tested in sodium chloride 0.9%.
[c]Refer to Appendix I for the composition of parenteral nutrition solutions. TPN indicates a 2-in-1 admixture.
[d]Run at 21 mL/hr.
[e]Given over five minutes by syringe pump.
[f]Run at 94 mL/hr.

CHLOROTHIAZIDE SODIUM
AHFS 40:28.20

Products — Chlorothiazide sodium is supplied in vials containing lyophilized drug equivalent to 500 mg of chlorothiazide with mannitol 250 mg and sodium hydroxide to adjust the pH. Reconstitute with 18 mL of sterile water for injection to obtain an isotonic solution yielding a concentration of 28 mg/mL of drug. No less than 18 mL should be used for reconstitution. (1; 4; 7)

pH — From 9.2 to 10. (4; 7)

Sodium Content — Each 500-mg vial of chlorothiazide sodium contains approximately 2.5 mEq of sodium. (4)

Trade Name(s) — Sodium Diuril.

Administration — Chlorothiazide sodium is administered intravenously by direct injection or infusion. It must not be administered intramuscularly or subcutaneously, and extravasation must be avoided. (1; 4)

Stability — Intact vials should be stored between 2 and 25 °C. (1) The reconstituted solution is intended for single use and unused solution should be discarded. (1; 4) However, the reconstituted solution has been stated to be stable for 24 hours. (7)

pH Effects — Chlorothiazide sodium appears to be stable at pH 7.5 to 9.5 in dextrose 5%. No loss of potency was noted over a 24-hour study period. (7)

The solubility of chlorothiazide sodium is very pH sensitive. Depending on concentration, precipitation occurs at approximately pH 7.4 and below. Additives that result in a final pH in this range should not be mixed. Chlorothiazide sodium is sufficiently alkaline to raise the pH of unbuffered solutions such as dextrose, saline, and their combinations. But if an acidic buffer is present, such as lactate or acetate buffers, the resultant pH may fall below pH 7.4, causing precipitation. (7)

Chlorothiazide sodium possesses some alkalizing power. Therefore, it should not be combined with drugs known to be unstable in alkaline media. (7)

Compatibility Information

Solution Compatibility

Chlorothiazide sodium

Solution	Mfr	Mfr	Conc/L	Remarks	Ref	C/I
Dextrose–Ringer's injection combinations	AB	MSD	2 g	Physically compatible	3	C
Dextrose–Ringer's injection, lactated, combinations	AB	MSD	2 g	Physically compatible	3	C
Dextrose–saline combinations	AB	MSD	2 g	Physically compatible	3	C
Dextrose 5% in sodium chloride 0.9%	AB	MSD	1 g	Stable for 24 hr	7	C
Dextrose 2.5%	AB	MSD	2 g	Physically compatible	3	C
Dextrose 5%	AB	MSD	1 g	Stable for 24 hr	7	C
	AB	MSD	2 g	Physically compatible	3	C
Dextrose 10%	AB	MSD	2 g	Physically compatible	3	C
Ionosol B in dextrose 5%	AB	MSD	500 mg	Physically incompatible	15	I
	AB	MSD	2 g	Precipitate forms after 6 hr	7	I
	AB	MSD	2 g	Haze or precipitate forms within 24 hr	3	I
Ionosol MB in dextrose 5%	AB	MSD	2 g	Physically compatible	3	C
Ionosol T in dextrose 5%	AB	MSD	2 g	Physically compatible	3	C
Normosol M in dextrose 5%	AB	MSD	2 g	Precipitate forms after 6 hr	7	I
Normosol R in dextrose 5%	AB	MSD	2 g	Precipitate forms after 6 hr	7	I
Ringer's injection	AB	MSD	1 g	Stable for 24 hr	7	C
	AB	MSD	2 g	Physically compatible	3	C
Ringer's injection, lactated	AB	MSD	1 g	Stable for 24 hr	7	C
	AB	MSD	2 g	Physically compatible	3	C
Sodium chloride 0.45%	AB	MSD	2 g	Physically compatible	3	C
Sodium chloride 0.9%	AB	MSD	1 g	Stable for 24 hr	7	C
	AB	MSD	2 g	Physically compatible	3	C
Sodium lactate ⅙ M	AB	MSD	2 g	Physically compatible	3	C

Additive Compatibility

Chlorothiazide sodium

Drug	Mfr	Conc/L	Mfr	Conc/L	Test Soln	Remarks	Ref	C/I
Amikacin sulfate	BR	5 g	MSD	10 mg	D5LR, D5R, D5S, D5W, D10W, LR, NS, R, SL	Precipitate forms within 4 hr at 25 °C	294	I
Chlorpromazine HCl	BP	200 mg	BP	2 g	D5W, NS	Precipitates immediately	26	I
Hydralazine HCl	BP	80 mg	BP	2 g	D5W, NS	Yellow color with precipitate in 3 hr	26	I
Lidocaine HCl	AST	2 g	MSD	500 mg		Physically compatible	24	C
Nafcillin sodium	WY	500 mg	MSD	500 mg		Physically compatible	27	C
Polymyxin B sulfate	BP	20 mg	BP	2 g	D5W	Yellow color produced	26	I
Prochlorperazine mesylate	BP	100 mg	BP	2 g	D5W	Precipitates immediately	26	I
	BP	100 mg	BP	2 g	NS	Haze develops over 3 hr	26	I
Promethazine HCl	BP	100 mg	BP	2 g	D5W, NS	Precipitates immediately	26	I
Ranitidine HCl	GL	50 mg and 2 g		5 g	D5W	Physically compatible. Ranitidine stable for 24 hr at 25 °C. Chlorothiazide not tested	1515	C

Y-Site Injection Compatibility (1:1 Mixture)

Chlorothiazide sodium

Drug	Mfr	Conc	Mfr	Conc	Remarks	Ref	C/I
Alprostadil	BED	7.5 mcg/mL[c]	ME	25 mg/mL[b]	Visually compatible for 1 hr	2746	C
TPN #203, #204[a]			ME	28 mg/mL	White precipitate forms immediately	1974	I

[a]*Refer to Appendix I for the composition of the parenteral nutrition solutions. TPN indicates a 2-in-1 admixture.*
[b]*Tested in either dextrose 5% or in sodium chloride 0.9%, but the report did not specify which solution.*
[c]*Tested in a 1:1 mixture of (1) dextrose 5% and dextrose 5% in sodium chloride 0.45% with and without potassium chloride 20 mEq/L and also in (2) dextrose 10% in sodium chloride 0.45% with and without potassium chloride 20 mEq/L.*

CHLORPROMAZINE HYDROCHLORIDE
AHFS 28:16.08.24

Products — Chlorpromazine hydrochloride 25 mg/mL is available in 1- and 2-mL ampuls and vials. Each milliliter of solution also contains ascorbic acid 2 mg, sodium metabisulfite 1 mg, sodium sulfite 1 mg, and sodium chloride 6 mg in water for injection. (1):

pH — From 3.4 to 5.4. (1; 17)

Administration — Chlorpromazine hydrochloride may be administered slowly by deep intramuscular injection into the upper outer quadrant of the buttock. Dilution with sodium chloride 0.9% or procaine hydrochloride 2% has been recommended for intramuscular injection if local irritation is a problem. Subcutaneous injection is not recommended. The drug may be diluted to 1 mg/mL with sodium chloride 0.9% and administered by direct intravenous injection at a rate of 1 mg/min to adults and 0.5 mg/min to children. For infusion, it may be diluted in 500 to 1000 mL of sodium chloride 0.9%. (1; 4)

Stability — Intact containers should be stored at controlled room temperature. Freezing should be avoided. Protect the solution from light during storage or it may discolor. A slightly yellowed solution does not indicate potency loss. However, a markedly discolored solution should be discarded. (1)

pH Effects — The pH of maximum stability is 6. (67) Oxidation of chlorpromazine hydrochloride occurs in alkaline media. (4) The titration of chlorpromazine hydrochloride in sodium chloride 0.9% with alkali resulted in precipitation of chlorpromazine base at pH 6.7 to 6.8. (138)

Precipitation may occur if chlorpromazine hydrochloride is admixed with alkaline drugs or solutions.

Light Effects — Chlorpromazine hydrochloride ampuls and vials should be protected from light during storage. (1; 4) However, chlorpromazine hydrochloride infusion solutions in PVC bags exposed to light during administration lost less than 2% of the drug over a six-hour administration period. Light protection of infusion sets during administration was found not to be necessary. (2280)

Sorption — Chlorpromazine hydrochloride (May & Baker) 9 mg/L in sodium chloride 0.9% (Travenol) in PVC bags exhibited only about 5% sorption to the plastic bag during one week of storage at room temperature (15 to 20 °C). However, when the solution was buffered from its initial pH of 5 to pH 7.4, approximately 86% of the drug was lost in one week due to sorption. (536)

Chlorpromazine hydrochloride (May & Baker) 9 mg/L in sodium chloride 0.9% exhibited a cumulative 41% loss due to sorption during a seven-hour simulated infusion through an infusion set (Travenol) consisting of a cellulose propionate burette chamber and 170 cm of PVC tubing. Both the burette chamber and the tubing contributed to the loss. The extent of sorption was found to be independent of concentration. (606)

The drug was also tested as a simulated infusion over at least one hour by a syringe pump system. A glass syringe on a syringe pump was fitted with 20 cm of polyethylene tubing or 50 cm of Silastic tubing. A negligible amount of drug was lost with the polyethylene tubing, but a cumulative loss of 79% occurred during the one-hour infusion through the Silastic tubing. (606)

A 25-mL aliquot of chlorpromazine hydrochloride 9 mg/L in sodium chloride 0.9% was stored in all-plastic syringes composed of polypropylene barrels and polyethylene plungers for 24 hours at room temperature in the dark. The solution did not exhibit any loss due to sorption. (606)

In a continuation of this work, chlorpromazine hydrochloride (May & Baker) 90 mg/L in sodium chloride 0.9% in a glass bottle was delivered through a polyethylene administration set (Tridilset) over eight hours at 15 to 20 °C. The flow rate was set at 1 mL/min. No appreciable loss due to sorption occurred. (769) This finding is in contrast to a 41% loss using a conventional administration set. (606)

Central Venous Catheter — Chlorpromazine hydrochloride (Elkin-Sinn) 2 mg/mL in dextrose 5% was found to be compatible with the ARROWg+ard Blue Plus (Arrow International) chlorhexidine-bearing triple-lumen central catheter. Essentially complete delivery of the drug was found with little or no drug loss occurring. Furthermore, chlorhexidine delivered from the catheter remained at trace amounts with no substantial increase due to the delivery of the drug through the catheter. (2335)

Compatibility Information

Solution Compatibility

Chlorpromazine HCl

Solution	Mfr	Mfr	Conc/L	Remarks	Ref	C/I
Dextrose–Ringer's injection combinations	AB	SKF	50 mg	Physically compatible	3	C
Dextrose–Ringer's injection, lactated, combinations	AB	SKF	50 mg	Physically compatible	3	C
Dextrose–saline combinations	AB	SKF	50 mg	Physically compatible	3	C
Dextrose 2.5%	AB	SKF	50 mg	Physically compatible	3	C
Dextrose 5%	AB	SKF	50 mg	Physically compatible	3	C
Dextrose 10%	AB	SKF	50 mg	Physically compatible	3	C
Ionosol products	AB	SKF	50 mg	Physically compatible	3	C
Ringer's injection	AB	SKF	50 mg	Physically compatible	3	C
Ringer's injection, lactated	AB	SKF	50 mg	Physically compatible	3	C
Sodium chloride 0.45%	AB	SKF	50 mg	Physically compatible	3	C
Sodium chloride 0.9%	AB	SKF	50 mg	Physically compatible	3	C
		SKF	1 g	Variable assay results over 30 days at 23 °C	1083	?
Sodium lactate ⅙ M	AB	SKF	50 mg	Physically compatible	3	C

Additive Compatibility

Chlorpromazine HCl

Drug	Mfr	Conc/L	Mfr	Conc/L	Test Soln	Remarks	Ref	C/I
Aminophylline	BP	1 g	BP	200 mg	D5W, NS	Precipitates immediately	26	I
Amphotericin B		200 mg	BP	200 mg	D5W	Precipitates immediately	26	I
Ampicillin sodium	BP	2 g	BP	200 mg	D5W, NS	Precipitates immediately	26	I
Ascorbic acid	UP	500 mg	SKF	250 mg	D5W	Physically compatible	15	C
Chloramphenicol sodium succinate	BP	4 g	BP	200 mg	D5W	Precipitates immediately	26	I
	BP	4 g	BP	200 mg	NS	Haze develops over 3 hr	26	I
Chlorothiazide sodium	BP	2 g	BP	200 mg	D5W, NS	Precipitates immediately	26	I
Cloxacillin sodium	BP	1 g	BP	200 mg	NS	Haze forms over 3 hr	26	I
Ethacrynate sodium	MSD	50 mg	SKF	50 mg	NS	Little alteration of UV spectra within 8 hr at room temperature	16	C
Floxacillin sodium	BE	20 g	ANT	5 g	W	Yellow precipitate forms immediately	1479	I
Furosemide	HO	1 g	ANT	5 g	W	Precipitates immediately	1479	I
Methohexital sodium	BP	2 g	BP	200 mg	D5W, NS	Precipitates immediately	26	I
Penicillin G potassium	BP	10 million units	BP	200 mg	NS	Haze develops over 3 hr	26	I
Penicillin G sodium	BP	10 million units	BP	200 mg	NS	Haze develops over 3 hr	26	I
Phenobarbital sodium	BP	800 mg	BP	200 mg	D5W, NS	Precipitates immediately	26	I
Theophylline		2 g		200 mg	D5W	Visually compatible. 7% chlorpromazine and no theophylline loss in 48 hr	1909	C

Drugs in Syringe Compatibility

Chlorpromazine HCl

Drug (in syringe)	Mfr	Amt	Mfr	Amt	Remarks	Ref	C/I
Atropine sulfate		0.6 mg/ 1.5 mL	SKF	50 mg/ 2 mL	Physically compatible for at least 15 min	14	C
	ST	0.4 mg/ 1 mL	PO	50 mg/ 2 mL	Physically compatible for at least 15 min	326	C
Benztropine mesylate	MSD	2 mg/ 2 mL	STS	50 mg/ 2 mL	Visually compatible for 60 min	1784	C
Butorphanol tartrate	BR	4 mg/ 2 mL	MB	25 mg/ 1 mL	Physically compatible for 30 min at room temperature	566	C
Dimenhydrinate	HR	50 mg/ 1 mL	PO	50 mg/ 2 mL	Physically incompatible within 15 min	326	I
		10 mg/ 1 mL		25 mg/ 1 mL	Clear solution	2569	C
Diphenhydramine HCl	PD	50 mg/ 1 mL	PO	50 mg/ 2 mL	Physically compatible for at least 15 min	326	C
	ES	100 mg/ 2 mL	STS	50 mg/ 2 mL	Visually compatible for 60 min	1784	C

Drugs in Syringe Compatibility (Cont.)

Chlorpromazine HCl

Drug (in syringe)	Mfr	Amt	Mfr	Amt	Remarks	Ref	C/I
Doxapram HCl	RB	400 mg/ 20 mL		250 mg/ 5 mL	Physically compatible with no doxapram loss in 24 hr	1177	C
Droperidol	MN	2.5 mg/ 1 mL	PO	50 mg/ 2 mL	Physically compatible for at least 15 min	326	C
Fentanyl citrate	MN	0.05 mg/ 1 mL	PO	50 mg/ 2 mL	Physically compatible for at least 15 min	326	C
Glycopyrrolate	RB	0.2 mg/ 1 mL	SKF	25 mg/ 1 mL	Physically compatible. pH in glycopyrrolate stability range for 48 hr at 25 °C	331	C
	RB	0.2 mg/ 1 mL	SKF	50 mg/ 2 mL	Physically compatible. pH in glycopyrrolate stability range for 48 hr at 25 °C	331	C
	RB	0.4 mg/ 2 mL	SKF	25 mg/ 1 mL	Physically compatible. pH in glycopyrrolate stability range for 48 hr at 25 °C	331	C
Heparin sodium		2500 units/ 1 mL		50 mg/ 2 mL	Turbidity or precipitate forms within 5 min	1053	I
Hydromorphone HCl	KN	4 mg/ 2 mL	ES	25 mg/ 1 mL	Physically compatible for 30 min	517	C
Hydroxyzine HCl	PF	50 mg/ 1 mL	PO	50 mg/ 2 mL	Physically compatible for at least 15 min	326	C
	ES	100 mg/ 2 mL	STS	50 mg/ 2 mL	Visually compatible for 60 min	1784	C
Meperidine HCl	WY	100 mg/ 1 mL	SKF	50 mg/ 2 mL	Physically compatible for at least 15 min	14	C
	WI	50 mg/ 1 mL	PO	50 mg/ 2 mL	Physically compatible for at least 15 min	326	C
Metoclopramide HCl	NO	10 mg/ 2 mL	MB	25 mg/ 1 mL	Physically compatible for 15 min at room temperature	565	C
Midazolam HCl	RC	5 mg/ 1 mL	SKF	50 mg/ 2 mL	Physically compatible for 4 hr at 25 °C	1145	C
Morphine sulfate	WY	15 mg/ 1 mL	SKF	50 mg/ 2 mL	Physically compatible for at least 15 min	14	C
	ST	15 mg/ 1 mL	PO	50 mg/ 2 mL	Physically compatible for at least 15 min	326	C
Pantoprazole sodium	[a]	4 mg/ 1 mL		25 mg/ 1 mL	Precipitates immediately	2574	I
Pentazocine lactate	WI	30 mg/ 1 mL	SKF	50 mg/ 2 mL	Physically compatible for at least 15 min	14	C
	WI	30 mg/ 1 mL	PO	50 mg/ 2 mL	Physically compatible for at least 15 min	326	C
Pentobarbital sodium	WY	100 mg/ 2 mL	SKF	50 mg/ 2 mL	Precipitate forms within 15 min	14	I
	AB	500 mg/ 10 mL	SKF	50 mg/ 2 mL	Physically incompatible	55	I
	AB	50 mg/ 1 mL	PO	50 mg/ 2 mL	Physically incompatible within 15 min	326	I
Prochlorperazine edisylate	SKF		SKF	50 mg/ 2 mL	Physically compatible for at least 15 min	14	C
	PO	5 mg/ 1 mL	PO	50 mg/ 2 mL	Physically compatible for at least 15 min	326	C

Drugs in Syringe Compatibility (Cont.)

Chlorpromazine HCl

Drug (in syringe)	Mfr	Amt	Mfr	Amt	Remarks	Ref	C/I
Promethazine HCl	PO	50 mg/ 2 mL	PO	50 mg/ 2 mL	Physically compatible for at least 15 min	326	C
Ranitidine HCl	GL	50 mg/ 2 mL	RP	25 mg/ 1 mL	Physically compatible for 1 hr at 25 °C	978	C
	GL	50 mg/ 5 mL	RP	25 mg	Gas formation	1151	I
Scopolamine HBr		0.6 mg/ 1.5 mL	SKF	50 mg/ 2 mL	Physically compatible for at least 15 min	14	C
	ST	0.4 mg/ 1 mL	PO	50 mg/ 2 mL	Physically compatible for at least 15 min	326	C

[a]Test performed using the formulation WITHOUT edetate disodium.

Y-Site Injection Compatibility (1:1 Mixture)

Chlorpromazine HCl

Drug	Mfr	Conc	Mfr	Conc	Remarks	Ref	C/I
Allopurinol sodium	BW	3 mg/mL[b]	RU	2 mg/mL[b]	White precipitate forms immediately	1686	I
Amifostine	USB	10 mg/mL[a]	SCN	2 mg/mL[a]	Subvisible haze forms immediately	1845	I
Amphotericin B cholesteryl sulfate complex	SEQ	0.83 mg/mL[a]	ES	2 mg/mL[a]	Gross precipitate forms	2117	I
Amsacrine	NCI	1 mg/mL[a]	ES	2 mg/mL[a]	Visually compatible for 4 hr at 22 °C	1381	C
Aztreonam	SQ	40 mg/mL[a]	SCN	2 mg/mL[a]	Dense white turbidity forms immediately	1758	I
Bivalirudin	TMC	5 mg/mL[a]	ES	2 mg/mL[a]	Gross white precipitate forms immediately	2373	I
Cisatracurium besylate	GW	0.1, 2, 5 mg/ mL[a]	SCN	2 mg/mL[a]	Physically compatible for 4 hr at 23 °C	2074	C
Cladribine	ORT	0.015[b] and 0.5[c] mg/mL	SCN	2 mg/mL[b]	Physically compatible for 4 hr at 23 °C	1969	C
Dexmedetomidine HCl	AB	4 mcg/mL[b]	ES	2 mg/mL[b]	Physically compatible for 4 hr at 23 °C	2383	C
Docetaxel	RPR	0.9 mg/mL[a]	SCN	2 mg/mL[a]	Physically compatible for 4 hr at 23 °C	2224	C
Doxorubicin HCl liposomal	SEQ	0.4 mg/mL[a]	ES	2 mg/mL[a]	Physically compatible for 4 hr at 23 °C	2087	C
Etoposide phosphate	BR	5 mg/mL[a]	ES	2 mg/mL[a]	Cloudy solution forms immediately with particulates in 4 hr	2218	I
Famotidine	ME	2 mg/mL[b]		2 mg/mL[a]	Visually compatible for 4 hr at 22 °C	1936	C
Fenoldopam mesylate	AB	80 mcg/mL[b]	ES	2 mg/mL[b]	Physically compatible for 4 hr at 23 °C	2467	C
Filgrastim	AMG	30 mcg/mL[a]	RU	2 mg/mL[a]	Physically compatible for 4 hr at 22 °C	1687	C
Fluconazole	RR	2 mg/mL	ES	25 mg/mL	Physically compatible for 24 hr at 25 °C	1407	C
Fludarabine phosphate	BX	1 mg/mL[a]	ES	2 mg/mL[a]	Initial light haze intensifies within 30 min	1439	I
Furosemide	HMR	2.6 mg/mL[a]	RPR	0.13 mg/mL[a]	Precipitate forms immediately	2244	I
Gemcitabine HCl	LI	10 mg/mL[b]	ES	2 mg/mL[b]	Physically compatible for 4 hr at 23 °C	2226	C
Granisetron HCl	SKB	0.05 mg/mL[a]	SCN	2 mg/mL[a]	Physically compatible for 4 hr at 23 °C	2000	C
Heparin sodium	UP	1000 units/L[d]	SKF	25 mg/mL	Physically compatible for 4 hr at room temperature	534	C
	NOV	29.2 units/ mL[a]	RPR	0.13 mg/mL[a]	Visually compatible for 150 min	2244	C

Y-Site Injection Compatibility (1:1 Mixture) (Cont.)

Chlorpromazine HCl

Drug	Mfr	Conc	Mfr	Conc	Remarks	Ref	C/I
Hetastarch in lactated electrolyte	AB	6%	ES	2 mg/mL[a]	Physically compatible for 4 hr at 23 °C	2339	C
Hydrocortisone sodium succinate	UP	10 mg/L[d]	SKF	25 mg/mL	Physically compatible for 4 hr at room temperature	534	C
Linezolid	PHU	2 mg/mL	ES	2 mg/mL[a]	Measured haze level increases immediately	2264	I
Melphalan HCl	BW	0.1 mg/mL[b]	ES	2 mg/mL[b]	Large increase in measured turbidity occurs within 1 hr and grows over 3 hr	1557	I
Ondansetron HCl	GL	1 mg/mL[b]	ES	2 mg/mL[a]	Visually compatible for 4 hr at 22 °C	1365	C
Oxaliplatin	SS	0.5 mg/mL[a]	ES	2 mg/mL[a]	Physically compatible for 4 hr at 23 °C	2566	C
Paclitaxel	NCI	1.2 mg/mL[a]	ES	2 mg/mL[a]	Normal inherent haze from paclitaxel decreases immediately	1556	I
Pemetrexed disodium	LI	20 mg/mL[b]	ES	2 mg/mL[a]	Cloudy precipitate forms immediately	2564	I
Piperacillin sodium–tazobactam sodium	LE[e]	40 + 5 mg/mL[a]	RU	2 mg/mL[a]	Heavy white turbidity forms immediately. White precipitate forms in 4 hr	1688	I
Potassium chloride	AB	40 mEq/L[d]	SKF	25 mg/mL	Physically compatible for 4 hr at room temperature	534	C
	BRN	0.625 mEq/mL[a]	RPR	0.13 mg/mL[a]	Visually compatible for 150 min	2244	C
Propofol	ZEN	10 mg/mL	SCN	2 mg/mL[a]	Physically compatible for 1 hr at 23 °C	2066	C
Remifentanil HCl	GW	0.025 mg/mL[b]	SCN	2 mg/mL[a]	Slight haze forms in 1 hr	2075	I
	GW	0.25 mg/mL[b]	SCN	2 mg/mL[a]	Physically compatible for 4 hr at 23 °C	2075	C
Sargramostim	IMM	10 mcg/mL[b]	ES	2 mg/mL[b]	Slight haze forms immediately	1436	I
Teniposide	BR	0.1 mg/mL[a]	SCN	2 mg/mL[a]	Physically compatible for 4 hr at 23 °C	1725	C
Thiotepa	IMM[f]	1 mg/mL[a]	SCN	2 mg/mL[a]	Physically compatible for 4 hr at 23 °C	1861	C
Tigecycline	WY	1 mg/mL[b]		1 mg/mL[b]	Precipitates immediately	2714	I
TNA #218 to #226[g]			SCN	2 mg/mL[a]	Visually compatible for 4 hr at 23 °C	2215	C
TPN #212 to #215[g]			SCN	2 mg/mL[a]	Physically compatible for 4 hr at 23 °C	2109	C
Vinorelbine tartrate	BW	1 mg/mL[b]	RU	2 mg/mL[b]	Physically compatible for 4 hr at 22 °C	1558	C

[a]*Tested in dextrose 5%.*
[b]*Tested in sodium chloride 0.9%.*
[c]*Tested in bacteriostatic sodium chloride 0.9% preserved with benzyl alcohol 0.9%.*
[d]*Tested in dextrose 5% in Ringer's injection, dextrose 5% in Ringer's injection, lactated, dextrose 5%, Ringer's injection, lactated, and sodium chloride 0.9%.*
[e]*Test performed using the formulation WITHOUT edetate disodium.*
[f]*Lyophilized formulation tested.*
[g]*Refer to Appendix I for the composition of parenteral nutrition solutions. TNA indicates a 3-in-1 admixture, and TPN indicates a 2-in-1 admixture.*

Additional Compatibility Information

Hydroxyzine and Meperidine — Chlorpromazine hydrochloride (Elkins-Sinn) 6.25 mg/mL, hydroxyzine hydrochloride (Pfizer) 12.5 mg/mL, and meperidine hydrochloride (Winthrop) 25 mg/mL, in both glass and plastic syringes, have been reported to be physically compatible and chemically stable for at least one year at 4 and 25 °C when protected from light. (989)

Meperidine and Promethazine — Chlorpromazine hydrochloride, meperidine hydrochloride, and promethazine hydrochloride combined as an extemporaneous mixture for preoperative sedation, developed a brownish-yellow color after two weeks of storage with protection from light. The discoloration was attributed to the metacresol preservative content of the meperidine hydrochloride product used. Use of meperidine hydrochloride which contains a different preservative resulted in a solution that remained clear and colorless for at least three months when protected from light. (1148)

Chlorocresol — Chlorpromazine hydrochloride is incompatible with chlorocresol preservative. (467; 468)

CIDOFOVIR
AHFS 8:18.32

Products — Cidofovir is available in 5-mL vials. Each milliliter contains cidofovir 75 mg with sodium hydroxide and/or hydrochloric acid to adjust pH. (1) The product must be diluted in sodium chloride 0.9% for administration. (1; 4)

Appropriate safety precautions for handling mutagenic substances should be taken; preparation in a biological safety cabinet and wearing of suitable gloves and gowns with knit cuffs are recommended. If cidofovir solution contacts skin or mucosa, wash the affected area immediately with soap and water. (1; 4)

Partially used vials, diluted solutions, and materials used in admixture preparation and administration should be sealed in leak- and puncture-proof containers and incinerated at high temperature. (1; 4)

pH — Cidofovir has a pH adjusted to 7.4. (1)

The pH values of cidofovir admixtures in three infusion solutions were (1963):

Solution	Concentration	pH
Dextrose 5% in sodium chloride 0.45%	0.085 and 3.51 mg/mL	6.7 to 7.0
Dextrose 5%	0.21 and 8.12 mg/mL	7.2 to 7.6
Sodium chloride 0.9%	0.21 and 8.12 mg/mL	7.1 to 7.5

Osmolality — Cidofovir is hypertonic and is diluted for administration. The osmolalities of cidofovir admixtures in three infusion solutions were (1963):

Solution	Concentration	Osmolality (mOsm/kg)
Dextrose 5% in sodium chloride 0.45%	0.085 and 3.51 mg/mL	382 and 392
Dextrose 5%	0.21 and 8.12 mg/mL	241 and 286
Sodium chloride 0.9%	0.21 and 8.12 mg/mL	275 and 315

Trade Name(s) — Vistide.

Administration — Cidofovir is administered by intravenous infusion in 100 mL of sodium chloride 0.9% at a constant rate over a one-hour period using an infusion-control pump. Shorter periods must not be used. Patients must be prehydrated with sodium chloride 0.9% and treated with probenecid. Intraocular administration is contraindicated. (1; 4)

Stability — Cidofovir should be stored at controlled room temperature. The manufacturer states that, diluted in 100 mL of sodium chloride 0.9% for administration, cidofovir should be used within 24 hours of preparation. Admixtures not used immediately should be stored under refrigeration at 2 to 8 °C but should still be used within 24 hours of preparation. Refrigeration or freezing should not be used to extend beyond the 24-hour limit. (1; 4)

Syringes — Cidofovir 6.25 mg/mL in sodium chloride 0.9% packaged in polypropylene syringes (Becton Dickinson) has been reported to be stable by HPLC analysis for 150 days at room and refrigeration temperatures. (2607)

Sorption — Cidofovir is stated to be compatible with glass, PVC, and ethylene/propylene copolymer infusion solution containers. (1)

Compatibility Information

Solution Compatibility

Cidofovir

Solution	Mfr	Mfr	Conc/L	Remarks	Ref	C/I
Dextrose 5% in sodium chloride 0.45%	AB[a], BA[a], MG[b]	GIL	85 mg and 3.51 g	Physically compatible with no increase in subvisual particulates in 24 hr at 4 and 30 °C	1963	C
Dextrose 5%	AB[a], BA[a], MG[b]	GIL	210 mg and 8.12 g	Physically compatible with no increase in subvisual particulates and no loss by HPLC in 24 hr at 4 and 30 °C	1963	C
Sodium chloride 0.9%	AB[a], BA[a], MG[b]	GIL	210 mg and 8.12 g	Physically compatible with no increase in subvisual particulates and no loss by HPLC in 24 hr at 4 and 30 °C	1963	C
	AB[a], BA[a], MG[b]	GIL	200 mg and 8.1 g	Physically compatible with no increase in subvisual particulates and no loss by HPLC in 5 days at 4 and −20 °C	2076	C

[a]Tested in PVC containers.
[b]Tested in polyolefin containers.

CIPROFLOXACIN
AHFS 8:12.18

Products — Ciprofloxacin is available as a premixed, ready-to-use solution in 100- and 200-mL PVC containers. Each milliliter contains 2 mg of ciprofloxacin with dextrose 5%, lactic acid as a solubilizer, and hydrochloric acid to adjust the pH. (1)

pH — From 3.5 to 4.6. (1; 17)

Trade Name(s) — Cipro I.V.

Administration — Ciprofloxacin is administered at a concentration of 1 to 2 mg/mL by intravenous infusion into a large vein slowly over 60 minutes. When given intermittently through a Y-site, the primary solution should be discontinued temporarily. (1; 4)

Stability — Ciprofloxacin is a clear, colorless to slightly yellow solution. It should be stored between 5 and 25 °C and protected from light and freezing. (1; 4)

Ciprofloxacin 25 mg/L in Dianeal 137 peritoneal dialysis solution exhibited little or no loss after 42 days at 4, 22, and 37 °C when protected from light. (1585) At 37 °C over 48 hours, losses of up to

10% occurred in the Dianeal PD-1 with dextrose 1.5%; losses of up to 7% occurred in the Dianeal PD-1 with dextrose 4.5%. (1826) Ciprofloxacin 25 and 50 mg/L in Dianeal PD-2 with dextrose 1.5, 2.5, and 4.25% and Extraneal, all solutions both with and without heparin, were found to be stable for four days at 38 °C. (2686)

pH Effects — Ciprofloxacin in aqueous solution is stated to be stable for up to 14 days at room temperature in the pH range of 1.5 to 7.5. (4) However, Teraoka et al. reported substantial loss of ciprofloxacin content in admixtures with a pH over 6. (1924)

Light Effects — Ciprofloxacin undergoes slow degradation when exposed to natural daylight. Exposure to mixed natural daylight and fluorescent light resulted in about 2% loss after 12 hours of exposure and about 9% loss after about 96 hours of exposure. (2399)

Central Venous Catheter — Ciprofloxacin (Bayer) 1 mg/mL in dextrose 5% was found to be compatible with the ARROWg+ard Blue Plus (Arrow International) chlorhexidine-bearing triple-lumen central catheter. Essentially complete delivery of the drug was found with little or no drug loss occurring. Furthermore, chlorhexidine delivered from the catheter remained at trace amounts with no substantial increase due to the delivery of the drug through the catheter. (2335)

Compatibility Information

Solution Compatibility

Ciprofloxacin

Solution	Mfr	Mfr	Conc/L	Remarks	Ref	C/I
Dextrose 5% in sodium chloride 0.225%		MI	0.5 to 2 g	Stable for 14 days at 5 and 25 °C	888	C
Dextrose 5% in sodium chloride 0.45%		MI	0.5 to 2 g	Stable for 14 days at 5 and 25 °C	888	C
Dextrose 5%	AB[a]	MI	1.5 g	Visually compatible with no loss in 48 hr at 25 °C under fluorescent light	1541	C
	[a]	BAY	800 mg	Visually compatible with no significant loss in 6 hr at 22 °C exposed to light	1698	C
		MI	0.5 to 2 g	Stable for 14 days at 5 and 25 °C	888	C
	BA[a]	MI	2.86 g	Visually compatible with no loss in 90 days at room temperature and 5 °C	1891	C
Dextrose 10%		MI	0.5 to 2 g	Stable for 14 days at 5 and 25 °C	888	C
Ringer's injection		MI	0.5 to 1 g	Stable for 14 days at 5 and 25 °C	888	C
Ringer's injection, lactated		MI	0.5 to 2 g	Stable for 14 days at 5 and 25 °C	888	C
Sodium chloride 0.9%	AB[a]	MI	1.5 g	Visually compatible with no loss in 48 hr at 25 °C under fluorescent light	1541	C
	[a]	BAY	800 mg	Visually compatible with no significant loss in 6 hr at 22 °C exposed to light	1698	C

Solution Compatibility (Cont.)

Ciprofloxacin

Solution	Mfr	Mfr	Conc/L	Remarks	Ref	C/I
		MI	0.5 to 2 g	Stable for 14 days at 5 and 25 °C	888	C
	BA[a]	MI	2.86 g	Visually compatible with no loss in 90 days at room temperature and 5 °C	1891	C
	AB	BAY	2 g	Visually compatible with no loss in 24 hr at 25 °C	1934	C

[a]Tested in PVC containers.

Additive Compatibility

Ciprofloxacin

Drug	Mfr	Conc/L	Mfr	Conc/L	Test Soln	Remarks	Ref	C/I
Amikacin sulfate	BR	4.1 g	MI	1.6 g	D5W, NS	Visually compatible and both stable for 48 hr at 25 °C under fluorescent light	1541	C
	APC	4.9 g	BAY	2 g	D5W	Visually compatible with no loss of ciprofloxacin in 24 hr at 22 °C under fluorescent light. Amikacin not tested	2413	C
Aminophylline	LY	2 g	MI	1.6 g	D5W, NS	Precipitate forms in 4 hr at 4 and 25 °C	1541	I
						Physically incompatible with loss of ciprofloxacin reported due to pH over 6.0	1924	I
Amoxicillin sodium		10 g		2 g	a	Precipitates immediately	1473	I
Amoxicillin sodium–clavulanate potassium		10 + 2 g		2 g	a	Precipitates immediately	1473	I
Amphotericin B		100 mg	MI	2 g	D5W	Physically incompatible	888	I
	APC	100 mg	BAY	2 g	D5W	Precipitates immediately	2413	I
Ampicillin sodium–sulbactam sodium		20 + 10 g	MI	2 g	D5W	Physically incompatible	888	I
	RR	20 + 10 g	BAY	2 g	D5W	Precipitates immediately	2413	I
Atracurium besylate	GW	2 g	BAY	1.6 g	D5W	Visually compatible with no loss of ciprofloxacin in 24 hr at 22 °C under fluorescent light. Atracurium not tested	2413	C
Azithromycin						Physically incompatible with loss of ciprofloxacin reported due to pH over 6.0	1924	I
Aztreonam	SQ	39.7 g	BAY	1.6 g	D5W	Visually compatible with no loss of ciprofloxacin in 24 hr at 22 °C under fluorescent light. Aztreonam not tested	2413	C
Ceftazidime		20 g	MI	2 g	D5W	Physically incompatible	888	I
	SKB	19.8 g	BAY	2 g	D5W	Visually compatible but pH changed by more than 1 unit	2413	?
Cefuroxime sodium		30 g	MI	2 g	D5W	Physically incompatible	888	I
	GW	30 g	BAY	2 g	D5W	Visually compatible for 6 hr, but small particles appeared by 24 hr at about 22 °C	2413	I
Clindamycin phosphate	LY	7.1 g	MI	1.6 g	D5W, NS	Precipitate forms immediately	1541	I
Cyclosporine	SZ	500 mg	BAY	2 g	NS	Visually compatible with 8% ciprofloxacin loss in 24 hr at 25 °C. Cyclosporine not tested	1934	C

Additive Compatibility (Cont.)

Ciprofloxacin

Drug	Mfr	Conc/L	Mfr	Conc/L	Test Soln	Remarks	Ref	C/I
Dobutamine HCl	LI	2 g	BAY	1.7 g	D5W	Visually compatible with no loss of ciprofloxacin in 24 hr at 22 °C under fluorescent light. Dobutamine not tested	2413	C
Dopamine HCl		400 mg	MI	2 g	NS	Compatible for 24 hr at 25 °C	888	C
		1.04 g	MI	2 g	NS	Compatible for 24 hr at 25 °C	888	C
Floxacillin sodium		10 g		2 g	[a]	Precipitates immediately	1473	I
Fluconazole	RR	1 g	BAY	1 g		Visually compatible with no loss of ciprofloxacin in 24 hr at 22 °C under fluorescent light. Fluconazole not tested	2413	C
Fluorouracil						Physically incompatible with loss of ciprofloxacin reported due to pH over 6.0	1924	I
Gentamicin sulfate	LY	1 g	MI	1.6 g	D5W, NS	Visually compatible and both drugs stable for 48 hr at 25 °C under fluorescent light and 4 °C in the dark	1541	C
	SC	10 g	BAY	2 g	NS	Visually compatible. Little ciprofloxacin loss in 24 hr at 25 °C. Gentamicin not tested	1934	C
	SC	1.6 g	BAY	2 g	D5W	Visually compatible with no loss of ciprofloxacin in 24 hr at 22 °C under fluorescent light. Gentamicin not tested	2413	C
Heparin sodium	CP	10,000, 100,000, 1 million units	BAY	2 g	NS	White precipitate forms immediately	1934	I
		4100 units	MI	2 g	NS	Physically incompatible	888	I
		8300 units	MI	2 g	NS	Physically incompatible	888	I
Lidocaine HCl		1 g	MI	2 g	NS	Compatible for 24 hr at 25 °C	888	C
		1.5 g	MI	2 g	NS	Compatible for 24 hr at 25 °C	888	C
Linezolid	PHU	2 g	BAY	4 g	[b]	Physically compatible with little or no loss of either drug in 7 days at 23 °C protected from light. Refrigeration results in precipitation after 1 day	2334	C
Metronidazole		5 g		2 g		No loss of either drug in 4 hr at 24 °C	1346	C
	SE	4.2 g	MI	1.6 g		Visually compatible. Both drugs stable for 48 hr at 25 °C in light and 4 °C in dark	1541	C
	RPR	2.5 g		1 g		Under 3% metronidazole loss in 24 hr at 25 °C in light or dark. Ciprofloxacin not tested	2361	C
	SCS	2.5 g	BAY	1 g		Visually compatible. No ciprofloxacin loss in 24 hr at 22 °C in light. Metronidazole not tested	2413	C
Midazolam HCl	RC	200 mg	BAY	2 g	D5W	Visually compatible. No ciprofloxacin loss in 24 hr at 22 °C in light. Midazolam not tested	2413	C
Norepinephrine bitartrate	SW	64 mg	BAY	2 g	D5W	Visually compatible. No ciprofloxacin loss in 24 hr at 22 °C in light. Norepinephrine not tested	2413	C

Additive Compatibility (Cont.)

					Ciprofloxacin			
Drug	Mfr	Conc/L	Mfr	Conc/L	Test Soln	Remarks	Ref	C/I
Pancuronium bromide	OR	200 mg	BAY	1.6 g	D5W	Visually compatible with no loss of cipro-floxacin in 24 hr at 22 °C under fluores-cent light. Pancuronium not tested	2413	C
Potassium chloride	AB	40 mEq	BAY	2 g	NS	Visually compatible with little or no cipro-floxacin loss in 24 hr at 25 °C	1934	C
		40 mEq	MI	2 g	NS	Compatible for 24 hr at 25 °C	888	C
	LY	2.9 g	BAY	2 g	D5W	Visually compatible with no loss of cipro-floxacin in 24 hr at 22 °C under fluores-cent light. Potassium chloride not tested	2413	C
Potassium phosphates		60 mg		2 g	D5W	Precipitation occurs	671	I
Ranitidine HCl	GL	500 mg and 1 g	BAY	2 g	NS	Visually compatible. Little ciprofloxacin loss in 24 hr at 25 °C. Ranitidine not tested	1934	C
Sodium bicarbonate		[c]	MI	2 g	D5W	Physically incompatible	888	I
	AST	4 g	BAY	2 g	D5W	Precipitates immediately	2413	I
Ticarcillin disodium–clavulanate potassium	SKB	30 g	BAY	2 g	D5W	Visually compatible but pH changed by more than 1 unit	2413	?
Tobramycin sulfate	LI	1 g	MI	1.6 g	D5W, NS	Visually compatible and both drugs stable for 48 hr at 25 °C under fluorescent light and 4 °C in the dark	1541	C
	LI	1.6 g	BAY	2 g	D5W	Visually compatible with no loss of cip-rofloxacin in 24 hr at 22 °C under fluo-rescent light. Tobramycin not tested	2413	C
Vecuronium bromide	OR	200 mg	BAY	1.6 g	D5W	Visually compatible with no loss of cipro-floxacin in 24 hr at 22 °C under fluores-cent light. Vecuronium not tested	2413	C

[a] Drug added to ciprofloxacin solution.
[b] Admixed in the linezolid infusion container.
[c] Final sodium bicarbonate concentration not specified.

Drugs in Syringe Compatibility

					Ciprofloxacin		
Drug (in syringe)	Mfr	Amt	Mfr	Amt	Remarks	Ref	C/I
Pantoprazole sodium	[a]	4 mg/1 mL		2 mg/1 mL	Precipitates immediately	2574	I

[a] Test performed using the formulation WITHOUT edetate disodium.

Y-Site Injection Compatibility (1:1 Mixture)

					Ciprofloxacin		
Drug	Mfr	Conc	Mfr	Conc	Remarks	Ref	C/I
Amifostine	USB	10 mg/mL[a]	MI	1 mg/mL[a]	Physically compatible for 4 hr at 23 °C	1845	C
Amino acids, dextrose	AB	AA 5%, D 25%	MI	2 mg/mL[a]	Visually compatible for 2 hr at 25 °C	1628	C

Y-Site Injection Compatibility (1:1 Mixture) (Cont.)

Ciprofloxacin

Drug	Mfr	Conc	Mfr	Conc	Remarks	Ref	C/I
Aminophylline	AB	2 mg/mL[a,b]	MI	2 mg/mL[a,b]	Fine white crystals form in 20 min in D5W and 2 min in NS	1655	I
Amiodarone HCl	WY	6 mg/mL[a]	BAY	2 mg/mL[a]	Visually compatible for 24 hr at 22 °C	2352	C
Ampicillin sodium–sulbactam sodium		3 + 1.5 g[c]		400 mg[c]	White crystals form immediately when administered sequentially through a Y-site into running D5S	1887	I
Anidulafungin	VIC	0.5 mg/mL[a]	AB	2 mg/mL[a]	Physically compatible for 4 hr at 23 °C	2617	C
Azithromycin	PF	2 mg/mL[b]	BAY	2 mg/mL[d,e]	Amber microcrystals found	2368	I
Aztreonam	SQ	20 mg/mL[a,b]	MI	1 mg/mL[a]	Physically compatible for 24 hr at 22 °C	1189	C
	SQ	40 mg/mL[a]	MI	1 mg/mL[a]	Physically compatible for 4 hr at 23 °C	1758	C
Bivalirudin	TMC	5 mg/mL[a]	BAY	2 mg/mL[a]	Physically compatible for 4 hr at 23 °C	2373	C
Calcium gluconate	LY	10%	MI	2 mg/mL[a]	Visually compatible for 2 hr at 25 °C	1628	C
Caspofungin acetate	ME	0.7 mg/mL[b]	HOS	2 mg/mL[b]	Physically compatible for 4 hr at room temperature	2758	C
	ME	0.5 mg/mL[b]	BAY	2 mg/mL[j]	Physically compatible over 60 min	2766	C
Ceftaroline fosamil	FOR	2.22 mg/mL[a,b,k]	BED	2 mg/mL[a,b,k]	Physically compatible for 4 hr at 23 °C	2826	C
Ceftazidime	SKF	20 mg/mL[a,b]	MI	1 mg/mL[a]	Physically compatible for 24 hr at 22 °C	1189	C
Cisatracurium besylate	GW	0.1, 2, 5 mg/mL[a]	BAY	1 mg/mL[a]	Physically compatible for 4 hr at 23 °C	2074	C
Clarithromycin	AB	4 mg/mL[a]	BAY	2 mg/mL[a]	Visually compatible for 72 hr at both 30 and 17 °C	2174	C
Dexamethasone sodium phosphate	LY	4 mg/mL	MI	2 mg/mL[a,b]	Cloudiness rapidly dissipates. White crystals form in 1 hr at 24 °C	1655	I
Dexmedetomidine HCl	AB	4 mcg/mL[b]	BAY	1 mg/mL[b]	Physically compatible for 4 hr at 23 °C	2383	C
Digoxin	ES	0.25 mg/mL	MI	2 mg/mL[a,b]	Visually compatible for 24 hr at 24 °C	1655	C
	BW	0.25 mg/mL	BAY	2 mg/mL[b]	Visually compatible with no ciprofloxacin loss in 15 min. Digoxin not tested	1934	C
Diltiazem HCl	MMD	5 mg/mL	MI	2 and 10 mg/mL[b]	Visually compatible	1807	C
Dimenhydrinate		10 mg/mL		2 mg/mL	Clear solution	2569	C
Diphenhydramine HCl	ES	50 mg/mL	MI	2 mg/mL[a,b]	Visually compatible for 24 hr at 24 °C	1655	C
Dobutamine HCl	LI	250 mcg/mL[a,b]	MI	2 mg/mL[a,b]	Visually compatible for 24 hr at 24 °C	1655	C
Docetaxel	RPR	0.9 mg/mL[a]	BAY	1 mg/mL[a]	Physically compatible for 4 hr at 23 °C	2224	C
Dopamine HCl	AB	1.6 mg/mL[a,b]	MI	2 mg/mL[a,b]	Visually compatible for 24 hr at 24 °C	1655	C
Doripenem	JJ	5 mg/mL[a,b]	BED	2 mg/mL[a,b]	Physically compatible for 4 hr at 23 °C	2743	C
Doxorubicin HCl liposomal	SEQ	0.4 mg/mL[a]	BAY	1 mg/mL[a]	Physically compatible for 4 hr at 23 °C	2087	C
Etoposide phosphate	BR	5 mg/mL[a]	BAY	1 mg/mL[a]	Physically compatible for 4 hr at 23 °C	2218	C
Fenoldopam mesylate	AB	80 mcg/mL[b]	BAY	2 mg/mL[b]	Physically compatible for 4 hr at 23 °C	2467	C
Furosemide	AB	10 mg/mL	MI	2 mg/mL[a,b]	Precipitates immediately	1655	I
	DMX	5 mg/mL	BAY	2 mg/mL[b]	White precipitate forms immediately	1934	I
Gallium nitrate	FUJ	1 mg/mL[b]	MI	2 mg/mL[b]	Visually compatible for 24 hr at 25 °C	1673	C
Gemcitabine HCl	LI	10 mg/mL[b]	BAY	1 mg/mL[b]	Physically compatible for 4 hr at 23 °C	2226	C

Y-Site Injection Compatibility (1:1 Mixture) (Cont.)

Ciprofloxacin

Drug	Mfr	Conc	Mfr	Conc	Remarks	Ref	C/I
Gentamicin sulfate	LY	1.6 mg/mL[a,b]	MI	2 mg/mL[a,b]	Visually compatible for 24 hr at 24 °C	1655	C
Granisetron HCl	SKB	0.05 mg/mL[a]	MI	1 mg/mL[a]	Physically compatible for 4 hr at 23 °C	2000	C
Heparin sodium		10 units/mL		2 mg/mL	Turbidity forms rapidly with subsequent white precipitate	1483	I
	LY	100 units/mL[a,b]	MI	2 mg/mL[a,b]	Crystals form immediately	1655	I
	CP	10, 100, 1000 units/mL[b]	BAY	2 mg/mL[b]	White precipitate forms immediately	1934	I
Hetastarch in lactated electrolyte	AB	6%	BAY	2 mg/mL[a]	Physically compatible for 4 hr at 23 °C	2339	C
Hydrocortisone sodium succinate	UP	50 mg/mL	MI	2 mg/mL[a,b]	Transient cloudiness rapidly dissipates. Crystals form in 1 hr at 24 °C	1655	I
Hydroxyethyl starch 130/0.4 in sodium chloride 0.9%	FRK	6%	AB	0.5, 1, 2 mg/mL[a]	Visually compatible for 24 hr at room temperature	2770	C
Hydroxyzine HCl	ES	50 mg/mL	MI	2 mg/mL[a,b]	Visually compatible for 24 hr at 24 °C	1655	C
Lidocaine HCl	AB	4[a] and 20 mg/mL	MI	2 mg/mL[a,b]	Visually compatible for 24 hr at 24 °C	1655	C
Linezolid	PHU	2 mg/mL	BAY	1 mg/mL[a]	Physically compatible for 4 hr at 23 °C	2264	C
Lorazepam	WY	0.33 mg/mL[b]	BAY	2 mg/mL	Visually compatible for 24 hr at 22 °C	1855	C
Magnesium sulfate	AB	4 mEq/mL	MI	2 mg/mL[a,b]	Precipitate forms in 4 hr in D5W and 1 hr in NS at 24 °C	1655	I
	LY	50%	MI	2 mg/mL[a]	Visually compatible for 2 hr at 25 °C	1628	C
Methylprednisolone sodium succinate	UP	62.5 mg/mL	MI	2 mg/mL[a,b]	Transient cloudiness rapidly dissipates. Crystals form in 2 hr at 24 °C	1655	I
Metoclopramide HCl	DU	5 mg/mL	MI	2 mg/mL[a,b]	Visually compatible for 24 hr at 24 °C	1655	C
		5 mg/mL	BAY	2 mg/mL[b]	Visually compatible. No ciprofloxacin loss in 15 min. Metoclopramide not tested	1934	C
Midazolam HCl	RC	5 mg/mL	BAY	2 mg/mL	Visually compatible for 24 hr at 22 °C	1855	C
Milrinone lactate	SS	0.2 mg/mL[a]	BAY	2 mg/mL	Visually compatible for 4 hr at 25 °C	2381	C
Pemetrexed disodium	LI	20 mg/mL[b]	BAY	2 mg/mL[a]	Slight color darkening occurs over 4 hr	2564	I
Phenytoin sodium	PD	50 mg/mL	MI	2 mg/mL[a,b]	Immediate crystal formation	1655	I
Potassium acetate	LY	2 mEq/mL	MI	2 mg/mL[a]	Visually compatible for 2 hr at 25 °C	1628	C
Potassium chloride	LY	0.04 mEq/mL	MI	2 mg/mL[a,b]	Visually compatible for 24 hr at 24 °C	1655	C
	AMR	2 mEq/mL	MI	2 mg/mL[a]	Visually compatible for 2 hr at 25 °C	1628	C
Promethazine HCl	ES	25 mg/mL	MI	2 mg/mL[a,b]	Visually compatible for 24 hr at 24 °C	1655	C
Quinupristin–dalfopristin	AVE	2 mg/mL[a]		1 mg/mL[a]	Physically compatible	1	C
Ranitidine HCl	GL	0.5 mg/mL[a,b]	MI	2 mg/mL[a,b]	Visually compatible for 24 hr at 24 °C	1655	C
Remifentanil HCl	GW	0.025 and 0.25 mg/mL[b]	BAY	1 mg/mL[a]	Physically compatible for 4 hr at 23 °C	2075	C
Sodium bicarbonate	AB	1 mEq/mL	MI	2 mg/mL[a]	Visually compatible for 24 hr at 24 °C	1655	C
	AB	1 mEq/mL	MI	2 mg/mL[b]	Very fine crystals form in 20 min in NS	1655	I
	AB	1 mEq/mL	MI	2 mg/mL[a]	Physically compatible for 4 hr at 23 °C	1869	C

Y-Site Injection Compatibility (1:1 Mixture) (Cont.)

Ciprofloxacin

Drug	Mfr	Conc	Mfr	Conc	Remarks	Ref	C/I
	AB	0.1 mEq/mL[a]	MI	2 mg/mL[a]	Subvisible haze forms immediately. Crystalline precipitate in 4 hr at 23 °C	1869	I
	AB	1 and 0.75[a] mEq/mL	BAY	1 and 2 mg/mL[a]	Physically compatible for 4 hr at 23 °C	2065	C
	AB	1 and 0.75[b] mEq/mL	BAY	1 mg/mL[b]	Physically compatible for 4 hr at 23 °C	2065	C
	AB	1 and 0.75[b] mEq/mL	BAY	2 mg/mL[b]	Particles form immediately, becoming more numerous over 4 hr at 23 °C	2065	I
	AB	0.5, 0.25, 0.1 mEq/mL[a]	BAY	1 and 2 mg/mL[a]	Particles form immediately, becoming more numerous over 4 hr at 23 °C	2065	I
	AB	0.5, 0.25, 0.1 mEq/mL[b]	BAY	1 mg/mL[b]	Particles form immediately, becoming more numerous over 4 hr at 23 °C	2065	I
	AB	0.5, 0.25, 0.1 mEq/mL[b]	BAY	2 mg/mL[b]	Precipitate forms immediately	2065	I
Sodium chloride	AMR	4 mEq/mL	MI	2 mg/mL[a]	Visually compatible for 2 hr at 25 °C	1628	C
Sodium phosphates	AB	3 mmol/mL	BAY	2 mg/mL[a]	Microcrystals form in 1 hr at 23 °C	1972	I
	AB	3 mmol/mL	BAY	2 mg/mL[f]	White crystalline precipitate forms immediately	1971; 1972	I
Tacrolimus	FUJ	1 mg/mL[b]	MI	1 mg/mL[a]	Visually compatible for 24 hr at 25 °C	1630	C
Teicoplanin	GRP	60 mg/mL	BAY	2 mg/mL[b]	White precipitate forms immediately but disappears with shaking	1934	?
Telavancin HCl	ASP	7.5 mg/mL[a]	BED	2 mg/mL[a]	Physically compatible for 2 hr	2830	C
Teniposide	BR	0.1 mg/mL[a]	MI	2 mg/mL[a]	Physically compatible for 4 hr at 23 °C	1725	C
Thiotepa	IMM[g]	1 mg/mL[a]	MI	1 mg/mL[a]	Physically compatible for 4 hr at 23 °C	1861	C
Tigecycline	WY	1 mg/mL[b]		1 mg/mL[b]	Physically compatible for 4 hr	2714	C
TNA #218 to #226[i]			BAY	1 mg/mL[a]	Visually compatible for 4 hr at 23 °C	2215	C
Tobramycin sulfate	LI	1.6 mg/mL[a,b]	MI	1 mg/mL[a]	Physically compatible for 24 hr at 22 °C	1189	C
TPN #212 to #215[i]			MI	1 mg/mL[a]	Amber discoloration forms in 1 to 4 hr	2109	I
Vasopressin	APP	0.2 unit/mL[b]	BAY	2 mg/mL[a]	Physically compatible	2641	C
Verapamil HCl	KN	2.5 mg/mL	MI	2 mg/mL[a,b]	Visually compatible for 24 hr at 24 °C	1655	C
Warfarin sodium	DU	2 mg/mL[h]	MI	2 mg/mL[a]	Immediate haze; crystals form in 1 hr	2010	I
	DME	2 mg/mL[h]	MI	2 mg/mL[a]	Immediate haze; crystals form in 1 hr	2078	I

[a]*Tested in dextrose 5%.*
[b]*Tested in sodium chloride 0.9%.*
[c]*Concentration and volume not specified.*
[d]*Tested in sodium chloride 0.45%.*
[e]*Injected via Y-site into an administration set running azithromycin.*
[f]*Tested in both sodium chloride 0.9% and 0.45%.*
[g]*Lyophilized formulation tested.*
[h]*Tested in sterile water for injection.*
[i]*Refer to Appendix I for the composition of parenteral nutrition solutions. TNA indicates a 3-in-1 admixture, and TPN indicates a 2-in-1 admixture.*
[j]*Tested as the premixed infusion solution.*
[k]*Tested in Ringer's injection, lactated.*

CISATRACURIUM BESYLATE
AHFS 12:20.20

Products — Cisatracurium besylate is available as a 2-mg/mL solution in 5- and 10-mL vials. The drug is also available as a 10-mg/mL solution in 20-mL vials intended for use in intensive care units only. The pH is adjusted with benzenesulfonic acid. The 2-mg/mL concentration in 10-mL vials also contains benzyl alcohol 0.9%. The other dosage forms have no preservative and are for single use only. (1)

pH — From 3.25 to 3.65. (1)

Trade Name(s) — Nimbex.

Administration — Cisatracurium besylate is administered intravenously only. Both initial bolus doses and continuous intravenous infusion have been used. Rates of administration depend on the drug concentration in the solution, desired dose, and patient weight. Avoid contact with alkaline drugs during administration. (1)

Stability — Cisatracurium besylate injection is a colorless to slightly yellow or greenish-yellow solution. Intact vials of cisatracurium besylate should be stored at 2 to 8 °C protected from light and freezing. Potency losses of 5% per year occur under refrigeration. However, at 25 °C, potency losses increase to about 5% per month. The manufac-

turer recommends that vials that have been warmed to room temperature be used within 21 days even if rerefrigerated. (1)

In an independent study, cisatracurium besylate 2 mg/mL in 5- and 10-mL vials and the 10-mg/mL solution in 20-mL vials was stored at 4 and 23 °C both protected from light and exposed to fluorescent light. All the samples remained physically stable throughout the 90-day study period. Samples stored under refrigeration exhibited little or no drug loss in 90 days whether exposed to or protected from light. At 23 °C, samples were stable through 45 days of storage with losses near 5 to 7% in most samples. However, most samples became unacceptable after 90 days of storage at 23 °C, exhibiting losses of 9 to 14%. (2116)

pH Effects — The manufacturer indicates that cisatracurium besylate may not be compatible with barbiturates and other alkaline solutions having a pH greater than 8.5. (1)

Syringes — Cisatracurium besylate 2 mg/mL was repackaged in 3-mL plastic syringes (Becton-Dickinson) and sealed with tip caps (Red Cap, Burron). The syringes were stored at 4 and 23 °C both protected from light and exposed to fluorescent light. All of the samples remained physically stable throughout the 30-day study period. Little or no loss occurred when stored under refrigeration, whereas samples stored at 23 °C exhibited 4 to 7% loss in 30 days. (2116)

Compatibility Information

Solution Compatibility

Cisatracurium besylate

Solution	Mfr	Mfr	Conc/L	Remarks	Ref	C/I
Dextrose 5%			100 mg	Stable for 24 hr at 4 and 25 °C	1	C
	BAª	GW	100 mg	Physically compatible with 8% loss in 7 days and 15% loss in 14 days at 23 °C under fluorescent light. Little loss in 30 days at 4 °C	2116	C
	BAª	GW	2 g	Physically compatible with 10% loss in 14 days and 14% loss in 30 days at 23 °C under fluorescent light. Little loss in 30 days at 4 °C	2116	C
	BAª	GW	5 g	Physically compatible with 4% loss in 30 days at 23 °C under fluorescent light. Little loss in 30 days at 4 °C	2116	C
Dextrose 5% in Ringer's injection, lactated			100 to 200 mg	Stable for 24 hr at 4 °C	1	C
Dextrose 5% in sodium chloride 0.9%			100 mg	Stable for 24 hr at 4 and 25 °C	1	C
Ringer's injection, lactated				Cisatracurium unstable	1	I
Sodium chloride 0.9%			100 mg	Stable for 24 hr at 4 and 25 °C	1	C
	BAª	GW	100 mg	Physically compatible with 8% loss in 14 days and 14% loss in 30 days at 23 °C under fluorescent light. Little loss in 30 days at 4 °C	2116	C
	BAª	GW	2 g	Physically compatible with 6% loss in 30 days at 23 °C under fluorescent light. Little loss in 30 days at 4 °C	2116	C
	BAª	GW	5 g	Physically compatible with 3% loss in 30 days at 23 °C under fluorescent light. Little loss in 30 days at 4 °C	2116	C

ªTested in PVC containers.

Y-Site Injection Compatibility (1:1 Mixture)

Cisatracurium besylate

Drug	Mfr	Conc	Mfr	Conc	Remarks	Ref	C/I
Acyclovir sodium	BW	7 mg/mL[a]	GW	0.1 and 2 mg/mL[a]	Physically compatible for 4 hr at 23 °C	2074	C
	BW	7 mg/mL[a]	GW	5 mg/mL[a]	White cloudiness forms immediately	2074	I
Alfentanil HCl	JN	0.125 mg/mL[a]	GW	0.1, 2, 5 mg/mL[a]	Physically compatible for 4 hr at 23 °C	2074	C
Amikacin sulfate	AB	5 mg/mL[a]	GW	0.1, 2, 5 mg/mL[a]	Physically compatible for 4 hr at 23 °C	2074	C
Aminophylline	AB	2.5 mg/mL[a]	GW	0.1 and 2 mg/mL[a]	Physically compatible for 4 hr at 23 °C	2074	C
	AB	2.5 mg/mL[a]	GW	5 mg/mL[a]	Gray subvisible haze forms in 1 hr	2074	I
Amphotericin B	PH	0.6 mg/mL[a]	GW	0.1 mg/mL[a]	Physically compatible for 4 hr at 23 °C	2074	C
	PH	0.6 mg/mL[a]	GW	2 mg/mL[a]	Cloudiness forms immediately; gel-like precipitate forms in 1 hr	2074	I
	PH	0.6 mg/mL[a]	GW	5 mg/mL[a]	Turbidity forms immediately	2074	I
Amphotericin B cholesteryl sulfate complex	SEQ	0.83 mg/mL[a]	GW	2 mg/mL[a]	Gross precipitate forms	2117	I
Ampicillin sodium	SKB	20 mg/mL[b]	GW	0.1 and 2 mg/mL[a]	Physically compatible for 4 hr at 23 °C	2074	C
	SKB	20 mg/mL[b]	GW	5 mg/mL[a]	Gray subvisible haze forms in 1 hr	2074	I
Ampicillin sodium–sulbactam sodium	RR	20 + 10 mg/mL[b]	GW	0.1 and 2 mg/mL[a]	Physically compatible for 4 hr at 23 °C	2074	C
	RR	20 + 10 mg/mL[b]	GW	5 mg/mL[a]	Subvisible haze develops in 15 min	2074	I
Aztreonam	SQ	40 mg/mL[a]	GW	0.1, 2, 5 mg/mL[a]	Physically compatible for 4 hr at 23 °C	2074	C
Bumetanide	BV	0.04 mg/mL[a]	GW	0.1, 2, 5 mg/mL[a]	Physically compatible for 4 hr at 23 °C	2074	C
Buprenorphine HCl	RKC	0.04 mg/mL[a]	GW	0.1, 2, 5 mg/mL[a]	Physically compatible for 4 hr at 23 °C	2074	C
Butorphanol tartrate	APC	0.04 mg/mL[a]	GW	0.1, 2, 5 mg/mL[a]	Physically compatible for 4 hr at 23 °C	2074	C
Calcium gluconate	AB	40 mg/mL[a]	GW	0.1, 2, 5 mg/mL[a]	Physically compatible for 4 hr at 23 °C	2074	C
Cefazolin sodium	SKB	20 mg/mL[a]	GW	0.1 mg/mL[a]	Physically compatible for 4 hr at 23 °C	2074	C
	SKB	20 mg/mL[a]	GW	2 mg/mL[a]	Gray subvisible haze forms immediately	2074	I
	SKB	20 mg/mL[a]	GW	5 mg/mL[a]	Gray haze forms immediately	2074	I
Cefotaxime sodium	HO	20 mg/mL[a]	GW	0.1 mg/mL[a]	Physically compatible for 4 hr at 23 °C	2074	C
	HO	20 mg/mL[a]	GW	2 mg/mL[a]	Subvisible haze forms in 4 hr	2074	I
	HO	20 mg/mL[a]	GW	5 mg/mL[a]	Subvisible haze forms immediately	2074	I
Cefoxitin sodium	ME	20 mg/mL[a]	GW	0.1 mg/mL[a]	Physically compatible for 4 hr at 23 °C	2074	C
	ME	20 mg/mL[a]	GW	2 and 5 mg/mL[a]	Subvisible haze forms immediately	2074	I
Ceftaroline fosamil	FOR	2.22 mg/mL[a,b,c]	HOS	0.5 mg/mL[a,b,c]	Physically compatible for 4 hr at 23 °C	2826	C
Ceftazidime	SKB	40 mg/mL[a]	GW	0.1 and 2 mg/mL[a]	Physically compatible for 4 hr at 23 °C	2074	C
	SKB	40 mg/mL[a]	GW	5 mg/mL[a]	Subvisible haze forms immediately	2074	I

Y-Site Injection Compatibility (1:1 Mixture) (Cont.)

Cisatracurium besylate

Drug	Mfr	Conc	Mfr	Conc	Remarks	Ref	C/I
Ceftriaxone sodium	RC	20 mg/mL[a]	GW	0.1, 2, 5 mg/mL[a]	Physically compatible for 4 hr at 23 °C	2074	C
Cefuroxime sodium	LI	30 mg/mL[a]	GW	0.1 mg/mL[a]	Physically compatible for 4 hr at 23 °C	2074	C
	LI	30 mg/mL[a]	GW	2 mg/mL[a]	White cloudiness forms immediately	2074	I
	LI	30 mg/mL[a]	GW	5 mg/mL[a]	Turbidity forms immediately	2074	I
Chlorpromazine HCl	SCN	2 mg/mL[a]	GW	0.1, 2, 5 mg/mL[a]	Physically compatible for 4 hr at 23 °C	2074	C
Ciprofloxacin	BAY	1 mg/mL[a]	GW	0.1, 2, 5 mg/mL[a]	Physically compatible for 4 hr at 23 °C	2074	C
Clindamycin phosphate	AST	10 mg/mL[a]	GW	0.1, 2, 5 mg/mL[a]	Physically compatible for 4 hr at 23 °C	2074	C
Dexamethasone sodium phosphate	FUJ	2 mg/mL[a]	GW	0.1, 2, 5 mg/mL[a]	Physically compatible for 4 hr at 23 °C	2074	C
Dexmedetomidine HCl	AB	4 mcg/mL[b]	GW	0.5 mg/mL[b]	Physically compatible for 4 hr at 23 °C	2383	C
Diazepam	ES	5 mg/mL	GW	0.1, 2, 5 mg/mL[a]	White turbidity forms immediately	2074	I
	ES	0.25 mg/mL[a]	GW	0.1, 2, 5 mg/mL[a]	Physically compatible for 4 hr at 23 °C	2074	C
Digoxin	ES	0.25 mg/mL	GW	0.1, 2, 5 mg/mL[a]	Physically compatible for 4 hr at 23 °C	2074	C
Diphenhydramine HCl	SCN	2 mg/mL[a]	GW	0.1, 2, 5 mg/mL[a]	Physically compatible for 4 hr at 23 °C	2074	C
Dobutamine HCl	LI	4 mg/mL[a]	GW	0.1, 2, 5 mg/mL[a]	Physically compatible for 4 hr at 23 °C	2074	C
Dopamine HCl	AB	3.2 mg/mL[a]	GW	0.1, 2, 5 mg/mL[a]	Physically compatible for 4 hr at 23 °C	2074	C
Doxycycline hyclate	FUJ	1 mg/mL[a]	GW	0.1, 2, 5 mg/mL[a]	Physically compatible for 4 hr at 23 °C	2074	C
Droperidol	AB	2.5 mg/mL	GW	0.1, 2, 5 mg/mL[a]	Physically compatible for 4 hr at 23 °C	2074	C
Enalaprilat	ME	0.1 mg/mL[a]	GW	0.1, 2, 5 mg/mL[a]	Physically compatible for 4 hr at 23 °C	2074	C
Epinephrine HCl	AMR	0.05 mg/mL[a]	GW	0.1, 2, 5 mg/mL[a]	Physically compatible for 4 hr at 23 °C	2074	C
Esmolol HCl	OHM	10 mg/mL[a]	GW	0.1, 2, 5 mg/mL[a]	Physically compatible for 4 hr at 23 °C	2074	C
Famotidine	ME	2 mg/mL[a]	GW	0.1, 2, 5 mg/mL[a]	Physically compatible for 4 hr at 23 °C	2074	C
Fenoldopam mesylate	AB	80 mcg/mL[b]	AB	0.5 mg/mL[b]	Physically compatible for 4 hr at 23 °C	2467	C
Fentanyl citrate	AB	12.5 mcg/mL[a]	GW	0.1, 2, 5 mg/mL[a]	Physically compatible for 4 hr at 23 °C	2074	C
Fluconazole	RR	2 mg/mL	GW	0.1, 2, 5 mg/mL[a]	Physically compatible for 4 hr at 23 °C	2074	C
Furosemide	AB	3 mg/mL[a]	GW	0.1 mg/mL[a]	Physically compatible for 4 hr at 23 °C	2074	C
	AB	3 mg/mL[a]	GW	2 and 5 mg/mL[a]	White cloudiness forms immediately	2074	I

Y-Site Injection Compatibility (1:1 Mixture) (Cont.)

Cisatracurium besylate

Drug	Mfr	Conc	Mfr	Conc	Remarks	Ref	C/I
Ganciclovir sodium	SY	20 mg/mL[a]	GW	0.1 and 2 mg/mL[a]	Physically compatible for 4 hr at 23 °C	2074	**C**
	SY	20 mg/mL[a]	GW	5 mg/mL[a]	White cloudiness forms immediately	2074	**I**
Gentamicin sulfate	ES	5 mg/mL[a]	GW	0.1, 2, 5 mg/mL[a]	Physically compatible for 4 hr at 23 °C	2074	**C**
Haloperidol lactate	MN	0.2 mg/mL[a]	GW	0.1, 2, 5 mg/mL[a]	Physically compatible for 4 hr at 23 °C	2074	**C**
Heparin sodium	AB	100 units/mL	GW	0.1 and 2 mg/mL[a]	Physically compatible for 4 hr at 23 °C	2074	**C**
	AB	100 units/mL	GW	5 mg/mL[a]	White cloudiness forms immediately	2074	**I**
Hetastarch in lactated electrolyte	AB	6%	GW	0.5 mg/mL[a]	Physically compatible for 4 hr at 23 °C	2339	**C**
Hydrocortisone sodium succinate	AB	1 mg/mL[a]	GW	0.1, 2, 5 mg/mL[a]	Physically compatible for 4 hr at 23 °C	2074	**C**
Hydromorphone HCl	ES	0.5 mg/mL[a]	GW	0.1, 2, 5 mg/mL[a]	Physically compatible for 4 hr at 23 °C	2074	**C**
Hydroxyzine HCl	ES	2 mg/mL[a]	GW	0.1, 2, 5 mg/mL[a]	Physically compatible for 4 hr at 23 °C	2074	**C**
Imipenem–cilastatin sodium	ME	10 mg/mL[b]	GW	0.1, 2, 5 mg/mL[a]	Physically compatible for 4 hr at 23 °C	2074	**C**
Isoproterenol HCl	AB	0.02 mg/mL[a]	GW	0.1, 2, 5 mg/mL[a]	Physically compatible for 4 hr at 23 °C	2074	**C**
Ketorolac tromethamine	RC	15 mg/mL[a]	GW	0.1, 2, 5 mg/mL[a]	Physically compatible for 4 hr at 23 °C	2074	**C**
Lidocaine HCl	AST	8 mg/mL[a]	GW	0.1, 2, 5 mg/mL[a]	Physically compatible for 4 hr at 23 °C	2074	**C**
Linezolid	PHU	2 mg/mL	GW	2 mg/mL	Physically compatible for 4 hr at 23 °C	2264	**C**
Lorazepam	WY	0.5 mg/mL[a]	GW	0.1, 2, 5 mg/mL[a]	Physically compatible for 4 hr at 23 °C	2074	**C**
Magnesium sulfate	AB	100 mg/mL[a]	GW	0.1, 2, 5 mg/mL[a]	Physically compatible for 4 hr at 23 °C	2074	**C**
Mannitol	BA	15%	GW	0.1, 2, 5 mg/mL[a]	Physically compatible for 4 hr at 23 °C	2074	**C**
Meperidine HCl	AST	4 mg/mL[a]	GW	0.1, 2, 5 mg/mL[a]	Physically compatible for 4 hr at 23 °C	2074	**C**
Methylprednisolone sodium succinate	AB	5 mg/mL[a]	GW	0.1 mg/mL[a]	Physically compatible for 4 hr at 23 °C	2074	**C**
	AB	5 mg/mL[a]	GW	2 mg/mL[a]	Subvisible haze forms immediately	2074	**I**
	AB	5 mg/mL[a]	GW	5 mg/mL[a]	Haze forms immediately	2074	**I**
Metoclopramide HCl	AB	5 mg/mL	GW	0.1, 2, 5 mg/mL[a]	Physically compatible for 4 hr at 23 °C	2074	**C**
Metronidazole	AB	5 mg/mL	GW	0.1, 2, 5 mg/mL[a]	Physically compatible for 4 hr at 23 °C	2074	**C**
Micafungin sodium	ASP	1.5 mg/mL[b]	AB	0.5 mg/mL[b]	Gross precipitate forms immediately	2683	**I**
Midazolam HCl	RC	1 mg/mL[a]	GW	0.1, 2, 5 mg/mL[a]	Physically compatible for 4 hr at 23 °C	2074	**C**

Y-Site Injection Compatibility (1:1 Mixture) (Cont.)

Cisatracurium besylate

Drug	Mfr	Conc	Mfr	Conc	Remarks	Ref	C/I
Morphine sulfate	AST	1 mg/mL[a]	GW	0.1, 2, 5 mg/mL[a]	Physically compatible for 4 hr at 23 °C	2074	C
Nalbuphine HCl	AST	10 mg/mL	GW	0.1, 2, 5 mg/mL[a]	Physically compatible for 4 hr at 23 °C	2074	C
Nitroglycerin	DU	0.4 mg/mL[a]	GW	0.1, 2, 5 mg/mL[a]	Physically compatible for 4 hr at 23 °C	2074	C
Norepinephrine bitartrate	SW	0.12 mg/mL[a]	GW	0.1, 2, 5 mg/mL[a]	Physically compatible for 4 hr at 23 °C	2074	C
Ondansetron HCl	CER	1 mg/mL[a]	GW	0.1, 2, 5 mg/mL[a]	Physically compatible for 4 hr at 23 °C	2074	C
Palonosetron HCl	MGI	50 mcg/mL	AB	0.5 mg/mL[a]	Physically compatible with no loss of either drug in 4 hr at room temperature	2764	C
Phenylephrine HCl	GNS	1 mg/mL[a]	GW	0.1, 2, 5 mg/mL[a]	Physically compatible for 4 hr at 23 °C	2074	C
Piperacillin sodium–tazobactam sodium	CY[d]	40 + 5 mg/mL[a]	GW	0.1 and 2 mg/mL[a]	Physically compatible for 4 hr at 23 °C	2074	C
	CY[d]	40 + 5 mg/mL[a]	GW	5 mg/mL[a]	Particles and subvisible haze within 4 hr	2074	I
Potassium chloride	AB	0.1 mEq/mL[a]	GW	0.1, 2, 5 mg/mL[a]	Physically compatible for 4 hr at 23 °C	2074	C
Procainamide HCl	ES	10 mg/mL[a]	GW	0.1, 2, 5 mg/mL[a]	Physically compatible for 4 hr at 23 °C	2074	C
Prochlorperazine edisylate	SO	0.5 mg/mL[a]	GW	0.1, 2, 5 mg/mL[a]	Physically compatible for 4 hr at 23 °C	2074	C
Promethazine HCl	ES	2 mg/mL[a]	GW	0.1, 2, 5 mg/mL[a]	Physically compatible for 4 hr at 23 °C	2074	C
Propofol	ASZ, BA	10 mg/mL	GW	5 mg/mL[a]	Emulsion disruption upon mixing	2336	I
	BA	10 mg/mL	GW	0.5 mg/mL[a]	Emulsion disruption upon mixing	2336	I
	ASZ	10 mg/mL	GW	0.5 mg/mL[a]	Physically compatible for at least 1 hr at room temperature	2336	C
Ranitidine HCl	GL	2 mg/mL[a]	GW	0.1, 2, 5 mg/mL[a]	Physically compatible for 4 hr at 23 °C	2074	C
Remifentanil HCl	GW	0.025 and 0.25 mg/mL[b]	GW	2 mg/mL[a]	Physically compatible for 4 hr at 23 °C	2075	C
Sodium bicarbonate	AB	1 mEq/mL	GW	0.1 mg/mL[a]	Physically compatible for 4 hr at 23 °C	2074	C
	AB	1 mEq/mL	GW	2 mg/mL[a]	Subvisible brown color and haze in 1 hr	2074	I
	AB	1 mEq/mL	GW	5 mg/mL[a]	Subvisible haze forms immediately with brown color and turbidity in 4 hr	2074	I
Sodium nitroprusside	AB	2 mg/mL[a]	GW	0.1 mg/mL[a]	Physically compatible for 4 hr at 23 °C protected from light	2074	C
	AB	2 mg/mL[a]	GW	2 and 5 mg/mL[a]	White cloudiness forms immediately	2074	I
Sufentanil citrate	ES	0.0125 mg/mL[a]	GW	0.1, 2, 5 mg/mL[a]	Physically compatible for 4 hr at 23 °C	2074	C
Theophylline	AB	3.2 mg/mL	GW	0.1, 2, 5 mg/mL[a]	Physically compatible for 4 hr at 23 °C	2074	C

Y-Site Injection Compatibility (1:1 Mixture) (Cont.)

Cisatracurium besylate

Drug	Mfr	Conc	Mfr	Conc	Remarks	Ref	C/I
Ticarcillin disodium–clavulanate potassium	SKB	31 mg/mL[a]	GW	0.1 and 2 mg/mL[a]	Physically compatible for 4 hr at 23 °C	2074	C
	SKB	31 mg/mL[a]	GW	5 mg/mL[a]	Subvisible haze forms immediately	2074	I
Tobramycin sulfate	AB	5 mg/mL[a]	GW	0.1, 2, 5 mg/mL[a]	Physically compatible for 4 hr at 23 °C	2074	C
Trimethoprim–sulfamethoxazole	ES	0.8 + 4 mg/mL[a]	GW	0.1 mg/mL[a]	Physically compatible for 4 hr at 23 °C	2074	C
	ES	0.8 + 4 mg/mL[a]	GW	2 mg/mL[a]	Subvisible haze forms in 1 hr	2074	I
	ES	0.8 + 4 mg/mL[a]	GW	5 mg/mL[a]	Subvisible haze forms immediately	2074	I
Vancomycin HCl	AB	10 mg/mL[a]	GW	0.1, 2, 5 mg/mL[a]	Physically compatible for 4 hr at 23 °C	2074	C
Zidovudine	BW	4 mg/mL[a]	GW	0.1, 2, 5 mg/mL[a]	Physically compatible for 4 hr at 23 °C	2074	C

[a]*Tested in dextrose 5%.*
[b]*Tested in sodium chloride 0.9%.*
[c]*Tested in Ringer's injection, lactated.*
[d]*Test performed using the formulation WITHOUT edetate disodium.*

CISPLATIN
AHFS 10:00

Products — Cisplatin is available as a sterile aqueous injection containing cisplatin 1 mg/mL and sodium chloride 9 mg/mL, with hydrochloric acid and/or sodium hydroxide to adjust the pH. This aqueous solution is available in 50-mL (50-mg), 100-mL (100-mg), and 200-mL (200-mg) vials. (1; 4)

pH — From 3.5 to 4.5. (1)

Osmolality — The aqueous injection has an osmolality of about 285 mOsm/kg. (4)

Sodium Content — Each 10 mg of cisplatin contains 1.54 mEq of sodium. (846; 869)

Administration — Cisplatin is administered by intravenous infusion with a regimen of hydration (with or without mannitol and/or furosemide) prior to therapy. One regimen consists of 1 to 2 L of fluid given over eight to 12 hours prior to cisplatin administration. In addition, adequate hydration and urinary output must be maintained for 24 hours after therapy. The official labeling recommends diluting the cisplatin dose in 2 L of compatible infusion solution containing mannitol 37.5 g and infusing over six to eight hours. (1; 4) Other dilutions and rates of administration have been used, including intravenous infusions over periods from 15 to 120 minutes and continuous infusion over one to five days. Intra-arterial infusion and intraperitoneal instillation have been used. (4)

Because of an interaction occurring between cisplatin and the metal aluminum, only administration equipment such as needles, syringes, catheters, and sets that contain no aluminum should be used for this drug. Aluminum in contact with cisplatin solution will result in a replacement oxidation–reduction reaction, forcing platinum from the cisplatin molecule out of solution and appearing as a black or brown precipitate. Other metal components such as stainless steel needles and plated brass hubs do not elicit an observable reaction within 24 hours. (1; 203; 204; 512; 988)

Stability — Intact vials of the clear, colorless aqueous injection should be stored between 20 and 25 °C and protected from light; they should not be refrigerated. (1; 4)

After initial vial entry, the aqueous cisplatin injection in amber vials is stable for 28 days if it is protected from light or for seven days if it is exposed to fluorescent room light. (1)

Concern has been expressed that storage of cisplatin solutions for several weeks might result in substantial amounts of the toxic mono- and di-aquo species. (1199) However, the solution's chloride content, rather than extended storage time periods, appears to determine the extent of aquated product formation. (See Effect of Chloride Ion below.)

Kristjansson et al. evaluated the long-term stability of cisplatin 1 mg/mL in an aqueous solution containing sodium chloride 9 mg/mL and mannitol 10 mg/mL in glass vials. After 22 months at 5 °C, the 4% loss of cisplatin could be explained as the expected equilibrium between cisplatin and its aquated products. Furthermore, a precipitate formed and required sonication at 40 °C for about 20 to 30 minutes to redissolve. Storage of the cisplatin solution at 40 °C for

10 months resulted in no physical change. After an additional one year at 5 °C, these samples exhibited an average 15% loss, which the authors concluded was not the result of the formation of aquated species or the toxic and inactive oligomeric species. These proposed degradation products were not present in the 40 °C sample. (1246)

Theuer et al. reported little or no loss of cisplatin potency, after 27 days at room temperature with protection from light, from a solution of cisplatin 500 mcg/mL in sodium chloride 0.9% at pH 4.75 and 3.25. (1605)

Cisplatin may react with sodium thiosulfate, sodium metabisulfite, and sodium bisulfite in solution, rapidly and completely inactivating the cisplatin. (4; 1089; 1175)

Cisplatin 1 mg/mL did not support the growth of several microorganisms and may impart an antimicrobial effect at this concentration. Loss of viability was observed for *Staphylococcus aureus*, *Escherichia coli*, *Pseudomonas aeruginosa*, *Pseudomonas cepacia*, *Candida albicans*, and *Aspergillus niger*. (1187)

pH Effects — The pH of maximum stability is 3.5 to 5.5. Alkaline media should be avoided because of increased hydrolysis. (1379)

In the dark at pH 6.3, cisplatin (Bristol) 1 mg/mL in sodium chloride 0.9% reached the maximum amount of decomposition product permitted in the *USP* in 34 days. Half of that amount was formed in 96 days at pH 4.3. (1647)

Cisplatin degradation results in ammonia formation, which increases the solution pH. Thus, the initial cisplatin degradation rate may be slow but increases with time. (1647)

Temperature Effects — It is recommended that cisplatin not be refrigerated because of the formation of a crystalline precipitate. (1; 4; 633; 636; 1246) In a study of cisplatin at concentrations of 0.4 to 1 mg/mL in sodium chloride 0.9%, it was found that at 0.6 mg/mL or greater a precipitate formed on refrigeration at 2 to 6 °C. At 1 mg/mL the precipitation was noted in one hour. However, the 0.6-mg/mL solution did not have a precipitate until after 48 hours under refrigeration. The 0.5-mg/mL and lower solutions did not precipitate for up to 72 hours at 2 to 6 °C. In solutions where precipitate did form, redissolution occurred very slowly with warming back to room temperature. (317) Sonication at 40 °C has been used to redissolve the precipitate in about 20 to 30 minutes. (1246) The warming of precipitated cisplatin solutions to effect redissolution is not recommended, however. Solutions containing a precipitate should not be used. (4; 633)

Freezing Solutions — Cisplatin (Bristol) 50 and 200 mg/L in dextrose 5% in sodium chloride 0.45% in PVC bags and admixed with either mannitol 18.75 g/L or magnesium sulfate 1 or 2 g/L is reportedly stable for 30 days when frozen at −15 °C followed by an additional 48 hours at 25 °C. (1088)

Light Effects — Although changes in the UV spectra of cisplatin solutions on exposure to intense light have long been recognized (317), their significance was questioned. It was reported that exposure to normal laboratory light for 72 hours had no significant effect on cisplatin's stability. (635)

More recently, however, Zieske et al. reported substantial cisplatin decomposition after exposure to typical laboratory light, a mixture of incandescent and fluorescent illumination. As much as 12% degraded to trichloroammineplatinate (II) after 25 hours. Cisplatin was most sensitive to light in the UV to blue region and had little sensitivity to yellow or red light. It was protected from light-induced degradation by low-actinic amber glass flasks but not by PVC bags, clear glass vials, or polyethylene syringes. The authors concluded that exposure to moderately intense white light for more than one hour should be avoided. (1647)

The manufacturer recommends that a cisplatin solution removed from its amber vial be protected from light if it is not used within six hours. Even in the amber vial, the cisplatin solution should be discarded after seven days if exposed to fluorescent room light. (1)

Chloride Ion Effects — The stability of cisplatin in solution is dependent on the chloride ion concentration present. Cisplatin is stable in solutions containing an adequate amount of chloride ion but is incompatible in solutions having a low chloride content. (4; 316; 317; 634; 635; 637) In solutions with an inadequate chloride content, one or both chloride ions in the cisplatin molecule are displaced by water, forming mono- and diaquo species. The minimum acceptable chloride ion concentration is about 0.040 mol/L, the equivalent of about 0.2% sodium chloride. (317; 634; 635)

At a cisplatin concentration of 200 mg/L in sodium chloride 0.9% with the pH adjusted to 4, about 3% decomposition occurs in less than one hour at room temperature. An equilibrium is then reached, with the cisplatin remaining stable thereafter. At lesser concentrations of chloride ion, greater decomposition of cisplatin occurs. In sodium chloride 0.45 and 0.2%, approximately 4 and 7% decomposition occurred at equilibrium, respectively. In very low chloride-containing solutions, most of the drug may be decomposed. The decomposition appears to be reversible, with cisplatin being reformed in the presence of high chloride concentrations. (317)

In another study, the stability of cisplatin 50 and 500 mg/L was evaluated in aqueous solutions containing sodium chloride 0.9, 0.45, and 0.1% and also in water over 24 hours at 25 °C exposed to light. Approximately 2 and 4% of the cisplatin were lost in the sodium chloride 0.9 and 0.45% solutions, respectively. In the 0.1% solution, about 4 to 10% decomposition occurred in four to six hours, increasing to approximately 11 to 15% at both 12 and 24 hours. In aqueous solution with no chloride content, cisplatin decomposed rapidly, with about a 30 to 35% loss in four hours increasing to a 70 to 80% loss in 24 hours. (635)

Ambulatory Pumps — Cisplatin (David Bull) reconstituted to concentrations of 1 and 1.6 mg/mL with sterile water for injection was evaluated for stability for 14 days protected from light in Pharmacia Deltec medication cassettes at 24 and 37 °C. The 1.6-mg/mL concentration developed a yellow crystalline precipitate rendering it unfit for use. For the 1-mg/mL concentration, little change in cisplatin concentration was found, but water loss due to evaporation was found to be about 1% at 24 °C and 3% at 37 °C in 14 days. (2319)

Filtration — Cisplatin 10 to 300 mcg/mL exhibited no loss due to sorption to cellulose nitrate/cellulose acetate ester (Millex OR) or Teflon (Millex FG) filters. (1415; 1416)

Compatibility Information

Solution Compatibility

Cisplatin

Solution	Mfr	Mfr	Conc/L	Remarks	Ref	C/I
Dextrose 5% in sodium chloride 0.225%	AB[a]	NCI	300 mg	3% loss in 23 hr at 25 °C under fluorescent light	1087	C
Dextrose 5% in sodium chloride 0.45%		BV	50 and 500 mg	Less than 10% loss in 24 hr at room temperature	234	C
	AB[b]	NCI	300 mg	2% loss in 23 hr at 25 °C under fluorescent light	1087	C
Dextrose 5% in sodium chloride 0.9%		BV	50 and 500 mg	Less than 10% loss in 24 hr at room temperature	234	C
			500 mg	2% loss in 24 hr at 25 °C	635	C
	AB[a]	NCI	300 mg	1% loss in 23 hr at 25 °C under fluorescent light	1087	C
Dextrose 5% in sodium chloride 0.45%[f]		BR	50, 100, 200 mg	Physically compatible. Stable for 72 hr at 25 and 4 °C plus 8-hr infusion with 2 to 10% loss	636	C
Dextrose 5% in sodium chloride 0.33%[f,g]		BR	50, 100, 200 mg	Physically compatible. Stable for 72 hr at 25 and 4 °C plus 8-hr infusion with 0 to 8% loss	636	C
Dextrose 5%	TR	BV	100 mg	Decomposition occurs in under 2 hr	316	I
	AB[a]	NCI	300 mg	4% loss in 2 hr and 6% in 23 hr at 25 °C	1087	C
	AB[a]	NCI	75 mg	10% loss in 2 hr and 16% in 6 hr at 25 °C	1087	I
Sodium chloride 0.9%			50 and 500 mg	2% loss in 24 hr at 25 °C	635	C
	TR	BV	100 mg	No loss in 24 hr at room temperature	316	C
		BV	200 mg	2 to 3% loss in 1 hr and no further loss for 24 hr at room temperature and pH adjusted to 4	317	C
	AB[a]	NCI	300 mg	1% loss in 23 hr at 25 °C under fluorescent light	1087	C
	[c]	BEL	600 mg	Little loss in 9 days at 23 °C in dark	1757	C
	[d]	BEL	500 and 900 mg	Little loss in 28 days at 22 and 35 °C in dark	1827	C
	[e]	WAS	167 mg	Little loss in 14 days at 30 °C in dark	1828	C
		EBE	100 mg	9% loss in 5 days and 13% loss in 6 days at 22 °C in dark. 3% loss in 7 days at 4 °C in dark	2293	C
Sodium chloride 0.45%			50 and 500 mg	Approximately 4% loss in 24 hr at 25 °C	635	C
		BV	200 mg	4 to 5% loss in 1 hr and no further loss for 24 hr at room temperature and pH adjusted to 4	317	C
Sodium chloride 0.3%		BR	50, 100, 200 mg	Physically compatible and 2 to 3% loss over 72 hr at 25 and 4 °C	636	C
Sodium chloride 0.225%		BR	50, 100, 200 mg	Physically compatible and 2 to 5% loss over 72 hr at 25 and 4 °C	636	C

[a]Tested in glass containers.
[b]Tested in both glass and PVC containers.
[c]Tested in PVC containers.
[d]Tested in ethylene vinyl acetate containers.
[e]Tested in glass, PVC, polyethylene, and polypropylene containers.
[f]Tested with mannitol 1.875% present.
[g]Tested with and without potassium chloride 20 mEq/L present.

Additive Compatibility

Cisplatin

Drug	Mfr	Conc/L	Mfr	Conc/L	Test Soln	Remarks	Ref	C/I
Carboplatin		1 g		200 mg	NS	Under 10% drug loss in 7 days at 23 °C	1954	C
Cyclophosphamide with etoposide		2 g 200 mg		200 mg	NS	All drugs stable for 7 days at room temperature	1379	C
Etoposide	BR	200 and 400 mg	BR	200 mg	NS[a]	Physically compatible. Under 10% loss of both drugs in 24 hr at 22 °C	1329	C
	BR	200 and 400 mg	BR	200 mg	D5½S[a]	Physically compatible. Under 10% loss of both drugs in 24 hr at 22 °C	1329	C
		400 mg		200 mg	NS	10% etoposide loss and no cisplatin loss in 7 days at room temperature	1388	C
		200 mg		200 mg	NS	Both drugs stable for 14 days at room temperature protected from light	1379	C
Etoposide[e]	BR	400 mg	BR	200 mg	D5½S, NS[a]	Physically compatible. Drugs stable for 8 hr at 22 °C. Precipitate within 24 to 48 hr	1329	I
Etoposide with cyclophosphamide		200 mg 2 g		200 mg	NS	All drugs stable for 7 days at room temperature	1379	C
Etoposide with floxuridine		300 mg 700 mg		200 mg	NS	All drugs stable for 7 days at room temperature	1379	C
Etoposide with ifosfamide		200 mg		2 g 200 mg	NS	All drugs stable for 5 days at room temperature	1379	C
Floxuridine	RC	10 g	BR	500 mg	NS	13% floxuridine loss in 7 days at room temperature in dark	1386	C
Floxuridine with etoposide		700 mg 300 mg		200 mg	NS	All drugs stable for 7 days at room temperature	1379	C
Floxuridine with leucovorin calcium		700 mg 140 mg		200 mg	NS	All drugs stable for 7 days at room temperature	1379	C
Fluorouracil	SO	1 g	BR	200 mg	NS[b]	10% cisplatin loss in 1.5 hr and 25% loss in 4 hr at 25 °C	1339	I
	SO	10 g	BR	500 mg	NS[b]	10% cisplatin loss in 1.2 hr and 25% loss in 3 hr at 25 °C	1339	I
	AD	10 g	BR	500 mg	NS	80% cisplatin loss in 24 hr at room temperature due to low pH	1386	I
Hydroxyzine HCl	LY	500 mg	BR	200 mg	NS[c]	Physically compatible for 48 hr	1190	C
Ifosfamide		2 g		200 mg	NS	Both drugs stable for 7 days at room temperature	1379	C
Ifosfamide with etoposide		2 g 200 mg		200 mg	NS	All drugs stable for 5 days at room temperature	1379	C
Leucovorin calcium		140 mg		200 mg	NS	Both drugs stable for 15 days at room temperature protected from light	1379	C
Leucovorin calcium with floxuridine		140 mg 700 mg		200 mg	NS	All drugs stable for 7 days at room temperature	1379	C
Magnesium sulfate		1 and 2 g	BR	50 and 200 mg	D5½S[b]	Compatible for 48 hr at 25 °C and 96 hr at 4 °C followed by 48 hr at 25 °C	1088	C
Mannitol		18.75 g	BR	50 and 200 mg	D5½S[b]	Compatible for 48 hr at 25 °C and 96 hr at 4 °C followed by 48 hr at 25 °C	1088	C
Mesna		3.33 g		67 mg	NS	Cisplatin not detectable after 1 hr	1291	I
		110 mg		67 mg	NS	Cisplatin weakly detected after 1 hr	1291	I

Additive Compatibility (Cont.)

Cisplatin

Drug	Mfr	Conc/L	Mfr	Conc/L	Test Soln	Remarks	Ref	C/I
Ondansetron HCl	GL	1.031 g	BR	485 mg	NS[b]	Physically compatible. Little loss of drugs in 24 hr at 4 °C then 7 days at 30 °C	1846	**C**
	GL	479 mg	BR	219 mg	NS[d]	Physically compatible. Little loss of drugs in 7 days at 4 °C then 24 hr at 30 °C	1846	**C**
Paclitaxel	BMS	300 mg	BMS	200 mg	NS	No paclitaxel loss and cisplatin losses of 1, 4, and 5% at 4, 24, and 32 °C, respectively, in 24 hr. Physically compatible for 24 hr but microparticles of paclitaxel form after 3 to 5 days	2094	**C**
	BMS	1.2 g	BMS	200 mg	NS	No paclitaxel loss but cisplatin losses of 10, 19, and 22% at 4, 24, and 32 °C, respectively, in 24 hr. Physically compatible for 24 hr but microparticles of paclitaxel form after 3 to 5 days	2094	**I**
Sodium bicarbonate[c]		5%		50 and 500 mg		Bright gold precipitate forms in 8 to 24 hr at 25 °C	635	**I**
Thiotepa		1 g		200 mg	NS	Yellow precipitation	1379	**I**

[a]*Tested in both glass and PVC containers.*
[b]*Tested in PVC containers.*
[c]*Tested in glass containers.*
[d]*Tested in polyisoprene reservoirs (Travenol Infusors).*
[e]*Tested with mannitol 1.875% and potassium chloride 20 mEq/L present.*

Drugs in Syringe Compatibility

Cisplatin

Drug (in syringe)	Mfr	Amt	Mfr	Amt	Remarks	Ref	C/I
Bleomycin sulfate		1.5 units/ 0.5 mL		0.5 mg/ 0.5 mL	Physically compatible for 5 min at room temperature followed by 8 min of centrifugation	980	**C**
Cyclophosphamide		10 mg/ 0.5 mL		0.5 mg/ 0.5 mL	Physically compatible for 5 min at room temperature followed by 8 min of centrifugation	980	**C**
Doxapram HCl	RB	400 mg/ 20 mL		10 mg/ 20 mL	Physically compatible with no doxapram loss in 24 hr	1177	**C**
Doxorubicin HCl		1 mg/ 0.5 mL		0.5 mg/ 0.5 mL	Physically compatible for 5 min at room temperature followed by 8 min of centrifugation	980	**C**
Doxorubicin HCl with mitomycin	BED BMS	25 mg 5 mg	BMS	50 mg	Brought to a 5-mL final volume with NS. Visually compatible but more than 10% loss of mitomycin in 4 hr at 25 °C. At 4 °C, less than 10% loss of all three drugs in 12 hr, but about 16% mitomycin loss in 24 hr	2423	**I**
Droperidol		1.25 mg/ 0.5 mL		0.5 mg/ 0.5 mL	Physically compatible for 5 min at room temperature followed by 8 min of centrifugation	980	**C**
Fluorouracil		25 mg/ 0.5 mL		0.5 mg/ 0.5 mL	Physically compatible for 5 min at room temperature followed by 8 min of centrifugation	980	**C**
Furosemide		5 mg/ 0.5 mL		0.5 mg/ 0.5 mL	Physically compatible for 5 min at room temperature followed by 8 min of centrifugation	980	**C**

Drugs in Syringe Compatibility (Cont.)

Cisplatin

Drug (in syringe)	Mfr	Amt	Mfr	Amt	Remarks	Ref	C/I
Heparin sodium		500 units/ 0.5 mL		0.5 mg/ 0.5 mL	Physically compatible for 5 min at room temperature followed by 8 min of centrifugation	980	**C**
Leucovorin calcium		5 mg/ 0.5 mL		0.5 mg/ 0.5 mL	Physically compatible for 5 min at room temperature followed by 8 min of centrifugation	980	**C**
Methotrexate sodium		12.5 mg/ 0.5 mL		0.5 mg/ 0.5 mL	Physically compatible for 5 min at room temperature followed by 8 min of centrifugation	980	**C**
Metoclopramide HCl		2.5 mg/ 0.5 mL		0.5 mg/ 0.5 mL	Physically compatible for 5 min at room temperature followed by 8 min of centrifugation	980	**C**
Mitomycin		0.25 mg/ 0.5 mL		0.5 mg/ 0.5 mL	Physically compatible for 5 min at room temperature followed by 8 min of centrifugation	980	**C**
Mitomycin with doxorubicin HCl	BMS BED	5 mg 25 mg	BMS	50 mg	Brought to a 5-mL final volume with NS. Visually compatible but more than 10% loss of mitomycin in 4 hr at 25 °C. At 4 °C, less than 10% loss of all three drugs in 12 hr, but about 16% mitomycin loss in 24 hr	2423	**I**
Vinblastine sulfate		0.5 mg/ 0.5 mL		0.5 mg/ 0.5 mL	Physically compatible for 5 min at room temperature followed by 8 min of centrifugation	980	**C**
Vincristine sulfate		0.5 mg/ 0.5 mL		0.5 mg/ 0.5 mL	Physically compatible for 5 min at room temperature followed by 8 min of centrifugation	980	**C**

Y-Site Injection Compatibility (1:1 Mixture)

Cisplatin

Drug	Mfr	Conc	Mfr	Conc	Remarks	Ref	C/I
Allopurinol sodium	BW	3 mg/mL[b]	BR	1 mg/mL	Physically compatible for 4 hr at 22 °C	1686	**C**
Amifostine	USB	10 mg/mL[a]	BR	1 mg/mL	Subvisible haze forms in 4 hr	1845	**I**
Amphotericin B cholesteryl sulfate complex	SEQ	0.83 mg/mL[a]	BR	1 mg/mL	Gross precipitate forms	2117	**I**
Anidulafungin	VIC	0.5 mg/mL[a]	SIC	1 mg/mL[b]	Physically compatible for 4 hr at 23 °C	2617	**C**
Aztreonam	SQ	40 mg/mL[a]	BMS	1 mg/mL	Physically compatible for 4 hr at 23 °C	1758	**C**
Bleomycin sulfate		3 units/mL		1 mg/mL	Drugs injected sequentially in Y-site with no flush. No precipitate seen	980	**C**
Caspofungin acetate	ME	0.7 mg/mL[b]	APP	0.5 mg/mL[b]	Physically compatible for 4 hr at room temperature	2758	**C**
Cladribine	ORT	0.015[b] and 0.5[c] mg/mL	BR	1 mg/mL	Physically compatible for 4 hr at 23 °C	1969	**C**
Cyclophosphamide		20 mg/mL		1 mg/mL	Drugs injected sequentially in Y-site with no flush. No precipitate seen	980	**C**
Doripenem	JJ	5 mg/mL[a,b]	SIC	0.5 mg/mL[b]	Physically compatible for 4 hr at 23 °C	2743	**C**
Doxorubicin HCl		2 mg/mL		1 mg/mL	Drugs injected sequentially in Y-site with no flush. No precipitate seen	980	**C**
Doxorubicin HCl liposomal	SEQ	0.4 mg/mL[a]	BR	1 mg/mL	Physically compatible for 4 hr at 23 °C	2087	**C**
Droperidol		2.5 mg/mL		1 mg/mL	Drugs injected sequentially in Y-site with no flush. No precipitate seen	980	**C**

Y-Site Injection Compatibility (1:1 Mixture) (Cont.)

Cisplatin

Drug	Mfr	Conc	Mfr	Conc	Remarks	Ref	C/I
Etoposide phosphate	BR	5 mg/mL[a]	BR	1 mg/mL	Physically compatible for 4 hr at 23 °C	2218	C
Filgrastim	AMG	30 mcg/mL[a]	BR	1 mg/mL	Physically compatible for 4 hr at 22 °C	1687	C
Fludarabine phosphate	BX	1 mg/mL[a]	BR	1 mg/mL	Visually compatible for 4 hr at 22 °C	1439	C
Fluorouracil		50 mg/mL		1 mg/mL	Drugs injected sequentially in Y-site with no flush. No precipitate seen	980	C
Furosemide		10 mg/mL		1 mg/mL	Drugs injected sequentially in Y-site with no flush. No precipitate seen	980	C
Gallium nitrate	FUJ	1 mg/mL[b]	BR	1 mg/mL	Precipitates immediately	1673	I
Gemcitabine HCl	LI	10 mg/mL[b]	BR	1 mg/mL	Physically compatible for 4 hr at 23 °C	2226	C
Granisetron HCl	SKB	1 mg/mL	BR	0.05 mg/mL[b]	Physically compatible with little or no granisetron loss in 4 hr at 22 °C	1883	C
	SKB	1 mg/mL	BR	1 mg/mL	Physically compatible with little or no loss of either drug in 4 hr at 22 °C	1883	C
Heparin sodium		1000 units/ mL		1 mg/mL	Drugs injected sequentially in Y-site with no flush. No precipitate seen	980	C
Leucovorin calcium		10 mg/mL		1 mg/mL	Drugs injected sequentially in Y-site with no flush. No precipitate seen	980	C
Linezolid	PHU	2 mg/mL	BR	1 mg/mL	Physically compatible for 4 hr at 23 °C	2264	C
Melphalan HCl	BW	0.1 mg/mL[b]	BR	1 mg/mL	Physically compatible for 3 hr at 22 °C	1557	C
Methotrexate sodium		25 mg/mL		1 mg/mL	Drugs injected sequentially in Y-site with no flush. No precipitate seen	980	C
Metoclopramide HCl		5 mg/mL		1 mg/mL	Drugs injected sequentially in Y-site with no flush. No precipitate seen	980	C
Mitomycin		0.5 mg/mL		1 mg/mL	Drugs injected sequentially in Y-site with no flush. No precipitate seen	980	C
Ondansetron HCl	GL	1 mg/mL[b]	BR	1 mg/mL	Visually compatible for 4 hr at 22 °C	1365	C
	GL	16 to 160 mcg/mL		0.48 mg/mL	Physically compatible when cisplatin given over 1 to 8 hr via Y-site	1366	C
Paclitaxel	NCI	1.2 mg/mL[a]		1 mg/mL	Physically compatible for 4 hr at 22 °C	1528	C
Palonosetron HCl	MGI	50 mcg/mL	BMS	0.5 mg/mL[b]	Physically compatible. No palonosetron and 5% cisplatin loss in 4 hr	2579	C
Pemetrexed disodium	LI	20 mg/mL[b]	BMS	0.5 mg/mL[b]	Physically compatible for 4 hr at 23 °C	2564	C
Piperacillin sodium–tazobactam sodium	LE[f]	40 + 5 mg/ mL[a]	BR	1 mg/mL	Haze and particles form in 1 hr	1688	I
Propofol	ZEN	10 mg/mL	BR	1 mg/mL	Physically compatible for 1 hr at 23 °C	2066	C
Sargramostim	IMM	10 mcg/mL[b]	BR	1 mg/mL	Visually compatible for 4 hr at 22 °C	1436	C
Teniposide	BR	0.1 mg/mL[a]	BR	1 mg/mL	Physically compatible for 4 hr at 23 °C	1725	C
Thiotepa	IMM[d]	1 mg/mL[a]	BMS	1 mg/mL	White cloudiness appears in 4 hr at 23 °C	1861	I
TNA #218 to #226[e]			BMS	1 mg/mL	Visually compatible for 4 hr at 23 °C	2215	C
Topotecan HCl	SKB	56 mcg/mL[b]	BR	0.168 mg/ mL[b]	Visually compatible. Little loss of either drug in 4 hr at 22 °C	2245	C
TPN #212 to #215[e]			BMS	1 mg/mL	Amber discoloration formed in 1 to 4 hr	2109	I
Vinblastine sulfate		1 mg/mL		1 mg/mL	Drugs injected sequentially in Y-site with no flush. No precipitate seen	980	C

Y-Site Injection Compatibility (1:1 Mixture) (Cont.)

Cisplatin

Drug	Mfr	Conc	Mfr	Conc	Remarks	Ref	C/I
Vincristine sulfate		1 mg/mL		1 mg/mL	Drugs injected sequentially in Y-site with no flush. No precipitate seen	980	C
Vinorelbine tartrate	BW	1 mg/mLᵇ	BR	1 mg/mL	Physically compatible for 4 hr at 22 °C	1558	C

ᵃTested in dextrose 5%.
ᵇTested in sodium chloride 0.9%.
ᶜTested in bacteriostatic sodium chloride 0.9% preserved with benzyl alcohol 0.9%.
ᵈLyophilized formulation tested.
ᵉRefer to Appendix I for the composition of parenteral nutrition solutions. TNA indicates a 3-in-1 admixture, and TPN indicates a 2-in-1 admixture.
ᶠTest performed using the formulation WITHOUT edetate disodium.

CLADRIBINE
AHFS 10:00

Products — Cladribine is available as a solution in 10-mL single-use vials. Each milliliter of the solution contains cladribine 1 mg, sodium chloride 9 mg, and phosphoric acid and/or dibasic sodium phosphate to adjust the pH. The injection is a concentrate that must be diluted for administration. (1; 4)

pH — From 5.5 to 8. (1)

Tonicity — Cladribine injection is isotonic. (1)

Sodium Content — Each milliliter of cladribine injection contains 0.15 mEq of sodium. (1)

Trade Name(s) — Leustatin.

Administration — Cladribine is administered by continuous intravenous infusion after dilution in 500 mL of sodium chloride 0.9% for repeated single daily doses. Alternatively, cladribine may be diluted in bacteriostatic sodium chloride 0.9% containing benzyl alcohol 0.9% for a seven-day continuous infusion. The seven-day solution should be prepared by adding both the drug and solution to the pump reservoir through 0.22-μm filters, bringing the final volume to 100 mL. Remove air in the reservoirs by aspiration using a syringe and filter or vent-filter assembly. The finished preserved solution is then administered continuously over seven days. (1; 4)

The use of dextrose 5% as a diluent is not recommended because of an increased rate of cladribine degradation. (1)

Stability — Intact cladribine vials should be stored under refrigeration and protected from light. The solution is clear and colorless. A precipitate may develop upon low-temperature storage; the precipitate may be redissolved by allowing the solution to warm to room temperature with vigorous shaking. (1) Heating the solution is not recommended. However, less than 5% loss is reported to occur in seven days when the solution is stored at 37 °C. (1369) Freezing does not adversely affect stability of the product. Thawing should be allowed to occur naturally by exposure to room temperature. The vials should not be heated or exposed to microwaves. After thawing, the vial contents are stable under refrigeration until expiration. Thawed vials should not be refrozen. (1)

Cladribine (Ortho Biotech) 0.025 mg/mL in sodium chloride 0.9% did not exhibit an antimicrobial effect on *Enterococcus faecium*, *Staphylococcus aureus*, *Pseudomonas aeruginosa*, and *Candida albicans* inoculated into the solution. Admixtures should be stored under refrigeration whenever possible, and the potential for microbiological growth should be considered when assigning expiration periods. (2160)

Ambulatory Pumps — Prepared in bacteriostatic sodium chloride 0.9% preserved with benzyl alcohol 0.9%, cladribine exhibits both chemical and physical stability for at least seven days in Sims Deltec ambulatory infusion pump reservoirs. Preservative effectiveness may be reduced in solutions prepared for patients weighing more than 85 kg due to greater benzyl alcohol dilution. (1) In concentrations of 0.15 to 0.3 mg/mL in bacteriostatic sodium chloride 0.9% containing benzyl alcohol, the drug is stated to be stable for at least 14 days. (1369)

Compatibility Information

Solution Compatibility

Cladribine

Solution	Mfr	Mfr	Conc/L	Remarks	Ref	C/I
Dextrose 5%				Increased cladribine decomposition	1	**I**
Sodium chloride 0.9%				Stable for 24 hr at room temperature exposed to light, but use in 8 hr is recommended	1	**C**
	a,b	JC	16 mg	Visually compatible and little or no loss in 30 days at 4 and 18 °C	2154	**C**
	c		24 mg	No loss of drug in 2 weeks at 4 °C	2398	**C**

[a]Tested in PVC containers.
[b]Tested in polyethylene-lined trilayer (Clearflex) containers.
[c]Tested in glass infusion bottles.

Y-Site Injection Compatibility (1:1 Mixture)

Cladribine

Drug	Mfr	Conc	Mfr	Conc	Remarks	Ref	C/I
Aminophylline	AMR	2.5 mg/mL[a]	ORT	0.015[a] and 0.5[b] mg/mL	Physically compatible for 4 hr at 23 °C	1969	C
Bumetanide	RC	0.04 mg/mL[a]	ORT	0.015[a] and 0.5[b] mg/mL	Physically compatible for 4 hr at 23 °C	1969	C
Buprenorphine HCl	RKC	0.04 mg/mL[a]	ORT	0.015[a] and 0.5[b] mg/mL	Physically compatible for 4 hr at 23 °C	1969	C
Butorphanol tartrate	APC	0.04 mg/mL[a]	ORT	0.015[a] and 0.5[b] mg/mL	Physically compatible for 4 hr at 23 °C	1969	C
Calcium gluconate	AMR	40 mg/mL[a]	ORT	0.015[a] and 0.5[b] mg/mL	Physically compatible for 4 hr at 23 °C	1969	C
Carboplatin	BR	5 mg/mL[a]	ORT	0.015[a] and 0.5[b] mg/mL	Physically compatible for 4 hr at 23 °C	1969	C
Chlorpromazine HCl	SCN	2 mg/mL[a]	ORT	0.015[a] and 0.5[b] mg/mL	Physically compatible for 4 hr at 23 °C	1969	C
Cisplatin	BR	1 mg/mL	ORT	0.015[a] and 0.5[b] mg/mL	Physically compatible for 4 hr at 23 °C	1969	C
Cyclophosphamide	MJ	10 mg/mL[a]	ORT	0.015[a] and 0.5[b] mg/mL	Physically compatible for 4 hr at 23 °C	1969	C
Cytarabine	CHI	50 mg/mL	ORT	0.015[a] and 0.5[b] mg/mL	Physically compatible for 4 hr at 23 °C	1969	C
Dexamethasone sodium phosphate	AMR	1 mg/mL[a]	ORT	0.015[a] and 0.5[b] mg/mL	Physically compatible for 4 hr at 23 °C	1969	C
Diphenhydramine HCl	SCN	2 mg/mL[a]	ORT	0.015[a] and 0.5[b] mg/mL	Physically compatible for 4 hr at 23 °C	1969	C
Dobutamine HCl	LI	4 mg/mL[a]	ORT	0.015[a] and 0.5[b] mg/mL	Physically compatible for 4 hr at 23 °C	1969	C
Dopamine HCl	AST	3.2 mg/mL[a]	ORT	0.015[a] and 0.5[b] mg/mL	Physically compatible for 4 hr at 23 °C	1969	C
Doxorubicin HCl	CHI	2 mg/mL	ORT	0.015[a] and 0.5[b] mg/mL	Physically compatible for 4 hr at 23 °C	1969	C

Y-Site Injection Compatibility (1:1 Mixture) (Cont.)

Cladribine

Drug	Mfr	Conc	Mfr	Conc	Remarks	Ref	C/I
Droperidol	JN	0.4 mg/mL[a]	ORT	0.015[a] and 0.5[b] mg/mL	Physically compatible for 4 hr at 23 °C	1969	C
Enalaprilat	MSD	0.1 mg/mL[a]	ORT	0.015[a] and 0.5[b] mg/mL	Physically compatible for 4 hr at 23 °C	1969	C
Etoposide	BR	0.4 mg/mL[a]	ORT	0.015[a] and 0.5[b] mg/mL	Physically compatible for 4 hr at 23 °C	1969	C
Famotidine	ME	2 mg/mL[a]	ORT	0.015[a] and 0.5[b] mg/mL	Physically compatible for 4 hr at 23 °C	1969	C
Furosemide	AB	3 mg/mL[a]	ORT	0.015[a] and 0.5[b] mg/mL	Physically compatible for 4 hr at 23 °C	1969	C
Gallium nitrate	FUJ	0.4 mg/mL[b]	ORT	0.015[a] and 0.5[b] mg/mL	Physically compatible for 4 hr at 23 °C	1969	C
Granisetron HCl	SKB	0.05 mg/mL[a]	ORT	0.015[a] and 0.5[b] mg/mL	Physically compatible for 4 hr at 23 °C	1969	C
Haloperidol lactate	MN	0.2 mg/mL[a]	ORT	0.015[a] and 0.5[b] mg/mL	Physically compatible for 4 hr at 23 °C	1969	C
Heparin sodium	WY	100 units/mL[a]	ORT	0.015[a] and 0.5[b] mg/mL	Physically compatible for 4 hr at 23 °C	1969	C
Hydrocortisone sodium succinate	UP	1 mg/mL[a]	ORT	0.015[a] and 0.5[b] mg/mL	Physically compatible for 4 hr at 23 °C	1969	C
Hydromorphone HCl	KN	0.5 mg/mL[a]	ORT	0.015[a] and 0.5[b] mg/mL	Physically compatible for 4 hr at 23 °C	1969	C
Hydroxyzine HCl	ES	4 mg/mL[a]	ORT	0.015[a] and 0.5[b] mg/mL	Physically compatible for 4 hr at 23 °C	1969	C
Idarubicin HCl	AD	0.5 mg/mL[a]	ORT	0.015[a] and 0.5[b] mg/mL	Physically compatible for 4 hr at 23 °C	1969	C
Leucovorin calcium	IMM	2 mg/mL[a]	ORT	0.015[a] and 0.5[b] mg/mL	Physically compatible for 4 hr at 23 °C	1969	C
Lorazepam	WY	0.1 mg/mL[a]	ORT	0.015[a] and 0.5[b] mg/mL	Physically compatible for 4 hr at 23 °C	1969	C
Mannitol	BA	15%	ORT	0.015[a] and 0.5[b] mg/mL	Physically compatible for 4 hr at 23 °C	1969	C
Meperidine HCl	WY	4 mg/mL[a]	ORT	0.015[a] and 0.5[b] mg/mL	Physically compatible for 4 hr at 23 °C	1969	C
Mesna	MJ	10 mg/mL[a]	ORT	0.015[a] and 0.5[b] mg/mL	Physically compatible for 4 hr at 23 °C	1969	C
Methylprednisolone sodium succinate	AB	5 mg/mL[a]	ORT	0.015[a] and 0.5[b] mg/mL	Physically compatible for 4 hr at 23 °C	1969	C
Metoclopramide HCl	RB	5 mg/mL	ORT	0.015[a] and 0.5[b] mg/mL	Physically compatible for 4 hr at 23 °C	1969	C
Mitoxantrone HCl	LE	0.5 mg/mL[a]	ORT	0.015[a] and 0.5[b] mg/mL	Physically compatible for 4 hr at 23 °C	1969	C
Morphine sulfate	AST	1 mg/mL[a]	ORT	0.015[a] and 0.5[b] mg/mL	Physically compatible for 4 hr at 23 °C	1969	C
Nalbuphine HCl	AST	10 mg/mL	ORT	0.015[a] and 0.5[b] mg/mL	Physically compatible for 4 hr at 23 °C	1969	C

Y-Site Injection Compatibility (1:1 Mixture) (Cont.)

Cladribine

Drug	Mfr	Conc	Mfr	Conc	Remarks	Ref	C/I
Ondansetron HCl	CER	1 mg/mL[a]	ORT	0.015[a] and 0.5[b] mg/mL	Physically compatible for 4 hr at 23 °C	1969	C
Paclitaxel	BR	0.6 mg/mL[a]	ORT	0.015[a] and 0.5[b] mg/mL	Physically compatible for 4 hr at 23 °C	1969	C
Potassium chloride	AB	0.1 mEq/mL[a]	ORT	0.015[a] and 0.5[b] mg/mL	Physically compatible for 4 hr at 23 °C	1969	C
Prochlorperazine edisylate	SCN	0.5 mg/mL[a]	ORT	0.015[a] and 0.5[b] mg/mL	Physically compatible for 4 hr at 23 °C	1969	C
Promethazine HCl	SCN	2 mg/mL[a]	ORT	0.015[a] and 0.5[b] mg/mL	Physically compatible for 4 hr at 23 °C	1969	C
Ranitidine HCl	GL	2 mg/mL[a]	ORT	0.015[a] and 0.5[b] mg/mL	Physically compatible for 4 hr at 23 °C	1969	C
Sodium bicarbonate	AB	1 mEq/mL	ORT	0.015[a] and 0.5[b] mg/mL	Physically compatible for 4 hr at 23 °C	1969	C
Teniposide	BR	0.1 mg/mL[a]	ORT	0.015[a] and 0.5[b] mg/mL	Physically compatible for 4 hr at 23 °C	1969	C
Vincristine sulfate	LI	0.05 mg/mL[a]	ORT	0.015[a] and 0.5[b] mg/mL	Physically compatible for 4 hr at 23 °C	1969	C

[a]*Tested in sodium chloride 0.9%.*
[b]*Tested in bacteriostatic sodium chloride 0.9% preserved with benzyl alcohol 0.9%.*

CLARITHROMYCIN
AHFS 8:12.12.92

Products — Clarithromycin is available in 500-mg vials with lactobionic acid as a solubilizing agent and sodium hydroxide to adjust pH. Reconstitute with 10 mL of sterile water for injection, and shake to dissolve the powder. Do not use diluents containing preservatives or inorganic salts. Each milliliter of the resultant solution contains 50 mg of clarithromycin. This solution must be diluted before use. See Administration below. (38; 115)

Trade Name(s) — Klacid, Klaricid, Zeclar.

Administration — Clarithromycin is administered by intravenous infusion after dilution in an appropriate infusion solution. It should not be given by intravenous bolus or intramuscular injection. The reconstituted drug solution (500 mg) is added to 250 mL of compatible infusion solution yielding a 2-mg/mL final solution. The final diluted solution is administered by intravenous infusion over 60 minutes into one of the larger proximal veins. (38; 115)

Stability — Intact containers of the white to off-white lyophilized powder should be stored at 30 °C or below and protected from light. When reconstituted as directed, the 50-mg/mL solution should be used within 24 hours stored at room temperature of 25 °C (38; 115) and 48 hours stored under refrigeration at 5 °C. (115)

Compatibility Information

Solution Compatibility

Clarithromycin

Solution	Mfr	Mfr	Conc/L	Remarks	Ref	C/I
Dextrose 5%			2 g	Use within 6 hr at 25 °C or 48 hr at 5 °C	115	C
Dextrose 5% in Ringer's injection, lactated			2 g	Use within 6 hr at 25 °C or 48 hr at 5 °C	115	C
Dextrose 5% in sodium chloride 0.45%			2 g	Use within 6 hr at 25 °C or 48 hr at 5 °C	115	C

Solution Compatibility (Cont.)

Clarithromycin

Solution	Mfr	Mfr	Conc/L	Remarks	Ref	C/I
Normosol M in dextrose 5%			2 g	Use within 6 hr at 25 °C or 48 hr at 5 °C	115	C
Normosol R in dextrose 5%			2 g	Use within 6 hr at 25 °C or 48 hr at 5 °C	115	C
Ringer's injection, lactated			2 g	Use within 6 hr at 25 °C or 48 hr at 5 °C	115	C
Sodium chloride 0.9%			2 g	Use within 6 hr at 25 °C or 48 hr at 5 °C	115	C

Y-Site Injection Compatibility (1:1 Mixture)

Clarithromycin

Drug	Mfr	Conc	Mfr	Conc	Remarks	Ref	C/I
Aminophylline	EV	2 mg/mL[a]	AB	4 mg/mL[a]	Needle-like crystals form in 2 hr at 30 °C and 4 hr at 17 °C	2174	I
Amiodarone HCl	SW	3 mg/mL[a]	AB	4 mg/mL[a]	Visually compatible for 72 hr at both 30 and 17 °C	2174	C
Amoxicillin sodium–clavulanate potassium	BE	20 + 4 mg/mL[a]	AB	4 mg/mL[a]	Visually compatible for 72 hr at both 30 and 17 °C	2174	C
Ampicillin sodium	BE	40 mg/mL[a]	AB	4 mg/mL[a]	Visually compatible for 72 hr at both 30 and 17 °C	2174	C
Atracurium besylate	GW	1 mg/mL[a]	AB	4 mg/mL[a]	Visually compatible for 72 hr at both 30 and 17 °C	2174	C
Bumetanide	LEO	0.5 mg/mL	AB	4 mg/mL[a]	Visually compatible for 72 hr at both 30 and 17 °C	2174	C
Cefepime HCl	BMS	120 mg/mL[b]		50 mg/mL	Physically compatible with less than 10% cefepime loss. Clarithromycin not tested	2513	C
Ceftazidime	SKB	125 mg/mL		50 mg/mL	Precipitates immediately	2434	I
	SKB	125 mg/mL		10 mg/mL	Trace precipitation	2434	I
	GSK	120 mg/mL[b]		50 mg/mL	Precipitates	2513	I
Cefuroxime sodium	GW	60 mg/mL[a]	AB	4 mg/mL[a]	White precipitate forms in 3 hr at 30 °C and 24 hr at 17 °C	2174	I
Ciprofloxacin	BAY	2 mg/mL[a]	AB	4 mg/mL[a]	Visually compatible for 72 hr at both 30 and 17 °C	2174	C
Dobutamine HCl	BI	2 mg/mL[a]	AB	4 mg/mL[a]	Visually compatible for 72 hr at both 30 and 17 °C	2174	C
Dopamine HCl	DB	3.2 mg/mL[a]	AB	4 mg/mL[a]	Visually compatible for 72 hr at both 30 and 17 °C	2174	C
Floxacillin sodium	BE	40 mg/mL[a]	AB	4 mg/mL[a]	Translucent precipitate in 1 to 2 hr becoming a gel in 3 hr at 30 and 17 °C	2174	I
Furosemide	ANT	10 mg/mL	AB	4 mg/mL[a]	White cloudiness forms immediately, becoming an obvious precipitate in 15 min	2174	I
Gentamicin sulfate	RS	40 mg/mL	AB	4 mg/mL[a]	Visually compatible for 72 hr at both 30 and 17 °C	2174	C
Heparin sodium	CPP	1000 units/mL[a]	AB	4 mg/mL[a]	White cloudiness forms immediately	2174	I
Insulin, human	NOV	4 units/mL[a]	AB	4 mg/mL[a]	Visually compatible for 72 hr at both 30 and 17 °C	2174	C

Y-Site Injection Compatibility (1:1 Mixture) (Cont.)

Clarithromycin

Drug	Mfr	Conc	Mfr	Conc	Remarks	Ref	C/I
Lidocaine HCl	ANT	4 mg/mL[a]	AB	4 mg/mL[a]	Visually compatible for 72 hr at both 30 and 17 °C	2174	C
Metoclopramide HCl	ANT	5 mg/mL	AB	4 mg/mL[a]	Visually compatible for 72 hr at both 30 and 17 °C	2174	C
Metronidazole	PRK	5 mg/mL	AB	4 mg/mL[a]	Visually compatible for 72 hr at both 30 and 17 °C	2174	C
Penicillin G sodium	BRT	24 mg/mL[a]	AB	4 mg/mL[a]	Visually compatible for 72 hr at both 30 and 17 °C	2174	C
Phenytoin sodium	ANT	20 mg/mL[a]	AB	4 mg/mL[a]	White cloudy precipitate in 1 hr at both 30 and 17 °C	2174	I
Prochlorperazine mesylate	ANT	12.5 mg/mL	AB	4 mg/mL[a]	Visually compatible for 72 hr at both 30 and 17 °C	2174	C
Potassium chloride	ANT	0.08 mmol/mL[a]	AB	4 mg/mL[a]	Visually compatible for 72 hr at both 30 and 17 °C	2174	C
Ranitidine HCl	GW	5 mg/mL[a]	AB	4 mg/mL[a]	Visually compatible for 72 hr at both 30 and 17 °C	2174	C
Ticarcillin disodium–clavulanate potassium	BE	32 mg/mL[a]	AB	4 mg/mL[a]	Visually compatible for 72 hr at both 30 and 17 °C	2174	C
Vancomycin HCl	DB	10 mg/mL[a]	AB	4 mg/mL[a]	Visually compatible for 72 hr at both 30 and 17 °C	2174	C
Vecuronium bromide	OR	2 mg/mL[a]	AB	4 mg/mL[a]	Visually compatible for 72 hr at both 30 and 17 °C	2174	C
Verapamil HCl	BKN	2.5 mg/mL	AB	4 mg/mL[a]	Visually compatible for 72 hr at both 30 and 17 °C	2174	C

[a]*Tested in dextrose 5%.*
[b]*Tested in sterile water for injection.*

CLINDAMYCIN PHOSPHATE
AHFS 8:12.28.20

Products — Clindamycin phosphate 150 mg/mL is available in 2-, 4-, and 6-mL vials and a 60-mL pharmacy bulk container. Each milliliter of solution also contains benzyl alcohol 9.45 mg, disodium edetate 0.5 mg, and sodium hydroxide and/or hydrochloric acid to adjust pH in water for injection. (1; 4):

Clindamycin phosphate also is available in 50-mL bags containing 300, 600, or 900 mg of drug in dextrose 5%. Disodium edetate 0.04 mg/mL and sodium hydroxide and/or hydrochloric acid are also present to adjust the pH. (1)

pH — The product pH may range from 5.5 to 7 (4) but is usually about 6 to 6.3. (102; 103)

Osmolality — Clindamycin phosphate (Upjohn) 150 mg/mL has been reported to have an osmolality of 795 mOsm/kg (50) or 835 mOsm/kg (1071) as determined by freezing-point depression. However, the manufacturer has stated that the osmolality is usually 825 to 880 mOsm/kg. (1705)

The osmolality of clindamycin phosphate (Upjohn) 12 mg/mL was determined to be 293 mOsm/kg in dextrose 5% and 309 mOsm/kg in sodium chloride 0.9%. (1375)

The osmolalities of the 300-, 600-, and 900-mg premixed infusion solutions in dextrose 5% are 296, 322, and 339 mOsm/kg, respectively. (4)

The osmolality of clindamycin phosphate 600 mg was calculated for the following dilutions (1054):

	Osmolality (mOsm/kg)	
Diluent	50 mL	100 mL
Dextrose 5%	279	268
Sodium chloride 0.9%	306	294

Trade Name(s) — Cleocin Phosphate.

Administration — Clindamycin phosphate is administered by intramuscular injection; single injections greater than 600 mg are not recommended. It may also be administered by intermittent intravenous infusion in concentrations not exceeding 18 mg/mL. Intermittent infusions should be infused over 10 to 60 minutes at a rate not exceeding 30 mg/min. Intravenous doses under 900 mg may be diluted in 50 mL of a compatible diluent; doses of 900 mg or more should be diluted in 100 mL of diluent. Not more than 1200 mg of clindamycin phosphate should be given in a one-hour period. The drug should not be given undiluted as a bolus. (1; 4)

Alternatively, following an initial single rapid infusion, continuous intravenous infusion at rates of 0.75 to 1.25 mg/min have been suggested. (1; 4)

Stability — Intact containers of clindamycin phosphate should be stored at controlled room temperature; temperatures above 30 °C should be avoided. (1) Less than 10% decomposition occurs in two years at 25 °C at pH 3.5 to 6.5. (102; 103) Crystallization may occur on refrigeration; the crystals resolubilize on warming to room temperature, but care should be exercised to ensure that all crystals have redissolved. This would also apply if the product is frozen. (102)

Clindamycin phosphate (Upjohn) 10 mg/L stability in peritoneal dialysis solutions (Dianeal 137 and PD2) with heparin sodium 500 units/L was evaluated. Approximately 102 ± 9% activity remained after 24 hours at 25 °C. (1228)

pH Effects — Maximum stability occurs at pH 4, but an acceptable long-term shelf life is attained at pH 1 to 6.5. (1072)

Syringes — Clindamycin phosphate 900 mg/6 mL in polypropylene syringes (Becton-Dickinson) retained more than 95% of the initial concentration over at least 48 hours at room temperature. (172) Diluted with sterile water for injection to concentrations of 20, 40, 60, and 120 mg/mL and stored in Monoject plastic syringes or glass vials, clindamycin phosphate exhibited little change in concentration and was free of particulate matter over 30 days at 25 °C and 60 days at −15 °C. (173)

Clindamycin phosphate (Upjohn) 900 mg/6 mL showed no more than a 4 to 5% loss when stored in polypropylene syringes (Becton-Dickinson) for 48 hours at 25 °C under fluorescent light. (1159)

Clindamycin phosphate (Upjohn) 600 mg stored in polypropylene syringes (3M) at 25 °C under fluorescent light exhibited no loss in 48 hours. (1164)

Vials — Dilution of clindamycin phosphate 300 and 900 mg in glass vials containing 20 mL of dextrose 10% resulted in no visual changes and less than a 10% loss after 30 days of refrigeration at 10 °C. (1604)

Clindamycin phosphate (Abbott) injection was diluted with sterile water for injection to a concentration of 15 mg/mL for use in minimizing measurement errors in pediatric dosing. The dilution was packaged in glass vials, and samples were stored at 22 and 4 °C. The dilution remained visually free of particulate matter at both storage conditions throughout the study. No clindamycin loss after 91 days at either 4 or 22 °C. (1714)

Clindamycin phosphate is incompatible with natural rubber closures because of the extraction of crystalline particulate matter, primarily β-sitosterol and stigmasterol. Simple cleaning procedures for the closures do not effectively remove the source of contamination. It is recommended that if clindamycin phosphate is repackaged in vials or disposable syringes, storage at room temperature should be limited to a few days. (102)

Central Venous Catheter — Clindamycin phosphate (Upjohn) 2 mg/mL in dextrose 5% was found to be compatible with the ARROWg+ard Blue Plus (Arrow International) chlorhexidine-bearing triple-lumen central catheter. Essentially complete delivery of the drug was found with little or no drug loss occurring. Furthermore, chlorhexidine delivered from the catheter remained at trace amounts with no substantial increase due to the delivery of the drug through the catheter. (2335)

Compatibility Information

Solution Compatibility

Clindamycin phosphate

Solution	Mfr	Mfr	Conc/L	Remarks	Ref	C/I
Amino acids 4.25%, dextrose 25%	MG	UP	600 mg	No increase in particulate matter in 24 hr at 5 °C	349	C
Dextrose 2.5% in Ringer's injection, lactated		UP	600 mg	Physically compatible and stable for 24 hr at room temperature	104	C
Dextrose 5% in Ringer's injection		UP	600 mg	Physically compatible and stable for 24 hr at room temperature	104	C
Dextrose 5% in sodium chloride 0.45%		UP	600 mg	Stable for 24 hr	101	C
Dextrose 5% in sodium chloride 0.9%	MG	UP	250 mg	Stable for 24 hr at 4 and 25 °C	105	C
		UP	600 mg	Physically compatible and stable for 24 hr at room temperature	104	C
Dextrose 5%	MG	UP	250 mg	Stable for 24 hr at 4 and 25 °C	105	C
		UP	600 mg	Physically compatible and stable for 24 hr at room temperature	104	C
		UP	6, 9, 12 g	Stable for 24 hr	101	C

Solution Compatibility (Cont.)

Clindamycin phosphate

Solution	Mfr	Mfr	Conc/L	Remarks	Ref	C/I
			6 g	3% loss in 79 days frozen at −10 °C	174	C
	TR[a]	UP	6 g	Physically compatible and 9% loss in 24 hr at room temperature. No loss in 340 days at −10 °C	555	C
	TR[a,b]	UP	6, 9, 12 g	Physically compatible and stable for16 days at 25 °C, 32 days at 4 °C, and 56 days at −10 °C	753	C
	AB[a,b]	UP	9 g	Physically compatible and no loss in 24 hr at 25 °C	994	C
	AB[a]	UP	18 g	3% loss in 28 days frozen at −20 °C	981	C
	TR[a]	QU	6 and 12 g	Physically compatible with no loss in 22 days at 25 °C, 54 days at 5 °C, and 68 days at −10 °C	1351	C
	MG[c]	UP	7.6 g	Visually compatible with no loss in 30 days at −20 °C then 14 days at 4 °C	1539	C
	BA[a], BRN[b,c]	GW	3 g	Visually compatible with little loss in 24 hr at 4 and 22 °C	2289	C
	BA[f]	SZ	1 and 12 g	Little loss in 7 days at 23 °C and 21 days at 4 °C	2819	C
Dextrose 10%	MG	UP	250 mg	Stable for 24 hr at 4 and 25 °C	105	C
Isolyte M in dextrose 5%	MG	UP	250 mg	Stable for 24 hr at 4 and 25 °C	105	C
Isolyte P in dextrose 5%	MG	UP	250 mg	Stable for 24 hr at 4 and 25 °C	105	C
Normosol R	AB	UP	1.2 g	Stable for 24 hr	101	C
Ringer's injection, lactated	MG	UP	250 mg	Stable for 24 hr at 4 and 25 °C	105	C
	TR[a,b]	UP	6, 9, 12 g	Physically compatible with no loss in 16 days at 25 °C, 32 days at 5 °C, and 56 days at −10 °C	753	C
Sodium chloride 0.9%		UP	600 mg	Physically compatible and stable for 24 hr at room temperature	104	C
		UP	6 g	Stable for 24 hr	101	C
	MG	UP	250 mg	Stable for 24 hr at 4 and 25 °C	105	C
	TR[a,b]	UP	6, 9, 12 g	Physically compatible with no loss in 16 days at 25 °C, 32 days at 4 °C, and 56 days at −10 °C	753	C
	AB[a,b]	UP	9 g	Physically compatible and no loss in 24 hr at 25 °C	994	C
	AB[a]	UP	18 g	4% loss in 28 days frozen at −20 °C	981	C
	TR[a]	QU	6 and 12 g	Physically compatible with no loss in 22 days at 25 °C, 54 days at 5 °C, and 68 days at −10 °C	1351	C
	BR[a], BRN[b,c]	GW	3 g	Visually compatible with little loss in 24 hr at 4 and 22 °C	2289	C
	HOS[f]	SZ	1 and 12 g	Little loss in 7 days at 23 °C and 21 days at 4 °C	2819	C
TPN #21[d]		UP	250 mg	Stable for 24 hr at 4 and 25 °C	87	C
TPN #22[d]		UP	3 g	Physically compatible with no loss in 24 hr at 22 °C in the dark	837	C
TPN #107[d]			400 mg[e]	Stable for 24 hr at 21 °C	1326	C

[a]*Tested in PVC containers.*
[b]*Tested in glass containers.*
[c]*Tested in polyolefin containers.*
[d]*Refer to Appendix I for the composition of parenteral nutrition solutions. TPN indicates a 2-in-1 admixture.*
[e]*As clindamycin base.*
[f]*Tested in Accufusor reservoirs.*

Additive Compatibility

Clindamycin phosphate

Drug	Mfr	Conc/L	Mfr	Conc/L	Test Soln	Remarks	Ref	C/I
Amikacin sulfate	BR	5 g	UP	6 g	D5LR, D5R, D5S, D5W, D10W, LR, NS, R, SL	Physically compatible and amikacin stable for 24 hr at 25 °C. Clindamycin not analyzed	293	C
	BR	4 g	UP	9 g	D5W, NS[a]	Both stable for 48 hr at 25 °C under fluorescent light	981	C
Aminophylline	SE	600 mg	UP	600 mg		Physically incompatible	101	I
Ampicillin sodium	WY	10 and 20 g	UP	24 g	NS	Physically compatible	1035	C
	WY	3.7 g	UP	3 g	NS	Physically compatible with 4% ampicillin loss in 1 day at 24 °C	1035	C
Aztreonam	SQ	10 and 20 g	UP	3 and 6 g	D5W, NS[b]	Physically compatible with little or no loss of either drug in 48 hr at 25 °C and 7 days at 4 °C	1002	C
	SQ	20 g	UP	9 g	D5W[a]	Physically compatible with 3% clindamycin loss and 5% aztreonam loss in 48 hr at 25 °C under fluorescent light	1026	C
	SQ	20 g	UP	9 g	NS[a]	Physically compatible with 2% clindamycin loss and no aztreonam loss in 48 hr at 25 °C under fluorescent light	1026	C
Cefazolin sodium	SKF	10 g	UP	9 g	D5W[a]	Physically compatible with no clindamycin loss and 8% cefazolin loss in 48 hr at room temperature under fluorescent light	983	C
	SKF	10 g	UP	9 g	NS[a]	Physically compatible with no clindamycin loss and 3% cefazolin loss in 48 hr at room temperature under fluorescent light	983	C
Cefazolin sodium[f]	SKF	10 g	UP	9 g	D5W, NS[a]	10% cefazolin loss in 4 hr in D5W and 12 hr in NS at 25 °C. No clindamycin and gentamicin loss in 24 hr	1328	I
Cefepime HCl	BR	40 g	UP	0.25 g	D5W, NS	7% or less cefepime loss in 24 hr at room temperature and 10% or less loss in 7 days at 5 °C. No clindamycin loss in 24 hr at room temperature and 8% or less loss in 7 days at 5 °C	1682	C
	BR	4 g	UP	6 g	D5W, NS	7% or less cefepime loss in 24 hr at room temperature and 10% or less loss in 7 days at 5 °C. No clindamycin loss in 24 hr at room temperature and 8% or less loss in 7 days at 5 °C	1682	C
Cefotaxime sodium	HO	20 g	UP	9 g	D5W, NS[c]	Physically compatible with no clindamycin loss and 3% cefotaxime loss in 24 hr at 25 °C	994	C
Cefoxitin sodium	MSD	20 g	UP	9 g	D5W[a]	Physically compatible with no loss of either drug in 48 hr at room temperature	983	C
	MSD	20 g	UP	9 g	NS[a]	Physically compatible with no clindamycin loss and 7% cefoxitin loss in 48 hr at room temperature	983	C

Additive Compatibility (Cont.)

Clindamycin phosphate

Drug	Mfr	Conc/L	Mfr	Conc/L	Test Soln	Remarks	Ref	C/I
Ceftazidime	GL	20 g	UP	9 g	D5W[a]	Physically compatible with 9% clindamycin loss and 11% ceftazidime loss in 48 hr at 25 °C under fluorescent light	1026	C
	GL	20 g	UP	9 g	NS[a]	Physically compatible with 5% clindamycin loss and 7% ceftazidime loss in 48 hr at 25 °C under fluorescent light	1026	C
Ceftriaxone sodium	RC	20 g	UP	12 g	D5W[a]	10% ceftriaxone loss in 4 hr and 17% in 24 hr at 25 °C under fluorescent light. No clindamycin loss in 48 hr	1026	I
	RC	20 g	UP	12 g	NS[a]	10% ceftriaxone loss in 1 hr and 12% in 24 hr at 25 °C under fluorescent light. 6% clindamycin loss in 48 hr	1026	I
Cefuroxime sodium	GL	15 g	UP	9 g	D5W	Physically compatible with 4% clindamycin loss and 6 to 8% cefuroxime loss in 48 hr at 25 °C under fluorescent light	1164	C
	GL	15 g	UP	9 g	NS	Physically compatible with 9% clindamycin and cefuroxime losses in 48 hr at 25 °C under fluorescent light	1164	C
Ciprofloxacin	MI	1.6 g	LY	7.1 g	D5W, NS	Precipitate forms immediately	1541	I
Fluconazole	PF	1 g	AST	6 g	D5W	Visually compatible with no fluconazole loss in 72 hr at 25 °C under fluorescent light. Clindamycin not tested	1677	C
Gentamicin sulfate		120 mg	UP	2.4 g	D5W	Physically compatible. Clindamycin stable for 24 hr at room temperature	104	C
		60 mg	UP	1.2 g	D5W	Physically compatible. Clindamycin stable for 24 hr at room temperature	104	C
		600 mg	UP	12 g	D5W	Physically compatible	101	C
		800 mg	UP	9 g	D5W	Clindamycin stable for 24 hr	101	C
	AB	1 g	UP	9 g	D5W, NS[c]	Physically compatible and both drugs stable for 48 hr at room temperature exposed to light and 1 week frozen	174	C
	LY	1.2 g	UP	9 g	D5W[a]	Physically compatible and both drugs stable for 7 days at 4 and 25 °C	174	C
	LY	1.2 g	UP	9 g	NS[a]	Physically compatible and both drugs stable for 14 days at 4 and 25 °C	174	C
	LY	2.4 g	UP	18 g	D5W, NS[c]	Physically compatible and both drugs stable for 14 days at 4 and 25 °C	174	C
	ES	1.2 g	UP	9 g	D5W, NS[a]	Physically compatible and both drugs stable for 28 days frozen at −20 °C	174	C
	ES	2.4 g	UP	18 g	D5W, NS[b]	Both drugs stable for 28 days frozen at −20 °C	981	C
	ES	667 mg	UP	6 g	D5W[b]	Physically compatible with no clindamycin loss and 9% gentamicin loss in 24 hr at room temperature	995	C
		75 mg		400 mg[d]	TPN #107[e]	19% gentamicin loss and 15% clindamycin loss in 24 hr at 21 °C	1326	I

Additive Compatibility (Cont.)

Clindamycin phosphate

Drug	Mfr	Conc/L	Mfr	Conc/L	Test Soln	Remarks	Ref	C/I
Gentamicin sulfate[g]	ES	800 mg	UP	9 g	D5W, NS[a]	10% cefazolin loss in 4 hr in D5W and 12 hr in NS at 25 °C. No clindamycin and gentamicin loss in 24 hr	1328	I
Heparin sodium		100,000 units	UP	9 g	D5W	Clindamycin stable for 24 hr	101	C
Hydrocortisone sodium succinate	UP	1 g	UP	1.2 g	W	Clindamycin stable for 24 hr	101	C
Methylprednisolone sodium succinate	UP	500 mg	UP	1.2 g	D5W, W	Clindamycin stable for 24 hr	101	C
Metoclopramide HCl	RB	100 and 200 mg	UP	6 g		Physically compatible for 24 hr at 25 °C	1167	C
	RB	1.9 g	UP	3.5 g		Physically compatible for 24 hr at 25 °C	1167	C
	RB	1.2 g	UP	4.4 g		Physically compatible for 24 hr at 25 °C	1167	C
Potassium chloride		40 mEq	UP	600 mg	D5½S	Physically compatible and clindamycin stable for 24 hr at room temperature	104	C
		100 mEq	UP	600 mg	D5W, NS	Physically compatible	101	C
		400 mEq	UP	6 g	D5½S	Clindamycin stable for 24 hr	101	C
Ranitidine HCl	GL	100 mg	UP	1.2 g	D5W	Color change and gas formation	1151	I
	GL	50 mg and 2 g		1.2 g	D5W, NS	Physically compatible. Ranitidine stable for 24 hr at 25 °C. Clindamycin not tested	1515	C
Sodium bicarbonate		44 mEq	UP	1.2 g	D5S, D5W	Clindamycin stable for 24 hr	101	C
Tobramycin sulfate	DI	1 g	UP	9 g	D5W, NS[c]	Physically compatible and both drugs stable for 48 hr at room temperature exposed to light and for 1 week frozen	174	C
	DI	1.2 g	UP	9 g	D5W[a]	Physically compatible and clindamycin stable for 28 days frozen. 8% tobramycin loss in 14 days and 17% in 28 days	174	C
	DI	1.2 g	UP	9 g	NS[a]	Physically compatible and both drugs stable for 28 days frozen	174	C
	DI	2.4 g	UP	18 g	D5W[b]	8% tobramycin lost in 14 days and 17% in 28 days at −20 °C. Clindamycin stable	981	C
	DI	2.4 g	UP	18 g	NS[b]	Both drugs stable for 28 days frozen at −20 °C	981	C
Tramadol HCl	GRU	400 mg	AB	6 g	NS	Tramadol losses of 20% in 4 hr at room temperature with precipitate	2652	I
Verapamil HCl	KN	80 mg	UP	1.2 g	D5W, NS	Physically compatible for 24 hr	764	C

[a]*Tested in glass containers.*
[b]*Tested in PVC containers.*
[c]*Tested in both glass and PVC containers.*
[d]*Present as clindamycin base.*
[e]*Refer to Appendix I for the composition of parenteral nutrition solutions. TPN indicates a 2-in-1 admixture.*
[f]*Tested in combination with gentamicin sulfate 800 mg/L.*
[g]*Tested in combination with cefazolin sodium 10 g/L.*

Drugs in Syringe Compatibility

Clindamycin phosphate

Drug (in syringe)	Mfr	Amt	Mfr	Amt	Remarks	Ref	C/I
Amikacin sulfate	BR	750 mg/ 4 mL[a]	UP	900 mg/ 6 mL	Physically compatible with little loss of either drug in 48 hr at 25 °C	1159	C
Aztreonam	SQ	2 g	UP	600 mg/ 4 mL	Physically compatible with 2% clindamycin loss and 8% aztreonam loss in 48 hr at 25 °C under fluorescent light	1164	C
Caffeine citrate		20 mg/ 1 mL	UP	150 mg/ 1 mL	Visually compatible for 4 hr at 25 °C	2440	C
Dimenhydrinate		10 mg/ 1 mL		150 mg/ 1 mL	Clear solution	2569	C
Gentamicin sulfate	ES	120 mg/ 4 mL[a]	UP	900 mg/ 6 mL	Physically compatible with little loss of either drug for 48 hr at 25 °C	1159	C
Heparin sodium		2500 units/ 1 mL	UP	300 mg	Physically compatible for at least 5 min	1053	C
Pantoprazole sodium	[b]	4 mg/ 1 mL		150 mg/ 1 mL	Precipitates within 1 hr	2574	I
Tobramycin sulfate	DI	120 mg/ 4 mL[a]	UP	900 mg/ 6 mL	Cloudy white precipitate forms immediately and changes to gel-like precipitate	1159	I

[a]Diluted to 4 mL with 1 mL of sodium chloride 0.9%.
[b]Test performed using the formulation WITHOUT edetate disodium.

Y-Site Injection Compatibility (1:1 Mixture)

Clindamycin phosphate

Drug	Mfr	Conc	Mfr	Conc	Remarks	Ref	C/I
Acyclovir sodium	BW	5 mg/mL[a]	UP	12 mg/mL[a]	Physically compatible for 4 hr at 25 °C	1157	C
Allopurinol sodium	BW	3 mg/mL[b]	AB	10 mg/mL[b]	Tiny particles form immediately and become more numerous over 4 hr	1686	I
Amifostine	USB	10 mg/mL[a]	AST	10 mg/mL[a]	Physically compatible for 4 hr at 23 °C	1845	C
Amiodarone HCl	LZ	4 mg/mL[c]	UP	6 mg/mL[c]	Physically compatible for 4 hr at room temperature	1444	C
Amphotericin B cholesteryl sulfate complex	SEQ	0.83 mg/mL[a]	UP	10 mg/mL[a]	Physically compatible for 4 hr at 23 °C	2117	C
Amsacrine	NCI	1 mg/mL[a]	UP	10 mg/mL[a]	Visually compatible for 4 hr at 22 °C	1381	C
Anakinra	SYN	4 and 36 mg/ mL[b]	AST	12 mg/mL[b]	Physically compatible with little or no loss of either drug in 4 hr at 22 °C	2510	C
Anidulafungin	VIC	0.5 mg/mL[a]	AB	10 mg/mL[a]	Physically compatible for 4 hr at 23 °C	2617	C
Azithromycin	PF	2 mg/mL[b]	PHU	30 mg/mL[k,l]	Amber and white microcrystals found	2368	I
Aztreonam	SQ	40 mg/mL[a]	AST	10 mg/mL[a]	Physically compatible for 4 hr at 23 °C	1758	C
Bivalirudin	TMC	5 mg/mL[a]	AB	10 mg/mL[a]	Physically compatible for 4 hr at 23 °C	2373	C
Caspofungin acetate	ME	0.7 mg/mL[b]	BED	10 mg/mL[b]	Immediate white turbid precipitate forms	2758	I
	ME	0.5 mg/mL[b]	HOS	60 mg/mL[k]	Fine white crystals reported	2766	I
Ceftaroline fosamil	FOR	2.22 mg/ mL[a,b,m]	BED	10 mg/mL[a,b,m]	Physically compatible for 4 hr at 23 °C	2826	C

Y-Site Injection Compatibility (1:1 Mixture) (Cont.)

Clindamycin phosphate

Drug	Mfr	Conc	Mfr	Conc	Remarks	Ref	C/I
Cisatracurium besylate	GW	0.1, 2, 5 mg/mL[a]	AST	10 mg/mL[a]	Physically compatible for 4 hr at 23 °C	2074	C
Cyclophosphamide	MJ	20 mg/mL[a]	UP	12 mg/mL[a]	Physically compatible for 4 hr at 25 °C	1194	C
Dexmedetomidine HCl	AB	4 mcg/mL[b]	AB	10 mg/mL[b]	Physically compatible for 4 hr at 23 °C	2383	C
Diltiazem HCl	MMD	5 mg/mL	UP	12[b] and 150 mg/mL	Visually compatible	1807	C
Docetaxel	RPR	0.9 mg/mL[a]	AST	10 mg/mL[a]	Physically compatible for 4 hr at 23 °C	2224	C
Doxapram HCl	RB	2 mg/mL[a]	PHU	10 mg/mL[a]	Gas bubbles evolve immediately	2470	I
Doxorubicin HCl liposomal	SEQ	0.4 mg/mL[a]	AST	10 mg/mL[a]	Physically compatible for 4 hr at 23 °C	2087	C
Enalaprilat	MSD	0.05 mg/mL[b]	UP	9 mg/mL[a]	Physically compatible for 24 hr at room temperature under fluorescent light	1355	C
Esmolol HCl	DCC	10 mg/mL[a]	UP	9 mg/mL[a]	Physically compatible for 24 hr at 22 °C	1169	C
Etoposide phosphate	BR	5 mg/mL[a]	AST	10 mg/mL[a]	Physically compatible for 4 hr at 23 °C	2218	C
Fenoldopam mesylate	AB	80 mcg/mL[b]	AB	10 mg/mL[b]	Physically compatible for 4 hr at 23 °C	2467	C
Filgrastim	AMG	30 mcg/mL[a]	AB	10 mg/mL[a]	Particles and filaments form immediately	1687	I
Fluconazole	RR	2 mg/mL	AB	24 mg/mL	Precipitates immediately	1407	I
Fludarabine phosphate	BX	1 mg/mL[a]	LY	10 mg/mL[a]	Visually compatible for 4 hr at 22 °C	1439	C
Foscarnet sodium	AST	24 mg/mL	AB	24 mg/mL	Physically compatible for 24 hr at room temperature under fluorescent light	1335	C
	AST	24 mg/mL	UP	12 mg/mL[c]	Physically compatible for 24 hr at 25 °C under fluorescent light	1393	C
Gemcitabine HCl	LI	10 mg/mL[b]	AST	10 mg/mL[b]	Physically compatible for 4 hr at 23 °C	2226	C
Granisetron HCl	SKB	0.05 mg/mL[a]	AB	10 mg/mL[a]	Physically compatible for 4 hr at 23 °C	2000	C
Heparin sodium	TR	50 units/mL	UP	12 mg/mL[a]	Visually compatible for 4 hr at 25 °C	1793	C
Hetastarch in lactated electrolyte	AB	6%	PHU	10 mg/mL[a]	Physically compatible for 4 hr at 23 °C	2339	C
Hydromorphone HCl	WY	0.2 mg/mL[a]	UP	12 mg/mL[a]	Physically compatible for 4 hr at 25 °C	987	C
Hydroxyethyl starch 130/0.4 in sodium chloride 0.9%	FRK	6%	SZ	6, 12, 24 mg/mL[a]	Visually compatible for 24 hr at room temperature	2770	C
Idarubicin HCl	AD	1 mg/mL[b]	AST	12 mg/mL[a]	Haze and precipitate form immediately	1525	I
Labetalol HCl	SC	1 mg/mL[a]	UP	9 mg/mL[a]	Physically compatible for 24 hr at 18 °C	1171	C
Levofloxacin	OMN	5 mg/mL[a]	UP	150 mg/mL	Visually compatible for 4 hr at 24 °C	2233	C
Linezolid	PHU	2 mg/mL	UP	10 mg/mL[a]	Physically compatible for 4 hr at 23 °C	2264	C
Magnesium sulfate	IX	16.7, 33.3, 66.7, 100 mg/mL[a]	UP	12 mg/mL[a]	Physically compatible for at least 4 hr at 32 °C	813	C
Melphalan HCl	BW	0.1 mg/mL[b]	AB	10 mg/mL[b]	Physically compatible for 3 hr at 22 °C	1557	C
Meperidine HCl	WY	10 mg/mL[a]	UP	12 mg/mL[a]	Physically compatible for 4 hr at 25 °C	987	C
Midazolam HCl	RC	1 mg/mL[a]	UP	9 mg/mL[a]	Visually compatible for 24 hr at 23 °C	1847	C
Milrinone lactate	SS	0.2 mg/mL[a]	PHU	18 mg/mL[a]	Visually compatible for 4 hr at 25 °C	2381	C
Morphine sulfate	WI	1 mg/mL[a]	UP	12 mg/mL[a]	Physically compatible for 4 hr at 25 °C	987	C
Multivitamins	USV	5 mL/L[a]	UP	600 mg/100 mL[a]	Physically compatible for 24 hr at room temperature	323	C

Y-Site Injection Compatibility (1:1 Mixture) (Cont.)

Clindamycin phosphate

Drug	Mfr	Conc	Mfr	Conc	Remarks	Ref	C/I
Nicardipine HCl	DCC	0.1 mg/mL[a]	UP	9 mg/mL[a]	Visually compatible for 24 hr at room temperature	235	C
Ondansetron HCl	GL	1 mg/mL[b]	LY	10 mg/mL[a]	Visually compatible for 4 hr at 22 °C	1365	C
Pemetrexed disodium	LI	20 mg/mL[b]	PHU	10 mg/mL[a]	Physically compatible for 4 hr at 23 °C	2564	C
Piperacillin sodium–tazobactam sodium	LE[d]	40 + 5 mg/mL[a]	AB	10 mg/mL[a]	Physically compatible for 4 hr at 22 °C	1688	C
Propofol	ZEN	10 mg/mL	AST	10 mg/mL[a]	Physically compatible for 1 hr at 23 °C	2066	C
Remifentanil HCl	GW	0.025 and 0.25 mg/mL[b]	AST	10 mg/mL[a]	Physically compatible for 4 hr at 23 °C	2075	C
Sargramostim	IMM	10 mcg/mL[b]	LY	10 mg/mL[b]	Visually compatible for 4 hr at 22 °C	1436	C
Tacrolimus	FUJ	1 mg/mL[b]	ES	12 mg/mL[a]	Visually compatible for 24 hr at 25 °C	1630	C
Teniposide	BR	0.1 mg/mL[a]	AST	10 mg/mL[a]	Physically compatible for 4 hr at 23 °C	1725	C
Theophylline	TR	4 mg/mL	UP	12 mg/mL[a]	Visually compatible for 6 hr at 25 °C	1793	C
Thiotepa	IMM[e]	1 mg/mL[a]	AST	10 mg/mL[a]	Physically compatible for 4 hr at 23 °C	1861	C
TNA #73[f]		32.5 mL[g]	UP	12 mg/mL[a]	Visually compatible for 4 hr at 25 °C	1008	C
TNA #218 to #226[f]			AST	10 mg/mL[a]	Visually compatible for 4 hr at 23 °C	2215	C
TPN #61[f]		[h]	UP	50 mg/0.33 mL[i]	Physically compatible	1012	C
		[j]	UP	300 mg/2 mL[i]	Physically compatible	1012	C
TPN #212 to #215[f]			AB	10 mg/mL[a]	Physically compatible for 4 hr at 23 °C	2109	C
Vinorelbine tartrate	BW	1 mg/mL[b]	AB	10 mg/mL[b]	Physically compatible for 4 hr at 22 °C	1558	C
Zidovudine	BW	4 mg/mL[a]	UP	12 mg/mL[a]	Physically compatible for 4 hr at 25 °C	1193	C

[a]*Tested in dextrose 5%.*
[b]*Tested in sodium chloride 0.9%.*
[c]*Tested in both dextrose 5% and sodium chloride 0.9%.*
[d]*Test performed using the formulation WITHOUT edetate disodium.*
[e]*Lyophilized formulation tested.*
[f]*Refer to Appendix I for the composition of parenteral nutrition solutions. TNA indicates a 3-in-1 admixture, and TPN indicates a 2-in-1 admixture.*
[g]*A 32.5-mL sample of parenteral nutrition solution mixed with 50 mL of antibiotic solution.*
[h]*Run at 21 mL/hr.*
[i]*Given over 10 minutes by syringe pump.*
[j]*Run at 94 mL/hr.*
[k]*Tested in sodium chloride 0.45%.*
[l]*Injected via Y-site into an administration set running azithromycin.*
[m]*Tested in Ringer's injection, lactated.*

CLONAZEPAM
AHFS 28:12.08

Products — Clonazepam is available in 1-mL ampuls containing 1 mg of drug in a solvent composed of absolute alcohol, glacial acetic acid, benzyl alcohol, and propylene glycol. An ampul containing 1 mL of sterile water for injection is included as a diluent. (38; 115)

pH — Clonazepam (Roche) 0.125, 0.222, and 0.5 mg/mL in sodium chloride 0.9% for continuous subcutaneous infusion had pH values of 3.6, 3.5, and 3.6, respectively. (2161)

Trade Name(s) — Rivotril.

Administration — Clonazepam is administered by slow intravenous injection. For bolus administration, the content of the diluent ampul is added to the drug immediately before administration. The injection is administered at a rate not exceeding 0.25 to 0.5 mg/min into a large vein of the antecubital fossa. Clonazepam is also administered as a slow intravenous infusion; up to 3 mg of clonazepam is added to 250 mL of dextrose 5 or 10%, sodium chloride 0.9%, or dextrose 2.5% in sodium chloride 0.45%. In exceptional cases and if intravenous administration is not possible, intramuscular injection has been cited. (38; 115)

Stability — The colorless to slightly greenish-yellow solution in intact ampuls should be stored below 30 °C and protected from light. The manufacturer recommends that the drug be used immediately after mixing with the supplied diluent. After dilution in a recommended infusion solution in a glass container, the infusion should be completed within 24 hours. If prepared in an infusion solution in a PVC container, the infusion should be completed without delay after preparation, usually within four hours of addition to the container due to sorption loss. (38; 115)

Clonazepam should not be mixed with sodium bicarbonate because of the potential for precipitation. (38; 115)

Syringes — Clonazepam (Roche) 5 and 10 mg, diluted to 48 mL with sodium chloride 0.9% and stored in polyethylene syringes, was physically compatible and exhibited no clonazepam loss in 10 hours at room temperature. (1708)

Reconstituted clonazepam (Roche) 0.5 mg/mL packaged in polypropylene syringes was evaluated. Less than 2% clonazepam loss occurred in 48 hours stored at room temperature exposed to normal room light. (2172)

Sorption — Clonazepam shows sorption losses in contact with PVC. It is recommended that glass containers be used for infusions. If PVC bags are used, the admixture should be infused without delay after preparation, and usually over no longer than four hours. (38; 115)

Hooymans et al. compared losses of clonazepam to PVC and polyethylene-lined infusion tubing. Clonazepam (Roche) 5 and 10 mg, diluted in sodium chloride 0.9% to a final volume of 48 mL in polyethylene syringes, was delivered at room temperature through tubing at flow rates of 2 or 4 mL/hr (5 mg in 48 mL) and 2 mL/hr (10 mg in 48 mL). No losses were observed in the plastic syringes or to the polyethylene-lined tubing over 10 hours. Losses to the PVC tubing depended on the flow rate and concentration, being greater at 2 mL/hr and at 5 mg/48 mL, respectively. Potency decreased to approximately 40 and 55% of the original strength after 0.6 hour for the 5-mg/48 mL concentration at 2 and 4 mL/hr, respectively. After 0.6 hour, the 10-mg/48 mL concentration was at 55% of original potency when delivered at 2 mL/hr. Effluent concentrations gradually increased after the first hour, reaching approximately 80 to 90% of original concentrations after 10 hours. (1708)

Clonazepam (Roche) (concentration unspecified) in dextrose 5% in PVC containers was delivered over four hours through PVC administration sets. Losses due to sorption ranged from about 13 to 18% determined by UV spectroscopy. (2045)

Compatibility Information

Solution Compatibility

Clonazepam

Solution	Mfr	Mfr	Conc/L	Remarks	Ref	C/I
Dextrose 5%	AB[a]	RC	6 mg	Physically compatible with no loss in 10 hr	1707	C
	TR[b]	RC	6 mg	7% loss in 7 hr, 17 to 20% loss in 24 hr, and 31 to 33% loss in 6 days at room temperature protected from light	1707	I
Sodium chloride 0.9%	AB[a]	RC	6 mg	Physically compatible with no loss in 10 hr	1707	C
	TR[b]	RC	6 mg	14% loss in 7 hr, 17 to 20% loss in 24 hr, and 31 to 33% loss in 6 days at room temperature protected from light	1707	I

[a] Tested in glass containers.
[b] Tested in PVC containers.

Drugs in Syringe Compatibility

Clonazepam

Drug (in syringe)	Mfr	Amt	Mfr	Amt	Remarks	Ref	C/I
Heparin sodium		2500 units/ 1 mL	RC	1 mg/ 2 mL	Visually compatible for at least 5 min	1053	C

Y-Site Injection Compatibility (1:1 Mixture)

Clonazepam

Drug	Mfr	Conc	Mfr	Conc	Remarks	Ref	C/I
TPN #189[a]			RC	10 mg/mL[b]	Visually compatible for 24 hr at 22 °C	1767	C

[a]*Refer to Appendix I for the composition of parenteral nutrition solutions. TPN indicates a 2-in-1 admixture.*
[b]*Tested in sterile water for injection.*

CLONIDINE HYDROCHLORIDE
AHFS 24:08.16

Products — Clonidine hydrochloride is available in concentrations of 0.1 mg/mL (100 mcg/mL) and 0.5 mg/mL (500 mcg/mL) in 10-mL vials. Each milliliter of the preservative-free solution also contains sodium chloride 9 mg in water for injection. Hydrochloric acid and/or sodium hydroxide may have been added to adjust the pH. (1)

pH — From 5 to 7. (1)

Trade Name(s) — Duraclon.

Administration — Clonidine hydrochloride injection is administered by continuous epidural infusion using an appropriate epidural infusion device. The 0.5-mg/mL concentration must be diluted with sodium chloride 0.9% to 0.1 mg/mL for use. Clonidine hydrochloride injection must not be used with a preservative. (1)

Stability — Intact vials containing the clear, colorless solution should be stored at controlled room temperature. (1) They are stable for six months stored at an elevated temperature of 40 °C, remaining clear and colorless with no loss of clonidine hydrochloride. (2069) Clonidine hydrochloride (Roxane) 100 mcg/mL was filled into plastic syringes (Becton-Dickinson), pump reservoirs (Bard), and glass vials and stored at 22 to 27 °C for seven days. The solution was also filled into administration set tubing (Kendall McGaw) and stored under the same conditions. In all cases, the solution remained clear and colorless and no loss of potency was found. (2069)

Clonidine hydrochloride 100 mcg/mL was delivered at a rate of 0.1 mL/hr for seven days through two epidural catheter sets, Epi-Cath (Abbott) and Port-A-Cath (Pharmacia Deltec). The temperature was maintained at 37 °C to simulate internal use of the set. The delivered solution remained clear and colorless throughout the study. Furthermore, the solution delivered through the Epi-Cath resulted in little or no loss. With the Port-A-Cath, a concentrating effect due to a loss of water was countered by a small clonidine hydrochloride loss of drug (about 5%). The net effect was delivery of about 95% of the clonidine hydrochloride dose. (2069)

Syringes — Clonidine hydrochloride (Boehringer Ingelheim) 9 mcg/mL in sodium chloride 0.9% was packaged in two types of polypropylene syringes. The Omnifix (B. Braun) syringes had polyisoprene piston tips while the Terumo syringes had no natural or synthetic rubber in the product. Stored at 4, 21, and 35 °C for 30 days, the test solutions in Terumo syringes exhibited no visual changes or changes in measured pH. Stored at 4, 21, and 35 °C for 30 days, the test solutions in Omnifix syringes exhibited no visual changes but substantial changes in measured pH occurred in some samples. An acceptable pH was maintained for 30 days at 4 °C, 5 days at 21 °C, and less than 1 day at 35 °C. Although the pH remained within the stability range for the drug in most of the samples, this does not definitively demonstrate stability. (2387)

Implantable Pumps — An admixture of bupivacaine hydrochloride 25 mg/mL, clonidine hydrochloride 2 mg/mL, and morphine sulfate 50 mg/mL in sterile water for injection was reported to be physically and chemically stable for 90 days at 37 °C in SynchroMed implantable pumps. Little or no loss of any drug occurred. (2585)

Clonidine hydrochloride and morphine sulfate powders were dissolved in ziconatide acetate (Elan) injection to yield concentrations of 2 and 35 mg/mL and 25 mcg/mL, respectively. Stored at 37 °C, 11% ziconotide loss in 7 days, 4% clonidine loss in 20 days, and no morphine loss in 28 days occurred. (2752)

Morphine sulfate (Infumorph) 20 mg/mL with clonidine hydrochloride (Boehringer Ingelheim) 50 mcg/mL and morphine sulfate 2 mg/mL with clonidine hydrochloride 1.84 mg/mL were evaluated in SynchroMed EL (Medtronic) implantable pumps with silicone elastomer intrathecal catheters at 37 °C for three months. No visible incompatibilities were observed, and delivered concentrations of both drugs were in the range of 94.0 to 99.6% of the theoretical concentrations throughout the study. Furthermore, no impairment of mechanical performance of the pump or any of its components was found. (2477)

Compatibility Information

Solution Compatibility

Clonidine HCl

Solution	Mfr	Mfr	Conc/L	Remarks	Ref	C/I
Sodium chloride 0.9%	BA		200 mg	Visually compatible with no loss of drug in 10 weeks at 37 °C protected from light	2359	C

Additive Compatibility

Clonidine HCl

Drug	Mfr	Conc/L	Mfr	Conc/L	Test Soln	Remarks	Ref	C/I
Baclofen		1 g		0.2 g	NS	Visually compatible with no loss of either drug in 10 weeks at 37 °C in dark	2359	C
Bupivacaine HCl with fentanyl citrate	AST JN	1 g 35 mg	BI	9 mg	NS[a]	Visually compatible with less than 10% change of any drug in 28 days at 4 °C and 24 days at 25 °C in the dark	2437	C
Fentanyl citrate with bupivacaine HCl	JN AST	35 mg 1 g	BI	9 mg	NS[a]	Visually compatible with less than 10% change of any drug in 28 days at 4 °C and 24 days at 25 °C in the dark	2437	C
Hydromorphone HCl		25 mg	BI	150 mg	[c]	No clonidine loss in 35 days at 37 °C	2593	C
Meperidine HCl		8 g	BI	3 mg	NS[a]	Visually compatible with no loss of either drug in 21 days at room temperature	2710	C
Ropivacaine HCl	ASZ	1 g	BI	5 and 50 mg	NS[b]	Physically compatible. No loss of either drug in 30 days at 30 °C in the dark	2433	C
	ASZ	2 g	BI	5 mg	[b]	Physically compatible. No loss of either drug in 30 days at 30 °C in the dark	2433	C
Ziconotide acetate	ELN	25 mg[d]	BB	2 g[e]		No loss of either drug in 28 days at 37 °C	2703	C

[a]Tested in PVC containers.
[b]Tested in polypropylene bags (Mark II Polybags).
[c]Tested in SynchroMed implantable pumps.
[d]Tested in SynchroMed II implantable pumps.
[e]Clonidine HCl powder dissolved in ziconotide acetate injection.

Drugs in Syringe Compatibility

Clonidine HCl

Drug (in syringe)	Mfr	Amt	Mfr	Amt	Remarks	Ref	C/I
Bupivacaine HCl	SAN	3.75 mg/ 1 mL	FUJ	100 mcg/ 1 mL	Physically and chemically stable for 14 days at room temperature	2069	C
	SAN	60 mg/ 8 mL	FUJ	100 mcg/ 1 mL	Physically and chemically stable for 14 days at room temperature	2069	C
Bupivacaine HCl with fentanyl citrate	AST JN	50 mg 1.75 mg	BI	0.45 mg	Diluted to 50 mL with NS. Visually compatible with less than 10% loss of any drug in 25 days at 4 and 25 °C in the dark	2437	C
Bupivacaine HCl with morphine sulfate	SW ES	1.5 mg/ mL 0.2 mg/ mL	BI	0.03 mg/ mL	Diluted to 5 mL with NS. Visually compatible with no new GC/MS peaks in 1 hr at room temperature	1956	C

Drugs in Syringe Compatibility (Cont.)

Clonidine HCl

Drug (in syringe)	Mfr	Amt	Mfr	Amt	Remarks	Ref	C/I
Fentanyl citrate with bupivacaine HCl	JN AST	1.75 mg 50 mg	BI	0.45 mg	Diluted to 50 mL with NS. Visually compatible with less than 10% loss of any drug in 25 days at 4 and 25 °C in the dark	2437	C
Fentanyl citrate with lidocaine HCl	JN AST	0.01 mg/mL 2 mg/mL	BI	0.03 mg/mL	Diluted to 5 mL with NS. Visually compatible with no new GC/MS peaks in 1 hr at room temperature	1956	C
Heparin sodium		2500 units/1 mL	BI	0.15 mg/1 mL	Visually compatible for at least 5 min	1053	C
Ketamine HCl with tetracaine HCl	PD SW	2 mg/mL 2 mg/mL	BI	0.03 mg/mL	Diluted to 5 mL with NS. Visually compatible with no new GC/MS peaks in 1 hr at room temperature	1956	C
Lidocaine HCl with fentanyl citrate	AST JN	2 mg/mL 0.01 mg/mL	BI	0.03 mg/mL	Diluted to 5 mL with NS. Visually compatible with no new GC/MS peaks in 1 hr at room temperature	1956	C
Morphine sulfate	ES	10 mg/1 mL	FUJ	100 mcg/1 mL	Physically and chemically stable for 14 days at room temperature	2069	C
	[a]	5 mg/mL[b]	[a]	0.25 mg/mL[b]	Physically compatible. Little morphine or clonidine loss in 60 days at 23 °C in light and at 4 °C in dark	2380	C
	[a]	50 mg/mL[c]	[a]	4 mg/mL[c]	Physically compatible. Little morphine or clonidine loss in 60 days at 23 °C in light and at 4 °C in dark. Slight yellow discoloration at 23 °C not indicative of decomposition	2380	C
Morphine sulfate with bupivacaine HCl	ES SW	0.2 mg/mL 1.5 mg/mL	BI	0.03 mg/mL	Diluted to 5 mL with NS. Visually compatible with no new GC/MS peaks in 1 hr at room temperature	1956	C
Tetracaine HCl with ketamine HCl	SW PD	2 mg/mL 2 mg/mL	BI	0.03 mg/mL	Diluted to 5 mL with NS. Visually compatible with no new GC/MS peaks in 1 hr at room temperature	1956	C
Ziconotide acetate	ELN	25 mcg/mL	BB	2 mg/mL[d]	No loss of either drug in 28 days at 5 °C	2703	C

[a]Extemporaneously compounded from morphine sulfate and clonidine hydrochloride powder.
[b]Tested in sodium chloride 0.9%.
[c]Tested in sterile water for injection.
[d]Clonidine HCl powder dissolved in ziconotide acetate.

Y-Site Injection Compatibility (1:1 Mixture)

Clonidine HCl

Drug	Mfr	Conc	Mfr	Conc	Remarks	Ref	C/I
Aminophylline	NYC	0.9 mg/mL[b]	BI	18 mcg/mL[b]	Visually compatible	2642	C
Dobutamine HCl	LI	2 mg/mL[a]	BI	18 mcg/mL[b]	Visually compatible	2642	C
Dopamine HCl	NYC	2 mg/mL[a]	BI	18 mcg/mL[b]	Visually compatible	2642	C
Epinephrine HCl	NYC	20 mcg/mL[a]	BI	18 mcg/mL[b]	Visually compatible	2642	C
Fentanyl citrate	ALP	50 mcg/mL	BI	18 mcg/mL[b]	Visually compatible	2642	C
Labetalol HCl	GSK	1 mg/mL[a,b]	BI	18 mcg/mL[b]	Visually compatible	2642	C

Y-Site Injection Compatibility (1:1 Mixture) (Cont.)

Clonidine HCl

Drug	Mfr	Conc	Mfr	Conc	Remarks	Ref	C/I
Lorazepam	WY	0.33 mg/mL[b]	BI	0.015 mg/mL	Visually compatible for 24 hr at 22 °C	1855	C
Magnesium sulfate	BRN	9.6 mg/mL[a]	BI	18 mcg/mL[b]	Visually compatible	2642	C
Midazolam HCl	RC	5 mg/mL	BI	0.015 mg/mL	Orange color in 24 hr at 22 °C	1855	I
	ALP	1 mg/mL	BI	18 mcg/mL[b]	Visually compatible	2642	C
Nitroglycerin	NYC	0.4 mg/mL[a]	BI	18 mcg/mL[b]	Visually compatible	2642	C
Norepinephrine bitartrate	APO	20 mcg/mL[a]	BI	18 mcg/mL[b]	Visually compatible	2642	C
Potassium chloride	BRN	1 mEq/mL	BI	18 mcg/mL[b]	Visually compatible	2642	C
Theophylline	ASZ	1 mg/mL	BI	18 mcg/mL[b]	Visually compatible	2642	C
Verapamil HCl	AB	2.5 mg/mL	BI	18 mcg/mL[b]	Visually compatible	2642	C

[a]Tested in dextrose 5%.
[b]Tested in sodium chloride 0.9%.

CLOXACILLIN SODIUM
AHFS 8:12.16.12

Products — Cloxacillin sodium is available as a dry powder in vials containing 250 mg, 500 mg, 1 g, and 2 g of cloxacillin as the sodium salt. (1)

For intramuscular use, add 1.9 or 1.7 mL of sterile water for injection to the 250- or 500-mg vials, respectively, and shake well to yield nominal concentrations of 125 or 250 mg/mL, respectively. (1)

For intravenous use, reconstitute the 250-mg vials with 4.9 mL of sterile water for injection and shake well to yield a 50-mg/mL concentration. Reconstitute the 500-mg or 1-g vials with 4.8 or 9.6 mL of sterile water for injection, respectively, and shake well to yield a 100-mg/mL concentration. (1)

For intravenous infusion, reconstitute the 1- or 2-g vial with 3.4 or 6.8 mL of sterile water for injection, respectively, and shake well to yield a 250-mg/mL concentration that is then added to an appropriate infusion solution for administration. (1)

Sodium Content — Each gram of cloxacillin sodium contains approximately 50 mg of sodium. (1)

Administration — Cloxacillin sodium may be administered by intramuscular injection, direct intravenous injection slowly over two to four minutes, and intravenous infusion over 30 to 40 minutes. (1)

Stability — Intact vials containing the drug in dry form are stored at controlled room temperature not exceeding 25 °C. After reconstitution with sterile water for injection, cloxacillin sodium solutions are stable for up to 24 hours at controlled room temperature not exceeding 25 °C or 48 hours under refrigeration. (1)

Cloxacillin sodium (Beecham) 250 mg reconstituted with 1.5 mL and 500 mg reconstituted with 2 mL of sterile water for injection exhibited a 5% loss in seven days at 5 °C and a 15% loss in four days at 23 °C. (99)

Cloxacillin sodium (Ayerst) 20 g/L in sodium chloride 0.9% or dextrose 5% was stored in PVC minibags (Travenol) or glass bottles (Travenol) for 24 hours at 5 and 22 °C. No significant decrease in antibiotic stability was observed at 24 hours in sodium chloride 0.9% in either container. With dextrose 5%, a decrease in cloxacillin was observed at 24 hours. The results indicated that cloxacillin sodium was stable for 24 hours in sodium chloride 0.9% and for eight hours in dextrose 5%. (298)

pH Effects — Cloxacillin sodium is most stable at pH 5.5 to 7, with a minimum decomposition rate at pH 6.3. (1476; 1477)

Freezing Solutions — Cloxacillin sodium (Beecham) at concentrations of 1 to 10%, buffered to pH 6.05, loses not more than 1% potency in one month when frozen at −20 °C. (99)

Cloxacillin sodium (Beecham) 1 g/50 mL of dextrose 5% or sodium chloride 0.9% in PVC containers (Travenol) was frozen at −20 °C for 30 days, followed by natural thawing and storage at 5 °C for 21 hours. The cloxacillin concentration was retained for the duration of the study. (299)

Cloxacillin sodium 2 g/100 mL in dextrose 5% or sodium chloride 0.9% in PVC containers was frozen at −27 °C for up to nine months and then thawed by microwave. The results indicated that at least 90% of the concentration was retained. A distinct yellow discoloration was observed in solutions in dextrose 5% stored for six months. Consequently, the authors recommended that such frozen solutions be stored for not more than three months. (1176)

Cloxacillin sodium (Beecham) 500 mg in 50-mL PVC bags (Travenol) stored at −20 °C and thawed under natural conditions was stable for at least 100 days. In addition, the drug was stable under refrigeration for four days followed by 24 hours at room temperature after thawing. (1478)

Sorption—Cloxacillin sodium was shown not to exhibit sorption to PVC bags and tubing, polyethylene tubing, Silastic tubing, and polypropylene syringes. (536; 606)

Filtration—Cloxacillin sodium (Beecham) 1.97 mg/mL in sodium chloride 0.9% or dextrose 5% was filtered through a 0.22-μm cellulose acetate membrane filter (Ivex-HP, Millipore) over six hours. No significant loss due to binding was noted. (1034)

Compatibility Information

Solution Compatibility

Cloxacillin sodium

Solution	Mfr	Mfr	Conc/L	Remarks	Ref	C/I
Dextrose 5%		BE	10 g	Less than 5% loss in 24 hr at room temperature	99	**C**
	TR[a]	AY	20 g	Potency retained for 24 hr at 5 °C	298	**C**
	TR[b]	AY	20 g	3% loss in 1 hr and 12% loss in 24 hr at 22 °C	298	**I**
	BA[b]	AY	20 g	1 to 7% loss in 8 hr and 13 to 15% loss in 24 hr at 5 and 22 °C	298	**I**
		AST	2.25 g	Less than 4% cloxacillin loss in 48 hr at 25 °C	1476	**C**
	BA[a]	NVP	5 to 50 g	Physically compatible with less than 7% loss in 18 days at 4 °C	2372	**C**
	BA[a]	NVP	5 g	Physically compatible with 10% loss calculated in 3.8 days at 23 °C	2372	**C**
	BA[a]	NVP	10 g	Physically compatible with 10% loss calculated in 3 days at 23 °C	2372	**C**
	BA[a]	NVP	20 g	Physically compatible with 10% loss calculated in 2.6 days at 23 °C	2372	**C**
	BA[a]	NVP	40 g	Physically compatible with 10% loss calculated in 1.9 days at 23 °C	2372	**C**
	BA[a]	NVP	50 g	Physically compatible with 10% loss calculated in 1.7 days at 23 °C	2372	**C**
Ringer's injection		BE	10 g	Less than 10% loss in 24 hr at room temperature	99	**C**
Sodium chloride 0.9%		BE	10 g	Less than 5% loss in 24 hr at room temperature	99	**C**
	TR[b], BA[a]	AY	20 g	Potency retained for 24 hr at 5 and 22 °C	298	**C**
	BA[a]	NVP	5 to 50 g	Physically compatible with less than 7% loss in 18 days at 4 °C	2372	**C**
	BA[a]	NVP	5 g	Physically compatible with 10% loss calculated in 2.1 days at 23 °C	2372	**C**
	BA[a]	NVP	10 g	Physically compatible with 10% loss calculated in 1.9 days at 23 °C	2372	**C**
	BA[a]	NVP	20 g	Physically compatible with 10% loss calculated in 1.9 days at 23 °C	2372	**C**
	BA[a]	NVP	40 g	Physically compatible with 10% loss calculated in 1.5 days at 23 °C	2372	**C**
	BA[a]	NVP	50 g	Physically compatible with 10% loss calculated in 1.5 days at 23 °C	2372	**C**
Sodium lactate ⅙ M		BE	10 g	15% loss in 24 hr at room temperature	99	**I**
		AST	2.25 g	10% cloxacillin loss in 7 hr at 25 °C	1476	**I**
TPN #22[c]		AY	10 g	Physically compatible with no activity loss in 24 hr at 22 °C in the dark	837	**C**

[a]*Tested in PVC containers.*
[b]*Tested in glass containers.*
[c]*Refer to Appendix I for the composition of parenteral nutrition solutions. TPN indicates a 2-in-1 admixture.*

Additive Compatibility

Cloxacillin sodium

Drug	Mfr	Conc/L	Mfr	Conc/L	Test Soln	Remarks	Ref	C/I
Amikacin sulfate	BR	5 g	BR	10 g	D5LR, D5R, D5S, D5W, D10W, LR, NS, R, SL	Physically compatible and both stable for 24 hr at 25 °C	293	C
Chlorpromazine HCl	BP	200 mg	BP	1 g	NS	Haze forms over 3 hr	26	I
Dextran 40	PH	10%	AST	2.25 g	D5W	Under 4% cloxacillin loss in 48 hr at 25 °C	1476	C
	PH	10%	BE	4 g	D5W	2% cloxacillin loss in 24 hr at 20 °C	834	C
	PH	10%	BE	8 g	D5W, NS	Under 5% loss in 24 hr at room temperature	99	C
Fat emulsion, intravenous		10%		10 g		Aggregation of oil droplets	37	I
Floxacillin sodium	BE	20 g	BE	20 g	NS	Physically compatible for 24 hr at 15 and 30 °C. Haze forms in 48 hr at 30 °C. No change at 15 °C	1479	C
Furosemide	HO	1 g	BE	20 g	NS	Physically compatible for 72 hr at 15 and 30 °C	1479	C
Gentamicin sulfate	RS	160 mg	BE	4 g	D5¼S, D5W, NS	Precipitate forms	157	I
Heparin sodium		32,000 units		2 g	NS	Physically compatible and heparin stable for 24 hr	57	C
Hydrocortisone sodium succinate	GL	200 mg	BE	20 g	D5S, D5W, NS	Physically compatible and cloxacillin stable for 24 hr at 25 °C	89	C
Potassium chloride		60 mEq	AST	2.25 g	D5W	10% cloxacillin loss in 48 hr at 25 °C	1476	C

Drugs in Syringe Compatibility

Cloxacillin sodium

Drug (in syringe)	Mfr	Amt	Mfr	Amt	Remarks	Ref	C/I
Chloramphenicol sodium succinate	PD	250 and 400 mg/ 1.5 to 2 mL	BE	250 mg	No precipitate or color change within 1 hr at room temperature	99	C
	PD	250 and 400 mg/ mL	AY	250 mg	Physically compatible for 1 hr at room temperature	300	C
Colistimethate sodium	PX	40 mg/ 2 mL	BE	250 mg	No precipitate or color change within 1 hr at room temperature	99	C
	PX	500 mg/ 2 mL	AY	250 mg	Physically compatible for 1 hr at room temperature	300	C
Dimenhydrinate		10 mg/ 1 mL		100 mg/ 1 mL	Clear solution	2569	C
Erythromycin lactobionate	AB	300 mg/ 6 mL	AY	250 mg	Precipitate forms within 1 hr at room temperature	300	I
Gentamicin sulfate		80 mg/ 2 mL	BE	250 mg	Physically incompatible within 1 hr at room temperature	99	I

Drugs in Syringe Compatibility (Cont.)

Cloxacillin sodium

Drug (in syringe)	Mfr	Amt	Mfr	Amt	Remarks	Ref	C/I
Hydromorphone HCl	KN	2, 10, 40 mg/ 1 mL	AY	250 mg/ 1 mL	Precipitate forms but dissipates with shaking. Under 10% loss of both drugs in 24 hr at room temperature	2082	?
Lidocaine HCl			BE		Physically compatible	89	C
Lincomycin HCl	UP	600 mg/ 2 mL	BE	250 mg	No precipitate or color change within 1 hr at room temperature	99	C
	UP	600 mg/ 2 mL	AY	250 mg	Physically compatible for 1 hr at room temperature	300	C
Pantoprazole sodium	a	4 mg/ 1 mL		100 mg/ 1 mL	Precipitates immediately	2574	I
Polymyxin B sulfate	BE	250,000 units/1.5 to 2 mL	BE	250 mg	Physically incompatible within 1 hr at room temperature	99	I
Streptomycin sulfate		1 g/2 mL	BE	250 mg	No precipitate or color change within 1 hr at room temperature	99	C
	BP	1 g/2 mL	AY	250 mg	Physically compatible for 1 hr at room temperature	300	C
	BP	1 g/ 1.5 mL	AY	250 mg	Syrupy solution forms	300	I
	BP	750 mg/ 1.5 mL	AY	250 mg	Precipitate forms within 1 hr at room temperature	300	I

[a]*Test performed using the formulation WITHOUT edetate disodium.*

Y-Site Injection Compatibility (1:1 Mixture)

Cloxacillin sodium

Drug	Mfr	Conc	Mfr	Conc	Remarks	Ref	C/I
Hydromorphone HCl	KN	2, 10, 40 mg/ mL	AY	250 mg/mL	Turbidity forms but dissipates with shaking and solution remains clear. Both drugs stable for 24 hr	1532	?
	KN	2, 10, 40 mg/ mL	AY	40 mg/mL[a]	Turbidity forms immediately and cloxacillin precipitate develops	1532	I
	KN	2, 10, 40 mg/ mL	AY	27 mg/mL[a]	Turbidity forms immediately	1532	I
	KN	2, 10, 40 mg/ mL	AY	12 mg/mL[a]	Visually compatible for 24 hr; precipitate forms in 96 hr	1532	C

[a]*Tested in dextrose 5%.*

COLISTIMETHATE SODIUM
AHFS 8:12.28.28

Products — Colistimethate sodium parenteral is available in vials containing the equivalent of 150 mg of colistin base. The 150-mg vial should be reconstituted with 2 mL of sterile water for injection to yield a solution containing 75 mg/mL of colistin base activity. During reconstitution, the contents of the vials should be gently swirled to avoid frothing. (1; 4)

pH — The pH of the reconstituted solution is 7 to 8. (4)

Trade Name(s) — Coly-Mycin M Parenteral.

Administration — Colistimethate sodium parenteral may be administered by intramuscular injection, by direct intravenous injection injected slowly over three to five minutes, or by continuous intravenous infusion of half the daily dose at a rate of 5 to 6 mg/hr begun one to two hours after an initial half-daily dose by direct intravenous injection. (4)

Stability — Intact vials should be stored at controlled room temperature. Reconstituted solutions are stable for seven days when stored under refrigeration at 2 to 8 °C or at controlled room temperature. Dilutions for infusion should be discarded after 24 hours. (1; 4) FDA's MedWatch reported a possible fatality from a decomposed colistimethate sodium inhalation solution premixed with sterile water for injection.

Filtration — Colistimethate sodium (R. Bellon) 0.16 mg/mL in dextrose 5% and sodium chloride 0.9% was filtered through a 0.22-μm cellulose ester member filter (Ivex-HP, Millipore) over six hours. No significant drug loss due to binding to the filter was noted. (1034)

Compatibility Information

Solution Compatibility

Colistimethate sodium

Solution	Mfr	Mfr	Conc/L	Remarks	Ref	C/I
Dextrose 5%				Compatible and stable for 24 hr	1	C
Dextrose–saline combinations				Compatible and stable for 24 hr	1	C
Ringer's injection, lactated				Compatible and stable for 24 hr	1	C
Sodium chloride 0.9%				Compatible and stable for 24 hr	1	C

Additive Compatibility

Colistimethate sodium

Drug	Mfr	Conc/L	Mfr	Conc/L	Test Soln	Remarks	Ref	C/I
Amikacin sulfate	BR	5 g	WC	500 mg	D5LR, D5R, D5S, D5W, D10W, LR, NS, R, SL	Physically compatible and amikacin stable for 24 hr at 25 °C. Colistimethate not analyzed	293	C
Ascorbic acid	UP	500 mg	WC	500 mg	D5W	Physically compatible	15	C
Chloramphenicol sodium succinate	PD	10 g	WC	500 mg	D5W	Physically compatible	15	C
	PD	10 g	WC	500 mg		Physically compatible	6	C
Diphenhydramine HCl	PD	80 mg	WC	500 mg	D5W	Physically compatible	15	C
Erythromycin lactobionate	AB	5 g	WC	500 mg	D5W	Physically incompatible	15	I
	AB	1 g	WC	500 mg	D	Precipitate forms within 1 hr	20	I
Heparin sodium	UP	4000 units	WC	500 mg	D5W	Physically compatible	15	C
	AB	20,000 units	WC	500 mg	D	Physically compatible	21	C
Hydrocortisone sodium succinate	UP	500 mg	WC	500 mg	D5W	Physically incompatible	15	I

Additive Compatibility (Cont.)

Colistimethate sodium

Drug	Mfr	Conc/L	Mfr	Conc/L	Test Soln	Remarks	Ref	C/I
Penicillin G potassium	SQ	20 million units	WC	500 mg	D5W	Physically compatible	15	C
	SQ	5 million units	WC	500 mg	D	Physically compatible	47	C
Penicillin G sodium	UP	20 million units	WC	500 mg	D5W	Physically compatible	15	C
Phenobarbital sodium	WI	200 mg	WC	500 mg	D5W	Physically compatible	15	C
Polymyxin B sulfate	BW	200 mg	WC	500 mg	D5W	Physically compatible	15	C
Ranitidine HCl	GL	50 mg and 2 g		1.5 g	D5W	Physically compatible. Ranitidine stable for 24 hr at 25 °C. Colistimethate not tested	1515	C

Drugs in Syringe Compatibility

Colistimethate sodium

Drug (in syringe)	Mfr	Amt	Mfr	Amt	Remarks	Ref	C/I
Ampicillin sodium	AY	500 mg	PX	40 mg/ 2 mL	No precipitate or color change within 1 hr at room temperature	99	C
	AY	500 mg	PX	500 mg/ 2 mL	Physically compatible for 1 hr at room temperature	300	C
Cloxacillin sodium	BE	250 mg	PX	40 mg/ 2 mL	No precipitate or color change within 1 hr at room temperature	99	C
	AY	250 mg	PX	500 mg/ 2 mL	Physically compatible for 1 hr at room temperature	300	C
Penicillin G sodium		1 million units	PX	40 mg/ 2 mL	No precipitate or color change within 1 hr at room temperature	99	C

Y-Site Injection Compatibility (1:1 Mixture)

Colistimethate sodium

Drug	Mfr	Conc	Mfr	Conc	Remarks	Ref	C/I
Telavancin HCl	ASP	7.5 mg/mL[a]	PAD	4.5 mg/mL[a]	Visible turbidity formed	2830	I
	ASP	7.5 mg/mL[b,c]	PAD	4.5 mg/mL[b,c]	Physically compatible for 2 hr	2830	C

[a]Tested in dextrose 5%.
[b]Tested in sodium chloride 0.9%.
[c]Tested in Ringer's injection, lactated.

CYANOCOBALAMIN
AHFS 88:08

Products — Cyanocobalamin is available in concentrations of 100 mcg/mL and 1 mg/mL with sodium chloride 0.9%, benzyl alcohol 1.5%, and sodium hydroxide and/or hydrochloric acid to adjust pH during manufacturing. (1; 4)

pH — From 4.5 to 7. (1)

Administration — Cyanocobalamin is administered by intramuscular or deep subcutaneous injection. The intravenous route is not recommended because the drug is excreted more rapidly and almost all of the cyanocobalamin is lost in the urine. (1; 4)

Stability — The clear pink to red solutions are stable at room temperature and may be autoclaved at 121 °C for short periods such as 15 to 20 minutes. Cyanocobalamin is light sensitive, so protection from light is recommended. (1; 4) Exposure to light results in the organometallic bond being cleaved, with the extent of degradation generally increasing with increasing light intensity. (1072)

The vitamins in Cernevit (Baxter) diluted in three 2-in-1 parenteral nutrition admixtures were tested for stability over 48 hours. Most of the vitamins, including cyanocobalamin, retained their initial concentrations. (2796)

pH Effects — Cyanocobalamin is stable at pH 3 to 7 but is most stable at pH 4.5 to 5. (1072) It is stated to be incompatible with alkaline and strongly acidic solutions. (4)

Sorption — Cyanocobalamin (Organon) 30 mg/L did not display significant sorption to a PVC plastic test strip in 24 hours. (12)

Filtration — Cyanocobalamin (Wyeth) 1 mg/L in dextrose 5% and in sodium chloride 0.9% was filtered at a rate of 120 mL/hr for six hours through a 0.22-μm cellulose ester membrane filter (Ivex-2). No significant reduction in potency due to binding to the filter was noted. (533)

Compatibility Information

Solution Compatibility

Cyanocobalamin

Solution	Mfr	Mfr	Conc/L	Remarks	Ref	C/I
Dextrose–Ringer's injection combinations	AB	AB	1 mg	Physically compatible	3	C
Dextrose–Ringer's injection, lactated, combinations	AB	AB	1 mg	Physically compatible	3	C
Dextrose–saline combinations	AB	AB	1 mg	Physically compatible	3	C
Dextrose 2.5%	AB	AB	1 mg	Physically compatible	3	C
Dextrose 5%	AB	AB	1 mg	Physically compatible	3	C
Dextrose 10%	AB	AB	1 mg	Physically compatible	3	C
Ionosol products	AB	AB	1 mg	Physically compatible	3	C
Ringer's injection	AB	AB	1 mg	Physically compatible	3	C
Ringer's injection, lactated	AB	AB	1 mg	Physically compatible	3	C
Sodium chloride 0.45%	AB	AB	1 mg	Physically compatible	3	C
Sodium chloride 0.9%	AB	AB	1 mg	Physically compatible	3	C
Sodium lactate ⅙ M	AB	AB	1 mg	Physically compatible	3	C

Additive Compatibility

Cyanocobalamin

Drug	Mfr	Conc/L	Mfr	Conc/L	Test Soln	Remarks	Ref	C/I
Ascorbic acid	AB	1 g	AB	1 mg		Physically compatible	3	C
Chloramphenicol sodium succinate	PD	1 g	AB	1 mg		Physically compatible	6	C

Y-Site Injection Compatibility (1:1 Mixture)

		Cyanocobalamin					
Drug	*Mfr*	*Conc*	*Mfr*	*Conc*	*Remarks*	*Ref*	*C/I*
Heparin sodium	UP	1000 units/L[a]	PD	0.1 mg/mL	Physically compatible for 4 hr at room temperature	534	C
Hydrocortisone sodium succinate	UP	10 mg/L[a]	PD	0.1 mg/mL	Physically compatible for 4 hr at room temperature	534	C
Potassium chloride	AB	40 mEq/L[a]	PD	0.1 mg/mL	Physically compatible for 4 hr at room temperature	534	C

[a]*Tested in dextrose 5% in Ringer's injection, dextrose 5% in Ringer's injection, lactated, dextrose 5%, Ringer's injection, lactated, and sodium chloride 0.9%.*

CYCLIZINE LACTATE
AHFS 56:22.08

Products — Cyclizine lactate is available in 1-mL ampuls containing 50 mg of drug in water for injection. (38; 115)

pH — From 3.3 to 3.7. (176)

Trade Name(s) — Valoid.

Administration — Cyclizine lactate is administered by intramuscular or intravenous injection. When administered intravenously, it should be injected slowly, with minimal withdrawal of blood in the syringe. (38; 115)

Stability — Cyclizine lactate injection, a colorless solution, should be stored below 25 °C and protected from light. (38; 115)

Crystallization — Cyclizine lactate has an aqueous solubility of 8 mg/mL. When the drug was diluted to concentrations of 7.5 and 3.75 mg/mL in water or dextrose 5%, it remained in solution for at least 24 hours at 23 °C. However, when these dilutions were made with sodium chloride 0.9%, crystals formed within 24 hours at 23 °C. (1761)

Compatibility Information

Additive Compatibility

			Cyclizine lactate					
Drug	*Mfr*	*Conc/L*	*Mfr*	*Conc/L*	*Test Soln*	*Remarks*	*Ref*	*C/I*
Oxycodone HCl	NAP	1 g	GW	1 g	NS	Crystals form in a few hours	2600	I
	NAP	1 g	GW	1 g	W	Visually compatible. Under 4% concentration change in 24 hr at 25 °C	2600	C
	NAP	1 g	GW	500 mg	NS	Crystals form in a few hours	2600	I
	NAP	1 g	GW	500 mg	W	Visually compatible. Under 4% concentration change in 24 hr at 25 °C	2600	C

Drugs in Syringe Compatibility

			Cyclizine lactate				
Drug (in syringe)	*Mfr*	*Amt*	*Mfr*	*Amt*	*Remarks*	*Ref*	*C/I*
Diamorphine HCl	MB	20, 50, 100 mg/1 mL	CA	5 mg/1 mL[a]	Physically compatible and diamorphine stable for 24 hr at room temperature	1454	C
	EV	15 mg/1 mL	CA	15 mg/1 mL	Physically compatible for 24 hr at room temperature	1455	C

Drugs in Syringe Compatibility (Cont.)

Cyclizine lactate

Drug (in syringe)	Mfr	Amt	Mfr	Amt	Remarks	Ref	C/I
	EV	37.5 to 150 mg/ 1 mL	CA	12.5 to 50 mg/ 1 mL	Precipitate forms within 24 hr	1455	I
	HC	25 to 100 mg/ mL	CA	10 mg/ mL	Visually incompatible	1672	I
	HC	20 mg/ mL	CA	10 mg/ mL	Visually compatible for 48 hr at 5 and 20 °C	1672	C
	HC	100 mg/ mL	CA	6.7 mg/ mL	Visually compatible for 48 hr at 5 and 20 °C	1672	C
	HC	2 mg/mL	CA	6.7 mg/ mL	5% diamorphine loss in 9.9 days at 20 °C. Cyclizine stable for 45 days	1672	C
	HC	20 mg/ mL	CA	6.7 mg/ mL	5% diamorphine loss in 13.6 days at 20 °C. Cyclizine stable for 45 days	1672	C
	BP	6 mg/mL	WEL	51 mg/ mL	Physically compatible. 10% diamorphine loss in 1.7 days. Little cyclizine loss at 23 °C	2071	C
	BP	9 mg/mL	WEL	32 mg/ mL	Physically compatible. Under 10% diamorphine loss and little cyclizine loss in 4 days at 23 °C	2071	C
	BP	10 mg/ mL	WEL	39 mg/ mL	Physically compatible. Under 10% diamorphine loss and little cyclizine loss in 4 days at 23 °C	2071	C
	BP	10 mg/ mL	WEL	28 mg/ mL	Physically compatible. 10% diamorphine loss in 3.1 days and little cyclizine loss at 23 °C	2071	C
	BP	12 mg/ mL	WEL	51 mg/ mL	Physically compatible. 10% diamorphine loss in 2.2 days and little cyclizine loss at 23 °C	2071	C
	BP	14 mg/ mL	WEL	40 mg/ mL	Crystals form	2071	I
	BP	17 mg/ mL	WEL	26 mg/ mL	Physically compatible. 10% diamorphine loss in 1.1 days and 10% cyclizine loss in 2.5 days at 23 °C	2071	C
	BP	18 mg/ mL	WEL	52 mg/ mL	Crystals form	2071	I
	BP	20 mg/ mL	WEL	10 mg/ mL	Physically compatible. Under 10% diamorphine loss and little cyclizine loss in 7 days at 23 °C	2071	C
	BP	20 mg/ mL	WEL	15 mg/ mL	Physically compatible. Little diamorphine loss and 10% cyclizine loss in 0.5 days at 23 °C	2071	I
	BP	21 mg/ mL	WEL	26 mg/ mL	Physically compatible. 10% diamorphine loss in 4.9 days. 10% cyclizine loss in 3.2 days at 23 °C	2071	C
	BP	23 mg/ mL	WEL	18 mg/ mL	Physically compatible. Little diamorphine loss and 10% cyclizine loss in 3.2 days at 23 °C	2071	C
	BP	26 mg/ mL	WEL	23 mg/ mL	Physically compatible. 10% diamorphine loss in 1.9 days. 10% cyclizine loss in 9 hr at 23 °C	2071	I
	BP	30 mg/ mL	WEL	30 mg/ mL	Physically compatible. 10% diamorphine loss in 21 hr and 10% cyclizine loss in 9 hr at 23 °C	2071	I
	BP	49 mg/ mL	WEL	10 mg/ mL	Physically compatible. Little diamorphine loss and 10% cyclizine loss in 5.5 days at 23 °C	2071	C
	BP	51 mg/ mL	WEL	4 mg/mL	Physically compatible. Little diamorphine or cyclizine loss in 7 days at 23 °C	2071	C
	BP	61 mg/ mL	WEL	8 mg/mL	Physically compatible. 10% diamorphine loss in 1.4 days. 10% cyclizine loss in 1.1 days at 23 °C	2071	C

Drugs in Syringe Compatibility (Cont.)

Cyclizine lactate

Drug (in syringe)	Mfr	Amt	Mfr	Amt	Remarks	Ref	C/I
	BP	65 mg/mL	WEL	13 mg/mL	Physically compatible. 10% diamorphine loss in 1.6 days. 10% cyclizine loss in 12 hr at 23 °C	2071	I
	BP	92 mg/mL	WEL	10 mg/mL	Physically compatible. Little diamorphine loss and 10% cyclizine loss in 2.4 days at 23 °C	2071	C
	BP	99 mg/mL	WEL	4 mg/mL	Physically compatible. Little diamorphine or cyclizine loss in 7 days at 23 °C	2071	C
Diamorphine HCl with haloperidol lactate	BP JC	11 mg/mL 2.2 mg/mL	WEL	16 mg/mL	Physically compatible with less than 10% loss of any drug in 7 days at 23 °C	2071	C
Diamorphine HCl with haloperidol lactate	BP JC	16 mg/mL 2.2 mg/mL	WEL	25 mg/mL	Physically compatible with less than 10% loss of any drug in 7 days at 23 °C	2071	C
Diamorphine HCl with haloperidol lactate	BP JC	40 mg/mL 2.2 mg/mL	WEL	11 mg/mL	Physically compatible with less than 10% loss of any drug in 7 days at 23 °C	2071	C
Diamorphine HCl with haloperidol lactate	BP JC	42 mg/mL 2.1 mg/mL	WEL	13 mg/mL	Physically compatible with less than 10% loss of any drug in 7 days at 23 °C	2071	C
Diamorphine HCl with haloperidol lactate	BP JC	55 mg/mL 2.1 mg/mL	WEL	9 mg/mL	Physically compatible with less than 10% loss of any drug in 7 days at 23 °C	2071	C
Diamorphine HCl with haloperidol lactate	BP JC	56 mg/mL 2.1 mg/mL	WEL	13 mg/mL	Physically compatible with less than 10% loss of any drug in 7 days at 23 °C	2071	C
Haloperidol lactate	SE	1.5 mg/0.3 mL	WEL	150 mg/3 mL	Diluted with 17 mL of NS. Crystals of cyclizine form within 24 hr at 25 °C	1761	I
	SE	1.5 mg/0.3 mL	WEL	150 mg/3 mL	Diluted with 17 mL of D5W or W. Visually compatible for 24 hr at 25 °C	1761	C
Haloperidol lactate with diamorphine HCl	JC BP	2.2 mg/mL 11 mg/mL	WEL	16 mg/mL	Physically compatible with less than 10% loss of any drug in 7 days at 23 °C	2071	C
Haloperidol lactate with diamorphine HCl	JC BP	2.2 mg/mL 16 mg/mL	WEL	25 mg/mL	Physically compatible with less than 10% loss of any drug in 7 days at 23 °C	2071	C
Haloperidol lactate with diamorphine HCl	JC BP	2.2 mg/mL 40 mg/mL	WEL	11 mg/mL	Physically compatible with less than 10% loss of any drug in 7 days at 23 °C	2071	C
Haloperidol lactate with diamorphine HCl	JC BP	2.1 mg/mL 42 mg/mL	WEL	13 mg/mL	Physically compatible with less than 10% loss of any drug in 7 days at 23 °C	2071	C
Haloperidol lactate with diamorphine HCl	JC BP	2.1 mg/mL 55 mg/mL	WEL	9 mg/mL	Physically compatible with less than 10% loss of any drug in 7 days at 23 °C	2071	C

Drugs in Syringe Compatibility (Cont.)

Cyclizine lactate

Drug (in syringe)	Mfr	Amt	Mfr	Amt	Remarks	Ref	C/I
Haloperidol lactate with	JC	2.1 mg/ mL	WEL	13 mg/ mL	Physically compatible with less than 10% loss of any drug in 7 days at 23 °C	2071	C
diamorphine HCl	BP	56 mg/ mL					
Ketorolac tromethamine	RC	30 mg/ mL	WEL	50 mg/ mL	White precipitate forms	2495	I
Oxycodone HCl	NAP	200 mg/ 20 mL	GW	150 mg/ 3 mL	Crystals form in 5 hr	2600	I
	NAP	70 mg/ 7 mL	GW	50 mg/ 1 mL	Crystals form in 5 hr	2600	I
	NAP	100 mg/ 10 mL	GW	50 mg/ 1 mL	Visually compatible. Under 4% concentration change in 24 hr at 25 °C	2600	C
	NAP	150 mg/ 15 mL	GW	50 mg/ 1 mL	Visually compatible. Under 4% concentration change in 24 hr at 25 °C	2600	C
	NAP	200 mg/ 20 mL	GW	50 mg/ 1 mL	Visually compatible. Under 4% concentration change in 24 hr at 25 °C	2600	C
	NAP	200 mg/ 20 mL	GW	100 mg/ 2 mL	Visually compatible. Under 4% concentration change in 24 hr at 25 °C	2600	C
Ranitidine HCl	GL	50 mg/ 2 mL	CA	50 mg/ 1 mL	Physically compatible for 1 hr at 25 °C	978	C

ᵃDiluted with sterile water for injection.

CYCLOPHOSPHAMIDE
AHFS 10:00

Products — Cyclophosphamide is available as a dry powder in vials containing 500 mg, 1 g, and 2 g. Reconstitute the vials with 25, 50, and 100 mL, respectively, of sodium chloride 0.9%. Sterile water for injection may be used for reconstitution if the dose is to be diluted in an intravenous infusion solution for administration. Shake the vials to dissolve the powder, yielding a solution containing cyclophosphamide concentrations of 20 mg/mL. (1)

pH — Reconstituted solutions have a pH of 3 to 9. (17) A 22-mg/mL solution was found to have a pH of 6.87. (126)

Osmolarity — Cyclophosphamide solution has an osmolality of 374 mOsm/kg if sodium chloride 0.9% is used for the reconstitution. However, if reconstituted with sterile water for injection, the solution is very hypotonic, having an osmolality of 74 mOsm/kg. This solution is to be used by diluting the dose in an intravenous infusion solution for administration. (1)

Administration — Cyclophosphamide reconstituted with sodium chloride 0.9% may be administered intramuscularly, intraperitoneally, intrapleurally, by direct intravenous injection, or by continuous or intermittent intravenous infusion. (1)

Cyclophosphamide reconstituted with sterile water for injection is very hypotonic and not suitable for direct intravenous injection. The dose must be diluted in a compatible intravenous infusion solution for intravenous administration. (1)

Stability — Cyclophosphamide products should not be stored at temperatures above 25 °C, although they will withstand brief exposures to temperatures up to 30 °C. Reconstituted solutions should be used within 24 hours if stored at room temperature or within six days if stored under refrigeration. (1; 4) When reconstituted with sterile water for injection or paraben-preserved bacteriostatic water for injection to a concentration of 21 mg/mL, less than 1.5% cyclophosphamide decomposition will occur within eight hours at 24 to 27 °C and within six days at 5 °C. The rate constant for decomposition of cyclophosphamide when reconstituted with benzyl alcohol-preserved bacteriostatic water for injection is significantly higher than with sterile water for injection. It was suggested that benzyl alcohol may catalyze somewhat the decomposition of cyclophosphamide. (125)

The stability of cyclophosphamide 20 mg/mL, reconstituted with sterile water for injection and stored in various containers at several temperatures was evaluated. In glass ampuls at 20 to 23 °C, approximately 13 and 35% were lost in one and four weeks, respectively. Under refrigeration at 4 °C or frozen at −20 °C, the solution lost not more than 3% over four weeks. (1090)

Cyclophosphamide (Bristol-Myers Squibb) reconstituted with sterile water for injection to a concentration of 20 mg/mL was found to undergo about 10% degradation in 4 days at 25 °C. When the solutions were stored under refrigeration at 5 °C, approximately 6% loss occurred in 52 days and 10 to 12% loss occurred in 119 days. (2255)

Immersion of a needle with an aluminum component in cyclophosphamide (Adria) 20 mg/mL resulted in a slight darkening of the aluminum and gas production after a few days at 24 °C with protection from light. (988)

pH Effects — Cyclophosphamide exhibits maximum solution stability over the range of 2 to 10 or 11; the rate of decomposition is essentially the same over this broad pH range. At pH values less than 2 and above 11, increased rates of decomposition have been observed. (1369; 2002)

Syringes — In polypropylene syringes (Plastipak, Becton Dickinson) sealed with blind Luer locking hubs, the 20-mg/mL cyclophosphamide solution similarly lost about 3% in four weeks at 4 °C and about 10% in 11 to 14 weeks. When frozen at −20 °C (with microwave thawing), the solution lost about 4% in 19 weeks. However, the syringe plungers contracted markedly during freezing, resulting in drug solution seeping past the plunger onto the inner surface of the barrel. This seeping poses the risk of bacterial contamination. Furthermore, cyclophosphamide precipitated during microwave thawing and required vigorous shaking for five minutes to redissolve. This precipitation during thawing appears not to occur at concentrations less than 8 mg/mL. (1090)

Central Venous Catheter — Cyclophosphamide (Mead Johnson) 2 mg/mL in dextrose 5% was found to be compatible with the ARROWg+ard Blue Plus (Arrow International) chlorhexidine-bearing triple-lumen central catheter. Essentially complete delivery of the drug was found with little or no drug loss occurring. Furthermore, chlorhexidine delivered from the catheter remained at trace amounts with no substantial increase due to the delivery of the drug through the catheter. (2335)

Compatibility Information

Solution Compatibility

Cyclophosphamide

Solution	Mfr	Mfr	Conc/L	Remarks	Ref	C/I
Amino acids 4.25%, dextrose 25%	MG	MJ	500 mg	No increase in particulate matter in 24 hr at 5 °C	349	C
Dextrose 5% in Ringer's injection, lactated				Manufacturer recommended solution	1	C
Dextrose 5% in sodium chloride 0.9%				Manufacturer recommended solution	1	C
	CU	MJ	100 mg	1.5% loss in 8 hr at 27 °C and 6 days at 5 °C	125	C
	CU	MJ	3.1 g	1.5% loss in 8 hr at 27 °C and 6 days at 5 °C	125	C
Dextrose 5%				Manufacturer recommended solution	1	C
	CU	MJ	100 mg	1.5% loss in 8 hr at 27 °C and 6 days at 5 °C	125	C
	CU	MJ	3.1 g	1.5% loss in 8 hr at 27 °C and 6 days at 5 °C	125	C
	TR[a]	MJ	6.6 g	Less than 10% loss in 24 hr at room temperature	519	C
	MG, TR[b]		6.7 g	Less than 10% loss in 24 hr at room temperature exposed to light	1658	C
Ringer's injection, lactated				Manufacturer recommended solution	1	C
Sodium chloride 0.45%				Manufacturer recommended solution	1	C
Sodium chloride 0.9%		MJ	4 g	3.5% loss in 24 hr at room temperature	127	C
		MJ	4 g	1% loss in 4 weeks under refrigeration	127	C
	TR	CE	4 g[c]	Physically compatible with no loss in 4 weeks and 8% in 19 weeks at 4 and −20 °C	1090	C
		BMS	400 mg	8% loss in 6 days at 23 °C. Less than 2% loss in 14 days at 4 °C	2255	C
Sodium lactate ⅙ M				Manufacturer recommended solution	1	C

[a]*Tested in both glass and PVC containers.*
[b]*Tested in glass, PVC, and polyolefin containers.*
[c]*Tested in PVC containers.*

Additive Compatibility

Cyclophosphamide

Drug	Mfr	Conc/L	Mfr	Conc/L	Test Soln	Remarks	Ref	C/I
Cisplatin with etoposide		200 mg 200 mg		2 g	NS	All drugs stable for 7 days at room temperature	1379	C
Etoposide with cisplatin		200 mg 200 mg		2 g	NS	All drugs stable for 7 days at room temperature	1379	C
Fluorouracil		8.3 g		1.67 g	NS	Both drugs stable for 14 days at room temperature	1389	C
Fluorouracil with methotrexate sodium		8.3 g 25 mg		1.67 g	NS	9.3% cyclophosphamide loss in 7 days at room temperature. No loss of other drugs observed	1389	C
Hydroxyzine HCl	LY	500 mg	AD	1 g	D5W[a]	Physically compatible for 48 hr	1190	C
Mesna	AM	3.2 g	AM	10.8 g	D5W	Physically compatible with about 5% loss of both drugs in 24 hr at 22 °C. 7% cyclophosphamide loss and 10% mesna loss occurred in 72 hr at 4 °C	2486	C
	AM	540 mg	AM	1.8 g	D5W	Physically compatible with about 10% loss of both drugs in 12 hr at 22 °C	2486	I
	AM	540 mg	AM	1.8 g	D5W	Physically compatible with about 9% loss of both drugs in 72 hr at 4 °C	2486	C
Methotrexate sodium		25 mg		1.67 g	NS	6.6% cyclophosphamide loss in 14 days at room temperature	1379; 1389	C
Methotrexate sodium with fluorouracil		25 mg 8.3 g		1.67 g	NS	9.3% cyclophosphamide loss in 7 days at room temperature. No loss of other drugs observed	1389	C
Mitoxantrone HCl	LE	500 mg	AD	10 g	D5W	Visually compatible. Mitoxantrone stable for 24 hr at room temperature. Cyclophosphamide not tested	1531	C
Ondansetron HCl	GL	50 mg	MJ	300 mg	D5W[b], NS[b]	Visually compatible with 9 to 10% cyclophosphamide loss and no ondansetron loss in 5 days at 24 °C. No loss of either drug in 8 days at 4 °C	1812	C
	GL	400 mg	MJ	2 g	D5W[b], NS[b]	Visually compatible with 10% cyclophosphamide loss and no ondansetron loss in 5 days at 24 °C. No loss of either drug in 8 days at 4 °C	1812	C

[a]*Tested in glass containers.*
[b]*Tested in PVC containers.*

Drugs in Syringe Compatibility

Cyclophosphamide

Drug (in syringe)	Mfr	Amt	Mfr	Amt	Remarks	Ref	C/I
Bleomycin sulfate		1.5 units/ 0.5 mL		10 mg/ 0.5 mL	Physically compatible for 5 min at room temperature followed by 8 min of centrifugation	980	C
Cisplatin		0.5 mg/ 0.5 mL		10 mg/ 0.5 mL	Physically compatible for 5 min at room temperature followed by 8 min of centrifugation	980	C
Doxapram HCl	RB	400 mg/ 20 mL		100 mg/ 5 mL	Physically compatible with 2% doxapram loss in 24 hr	1177	C

Drugs in Syringe Compatibility (Cont.)

Cyclophosphamide

Drug (in syringe)	Mfr	Amt	Mfr	Amt	Remarks	Ref	C/I
Doxorubicin HCl		1 mg/ 0.5 mL		10 mg/ 0.5 mL	Physically compatible for 5 min at room temperature followed by 8 min of centrifugation	980	C
Droperidol		1.25 mg/ 0.5 mL		10 mg/ 0.5 mL	Physically compatible for 5 min at room temperature followed by 8 min of centrifugation	980	C
Fluorouracil		25 mg/ 0.5 mL		10 mg/ 0.5 mL	Physically compatible for 5 min at room temperature followed by 8 min of centrifugation	980	C
Furosemide		5 mg/ 0.5 mL		10 mg/ 0.5 mL	Physically compatible for 5 min at room temperature followed by 8 min of centrifugation	980	C
Heparin sodium		500 units/ 0.5 mL		10 mg/ 0.5 mL	Physically compatible for 5 min at room temperature followed by 8 min of centrifugation	980	C
Leucovorin calcium		5 mg/ 0.5 mL		10 mg/ 0.5 mL	Physically compatible for 5 min at room temperature followed by 8 min of centrifugation	980	C
Methotrexate sodium		12.5 mg/ 0.5 mL		10 mg/ 0.5 mL	Physically compatible for 5 min at room temperature followed by 8 min of centrifugation	980	C
Metoclopramide HCl		2.5 mg/ 0.5 mL		10 mg/ 0.5 mL	Physically compatible for 5 min at room temperature followed by 8 min of centrifugation	980	C
	RB	10 mg/ 2 mL	MJ	40 mg/ 2 mL	Physically compatible for 24 hr at 25 °C	1167	C
	RB	10 mg/ 2 mL	MJ	1 g/ 50 mL	Physically compatible for 24 hr at 25 °C	1167	C
	RB	160 mg/ 32 mL	MJ	1 g/ 50 mL	Physically compatible for 24 hr at 25 °C	1167	C
Mitomycin		0.25 mg/ 0.5 mL		10 mg/ 0.5 mL	Physically compatible for 5 min at room temperature followed by 8 min of centrifugation	980	C
Vinblastine sulfate		0.5 mg/ 0.5 mL		10 mg/ 0.5 mL	Physically compatible for 5 min at room temperature followed by 8 min of centrifugation	980	C
Vincristine sulfate		0.5 mg/ 0.5 mL		10 mg/ 0.5 mL	Physically compatible for 5 min at room temperature followed by 8 min of centrifugation	980	C

Y-Site Injection Compatibility (1:1 Mixture)

Cyclophosphamide

Drug	Mfr	Conc	Mfr	Conc	Remarks	Ref	C/I
Allopurinol sodium	BW	3 mg/mL[b]	MJ	10 mg/mL[b]	Physically compatible for 4 hr at 22 °C	1686	C
Amifostine	USB	10 mg/mL[a]	MJ	10 mg/mL[a]	Physically compatible for 4 hr at 23 °C	1845	C
Amikacin sulfate	BR	5 mg/mL[a]	MJ	20 mg/mL[a]	Physically compatible for 4 hr at 25 °C	1194	C
Amphotericin B cholesteryl sulfate complex	SEQ	0.83 mg/mL[a]	MJ	10 mg/mL[a]	Increased turbidity forms immediately	2117	I
Ampicillin sodium	BR	20 mg/mL[b]	MJ	20 mg/mL[a]	Physically compatible for 4 hr at 25 °C	1194	C
Anidulafungin	VIC	0.5 mg/mL[a]	MJ	10 mg/mL[a]	Physically compatible for 4 hr at 23 °C	2617	C
Aztreonam	SQ	40 mg/mL[a]	MJ	10 mg/mL[a]	Physically compatible for 4 hr at 23 °C	1758	C
Bleomycin sulfate		3 units/mL		20 mg/mL	Drugs injected sequentially in Y-site with no flush. No precipitate seen	980	C
Cefazolin sodium	SKF	20 mg/mL[a]	MJ	20 mg/mL[a]	Physically compatible for 4 hr at 25 °C	1194	C

Y-Site Injection Compatibility (1:1 Mixture) (Cont.)

Cyclophosphamide

Drug	Mfr	Conc	Mfr	Conc	Remarks	Ref	C/I
Cefotaxime sodium	HO	20 mg/mL[a]	MJ	20 mg/mL[a]	Physically compatible for 4 hr at 25 °C	1194	C
Cefoxitin sodium	MSD	20 mg/mL[a]	MJ	20 mg/mL[a]	Physically compatible for 4 hr at 25 °C	1194	C
Cefuroxime sodium	GL	30 mg/mL[a]	MJ	20 mg/mL[a]	Physically compatible for 4 hr at 25 °C	1194	C
Chloramphenicol sodium succinate	ES	20 mg/mL[a]	MJ	20 mg/mL[a]	Physically compatible for 4 hr at 25 °C	1194	C
Cisplatin		1 mg/mL		20 mg/mL	Drugs injected sequentially in Y-site with no flush. No precipitate seen	980	C
Cladribine	ORT	0.015[b] and 0.5[c] mg/mL	MJ	10 mg/mL[b]	Physically compatible for 4 hr at 23 °C	1969	C
Clindamycin phosphate	UP	12 mg/mL[a]	MJ	20 mg/mL[a]	Physically compatible for 4 hr at 25 °C	1194	C
Doripenem	JJ	5 mg/mL[a,b]	BMS	10 mg/mL[a,b]	Physically compatible for 4 hr at 23 °C	2743	C
Doxorubicin HCl		2 mg/mL		20 mg/mL	Drugs injected sequentially in Y-site with no flush. No precipitate seen	980	C
Doxorubicin HCl liposomal	SEQ	0.4 mg/mL[a]	MJ	10 mg/mL[a]	Physically compatible for 4 hr at 23 °C	2087	C
Doxycycline hyclate	ES	1 mg/mL[a]	MJ	20 mg/mL[a]	Physically compatible for 4 hr at 25 °C	1194	C
Droperidol		2.5 mg/mL		20 mg/mL	Drugs injected sequentially in Y-site with no flush. No precipitate seen	980	C
Erythromycin lactobionate	AB	5 mg/mL[a]	MJ	20 mg/mL[a]	Physically compatible for 4 hr at 25 °C	1194	C
Etoposide phosphate	BR	5 mg/mL[a]	MJ	10 mg/mL[a]	Physically compatible for 4 hr at 23 °C	2218	C
Filgrastim	AMG	30 mcg/mL[a]	MJ	10 mg/mL[a]	Physically compatible for 4 hr at 22 °C	1687	C
Fludarabine phosphate	BX	1 mg/mL[a]	MJ	10 mg/mL[a]	Visually compatible for 4 hr at 22 °C	1439	C
Fluorouracil		50 mg/mL		20 mg/mL	Drugs injected sequentially in Y-site with no flush. No precipitate seen	980	C
Furosemide		10 mg/mL		20 mg/mL	Drugs injected sequentially in Y-site with no flush. No precipitate seen	980	C
Gallium nitrate	FUJ	1 mg/mL[b]	MJ	20 mg/mL	Visually compatible for 24 hr at 25 °C	1673	C
Gemcitabine HCl	LI	10 mg/mL[b]	BR	10 mg/mL[b]	Physically compatible for 4 hr at 23 °C	2226	C
Gentamicin sulfate	TR	1.6 mg/mL[a]	MJ	20 mg/mL[a]	Physically compatible for 4 hr at 25 °C	1194	C
Granisetron HCl	SKB	1 mg/mL	MJ	2 mg/mL[b]	Physically compatible with little loss of either drug in 4 hr at 22 °C	1883	C
Heparin sodium		1000 units/mL		20 mg/mL	Drugs injected sequentially in Y-site with no flush. No precipitate seen	980	C
Idarubicin HCl	AD	1 mg/mL[b]	AD	4 mg/mL[a]	Visually compatible for 24 hr at 25 °C	1525	C
Leucovorin calcium		10 mg/mL		20 mg/mL	Drugs injected sequentially in Y-site with no flush. No precipitate seen	980	C
Linezolid	PHU	2 mg/mL	MJ	10 mg/mL[a]	Physically compatible for 4 hr at 23 °C	2264	C
Melphalan HCl	BW	0.1 mg/mL[b]	BR	10 mg/mL[b]	Physically compatible for 3 hr at 22 °C	1557	C
Methotrexate sodium		25 mg/mL		20 mg/mL	Drugs injected sequentially in Y-site with no flush. No precipitate seen	980	C
		30 mg/mL		20 mg/mL[a]	Visually compatible for 4 hr at room temperature	1788	C
Metoclopramide HCl		5 mg/mL		20 mg/mL	Drugs injected sequentially in Y-site with no flush. No precipitate seen	980	C

Y-Site Injection Compatibility (1:1 Mixture) (Cont.)

Cyclophosphamide

Drug	Mfr	Conc	Mfr	Conc	Remarks	Ref	C/I
Metronidazole	SE	5 mg/mL	MJ	20 mg/mL[a]	Physically compatible for 4 hr at 25 °C	1194	C
Mitomycin		0.5 mg/mL		20 mg/mL	Drugs injected sequentially in Y-site with no flush. No precipitate seen	980	C
Nafcillin sodium	WY	20 mg/mL[a]	MJ	20 mg/mL[a]	Physically compatible for 4 hr at 25 °C	1194	C
Ondansetron HCl	GL	1 mg/mL[b]	MJ	10 mg/mL[a]	Visually compatible for 4 hr at 22 °C	1365	C
	GL	16 to 160 mcg/mL		20 mg/mL	Physically compatible when cyclophosphamide given as 5-min bolus via Y-site	1366	C
Oxacillin sodium	BE	20 mg/mL[a]	MJ	20 mg/mL[a]	Physically compatible for 4 hr at 25 °C	1194	C
Oxaliplatin	SS	0.5 mg/mL[a]	MJ	10 mg/mL[a]	Physically compatible for 4 hr at 23 °C	2566	C
Paclitaxel	NCI	1.2 mg/mL[a]		10 mg/mL[a]	Physically compatible for 4 hr at 22 °C	1528	C
Palonosetron HCl	MGI	50 mcg/mL	MJ	10 mg/mL[a]	Physically compatible and no loss of either drug in 4 hr	2640	C
Pemetrexed disodium	LI	20 mg/mL[b]	MJ	10 mg/mL[a]	Physically compatible for 4 hr at 23 °C	2564	C
Penicillin G potassium	PF	100,000 units/mL[a]	MJ	20 mg/mL[a]	Physically compatible for 4 hr at 25 °C	1194	C
Piperacillin sodium–tazobactam sodium	LE[f]	40 + 5 mg/mL[a]	MJ	10 mg/mL[a]	Physically compatible for 4 hr at 22 °C	1688	C
Propofol	ZEN	10 mg/mL	MJ	10 mg/mL[a]	Physically compatible for 1 hr at 23 °C	2066	C
Sargramostim	IMM	10 mcg/mL[b]	MJ	10 mg/mL[b]	Visually compatible for 4 hr at 22 °C	1436	C
Sodium bicarbonate		1.4%		20 mg/mL[a]	Visually compatible for 4 hr at room temperature	1788	C
Teniposide	BR	0.1 mg/mL[a]	MJ	10 mg/mL[a]	Physically compatible for 4 hr at 23 °C	1725	C
Thiotepa	IMM[d]	1 mg/mL[a]	MJ	10 mg/mL[a]	Physically compatible for 4 hr at 23 °C	1861	C
Ticarcillin disodium–clavulanate potassium	BE	31 mg/mL[a]	MJ	20 mg/mL[a]	Physically compatible for 4 hr at 25 °C	1194	C
TNA #218 to #226[e]			MJ	10 mg/mL[a]	Visually compatible for 4 hr at 23 °C	2215[e]	C
Tobramycin sulfate	DI	0.8 mg/mL[a]	MJ	20 mg/mL[a]	Physically compatible for 4 hr at 25 °C	1194	C
Topotecan HCl	SKB	56 mcg/mL[a,b]	MJ	20 mg/mL	Visually compatible. Little loss of either drug in 4 hr at 22 °C	2245	C
TPN #212 to #215[e]			MJ	10 mg/mL[a]	Physically compatible for 4 hr at 23 °C	2109	C
Trimethoprim–sulfamethoxazole	BW	0.8 + 4 mg/mL[a]	MJ	20 mg/mL[a]	Physically compatible for 4 hr at 25 °C	1194	C
Vancomycin HCl	LI	5 mg/mL[a]	MJ	20 mg/mL[a]	Physically compatible for 4 hr at 25 °C	1194	C
Vinblastine sulfate		1 mg/mL		20 mg/mL	Drugs injected sequentially in Y-site with no flush. No precipitate seen	980	C
Vincristine sulfate		1 mg/mL		20 mg/mL	Drugs injected sequentially in Y-site with no flush. No precipitate seen	980	C
Vinorelbine tartrate	BW	1 mg/mL[b]	MJ	10 mg/mL[b]	Physically compatible for 4 hr at 22 °C	1558	C

[a]Tested in dextrose 5%.
[b]Tested in sodium chloride 0.9%.
[c]Tested in bacteriostatic sodium chloride 0.9% preserved with benzyl alcohol 0.9%.
[d]Lyophilized formulation tested.
[e]Refer to Appendix I for the composition of parenteral nutrition solutions. TNA indicates a 3-in-1 admixture, and TPN indicates a 2-in-1 admixture.
[f]Test performed using the formulation WITHOUT edetate disodium.

CYCLOSPORINE
AHFS 92:44

Products — Cyclosporine is available as a concentrate in 5-mL ampuls. Each milliliter of the sterile solution contains cyclosporine 50 mg, polyoxyethylated castor oil (Cremophor EL) 650 mg, and alcohol 278 mg (32.9%). (1; 874)

Cyclosporine concentrate must be diluted before administration. (1; 874)

Trade Name(s) — Sandimmune.

Administration — Cyclosporine concentrate for injection is administered over two to six hours by intravenous infusion after dilution. Each milliliter of concentrate should be diluted in 20 to 100 mL of dextrose 5% or sodium chloride 0.9%. (1; 4)

Stability — Cyclosporine injection is a clear, faintly brown-yellow solution. It should be stored at 20 to 25 °C and protected from light and freezing. (1; 4; 874) Light protection is not required for intravenous admixtures of cyclosporine. (4; 1091) Cyclosporine diluted for infusion should be discarded after 24 hours. (1)

Sorption — Simulated infusion studies of cyclosporine (Sandoz) 2 mg/mL in dextrose 5% and sodium chloride 0.9% were performed at a rate of 0.67 mg/mL over 75 minutes through 70-inch microdrip administration sets (Abbott). Significant amounts of cyclosporine were lost, presumably as a result of sorption to the tubing. Approximately 7% of the dose was lost from the dextrose 5% admixture, and about 13% was lost from the sodium chloride 0.9% admixture. The authors noted that as much as 30% of a pediatric dose could be lost. (1091)

In contrast, no significant cyclosporine loss occurred when 2.38 and 0.495 mg/mL in dextrose 5% and sodium chloride 0.9%, in either glass or PVC containers, were delivered over six hours by an electronic infusion pump. (1154)

Cyclosporine 0.495 mg/mL in sodium chloride 0.9%, dextrose 5%, maltose 10%, and an electrolyte maintenance solution exhibited loss of delivered cyclosporine due to sorption when run through PVC administration tubing. The delivered cyclosporine concentrations were reduced to about 70% during the first two to four hours but rose to over 90% after 8 to 24 hours. The extent of sorption was somewhat higher in the electrolyte solutions compared to the sugar solutions.

No loss occurred when the cyclosporine solutions were run through polybutadiene administration tubing. (2443)

Plasticizer Leaching — Polyoxyethylated castor oil (Cremophor EL), a nonionic surfactant, may leach phthalate from PVC containers such as bags of infusion solutions. (1; 4) An acceptability limit of no more than 5 parts per million (5 mcg/mL) for diethylhexyl phthalate (DEHP) plasticizer leached from PVC containers, etc. has been proposed. The limit was proposed based on a review of metabolic and toxicologic considerations. (2185)

Cyclosporine (Sandoz) 3 mg/mL in dextrose 5% leached relatively large amounts of DEHP plasticizer from PVC bags. This leaching was due to the surfactant Cremophor EL in the formulation. After four hours at 24 °C, the DEHP concentration in 50-mL bags of infusion solution was as much as 13 mcg/mL and it increased through 24 hours to 104 mcg/mL. This finding is consistent with the high surfactant concentration (3.9%) in the final admixture solution. The actual amount of DEHP leached from PVC containers and administration sets may vary in clinical situations, depending on surfactant concentration, bag size, and contact time. Non-PVC containers and administration sets should be used to administer cyclosporine solutions. (1683)

Storage of cyclosporine (Sandoz) 3 mg/mL in dextrose 5% in PVC bags at 24 °C was shown to cause leaching of significant amounts of DEHP due to the vehicle containing Cremophor EL and alcohol. Use of glass containers and tubing that does not contain DEHP to administer cyclosporine was recommended. (1092)

Cyclosporine 0.495 mg/mL in sodium chloride 0.9%, dextrose 5%, maltose 10%, and an electrolyte maintenance solution leached relatively large amounts of DEHP plasticizer when run through PVC administration tubing. The bulk of the leaching occurred during the first four hours but reached a plateau after 8 hours. About 94 mcg/mL was delivered over 12 hours in the saline solution. The cyclosporine admixtures in electrolyte solutions leached a greater amount of DEHP than those prepared in sugar-containing solutions. (2443)

Filtration — Use of either a 0.22- or 0.45-μm filter reduced the delivered cyclosporine concentration from 2.38- and 0.495-mg/mL solutions in dextrose 5% and sodium chloride 0.9%. A significant (but unspecified) decrease was found in the first sample, taken at one minute. At the six-hour time point, the concentration had returned to the original concentration. The total amount of drug delivered over six hours was not quantified. (1154)

Compatibility Information

Solution Compatibility

Cyclosporine

Solution	Mfr	Mfr	Conc/L	Remarks	Ref	C/I
Amino acids 5%, dextrose 25%	MG	SZ	150 mg	Visually compatible with no cyclosporine loss in 72 hr at 21 °C	1616	**C**
Dextrose 5%	AB[a]	SZ	2 g	Physically compatible with no cyclosporine loss in 24 hr at 24 °C in the dark or light	1091	**C**
	AB[b]	SZ	2 g	Physically compatible with 5% cyclosporine loss in 48 hr at 24 °C under fluorescent light and refrigerated at 6 °C	1330	**C**
	BA	SZ	1 g	Visually compatible with no cyclosporine loss in 72 hr at 21 °C	1616	**C**

Solution Compatibility (Cont.)

Cyclosporine

Solution	Mfr	Mfr	Conc/L	Remarks	Ref	C/I
			2 g	Physically compatible with little or no loss in 24 hr at room temperature or refrigerated	2503	**C**
Sodium chloride 0.9%	AB[a]	SZ	2 g	Physically compatible with 7 to 8% cyclosporine loss in 24 hr at 24 °C in the dark or light	1091	**C**
			2 g	Physically compatible with little loss in 24 hr at room temperature or refrigerated	2503	**C**

[a]Tested in both glass and PVC containers.
[b]Tested in glass containers.

Additive Compatibility

Cyclosporine

Drug	Mfr	Conc/L	Mfr	Conc/L	Test Soln	Remarks	Ref	C/I
Ciprofloxacin	BAY	2 g	SZ	500 mg	NS	Visually compatible with 8% ciprofloxacin loss in 24 hr at 25 °C. Cyclosporine not tested	1934	**C**
Fat emulsion, intravenous	AB	10%	SZ	400 mg		No cyclosporine loss in 72 hr at 21 °C	1616	**C**
	KA	10 and 20%	SZ	500 mg and 2 g		Physically compatible with no cyclosporine loss in 48 hr at 24 °C under fluorescent light	1625	**C**
Magnesium sulfate	LY	30 g	SZ	2 g	D5W	Transient turbidity upon preparation. 5% cyclosporine loss in 6 hr and 10% loss in 12 hr at 24 °C under fluorescent light	1629	**I**

Drugs in Syringe Compatibility

Cyclosporine

Drug (in syringe)	Mfr	Amt	Mfr	Amt	Remarks	Ref	C/I
Dimenhydrinate		10 mg/ 1 mL		50 mg/ 1 mL	Clear solution	2569	**C**
Pantoprazole sodium	[a]	4 mg/ 1 mL		50 mg/ 1 mL	Precipitates	2574	**I**

[a]Test performed using the formulation WITHOUT edetate disodium.

Y-Site Injection Compatibility (1:1 Mixture)

Cyclosporine

Drug	Mfr	Conc	Mfr	Conc	Remarks	Ref	C/I
Acyclovir sodium	BV	5 mg/mL[b]	BED	1 mg/mL[a]	Crystals form	2794	**I**
Amphotericin B cholesteryl sulfate complex	SEQ	0.83 mg/mL[a]	SZ	5 mg/mL[a]	Decreased natural turbidity occurs	2117	**I**
Anidulafungin	VIC	0.5 mg/mL[a]	NOV	5 mg/mL[a]	Physically compatible for 4 hr at 23 °C	2617	**C**
Caspofungin acetate	ME	0.7 mg/mL[b]	BED	5 mg/mL[b]	Physically compatible for 4 hr at room temperature	2758	**C**

Y-Site Injection Compatibility (1:1 Mixture) (Cont.)

			Cyclosporine				
Drug	Mfr	Conc	Mfr	Conc	Remarks	Ref	C/I
Ceftaroline fosamil	FOR	2.22 mg/mL[a,b,e]	BED	5 mg/mL[a,b,e]	Physically compatible for 4 hr at 23 °C	2826	C
Doripenem	JJ	5 mg/mL[a,b]	BED	5 mg/mL[a,b]	Physically compatible for 4 hr at 23 °C	2743	C
Linezolid	PHU	2 mg/mL	SZ	5 mg/mL[a]	Physically compatible for 4 hr at 23 °C	2264	C
Meropenem	ASZ	10 mg/mL[b]	BED	1 mg/mL[a]	Physically compatible	2794	C
Micafungin sodium	ASP	1.5 mg/mL[b]	BED	5 mg/mL[b]	Physically compatible for 4 hr at 23 °C	2683	C
Mycophenolate mofetil HCl	RC	5.9 mg/mL[a]	BED	1 mg/mL[a]	Effervescence reported. No mycophenolate mofetil loss in 4 hr	2738	?
Propofol	ZEN	10 mg/mL	SZ	5 mg/mL[a]	Physically compatible for 1 hr at 23 °C	2066	C
Sargramostim	IMM	6[c] and 15[b] mcg/mL	SZ	5 mg/mL[b]	Visually compatible for 2 hr	1618	C
Telavancin HCl	ASP	7.5 mg/mL[a]	BED	5 mg/mL[a]	Physically compatible for 2 hr	2830	C
	ASP	7.5 mg/mL[b,e]	BED	5 mg/mL[b,e]	Increase in measured turbidity	2830	I
TNA #220, #223[d]			SZ	5 mg/mL[a]	Small amount of precipitate forms immediately	2215	I
TNA #218, #219, #221, #222, #224 to #226[d]			SZ	5 mg/mL[a]	Visually compatible for 4 hr at 23 °C	2215	C
TPN #212, #213[d]			SZ	5 mg/mL[a]	Physically compatible for 4 hr at 23 °C	2109	C
TPN #214, #215[d]			SZ	5 mg/mL[a]	Small amount of subvisible precipitate forms in 4 hr	2109	I

[a]Tested in dextrose 5%.
[b]Tested in sodium chloride 0.9%.
[c]Tested in sodium chloride 0.9% with albumin human 0.1%.
[d]Refer to Appendix I for the composition of parenteral nutrition solutions. TNA indicates a 3-in-1 admixture, and TPN indicates a 2-in-1 admixture.
[e]Tested in Ringer's injection, lactated.

CYTARABINE
(CYTOSINE ARABINOSIDE)
AHFS 10:00

Products — Cytarabine for injection is available as lyophilized products in 100-mg, 500-mg, and 1-g vials. For intravenous or subcutaneous use, reconstitute the vials with bacteriostatic water for injection containing benzyl alcohol in the following amounts (1):

Vial Size	Volume of Diluent	Concentration
100 mg	5 mL	20 mg/mL
500 mg	10 mL	50 mg/mL
1 g	10 mL	100 mg/mL

For intrathecal injection, *only* a preservative-free diluent should be used. (1; 4)

Hydrochloric acid and/or sodium hydroxide may have been added to adjust the pH. (1; 4)

Cytarabine injection is available as a 20-mg/mL solution in 5-, 25-, and 50-mL vials with sodium chloride 6.8 mg/mL in water for injection. Hydrochloric acid and/or sodium hydroxide may have been added during manufacturing to adjust pH. (1)

Cytarabine injection is available as a 100-mg/mL solution in 20-mL vials in water for injection. Hydrochloric acid and/or sodium hydroxide may have been added during manufacturing to adjust pH. (1)

pH — After reconstitution of the lyophilized products, the USP specifies a pH range of 4 to 6. (17) Cytarabine injection has a pH of about 7.4, with a range of 7 to 9. (1; 4)

Sodium Content — Cytarabine 20 mg/mL injection contains 0.12 mEq of sodium per milliliter. (1; 4)

Administration — Cytarabine may be administered by subcutaneous, intrathecal (prepared in preservative-free diluent), or direct intravenous injection and by continuous or intermittent intravenous infusion. (1; 4) Some forms may contain preservatives and should not be used for intrathecal administration. It has been administered by intramuscular injection and continuous subcutaneous infusion as well. (4)

Stability — Intact vials of lyophilized cytarabine for injection and cytarabine injection should be stored at controlled room temperature. (1)

Cytarabine reconstituted with bacteriostatic water for injection containing benzyl alcohol may be stored at a controlled room temperature for up to 48 hours. Solutions with a slight haze should be discarded. (4) However, a stability study of cytarabine in aqueous solution showed maximum stability in the neutral pH range. It was calculated to retain 90% for six and a half months at pH 6.9 at 25 °C. The rate of decomposition of cytarabine in alkaline solutions is about 10 times as great as in acid solutions. (82)

The manufacturer indicates that for concentrations of 20 and 250 mg/mL in bacteriostatic water for injection, greater than 99% is retained after five days of storage at room temperature. (174) However, cytarabine has an aqueous solubility of 100 mg/mL (4; 1369), and precipitation from more highly concentrated solutions has been observed in varying time frames. In another test, concentrations of 40 and 80 mg/mL in bacteriostatic water for injection were stored in plastic syringes (Becton Dickinson) at 37, 25, 4, and −20 °C. Cytarabine remained stable for at least 15 days at 25 and 4 °C and for seven days at 37 °C. However, storage at −20 °C resulted in a precipitate. (174)

In another report, reconstituted 100- and 500-mg vials retained between 89.2 and 92% at 17 days after reconstitution when stored at 25 °C. (189)

Immersion of a needle with an aluminum component in cytarabine (Upjohn) 20 mg/mL resulted in no visually apparent reaction after seven days at 24 °C. (988)

Cytarabine 12.5 mg/mL in sodium chloride 0.9% did not inhibit the growth of inoculated *Staphylococcus epidermidis* during 21 days at 35 °C. At a concentration of 50 mg/mL in sodium chloride, the viability was reduced but not eliminated. (1659) The potential for microbiological growth should be considered when assigning expiration periods.

Syringes — Cytarabine (Upjohn) 50 mg/mL in polypropylene syringes containing 5, 10, and 20 mL was stable for 29 days at 8 and 21 °C in the dark, exhibiting losses of 8.5% or less. (1566)

Reconstituted solutions containing 20 and 50 mg/mL of cytarabine (Upjohn) were stored in plastic syringes (Pharmaseal) at 22, 8, and −10 °C. No decomposition occurred during one week of storage at these temperatures. (748)

Cytarabine (Upjohn) 50 mg/2.5 mL was stored at 5 and 25 °C in 5-mL plastic syringes (Becton Dickinson) with rubber tip caps and in glass flasks covered with parafilm. After seven days, samples in the plastic syringes showed a 2 to 3% loss of cytarabine at both temperatures. The 25 °C sample in glass also showed a 2% loss, but the 5 °C sample in glass showed no loss after seven days. (759)

Intrathecal Injections — In a study of solutions for intrathecal injection, cytarabine (Upjohn) was reconstituted to a concentration of 5 mg/mL with Elliott's B solution (artificial cerebrospinal fluid), sodium chloride 0.9%, and Ringer's injection, lactated. In Elliott's B solution and Ringer's injection, lactated, cytarabine exhibited no change in concentration over seven days at room temperature under fluorescent light and at 30 °C. In sodium chloride 0.9%, no decomposition was noted in 24 hours, but a 3% loss was observed at room temperature and 6% at 30 °C over seven days. (327)

Bacterially contaminated intrathecal solutions could pose very grave risks; consequently, such solutions should be administered as soon as possible after preparation. (328)

The osmolarity and pH of cytarabine in these three solutions at a concentration of 2.5 mg/mL were as follows (327):

In Elliott's B solution	299 mOsm/kg, pH 7.3
In Ringer's injection, lactated	262 mOsm/kg, pH 5.6
In sodium chloride 0.9%	299 mOsm/kg, pH 5.3

In another study, the stability and compatibility of cytarabine (Upjohn), methotrexate (NCI), and hydrocortisone (Upjohn), mixed together in intrathecal injections, were evaluated. Two combinations were tested: (1) cytarabine 50 mg, methotrexate 12 mg (as the sodium salt), and hydrocortisone 25 mg (as the sodium succinate salt); and (2) cytarabine 30 mg, methotrexate 12 mg (as the sodium salt), and hydrocortisone 15 mg (as the sodium succinate salt). Each drug combination was added to 12 mL of Elliott's B solution (NCI), sodium chloride 0.9% (Abbott), dextrose 5% (Abbott), and Ringer's injection, lactated (Abbott), and stored for 24 hours at 25 °C. Cytarabine and methotrexate were both chemically stable, with no drug loss after the full 24 hours in all solutions. Hydrocortisone was also stable in the sodium chloride 0.9%, dextrose 5%, and Ringer's injection, lactated, with about a 2% drug loss. However, in Elliott's B solution, hydrocortisone was significantly less stable, with a 6% loss in the 25-mg concentration over 24 hours. The 15-mg concentration was worse, with a 5% loss in 10 hours and a 13% loss in 24 hours. The higher pH of Elliott's B solution and the lower concentration of hydrocortisone may have been factors in this increased decomposition. All mixtures were physically compatible during this study, but a precipitate formed after several days of storage. (819)

Elliott's B solution has been recommended as a diluent for cytosine arabinoside for intrathecal administration because it is more nearly physiologic. (435) The patient's own spinal fluid has been recommended also. (830)

Cytarabine (Upjohn) 3 mg/mL diluted in Elliott's B solution (Orphan Medical) was packaged as 20 mL in 30-mL glass vials and 20-mL plastic syringes (Becton Dickinson) with Red Cap (Burron) Luer-Lok syringe tip caps. The solution was physically compatible and was chemically stable, exhibiting little or no loss during storage for 48 hours at 4 and 23 °C. (1976)

Implantable Pumps — Cytarabine (Upjohn) 1 mg/mL in Elliott's B solution was evaluated for stability in an implantable infusion pump (Infusaid model 400). In this in vitro assessment, no cytarabine loss occurred in 15 days at 37 °C with mild agitation. (767)

Sorption — Cytarabine (Mack) 0.144 mg/mL in dextrose 5% and in sodium chloride 0.9% exhibited little or no loss due to sorption in polyethylene and PVC containers compared to glass containers over 72 hours at room and refrigeration temperatures. (2420; 2430)

Filtration — Cytarabine 100 mg/15 mL was injected as a bolus through a 0.2-μm nylon, air-eliminating filter (Ultipor, Pall) to evaluate the effect of filtration on simulated intravenous push delivery. Spectrophotometric evaluation showed that about 96% of the drug was delivered through the filter after flushing with 10 mL of sodium chloride 0.9%. (809)

Cytarabine 10 to 100 mcg/mL exhibited no loss due to sorption to either cellulose nitrate/cellulose acetate ester (Millex OR) or polytetrafluoroethylene (Millex FG) filters. (1416)

Central Venous Catheter — Cytarabine (Fujisawa) 5 mg/mL in dextrose 5% was found to be compatible with the ARROWg+ard Blue Plus (Arrow International) chlorhexidine-bearing triple-lumen central catheter. Essentially complete delivery of the drug was found with little or no drug loss occurring. Furthermore, chlorhexidine delivered from the catheter remained at trace amounts with no substantial increase due to the delivery of the drug through the catheter. (2335)

Compatibility Information

Solution Compatibility

Cytarabine

Solution	Mfr	Mfr	Conc/L	Remarks	Ref	C/I
Amino acids 4.25%, dextrose 25%	MG	UP	100 mg	No increase in particulate matter in 24 hr at 5 °C	349	C
Dextrose 5% in Ringer's injection, lactated	TR[a]	UP	500 mg	Stable for 24 hr at 5 °C	282	C
Dextrose 5% in sodium chloride 0.2%	[a]	UP	8, 24, 32 g	No loss in 7 days at room temperature or 4 or −20 °C	174	C
Dextrose 5% in sodium chloride 0.9%	TR[a]	UP	500 mg	Stable for 24 hr at 5 °C	282	C
		UP	3.6 g	Physically compatible	174	C
Dextrose 10% in sodium chloride 0.9%		UP	3.6 g	Physically compatible	174	C
Dextrose 5%			500 mg	Stable for 8 days at room temperature	1	C
	TR[a]	UP	500 mg	Stable for 24 hr at 5 °C	282	C
	TR[a]	UP	1.87 g	Under 10% loss in 24 hr at room temperature	519	C
		UP	500 mg	Stable for 7 days at room temperature	174	C
	[a]	UP	8, 24, 32 g	No loss in 7 days at room temperature or 4 or −20 °C	174	C
			0.5 to 5 g	Under 10% loss in 14 days at room temperature	1379	C
	[b]	UP	1.25 and 25 g	Visually compatible with less than 6% cytarabine loss in 28 days at 4 and 22 °C and 7 days at 35 °C protected from light. Excessive decomposition products in 14 days at 35 °C	1548	C
	MG, TR[a]		1.83 g	Less than 10% cytarabine loss in 24 hr at room temperature exposed to light	1658	C
		UP	157 mg	Less than 2% loss in 48 hr at room temperature, exposed to light and in the dark, and at 4 °C	1955	C
Ringer's injection		UP	3.6 g	Physically compatible	174	C
			0.5 to 5 g	Under 10% loss in 14 days at room temperature	1379	C
Ringer's injection, lactated	TR[a]	UP	500 mg	Stable for 24 hr at 5 °C	282	C
Sodium chloride 0.9%			500 mg	Stable for 8 days at room temperature	1	C
	TR[a]	UP	500 mg	Stable for 24 hr at 5 °C	282	C
		UP	500 mg	Stable for 7 days at room temperature	174	C
	[a]	UP	8, 24, 32 g	No loss in 7 days at room temperature or 4 or −20 °C	174	C
		UP	3.6 g	Physically compatible	174	C
			0.5 to 5 g	Under 10% loss in 14 days at room temperature	1379	C
	[b]	UP	1.25 and 25 g	Visually compatible with less than 6% cytarabine loss in 28 days at 4 and 22 °C and 7 days at 35 °C protected from light. Excessive decomposition products in 14 days at 35 °C	1548	C
Sodium lactate ⅙ M		UP	3.6 g	Physically compatible	174	C

Solution Compatibility (Cont.)

Cytarabine

Solution	Mfr	Mfr	Conc/L	Remarks	Ref	C/I
TPN #57[c]		UP	50 mg	Physically compatible with no loss in 48 hr at 25 or 8 °C	996	**C**

[a]*Tested in both glass and PVC containers.*
[b]*Tested in ethylene vinyl acetate (EVA) containers.*
[c]*Refer to Appendix I for the composition of parenteral nutrition solutions. TPN indicates a 2-in-1 admixture.*

Additive Compatibility

Cytarabine

Drug	Mfr	Conc/L	Mfr	Conc/L	Test Soln	Remarks	Ref	C/I
Daunorubicin HCl with etoposide	RP BR	33 mg 400 mg	UP	267 mg	D5½S	Physically compatible with about 6% cytarabine loss and no loss of other drugs in 72 hr at 20 °C	1162	**C**
Daunorubicin HCl with etoposide	BEL SZ	15.7 mg 157 mg	UP	157 mg	D5W	Less than 10% loss of any drug in 48 hr at room temperature, exposed to light and in the dark, and at 4 °C	1955	**C**
Etoposide with daunorubicin HCl	BR RP	400 mg 33 mg	UP	267 mg	D5½S	Physically compatible with about 6% cytarabine loss and no loss of other drugs in 72 hr at 20 °C	1162	**C**
Etoposide with daunorubicin HCl	SZ BEL	157 mg 15.7 mg	UP	157 mg	D5W	Less than 10% loss of any drug in 48 hr at room temperature, exposed to light and in the dark, and at 4 °C	1955	**C**
Fluorouracil	RC	250 mg	UP	400 mg	D5W	Altered UV spectra for cytarabine within 1 hr at room temperature	207	**I**
Gentamicin sulfate		80 mg 240 mg	UP UP	100 mg 300 mg	D5W D5W	Physically compatible for 24 hr / Physically incompatible	174 174	**C** **I**
Heparin sodium		10,000 units 20,000 units	UP UP	500 mg 100 mg	NS D5W	Haze formation / Haze formation	174 174	**I** **I**
Hydrocortisone sodium succinate	UP UP	500 mg 500 mg	UP UP	360 mg 360 mg	D5S, D10S R, SL	Physically compatible for 40 hr / Physically incompatible	174 174	**C** **I**
Hydroxyzine HCl	LY	500 mg	UP	1 g	D5W[a]	Physically compatible for 48 hr	1190	**C**
Insulin, regular		40 units	UP	100 and 500 mg	D5W	Fine precipitate forms	174	**I**
Lincomycin HCl		1, 1.5, 2, 2.4, 3 g	UP	500 mg		Physically compatible for 48 hr	174	**C**
Methotrexate sodium	LE	200 mg	UP	400 mg	D5W	Physically compatible. Very little change in UV spectra in 8 hr at room temperature	207	**C**
Methylprednisolone sodium succinate	UP UP	250 mg 250 mg	UP UP	360 mg 360 mg	D5S, D10S, NS R, SL	Clear solution for 24 hr / Physically incompatible	329 329	**C** **I**
Mitoxantrone HCl	LE	500 mg	UP	500 mg	D5W	Visually compatible. Mitoxantrone stable for 24 hr at room temperature. Cytarabine not tested	1531	**C**

Additive Compatibility (Cont.)

Cytarabine

Drug	Mfr	Conc/L	Mfr	Conc/L	Test Soln	Remarks	Ref	C/I
Nafcillin sodium		4 g	UP	100 mg	D5W	Heavy crystalline precipitation	174	I
Ondansetron HCl	GL	30 and 300 mg	UP	200 mg	D5W[b]	Physically compatible with little loss of either drug in 48 hr at 23 °C	1876	C
	GL	30 and 300 mg	UP	40 g	D5W[b]	Physically compatible with little loss of either drug in 48 hr at 23 °C	1876	C
Oxacillin sodium		2 g	UP	100 mg	D5W	pH outside stability range for oxacillin	174	I
Penicillin G sodium		2 million units	UP	200 mg	D5W	pH outside stability range for penicillin G	174	I
Potassium chloride		80 mEq	UP	170 mg	D5S	Physically compatible for 24 hr	174	C
		100 mEq	UP	2 g	D5S	Physically compatible. Stable for 8 days	174	C
Sodium bicarbonate	AB	50 mEq	UP	200 mg and 1 g	D5W[c]	Physically compatible with no cytarabine loss in 7 days at 8 and 22 °C	748	C
	AB	50 mEq	UP	200 mg	D5¼S[c]	Physically compatible with no cytarabine loss in 7 days at 8 and 22 °C	748	C
Vincristine sulfate	LI	4 mg	UP	16 mg	D5W	Physically compatible. No alteration in UV spectra in 8 hr at room temperature	207	C

[a]*Tested in glass containers.*
[b]*Tested in PVC containers.*
[c]*Tested in both glass and PVC containers.*

Drugs in Syringe Compatibility

Cytarabine

Drug (in syringe)	Mfr	Amt	Mfr	Amt	Remarks	Ref	C/I
Metoclopramide HCl	RB	10 mg/2 mL	UP	50 mg/1 mL	Physically compatible for 48 hr at 25 °C	1167	C
	RB	160 mg/32 mL	UP	500 mg/10 mL	Physically compatible for 48 hr at 25 °C	1167	C

Y-Site Injection Compatibility (1:1 Mixture)

Cytarabine

Drug	Mfr	Conc	Mfr	Conc	Remarks	Ref	C/I
Allopurinol sodium	BW	3 mg/mL[b]	SCN	50 mg/mL	Tiny particles form within 4 hr	1686	I
Amifostine	USB	10 mg/mL[a]	CET	50 mg/mL	Physically compatible for 4 hr at 23 °C	1845	C
Amphotericin B cholesteryl sulfate complex	SEQ	0.83 mg/mL[a]	BED	50 mg/mL	Physically compatible for 4 hr at 23 °C	2117	C
Amsacrine	NCI	1 mg/mL[a]	QU	50 mg/mL	Visually compatible for 4 hr at 22 °C	1381	C
Anidulafungin	VIC	0.5 mg/mL[a]	BED	50 mg/mL	Physically compatible for 4 hr at 23 °C	2617	C
Aztreonam	SQ	40 mg/mL[a]	CET	50 mg/mL	Physically compatible for 4 hr at 23 °C	1758	C
Caspofungin acetate	ME	0.7 mg/mL[b]	MAY	50 mg/mL	Microparticles form within 4 hr	2758	I
Cladribine	ORT	0.015[b] and 0.5[c] mg/mL	CHI	50 mg/mL	Physically compatible for 4 hr at 23 °C	1969	C

Y-Site Injection Compatibility (1:1 Mixture) (Cont.)

Cytarabine

Drug	Mfr	Conc	Mfr	Conc	Remarks	Ref	C/I
Doxorubicin HCl liposomal	SEQ	0.4 mg/mL[a]	CHI	50 mg/mL	Physically compatible for 4 hr at 23 °C	2087	C
Etoposide phosphate	BR	5 mg/mL[a]	BED	50 mg/mL	Physically compatible for 4 hr at 23 °C	2218	C
Filgrastim	AMG	30 mcg/mL[a]	CET	50 mg/mL	Physically compatible for 4 hr at 22 °C	1687	C
Fludarabine phosphate	BX	1 mg/mL[a]	UP	50 mg/mL	Visually compatible for 4 hr at 22 °C	1439	C
Gallium nitrate	FUJ	1 mg/mL[b]	CET	50 mg/mL	Precipitates immediately	1673	I
Gemcitabine HCl	LI	10 mg/mL[b]	BED	50 mg/mL	Physically compatible for 4 hr at 23 °C	2226	C
Gentamicin sulfate	GNS	15 mg/mL[d]	UP	16 mg/mL[b]	Visually compatible for 24 hr at room temperature in test tubes. No precipitate found on filter from Y-site delivery	2063	C
Granisetron HCl	SKB	1 mg/mL	UP	2 mg/mL[b]	Physically compatible with little loss of either drug in 4 hr at 22 °C	1883	C
	SKB	0.05 mg/mL[a]	UP	50 mg/mL	Physically compatible for 4 hr at 23 °C	2000	C
Hydrocortisone sodium succinate	UP	125 mg/mL	UP	16 mg/mL[b]	Visually compatible for 24 hr at room temperature in test tubes. No precipitate found on filter from Y-site delivery	2063	C
Idarubicin HCl	AD	1 mg/mL[b]	CET	6 mg/mL[a]	Visually compatible for 24 hr at 25 °C	1525	C
Linezolid	PHU	2 mg/mL	BED	50 mg/mL	Physically compatible for 4 hr at 23 °C	2264	C
Melphalan HCl	BW	0.1 mg/mL[b]	UP	50 mg/mL	Physically compatible for 3 hr at 22 °C	1557	C
Methotrexate sodium		30 mg/mL	UP	0.6 mg/mL[a]	Visually compatible for 4 hr at room temperature	1788	C
Methylprednisolone sodium succinate	UP	5 mg/mL[a]	UP	16 mg/mL[b]	Visually compatible for 24 hr at room temperature in test tubes. No precipitate found on filter from Y-site delivery	2063	C
Ondansetron HCl	GL	1 mg/mL[b]	UP	50 mg/mL	Visually compatible for 4 hr at 22 °C	1365	C
Paclitaxel	NCI	1.2 mg/mL[a]		50 mg/mL	Physically compatible for 4 hr at 22 °C	1528	C
Pemetrexed disodium	LI	20 mg/mL[b]	PHU	50 mg/mL	Physically compatible for 4 hr at 23 °C	2564	C
Piperacillin sodium–tazobactam sodium	LE[g]	40 + 5 mg/mL[a]	SCN	50 mg/mL	Physically compatible for 4 hr at 22 °C	1688	C
Propofol	ZEN	10 mg/mL	CHI	50 mg/mL	Physically compatible for 1 hr at 23 °C	2066	C
Sargramostim	IMM	10 mcg/mL[b]	SCN	50 mg/mL	Visually compatible for 4 hr at 22 °C	1436	C
Sodium bicarbonate		1.4%	UP	0.6 mg/mL[a]	Visually compatible for 4 hr at room temperature	1788	C
Teniposide	BR	0.1 mg/mL[a]	CET	50 mg/mL	Physically compatible for 4 hr at 23 °C	1725	C
Thiotepa	IMM[e]	1 mg/mL[a]	CET	50 mg/mL	Physically compatible for 4 hr at 23 °C	1861	C
TNA #218 to #226[f]			BED	50 mg/mL	Visually compatible for 4 hr at 23 °C	2215	C
TPN #212 to #215[f]			CHI	50 mg/mL	Substantial loss of natural subvisible turbidity occurs immediately	2109	I
Vinorelbine tartrate	BW	1 mg/mL[b]	CET	50 mg/mL	Physically compatible for 4 hr at 22 °C	1558	C

[a]Tested in dextrose 5%.
[b]Tested in sodium chloride 0.9%.
[c]Tested in bacteriostatic sodium chloride 0.9% preserved with benzyl alcohol 0.9%.
[d]Tested in sodium chloride 0.45%.
[e]Lyophilized formulation tested.
[f]Refer to Appendix I for the composition of parenteral nutrition solutions. TNA indicates a 3-in-1 admixture, and TPN indicates a 2-in-1 admixture.
[g]Test performed using the formulation WITHOUT edetate disodium.

DACARBAZINE
AHFS 10:00

Products — Dacarbazine is available in vials containing 100 and 200 mg of drug along with anhydrous citric acid and mannitol. Reconstitute the 100- and 200-mg vials with 9.9 and 19.7 mL of sterile water for injection, respectively, to yield solutions containing 10 mg/mL of dacarbazine. (1)

pH — From 3 to 4. (1)

Administration — Dacarbazine is administered as a direct intravenous injection over one minute and as an intravenous infusion in up to 250 mL of dextrose 5% or sodium chloride 0.9% over 15 to 30 minutes. (4) Extravasation may result in severe pain and tissue damage. (1; 4; 377)

In the event of spills or leaks, the manufacturer recommends the use of sulfuric acid 10% in contact for 24 hours to inactivate dacarbazine. (1200)

Stability — Intact vials of dacarbazine should be stored at 2 to 8 °C and protected from light. (1; 4) However, dacarbazine in intact vials stored at controlled room temperature has been stated to be stable for periods of four weeks (1239; 1433) to three months. (1433; 2745) The manufacturer also recommends storage of reconstituted solutions for up to eight hours at normal room temperatures and light or up to 72 hours at 4 °C. (1) However, it has been reported that solutions are stable for at least 24 hours at room temperature (1% decomposition) and at least 96 hours under refrigeration (less than 1% decomposition) when protected from light. (285) A change in color from pale yellow or ivory to pink or red is a sign of decomposition. (4; 285; 1093)

Immersion of a needle with an aluminum component in dacarbazine (Miles) 10 mg/mL resulted in no visually apparent unexpected reaction after seven days at 24 °C. (988)

Light Effects — Administration of dacarbazine in a room illuminated only with a red photographic light apparently reduced the incidence of disagreeable side effects. The authors attributed this result to a reduced amount of photodegradation of dacarbazine. (469)

Multiple photodegradation products of dacarbazine have been identified and specific concentrations of each are crucially dependent on the pH of the solution. (496)

The effects of daylight and fluorescent light on dacarbazine (Bayer) 4 mg/mL in sodium chloride 0.9% were reported. Exposure to direct sunlight resulted in up to a 12% loss in 30 minutes, and a pink color formed in 35 to 40 minutes. Exposure to indirect daylight resulted in less than a 2% loss in 30 minutes. Solutions protected from light or exposed to fluorescent light lost about 4% of their dacarbazine in 24 hours. (1248)

The photostability of dacarbazine has been shown to increase with the addition of reduced glutathione at about 5 mg/100 mL. (1829)

Dacarbazine (Aventis) 11 mg/mL reconstituted with sterile water for injection in original amber glass vials stored at room temperature exposed to fluorescent light formed a visible precipitate and became yellow in 24 hours and turned pink after 96 hours. About 4% dacarbazine loss occurred in 96 hours, but precipitation limited the utility period to 24 hours. Formation of 2-azahypoxanthine, a potentially toxic decomposition product, was also noted. Under refrigeration protected from light, no precipitation was seen, but red discoloration appeared after 96 hours; little or no loss of dacarbazine occurred in seven days. Reconstituted dacarbazine was stated to be stable for 24 hours at room temperature under fluorescent light and 96 hours refrigerated in the dark. (2386)

Dacarbazine (Aventis) 1.4 mg/mL in dextrose 5% in PVC bags (Fresenius) was stored under a variety of temperature and light conditions. In PVC bags exposed to natural sunlight, the solution turned pink in six hours and red in 48 hours; it developed a precipitate in 96 hours. About 11% dacarbazine loss in three hours and 35% loss in 24 hours. Exposed to or protected from fluorescent light at room temperature and refrigerated, no visible changes occurred in seven days. At room temperature, dacarbazine losses were about 6% in 24 hours exposed to fluorescent light and 7% in 48 hours protected from light. Refrigerated samples protected from light exhibited little or no loss in seven days. (2386)

Simulated infusion of the dacarbazine 1.4-mg/mL solution through transparent (Baxter) and opaque (Codan) infusion tubing over about 110 minutes exposed to light resulted in the delivery of 94% (transparent tubing) and 98% (opaque tubing) of the dacarbazine. (2386)

Sorption — Dacarbazine (Medac) 0.64 mg/mL in sodium chloride 0.9% exhibited no loss due to sorption in polyethylene and PVC containers compared to glass containers over 48 hours at refrigeration temperature. (2420; 2430)

Compatibility Information

Solution Compatibility

Dacarbazine

Solution	Mfr	Mfr	Conc/L	Remarks	Ref	C/I
Dextrose 5%	a		1.7 g	Less than 10% loss in 24 hr at room temperature	519	C
	MG, TR[b]		1.7 g	Less than 10% loss in 24 hr at room temperature exposed to light	1658	C
	BA[c]	MI	1 and 3 g	Physically compatible with 4% loss in 8 hr and 10 to 15% loss in 24 hr at 23 °C	1876	I
	FRE[c]	AVE	1.4 g	Exposed to sunlight, pink color formed in 3 hr and red color in 6 hr with precipitation in 96 hr at 23 °C. 11% loss in 3 hr	2386	I

Solution Compatibility (Cont.)

Dacarbazine

Solution	Mfr	Mfr	Conc/L	Remarks	Ref	C/I
	FRE[c]	AVE	1.4 g	Exposed to or protected from fluorescent light, visually compatible for 7 days. 6% loss in 24 hr exposed to fluorescent light and 7% loss in 48 hr in the dark. Little loss at 4 °C in 7 days	2386	C

[a]*Tested in both glass and PVC containers.*
[b]*Tested in glass, PVC, and polyolefin containers.*
[c]*Tested in PVC containers.*

Additive Compatibility

Dacarbazine

Drug	Mfr	Conc/L	Mfr	Conc/L	Test Soln	Remarks	Ref	C/I
Doxorubicin HCl with ondansetron HCl	AD GL	800 mg 640 mg	LY	8 g	D5W[a]	Visually compatible. Under 10% ondansetron and doxorubicin loss in 24 hr at 30 °C and 7 days at 4 °C then 24 hr at 30 °C. Dacarbazine stable for 8 hr but 13% loss in 24 hr	2092	I
Doxorubicin HCl with ondansetron HCl	AD GL	800 mg 640 mg	LY	8 g	D5W[b]	Visually compatible. Under 10% loss of all drugs in 24 hr at 30 °C and 7 days at 4 °C then 24 hr at 30 °C	2092	C
Doxorubicin HCl with ondansetron HCl	AD GL	1.5 g 640 mg	LY	20 g	D5W[a,b]	Visually compatible. Under 10% loss of all drugs in 24 hr at 30 °C and 7 days at 4 °C then 24 hr at 30 °C	2092	C
Ondansetron HCl	GL	30 and 300 mg	MI	1 g	D5W[a]	Physically compatible with little loss of ondansetron in 48 hr at 23 °C. 8 to 12% dacarbazine loss in 24 hr and 20% loss in 48 hr at 23 °C	1876	C
	GL	30 and 300 mg	MI	3 g	D5W[a]	Physically compatible with little loss of ondansetron in 48 hr at 23 °C. 8% dacarbazine loss in 24 hr and 15% loss in 48 hr at 23 °C	1876	C
Ondansetron HCl with doxorubicin HCl	GL AD	640 mg 800 mg	LY	8 g	D5W[a]	Visually compatible. Under 10% ondansetron and doxorubicin loss in 24 hr at 30 °C and 7 days at 4 °C then 24 hr at 30 °C. Dacarbazine stable for 8 hr but 13% loss in 24 hr	2092	I
Ondansetron HCl with doxorubicin HCl	GL AD	640 mg 800 mg	LY	8 g	D5W[b]	Visually compatible. Under 10% loss of all drugs in 24 hr at 30 °C and 7 days at 4 °C then 24 hr at 30 °C	2092	C
Ondansetron HCl with doxorubicin HCl	GL AD	640 mg 1.5 g	LY	20 g	D5W[a,b]	Visually compatible. Under 10% loss of all drugs in 24 hr at 30 °C and 7 days at 4 °C then 24 hr at 30 °C	2092	C

[a]*Tested in PVC containers.*
[b]*Tested in polyisoprene infusion pump reservoirs.*

Y-Site Injection Compatibility (1:1 Mixture)

Dacarbazine

Drug	Mfr	Conc	Mfr	Conc	Remarks	Ref	C/I
Allopurinol sodium	BW	3 mg/mL[b]	MI	4 mg/mL[b]	Small particles form within 1 hr and become large pink pellets in 24 hr	1686	I
Amifostine	USB	10 mg/mL[a]	MI	4 mg/mL[a]	Physically compatible for 4 hr at 23 °C	1845	C
Aztreonam	SQ	40 mg/mL[a]	MI	4 mg/mL[a]	Physically compatible for 4 hr at 23 °C	1758	C
Doxorubicin HCl liposomal	SEQ	0.4 mg/mL[a]	MI	4 mg/mL[a]	Physically compatible for 4 hr at 23 °C	2087	C
Etoposide phosphate	BR	5 mg/mL[a]	MI	4 mg/mL[a]	Physically compatible for 4 hr at 23 °C	2218	C
Filgrastim	AMG	30 mcg/mL[a]	MI	4 mg/mL[a]	Physically compatible for 4 hr at 22 °C	1687	C
Fludarabine phosphate	BX	1 mg/mL[a]	MI	4 mg/mL[a]	Visually compatible for 4 hr at 22 °C	1439	C
Granisetron HCl	SKB	1 mg/mL	MI	1.7 mg/mL[b]	Physically compatible with little loss of either drug in 4 hr at 22 °C	1883	C
Heparin sodium	WY	100 units/mL	MI	25 mg/mL[b]	White precipitate forms immediately[c]	1158	I
	WY	100 units/mL	MI	10 mg/mL[b]	No observable precipitation[c]	1158	C
Hydrocortisone sodium succinate					Pink precipitate forms immediately	524	I
Melphalan HCl	BW	0.1 mg/mL[b]	MI	4 mg/mL[b]	Physically compatible for 3 hr at 22 °C	1557	C
Ondansetron HCl	GL	1 mg/mL[b]	MI	4 mg/mL[a]	Visually compatible for 4 hr at 22 °C	1365	C
Paclitaxel	NCI	1.2 mg/mL[a]	MI	4 mg/mL[a]	Physically compatible for 4 hr at 22 °C	1556	C
Palonosetron HCl	MGI	50 mcg/mL	BV	4 mg/mL[a]	Physically compatible and no loss of either drug in 4 hr	2681	C
Piperacillin sodium–tazobactam sodium	LE[e]	40 + 5 mg/mL[a]	MI	4 mg/mL[a]	Turbidity and particles form immediately and increase over 4 hr	1688	I
Sargramostim	IMM	10 mcg/mL[b]	MI	4 mg/mL[b]	Visually compatible for 4 hr at 22 °C	1436	C
Teniposide	BR	0.1 mg/mL[a]	MI	4 mg/mL[a]	Physically compatible for 4 hr at 23 °C	1725	C
Thiotepa	IMM[d]	1 mg/mL[a]	MI	4 mg/mL[a]	Physically compatible for 4 hr at 23 °C	1861	C
Vinorelbine tartrate	BW	1 mg/mL[b]	MI	4 mg/mL[b]	Physically compatible for 4 hr at 22 °C	1558	C

[a]*Tested in dextrose 5%.*
[b]*Tested in sodium chloride 0.9%.*
[c]*Dacarbazine in intravenous tubing flushed with heparin sodium.*
[d]*Lyophilized formulation tested.*
[e]*Test performed using the formulation WITHOUT edetate disodium.*

DACTINOMYCIN
(ACTINOMYCIN D)
AHFS 10:00

Products — Dactinomycin is available in vials containing 0.5 mg of drug with mannitol 20 mg. Reconstitute with 1.1 mL of sterile water for injection *without* preservatives to yield a gold-colored solution containing 0.5 mg/mL of dactinomycin. Other solvents, especially those containing preservatives such as bacteriostatic water for injection (benzyl alcohol or parabens), may cause precipitation. (1; 4)

pH — The pH of the reconstituted solution is 5.5 to 7. (4)

Trade Name(s) — Cosmegen.

Administration — Dactinomycin may be administered by direct intravenous injection, intravenous infusion, and isolation perfusion technique. It must *not* be given intramuscularly or subcutaneously. (1; 4) Extravasation should be avoided because of possible corrosion of soft tissue. (1; 4; 377) An inline cellulose ester membrane filter should not be used for administration of dactinomycin. See Filtration below.

In the event of spills or leaks, the manufacturer recommends the use of trisodium phosphate 5% to inactivate dactinomycin. (1200)

Stability — Intact vials of dactinomycin should be stored at controlled room temperature and protected from light and humidity. (1) The clear, gold-colored, reconstituted solution is stable at room temperature; however, this solution contains no preservative so it has been suggested that unused portions of the injection be discarded. (1; 4) The drug is reported to be most stable at pH 5 to 7. (1369) A 30-mcg/mL concentration at this pH range exhibits about a 2 to 3% loss in six hours at 25 °C; at pH 9, an 80% loss occurs under these conditions. (51)

Dactinomycin, reconstituted according to the manufacturer's instructions, was cultured with human lymphoblasts to determine whether its cytotoxic activity was retained. The solution retained cytotoxicity for 24 hours at 4 °C and room temperature. (1575)

Filtration — Dactinomycin may exhibit considerable binding to cellulose acetate/nitrate (Millex OR) and polytetrafluoroethylene (Millex GV) filters. (1249)

Dactinomycin (MSD) 0.5 mg/L in dextrose 5%, sodium chloride 0.9%, and Ringer's injection, lactated, was filtered over 12 hours through a 5-μm stainless steel depth filter (Argyle Filter Connector), a 0.22-μm cellulose ester membrane filter (Ivex-2 Filter Set), and a 0.22-μm polycarbonate membrane filter (In-Sure Filter Set). No significant reduction in potency due to binding was observed with the stainless steel filter. Approximately 25% of the drug delivered through the polycarbonate filter in the first 10 mL of solution was bound, but binding decreased rapidly thereafter, resulting in only 0.3% of the total delivered dose in 12 hours being bound. (320)

In contrast, filtration through the cellulose ester filter resulted in the binding of about 95 to 99% of the drug in the first 10 mL, with the total cumulative amount of drug bound in 12 hours being 13%. Approximately half of the bound drug was released by rinsing three times with 100 mL of the same intravenous solutions used in the admixtures. (320)

A filter material specially treated with a proprietary agent was evaluated for a reduction in dactinomycin binding. Dactinomycin (MSD) 0.5 mg/L in dextrose 5% and sodium chloride 0.9% was run at a rate of 2 mL/min through an administration set with a treated 0.22-μm cellulose ester inline filter. Cumulative dactinomycin losses of less than 3% occurred from both solutions, compared to much higher losses previously reported for untreated cellulose ester filter material. Furthermore, equilibrium binding studies showed a sixfold reduction in binding from both solutions. (904) All Abbott Ivex integral filter and extension sets currently use this treated filter material. (1074)

In another study, dactinomycin 0.5 mg/1 mL was injected as a bolus through a 0.2-μm nylon, air-eliminating, filter (Ultipor, Pall) to evaluate the effect of filtration on simulated intravenous push delivery. Spectrophotometric evaluation showed that about 87% of the drug was delivered through the filter after flushing with 10 mL of sodium chloride 0.9%. (809)

Dactinomycin 4 to 50 mcg/mL exhibited a greater than 95% loss due to sorption to cellulose nitrate/cellulose acetate ester filters (Millex OR) and a 50 to 60% loss with polytetrafluoroethylene filters (Millex FG). (1415; 1416)

Compatibility Information

Solution Compatibility

Dactinomycin

Solution	Mfr	Mfr	Conc/L	Remarks	Ref	C/I
Dextrose 5%				Manufacturer recommended solution	1	C
	a	MSD	9.8 mg	Less than 10% loss in 24 hr at room temperature	519	C
	MG, TR[a]	MSD	9.8 mg	Less than 10% loss in 24 hr at room temperature exposed to light	1658	C
	MG, TR[b]	MSD	7.5 mg	Less than 10% loss in 24 hr at room temperature exposed to light	1658	C
Sodium chloride 0.9%				Manufacturer recommended solution	1	C

[a]Tested in both glass and PVC containers.
[b]Tested in both glass and polyolefin containers.

Y-Site Injection Compatibility (1:1 Mixture)

Dactinomycin

Drug	Mfr	Conc	Mfr	Conc	Remarks	Ref	C/I
Allopurinol sodium	BW	3 mg/mL[b]	MSD	0.01 mg/mL[b]	Physically compatible for 4 hr at 22 °C	1686	C
Amifostine	USB	10 mg/mL[a]	ME	0.01 mg/mL[a]	Physically compatible for 4 hr at 23 °C	1845	C
Aztreonam	SQ	40 mg/mL[a]	ME	0.01 mg/mL[a]	Physically compatible for 4 hr at 23 °C	1758	C
Etoposide phosphate	BR	5 mg/mL[a]	ME	0.01 mg/mL[a]	Physically compatible for 4 hr at 23 °C	2218	C
Filgrastim	AMG	30 mcg/mL[a]	MSD	0.01 mg/mL[a]	Particles and filaments form immediately	1687	I
Fludarabine phosphate	BX	1 mg/mL[a]	MSD	0.01 mg/mL[a]	Visually compatible for 4 hr at 22 °C	1439	C
Gemcitabine HCl	LI	10 mg/mL[b]	ME	0.01 mg/mL[b]	Physically compatible for 4 hr at 23 °C	2226	C

Y-Site Injection Compatibility (1:1 Mixture) (Cont.)

Dactinomycin

Drug	Mfr	Conc	Mfr	Conc	Remarks	Ref	C/I
Granisetron HCl	SKB	0.05 mg/mL[a]	ME	0.01 mg/mL[a]	Physically compatible for 4 hr at 23 °C	2000	C
Melphalan HCl	BW	0.1 mg/mL[b]	MSD	0.01 mg/mL[b]	Physically compatible for 3 hr at 22 °C	1557	C
Ondansetron HCl	GL	1 mg/mL[b]	MSD	0.01 mg/mL[a]	Visually compatible for 4 hr at 22 °C	1365	C
Sargramostim	IMM	10 mcg/mL[b]	MSD	0.01 mg/mL[b]	Visually compatible for 4 hr at 22 °C	1436	C
Teniposide	BR	0.1 mg/mL[a]	MSD	0.01 mg/mL[a]	Physically compatible for 4 hr at 23 °C	1725	C
Thiotepa	IMM[c]	1 mg/mL[a]	ME	0.01 mg/mL[a]	Physically compatible for 4 hr at 23 °C	1861	C
Vinorelbine tartrate	BW	1 mg/mL[b]	MSD	0.01 mg/mL[b]	Physically compatible for 4 hr at 22 °C	1558	C

[a]Tested in dextrose 5%.
[b]Tested in sodium chloride 0.9%.
[c]Lyophilized formulation tested.

DALTEPARIN SODIUM
AHFS 20:12.04.16

Products — Dalteparin is available in multiple-dose vials, providing 10,000 and 25,000 anti-Factor Xa units/mL (64 and 160 mg/mL). It is also available in 0.2-mL prefilled syringes, providing 2500, 5000, 7500, 10,000, 12,500, 15,000, and 18,000 anti-Factor Xa units per syringe (16, 32, 48, 64, 80, 96, and 115.2 mg/0.2-mL syringe). Also present in the syringe products are sodium chloride and water for injection. The multiple-dose vials contain benzyl alcohol 14 mg/mL as a preservative. (1)

pH — From 5 to 7.5. (1)

Units — Each milligram of dalteparin sodium is equivalent to 156.25 anti-Factor Xa units. (4)

Trade Name(s) — Fragmin.

Administration — Dalteparin is administered by deep subcutaneous injection to patients who are seated or lying down. It must not be administered by intramuscular injection.

Stability — Intact containers of dalteparin sodium should be stored at controlled room temperature. (1)

Syringes — Dalteparin sodium (Pharmacia & Upjohn) 10,000 units/mL was packaged in 1-mL tuberculin syringes (Becton Dickinson), apparently with the needles left attached, and stored at room temperature of about 25 °C exposed to fluorescent light and under refrigeration at about 4 °C for 15 days. Chromogenic assays of the dalteparin activity were variable, but there was no indication of substantial loss of activity. Dalteparin activity remained at 95% or above of the initial level throughout. An 8% loss of the benzyl alcohol preservative occurred in 10 days and a 10% loss in 15 days in the room temperature samples. Benzyl alcohol losses from refrigerated samples were minimal. Unfortunately, many syringes became non-functional during the study with the fluid unable to be expressed through the attached needles, thus necessitating removal of the needles. The cause of this needle blockage was not addressed. (2323) However, evaporation from the needle tip opening, leaving dried material that blocked the fluid flow, is a possibility.

Dalteparin (Pharmacia) 10,000 and 25,000 units/mL was packaged in 1-mL (Becton Dickinson) and 3-mL (Sherwood) plastic syringes and stored for 30 days at room temperature and 4 °C. No loss of activity was found. (2484)

In another report, the stability of dalteparin 25,000 units/mL packaged in 1-mL polypropylene tuberculin syringes was evaluated over 10 days stored at 22 and 4 °C. Losses of 7 and 4%, respectively, were found at the two storage temperatures. However, eight of 45 test syringes stored at room temperature could not be operated to eject the dalteparin. None of the refrigerated samples exhibited this failure. The authors speculated that precipitation had resulted in blockage. (2546)

Dalteparin injection diluted in sodium chloride 0.9% to 2500 units/mL was packaged in tuberculin syringes and stored for 28 days under refrigeration at 4 °C. Anti-Xa activity determined by chromogenic assay found no significant differences over the course of 28 days. (2774)

Compatibility Information

Solution Compatibility

Dalteparin sodium

Solution	Mfr	Mfr	Conc/L	Remarks	Ref	C/I
Sodium chloride 0.9%			250,000 units	Activity retained for 28 days at 4 °C	2774	C

DAPTOMYCIN
AHFS 8:12.28.12

Products — Daptomycin is available in 500-mg vials with sodium hydroxide to adjust the pH. Reconstitute with 10 mL of sodium chloride 0.9% transferred into the vial slowly directing the stream against the vial wall. Rotate the vial ensuring that the entire daptomycin powder becomes wetted. Allow the reconstituted vial to stand undisturbed for 10 minutes. Then gently rotate or swirl the vial contents to ensure complete dissolution of the powder. Vigorous agitation or shaking of the vial should be avoided to minimize foaming. (1)

Trade Name(s) — Cubicin.

Administration — Reconstituted daptomycin is administered by intravenous injection over two minutes or by intravenous infusion over 30 minutes when diluted in sodium chloride 0.9% to a concentration not exceeding 20 mg/mL. (1; 4)

Stability — Intact vials of daptomycin should be stored under refrigeration at 2 to 8 °C. (1) Although refrigerated storage is required, the manufacturer has stated the drug may be stored at room temperature for 12 months. (2745)

Daptomycin reconstituted as directed is stable for 12 hours at room temperature and 48 hours under refrigeration. Diluted for infusion, daptomycin is also stable for 12 hours at room temperature and 48 hours under refrigeration. However, the time after reconstitution in the vial and after dilution for infusion in the bag together should not exceed a combined time of 12 hours at room temperature and 48 hours under refrigeration. (1)

Compatibility Information

Solution Compatibility

Daptomycin

Solution	Mfr	Mfr	Conc/L	Remarks	Ref	C/I
Dextrose 5%				Incompatible in dextrose solutions	1	I
Ringer's injection, lactated				Compatible	1	C
Sodium chloride 0.9%				Compatible	1	C

Y-Site Injection Compatibility (1:1 Mixture)

Daptomycin

Drug	Mfr	Conc	Mfr	Conc	Remarks	Ref	C/I
Aztreonam	BMS	16.7 mg/mL[a,b]	CUB	16.7 mg/mL[a,b]	Physically compatible with little loss of either drug in 2 hr at 25 °C	2553	C
Caspofungin acetate	ME	0.7 mg/mL[b]	CUB	10 mg/mL[b]	Physically compatible for 4 hr at room temperature	2758	C
Ceftazidime	GSK	16.7 mg/mL[a,b]	CUB	16.7 mg/mL[a,b]	Physically compatible with no loss of either drug in 2 hr at 25 °C	2553	C
Ceftriaxone sodium	RC	16.7 mg/mL[a,b]	CUB	16.7 mg/mL[a,b]	Physically compatible with 4 to 5% loss of both drugs in 2 hr at 25 °C	2553	C

Y-Site Injection Compatibility (1:1 Mixture) (Cont.)

Daptomycin

Drug	Mfr	Conc	Mfr	Conc	Remarks	Ref	C/I
Dopamine HCl	AMR	3.6 mg/mL[a]	CUB	18.2 mg/mL[a,b]	Physically compatible with no loss of either drug in 2 hr at 25 °C	2553	C
Doripenem	JJ	5 mg/mL[a,b]	CUB	10 mg/mL[b]	Physically compatible for 4 hr at 23 °C	2743	C
Fluconazole	PF	1.3 mg/mL[a]	CUB	6.3 mg/mL[a,b]	Physically compatible. No daptomycin loss and 4% fluconazole loss in 2 hr at 25 °C	2553	C
Gentamicin sulfate	AB	1.5 mg/mL[a]	CUB	19.2 mg/mL[a,b]	Physically compatible with no loss of either drug in 2 hr at 25 °C	2553	C
Heparin sodium	ES	98 units/mL[a,b]	CUB	19.6 mg/mL[a,b]	Physically compatible with no loss of either drug in 2 hr at 25 °C	2553	C
Levofloxacin	OMN	7.1 mg/mL[a,b]	CUB	14.3 mg/mL[a,b]	Physically compatible with no loss of either drug in 2 hr at 25 °C	2553	C
Lidocaine HCl	ASZ	3.3 mg/mL[a,b]	CUB	16.7 mg/mL[a,b]	Physically compatible with no loss of either drug in 2 hr at 25 °C	2553	C

[a]*Final concentration after mixing.*
[b]*Tested in sodium chloride 0.9%.*

DAUNORUBICIN HYDROCHLORIDE
AHFS 10:00

Products — Daunorubicin hydrochloride is available in vials containing daunorubicin base 20 mg (21.4 mg as the hydrochloride salt) with mannitol 100 mg. Reconstitute with 4 mL of sterile water for injection to yield a solution containing 5 mg/mL of daunorubicin. (1)

pH — From 4.5 to 6.5. (1; 4)

Trade Name(s) — Cerubidine.

Administration — Daunorubicin hydrochloride is administered intravenously *only*. Extravasation will result in severe tissue damage. The dose may be diluted with 10 to 15 mL of sodium chloride 0.9% and injected over two or three minutes into the sidearm or tubing of a rapidly flowing intravenous infusion of dextrose 5% or sodium chloride 0.9%. (1; 4) Alternatively, the dose has been diluted in 100 mL and infused over 30 to 45 minutes. (4)

In the event of spills or leaks, Wyeth-Ayerst recommends the use of sodium hypochlorite 5% (household bleach) until a colorless liquid results to inactivate daunorubicin hydrochloride. (1200)

Stability — Intact vials of daunorubicin hydrochloride should be stored at controlled room temperature protected from light. The manufacturer states that the reconstituted solution is stable for 24 hours at controlled room temperature and 48 hours under refrigeration. (1; 4)

Immersion of a needle with an aluminum component in daunorubicin hydrochloride (Ives) 5 mg/mL resulted in a darkening of the solution, with black patches forming on the aluminum in 12 to 24 hours at 24 °C with protection from light. (988)

pH Effects — Daunorubicin hydrochloride appears to have pH-dependent stability in solution. (526; 1250) Solutions of daunorubicin hydrochloride are less stable at pH values above 8. Decomposition occurs, as indicated by a color change from red to blue-purple. The drug becomes progressively more stable as the pH of drug–infusion solution admixtures becomes more acidic from 7.4 down to 4.5. (526) The pH range of maximum stability was reported to be approximately 4.5 to 5.5. Below pH 4, decomposition increases substantially. (1207)

Light Effects — Protection of the reconstituted solution from sunlight has been recommended. (1) Photoinactivation of daunorubicin hydrochloride exposed to radiation of 366 nm and fluorescent light has been reported. (1094) One source indicates that significant losses due to light exposure for a sufficient time may occur in concentrations below 100 mcg/mL. However, in clinical concentrations at or above 500 mcg/mL, no special light protection is required. (1369)

Syringes — Daunorubicin hydrochloride (Rhone-Poulenc) 2 mg/mL in polypropylene syringes exhibited little loss in 43 days at 4 °C. (1460)

Filtration — Daunorubicin hydrochloride binds only slightly to cellulose acetate/nitrate (Millex OR) and polytetrafluoroethylene (Millex FG) filters. (1249; 1415; 1416)

Compatibility Information

Solution Compatibility

Daunorubicin HCl

Solution	Mfr	Mfr	Conc/L	Remarks	Ref	C/I
Dextrose 3.3% in sodium chloride 0.3%		RP	100 mg	5% or less loss in 4 weeks at 25 °C in the dark	1007	C
Dextrose 5%	AB	NCI	20 mg	Physically compatible with 2% loss in 24 hr at 21 °C	526	C
		RP	100 mg	5% or less loss in 4 weeks at 25 °C in the dark	1007	C
	[a]	BEL	16 mg	No loss in 7 days at 4 °C protected from light	1700	C
	TR[a]	RP	100 mg	7% or less loss in 43 days at 4 and 25 °C in the dark and at −20 °C	1460	C
		BEL	15.7 mg	5 to 8% loss in 48 hr at room temperature, exposed to light and in the dark, and at 4 °C	1955	C
Ringer's injection, lactated	AB	NCI	20 mg	Physically compatible. 5% loss in 24 hr at 21 °C	526	C
		RP	100 mg	5% or less loss in 4 weeks at 25 °C in the dark	1007	C
Sodium chloride 0.9%	AB	NCI	20 mg	Physically compatible. 3% loss in 24 hr at 21 °C	526	C
		RP	100 mg	5% or less loss in 4 weeks at 25 °C in the dark	1007	C
	[a]	BEL	16 mg	No loss in 7 days at 4 °C protected from light	1700	C
	TR[a]	RP	100 mg	10% or less loss in 43 days at 4 and 25 °C in the dark and at −20 °C	1460	C

[a] Tested in PVC containers.

Additive Compatibility

Daunorubicin HCl

Drug	Mfr	Conc/L	Mfr	Conc/L	Test Soln	Remarks	Ref	C/I
Cytarabine with etoposide	UP BR	267 mg 400 mg	RP	33 mg	D5½S	Physically compatible with about 6% cytarabine loss and no loss of other drugs in 72 hr at 20 °C	1162	C
Cytarabine with etoposide	UP SZ	157 mg 157 mg	BEL	15.7 mg	D5W	Less than 10% loss of any drug in 48 hr at room temperature, exposed to light and in the dark, and at 4 °C	1955	C
Dexamethasone sodium phosphate						Immediate milky precipitation	524	I
Etoposide with cytarabine	BR UP	400 mg 267 mg	RP	33 mg	D5½S	Physically compatible with about 6% cytarabine loss and no loss of other drugs in 72 hr at 20 °C	1162	C
Etoposide with cytarabine	SZ UP	157 mg 157 mg	BEL	15.7 mg	D5W	Less than 10% loss of any drug in 48 hr at room temperature, exposed to light and in the dark, and at 4 °C	1955	C
Heparin sodium	UP	4000 units	FA	200 mg	D5W	Physically incompatible	15	I
Hydrocortisone sodium succinate	UP	500 mg	FA	200 mg	D5W	Physically compatible	15	C

Y-Site Injection Compatibility (1:1 Mixture)

Daunorubicin HCl

Drug	Mfr	Conc	Mfr	Conc	Remarks	Ref	C/I
Allopurinol sodium	BW	3 mg/mL[b]	WY	1 mg/mL[b]	Reddish-purple color and haze form immediately. Reddish-brown particles form within 1 hr	1686	I
Amifostine	USB	10 mg/mL[a]	WY	1 mg/mL[a]	Physically compatible for 4 hr at 23 °C	1845	C
Anidulafungin	VIC	0.5 mg/mL[a]	BED	1 mg/mL[a]	Physically compatible for 4 hr at 23 °C	2617	C
Aztreonam	SQ	40 mg/mL[a]	WY	1 mg/mL[a]	Haze forms immediately	1758	I
Caspofungin acetate	ME	0.7 mg/mL[b]	BED	1 mg/mL[b]	Physically compatible for 4 hr at room temperature	2758	C
Etoposide phosphate	BR	5 mg/mL[a]	BED	1 mg/mL[a]	Physically compatible for 4 hr at 23 °C	2218	C
Filgrastim	AMG	30 mcg/mL[a]	WY	1 mg/mL[a]	Physically compatible for 4 hr at 22 °C	1687	C
Fludarabine phosphate	BX	1 mg/mL[a]	WY	2 mg/mL[a]	Slight haze forms in 4 hr at 22 °C	1439	I
Gemcitabine HCl	LI	10 mg/mL[b]	BED	1 mg/mL[b]	Physically compatible for 4 hr at 23 °C	2226	C
Granisetron HCl	SKB	0.05 mg/mL[a]	CHI	1 mg/mL[a]	Physically compatible for 4 hr at 23 °C	2000	C
Melphalan HCl	BW	0.1 mg/mL[b]	WY	1 mg/mL[b]	Physically compatible for 3 hr at 22 °C	1557	C
Methotrexate sodium		30 mg/mL	BEL	0.52 mg/mL[a]	Visually compatible for 4 hr at room temperature	1788	C
Ondansetron HCl	GL	1 mg/mL[b]	WY	2 mg/mL[a]	Visually compatible for 4 hr at 22 °C	1365	C
Piperacillin sodium–tazobactam sodium	LE[d]	40 + 5 mg/mL[a]	WY	1 mg/mL[a]	Turbidity increases immediately	1688	I
Sodium bicarbonate		1.4%	BEL	0.52 mg/mL[a]	Visually compatible for 4 hr at room temperature	1788	C
Teniposide	BR	0.1 mg/mL[a]	WY	1 mg/mL[a]	Physically compatible for 4 hr at 23 °C	1725	C
Thiotepa	IMM[c]	1 mg/mL[a]	WY	1 mg/mL[a]	Physically compatible for 4 hr at 23 °C	1861	C
Vinorelbine tartrate	BW	1 mg/mL[b]	WY	1 mg/mL[b]	Physically compatible for 4 hr at 22 °C	1558	C

[a]*Tested in dextrose 5%.*
[b]*Tested in sodium chloride 0.9%.*
[c]*Lyophilized formulation tested.*
[d]*Test performed using the formulation WITHOUT edetate disodium.*

DEFEROXAMINE MESYLATE
AHFS 64:00

Products — Deferoxamine mesylate is available in vials containing 500 mg and 2 g of sterile drug in dry form. For intramuscular injection, reconstitute the 500-mg and 2-g vials with 2 and 8 mL, respectively, to yield solutions providing deferoxamine mesylate 213 mg/mL. For intravenous and subcutaneous infusion, reconstitute the 500-mg and 2-g vials with 5 and 20 mL, respectively, to yield solutions providing deferoxamine mesylate 95 mg/mL. (1)

Tonicity — Reconstituted deferoxamine 95 mg/mL is isotonic. (1)

Trade Name(s) — Desferal.

Administration — Deferoxamine mesylate is administered by intramuscular injection, subcutaneous infusion using a portable infusion control device, and by slow intravenous infusion after dilution at an initial rate not exceeding 15 mg/kg/hr for the first 1000 mg. Subsequent dosing should be at a decreased rate not exceeding 125 mg/hr. (1)

Stability — Store the intact vials at temperatures not exceeding 25 °C. Deferoxamine mesylate is a white to off-white powder that forms a clear colorless to yellow solution when reconstituted with sterile water for injection. The manufacturer states that reconstitution with other diluents may result in precipitation. Turbid solutions should not be used. The reconstituted solution is stable for 24 hours at room temperature. The solution should not be refrigerated. (1)

For intravenous infusion, sodium chloride 0.9%, dextrose 5%, or lactated Ringer's injection are recommended for use as diluents. (1)

Syringes — Deferoxamine mesylate (Ciba-Geigy) 250 mg/mL in sterile water for injection 3 mL in 10-mL polypropylene infusion pump syringes (Pharmacia Deltec) had little loss in 14 days of storage at 30 °C. (1967)

Ambulatory Pumps — Deferoxamine mesylate stability was evaluated at concentrations of 210, 285, and 370 mg/mL in sterile water for injection in PVC infusion cassette reservoirs (Pharmacia Deltec) stored at 20 to 23 °C. Analysis was inconclusive because of an inordinate degree of assay variation. However, a white precipitate formed in varying time periods, depending on the concentration. Higher concentrations precipitated more rapidly than lower concentrations. In the 370-mg/mL concentration, precipitation was observed in as little as one day while the 285- and 210-mg/mL concentrations developed precipitation in 9 and 17 days, respectively. This study's inordinate degree of assay variability coupled with the propensity for precipitation preclude a reasonable determination of stability for these high concentrations of deferoxamine mesylate. (672)

Elastomeric Reservoir Pumps — Deferoxamine mesylate (Ciba-Geigy) 5 mg/mL in both dextrose 5% and sodium chloride 0.9% was evaluated for binding potential to natural rubber elastomeric reservoirs (Baxter). No binding was found after storage for two weeks at 35 °C with gentle agitation. (2014)

DEXAMETHASONE SODIUM PHOSPHATE
AHFS 68:04

Products — Dexamethasone sodium phosphate is available as dexamethasone phosphate 4 mg/mL with sodium sulfite 1 mg/mL, benzyl alcohol 10 mg/mL, sodium citrate for isotonicity, and citric acid and sodium hydroxide to adjust pH in water for injection. It is also available as dexamethasone phosphate 10 mg/mL with sodium metabisulfite 1 mg/mL, benzyl alcohol 10 mg/mL, sodium citrate 10 mg/mL, and citric acid and sodium hydroxide to adjust pH in water for injection. (1)

pH — Dexamethasone sodium phosphate injections have a pH range from 7 to 8.5. (1; 17) Dexamethasone sodium phosphate (David Bull) 0.5, 1, and 2 mg/mL in sodium chloride 0.9% for continuous subcutaneous infusion had pH values of 7.3, 7.3, and 7.5, respectively. (2161)

Osmolality — The osmolality of the 4-mg/mL concentration of dexamethasone sodium phosphate (Elkins-Sinn) was determined by freezing-point depression to be 356 mOsm/kg. (1071) Another study reported the osmolality of a dexamethasone injection (manufacturer not noted) to be 255 mOsm/kg. (1233)

Dexamethasone sodium phosphate (David Bull) 0.5, 1, and 2 mg/mL in sodium chloride 0.9% for continuous subcutaneous infusion had osmolalities of 269, 260, and 238 mOsm/kg, respectively. (2161)

Administration — Dexamethasone sodium phosphate 4- and 10-mg/mL may be administered intravenously by direct injection slowly over one to several minutes or by continuous or intermittent intravenous infusion and by intramuscular, intra-articular, intrasynovial, intralesional, or soft-tissue injection. (1; 4)

Stability — The injections should be protected from light and freezing. In addition, dexamethasone sodium phosphate is heat labile and should not be autoclaved to sterilize the vial's exterior. (1; 4)

Dexamethasone sodium phosphate (Lyphomed) was diluted to a concentration of 1 mg/mL with bacteriostatic sodium chloride 0.9% and packaged in 10-mL sterile glass vials. The dilutions remained clear and colorless, and little or no loss of dexamethasone was found after 28 days of storage at 4 and 22 °C. (1940)

Dexamethasone sodium phosphate under simulated summer conditions in paramedic vehicles was exposed to temperatures ranging from 26 to 38 °C over 4 weeks. Analysis found no loss of the drug under these conditions. (2562)

Syringes — The stability of dexamethasone sodium phosphate (Organon Teknica) 10 mg/mL repackaged into 1- and 2.5-mL Glaspak (Becton Dickinson) and 1- and 3-mL plastic (Monoject, Sherwood) syringes was reported. Samples in the Glaspak syringes were stored at 4 and 23 °C, exposed to light and both shaken and unshaken during storage. Samples in plastic syringes were stored only at 23 °C. Not more than 5% loss occurred in the Glaspak syringes after 91 days at either temperature. Similarly, losses in the 3-mL plastic syringes were 7% or less after 55 days while losses in the 1-mL plastic syringes were 3% or less in 35 days; these time periods were the maximum that the plastic syringes were evaluated in this study. No contamination by the rubber components was found to leach into the drug solution. (1897)

Sorption — Dexamethasone sodium phosphate was shown not to exhibit sorption to PVC bags and tubing, polyethylene tubing, Silastic tubing, and polypropylene syringes. (536; 606)

Filtration — Dexamethasone sodium phosphate (MSD) 4 mg/L in dextrose 5%, sodium chloride 0.9%, and Ringer's injection, lactated, filtered over 12 hours through a 5-μm stainless steel depth filter (Argyle Filter Connector), a 0.22-μm cellulose ester membrane filter (Ivex-2 Filter Set), and a 0.22-μm polycarbonate membrane filter (In-Sure Filter Set), showed no significant reduction due to binding to the filters. (320)

In another study, dexamethasone sodium phosphate (MSD) 4 mg/L in dextrose 5% and sodium chloride 0.9% did not display significant sorption to a 0.45-μm cellulose membrane filter (Abbott S-A-I-F) during an eight-hour simulated infusion. (567)

Central Venous Catheter — Dexamethasone sodium phosphate (American Regent) 0.5 mg/mL in dextrose 5% was found to be compatible with the ARROWg+ard Blue Plus (Arrow International) chlorhexidine-bearing triple-lumen central catheter. Essentially complete delivery of the drug was found with little or no drug loss occurring. Furthermore, chlorhexidine delivered from the catheter remained at trace amounts with no substantial increase due to the delivery of the drug through the catheter. (2335)

Compatibility Information

Solution Compatibility

Dexamethasone sodium phosphate

Solution	Mfr	Mfr	Conc/L	Remarks	Ref	C/I
Dextrose 5%	a	AMR	94 and 658 mg	Visually compatible with no loss in 14 days stored at 24 °C protected from light	1875	**C**
Sodium chloride 0.9%	a	AMR	92 and 660 mg	Visually compatible with no loss in 14 days stored at 24 °C protected from light	1875	**C**
	BA[a]	ES	200 and 400 mg	Visually compatible with no loss in 30 days at 4 °C then 2 days at 23 °C	1882	**C**
	BA	APP	0.1 and 1 g[b]	Visually compatible with less than 3% loss in 22 days at 25 °C	2392	**C**
	BA	DB	250 and 500 mg	Visually compatible with 3% or less loss in 48 hr at room temperature	2531	**C**

[a]Tested in PVC containers.
[b]Tested in polypropylene syringes.

Additive Compatibility

Dexamethasone sodium phosphate

Drug	Mfr	Conc/L	Mfr	Conc/L	Test Soln	Remarks	Ref	C/I
Amikacin sulfate	BR	5 g	MSD	40 mg	D5LR, D5R, D5S, D5W, D10W, LR, NS, R, SL	Physically compatible and both stable for 24 hr at 25 °C	294	**C**
	BR	5 g	MSD	40 mg	D2.5S	16% dexamethasone loss in 4 hr at 25 °C	294	**I**
Aminophylline		625 mg		30 mg	D5W	Physically compatible and chemically stable for 24 hr at 4 and 30 °C	521	**C**
Bleomycin sulfate	BR	20 and 30 units	MSD	50 mg	NS	Physically compatible and bleomycin activity retained for 1 week at 4 °C. Dexamethasone not tested	763	**C**
Daunorubicin HCl						Immediate milky precipitation	524	**I**
Diphenhydramine HCl with lorazepam and metoclopramide HCl	ES WY DU	2 g 40 mg 4 g	AMR	400 mg	NS[a]	Rapid lorazepam losses of 8, 10, and 15% at 3, 23, and 30 °C, respectively, in 24 hr. Other drugs stable for 14 days at all three storage temperatures	1733	**I**
Floxacillin sodium	BE	20 g	MSD	4 g	NS	Physically compatible for 72 hr at 15 and 30 °C	1479	**C**
Furosemide	HO	1 g	MSD	4 g	NS	Physically compatible for 72 hr at 15 and 30 °C	1479	**C**
Granisetron HCl	SKB	10 and 40 mg	AMR	92 mg	D5W, NS[b]	Visually compatible. Little loss of either drug in 14 days at 4 and 24 °C in dark	1875	**C**
	SKB	10 and 40 mg	AMR	660 mg	D5W, NS[b]	Visually compatible. Little dexamethasone and 8% granisetron loss in 14 days at 4 and 24 °C in dark	1875	**C**
	BE	55 and 51 mg	MSD	75 and 345 mg	D5W, NS[b]	Visually compatible. Little loss of either drug in 72 hr at room temperature	1884	**C**
Lidocaine HCl	AST	2 g	MSD	4 mg		Physically compatible	24	**C**

Additive Compatibility (Cont.)

Dexamethasone sodium phosphate

Drug	Mfr	Conc/L	Mfr	Conc/L	Test Soln	Remarks	Ref	C/I
Lorazepam with diphenhydramine HCl and metoclopramide HCl	WY ES DU	40 mg 2 g 4 g	AMR	400 mg	NS[a]	Rapid lorazepam losses of 8, 10, and 15% at 3, 23, and 30 °C, respectively, in 24 hr. Other drugs stable for 14 days at all three storage temperatures	1733	I
Meropenem	ZEN	1 and 20 g	MSD	4 g	NS	Visually compatible for 4 hr at room temperature	1994	C
Metoclopramide HCl with diphenhydramine HCl and lorazepam	DU ES WY	4 g 2 g 40 mg	AMR	400 mg	NS[a]	Rapid lorazepam losses of 8, 10, and 15% at 3, 23, and 30 °C, respectively, in 24 hr. Other drugs stable for 14 days at all three storage temperatures	1733	I
Mitomycin	BR	100 mg	LY	5 g	NS[c]	Visually compatible. 10% calculated loss of mitomycin in 68 hr and dexamethasone in 250 hr at 25 °C	1866	C
	BR	100 mg	LY	5 g	NS[b]	Visually compatible. 10% calculated loss of mitomycin in 91 hr and dexamethasone in 154 hr at 25 °C	1866	C
	BR	100 mg	LY	5 g	NS[c]	Visually compatible. 10% calculated loss of mitomycin in 211 hr and dexamethasone in 98 hr at 4 °C	1866	C
	BR	100 mg	LY	5 g	NS[b]	Visually compatible. 10% calculated loss of mitomycin in 238 hr and dexamethasone in 355 hr at 4 °C	1866	C
Nafcillin sodium	WY	500 mg	MSD	4 mg		Physically compatible	27	C
Ondansetron HCl	GL	48 mg		20 and 40 mg	D5W, NS	Visually compatible for 24 hr at 22 °C	1608	C
	GL	160 mg		200 and 400 mg	NS	Visually compatible for 24 hr at 22 °C	1608	C
	CER	100 mg	ES	200 mg	NS[b]	Visually compatible. No dexamethasone and 8% ondansetron loss in 30 days at 4 °C then 2 days at 23 °C	1882	C
	CER	100 and 200 mg	ES	400 mg	NS[b]	Visually compatible. No dexamethasone and 7 to 10% ondansetron loss in 30 days at 4 °C then 2 days at 23 °C	1882	C
	CER	200, 400, 640 mg	ES	200 mg	NS[b]	Visually compatible. No dexamethasone and 5% ondansetron loss in 30 days at 4 °C then 2 days at 23 °C	1882	C
	CER	400 and 640 mg	ES	400 mg	NS[b]	Visually compatible. No dexamethasone and 3% ondansetron loss in 30 days at 4 °C then 2 days at 23 °C	1882	C
	CER	640 mg	ES	200 and 400 mg	D5W[d]	Visually compatible. 7% dexamethasone and no ondansetron loss in 30 days at 4 °C then 2 days at 23 °C	1882	C
	GL	150 mg	MSD	400 mg	NS[b]	Visually compatible. 4% or less loss of either drug in 28 days at 4 and 22 °C	2084	C
	GL	150 mg	MSD	400 mg	D5W[b]	Visually compatible. 4% or less loss of either drug in 28 days at 4 °C. 10% ondansetron loss in 3 days at 22 °C	2084	C
	GL	750 mg	MSD	230 mg	NS[b]	Visually compatible. 4% or less loss of either drug in 28 days at 4 °C. 10% ondansetron loss in 7 days at 22 °C	2084	C
	GL	750 mg	MSD	230 mg	D5W[b]	Visually compatible. Up to 13% ondansetron loss in 3 days at 4 and 22 °C	2084	?

Additive Compatibility (Cont.)

Dexamethasone sodium phosphate

Drug	Mfr	Conc/L	Mfr	Conc/L	Test Soln	Remarks	Ref	C/I
	GSK	80 mg	OR	100 mg	D5W[f]	Visually compatible. Under 3% ondansetron and 8% dexamethasone loss when frozen for 3 months then stored refrigerated for 30 days	2822	C
Oxycodone HCl	NAP	0.8 g	FAU	0.8 g	NS, W	Visually compatible. Under 4% concentration change in 24 hr at 25 °C	2600	C
Palonosetron HCl	MGI	5 mg	AMR	200 and 400 mg	D5W, NS[b]	Physically compatible. Little loss of either drug in 48 hr at 23 °C in light and 14 days at 4 °C	2552	C
Prochlorperazine edisylate	SKF	100 mg	MSD	20 mg	D5W	Physically compatible	15	C
Ranitidine HCl	GL	50 mg and 2 g		40 mg	D5W	Physically compatible. Ranitidine stable for 24 hr at 25 °C. Dexamethasone not tested	1515	C
Tramadol HCl	AND	11.18 g	ME	440 mg	NS[e]	Visually compatible for 7 days at 25 °C protected from light	2701	C
	AND	33.3 g	ME	1.33 g	NS[e]	Visually compatible for 7 days at 25 °C protected from light	2701	C
Verapamil HCl	KN	80 mg	MSD	40 mg	D5W, NS	Physically compatible for 24 hr	764	C

[a]Tested in Pharmacia-Deltec PVC pump reservoirs.
[b]Tested in PVC containers.
[c]Tested in glass containers.
[d]Tested in ondansetron hydrochloride ready-to-use CR3 polyester bags.
[e]Tested in elastomeric pump reservoirs (Baxter).
[f]Tested in polyolefin containers.

Drugs in Syringe Compatibility

Dexamethasone sodium phosphate

Drug (in syringe)	Mfr	Amt	Mfr	Amt	Remarks	Ref	C/I
Caffeine citrate		20 mg/1 mL	ES	4 mg/1 mL	Visually compatible for 4 hr at 25 °C	2440	C
Dimenhydrinate		10 mg/1 mL		10 mg/1 mL	Clear solution	2569	C
Diphenhydramine HCl	PD	50 mg/mL[a]	DB, SX	4 and 10 mg/mL[a]	White turbidity and precipitate form immediately	1542	I
	PD	4.54 mg/mL[b]	DB	9.52 mg/mL[b]	Visually compatible for 24 hr at 24 °C	1542	C
	PD	4.54 to 15 mg/mL[b]	DB	5 to 9.02 mg/mL[b]	Precipitate forms	1542	I
	PD	34.8 to 40 mg/mL[b]	SX	2 mg/mL[b]	Visually compatible for 24 hr at 24 °C	1542	C
	PD	25 mg/mL[b]	SX	1 mg/mL[b]	Precipitate forms	1542	I
Doxapram HCl	RB	400 mg/20 mL	MSD	3.3 mg/1 mL	Immediate turbidity and precipitation	1177	I

Drugs in Syringe Compatibility (Cont.)

Dexamethasone sodium phosphate

Drug (in syringe)	Mfr	Amt	Mfr	Amt	Remarks	Ref	C/I
Furosemide	HO	3.33 to 10 mg/mL	ME	0.33 to 3.33 mg/mL	Tested in NS. No visible precipitation with under 10% loss of either drug in 5 days at 4 and 25 °C. Precipitation with over 10% drug loss in 15 days	2711	**C**
Glycopyrrolate	RB	0.2 mg/1 mL	MSD	4 mg/1 mL	Physically compatible for 48 hr at 25 °C. pH >6.0. 5% glycopyrrolate loss may occur in 4 to 7 hr	331	**I**
	RB	0.2 mg/1 mL	MSD	8 mg/2 mL	Physically compatible for 48 hr at 25 °C. pH >6.0. 5% glycopyrrolate loss may occur in 4 to 7 hr	331	**I**
	RB	0.4 mg/2 mL	MSD	4 mg/1 mL	Physically compatible for 48 hr at 25 °C. pH >6.0. 5% glycopyrrolate loss may occur in 4 to 7 hr	331	**I**
	RB	0.2 mg/1 mL	MSD	24 mg/1 mL	Physically compatible for 48 hr at 25 °C. pH >6.0. 5% glycopyrrolate loss may occur in 4 to 7 hr	331	**I**
	RB	0.2 mg/1 mL	MSD	48 mg/2 mL	Physically compatible for 48 hr at 25 °C. pH >6.0. 5% glycopyrrolate loss may occur in 4 to 7 hr	331	**I**
	RB	0.4 mg/2 mL	MSD	24 mg/1 mL	Physically compatible for 48 hr at 25 °C. pH >6.0. 5% glycopyrrolate loss may occur in 4 to 7 hr	331	**I**
Granisetron HCl	BE	0.15 mg/mL[c]	MSD	0.2 and 1 mg/mL[c]	Visually compatible. Little loss of either drug in 72 hr at room temperature	1884	**C**
Hydromorphone HCl	KN	2, 10, 40 mg/mL[a]	SX	4 mg/mL[a]	Visually compatible and both drugs stable for 24 hr at 24 °C	1542	**C**
	KN	2 and 10 mg/mL[a]	DB	10 mg/mL[a]	Visually compatible and both drugs stable for 24 hr at 24 °C	1542	**C**
	KN	40 mg/mL[a]	DB	10 mg/mL[a]	White turbidity forms immediately	1542	**I**
	KN	11.6 mg/mL[b]	DB	7.1 mg/mL[b]	Visually compatible for 24 hr at 24 °C	1542	**C**
	KN	13.3 to 17.5 mg/mL[b]	DB	5.5 to 6.6 mg/mL[b]	Precipitate forms	1542	**I**
	KN	10.5 mg/mL[b]	DB	4.75 mg/mL[b]	Visually compatible for 24 hr at 24 °C	1542	**C**
	KN	14.75 to 25 mg/mL[b]	DB	3 to 4.1 mg/mL[b]	Precipitate forms	1542	**I**
	KN	26.66 mg/mL[b]	SX	3.34 mg/mL[b]	Visually compatible for 24 hr at 24 °C	1542	**C**
Ketamine HCl	PF	1 mg	OR	50 and 600 mg	Diluted to 14 mL with NS. Physically compatible with no loss of either drug in 8 days at 4 and 23 °C	2677	**C**
Metoclopramide HCl	RB	10 mg/2 mL	ES, MSD	8 mg/2 mL	Physically compatible for 48 hr at 25 °C	1167	**C**
	RB	160 mg/32 mL	ES, MSD	8 mg/2 mL	Physically compatible for 48 hr at 25 °C	1167	**C**

Drugs in Syringe Compatibility (Cont.)

Dexamethasone sodium phosphate

Drug (in syringe)	Mfr	Amt	Mfr	Amt	Remarks	Ref	C/I
Midazolam HCl	RC	2.5 mg/ 8 mL	DB	2 mg/ 8 mL	Diluted in NS. Visually clear. No dexamethasone loss in 48 hr. Midazolam losses over 10% beyond 24 hr at room temperature	2531	C
	RC	5 mg/ 8 mL	DB	2 mg/ 8 mL	Diluted in NS. Visually clear. No dexamethasone loss in 48 hr. Midazolam losses were 7% in 48 hr at room temperature	2531	C
	RC	5 mg/ 8 mL	DB	4 mg/ 8 mL	Diluted in NS. Cloudiness forms immediately	2531	I
	RC	7.5 mg/ 8 mL	DB	4 mg/ 8 mL	Diluted in NS. Cloudiness forms immediately	2531	I
	RC	7.5 mg/ 8 mL	DB	2 mg/ 8 mL	Diluted in NS. Crystals form in some samples within 24 hr	2531	I
Ondansetron HCl	CER	0.17 mg/ mL[d]	ES	0.33 and 0.67 mg/ mL[d]	Visually compatible. No loss of either drug in 30 days at 4 °C then 2 days at 23 °C	1882	C
	CER	0.25 mg/ mL[d]	ES	0.5 mg/ mL[d]	Visually compatible. No loss of either drug in 30 days at 4 °C then 2 days at 23 °C	1882	C
	CER	0.25 mg/ mL[d]	ES	1 mg/ mL[d]	Visually compatible for 3 days at 4 °C. Precipitation of ondansetron observed at 7 days as opaque white ring	1882	C
	CER	0.33 mg/ mL[d]	ES	0.33 and 0.67 mg/ mL[d]	Visually compatible. No loss of either drug in 30 days at 4 °C then 2 days at 23 °C	1882	C
	CER	0.5 mg/ mL[d]	ES	0.5 mg/ mL[d]	Visually compatible. No loss of either drug in 30 days at 4 °C then 2 days at 23 °C	1882	C
	CER	0.5 mg/ mL[d]	ES	1 mg/ mL[d]	Visually compatible for 3 days at 4 °C. Precipitation of ondansetron observed at 5 days as opaque white ring	1882	C
	CER	0.67 mg/ mL[d]	ES	0.33 and 0.67 mg/ mL[d]	Visually compatible. No loss of either drug in 30 days at 4 °C then 2 days at 23 °C	1882	C
	CER	1.07 mg/ mL[d]	ES	0.33 mg/ mL[d]	Visually compatible. No loss of either drug in 30 days at 4 °C then 2 days at 23 °C	1882	C
	CER	1.07 mg/ mL[d]	ES	0.67 mg/ mL[d]	Heavy white precipitate in 72 hr at 4 °C. 25 to 30% loss of both drugs	1882	I
		4 mg/ 2 mL	OM[h]	4 mg/ 1 mL	Physically incompatible within 3 min	2767	I
		4 mg/ 2 mL	[i]	4 mg/ 1 mL	Physically compatible	2767	C
Oxycodone HCl	NAP	200 mg/ 20 mL	FAU	40 mg/ 10 mL	Visually compatible. Under 4% concentration change in 24 hr at 25 °C	2600	C
Palonosetron HCl	MGI	0.25 mg/ 5 mL	AMR	3.3 mg/ 5 mL[e,f]	Physically compatible. Little loss of either drug in 48 hr at 23 °C in light and 14 days at 4 °C	2552	C
Pantoprazole sodium	[g]	4 mg/ 1 mL		10 mg/ 1 mL	Precipitates immediately	2574	I
Ranitidine HCl	GL	50 mg/ 5 mL	ME	4 mg	Physically compatible for 4 hr at ambient temperature under fluorescent light	1151	C

Drugs in Syringe Compatibility (Cont.)

Dexamethasone sodium phosphate

Drug (in syringe)	Mfr	Amt	Mfr	Amt	Remarks	Ref	C/I
Tramadol HCl	GRU	33.33, 16.66, 8.33 mg/mL[f]	ME	3.33, 1.67, 1.33, 0.33 mg/mL[f]	Physically compatible and both drugs chemically stable for 5 days at 25 °C protected from light	2747	C

[a] Mixed in equal quantities. Final concentration is one-half the indicated concentration.
[b] Mixed in varying quantities to yield the final concentrations noted.
[c] Diluted with water.
[d] Diluted with sodium chloride 0.9% drawn into a syringe prior to drugs to yield the concentrations cited.
[e] Tested in dextrose 5%.
[f] Tested in sodium chloride 0.9%.
[g] Test performed using the formulation WITHOUT edetate disodium.
[h] Contained benzyl alcohol as a preservative.
[i] Contained parabens as preservatives.

Y-Site Injection Compatibility (1:1 Mixture)

Dexamethasone sodium phosphate

Drug	Mfr	Conc	Mfr	Conc	Remarks	Ref	C/I
Acyclovir sodium	BW	5 mg/mL[a]	ES	0.2 mg/mL[a]	Physically compatible for 4 hr at 25 °C	1157	C
	BV	5 mg/mL[b]	APP	4 mg/mL	Physically compatible	2794	C
Allopurinol sodium	BW	3 mg/mL[b]	LY	1 mg/mL[b]	Physically compatible for 4 hr at 22 °C	1686	C
Amifostine	USB	10 mg/mL[a]	AMR	1 mg/mL[a]	Physically compatible for 4 hr at 23 °C	1845	C
Amikacin sulfate	SQ	50 mg/mL[c]	AMR	4 mg/mL	Visually compatible for 24 hr at room temperature in test tubes. No precipitate found on filter from Y-site delivery	2063	C
Amphotericin B cholesteryl sulfate complex	SEQ	0.83 mg/mL[a]	ES	2 mg/mL[a]	Physically compatible for 4 hr at 23 °C	2117	C
Amsacrine	NCI	1 mg/mL[a]	QU	1 mg/mL[a]	Visually compatible for 4 hr at 22 °C	1381	C
Anidulafungin	VIC	0.5 mg/mL[a]	AMR	1 mg/mL[a]	Physically compatible for 4 hr at 23 °C	2617	C
Aztreonam	SQ	40 mg/mL[a]	AMR	1 mg/mL[a]	Physically compatible for 4 hr at 23 °C	1758	C
Bivalirudin	TMC	5 mg/mL[a]	APP	1 mg/mL[a]	Physically compatible for 4 hr at 23 °C	2373	C
Ceftaroline fosamil	FOR	2.22 mg/mL[g]	SIC	1 mg/mL[g]	Physically compatible for 4 hr at 23 °C	2826	C
Ciprofloxacin	MI	2 mg/mL[e]	LY	4 mg/mL	Cloudiness rapidly dissipates. White crystals form in 1 hr at 24 °C	1655	I
Cisatracurium besylate	GW	0.1, 2, 5 mg/mL[a]	FUJ	2 mg/mL[a]	Physically compatible for 4 hr at 23 °C	2074	C
Cladribine	ORT	0.015[b] and 0.5[f] mg/mL	AMR	1 mg/mL[b]	Physically compatible for 4 hr at 23 °C	1969	C
Dexmedetomidine HCl	AB	4 mcg/mL[b]	AMR	1 mg/mL[b]	Physically compatible for 4 hr at 23 °C	2383	C
Docetaxel	RPR	0.9 mg/mL[a]	ES	2 mg/mL[a]	Physically compatible for 4 hr at 23 °C	2224	C
Doripenem	JJ	5 mg/mL[a,b]	APP	1 mg/mL[a,b]	Physically compatible for 4 hr at 23 °C	2743	C
Doxorubicin HCl liposomal	SEQ	0.4 mg/mL[a]	ES	2 mg/mL[a]	Physically compatible for 4 hr at 23 °C	2087	C
Etoposide phosphate	BR	5 mg/mL[a]	ES	1 mg/mL[a]	Physically compatible for 4 hr at 23 °C	2218	C
Famotidine	MSD	0.2 mg/mL[a]	ES	10 mg/mL	Physically compatible for 14 hr	1196	C
	ME	2 mg/mL[b]		1 mg/mL[a]	Visually compatible for 4 hr at 22 °C	1936	C
Fenoldopam mesylate	AB	80 mcg/mL[b]	AMR	1 mg/mL[b]	Trace haze forms immediately	2467	I

Y-Site Injection Compatibility (1:1 Mixture) (Cont.)

Dexamethasone sodium phosphate

Drug	Mfr	Conc	Mfr	Conc	Remarks	Ref	C/I
Fentanyl citrate	JN	0.025 mg/mL[a]	AMR	1 mg/mL[a]	Physically compatible for 48 hr at 22 °C	1706	C
Filgrastim	AMG	30 mcg/mL[a]	LY	1 mg/mL[a]	Physically compatible for 4 hr at 22 °C	1687	C
Fluconazole	RR	2 mg/mL	ES	4 mg/mL	Physically compatible for 24 hr at 25 °C	1407	C
Fludarabine phosphate	BX	1 mg/mL[a]	MSD	1 mg/mL[a]	Visually compatible for 4 hr at 22 °C	1439	C
Foscarnet sodium	AST	24 mg/mL	OR	10 mg/mL	Physically compatible for 24 hr at room temperature under fluorescent light	1335	C
Gallium nitrate	FUJ	1 mg/mL[b]	AMR	4 mg/mL	Visually compatible for 24 hr at 25 °C	1673	C
Gemcitabine HCl	LI	10 mg/mL[b]	ES	1 mg/mL[b]	Physically compatible for 4 hr at 23 °C	2226	C
Granisetron HCl	SKB	1 mg/mL	ME	0.24 mg/mL[b]	Physically compatible with little or no loss of either drug in 4 hr at 22 °C	1883	C
Heparin sodium	TR	50 units/mL	ES	0.08 mg/mL[a]	Visually compatible for 4 hr at 25 °C	1793	C
Heparin sodium[m]	RI	1000 units/L[g]	MSD	4 mg/mL	Physically compatible for 4 hr at room temperature	322	C
Hetastarch in lactated electrolyte	AB	6%	APP	1 mg/mL[a]	Physically compatible for 4 hr at 23 °C	2339	C
Hydrocortisone sodium succinate[n]	UP	100 mg/L[g]	MSD	4 mg/mL	Physically compatible for 4 hr at room temperature	322	C
Hydromorphone HCl	AST	0.5 mg/mL[a]	AMR	1 mg/mL[a]	Physically compatible for 48 hr at 22 °C	1706	C
Idarubicin HCl	AD	1 mg/mL[b]	OR	10 mg/mL	Haze forms immediately and precipitate forms in 20 min	1525	I
	AD	1 mg/mL[b]	AMR	0.2 mg/mL[b]	Haze forms in 20 min	1525	I
Levofloxacin	OMN	5 mg/mL[a]	ES	4 mg/mL	Visually compatible for 4 hr at 24 °C	2233	C
Linezolid	PHU	2 mg/mL	FUJ	1 mg/mL[a]	Physically compatible for 4 hr at 23 °C	2264	C
Lorazepam	WY	0.33 mg/mL[b]		4 mg/mL	Visually compatible for 24 hr at 22 °C	1855	C
Melphalan HCl	BW	0.1 mg/mL[b]	LY	1 mg/mL[b]	Physically compatible for 3 hr at 22 °C	1557	C
Meperidine HCl	AB	10 mg/mL	LY	0.2 mg/mL[a]	Physically compatible for 4 hr at 25 °C	1397	C
Meropenem	ZEN	1 and 50 mg/mL[b]	MSD	10 mg/mL[h]	Visually compatible for 4 hr at room temperature	1994	C
Methadone HCl	LI	1 mg/mL[a]	AMR	1 mg/mL[a]	Physically compatible for 48 hr at 22 °C	1706	C
Methotrexate sodium		30 mg/mL	MSD	4 mg/mL	Visually compatible for 2 hr at room temperature. Precipitate forms in 4 hr	1788	I
Midazolam HCl	RC	1 mg/mL[a]	ES	4 mg/mL	Immediate haze. Precipitate in 8 hr	1847	I
	RC	5 mg/mL		4 mg/mL	White precipitate forms immediately	1855	I
Milrinone lactate	SS	0.2 mg/mL[a]	ES	10 mg/mL[a]	Visually compatible for 4 hr at 25 °C	2381	C
Morphine sulfate	AB	1 mg/mL	LY	0.2 mg/mL[a]	Physically compatible for 4 hr at 25 °C	1397	C
	AST	1 mg/mL[a]	AMR	1 mg/mL[a]	Physically compatible for 48 hr at 22 °C	1706	C
Ondansetron HCl	GL	1 mg/mL[b]	MSD	1 mg/mL[a]	Visually compatible for 4 hr at 22 °C	1365	C
Oxaliplatin	SS	0.5 mg/mL[a]	AMR	1 mg/mL[a]	Physically compatible for 4 hr at 23 °C	2566	C
Paclitaxel	NCI	1.2 mg/mL[a]		1 mg/mL[a]	Physically compatible for 4 hr at 22 °C	1528	C
Pemetrexed disodium	LI	20 mg/mL[b]	AMR	1 mg/mL[a]	Physically compatible for 4 hr at 23 °C	2564	C
Piperacillin sodium–tazobactam sodium	LE[l]	40 + 5 mg/mL[a]	LY	1 mg/mL[a]	Physically compatible for 4 hr at 22 °C	1688	C

Y-Site Injection Compatibility (1:1 Mixture) (Cont.)

Dexamethasone sodium phosphate

Drug	Mfr	Conc	Mfr	Conc	Remarks	Ref	C/I
Potassium chloride		40 mEq/L[g]	MSD	4 mg/mL	Physically compatible for 4 hr at room temperature	322	C
Propofol	ZEN	10 mg/mL	AMR	1 mg/mL[a]	Physically compatible for 1 hr at 23 °C	2066	C
Remifentanil HCl	GW	0.025 and 0.25 mg/mL[b]	FUJ	2 mg/mL[a]	Physically compatible for 4 hr at 23 °C	2075	C
Sargramostim	IMM	10 mcg/mL[b]	ES	1 mg/mL[b]	Visually compatible for 4 hr at 22 °C	1436	C
Sodium bicarbonate		1.4%	MSD	4 mg/mL	Visually compatible for 4 hr at room temperature	1788	C
Tacrolimus	FUJ	1 mg/mL[b]	ES	4 mg/mL[a]	Visually compatible for 24 hr at 25 °C	1630	C
Telavancin HCl	ASP	7.5 mg/mL[g]	AMR	1 mg/mL[g]	Physically compatible for 2 hr	2830	C
Teniposide	BR	0.1 mg/mL[a]	LY	1 mg/mL[a]	Physically compatible for 4 hr at 23 °C	1725	C
Theophylline	TR	4 mg/mL	ES	0.08 mg/mL[a]	Visually compatible for 6 hr at 25 °C	1793	C
Thiotepa	IMM[j]	1 mg/mL[a]	AMR	1 mg/mL[a]	Physically compatible for 4 hr at 23 °C	1861	C
TNA #218 to #226[k]			FUJ, ES	1 mg/mL[a]	Visually compatible for 4 hr at 23 °C	2215	C
Topotecan HCl	SKB	56 mcg/mL[b]	RU	4 mg/mL	Haze and color change to intense yellow occur immediately	2245	I
TPN #203, #204[k]			AMR	4 mg/mL	Visually compatible for 2 hr at 23 °C	1974	C
TPN #212 to #215[k]			AMR	1 mg/mL[a]	Physically compatible for 4 hr at 23 °C	2109	C
Vinorelbine tartrate	BW	1 mg/mL[b]	LY	1 mg/mL[b]	Physically compatible for 4 hr at 22 °C	1558	C
Zidovudine	BW	4 mg/mL[a]	ES	0.16 mg/mL[a]	Physically compatible for 4 hr at 25 °C	1193	C

[a]*Tested in dextrose 5%.*
[b]*Tested in sodium chloride 0.9%.*
[c]*Tested in sodium chloride 0.45%.*
[d]*Tested in dextrose 5%, Ringer's injection, lactated, sodium chloride 0.45%, and sodium chloride 0.9%.*
[e]*Tested in both dextrose 5% and sodium chloride 0.9%.*
[f]*Tested in bacteriostatic sodium chloride 0.9% preserved with benzyl alcohol 0.9%.*
[g]*Tested in dextrose 5%, Ringer's injection, lactated, and sodium chloride 0.9%.*
[h]*Tested in sterile water for injection.*
[i]*Tested in dextrose 5% with sodium bicarbonate 0.05 mEq/mL.*
[j]*Lyophilized formulation tested.*
[k]*Refer to Appendix I for the composition of the parenteral nutrition solutions. TNA indicates a 3-in-1 admixture, and TPN indicates a 2-in-1 admixture.*
[l]*Test performed using the formulation WITHOUT edetate disodium.*
[m]*Tested in combination with hydrocortisone sodium succinate (Upjohn) 100 mg/L.*
[n]*Tested in combination with heparin sodium (Riker) 1000 units/L.*

DEXMEDETOMIDINE HYDROCHLORIDE
AHFS 28:24.92

Products — Dexmedetomidine hydrochloride is available as a concentrate providing 100 mcg/mL of dexmedetomidine as the hydrochloride in 2-mL (200-mcg) vials. Each milliliter also contains sodium chloride 9 mg in water for injection. The drug must be diluted in sodium chloride 0.9% for administration. (1)

pH — From 4.5 to 7.0. (1)

Trade Name(s) — Precedex.

Administration — Dexmedetomidine hydrochloride is administered by slow intravenous infusion using a controlled infusion device over periods not exceeding 24 hours. To prepare a 4-mcg/mL dilution, the manufacturer recommends adding 2 mL of the injection to 48 mL of sodium chloride 0.9% and shake gently to mix. (1; 4)

Stability — Intact single-use vials of the clear, colorless injection should be stored at controlled room temperature. (1)

Sorption — Dexmedetomidine hydrochloride is known to undergo sorption to some types of natural rubber. Although the drug is dosed to effect, the manufacturer recommends the use of administration equipment with synthetic rubber or coated natural rubber gaskets. (1)

Compatibility Information

Solution Compatibility

Dexmedetomidine HCl

Solution	Mfr	Mfr	Conc/L	Remarks	Ref	C/I
Dextrose 5%		HOS		Stated to be compatible	1	C
Ringer's injection, lactated		HOS		Stated to be compatible	1	C
Sodium chloride 0.9%		HOS		Stated to be compatible	1	C

Y-Site Injection Compatibility (1:1 Mixture)

Dexmedetomidine HCl

Drug	Mfr	Conc	Mfr	Conc	Remarks	Ref	C/I
Alfentanil HCl	TAY	0.5 mg/mL	AB	4 mcg/mL[b]	Physically compatible for 4 hr at 23 °C	2383	C
Amikacin sulfate	APO	5 mg/mL[b]	AB	4 mcg/mL[b]	Physically compatible for 4 hr at 23 °C	2383	C
Aminophylline	AB	2.5 mg/mL[b]	AB	4 mcg/mL[b]	Physically compatible for 4 hr at 23 °C	2383	C
Amiodarone HCl	WAY	4 mg/mL[b]	AB	4 mcg/mL[b]	Physically compatible for 4 hr at 23 °C	2383	C
Amphotericin B	APO	0.6 mg/mL[a]	AB	4 mcg/mL[b]	Yellow precipitate forms immediately	2383	I
Ampicillin sodium	APO	20 mg/mL[b]	AB	4 mcg/mL[b]	Physically compatible for 4 hr at 23 °C	2383	C
Ampicillin sodium–sulbactam sodium	PF	20 + 10 mg/mL[b]	AB	4 mcg/mL[b]	Physically compatible for 4 hr at 23 °C	2383	C
Atracurium besylate			HOS		Stated to be compatible	1	C
Atropine sulfate			HOS		Stated to be compatible	1	C
Azithromycin	PF	2 mg/mL[b]	AB	4 mcg/mL[b]	Physically compatible for 4 hr at 23 °C	2383	C
Aztreonam	BMS	40 mg/mL[b]	AB	4 mcg/mL[b]	Physically compatible for 4 hr at 23 °C	2383	C
Bumetanide	BED	40 mcg/mL[b]	AB	4 mcg/mL[b]	Physically compatible for 4 hr at 23 °C	2383	C
Butorphanol tartrate	APO	40 mcg/mL[b]	AB	4 mcg/mL[b]	Physically compatible for 4 hr at 23 °C	2383	C
Calcium gluconate	APP	40 mg/mL[b]	AB	4 mcg/mL[b]	Physically compatible for 4 hr at 23 °C	2383	C
Cefazolin sodium	LI	20 mg/mL[b]	AB	4 mcg/mL[b]	Physically compatible for 4 hr at 23 °C	2383	C
Cefepime HCl	BMS	20 mg/mL[b]	AB	4 mcg/mL[b]	Physically compatible for 4 hr at 23 °C	2383	C
Cefotaxime sodium	HO	20 mg/mL[b]	AB	4 mcg/mL[b]	Physically compatible for 4 hr at 23 °C	2383	C
Cefotetan disodium	ZEN	20 mg/mL[b]	AB	4 mcg/mL[b]	Physically compatible for 4 hr at 23 °C	2383	C
Cefoxitin sodium	ME	20 mg/mL[b]	AB	4 mcg/mL[b]	Physically compatible for 4 hr at 23 °C	2383	C
Ceftazidime	GW	40 mg/mL[b]	AB	4 mcg/mL[b]	Physically compatible for 4 hr at 23 °C	2383	C
Ceftriaxone sodium	RC	20 mg/mL[b]	AB	4 mcg/mL[b]	Physically compatible for 4 hr at 23 °C	2383	C
Cefuroxime sodium	GW	30 mg/mL[b]	AB	4 mcg/mL[b]	Physically compatible for 4 hr at 23 °C	2383	C
Chlorpromazine HCl	ES	2 mg/mL[b]	AB	4 mcg/mL[b]	Physically compatible for 4 hr at 23 °C	2383	C
Ciprofloxacin	BAY	1 mg/mL[b]	AB	4 mcg/mL[b]	Physically compatible for 4 hr at 23 °C	2383	C
Cisatracurium besylate	GW	0.5 mg/mL[b]	AB	4 mcg/mL[b]	Physically compatible for 4 hr at 23 °C	2383	C
Clindamycin phosphate	AB	10 mg/mL[b]	AB	4 mcg/mL[b]	Physically compatible for 4 hr at 23 °C	2383	C
Dexamethasone sodium phosphate	AMR	1 mg/mL[b]	AB	4 mcg/mL[b]	Physically compatible for 4 hr at 23 °C	2383	C
Diazepam	AB	5 mg/mL	AB	4 mcg/mL[b]	White turbid precipitate forms immediately	2383	I
Digoxin	ES	0.25 mg/mL	AB	4 mcg/mL[b]	Physically compatible for 4 hr at 23 °C	2383	C

Y-Site Injection Compatibility (1:1 Mixture) (Cont.)

Dexmedetomidine HCl

Drug	Mfr	Conc	Mfr	Conc	Remarks	Ref	C/I
Diltiazem HCl	BA	5 mg/mL	AB	4 mcg/mL[b]	Physically compatible for 4 hr at 23 °C	2383	C
Diphenhydramine HCl	PD	2 mg/mL[b]	AB	4 mcg/mL[b]	Physically compatible for 4 hr at 23 °C	2383	C
Dobutamine HCl	AST	4 mg/mL[b]	AB	4 mcg/mL[b]	Physically compatible for 4 hr at 23 °C	2383	C
Dolasetron mesylate	HO	2 mg/mL[b]	AB	4 mcg/mL[b]	Physically compatible for 4 hr at 23 °C	2383	C
Dopamine HCl	AB	3.2 mg/mL[b]	AB	4 mcg/mL[b]	Physically compatible for 4 hr at 23 °C	2383	C
Doxycycline hyclate	APP	1 mg/mL[b]	AB	4 mcg/mL[b]	Physically compatible for 4 hr at 23 °C	2383	C
Droperidol	AMR	2.5 mg/mL	AB	4 mcg/mL[b]	Physically compatible for 4 hr at 23 °C	2383	C
Enalaprilat	BED	0.1 mg/mL[b]	AB	4 mcg/mL[b]	Physically compatible for 4 hr at 23 °C	2383	C
Ephedrine sulfate	TAY	5 mg/mL[b]	AB	4 mcg/mL[b]	Physically compatible for 4 hr at 23 °C	2383	C
Epinephrine HCl	AMR	50 mcg/mL[b]	AB	4 mcg/mL[b]	Physically compatible for 4 hr at 23 °C	2383	C
Erythromycin lactobionate	AB	5 mg/mL[b]	AB	4 mcg/mL[b]	Physically compatible for 4 hr at 23 °C	2383	C
Esmolol HCl	BA	10 mg/mL[b]	AB	4 mcg/mL[b]	Physically compatible for 4 hr at 23 °C	2383	C
Etomidate			HOS		Stated to be compatible	1	C
Famotidine	ME	2 mg/mL[b]	AB	4 mcg/mL[b]	Physically compatible for 4 hr at 23 °C	2383	C
Fenoldopam mesylate	AB	80 mcg/mL[b]	AB	4 mcg/mL[b]	Physically compatible for 4 hr at 23 °C	2383	C
Fentanyl citrate			HOS		Stated to be compatible	1	C
Fluconazole	PF	2 mg/mL	AB	4 mcg/mL[b]	Physically compatible for 4 hr at 23 °C	2383	C
Furosemide	AMR	3 mg/mL[b]	AB	4 mcg/mL[b]	Physically compatible for 4 hr at 23 °C	2383	C
Gentamicin sulfate	APP	5 mg/mL[b]	AB	4 mcg/mL[b]	Physically compatible for 4 hr at 23 °C	2383	C
Glycopyrrolate			HOS		Stated to be compatible	1	C
Granisetron HCl	SKB	50 mcg/mL[b]	AB	4 mcg/mL[b]	Physically compatible for 4 hr at 23 °C	2383	C
Haloperidol lactate	MN	0.2 mg/mL[b]	AB	4 mcg/mL[b]	Physically compatible for 4 hr at 23 °C	2383	C
Heparin sodium	AB	100 units/mL	AB	4 mcg/mL[b]	Physically compatible for 4 hr at 23 °C	2383	C
Hydromorphone HCl	AST	0.5 mg/mL[b]	AB	4 mcg/mL[b]	Physically compatible for 4 hr at 23 °C	2383	C
Hydroxyzine HCl	ES	2 mg/mL[b]	AB	4 mcg/mL[b]	Physically compatible for 4 hr at 23 °C	2383	C
Isoproterenol HCl	AB	20 mcg/mL[b]	AB	4 mcg/mL[b]	Physically compatible for 4 hr at 23 °C	2383	C
Ketorolac tromethamine	AB	15 mg/mL	AB	4 mcg/mL[b]	Physically compatible for 4 hr at 23 °C	2383	C
Labetalol HCl	AB	2 mg/mL[b]	AB	4 mcg/mL[b]	Physically compatible for 4 hr at 23 °C	2383	C
Levofloxacin	ORT	5 mg/mL[b]	AB	4 mcg/mL[b]	Physically compatible for 4 hr at 23 °C	2383	C
Lidocaine HCl	AST	10 mg/mL[b]	AB	4 mcg/mL[b]	Physically compatible for 4 hr at 23 °C	2383	C
Linezolid	PHU	2 mg/mL	AB	4 mcg/mL[b]	Physically compatible for 4 hr at 23 °C	2383	C
Lorazepam	ESL	0.5 mg/mL[b]	AB	4 mcg/mL[b]	Physically compatible for 4 hr at 23 °C	2383	C
Magnesium sulfate	APP	100 mg/mL[b]	AB	4 mcg/mL[b]	Physically compatible for 4 hr at 23 °C	2383	C
Meperidine HCl	AST	10 mg/mL[b]	AB	4 mcg/mL[b]	Physically compatible for 4 hr at 23 °C	2383	C
Methylprednisolone sodium succinate	PHU	5 mg/mL[b]	AB	4 mcg/mL[b]	Physically compatible for 4 hr at 23 °C	2383	C
Metoclopramide HCl	FAU	5 mg/mL	AB	4 mcg/mL[b]	Physically compatible for 4 hr at 23 °C	2383	C
Metronidazole	BA	5 mg/mL	AB	4 mcg/mL[b]	Physically compatible for 4 hr at 23 °C	2383	C
Midazolam HCl			HOS		Stated to be compatible	1	C

Y-Site Injection Compatibility (1:1 Mixture) (Cont.)

Dexmedetomidine HCl

Drug	Mfr	Conc	Mfr	Conc	Remarks	Ref	C/I
Milrinone lactate	SAN	0.2 mg/mL[b]	AB	4 mcg/mL[b]	Physically compatible for 4 hr at 23 °C	2383	C
Morphine sulfate			HOS		Stated to be compatible	1	C
Nalbuphine HCl	AST	10 mg/mL	AB	4 mcg/mL[b]	Physically compatible for 4 hr at 23 °C	2383	C
Nitroglycerin	AMR	0.4 mg/mL[b]	AB	4 mcg/mL[b]	Physically compatible for 4 hr at 23 °C	2383	C
Norepinephrine bitartrate	AB	0.12 mg/mL[b]	AB	4 mcg/mL[b]	Physically compatible for 4 hr at 23 °C	2383	C
Ondansetron HCl	GW	1 mg/mL[b]	AB	4 mcg/mL[b]	Physically compatible for 4 hr at 23 °C	2383	C
Pancuronium bromide			HOS		Stated to be compatible	1	C
Phenylephrine HCl			HOS		Stated to be compatible	1	C
Piperacillin sodium–tazobactam sodium	LE[c]	40 + 5 mg/mL[b]	AB	4 mcg/mL[b]	Physically compatible for 4 hr at 23 °C	2383	C
Potassium chloride	AB	0.1 mEq/mL[b]	AB	4 mcg/mL[b]	Physically compatible for 4 hr at 23 °C	2383	C
Procainamide HCl	ES	10 mg/mL[b]	AB	4 mcg/mL[b]	Physically compatible for 4 hr at 23 °C	2383	C
Prochlorperazine edisylate	SKB	0.5 mg/mL[b]	AB	4 mcg/mL[b]	Physically compatible for 4 hr at 23 °C	2383	C
Promethazine HCl	ES	2 mg/mL[b]	AB	4 mcg/mL[b]	Physically compatible for 4 hr at 23 °C	2383	C
Propofol	ASZ	10 mg/mL	AB	4 mcg/mL[b]	Physically compatible for 4 hr at 23 °C	2383	C
Ranitidine HCl	GW	2 mg/mL[b]	AB	4 mcg/mL[b]	Physically compatible for 4 hr at 23 °C	2383	C
Remifentanil HCl	AB	0.25 mg/mL[b]	AB	4 mcg/mL[b]	Physically compatible for 4 hr at 23 °C	2383	C
Rocuronium bromide	OR	1 mg/mL[b]	AB	4 mcg/mL[b]	Physically compatible for 4 hr at 23 °C	2383	C
Sodium bicarbonate	AMR	1 mEq/mL	AB	4 mcg/mL[b]	Physically compatible for 4 hr at 23 °C	2383	C
Sodium nitroprusside	BA	2 mg/mL[b]	AB	4 mcg/mL[b]	Physically compatible for 4 hr at 23 °C protected from light	2383	C
Succinylcholine chloride			HOS		Stated to be compatible	1	C
Sufentanil citrate	AB	50 mcg/mL	AB	4 mcg/mL[b]	Physically compatible for 4 hr at 23 °C	2383	C
Theophylline	AB	4 mg/mL[a]	AB	4 mcg/mL[b]	Physically compatible for 4 hr at 23 °C	2383	C
Ticarcillin disodium–clavulanate potassium	SKB	31 mg/mL[b]	AB	4 mcg/mL[b]	Physically compatible for 4 hr at 23 °C	2383	C
Tobramycin sulfate	GNS	5 mg/mL[b]	AB	4 mcg/mL[b]	Physically compatible for 4 hr at 23 °C	2383	C
Trimethoprim–sulfamethoxazole	GNS	0.8 + 4 mg/mL[b]	AB	4 mcg/mL[b]	Physically compatible for 4 hr at 23 °C	2383	C
Vancomycin HCl	AB	10 mg/mL[b]	AB	4 mcg/mL[b]	Physically compatible for 4 hr at 23 °C	2383	C
Vecuronium bromide			HOS		Stated to be compatible	1	C
Verapamil HCl	AB	1.25 mg/mL[b]	AB	4 mcg/mL[b]	Physically compatible for 4 hr at 23 °C	2383	C

[a]Tested in dextrose 5%.
[b]Tested in sodium chloride 0.9%.
[c]Test performed using the formulation WITHOUT edetate disodium.

DEXRAZOXANE
AHFS 92:56

Products — Dexrazoxane is available as a lyophilized powder in vials containing 250 or 500 mg of drug. Each vial is packaged with a 25- or 50-mL vial, respectively, of 0.167 M sodium lactate injection for use as a diluent. Reconstitution with the diluent provided results in a dexrazoxane 10-mg/mL solution. The pH has been adjusted during manufacturing with hydrochloric acid. (1)

pH — From 3.5 to 5.5. (1)

Trade Name(s) — Zinecard.

Administration — Dexrazoxane is administered by slow intravenous push of the reconstituted solution or rapid intravenous infusion after dilution. (1)

Stability — Intact vials are stored at controlled room temperature. The manufacturer indicates that reconstituted solutions are stable for only six hours at room temperature or under refrigeration and recommends discarding unused solutions. (1)

However, reconstituted solutions of dexrazoxane 10 mg/mL were found to be stable for about 24 hours at 21 °C exposed to or protected from fluorescent light; about 7% loss occurred when reconstituted with dextrose 5% and about 9% loss occurred when reconstituted with sodium chloride 0.9%. Refrigeration resulted in precipitation after one day. (2395)

pH Effects — Dexrazoxane is most stable at acidic pH and is highly unstable in alkaline solutions. More than 10% loss occurs in less than two hours at pH values above 7. (2395)

Light Effects — No adverse effect on drug stability was found in 1- and 10-mg/mL solutions when exposed to fluorescent light. (2395)

Compatibility Information

Solution Compatibility

Dexrazoxane

Solution	Mfr	Mfr	Conc/L	Remarks	Ref	C/I
Dextrose 5%			1.3 to 5 g	Compatible and stable for 6 hr at room temperature or refrigerated	1	C
	a	NCI	1 g	Visually compatible with less than 10% loss in 24 hr at 21 °C exposed to and protected from light and in 3 days at 4 °C in the dark	2395	C
Sodium chloride 0.9%			1.3 to 5 g	Compatible and stable for 6 hr at room temperature or refrigerated	1	C
	a	NCI	1 g	Visually compatible with less than 10% loss in 24 hr at 21 °C exposed to and protected from light and in 3 days at 4 °C in the dark	2395	C

a Tested in both glass and PVC containers.

Y-Site Injection Compatibility (1:1 Mixture)

Dexrazoxane

Drug	Mfr	Conc	Mfr	Conc	Remarks	Ref	C/I
Gemcitabine HCl	LI	10 mg/mL[b]	PH	5 mg/mL[b]	Physically compatible for 4 hr at 23 °C	2226	C
Pemetrexed disodium	LI	20 mg/mL[b]	PHU	5 mg/mL[a]	Physically compatible for 4 hr at 23 °C	2564	C

a Tested in dextrose 5%.
b Tested in sodium chloride 0.9%.

DEXTRAN 40
AHFS 40:12

Products — Dextran 40 products are available as 10% injections in dextrose 5% or sodium chloride 0.9% in 500-mL containers. The colloidal products contain low molecular weight dextran (average molecular weight of 40,000) with either dextrose, hydrous, 5 g/100 mL or sodium chloride 0.9 g/100 mL in water for injection. (1; 4)

pH — The pH of dextran 40 10% in dextrose 5% ranges from 3 to 7. The pH of dextran 40 10% in sodium chloride 0.9% ranges from 3.5 to 7. (1; 4)

Osmolarity — Dextran 40 10% in dextrose 5% has a calculated osmolarity of 255 mOsm/L. Dextran 40 10% in sodium chloride 0.9% has a calculated osmolarity of 310 mOsm/L. (1)

Sodium Content — Dextran 40 10% in sodium chloride 0.9% provides 77 mEq of sodium per 500-mL bottle. (1; 4)

Trade Name(s) — LMD.

Administration — Dextran 40 10% injection is administered by intravenous infusion. (1; 4)

Stability — Dextran 40 products should not be administered unless they are clear. Long periods of storage or exposure to temperature fluctuations may cause the formation of dextran flakes or crystals. Therefore, solutions should be stored at a constant temperature, preferably 25 °C, and protected from freezing and extreme heat. Do not use dextran solutions that contain crystals. (1) However, if flakes or crystals do appear, they can be dissolved by heating in a water bath at 100 °C or autoclaving at 110 °C for 15 minutes. (4; 1484; 1485) Because no antibacterial preservative is present, partially used containers should be discarded. (4)

Compatibility Information

Additive Compatibility

Dextran 40

Drug	Mfr	Conc/L	Mfr	Conc/L	Test Soln	Remarks	Ref	C/I
Amoxicillin sodium		10, 20, 50 g		10%	D5W	9, 12, and 12% amoxicillin loss at 10, 20, and 50 g/L, respectively, in 1 hr at 25 °C	1469	I
		10, 20, 50 g		10%	NS	12, 14, and 20% amoxicillin loss at 10, 20, and 50 g/L, respectively, in 3 hr at 25 °C	1469	I
Ampicillin sodium		4 g		10%	D5W	46% ampicillin loss in 24 hr at 20 °C	834	I
	AY	8 g	PH	10%	D5W	50% loss in 24 hr at room temperature	99	I
	BAY	15 g	PH	10%	D5W	10% ampicillin loss in 1.5 hr at 25 °C	604	I
	BAY	2 g	PH	10%	D5W	10% ampicillin loss in 3.5 hr at 25 °C	604	I
	BAY	5 g	PH	10%	D5W	10% ampicillin loss in 2.3 hr at 25 °C	604	I
	AY	8 g	PH	10%	NS	25% loss in 24 hr at room temperature	99	I
	BAY	15 g	PH	10%	NS	10% ampicillin loss in 2.3 hr at 25 °C	604	I
	BAY	2 g	PH	10%	NS	10% ampicillin loss in 2.8 hr at 25 °C	604	I
	BAY	5 g	PH	10%	NS	10% ampicillin loss in 2.5 hr at 25 °C	604	I
Cloxacillin sodium	AST	2.25 g	PH	10%	D5W	Under 4% cloxacillin loss in 48 hr at 25 °C	1476	C
	BE	4 g	PH	10%	D5W	2% cloxacillin loss in 24 hr at 20 °C	834	C
	BE	8 g	PH	10%	D5W, NS	Under 5% loss in 24 hr at room temperature	99	C
Enalaprilat	MSD	25 mg	TR	10%	D5W	Physically compatible for 24 hr at room temperature under fluorescent light	1355	C
Floxacillin sodium				10%	D5W, NS	Under 10% loss in 24 hr at room temperature	1475	C
Gentamicin sulfate				10%	D5W	Gentamicin stable for 24 hr at room temperature	227	C
Nafcillin sodium	WY	2 and 30 g	PH	10%	D5W	Physically compatible and stable for 24 hr at 25 °C	27	C
Oxacillin sodium		4 g		10%	D5W	3% loss in 24 hr at 20 °C	834	C
Penicillin G potassium		6 million units		10%	D5W	34% loss in 24 hr at 20 °C	834	I

Additive Compatibility (Cont.)

Dextran 40

Drug	Mfr	Conc/L	Mfr	Conc/L	Test Soln	Remarks	Ref	C/I
Penicillin G sodium	KA	6 million units	PH	10%		Stable for 24 hr at 25 °C	131	C
Tobramycin sulfate	LI	200 mg and 1 g	TR	10%	D5W	Physically compatible and stable for 24 hr at 25 °C. Not more than 9% loss	147	C
Verapamil HCl	KN	80 mg	TR	10%	NS	Physically compatible for 24 hr	764	C

Y-Site Injection Compatibility (1:1 Mixture)

Dextran 40

Drug	Mfr	Conc	Mfr	Conc	Remarks	Ref	C/I
Enalaprilat	MSD	0.05 mg/mL[b]	TR	100 mg/mL[a]	Physically compatible for 24 hr at room temperature under fluorescent light	1355	C
Famotidine	MSD	0.2 mg/mL[a]	PH	100 mg/mL[a]	Physically compatible for 4 hr at 25 °C	1188	C
Nicardipine HCl	DCC	0.1 mg/mL[a]	TR	10%	Visually compatible for 24 hr at room temperature	235	C

[a]*Tested in dextrose 5%.*
[b]*Tested in sodium chloride 0.9%.*

DIAMORPHINE HYDROCHLORIDE
(DIACETYLMORPHINE HCL)
AHFS 28:08.08

Products — Diamorphine hydrochloride is available as a lyophilized product in 10-, 30-, 100-, and 500-mg ampuls. (38)

Diamorphine hydrochloride is very soluble in water. Up to 100 mg can be reconstituted in 1 mL of diluent; a minimum of 2 mL of diluent is recommended for the 500-mg size. The preferred diluent is dextrose 5%, but sodium chloride 0.9% also may be used. (1442)

Administration — Diamorphine hydrochloride is given by intramuscular, intravenous, or subcutaneous injection. Administration can also be by slow continuous subcutaneous or intravenous injection with an infusion control device. (38)

Stability — Ampuls of lyophilized diamorphine hydrochloride should be stored at or below 25 °C and protected from light. (38)

Diamorphine hydrochloride 1 mg/mL as an aqueous solution in flint glass ampuls stored at 25 °C exhibited 10% loss in 50 days. (1958)

In another study, diamorphine hydrochloride up to 25 mg/mL in sterile water for injection was stable for up to 24 hours at ambient temperature when protected from light. (1454)

pH Effects — The stability of the reconstituted injection depends on its pH; it is most stable at acidic pH, around 3.8 to 4.4 (1442) to pH 4.5 (1958). Degradation increases greatly at neutral or basic pH (1448).

Diamorphine hydrochloride exhibits a pH-dependent incompatibility in sodium chloride injection. To remain in solution, the pH must be below 6. (1458) Solutions containing up to 250 mg/mL of diamorphine hydrochloride have been shown to be compatible in sodium chloride 0.9%. (1457; 1458; 1459)

Temperature Effects — Solutions of diamorphine hydrochloride in sterile water for injection at concentrations greater than 15 mg/mL exhibited precipitation when stored at 21 and 37 °C for longer than two weeks. At concentrations of 1 to 250 mg/mL in sterile water for injection in glass containers, diamorphine hydrochloride was stable for eight weeks at −20 °C, exhibiting less than 10% degradation. At 4 °C, degradation was inversely related to concentration. Diamorphine hydrochloride 31 and 250 mg/mL was stable, but solutions containing 1 and 7.81 mg/mL showed 15 and 12% losses, respectively, after eight weeks of storage. (1452)

Syringes — The stability of diamorphine hydrochloride solutions containing 1 and 20 mg/mL in sodium chloride 0.9% in glass syringes was determined. At ambient temperature, diamorphine hydrochloride in glass syringes was stable for seven days at 1 mg/mL and for 12 days at 20 mg/mL. This was somewhat less than the drug's stability at these concentrations in PVC containers; adequate stability was maintained for at least 15 days in PVC containers. (1449)

Diamorphine hydrochloride stability in plastic syringes was reported to be 14 days at room temperature and greater than 40 days at 4 °C. (982)

Diamorphine hydrochloride (Hillcross) 2 and 20 mg/mL in water for injection was stored in plastic syringes (Becton-Dickinson) sealed with blind hubs. A 5% loss occurred in 18 days at 20 °C. (1672)

Infusion Pumps — Solutions containing diamorphine hydrochloride 250 mg/mL in an Act-a-Pump (Pharmacia) reservoir were stable for at least 14 days during simulated patient use. (1450) Degradation was both temperature and concentration dependent. Solutions of diamorphine hydrochloride 1 mg/mL in water stored at 21 °C for 42 days showed 10.6% degradation. At 37 °C, 32.6% degradation occurred. (1451)

However, at a concentration of 250 mg/mL, diamorphine hydrochloride losses of 11 and 85.8% at 21 and 37 °C, respectively (1451), were partially attributed to precipitation. (1452)

Diamorphine hydrochloride (Evans Medical) 5 mg/mL in sterile water for injection was stable in Parker Micropump PVC reservoirs for 14 days at 4 °C, exhibiting no loss. At 37 °C, about a 2% loss occurred in seven days and a 7% loss occurred in 14 days. (1696)

Elastomeric Reservoir Pumps — Diamorphine hydrochloride 1 and 20 mg/mL in sodium chloride 0.9% was evaluated for stability in two elastomeric disposable infusion devices, Infusor (Travenol) and Intermate 200 (I.S.C.). The drug was stable for 15 days in most cases. However, solutions containing diamorphine hydrochloride 1 mg/mL in the Intermate reservoir stored at 31 °C were only stable for two days. (1449)

Compatibility Information

Solution Compatibility

Diamorphine HCl

Solution	Mfr	Mfr	Conc/L	Remarks	Ref	C/I
Sodium chloride 0.9%	TR[a]	EV	1 and 20 g	Little or no loss in 15 days at 4 and 24 °C	1449	C

[a]*Tested in PVC containers.*

Additive Compatibility

Diamorphine HCl

Drug	Mfr	Conc/L	Mfr	Conc/L	Test Soln	Remarks	Ref	C/I
Bupivacaine HCl	GL	1.25 g		0.125 g	NS	Visually compatible with 8% diamorphine loss and no bupivacaine loss in 28 days at room temperature	1791	C
	AST	150 mg	NAP	20 mg	NS[a]	5% diamorphine and no bupivacaine loss in 14 days at 7 °C. Both drugs were stable for 6 months at −20 °C	2070	C
Floxacillin sodium	BE	20 g	EV	500 mg	W	Physically compatible for 24 hr at 15 and 30 °C. Haze forms in 48 hr at 30 °C. No change at 15 °C	1479	C
Furosemide	HO	1 g	EV	500 mg	W	Physically compatible for 72 hr at 15 and 30 °C	1479	C
Ropivacaine HCl	ASZ	2 g		25 mg	a	No ropivacaine and 10% diamorphine loss in 70 days at 4 °C and 28 days at 21 °C	2517	C

[a]*Tested in PVC containers.*

Drugs in Syringe Compatibility

Diamorphine HCl

Drug (in syringe)	Mfr	Amt	Mfr	Amt	Remarks	Ref	C/I
Bupivacaine HCl	AST	0.5%	EV	1 and 10 mg/mL	10 to 11% diamorphine loss in 5 weeks at 20 °C and 3 to 7% loss in 8 weeks at 6 °C. No bupivacaine loss at 6 or 20 °C in 8 weeks	1952	C

Drugs in Syringe Compatibility (Cont.)

Diamorphine HCl

Drug (in syringe)	Mfr	Amt	Mfr	Amt	Remarks	Ref	C/I
Cyclizine lactate	CA	5 mg/ 1 mL[a]	MB	20, 50, 100 mg/ 1 mL	Physically compatible and diamorphine stable for 24 hr at room temperature	1454	**C**
	CA	15 mg/ 1 mL	EV	15 mg/ 1 mL	Physically compatible for 24 hr at room temperature	1455	**C**
	CA	12.5 to 50 mg/ 1 mL	EV	37.5 to 150 mg/ 1 mL	Precipitate forms within 24 hr	1455	**I**
	CA	10 mg/ mL	HC	25 to 100 mg/ mL	Visually incompatible	1672	**I**
	CA	10 mg/ mL	HC	20 mg/ mL	Visually compatible for 48 hr at 5 and 20 °C	1672	**C**
	CA	6.7 mg/ mL	HC	100 mg/ mL	Visually compatible for 48 hr at 5 and 20 °C	1672	**C**
	CA	6.7 mg/ mL	HC	2 mg/mL	5% diamorphine loss in 9.9 days at 20 °C. Cyclizine stable for 45 days	1672	**C**
	CA	6.7 mg/ mL	HC	20 mg/ mL	5% diamorphine loss in 13.6 days at 20 °C. Cyclizine stable for 45 days	1672	**C**
	WEL	51 mg/ mL	BP	6 mg/mL	Physically compatible. 10% diamorphine loss in 1.7 days. Little cyclizine loss at 23 °C	2071	**C**
	WEL	32 mg/ mL	BP	9 mg/mL	Physically compatible. Under 10% diamorphine loss and little cyclizine loss in 4 days at 23 °C	2071	**C**
	WEL	39 mg/ mL	BP	10 mg/ mL	Physically compatible. Under 10% diamorphine loss and little cyclizine loss in 4 days at 23 °C	2071	**C**
	WEL	28 mg/ mL	BP	10 mg/ mL	Physically compatible. 10% diamorphine loss in 3.1 days and little cyclizine loss at 23 °C	2071	**C**
	WEL	51 mg/ mL	BP	12 mg/ mL	Physically compatible. 10% diamorphine loss in 2.2 days and little cyclizine loss at 23 °C	2071	**C**
	WEL	40 mg/ mL	BP	14 mg/ mL	Crystals form	2071	**I**
	WEL	26 mg/ mL	BP	17 mg/ mL	Physically compatible. 10% diamorphine loss in 1.1 days and 10% cyclizine loss in 2.5 days at 23 °C	2071	**C**
	WEL	52 mg/ mL	BP	18 mg/ mL	Crystals form	2071	**I**
	WEL	10 mg/ mL	BP	20 mg/ mL	Physically compatible. Under 10% diamorphine loss and little cyclizine loss in 7 days at 23 °C	2071	**C**
	WEL	15 mg/ mL	BP	20 mg/ mL	Physically compatible. Little diamorphine loss and 10% cyclizine loss in 0.5 days at 23 °C	2071	**I**
	WEL	26 mg/ mL	BP	21 mg/ mL	Physically compatible. 10% diamorphine loss in 4.9 days. 10% cyclizine loss in 3.2 days at 23 °C	2071	**C**
	WEL	18 mg/ mL	BP	23 mg/ mL	Physically compatible. Little diamorphine loss and 10% cyclizine loss in 3.2 days at 23 °C	2071	**C**
	WEL	23 mg/ mL	BP	26 mg/ mL	Physically compatible. 10% diamorphine loss in 1.9 days. 10% cyclizine loss in 9 hr at 23 °C	2071	**I**
	WEL	30 mg/ mL	BP	30 mg/ mL	Physically compatible. 10% diamorphine loss in 21 hr and 10% cyclizine loss in 9 hr at 23 °C	2071	**I**
	WEL	10 mg/ mL	BP	49 mg/ mL	Physically compatible. Little diamorphine loss and 10% cyclizine loss in 5.5 days at 23 °C	2071	**C**

Drugs in Syringe Compatibility (Cont.)

Diamorphine HCl

Drug (in syringe)	Mfr	Amt	Mfr	Amt	Remarks	Ref	C/I
	WEL	4 mg/mL	BP	51 mg/mL	Physically compatible. Little diamorphine or cyclizine loss in 7 days at 23 °C	2071	C
	WEL	8 mg/mL	BP	61 mg/mL	Physically compatible. 10% diamorphine loss in 1.4 days. 10% cyclizine loss in 1.1 days at 23 °C	2071	C
	WEL	13 mg/mL	BP	65 mg/mL	Physically compatible. 10% diamorphine loss in 1.6 days. 10% cyclizine loss in 12 hr at 23 °C	2071	I
	WEL	10 mg/mL	BP	92 mg/mL	Physically compatible. Little diamorphine loss and 10% cyclizine loss in 2.4 days at 23 °C	2071	C
	WEL	4 mg/mL	BP	99 mg/mL	Physically compatible. Little diamorphine or cyclizine loss in 7 days at 23 °C	2071	C
Cyclizine lactate with haloperidol lactate	WEL JC	16 mg/mL 2.2 mg/mL	BP	11 mg/mL	Physically compatible with less than 10% loss of any drug in 7 days at 23 °C	2071	C
Cyclizine lactate with haloperidol lactate	WEL JC	25 mg/mL 2.2 mg/mL	BP	16 mg/mL	Physically compatible with less than 10% loss of any drug in 7 days at 23 °C	2071	C
Cyclizine lactate with haloperidol lactate	WEL JC	11 mg/mL 2.2 mg/mL	BP	40 mg/mL	Physically compatible with less than 10% loss of any drug in 7 days at 23 °C	2071	C
Cyclizine lactate with haloperidol lactate	WEL JC	13 mg/mL 2.1 mg/mL	BP	42 mg/mL	Physically compatible with less than 10% loss of any drug in 7 days at 23 °C	2071	C
Cyclizine lactate with haloperidol lactate	WEL JC	9 mg/mL 2.1 mg/mL	BP	55 mg/mL	Physically compatible with less than 10% loss of any drug in 7 days at 23 °C	2071	C
Cyclizine lactate with haloperidol lactate	WEL JC	13 mg/mL 2.1 mg/mL	BP	56 mg/mL	Physically compatible with less than 10% loss of any drug in 7 days at 23 °C	2071	C
Haloperidol lactate	SE	1.5 mg/1 mL[a]	MB	10, 25, 50 mg/1 mL	Physically compatible and diamorphine content retained for 24 hr at room temperature	1454	C
	SE	2 mg/1 mL	EV	20 mg/1 mL	Crystallization with 58% haloperidol loss in 7 days at room temperature	1455	I
	SE	5 mg/1 mL	EV	50 and 150 mg/1 mL	Precipitates immediately	1455	I
	SE	2.5 mg/8 mL	EV	100 mg/8 mL	Physically compatible for 24 hr at room temperature and 7 days at 6 °C	1456	C
	SE	0.75 mg/mL	HC	20 to 100 mg/mL	Visually compatible for 48 hr at 5 and 20 °C	1672	C
	SE	0.75 mg/mL	HC	2 mg/mL	5% diamorphine loss in 14.8 days at 20 °C. Haloperidol stable for 45 days	1672	C
	SE	0.75 mg/mL	HC	20 mg/mL	5% diamorphine loss in 20.7 days at 20 °C. Haloperidol stable for 45 days	1672	C
	JC	2 and 3 mg/mL	BP	20, 50, 100 mg/mL	Physically compatible with less than 10% loss of either drug in 7 days at 23 °C	2071	C

Drugs in Syringe Compatibility (Cont.)

Diamorphine HCl

Drug (in syringe)	Mfr	Amt	Mfr	Amt	Remarks	Ref	C/I
	JC	4 mg/mL	BP	20 and 50 mg/mL	Physically compatible with less than 10% loss of either drug in 7 days at 23 °C	2071	C
Haloperidol lactate with cyclizine lactate	JC WEL	2.2 mg/mL 16 mg/mL	BP	11 mg/mL	Physically compatible with less than 10% loss of any drug in 7 days at 23 °C	2071	C
Haloperidol lactate with cyclizine lactate	JC WEL	2.2 mg/mL 25 mg/mL	BP	16 mg/mL	Physically compatible with less than 10% loss of any drug in 7 days at 23 °C	2071	C
Haloperidol lactate with cyclizine lactate	JC WEL	2.2 mg/mL 11 mg/mL	BP	40 mg/mL	Physically compatible with less than 10% loss of any drug in 7 days at 23 °C	2071	C
Haloperidol lactate with cyclizine lactate	JC WEL	2.1 mg/mL 13 mg/mL	BP	42 mg/mL	Physically compatible with less than 10% loss of any drug in 7 days at 23 °C	2071	C
Haloperidol lactate with cyclizine lactate	JC WEL	2.1 mg/mL 9 mg/mL	BP	55 mg/mL	Physically compatible with less than 10% loss of any drug in 7 days at 23 °C	2071	C
Haloperidol lactate with cyclizine lactate	JC WEL	2.1 mg/mL 13 mg/mL	BP	56 mg/mL	Physically compatible with less than 10% loss of any drug in 7 days at 23 °C	2071	C
Methotrimeprazine HCl	MB	1.25 and 2.5 mg/1 mL[a]	MB	50 mg/1 mL	Physically compatible and diamorphine stable for 24 hr at room temperature	1454	C
Metoclopramide HCl	BK	5 mg/1 mL	MB	10, 25, 50 mg/1 mL	Physically compatible and diamorphine stable for 24 hr at room temperature	1454	C
	LA	5 mg/1 mL	EV	50 and 150 mg/1 mL	Slight discoloration with 8% metoclopramide loss and 9% diamorphine loss in 7 days at room temperature	1455	C
Midazolam HCl	RC	10[b] and 75[c] mg	EV	10 mg	Visually compatible. 10% diamorphine and no midazolam loss in 15.9 days at 22 °C	1792	C
	RC	10[b] and 75[c] mg	EV	500 mg	Visually compatible. 10% diamorphine and no midazolam loss in 22.2 days at 22 °C	1792	C
Octreotide acetate	NVA	300 mcg/8 mL[a]	EV	50 mg/8 mL[a]	Visually compatible with no octreotide loss in 48 hr. Diamorphine not tested	2709	C
	NVA	600 mcg/8 mL[a]	EV	50 mg/8 mL[a]	Visually compatible with no octreotide loss in 48 hr. Diamorphine not tested	2709	C
	NVA	900 mcg/8 mL[a]	EV	50 mg/8 mL[a]	Visually compatible with 1% octreotide loss in 48 hr. Diamorphine not tested	2709	C
	NVA	300 mcg/8 mL[a]	EV	100 mg/8 mL[a]	Visually compatible with 4% octreotide loss in 48 hr. Diamorphine not tested	2709	C
	NVA	600 mcg/8 mL[a]	EV	100 mg/8 mL[a]	Visually compatible with 6% octreotide loss in 48 hr. Diamorphine not tested	2709	C
	NVA	900 mcg/8 mL[a]	EV	100 mg/8 mL[a]	Visually compatible with 5% octreotide loss in 48 hr. Diamorphine not tested	2709	C
	NVA	600 mcg/8 mL[a]	EV	200 mg/8 mL[a]	Visually compatible with 6% octreotide loss in 48 hr. Diamorphine not tested	2709	C

Drugs in Syringe Compatibility (Cont.)

Diamorphine HCl

Drug (in syringe)	Mfr	Amt	Mfr	Amt	Remarks	Ref	C/I
Prochlorperazine edisylate	MB	1.25 mg/ 1 mL[a]	MB	10, 25, 50 mg/ 1 mL	Physically compatible and diamorphine content retained for 24 hr at room temperature	1454	C
Ropivacaine HCl	ASZ	10 g		45 mg	No ropivacaine loss and 10% diamorphine loss in 30 days at 4 °C and 16 days at 21 °C	2517	C
Scopolamine butylbromide	BI	20 mg/ 1 mL	EV	50 and 150 mg/ 1 mL	Physically compatible with no scopolamine loss and 4% diamorphine loss in 7 days at room temperature	1455	C
Scopolamine HBr	EV	60 mcg/ 1 mL[a]	MB	10, 25, 50 mg/ 1 mL	Physically compatible and diamorphine stable for 24 hr at room temperature	1454	C
	EV	0.4 mg/ 1 mL	EV	50 and 150 mg/ 1 mL	Physically compatible with 7% diamorphine loss in 7 days at room temperature	1455	C

[a] *Diluted with sterile water for injection.*
[b] *Diluted with sterile water to 15 mL.*
[c] *Diamorphine hydrochloride reconstituted with midazolam injection.*

DIAZEPAM
AHFS 28:24.08

Products — Diazepam 5 mg/mL is available in 2-mL ampuls and vials, 10-mL vials, and 2-mL syringe cartridges. Each milliliter of solution also contains propylene glycol 40%, ethanol 10%, sodium benzoate and benzoic acid 5%, and benzyl alcohol 1.5%. (1)

pH — From 6.2 to 6.9. (17)

Osmolality — The osmolality of diazepam (Roche) was determined to be 7775 mOsm/kg. Diazemuls (Kabi) has an osmolality of 349 mOsm/kg. (1233)

Administration — Diazepam is administered by direct intravenous injection into a large vein (1; 4) or, if necessary, into the tubing of a running infusion solution. (4) Extravasation should be avoided. It is recommended that the rate of administration in adults not exceed 5 mg/min; for children, it is recommended that the dose be administered over not less than three minutes. Diazepam can be given by deep intramuscular injection (1; 4), but this route may yield low or erratic plasma levels. (4; 121; 638) Intravenous infusion of diazepam diluted in infusion solutions has been performed but is not recommended. (1; 4)

Stability — The commercial product should be stored at controlled room temperature and protected from light. (1)

The drug is most stable at pH 4 to 8 and is subject to acid-catalyzed hydrolysis below pH 3. (643)

In tropical climates, diazepam injection is subject to discoloration from degradation by an oxidative hydrolytic mechanism. The rate of degradation leading to discoloration is dependent on various factors including the polarity/dielectric constant of the vehicle, pH, oxygen and electrolyte content, access to light, and storage temperature. (1749)

Diazepam injection under simulated summer conditions in paramedic vehicles was exposed to temperatures ranging from 26 to 38 °C over 4 weeks. Analysis found no loss of the drug under these conditions. (2562)

Syringes — Diazepam 5 mg/mL was filled into 3-mL plastic syringes (Becton Dickinson, Sherwood Monoject, and Terumo) and stored at −20, 4, and 25 °C in the dark. Losses, presumably due to sorption to surfaces and/or the elastomeric plunger seal, ranged from 6% at 25 °C to 2 or 3% at 4 °C to 1% or less at −20 °C in one day. Storage for seven days at 4 °C and 30 days at −20 °C resulted in losses of 4 to 8% and 5 to 13%, respectively. (1562)

Diazepam (Roche) 10 mg/2 mL stored in plastic syringes composed of polypropylene and polyethylene exhibited no loss of diazepam in four hours. (351)

Diazepam (Roche) 5 mg/mL was stored in 1.5-mL disposable glass syringes with slit rubber plunger-stoppers (Hy-Pod) for 90 days at 30 and 4 °C in light-resistant bags. Diazepam was gradually lost from the solution, with the disappearance being essentially complete in 60 days. At 4 °C, about 5% was lost at the 60- and 90-day intervals; about 9 to 10% was lost at 30 °C in this period. The loss was attributed to sorption to the rubber plunger-stoppers. (794)

Sorption — The stability of diazepam in several infusion fluids in glass containers (321) does not extend to the solutions in PVC bags in which substantial sorption occurs. At 10 mg in 100 and 200 mL, over 24% loss occurred in 30 minutes and 80 to 90% loss occurred in 24 hours. (330)

Diazepam 8 mg/L in sodium chloride 0.9% in PVC bags exhibited 20% loss in 24 hours and 32% loss in one week at 15 to 20 °C due to sorption. (536)

The sorption of diazepam to PVC infusion bags was evaluated at concentrations of 5 and 20 mg/100 mL in dextrose 5% and sodium chloride 0.9%. Diazepam concentration was under 45% in two hours and 20 to 25% in eight hours. (647)

Diazepam sorption that results from plastic infusion sets was evaluated. Dilutions of 7.5 and 30 mg in 150 mL of dextrose 5% and sodium chloride 0.9% were prepared in the burette chamber of a Buretrol. The solutions flowed through the tubing at 30 mL/hr for two hours. Less than 10% decrease in diazepam occurred in the burette chamber. However, running the solution through the tubing resulted in steep declines to 43% of the initial amount. When diazepam 25 and 100 mg/500 mL of dextrose 5% and sodium chloride 0.9% prepared in glass bottles and 100-mL aliquots were run through the Buretrol over one hour, only about 60 to 70% of the diazepam was delivered. The presence of a 0.5-μm inline filter did not affect the concentration delivered. (647)

Over 90% loss due to sorption to the administration set (Abbott) and the extension tubing (Extracorporeal) both with and without a 0.22-μm inline filter (Abbott) was reported. Diazepam 0.02 to 0.04 mg/mL in dextrose 5% had no precipitation, and solutions in glass bottles were stable over 24 hours. However, the amount delivered through the tubing was only 40 to 55% at time zero, and this amount dropped to 2 to 7% at 24 hours. No difference was noted from the inline filter. (645)

The sorption of diazepam to administration sets from solutions of diazepam 25 and 50 mg/500 mL in glass bottles of dextrose 5% and Ringer's injection, lactated, or 12.5 and 25 mg/250 mL of these same solutions in Soluset burette chambers was tested. The admixtures showed no evidence of physical incompatibility over four hours at room temperature. The solutions in glass bottles were run through Venosets composed of PVC drip chambers and tubing at 2.5 and 5 mg/hr. The solutions stored in the cellulose propionate burette chambers of the Solusets were also run through their PVC tubing at the same rates. The solution delivered through the Venosets contained about 91 to 97% of the initial concentration, with the more dilute solution having slightly more drug remaining. However, the Soluset delivered only about 50 to 60% in two hours and about 35 to 45% of the initial concentration after four hours. Most of the loss was due to sorption to the cellulose propionate burette chamber. This result was attributed to the larger surface area of the burette compared with the tubing and/or the difference in plastic composition. Almost all of the lost diazepam could be recovered through desorption from the burettes. The use of 0.45-μm inline filters had no effect on the drug concentration. (646)

Diazepam 50-mg/500 mL solution in dextrose 5% prepared in glass bottles and run through an administration set (Travenol) at 100 mL/hr was assessed. Only 63% of the diazepam was initially delivered but gradually climbed to 81% at the end of five hours. (649)

A 27 to 33% diazepam loss was noted from admixtures in both dextrose 5% and sodium chloride 0.9% in PVC bags. Diazepam concentrations ranged from 0.05 to 0.2 mg/mL. No drug decomposition could be detected. Diazepam solutions in dextrose 5% were also run through a 70-inch Travenol set. A steep decline to under 70% was delivered during the first 15 minutes, after which the delivered amount increased to between 80 and 90% over the next 85 minutes as saturation of the tubing occurred. A quantitatively smaller, but qualitatively similar, effect was observed when diazepam was administered by intravenous push through an intravenous catheter (Abbott Veno-

cath-18) of 11.5-inch total length. The decline in delivered diazepam reached a nadir of 95% in about eight minutes before returning to 100% at 10 minutes. The smaller effect of the intravenous catheter relates to its relatively shorter length. (650)

Diazepam 8 mg/L in sodium chloride 0.9% in glass bottles exhibited a cumulative 7% loss due to sorption during a seven-hour simulated infusion through an infusion set (Travenol). The set consisted of a cellulose propionate burette chamber and 170 cm of PVC tubing. Diazepam sorption was attributed mainly to the tubing. The extent of sorption was found to be independent of concentration. (606)

Diazepam was also tested as a simulated infusion over at least one hour by a syringe pump system. A glass syringe on a syringe pump was fitted with 20 cm of polyethylene tubing or 50 cm of Silastic tubing. A negligible amount of drug was lost with the polyethylene tubing, but a cumulative loss of 21% occurred during the one-hour infusion through the Silastic tubing. (606)

Storage of a 25-mL aliquot of the 8-mg/L diazepam solution in all-plastic syringes composed of polypropylene barrels and polyethylene plungers for 24 hours at room temperature in the dark did not result in any drug loss due to sorption. (606)

Diazepam 20 mg/500 mL in dextrose 5% was delivered at 4 mL/hr through PVC tubing by means of an infusion pump. Under 20% of the diazepam was delivered at any time point over 24 hours. Increasing the concentration to 50 mg/500 mL in dextrose 5% and increasing the infusion rate to 20 mL/hr decreased the amount of diazepam lost from the solution. After 30 minutes of solution delivery, the diazepam in the tubing effluent was about 30% of the initial concentration. Subsequently, the delivered diazepam concentration climbed to about 60% over 24 hours. (351)

The partition coefficients of diazepam with various plastics from intravenous containers and administration sets were determined. PVC bags and tubings from a variety of suppliers were all similar in partitioning and hundreds of times greater than polyolefin containers. Volume-control chambers made from cellulose propionate had partition coefficients smaller than those of PVC but still sufficient to cause serious depletion of diazepam from the chambers. (644)

The uptake of diazepam into PVC is absorption into the plastic matrix rather than adsorption to the surface. The absorption is independent of concentration but related to contact time with the plastic. Decreasing the flow rate or increasing the tubing length increases the amount of diazepam absorbed.

Increasing the flow rate from 10 to 264 mL/hr through 198 cm of PVC tubing decreased the amount of diazepam absorbed from 88 down to 28%. Increasing the tubing length from 100 to 350 cm increased the amount absorbed from 17 to 59%. However, it was noted that absorption is not markedly affected by tubing length within the range of lengths commercially available. (644)

Diazepam 50 mg/L in sodium chloride 0.9% in a glass bottle was delivered through a polyethylene administration set (Tridilset) over eight hours at 15 to 20 °C. The flow rate was 1 mL/min. No appreciable loss due to sorption occurred. This finding is in contrast to a 20% loss using a conventional administration set. (769)

The sorption of diazepam 40 and 120 mg/L in sodium chloride 0.9% was evaluated in 100- and 500-mL PVC infusion bags. After eight hours at 20 to 24 °C, 58 to 60% of the diazepam was lost in the 100-mL bag and 31% was lost in the 500-mL bag. The extent of sorption was independent of concentration but was influenced by the size of the PVC container. This difference results from the ratio of the surface area of plastic to the volume of solution. As the volume of solution in the bag decreases, the extent of sorption increases. (770)

Diazepam showed negligible (<3%) loss when aqueous solutions were stored in polypropylene bags. (770)

Extensive sorption of diazepam in dextrose 5% and sodium chloride 0.9% to PVC containers was found. Solutions of 10 to 80 mg/L showed a 12 to 20% diazepam loss in one hour. In six hours, the loss was 30% at 5 °C and 40% at room temperature. Over 30% of the missing diazepam could be recovered by washing the PVC with methanol. Sorption did not occur to glass or polyethylene containers, which showed losses of about 6 to 8% in 24 hours. (796)

No loss of diazepam occurred to glass or polyethylene containers in 200-mg/L concentrations in dextrose 5% or sodium chloride 0.9%. In PVC containers, drug losses of 37 to 43% occurred in 24 hours at 25 °C. (797)

Testing the administration of diazepam with a glass syringe on an infusion pump connected with high-density polyethylene tubing resulted in negligible drug loss. (795)

Plastic syringes having polypropylene barrels and polyethylene plungers (Pharma-Plast, AHS Australia) and all-glass containers were compared for the possible sorption of diazepam. After 24 hours of storage, no drug loss was found in either container. The authors indicated that these plastic syringes could be used with syringe pumps. (782)

The effect of several factors on the rate and extent of sorption of diazepam by PVC was evaluated. Sorption proved to be independent of changes in ethanol–propylene glycol concentrations in the vehicle, pH changes in the admixtures over 4.2 to 7.5, and the diazepam concentration. The rate and extent of sorption could be minimized by decreasing the storage temperature, minimizing the storage time, and increasing the surface area to volume ratio by storing the largest possible fluid volume in a given PVC bag and using short lengths of small diameter infusion tubing. Use of glass or polyolefin solution bottles and polyolefin infusion tubing avoids the loss of diazepam. (880)

The sorption of diazepam 20 mg/500 mL in sodium chloride 0.9%, run at 1 mL/min through PVC and polybutadiene (PBD) administration sets (Avon Medicals, U.K.), was reported. The delivered concentration through the PVC set was 80% initially and then climbed to 90% after four hours. For a concentration of 10 mg/120 mL prepared in a cellulose propionate burette, 10 to 15% sorption occurred in the burette. Use of the PBD set, with or without a methacrylate butadiene styrene burette chamber, resulted in no loss of diazepam. (1027)

The delivery of diazepam 50 and 100 mg/500 mL in dextrose 5% and sodium chloride 0.9% through a PVC administration set (Accuset 9210, IMED) and a set composed of ethylene vinyl acetate with a polyethylene inner wall (Accuset 9630, IMED) was evaluated. The solutions were run through the sets at 50 and 100 mL/hr. The delivered diazepam concentration varied between 44 and 71% at 50 mL/hr and between 62 and 89% at 100 mL/hr, increasing from the lower to the higher percentage over the five-hour study period. The non-PVC set exhibited no sorption of diazepam, delivering 100% of the diazepam. (1096)

The percentage of diazepam delivered through PVC administration sets varied with the length of the tubing; the longer the tubing, the smaller was the percentage delivered. For a 25-mg/500 mL admixture in sodium chloride 0.9%, delivery through PVC tubing in lengths from 23 to 185 cm varied from 88% of the theoretical amount for the shortest length to 53% for the 185-cm length. (1097)

The effect of container type and flow rate on the sorption of diazepam was evaluated. Glass and polyethylene containers showed 0 and 5% sorption, respectively, of the diazepam content of a 25-mg/500 mL admixture in sodium chloride 0.9% in seven days at 25 °C. PVC containers showed a 75% loss in this time period. Simulated infusion of this solution from glass bottles through PVC sets at flow rates of 30 to 120 mL/hr showed that a greater percentage of diazepam was lost at the slower infusion rates. At 30 mL/hr, 63% was lost after four hours, while only 23% was lost after four hours at 120 mL/hr. (1098)

A rapid diazepam loss from a 40-mcg/mL solution in sodium chloride 0.9% in a PVC container at 21 °C was reported. A 15% loss occurred in two hours, and a 55% loss occurred in 24 hours. Little or no diazepam loss occurred in 24 hours in glass bottles or polyethylene-lined laminated bags. (1392)

Diazepam 100 mcg/mL in sodium chloride 0.9% exhibited no loss due to sorption in 24 hours at 21 °C in glass bottles and polypropylene trilayer bags (Softbag, Orion). However, about a 70% loss occurred due to sorption in PVC bags. (1796)

Diazepam 40 mcg/mL in 0.9% sodium chloride and in pH 7 buffer also underwent sorption to ethylene vinyl acetate (EVA) plastic bags. Losses exceeding 25% occurred within 24 hours stored at 30 °C. The solutions appeared to reach equilibrium after 96 hours of storage. (1917)

Diazepam 0.04 mg/mL in dextrose 5% and sodium chloride 0.9% in PVC, polyethylene, and glass containers exhibited only 4 to 5% loss in glass and polyethylene containers but 66% loss due to sorption in PVC containers stored at 4 and 22 °C for 24 hours. (2289)

To minimize the sorption of diazepam, glass or polyolefin containers should be used. If PVC bags are used, the lowest possible surface-to-volume ratio should be selected and storage time should be minimized. The use of non-PVC administration sets will reduce loss. If PVC tubing is used, it should be the shortest possible length with a small diameter, and the set should not contain a burette chamber. More rapid flow rates (consistent with safe clinical use) will also reduce the loss of diazepam.

Filtration — Diazepam (Roche) 50 mcg/mL in dextrose 5% and sodium chloride 0.9% was delivered over seven hours through four kinds of 0.2-μm membrane filters varying in size and composition. Diazepam concentration losses of 7 to 17% were found during the first 60 minutes; subsequent diazepam levels returned to the original concentration when the binding sites became saturated. (1399)

Compatibility Information

Solution Compatibility

	Diazepam					
Solution	Mfr	Mfr	Conc/L	Remarks	Ref	C/I
Dextrose 5%	BA[a]	RC	>250 mg	Immediate white precipitation	321	I
	BA[a]	RC	250 mg	No precipitate in 24 hr. 6% loss in 4 hr	321	I
	BA[a]	RC	100 and 125 mg	No precipitate and 8 to 10% loss in 24 hr	321	C
	BA[a]	RC	50 and 67 mg	No precipitate and 0 to 1% loss in 24 hr	321	C
	BA[b]	RC	100 mg	35% loss in 30 min. 90% loss in 24 hr at room temperature	330	I
	BA[b]	RC	50 mg	35% loss in 30 min. 77% loss in 24 hr at room temperature	330	I
		RC	370 mg	Precipitate formed	640	I
	TR[b]	RC	50 and 200 mg	Solution initially cloudy but clears. 55 to 60% loss within 2 hr	647	I
	BT[b]	RC	40 mg	No precipitate but 12 to 14% loss in 1 hr at room temperature and 5 °C	796	I
	BT[c]	RC	40 mg	No precipitate and about 10% loss in 24 hr at room temperature	796	C
	ON[a,c]	ON	200 mg	No precipitate and negligible loss in 24 hr at 25 °C	797	C
	[b]	ON	200 mg	No precipitate but about 10% loss in 3.5 hr and about 37% in 24 hr at 25 °C	797	I
	BA[b]	BRN	40 mg	Visually compatible but 66% loss due to sorption to the PVC container in 24 hr at 4 and 22 °C	2289	I
	BRN[a,c]	BRN	40 mg	Visually compatible with 4 to 5% loss in 24 hr at 4 and 22 °C	2289	C
Ringer's injection	BA[a]	RC	>250 mg	Immediate white precipitation	321	I
	BA[a]	RC	250 mg	White precipitate in 6 to 8 hr. 8% loss in 4 hr	321	I
	BA[a]	RC	100 and 125 mg	No precipitate and 7 to 12% loss in 24 hr	321	C
	BA[a]	RC	50 and 67 mg	No precipitate and 0 to 3% loss in 24 hr	321	C
	BA[b]	RC	100 mg	38% loss in 30 min. 89% loss in 24 hr at room temperature	330	I
	BA[b]	RC	50 mg	29% loss in 30 min. 78% loss in 24 hr at room temperature	330	I
Ringer's injection, lactated	BA[a]	RC	>250 mg	Immediate white precipitation	321	I
	BA[a]	RC	250 mg	White precipitate in 8 to 12 hr. 5% loss in 4 hr	321	I
		RC	200 mg	Transient cloudiness followed by clear solution	392	?
	BA[a]	RC	100 and 125 mg	No precipitate and 8 to 10% loss in 24 hr	321	C
	BA[a]	RC	50 and 67 mg	No precipitate and 6% loss in 24 hr	321	C
	BA[b]	RC	100 mg	35% loss in 30 min. 89% loss in 24 hr at room temperature	330	I
	BA[b]	RC	50 mg	40% loss in 30 min. 78% loss in 24 hr at room temperature	330	I
Sodium chloride 0.9%	BA[a]	RC	>250 mg	Immediate white precipitation	321	I
	BA[a]	RC	250 mg	No precipitate in 24 hr. 6% loss in 4 hr	321	I
	BA[a]	RC	125 mg	No precipitate and 6% loss in 24 hr	321	C

Solution Compatibility (Cont.)

Diazepam

Solution	Mfr	Mfr	Conc/L	Remarks	Ref	C/I
	BA[a]	RC	100 mg	No precipitate and 4 to 5% loss in 24 hr	321; 330	C
	BA[a]	RC	67 mg	No precipitate and 6% loss in 24 hr	321	C
	BA[a]	RC	50 mg	No precipitate and 1 to 3% loss in 24 hr	321; 330	C
	BA[b]	RC	100 mg	29% loss in 30 min. 89% loss in 24 hr at room temperature	330	I
	BA[b]	RC	50 mg	24% loss in 30 min. 80% loss in 24 hr at room temperature	330	I
	TR[b]	RC	50 and 200 mg	Solution initially cloudy but clears. 55 to 60% loss within 2 hr	647	I
	[a]	RC	40 mg	No precipitate and 6% loss in 24 hr at room temperature	796	C
	BT, TR[b]	RC	10 to 80 mg	No precipitate but 12 to 20% loss in 1 hr at room temperature and 5 °C	796	I
	BT[c]	RC	10 to 80 mg	No precipitate and 2 to 8% loss in 24 hr at room temperature and 5 °C	796	C
	ON[a,c]	ON	200 mg	No precipitate and negligible loss in 24 hr at 25 °C	797	C
	[b]	ON	200 mg	No precipitate but 10% loss in 1 hr and 43% in 24 hr at 25 °C	797	I
	[a]		400 mg	Precipitate forms immediately or within 1 min	1095	I
	[a]		333 mg	Precipitate forms after 30 min	1095	I
	[a]		100 and 200 mg	Remained clear for 10 days	1095	C
	[a]		50 mg	No diazepam loss in 7 days at 25 °C	1098	C
	[b]		50 mg	Over 40% loss in 1 day and 75% in 7 days at 25 °C	1098	I
	[c]		50 mg	5% loss in 7 days at 25 °C	1098	C
	[b]		40 mg	15% diazepam loss in 2 hr and 55% loss in 24 hr at 21 °C in dark	1392	I
	[a,c]		40 mg	Little diazepam loss in 24 hr at 21 °C in dark	1392	C
	ON[d]	ON	100 mg	Visually compatible with no loss in 24 hr at 21 °C	1796	C
	ON[b]	ON	100 mg	Visually compatible but 70% loss due to sorption in 24 hr at 21 °C	1796	I
	BA[b]	BRN	40 mg	Visually compatible but 66% loss due to sorption to the PVC container in 24 hr at 4 and 22 °C	2289	I
	BRN[a,c]	BRN	40 mg	Visually compatible with 4 to 5% loss in 24 hr at 4 and 22 °C	2289	C

[a]Tested in glass containers.
[b]Tested in PVC containers.
[c]Tested in polyethylene containers.
[d]Tested in glass containers and polypropylene trilayer containers.

Additive Compatibility

Diazepam

Drug	Mfr	Conc/L	Mfr	Conc/L	Test Soln	Remarks	Ref	C/I
Bleomycin sulfate	BR	20 and 30 units	RC	50 and 100 mg	NS	Physically incompatible	763	I
Dobutamine HCl	LI	1 g	RC	2.5 g	D5W, NS	Rapid clouding of solution with yellow precipitate within 24 hr at 21 °C	812	I
Doxorubicin HCl	AD		RC			Precipitates immediately	524	I

Additive Compatibility (Cont.)

Diazepam

Drug	Mfr	Conc/L	Mfr	Conc/L	Test Soln	Remarks	Ref	C/I
Floxacillin sodium	BE	20 g	PHX	1 g	D5W	Haze forms in 7 hr at 30 °C and 48 hr at 15 °C	1479	I
Fluorouracil			RC			Precipitates immediately	524	I
Furosemide	HO	1 g	PHX	1 g	D5W	Precipitates immediately	1479	I
Verapamil HCl	KN	80 mg	RC	20 mg	D5W, NS	Physically compatible for 24 hr	764	C

Drugs in Syringe Compatibility

Diazepam

Drug (in syringe)	Mfr	Amt	Mfr	Amt	Remarks	Ref	C/I
Buprenorphine HCl					Incompatible	4	I
Dimenhydrinate		10 mg/ 1 mL		5 mg/ 1 mL	Loss of clarity	2569	I
Doxapram HCl	RB	400 mg/ 20 mL		10 mg/ 2 mL	Immediate turbidity and precipitation	1177	I
Glycopyrrolate	RB	0.2 mg/ 1 mL	RC	5 mg/ 1 mL	Precipitates immediately	331	I
	RB	0.2 mg/ 1 mL	RC	10 mg/ 2 mL	Precipitates immediately	331	I
	RB	0.4 mg/ 2 mL	RC	5 mg/ 1 mL	Precipitates immediately	331	I
Heparin sodium		2500 units/ 1 mL		10 mg/ 2 mL	Turbidity or precipitate forms within 5 min	1053	I
Hydromorphone HCl	KN	2, 10, 40 mg/ 1 mL	SX	5 mg/ 1 mL	Diazepam precipitate forms immediately due to aqueous dilution	2082	I
Ketorolac tromethamine	SY	180 mg/ 6 mL	ES	15 mg/ 3 mL	Visually compatible for 4 hr at 24 °C. Increase in absorbance occurs immediately, persists for 30 min, and dissipates by 1 hr	1703	?
Nalbuphine HCl	EN	10 mg/ 1 mL	RC	5 mg/ 1 mL	Immediate milky precipitate that persists for 36 hr at 27 °C	762	I
	EN	5 mg/ 0.5 mL	RC	5 mg/ 1 mL	Immediate milky precipitate that clears upon shaking. Clear for 36 hr at 27 °C	762	?
	EN	2.5 mg/ 0.25 mL	RC	5 mg/ 1 mL	Immediate milky precipitate that clears upon shaking. Clear for 36 hr at 27 °C	762	?
	DU	10 mg/ 1 mL	RC	10 mg/ 2 mL	Physically incompatible	128	I
	DU	20 mg/ 1 mL	RC	10 mg/ 2 mL	Physically incompatible	128	I
Pantoprazole sodium	[a]	4 mg/ 1 mL		5 mg/ 1 mL	Red precipitate forms immediately	2574	I
Ranitidine HCl	GL	50 mg/ 2 mL	RC	10 mg/ 2 mL	Immediate white haze that disappears following vortex mixing	978	?
	GL	50 mg/ 5 mL		10 mg	Physically compatible for 4 hr at ambient temperature under fluorescent light	1151	C

[a]Test performed using the formulation WITHOUT edetate disodium.

Y-Site Injection Compatibility (1:1 Mixture)

Diazepam

Drug	Mfr	Conc	Mfr	Conc	Remarks	Ref	C/I
Amphotericin B cholesteryl sulfate complex	SEQ	0.83 mg/mL[a]	SW	5 mg/mL	Gross precipitate forms	2117	I
Atracurium besylate	BW	0.5 mg/mL[a]	ES	5 mg/mL	Cloudy solution forms immediately	1337	I
Bivalirudin	TMC	5 mg/mL[a]	AB	5 mg/mL	Yellowish precipitate forms immediately	2373	I
Ceftaroline fosamil	FOR	2.22 mg/mL[a,b,d]	HOS	5 mg/mL	Turbid precipitation forms	2826	I
Cisatracurium besylate	GW	0.1, 2, 5 mg/mL[a]	ES	5 mg/mL	White turbidity forms immediately	2074	I
	GW	0.1, 2, 5 mg/mL[a]	ES	0.25 mg/mL[a]	Physically compatible for 4 hr at 23 °C	2074	C
Dexmedetomidine HCl	AB	4 mcg/mL[b]	AB	5 mg/mL	White turbid precipitate forms immediately	2383	I
Diltiazem HCl	MMD	1[b] and 5 mg/mL	ES	5 mg/mL	Cloudiness and precipitate form	1807	I
Dobutamine HCl	LI	4 mg/mL[a,b]	ES	0.2 mg/mL[a,b]	Physically compatible for 3 hr	1316	C
Doripenem	JJ	5 mg/mL[a,b]	HOS	5 mg/mL	Gross white turbid precipitate forms	2743	I
Fenoldopam mesylate	AB	80 mcg/mL[b]	AB	5 mg/mL	Gross white turbidity forms immediately	2467	I
Fentanyl citrate	JN	0.025 mg/mL[a]	ES	0.5 mg/mL[a]	Physically compatible for 48 hr at 22 °C	1706	C
Fluconazole	RR	2 mg/mL	ES	5 mg/mL	Precipitates immediately	1407	I
Foscarnet sodium	AST	24 mg/mL	ES	5 mg/mL	Gas production	1335	I
Heparin sodium[f]	RI	1000 units/L[a,b,d]	RC	5 mg/mL	Immediate haziness and globule formation	322	I
Hetastarch in lactated electrolyte	AB	6%	AB	5 mg/mL	White turbidity forms immediately	2339	I
Hydrocortisone sodium succinate[g]	UP	100 mg/L[a,b,d]	RC	5 mg/mL	Immediate haziness and globule formation	322	I
Hydromorphone HCl	KN	2, 10, 40 mg/mL	SX	5 mg/mL	Turbidity forms immediately and diazepam precipitate develops	1532	I
	AST	0.5 mg/mL[a]	ES	0.5 mg/mL[a]	Physically compatible for 48 hr at 22 °C	1706	C
Linezolid	PHU	2 mg/mL	AB	5 mg/mL	Turbid precipitate forms immediately	2264	I
Meropenem	ZEN	1 and 50 mg/mL[b]	RC	5 mg/mL	White precipitate forms immediately	1994	I
Methadone HCl	LI	1 mg/mL[a]	ES	0.5 mg/mL[a]	Physically compatible for 48 hr at 22 °C	1706	C
Morphine sulfate	AST	1 mg/mL[a]	ES	0.5 mg/mL[a]	Physically compatible for 48 hr at 22 °C	1706	C
Nafcillin sodium	WY	33 mg/mL[b]		5 mg/mL	No precipitation	547	C
Oxaliplatin	SS	0.5 mg/mL[a]	AB	5 mg/mL	Gross white turbidity forms immediately	2566	I
Pancuronium bromide	ES	0.05 mg/mL[a]	ES	5 mg/mL	Cloudy solution forms immediately	1337	I
Potassium chloride		40 mEq/L[a,b,d]	RC	5 mg/mL	Immediate haziness and globule formation	322	I
Propofol	ZEN	10 mg/mL	ES	5 mg/mL	Emulsion broke and oiled out	2066	I
Quinidine gluconate	LI	6 mg/mL[a,b]	ES	0.2 mg/mL[a,b]	Physically compatible for 3 hr	1316	C
Remifentanil HCl	GW	0.025 and 0.25 mg/mL[b]	ES	5 mg/mL	White turbidity forms immediately	2075	I
	GW	0.025 and 0.25 mg/mL[b]	ES	0.25 mg/mL[a]	Physically compatible for 4 hr at 23 °C	2075	C

Y-Site Injection Compatibility (1:1 Mixture) (Cont.)

Diazepam

Drug	Mfr	Conc	Mfr	Conc	Remarks	Ref	C/I
Tirofiban HCl	ME	50 mcg/mL[a,b]	ES	5 mg/mL	Precipitate forms immediately	2356	**I**
Vecuronium bromide	OR	0.1 mg/mL[a]	ES	5 mg/mL	Cloudy solution forms immediately	1337	**I**

[a]*Tested in dextrose 5%.*
[b]*Tested in sodium chloride 0.9%.*
[c]*Given over three minutes via a Y-site into the running heparin admixture.*
[d]*Tested in Ringer's injection, lactated.*
[e]*Refer to Appendix I for the composition of parenteral nutrition solutions. TPN indicates a 2-in-1 admixture.*
[f]*Tested in combination with hydrocortisone sodium succinate (Upjohn) 100 mg/L.*
[g]*Tested in combination with heparin sodium (Riker) 1000 units/L.*

Additional Compatibility Information

Infusion Solutions — Although the package insert for diazepam contains a caveat against dilution of the product before intravenous administration (1), interest in the intravenous administration of diluted diazepam has been expressed repeatedly in the literature.

Roche indicated that an ampul of diazepam should be diluted in no more than 5 mL or, alternatively, all the way to 20 mL to avoid precipitation. Between these concentrations, a fine white precipitate may occur. (379)

Dilution of diazepam in a volume of 25% or more of the diazepam volume is stated to result in the immediate precipitation of diazepam. No precipitation was observed if aqueous dilution was made with a volume of less than 25% of the diazepam volume. (2082)

Diazepam injection added to sodium chloride 0.9% caused the immediate formation of a light yellow to white precipitate. The maximum dilution that produced such a precipitate was 15-fold, representing a mixture of about 0.3 to 0.4 mg/mL. Analysis of the diazepam injection–sodium chloride 0.9% precipitate showed that it was almost entirely diazepam. A precipitate also formed in human plasma. A solution composed of all ingredients of diazepam injection except diazepam was tried, but dilution yielded no precipitate. It was estimated that injection of 5 mg/min into the tubing of an intravenous infusion of sodium chloride 0.9% would result in a precipitate unless the solution rate exceeded 17 mL/min. (381)

It was determined that the precipitate induced by adding 2 mL of sterile water for injection to 1 mL of diazepam injection is only diazepam. The precipitate appeared to be oily and adhered to the walls of the container, leaving a clear solution. This may explain the reports of the clearing of cloudy solutions with time. (641; 642)

As little as 10 mg of diazepam in 100 mL of dextrose 5% resulted in a precipitate. It was also found that an infusion rate of over 15 to 20 mL/min was required to prevent precipitation of diazepam being injected at a rate of 5 mg/min in running infusions of dextrose 5% and sodium chloride 0.9%. (382)

Nevertheless, interest in infusing diazepam has persisted because of bioavailability problems associated with intramuscular injection (121; 383; 384; 638) and a belief in the utility of diazepam infusions. (386; 387; 388; 389; 390; 391; 392; 1099)

Diazepam 10 mg in 250 mL and 5 mg in 50 mL of sodium chloride 0.9% resulted in no observable precipitate. (385)

A transient cloudiness occurred when 100 mg of diazepam was added to 500 mL of Ringer's injection, lactated. The solution thereafter remained clear, and the clinical response to the diazepam infusion was good. (392)

A study was conducted on the compatibility and stability of diazepam in a variety of intravenous infusion solutions. Results indicate that a visible precipitate is produced in dilutions of 1:1 to 1:10. Haziness was reported at 1:15, and delayed precipitates forming after six to eight hours were seen in some solutions at 1:20. Dilutions of 1:40 to 1:100 remained clear for 24 hours. Further, the concentration of the 1:40 to 1:100 dilutions was retained for 24 hours. (321)

The equilibrium solubilities of diazepam in water for injection, sodium chloride 0.9%, dextrose 5%, and Ringer's injection, lactated were determined. The equilibrium solubilities were found to be about 0.04 to 0.05 mg/mL in all of the solutions at 25 °C. This finding corroborated the work of others which indicated the solubility to be about 0.05 to 0.06 mg/mL. It was concluded that a more conservative 1:100 dilution should be used for diazepam infusion to guarantee solubility for 24 hours. (643)

The aqueous solubility of diazepam over a pH range of approximately 3 to 8 in phosphate buffer adjusted with hydrochloric acid or sodium hydroxide as well as dextrose 5%, sodium chloride 0.9%, and Ringer's injection, lactated was determined. In the pH range of 4 to 8, which included all three infusion solutions, the solubility was approximately 0.05 to 0.06 mg/mL at 25 °C. Dilution to at least 0.04 mg/mL was recommended to ensure rapid and complete resolution upon addition to the infusion solution. (644)

Various dilutions of diazepam in water for injection and sodium chloride 0.9% were tested. The observations are tabulated here (1095):

Diazepam Concentration	Diluent	Observation
10 mg/5 mL	W, NS	Clear for 1 min but then precipitate forms
10 mg/10 mL	W, NS	Precipitates immediately
10 mg/20 mL	NS	Precipitates immediately
10 mg/25 mL	NS	Precipitates immediately
10 mg/30 mL	NS	Clear for 30 min but then precipitate forms
10 mg/50 mL	NS	Clear for 10 days
10 mg/100 mL	NS	Clear for 10 days

Order of Mixing — It has been reported that addition of diazepam to dextrose 5% and sodium chloride 0.9% to form concentrations of 50 and 200 mg/L results in an immediate and persistent yellow precipitate. However, addition of the diluent to the diazepam injection to these same concentrations results initially in a cloudy solution which clears before the completion of admixture. It was recommended that admixtures of diazepam be prepared by adding the infusion solution to the diazepam injection. (647; 648)

DIGOXIN
AHFS 24:04.08

Products — Digoxin is available in 1- and 2-mL ampuls and vials containing 0.25 mg/mL in propylene glycol 40% and alcohol 10%, along with sodium phosphate 0.17% and citric acid 0.08%. (1)

Digoxin pediatric injection is available in 1-mL ampuls containing 0.1 mg/mL in propylene glycol 40% and alcohol 10%, along with sodium phosphate 0.17% and citric acid 0.08%. (1)

pH — From 6.8 to 7.2. (1)

Osmolality — The osmolality of digoxin pediatric injection (Burroughs Wellcome) was determined to be 9105 mOsm/kg by freezing-point depression and 5885 mOsm/kg by vapor pressure. (1071)

Trade Name(s) — Lanoxin.

Administration — Digoxin is administered by direct intravenous injection slowly over a minimum of five minutes or longer given undiluted or diluted with a fourfold or greater volume of sterile water for injection, dextrose 5%, or sodium chloride 0.9%. If a tuberculin syringe is used for very small doses, the possibility of inadvertent overdosage exists. Following intravenous administration, the syringe should not be flushed with parenteral solution. (1; 4) Deep intramuscular injection of not more than 2 mL at a single site followed by massage has been performed. However, it is painful and causes severe local irritation. (4)

Stability — Intact containers of digoxin should be stored at controlled room temperature and protected from light. (1)

pH Effects — Digoxin is hydrolyzed in acidic solutions with a pH less than 3. At pH 5 to 8, however, digoxin is not hydrolyzed in aqueous solutions. (798; 799; 800; 801)

Plasticizer Leaching — Digoxin (Elkins-Sinn) 0.04 mg/mL in dextrose 5% did not leach diethylhexyl phthalate (DEHP) plasticizer from 50-mL PVC bags in 24 hours at 24 °C. (1683)

Filtration — Digoxin (Burroughs Wellcome) 1 mg/L in dextrose 5%, sodium chloride 0.9%, and Ringer's injection, lactated, filtered over 12 hours through a 5-μm stainless steel depth filter (Argyle Filter Connector), a 0.22-μm cellulose ester membrane filter (Ivex-2 Filter Set), and a 0.22-μm polycarbonate membrane filter (In-Sure Filter Set), showed no significant reduction due to binding to the filters. (320)

In another evaluation, digoxin (Burroughs Wellcome) 3 mg/L in dextrose 5% and sodium chloride 0.9% did not display significant sorption to a 0.45-μm cellulose membrane filter (Abbott S-A-I-F) during an eight-hour simulated infusion. (567)

Digoxin (Wellcome) 1 mcg/mL in dextrose 5% and sodium chloride 0.9% was delivered over eight hours through four kinds of 0.2-μm membrane filters varying in size and composition. In the first 20 minutes, digoxin concentration losses were 10 to 23% through the Sterifix filter and 24 to 32% through the Pall ELD-96LL filter. However, losses of 63 to 73% occurred in the first 20 minutes with the Ivex-HP and Pall FAE-020LL filters. Subsequent digoxin levels returned to the original concentration when the binding sites became saturated. (1399)

Compatibility Information

Solution Compatibility

Digoxin

Solution	Mfr	Mfr	Conc/L	Remarks	Ref	C/I
Dextrose 5%	AB	BW	2.5 mg	Physically compatible with no loss of digoxin in 48 hr at 4 and 23 °C	778	C
Dextrose 5% in sodium chloride 0.45%[a]	AB	BW	2.5 mg	Physically compatible with no loss of digoxin in 6-hr study period at 23 °C	778	C
Ringer's injection, lactated	AB	BW	2.5 mg	Physically compatible with no loss of digoxin in 6-hr study period at 23 °C	778	C
Sodium chloride 0.45%		ES	125 mg	Physically compatible with no loss of digoxin in 4 hr at 22 °C	1419	C
Sodium chloride 0.9%	AB	BW	2.5 mg	Physically compatible with no loss of digoxin in 48 hr at 4 and 23 °C	778	C

[a]*Tested in combination with potassium chloride 20 mEq/L.*

Additive Compatibility

Digoxin

Drug	Mfr	Conc/L	Mfr	Conc/L	Test Soln	Remarks	Ref	C/I
Dobutamine HCl	LI	1 g	BW	4 mg	D5W, NS	Slightly pink in 24 hr at 25 °C	789	I
Floxacillin sodium	BE	20 g	BW	25 mg	NS	Physically compatible for 72 hr at 15 and 30 °C	1479	C
Furosemide	HO	1 g	BW	25 mg	NS	Physically compatible for 72 hr at 15 and 30 °C	1479	C
Lidocaine HCl	AST	2 g	ES	1 mg	D5W, LR, NS	Physically compatible for 24 hr at 25 °C	775	C
Ranitidine HCl	GL	50 mg and 2 g		2.5 mg	D5W	Physically compatible. Ranitidine stable for 24 hr at 25 °C. Digoxin not tested	1515	C
Verapamil HCl	KN	80 mg	BW	2 mg	D5W, NS	Physically compatible for 48 hr	739	C

Drugs in Syringe Compatibility

Digoxin

Drug (in syringe)	Mfr	Amt	Mfr	Amt	Remarks	Ref	C/I
Dimenhydrinate		10 mg/ 1 mL		0.05 mg/ 1 mL	Clear solution	2569	C
Doxapram HCl	RB	400 mg/ 20 mL		0.25 mg/ 1 mL	10% doxapram loss in 9 hr and 17% in 24 hr	1177	I
Heparin sodium		2500 units/ 1 mL		0.25 mg/ 1 mL	Physically compatible for at least 5 min	1053	C
Milrinone lactate	WI	3.5 mg/ 3.5 mL	BW	0.5 mg/ 2 mL	Brought to 10-mL total volume with D5W. Physically compatible with no loss of either drug in 4 hr at 23 °C	1191	C
Pantoprazole sodium	[a]	4 mg/ 1 mL		0.05 mg/ 1 mL	Precipitates within 4 hr	2574	I

[a]*Test performed using the formulation without edetate disodium.*

Y-Site Injection Compatibility (1:1 Mixture)

Digoxin

Drug	Mfr	Conc	Mfr	Conc	Remarks	Ref	C/I
Amiodarone HCl	WY	6 mg/mL[a]	ES	0.25 mg/mL	Immediate opaque white turbidity	2352	I
Amphotericin B cholesteryl sulfate complex	SEQ	0.83 mg/mL[a]	WY	0.25 mg/mL	Microprecipitate forms in 4 hr at 23 °C	2117	I
Anidulafungin	VIC	0.5 mg/mL[a]	GW	0.25 mg/mL	Physically compatible for 4 hr at 23 °C	2617	C
Bivalirudin	TMC	5 mg/mL[a]	GW	0.25 mg/mL	Physically compatible for 4 hr at 23 °C	2373	C
Ceftaroline fosamil	FOR	2.22 mg/mL[d]	BA	0.25 mg/mL	Physically compatible for 4 hr at 23 °C	2826	C
Ciprofloxacin	MI	2 mg/mL[c]	ES	0.25 mg/mL	Visually compatible for 24 hr at 24 °C	1655	C
	BAY	2 mg/mL[b]	BW	0.25 mg/mL	Visually compatible with no ciprofloxacin loss in 15 min. Digoxin not tested	1934	C
Cisatracurium besylate	GW	0.1, 2, 5 mg/ mL[a]	ES	0.25 mg/mL	Physically compatible for 4 hr at 23 °C	2074	C

Y-Site Injection Compatibility (1:1 Mixture) (Cont.)

Digoxin

Drug	Mfr	Conc	Mfr	Conc	Remarks	Ref	C/I
Dexmedetomidine HCl	AB	4 mcg/mL[b]	ES	0.25 mg/mL	Physically compatible for 4 hr at 23 °C	2383	C
Diltiazem HCl	MMD	1[b] and 5 mg/mL	ES	0.5 mg/mL	Visually compatible	1807	C
Doripenem	JJ	5 mg/mL[a,b]	BA	0.25 mg/mL	Physically compatible for 4 hr at 23 °C	2743	C
Famotidine	MSD	0.2 mg/mL[a]	ES	0.25 mg/mL	Physically compatible for 14 hr	1196	C
Fenoldopam mesylate	AB	80 mcg/mL[b]	ES	0.25 mg/mL	Physically compatible for 4 hr at 23 °C	2467	C
Fluconazole	RR	2 mg/mL	BW	0.25 mg/mL	Gas production	1407	I
Foscarnet sodium	AST	24 mg/mL	WY	0.25 mg/mL	Gas production	1335	I
Heparin sodium[f]	RI	1000 units/L[d]	BW	0.25 mg/mL	Physically compatible for 4 hr at room temperature	322	C
Hetastarch in lactated electrolyte	AB	6%	ES	0.25 mg/mL	Physically compatible for 4 hr at 23 °C	2339	C
Hydrocortisone sodium succinate[g]	UP	100 mg/L[d]	BW	0.25 mg/mL	Physically compatible for 4 hr at room temperature	322	C
Insulin, regular	LI	1 unit/mL[b]	ES	0.005 mg/mL[b]	Physically compatible for 3 hr	1316	C
	LI	1 unit/mL[a]	ES	0.005 mg/mL[a]	Slight haze in 1 hr	1316	I
Linezolid	PHU	2 mg/mL	ES	0.25 mg/mL	Physically compatible for 4 hr at 23 °C	2264	C
Meperidine HCl	AB	10 mg/mL	BW	0.25 mg/mL	Physically compatible for 4 hr at 25 °C	1397	C
Meropenem	ZEN	1 and 50 mg/mL[b]	BW	0.25 mg/mL	Visually compatible for 4 hr at room temperature	1994	C
Midazolam HCl	RC	1 mg/mL[a]	BW	0.1 mg/mL	Visually compatible for 24 hr at 23 °C	1847	C
Milrinone lactate	WI	200 mcg/mL[a]	BW	0.25 mg/mL	Physically compatible with no loss of either drug in 4 hr at 23 °C	1191	C
Morphine sulfate	AB	1 mg/mL	BW	0.25 mg/mL	Physically compatible for 4 hr at 25 °C	1397	C
Nesiritide	SCI	50 mcg/mL[a,b]		0.25 mg/mL	Physically compatible for 4 hr	2625	C
Potassium chloride		40 mEq/L[d]	BW	0.25 mg/mL	Physically compatible for 4 hr at room temperature	322	C
Remifentanil HCl	GW	0.025 and 0.25 mg/mL[b]	ES	0.25 mg/mL	Physically compatible for 4 hr at 23 °C	2075	C
Tacrolimus	FUJ	1 mg/mL[b]	WY	0.25 mg/mL	Visually compatible for 24 hr at 25 °C	1630	C
Telavancin HCl	ASP	7.5 mg/mL[d]	BA	0.25 mg/mL	Visible turbidity formed	2830	I
TNA #73[e]			BW	12.5 mcg/mL[c]	Visually compatible for 4 hr	1009	C
TNA #218 to #226[e]			ES, WY	0.25 mg/mL	Visually compatible for 4 hr at 23 °C	2215	C
TPN #212 to #215[e]			BW	0.25 mg/mL	Physically compatible for 4 hr at 23 °C	2109	C

[a]Tested in dextrose 5%.
[b]Tested in sodium chloride 0.9%.
[c]Tested in both dextrose 5% and sodium chloride 0.9%.
[d]Tested in dextrose 5%, Ringer's injection, lactated, and sodium chloride 0.9%.
[e]Refer to Appendix I for the composition of parenteral nutrition solutions. TNA indicates a 3-in-1 admixture, and TPN indicates a 2-in-1 admixture.
[f]Tested in combination with hydrocortisone sodium succinate (Upjohn) 100 mg/L.
[g]Tested in combination with heparin sodium (Riker) 1000 units/L.

DILTIAZEM HYDROCHLORIDE
AHFS 24:28.92

Products — Diltiazem hydrochloride is available as a 5-mg/mL solution in 5-mL (25-mg), 10-mL (50-mg), and 25-mL (125-mg) vials. Also present in each milliliter of solution are citric acid 0.75 mg, sodium citrate dihydrate 0.65 mg, sorbitol solution 71.4 mg, and water for injection. Sodium hydroxide or hydrochloric acid may be used to adjust the pH. (1)

pH — From 3.7 to 4.1. (1)

Administration — Diltiazem hydrochloride is administered by direct intravenous injection over two minutes and by continuous intravenous infusion after dilution. (1)

Stability — Intact vials of the liquid injection should be stored under refrigeration and protected from freezing. Diltiazem hydrochloride may be stored for up to one month at room temperature but should then be destroyed. (1)

pH Effects — An increased rate of diltiazem hydrochloride hydrolysis occurs with increasing pH. Hydrolysis was lowest at pH 5 and 6 but increased substantially at pH 7 and 8. Diltiazem hydrochloride 100 mcg/mL in sodium chloride 0.9% with a pH between 5 and 6 exhibited no loss in 24 hours. Buffered to pH 7, losses of 3 to 4% in 24 hours were found. (1915)

Light Effects — Diltiazem hydrochloride reconstituted with distilled water to a concentration of 10 mg/mL was exposed to UVA-UVB radiation with a solar simulator for 28 hours. Only 5.6% degradation occurred under this intense light exposure. The drug maintained adequate stability and light protection was not required. (2432)

Sorption — A pH-dependent loss of diltiazem hydrochloride occurs due to sorption to PVC containers and administration sets. Diltiazem hydrochloride 100 mcg/mL in sodium chloride 0.9% buffered to neutrality exhibits a loss of 11% in 24 hours in PVC containers but only 3 to 4% in glass and polypropylene containers. Similar results were found with PVC administration sets. Buffered to pH 8, diltiazem hydrochloride concentration was initially reduced to about 83% when delivered at 0.52 mL/min through a 100-cm PVC administration set. At pH 6 and 7, initial losses were much less, about 1 and 5%, respectively. Delivered diltiazem hydrochloride returned to full concentration in less than one hour at pH 6 and 7 but at pH 8 was only about 93% in two hours. (1915)

Diltiazem hydrochloride 0.05 mg/mL in dextrose 5% and sodium chloride 0.9% packaged in PVC, polyethylene, and glass containers exhibited little or no loss due to sorption to any of the container types when stored at 4 and 22 °C for 24 hours protected from light. (2289)

Diltiazem hydrochloride (Synthelabo) 1 g/L in dextrose 5% and in sodium chloride 0.9% was evaluated for loss due to sorption to a variety of polymer container types compared to glass containers. No significant loss due to sorption was found at 21 °C after 48 hours of contact time to PVC and polyethylene containers and 24 hours of contact time to polyamide containers. (274)

Similarly, no significant loss of diltiazem hydrochloride occurred from 1-g/L solutions in dextrose 5% and in sodium chloride 0.9% in cellulose propionate (Abbott), butadiene styrene (B. Braun), and metacrylate butadiene styrene (Avon) burettes for 24 hours at 21 °C and when delivered over 5 hours through PVC (Abbott and Baxter), PVC/polyethylene double polymer (Abbott), and polybutadiene (Avon) administration tubing. (274)

Filtration — Cellulose ester filters (B. Braun and Millipore) were found to result in a temporary reduction in the concentration of delivered diltiazem hydrochloride from a 1-g/L solution in sodium chloride 0.9%. The concentration of delivered diltiazem hydrochloride returned to near 100% after about one to two hours of infusion through the filter. No reduction in delivered concentration was found if dextrose 5% was used as the vehicle. No loss occurred in either infusion solution with polyamide (Pall) filters. (274)

Compatibility Information

Solution Compatibility

Diltiazem HCl

Solution	Mfr	Mfr	Conc/L	Remarks	Ref	C/I
Dextrose 5%			1 g	Compatible and stable for 24 hr at room and refrigeration temperatures	1	C
	BA[a]	GO	50 mg	Visually compatible. 4% loss in 24 hr at 22 °C and little loss at 4 °C	2289	C
	BRN[b]	GO	50 mg	Visually compatible. Little loss in 24 hr at 4 and 22 °C	2289	C
		SYO	1 g	No loss occurred in 48 hr at 21 °C	274	C
	GRI[a]	BED	1 g	Physically compatible. No loss in 90 days at 25 and 5 °C	2750	C
Dextrose 5% in sodium chloride 0.45%			1 g	Compatible and stable for 24 hr at room and refrigeration temperatures	1	C
Sodium chloride 0.9%			1 g	Compatible and stable for 24 hr at room and refrigeration temperatures	1	C
	BA[a]	GO	50 mg	Visually compatible. 4% loss in 24 hr at 22 °C and little or no loss at 4 °C	2289	C

Solution Compatibility (Cont.)

Diltiazem HCl

Solution	Mfr	Mfr	Conc/L	Remarks	Ref	C/I
	BRN[b]	GO	50 mg	Visually compatible. Little loss in 24 hr at 4 and 22 °C	2289	C
		SYO	1 g	No loss occurred in 48 hr at 21 °C	274	C
	GRI[a]	BED	1 g	Physically compatible. No loss in 90 days at 25 and 5 °C	2750	C

[a]Tested in PVC containers.
[b]Tested in polyethylene and glass containers.

Y-Site Injection Compatibility (1:1 Mixture)

Diltiazem HCl

Drug	Mfr	Conc	Mfr	Conc	Remarks	Ref	C/I
Acetazolamide sodium	LE	100 mg/mL	MMD	5 mg/mL	Precipitate forms	1807	I
	LE	100 mg/mL	MMD	1 mg/mL[b]	Visually compatible	1807	C
Acyclovir sodium	BW	5[a] and 7[b] mg/mL	MMD	5 mg/mL	Cloudiness and precipitate form	1807	I
	BW	5[a] and 7[b] mg/mL	MMD	1 mg/mL[b]	Visually compatible	1807	C
Albumin human	AR, AT	5 and 25%	MMD	5 mg/mL	Visually compatible	1807	C
Amikacin sulfate	BR	5[b] and 250 mg/mL	MMD	5 mg/mL	Visually compatible	1807	C
Aminophylline	AMR	25 mg/mL[b]	MMD	5 mg/mL	Cloudiness forms	1807	I
	AMR	25 mg/mL[b]	MMD	1 mg/mL[b]	Visually compatible	1807	C
	AMR	2 mg/mL[a,b]	MMD	5 mg/mL	Visually compatible	1807	C
Amphotericin B	SQ	0.1 mg/mL[a]	MMD	5 mg/mL	Visually compatible	1807	C
Ampicillin sodium	WY	100 mg/mL[b]	MMD	5 mg/mL	Cloudiness forms	1807	I
	WY	100 mg/mL[b]	MMD	1 mg/mL[b]	Visually compatible	1807	C
	WY	10 and 20 mg/mL[b]	MMD	5 mg/mL	Visually compatible	1807	C
Ampicillin sodium–sulbactam sodium	RR	45 + 22.5 mg/mL[b]	MMD	5 mg/mL	Cloudiness forms	1807	I
	RR	45 + 22.5 mg/mL[b]	MMD	1 mg/mL[b]	Visually compatible	1807	C
	RR	2 + 1 and 15 + 7.5 mg/mL[b]	MMD	5 mg/mL	Visually compatible	1807	C
Argatroban	GSK	1 mg/mL[b]	BV	5 mg/mL	Visually compatible for 24 hr at 23 °C	2391	C
Aztreonam	SQ	20 and 333 mg/mL[b]	MMD	5 mg/mL	Visually compatible	1807	C
	SQ	333 mg/mL[b]	MMD	1 mg/mL[b]	Visually compatible	1807	C
Bivalirudin	TMC	5 mg/mL[a]	BA	5 mg/mL	Physically compatible for 4 hr at 23 °C	2373	C
	TMC	5 mg/mL[a,b]	BV	5 mg/mL	Visually compatible for 6 hr at 23 °C	2680	C
Bumetanide	RC	0.25 mg/mL	MMD	1[b] and 5 mg/mL	Visually compatible	1807	C
Caspofungin acetate	ME	0.7 mg/mL[b]	HOS	5 mg/mL	Physically compatible for 4 hr at room temperature	2758	C
Cefazolin sodium	LI	20 and 200 mg/mL[b]	MMD	5 mg/mL	Visually compatible	1807	C

Y-Site Injection Compatibility (1:1 Mixture) (Cont.)

Diltiazem HCl

Drug	Mfr	Conc	Mfr	Conc	Remarks	Ref	C/I
	LI	200 mg/mL[b]	MMD	1 mg/mL[b]	Visually compatible	1807	C
Cefotaxime sodium	HO	10 and 180 mg/mL[b]	MMD	5 mg/mL	Visually compatible	1807	C
	HO	180 mg/mL[b]	MMD	1 mg/mL[b]	Visually compatible	1807	C
Cefotetan disodium	STU	10 and 200 mg/mL[b]	MMD	5 mg/mL	Visually compatible	1807	C
	STU	200 mg/mL[b]	MMD	1 mg/mL[b]	Visually compatible	1807	C
Cefoxitin sodium	MSD	10 and 200 mg/mL[b]	MMD	5 mg/mL	Visually compatible	1807	C
	MSD	200 mg/mL[b]	MMD	1 mg/mL[b]	Visually compatible	1807	C
Ceftaroline fosamil	FOR	2.22 mg/mL[a,b,f]	HOS	5 mg/mL	Physically compatible for 4 hr at 23 °C	2826	C
Ceftazidime	GL	10 and 170 mg/mL[b]	MMD	5 mg/mL	Visually compatible	1807	C
	GL	170 mg/mL[b]	MMD	1 mg/mL[b]	Visually compatible	1807	C
Ceftriaxone sodium	RC	40 mg/mL[b]	MMD	5 mg/mL	Visually compatible	1807	C
Cefuroxime sodium	LI	15 and 100 mg/mL[b]	MMD	5 mg/mL	Visually compatible	1807	C
	LI	100 mg/mL[b]	MMD	1 mg/mL[b]	Visually compatible	1807	C
Ciprofloxacin	MI	2 and 10 mg/mL[b]	MMD	5 mg/mL	Visually compatible	1807	C
Clindamycin phosphate	UP	12[b] and 150 mg/mL	MMD	5 mg/mL	Visually compatible	1807	C
Dexmedetomidine HCl	AB	4 mcg/mL[b]	BA	5 mg/mL	Physically compatible for 4 hr at 23 °C	2383	C
Diazepam	ES	5 mg/mL	MMD	1[b] and 5 mg/mL	Cloudiness and precipitate form	1807	I
Digoxin	ES	0.5 mg/mL	MMD	1[b] and 5 mg/mL	Visually compatible	1807	C
Dobutamine HCl	LI	2 mg/mL[a]	MMD	1 mg/mL[a]	Visually compatible for 24 hr at 25 °C	1530	C
	LI	1 mg/mL[c]	MMD	5 mg/mL	Visually compatible	1807	C
	LI	4 mg/mL[a]	MMD	1 mg/mL[a]	Visually compatible for 4 hr at 27 °C	2062	C
Dopamine HCl	AB	1.6 mg/mL[a]	MMD	1 mg/mL[a]	Visually compatible for 24 hr at 25 °C	1530	C
	AB, SO	0.8 mg/mL[c]	MMD	5 mg/mL	Visually compatible	1807	C
	AB	3.2 mg/mL[a]	MMD	1 mg/mL[a]	Visually compatible for 4 hr at 27 °C	2062	C
Doripenem	JJ	5 mg/mL[a,b]	BED	5 mg/mL	Physically compatible for 4 hr at 23 °C	2743	C
Doxycycline hyclate	RR	1 and 10 mg/mL[b]	MMD	5 mg/mL	Visually compatible	1807	C
Epinephrine HCl	PD	0.004 and 0.05 mg/mL[b]	MMD	5 mg/mL	Visually compatible	1807	C
	PD	0.05 mg/mL[b]	MMD	1 mg/mL[b]	Visually compatible	1807	C
	AB	0.02 mg/mL[a]	MMD	1 mg/mL[a]	Visually compatible for 4 hr at 27 °C	2062	C
Erythromycin lactobionate	ES	5 and 50 mg/mL[b]	MMD	5 mg/mL	Visually compatible	1807	C
Esmolol HCl	DU	10 mg/mL[a]	MMD	1 mg/mL[a]	Visually compatible for 24 hr at 25 °C	1530	C
Fenoldopam mesylate	AB	80 mcg/mL[b]	BA	5 mg/mL	Physically compatible for 4 hr at 23 °C	2467	C

Y-Site Injection Compatibility (1:1 Mixture) (Cont.)

Diltiazem HCl

Drug	Mfr	Conc	Mfr	Conc	Remarks	Ref	C/I
Fentanyl citrate	ES	0.05 mg/mL	MMD	1 mg/mL[a]	Visually compatible for 4 hr at 27 °C	2062	C
Fluconazole	RR	2 mg/mL	MMD	5 mg/mL	Visually compatible	1807	C
Furosemide	AMR	10 mg/mL	MMD	1[b] and 5 mg/mL	Heavy precipitate forms	1807	I
	AMR	10 mg/mL	MMD	1 mg/mL[a]	Precipitate forms immediately	2062	I
Gentamicin sulfate	SC	2.4[b] and 40 mg/mL	MMD	1[b] and 5 mg/mL	Visually compatible	1807	C
Heparin sodium	LY	20,000 units/mL	MMD	5 mg/mL	Precipitate forms	1807	I
	LY	20,000 units/mL	MMD	1 mg/mL[b]	Visually compatible	1807	C
	SCN	5000 and 10,000 units/mL	MMD	1[b] and 5 mg/mL	Visually compatible	1807	C
	LY, SCN	80 units/mL[c]	MMD	5 mg/mL	Visually compatible	1807	C
	ES	100 units/mL[a]	MMD	1 mg/mL[a]	Visually compatible for 4 hr at 27 °C	2062	C
Hetastarch in lactated electrolyte	AB	6%	BA	5 mg/mL	Physically compatible for 4 hr at 23 °C	2339	C
Hetastarch in sodium chloride 0.9%	DU	6%	MMD	5 mg/mL	Visually compatible	1807	C
Hydrocortisone sodium succinate	UP	50 and 125 mg/mL	MMD	5 mg/mL	Precipitate forms but clears with swirling	1807	?
	UP	50 and 125 mg/mL	MMD	1 mg/mL[b]	Visually compatible	1807	C
	UP	1[b] and 2[a] mg/mL	MMD	5 mg/mL	Visually compatible	1807	C
Hydromorphone HCl	KN	1 mg/mL	MMD	1 mg/mL[a]	Visually compatible for 4 hr at 27 °C	2062	C
Imipenem–cilastatin sodium	MSD	5 mg/mL[c]	MMD	5 mg/mL	Visually compatible	1807	C
Labetalol HCl	AH	2 mg/mL[a]	MMD	1 mg/mL[a]	Visually compatible for 4 hr at 27 °C	2062	C
Lidocaine HCl	AST	8 mg/mL[a]	MMD	1 mg/mL[a]	Visually compatible for 24 hr at 25 °C	1530	C
	AB	10 mg/mL[b]	MMD	1[b] and 5 mg/mL	Visually compatible	1807	C
	AB, SCN	4 and 8 mg/mL[a]	MMD	5 mg/mL	Visually compatible	1807	C
Lorazepam	WY	4 mg/mL	MMD	5 mg/mL	Visually compatible	1807	C
	WY	2 mg/mL[b]	MMD	1 mg/mL[b]	Visually compatible	1807	C
	WY	0.5 mg/mL[a]	MMD	1 mg/mL[a]	Visually compatible for 4 hr at 27 °C	2062	C
Meperidine HCl	WY	100 mg/mL	MMD	1[b] and 5 mg/mL	Visually compatible	1807	C
	WY	10 mg/mL[b]	MMD	5 mg/mL	Visually compatible	1807	C
Methylprednisolone sodium succinate	UP	2.5[a], 20[b], 62.5 mg/mL	MMD	1 mg/mL[b]	Visually compatible	1807	C
	UP	2.5 mg/mL[a]	MMD	5 mg/mL	Cloudiness forms	1807	I
	UP	20 mg/mL[b]	MMD	5 mg/mL	Precipitate forms	1807	I
	UP	62.5 mg/mL	MMD	5 mg/mL	Cloudiness forms but clears with swirling	1807	?
Metoclopramide HCl	RB	5 mg/mL	MMD	1[b] and 5 mg/mL	Visually compatible	1807	C
	RB	0.2 mg/mL[b]	MMD	5 mg/mL	Visually compatible	1807	C

Y-Site Injection Compatibility (1:1 Mixture) (Cont.)

Diltiazem HCl

Drug	Mfr	Conc	Mfr	Conc	Remarks	Ref	C/I
Metoprolol tartrate	BED	1 mg/mL	NVP	1 mg/mL[a]	Visually compatible for 24 hr at 19 °C	2795	C
Metronidazole	SE	5 mg/mL	MMD	5 mg/mL	Visually compatible	1807	C
Micafungin sodium	ASP	1.5 mg/mL[b]	BA	5 mg/mL	Gross precipitate forms immediately	2683	I
Midazolam HCl	RC	2 mg/mL[a]	MMD	1 mg/mL[a]	Visually compatible for 4 hr at 27 °C	2062	C
Milrinone lactate	SW	0.2 mg/mL[a]	MMD	1 mg/mL[a]	Visually compatible for 4 hr at 27 °C	2062	C
	SW	0.4 mg/mL[a]	MMD	1 mg/mL[a]	Visually compatible with little loss of either drug in 4 hr at 23 °C	2214	C
Morphine sulfate	SCN	15 mg/mL	MMD	1[b] and 5 mg/mL	Visually compatible	1807	C
	SCN	0.4 mg/mL[b]	MMD	5 mg/mL	Visually compatible	1807	C
	SCN	2 mg/mL[a]	MMD	1 mg/mL[a]	Visually compatible for 4 hr at 27 °C	2062	C
Multivitamins		[d]	MMD	5 mg/mL	Visually compatible	1807	C
Nafcillin sodium	WY	10 mg/mL[b]	MMD	5 mg/mL	Cloudiness forms and persists	1807	I
	WY	200 mg/mL[b]	MMD	5 mg/mL	Cloudiness forms but clears with swirling	1807	?
	WY	10 and 200 mg/mL[b]	MMD	1 mg/mL[b]	Visually compatible	1807	C
Nesiritide	SCI	50 mcg/mL[a,b]		5 mg/mL	Physically compatible for 4 hr	2625	C
Nicardipine HCl	WY	1 mg/mL[a]	MMD	1 mg/mL[a]	Visually compatible for 4 hr at 27 °C	2062	C
Nitroglycerin	DU	0.032 mg/mL[a]	MMD	1 mg/mL[a]	Visually compatible for 24 hr at 25 °C	1530	C
	DU	400 mcg/mL[b]	MMD	1[b] and 5 mg/mL	Visually compatible	1807	C
	DU	400 mcg/mL[a]	MMD	5 mg/mL	Visually compatible	1807	C
	AB	0.4 mg/mL[a]	MMD	1 mg/mL[a]	Visually compatible for 4 hr at 27 °C	2062	C
Norepinephrine bitartrate	WI	0.12 mg/mL[a]	MMD	1 mg/mL[a]	Visually compatible for 24 hr at 25 °C	1530	C
	AB	0.128 mg/mL[a]	MMD	1 mg/mL[a]	Visually compatible for 4 hr at 27 °C	2062	C
Oxacillin sodium		100 mg/mL[b]	MMD	1[b] and 5 mg/mL	Visually compatible	1807	C
		10 mg/mL[b]	MMD	5 mg/mL	Visually compatible	1807	C
Penicillin G potassium	RR	1 million units/mL	MMD	1[b] and 5 mg/mL	Visually compatible	1807	C
	RR	100,000 units/mL[b]	MMD	5 mg/mL	Visually compatible	1807	C
Pentamidine isethionate	LY	6 and 30 mg/mL[a]	MMD	5 mg/mL	Visually compatible	1807	C
Phenytoin sodium	PD	50 mg/mL	MMD	1 mg/mL[b]	Precipitate forms	1807	I
Potassium chloride	LY	0.08[a] and 2 mEq/mL	MMD	5 mg/mL	Visually compatible	1807	C
Potassium phosphates	AMR	0.015 mmol/mL	MMD	5 mg/mL	Visually compatible	1807	C
Procainamide HCl	ES	500 mg/mL	MMD	5 mg/mL	Cloudiness forms but clears within 2 min	1807	?
	ES	50 mg/mL[a]	MMD	1 mg/mL[b]	Visually compatible	1807	C
	ES	2 mg/mL[a]	MMD	5 mg/mL	Visually compatible	1807	C

Y-Site Injection Compatibility (1:1 Mixture) (Cont.)

Diltiazem HCl

Drug	Mfr	Conc	Mfr	Conc	Remarks	Ref	C/I
Ranitidine HCl	GL	25 mg/mL	MMD	1[b] and 5 mg/mL	Visually compatible	1807	C
	GL	0.5[e] and 1[b] mg/mL	MMD	5 mg/mL	Visually compatible	1807	C
	GL	1 mg/mL[a]	MMD	1 mg/mL[a]	Visually compatible for 4 hr at 27 °C	2062	C
Rifampin	MMD	6 mg/mL[b]	MMD	1[b] and 5 mg/mL	Precipitate forms	1807	I
Sodium bicarbonate	LY	1 mEq/mL	MMD	5 mg/mL	Precipitate forms	1807	I
	LY	1 mEq/mL	MMD	1 mg/mL[b]	Visually compatible	1807	C
	AMR	0.05 mEq/mL[a]	MMD	5 mg/mL	Visually compatible	1807	C
Sodium nitroprusside	AB	0.2 mg/mL[a]	MMD	5 mg/mL	Visually compatible	1807	C
Telavancin HCl	ASP	7.5 mg/mL[a,b,f]	BED	5 mg/mL	Physically compatible for 2 hr	2830	C
Theophylline	AB	0.8 mg/mL[a]	MMD	5 mg/mL	Visually compatible	1807	C
Ticarcillin disodium–clavulanate potassium	BE	200 mg/mL[b]	MMD	1[b] and 5 mg/mL	Visually compatible	1807	C
	BE	10 mg/mL[b]	MMD	5 mg/mL	Visually compatible	1807	C
Tobramycin sulfate	LI	2.4[b] and 40 mg/mL	MMD	5 mg/mL	Visually compatible	1807	C
Trimethoprim–sulfamethoxazole	BW, RC	0.21 + 1 and 0.63 + 3.2 mg/mL[a]	MMD	5 mg/mL	Visually compatible	1807	C
Vancomycin HCl	LI	5 and 50 mg/mL[b]	MMD	5 mg/mL	Visually compatible	1807	C
Vasopressin	AMR	2 and 4 units/mL[b]	NVP	1 mg/mL[b]	Physically compatible with vasopressin pushed through a Y-site over 5 sec	2478	C
Vecuronium bromide	OR	1 mg/mL	MMD	1 mg/mL[a]	Visually compatible for 4 hr at 27 °C	2062	C

[a]Tested in dextrose 5%.
[b]Tested in sodium chloride 0.9%.
[c]Tested in both dextrose 5% and sodium chloride 0.9%.
[d]Concentration not specified.
[e]Tested in sodium chloride 0.45%.
[f]Tested in Ringer's injection, lactated.

DIMENHYDRINATE
AHFS 56:22.08

Products — Dimenhydrinate is available in 1-mL and 10-mL vials containing dimenhydrinate 50 mg/mL in propylene glycol 50% and water. Sodium hydroxide and/or hydrochloric acid may be used to adjust the pH and benzyl alcohol is present in multiple-dose vials as a preservative. Dimenhydrinate contains 53 to 55.5% of diphenhydramine and 44 to 47% of 8-chlorotheophylline. (1; 4)

pH — From 6.4 to 7.2. (1; 4)

Administration — Dimenhydrinate is administered by intramuscular injection or by intravenous injection over two minutes after dilution with 10 mL of sodium chloride 0.9%. (1; 4)

Stability — Intact containers should be stored at controlled room temperature and protected from freezing. (1; 4)

pH Effects — A test of dimenhydrinate solutions at pH 2 to 10 showed no separation or precipitation at pH 5.4 to 8.6 on extended room temperature storage. Below pH 5.4, a white powdery precipitate of 8-chlorotheophylline formed within 24 hours. Above pH 8.6, an oily liquid separated within 30 minutes. (279)

Compatibility Information

Solution Compatibility

Dimenhydrinate

Solution	Mfr	Mfr	Conc/L	Remarks	Ref	C/I
Dextrose–Ringer's injection combinations	AB	SE	50 mg	Physically compatible	3	C
Dextrose–Ringer's injection, lactated, combinations	AB	SE	50 mg	Physically compatible	3	C
Dextrose–saline combinations	AB	SE	50 mg	Physically compatible	3	C
Dextrose 5% in sodium chloride 0.9%		SE	50 mg	Physically compatible	74	C
Dextrose 2.5%	AB	SE	50 mg	Physically compatible	3	C
Dextrose 5%	AB	SE	50 mg	Physically compatible	3	C
		SE	50 mg	Physically compatible	74	C
				Stable for 10 days at room temperature	279	C
Dextrose 10%	AB	SE	50 mg	Physically compatible	3	C
Ionosol products	AB	SE	50 mg	Physically compatible	3	C
Ringer's injection	AB	SE	50 mg	Physically compatible	3	C
Ringer's injection, lactated	AB	SE	50 mg	Physically compatible	3	C
		SE	50 mg	Physically compatible	74	C
Sodium chloride 0.45%	AB	SE	50 mg	Physically compatible	3	C
Sodium chloride 0.9%	AB	SE	50 mg	Physically compatible	3	C
		SE	50 mg	Physically compatible	74	C
				Stable for 10 days at room temperature	279	C
Sodium lactate ⅙ M	AB	SE	50 mg	Physically compatible	3	C

Additive Compatibility

Dimenhydrinate

Drug	Mfr	Conc/L	Mfr	Conc/L	Test Soln	Remarks	Ref	C/I
Amikacin sulfate	BR	5 g	SE	100 mg	D5LR, D5R, D5S, D5W, D10W, LR, NS, R, SL	Physically compatible and both stable for 24 hr at 25 °C	294	C

Additive Compatibility (Cont.)

Dimenhydrinate

Drug	Mfr	Conc/L	Mfr	Conc/L	Test Soln	Remarks	Ref	C/I
Aminophylline		250 mg	SE	50 mg	D5W	Physically compatible	74	C
	SE	1 g	SE	500 mg	D5W	Physically incompatible	15	I
Ammonium chloride	AB	20 g	SE	500 mg	D5W	Physically compatible	15	C
Chloramphenicol sodium succinate	PD	500 mg	SE	50 mg	D5W	Physically compatible	74	C
Heparin sodium		12,000 units	SE	50 mg	D5W	Physically compatible	74	C
	UP	4000 units	SE	500 mg	D5W	Physically compatible	15	C
	AB	20,000 units	SE	50 mg	D	Physically compatible	21	C
Hydrocortisone sodium succinate	UP	100 mg	SE	50 mg	D5W	Physically compatible	74	C
	UP	500 mg	SE	500 mg	D5W	Physically incompatible	15	I
Hydroxyzine HCl	RR	250 mg	SE	500 mg	D5W	Physically compatible	15	C
Norepinephrine bitartrate	WI	8 mg	SE	50 mg	D5W	Physically compatible	74	C
Penicillin G potassium		1 million units	SE	50 mg	D5W	Physically compatible	74	C
Pentobarbital sodium	AB	1 g	SE	500 mg	D5W	Physically compatible	15	C
Phenobarbital sodium	WI	200 mg	SE	500 mg	D5W	Physically compatible	15	C
Potassium chloride		3 g	SE	50 mg	D5W	Physically compatible	74	C
Prochlorperazine edisylate	SKF	100 mg	SE	500 mg	D5W	Physically compatible	15	C
Vancomycin HCl	LI	1 g	SE	50 mg	D5W	Physically compatible	74	C

Drugs in Syringe Compatibility

Dimenhydrinate

Drug (in syringe)	Mfr	Amt	Mfr	Amt	Remarks	Ref	C/I
Aminophylline		50 mg/ 1 mL		10 mg/ 1 mL	Light cloudiness forms immediately	2569	I
Ampicillin sodium		50 mg/ 1 mL		10 mg/ 1 mL	Clear solution	2569	C
Atropine sulfate	ST	0.4 mg/ 1 mL	HR	50 mg/ 1 mL	Physically compatible for at least 15 min	326	C
Butorphanol tartrate	BR	4 mg/ 2 mL	HR	50 mg/ 1 mL	Gas evolves	761	I
Caffeine citrate		10 mg/ 1 mL		10 mg/ 1 mL	Clear solution	2569	C
Calcium gluconate		100 mg/ 1 mL		10 mg/ 1 mL	Clear solution	2569	C
Cefazolin sodium		100 mg/ 1 mL		10 mg/ 1 mL	Clear solution	2569	C
Cefotaxime sodium		100 mg/ 1 mL		10 mg/ 1 mL	Clear solution	2569	C

Drugs in Syringe Compatibility (Cont.)

Dimenhydrinate

Drug (in syringe)	Mfr	Amt	Mfr	Amt	Remarks	Ref	C/I
Ceftazidime		100 mg/ 1 mL		10 mg/ 1 mL	Clear solution	2569	C
Cefuroxime sodium		100 mg/ 1 mL		10 mg/ 1 mL	Clear solution	2569	C
Chlorpromazine HCl	PO	50 mg/ 2 mL	HR	50 mg/ 1 mL	Physically incompatible within 15 min	326	I
		25 mg/ 1 mL		10 mg/ 1 mL	Clear solution	2569	C
Clindamycin phosphate		150 mg/ 1 mL		10 mg/ 1 mL	Clear solution	2569	C
Cloxacillin sodium		100 mg/ 1 mL		10 mg/ 1 mL	Clear solution	2569	C
Cyclosporine		50 mg/ 1 mL		10 mg/ 1 mL	Clear solution	2569	C
Dexamethasone sodium phosphate		10 mg/ 1 mL		10 mg/ 1 mL	Clear solution	2569	C
Diazepam		5 mg/ 1 mL		10 mg/ 1 mL	Loss of clarity	2569	I
Digoxin		0.05 mg/ 1 mL		10 mg/ 1 mL	Clear solution	2569	C
Diphenhydramine HCl	PD	50 mg/ 1 mL	HR	50 mg/ 1 mL	Physically compatible for at least 15 min	326	C
Dobutamine HCl		12.5 mg/ 1 mL		10 mg/ 1 mL	Clear solution	2569	C
Droperidol	MN	2.5 mg/ 1 mL	HR	50 mg/ 1 mL	Physically compatible for at least 15 min	326	C
Fentanyl citrate	MN	0.05 mg/ 1 mL	HR	50 mg/ 1 mL	Physically compatible for at least 15 min	326	C
Furosemide		10 mg/ 1 mL		10 mg/ 1 mL	Precipitate forms	2569	I
Gentamicin sulfate		10 mg/ 1 mL		10 mg/ 1 mL	Clear solution	2569	C
		40 mg/ 1 mL		10 mg/ 1 mL	Clear solution	2569	C
Glycopyrrolate	RB	0.2 mg/ 1 mL	SE	50 mg/ 1 mL	Precipitates immediately	331	I
	RB	0.2 mg/ 1 mL	SE	100 mg/ 2 mL	Precipitates immediately	331	I
	RB	0.4 mg/ 2 mL	SE	50 mg/ 1 mL	Precipitates immediately	331	I
Heparin sodium		2500 units/ 1 mL		65 mg/ 10 mL	Physically compatible for at least 5 min	1053	C
		25,000 units/ 1 mL		10 mg/ 1 mL	Precipitate forms	2569	I
Hydrocortisone sodium succinate		125 mg/ 1 mL		10 mg/ 1 mL	Clear solution	2569	C

Drugs in Syringe Compatibility (Cont.)

Dimenhydrinate

Drug (in syringe)	Mfr	Amt	Mfr	Amt	Remarks	Ref	C/I
Hydromorphone HCl	KN	2, 10, 40 mg/ 1 mL	SQ	50 mg/ 1 mL	Visually compatible with both drugs stable for 24 hr at 4, 23, and 37 °C. Precipitate forms after 24 hr	1776	C
		50 mg/ 1 mL		10 mg/ 1 mL	Precipitate forms in about 2 hr	2569	I
Hydroxyzine HCl	PF	50 mg/ 1 mL	HR	50 mg/ 1 mL	Physically incompatible within 15 min	326	I
Iodipamide meglumine	SQ	52%, 40 mL	SE	50 mg/ 1 mL	Forms a precipitate initially but clears within 1 hr and remains clear for 48 hr	530	?
	SQ	52%, 20 to 1 mL	SE	50 mg/ 1 mL	Forms a precipitate initially but clears within 1 hr. Precipitate reforms on standing	530	I
Iothalamate meglumine	MA	60%, 40 to 1 mL	SE	50 mg/ 1 mL	Physically compatible for 48 hr	530	C
Lorazepam		4 mg/ 1 mL		10 mg/ 1 mL	Clear solution	2569	C
Magnesium sulfate		500 mg/ 1 mL		10 mg/ 1 mL	Clear solution	2569	C
Meperidine HCl	WI	50 mg/ 1 mL	HR	50 mg/ 1 mL	Physically compatible for at least 15 min	326	C
Metoclopramide HCl	NO	10 mg/ 2 mL	HR	50 mg/ 1 mL	Physically compatible for 15 min at room temperature	565	C
Midazolam HCl	RC	5 mg/ 1 mL	SE	50 mg/ 1 mL	White precipitate forms immediately	1145	I
Morphine sulfate	ST	15 mg/ 1 mL	HR	50 mg/ 1 mL	Physically compatible for at least 15 min	326	C
Naloxone HCl		0.4 mg/ 1 mL		10 mg/ 1 mL	Clear solution	2569	C
Octreotide acetate		0.5 mg/ 1 mL		10 mg/ 1 mL	Precipitate forms in about 1 hr	2569	I
Oxytocin		10 units/ 1 mL		10 mg/ 1 mL	Precipitate forms	2569	I
Pantoprazole sodium	a	4 mg/ 1 mL		50 mg/ 1 mL	White precipitate	2574	I
Penicillin G sodium		500,000 units/ 1 mL		10 mg/ 1 mL	Clear solution	2569	C
Pentazocine lactate	WI	30 mg/ 1 mL	HR	50 mg/ 1 mL	Physically compatible for at least 15 min	326	C
Pentobarbital sodium	AB	500 mg/ 10 mL	SE	50 mg/ 1 mL	Physically incompatible	55	I
	AB	50 mg/ 1 mL	HR	50 mg/ 1 mL	Physically incompatible within 15 min	326	I
Piperacillin sodium–tazobactam sodium	a	200 + 25 mg/ 1 mL		10 mg/ 1 mL	Clear solution	2569	C
Potassium chloride		2 mEq/ 1 mL		10 mg/ 1 mL	Precipitate forms in about 1 hr	2569	I

Drugs in Syringe Compatibility (Cont.)

Dimenhydrinate

Drug (in syringe)	Mfr	Amt	Mfr	Amt	Remarks	Ref	C/I
Prochlorperazine edisylate	PO	5 mg/ 1 mL	HR	50 mg/ 1 mL	Physically incompatible within 15 min	326	I
Promethazine HCl	PO	50 mg/ 2 mL	HR	50 mg/ 1 mL	Physically incompatible within 15 min	326	I
		25 mg/ 1 mL		10 mg/ 1 mL	Solution discolors	2569	I
Ranitidine HCl	GL	50 mg/ 2 mL	HR	50 mg/ 1 mL	Physically compatible for 1 hr at 25 °C	978	C
Salbutamol		1 mg/ 1 mL		10 mg/ 1 mL	Precipitate forms	2569	I
Scopolamine HBr	ST	0.4 mg/ 1 mL	HR	50 mg/ 1 mL	Physically compatible for at least 15 min	326	C
Sodium bicarbonate		1 mEq/ 1 mL		10 mg/ 1 mL	Precipitates immediately	2569	I
Tobramycin sulfate		40 mg/ 1 mL		10 mg/ 1 mL	Clear solution	2569	C
Trimethoprim–sulfamethoxazole		16 + 80 mg/ 1 mL		10 mg/ 1 mL	Clear solution	2569	C
Vancomycin HCl		50 mg/ 1 mL		10 mg/ 1 mL	Precipitate forms	2569	I
Verapamil HCl		2.5 mg/ 1 mL		10 mg/ 1 mL	Clear solution	2569	C

[a]Test performed using the formulation WITHOUT edetate disodium.

Y-Site Injection Compatibility (1:1 Mixture)

Dimenhydrinate

Drug	Mfr	Conc	Mfr	Conc	Remarks	Ref	C/I
Acyclovir sodium	BW	5 mg/mL[a]	SE	1 mg/mL[a]	Physically compatible for 4 hr at 25 °C	1157	C
Ciprofloxacin		2 mg/mL		10 mg/mL	Clear solution	2569	C
Fluconazole		2 mg/mL		10 mg/mL	Clear solution	2569	C
Hydroxyethyl starch 130/0.4 in sodium chloride 0.9%	FRK	6%	SZ	0.5, 0.75, 1 mg/mL[a]	Visually compatible for 24 hr at room temperature	2770	C
Metronidazole		5 mg/mL		10 mg/mL	Clear solution	2569	C
Pantoprazole sodium	ALT[c]	0.16 to 0.8 mg/mL[b]	AST	0.5 to 1 mg/ mL[a]	Visually compatible for 12 hr at 23 °C	2603	C

[a]Tested in dextrose 5%.
[b]Tested in sodium chloride 0.9%.
[c]Test performed using the formulation WITHOUT edetate disodium.

DIPHENHYDRAMINE HYDROCHLORIDE
AHFS 4:04

Products — Diphenhydramine hydrochloride is available as a 50-mg/mL solution in 1-mL vials and disposable syringes. Also present in the vials is 0.1 mg/mL of benzethonium chloride. The pH may have been adjusted with sodium hydroxide or hydrochloric acid. (1)

pH — From 4 to 6.5. (17)

Trade Name(s) — Benadryl.

Administration — Diphenhydramine hydrochloride is administered by deep intramuscular injection, slow direct intravenous injection, or continuous or intermittent intravenous infusion. (1; 4) Subcutaneous or perivascular injection should be avoided due to irritation. (4)

Stability — Diphenhydramine hydrochloride in intact containers should be stored in light-resistant containers at controlled room temperature. Freezing should be avoided. (1; 4)

Diphenhydramine hydrochloride under simulated summer conditions in paramedic vehicles was exposed to temperatures ranging from 26 to 38 °C over 4 weeks. Analysis found no loss of the drug under these conditions. (2562)

Central Venous Catheter — Diphenhydramine hydrochloride (Schein) 2 mg/mL in dextrose 5% was found to be compatible with the ARROWg+ard Blue Plus (Arrow International) chlorhexidine-bearing triple-lumen central catheter. Essentially complete delivery of the drug was found with little or no drug loss occurring. Furthermore, chlorhexidine delivered from the catheter remained at trace amounts with no substantial increase due to the delivery of the drug through the catheter. (2335)

Compatibility Information

Solution Compatibility

Diphenhydramine HCl

Solution	Mfr	Mfr	Conc/L	Remarks	Ref	C/I
Dextrose–Ringer's injection combinations	AB	PD	100 mg	Physically compatible	3	C
Dextrose–Ringer's injection, lactated, combinations	AB	PD	100 mg	Physically compatible	3	C
Dextrose–saline combinations	AB	PD	100 mg	Physically compatible	3	C
Dextrose 2.5%	AB	PD	100 mg	Physically compatible	3	C
Dextrose 5%	AB	PD	100 mg	Physically compatible	3	C
Dextrose 10%	AB	PD	100 mg	Physically compatible	3	C
Ionosol products	AB	PD	100 mg	Physically compatible	3	C
Ringer's injection	AB	PD	100 mg	Physically compatible	3	C
Ringer's injection, lactated	AB	PD	100 mg	Physically compatible	3	C
Sodium chloride 0.45%	AB	PD	100 mg	Physically compatible	3	C
Sodium chloride 0.9%	AB	PD	100 mg	Physically compatible	3	C
Sodium lactate ⅙ M	AB	PD	100 mg	Physically compatible	3	C

Additive Compatibility

Diphenhydramine HCl

Drug	Mfr	Conc/L	Mfr	Conc/L	Test Soln	Remarks	Ref	C/I
Amikacin sulfate	BR	5 g	PD	100 mg	D5LR, D5R, D5S, D5W, D10W, LR, NS, R, SL	Physically compatible and both stable for 24 hr at 25 °C	294	C
Aminophylline	SE	500 mg	PD	50 mg		Physically compatible	6	C
Amphotericin B	SQ	100 mg	PD	80 mg	D5W	Physically incompatible	15	I
Ascorbic acid	UP	500 mg	PD	80 mg	D5W	Physically compatible	15	C

Additive Compatibility (Cont.)

Diphenhydramine HCl

Drug	Mfr	Conc/L	Mfr	Conc/L	Test Soln	Remarks	Ref	C/I
Bleomycin sulfate	BR	20 and 30 units	PD	100 mg	NS	Physically compatible and bleomycin activity retained for 1 week at 4 °C. Diphenhydramine not tested	763	C
Colistimethate sodium	WC	500 mg	PD	80 mg	D5W	Physically compatible	15	C
Dexamethasone sodium phosphate with lorazepam and metoclopramide HCl	AMR WY DU	400 mg 40 mg 4 g	ES	2 g	NSa	Rapid lorazepam losses of 8, 10, and 15% at 3, 23, and 30 °C, respectively, in 24 hr. Other drugs stable for 14 days at all three storage temperatures	1733	I
Erythromycin lactobionate	AB	1 g	PD	50 mg		Physically compatible. Erythromycin stable for 24 hr at 25 °C	20	C
	AB	1 g	PD	50 mg	D5W	Erythromycin stable for 24 hr at 25 °C	48	C
Fat emulsion, intravenous	VT	10%	PD	100 mg		Physically compatible for 48 hr at 4 °C and room temperature	32	C
Iodipamide meglumine	SQ		PD	20 to 200 mg	NS	Dense putty-like white precipitate forms immediately	309	I
Lidocaine HCl	AST	2 g	PD	50 mg		Physically compatible	24	C
Lorazepam with dexamethasone sodium phosphate and metoclopramide HCl	WY AMR DU	40 mg 400 mg 4 g	ES	2 g	NSa	Rapid lorazepam losses of 8, 10, and 15% at 3, 23, and 30 °C, respectively, in 24 hr. Other drugs stable for 14 days at all three storage temperatures	1733	I
Methyldopate HCl	MSD	1 g	PD	50 mg	D, D–S, S	Physically compatible	23	C
Metoclopramide HCl with dexamethasone sodium phosphate and lorazepam	DU AMR WY	4 g 400 mg 40 mg	ES	2 g	NSa	Rapid lorazepam losses of 8, 10, and 15% at 3, 23, and 30 °C, respectively, in 24 hr. Other drugs stable for 14 days at all three storage temperatures	1733	I
Nafcillin sodium	WY	500 mg	PD	50 mg		Physically compatible	27	C
Penicillin G potassium	SQ	20 million units	PD	80 mg	D5W	Physically compatible	15	C
	SQ	1 million units	PD	50 mg	D5W	Physically compatible. Penicillin stable for 24 hr at 25 °C	47	C
Penicillin G sodium	UP	20 million units	PD	80 mg	D5W	Physically compatible	15	C
Polymyxin B sulfate	BW	200 mg	PD	80 mg	D5W	Physically compatible	15	C

[a]Tested in Pharmacia-Deltec PVC pump reservoirs.

Drugs in Syringe Compatibility

Diphenhydramine HCl

Drug (in syringe)	Mfr	Amt	Mfr	Amt	Remarks	Ref	C/I
Atropine sulfate	ST	0.4 mg/ 1 mL	PD	50 mg/ 1 mL	Physically compatible for at least 15 min	326	C
Buprenorphine HCl					Physically and chemically compatible	4	C

Drugs in Syringe Compatibility (Cont.)

Diphenhydramine HCl

Drug (in syringe)	Mfr	Amt	Mfr	Amt	Remarks	Ref	C/I
Butorphanol tartrate	BR	4 mg/ 2 mL	PD	50 mg/ 1 mL	Physically compatible for 30 min at room temperature	566	C
Chlorpromazine HCl	PO	50 mg/ 2 mL	PD	50 mg/ 1 mL	Physically compatible for at least 15 min	326	C
	STS	50 mg/ 2 mL	ES	100 mg/ 2 mL	Visually compatible for 60 min	1784	C
Dexamethasone sodium phosphate	DB, SX	4 and 10 mg/ mL[a]	PD	50 mg/ mL[a]	White turbidity and precipitate form immediately	1542	I
	DB	9.52 mg/ mL[b]	PD	4.54 mg/ mL[b]	Visually compatible for 24 hr at 24 °C	1542	C
	DB	5 to 9.02 mg/ mL[b]	PD	4.54 to 15 mg/ mL[b]	Precipitate forms	1542	I
	SX	2 mg/ mL[b]	PD	34.8 to 40 mg/ mL[b]	Visually compatible for 24 hr at 24 °C	1542	C
	SX	1 mg/ mL[b]	PD	25 mg/ mL[b]	Precipitate forms	1542	I
Dimenhydrinate	HR	50 mg/ 1 mL	PD	50 mg/ 1 mL	Physically compatible for at least 15 min	326	C
Droperidol	MN	2.5 mg/ 1 mL	PD	50 mg/ 1 mL	Physically compatible for at least 15 min	326	C
Fentanyl citrate	MN	0.05 mg/ 1 mL	PD	50 mg/ 1 mL	Physically compatible for at least 15 min	326	C
Fluphenazine HCl	LY	5 mg/ 2 mL	ES	100 mg/ 2 mL	Visually compatible for 60 min	1784	C
Glycopyrrolate	RB	0.2 mg/ 1 mL	PD	10 mg/ 1 mL	Physically compatible. pH in glycopyrrolate stability range for 48 hr at 25 °C	331	C
	RB	0.2 mg/ 1 mL	PD	20 mg/ 2 mL	Physically compatible. pH in glycopyrrolate stability range for 48 hr at 25 °C	331	C
	RB	0.4 mg/ 2 mL	PD	10 mg/ 1 mL	Physically compatible. pH in glycopyrrolate stability range for 48 hr at 25 °C	331	C
	RB	0.2 mg/ 1 mL	PD	50 mg/ 1 mL	Physically compatible. pH in glycopyrrolate stability range for 48 hr at 25 °C	331	C
	RB	0.2 mg/ 1 mL	PD	100 mg/ 2 mL	Physically compatible. pH in glycopyrrolate stability range for 48 hr at 25 °C	331	C
	RB	0.4 mg/ 2 mL	PD	50 mg/ 1 mL	Physically compatible. pH in glycopyrrolate stability range for 48 hr at 25 °C	331	C
Haloperidol lactate	MN	10 mg/ 2 mL	ES	100 mg/ 2 mL	White precipitate forms within 5 min	1784	I
	MN	5 mg/ 1 mL	ES	50 mg/ 1 mL	White cloudy precipitate forms in 2 hr at room temperature	1886	I
Hydromorphone HCl	KN	4 mg/ 2 mL	PD	50 mg/ 1 mL	Physically compatible for 30 min	517	C
Hydroxyzine HCl	PF	50 mg/ 1 mL	PD	50 mg/ 1 mL	Physically compatible for at least 15 min	326	C
Iodipamide meglumine	SQ		PD	5 mg/ 0.1 mL to 50 mg/ 1 mL	Dense putty-like white precipitate forms immediately	309	I

Drugs in Syringe Compatibility (Cont.)

Diphenhydramine HCl

Drug (in syringe)	Mfr	Amt	Mfr	Amt	Remarks	Ref	C/I
	SQ	52%, 40 to 1 mL	PD	1 mL[c]	Forms a precipitate initially but clears within 1 hr and remains clear for 48 hr	530	?
Iohexol	WI	64.7%, 5 mL	PD	12.5 mg/ 0.25 mL	Physically compatible for at least 2 hr	1438	C
Iopamidol	SQ	61%, 5 mL	PD	12.5 mg/ 0.25 mL	Physically compatible for at least 2 hr	1438	C
Iothalamate meglumine	MA	5 mL	PD	50 mg/ 1 mL	No precipitate observed	309	C
	MA	60%, 40 to 1 mL	PD	1 mL[c]	Physically compatible for 48 hr	530	C
	MA	60%, 5 mL	PD	12.5 mg/ 0.25 mL	Physically compatible for at least 2 hr	1438	C
Ioxaglate meglumine–ioxaglate sodium	MA	5 mL	PD	12.5 mg/ 0.25 mL	Precipitate forms immediately and persists for at least 2 hr	1438	I
Meperidine HCl	WY	100 mg/ 1 mL	PD	50 mg/ 1 mL	Physically compatible for at least 15 min	14	C
	WI	50 mg/ 1 mL	PD	50 mg/ 1 mL	Physically compatible for at least 15 min	326	C
Metoclopramide HCl	NO	10 mg/ 2 mL	PD	50 mg/ 1 mL	Physically compatible for 15 min at room temperature	565	C
	RB	10 mg/ 2 mL	PD	50 mg/ 5 mL	Physically compatible for 48 hr at 25 °C	1167	C
	RB	10 mg/ 2 mL	PD	250 mg/ 25 mL	Physically compatible for 48 hr at 25 °C	1167	C
	RB	160 mg/ 32 mL	PD	40 mg/ 4 mL	Physically compatible for 48 hr at 25 °C	1167	C
	RB	160 mg/ 32 mL	PD	200 mg/ 20 mL	Physically compatible for 48 hr at 25 °C	1167	C
Midazolam HCl	RC	5 mg/ 1 mL	ES	50 mg/ 1 mL	Physically compatible for 4 hr at 25 °C	1145	C
Morphine sulfate	WY	15 mg/ 1 mL	PD	50 mg/ 1 mL	Physically compatible for at least 15 min	14	C
	ST	15 mg/ 1 mL	PD	50 mg/ 1 mL	Physically compatible for at least 15 min	326	C
Nalbuphine HCl	DU	10 mg/ 1 mL	PD	50 mg/ 1 mL	Physically compatible for 48 hr	128	C
	DU	20 mg/ 1 mL	PD	50 mg/ 1 mL	Physically compatible for 48 hr	128	C
Pantoprazole sodium	[d]	4 mg/ 1 mL		50 mg/ 1 mL	Precipitates immediately	2574	I
Pentazocine lactate	WI	30 mg/ 1 mL	PD	50 mg/ 1 mL	Physically compatible for at least 15 min	326	C
Pentobarbital sodium	WY	100 mg/ 2 mL	PD	50 mg/ 1 mL	Precipitate observed within 15 min	14	I
	AB	500 mg/ 10 mL	PD	50 mg/ 1 mL	Physically incompatible	55	I
	AB	50 mg/ 1 mL	PD	50 mg/ 1 mL	Physically incompatible within 15 min	326	I
Prochlorperazine edisylate	PO	5 mg/ 1 mL	PD	50 mg/ 1 mL	Physically compatible for at least 15 min	326	C

Drugs in Syringe Compatibility (Cont.)

Diphenhydramine HCl

Drug (in syringe)	Mfr	Amt	Mfr	Amt	Remarks	Ref	C/I
Promethazine HCl	WY	50 mg/ 2 mL	PD	50 mg/ 1 mL	Physically compatible for at least 15 min	14	**C**
	PO	50 mg/ 2 mL	PD	50 mg/ 1 mL	Physically compatible for at least 15 min	326	**C**
Ranitidine HCl	GL	50 mg/ 2 mL	PD	50 mg/ 1 mL	Physically compatible for 1 hr at 25 °C	978	**C**
Scopolamine HBr	ST	0.4 mg/ 1 mL	PD	50 mg/ 1 mL	Physically compatible for at least 15 min	326	**C**

[a] Mixed in equal quantities. Final concentration is one-half the indicated concentration.
[b] Mixed in varying quantities to yield the final concentrations noted.
[c] Diphenhydramine hydrochloride concentration unspecified.
[d] Test performed using the formulation WITHOUT edetate disodium.

Y-Site Injection Compatibility (1:1 Mixture)

Diphenhydramine HCl

Drug	Mfr	Conc	Mfr	Conc	Remarks	Ref	C/I
Abciximab	LI	36 mcg/mL[a]	ES	25 mg/mL	Visually compatible for 12 hr at 23 °C	2374	**C**
Acyclovir sodium	BW	5 mg/mL[a]	ES	1 mg/mL[a]	Physically compatible for 4 hr at 25 °C	1157	**C**
	BV	5 mg/mL[b]	BA	50 mg/mL	Cloudy upon mixing	2794	**I**
Aldesleukin	CHI	33,800 I.U./ mL[a]	SCN	50 mg/mL	Visually compatible for 2 hr	1857	**C**
Allopurinol sodium	BW	3 mg/mL[b]	PD	2 mg/mL[b]	White precipitate forms immediately	1686	**I**
Amifostine	USB	10 mg/mL[a]	PD	2 mg/mL[a]	Physically compatible for 4 hr at 23 °C	1845	**C**
Amphotericin B cholesteryl sulfate complex	SEQ	0.83 mg/mL[a]	SCN	2 mg/mL[a]	Microprecipitate and increased turbidity form immediately	2117	**I**
Amsacrine	NCI	1 mg/mL[a]	PD	2 mg/mL[a]	Visually compatible for 4 hr at 22 °C	1381	**C**
Argatroban	GSK	1 mg/mL[b]	ES	50 mg/mL	Visually compatible for 24 hr at 23 °C	2391	**C**
Azithromycin	PF	2 mg/mL[b]	ES	50 mg/mL[i]	Visually compatible	2368	**C**
Aztreonam	SQ	40 mg/mL[a]	PD	2 mg/mL[a]	Physically compatible for 4 hr at 23 °C	1758	**C**
Bivalirudin	TMC	5 mg/mL[a]	ES	2 mg/mL[a]	Physically compatible for 4 hr at 23 °C	2373	**C**
Caspofungin acetate	ME	0.5 mg/mL[b]	BA	50 mg/mL	Physically compatible with diphenhydramine HCl given i.v. push over 2 to 5 min	2766	**C**
Ceftaroline fosamil	FOR	2.22 mg/ mL[a,b,k]	BA	2 mg/mL[a,b,k]	Physically compatible for 4 hr at 23 °C	2826	**C**
Ciprofloxacin	MI	2 mg/mL[c]	ES	50 mg/mL	Visually compatible for 24 hr at 24 °C	1655	**C**
Cisatracurium besylate	GW	0.1, 2, 5 mg/ mL[a]	SCN	2 mg/mL[a]	Physically compatible for 4 hr at 23 °C	2074	**C**
Cladribine	ORT	0.015[b] and 0.5[d] mg/mL	SCN	2 mg/mL[b]	Physically compatible for 4 hr at 23 °C	1969	**C**

Y-Site Injection Compatibility (1:1 Mixture) (Cont.)

Diphenhydramine HCl

Drug	Mfr	Conc	Mfr	Conc	Remarks	Ref	C/I
Dexmedetomidine HCl	AB	4 mcg/mL[b]	PD	2 mg/mL[b]	Physically compatible for 4 hr at 23 °C	2383	**C**
Docetaxel	RPR	0.9 mg/mL[a]	ES	2 mg/mL[a]	Physically compatible for 4 hr at 23 °C	2224	**C**
Doripenem	JJ	5 mg/mL[a,b]	BA	2 mg/mL[a,b]	Physically compatible for 4 hr at 23 °C	2743	**C**
Doxorubicin HCl liposomal	SEQ	0.4 mg/mL[a]	SCN	2 mg/mL[a]	Physically compatible for 4 hr at 23 °C	2087	**C**
Etoposide phosphate	BR	5 mg/mL[a]	ES	2 mg/mL[a]	Physically compatible for 4 hr at 23 °C	2218	**C**
Famotidine	ME	2 mg/mL[b]		2 mg/mL[a]	Visually compatible for 4 hr at 22 °C	1936	**C**
Fenoldopam mesylate	AB	80 mcg/mL[b]	ES	2 mg/mL[b]	Physically compatible for 4 hr at 23 °C	2467	**C**
Fentanyl citrate	JN	0.025 mg/mL[a]	SCN	2 mg/mL[a]	Physically compatible for 48 hr at 22 °C	1706	**C**
Filgrastim	AMG	30 mcg/mL[a]	ES	2 mg/mL[a]	Physically compatible for 4 hr at 22 °C	1687	**C**
Fluconazole	RR	2 mg/mL	ES	50 mg/mL	Physically compatible for 24 hr at 25 °C	1407	**C**
Fludarabine phosphate	BX	1 mg/mL[a]	WY	2 mg/mL[a]	Visually compatible for 4 hr at 22 °C	1439	**C**
Foscarnet sodium	AST	24 mg/mL	PD	50 mg/mL	Cloudy solution	1335	**I**
Gallium nitrate	FUJ	1 mg/mL[b]	ES	50 mg/mL	Visually compatible for 24 hr at 25 °C	1673	**C**
Gemcitabine HCl	LI	10 mg/mL[b]	SCN	2 mg/mL[b]	Physically compatible for 4 hr at 23 °C	2226	**C**
Granisetron HCl	SKB	1 mg/mL	PD	1 mg/mL[b]	Physically compatible with little loss of either drug in 4 hr at 22 °C	1883	**C**
	SKB	0.05 mg/mL[a]	SCN	2 mg/mL[a]	Physically compatible for 4 hr at 23 °C	2000	**C**
Heparin sodium	UP	1000 units/L[e]	PD	50 mg/mL	Physically compatible for 4 hr at room temperature	534	**C**
Hetastarch in lactated electrolyte	AB	6%	SCN	2 mg/mL[a]	Physically compatible for 4 hr at 23 °C	2339	**C**
Hydrocortisone sodium succinate	UP	10 mg/L[e]	PD	50 mg/mL	Physically compatible for 4 hr at room temperature	534	**C**
Hydromorphone HCl	AST	0.5 mg/mL[a]	SCN	2 mg/mL[a]	Physically compatible for 48 hr at 22 °C	1706	**C**
Idarubicin HCl	AD	1 mg/mL[b]	ES	1[a] and 50 mg/mL	Visually compatible for 24 hr at 25 °C	1525	**C**
Linezolid	PHU	2 mg/mL	ES	2 mg/mL[a]	Physically compatible for 4 hr at 23 °C	2264	**C**
Melphalan HCl	BW	0.1 mg/mL[b]	WY	2 mg/mL[b]	Physically compatible for 3 hr at 22 °C	1557	**C**
Meperidine HCl	AB	10 mg/mL	ES	1[a] and 50 mg/mL	Physically compatible for 4 hr at 25 °C	1397	**C**
Meropenem	ZEN	1 and 50 mg/mL[b]	PD	50 mg/mL	Visually compatible for 4 hr at room temperature	1994	**C**
Methadone HCl	LI	1 mg/mL[a]	SCN	2 mg/mL[a]	Physically compatible for 48 hr at 22 °C	1706	**C**
Morphine sulfate	AST	1 mg/mL[a]	SCN	2 mg/mL[a]	Physically compatible for 48 hr at 22 °C	1706	**C**
Ondansetron HCl	GL	1 mg/mL[b]	PD	2 mg/mL[a]	Visually compatible for 4 hr at 22 °C	1365	**C**
Oxaliplatin	SS	0.5 mg/mL[a]	ES	2 mg/mL[a]	Physically compatible for 4 hr at 23 °C	2566	**C**
Paclitaxel	NCI	1.2 mg/mL[a]		2 mg/mL[a]	Physically compatible for 4 hr at 22 °C	1528	**C**
Pemetrexed disodium	LI	20 mg/mL[b]	ES	2 mg/mL[a]	Physically compatible for 4 hr at 23 °C	2564	**C**
Piperacillin sodium–tazobactam sodium	LE[j]	40 + 5 mg/mL[a]	WY	2 mg/mL[a]	Physically compatible for 4 hr at 22 °C	1688	**C**
Potassium chloride	AB	40 mEq/L[e]	PD	50 mg/mL	Physically compatible for 4 hr at room temperature	534	**C**

Y-Site Injection Compatibility (1:1 Mixture) (Cont.)

Diphenhydramine HCl

Drug	Mfr	Conc	Mfr	Conc	Remarks	Ref	C/I
Propofol	ZEN	10 mg/mL	SCN	2 mg/mL[a]	Physically compatible for 1 hr at 23 °C	2066	C
Remifentanil HCl	GW	0.025 and 0.25 mg/mL[b]	SCN	2 mg/mL[a]	Physically compatible for 4 hr at 23 °C	2075	C
Sargramostim	IMM	10 mcg/mL[b]	RU	1 mg/mL[b]	Visually compatible for 4 hr at 22 °C	1436	C
Tacrolimus	FUJ	1 mg/mL[b]	ES	1 mg/mL[a]	Visually compatible for 24 hr at 25 °C	1630	C
Teniposide	BR	0.1 mg/mL[a]	ES	2 mg/mL[a]	Physically compatible for 4 hr at 23 °C	1725	C
Thiotepa	IMM[g]	1 mg/mL[a]	WY	2 mg/mL[a]	Physically compatible for 4 hr at 23 °C	1861	C
TNA #218 to #226[h]			SCN, PD	2[a] and 50 mg/mL	Visually compatible for 4 hr at 23 °C	2215	C
TPN #212 to #215[h]			SCN	2[a] and 50 mg/mL	Physically compatible for 4 hr at 23 °C	2109	C
Vinorelbine tartrate	BW	1 mg/mL[b]	ES	2 mg/mL[b]	Physically compatible for 4 hr at 22 °C	1558	C

[a] *Tested in dextrose 5%.*
[b] *Tested in sodium chloride 0.9%.*
[c] *Tested in both dextrose 5% and sodium chloride 0.9%.*
[d] *Tested in bacteriostatic sodium chloride 0.9% preserved with benzyl alcohol 0.9%.*
[e] *Tested in dextrose 5% in Ringer's injection, dextrose 5% in Ringer's injection, lactated, dextrose 5%, Ringer's injection, lactated, and sodium chloride 0.9%.*
[f] *Tested in dextrose 5% with sodium bicarbonate 0.05 mEq/mL.*
[g] *Lyophilized formulation tested.*
[h] *Refer to Appendix I for the composition of parenteral nutrition solutions. TNA indicates a 3-in-1 admixture, and TPN indicates a 2-in-1 admixture.*
[i] *Injected via Y-site into an administration set running azithromycin.*
[j] *Test performed using the formulation WITHOUT edetate disodium.*
[k] *Tested in Ringer's injection, lactated.*

DOBUTAMINE HYDROCHLORIDE
AHFS 12:12.08.08

Products — Dobutamine hydrochloride is available in 20-, 40-, and 100-mL single-dose vials as a concentrate for injection. Each milliliter contains 12.5 mg of dobutamine (as the hydrochloride), sodium bisulfite 0.24 mg, and hydrochloric acid and/or sodium hydroxide to adjust the pH. Dobutamine hydrochloride concentrate for injection must be diluted further to a concentration not greater than 5 mg/mL before administration. (1; 4)

Dobutamine hydrochloride is also available in plastic bags as premixed solutions in concentrations of 1, 2, and 4 mg/mL in dextrose 5%. Sodium metabisulfite and edetate disodium dihydrate may also be present. (4)

pH — From 2.5 to 5.5. (1; 4; 17) The premixed infusion solutions in dextrose 5% have a pH range of 2.5 to 5.5. (4)

Osmolality — The osmolality of dobutamine hydrochloride injection (Lilly) was determined to be 273 mOsm/kg by freezing-point depression and vapor pressure. (1071) At a concentration of 5 mg/mL (manufacturer and diluent unstated), the osmolality was determined to be 361 mOsm/kg by freezing-point depression. (1233)

The premixed infusion solutions in dextrose 5% have osmolalities ranging from 260 to 284 mOsm/kg for the four concentrations available. (4)

Administration — Dobutamine hydrochloride is administered by intravenous infusion after dilution to a concentration no greater than 5 mg/mL. The concentration used is dependent on the patient's dosage and fluid requirements. An infusion pump or other infusion control device should be used to control the flow rate. (1; 4)

Stability — Intact containers should be stored at controlled room temperature and protected from excessive heat and freezing. Solutions that are further diluted for intravenous infusion should be used within 24 hours. (1; 4)

Dobutamine hydrochloride concentrate for injection is a clear, colorless to pale straw-colored solution. Solutions of dobutamine hydrochloride may have a pink discoloration. This discoloration, which will increase with time, results from a slight oxidation of the drug. However, there is no significant loss of drug within the recommended storage times for solutions of the drug. (4)

Dobutamine hydrochloride has been stated to be incompatible with alkaline solutions. (1; 4)

Dobutamine hydrochloride (Lilly) 2.5, 5, and 7.5 mcg/mL in Dianeal PD-1 (Baxter) with dextrose 1.5 and 4.25% retained at least 90% when stored for 24 hours at 4, 26, and 37 °C. (1417; 1702)

Syringes — Dobutamine hydrochloride (Lilly) 250 mg/50 mL in dextrose 5% exhibited no change in appearance and no drug loss when stored in 60-mL plastic syringes (Becton Dickinson) for 24 hours at 25 °C. (1579)

Dobutamine hydrochloride (Lilly) 5 mg/mL in dextrose 5% was packaged in 50-mL polypropylene syringes (Becton Dickinson) and stored at 4 and 24 °C in the dark and exposed to room light for 48 hours. Dobutamine losses were less than 10% throughout the study. (1961)

Sorption — Delivering dobutamine hydrochloride (Lilly) 5 mg/mL in dextrose 5% by syringe pump over 12 hours at 24 °C through PVC and polyethylene tubing did not result in substantial dobutamine losses. (1961)

Filtration — Dobutamine hydrochloride (Lilly) 0.5 mg/mL in dextrose 5% and sodium chloride 0.9% was filtered through a 0.22-μm cellulose ester membrane filter (Ivex-HP, Millipore) over six hours. No significant drug loss due to binding to the filter was noted. (1034)

Central Venous Catheter — Dobutamine hydrochloride (Astra) 4 mg/mL in dextrose 5% was found to be compatible with the ARROWg+ard Blue Plus (Arrow International) chlorhexidine-bearing triple-lumen central catheter. Essentially complete delivery of the drug was found with little or no drug loss occurring. Furthermore, chlorhexidine delivered from the catheter remained at trace amounts with no substantial increase due to the delivery of the drug through the catheter. (2335)

Compatibility Information

Solution Compatibility

Dobutamine HCl

Solution	Mfr	Mfr	Conc/L	Remarks	Ref	C/I
Dextrose 2.5% in half-strength Ringer's injection, lactated	MG[a]	LI	1 g	No loss in 48 hr at 25 °C. Slight pink color at 8 hr becoming slightly brown at 24 hr	789	C
Dextrose 5% in Ringer's injection, lactated				Use within 24 hr	1	C
	MG[a]	LI	1 g	No loss in 48 hr at 25 °C. Slight pink color at 8 hr becoming slightly brown at 48 hr	789	C
Dextrose 2.5% in sodium chloride 0.45%	MG[a]	LI	1 g	No loss in 48 hr at 25 °C. Slight pink color at 24 hr becoming slightly brown at 48 hr	789	C
Dextrose 5% in sodium chloride 0.45%				Use within 24 hr	1	C
	AB[b], CU[a]	LI	1 g	No loss in 48 hr at 25 °C. Slight pink color at 24 hr becoming slightly brown at 48 hr	749	C
Dextrose 5% in sodium chloride 0.9%				Use within 24 hr	1	C
	MG[b]	LI	1 g	No loss in 48 hr at 25 °C. Slight pink color at 24 hr becoming slightly brown at 48 hr	789	C
Dextrose 5%				Use within 24 hr	1	C
	CU[a], TR[b]	LI	1 g	No loss in 48 hr at 25 °C. Slight pink color at 24 hr becoming slightly brown at 48 hr	749	C
	TR[b]	LI	250 mg	Physically compatible with no loss in 48 hr at 24 °C. Transient light pink color. No loss after 7 days at 5 °C	811	C
	[a]		2 to 8 g	Pale pink discoloration with 4% or less dobutamine loss in 24 hr exposed to light	1412	C
	BA[b]	LI	5 g	5% loss in 100 days at 5 °C protected from light	1610	C
	BA[b]	LI	1 g	5% loss in 234.7 days at 5 °C protected from light	1610	C
	TR[b]	LI	0.25 and 1 g	Visually compatible with no dobutamine loss in 48 hr at room temperature	1802	C
	AB[b]	AB	4 g	Visually compatible with no loss in 30 days at 4 and 23 °C protected from light	2241	C
	BA[b], BRN[a,c]	GIU	0.5 g	Visually compatible with little loss in 24 hr at 4 and 22 °C	2289	C
Dextrose 10%				Use within 24 hr	1	C
Normosol M in dextrose 5%				Use within 24 hr	1	C

Solution Compatibility (Cont.)

Dobutamine HCl

Solution	Mfr	Mfr	Conc/L	Remarks	Ref	C/I
Ringer's injection, lactated				Use within 24 hr	1	C
	CU[a], TR[b]	LI	1 g	No loss in 48 hr at 25 °C. Slight pink color at 3 hr becoming slightly brown at 48 hr	749	C
Sodium chloride 0.45%	MG[a]	LI	1 g	No loss in 48 hr at 25 °C. Slight pink color at 24 hr becoming slightly brown at 48 hr	789	C
Sodium chloride 0.9%				Use within 24 hr	1	C
		LI	200 mg	Physically compatible for 24 hr	552	C
	CU[a], TR[b]	LI	1 g	No loss in 48 hr at 25 °C. Slight pink color at 24 hr becoming slightly brown at 48 hr	749	C
	TR[b]	LI	250 mg	About 3% dobutamine loss in 48 hr at 24 °C. Initially colorless solution becomes pink with time. No decomposition after 7 days at 5 °C	811	C
	[a]		2 to 8 g	Pale pink discoloration with 3% or less dobutamine loss in 24 hr exposed to light	1412	C
	TR[a]	LI	0.25 and 1 g	Visually compatible with no loss in 48 hr at room temperature	1802	C
	BA[b], BRN[a,c]	GIU	0.5 g	Visually compatible with little loss in 24 hr at 4 and 22 °C	2289	C
Sodium lactate ⅙ M				Use within 24 hr	1	C

[a]Tested in glass containers.
[b]Tested in PVC containers.
[c]Tested in polyethylene containers.

Additive Compatibility

Dobutamine HCl

Drug	Mfr	Conc/L	Mfr	Conc/L	Test Soln	Remarks	Ref	C/I
Acyclovir sodium	BW	2.5 g	LI	0.5 g	D5W	Discoloration in 25 min. Cloudiness and brown color in 2 hr due to dobutamine oxidation. No acyclovir loss	1343	I
Alteplase	GEN	0.5 g	LI	5 g	D5W, NS	Yellow discoloration and precipitate form	1856	I
Aminophylline	SE	1 g	LI	1 g	D5W, NS	Cloudy in 6 hr at 25 °C	789	I
	ES	2.5 g	LI	1 g	D5W, NS	White precipitate in 12 hr at 21 °C	812	I
Amiodarone HCl	LZ	2.5 g	LI	1 g	D5W, NS	Physically compatible for 24 hr at 21 °C	812	C
Atracurium besylate	BW	500 mg		1 g	D5W	Physically compatible and atracurium stable for 24 hr at 5 and 30 °C	1694	C
Atropine sulfate	AB	16.7 mg	LI	167 mg	NS	Physically compatible for 24 hr	552	C
	ES	50 mg	LI	1 g	D5W, NS	Physically compatible for 24 hr at 21 °C	812	C
Bumetanide	RC	125 mg	LI	1 g	D5W, NS	Immediate yellow discoloration with yellow precipitate within 6 hr at 21 °C	812	I
Calcium chloride	UP	9 g	LI	182 mg	NS	Physically compatible for 20 hr. Haze forms at 24 hr	552	I
	ES	2 g	LI	1 g	D5W, NS	Deeply pink in 24 hr at 25 °C	789	I
	ES	50 g	LI	1 g	D5W, NS	Physically compatible for 24 hr at 21 °C	812	C
Calcium gluconate	VI	9 g	LI	182 mg	NS	Small particles form within 4 hr. White precipitate and haze after 15 hr	552	I
	ES	2 g	LI	1 g	D5W, NS	Deeply pink in 24 hr at 25 °C	789	I
	IX	50 g	LI	1 g	D5W, NS	Small white particles in 24 hr at 21 °C	812	I

Additive Compatibility (Cont.)

Dobutamine HCl

Drug	Mfr	Conc/L	Mfr	Conc/L	Test Soln	Remarks	Ref	C/I
Ciprofloxacin	BAY	1.7 g	LI	2 g	D5W	Visually compatible with no loss of ciprofloxacin in 24 hr at 22 °C under fluorescent light. Dobutamine not tested	2413	**C**
Diazepam	RC	2.5 g	LI	1 g	D5W, NS	Rapid clouding of solution with yellow precipitate within 24 hr at 21 °C	812	**I**
Digoxin	BW	4 mg	LI	1 g	D5W, NS	Slightly pink in 24 hr at 25 °C	789	**I**
Dopamine HCl	AS	5.5 g	LI	172 mg	NS	Physically compatible for 24 hr	552	**C**
	ACC	1.6 g	LI	1 g	D5W, NS	Physically compatible with no color change in 24 hr at 25 °C	789	**C**
	ES	800 mg	LI	1 g	D5W, NS	Physically compatible for 24 hr at 21 °C	812	**C**
Enalaprilat	MSD	12 mg	LI	1 g	D5W[a]	Visually compatible. Little enalaprilat loss in 24 hr at room temperature under fluorescent light. Dobutamine not tested	1572	**C**
Epinephrine HCl	BR	50 mg	LI	1 g	D5W, NS	Physically compatible for 24 hr at 21 °C	812	**C**
Floxacillin sodium	BE	20 g	LI	500 mg	NS	Haze forms immediately and precipitate forms in 24 to 48 hr at 15 and 30 °C	1479	**I**
Flumazenil	RC	20 mg	LI	2 g	D5W[a]	Visually compatible. No flumazenil loss in 24 hr at 23 °C in fluorescent light. Dobutamine not tested	1710	**C**
Furosemide	HO	1 g	LI	1 g	D5W, NS	Cloudy in 1 hr at 25 °C	789	**I**
	WY	5 g	LI	1 g	D5W, NS	Immediate white precipitate	812	**I**
	HO	1 g	LI	500 mg	NS	Haze forms immediately	1479	**I**
Heparin sodium	ES	40,000 units	LI	1 g	D5W, NS	Physically compatible with no color change in 24 hr at 25 °C	789	**C**
	LY	50,000 units	LI	1 g	D5W, NS	Physically compatible for 24 hr at 21 °C	812	**C**
	ES	5 million units	LI	1 g	D5W, NS	Pink discoloration within 6 hr at 21 °C	812	**I**
	ES	50,000 units	LI	1 g	D5W	Precipitate forms within 3 min	841	**I**
	LY	50,000 units	LI	1.5 g	D5W, NS	Obvious precipitation	1318	**I**
	LY	50,000 units	LI	900 mg	D5W, W	Physically compatible for 4 hr, but heat of reaction detected by microcalorimetry	1318	**I**
	LY	50,000 units	LI	900 mg	NS	Physically compatible for 4 hr with no heat of reaction detected by microcalorimetry	1318	**C**
Hydralazine HCl	CI	200 mg	LI	200 mg	NS	Physically compatible for 24 hr	552	**C**
Isoproterenol HCl	ES	2 mg	LI	1 g	D5W, NS	Physically compatible for 24 hr at 21 °C	812	**C**
Lidocaine HCl	ES	4 g	LI	1 g	D5W, NS	Visually compatible for 24 hr at 25 °C	789	**C**
	AST	4 and 10 g	LI	1 g	D5W, NS	Physically compatible for 24 hr at 21 °C	812	**C**
Magnesium sulfate	TO	2 g	LI	1 g	D5W, NS	Slightly pink in 24 hr at 25 °C	789	**I**
	ES	83 g[b]	LI	167 mg	NS	Haze forms between 20 and 24 hr	552	**I**
Meperidine HCl	ES	50 g	LI	1 g	D5W, NS	Physically compatible for 24 hr at 21 °C	812	**C**
Meropenem	ZEN	1 and 20 g	LI	1 g	NS	Visually compatible for 4 hr at room temperature	1994	**C**

Additive Compatibility (Cont.)

Dobutamine HCl

Drug	Mfr	Conc/L	Mfr	Conc/L	Test Soln	Remarks	Ref	C/I
Morphine sulfate	ES	5 g	LI	1 g	D5W, NS	Physically compatible for 24 hr at 21 °C	812	C
Nitroglycerin	AB	120 mg	LI	1 g	D5W, NS	Physically compatible for 24 hr at 21 °C	812	C
	ACC	100 mg	LI	500 mg	D5S	Stable with no loss of either drug after 24 hr at 25 °C. Pink color after 4 hr	990	C
Nitroglycerin with sodium nitroprusside		200 to 800 mg 200 to 800 mg		2 to 8 g	D5W[c]	Pink color with small amount of dark brown precipitate and 11 to 19% nitroglycerin loss in 24 hr exposed to light	1412	I
Nitroglycerin with sodium nitroprusside		200 to 800 mg 200 to 800 mg		2 to 8 g	NS[c]	Pink color with 8% or less loss for any drug for 24 hr exposed to light	1412	C
Norepinephrine bitartrate	BN	32 mg	LI	1 g	D5W, NS	Physically compatible for 24 hr at 21 °C	812	C
Phentolamine mesylate	CI	20 mg	LI	1 g	D5W, NS	Physically compatible for 24 hr at 21 °C	812	C
Phenylephrine HCl	WI	20 mg	LI	1 g	D5W, NS	Physically compatible for 24 hr at 21 °C	812	C
Phenytoin sodium	AHP	25 g	LI	1 g	D5W, NS	White precipitate forms rapidly, with brown solution in 6 hr at 21 °C	812	I
	ES	1 g	LI	1 g	D5W, NS	White precipitate forms within 5 to 10 min	789	I
Potassium chloride	ES	160 mEq	LI	1 g	D5W, NS	Slightly pink in 24 hr at 25 °C	789	I
	AB	20 mEq	LI	1 g	D5W, NS	Physically compatible for 24 hr at 21 °C	812	C
Potassium phosphates	AB	100 mmol	LI	200 mg	NS	Small particles form after 1 hr. White precipitate noted after 15 hr	552	I
Procainamide HCl	SQ	1 g	LI	1 g	D5W, NS	Physically compatible with no color change in 24 hr at 25 °C	789	C
	AHP	4 and 50 g	LI	1 g	D5W, NS	Physically compatible for 24 hr at 21 °C	812	C
Propranolol HCl	AY	50 mg	LI	1 g	D5W, NS	Physically compatible for 24 hr at 21 °C	812	C
Ranitidine HCl	GL	2 g	LI	250 mg and 1 g	D5W, NS[a]	Physically compatible. No ranitidine loss in 48 hr at room temperature in light. Dobutamine not tested	1361	C
	GL	50 mg	LI	250 mg and 1 g	D5W[a]	Physically compatible. 7% ranitidine loss in 48 hr at room temperature in light. Dobutamine not tested	1361	C
	GL	50 mg	LI	250 mg and 1 g	NS[a]	Physically compatible. No ranitidine loss in 48 hr at room temperature in light. Dobutamine not tested	1361	C
	GL	50 mg and 2 g	LI	0.25 and 1 g	D5W, NS[a]	Visually compatible. Little loss of either drug in 48 hr at room temperature	1802	C
Sodium bicarbonate	MG	5%	LI	1 g		Cloudy brown with precipitate in 3 hr at 25 °C. 18% dobutamine loss in 24 hr	789	I
	IX	500 mEq	LI	1 g	D5W, NS	White precipitate in 6 hr at 21 °C	812	I

Additive Compatibility (Cont.)

Dobutamine HCl

Drug	Mfr	Conc/L	Mfr	Conc/L	Test Soln	Remarks	Ref	C/I
Sodium nitroprusside with nitroglycerin		200 to 800 mg 200 to 800 mg		2 to 8 g	D5W[c]	Pink color with small amount of dark brown precipitate and 11 to 19% nitroglycerin loss in 24 hr exposed to light	1412	I
Sodium nitroprusside with nitroglycerin		200 to 800 mg 200 to 800 mg		2 to 8 g	NS[c]	Pink color with 8% or less loss for any drug for 24 hr exposed to light	1412	C
Verapamil HCl	KN	80 mg	LI	500 mg	D5W, NS	Slight pink color develops after 24 hr because of dobutamine oxidation	764	I
	KN	160 mg	LI	250 mg	D5W	No loss of either drug in 48 hr at 24 °C or 7 days at 5 °C. Transient pink color	811	C
	KN	160 mg	LI	250 mg	NS	Pink color and no verapamil and 3% dobutamine loss in 48 hr at 24 °C. At 5 °C, no loss of either drug in 7 days	811	C
	KN	1.25 g	LI	1 g	D5W, NS	Physically compatible for 24 hr at 21 °C	812	C
Zidovudine	GW	2 g	AB	1 g	D5W	No more than 5% loss for either drug at 23 °C and 2% loss at 4 °C in 24 hr	2489	C
	GW	2 g	AB	1 g	NS	No more than 4% loss for either drug at 23 °C and 2% loss at 4 °C in 24 hr	2489	C

[a]Tested in PVC containers.
[b]Tested as 1 g/12 mL final concentration.
[c]Tested in glass containers.

Drugs in Syringe Compatibility

Dobutamine HCl

Drug (in syringe)	Mfr	Amt	Mfr	Amt	Remarks	Ref	C/I
Caffeine citrate		20 mg/ 1 mL	GNS	12.5 mg/ 1 mL	Visually compatible for 4 hr at 25 °C	2440	C
Dimenhydrinate		10 mg/ 1 mL		12.5 mg/ 1 mL	Clear solution	2569	C
Doxapram HCl	RB	400 mg/ 20 mL	LI	100 mg/ 10 mL	5% doxapram loss in 3 hr and 11% in 24 hr	1177	I
Heparin sodium		2500 units/ 1 mL	LI	250 mg/ 10 mL	Physically compatible for at least 5 min	1053	C
Pantoprazole sodium	a	4 mg/ 1 mL		12.5 mg/ 1 mL	White precipitate forms within 1 hr	2574	I
Ranitidine HCl	GL	50 mg/ 5 mL	LI	25 mg	Physically compatible for 4 hr at ambient temperature under fluorescent light	1151	C

[a]Test performed using the formulation WITHOUT edetate disodium.

Y-Site Injection Compatibility (1:1 Mixture)

Dobutamine HCl

Drug	Mfr	Conc	Mfr	Conc	Remarks	Ref	C/I
Acyclovir sodium	BW	5 mg/mL[a]	LI	1 mg/mL[a]	Cloudy and brown in 1 hr at 25 °C	1157	I
Alprostadil	BED	7.5 mcg/mL[p,q]	AB	3 mg/mL[o]	Visually compatible for 1 hr	2746	C
Alteplase	GEN	1 mg/mL	LI	2 mg/mL[a]	Haze in 20 min spectrophotometrically and in 2 hr visually	1340	I
Amifostine	USB	10 mg/mL[a]	LI	4 mg/mL[a]	Physically compatible for 4 hr at 23 °C	1845	C
Aminophylline	ES	4 mg/mL[c]	LI	4 mg/mL[c]	Slight precipitate and color change in 1 hr	1316	I
Amiodarone HCl	LZ	4 mg/mL[c]	LI	2 mg/mL[c]	Physically compatible for 24 hr at 21 °C	1032	C
Amphotericin B cholesteryl sulfate complex	SEQ	0.83 mg/mL[a]	AST	4 mg/mL[a]	Gross precipitate forms	2117	I
Anidulafungin	VIC	0.5 mg/mL[a]	AB	4 mg/mL[a]	Physically compatible for 4 hr at 23 °C	2617	C
Argatroban	GSK	1 mg/mL[b]	LI	12.5 mg/mL	Visually compatible for 24 hr at 23 °C	2391	C
Atracurium besylate	BW	0.5 mg/mL[a]	LI	1 mg/mL[a]	Physically compatible for 24 hr at 28 °C	1337	C
Aztreonam	SQ	40 mg/mL[a]	LI	4 mg/mL[a]	Physically compatible for 4 hr at 23 °C	1758	C
Bivalirudin	TMC	5 mg/mL[a]	AB	4 mg/mL[a]	Physically compatible for 4 hr at 23 °C	2373	C
	TMC	5 mg/mL[a,b]	BV	12.5 mg/mL	Cloudiness forms immediately	2680	I
Calcium chloride	AB	4 mg/mL[c]	LI	4 mg/mL[c]	Physically compatible for 3 hr	1316	C
Calcium gluconate	AST	4 mg/mL[c]	LI	4 mg/mL[c]	Physically compatible for 3 hr	1316	C
Caspofungin acetate	ME	0.7 mg/mL[b]	HOS	4 mg/mL[b]	Physically compatible for 4 hr at room temperature	2758	C
	ME	0.5 mg/mL[b]	BA	1 mg/mL[f]	Physically compatible over 60 min	2766	C
Cefepime HCl	BMS	120 mg/mL[c]		1 mg/mL	Physically compatible with less than 10% cefepime loss. Dobutamine not tested	2513	C
	BMS	120 mg/mL[c]		250 mg/mL	Precipitates	2513	I
Ceftaroline fosamil	FOR	2.22 mg/mL[a]	HOS	4 mg/mL[a]	Haze increases and particulates appear	2826	I
	FOR	2.22 mg/mL[b,l]	HOS	4 mg/mL[b,l]	Physically compatible for 4 hr at 23 °C	2826	C
Ceftazidime	GSK	120 mg/mL[d]		1 mg/mL	Physically compatible with less than 10% ceftazidime loss. Dobutamine not tested	2513	C
	GSK	120 mg/mL[d]		250 mg/mL	Precipitates	2513	I
Ciprofloxacin	MI	2 mg/mL[c]	LI	250 mcg/mL[c]	Visually compatible for 24 hr at 24 °C	1655	C
Cisatracurium besylate	GW	0.1, 2, 5 mg/mL[a]	LI	4 mg/mL[a]	Physically compatible for 4 hr at 23 °C	2074	C
Cladribine	ORT	0.015[b] and 0.5[e] mg/mL	LI	4 mg/mL[b]	Physically compatible for 4 hr at 23 °C	1969	C
Clarithromycin	AB	4 mg/mL[a]	BI	2 mg/mL[a]	Visually compatible for 72 hr at both 30 and 17 °C	2174	C
Clonidine HCl	BI	18 mcg/mL[b]	LI	2 mg/mL[a]	Visually compatible	2642	C
Dexmedetomidine HCl	AB	4 mcg/mL[b]	AST	4 mg/mL[b]	Physically compatible for 4 hr at 23 °C	2383	C
Diazepam	ES	0.2 mg/mL[c]	LI	4 mg/mL[c]	Physically compatible for 3 hr	1316	C
Diltiazem HCl	MMD	1 mg/mL[a]	LI	2 mg/mL[a]	Visually compatible for 24 hr at 25 °C	1530	C
	MMD	5 mg/mL	LI	1 mg/mL[c]	Visually compatible	1807	C
	MMD	1 mg/mL[a]	LI	4 mg/mL[a]	Visually compatible for 4 hr at 27 °C	2062	C
Docetaxel	RPR	0.9 mg/mL[a]	AST	4 mg/mL[a]	Physically compatible for 4 hr at 23 °C	2224	C
Dopamine HCl	DCC	3.2 mg/mL[c]	LI	4 mg/mL[c]	Physically compatible for 3 hr	1316	C

Y-Site Injection Compatibility (1:1 Mixture) (Cont.)

Dobutamine HCl

Drug	Mfr	Conc	Mfr	Conc	Remarks	Ref	C/I
	AB	3.2 mg/mL[a]	LI	4 mg/mL[a]	Visually compatible for 4 hr at 27 °C	2062	C
Dopamine HCl with lidocaine HCl	DCC AB	3.2 mg/mL[c] 8 mg/mL[c]	LI	4 mg/mL[c]	Physically compatible for 3 hr	1316	C
Dopamine HCl with nitroglycerin	DCC LY	3.2 mg/mL[c] 0.4 mg/mL[c]	LI	4 mg/mL[c]	Physically compatible for 3 hr	1316	C
Dopamine HCl with sodium nitroprusside	DCC ES	3.2 mg/mL[c] 0.4 mg/mL[c]	LI	4 mg/mL[c]	Physically compatible for 3 hr	1316	C
Doripenem	JJ	5 mg/mL[a,b]	HOS	4 mg/mL[a,b]	Physically compatible for 4 hr at 23 °C	2743	C
Doxorubicin HCl liposomal	SEQ	0.4 mg/mL[a]	BA	4 mg/mL[a]	Physically compatible for 4 hr at 23 °C	2087	C
Enalaprilat	MSD	0.05 mg/mL[b]	LI	1 mg/mL[a]	Physically compatible for 24 hr at room temperature under fluorescent light	1355	C
Epinephrine HCl	AB	0.02 mg/mL[a]	LI	4 mg/mL[a]	Visually compatible for 4 hr at 27 °C	2062	C
Etoposide phosphate	BR	5 mg/mL[a]	AST	4 mg/mL[a]	Physically compatible for 4 hr at 23 °C	2218	C
Famotidine	MSD ME	0.2 mg/mL[a] 2 mg/mL[b]	LI	1 mg/mL[a] 4 mg/mL[a]	Physically compatible for 4 hr at 25 °C Visually compatible for 4 hr at 22 °C	1188 1936	C C
Fenoldopam mesylate	AB	80 mcg/mL[b]	BED	4 mg/mL[b]	Physically compatible for 4 hr at 23 °C	2467	C
Fentanyl citrate	ES	0.05 mg/mL	LI	4 mg/mL[a]	Visually compatible for 4 hr at 27 °C	2062	C
Fluconazole	RR	2 mg/mL	LI	2 mg/mL[a]	Visually compatible for 24 hr at 28 °C under fluorescent light	1760	C
Foscarnet sodium	AST	24 mg/mL	LI	12.5 mg/mL	Delayed formation of muddy precipitate	1335	I
Furosemide	ES ES AMR	1 mg/mL[b] 1 mg/mL[a] 10 mg/mL	LI LI LI	4 mg/mL[b] 4 mg/mL[a] 4 mg/mL[a]	Physically compatible for 3 hr Slight precipitate in 1 hr Precipitate forms immediately	1316 1316 2062	C I I
Gemcitabine HCl	LI	10 mg/mL[b]	AST	4 mg/mL[b]	Physically compatible for 4 hr at 23 °C	2226	C
Granisetron HCl	SKB	0.05 mg/mL[a]	BA	4 mg/mL[a]	Physically compatible for 4 hr at 23 °C	2000	C
Haloperidol lactate	MN	0.5[a] and 5 mg/mL	LI	4 mg/mL[a]	Visually compatible for 24 hr at 21 °C	1523	C
Heparin sodium	ES ES TR OR ES	50 units/mL[b] 50 units/mL[a] 50 units/mL 100 units/mL[a] 100 units/mL[a]	LI LI LI LI LI	4 mg/mL[b] 4 mg/mL[a] 1 mg/mL[a] 4 mg/mL[a] 4 mg/mL[a]	Physically compatible for 3 hr Immediate gross precipitation Visually compatible for 4 hr at 25 °C Haze and white precipitate form Precipitate forms in 4 hr at 27 °C	1316 1316 1793 1877 2062	C I C I I
Hetastarch in lactated electrolyte	AB	6%	AST	4 mg/mL[a]	Physically compatible for 4 hr at 23 °C	2339	C
Hydromorphone HCl	KN	1 mg/mL	LI	4 mg/mL[a]	Visually compatible for 4 hr at 27 °C	2062	C
Hydroxyethyl starch 130/0.4 in sodium chloride 0.9%	FRK	6%	SZ	1, 2, 4 mg/mL[a]	Visually compatible for 24 hr at room temperature	2770	C
Indomethacin sodium trihydrate	MSD	1 mg/mL[b]	LI	1.2 mg/mL[a]	Hazy precipitate forms immediately	1527	I
Insulin, regular	LI	1 unit/mL[c]	LI	4 mg/mL[c]	Physically compatible for 3 hr	1316	C
Labetalol HCl	GL GL AH	1 mg/mL[a] 5 mg/mL 2 mg/mL[a]	LI LI LI	2.5 mg/mL[a] 4 mg/mL[a] 4 mg/mL[a]	Visually compatible. Little loss of either drug in 4 hr at room temperature Visually compatible for 24 hr at 23 °C Visually compatible for 4 hr at 27 °C	1762 1877 2062	C C C
Levofloxacin	OMN	5 mg/mL[a]	AB	12.5 mg/mL	Visually compatible for 4 hr at 24 °C	2233	C

Y-Site Injection Compatibility (1:1 Mixture) (Cont.)

Dobutamine HCl

Drug	Mfr	Conc	Mfr	Conc	Remarks	Ref	C/I
Lidocaine HCl	AB	8 mg/mL[c]	LI	4 mg/mL[c]	Physically compatible for 3 hr	1316	C
Lidocaine HCl with dopamine HCl	AB DCC	8 mg/mL[c] 3.2 mg/mL[c]	LI	4 mg/mL[c]	Physically compatible for 3 hr	1316	C
Lidocaine HCl with nitroglycerin	AB LY	8 mg/mL[c] 0.4 mg/mL[c]	LI	4 mg/mL[c]	Physically compatible for 3 hr	1316	C
Lidocaine HCl with sodium nitroprusside	AB ES	8 mg/mL[c] 0.4 mg/mL[c]	LI	4 mg/mL[c]	Physically compatible for 3 hr	1316	C
Linezolid	PHU	2 mg/mL	AST	4 mg/mL[a]	Physically compatible for 4 hr at 23 °C	2264	C
Lorazepam	WY	0.5 mg/mL[a]	LI	4 mg/mL[a]	Visually compatible for 4 hr at 27 °C	2062	C
Magnesium sulfate	LY	40 mg/mL[c]	LI	4 mg/mL[c]	Physically compatible for 3 hr	1316	C
Meperidine HCl	AB	10 mg/mL	LI	1 mg/mL[a]	Physically compatible for 4 hr at 25 °C	1397	C
Micafungin sodium	ASP	1.5 mg/mL[b]	AB	4 mg/mL[b]	Gross precipitate forms immediately	2683	I
Midazolam HCl	RC RC RC	1 mg/mL[a] 1 mg/mL[a] 2 mg/mL[a]	GNS LI LI	2 mg/mL[a] 4 mg/mL[a] 4 mg/mL[a]	Particles form in 8 hr Visually compatible for 24 hr at 23 °C Visually compatible for 4 hr at 27 °C	1847 1877 2062	I C C
Milrinone lactate	SW SW	0.2 mg/mL[a] 0.4 mg/mL[a]	LI GEN	4 mg/mL[a] 8 mg/mL[a]	Visually compatible for 4 hr at 27 °C Visually compatible. Little loss of either drug in 4 hr at 23 °C	2062 2214	C C
Morphine sulfate	SCN	2 mg/mL[a]	LI	4 mg/mL[a]	Visually compatible for 4 hr at 27 °C	2062	C
Nesiritide	SCI	50 mcg/mL[a,b]		12.5 mg/mL	Physically compatible for 4 hr. May be chemically incompatible with nesiritide[m]	2625	?
Nicardipine HCl	WY DCC	1 mg/mL[a] 0.1 mg/mL[a]	LI LI	4 mg/mL[a] 1 mg/mL[a]	Visually compatible for 4 hr at 27 °C Visually compatible for 24 hr at room temperature	2062 235	C C
Nitroglycerin	LY AB	0.4 mg/mL[c] 0.4 mg/mL[a]	LI LI	4 mg/mL[c] 4 mg/mL[a]	Physically compatible for 3 hr Visually compatible for 4 hr at 27 °C	1316 2062	C C
Nitroglycerin with dopamine HCl	LY DCC	0.4 mg/mL[c] 3.2 mg/mL[c]	LI	4 mg/mL[c]	Physically compatible for 3 hr	1316	C
Nitroglycerin with lidocaine HCl	LY AB	0.4 mg/mL[c] 8 mg/mL[c]	LI	4 mg/mL[c]	Physically compatible for 3 hr	1316	C
Nitroglycerin with sodium nitroprusside	LY ES	0.4 mg/mL[c] 0.4 mg/mL[c]	LI	4 mg/mL[c]	Physically compatible for 3 hr	1316	C
Norepinephrine bitartrate	AB	0.128 mg/mL[a]	LI	4 mg/mL[a]	Visually compatible for 4 hr at 27 °C	2062	C
Oxaliplatin	SS	0.5 mg/mL[a]	BED	4 mg/mL[a]	Physically compatible for 4 hr at 23 °C	2566	C
Pancuronium bromide	ES	0.05 mg/mL[a]	LI	1 mg/mL[a]	Physically compatible for 24 hr at 28 °C	1337	C
Pantoprazole sodium	ALT[n]	0.16 to 0.8 mg/mL[b]	LI	1 to 4 mg/mL[a]	Cloudiness forms over time	2603	I
Pemetrexed disodium	LI	20 mg/mL[b]	AB	4 mg/mL[a]	White cloudy precipitate with microparticulates forms immediately	2564	I
Phytonadione	MSD	0.4 mg/mL[c]	LI	4 mg/mL[c]	Slight haze in 3 hr	1316	I
Piperacillin sodium–tazobactam sodium	LE[n]	40 + 5 mg/mL[a]	LI	4 mg/mL[a]	Heavy white turbidity forms immediately	1688	I

Y-Site Injection Compatibility (1:1 Mixture) (Cont.)

Dobutamine HCl

Drug	Mfr	Conc	Mfr	Conc	Remarks	Ref	C/I
Potassium chloride	AB	0.06 mEq/mL[c]	LI	4 mg/mL[c]	Physically compatible for 3 hr	1316	C
Propofol	ZEN	10 mg/mL	LI	4 mg/mL[a]	Physically compatible for 1 hr at 23 °C	2066	C
Ranitidine HCl	GL	0.5 mg/mL[f]	LI	1 mg/mL[a]	Physically compatible for 24 hr	1323	C
	GL	1 mg/mL[a]	LI	4 mg/mL[a]	Visually compatible for 4 hr at 27 °C	2062	C
Remifentanil HCl	GW	0.025 and 0.25 mg/mL[b]	LI	4 mg/mL[a]	Physically compatible for 4 hr at 23 °C	2075	C
Sodium nitroprusside	ES	0.4 mg/mL[c]	LI	4 mg/mL[c]	Physically compatible for 3 hr	1316	C
	RC	0.3, 1.2, 3 mg/mL[a]	LI	1.5 mg/mL[k]	Visually compatible for 48 hr at 24 °C protected from light	2357	C
	RC	1.2 and 3 mg/mL[a]	LI	6 mg/mL[k]	Color darkening occurs over 48 hr at 24 °C protected from light	2357	?
	RC	0.3 and 1.2 mg/mL[a]	LI	12.5 mg/mL[k]	Visually compatible for 48 hr at 24 °C protected from light	2357	C
	RC	3 mg/mL[a]	LI	12.5 mg/mL[k]	Color darkening occurs over 48 hr at 24 °C protected from light	2357	?
Sodium nitroprusside with dopamine HCl	ES DCC	0.4 mg/mL[c] 3.2 mg/mL[c]	LI	4 mg/mL[c]	Physically compatible for 3 hr	1316	C
Sodium nitroprusside with lidocaine HCl	ES AB	0.4 mg/mL[c] 8 mg/mL[c]	LI	4 mg/mL[c]	Physically compatible for 3 hr	1316	C
Sodium nitroprusside with nitroglycerin	ES LY	0.4 mg/mL[c] 0.4 mg/mL[c]	LI	4 mg/mL[c]	Physically compatible for 3 hr	1316	C
Tacrolimus	FUJ	1 mg/mL[b]	LI	1 mg/mL[a]	Visually compatible for 24 hr at 25 °C	1630	C
Telavancin HCl	ASP	7.5 mg/mL[a,b,l]	HOS	4 mg/mL[a,b,l]	Physically compatible for 2 hr	2830	C
Theophylline	TR	4 mg/mL	LI	1 mg/mL[a]	Visually compatible for 6 hr at 25 °C	1793	C
Thiotepa	IMM[g]	1 mg/mL[a]	LI	4 mg/mL[a]	Physically compatible for 4 hr at 23 °C	1861	C
Tigecycline	WY	1 mg/mL[b]		0.2 and 1 mg/mL[b]	Physically compatible for 4 hr	2714	C
Tirofiban HCl	ME	50 mcg/mL[a,b]	AB	0.25 and 5 mg/mL[a,b]	Physically compatible with no loss of either drug in 4 hr at 23 °C	2356	C
TNA #218 to #226[h]			AST	4 mg/mL[a]	Visually compatible for 4 hr at 23 °C	2215	C
TPN #91[h]		[i]	LI	1 mg/mL[j]	Physically compatible	1170	C
TPN #189[h]			LI	50 mg/mL[b]	Visually compatible for 24 hr at 22 °C	1767	C
TPN #203, #204[h]			LI	5 mg/mL	Visually compatible for 4 hr at 23 °C	1974	C
TPN #212 to #215[h]			LI	4 mg/mL[a]	Physically compatible for 4 hr at 23 °C	2109	C
Vasopressin	AMR	2 and 4 units/mL[b]	AB	4.2 mg/mL[a]	Physically compatible with vasopressin pushed through a Y-site over 5 sec	2478	C
Vecuronium bromide	OR	0.1 mg/mL[a]	LI	1 mg/mL[a]	Physically compatible for 24 hr at 28 °C	1337	C
	OR	1 mg/mL	LI	4 mg/mL[a]	Visually compatible for 4 hr at 27 °C	2062	C
Verapamil HCl	LY	0.2 mg/mL[c]	LI	4 mg/mL[c]	Physically compatible for 3 hr	1316	C

Y-Site Injection Compatibility (1:1 Mixture) (Cont.)

Dobutamine HCl

Drug	Mfr	Conc	Mfr	Conc	Remarks	Ref	C/I
Warfarin sodium	DU	2 mg/mL[d]	LI	1 mg/mL[a]	Haze and precipitate form immediately	2010	I
	DME	2 mg/mL[d]	LI	1 mg/mL[a]	Haze and precipitate form immediately	2078	I
Zidovudine	BW	4 mg/mL[a]	LI	5 mg/mL[a]	Physically compatible for 4 hr at 25 °C	1193	C

[a]*Tested in dextrose 5%.*
[b]*Tested in sodium chloride 0.9%.*
[c]*Tested in both dextrose 5% and sodium chloride 0.9%.*
[d]*Tested in sterile water for injection.*
[e]*Tested in bacteriostatic sodium chloride 0.9% preserved with benzyl alcohol 0.9%.*
[f]*Premixed infusion solution.*
[g]*Lyophilized formulation tested.*
[h]*Refer to Appendix I for the composition of parenteral nutrition solutions. TNA indicates a 3-in-1 admixture, and TPN indicates a 2-in-1 admixture.*
[i]*Run at 10 mL/hr.*
[j]*In dextrose 5% infused at 1.2 mL/hr.*
[k]*Tested in dextrose 5% in sodium chloride 0.45%.*
[l]*Tested in Ringer's injection, lactated.*
[m]*Nesiritide is incompatible with bisulfite antioxidants used in some drug formulations. The specific formulation of the product to be used should be checked to assure that no sulfite antioxidants are present.*
[n]*Test performed using the formulation WITHOUT edetate disodium.*
[o]*Tested in either dextrose 5% or in sodium chloride 0.9%, but the report did not specify which solution.*
[p]*Tested in a 1:1 mixture of (1) dextrose 5% and dextrose 5% in sodium chloride 0.45% with and without potassium chloride 20 mEq/L and also in (2) dextrose 10% in sodium chloride 0.45% with and without potassium chloride 20 mEq/L.*
[q]*Tested in a 1:1 mixture of dextrose 5% and TPN #274 (see Appendix I).*

DOCETAXEL
AHFS 10:00

Products — Several different dosage forms of docetaxel injection are available. **CAUTION: Care should be taken to ensure that the correct drug product, dose, and preparation procedure are used and that no confusion among differing products and concentrations occurs.**

Docetaxel is available in a two-vial formulation as a concentrate in polysorbate 80 in single-use vials containing 20 mg (0.5 mL) and 80 mg (2 mL). Each size vial is packaged with a vial of special diluent composed of ethanol 13% in water for injection. Both the docetaxel vials and the accompanying diluent contain an overfill. (1)

The preparation of the product is a two-step procedure. The first step is the preparation of the premix solution. The premix solution is then further diluted prior to administration (step 2). (1)

To prepare the premix, allow the proper number of vials of docetaxel concentrate to stand at room temperature for about five minutes if they have been stored refrigerated. Then withdraw the entire contents of the accompanying diluent (approximately 1.8 mL for docetaxel 20 mg and approximately 7.1 mL for docetaxel 80 mg) and add to each vial of docetaxel concentrate. Using repeated inversions, mix each vial for about 45 seconds to ensure thorough mixing. Do not shake the vials. This final premix solution is a clear solution having a docetaxel concentration of 10 mg/mL. If foam appears from the surfactant in the formulation, allow the vials to stand until most of the foam has dissipated; it is not necessary for all of the foam to have dissipated before proceeding with the rest of the preparation steps. (1)

Withdraw the necessary amount of the docetaxel 10-mg/mL premix solution using a syringe and add it into a 250-mL glass or polyolefin (polyethylene or polypropylene) container of dextrose 5% or sodium chloride 0.9% to produce a final concentration between 0.3 and 0.74 mg/mL. It is necessary to use a larger volume of infusion solution if the docetaxel dose exceeds 200 mg so that the concentration does not exceed 0.74 mg/mL. The infusion admixture should be mixed thoroughly by rotation. (1)

Docetaxel is also available in one-vial formulations as concentrates of either 10 mg/mL or 20 mg/mL in an equal volume mixture of polysorbate 80 and ethanol in vials. Citric acid may be present in some forms. These are concentrates that must be diluted to a concentration between 0.3 and 0.74 mg/mL for intravenous administration. (1)

The use of gloves during preparation of docetaxel doses is recommended. If the docetaxel concentrate, premix solution, or admixture comes in contact with skin, the affected area should be washed thoroughly with soap and water. Contact with mucosa requires thorough flushing with water. (1)

Trade Name(s) — Taxotere.

Administration — Docetaxel is administered as a one-hour intravenous infusion at ambient temperature and light to patients adequately premedicated to control adverse effects. (1)

Stability — Docetaxel concentrate is a clear, viscous yellow to yellow-brown liquid. (1310) Intact containers of docetaxel with the accompanying special diluent should be stored under refrigeration or at controlled room temperature. Freezing of the concentrate does not adversely affect docetaxel. The vials should be left in the original packages to protect the drug from bright light. (1)

The manufacturer recommends that the premix solution and the fully diluted admixture in dextrose 5% or sodium chloride 0.9% be used as soon as possible after preparation. The premix solution is stable for at least eight hours after preparation under refrigeration or at room temperatures up to 25 °C according to the labeling. (1) Thiesen and Kramer evaluated the stability of docetaxel 10-mg/mL mixed concentrate over 28 days at 25 and 4 °C. The mixed concentrate remained visually clear with no color change and no docetaxel loss at either temperature. (2242)

The drug diluted in infusion solutions for administration has been stated to be stable for four hours at room temperature and is not light sensitive. (1310) The manufacturer recommends use of the dilution for infusion within four hours, including the one-hour period needed for infusion. (1)

Docetaxel 0.8 mg/mL in sodium chloride 0.9% did not exhibit an antimicrobial effect on *Enterococcus faecium*, *Staphylococcus aureus*, *Pseudomonas aeruginosa*, and *Candida albicans* inoculated into the solution. Diluted solutions should be stored under refrigeration whenever possible, and the potential for microbiological growth should be considered when assigning expiration periods. (2160)

Plasticizer Leaching — The surfactant (polysorbate 80) contained in the docetaxel formulation can leach plasticizer from diethylhexyl phthalate (DEHP)-plasticized PVC containers and administration sets. The amount leached is time and concentration dependent. (1683) The manufacturer recommends that docetaxel concentrate not be allowed to contact such containers and equipment. To minimize the amount of plasticizer exposure to the patient, the use of glass or polyolefin (such as polyethylene, polypropylene, etc.) containers and polyethylene-lined administration sets is recommended for the administration of docetaxel admixtures. (1)

Mazzo et al. evaluated the leaching of DEHP plasticizer by docetaxel 0.56 and 0.96 mg/mL in dextrose 5% and in sodium chloride 0.9%. PVC bags of the solutions were used to prepare the admixtures. The leaching of the plasticizer was found to be time and concentration dependent; however, there was little difference between the two infusion solutions. After storage for eight hours at 21 °C, leached DEHP was found in the range of 30 to 51 mcg/mL for the 0.96-mg/mL concentration and 25 to 36 mcg/mL for the 0.56-mg/mL concentration. During a simulated one-hour infusion, the amount of leached DEHP did not exceed 14 mcg/mL. (1825)

An acceptability limit of no more than 5 parts per million (5 mcg/mL) for DEHP plasticizer leached from PVC containers, etc. has been proposed. The limit was proposed based on a review of metabolic and toxicologic considerations. (2185)

A study was performed on the compatibility of docetaxel 0.31 and 0.88 mg/mL in dextrose 5% or sodium chloride 0.9% with various infusion sets. The docetaxel solutions were run through the administration sets and the effluent was analyzed for DEHP plasticizer. At the higher concentration of docetaxel (0.88 mg/mL), unacceptable amounts of DEHP were leached from the Baxter vented nitroglycerin

Table 1. Administration Sets Compatible with Docetaxel Infusions at Concentrations of 0.88 mg/mL or Less (2451)

Manufacturer	Administration Set
Abbott	LifeCare 5000 Plum non-polyvinyl chloride specialty set (11594)
	LifeCare model 4P specialty set, non-PVC (11434)
	Life Shield anesthesia pump set OL with cartridge (13503)
	Nitroglycerin primary i.v. pump set OL, vented (1772)
	Omni-Flow universal primary i.v. pump short mini-bore (40527)
Block Medical	Verifuse nonvented administration set with 0.22-μm filter, check valve, and non-DEHP PVC tubing (V021015)
I-Flow	Vivus-400 polyethylene-lined infusion set (5000-784)
IMED	Closed system non-PVC fluid path nonvented quick spike set (9630)
	Non-PVC set with inline filter (9986)
	Gemini 20 nonvented primary administration set for nitroglycerin and emulsions (2260)
IVAC	Universal set with low-sorbing tubing (52053, 59953, S75053)
	Reduced-PVC full set MiniMed Uni-Set macrobore (28190)
Ivion/Medex	WalkMed spike set (SP-06) with pump set (PS-401, PS-360, PS-560)
McGaw	Horizon pump vented nitroglycerin i.v. set (V7450)
	Intelligent pump vented nitroglycerin i.v. set (V7150)
SoloPak	Primary solution set with universal spike, 0.22-μm filter, and injection site (73600)

Table 2. Extension Sets Compatible with Docetaxel Infusions at Concentrations of 0.88 mg/mL or Less (2451)

Manufacturer	Administration Set
Abbott	IVEX-HP filter set (4524)
	IVEX-2 filter set (2679)
Baxter	Polyethylene-lined extension set with 0.22-μm air-eliminating filter (1C8363)
Becton Dickinson	E-Z infusion set (38-53121)
	E-Z infusion set shorty (38-53741)
	Intima i.v. catheter placement set (38-6918-1)
	J-loop connector (38-1252-2)
Braun	0.2-μm filter extension set (FE-2012L)
	Small-bore 0.2-μm filter extension set (PFE-2007)
	Small-bore extension set with T-fitting (ET-04T)
	Small-bore extension set with reflux valve (ET-116L)
	Whin-winged extension set 90° Huber needle (HW-2276)
	Whin extension set with Y-site and Huber needle (HW-2276 YHRF)
	Y-extension set with valve (ET-08-YL)
Gish Biomedical	VasTack noncoring portal-access needle system (VT 2022)
IMED	0.2-μm add-on filter set (9400XL)
IVAC	Spec-Sets extension set with 0.2-μm inline filter (C20028, C20350)
Pall	SetSaver extended-life disposable set with 0.2-μm filter (ELD-96P)
	SetSaver extended-life disposable set with 0.2-μm filter (ELD-96LL)
	SetSaver extended-life disposable microbore extension tubing with 0.2-μm Posidyne filter (ELD-96LYL)
	SetSaver extended-life disposable intravenous filter 0.2-μm with standard bore extension tubing with injection site (ELD-96LYLS)
Pfizer/Strato Medical	Lifeport vascular-access system infusion set with Y-site (LPS 3009)

set (2C7552S), the Baxter vented volumetric pump nitroglycerin set (2C1042), and the IMED standard PVC set (9210). At both low and high concentrations (0.31 and 0.88 mg/mL), unacceptable amounts of DEHP were leached from the IVAC MiniMed Uni-Set microbore (28026) and MiniMed Uni-Set macrobore full set (28034). The sets cited in Table 1 and Table 2 leached little or no DEHP. (2451)

With use of infusion bags and tubing that are free of DEHP plasticizer and the elimination of PVC precision flow regulators, a reduction in leached DEHP of up to 99% has been reported. (2679)

Docetaxel vehicle equivalent to docetaxel 0.74 mg/mL in dextrose 5% was tested in VISIV polyolefin bags at room temperature near 23 °C for 24 hours. No leached plastic components were found within the 24-hour study period. (2660; 2792)

Docetaxel in PVC containers leached 200 to 500 mcg/mL of DEHP in 48 hours stored under refrigeration and at room temperature, respectively. Use of nonplasticized containers such as polyethylene plastic containers was recommended. (2718)

Filtration — The use of inline filters for docetaxel administration is not required by the manufacturer. (4)

Compatibility Information

Solution Compatibility

Docetaxel

Solution	Mfr	Mfr	Conc/L	Remarks	Ref	C/I
Dextrose 5%	BRN[a]	RPR	0.3 and 0.9 g	Visually compatible with little or no loss in 28 days at 25 °C protected from light	2242	C
	BRN[b]	RPR	0.3 and 0.9 g	Visually compatible with little or no loss in 28 days at 25 °C protected from light	2242	C
	BR[c]	RPR	0.3 and 0.9 g	Visually compatible with little or no loss in 5 days at 25 °C protected from light. Precipitation and accompanying loss of drug occurred after 5 days in some samples	2242	C
Sodium chloride 0.9%	BRN[a]	RPR	0.3 and 0.9 g	Visually compatible with little or no loss in 28 days at 25 °C protected from light	2242	C
	BRN[d]	RPR	0.3 and 0.9 g	Visually compatible with little or no loss in 28 days at 25 °C protected from light	2242	C
	BR[c]	RPR	0.3 and 0.9 g	Visually compatible with little or no loss in 3 days at 25 °C protected from light. Precipitation and accompanying loss of drug occurred after 3 days in some samples	2242	C
	BRN[d], FRE[c]	SAA	740 mg	Precipitation when stored at 23 °C. No precipitation or loss of docetaxel in 48 hr when stored at 4 °C followed by 4 hr at 23 °C	2718	?
	BRN[e]	AVE	0.4 and 0.8 g	Visually compatible. No docetaxel loss in 35 days at 4 °C and at 23 °C exposed to fluorescent light	2761	C
	BA[b], GRI[a]	RP	0.3 and 0.9 g	Physically and chemically stable for 24 hr at 20 °C. Precipitation after that time	2804	C

[a]Tested in glass containers.
[b]Tested in polypropylene containers.
[c]Tested in PVC containers.
[d]Tested in polyethylene containers.
[e]Tested in polypropylene-polyethylene copolymer PAB bags.

Y-Site Injection Compatibility (1:1 Mixture)

Docetaxel

Drug	Mfr	Conc	Mfr	Conc	Remarks	Ref	C/I
Acyclovir sodium	GW	7 mg/mL[a]	RPR	0.9 mg/mL[a]	Physically compatible for 4 hr at 23 °C	2224	C
Amifostine	ALZ	10 mg/mL[b]	RPR	0.9 mg/mL[a]	Physically compatible for 4 hr at 23 °C	2224	C
Amikacin sulfate	AB	5 mg/mL[a]	RPR	0.9 mg/mL[a]	Physically compatible for 4 hr at 23 °C	2224	C
Aminophylline	AB	2.5 mg/mL[a]	RPR	0.9 mg/mL[a]	Physically compatible for 4 hr at 23 °C	2224	C
Amphotericin B	PH	0.6 mg/mL[a]	RPR	0.9 mg/mL[a]	Visible turbidity forms immediately	2224	I

Y-Site Injection Compatibility (1:1 Mixture) (Cont.)

Docetaxel

Drug	Mfr	Conc	Mfr	Conc	Remarks	Ref	C/I
Ampicillin sodium	SKB	20 mg/mL[b]	RPR	0.9 mg/mL[a]	Physically compatible for 4 hr at 23 °C	2224	C
Ampicillin sodium–sulbactam sodium	RR	20 + 10 mg/mL[b]	RPR	0.9 mg/mL[a]	Physically compatible for 4 hr at 23 °C	2224	C
Anidulafungin	VIC	0.5 mg/mL	AVE	2 mg/mL[a]	Physically compatible for 4 hr at 23 °C	2617	C
Aztreonam	BMS	40 mg/mL[a]	RPR	0.9 mg/mL[a]	Physically compatible for 4 hr at 23 °C	2224	C
Bumetanide	RC	0.04 mg/mL[a]	RPR	0.9 mg/mL[a]	Physically compatible for 4 hr at 23 °C	2224	C
Buprenorphine HCl	RKC	0.04 mg/mL[a]	RPR	0.9 mg/mL[a]	Physically compatible for 4 hr at 23 °C	2224	C
Butorphanol tartrate	APC	0.04 mg/mL[a]	RPR	0.9 mg/mL[a]	Physically compatible for 4 hr at 23 °C	2224	C
Calcium gluconate	FUJ	40 mg/mL[a]	RPR	0.9 mg/mL[a]	Physically compatible for 4 hr at 23 °C	2224	C
Cefazolin sodium	APC	20 mg/mL[a]	RPR	0.9 mg/mL[a]	Physically compatible for 4 hr at 23 °C	2224	C
Cefepime HCl	BMS	20 mg/mL[a]	RPR	0.9 mg/mL[a]	Physically compatible for 4 hr at 23 °C	2224	C
Cefotaxime sodium	HO	20 mg/mL[a]	RPR	0.9 mg/mL[a]	Physically compatible for 4 hr at 23 °C	2224	C
Cefotetan disodium	ZEN	20 mg/mL[a]	RPR	0.9 mg/mL[a]	Physically compatible for 4 hr at 23 °C	2224	C
Cefoxitin sodium	ME	20 mg/mL[a]	RPR	0.9 mg/mL[a]	Physically compatible for 4 hr at 23 °C	2224	C
Ceftazidime	SKB	40 mg/mL[a]	RPR	0.9 mg/mL[a]	Physically compatible for 4 hr at 23 °C	2224	C
Ceftriaxone sodium	RC	20 mg/mL[a]	RPR	0.9 mg/mL[a]	Physically compatible for 4 hr at 23 °C	2224	C
Cefuroxime sodium	LI	30 mg/mL[a]	RPR	0.9 mg/mL[a]	Physically compatible for 4 hr at 23 °C	2224	C
Chlorpromazine HCl	SCN	2 mg/mL[a]	RPR	0.9 mg/mL[a]	Physically compatible for 4 hr at 23 °C	2224	C
Ciprofloxacin	BAY	1 mg/mL[a]	RPR	0.9 mg/mL[a]	Physically compatible for 4 hr at 23 °C	2224	C
Clindamycin phosphate	AST	10 mg/mL[a]	RPR	0.9 mg/mL[a]	Physically compatible for 4 hr at 23 °C	2224	C
Dexamethasone sodium phosphate	ES	2 mg/mL[a]	RPR	0.9 mg/mL[a]	Physically compatible for 4 hr at 23 °C	2224	C
Diphenhydramine HCl	ES	2 mg/mL[a]	RPR	0.9 mg/mL[a]	Physically compatible for 4 hr at 23 °C	2224	C
Dobutamine HCl	AST	4 mg/mL[a]	RPR	0.9 mg/mL[a]	Physically compatible for 4 hr at 23 °C	2224	C
Dopamine HCl	AB	3.2 mg/mL[a]	RPR	0.9 mg/mL[a]	Physically compatible for 4 hr at 23 °C	2224	C
Doripenem	JJ	5 mg/mL[a,b]	SAA	0.8 mg/mL[a,b]	Physically compatible for 4 hr at 23 °C	2743	C
Doxorubicin HCl liposomal	SEQ	0.4 mg/mL[a]	RPR	2 mg/mL[a]	Partial loss of measured natural turbidity	2087	I
Doxycycline hyclate	FUJ	1 mg/mL[a]	RPR	0.9 mg/mL[a]	Physically compatible for 4 hr at 23 °C	2224	C
Droperidol	AST	0.4 mg/mL[a]	RPR	0.9 mg/mL[a]	Physically compatible for 4 hr at 23 °C	2224	C
Enalaprilat	ME	0.1 mg/mL[a]	RPR	0.9 mg/mL[a]	Physically compatible for 4 hr at 23 °C	2224	C
Famotidine	ME	2 mg/mL[a]	RPR	0.9 mg/mL[a]	Physically compatible for 4 hr at 23 °C	2224	C
Fluconazole	RR	2 mg/mL	RPR	0.9 mg/mL[a]	Physically compatible for 4 hr at 23 °C	2224	C
Furosemide	AMR	3 mg/mL[a]	RPR	0.9 mg/mL[a]	Physically compatible for 4 hr at 23 °C	2224	C
Ganciclovir sodium	RC	20 mg/mL[a]	RPR	0.9 mg/mL[a]	Physically compatible for 4 hr at 23 °C	2224	C
Gemcitabine HCl	LI	10 mg/mL[b]	RPR	2 mg/mL[a]	Physically compatible for 4 hr at 23 °C	2226	C
Gentamicin sulfate	AB	5 mg/mL[a]	RPR	0.9 mg/mL[a]	Physically compatible for 4 hr at 23 °C	2224	C
Granisetron HCl	SKB	0.05 mg/mL[a]	RPR	0.9 mg/mL[a]	Physically compatible for 4 hr at 23 °C	2224	C
Haloperidol lactate	MN	0.2 mg/mL[a]	RPR	0.9 mg/mL[a]	Physically compatible for 4 hr at 23 °C	2224	C
Heparin sodium	ES	100 units/mL	RPR	0.9 mg/mL[a]	Physically compatible for 4 hr at 23 °C	2224	C

Y-Site Injection Compatibility (1:1 Mixture) (Cont.)

Docetaxel

Drug	Mfr	Conc	Mfr	Conc	Remarks	Ref	C/I
Hydrocortisone sodium succinate	AB	1 mg/mL[a]	RPR	0.9 mg/mL[a]	Physically compatible for 4 hr at 23 °C	2224	C
Hydromorphone HCl	AST	0.5 mg/mL[a]	RPR	0.9 mg/mL[a]	Physically compatible for 4 hr at 23 °C	2224	C
Hydroxyzine HCl	ES	2 mg/mL[a]	RPR	0.9 mg/mL[a]	Physically compatible for 4 hr at 23 °C	2224	C
Imipenem–cilastatin sodium	ME	10 mg/mL[b]	RPR	0.9 mg/mL[a]	Physically compatible for 4 hr at 23 °C	2224	C
Leucovorin calcium	ES	2 mg/mL[a]	RPR	0.9 mg/mL[a]	Physically compatible for 4 hr at 23 °C	2224	C
Lorazepam	WY	0.5 mg/mL[a]	RPR	0.9 mg/mL[a]	Physically compatible for 4 hr at 23 °C	2224	C
Magnesium sulfate	AST	100 mg/mL[a]	RPR	0.9 mg/mL[a]	Physically compatible for 4 hr at 23 °C	2224	C
Mannitol	BA	15%	RPR	0.9 mg/mL[a]	Physically compatible for 4 hr at 23 °C	2224	C
Meperidine HCl	AST	4 mg/mL[a]	RPR	0.9 mg/mL[a]	Physically compatible for 4 hr at 23 °C	2224	C
Meropenem	ZEN	20 mg/mL[b]	RPR	0.9 mg/mL[a]	Physically compatible for 4 hr at 23 °C	2224	C
Mesna	MJ	10 mg/mL[a]	RPR	0.9 mg/mL[a]	Physically compatible for 4 hr at 23 °C	2224	C
Methylprednisolone sodium succinate	PHU	5 mg/mL[a]	RPR	0.9 mg/mL[a]	Partial loss of measured natural turbidity occurs immediately	2224	I
Metoclopramide HCl	AB	5 mg/mL	RPR	0.9 mg/mL[a]	Physically compatible for 4 hr at 23 °C	2224	C
Metronidazole	BA	5 mg/mL	RPR	0.9 mg/mL[a]	Physically compatible for 4 hr at 23 °C	2224	C
Morphine sulfate	ES	1 mg/mL[a]	RPR	0.9 mg/mL[a]	Physically compatible for 4 hr at 23 °C	2224	C
Nalbuphine HCl	AST	10 mg/mL	RPR	0.9 mg/mL[a]	Increase in measured subvisible turbidity occurs immediately	2224	I
Ondansetron HCl	GW	1 mg/mL[a]	RPR	0.9 mg/mL[a]	Physically compatible for 4 hr at 23 °C	2224	C
Oxaliplatin	SS	0.5 mg/mL[a]	AVE	2 mg/mL[a]	Physically compatible for 4 hr at 23 °C	2566	C
Palonosetron HCl	MGI	50 mcg/mL	AVE	0.8 mg/mL[a]	Physically compatible and no loss of either drug in 4 hr	2533	C
Pemetrexed disodium	LI	20 mg/mL[b]	AVE	0.8 mg/mL[a]	Physically compatible for 4 hr at 23 °C	2564	C
Piperacillin sodium–tazobactam sodium	CY[c]	40 + 5 mg/mL[a]	RPR	0.9 mg/mL[a]	Physically compatible for 4 hr at 23 °C	2224	C
Potassium chloride	AB	0.1 mEq/mL[a]	RPR	0.9 mg/mL[a]	Physically compatible for 4 hr at 23 °C	2224	C
Prochlorperazine edisylate	SO	0.5 mg/mL[a]	RPR	0.9 mg/mL[a]	Physically compatible for 4 hr at 23 °C	2224	C
Promethazine HCl	SCN	2 mg/mL[a]	RPR	0.9 mg/mL[a]	Physically compatible for 4 hr at 23 °C	2224	C
Ranitidine HCl	GL	2 mg/mL[a]	RPR	0.9 mg/mL[a]	Physically compatible for 4 hr at 23 °C	2224	C
Sodium bicarbonate	AB	1 mEq/mL	RPR	0.9 mg/mL[a]	Physically compatible for 4 hr at 23 °C	2224	C
Ticarcillin disodium–clavulanate potassium	SKB	31 mg/mL[a]	RPR	0.9 mg/mL[a]	Physically compatible for 4 hr at 23 °C	2224	C
Tobramycin sulfate	LI	5 mg/mL[a]	RPR	0.9 mg/mL[a]	Physically compatible for 4 hr at 23 °C	2224	C
Trimethoprim–sulfamethoxazole	ES	0.8 + 4 mg/mL[a]	RPR	0.9 mg/mL[a]	Physically compatible for 4 hr at 23 °C	2224	C
Vancomycin HCl	LI	10 mg/mL[a]	RPR	0.9 mg/mL[a]	Physically compatible for 4 hr at 23 °C	2224	C
Zidovudine	GW	4 mg/mL[a]	RPR	0.9 mg/mL[a]	Physically compatible for 4 hr at 23 °C	2224	C

[a] Tested in dextrose 5%.
[b] Tested in sodium chloride 0.9%.
[c] Test performed using the formulation WITHOUT edetate disodium.

DOLASETRON MESYLATE
AHFS 56:22.20

Products — Dolasetron mesylate is available in 0.625-mL (12.5-mg) single-use ampuls and 5-mL (100-mg) single-use vials. Each milliliter of solution contains 20 mg of dolasetron mesylate and 38.2 mg of mannitol with acetate buffer in water for injection. (1)

Dolasetron mesylate is also available in 25-mL (500-mg) multidose vials. Each milliliter of solution contains 20 mg of dolasetron mesylate, 29 mg of mannitol, and 5 mg of phenol with acetate buffer in water for injection. (1)

pH — From 3.2 to 3.8. (1)

Trade Name(s) — Anzemet.

Administration — Dolasetron mesylate is administered intravenously undiluted up to a rate of 100 mg/30 seconds or diluted in a compatible infusion solution to a volume of 50 mL for infusion over 15 minutes. The administration line should be flushed both before and after dolasetron mesylate administration. (1)

Stability — Dolasetron mesylate injection is a clear, colorless solution. Intact containers should be stored at controlled room temperature and protected from light. (1)

Syringes — Dolasetron mesylate (Aventis) 12.5 mg/0.63 mL was packaged in 1-mL syringes sealed with tip caps. No loss of dolasetron mesylate occurred after 240 days of storage at 22 °C. (2626)

Compatibility Information

Solution Compatibility

Dolasetron mesylate

Solution	Mfr	Mfr	Conc/L	Remarks	Ref	C/I
Dextrose 5% in Ringer's injection, lactated				Stable for 24 hr at room temperature and 48 hr refrigerated	1	C
Dextrose 5% in sodium chloride 0.45%				Stable for 24 hr at room temperature and 48 hr refrigerated	1	C
Dextrose 5%				Stable for 24 hr at room temperature and 48 hr refrigerated	1	C
	HMR		10 g	Physically compatible with no loss in 31 days at 4 and 23 °C	2675	C
Ringer's injection, lactated				Stable for 24 hr at room temperature and 48 hr refrigerated	1	C
Sodium chloride 0.9%				Stable for 24 hr at room temperature and 48 hr refrigerated	1	C
	HMR		10 g	Physically compatible with no loss in 31 days at 4 and 23 °C	2675	C
			12.5 g[a]	Visually compatible and no loss in 31 days at room temperature	2736	C

[a]*Tested in polypropylene syringes.*

Y-Site Injection Compatibility (1:1 Mixture)

Dolasetron mesylate

Drug	Mfr	Conc	Mfr	Conc	Remarks	Ref	C/I
Azithromycin	PF	2 mg/mL[b]	HMR	20 mg/mL[c]	Visually compatible	2368	C
Caspofungin acetate	ME	0.5 mg/mL[b]	SAA	20 mg/mL	Physically compatible with dolasetron mesylate given i.v. push over 2 to 5 min	2766	C
Dexmedetomidine HCl	AB	4 mcg/mL[b]	HO	2 mg/mL[b]	Physically compatible for 4 hr at 23 °C	2383	C
Fenoldopam mesylate	AB	80 mcg/mL[b]	AVE	2 mg/mL[b]	Physically compatible for 4 hr at 23 °C	2467	C
Hetastarch in lactated electrolyte	AB	6%	HO	2 mg/mL[a]	Physically compatible for 4 hr at 23 °C	2339	C
Oxaliplatin	SS	0.5 mg/mL[a]	AVE	2 mg/mL[a]	Physically compatible for 4 hr at 23 °C	2566	C

[a]*Tested in dextrose 5%.*
[b]*Tested in sodium chloride 0.9%.*
[c]*Injected via Y-site into an administration set running azithromycin.*

DOPAMINE HYDROCHLORIDE
AHFS 12:12.08.08

Products — Dopamine hydrochloride is available in 200-mg (40 mg/mL), 400-mg (40 mg/mL), 400-mg (80 mg/mL), 800-mg (80 mg/mL), and 800-mg (160 mg/mL) vials and prefilled syringes. The solutions also contain sodium metabisulfite 0.9% as an antioxidant, citric acid and sodium citrate buffer, and hydrochloric acid or sodium hydroxide to adjust the pH in water for injection. (1; 4)

Dopamine hydrochloride is available premixed for infusion in concentrations of 0.8, 1.6, and 3.2 mg/mL in dextrose 5%. Also present are sodium metabisulfite 0.5 mg/mL and hydrochloric acid and/or sodium hydroxide for pH adjustment. (1)

pH — Dopamine hydrochloride injection has a pH of about 3.3 (range 2.5 to 5). The premixed dopamine hydrochloride infusions have a pH of about 3.3 to 3.8 (range 2.5 to 4.5). (1; 4)

Osmotic Values — The osmolality of dopamine hydrochloride 40 mg/mL was 619 mOsm/kg by freezing-point depression and 581 mOsm/kg by vapor pressure. (1071) At a concentration of 10 mg/mL (diluent unspecified), the osmolality was determined to be 277 mOsm/kg. (1233) The osmolarity of Hospira's premixed dopamine hydrochloride in dextrose 5% is 261, 269, and 286 mOsm/L for the 0.8-, 1.6-, and 3.2-mg/mL concentrations, respectively. (1; 4)

Administration — Dopamine hydrochloride is administered by intravenous infusion into a large vein using an infusion pump or other infusion control device. The premixed infusion solutions are suitable for administration without dilution, but the concentrated injection must be diluted for use. Often the dose of concentrate is added to 250 or 500 mL of compatible solution. The concentration used depends on the patient's requirements. Concentrations as high as 3200 mcg/mL have been used. (1; 4)

Stability — Intact containers of dopamine hydrochloride should be stored at controlled room temperature. The injections should be protected from excessive heat and from freezing. (1; 4) Do not use the injection if it is darker than slightly yellow or discolored in any other way. (1)

Dopamine hydrochloride under simulated summer conditions in paramedic vehicles was exposed to temperatures ranging from 26 to 38 °C over 4 weeks. Analysis found no loss of the drug under these conditions. (2562)

pH Effects — The pH of the solution is one of the most critical factors determining dopamine hydrochloride stability. Dopamine hydrochloride is stable over a pH range of 4 to 6.4 when mixed with other drugs in dextrose 5% (312), but it is most stable at pH 5 or below. (79) In alkaline solutions, the catechol moieties are oxidized, cyclized, and polymerized to colored materials (312), forming a pink to violet color. (78) Decomposition is also indicated by the formation of a yellow or brown discoloration of the solution. (4) Discolored solutions should not be used. (1; 4; 312)

Freezing Solutions — Dopamine hydrochloride 0.5 mg/mL in dextrose 5% in polypropylene syringes (Codan Medical and B. Braun) were frozen at –20 °C for 6 months. No visible precipitation or color change was observed. However, layering or stratification occurred in the frozen samples. Repeated inversion of the syringes was required to yield a clear and uniform solution. Less than 2% dopamine loss occurred in 6 months to samples in the Codan syringes. However, samples frozen in the Braun syringes were less stable with dopamine losses up to 14%. The Braun syringes when frozen allowed air to enter into the product, which could compromise sterility as well as stability. (2530)

Light Effects — Exposure of dopamine hydrochloride 100 mg/100 mL in dextrose 5% to fluorescent and blue phototherapy light for 36 hours at 25 °C, while static or flowing through tubing at 2 mL/hr, resulted in no significant difference in drug concentration compared to controls stored in the dark. Because no unacceptable loss occurs, protection of dopamine hydrochloride infusions from blue phototherapy lights is not necessary. (1100)

Syringes — Dopamine hydrochloride (Abbott) 200 mg/50 mL in dextrose 5% exhibited no change in appearance and no drug loss when stored in 60-mL plastic syringes (Becton Dickinson) for 24 hours at 25 °C. (1579)

Dopamine hydrochloride (Therabel Lucien Pharma) 4 mg/mL in dextrose 5% was packaged in 50-mL polypropylene syringes (Becton Dickinson) and stored at 4 and 24 °C in the dark and exposed to room light for 48 hours. Dopamine losses were less than 10% throughout the study. (1961)

Sorption — Dopamine hydrochloride has been shown not to exhibit sorption to PVC bags and tubing, polyethylene tubing, polypropylene syringes, and polypropylene-polystyrene syringes. (536; 784; 1961)

Filtration — Dopamine hydrochloride 100 mcg/mL in dextrose 5% or sodium chloride 0.9% was delivered over five hours through four kinds of 0.2-μm membrane filters varying in size and composition. Dopamine concentration losses of 3 to 5% were found during the first 60 minutes; subsequent dopamine levels returned to the original concentration when the binding sites became saturated. (1399)

Central Venous Catheter — Dopamine hydrochloride (Abbott) 3.2 mg/mL in dextrose 5% was found to be compatible with the ARROWg+ard Blue Plus (Arrow International) chlorhexidine-bearing triple-lumen central catheter. Essentially complete delivery of the drug was found with little or no drug loss occurring. Furthermore, chlorhexidine delivered from the catheter remained at trace amounts with no substantial increase due to the delivery of the drug through the catheter. (2335)

Compatibility Information

Solution Compatibility

Dopamine HCl

Solution	Mfr	Mfr	Conc/L	Remarks	Ref	C/I
Amino acids 4.25%, dextrose 25%	MG	AS	400 mg	No increase in particulate matter in 24 hr at 4 °C	349	**C**
Dextrose 5% in Ringer's injection, lactated	MG	AS	800 mg	Less than 5% loss in 48 hr at 25 °C	79	**C**
Dextrose 5% in sodium chloride 0.45%	MG	AS	800 mg	Less than 5% loss in 48 hr at 25 °C	79	**C**
Dextrose 5% in sodium chloride 0.9%	MG	AS	800 mg	Less than 5% loss in 48 hr at 25 °C	79	**C**
Dextrose 10% in sodium chloride 0.18%	TR[a]		300 mg	Visually compatible with no loss in 96 hr at room temperature under fluorescent light	1569	**C**
Dextrose 5%	MG	AS	800 mg	Less than 5% loss in 48 hr at 25 °C	79	**C**
	TR[a]	AS	800 mg	Stable for 24 hr at 25 °C	79	**C**
		AS	800 mg	Stable for 7 days at 5 °C	79	**C**
	AB	ACC	800 mg	Physically compatible. 10% loss calculated to occur after 142 hr at 25 °C	527	**C**
	BA[a]	DB	3.2 g	5% loss in 14.75 days at 5 °C protected from light	1610	**C**
	TR[a]	ES	0.4 and 3.2 g	Visually compatible with no loss in 48 hr at room temperature	1802	**C**
	BA[a]	SO	6.1 g	3% loss in 24 hr at 23 °C	2085	**C**
	FRE	NYC	500 mg	Visually compatible. Losses of 4% in 7 days at room temperature and 2% in 3 months refrigerated	2530	**C**
Dextrose 10%	TR[a]		300 mg	Visually compatible with no loss in 96 hr at room temperature under fluorescent light	1569	**C**
Ringer's injection, lactated	MG	AS	800 mg	Less than 5% loss in 48 hr at 25 °C	79	**C**
Sodium chloride 0.9%	MG	AS	800 mg	Less than 5% loss in 48 hr at 25 °C	79	**C**
	TR[a]	ES	0.4 and 3.2 g	Visually compatible. 5% loss in 48 hr at room temperature	1802	**C**
Sodium lactate ⅙ M	MG	AS	800 mg	Less than 5% loss in 48 hr at 25 °C	79	**C**

[a]Tested in PVC containers.

Additive Compatibility

Dopamine HCl

Drug	Mfr	Conc/L	Mfr	Conc/L	Test Soln	Remarks	Ref	C/I
Acyclovir sodium	BW	2.5 g	SO	0.8 g	D5W	Yellow color developed in 1.5 hr due to dopamine oxidation. No acyclovir loss	1343	**I**
Alteplase	GEN	0.5 g	ACC	5 g	D5W, NS	About 30% alteplase clot-lysis activity loss in 24 hr at 25 °C	1856	**I**
Aminophylline	SE	500 mg	ACC	800 mg	D5W	Physically compatible. At 25 °C, 10% dopamine decomposition occurs in 111 hr	527	**C**
Amphotericin B	SQ	200 mg	AS	800 mg	D5W	Precipitates immediately	78	**I**
Ampicillin sodium	BR	4 g	AS	800 mg	D5W	Color change. 36% ampicillin loss in 6 hr at 23 to 25 °C. Dopamine loss in 6 hr	78	**I**
Atracurium besylate	BW	500 mg		1.6 g	D5W	Physically compatible and atracurium stable for 24 hr at 5 and 30 °C	1694	**C**
Calcium chloride	UP		AS	800 mg	D5W	No dopamine loss in 24 hr at 25 °C	312	**C**

Additive Compatibility (Cont.)

Dopamine HCl

Drug	Mfr	Conc/L	Mfr	Conc/L	Test Soln	Remarks	Ref	C/I
Chloramphenicol sodium succinate	PD	4 g	AS	800 mg	D5W	Both drugs stable for 24 hr at 25 °C	78	C
Ciprofloxacin	MI	2 g		400 mg	NS	Compatible for 24 hr at 25 °C	888	C
	MI	2 g		1.04 g	NS	Compatible for 24 hr at 25 °C	888	C
Dobutamine HCl	LI	172 mg	AS	5.5 g	NS	Physically compatible for 24 hr	552	C
	LI	1 g	ACC	1.6 g	D5W, NS	Physically compatible with no color change in 24 hr at 25 °C	789	C
	LI	1 g	ES	800 mg	D5W, NS	Physically compatible for 24 hr at 21 °C	812	C
Enalaprilat	MSD	12 mg	AMR	1.6 g	D5W[b]	Visually compatible. 5% enalaprilat loss in 24 hr at room temperature under fluorescent light. Dopamine not tested	1572	C
Flumazenil	RC	20 mg	AB	3.2 g	D5W[b]	Visually compatible. 7% flumazenil loss in 24 hr at 23 °C in fluorescent light. Dopamine not tested	1710	C
Gentamicin sulfate	SC	2 g	AS	800 mg	D5W	No dopamine and 7% gentamicin loss in 24 hr at 25 °C	312	C
	SC	320 mg	AS	800 mg	D5W	Gentamicin stable through 6 hr. 80% gentamicin loss in 24 hr at 25 °C. Dopamine stable for 24 hr	78	I
Heparin sodium	AB	200,000 units	AS	800 mg	D5W	No dopamine or heparin loss in 24 hr at 25 °C	312	C
Hydrocortisone sodium succinate	UP	1 g	AS	800 mg	D5W	No dopamine loss in 18 hr at 25 °C	312	C
Lidocaine HCl	AST	4 g	AS	800 mg	D5W[b]	No dopamine or lidocaine loss in 24 hr at 25 °C	312	C
	AST	2 g	ACC	800 mg	D5W, LR, NS	Physically compatible for 24 hr at 25 °C	775	C
Mannitol	MG	20%	AS	800 mg		Under 5% dopamine loss in 48 hr at 25 °C	79	C
Meropenem	ZEN	1 and 20 g	DU	800 mg	NS	Visually compatible for 4 hr at room temperature	1994	C
Methylprednisolone sodium succinate	UP	500 mg	AS	800 mg	D5W	No dopamine loss in 18 hr at 25 °C	312	C
	UP	500 mg	AS	800 mg	D5W	Clear solution for 24 hr	329	C
Nitroglycerin	ACC	400 mg	ACC	800 mg	D5W, NS[c]	Physically compatible with little or no nitroglycerin loss in 48 hr at 23 °C. Dopamine not tested	929	C
Oxacillin sodium	BR	2 g	AS	800 mg	D5W	No dopamine and 2% oxacillin loss in 24 hr at 25 °C	312	C
Penicillin G potassium	LI	20 million units	AS	800 mg	D5W	14% penicillin loss in 24 hr at 25 °C. Dopamine stable for 24 hr	78	I
Potassium chloride	MG		AS	800 mg	D5W	No dopamine loss in 24 hr at 25 °C	312	C
Ranitidine HCl	GL	50 mg and 2 g	ES	400 mg and 3.2 g	D5W, NS[b]	Physically compatible. 6% ranitidine loss in 48 hr at room temperature in light. Dopamine not tested	1361	C
	GL	50 mg and 2 g	ES	0.4 and 3.2 g	D5W, NS[a]	Visually compatible. No dopamine and 7% ranitidine loss in 48 hr at room temperature	1802	C

Additive Compatibility (Cont.)

Dopamine HCl

Drug	Mfr	Conc/L	Mfr	Conc/L	Test Soln	Remarks	Ref	C/I
Sodium bicarbonate	MG	5%	AS	800 mg		Color change 5 min after mixing	79	I
Verapamil HCl	KN	80 mg	ES	400 mg	D5W, NS	Physically compatible for 24 hr	764	C

[a]Tested in both glass and PVC containers.
[b]Tested in PVC containers.
[c]Tested in glass containers.

Drugs in Syringe Compatibility

Dopamine HCl

Drug (in syringe)	Mfr	Amt	Mfr	Amt	Remarks	Ref	C/I
Caffeine citrate		20 mg/ 1 mL	SO	80 mg/ 1 mL	Visually compatible for 4 hr at 25 °C	2440	C
Doxapram HCl	RB	400 mg/ 20 mL		100 mg/ 5 mL	Physically compatible with 3% doxapram loss in 24 hr	1177	C
Heparin sodium		2500 units/ 1 mL		50 mg/ 5 mL	Physically compatible for at least 5 min	1053	C
Pantoprazole sodium	[a]	4 mg/ 1 mL		40 mg/ 1 mL	Whitish precipitate forms within 1 hr	2574	I
Ranitidine HCl	GL	50 mg/ 5 mL		40 mg	Physically compatible for 4 hr at ambient temperature under fluorescent light	1151	C

[a]Test performed using the formulation WITHOUT edetate disodium.

Y-Site Injection Compatibility (1:1 Mixture)

Dopamine HCl

Drug	Mfr	Conc	Mfr	Conc	Remarks	Ref	C/I
Acyclovir sodium	BW	5 mg/mL[a]	AB	1.6 mg/mL[a]	Solution turns dark brown in 2 hr at 25 °C	1157	I
Aldesleukin	CHI	33,800 I.U./ mL[a]	ES	1.6 mg/mL[a]	Visually compatible with little or no loss of aldesleukin activity	1857	C
	CHI[i]	[a]			Unacceptable loss of aldesleukin activity	1890	I
Alprostadil	BED	7.5 mcg/mL[t,u]	AB	3 mg/mL[s]	Visually compatible for 1 hr	2746	C
Alteplase	GEN	1 mg/mL	DU	8 mg/mL[a]	Haze noted in 4 hr	1340	I
Amifostine	USB	10 mg/mL[a]	AST	3.2 mg/mL[a]	Physically compatible for 4 hr at 23 °C	1845	C
Amiodarone HCl	LZ	4 mg/mL[c]	ES	1.6 mg/mL[c]	Physically compatible for 24 hr at 21 °C	1032	C
Amphotericin B cholesteryl sulfate complex	SEQ	0.83 mg/mL[a]	AB	3.2 mg/mL[a]	Gross precipitate forms	2117	I
Anidulafungin	VIC	0.5 mg/mL[a]	AMR	3.2 mg/mL[a]	Physically compatible for 4 hr at 23 °C	2617	C
Argatroban	GSK	1 mg/mL[b]	AMR	80 mg/mL	Visually compatible for 24 hr at 23 °C	2391	C
Atracurium besylate	BW	0.5 mg/mL[a]	SO	1.6 mg/mL[a]	Physically compatible for 24 hr at 28 °C	1337	C
Aztreonam	SQ	40 mg/mL[a]	AST	3.2 mg/mL[a]	Physically compatible for 4 hr at 23 °C	1758	C
Bivalirudin	TMC	5 mg/mL[a]	AB	3.2 mg/mL[a]	Physically compatible for 4 hr at 23 °C	2373	C
	TMC	5 mg/mL[a,b]	AMR	80 mg/mL	Visually compatible for 6 hr at 23 °C	2680	C

Y-Site Injection Compatibility (1:1 Mixture) (Cont.)

Dopamine HCl

Drug	Mfr	Conc	Mfr	Conc	Remarks	Ref	C/I
Caffeine citrate		20 mg/mL		0.6 mg/mL[a]	Compatible and stable for 24 hr at room temperature	1	C
Caspofungin acetate	ME	0.7 mg/mL[b]	AMR	3.2 mg/mL[b]	Physically compatible for 4 hr at room temperature	2758	C
	ME	0.5 mg/mL[b]	BA	3.2 mg/mL[r]	Physically compatible over 60 min	2766	C
Cefepime HCl	BMS	120 mg/mL[d]		0.4 mg/mL	Physically compatible with less than 10% cefepime loss. Dopamine not tested	2513	C
Ceftaroline fosamil	FOR	2.22 mg/mL[a,b,n]	HOS	3.2 mg/mL[a,b,n]	Physically compatible for 4 hr at 23 °C	2826	C
Ceftazidime	GSK	120 mg/mL[d]		0.4 mg/mL	Physically compatible with less than 10% ceftazidime loss. Dopamine not tested	2513	C
Ciprofloxacin	MI	2 mg/mL[c]	AB	1.6 mg/mL[c]	Visually compatible for 24 hr at 24 °C	1655	C
Cisatracurium besylate	GW	0.1, 2, 5 mg/mL[a]	AB	3.2 mg/mL[a]	Physically compatible for 4 hr at 23 °C	2074	C
Cladribine	ORT	0.015[b] and 0.5[f] mg/mL	AST	3.2 mg/mL[b]	Physically compatible for 4 hr at 23 °C	1969	C
Clarithromycin	AB	4 mg/mL[a]	DB	3.2 mg/mL[a]	Visually compatible for 72 hr at both 30 and 17 °C	2174	C
Clonidine HCl	BI	18 mcg/mL[b]	NYC	2 mg/mL[a]	Visually compatible	2642	C
Daptomycin	CUB	18.2 mg/mL[b,o]	AMR	3.6 mg/mL[o]	Physically compatible with no loss of either drug in 2 hr at 25 °C	2553	C
Dexmedetomidine HCl	AB	4 mcg/mL[b]	AB	3.2 mg/mL[b]	Physically compatible for 4 hr at 23 °C	2383	C
Diltiazem HCl	MMD	1 mg/mL[a]	AB	1.6 mg/mL[a]	Visually compatible for 24 hr at 25 °C	1530	C
	MMD	5 mg/mL	AB, SO	0.8 mg/mL[c]	Visually compatible	1807	C
	MMD	1 mg/mL[a]	AB	3.2 mg/mL[a]	Visually compatible for 4 hr at 27 °C	2062	C
Dobutamine HCl	LI	4 mg/mL[b]	DCC	3.2 mg/mL[c]	Physically compatible for 3 hr	1316	C
	LI	4 mg/mL[a]	AB	3.2 mg/mL[a]	Visually compatible for 4 hr at 27 °C	2062	C
Dobutamine HCl with lidocaine HCl	LI AB	4 mg/mL[c] 8 mg/mL[c]	DCC	3.2 mg/mL[c]	Physically compatible for 3 hr	1316	C
Dobutamine HCl with nitroglycerin	LI LY	4 mg/mL[c] 0.4 mg/mL[c]	DCC	3.2 mg/mL[c]	Physically compatible for 3 hr	1316	C
Dobutamine HCl with sodium nitroprusside	LI ES	4 mg/mL[c] 0.4 mg/mL[c]	DCC	3.2 mg/mL[c]	Physically compatible for 3 hr	1316	C
Docetaxel	RPR	0.9 mg/mL[a]	AB	3.2 mg/mL[a]	Physically compatible for 4 hr at 23 °C	2224	C
Doripenem	JJ	5 mg/mL[a,b]	AMR	3.2 mg/mL[a,b]	Physically compatible for 4 hr at 23 °C	2743	C
Doxorubicin HCl liposomal	SEQ	0.4 mg/mL[a]	AB	3.2 mg/mL[a]	Physically compatible for 4 hr at 23 °C	2087	C
Enalaprilat	MSD	0.05 mg/mL[b]	IMS	1.6 mg/mL[a]	Physically compatible for 24 hr at room temperature under fluorescent light	1355	C
Epinephrine HCl	AB	0.02 mg/mL[a]	AB	3.2 mg/mL[a]	Visually compatible for 4 hr at 27 °C	2062	C
Esmolol HCl	DCC	10 mg/mL[a]	IMS	1.6 mg/mL[a]	Physically compatible for 24 hr at 22 °C	1169	C
Etoposide phosphate	BR	5 mg/mL[a]	AST	3.2 mg/mL[a]	Physically compatible for 4 hr at 23 °C	2218	C
Famotidine	MSD	0.2 mg/mL[a]	TR	1.6 mg/mL[a]	Physically compatible for 4 hr at 25 °C	1188	C
	ME	2 mg/mL[b]		1.6 mg/mL[a]	Visually compatible for 4 hr at 22 °C	1936	C

Y-Site Injection Compatibility (1:1 Mixture) (Cont.)

Dopamine HCl

Drug	Mfr	Conc	Mfr	Conc	Remarks	Ref	C/I
Fenoldopam mesylate	AB	80 mcg/mL[b]	AB	3.2 mg/mL[b]	Physically compatible for 4 hr at 23 °C	2467	C
Fentanyl citrate	ES	0.05 mg/mL	AB	3.2 mg/mL[a]	Visually compatible for 4 hr at 27 °C	2062	C
Fluconazole	RR	2 mg/mL	AMR	1.6 mg/mL[a]	Visually compatible for 24 hr at 28 °C under fluorescent light	1760	C
Foscarnet sodium	AST	24 mg/mL	DU	80 mg/mL	Physically compatible for 24 hr at room temperature under fluorescent light	1335	C
Furosemide	AB, AMR	5 mg/mL	AST, DU	12.8 mg/mL	Physically compatible for 3 hr at room temperature	1978	C
	AB, AMR	5 mg/mL	AB, AMR	12.8 mg/mL	White precipitate forms immediately	1978	I
	AMR	10 mg/mL	AB	3.2 mg/mL[a]	Precipitate forms in 4 hr at 27 °C	2062	I
Gemcitabine HCl	LI	10 mg/mL[b]	AB	3.2 mg/mL[b]	Physically compatible for 4 hr at 23 °C	2226	C
Granisetron HCl	SKB	0.05 mg/mL[a]	AB	3.2 mg/mL[a]	Physically compatible for 4 hr at 23 °C	2000	C
Haloperidol lactate	MN	0.5[a] and 5 mg/mL	DU	1.6 mg/mL[a]	Visually compatible for 24 hr at 21 °C	1523	C
Heparin sodium	UP	1000 units/L[g]	ACC	40 mg/mL	Physically compatible for 4 hr at room temperature	534	C
	ES	100 units/mL[a]	AB	3.2 mg/mL[a]	Visually compatible for 4 hr at 27 °C	2062	C
	TR	50 units/mL	BA	1.6 mg/mL	Visually compatible for 4 hr at 25 °C	1793	C
Hetastarch in lactated electrolyte	AB	6%	AB	3.2 mg/mL[a]	Physically compatible for 4 hr at 23 °C	2339	C
Hydrocortisone sodium succinate	UP	10 mg/L[g]	ACC	40 mg/mL	Physically compatible for 4 hr at room temperature	534	C
Hydromorphone HCl	KN	1 mg/mL	AB	3.2 mg/mL[a]	Visually compatible for 4 hr at 27 °C	2062	C
Hydroxyethyl starch 130/0.4 in sodium chloride 0.9%	FRK	6%	BMS	0.8, 3.2, 6.4 mg/mL[a]	Visually compatible for 24 hr at room temperature	2770	C
Indomethacin sodium trihydrate	MSD	1 mg/mL[b]	AB	1.2 mg/mL[a]	Hazy precipitate forms immediately	1527	I
Insulin, regular	LI	1 unit/mL[a]	DU	3.2 mg/mL[a]	White precipitate forms immediately, dissolves quickly, and reforms in 24 hr at 23 °C	1877	I
Labetalol HCl	SC	1 mg/mL[a]	IMS	1.6 mg/mL[a]	Physically compatible for 24 hr at 18 °C	1171	C
	GL	1 mg/mL[a]	ES	1.6 mg/mL[a]	Visually compatible. Little loss of either drug in 4 hr at room temperature	1762	C
	AH	2 mg/mL[a]	AB	3.2 mg/mL[a]	Visually compatible for 4 hr at 27 °C	2062	C
Levofloxacin	OMN	5 mg/mL[a]	AMR	80 mg/mL	Visually compatible for 4 hr at 24 °C	2233	C
Lidocaine HCl	AB	8 mg/mL[c]	DCC	3.2 mg/mL[c]	Physically compatible for 3 hr	1316	C
Lidocaine HCl with dobutamine HCl	AB LI	8 mg/mL[c] 4 mg/mL[c]	DCC	3.2 mg/mL[c]	Physically compatible for 3 hr	1316	C
Lidocaine HCl with nitroglycerin	AB LY	8 mg/mL[c] 0.4 mg/mL[c]	DCC	3.2 mg/mL[c]	Physically compatible for 3 hr	1316	C
Lidocaine HCl with sodium nitroprusside	AB ES	8 mg/mL[c] 0.4 mg/mL[c]	DCC	3.2 mg/mL[c]	Physically compatible for 3 hr	1316	C
Linezolid	PHU	2 mg/mL	AB	3.2 mg/mL[a]	Physically compatible for 4 hr at 23 °C	2264	C
Lorazepam	WY	0.5 mg/mL[a]	AB	3.2 mg/mL[a]	Visually compatible for 4 hr at 27 °C	2062	C

Y-Site Injection Compatibility (1:1 Mixture) (Cont.)

Dopamine HCl

Drug	Mfr	Conc	Mfr	Conc	Remarks	Ref	C/I
Meperidine HCl	AB	10 mg/mL	AB	1.6 mg/mL[a]	Physically compatible for 4 hr at 25 °C	1397	C
Methylprednisolone sodium succinate	UP	5 mg/mL[a]	AB	0.8 mg/mL[a]	Visually compatible for 24 hr at room temperature in test tubes. No precipitate found on filter from Y-site delivery	2063	C
Metronidazole	MG	5 mg/mL	AB	0.8 mg/mL[a]	Visually compatible for 24 hr at room temperature in test tubes. No precipitate found on filter from Y-site delivery	2063	C
Micafungin sodium	ASP	1.5 mg/mL[b]	AMR	3.2 mg/mL[b]	Physically compatible for 4 hr at 23 °C	2683	C
Midazolam HCl	RC	1 mg/mL[a]	AB	1.6 mg/mL[a]	Visually compatible for 24 hr at 23 °C	1847	C
	RC	1 mg/mL[a]	DU	3.2 mg/mL[a]	Visually compatible for 24 hr at 23 °C	1877	C
	RC	2 mg/mL[a]	AB	3.2 mg/mL[a]	Visually compatible for 4 hr at 27 °C	2062	C
Milrinone lactate	SW	0.2 mg/mL[a]	AB	3.2 mg/mL[a]	Visually compatible for 4 hr at 27 °C	2062	C
	SW	0.4 mg/mL[a]	SO	6.4 mg/mL[a]	Visually compatible. Little loss of either drug in 4 hr at 23 °C	2214	C
Morphine sulfate	AB	1 mg/mL	AB	1.6 mg/mL[a]	Physically compatible for 4 hr at 25 °C	1397	C
	SCN	2 mg/mL[a]	AB	3.2 mg/mL[a]	Visually compatible for 4 hr at 27 °C	2062	C
Mycophenolate mofetil HCl	RC	5.9 mg/mL[a]	AMR	4 mg/mL[a]	Physically compatible and 4% mycophenolate mofetil loss in 4 hr	2738	C
Nesiritide	SCI	50 mcg/mL[a,b]		80 mg/mL	Physically compatible for 4 hr. May be chemically incompatible with nesiritide[p]	2625	?
Nicardipine HCl	WY	1 mg/mL[a]	AB	3.2 mg/mL[a]	Visually compatible for 4 hr at 27 °C	2062	C
	DCC	0.1 mg/mL[a]	IMS	1.6 mg/mL[a]	Visually compatible for 24 hr at room temperature	235	C
Nitroglycerin	LY	0.4 mg/mL[c]	DCC	3.2 mg/mL[c]	Physically compatible for 3 hr	1316	C
	AB	0.4 mg/mL[a]	AB	3.2 mg/mL[a]	Visually compatible for 4 hr at 27 °C	2062	C
Nitroglycerin with dobutamine HCl	LY LI	0.4 mg/mL[c] 4 mg/mL[c]	DCC	3.2 mg/mL[c]	Physically compatible for 3 hr	1316	C
Nitroglycerin with lidocaine HCl	LY AB	0.4 mg/mL[c] 8 mg/mL[c]	DCC	3.2 mg/mL[c]	Physically compatible for 3 hr	1316	C
Nitroglycerin with sodium nitroprusside	LY ES	0.4 mg/mL[c] 0.4 mg/mL[c]	DCC	3.2 mg/mL[c]	Physically compatible for 3 hr	1316	C
Norepinephrine bitartrate	STR	0.064 mg/mL[a]	DU	3.2 mg/mL[a]	Visually compatible for 24 hr at 23 °C	1877	C
	AB	0.128 mg/mL[a]	AB	3.2 mg/mL[a]	Visually compatible for 4 hr at 27 °C	2062	C
Ondansetron HCl	GL	0.32 mg/mL[b]	AB	0.8 mg/mL[a]	Visually compatible for 24 hr at room temperature in test tubes. No precipitate found on filter from Y-site delivery	2063	C
Oxaliplatin	SS	0.5 mg/mL[a]	AB	3.2 mg/mL[a]	Physically compatible for 4 hr at 23 °C	2566	C
Pancuronium bromide	ES	0.05 mg/mL[a]	SO	1.6 mg/mL[a]	Physically compatible for 24 hr at 28 °C	1337	C
Pantoprazole sodium	ALT[q]	0.16 to 0.8 mg/mL[b]	DU	0.8 to 3.2 mg/mL[a]	Visually compatible for 12 hr at 23 °C	2603	C
Pemetrexed disodium	LI	20 mg/mL[b]	AB	3.2 mg/mL[a]	Physically compatible for 4 hr at 23 °C	2564	C

Y-Site Injection Compatibility (1:1 Mixture) (Cont.)

Dopamine HCl

Drug	Mfr	Conc	Mfr	Conc	Remarks	Ref	C/I
Piperacillin sodium–tazobactam sodium	LE[q]	40 + 5 mg/mL[a]	AST	3.2 mg/mL[a]	Physically compatible for 4 hr at 22 °C	1688	C
Potassium chloride	AB	40 mEq/L[g]	ACC	40 mg/mL	Physically compatible for 4 hr at room temperature	534	C
Propofol	ZEN	10 mg/mL	AST	3.2 mg/mL[a]	Physically compatible for 1 hr at 23 °C	2066	C
Ranitidine HCl	GL	0.5 mg/mL[h]	ES	1.6 mg/mL[a]	Physically compatible for 24 hr	1323	C
	GL	1 mg/mL[a]	AB	3.2 mg/mL[a]	Visually compatible for 4 hr at 27 °C	2062	C
Remifentanil HCl	GW	0.025 and 0.25 mg/mL[b]	AB	3.2 mg/mL[a]	Physically compatible for 4 hr at 23 °C	2075	C
Sargramostim	IMM	6[b,i] and 15[b] mcg/mL	DU	1.6 mg/mL[c]	Visually compatible for 2 hr	1618	C
Sodium nitroprusside	ES	0.4 mg/mL[c]	DCC	3.2 mg/mL[c]	Physically compatible for 3 hr	1316	C
	RC	0.3, 1.2, 3 mg/mL[a]	DU	1.5, 6, 15 mg/mL[m]	Visually compatible for 48 hr at 24 °C protected from light	2357	C
Sodium nitroprusside with dobutamine HCl	ES LI	0.4 mg/mL[c] 4 mg/mL[c]	DCC	3.2 mg/mL[c]	Physically compatible for 3 hr	1316	C
Sodium nitroprusside with lidocaine HCl	ES AB	0.4 mg/mL[c] 8 mg/mL[c]	DCC	3.2 mg/mL[c]	Physically compatible for 3 hr	1316	C
Sodium nitroprusside with nitroglycerin	ES LY	0.4 mg/mL[c] 0.4 mg/mL[c]	DCC	3.2 mg/mL[c]	Physically compatible for 3 hr	1316	C
Tacrolimus	FUJ	1 mg/mL[b]	ES	1.6 mg/mL[a]	Visually compatible for 24 hr at 25 °C	1630	C
Telavancin HCl	ASP	7.5 mg/mL[a,b,n]	HOS	3.2 mg/mL[a,b,n]	Physically compatible for 2 hr	2830	C
Theophylline	TR	4 mg/mL	BA	1.6 mg/mL	Visually compatible for 6 hr at 25 °C	1793	C
Thiotepa	IMM[j]	1 mg/mL[a]	AST	3.2 mg/mL[a]	Physically compatible for 4 hr at 23 °C	1861	C
Tigecycline	WY	1 mg/mL[b]		1.6 mg/mL[b]	Physically compatible for 4 hr	2714	C
Tirofiban HCl	ME	0.05 mg/mL[a,b]	AMR	0.2 and 3.2 mg/mL[a,b]	Physically compatible. Little loss of either drug in 4 hr at room temperature	2250	C
TNA #73[k]			AB	1.6 mg/mL[c]	Visually compatible for 4 hr	1009	C
TNA #222, #223[k]			AB	3.2 mg/mL[a]	Precipitate forms immediately	2215	I
TNA #218 to #221, #224 to #226[k]			AB	3.2 mg/mL[a]	Visually compatible for 4 hr at 23 °C	2215	C
TPN #189[k]			DB	1.6 mg/mL[b]	Visually compatible for 24 hr at 22 °C	1767	C
TPN #203, #204[k]			AMR	3.2 mg/mL	Visually compatible for 4 hr at 23 °C	1974	C
TPN #212 to #215[k]			AB	3.2 mg/mL[a]	Physically compatible for 4 hr at 23 °C	2109	C
Vasopressin	AMR	2 and 4 units/mL[b]	AMR	4.2 mg/mL[a]	Physically compatible with vasopressin pushed through a Y-site over 5 sec	2478	C
	APP	0.2 unit/mL[b]	BA	3.2 mg/mL[a]	Physically compatible	2641	C
Vecuronium bromide	OR	0.1 mg/mL[a]	SO	1.6 mg/mL[a]	Physically compatible for 24 hr at 28 °C	1337	C
	OR	1 mg/mL	AB	3.2 mg/mL[a]	Visually compatible for 4 hr at 27 °C	2062	C
Verapamil HCl			[l]		Physically compatible	840	C

Y-Site Injection Compatibility (1:1 Mixture) (Cont.)

Dopamine HCl

Drug	Mfr	Conc	Mfr	Conc	Remarks	Ref	C/I
Warfarin sodium	DU	2 mg/mL[d]	FAU	1.6 mg/mL[a]	Visually compatible with no warfarin loss in 30 min	2010	C
	DME	2 mg/mL[d]	DU	1.6 mg/mL[a]	Visually compatible for 24 hr at 24 °C	2078	C
Zidovudine	BW	4 mg/mL[a]	AB	1.6 mg/mL[a]	Physically compatible for 4 hr at 25 °C	1193	C

[a]*Tested in dextrose 5%.*
[b]*Tested in sodium chloride 0.9%.*
[c]*Tested in both dextrose 5% and sodium chloride 0.9%.*
[d]*Tested in sterile water for injection.*
[e]*Tested in dextrose 5%, Ringer's injection, lactated, sodium chloride 0.45%, and sodium chloride 0.9%.*
[f]*Tested in bacteriostatic sodium chloride 0.9% preserved with benzyl alcohol 0.9%.*
[g]*Tested in dextrose 5% in Ringer's injection, dextrose 5% in Ringer's injection, lactated, dextrose 5%, Ringer's injection, lactated, and sodium chloride 0.9%.*
[h]*Tested in premixed infusion solution.*
[i]*Tested with albumin human 0.1%.*
[j]*Lyophilized formulation tested.*
[k]*Refer to Appendix I for the composition of parenteral nutrition solutions. TNA indicates a 3-in-1 admixture, and TPN indicates a 2-in-1 admixture.*
[l]*Injected into a line being used to infuse dopamine hydrochloride in dextrose 5% in sodium chloride 0.3% with potassium chloride 20 mEq.*
[m]*Tested in dextrose 5% in sodium chloride 0.45%.*
[n]*Tested in Ringer's injection, lactated.*
[o]*Final concentration after mixing.*
[p]*Nesiritide is incompatible with bisulfite antioxidants used in some drug formulations. The specific formulation of the product to be used should be checked to assure that no sulfite antioxidants are present.*
[q]*Test performed using the formulation WITHOUT edetate disodium.*
[r]*Tested as the premixed infusion solution.*
[s]*Tested in either dextrose 5% or in sodium chloride 0.9%, but the report did not specify which solution.*
[t]*Tested in a 1:1 mixture of (1) dextrose 5% and dextrose 5% in sodium chloride 0.45% with and without potassium chloride 20 mEq/L and also in (2) dextrose 10% in sodium chloride 0.45% with and without potassium chloride 20 mEq/L.*
[u]*Tested in a 1:1 mixture of dextrose 5% and TPN #274 (see Appendix I).*

DORIPENEM
AHFS 8:12.07.08

Products — Doripenem is available in vials containing doripenem 500 mg on the anhydrous basis. Reconstitute each vial with 10 mL of sterile water for injection or sodium chloride 0.9% and gently shake to form a 50-mg/mL suspension. This suspension is ***not*** suitable for administration. (1)

For a 500-mg dose, the suspension should be withdrawn from the vial using a syringe with a 21-gauge needle and added to a 100-mL bag of dextrose 5% or sodium chloride 0.9%. The bag should be gently shaken until the solution is clear, forming a doripenem 4.5-mg/mL solution suitable for intravenous infusion. (1)

For a 250-mg dose, the suspension should be withdrawn from the vial using a syringe with a 21-gauge needle and added to a 100-mL bag of dextrose 5% or sodium chloride 0.9%. The bag should be gently shaken until the solution is clear, forming a doripenem 4.5-mg/mL solution suitable for intravenous infusion. Remove 55 mL of this solution and discard. The remaining solution delivers 250 mg of doripenem. (1)

Trade Name(s) — Doribax.

Administration — Doripenem is administered by intravenous administration over one hour as a 4.5-mg/mL solution in dextrose 5% or sodium chloride 0.9%. (1)

Stability — Intact vials of doripenem should be stored at controlled room temperature. After initial reconstitution, the suspension may be stored for up to one hour prior to adding to the intravenous solution. After addition to dextrose 5% or sodium chloride 0.9%, the solution may be colorless to slightly yellow; slight variations in color within this range are not indications of differences in drug stability. The manufacturer states that doripenem is stable for four hours in dextrose 5% and eight hours in sodium chloride 0.9%. If stored under refrigeration, doripenem is stated to be stable for 24 hours. These time frames include both storage and administration. (1)

Freezing Solutions — The manufacturer states that the initial reconstituted doripenem suspension and also dilutions in infusion solutions should not be frozen. (1)

Doripenem 5 and 10 mg/mL in sodium chloride 0.9% was frozen at −20 °C. Upon thawing a visible white precipitate was found. Vigorous shaking for three to 12 minutes resulted in the precipitate no longer being visible. Not more than 5% doripenem loss occurred upon 14 days of frozen storage followed by 24 hours of thawing under refrigeration and then two hours at room temperature; a similar amount of loss occurred upon 28 days of frozen storage followed by 4 to 6 hours of thawing at room temperature. (2809)

Compatibility Information

Solution Compatibility

Doripenem

Solution	Mfr	Mfr	Conc/L	Remarks	Ref	C/I
Dextrose 5%		JJ	5 g	Physically compatible and less than 5% loss in 4 hr at 25 °C and 48 hr at 4 °C	2757	C
	a,b	OMN	1 and 10 g	Visually compatible. Up to 3.6% loss in 8 hr at 25 °C under fluorescent light and 48 hr at 4 °C	2801	C
	a	OMN	5 and 10 g	Visually compatible. 8 to 10% loss in 18 hr at 23 °C in dark	2808	C
	c	OMN	5 and 10 g	Visually compatible. 6 to 8% loss in 18 hr and 10 to 12% loss in 24 hr at 23 °C in dark	2808	C
	a,c	OMN	5 g	Visually compatible. Up to 10% loss in 16 hours at 25 °C and 10 days at 4 °C	2809	C
	a,c	OMN	10 g	Visually compatible. Up to 10% loss in 16 hours at 25 °C and 7 days at 4 °C	2809	C
Sodium chloride 0.9%		JJ	5 g	Physically compatible and less than 8% loss in 12 hr at 25 °C and 72 hr at 4 °C	2757	C
	a,b	OMN	1 and 10 g	Visually compatible. Up to 6.8% loss in 12 hr at 25 °C under fluorescent light and 72 hr at 4 °C	2801	C
	a,c	OMN	5 and 10 g	Visually compatible. 8 to 10% loss in 24 hr at 23 °C in dark	2809	C
	a,c	OMN	5 g	Visually compatible. Up to 10% loss in 24 hours at 25 °C and 10 days at 4 °C	2809	C
	a,c	OMN	10 g	Visually compatible. Up to 10% loss in 24 hours at 25 °C and 7 days at 4 °C	2809	C

[a] Tested in PVC bags.
[b] Tested in polyethylene bags.
[c] Tested in Eclipse elastomeric containers.

Y-Site Injection Compatibility (1:1 Mixture)

Doripenem

Drug	Mfr	Conc	Mfr	Conc	Remarks	Ref	C/I
Acyclovir sodium	BED	7 mg/mL[a,b]	JJ	5 mg/mL[a,b]	Physically compatible for 4 hr at 23 °C	2743	C
Amikacin sulfate	BED	5 mg/mL[a,b]	JJ	5 mg/mL[a,b]	Physically compatible for 4 hr at 23 °C	2743	C
Aminophylline	AMR	2.5 mg/mL[a,b]	JJ	5 mg/mL[a,b]	Physically compatible for 4 hr at 23 °C	2743	C
Amiodarone HCl	BED	4 mg/mL[a,b]	JJ	5 mg/mL[a,b]	Physically compatible for 4 hr at 23 °C	2743	C
Amphotericin B	XGN	0.6 mg/mL[a]	JJ	5 mg/mL[a]	Physically compatible for 4 hr at 23 °C	2743	C
	XGN	0.6 mg/mL[a]	JJ	5 mg/mL[b]	Yellow precipitate forms immediately	2743	I
Amphotericin B cholesteryl sulfate complex	INT	0.83 mg/mL[a]	JJ	5 mg/mL[a]	Physically compatible for 4 hr at 23 °C	2743	C
	INT	0.83 mg/mL[a]	JJ	5 mg/mL[b]	Microprecipitate forms	2743	I
Amphotericin B lipid complex	ENZ	1 mg/mL[a]	JJ	5 mg/mL[a]	Physically compatible for 4 hr at 23 °C	2743	C
	ENZ	1 mg/mL[a]	JJ	5 mg/mL[b]	Measured haze increases immediately	2743	I
Amphotericin B liposomal	ASP	1 mg/mL[a]	JJ	5 mg/mL[a]	Physically compatible for 4 hr at 23 °C	2743	C
	ASP	1 mg/mL[a]	JJ	5 mg/mL[b]	Measured haze increases immediately	2743	I
Anidulafungin	PF	0.5 mg/mL[a,b]	JJ	5 mg/mL[a,b]	Physically compatible for 4 hr at 23 °C	2743	C
Atropine sulfate	BA	0.4 mg/mL	JJ	5 mg/mL[a,b]	Physically compatible for 4 hr at 23 °C	2743	C
Azithromycin	BA	2 mg/mL[a,b]	JJ	5 mg/mL[a,b]	Physically compatible for 4 hr at 23 °C	2743	C

Y-Site Injection Compatibility (1:1 Mixture) (Cont.)

Doripenem

Drug	Mfr	Conc	Mfr	Conc	Remarks	Ref	C/I
Bumetanide	BED	0.04 mg/mL[a,b]	JJ	5 mg/mL[a,b]	Physically compatible for 4 hr at 23 °C	2743	C
Calcium gluconate	AMR	40 mg/mL[a,b]	JJ	5 mg/mL[a,b]	Physically compatible for 4 hr at 23 °C	2743	C
Carboplatin	SIC	5 mg/mL[a,b]	JJ	5 mg/mL[a,b]	Physically compatible for 4 hr at 23 °C	2743	C
Caspofungin acetate	ME	0.5 mg/mL[b]	JJ	5 mg/mL[a,b]	Physically compatible for 4 hr at 23 °C	2743	C
Ceftaroline fosamil	FOR	2.22 mg/mL[a,b,d]	SHI	5 mg/mL[b]	Physically compatible for 4 hr at 23 °C	2826	C
Ciprofloxacin	BED	2 mg/mL[a,b]	JJ	5 mg/mL[a,b]	Physically compatible for 4 hr at 23 °C	2743	C
Cisplatin	SIC	0.5 mg/mL[b]	JJ	5 mg/mL[a,b]	Physically compatible for 4 hr at 23 °C	2743	C
Cyclophosphamide	BMS	10 mg/mL[a,b]	JJ	5 mg/mL[a,b]	Physically compatible for 4 hr at 23 °C	2743	C
Cyclosporine	BED	5 mg/mL[a,b]	JJ	5 mg/mL[a,b]	Physically compatible for 4 hr at 23 °C	2743	C
Daptomycin	CUB	10 mg/mL[b]	JJ	5 mg/mL[a,b]	Physically compatible for 4 hr at 23 °C	2743	C
Dexamethasone sodium phosphate	APP	1 mg/mL[a,b]	JJ	5 mg/mL[a,b]	Physically compatible for 4 hr at 23 °C	2743	C
Diazepam	HOS	5 mg/mL	JJ	5 mg/mL[a,b]	Gross white turbid precipitate forms	2743	I
Digoxin	BA	0.25 mg/mL	JJ	5 mg/mL[a,b]	Physically compatible for 4 hr at 23 °C	2743	C
Diltiazem HCl	BED	5 mg/mL	JJ	5 mg/mL[a,b]	Physically compatible for 4 hr at 23 °C	2743	C
Diphenhydramine HCl	BA	2 mg/mL[a,b]	JJ	5 mg/mL[a,b]	Physically compatible for 4 hr at 23 °C	2743	C
Dobutamine HCl	HOS	4 mg/mL[a,b]	JJ	5 mg/mL[a,b]	Physically compatible for 4 hr at 23 °C	2743	C
Docetaxel	SAA	0.8 mg/mL[a,b]	JJ	5 mg/mL[a,b]	Physically compatible for 4 hr at 23 °C	2743	C
Dopamine HCl	AMR	3.2 mg/mL[a,b]	JJ	5 mg/mL[a,b]	Physically compatible for 4 hr at 23 °C	2743	C
Doxorubicin HCl	BED	1 mg/mL[a,b]	JJ	5 mg/mL[a,b]	Physically compatible for 4 hr at 23 °C	2743	C
Enalaprilat	SIC	0.1 mg/mL[a,b]	JJ	5 mg/mL[a,b]	Physically compatible for 4 hr at 23 °C	2743	C
Esmolol HCl	BED	10 mg/mL[a,b]	JJ	5 mg/mL[a,b]	Physically compatible for 4 hr at 23 °C	2743	C
Esomeprazole sodium	ASZ	0.4 mg/mL[b]	JJ	5 mg/mL[a,b]	Physically compatible for 4 hr at 23 °C	2743	C
Etoposide phosphate	SIC	5 mg/mL[a,b]	JJ	5 mg/mL[a,b]	Physically compatible for 4 hr at 23 °C	2743	C
Famotidine	BED	2 mg/mL[a,b]	JJ	5 mg/mL[a,b]	Physically compatible for 4 hr at 23 °C	2743	C
Fentanyl citrate	HOS	0.05 mg/mL	JJ	5 mg/mL[a,b]	Physically compatible for 4 hr at 23 °C	2743	C
Fluconazole	HAE	2 mg/mL	JJ	5 mg/mL[a,b]	Physically compatible for 4 hr at 23 °C	2743	C
Fluorouracil	ABX	16 mg/mL[a,b]	JJ	5 mg/mL[a,b]	Physically compatible for 4 hr at 23 °C	2743	C
Foscarnet sodium	HOS	24 mg/mL	JJ	5 mg/mL[a,b]	Physically compatible for 4 hr at 23 °C	2743	C
Furosemide	AMR	3 mg/mL[a,b]	JJ	5 mg/mL[a,b]	Physically compatible for 4 hr at 23 °C	2743	C
Gemcitabine HCl	LI	10 mg/mL[b]	JJ	5 mg/mL[a,b]	Physically compatible for 4 hr at 23 °C	2743	C
Gentamicin sulfate	HOS	5 mg/mL[a,b]	JJ	5 mg/mL[a,b]	Physically compatible for 4 hr at 23 °C	2743	C
Granisetron HCl	RC	0.05 mg/mL[a,b]	JJ	5 mg/mL[a,b]	Physically compatible for 4 hr at 23 °C	2743	C
Heparin sodium	HOS	100 units/mL	JJ	5 mg/mL[a,b]	Physically compatible for 4 hr at 23 °C	2743	C
Hydrocortisone sodium succinate	PHU	1 mg/mL[a,b]	JJ	5 mg/mL[a,b]	Physically compatible for 4 hr at 23 °C	2743	C
Hydromorphone HCl	BA	1 mg/mL[a,b]	JJ	5 mg/mL[a,b]	Physically compatible for 4 hr at 23 °C	2743	C
Ifosfamide	BMS	20 mg/mL[a,b]	JJ	5 mg/mL[a,b]	Physically compatible for 4 hr at 23 °C	2743	C

Y-Site Injection Compatibility (1:1 Mixture) (Cont.)

Doripenem

Drug	Mfr	Conc	Mfr	Conc	Remarks	Ref	C/I
Insulin, regular	NOV	1 unit/mL[a,b]	JJ	5 mg/mL[a,b]	Physically compatible for 4 hr at 23 °C	2743	C
Labetalol HCl	HOS	2 mg/mL[a,b]	JJ	5 mg/mL[a,b]	Physically compatible for 4 hr at 23 °C	2743	C
Levofloxacin	OMN	5 mg/mL[a,b]	JJ	5 mg/mL[a,b]	Physically compatible for 4 hr at 23 °C	2743	C
Linezolid	PHU	2 mg/mL	JJ	5 mg/mL[a,b]	Physically compatible for 4 hr at 23 °C	2743	C
Lorazepam	BED	0.5 mg/mL[a,b]	JJ	5 mg/mL[a,b]	Physically compatible for 4 hr at 23 °C	2743	C
Magnesium sulfate	AMR	100 mg/mL[a,b]	JJ	5 mg/mL[a,b]	Physically compatible for 4 hr at 23 °C	2743	C
Mannitol	HOS	15%	JJ	5 mg/mL[a,b]	Physically compatible for 4 hr at 23 °C	2743	C
Meperidine HCl	HOS	10 mg/mL[a,b]	JJ	5 mg/mL[a,b]	Physically compatible for 4 hr at 23 °C	2743	C
Methotrexate sodium	BED	12.5 mg/mL[a,b]	JJ	5 mg/mL[a,b]	Physically compatible for 4 hr at 23 °C	2743	C
Methylprednisolone sodium succinate	PHU	5 mg/mL[a,b]	JJ	5 mg/mL[a,b]	Physically compatible for 4 hr at 23 °C	2743	C
Metoclopramide HCl	HOS	5 mg/mL	JJ	5 mg/mL[a,b]	Physically compatible for 4 hr at 23 °C	2743	C
Metronidazole	BA	5 mg/mL	JJ	5 mg/mL[a,b]	Physically compatible for 4 hr at 23 °C	2743	C
Micafungin sodium	ASP	1.5 mg/mL[a,b]	JJ	5 mg/mL[a,b]	Physically compatible for 4 hr at 23 °C	2743	C
Midazolam HCl	BED	2 mg/mL[a,b]	JJ	5 mg/mL[a,b]	Physically compatible for 4 hr at 23 °C	2743	C
Milrinone lactate	BA	0.2 mg/mL[a,b]	JJ	5 mg/mL[a,b]	Physically compatible for 4 hr at 23 °C	2743	C
Morphine sulfate	BA	15 mg/mL	JJ	5 mg/mL[a,b]	Physically compatible for 4 hr at 23 °C	2743	C
Moxifloxacin HCl	BAY	1.6 mg/mL	JJ	5 mg/mL[a,b]	Physically compatible for 4 hr at 23 °C	2743	C
Norepinephrine bitartrate	BED	0.128 mg/mL[a,b]	JJ	5 mg/mL[a,b]	Physically compatible for 4 hr at 23 °C	2743	C
Ondansetron HCl	WOC	1 mg/mL[a,b]	JJ	5 mg/mL[a,b]	Physically compatible for 4 hr at 23 °C	2743	C
Paclitaxel	MAY	0.6 mg/mL[a,b]	JJ	5 mg/mL[a,b]	Physically compatible for 4 hr at 23 °C	2743	C
Pantoprazole sodium	WY[c]	0.4 mg/mL[a,b]	JJ	5 mg/mL[a,b]	Physically compatible for 4 hr at 23 °C	2743	C
Phenobarbital sodium	BA	5 mg/mL[a,b]	JJ	5 mg/mL[a,b]	Physically compatible for 4 hr at 23 °C	2743	C
Phenylephrine HCl	GNS	1 mg/mL[a,b]	JJ	5 mg/mL[a,b]	Physically compatible for 4 hr at 23 °C	2743	C
Potassium chloride	APP	0.1 mEq/mL[a,b]	JJ	5 mg/mL[a,b]	Physically compatible for 4 hr at 23 °C	2743	C
Potassium phosphates	APP	0.5 mmol/mL[a,b]	JJ	5 mg/mL[a,b]	Measured haze increases after 1 hr	2743	I
Propofol	BED	10 mg/mL	JJ	5 mg/mL[a,b]	Precipitation forms immediately	2743	I
Ranitidine HCl	BED	2 mg/mL[a,b]	JJ	5 mg/mL[a,b]	Physically compatible for 4 hr at 23 °C	2743	C
Sodium bicarbonate	HOS	1 mEq/mL	JJ	5 mg/mL[a,b]	Physically compatible for 4 hr at 23 °C	2743	C
Sodium phosphates	AMR	0.5 mmol/mL[a,b]	JJ	5 mg/mL[a,b]	Physically compatible for 4 hr at 23 °C	2743	C
Tacrolimus	ASP	0.02 mg/mL[a,b]	JJ	5 mg/mL[a,b]	Physically compatible for 4 hr at 23 °C	2743	C
Telavancin HCl	ASP	7.5 mg/mL[a,b]	OMN	10 mg/mL[a,b]	Physically compatible for 2 hr	2830	C
Tigecycline	WY	1 mg/mL[a,b]	JJ	5 mg/mL[a,b]	Physically compatible for 4 hr at 23 °C	2743	C
Tobramycin sulfate	SIC	5 mg/mL[a,b]	JJ	5 mg/mL[a,b]	Physically compatible for 4 hr at 23 °C	2743	C

Y-Site Injection Compatibility (1:1 Mixture) (Cont.)

Doripenem

Drug	Mfr	Conc	Mfr	Conc	Remarks	Ref	C/I
Vancomycin HCl	HOS	10 mg/mL[a,b]	JJ	5 mg/mL[a,b]	Physically compatible for 4 hr at 23 °C	2743	C
Voriconazole	PF	4 mg/mL[a,b]	JJ	5 mg/mL[a,b]	Physically compatible for 4 hr at 23 °C	2743	C
Zidovudine	GSK	4 mg/mL[a,b]	JJ	5 mg/mL[a,b]	Physically compatible for 4 hr at 23 °C	2743	C

[a]*Tested in dextrose 5% in water.*
[b]*Tested in sodium chloride 0.9%.*
[c]*Test performed using the formulation WITH edetate disodium.*
[d]*Tested in Ringer's injection, lactated.*

DOXAPRAM HYDROCHLORIDE
AHFS 28:20.92

Products — Doxapram hydrochloride is available in 20-mL multiple-dose vials. Each milliliter of solution contains doxapram hydrochloride 20 mg and benzyl alcohol 0.9% in water for injection. (1)

pH — From 3.5 to 5. (1)

Trade Name(s) — Dopram.

Administration — Doxapram hydrochloride is administered by intravenous injection or infusion of a solution diluted to 1 or 2 mg/mL with a compatible diluent. (1; 4)

Stability — Doxapram hydrochloride injection should be stored at controlled room temperature and protected from freezing. (1; 4)

pH Effects — Doxapram hydrochloride in solution became turbid when the pH was adjusted from 3.8 to 5.7 with 0.1 N sodium hydroxide. When the pH was adjusted down to 1.9 with 0.1 N hydrochloride, no visible change occurred to the clear solution. (1177) The drug is stated to be incompatible with alkaline drugs. (4)

At pH 2.5 to 6.5, doxapram hydrochloride remained chemically stable for 24 hours. At pH 7.5 and above, a 10 to 15% doxapram hydrochloride loss occurred in about six hours. (1177)

Compatibility Information

Solution Compatibility

Doxapram HCl

Solution	Mfr	Mfr	Conc/L	Remarks	Ref	C/I
Dextrose 5%				Recommended solution	1	C
Dextrose 10%				Recommended solution	1	C
Sodium chloride 0.9%				Recommended solution	1	C

Drugs in Syringe Compatibility

Doxapram HCl

Drug (in syringe)	Mfr	Amt	Mfr	Amt	Remarks	Ref	C/I
Amikacin sulfate		100 mg/ 2 mL	RB	400 mg/ 20 mL	Physically compatible with no doxapram loss in 24 hr	1177	C
Aminophylline		250 mg/ 10 mL	RB	400 mg/ 20 mL	Immediate turbidity and precipitation	1177	I
Ascorbic acid		500 mg/ 2 mL	RB	400 mg/ 20 mL	Immediate turbidity changing to precipitation in 24 hr	1177	I

Drugs in Syringe Compatibility (Cont.)

Doxapram HCl

Drug (in syringe)	Mfr	Amt	Mfr	Amt	Remarks	Ref	C/I
Bumetanide		0.5 mg/ 1 mL	RB	400 mg/ 20 mL	Physically compatible with 3% doxapram loss in 24 hr	1177	C
Cefotaxime sodium		500 mg/ 4 mL	RB	400 mg/ 20 mL	Precipitates immediately	1177	I
Cefotetan disodium		1 g/ 10 mL	RB	400 mg/ 20 mL	Immediate turbidity	1177	I
Cefuroxime sodium	GL	750 mg/ 7 mL	RB	400 mg/ 20 mL	Immediate turbidity	1177	I
Chlorpromazine HCl		250 mg/ 5 mL	RB	400 mg/ 20 mL	Physically compatible with no doxapram loss in 24 hr	1177	C
Cisplatin		10 mg/ 20 mL	RB	400 mg/ 20 mL	Physically compatible with no doxapram loss in 24 hr	1177	C
Cyclophosphamide		100 mg/ 5 mL	RB	400 mg/ 20 mL	Physically compatible with 2% doxapram loss in 24 hr	1177	C
Dexamethasone sodium phosphate	MSD	3.3 mg/ 1 mL	RB	400 mg/ 20 mL	Immediate turbidity and precipitation	1177	I
Diazepam		10 mg/ 2 mL	RB	400 mg/ 20 mL	Immediate turbidity and precipitation	1177	I
Digoxin		0.25 mg/ 1 mL	RB	400 mg/ 20 mL	10% doxapram loss in 9 hr and 17% in 24 hr	1177	I
Dobutamine HCl	LI	100 mg/ 10 mL	RB	400 mg/ 20 mL	5% doxapram loss in 3 hr and 11% in 24 hr	1177	I
Dopamine HCl		100 mg/ 5 mL	RB	400 mg/ 20 mL	Physically compatible with 3% doxapram loss in 24 hr	1177	C
Doxycycline hyclate		100 mg/ 5 mL	RB	400 mg/ 20 mL	Physically compatible with 3% doxapram loss in 24 hr	1177	C
Epinephrine HCl		1 mg/ 1 mL	RB	400 mg/ 20 mL	Physically compatible with no doxapram loss in 24 hr	1177	C
Folic acid		15 mg/ 1 mL	RB	400 mg/ 20 mL	Immediate turbidity	1177	I
Furosemide	HO	100 mg/ 10 mL	RB	400 mg/ 20 mL	Immediate turbidity	1177	I
Hydrocortisone sodium succinate	UP	500 mg/ 2 mL	RB	400 mg/ 20 mL	Immediate turbidity and precipitation	1177	I
Hydroxyzine HCl		25 mg/ 1 mL	RB	400 mg/ 20 mL	Physically compatible with no doxapram loss in 24 hr	1177	C
Isoniazid		100 mg/ 2 mL	RB	400 mg/ 20 mL	Physically compatible with 2% doxapram loss in 24 hr	1177	C
Ketamine HCl	PD	200 mg/ 20 mL	RB	400 mg/ 20 mL	Physically compatible with no doxapram loss in 9 hr but 12% loss in 24 hr	1177	I
Lincomycin HCl		300 mg/ 1 mL	RB	400 mg/ 20 mL	Physically compatible with no doxapram loss in 24 hr	1177	C
Methotrexate sodium		50 mg/ 20 mL	RB	400 mg/ 20 mL	Physically compatible with 4% doxapram loss in 24 hr	1177	C
Methylprednisolone sodium succinate	UP	40 mg/ 2 mL	RB	400 mg/ 20 mL	Immediate turbidity and precipitation	1177	I

Drugs in Syringe Compatibility (Cont.)

Doxapram HCl

Drug (in syringe)	Mfr	Amt	Mfr	Amt	Remarks	Ref	C/I
Phytonadione		10 mg/ 1 mL	RB	400 mg/ 20 mL	Physically compatible with no doxapram loss in 24 hr	1177	C
Pyridoxine HCl		10 mg/ 1 mL	RB	400 mg/ 20 mL	Physically compatible with 6% doxapram loss in 24 hr	1177	C
Terbutaline sulfate		0.2 mg/ 1 mL	RB	400 mg/ 20 mL	Physically compatible with 6% doxapram loss in 24 hr	1177	C
Thiamine HCl		10 mg/ 2 mL	RB	400 mg/ 20 mL	Physically compatible with 6% doxapram loss in 24 hr	1177	C
Tobramycin sulfate		60 mg/ 1.5 mL	RB	400 mg/ 20 mL	Physically compatible with no doxapram loss in 24 hr	1177	C
Vincristine sulfate		1 mg/ 10 mL	RB	400 mg/ 20 mL	Physically compatible with 7% doxapram loss in 24 hr	1177	C

Y-Site Injection Compatibility (1:1 Mixture)

Doxapram HCl

Drug	Mfr	Conc	Mfr	Conc	Remarks	Ref	C/I
Ampicillin sodium	APO	50 mg/mL[b]	RB	2 mg/mL[a]	Visually compatible for 4 hr at 23 °C	2470	C
Caffeine citrate	BI	20 mg/mL	RB	2 mg/mL[a]	Visually compatible for 4 hr at 23 °C	2470	C
Calcium chloride	APP	100 mg/mL	RB	2 mg/mL[a]	Visually compatible for 4 hr at 23 °C	2470	C
Calcium gluconate	APP	100 mg/mL	RB	2 mg/mL[a]	Visually compatible for 4 hr at 23 °C	2470	C
Cefazolin sodium	APO	100 mg/mL[a]	RB	2 mg/mL[a]	Visually compatible for 4 hr at 23 °C	2470	C
Ceftazidime	GW	40 mg/mL[a]	RB	2 mg/mL[a]	Visually compatible for 4 hr at 23 °C	2470	C
Clindamycin phosphate	PHU	10 mg/mL[a]	RB	2 mg/mL[a]	Gas bubbles evolve immediately	2470	I
Erythromycin lactobionate	AB	5 mg/mL[a]	RB	2 mg/mL[a]	Visually compatible for 4 hr at 23 °C	2470	C
Fentanyl citrate	ESL	25 mcg/mL[a]	RB	2 mg/mL[a]	Visually compatible for 4 hr at 23 °C	2470	C
Gentamicin sulfate	APP	10 mg/mL[a]	RB	2 mg/mL[a]	Visually compatible for 4 hr at 23 °C	2470	C
Heparin sodium	APP	1 unit/mL[c]	RB	2 mg/mL[a]	Visually compatible for 4 hr at 23 °C	2470	C
Insulin, regular	NOV	1 unit/mL[c]	RB	2 mg/mL[a]	Visually compatible for 4 hr at 23 °C	2470	C
Metoclopramide HCl	AB	1 mg/mL	RB	2 mg/mL[a]	Visually compatible for 4 hr at 23 °C	2470	C
Metronidazole	AB	5 mg/mL	RB	2 mg/mL[a]	Visually compatible for 4 hr at 23 °C	2470	C
Oxacillin sodium	APO	20 mg/mL[a]	RB	2 mg/mL[a]	Visually compatible for 4 hr at 23 °C	2470	C
Phenobarbital sodium	ES	10 mg/mL[b]	RB	2 mg/mL[a]	Visually compatible for 4 hr at 23 °C	2470	C
Ranitidine HCl	GSK	5 mg/mL[a]	RB	2 mg/mL[a]	Visually compatible for 4 hr at 23 °C	2470	C
Vancomycin HCl	APP	5 mg/mL[a]	RB	2 mg/mL[a]	Visually compatible for 4 hr at 23 °C	2470	C

[a] Tested in dextrose 5%.
[b] Tested in sodium chloride 0.9%.
[c] Tested in sodium chloride 0.45%.

DOXORUBICIN HYDROCHLORIDE
AHFS 10:00

Products — Doxorubicin hydrochloride is available as a lyophilized product in 10-, 20-, and 50-mg single-dose glass vials with 50 mg of lactose for each 10 mg of doxorubicin hydrochloride. (1)

Reconstitution of the lyophilized products should be performed with sodium chloride 0.9%. Bacteriostatic diluents are not recommended. Add 5, 10, or 25 mL sodium chloride 0.9% to the 10-, 20-, or 50-mg vial, respectively. After the diluent is added, the vial should be shaken and the drug allowed to dissolve, forming a 2-mg/mL solution. (1)

Additionally, doxorubicin hydrochloride is available in 5-, 10-, 25-, and 100-mL vials as a 2-mg/mL solution without preservatives. The solution also contains sodium chloride 0.9% and hydrochloric acid to adjust the pH in water for injection. (1)

pH — The pH of lyophilized doxorubicin hydrochloride reconstituted with sodium chloride 0.9% is 3.8 to 6.5. (4) The pH of the solution products is adjusted to 3. (1)

Trade Name(s) — Adriamycin.

Administration — Doxorubicin hydrochloride is administered intravenously, preferably into the tubing of a running intravenous infusion of sodium chloride 0.9% or dextrose 5% over not less than three to five minutes. (1; 4) The drug should not be administered intramuscularly or subcutaneously, and extravasation should be avoided because of local tissue necrosis. (1)

In the event of spills or leaks, a doxorubicin hydrochloride manufacturer recommends the use of sodium hypochlorite 5% (household bleach) for inactivation. (1200)

Stability — Doxorubicin hydrochloride liquid injections should be stored under refrigeration and protected from light. Intact vials should be kept in their cartons until use. (1; 4)

The lyophilized products in intact vials should be stored at room temperature and protected from light. The manufacturer states that its reconstituted lyophilized products are stable for seven days at room temperature and 15 days under refrigeration. (1)

For 50-mcg/mL and 0.5-mg/mL doxorubicin hydrochloride solutions, Janssen et al. reported that a greater rate of decomposition occurred in the more concentrated solution. (1206) However, most other studies found no concentration dependence for the degradation rate. (489; 526; 1208; 1255)

A darkening of doxorubicin hydrochloride color has been noted when solutions of the drug contact aluminum metal. This change was initially noticed in the first small amount of drug to be injected through a needle with an aluminum hub. When solutions of doxorubicin hydrochloride containing aluminum are allowed to stand, the color becomes much darker than the control. Precipitation may also occur. As a precautionary measure, the author recommended not using any aluminum-containing apparatus for preparing or administering doxorubicin hydrochloride. (653)

In another evaluation, stainless steel needles with steel or plastic hubs and pieces of aluminum were immersed in doxorubicin hydrochloride 2 mg/mL in sterile water for injection or sodium chloride 0.9%. After 24 hours, the solutions containing the needles were unchanged in appearance and pH. The solution containing the aluminum was darker in color, and the pH had changed from 4.8 to 5.2. The concentrations of all solutions remained the same after six hours; but

after three days, the solution containing aluminum was down to 91.9% while the others were only down to 94.4%. The authors concluded that doxorubicin hydrochloride does react with aluminum but at a slow rate and without major loss. They recommended not storing the drug in syringes capped with aluminum-hubbed needles but thought that doxorubicin could be injected safely through aluminum-hubbed needles. (887)

Immersion of a needle with an aluminum component in doxorubicin hydrochloride (Adria) 2 mg/mL resulted in a darkening of the solution, with black patches forming on the aluminum in 12 to 24 hours at 24 °C with protection from light. (988)

Doxorubicin hydrochloride 0.5 mg/mL in sodium chloride 0.9% supported the growth of *Escherichia coli*, *Klebsiella pneumoniae*, *Pseudomonas aeruginosa*, and *Candida albicans*, which are implicated in nosocomial infections. The arbitrary extension of expiration dates to doxorubicin hydrochloride solutions is highly questionable. (827)

Doxorubicin hydrochloride, etoposide phosphate, and vincristine sulfate admixtures at a variety of concentrations were unable to pass the USP test for antimicrobial effectiveness. Mixtures of these drugs are not "self-preserving" and permit microbial growth. (2343) The potential for microbiological growth should be considered when assigning expiration periods.

pH Effects — Doxorubicin hydrochloride appears to have pH-dependent stability in solution. (526; 1007; 1037) It becomes progressively more stable as the pH of drug–infusion solution admixtures becomes more acidic at 7.4 to 4.5. (526) The pH range of maximum stability has been variously stated to be about 4 to 5 (1007; 1460), 3 to 4 (1037), and about 4. (1208) At a concentration of 0.1 mg/mL in buffer solutions stored at 4 °C, no significant doxorubicin loss occurred in 60 days at pH 4, but substantial decomposition occurred at pH 7.4. (1206) Doxorubicin hydrochloride is unstable at pH values less than 3 or greater than 7. (4) In acidic media, splitting of the glycosidic bond results in a red-colored, water-insoluble aglycone and a water-soluble amino sugar. (4) In alkaline media, a color change to deep purple is indicative of decomposition. This color change also occurs with other anthracyclines. (394) It is thought to reflect cleavage of the amino sugar, resulting in an ineffective moiety. (524)

Freezing Solutions — Hoffman et al. found that doxorubicin hydrochloride, reconstituted to 2 mg/mL with sterile water for injection and kept at 4 °C, exhibited a 1.5% loss in one month and a 10.5% loss in six months. Freezing the solutions at −20 °C resulted in no loss over 30 days. It was indicated that filtration of stored solutions through a 0.22-μm filter was appropriate to ensure sterility. (652)

Doxorubicin hydrochloride (Farmitalia) 70 mg/50 mL in PVC bags of sodium chloride 0.9% (Travenol) could be frozen at −20 °C for at least 30 days and thawed by exposure to microwave radiation for two minutes with no significant change in concentration. However, the doxorubicin hydrochloride concentration apparently began declining after the fourth repetition of the freeze-thaw treatment with a loss of about 5%. (818)

The stability of doxorubicin hydrochloride 1 mg/mL in sodium chloride 0.9% in PVC containers at −20 °C was evaluated. No drug loss occurred after two weeks of storage and thawing for 150 minutes at room temperature or 180 seconds in a microwave oven. Refreezing the solutions and rethawing at room temperature or in a microwave oven three weeks later (total of five weeks of frozen storage) resulted in 3% drug loss. (1256)

Although the thawing of frozen doxorubicin hydrochloride solutions in microwave ovens has been suggested (818; 1256), Williamson recommended only room temperature thawing because of the risks of drug decomposition from overheating and exposure if the bags burst. (1257)

Light Effects — Doxorubicin hydrochloride is sensitive to light, especially in very dilute solutions. (489; 1073; 1094) However, the photolability of dilute solutions is not observed with more concentrated solutions. A 10-fold difference in photolability half-life was found between concentrations of 0.01 and 0.1 mg/mL. (1594) The manufacturers recommend protecting the solutions from exposure to sunlight and that any unused solution be discarded. (1; 4)

An evaluation of etoposide phosphate (Bristol-Myers Squibb) 2 mg/mL, doxorubicin hydrochloride 0.4 mg/mL, and vincristine sulfate 0.016 mg/mL (16 mcg/mL) in sodium chloride 0.9% in polyolefin plastic bags (McGaw) found little or no effect of constant exposure to normal fluorescent room light for 124 hours. The admixtures were physically compatible, and all three drugs in the admixture remained stable throughout the time period stored at an elevated temperature of 35 to 40 °C. (2343)

Syringes — Doxorubicin hydrochloride (Farmitalia) 2 mg/mL repackaged in polypropylene syringes exhibited little loss after storage for 43 days at 4 °C. (1460)

Doxorubicin hydrochloride (Adria) 2 mg/mL in sodium chloride 0.9% in glass vials and plastic syringes (Monoject and Terumo) and also 1 mg/mL in sodium chloride 0.9% in plastic syringes (Monoject) exhibited no visual changes and little or no loss when stored at 4 and 23 °C while exposed to light for 124 days. Potential extractable materials from the syringes were not detected during the study period. (1594)

Implantable Pumps — Vogelzang et al. reported the stability of 3- and 5-mg/mL concentrations in sodium chloride 0.9% in the reservoir of a Medtronic DAD implantable pump at 37 °C. Losses of about 5 to 6% in one week and 9 to 11% in two weeks occurred. Analyses after longer periods continued to show about a 5 to 6% loss per week at 37 °C. (1255)

Sorption — Doxorubicin hydrochloride 16 mcg/mL in dextrose 5% and sodium chloride 0.9% in PVC containers was infused through PVC infusion sets at 21 mL/hr over 24 hours at 22 °C while exposed to light. No evidence of sorption was found. (1700)

Doxorubicin hydrochloride (Farmitalia) 1 mg/mL in sodium chloride 0.9% exhibited no loss due to sorption to PVC and polyethylene administration lines during simulated infusions at 0.875 mL/hr for 2.5 hours via a syringe pump. (1795)

Filtration — Although doxorubicin hydrochloride was reported to undergo considerable binding to cellulose ester and polytetrafluoroethylene filters (1249; 1415; 1416), other studies did not confirm unacceptable losses at clinical concentrations. Doxorubicin hydrochloride 2 mg/mL in sterile water for injection showed no loss due to filtration when filtered through a 0.22-μm Millex filter. (652)

In another study, doxorubicin hydrochloride (Adria) 30 mg/15 mL was injected as a bolus through a 0.2-μm nylon, air-eliminating filter (Ultipor, Pall) to evaluate the effect of filtration on simulated intravenous push delivery. About 92% of the drug was delivered through the filter after flushing with 10 mL of sodium chloride 0.9%. (809)

Doxorubicin hydrochloride 1 mg/mL in sodium chloride 0.9% exhibited little loss due to sorption to cellulose acetate (Minisart 45, Sartorius), polysulfone (Acrodisc 45, Gelman), and nylon (Nylaflo, Gelman) filters. However, a 20 to 25% loss due to sorption occurred during the first 60 minutes of infusion through nylon filters (Utipore, Pall). A 35% loss was found during the first 15 min using a nylon filter (Posidyne ELD96, Pall). Return to the full concentrations occurred gradually within 1.5 to 2.5 hours. (1795)

Central Venous Catheter — Doxorubicin hydrochloride (Pharmacia) 0.25 mg/mL in dextrose 5% was found to be compatible with the ARROWg+ard Blue Plus (Arrow International) chlorhexidine-bearing triple-lumen central catheter. Essentially complete delivery of the drug was found with little or no drug loss occurring. Furthermore, chlorhexidine delivered from the catheter remained at trace amounts with no substantial increase due to the delivery of the drug through the catheter. (2335)

Compatibility Information

Solution Compatibility

Doxorubicin HCl

Solution	Mfr	Mfr	Conc/L	Remarks	Ref	C/I
Dextrose 3.3% in sodium chloride 0.3%			100 mg	5% loss in 4 weeks at 25 °C in the dark	1007	C
Dextrose 5%	TR[a]	AD	180 mg	10% loss in 40 hr at room temperature along with a color change and an increase in pH	519	C
	TR[b]	AD	180 mg	No decrease in 48 hr at room temperature	519	C
	AB[a]	AD	10 and 20 mg	Physically compatible. 2% loss in 24 hr at 21 °C in fluorescent light	526	C
			100 mg	5% loss in 4 weeks at 25 °C in the dark	1007	C
	[c]	BEL	0.5 g	Visually compatible. 5% loss in 28 days at 4 °C and 14 days at 22 and 35 °C in the dark	1548	C
	[c]	BEL	1.25 g	Visually compatible. 5% loss in 28 days at 4 and 22 °C and 7 days at 35 °C in the dark	1548	C
	MG[d], TR[b]		180 mg	Less than 10% loss in 48 hr at room temperature in light	1658	C

Solution Compatibility (Cont.)

Doxorubicin HCl

Solution	Mfr	Mfr	Conc/L	Remarks	Ref	C/I
	b		40 mg	10% loss in 7 days at 4 °C in the dark	1700	C
	TR[b]	FA	100 mg	10% or less loss in 43 days at −20, 4, and 25 °C in the dark	1460	C
Ringer's injection, lactated	AB[a]	AD	10 and 20 mg	Physically compatible. 8% loss in 24 hr at 21 °C in fluorescent light	526	C
			100 mg	10% loss in 1.7 days at 25 °C in the dark	1007	C
Sodium chloride 0.9%	AB[a]	AD	10 and 20 mg	Physically compatible. 5% in 24 hr at 21 °C in fluorescent light	526	C
			100 mg	10% loss in 6 days at 25 °C in the dark	1007	C
	TR[b]	FA	100 mg	10% or less loss in 43 days at −20, 4, and 25 °C in the dark	1460	C
	BA[e]	CET	2 g	Stable for 14 days at 3 and 23 °C plus 28 days at 30 °C	1538	C
	c	BEL	0.5 g	Visually compatible. 5% or less loss in 14 days at 4 and 22 °C and 7 days at 35 °C in the dark	1548	C
	c	BEL	1.25 g	Visually compatible. 5% or less loss in 28 days at 4 and 22 °C and 7 days at 35 °C in the dark	1548	C
	b		40 mg	6% loss in 7 days at 4 °C in the dark	1700	C

[a]Tested in glass containers.
[b]Tested in PVC containers.
[c]Tested in ethylene vinyl acetate (EVA) containers.
[d]Tested in both glass and polyolefin containers.
[e]Tested in Pharmacia Deltec reservoirs.

Additive Compatibility

Doxorubicin HCl

Drug	Mfr	Conc/L	Mfr	Conc/L	Test Soln	Remarks	Ref	C/I
Aminophylline			AD			Discolors from red to purple	524	I
Dacarbazine with ondansetron HCl	LY GL	8 g 640 mg	AD	800 mg	D5W[a]	Visually compatible. Under 10% ondansetron and doxorubicin loss in 24 hr at 30 °C and 7 days at 4 °C then 24 hr at 30 °C. Dacarbazine stable for 8 hr but 13% loss in 24 hr	2092	I
Dacarbazine with ondansetron HCl	LY GL	8 g 640 mg	AD	800 mg	D5W[b]	Visually compatible. Under 10% loss of all drugs in 24 hr at 30 °C and 7 days at 4 °C then 24 hr at 30 °C	2092	C
Dacarbazine with ondansetron HCl	LY GL	20 g 640 mg	AD	1.5 g	D5W[a,b]	Visually compatible. Under 10% loss of all drugs in 24 hr at 30 °C and 7 days at 4 °C then 24 hr at 30 °C	2092	C
Diazepam	RC		AD			Precipitates immediately	524	I
Etoposide with vincristine sulfate	BMS LI	200 mg 1.6 mg	PHU	40 mg	NS[c]	Visually compatible. All drugs stable for 72 hr at 30 °C in the dark	2239	C
Etoposide with vincristine sulfate	BMS LI	125 mg 1 mg	PHU	25 mg	NS[c]	Visually compatible. All drugs stable for 96 hr at 24 °C in light or dark	2239	C
Etoposide with vincristine sulfate	BMS LI	175 mg 1.4 mg	PHU	35 mg	NS[c]	Visually compatible. All drugs stable for 96 hr at 24 °C in light or dark	2239	C
Etoposide with vincristine sulfate	BMS LI	250 mg 2 mg	PHU	50 mg	NS[c]	Visually compatible. All drugs stable for 48 hr at 24 °C in light or dark. Etoposide precipitate in 72 hr	2239	C

Additive Compatibility (Cont.)

Doxorubicin HCl

Drug	Mfr	Conc/L	Mfr	Conc/L	Test Soln	Remarks	Ref	C/I
Etoposide with vincristine sulfate	BMS LI	350 mg 2.8 mg	PHU	70 mg	NS[c]	Visually compatible. All drugs stable for 24 hr at 24 °C in light or dark. Etoposide precipitate in 36 hr	2239	C
Etoposide with vincristine sulfate	BMS LI	500 mg 4 mg	PHU	100 mg	NS[c]	Etoposide precipitate formed in 12 hr at 24 °C in light or dark	2239	I
Etoposide phosphate with vincristine sulfate	BMS LI	600 mg 5 mg	PHU	120 mg	NS[c]	Physically compatible. Little loss of any drug in 124 hr at 4 and 40 °C	2343	C
Etoposide phosphate with vincristine sulfate	BMS LI	1.2 g 10 mg	PHU	240 mg	NS[c]	Physically compatible. Little loss of any drug in 124 hr at 4 and 40 °C	2343	C
Etoposide phosphate with vincristine sulfate	BMS LI	2 g 16 mg	PHU	400 mg	NS[c]	Physically compatible. Under 4% loss of any drug in 124 hr at 4 and 40 °C	2343	C
Fluorouracil			AD			Discolors from red to blue-purple	524	I
	RC	250 mg	AD	10 mg	D5W	Color changes to deep purple	296	I
Ondansetron HCl	GL	30 and 300 mg	MJ	100 mg and 2 g	D5W[a]	Physically compatible with little loss of either drug in 48 hr at 23 °C	1876	C
Ondansetron HCl with dacarbazine	GL LY	640 mg 8 g	AD	800 mg	D5W[a]	Visually compatible. Under 10% ondansetron and doxorubicin loss in 24 hr at 30 °C and 7 days at 4 °C then 24 hr at 30 °C. Dacarbazine stable for 8 hr but 13% loss in 24 hr	2092	I
Ondansetron HCl with dacarbazine	GL LY	640 mg 8 g	AD	800 mg	D5W[b]	Visually compatible. Under 10% loss of all drugs in 24 hr at 30 °C and 7 days at 4 °C then 24 hr at 30 °C	2092	C
Ondansetron HCl with dacarbazine	GL LY	640 mg 20 g	AD	1.5 g	D5W[a,b]	Visually compatible. Under 10% loss of all drugs in 24 hr at 30 °C and 7 days at 4 °C then 24 hr at 30 °C	2092	C
Ondansetron HCl with vincristine sulfate	GL LI	480 mg 14 mg	AD	400 mg	D5W[b]	Visually compatible. Under 10% loss of all drugs in 5 days at 4 °C then 24 hr at 30 °C	2092	C
Ondansetron HCl with vincristine sulfate	GL LI	960 mg 28 mg	AD	800 mg	D5W[a]	Visually compatible. Under 10% loss of all drugs after 120 hr at 30 °C	2092	C
Paclitaxel	BMS	300 mg	PH	200 mg	D5W, NS	Visually compatible for 1 day with microprecipitation in 3 to 5 days and gross precipitation in 7 days at 4, 23, and 32 °C in the dark. No paclitaxel and under 8% doxorubicin loss in 7 days	2247	C
	BMS	1.2 g	PH	200 mg	D5W, NS	Visually compatible for 1 day with microprecipitation in 3 to 5 days and gross precipitation in 7 days at 4, 23, and 32 °C in the dark. No paclitaxel and less than 7% doxorubicin loss in 7 days	2247	C
Vinblastine sulfate	LI	75 mg	AD	500 mg	NS[a]	Physically compatible for 10 days at 8, 25, and 32 °C. Assays highly erratic	838	?
	LI	150 mg	AD	1.5 g	NS[a]	Physically compatible for 10 days at 8, 25, and 32 °C. Assays highly erratic	838	?
Vincristine sulfate	LI	33 mg	FA	1.4 g	D5½S, NS	Visually compatible. Less than 10% loss of both drugs for 14 days at 25, 30, and 37 °C	1030	C

Additive Compatibility (Cont.)

Doxorubicin HCl

Drug	Mfr	Conc/L	Mfr	Conc/L	Test Soln	Remarks	Ref	C/I
	LI	50 mg	FA	1.88 and 2.37 g	D5½S, NS	Visually compatible. Less than 10% loss of both drugs for 14 days at 25 and 30 °C. Up to 16% doxorubicin loss at 37 °C in 14 days	1030	C
	LI	36 mg	NYC	1.67 g	NS[a,b]	Visually compatible and both drugs stable for 7 days at 4 °C then 4 days at 37 °C	1874	C
	FAU	200 mg	PHU	2 g	W[d]	Physically compatible. No loss of either drug in 7 days at 37 °C. 4% loss of both drugs in 14 days at 4 °C	2288	C
	PHC	33 mg	PHC	1.4 g	D5½S	Physically compatible. Little loss of either drug in 14 days at 4 and 25 °C. 12% loss of both drugs at 37 °C	2674	C
	PHC	33 mg	PHC	1.4 g	NS	Physically compatible. Little loss of either drug in 14 days at 4 and 25 °C. 4% loss of both drugs at 37 °C	2674	C
	PHC	53 mg	PHC	1.4 g	D5½S	Physically compatible. Little loss of either drug in 14 days at 4 and 25 °C. 8% loss of both drugs at 37 °C	2674	C
	PHC	53 mg	PHC	1.4 g	NS	Physically compatible. Little loss of either drug in 14 days at 4 and 25 °C. 9% loss of both drugs at 37 °C	2674	C
Vincristine sulfate with etoposide	LI BMS	1.6 mg 200 mg	PHU	40 mg	NS[c]	Visually compatible. All drugs stable for 72 hr at 30 °C in the dark	2239	C
Vincristine sulfate with etoposide	LI BMS	1 mg 125 mg	PHU	25 mg	NS[c]	Visually compatible. All drugs stable for 96 hr at 24 °C in light or dark	2239	C
Vincristine sulfate with etoposide	LI BMS	1.4 mg 175 mg	PHU	35 mg	NS[c]	Visually compatible. All drugs stable for 96 hr at 24 °C in light or dark	2239	C
Vincristine sulfate with etoposide	LI BMS	2 mg 250 mg	PHU	50 mg	NS[c]	Visually compatible. All drugs stable for 48 hr at 24 °C in light or dark. Etoposide precipitate in 72 hr	2239	C
Vincristine sulfate with etoposide	LI BMS	2.8 mg 350 mg	PHU	70 mg	NS[c]	Visually compatible. All drugs stable for 24 hr at 24 °C in light or dark. Etoposide precipitate in 36 hr	2239	C
Vincristine sulfate with etoposide	LI BMS	4 mg 500 mg	PHU	100 mg	NS[c]	Etoposide precipitate formed in 12 hr at 24 °C in light or dark	2239	I
Vincristine sulfate with etoposide phosphate	LI BMS	5 mg 600 mg	PHU	120 mg	NS[c]	Physically compatible. Little loss of any drug in 124 hr at 4 and 40 °C	2343	C
Vincristine sulfate with etoposide phosphate	LI BMS	10 mg 1.2 g	PHU	240 mg	NS[c]	Physically compatible. Little loss of any drug in 124 hr at 4 and 40 °C	2343	C
Vincristine sulfate with etoposide phosphate	LI BMS	16 mg 2 g	PHU	400 mg	NS[c]	Physically compatible. Under 4% loss of any drug in 124 hr at 4 and 40 °C	2343	C
Vincristine sulfate with ondansetron HCl	LI GL	14 mg 480 mg	AD	400 mg	D5W[b]	Visually compatible. Under 10% loss of all drugs in 5 days at 4 °C then 24 hr at 30 °C	2092	C
Vincristine sulfate with ondansetron HCl	LI GL	28 mg 960 mg	AD	800 mg	D5W[a]	Visually compatible. Under 10% loss of all drugs after 120 hr at 30 °C	2092	C

[a]Tested in PVC containers.
[b]Tested in polyisoprene infusion pump reservoirs.
[c]Tested in polyolefin-lined plastic bags.
[d]Tested in PVC reservoirs for the Graseby 9000 ambulatory pumps.

Drugs in Syringe Compatibility

Doxorubicin HCl

Drug (in syringe)	Mfr	Amt	Mfr	Amt	Remarks	Ref	C/I
Bleomycin sulfate		1.5 units/ 0.5 mL		1 mg/ 0.5 mL	Physically compatible for 5 min at room temperature followed by 8 min of centrifugation	980	C
Cisplatin		0.5 mg/ 0.5 mL		1 mg/ 0.5 mL	Physically compatible for 5 min at room temperature followed by 8 min of centrifugation	980	C
Cisplatin with mitomycin	BMS BMS	50 mg 5 mg	BED	25 mg	Brought to a 5-mL final volume with NS. Visually compatible but more than 10% loss of mitomycin in 4 hr at 25 °C. At 4 °C, less than 10% loss of all three drugs in 12 hr, but about 16% mitomycin loss in 24 hr	2423	I
Cyclophosphamide		10 mg/ 0.5 mL		1 mg/ 0.5 mL	Physically compatible for 5 min at room temperature followed by 8 min of centrifugation	980	C
Droperidol		1.25 mg/ 0.5 mL		1 mg/ 0.5 mL	Physically compatible for 5 min at room temperature followed by 8 min of centrifugation	980	C
Fluorouracil		25 mg/ 0.5 mL		1 mg/ 0.5 mL	Physically compatible for 5 min at room temperature followed by 8 min of centrifugation	980	C
		500 mg/ 10 mL		5 and 10 mg/ 10 mL[a]	Precipitate forms within several hours of mixing	1564	I
Furosemide		5 mg/ 0.5 mL		1 mg/ 0.5 mL	Precipitates immediately	980	I
Heparin sodium		500 units/ 0.5 mL		1 mg/ 0.5 mL	Precipitates immediately	980	I
Leucovorin calcium		5 mg/ 0.5 mL		1 mg/ 0.5 mL	Physically compatible for 5 min at room temperature followed by 8 min of centrifugation	980	C
Methotrexate sodium		12.5 mg/ 0.5 mL		1 mg/ 0.5 mL	Physically compatible for 5 min at room temperature followed by 8 min of centrifugation	980	C
Metoclopramide HCl		2.5 mg/ 0.5 mL		1 mg/ 0.5 mL	Physically compatible for 5 min at room temperature followed by 8 min of centrifugation	980	C
	RB	10 mg/ 2 mL	AD	40 mg/ 20 mL	Physically compatible for 48 hr at 25 °C	1167	C
	RB	160 mg/ 32 mL	AD	90 mg/ 45 mL	Physically compatible for 48 hr at 25 °C	1167	C
Mitomycin		0.25 mg/ 0.5 mL		1 mg/ 0.5 mL	Physically compatible for 5 min at room temperature followed by 8 min of centrifugation	980	C
Mitomycin with cisplatin	BMS BMS	5 mg 50 mg	BED	25 mg	Brought to a 5-mL final volume with NS. Visually compatible but more than 10% loss of mitomycin in 4 hr at 25 °C. At 4 °C, less than 10% loss of all three drugs in 12 hr, but about 16% mitomycin loss in 24 hr	2423	I
Vinblastine sulfate	LI	4.5 mg/ 4.5 mL	AD	45 mg/ 22.5 mL	Brought to 30-mL total volume with NS. Physically compatible for 10 days at 8, 25, and 32 °C. Assays highly erratic	838	?
	LI	2.25 mg/ 2.25 mL	AD	15 mg/ 7.5 mL	Brought to 30-mL total volume with NS. Physically compatible for 10 days at 8, 25, and 32 °C. Assays highly erratic	838	?
		0.5 mg/ 0.5 mL		1 mg/ 0.5 mL	Physically compatible for 5 min at room temperature followed by 8 min of centrifugation	980	C

Drugs in Syringe Compatibility (Cont.)

Doxorubicin HCl

Drug (in syringe)	Mfr	Amt	Mfr	Amt	Remarks	Ref	C/I
Vincristine sulfate		0.5 mg/ 0.5 mL		1 mg/ 0.5 mL	Physically compatible for 5 min at room temperature followed by 8 min of centrifugation	980	C

[a]Diluted in sodium chloride 0.9%.

Y-Site Injection Compatibility (1:1 Mixture)

Doxorubicin HCl

Drug	Mfr	Conc	Mfr	Conc	Remarks	Ref	C/I
Allopurinol sodium	BW	3 mg/mL[b]	CET	2 mg/mL	Immediate dark red color and haze. Reddish-brown particles within 1 hr	1686	I
Amifostine	USB	10 mg/mL[a]	CET	2 mg/mL	Physically compatible for 4 hr at 23 °C	1845	C
Amphotericin B cholesteryl sulfate complex	SEQ	0.83 mg/mL[a]	CHI	2 mg/mL	Gross precipitate forms	2117	I
Anidulafungin	VIC	0.5 mg/mL[a]	GNS	2 mg/mL[a]	Physically compatible for 4 hr at 23 °C	2617	C
Aztreonam	SQ	40 mg/mL[a]	CET	2 mg/mL	Physically compatible for 4 hr at 23 °C	1758	C
Bleomycin sulfate		3 units/mL		2 mg/mL	Drugs injected sequentially in Y-site with no flush. No precipitate seen	980	C
Caspofungin acetate	ME	0.7 mg/mL[b]	BED	1 mg/mL[b]	Physically compatible for 4 hr at room temperature	2758	C
Cisplatin		1 mg/mL		2 mg/mL	Drugs injected sequentially in Y-site with no flush. No precipitate seen	980	C
Cladribine	ORT	0.015[b] and 0.5[c] mg/mL	CHI	2 mg/mL	Physically compatible for 4 hr at 23 °C	1969	C
Cyclophosphamide		20 mg/mL		2 mg/mL	Drugs injected sequentially in Y-site with no flush. No precipitate seen	980	C
Doripenem	JJ	5 mg/mL[a,b]	BED	1 mg/mL[a,b]	Physically compatible for 4 hr at 23 °C	2743	C
Droperidol		2.5 mg/mL		2 mg/mL	Drugs injected sequentially in Y-site with no flush. No precipitate seen	980	C
Etoposide phosphate	BR	5 mg/mL[a]	GEN	2 mg/mL	Physically compatible for 4 hr at 23 °C	2218	C
Filgrastim	AMG	30 mcg/mL[a]	CET	2 mg/mL	Physically compatible for 4 hr at 22 °C	1687	C
Fludarabine phosphate	BX	1 mg/mL[a]	CET	2 mg/mL	Visually compatible for 4 hr at 22 °C	1439	C
Fluorouracil		50 mg/mL		2 mg/mL	Drugs injected sequentially in Y-site with no flush. No precipitate seen	980	C
Furosemide		10 mg/mL		2 mg/mL	Drugs injected sequentially in Y-site with no flush. Precipitates immediately	980	I
Gallium nitrate	FUJ	1 mg/mL[b]	CET	2 mg/mL	Precipitates immediately	1673	I
Gemcitabine HCl	LI	10 mg/mL[b]	PH	2 mg/mL	Physically compatible for 4 hr at 23 °C	2226	C
Granisetron HCl	SKB	1 mg/mL	AD	0.2 mg/mL[b]	Physically compatible with little loss of either drug in 4 hr at 22 °C	1883	C
Heparin sodium		1000 units/ mL		2 mg/mL	Drugs injected sequentially in Y-site with no flush. Precipitates immediately	980	I
Leucovorin calcium		10 mg/mL		2 mg/mL	Drugs injected sequentially in Y-site with no flush. No precipitate seen	980	C
Linezolid	PHU	2 mg/mL	FUJ	2 mg/mL	Physically compatible for 4 hr at 23 °C	2264	C

Y-Site Injection Compatibility (1:1 Mixture) (Cont.)

Doxorubicin HCl

Drug	Mfr	Conc	Mfr	Conc	Remarks	Ref	C/I
Melphalan HCl	BW	0.1 mg/mL[b]	AD	2 mg/mL	Physically compatible for 3 hr at 22 °C	1557	C
Methotrexate sodium		25 mg/mL		2 mg/mL	Drugs injected sequentially in Y-site with no flush. No precipitate seen	980	C
		30 mg/mL	FA	0.4 mg/mL[a]	Visually compatible for 4 hr at room temperature	1788	C
Metoclopramide HCl		5 mg/mL		2 mg/mL	Drugs injected sequentially in Y-site with no flush. No precipitate seen	980	C
Mitomycin		0.5 mg/mL		2 mg/mL	Drugs injected sequentially in Y-site with no flush. No precipitate seen	980	C
Ondansetron HCl	GL	1 mg/mL[b]	CET	2 mg/mL	Visually compatible for 4 hr at 22 °C	1365	C
	GL	16 to 160 mcg/mL		2 mg/mL	Physically compatible when doxorubicin given as 5-min bolus via Y-site	1366	C
Oxaliplatin	SS	0.5 mg/mL[a]	APP	1 mg/mL[a]	Physically compatible for 4 hr at 23 °C	2566	C
Paclitaxel	NCI	1.2 mg/mL[a]		2 mg/mL	Physically compatible for 4 hr at 22 °C	1528	C
Pemetrexed disodium	LI	20 mg/mL[b]	BED	1 mg/mL[a]	Dark-red discoloration forms immediately	2564	I
Piperacillin sodium–tazobactam sodium	LE[f]	40 + 5 mg/mL[a]	CET	2 mg/mL	Turbidity forms immediately	1688	I
Sargramostim	IMM	10 mcg/mL[b]	CET	2 mg/mL	Visually compatible for 4 hr at 22 °C	1436	C
Sodium bicarbonate		1.4%	FA	0.4 mg/mL[a]	Visually compatible for 2 hr at room temperature	1788	C
Teniposide	BR	0.1 mg/mL[a]	CET	2 mg/mL	Physically compatible for 4 hr at 23 °C	1725	C
Thiotepa	IMM[d]	1 mg/mL[a]	CHI	2 mg/mL	Physically compatible for 4 hr at 23 °C	1861	C
TNA #218 to #226[e]			PH, GEN	2 mg/mL	Damage to emulsion occurs immediately with free oil formation possible	2215	I
Topotecan HCl	SKB	56 mcg/mL[a,b]	PH	2 mg/mL	Visually compatible. Little loss of either drug in 4 hr at 22 °C	2245	C
TPN #212 to #215[e]			PH	2 mg/mL	Substantial loss of natural subvisible haze occurs immediately	2109	I
Vinblastine sulfate		1 mg/mL		2 mg/mL	Drugs injected sequentially in Y-site with no flush. No precipitate seen	980	C
Vincristine sulfate		1 mg/mL		2 mg/mL	Drugs injected sequentially in Y-site with no flush. No precipitate seen	980	C
Vinorelbine tartrate	BW	1 mg/mL[b]	CET	2 mg/mL	Physically compatible for 4 hr at 22 °C	1558	C

[a]Tested in dextrose 5%.
[b]Tested in sodium chloride 0.9%.
[c]Tested in bacteriostatic sodium chloride 0.9% preserved with benzyl alcohol 0.9%.
[d]Lyophilized formulation tested.
[e]Refer to Appendix I for the composition of parenteral nutrition solutions. TNA indicates a 3-in-1 admixture, and TPN indicates a 2-in-1 admixture.
[f]Test performed using the formulation WITHOUT edetate disodium.

DOXORUBICIN HYDROCHLORIDE LIPOSOMAL
AHFS 10:00

Products — Doxorubicin hydrochloride liposomal is available as a red translucent liposomal dispersion providing 2 mg/mL of doxorubicin hydrochloride packaged in vials containing 20 and 50 mg of drug. (1)

Over 90% of the doxorubicin hydrochloride is provided inside liposome carriers composed of *N*-(carbonyl-methoxypolyethylene glycol 2000)-1,2-distearoyl-*sn*-glycero-3-phosphoethanolamine sodium, 3.19 mg/mL; fully hydrogenated soy phosphatidylcholine, 9.58 mg/mL; and cholesterol, 3.19 mg/mL. The product also contains about 2 mg/mL of ammonium sulfate, histidine as a buffer, hydrochloric acid and/or sodium hydroxide to adjust pH, and sucrose to adjust tonicity. (1)

Trade Name(s) — Doxil.

Administration — Doxorubicin hydrochloride liposomal is administered intravenously after dilution in dextrose 5%. Doses of 90 mg or less should be diluted in 250 mL, while doses exceeding 90 mg should be diluted in 500 mL of dextrose 5%. The product should not be administered as a bolus injection, as the undiluted dispersion, as a rapid infusion, or by other routes. Extravasation should be avoided; the drug is extremely irritating to tissues. The use of protective gloves during dose preparation is recommended. (1)

The functional properties of a drug incorporated into a liposomal dispersion like this one may differ substantially from the functional properties of the conventional aqueous formulation. (1) CAUTION: Care should be taken to ensure that the correct drug product, dose, and administration procedures are used and that no confusion with other products occurs.

Stability — Intact vials of doxorubicin hydrochloride liposomal should be stored under refrigeration at 2 to 8 °C. After dilution in dextrose 5% for administration, the drug should be stored under refrigeration and administered within 24 hours after preparation. Freezing should be avoided because prolonged freezing may adversely affect liposomal products. However, short-term freezing (less than one month) did not adversely affect this product. (1)

Doxorubicin hydrochloride liposomal 0.15 mg/mL in dextrose 5% did not result in the loss of viability of *Staphylococcus aureus*, *Enterococcus faecium*, *Pseudomonas aeruginosa*, and *Candida albicans* within 120 hours at 22 °C. Diluted solutions should be stored under refrigeration whenever possible, and the potential for microbiological growth should be considered when assigning expiration periods. (2740)

Filtration — Doxorubicin hydrochloride liposomal is a liposomal dispersion; filtration, including inline filtration, should not be performed. (1)

Compatibility Information

Solution Compatibility

Doxorubicin HCl liposomal

Solution	Mfr	Mfr	Conc/L	Remarks	Ref	C/I
Dextrose 5%				Store at 4 °C and use within 24 hr	1	C

Y-Site Injection Compatibility (1:1 Mixture)

Doxorubicin HCl liposomal

Drug	Mfr	Conc	Mfr	Conc	Remarks	Ref	C/I
Acyclovir sodium	GW	7 mg/mL[a]	SEQ	0.4 mg/mL[a]	Physically compatible for 4 hr at 23 °C	2087	C
Allopurinol sodium	BW	3 mg/mL[a]	SEQ	0.4 mg/mL[a]	Physically compatible for 4 hr at 23 °C	2087	C
Aminophylline	AB	2.5 mg/mL[a]	SEQ	0.4 mg/mL[a]	Physically compatible for 4 hr at 23 °C	2087	C
Amphotericin B	APC	0.6 mg/mL[a]	SEQ	0.4 mg/mL[a]	Fivefold increase in measured particulates in 4 hr	2087	I
Amphotericin B cholesteryl sulfate complex	SEQ	0.83 mg/mL[a]	SEQ	2 mg/mL[a]	Gross precipitate forms	2117	I
Ampicillin sodium	SKB	20 mg/mL[b]	SEQ	0.4 mg/mL[a]	Physically compatible for 4 hr at 23 °C	2087	C
Aztreonam	SQ	40 mg/mL[a]	SEQ	0.4 mg/mL[a]	Physically compatible for 4 hr at 23 °C	2087	C
Bleomycin sulfate	MJ	1 unit/mL[b]	SEQ	0.4 mg/mL[a]	Physically compatible for 4 hr at 23 °C	2087	C
Buprenorphine HCl	RKC	0.04 mg/mL[a]	SEQ	0.4 mg/mL[a]	Partial loss of measured natural turbidity	2087	I
Butorphanol tartrate	APC	0.04 mg/mL[a]	SEQ	0.4 mg/mL[a]	Physically compatible for 4 hr at 23 °C	2087	C
Calcium gluconate	AB	40 mg/mL[a]	SEQ	0.4 mg/mL[a]	Physically compatible for 4 hr at 23 °C	2087	C
Carboplatin	BR	5 mg/mL[a]	SEQ	0.4 mg/mL[a]	Physically compatible for 4 hr at 23 °C	2087	C

Y-Site Injection Compatibility (1:1 Mixture) (Cont.)

Doxorubicin HCl liposomal

Drug	Mfr	Conc	Mfr	Conc	Remarks	Ref	C/I
Cefazolin sodium	SKB	20 mg/mL[a]	SEQ	0.4 mg/mL[a]	Physically compatible for 4 hr at 23 °C	2087	C
Cefepime HCl	BMS	20 mg/mL[a]	SEQ	0.4 mg/mL[a]	Physically compatible for 4 hr at 23 °C	2087	C
Cefoxitin sodium	ME	20 mg/mL[a]	SEQ	0.4 mg/mL[a]	Physically compatible for 4 hr at 23 °C	2087	C
Ceftazidime	SKB	40 mg/mL[a]	SEQ	0.4 mg/mL[a]	Partial loss of measured natural turbidity	2087	I
Ceftriaxone sodium	RC	20 mg/mL[a]	SEQ	0.4 mg/mL[a]	Physically compatible for 4 hr at 23 °C	2087	C
Chlorpromazine HCl	ES	2 mg/mL[a]	SEQ	0.4 mg/mL[a]	Physically compatible for 4 hr at 23 °C	2087	C
Ciprofloxacin	BAY	1 mg/mL[a]	SEQ	0.4 mg/mL[a]	Physically compatible for 4 hr at 23 °C	2087	C
Cisplatin	BR	1 mg/mL	SEQ	0.4 mg/mL[a]	Physically compatible for 4 hr at 23 °C	2087	C
Clindamycin phosphate	AST	10 mg/mL[a]	SEQ	0.4 mg/mL[a]	Physically compatible for 4 hr at 23 °C	2087	C
Cyclophosphamide	MJ	10 mg/mL[a]	SEQ	0.4 mg/mL[a]	Physically compatible for 4 hr at 23 °C	2087	C
Cytarabine	CHI	50 mg/mL	SEQ	0.4 mg/mL[a]	Physically compatible for 4 hr at 23 °C	2087	C
Dacarbazine	MI	4 mg/mL[a]	SEQ	0.4 mg/mL[a]	Physically compatible for 4 hr at 23 °C	2087	C
Dexamethasone sodium phosphate	ES	2 mg/mL[a]	SEQ	0.4 mg/mL[a]	Physically compatible for 4 hr at 23 °C	2087	C
Diphenhydramine HCl	SCN	2 mg/mL[a]	SEQ	0.4 mg/mL[a]	Physically compatible for 4 hr at 23 °C	2087	C
Dobutamine HCl	BA	4 mg/mL[a]	SEQ	0.4 mg/mL[a]	Physically compatible for 4 hr at 23 °C	2087	C
Docetaxel	RPR	2 mg/mL[a]	SEQ	0.4 mg/mL[a]	Partial loss of measured natural turbidity	2087	I
Dopamine HCl	AB	3.2 mg/mL[a]	SEQ	0.4 mg/mL[a]	Physically compatible for 4 hr at 23 °C	2087	C
Droperidol	AST	0.4 mg/mL[a]	SEQ	0.4 mg/mL[a]	Physically compatible for 4 hr at 23 °C	2087	C
Enalaprilat	MSD	0.1 mg/mL[a]	SEQ	0.4 mg/mL[a]	Physically compatible for 4 hr at 23 °C	2087	C
Etoposide	BR	0.4 mg/mL[a]	SEQ	0.4 mg/mL[a]	Physically compatible for 4 hr at 23 °C	2087	C
Famotidine	ME	2 mg/mL[a]	SEQ	0.4 mg/mL[a]	Physically compatible for 4 hr at 23 °C	2087	C
Fluconazole	RR	2 mg/mL	SEQ	0.4 mg/mL[a]	Physically compatible for 4 hr at 23 °C	2087	C
Fluorouracil	PH	16 mg/mL[a]	SEQ	0.4 mg/mL[a]	Physically compatible for 4 hr at 23 °C	2087	C
Furosemide	AMR	3 mg/mL[a]	SEQ	0.4 mg/mL[a]	Physically compatible for 4 hr at 23 °C	2087	C
Ganciclovir sodium	RC	20 mg/mL[a]	SEQ	0.4 mg/mL[a]	Physically compatible for 4 hr at 23 °C	2087	C
Gentamicin sulfate	ES	5 mg/mL[a]	SEQ	0.4 mg/mL[a]	Physically compatible for 4 hr at 23 °C	2087	C
Granisetron HCl	SKB	0.05 mg/mL[a]	SEQ	0.4 mg/mL[a]	Physically compatible for 4 hr at 23 °C	2087	C
Haloperidol lactate	MN	0.2 mg/mL[a]	SEQ	0.4 mg/mL[a]	Physically compatible for 4 hr at 23 °C	2087	C
Heparin sodium	ES	1000 units/mL[a]	SEQ	0.4 mg/mL[a]	Physically compatible for 4 hr at 23 °C	2087	C
Hydrocortisone sodium succinate	AB	1 mg/mL[a]	SEQ	0.4 mg/mL[a]	Physically compatible for 4 hr at 23 °C	2087	C
Hydromorphone HCl	ES	0.5 mg/mL[a]	SEQ	0.4 mg/mL[a]	Physically compatible for 4 hr at 23 °C	2087	C
Hydroxyzine HCl	ES	2 mg/mL[a]	SEQ	0.4 mg/mL[a]	10-fold increase in particles ≥10 μm in 4 hr	2087	I
Ifosfamide	MJ	25 mg/mL[a]	SEQ	0.4 mg/mL[a]	Physically compatible for 4 hr at 23 °C	2087	C
Leucovorin calcium	IMM	2 mg/mL[a]	SEQ	0.4 mg/mL[a]	Physically compatible for 4 hr at 23 °C	2087	C
Lorazepam	WY	0.1 mg/mL[a]	SEQ	0.4 mg/mL[a]	Physically compatible for 4 hr at 23 °C	2087	C
Magnesium sulfate	AST	100 mg/mL[a]	SEQ	0.4 mg/mL[a]	Physically compatible for 4 hr at 23 °C	2087	C
Mannitol	BA	15%	SEQ	0.4 mg/mL[a]	Partial loss of measured natural turbidity	2087	I

Y-Site Injection Compatibility (1:1 Mixture) (Cont.)

Doxorubicin HCl liposomal

Drug	Mfr	Conc	Mfr	Conc	Remarks	Ref	C/I
Meperidine HCl	AST	4 mg/mL[a]	SEQ	0.4 mg/mL[a]	Increase in measured turbidity	2087	I
Mesna	MJ	10 mg/mL[a]	SEQ	0.4 mg/mL[a]	Physically compatible for 4 hr at 23 °C	2087	C
Methotrexate sodium	IMM	15 mg/mL[a]	SEQ	0.4 mg/mL[a]	Physically compatible for 4 hr at 23 °C	2087	C
Methylprednisolone sodium succinate	UP	5 mg/mL[a]	SEQ	0.4 mg/mL[a]	Physically compatible for 4 hr at 23 °C	2087	C
Metoclopramide HCl	GNS	5 mg/mL	SEQ	0.4 mg/mL[a]	Increase in measured turbidity	2087	I
Metronidazole	AB	5 mg/mL	SEQ	0.4 mg/mL[a]	Physically compatible for 4 hr at 23 °C	2087	C
Mitoxantrone HCl	IMM	0.5 mg/mL[a]	SEQ	0.4 mg/mL[a]	Partial loss of measured natural turbidity	2087	I
Morphine sulfate	ES	1 mg/mL[a]	SEQ	0.4 mg/mL[a]	Partial loss of measured natural turbidity	2087	I
Ondansetron HCl	CER	1 mg/mL[a]	SEQ	0.4 mg/mL[a]	Physically compatible for 4 hr at 23 °C	2087	C
Paclitaxel	MJ	0.6 mg/mL[a]	SEQ	0.4 mg/mL[a]	Partial loss of measured natural turbidity	2087	I
Piperacillin sodium–tazobactam sodium	CY[c]	40 + 5 mg/mL[a]	SEQ	0.4 mg/mL[a]	Partial loss of measured natural turbidity	2087	I
Potassium chloride	AB	0.1 mEq/mL[a]	SEQ	0.4 mg/mL[a]	Physically compatible for 4 hr at 23 °C	2087	C
Prochlorperazine edisylate	SO	0.5 mg/mL[a]	SEQ	0.4 mg/mL[a]	Physically compatible for 4 hr at 23 °C	2087	C
Promethazine HCl	ES	2 mg/mL[a]	SEQ	0.4 mg/mL[a]	Increase in measured turbidity	2087	I
Ranitidine HCl	GL	2 mg/mL[a]	SEQ	0.4 mg/mL[a]	Physically compatible for 4 hr at 23 °C	2087	C
Sodium bicarbonate	AB	1 mEq/mL	SEQ	0.4 mg/mL[a]	Partial loss of measured natural turbidity	2087	I
Ticarcillin disodium–clavulanate potassium	SKB	31 mg/mL[a]	SEQ	0.4 mg/mL[a]	Physically compatible for 4 hr at 23 °C	2087	C
Tobramycin sulfate	AB	5 mg/mL[a]	SEQ	0.4 mg/mL[a]	Physically compatible for 4 hr at 23 °C	2087	C
Trimethoprim–sulfamethoxazole	ES	0.8 + 4 mg/mL[a]	SEQ	0.4 mg/mL[a]	Physically compatible for 4 hr at 23 °C	2087	C
Vancomycin HCl	AB	10 mg/mL[a]	SEQ	0.4 mg/mL[a]	Physically compatible for 4 hr at 23 °C	2087	C
Vinblastine sulfate	FAU	0.12 mg/mL[a]	SEQ	0.4 mg/mL[a]	Physically compatible for 4 hr at 23 °C	2087	C
Vincristine sulfate	FAU	0.05 mg/mL[a]	SEQ	0.4 mg/mL[a]	Physically compatible for 4 hr at 23 °C	2087	C
Vinorelbine tartrate	BW	1 mg/mL[a]	SEQ	0.4 mg/mL[a]	Physically compatible for 4 hr at 23 °C	2087	C
Zidovudine	BW	4 mg/mL[a]	SEQ	0.4 mg/mL[a]	Physically compatible for 4 hr at 23 °C	2087	C

[a]Tested in dextrose 5%.
[b]Tested in sodium chloride 0.9%.
[c]Test performed using the formulation WITHOUT edetate disodium.

DOXYCYCLINE HYCLATE
AHFS 8:12.24

Products — Doxycycline hyclate (doxycycline hydrochloride hemiethanolate hemihydrate) is available in vials containing the equivalent of 100 mg of doxycycline with 480 mg of ascorbic acid, respectively. Mannitol is also present in products from some manufacturers. (1; 4)

Reconstitute the 100-mg vial with 10 mL of sterile water for injection or other compatible diluent. The resultant solution contains the equivalent of 10 mg/mL of doxycycline. This solution must be further diluted to a concentration of 0.1 to 1 mg/mL with a compatible infusion solution prior to use. (1; 4)

pH — The pH range for reconstituted solutions is 1.8 to 3.3. (4)

Osmolality — The osmolality of doxycycline hyclate (Elkins-Sinn) 1 mg/mL was determined to be 292 mOsm/kg in dextrose 5% and 310 mOsm/kg in sodium chloride 0.9%. (1375)

Administration — Doxycycline hyclate is administered by slow intravenous infusion, usually over one to four hours; rapid administration should be avoided. The reconstituted solution should be diluted further with a compatible infusion solution to a concentration of approximately 0.1 to 1 mg/mL. Other parenteral routes are not recommended, and extravasation should be avoided. (1; 4)

Stability — Store the vials at room temperature and protect from light. Solutions of doxycycline hyclate diluted for infusion must be protected from direct sunlight. (1)

Doxycycline hyclate 0.1- to 1-mg/mL solutions may be stored for up to 72 hours prior to starting the infusion when kept in the refrigerator and protected from both direct sunlight and artificial light in compatible infusion solutions. Infusion must then be completed within 12 hours. (1)

Because of the acidity of the solution, doxycycline hyclate may precipitate the free acids of barbiturate salts and sulfonamide derivatives. It may also adversely affect the stability of acid-labile drugs. (6; 20; 22; 27)

Freezing Solutions — The manufacturers state that at a concentration of 10 mg/mL in sterile water for injection, doxycycline hyclate is stable for eight weeks when frozen at −20 °C. Frozen solutions that have been completely thawed should not be heated. Thawed solutions should not be refrozen. (1; 4)

Doxycycline hyclate (Pfizer) 10 mg/mL in sterile water for injection was stable for eight weeks when frozen at −20 °C. At a concentration of 1 mg/mL in dextrose 5%, doxycycline hyclate also showed no significant decomposition over eight weeks at −20 °C. (310)

Sorption — Doxycycline hyclate was shown not to exhibit sorption to PVC bags and tubing, polyethylene tubing, Silastic tubing, and polypropylene syringes. (536; 606)

Central Venous Catheter — Doxycycline hyclate (Fujisawa) 0.5 mg/mL in dextrose 5% was found to be compatible with the ARROWg+ard Blue Plus (Arrow International) chlorhexidine-bearing triple-lumen central catheter. Essentially complete delivery of the drug was found with little or no drug loss occurring. Furthermore, chlorhexidine delivered from the catheter remained at trace amounts with no substantial increase due to the delivery of the drug through the catheter. (2335)

Compatibility Information

Solution Compatibility

Doxycycline hyclate

Solution	Mfr	Mfr	Conc/L	Remarks	Ref	C/I
Dextrose 5%			0.1 to 1 g	Compatible and stable for 72 hr at 4 °C and 48 hr at 25 °C	1	C
	BA[a]	PF	800 mg and 1 g	Visually compatible with 5 to 8% loss in 96 hr at 23 °C. 2% loss in 7 days at 4 °C	1928	C
Normosol M in dextrose 5%			0.1 to 1 g	Compatible and stable for 72 hr at 4 °C	1	C
Normosol R in dextrose 5%			0.1 to 1 g	Compatible and stable for 72 hr at 4 °C	1	C
Plasma-Lyte 56 in dextrose 5%			0.1 to 1 g	Compatible and stable for 72 hr at 4 °C	1	C
Plasma-Lyte 148 in dextrose 5%			0.1 to 1 g	Compatible and stable for 72 hr at 4 °C	1	C
Ringer's injection			0.1 to 1 g	Compatible and stable for 72 hr at 4 °C	1	C
Sodium chloride 0.9%			0.1 to 1 g	Compatible and stable for 72 hr at 4 °C and 48 hr at 25 °C	1	C
	AB[b]	ES	2 g	5% loss for freshly prepared solutions during 24-hr simulated administration at 30 °C. Stored at 5 °C for 24 hr, then at 30 °C, >5% loss in 6 hr	1779	C
	BA[a]	PF	800 mg and 1 g	Visually compatible with 8% loss in 96 hr at 23 °C. 4% or less loss in 7 days at 4 °C	1928	C

[a] Tested in PVC containers.
[b] Tested in portable pump reservoirs (Pharmacia Deltec).

Additive Compatibility

Doxycycline hyclate

Drug	Mfr	Conc/L	Mfr	Conc/L	Test Soln	Remarks	Ref	C/I
Meropenem	ZEN	1 g	RR	200 mg	NS	Visually compatible for 4 hr at room temperature	1994	C
	ZEN	20 g	RR	200 mg	NS	Brown discoloration forms in 1 hr at room temperature	1994	I
Ranitidine HCl	GL	100 mg	PF	200 mg	D5W	Physically compatible for 24 hr at ambient temperature in light	1151	C

Drugs in Syringe Compatibility

Doxycycline hyclate

Drug (in syringe)	Mfr	Amt	Mfr	Amt	Remarks	Ref	C/I
Doxapram HCl	RB	400 mg/ 20 mL		100 mg/ 5 mL	Physically compatible with 3% doxapram loss in 24 hr	1177	C

Y-Site Injection Compatibility (1:1 Mixture)

Doxycycline hyclate

Drug	Mfr	Conc	Mfr	Conc	Remarks	Ref	C/I
Acyclovir sodium	BW	5 mg/mL[a]	PF	1 mg/mL[a]	Physically compatible for 4 hr at 25 °C	1157	C
Allopurinol sodium	BW	3 mg/mL[b]	ES	1 mg/mL[b]	Immediate brown particles. Hazy brown solution with precipitate in 4 hr	1686	I
Amifostine	USB	10 mg/mL[a]	LY	1 mg/mL[a]	Physically compatible for 4 hr at 23 °C	1845	C
Amiodarone HCl	LZ	4 mg/mL[c]	ACC	0.25 mg/mL[c]	Physically compatible for 4 hr at room temperature	1444	C
Aztreonam	SQ	40 mg/mL[a]	ES	1 mg/mL[a]	Physically compatible for 4 hr at 23 °C	1758	C
Bivalirudin	TMC	5 mg/mL[a]	APP	1 mg/mL[a]	Physically compatible for 4 hr at 23 °C	2373	C
Cisatracurium besylate	GW	0.1, 2, 5 mg/ mL[a]	FUJ	1 mg/mL[a]	Physically compatible for 4 hr at 23 °C	2074	C
Cyclophosphamide	MJ	20 mg/mL[a]	ES	1 mg/mL[a]	Physically compatible for 4 hr at 25 °C	1194	C
Dexmedetomidine HCl	AB	4 mcg/mL[b]	APP	1 mg/mL[b]	Physically compatible for 4 hr at 23 °C	2383	C
Diltiazem HCl	MMD	5 mg/mL	RR	1 and 10 mg/ mL[b]	Visually compatible	1807	C
Docetaxel	RPR	0.9 mg/mL[a]	FUJ	1 mg/mL[a]	Physically compatible for 4 hr at 23 °C	2224	C
Etoposide phosphate	BR	5 mg/mL[a]	FUJ	1 mg/mL[a]	Physically compatible for 4 hr at 23 °C	2218	C
Fenoldopam mesylate	AB	80 mcg/mL[b]	APP	1 mg/mL[b]	Physically compatible for 4 hr at 23 °C	2467	C
Filgrastim	AMG	30 mcg/mL[a]	ES	1 mg/mL[a]	Physically compatible for 4 hr at 22 °C	1687	C
Fludarabine phosphate	BX	1 mg/mL[a]	ES	1 mg/mL[a]	Visually compatible for 4 hr at 22 °C	1439	C
Gemcitabine HCl	LI	10 mg/mL[b]	FUJ	1 mg/mL[b]	Physically compatible for 4 hr at 23 °C	2226	C
Granisetron HCl	SKB	0.05 mg/mL[a]	LY	1 mg/mL[a]	Physically compatible for 4 hr at 23 °C	2000	C
Heparin sodium	TR	50 units/mL	ES	1 mg/mL[a]	Visually incompatible within 4 hr at 25 °C	1793	I
Hetastarch in lactated electrolyte	AB	6%	APP	1 mg/mL[a]	Physically compatible for 4 hr at 23 °C	2339	C

Y-Site Injection Compatibility (1:1 Mixture) (Cont.)

Doxycycline hyclate

Drug	Mfr	Conc	Mfr	Conc	Remarks	Ref	C/I
Hetastarch in sodium chloride 0.9%	DCC	6%	LY	1 mg/mL[a]	Visually compatible for 4 hr at room temperature	1313	C
	DCC	6%	LY	1 mg/mL[a]	White particle in one of five tests. No incompatibility during Y-site infusion	1315	?
Hydromorphone HCl	WY	0.2 mg/mL[a]	ES	1 mg/mL[a]	Physically compatible for 4 hr at 25 °C	987	C
Linezolid	PHU	2 mg/mL	FUJ	1 mg/mL[a]	Physically compatible for 4 hr at 23 °C	2264	C
Magnesium sulfate	IX	16.7, 33.3, 66.7, 100 mg/mL[a]	PF	1 mg/mL[a]	Physically compatible for at least 4 hr at 32 °C	813	C
Melphalan HCl	BW	0.1 mg/mL[b]	LY	1 mg/mL[b]	Physically compatible for 3 hr at 22 °C	1557	C
Meperidine HCl	WY	10 mg/mL[a]	ES	1 mg/mL[a]	Physically compatible for 4 hr at 25 °C	987	C
Meropenem	ZEN	1 mg/mL[b]	RR	1 mg/mL[d]	Visually compatible for 4 hr at room temperature	1994	C
	ZEN	50 mg/mL[b]	RR	1 mg/mL[d]	Amber discoloration forms within 30 min	1994	I
Morphine sulfate	WI	1 mg/mL[a]	ES	1 mg/mL[a]	Physically compatible for 4 hr at 25 °C	987	C
Ondansetron HCl	GL	1 mg/mL[b]	ES	1 mg/mL[a]	Visually compatible for 4 hr at 22 °C	1365	C
Pemetrexed disodium	LI	20 mg/mL[b]	APP	1 mg/mL[a]	Cloudy precipitate forms immediately	2564	I
Piperacillin sodium–tazobactam sodium	LE[j]	40 + 5 mg/mL[a]	ES	1 mg/mL[a]	Heavy white turbidity forms immediately	1688	I
Propofol	ZEN	10 mg/mL	LY	1 mg/mL[a]	Physically compatible for 1 hr at 23 °C	2066	C
Remifentanil HCl	GW	0.025 and 0.25 mg/mL[b]	FUJ	1 mg/mL[a]	Physically compatible for 4 hr at 23 °C	2075	C
Sargramostim	IMM	10 mcg/mL[b]	LY	1 mg/mL[b]	Visually compatible for 4 hr at 22 °C	1436	C
Tacrolimus	FUJ	1 mg/mL[b]	RR	5 mg/mL[a]	Visually compatible for 24 hr at 25 °C	1630	C
Telavancin HCl	ASP	7.5 mg/mL[a,b,k]	APP	1 mg/mL[a,b,k]	Physically compatible for 2 hr	2830	C
Teniposide	BR	0.1 mg/mL[a]	LY	1 mg/mL[a]	Physically compatible for 4 hr at 23 °C	1725	C
Theophylline	TR	4 mg/mL	ES	1 mg/mL[a]	Visually compatible for 6 hr at 25 °C	1793	C
Thiotepa	IMM[e]	1 mg/mL[a]	LY	1 mg/mL[a]	Physically compatible for 4 hr at 23 °C	1861	C
TNA #218 to #226[f]			FUJ	1 mg/mL[a]	Damage to emulsion occurs immediately with free oil formation possible	2215	I
TPN #61[f]		[g]	PF	10 mg/mL[h]	Physically compatible	987	C
		[i]	PF	60 mg/6 mL[h]	Physically compatible	987	C
TPN #212 to #215[f]			LY	1 mg/mL[a]	Physically compatible for 4 hr at 23 °C	2109	C
Vinorelbine tartrate	BW	1 mg/mL[b]	ES	1 mg/mL[b]	Physically compatible for 4 hr at 22 °C	1558	C

[a]Tested in dextrose 5%.
[b]Tested in sodium chloride 0.9%.
[c]Tested in both dextrose 5% and sodium chloride 0.9%.
[d]Tested in sterile water for injection.
[e]Lyophilized formulation tested.
[f]Refer to Appendix I for the composition of parenteral nutrition solutions. TNA indicates a 3-in-1 admixture, and TPN indicates a 2-in-1 admixture.
[g]Run at 21 mL/hr.
[h]Given over 30 minutes by syringe pump.
[i]Run at 94 mL/hr.
[j]Test performed using the formulation WITHOUT edetate disodium.
[k]Tested in Ringer's injection, lactated.

DROPERIDOL
AHFS 28:24.92

Products — Droperidol is available from various manufacturers in 1- and 2-mL ampuls and 1- and 2-mL vials. Each milliliter of solution contains droperidol 2.5 mg with lactic acid to adjust the pH. (1)

pH — From 3 to 3.8. (1)

Osmolality — The osmolality of droperidol 2.5 mg/mL was determined to be 16 mOsm/kg. (1233)

Administration — Droperidol may be administered intramuscularly or slowly intravenously. Intravenous infusion has been used in high-risk patients. (1)

Stability — Intact ampuls and vials of droperidol should be stored at controlled room temperature and protected from light. (1)

Precipitation may occur if droperidol is mixed with barbiturates. (4)

Syringes — The stability of droperidol 2.5 mg/mL repackaged in polypropylene syringes was evaluated. Little change in concentration was found after four weeks at room temperature out of direct light. (2164)

Central Venous Catheter — Droperidol (Abbott) 0.4 mg/mL in dextrose 5% was found to be compatible with the ARROWg+ard Blue Plus (Arrow International) chlorhexidine-bearing triple-lumen central catheter. Essentially complete delivery of the drug was found with little or no drug loss occurring. Furthermore, chlorhexidine delivered from the catheter remained at trace amounts with no substantial increase due to the delivery of the drug through the catheter. (2335)

Compatibility Information

Solution Compatibility

Droperidol

Solution	Mfr	Mfr	Conc/L	Remarks	Ref	C/I
Dextrose 5%	AB[a], TR[b]	JN	20 mg	Physically compatible and stable for 7 days at 27 °C	750	C
Ringer's injection, lactated	TR[a]	JN	20 mg	Physically compatible and stable for 7 days at 27 °C	750	C
	TR[b]	JN	20 mg	Physically compatible. Stable with no loss for 24 hr at 27 °C. 15% loss in 48 hr attributed to sorption	750	C
Sodium chloride 0.9%	AB[a]	JN	20 mg	Physically compatible with about 5% drug loss in 7 days at 27 °C	750	C
	TR[b]	JN	20 mg	Physically compatible and stable for 7 days at 27 °C	750	C
	[c]	AMR	1.25 g	Compatible and stable for 24 hr at 23 °C. Droperidol precipitates if refrigerated	2199	C

[a]Tested in glass containers.
[b]Tested in PVC containers.
[c]Tested in polypropylene syringes.

Additive Compatibility

Droperidol

Drug	Mfr	Conc/L	Mfr	Conc/L	Test Soln	Remarks	Ref	C/I
Fentanyl citrate with ketamine HCl	DB JN	10 mg 1 g	JN	50 mg	NS[a]	Visually compatible. 5% increase in all drugs in 30 days at 4 and 25 °C due to water loss	2653	C
Fentanyl citrate with ketamine HCl	DB JN	10 mg 1 g	JN	50 mg	NS[b]	Visually compatible with little loss of the drugs in 30 days at 25 °C	2653	C
Ketamine HCl with fentanyl citrate	JN DB	1 g 10 mg	JN	50 mg	NS[a]	Visually compatible. 5% increase in all drugs in 30 days at 4 and 25 °C due to water loss	2653	C
Ketamine HCl with fentanyl citrate	JN DB	1 g 10 mg	JN	50 mg	NS[b]	Visually compatible with little loss of the drugs in 30 days at 25 °C	2653	C

[a]Tested in PVC containers.
[b]Tested in glass containers.

Drugs in Syringe Compatibility

Droperidol

Drug (in syringe)	Mfr	Amt	Mfr	Amt	Remarks	Ref	C/I
Atropine sulfate	ST	0.4 mg/ 1 mL	MN	2.5 mg/ 1 mL	Physically compatible for at least 15 min	326	C
Bleomycin sulfate		1.5 units/ 0.5 mL		1.25 mg/ 0.5 mL	Physically compatible for 5 min at room temperature followed by 8 min of centrifugation	980	C
Buprenorphine HCl					Physically and chemically compatible	4	C
Butorphanol tartrate	BR	4 mg/ 2 mL	MN	5 mg/ 2 mL	Physically compatible for 30 min at room temperature	566	C
Chlorpromazine HCl	PO	50 mg/ 2 mL	MN	2.5 mg/ 1 mL	Physically compatible for at least 15 min	326	C
Cisplatin		0.5 mg/ 0.5 mL		1.25 mg/ 0.5 mL	Physically compatible for 5 min at room temperature followed by 8 min of centrifugation	980	C
Cyclophosphamide		10 mg/ 0.5 mL		1.25 mg/ 0.5 mL	Physically compatible for 5 min at room temperature followed by 8 min of centrifugation	980	C
Dimenhydrinate	HR	50 mg/ 1 mL	MN	2.5 mg/ 1 mL	Physically compatible for at least 15 min	326	C
Diphenhydramine HCl	PD	50 mg/ 1 mL	MN	2.5 mg/ 1 mL	Physically compatible for at least 15 min	326	C
Doxorubicin HCl		1 mg/ 0.5 mL		1.25 mg/ 0.5 mL	Physically compatible for 5 min at room temperature followed by 8 min of centrifugation	980	C
Fentanyl citrate	MN	0.05 mg/ 1 mL	MN	2.5 mg/ 1 mL	Physically compatible for at least 15 min	326	C
Fluorouracil		25 mg/ 0.5 mL		1.25 mg/ 0.5 mL	Precipitates immediately	980	I
Furosemide		5 mg/ 0.5 mL		1.25 mg/ 0.5 mL	Precipitates immediately	980	I
Glycopyrrolate	RB	0.2 mg/ 1 mL	MN	2.5 mg/ 1 mL	Physically compatible. pH in glycopyrrolate stability range for 48 hr at 25 °C	331	C
	RB	0.2 mg/ 1 mL	MN	5 mg/ 2 mL	Physically compatible. pH in glycopyrrolate stability range for 48 hr at 25 °C	331	C
	RB	0.4 mg/ 2 mL	MN	2.5 mg/ 1 mL	Physically compatible. pH in glycopyrrolate stability range for 48 hr at 25 °C	331	C
Heparin sodium		500 units/ 0.5 mL		1.25 mg/ 0.5 mL	Precipitates immediately	980	I
		2500 units/ 1 mL	JN	5 mg/ 2 mL	Turbidity or precipitate forms within 5 min	1053	I
Hydroxyzine HCl	PF	50 mg/ 1 mL	MN	2.5 mg/ 1 mL	Physically compatible for at least 15 min	326	C
Leucovorin calcium		5 mg/ 0.5 mL		1.25 mg/ 0.5 mL	Precipitates immediately	980	I
Meperidine HCl	WI	50 mg/ 1 mL	MN	2.5 mg/ 1 mL	Physically compatible for at least 15 min	326	C
Methotrexate sodium		12.5 mg/ 0.5 mL		1.25 mg/ 0.5 mL	Precipitates immediately	980	I
Metoclopramide HCl	NO	10 mg/ 2 mL	MN	2.5 mg/ 1 mL	Physically compatible for 15 min at room temperature	565	C

Drugs in Syringe Compatibility (Cont.)

Droperidol

Drug (in syringe)	Mfr	Amt	Mfr	Amt	Remarks	Ref	C/I
		2.5 mg/ 0.5 mL		1.25 mg/ 0.5 mL	Physically compatible for 5 min at room temperature followed by 8 min of centrifugation	980	C
Midazolam HCl	RC	5 mg/ 1 mL	JN	2.5 mg/ 1 mL	Physically compatible for 4 hr at 25 °C	1145	C
Mitomycin		0.25 mg/ 0.5 mL		1.25 mg/ 0.5 mL	Physically compatible for 5 min at room temperature followed by 8 min of centrifugation	980	C
Morphine sulfate	ST	15 mg/ 1 mL	MN	2.5 mg/ 1 mL	Physically compatible for at least 15 min	326	C
Nalbuphine HCl	EN	5 mg/ 0.5 mL	JN	5 mg/ 2 mL	Physically compatible for 36 hr at 27 °C	762	C
	EN	10 mg/ 1 mL	JN	2.5 mg/ 1 mL	Physically compatible for 36 hr at 27 °C	762	C
	EN	5 mg/ 0.5 mL	JN	2.5 mg/ 1 mL	Physically compatible for 36 hr at 27 °C	762	C
	DU	10 mg/ 1 mL	JN	5 mg/ 2 mL	Physically compatible for 48 hr	128	C
	DU	20 mg/ 1 mL	JN	5 mg/ 2 mL	Physically compatible for 48 hr	128	C
Ondansetron HCl	GW	1 mg/mL[a]	AMR	1.25 mg/ mL[a]	Droperidol precipitates at 4 °C. At 23 °C, little or no loss of either drug in 8 hr, but droperidol precipitates after that time	2199	I
Pentazocine lactate	WI	30 mg/ 1 mL	MN	2.5 mg/ 1 mL	Physically compatible for at least 15 min	326	C
Pentobarbital sodium	AB	50 mg/ 1 mL	MN	2.5 mg/ 1 mL	Physically incompatible within 15 min	326	I
Prochlorperazine edisylate	PO	5 mg/ 1 mL	MN	2.5 mg/ 1 mL	Physically compatible for at least 15 min	326	C
Promethazine HCl	PO	50 mg/ 2 mL	MN	2.5 mg/ 1 mL	Physically compatible for at least 15 min	326	C
Scopolamine HBr	ST	0.4 mg/ 1 mL	MN	2.5 mg/ 1 mL	Physically compatible for at least 15 min	326	C
Vinblastine sulfate		0.5 mg/ 0.5 mL		1.25 mg/ 0.5 mL	Physically compatible for 5 min at room temperature followed by 8 min of centrifugation	980	C
Vincristine sulfate		0.5 mg/ 0.5 mL		1.25 mg/ 0.5 mL	Physically compatible for 5 min at room temperature followed by 8 min of centrifugation	980	C

[a]Tested in sodium chloride 0.9%.

Y-Site Injection Compatibility (1:1 Mixture)

Droperidol

Drug	Mfr	Conc	Mfr	Conc	Remarks	Ref	C/I
Acyclovir sodium	BV	5 mg/mL[b]	MDX	2.5 mg/mL	Physically compatible	2794	C
Allopurinol sodium	BW	3 mg/mL[b]	JN	0.4 mg/mL[b]	Immediate turbidity with particles	1686	I
Amifostine	USB	10 mg/mL[a]	JN	0.4 mg/mL[a]	Physically compatible for 4 hr at 23 °C	1845	C
Amphotericin B cholesteryl sulfate complex	SEQ	0.83 mg/mL[a]	AST	2.5 mg/mL	Gross precipitate forms	2117	I

Y-Site Injection Compatibility (1:1 Mixture) (Cont.)

Droperidol

Drug	Mfr	Conc	Mfr	Conc	Remarks	Ref	C/I
Azithromycin	PF	2 mg/mL[b]	AMR	2.5 mg/mL[i]	Visually compatible	2368	**C**
Aztreonam	SQ	40 mg/mL[a]	JN	0.4 mg/mL[a]	Physically compatible for 4 hr at 23 °C	1758	**C**
Bivalirudin	TMC	5 mg/mL[a]	AMR	2.5 mg/mL	Physically compatible for 4 hr at 23 °C	2373	**C**
Bleomycin sulfate		3 units/mL		2.5 mg/mL	Drugs injected sequentially in Y-site with no flush. No precipitate seen	980	**C**
Cisatracurium besylate	GW	0.1, 2, 5 mg/mL[a]	AB	2.5 mg/mL	Physically compatible for 4 hr at 23 °C	2074	**C**
Cisplatin		1 mg/mL		2.5 mg/mL	Drugs injected sequentially in Y-site with no flush. No precipitate seen	980	**C**
Cladribine	ORT	0.015[b] and 0.5[c] mg/mL	JN	0.4 mg/mL[b]	Physically compatible for 4 hr at 23 °C	1969	**C**
Cyclophosphamide		20 mg/mL		2.5 mg/mL	Drugs injected sequentially in Y-site with no flush. No precipitate seen	980	**C**
Dexmedetomidine HCl	AB	4 mcg/mL[b]	AMR	2.5 mg/mL	Physically compatible for 4 hr at 23 °C	2383	**C**
Docetaxel	RPR	0.9 mg/mL[a]	AST	0.4 mg/mL[a]	Physically compatible for 4 hr at 23 °C	2224	**C**
Doxorubicin HCl		2 mg/mL		2.5 mg/mL	Drugs injected sequentially in Y-site with no flush. No precipitate seen	980	**C**
Doxorubicin HCl liposomal	SEQ	0.4 mg/mL[a]	AST	0.4 mg/mL[a]	Physically compatible for 4 hr at 23 °C	2087	**C**
Etoposide phosphate	BR	5 mg/mL[a]	AST	0.4 mg/mL[a]	Physically compatible for 4 hr at 23 °C	2218	**C**
Famotidine	ME	2 mg/mL[b]		0.4 mg/mL[a]	Visually compatible for 4 hr at 22 °C	1936	**C**
Fenoldopam mesylate	AB	80 mcg/mL[b]	AB	2.5 mg/mL	Physically compatible for 4 hr at 23 °C	2467	**C**
Filgrastim	AMG	30 mcg/mL[a]	JN	0.4 mg/mL[a]	Physically compatible for 4 hr at 22 °C	1687	**C**
Fluconazole	RR	2 mg/mL	DU	2.5 mg/mL	Physically compatible for 24 hr at 25 °C	1407	**C**
Fludarabine phosphate	BX	1 mg/mL[a]	JN	0.4 mg/mL[a]	Visually compatible for 4 hr at 22 °C	1439	**C**
Fluorouracil		50 mg/mL		2.5 mg/mL	Drugs injected sequentially in Y-site with no flush. Precipitates immediately	980	**I**
Foscarnet sodium	AST	24 mg/mL	QU	2.5 mg/mL	Delayed formation of yellow precipitate	1335	**I**
Furosemide		10 mg/mL		2.5 mg/mL	Drugs injected sequentially in Y-site with no flush. Precipitates immediately	980	**I**
		10 mg/mL		2.5 mg/mL	Precipitate forms	977	**I**
Gemcitabine HCl	LI	10 mg/mL[b]	AST	0.4 mg/mL[b]	Physically compatible for 4 hr at 23 °C	2226	**C**
Granisetron HCl	SKB	0.05 mg/mL[a]	AB	0.4 mg/mL[a]	Physically compatible for 4 hr at 23 °C	2000	**C**
Heparin sodium		1000 units/mL		2.5 mg/mL	Drugs injected sequentially in Y-site with no flush. Precipitates immediately	980	**I**
	UP	1000 units/L[e]	CR	1.25 mg/mL	Physically compatible for 4 hr at room temperature	534	**C**
Hetastarch in lactated electrolyte	AB	6%	AMR	2.5 mg/mL	Physically compatible for 4 hr at 23 °C	2339	**C**
Hydrocortisone sodium succinate	UP	10 mg/L[e]	CR	1.25 mg/mL	Physically compatible for 4 hr at room temperature	534	**C**
Idarubicin HCl	AD	1 mg/mL[b]	AMR	0.04[a] and 2.5 mg/mL	Visually compatible for 24 hr at 25 °C	1525	**C**
Leucovorin calcium		10 mg/mL		2.5 mg/mL	Drugs injected sequentially in Y-site with no flush. Precipitates immediately	980	**I**

Y-Site Injection Compatibility (1:1 Mixture) (Cont.)

Droperidol

Drug	Mfr	Conc	Mfr	Conc	Remarks	Ref	C/I
Linezolid	PHU	2 mg/mL	AMR	0.4 mg/mL[a]	Physically compatible for 4 hr at 23 °C	2264	C
Melphalan HCl	BW	0.1 mg/mL[b]	JN	0.4 mg/mL[b]	Physically compatible for 3 hr at 22 °C	1557	C
Meperidine HCl	AB	10 mg/mL	AMR	2.5 mg/mL	Physically compatible for 4 hr at 25 °C	1397	C
Methotrexate sodium		25 mg/mL		2.5 mg/mL	Precipitate forms	977	I
		25 mg/mL		2.5 mg/mL	Drugs injected sequentially in Y-site with no flush. Precipitates immediately	980	I
Metoclopramide HCl		5 mg/mL		2.5 mg/mL	Drugs injected sequentially in Y-site with no flush. No precipitate seen	980	C
Mitomycin		0.5 mg/mL		2.5 mg/mL	Drugs injected sequentially in Y-site with no flush. No precipitate seen	980	C
Nafcillin sodium	WY	33 mg/mL[b]		2.5 mg/mL	Precipitate forms, probably free nafcillin	547	I
Ondansetron HCl	GL	1 mg/mL[b]	JN	0.4 mg/mL[a]	Visually compatible for 4 hr at 22 °C	1365	C
Oxaliplatin	SS	0.5 mg/mL[a]	AB	2.5 mg/mL	Physically compatible for 4 hr at 23 °C	2566	C
Paclitaxel	NCI	1.2 mg/mL[a]	JN	0.4 mg/mL[a]	Physically compatible for 4 hr at 22 °C	1556	C
Pemetrexed disodium	LI	20 mg/mL[b]	AB	2.5 mg/mL	Gross white precipitate forms immediately	2564	I
Piperacillin sodium–tazobactam sodium	LE[f]	40 + 5 mg/mL[a]	JN	0.4 mg/mL[a]	Heavy white turbidity with white precipitate forms immediately	1688	I
Potassium chloride	AB	40 mEq/L[e]	CR	1.25 mg/mL	Physically compatible for 4 hr at room temperature	534	C
Propofol	ZEN	10 mg/mL	JN	0.4 mg/mL[a]	Physically compatible for 1 hr at 23 °C	2066	C
Remifentanil HCl	GW	0.025 and 0.25 mg/mL[b]	AST	2.5 mg/mL	Physically compatible for 4 hr at 23 °C	2075	C
Sargramostim	IMM	10 mcg/mL[b]	DU	0.4 mg/mL[b]	Visually compatible for 4 hr at 22 °C	1436	C
Teniposide	BR	0.1 mg/mL[a]	JN	0.4 mg/mL[a]	Physically compatible for 4 hr at 23 °C	1725	C
Thiotepa	IMM[g]	1 mg/mL[a]	JN	0.4 mg/mL[a]	Physically compatible for 4 hr at 23 °C	1861	C
TNA #218 to #226[h]			AB	0.4 mg/mL[a]	Damage to emulsion occurs in 1 to 4 hr with free oil formation possible	2215	I
TPN #212 to #215[h]			AB	0.4 mg/mL[a]	Physically compatible for 4 hr at 23 °C	2109	C
Vinblastine sulfate		1 mg/mL		2.5 mg/mL	Drugs injected sequentially in Y-site with no flush. No precipitate seen	980	C
Vincristine sulfate		1 mg/mL		2.5 mg/mL	Drugs injected sequentially in Y-site with no flush. No precipitate seen	980	C
Vinorelbine tartrate	BW	1 mg/mL[b]	JN	0.4 mg/mL[b]	Physically compatible for 4 hr at 22 °C	1558	C

[a]Tested in dextrose 5%.
[b]Tested in sodium chloride 0.9%.
[c]Tested in bacteriostatic sodium chloride 0.9% preserved with benzyl alcohol 0.9%.
[d]Given over three minutes via a Y-site into a running infusion solution of heparin sodium in sodium chloride 0.9%.
[e]Tested in dextrose 5% in Ringer's injection, dextrose 5% in Ringer's injection, lactated, dextrose 5%, Ringer's injection, lactated, and sodium chloride 0.9%.
[f]Test performed using the formulation WITHOUT edetate disodium.
[g]Lyophilized formulation tested.
[h]Refer to Appendix I for the composition of parenteral nutrition solutions. TNA indicates a 3-in-1 admixture, and TPN indicates a 2-in-1 admixture.
[i]Injected via Y-site into an administration set running azithromycin.

EDETATE CALCIUM DISODIUM
AHFS 64:00

Products — Edetate calcium disodium is available in 2.5-mL ampuls containing 200 mg/mL of drug. (1)

pH — From 6.5 to 8. (4)

Sodium Content — Edetate calcium disodium contains approximately 5.3 mEq of sodium per gram of calcium EDTA. (4)

Trade Name(s) — Calcium Disodium Versenate.

Administration — Edetate calcium disodium may be administered by slow intermittent or continuous intravenous infusion after dilution with sodium chloride 0.9% or dextrose 5% to a concentration of 2 to 4 mg/mL. Infusions are made over eight to 12 (1; 4) or up to 24 hours. (4) Although a single, prolonged daily infusion is recommended by the manufacturer (1), the drug has been given in divided daily doses by intermittent intravenous infusions of 15 to 60 minutes in low-risk patients. (4)

The total daily drug dose may also be given by intramuscular injection in equally divided doses at eight- or 12-hour intervals. To minimize pain from intramuscular injection, it should be mixed in equal quantities with lidocaine hydrochloride 1% (e.g., 1 mL of local anesthetic for each milliliter of edetate calcium disodium) or 0.25 mL of lidocaine hydrochloride 10% can be added to 5 mL of edetate calcium disodium to yield a final local anesthetic concentration of 0.5%. (1; 4)

Stability — Edetate calcium disodium in intact ampuls should be stored at controlled room temperature. (1; 4)

Compatibility Information

Solution Compatibility

Edetate calcium disodium

Solution	Mfr	Mfr	Conc/L	Remarks	Ref	C/I
Dextrose 5%			2 to 4 g	Manufacturer recommended solution	1	**C**
Dextrose 10%				Physically incompatible	1	**I**
Ringer's injection				Physically incompatible	1	**I**
Ringer's injection, lactated				Physically incompatible	1	**I**
Sodium chloride 0.9%			2 to 4 g	Manufacturer recommended solution	1	**C**
Sodium lactate ⅙ M				Physically incompatible	1	**I**

Additive Compatibility

Edetate calcium disodium

Drug	Mfr	Conc/L	Mfr	Conc/L	Test Soln	Remarks	Ref	C/I
Amphotericin B		200 mg	RI	4 g	D5W	Haze develops over 3 hr	26	**I**
Hydralazine HCl	BP	80 mg	RI	4 g	D5W	Yellow color produced	26	**I**

EDROPHONIUM CHLORIDE
AHFS 36:56

Products — Edrophonium chloride is available in 15-mL multiple-dose vials. Each milliliter of solution contains edrophonium chloride 10 mg with sodium sulfite 0.2% and sodium citrate and citric acid as buffers. The multiple-dose vials also contain phenol 0.45%. (1)

pH — Approximately 5.4. (1)

Trade Name(s) — Enlon.

Administration — Edrophonium chloride may be given intramuscularly or subcutaneously but is usually given intravenously. (1; 4)

Stability — Intact containers should be stored at controlled room temperature. (1)

Compatibility Information

Y-Site Injection Compatibility (1:1 Mixture)

Edrophonium chloride

Drug	Mfr	Conc	Mfr	Conc	Remarks	Ref	C/I
Heparin sodium	UP	1000 units/L[a]	RC	10 mg/mL	Physically compatible for 4 hr at room temperature	534	C
Hydrocortisone sodium succinate	UP	10 mg/L[a]	RC	10 mg/mL	Physically compatible for 4 hr at room temperature	534	C
Potassium chloride	AB	40 mEq/L[a]	RC	10 mg/mL	Physically compatible for 4 hr at room temperature	534	C

[a]*Tested in dextrose 5% in Ringer's injection, dextrose 5% in Ringer's injection, lactated, dextrose 5%, Ringer's injection, lactated, and sodium chloride 0.9%.*

ENALAPRILAT
AHFS 24:32.04

Products — Enalaprilat is available in 1- and 2-mL vials. Each milliliter of solution contains enalaprilat 1.25 mg with sodium chloride to adjust tonicity, sodium hydroxide to adjust pH, and benzyl alcohol 9 mg in water for injection. (1)

Administration — Enalaprilat is slowly injected intravenously over at least five minutes if undiluted or infused in up to 50 mL of compatible intravenous infusion solution. (1; 4)

Stability — Enalaprilat is a clear, colorless solution. The product should be stored below 30 °C. (1; 4)

Central Venous Catheter — Enalaprilat (Merck) 0.1 mg/mL in dextrose 5% was found to be compatible with the ARROWg+ard Blue Plus (Arrow International) chlorhexidine-bearing triple-lumen central catheter. Essentially complete delivery of the drug was found with little or no drug loss occurring. Furthermore, chlorhexidine delivered from the catheter remained at trace amounts with no substantial increase due to the delivery of the drug through the catheter. (2335)

Compatibility Information

Solution Compatibility

Enalaprilat

Solution	Mfr	Mfr	Conc/L	Remarks	Ref	C/I
Dextrose 5%				Stable for 24 hr at room temperature	1	C
	TR[a]	MSD	12 mg	Visually compatible with no loss in 24 hr at room temperature under fluorescent light	1572	C
Dextrose 5% in Ringer's injection, lactated				Stable for 24 hr at room temperature	1	C
Dextrose 5% in sodium chloride 0.9%				Stable for 24 hr at room temperature	1	C
Normosol R	AB	MSD	25 mg	Physically compatible for 24 hr at room temperature under fluorescent light	1355	C
Sodium chloride 0.9%				Stable for 24 hr at room temperature	1	C

[a]*Tested in PVC containers.*

Additive Compatibility

Enalaprilat

Drug	Mfr	Conc/L	Mfr	Conc/L	Test Soln	Remarks	Ref	C/I
Dextran 40	TR	10%	MSD	25 mg	D5W	Physically compatible for 24 hr at room temperature under fluorescent light	1355	C
Dobutamine HCl	LI	1 g	MSD	12 mg	D5W[a]	Visually compatible. Little enalaprilat loss in 24 hr at room temperature under fluorescent light. Dobutamine not tested	1572	C
Dopamine HCl	AMR	1.6 g	MSD	12 mg	D5W[a]	Visually compatible. 5% enalaprilat loss in 24 hr at room temperature under fluorescent light. Dopamine not tested	1572	C
Heparin sodium	ES	50,000 units	MSD	12 mg	D5W[a]	Visually compatible. Little enalaprilat loss in 24 hr at room temperature under fluorescent light. Heparin not tested	1572	C
Hetastarch in sodium chloride 0.9%	DU	6%	MSD	25 mg		Physically compatible for 24 hr at room temperature under fluorescent light	1355	C
Meropenem	ZEN	1 and 20 g	MSD	50 mg	NS	Visually compatible for 4 hr at room temperature	1994	C
Nitroglycerin	DU	200 mg	MSD	12 mg	D5W[b]	Visually compatible. 4% enalaprilat loss in 24 hr at room temperature in light. Nitroglycerin not tested	1572	C
Potassium chloride	AB	3 g	MSD	12 mg	D5W[a]	Visually compatible. Little enalaprilat loss in 24 hr at room temperature in light	1572	C
Sodium nitroprusside	ES	1 g	MSD	12 mg	D5W[a]	Visually compatible. Little enalaprilat loss in 24 hr at room temperature under fluorescent light. Sodium nitroprusside not tested	1572	C

[a]Tested in PVC containers.
[b]Tested in glass containers.

Drugs in Syringe Compatibility

Enalaprilat

Drug (in syringe)	Mfr	Amt	Mfr	Amt	Remarks	Ref	C/I
Pantoprazole sodium	[a]	4 mg/1 mL		1.25 mg/1 mL	Precipitate forms within 1 hr	2574	I

[a]Test performed using the formulation WITHOUT edetate disodium.

Y-Site Injection Compatibility (1:1 Mixture)

Enalaprilat

Drug	Mfr	Conc	Mfr	Conc	Remarks	Ref	C/I
Allopurinol sodium	BW	3 mg/mL[b]	MSD	0.1 mg/mL[b]	Physically compatible for 4 hr at 22 °C	1686	C
Amifostine	USB	10 mg/mL[a]	MSD	0.1 mg/mL[a]	Physically compatible for 4 hr at 23 °C	1845	C
Amikacin sulfate	BR	2 mg/mL[a]	MSD	0.05 mg/mL[b]	Physically compatible for 24 hr at room temperature under fluorescent light	1355	C
Aminophylline	ES	1 mg/mL[a]	MSD	0.05 mg/mL[b]	Physically compatible for 24 hr at room temperature under fluorescent light	1355	C

Y-Site Injection Compatibility (1:1 Mixture) (Cont.)

Enalaprilat

Drug	Mfr	Conc	Mfr	Conc	Remarks	Ref	C/I
Amphotericin B	SQ	0.1 mg/mL[a]	MSD	1.25 mg/mL	Layered haze develops in 4 hr at 21 °C	1409	I
Amphotericin B cholesteryl sulfate complex	SEQ	0.83 mg/mL[a]	ME	0.1 mg/mL[a]	Decreased natural turbidity occurs	2117	I
Ampicillin sodium	BR	10 mg/mL[b]	MSD	0.05 mg/mL[b]	Physically compatible for 24 hr at room temperature under fluorescent light	1355	C
Ampicillin sodium–sulbactam sodium	PF	10 + 5 mg/mL[b]	MSD	0.05 mg/mL[b]	Physically compatible for 24 hr at room temperature under fluorescent light	1355	C
Aztreonam	SQ	10 mg/mL[a]	MSD	0.05 mg/mL[b]	Physically compatible for 24 hr at room temperature under fluorescent light	1355	C
	SQ	40 mg/mL[a]	MSD	0.1 mg/mL[a]	Physically compatible for 4 hr at 23 °C	1758	C
Bivalirudin	TMC	5 mg/mL[a]	BED	0.1 mg/mL[a]	Physically compatible for 4 hr at 23 °C	2373	C
Butorphanol tartrate	BR	0.4 mg/mL[a]	MSD	0.05 mg/mL[b]	Physically compatible for 24 hr at room temperature under fluorescent light	1355	C
Calcium gluconate	ES	0.092 mEq/mL[a]	MSD	0.05 mg/mL[b]	Physically compatible for 24 hr at room temperature	1355	C
Cefazolin sodium	SKF[c]	20 mg/mL	MSD	0.05 mg/mL[b]	Physically compatible for 24 hr at room temperature under fluorescent light	1355	C
Ceftaroline fosamil	FOR	2.22 mg/mL[a,b,i]	SIC	0.1 mg/mL[a,b,i]	Physically compatible for 4 hr at 23 °C	2826	C
Ceftazidime	GL	10 mg/mL[a]	MSD	0.05 mg/mL[b]	Physically compatible for 24 hr at room temperature under fluorescent light	1355	C
Chloramphenicol sodium succinate	PD	10 mg/mL[a]	MSD	0.05 mg/mL[b]	Physically compatible for 24 hr at room temperature under fluorescent light	1355	C
Cisatracurium besylate	GW	0.1, 2, 5 mg/mL[a]	ME	0.1 mg/mL[a]	Physically compatible for 4 hr at 23 °C	2074	C
Cladribine	ORT	0.015[b] and 0.5[d] mg/mL	MSD	0.1 mg/mL[b]	Physically compatible for 4 hr at 23 °C	1969	C
Clindamycin phosphate	UP	9 mg/mL[a]	MSD	0.05 mg/mL[b]	Physically compatible for 24 hr at room temperature under fluorescent light	1355	C
Dexmedetomidine HCl	AB	4 mcg/mL[b]	BED	0.1 mg/mL[b]	Physically compatible for 4 hr at 23 °C	2383	C
Dextran 40	TR	100 mg/mL[a]	MSD	0.05 mg/mL[b]	Physically compatible for 24 hr at room temperature under fluorescent light	1355	C
Dobutamine HCl	LI	1 mg/mL[a]	MSD	0.05 mg/mL[b]	Physically compatible for 24 hr at room temperature under fluorescent light	1355	C
Docetaxel	RPR	0.9 mg/mL[a]	ME	0.1 mg/mL[a]	Physically compatible for 4 hr at 23 °C	2224	C
Dopamine HCl	IMS	1.6 mg/mL[a]	MSD	0.05 mg/mL[b]	Physically compatible for 24 hr at room temperature under fluorescent light	1355	C
Doripenem	JJ	5 mg/mL[a,b]	SIC	0.1 mg/mL[a,b]	Physically compatible for 4 hr at 23 °C	2743	C
Doxorubicin HCl liposomal	SEQ	0.4 mg/mL[a]	MSD	0.1 mg/mL[a]	Physically compatible for 4 hr at 23 °C	2087	C
Erythromycin lactobionate	AB	5 mg/mL[a]	MSD	0.05 mg/mL[b]	Physically compatible for 24 hr at room temperature under fluorescent light	1355	C
Esmolol HCl	DU	10 mg/mL[a]	MSD	0.05 mg/mL[b]	Physically compatible for 24 hr at room temperature under fluorescent light	1355	C
Etoposide phosphate	BR	5 mg/mL[a]	ME	0.1 mg/mL[a]	Physically compatible for 4 hr at 23 °C	2218	C

Y-Site Injection Compatibility (1:1 Mixture) (Cont.)

Enalaprilat

Drug	Mfr	Conc	Mfr	Conc	Remarks	Ref	C/I
Famotidine	MSD	0.2 mg/mL[a]	MSD	0.05 mg/mL[b]	Physically compatible for 24 hr at room temperature under fluorescent light	1355	C
Fenoldopam mesylate	AB	80 mcg/mL[b]	BA	0.1 mg/mL[b]	Physically compatible for 4 hr at 23 °C	2467	C
Fentanyl citrate	ES	2 mcg/mL[a]	MSD	0.05 mg/mL[b]	Physically compatible for 24 hr at room temperature under fluorescent light	1355	C
Filgrastim	AMG	30 mcg/mL[a]	MSD	0.1 mg/mL[a]	Physically compatible for 4 hr at 22 °C	1687	C
Ganciclovir sodium	SY	5 mg/mL[e]	MSD	1.25 mg/mL	Physically compatible for 4 hr at 21 °C	1409	C
Gemcitabine HCl	LI	10 mg/mL[b]	ME	0.1 mg/mL[b]	Physically compatible for 4 hr at 23 °C	2226	C
Gentamicin sulfate	ES	0.8 mg/mL[a]	MSD	0.05 mg/mL[b]	Physically compatible for 24 hr at room temperature under fluorescent light	1355	C
Granisetron HCl	SKB	0.05 mg/mL[a]	MSD	0.1 mg/mL[a]	Physically compatible for 4 hr at 23 °C	2000	C
Heparin sodium	IX	40 units/mL[a]	MSD	0.05 mg/mL[b]	Physically compatible for 24 hr at room temperature under fluorescent light	1355	C
Hetastarch in lactated electrolyte	AB	6%	ME	0.1 mg/mL[a]	Physically compatible for 4 hr at 23 °C	2339	C
Hetastarch in sodium chloride 0.9%	DCC	6%	MSD	0.05 mg/mL[b]	Physically compatible for 24 hr at room temperature under fluorescent light	1355	C
Hydrocortisone sodium succinate	UP	2 mg/mL[a]	MSD	0.05 mg/mL[b]	Physically compatible for 24 hr at room temperature under fluorescent light	1355	C
Labetalol HCl	GL	1 mg/mL[a]	MSD	0.05 mg/mL[b]	Physically compatible for 24 hr at room temperature under fluorescent light	1355	C
Lidocaine HCl	AST	4 mg/mL[a]	MSD	0.05 mg/mL[b]	Physically compatible for 24 hr at room temperature under fluorescent light	1355	C
Linezolid	PHU	2 mg/mL	ME	0.1 mg/mL[a]	Physically compatible for 4 hr at 23 °C	2264	C
Magnesium sulfate	LY	10 mEq/mL[a]	MSD	0.05 mg/mL[b]	Physically compatible for 24 hr at room temperature under fluorescent light	1355	C
Melphalan HCl	BW	0.1 mg/mL[b]	MSD	0.1 mg/mL[b]	Physically compatible for 3 hr at 22 °C	1557	C
Meropenem	ZEN	1 and 50 mg/mL[b]	MSD	0.05 mg/mL[f]	Visually compatible for 4 hr at room temperature	1994	C
Methylprednisolone sodium succinate	UP	0.8 mg/mL[a]	MSD	0.05 mg/mL[b]	Physically compatible for 24 hr at room temperature under fluorescent light	1355	C
Metronidazole	SE	5 mg/mL	MSD	0.05 mg/mL[b]	Physically compatible for 24 hr at room temperature under fluorescent light	1355	C
Morphine sulfate	WY	0.2 mg/mL[a]	MSD	0.05 mg/mL[b]	Physically compatible for 24 hr at room temperature under fluorescent light	1355	C
Nafcillin sodium	BR	10 mg/mL[a]	MSD	0.05 mg/mL[b]	Physically compatible for 24 hr at room temperature under fluorescent light	1355	C
Nesiritide	SCI	50 mcg/mL[a,b]		1.25 mg/mL	Physically incompatible	2625	I
Nicardipine HCl	DU	0.1 mg/mL[a]	MSD	0.05 mg/mL[b]	Physically compatible for 24 hr at room temperature under fluorescent light	1355	C
	DCC	0.1 mg/mL[a]	MSD	0.5 mg/mL[a]	Visually compatible for 24 hr at room temperature	235	C
Oxaliplatin	SS	0.5 mg/mL[a]	BA	0.1 mg/mL[a]	Physically compatible for 4 hr at 23 °C	2566	C
Pemetrexed disodium	LI	20 mg/mL[b]	BED	0.1 mg/mL[a]	Physically compatible for 4 hr at 23 °C	2564	C
Penicillin G potassium	PF	50,000 units/mL[a]	MSD	0.05 mg/mL[b]	Physically compatible for 24 hr at room temperature under fluorescent light	1355	C

Y-Site Injection Compatibility (1:1 Mixture) (Cont.)

Enalaprilat

Drug	Mfr	Conc	Mfr	Conc	Remarks	Ref	C/I
Phenobarbital sodium	WY	0.32 mg/mL[e]	MSD	1.25 mg/mL	Physically compatible for 4 hr at 21 °C	1409	C
Phenytoin sodium	PD	1 mg/mL[b]	MSD	1.25 mg/mL	Crystalline precipitate forms immediately	1409	I
Piperacillin sodium–tazobactam sodium	LE[j]	40 + 5 mg/mL[a]	MSD	0.1 mg/mL[a]	Physically compatible for 4 hr at 22 °C	1688	C
Potassium chloride	LY	0.4 mEq/mL[a]	MSD	0.05 mg/mL[b]	Physically compatible for 24 hr at room temperature under fluorescent light	1355	C
Potassium phosphates	LY	0.44 mEq/mL[a]	MSD	0.05 mg/mL[b]	Physically compatible for 24 hr at room temperature under fluorescent light	1355	C
Propofol	ZEN	10 mg/mL	MSD	0.1 mg/mL[a]	Physically compatible for 1 hr at 23 °C	2066	C
Ranitidine HCl	GL	0.5 mg/mL[a]	MSD	0.05 mg/mL[b]	Physically compatible for 24 hr at room temperature under fluorescent light	1355	C
Remifentanil HCl	GW	0.025 and 0.25 mg/mL[b]	ME	0.1 mg/mL[a]	Physically compatible for 4 hr at 23 °C	2075	C
Sodium acetate	LY	0.4 mEq/mL[a]	MSD	0.05 mg/mL[b]	Physically compatible for 24 hr at room temperature under fluorescent light	1355	C
Sodium nitroprusside	LY	0.2 mg/mL[a]	MSD	0.05 mg/mL[b]	Physically compatible for 24 hr at room temperature protected from light	1355	C
Teniposide	BR	0.1 mg/mL[a]	MSD	0.1 mg/mL[a]	Physically compatible for 4 hr at 23 °C	1725	C
Thiotepa	IMM[g]	1 mg/mL[a]	ME	0.1 mg/mL[a]	Physically compatible for 4 hr at 23 °C	1861	C
TNA #218 to #226[h]			ME	0.1 mg/mL[a]	Visually compatible for 4 hr at 23 °C	2215	C
Tobramycin sulfate	LI	0.8 mg/mL[a]	MSD	0.05 mg/mL[b]	Physically compatible for 24 hr at room temperature under fluorescent light	1355	C
TPN #212 to #215[h]			MSD	0.1 mg/mL[a]	Physically compatible for 4 hr at 23 °C	2109	C
Trimethoprim–sulfamethoxazole	QU	0.16 + 0.8 mg/mL[a]	MSD	0.05 mg/mL[b]	Physically compatible for 24 hr at room temperature under fluorescent light	1355	C
Vancomycin HCl	LE	5 mg/mL[a]	MSD	0.05 mg/mL[b]	Physically compatible for 24 hr at room temperature under fluorescent light	1355	C
Vinorelbine tartrate	BW	1 mg/mL[b]	MSD	0.1 mg/mL[b]	Physically compatible for 4 hr at 22 °C	1558	C

[a]Tested in dextrose 5%.
[b]Tested in sodium chloride 0.9%.
[c]Tested in premixed infusion solution.
[d]Tested in bacteriostatic sodium chloride 0.9% preserved with benzyl alcohol 0.9%.
[e]Tested in both dextrose 5% and sodium chloride 0.9%.
[f]Tested in sterile water for injection.
[g]Lyophilized formulation tested.
[h]Refer to Appendix I for the composition of parenteral nutrition solutions. TNA indicates a 3-in-1 admixture, and TPN indicates a 2-in-1 admixture.
[i]Tested in Ringer's injection, lactated.
[j]Test performed using the formulation WITHOUT edetate disodium.

ENOXAPARIN SODIUM
AHFS 20:12.04.16

Products — Enoxaparin sodium is available in multiple-dose vials containing 300 mg/3 mL with 1.5% benzyl alcohol preservative and prefilled syringes containing 30 mg/0.3 mL, 40 mg/0.4 mL, 60 mg/0.6 mL, 80 mg/0.8 mL, 100 mg/1 mL, 120 mg/0.8 mL, and 150 mg/1 mL in water for injection. The solution in prefilled syringes is preservative-free and is a single-dose injection. (1)

pH — From 5.5 to 7.5. (1)

Units — The approximate anti-factor Xa activity is 1000 I.U. for every 10 mg of enoxaparin sodium. (1; 4)

Trade Name(s) — Lovenox.

Administration — Enoxaparin sodium is administered by deep sub-cutaneous injection, without dilution, alternating administration sites between the left and right anterolateral and left and right posterolateral abdominal wall. Enoxaparin sodium in multiple-dose vials may also be given by intravenous bolus administration into an intravenous line with careful flushing both before and after administration with dextrose 5% or sodium chloride 0.9%. The drug can be mixed in dextrose 5% or sodium chloride 0.9% for intravenous administration. Enoxaparin sodium is not intended for and must not be given by intramuscular administration. (1; 4)

Stability — Enoxaparin sodium injection is a clear, colorless to pale yellow solution. Intact containers should be stored at controlled room temperature of 15 to 25 °C. (1)

Syringes — Enoxaparin (Rhone-Poulenc Rorer) 100 mg/1 mL was packaged in 1-mL tuberculin syringes fitted with 27-gauge, ½-inch nee-dles. The syringes were stored at 22 and 3 °C for 10 days. Anticoagulant activity had a 7 to 8% loss in 10 days under refrigeration but 15 to 25% losses in as little as two days at room temperature. (2272)

However, the manufacturer of enoxaparin sodium has indicated that the undiluted injection at a concentration of 100 mg/1 mL repackaged in plastic syringes is stable for five days at room temperature. (31)

Enoxaparin sodium diluted to about 20 mg/mL in sterile water for injection has been reported to undergo little or no change in anti-Xa activity for 29 days at room temperature when the dilution was packaged in glass vials and for about 14 days packaged in polypropylene syringes at room and refrigerated temperatures. (2499)

The stability of enoxaparin 100 mg/mL packaged in 1-mL polypropylene tuberculin syringes was evaluated over 10 days stored at 22 and 4 °C. Enoxaparin losses did not exceed 10% at the two storage temperatures. However, seven of 45 test syringes stored at room temperature could not be operated to eject the enoxaparin. None of the refrigerated samples exhibited this failure. The authors speculated that precipitation had resulted in blockage. (2546)

Compatibility Information

Solution Compatibility

Enoxaparin sodium

Solution	Mfr	Mfr	Conc/L	Remarks	Ref	C/I
Sodium chloride 0.9%	AB[a]	RP	1.2 g	No loss of activity in 48 hr at 21 °C under fluorescent light	1871	C

[a]*Tested in PVC containers.*

EPHEDRINE SULFATE
AHFS 12:12.12

Products — Ephedrine sulfate is available in vials containing 50 mg/1 mL in water for injection. (1)

pH — From 4.5 to 7. (17)

Administration — Ephedrine sulfate may be administered subcutaneously, intramuscularly, or slowly intravenously. (1; 4)

Stability — Intact containers of ephedrine sulfate should be stored at controlled room temperature and protected from light. (1; 4)

Syringes — The stability of ephedrine (salt form unspecified) 10 mg/mL repackaged in polypropylene syringes was evaluated. Little or no change in concentration was found after four weeks of storage at room temperature not exposed to direct light. (2164)

Ephedrine sulfate (Ben Venue) 5 mg/mL in sodium chloride 0.9% was packaged in 10-mL polypropylene syringes (Becton Dickinson) and stored at 25 °C in fluorescent light and at 4 °C. Ephedrine sulfate losses were less than 3% after 60 days under both conditions. (2365)

Ephedrine sulfate 50 mg/mL packaged in Becton-Dickinson polypropylene syringes was stable for four days at room temperature. Analysis found little or no loss of ephedrine sulfate, and no change in solution appearance occurred. (2649)

Compatibility Information

Solution Compatibility

Ephedrine sulfate

Solution	Mfr	Mfr	Conc/L	Remarks	Ref	C/I
Dextrose–Ringer's injection combinations	AB		50 mg	Physically compatible	3	C
Dextrose–Ringer's injection, lactated, combinations	AB		50 mg	Physically compatible	3	C

Solution Compatibility (Cont.)

Ephedrine sulfate

Solution	Mfr	Mfr	Conc/L	Remarks	Ref	C/I
Dextrose–saline combinations	AB		50 mg	Physically compatible	3	C
Dextrose 2.5%	AB		50 mg	Physically compatible	3	C
Dextrose 5%	AB		50 mg	Physically compatible	3	C
Dextrose 10%	AB		50 mg	Physically compatible	3	C
Ionosol products	AB		50 mg	Physically compatible	3	C
Ringer's injection	AB		50 mg	Physically compatible	3	C
Ringer's injection, lactated	AB		50 mg	Physically compatible	3	C
Sodium chloride 0.45%	AB		50 mg	Physically compatible	3	C
Sodium chloride 0.9%	AB		50 mg	Physically compatible	3	C
Sodium lactate ⅙ M	AB		50 mg	Physically compatible	3	C

Additive Compatibility

Ephedrine sulfate

Drug	Mfr	Conc/L	Mfr	Conc/L	Test Soln	Remarks	Ref	C/I
Chloramphenicol sodium succinate	PD	1 g	AB	50 mg		Physically compatible	6	C
Lidocaine HCl	AST	2 g		50 mg		Physically compatible	24	C
Nafcillin sodium	WY	500 mg		50 mg		Physically compatible	27	C
Penicillin G potassium		1 million units		50 mg		Physically compatible	3	C
	SQ	5 million units	AB	50 mg		Physically compatible	47	C
Pentobarbital sodium	AB	1 g	LI	250 mg	D5W	Physically incompatible	15	I
Phenobarbital sodium	WI	200 mg	LI	250 mg	D5W	Physically incompatible	15	I

Drugs in Syringe Compatibility

Ephedrine sulfate

Drug (in syringe)	Mfr	Amt	Mfr	Amt	Remarks	Ref	C/I
Pentobarbital sodium	AB	500 mg/ 10 mL		50 mg/ 1 mL	Physically compatible	55	C

Y-Site Injection Compatibility (1:1 Mixture)

Ephedrine sulfate

Drug	Mfr	Conc	Mfr	Conc	Remarks	Ref	C/I
Bivalirudin	TMC	5 mg/mL[a]	TAY	5 mg/mL[a]	Physically compatible for 4 hr at 23 °C	2373	C
Dexmedetomidine HCl	AB	4 mcg/mL[b]	TAY	5 mg/mL[b]	Physically compatible for 4 hr at 23 °C	2383	C
Etomidate	AB	2 mg/mL	AB	50 mg/mL	Visually compatible for 7 days at 25 °C	1801	C

Y-Site Injection Compatibility (1:1 Mixture) (Cont.)

			Ephedrine sulfate				
Drug	*Mfr*	*Conc*	*Mfr*	*Conc*	*Remarks*	*Ref*	*C/I*
Fenoldopam mesylate	AB	80 mcg/mL[b]	BED	5 mg/mL[b]	Physically compatible for 4 hr at 23 °C	2467	C
Hetastarch in lactated electrolyte	AB	6%	TAY	5 mg/mL[a]	Physically compatible for 4 hr at 23 °C	2339	C
Propofol	ZEN	10 mg/mL	AB	5 mg/mL[a]	Physically compatible for 1 hr at 23 °C	2066	C

[a]*Tested in dextrose 5%.*
[b]*Tested in sodium chloride 0.9%.*

EPINEPHRINE HYDROCHLORIDE
AHFS 12:12.12

Products — Epinephrine hydrochloride 1 mg/mL is available in 1-mL ampuls, 30-mL vials, and 0.3-mL auto-injector syringes. Epinephrine hydrochloride is also available at a concentration of 0.1 mg/mL (1:10,000) in vials and prefilled syringes. Some products also contain sodium chloride, a bisulfite antioxidant, and an antibacterial preservative such as chlorobutanol. (1; 4)

pH — From 2.2 to 5.0. (4; 17)

Osmolality — The osmolality of epinephrine hydrochloride (Abbott) 0.1 mg/mL was determined to be 273 mOsm/kg by freezing-point depression. (1071) A 1-mg/mL solution was determined to have an osmolality of 348 mOsm/kg. (1233)

Trade Name(s) — Adrenalin Chloride, Epipen.

Administration — Epinephrine hydrochloride may be administered by subcutaneous, intramuscular, intravenous, or intracardiac injection. Intramuscular injection into the buttocks should be avoided. (1; 4) Intravenous infusion at a rate of 1 to 10 mcg/min has also been described. (4)

Stability — Epinephrine hydrochloride is sensitive to light and air. (4; 1259) Protection from light is recommended. Withdrawal of doses from multiple-dose vials introduces air, which results in oxidation. As epinephrine oxidizes, it changes from colorless to pink, as adrenochrome forms, to brown, as melanin forms. (4; 1072) Discolored solutions or solutions containing a precipitate should not be used. (4) The various epinephrine preparations have varying stabilities, depending on the form and the preservatives present. The manufacturer's recommendations should be followed with regard to storage. (4)

The stability of epinephrine hydrochloride in intact ampuls subjected to resterilization to provide a sterile outer surface was evaluated. Epinephrine hydrochloride (adrenalin injection, BP) ampuls were resterilized by the following methods:

1. Autoclaved at 121 °C for 15 minutes.
2. Autoclaved at 115 °C for 30 minutes.
3. Exposed to ethylene oxide–freon (12:88) at 55 °C for four hours followed by aeration at 50 °C for 12 hours.

No loss of epinephrine hydrochloride concentration was found in samples from any of these methods. However, if ampuls were resterilized by autoclaving two times at 121 °C for 15 minutes, 8% of the drug was lost. (803)

Epinephrine hydrochloride is rapidly destroyed by alkalies or oxidizing agents including sodium bicarbonate, halogens, permanganates, chromates, nitrates, nitrites, and salts of easily reducible metals such as iron, copper, and zinc. (4)

Visual inspection for color changes may be inadequate to assess compatibility of epinephrine hydrochloride admixtures. In one evaluation with aminophylline stored at 25 °C, a color change was not noted until eight hours had elapsed. However, only 40% of the initial epinephrine hydrochloride was still present in the admixture at 24 hours. (527)

pH Effects — The primary determinant of catecholamine stability in intravenous admixtures is the pH of the solution. (527) Epinephrine hydrochloride is unstable in dextrose 5% at a pH above 5.5. (48) The pH of optimum stability is 3 to 4. (1072) In one study, the decomposition rate increased twofold (from 5 to 10% in 200 days at 30 °C) when the pH was increased from 2.5 to 4.5. (1259)

When lidocaine hydrochloride is mixed with epinephrine hydrochloride, the buffering capacity of the lidocaine hydrochloride may raise the pH of intravenous admixtures above 5.5, the maximum necessary for stability of epinephrine hydrochloride. The final pH is usually about 6. Epinephrine hydrochloride will begin to deteriorate within several hours. Therefore, admixtures should be used promptly after preparation or the separate administration of the epinephrine hydrochloride should be considered. This restriction does not apply to commercial lidocaine–epinephrine combinations that have had the pH adjusted for epinephrine stability. (24)

Syringes — Epinephrine hydrochloride was diluted to 1 and 7 mg/10 mL with sterile water for injection and repackaged into 10-mL glass vials and plastic syringes with 18-gauge needles (Becton-Dickinson). The diluted injections were stored at room temperature protected from light. Epinephrine stability was evaluated over 56 days of storage. The 1-mg/10 mL samples had an epinephrine loss of 4 to 6% in seven days and 13% in 14 days. The 7-mg/10 mL samples lost 2% in the glass vials and 5% in the syringes in 56 days. (1902)

Epinephrine hydrochloride 1:10,000 in autoinjector syringes was evaluated for stability over 45 days under use conditions in paramedic vehicles. Temperatures fluctuated with locations and conditions and ranged from 6.5 °C (43.7 °F) to 52 °C (125.6 °F) in high desert conditions. No visually apparent changes occurred, and not more than 6% loss of epinephrine hydrochloride was found. Most samples exhibited no loss. (2548)

Epinephrine hydrochloride under simulated summer conditions in paramedic vehicles was exposed to temperatures ranging from 26 to 38 °C over 4 weeks. Analysis found no loss of the drug under these conditions. However, the buffer in the injection was altered, resulting in an increase in pH. (2562)

Central Venous Catheter — Epinephrine hydrochloride (American Regent) 0.1 mg/mL in dextrose 5% was found to be compatible with the ARROWg+ard Blue Plus (Arrow International) chlorhexidine-bearing triple-lumen central catheter. Essentially complete delivery of the drug was found with little or no drug loss occurring. Furthermore, chlorhexidine delivered from the catheter remained at trace amounts with no substantial increase due to the delivery of the drug through the catheter. (2335)

Compatibility Information

Solution Compatibility

Epinephrine HCl

Solution	Mfr	Mfr	Conc/L	Remarks	Ref	C/I
Dextrose–Ringer's injection combinations	AB	PD	4 mg	Physically compatible	3	C
Dextrose–Ringer's injection, lactated, combinations	AB	PD	4 mg	Physically compatible	3	C
Dextrose 5% in Ringer's injection, lactated	TR[a]	PD	1 mg	Stable for 24 hr at 5 °C	282	C
Dextrose–saline combinations	AB	PD	4 mg	Physically compatible	3	C
Dextrose 5% in sodium chloride 0.9%	TR[a]	PD	1 mg	Stable for 24 hr at 5 °C	282	C
Dextrose 2.5%	AB	PD	4 mg	Physically compatible	3	C
Dextrose 5%	AB	PD	4 mg	Physically compatible	3	C
	TR[a]	PD	1 mg	Stable for 24 hr at 5 °C	282	C
	AB	PD	4 mg	Physically compatible and stable. At 25 °C, 10% loss is calculated to occur in 50 hr in light and in 1000 hr in the dark	527	C
	BA[b]	ANT	16 mg	5% loss in 20.75 days at 5 °C protected from light	1610	C
	BA[a]	AMR	87 mg	No epinephrine loss in 24 hr at 23 °C protected from light	2085	C
Dextrose 10%	AB	PD	4 mg	Physically compatible	3	C
Ionosol products	AB	PD	4 mg	Physically compatible	3	C
Ionosol T in dextrose 5%	AB	PD	4 mg	Haze or precipitate within 6 to 24 hr	3	I
Ringer's injection	AB	PD	4 mg	Physically compatible	3	C
Ringer's injection, lactated	AB	PD	4 mg	Physically compatible	3	C
	TR[a]	PD	1 mg	Stable for 24 hr at 5 °C	282	C
Sodium chloride 0.9%	TR[a]	PD	1 mg	Stable for 24 hr at 5 °C	282	C
Sodium lactate ⅙ M	AB	PD	4 mg	Physically compatible	3	C

[a]Tested in both glass and PVC containers.
[b]Tested in PVC containers.

Additive Compatibility

Epinephrine HCl

Drug	Mfr	Conc/L	Mfr	Conc/L	Test Soln	Remarks	Ref	C/I
Amikacin sulfate	BR	5 g	PD	2.5 mg	D5LR, D5R, D5S, D5W, D10W, LR, NS, R, SL	Physically compatible and both stable for 24 hr at 25 °C	294	C

Additive Compatibility (Cont.)

Epinephrine HCl

Drug	Mfr	Conc/L	Mfr	Conc/L	Test Soln	Remarks	Ref	C/I
Aminophylline	SE	500 mg	PD	4 mg	D5W	At 25 °C, 10% epinephrine decomposition in 1.2 hr in light and 3 hr in dark	527	I
		500 mg		4 mg	D5W	Pink to brown discoloration in 8 to 24 hr at room temperature	845	I
Bupivacaine HCl with fentanyl citrate	WI JN	440 mg 1.25 mg	AB	0.69 mg	[b]	No bupivacaine and fentanyl loss and 10% epinephrine loss in 30 days at 3 and 23 °C then 48 hr at 30 °C	1627	C
Bupivacaine HCl with fentanyl citrate	IVX	1 g 2 mg	IVX	2 mg		Visually compatible with less than 10% loss of epinephrine and no loss of other drugs in 182 days at 4 and 22 °C	2613	C
Dobutamine HCl	LI	1 g	BR	50 mg	D5W, NS	Physically compatible for 24 hr at 21 °C	812	C
Fentanyl citrate with bupivacaine HCl	JN WI	1.25 mg 440 mg	AB	0.69 mg	[b]	No bupivacaine and fentanyl loss and 10% epinephrine loss in 30 days at 3 and 23 °C then 48 hr at 30 °C	1627	C
Fentanyl citrate with bupivacaine HCl	IVX	2 mg 1 g	IVX	2 mg		Visually compatible with less than 10% loss of epinephrine and no loss of other drugs in 182 days at 4 and 22 °C	2613	C
Floxacillin sodium	BE	20 g	ANT	8 mg	W	Physically compatible for 72 hr at 15 and 30 °C	1479	C
Furosemide	HO	1 g	ANT	8 mg	W	Physically compatible for 72 hr at 15 and 30 °C	1479	C
Ranitidine HCl	GL	50 mg and 2 g		50 mg	D5W	Physically compatible. Ranitidine stable for 24 hr at 25 °C. Epinephrine not tested	1515	C
Sodium bicarbonate	AB	2.4 mEq[a]		4 mg	D5W	Epinephrine inactivated	772	I
		5%		4 mg		Epinephrine rapidly decomposes. 58% loss immediately after mixing	48	I
Verapamil HCl	KN	80 mg	PD	2 mg	D5W, NS	Physically compatible for 24 hr	764	C

[a] One vial of Neut added to a liter of admixture.
[b] Tested in portable infusion pump reservoirs (Pharmacia Deltec).

Drugs in Syringe Compatibility

Epinephrine HCl

Drug (in syringe)	Mfr	Amt	Mfr	Amt	Remarks	Ref	C/I
Caffeine citrate		20 mg/ 1 mL	IMS	0.1 mg/ 1 mL	Visually compatible for 4 hr at 25 °C	2440	C
Doxapram HCl	RB	400 mg/ 20 mL		1 mg/ 1 mL	Physically compatible with no doxapram loss in 24 hr	1177	C
Heparin sodium		2500 units/ 1 mL		1 mg/ 1 mL	Physically compatible for at least 5 min	1053	C
Iohexol	WI	64.7%, 5 mL	PD	1 mg/ 1 mL	Physically compatible for at least 2 hr	1438	C
Iopamidol	SQ	61%, 5 mL	PD	1 mg/ 1 mL	Physically compatible for at least 2 hr	1438	C

Drugs in Syringe Compatibility (Cont.)

Epinephrine HCl

Drug (in syringe)	Mfr	Amt	Mfr	Amt	Remarks	Ref	C/I
Iothalamate meglumine	MA	60%, 5 mL	PD	1 mg/ 1 mL	Physically compatible for at least 2 hr	1438	**C**
Ioxaglate meglumine–ioxaglate sodium	MA	5 mL	PD	1 mg/ 1 mL	Physically compatible for at least 2 hr	1438	**C**
Milrinone lactate	STR	5.25 mg/ 5.25 mL	AB	0.5 mg/ 0.5 mL	Physically compatible. No loss of either drug in 20 min at 23 °C	1410	**C**
Pantoprazole sodium	[a]	4 mg/ 1 mL		1 mg/ 1 mL	Precipitates	2574	**I**

[a]*Test performed using the formulation WITHOUT edetate disodium.*

Y-Site Injection Compatibility (1:1 Mixture)

Epinephrine HCl

Drug	Mfr	Conc	Mfr	Conc	Remarks	Ref	C/I
Amiodarone HCl	WY	6 mg/mL[a]	AMR	1 mg/mL	Visually compatible for 24 hr at 22 °C	2352	**C**
Ampicillin sodium	WY	40 mg/mL[b]	ES	32 mcg/mL[c]	Slight color change in 3 hr	1316	**I**
Anidulafungin	VIC	0.5 mg/mL[a]	AMR	50 mcg/mL	Physically compatible for 4 hr at 23 °C	2617	**C**
Atracurium besylate	BW	0.5 mg/mL[a]	AB	4 mcg/mL[a]	Physically compatible for 24 hr at 28 °C	1337	**C**
Bivalirudin	TMC	5 mg/mL[a]	AMR	50 mcg/mL[a]	Physically compatible for 4 hr at 23 °C	2373	**C**
Calcium chloride	AB	4 mg/mL[c]	ES	0.032 mg/mL[c]	Physically compatible for 3 hr	1316	**C**
Calcium gluconate	AST	4 mg/mL[c]	ES	0.032 mg/mL[c]	Physically compatible for 3 hr	1316	**C**
Caspofungin acetate	ME	0.7 mg/mL[b]	AMP	0.05 mg/mL[b]	Physically compatible for 4 hr at room temperature	2758	**C**
Ceftazidime	GSK	120 mg/mL[e]		50 mcg/mL	Physically compatible with less than 10% ceftazidime loss. Epinephrine not tested	2513	**C**
Cisatracurium besylate	GW	0.1, 2, 5 mg/mL[a]	AMR	0.05 mg/mL[a]	Physically compatible for 4 hr at 23 °C	2074	**C**
Clonidine HCl	BI	18 mcg/mL[b]	NYC	20 mcg/mL[a]	Visually compatible	2642	**C**
Dexmedetomidine HCl	AB	4 mcg/mL[b]	AMR	50 mcg/mL[b]	Physically compatible for 4 hr at 23 °C	2383	**C**
Diltiazem HCl	MMD	5 mg/mL	PD	0.004 and 0.05 mg/mL[b]	Visually compatible	1807	**C**
	MMD	1 mg/mL[b]	PD	0.05 mg/mL[b]	Visually compatible	1807	**C**
	MMD	1 mg/mL[a]	AB	0.02 mg/mL[a]	Visually compatible for 4 hr at 27 °C	2062	**C**
Dobutamine HCl	LI	4 mg/mL[a]	AB	0.02 mg/mL[a]	Visually compatible for 4 hr at 27 °C	2062	**C**
Dopamine HCl	AB	3.2 mg/mL[a]	AB	0.02 mg/mL[a]	Visually compatible for 4 hr at 27 °C	2062	**C**
Famotidine	MSD	0.2 mg/mL[a]	ES	4 mcg/mL[a]	Physically compatible for 4 hr at 25 °C	1188	**C**
Fenoldopam mesylate	AB	80 mcg/mL[b]	AMR	50 mcg/mL[b]	Physically compatible for 4 hr at 23 °C	2467	**C**
Fentanyl citrate	ES	0.05 mg/mL	AB	0.02 mg/mL[a]	Visually compatible for 4 hr at 27 °C	2062	**C**
Furosemide	AMR	10 mg/mL	AB	0.02 mg/mL[a]	Visually compatible for 4 hr at 27 °C	2062	**C**
Heparin sodium	UP	1000 units/L[d]	AB	0.1 mg/mL	Physically compatible for 4 hr at room temperature	534	**C**

Y-Site Injection Compatibility (1:1 Mixture) (Cont.)

Epinephrine HCl

Drug	Mfr	Conc	Mfr	Conc	Remarks	Ref	C/I
	ES	100 units/mL[a]	AB	0.02 mg/mL[a]	Visually compatible for 4 hr at 27 °C	2062	C
Hetastarch in lactated electrolyte	AB	6%	AB	0.05 mg/mL[a]	Physically compatible for 4 hr at 23 °C	2339	C
Hydrocortisone sodium succinate	UP	10 mg/L[d]	AB	0.1 mg/mL	Physically compatible for 4 hr at room temperature	534	C
Hydromorphone HCl	KN	1 mg/mL	AB	0.02 mg/mL[a]	Visually compatible for 4 hr at 27 °C	2062	C
Hydroxyethyl starch 130/0.4 in sodium chloride 0.9%	FRK	6%	BIO	16, 24, 32 mcg/mL[a]	Color change within 4 hr	2770	I
Labetalol HCl	AH	2 mg/mL[a]	AB	0.02 mg/mL[a]	Visually compatible for 4 hr at 27 °C	2062	C
Levofloxacin	OMN	5 mg/mL[a]	AB	1 mg/mL	Visually compatible for 4 hr at 24 °C	2233	C
Lorazepam	WY	0.5 mg/mL[a]	AB	0.02 mg/mL[a]	Visually compatible for 4 hr at 27 °C	2062	C
Micafungin sodium	ASP	1.5 mg/mL[b]	AB	50 mcg/mL[b]	Microparticulates form in 4 hr	2683	I
Midazolam HCl	RC	2 mg/mL[a]	AB	0.02 mg/mL[a]	Visually compatible for 4 hr at 27 °C	2062	C
Milrinone lactate	SW	0.2 mg/mL[a]	AB	0.02 mg/mL[a]	Visually compatible for 4 hr at 27 °C	2062	C
	SW	0.4 mg/mL[a]	AB	0.064 mg/mL[a]	Visually compatible. Little loss of either drug in 4 hr at 23 °C	2214	C
Morphine sulfate	SCN	2 mg/mL[a]	AB	0.02 mg/mL[a]	Visually compatible for 4 hr at 27 °C	2062	C
Nesiritide	SCI	50 mcg/mL[a,b]		1 mg/mL	Physically compatible for 4 hr. May be chemically incompatible with nesiritide[j]	2625	?
Nicardipine HCl	WY	1 mg/mL[a]	AB	0.02 mg/mL[a]	Visually compatible for 4 hr at 27 °C	2062	C
Nitroglycerin	AB	0.4 mg/mL[a]	AB	0.02 mg/mL[a]	Visually compatible for 4 hr at 27 °C	2062	C
Norepinephrine bitartrate	AB	0.128 mg/mL[a]	AB	0.02 mg/mL[a]	Visually compatible for 4 hr at 27 °C	2062	C
Pancuronium bromide	ES	0.05 mg/mL[a]	AB	4 mcg/mL[a]	Physically compatible for 24 hr at 28 °C	1337	C
Pantoprazole sodium	ALT[i]	0.16 to 0.8 mg/mL[b]	AB	16 to 32 mcg/mL[a]	Visually compatible for 12 hr at 23 °C	2603	C
Phytonadione	MSD	0.4 mg/mL[c]	ES	0.032 mg/mL[c]	Physically compatible for 3 hr	1316	C
Potassium chloride	AB	40 mEq/L[d]	AB	0.1 mg/mL	Physically compatible for 4 hr at room temperature	534	C
Propofol	ZEN	10 mg/mL	AMR	0.1 mg/mL	Physically compatible for 1 hr at 23 °C	2066	C
Ranitidine HCl	GL	1 mg/mL[a]	AB	0.02 mg/mL[a]	Visually compatible for 4 hr at 27 °C	2062	C
Remifentanil HCl	GW	0.025 and 0.25 mg/mL[b]	AMR	0.05 mg/mL[a]	Physically compatible for 4 hr at 23 °C	2075	C
Sodium nitroprusside	RC	1.2 and 3 mg/mL[a]	AB	0.03, 0.12, 0.3 mg/mL[h]	Visually compatible for 48 hr at 24 °C protected from light	2357	C
Tigecycline	WY	1 mg/mL[b]		4 mcg/mL[b]	Physically compatible for 4 hr	2714	C
Tirofiban HCl	ME	50 mcg/mL[a,b]	AMR	2 and 100 mcg/mL[a,b]	Physically compatible. No loss of either drug in 4 hr at 23 °C	2356	C
TPN #189[f]			AST	0.2 mg/mL[b]	Visually compatible for 24 hr at 22 °C	1767	C
Vasopressin	AMR	2 and 4 units/mL[b]	AMR	4 mcg/mL[b]	Physically compatible with vasopressin pushed through a Y-site over 5 sec	2478	C
Vecuronium bromide	OR	0.1 mg/mL[a]	AB	4 mcg/mL[a]	Physically compatible for 24 hr at 28 °C	1337	C
	OR	1 mg/mL	AB	0.02 mg/mL[a]	Visually compatible for 4 hr at 27 °C	2062	C

Y-Site Injection Compatibility (1:1 Mixture) (Cont.)

Epinephrine HCl

Drug	Mfr	Conc	Mfr	Conc	Remarks	Ref	C/I
Warfarin sodium	DU	0.1ᶜ and 2ᵉ mg/mL	AMR	0.1 mg/mLᶜ	Physically compatible for 24 hr at 23 °C	2011	C

ᵃTested in dextrose 5%.
ᵇTested in sodium chloride 0.9%.
ᶜTested in both dextrose 5% and sodium chloride 0.9%.
ᵈTested in dextrose 5% in Ringer's injection, dextrose 5% in Ringer's injection, lactated, dextrose 5%, Ringer's injection, lactated, and sodium chloride 0.9%.
ᵉTested in sterile water for injection.
ᶠRefer to Appendix I for the composition of parenteral nutrition solutions. TPN indicates a 2-in-1 admixture.
ᵍTested in dextrose 5%, Ringer's injection, lactated, sodium chloride 0.45%, and sodium chloride 0.9%.
ʰTested in dextrose 5% in sodium chloride 0.45%.
ⁱTest performed using the formulation WITHOUT edetate disodium.
ʲNesiritide is incompatible with bisulfite antioxidants used in some drug formulations. The specific formulation of the product to be used should be checked to assure that no sulfite antioxidants are present.

EPIRUBICIN HYDROCHLORIDE
AHFS 10:00

Products — Epirubicin hydrochloride is available as a 2-mg/mL, preservative-free, ready-to-use solution in single-use polypropylene vials of 25 and 100 mL containing 50 and 200 mg of drug, respectively. The solution also contains sodium chloride and water for injection. The pH has been adjusted with hydrochloric acid. (1)

pH — The solution pH has been adjusted to 3. (1)

Trade Name(s) — Ellence.

Administration — Epirubicin hydrochloride is administered by intravenous infusion over three to five minutes; infusion into the tubing of a freely running intravenous infusion of sodium chloride 0.9% or dextrose 5% is recommended. Administration by direct push is not recommended because of the risk of extravasation. Extravasation may cause pain, severe tissue lesions, and necrosis and should be avoided. Burning or stinging may indicate extravasation, requiring immediate termination of the infusion and restarting in another vein. Epirubicin hydrochloride must *not* be given by intramuscular or subcutaneous injection. (1)

Personnel preparing and administering this drug should take protective measures to avoid contact with the solution, including use of disposable gloves, gowns, masks, and eye goggles. Dose preparation should be performed in a suitable laminar airflow device on a work surface protected by plastic-backed absorbent paper. All equipment and materials used in preparing and administering doses should be disposed of safely using high-temperature incineration. (1)

Spills or leakage of epirubicin hydrochloride solutions should be diluted with sodium hypochlorite having 1% available chlorine, preferably by soaking, and then diluted further with water. (1)

Stability — Epirubicin hydrochloride in intact vials should be stored under refrigeration at 2 to 8 °C and protected from freezing and exposure to light. The manufacturer recommends discarding any unused solution from the single-dose vials within 24 hours after initial puncture of the vial stopper. (1)

pH Effects — Epirubicin hydrochloride stability is pH dependent. It becomes progressively more stable at acid pH. Maximum stability is obtained at pH 4 to 5. (1007; 1460) Prolonged contact of epirubicin hydrochloride with any solution having an alkaline pH should be avoided because of the resulting hydrolysis of the drug. (1)

Light Effects — Although epirubicin hydrochloride is photosensitive, no special precautions are necessary to protect solutions containing epirubicin hydrochloride 500 mcg/mL or greater during intravenous administration (1463) even over periods extending to 14 days in room light. (2081)

Syringes — Epirubicin hydrochloride 2 mg/mL in sterile water for injection was stable for at least 43 days at 4 °C in Plastipak (Becton-Dickinson) plastic syringes. (1460)

Epirubicin hydrochloride 0.5 mg/mL in sodium chloride 0.9% was reported to be stable for at least 28 days at 4 and 20 °C when stored in plastic syringes. (1564)

Epirubicin hydrochloride 2 mg/mL in sodium chloride 0.9% in 50-mL polypropylene syringes with blind luer hubs was stored at 25 °C both in light and dark and at 4 °C in dark. About 2 to 4% loss occurred in 14 days at 25 °C whether in light or dark. No loss was found after 180 days of refrigerated storage. (2081)

Sorption — Although epirubicin hydrochloride was initially reported to undergo sorptive losses to PVC containers, subsequent studies have shown no loss to glass, PVC, and high density polyethylene containers, PVC, polyethylene, and polybutadiene infusion sets, and polypropylene syringes. (1460; 1577; 1700)

Filtration — Epirubicin hydrochloride 50 mg/1000 mL in dextrose 5% and sodium chloride 0.9% was infused over 24 hours and exhibited a drug loss during the initial period of filtration through cellulose ester and nylon filters. However, the concentrations returned to expected levels within minutes, and the total amount of drug lost was deemed negligible. (1577)

Compatibility Information

Solution Compatibility

Epirubicin HCl

Solution	Mfr	Mfr	Conc/L	Remarks	Ref	C/I
Dextrose 3.3% in sodium chloride 0.3%		FA	100 mg	5% or less loss in 4 weeks at 25 °C in the dark	1007	C
Dextrose 5%		FA	100 mg	5% or less loss in 4 weeks at 25 °C in the dark	1007	C
	TR[a]	FA	100 mg	10% or less loss in 43 days at −20, 4, and 25 °C in the dark	1460	C
	[b]	FA	50 mg	9% loss in 30 days at 4 °C in the dark	1577	C
	[a]	FA	40 mg	Stable for 7 days at 4 °C in the dark	1700	C
Ringer's injection, lactated		FA	100 mg	10% loss in 3 days at 25 °C in the dark	1007	C
Sodium chloride 0.9%		FA	100 mg	10% loss in 8 days at 25 °C in the dark	1007	C
	TR[a]	FA	100 mg	10% or less loss in 43 days at −20, 4, and 25 °C in the dark	1460	C
	RS[a]		1 g	Under 5% loss in 4 weeks at −20 °C	1462	C
	[b]	FA	50 mg	6% or less loss in 25 days at 4 °C in the dark	1577	C
	[a]	FA	40 mg	Stable for 7 days at 4 °C in the dark	1700	C
		PH	1 g	Physically stable. No loss in 84 days at 8 °C	2534	C

[a]Tested in PVC containers.
[b]Tested in glass, PVC, and high density polyethylene containers.

Additive Compatibility

Epirubicin HCl

Drug	Mfr	Conc/L	Mfr	Conc/L	Test Soln	Remarks	Ref	C/I
Fluorouracil		10 g		0.5 to 1 g	NS	Greater than 10% epirubicin loss in 1 day	1379	I
Heparin sodium						Potential precipitation	1	I
Ifosfamide		2.5 g		1 g	NS	Under 10% loss of either drug in 14 days	1379	C
Irinotecan HCl	RPR	640 mg	CE	560 mg	NS	UV spectrum changes immediately upon mixing	2670	I

Drugs in Syringe Compatibility

Epirubicin HCl

Drug (in syringe)	Mfr	Amt	Mfr	Amt	Remarks	Ref	C/I
Fluorouracil		500 mg/ 10 mL		5 and 10 mg/ 10 mL[a]	Precipitate forms within several hours of mixing	1564	I
Ifosfamide		50 mg/ mL[a]		1 mg/mL[a]	Little or no loss of either drug in 28 days at 4 and 20 °C	1564	C
Ifosfamide with mesna		50 mg/ mL[a] 40 mg/ mL[a]		1 mg/mL[a]	50% epirubicin loss in 7 days at 4 and 20 °C. No loss of other drugs in 7 days	1564	I
Mesna with ifosfamide		40 mg/ mL[a] 50 mg/ mL[a]		1 mg/mL[a]	50% epirubicin loss in 7 days at 4 and 20 °C. No loss of other drugs in 7 days	1564	I

[a]Tested in sodium chloride 0.9%.

Y-Site Injection Compatibility (1:1 Mixture)

Epirubicin HCl

Drug	Mfr	Conc	Mfr	Conc	Remarks	Ref	C/I
Oxaliplatin	SS	0.5 mg/mL[a]	PHU	0.5 mg/mL[a]	Physically compatible for 4 hr at 23 °C	2566	C

[a]*Tested in dextrose 5%.*

EPOETIN ALFA
AHFS 20:16

Products — Epoetin alfa is available in 1-mL single-use (unpreserved) vials containing 2000, 3000, 4000, and 10,000 units/mL. The solution also contains in each milliliter albumin human 2.5 mg, sodium citrate 5.8 mg, sodium chloride 5.8 mg, and citric acid 0.06 mg in water for injection. (1)

Preservative-free single-dose epoetin alfa is also available in 1-mL vials containing 40,000 units along with albumin human 2.5 mg, sodium phosphate monobasic monohydrate 1.2 mg, sodium phosphate dibasic anhydrate 1.8 mg, sodium citrate 0.7 mg, sodium chloride 5.8 mg, and citric acid 6.8 mg in water for injection. (1)

Epoetin alfa is also available in 2-mL multidose (preserved) vials containing 10,000 units/mL and 1-mL multidose (preserved) vials containing 20,000 units/mL. The solution also contains in each milliliter albumin human 2.5 mg, sodium citrate 1.3 mg, sodium chloride 8.2 mg, citric acid 0.11 mg, and benzyl alcohol 1% in water for injection. (1)

pH — Single-use vials: from 6.6 to 7.2. Multidose vials: from 5.8 to 6.4. (1)

Tonicity — The injection is isotonic. (1)

Trade Name(s) — Epogen, Procrit.

Administration — Epoetin alfa is administered by intravenous or subcutaneous injection. For subcutaneous injection, epoetin alfa (single-dose) may be diluted at the time of administration with an equal quantity of bacteriostatic sodium chloride 0.9% containing benzyl alcohol 0.9% to help ameliorate local discomfort at the subcutaneous injection site. (1; 4)

Stability — Epoetin alfa is a colorless solution. It should not be used if it contains particulate matter or is discolored. Intact vials should be stored under refrigeration and protected from freezing. (1) Although refrigerated storage is required, the manufacturer has stated the single-dose form may be stored at room temperature for 14 days while the multidose form may be stored at room temperature for seven days. (2745) To prevent foaming and inactivation, the product should not be shaken; vigorous prolonged shaking may denature the protein, inactivating it. (1; 4) However, a small amount of flocculated protein in the solution does not affect potency. In addition, exposure to light for less than 24 hours does not adversely affect the product. (4)

The single-dose vials have no preservative. After a single dose has been removed from this product, the vial should not be re-entered and should be discarded. (1) Drawn into plastic tuberculin syringes, the preservative-free products at 2000 or 10,000 units/mL are reported to be stable for two weeks at room temperature or under refrigeration. However, use shortly after drawing up in syringes is recommended because of the absence of preservative. (4)

Usually, epoetin alfa should not be diluted and transferred to new containers or admixed with other drugs and solutions because of possible protein loss from adsorption to PVC containers and tubing. However, when 10,000-unit/mL single-use product is diluted in the original vial with benzyl alcohol-preserved sodium chloride 0.9% injection to a concentration of 4000 units/mL for subcutaneous use, it is stated to be stable for at least 12 weeks stored at 5 and 30 °C. Furthermore, the final benzyl alcohol concentration of 0.54% enabled the dilution to pass the USP preservative effectiveness test. (1905) Restriction of this dilution to 28 days used as a multiple-dose vial has been recommended. (1906) Higher concentrations of epoetin alfa (e.g., 5000 units/mL), which would have lower benzyl alcohol concentrations, were found to fail the preservative effectiveness test. (1905)

Epoetin alfa (Amgen) 20,000 units/1 mL was packaged in 1-mL hubless Medsaver (Becton-Dickinson) plastic syringes and stored under refrigeration for six weeks. No loss of epoetin alfa biological activity was found. (2472)

The multidose vials contain a preservative and may be stored under refrigeration after initial dose removal. The vials should be discarded 21 days after initial entry. (1)

Compatibility Information

Solution Compatibility

Epoetin alfa

Solution	Mfr	Mfr	Conc/L	Remarks	Ref	C/I
Dextrose 10%[b]	[a]	ORT	100 units	40 to 50% of epoetin alfa lost over 24-hr delivery	1878	I

Solution Compatibility (Cont.)

Epoetin alfa

Solution	Mfr	Mfr	Conc/L	Remarks	Ref	C/I
Dextrose 10%[c]	a	ORT	100 units	96% of the epoetin alfa delivered over 24 hr	1878	C
Sodium chloride 0.9%	a	ORT	100 units	15% of epoetin alfa lost over 24-hr delivery	1878	I
TPN[d]	a	ORT	100 units	96% of the epoetin alfa delivered over 24 hr	1878	C

[a] Delivered from a syringe through microbore tubing, T-connector, and a Teflon neonatal 24-gauge intravenous catheter.
[b] Tested with and without albumin human 0.01%.
[c] Tested with albumin human 0.05 and 0.1%.
[d] TPN composed of amino acids (TrophAmine) 0.5% or 2.25% with dextrose 12.5%, vitamins, trace elements, magnesium sulfate, calcium gluconate, sodium chloride, potassium acetate, and heparin sodium.

EPOPROSTENOL SODIUM
AHFS 24:12.92

Products — Epoprostenol sodium is available as a lyophilized powder in vials containing 0.5 and 1.5 mg of epoprostenol along with glycine 3.76 mg, sodium chloride 2.93 mg, and mannitol 50 mg. Sodium hydroxide may have been added during manufacturing to adjust the pH. (1)

The vials are reconstituted using only the special diluent packaged in 50-mL vials containing glycine 94 mg, sodium chloride 73.3 mg, and sodium hydroxide to adjust pH in water for injection. The diluent volume should be selected to accommodate the maximum and minimum flow rates of the infusion pump. In general, a 3- to 10-mcg/mL concentration of epoprostenol sodium is used. (1)

The manufacturer's instructions for preparing various concentrations of the drug are as follows (1):

For 3 mcg/mL, reconstitute one 0.5-mg vial with 5 mL of special diluent. Withdraw 3 mL and add a sufficient amount of special diluent to make 100 mL.

For 5 mcg/mL, reconstitute one 0.5-mg vial with 5 mL of special diluent. Withdraw the entire contents and add a sufficient amount of special diluent to make 100 mL.

For 10 mcg/mL, reconstitute two 0.5-mg vials with 5 mL each of special diluent. Withdraw the entire contents of both vials and add sufficient amount of special diluent to make a total of 100 mL.

For 15 mcg/mL, reconstitute one 1.5-mg vial with 5 mL of special diluent. Withdraw the entire contents and sufficient special diluent to make a total of 100 mL.

pH — From 10.2 to 10.8. (1)

Trade Name(s) — Flolan.

Administration — Epoprostenol sodium reconstituted with the special diluent is administered without dilution by continuous intravenous infusion through a central catheter using an ambulatory infusion pump. The drug may be given temporarily by peripheral infusion until a central line can be established. The reservoirs used should be PVC, polypropylene, or glass. (1)

To facilitate extended ambulatory use at temperatures exceeding 25 °C, a cold pouch with frozen gel packs is suggested. The cold pouch that is used must be capable of maintaining the temperature of the epoprostenol sodium solution at 2 to 8 °C for 12 hours. (1)

Stability — Intact vials of epoprostenol sodium should be stored at controlled room temperature and protected from light. The vials of special diluent should also be stored at controlled room temperature and protected from freezing. Epoprostenol sodium is only stable when reconstituted with the special diluent. The drug should not be mixed with any other drugs or solutions prior to or during administration. (1)

After reconstitution and prior to use, epoprostenol sodium must be stored under refrigeration and protected from light and freezing; reconstituted solution that has been frozen must be discarded. Any reconstituted solution should be discarded after 48 hours of refrigerated storage. During use, the reconstituted solution may be administered at room temperature for up to eight hours, or it can be used with a cold pouch containing two frozen gel packs for up to 24 hours. (1)

For room temperature administration, the reconstituted solution should not have been stored for longer than 40 hours under refrigeration and should be administered over no longer than eight hours. To manage room temperature administration, a 100-mL daily dose may be divided into three equal portions; two portions are stored under refrigeration until needed while the other portion is administered at room temperature. (1)

For administration using a cold pouch, the reconstituted solutions should be stored for no more than 24 hours and may then be infused for no longer than 24 hours. The frozen gel packs should be changed every 12 hours. (1)

pH Effects — Epoprostenol sodium becomes increasingly unstable at pH values lower than the normal range of 10.2 to 10.8. (1)

Light Effects — Epoprostenol sodium should be protected from light during storage and should not be exposed to direct sunlight either during storage or in use. (1)

Filtration — An inline 0.22-μm filter was used during trials with this drug. (1)

Compatibility Information

Y-Site Injection Compatibility (1:1 Mixture)

Epoprostenol sodium

Drug	Mfr	Conc	Mfr	Conc	Remarks	Ref	C/I
Bivalirudin	TMC	5 mg/mLᵃ	GW	10 mcg/mLᵃ	Physically compatible for 4 hr at 23 °C	2373	C

ᵃTested in dextrose 5%.

EPTIFIBATIDE
AHFS 20:12.18

Products — Eptifibatide is available at a concentration of 2 mg/mL in 10- and 100-mL vials and at a concentration of 0.75 mg/mL in 100-mL vials. Each milliliter of injection also contains citric acid 5.25 mg and sodium hydroxide to adjust pH. (1)

pH — The pH is adjusted to near 5.35 during manufacturing. (1)

Trade Name(s) — Integrilin.

Administration — Eptifibatide is administered by intravenous bolus injection from a syringe over one to two minutes and by continuous intravenous infusion using an infusion pump. Light protection during administration is not required. For continuous infusion, the appropriate concentration of eptifibatide in 100-mL vials is spiked with a vented infusion set and administered directly. (1; 4)

Eptifibatide may be administered in an intravenous line running sodium chloride 0.9% or dextrose 5% in sodium chloride 0.9% with or without potassium chloride in a concentration up to 60 mEq/L. (1)

Stability — Intact vials of eptifibatide should be stored under refrigeration and protected from light. The drug may be stored for up to two months at room temperature; the cartons of the vials stored at room temperature should be marked with a "DISCARD BY" date no more than two months after transfer to room temperature storage or the expiration date, whichever comes first. (1) Vials left unrefrigerated only briefly such that vials remain cool to the touch may be returned to refrigerated storage without altering the expiration date. (4)

pH Effects — The minimum rate of decomposition occurs in the pH range of 5 to 6. (2417)

Sorption — No incompatibilities with administration sets have been observed. However, no compatibility studies with PVC bags have been conducted. (1)

Compatibility Information

Y-Site Injection Compatibility (1:1 Mixture)

Eptifibatide

Drug	Mfr	Conc	Mfr	Conc	Remarks	Ref	C/I
Amiodarone HCl	WY	6 mg/mLᵃ	KEY	0.75 mg/mL	Visually compatible for 24 hr at 22 °C	2352	C
	WY	6 mg/mLᵃ	KEY	2 mg/mL	Visually compatible for 24 hr at 22 °C	2352	C
Argatroban	GSK	1 mg/mLᵃ·ᵇ·ᶜ	COR	2 mg/mLᶜ	Physically compatible with no loss of either drug in 4 hr at 23 °C	2630	C
Bivalirudin	TMC	5 mg/mLᵃ	KEY	2 mg/mL	Physically compatible for 4 hr at 23 °C	2373	C
Metoprolol tartrate	BED	1 mg/mL	SC	0.75 mg/mL	Visually compatible for 24 hr at 19 °C	2795	C
Micafungin sodium	ASP	1.5 mg/mLᵇ	SC	0.75 mg/mL	Physically compatible for 4 hr at 23 °C	2683	C

ᵃTested in dextrose 5%.
ᵇTested in sodium chloride 0.9%.
ᶜMixed argatroban:eptifibatide 1:1 and 16:1.

Additional Compatibility Information

Other Drugs — Eptifibatide is stated by the manufacturer to be chemically and physically compatible when administered in the same intravenous administration line as alteplase, atropine sulfate, dobutamine hydrochloride, heparin sodium, lidocaine hydrochloride, meperidine hydrochloride, metoprolol tartrate, midazolam hydrochloride, morphine sulfate, nitroglycerin, and verapamil hydrochloride. (1; 4)

Furosemide — Eptifibatide is chemically and physically incompatible with furosemide. A precipitate appears within one hour of mixing the drugs, and greater than 40% loss of furosemide occurs in 24 hours. (1; 4)

ERTAPENEM SODIUM
AHFS 8:12.07.08

Products — Ertapenem is available as a lyophilized powder in 1-g vials as the sodium salt with sodium bicarbonate 175 mg and sodium hydroxide to adjust the pH. For intravenous administration, reconstitute the 1-g vial with 10 mL of sterile water for injection, bacteriostatic water for injection, or sodium chloride 0.9% and shake well, yielding a 100-mg/mL concentration. Upon dissolution, immediately transfer the reconstituted solution to 50 mL of sodium chloride 0.9% for adults. For pediatric patients, the dose of reconstituted ertapenem should be transferred to a volume of sodium chloride 0.9% to yield a final concentration of 20 mg/mL or less. (1)

For intramuscular injection, reconstitute the 1-g vial with 3.2 mL of lidocaine hydrochloride 1% (without epinephrine) and shake well, yielding a 280-mg/mL concentration. Upon dissolution, administer within one hour. Do NOT administer the reconstituted intramuscular injection intravenously. (1)

pH — 7.5. (1)

Sodium Content — Approximately 137 mg or 6 mEq. (1)

Trade Name(s) — Invanz.

Administration — Ertapenem sodium diluted in sodium chloride 0.9% may be administered by intravenous infusion over 30 minutes or by deep intramuscular injection into a large muscle mass such as the gluteal muscle or the lateral part of the thigh. (1)

Stability — Intact vials of ertapenem sodium should be stored at controlled room temperature not exceeding 25 °C. The reconstituted drug solution for intravenous administration should be diluted immediately in sodium chloride 0.9%. Dextrose-containing solutions should NOT be used to dilute ertapenem. (1; 2723). The drug diluted for infusion may be stored and used within six hours at room temperature or may be stored for 24 hours under refrigeration and used within four hours after removal from refrigeration. The drug prepared for intramuscular administration should be used within one hour. Solutions of ertapenem sodium should not be frozen. (1)

Compatibility Information

Solution Compatibility

Ertapenem (as sodium salt)

Solution	Mfr	Mfr	Conc/L	Remarks	Ref	C/I
Dextrose 5% in sodium chloride 0.225%	AB	ME	10 and 20 g	Visually compatible. 10% loss in 6 hr at 25 °C. 8% loss in 32 hr and 11% loss in 48 hr at 4 °C	2487	I
Dextrose 5% in sodium chloride 0.9%	AB	ME	10 and 20 g	Visually compatible. 11% loss in 6 hr at 25 °C and 10% loss in 32 hr at 4 °C	2487	I
Dextrose 5%	AB	ME	10 and 20 g	Visually compatible. 10% loss in 6 hr at 25 °C and 5 to 8% loss in 24 hr at 4 °C	2487	I
Ringer's injection	AB	ME	10 and 20 g	Visually compatible. 10 to 12% ertapenem loss in 20 hr at 25 °C and 11% loss in 5 days at 4 °C	2487	I[a]
Ringer's injection, lactated	AB	ME	10 and 20 g	Visually compatible. 18% loss in 20 hr at 25 °C and 9% loss in 3 days at 4 °C	2487	I
Sodium chloride 0.225%	AB	ME	10 and 20 g	Visually compatible. 9 to 12% loss in 20 hr at 25 °C and 8 to 11% loss in 5 days at 4 °C	2487	I[a]
Sodium chloride 0.9%	AB	ME	10 and 20 g	Visually compatible. 9 to 11% loss in 20 hr at 25 °C and 8 to 11% loss in 5 days at 4 °C	2487	I[a]
	[b]	ME	10 g	Physically compatible with less than 10% drug loss in 24 hr at 25 °C and 7 days at 5 °C	2723	C
	[c]	ME	10 g	Physically compatible with less than 10% drug loss in 30 hr at 25 °C and 8 days at 5 °C	2723	C
	[b]	ME	20 g	Physically compatible with less than 10% drug loss in 18 hr at 25 °C and 5 days at 5 °C	2723	C
	[c]	ME	20 g	Physically compatible with less than 10% drug loss in 24 hr at 25 °C and 7 days at 5 °C	2723	C
Sodium lactate ⅙ M	AB	ME	10 and 20 g	Visually compatible. 7 to 9% loss in 6 hr at 25 °C and 8 to 11% loss in 2 days at 4 °C	2487	I

[a]*Incompatible by conventional standards but recommended for dilution of ertapenem with use in shorter periods of time.*
[b]*Tested in the Homepump Eclipse elastomeric pump reservoirs.*
[c]*Tested in Intermate elastomeric pump reservoirs.*

Additive Compatibility

Ertapenem (as sodium salt)

Drug	Mfr	Conc/L	Mfr	Conc/L	Test Soln	Remarks	Ref	C/I
Mannitol	AB	5%	ME	10 and 20 g		Precipitate in <1 hr. 15% loss in 20 hr at 25 °C. 7% loss in 2 days at 4 °C	2487	I
	AB	20%	ME	10 and 20 g		Precipitate in <1 hr. 13% loss in 6 hr at 25 °C. 8% loss in 1 day at 4 °C	2487	I
Sodium bicarbonate	AB	5%	ME	10 and 20 g		Visually compatible. 11% loss in 3 hr at 25 °C. 16 to 19% loss in 1 day at 4 °C	2487	I

Y-Site Injection Compatibility (1:1 Mixture)

Ertapenem (as sodium salt)

Drug	Mfr	Conc	Mfr	Conc	Remarks	Ref	C/I
Anidulafungin	VIC	0.5 mg/mL[a]	ME	20 mg/mL[b]	Microparticulates form immediately	2617	I
Caspofungin acetate	ME	0.7 mg/mL[b]	ME	20 mg/mL[b]	Immediate white turbid precipitate forms	2758	I
Heparin sodium	APP	40 and 100 units/mL[a]	ME	10 mg/mL[b]	Visually compatible with about 4% ertapenem loss in 4 hr	2487	C
	APP	50 and 100 units/mL[b]	ME	10 mg/mL[b]	Visually compatible with about 3% ertapenem loss in 4 hr	2487	C
Hetastarch in sodium chloride 0.9%	AB	6%	ME	10 mg/mL[b]	Visually compatible with about 3% ertapenem loss in 8 hr	2487	C
Potassium chloride	AB	0.01 and 0.04 mEq/mL[c]	ME	10 mg/mL[b]	Visually compatible with about 2% ertapenem loss in 4 hr	2487	C
Telavancin HCl	ASP	7.5 mg/mL[b]	ME	20 mg/mL[b]	Physically compatible for 2 hr	2830	C
Tigecycline	WY	1 mg/mL[b]		20 mg/mL[b]	Physically compatible for 4 hr	2714	C

[a]Tested in dextrose 5%.
[b]Tested in sodium chloride 0.9%.
[c]Tested in sterile water for injection.

ERYTHROMYCIN LACTOBIONATE
AHFS 8:12.12.04

Products — Erythromycin lactobionate is available in vials containing the equivalent of 1 g of erythromycin and in vials containing the equivalent of 500 mg of erythromycin. Reconstitute the 1-g vials with at least 20 mL and the 500-mg vials with 10 mL of sterile water for injection without preservatives. The resultant concentration is 5% (50 mg/mL). The drug is also available in 500-mg and 1-g ADD-Vantage vials without preservative. (1; 4)

pH — Reconstitution with sterile water for injection to a 50-mg/mL concentration results in a solution with a pH of 6.5 to 7.5. (20)

Osmolality — Erythromycin lactobionate 50 mg/mL in sterile water for injection has an osmolality of 223 mOsm/kg. (50)

The osmolality of erythromycin lactobionate was calculated for the following dilutions (1054):

Diluent	Osmolality (mOsm/kg)	
	50 mL	100 mL
500 mg		
Dextrose 5%	273	265
Sodium chloride 0.9%	299	291
1 g		
Dextrose 5%	287	273
Sodium chloride 0.9%	313	300

Trade Name(s) — Erythrocin Lactobionate-I.V.

Administration — Erythromycin lactobionate may be administered by continuous or intermittent intravenous infusion; it must not be given by direct intravenous injection. To minimize venous irritation, slow continuous infusion of a 1-mg/mL concentration is recommended. By intermittent infusion, one-fourth of the daily dose at a concentration of 1 to 5 mg/mL in at least 100 mL of infusion solution may be given over 20 to 60 minutes every six hours. (1; 4)

Stability — Do not use sodium chloride 0.9% or other solutions containing inorganic ions in the initial reconstitution of the regular vials. Such solutions result in the formation of a precipitate. (4; 20) (Note: This restriction does not apply to the drug in ADD-Vantage containers.)

The commercial vials are stable at room temperature. (20) Reconstituted (5%) solutions are stable for 14 days when stored under refrigeration (20) or for 24 hours when kept at room temperature. (1)

pH Effects — The stability of erythromycin lactobionate is extremely pH dependent. It is most stable at pH 6 to 8 (20; 1935) or 9. (1101; 2596) Erythromycin lactobionate is unstable in acidic solutions. Decomposition occurs at an increasingly more rapid rate as the pH approaches 4. (20) A pH over 5.5 is recommended for the final diluted solution. At pH 5.5 or below and at pH 10 or above, erythromycin lactobionate is particularly unstable, with 10% decomposition occurring in about eight or nine hours. The following pH profile was determined for erythromycin in solution (1101):

Solution pH	Approximate Time for 10% Decomposition (t_{90})
5.0	2.5 hr
5.5	8.8 hr
6.0	1 day
7.0	4.6 days
8.0	7.3 days
9.0	2.6 days
10.0	8.8 hr
11.0	53 min

Erythromycin lactobionate can alter the pH of solutions and give itself some protection against decomposition for varying periods. The length of time is dependent on the initial pH and the buffer capacity of the solution. (48) The pH of unbuffered dextrose 5% is raised one pH unit by the addition of erythromycin lactobionate. (20) The use of admixtures with a pH of less than 5 is not recommended. If the admixture pH is 5 to 6, it should be used immediately. (48)

The effect of buffering erythromycin lactobionate (Abbott) solutions was evaluated. Erythromycin lactobionate 2 mg/mL in sodium chloride 0.9% (pH 7.15 to 7.25) exhibited 5% losses in about 20 days at 5 °C. However, buffering with sodium bicarbonate to pH 7.5 to 8 extended stability, with 5% losses occurring in about 85 days at 5 °C. (1587)

Freezing Solutions — Erythromycin lactobionate (Abbott) 500 mg/110 mL in sodium chloride 0.9% in PVC bags was frozen at −20 °C; no loss occurred after 12 months of storage followed by microwave thawing. Furthermore, the solution was physically compatible, with no increase in subvisible particles. In addition, no erythromycin loss was found after six months at −20 °C followed by three freeze–thaw cycles. (1612)

Compatibility Information

Solution Compatibility

Erythromycin lactobionate

Solution	Mfr	Mfr	Conc/L	Remarks	Ref	C/I
Dextrose 5% in Ringer's injection, lactated	AB	AB	1 g	10% loss in 3 hr at 25 °C	20	I
	TR[a]	AB	1 g	10 to 24% loss in 24 hr at 5 °C	282	I
Dextrose 5% in sodium chloride 0.9%	TR[a]	AB	1 g	Stable for 24 hr at 5 °C	282	C
	AB	AB	1 g	33% loss in 24 hr	46	I
		AB	1 g	12% loss in 6 hr at 25 °C	48	I
		AB	2 g	15% loss in 6 hr	109	I
Dextrose 5%	TR[a]	AB	1 g	Stable for 24 hr at 5 °C	282	C
	AB	AB	1 g	15% loss in 24 hr	46	I
	AB	AB	1 g	10% loss in 10 hr at 25 °C	20	I
		AB	1 g	15% loss in 24 hr at 25 °C	48	I
		AB	2 g	14% loss in 6 hr	109	I
	TR[b]	AB	4 g	21% loss in activity in 24 hr at room temperature	518	I

Solution Compatibility (Cont.)

Erythromycin lactobionate

Solution	Mfr	Mfr	Conc/L	Remarks	Ref	C/I
	TR[b,c]	AB	4 g	Physically compatible and stable for 24 hr at room temperature	518	**C**
Dextrose 10%		AB	2 g	14% loss in 6 hr	109	**I**
Normosol M in dextrose 5%	AB	AB	1 g	10% loss in 6 hr at 25 °C	20	**I**
Normosol R		AB	1 g	14% loss in 24 hr at 25 °C	48	**I**
Ringer's injection	AB	AB	1 g	10% loss in 11 hr at 25 °C	20	**I**
Ringer's injection, lactated	TR[a]	AB	1 g	Stable for 24 hr at 5 °C	282	**C**
	AB	AB	1 g	10% loss in 18 hr at 25 °C	20	**I**
Sodium chloride 0.9%		AB	1 g	Stable for 24 hr at 25 °C	48	**C**
		AB	2 g	Stable for 24 hr	109	**C**
	AB	AB	1 g	Stable for 24 hr	46	**C**
	AB	AB	1 g	10% loss in 22 hr at 25 °C	20	**C**
	TR[a]	AB	1 g	Stable for 24 hr at 5 °C	282	**C**
	TR[b]	AB	4 g	Physically compatible and stable for 24 hr at room temperature	518	**C**
	TR[b,c]	AB	4 g	Physically compatible and stable for 24 hr at room temperature	518	**C**
		AB	2 g	5% loss in about 20 days at 5 °C	1587	**C**
	BA[b]	AB	8.3 g	No more than 5% loss after 60 days at 5 °C	1597	**C**
	AB[d]	ES	20 g	Little or no loss with 24-hr storage at 5 °C followed by 24-hr simulated administration at 30 °C via portable pump	1779	**C**

[a]*Tested in both glass and PVC containers.*
[b]*Tested in PVC containers.*
[c]*Buffered with sodium bicarbonate 4% (Neut, Abbott).*
[d]*Tested in portable pump reservoirs (Pharmacia Deltec).*

Additive Compatibility

Erythromycin lactobionate

Drug	Mfr	Conc/L	Mfr	Conc/L	Test Soln	Remarks	Ref	C/I
Aminophylline	SE	500 mg	AB	1 g		Physically compatible. Erythromycin stable for 24 hr at 25 °C	20	**C**
Ampicillin sodium	WY	3.7 g	AB	3 g	NS	Physically compatible with 6% ampicillin loss in 1 day at 24 °C	1035	**C**
Ascorbic acid	AB	1 g	AB	1 g		Physically compatible	3	**C**
	UP	500 mg	AB	5 g	D5W	Physically incompatible	15	**I**
Chloramphenicol sodium succinate	PD		AB		D5W	May precipitate at some concentrations	15	**I**
Colistimethate sodium	WC	500 mg	AB	5 g	D5W	Physically incompatible	15	**I**
	WC	500 mg	AB	1 g	D	Precipitate forms within 1 hr	20	**I**
Diphenhydramine HCl	PD	50 mg	AB	1 g		Physically compatible. Erythromycin stable for 24 hr at 25 °C	20	**C**
	PD	50 mg	AB	1 g	D5W	Erythromycin stable for 24 hr at 25 °C	48	**C**
Floxacillin sodium	BE	20 g	AB	5 g	NS	Precipitates immediately. Crystals form in 5 hr at 15 °C	1479	**I**
Furosemide	HO	1 g	AB	5 g	NS	Precipitates immediately. Crystals form in 12 to 24 hr at 15 and 30 °C	1479	**I**

Additive Compatibility (Cont.)

Erythromycin lactobionate

Drug	Mfr	Conc/L	Mfr	Conc/L	Test Soln	Remarks	Ref	C/I
Fusidate sodium	LEO	1 g		5 g	D–S	Physically compatible and chemically stable for 48 hr at room temperature	1800	C
Heparin sodium	UP	4000 units	AB	5 g	D5W	Physically incompatible	15	I
	AB	1500 units	AB	1 g		Precipitate forms within 1 hr	20	I
	AB	20,000 units	AB	1 g		Precipitate forms within 1 hr	21	I
	OR	20,000 units	AB	1.5 g	D5W, NS	Precipitate forms	113	I
Hydrocortisone sodium succinate	UP	500 mg	AB	5 g	D5W	Physically compatible	15	C
	UP	250 mg	AB	1 g		Physically compatible	20	C
Lidocaine HCl	AST	2 g	AB	1 g		Physically compatible	24	C
Linezolid	PHU	2 g	AB	5 g	b	Erythromycin loss of 15% in 1 hr and 30% in 4 hr at 23 °C. Loss of 45% in 1 day at 4 °C	2333	I
Metoclopramide HCl	RB	400 mg	AB	4 g	NS	Incompatible. If mixed, use immediately	924	I
	RB	100 mg	AB	5 g	NS	Incompatible. If mixed, use immediately	924	I
	RB	416 mg	AB	4.1 g		Incompatible. If mixed, use immediately	1167	I
	RB	1.1 g	AB	3.5 g		Incompatible. If mixed, use immediately	1167	I
Penicillin G potassium		1 million units	AB	1 g		Physically compatible	3	C
	SQ	20 million units	AB	5 g	D5W	Physically compatible	15	C
	SQ	5 million units	AB	1 g		Physically compatible	20; 47	C
Penicillin G sodium	UP	20 million units	AB	5 g	D5W	Physically compatible	15	C
Pentobarbital sodium	AB	500 mg	AB	1 g		Physically compatible. Erythromycin stable for 24 hr at 25 °C	20	C
Polymyxin B sulfate	BW	200 mg	AB	5 g	D5W	Physically compatible	15	C
Potassium chloride	AB	40 mEq	AB	1 g		Physically compatible	20	C
Prochlorperazine edisylate	SKF	10 mg	AB	1 g		Physically compatible. Erythromycin stable for 24 hr at 25 °C	20	C
Ranitidine HCl	GL	50 mg and 2 g		5 g	NS	Physically compatible. Ranitidine stable for 24 hr at 25 °C. Erythromycin not tested	1515	C
Sodium bicarbonate	AB	3.75 g	AB	1 g		Physically compatible. Erythromycin stable for 24 hr at 25 °C	20	C
	AB	2.4 mEq[a]	AB	1 g	D5W	Physically compatible for 24 hr	772	C
Verapamil HCl	KN	80 mg	AB	2 g	D5W, NS	Physically compatible for 24 hr	764	C

[a] *One vial of Neut added to a liter of admixture.*
[b] *Admixed in the linezolid infusion container.*

Drugs in Syringe Compatibility

Erythromycin lactobionate

Drug (in syringe)	Mfr	Amt	Mfr	Amt	Remarks	Ref	C/I
Ampicillin sodium	AY	500 mg	AB	300 mg/6 mL	Precipitate forms in 1 hr at room temperature	300	**I**
Cloxacillin sodium	AY	250 mg	AB	300 mg/6 mL	Precipitate forms within 1 hr at room temperature	300	**I**
Heparin sodium	AB	20,000 units/1 mL	AB	1 g	Physically incompatible	21	**I**

Y-Site Injection Compatibility (1:1 Mixture)

Erythromycin lactobionate

Drug	Mfr	Conc	Mfr	Conc	Remarks	Ref	C/I
Acyclovir sodium	BW	5 mg/mL[a]	AB	4 mg/mL[a]	Physically compatible for 4 hr at 25 °C	1157	**C**
Amiodarone HCl	LZ	4 mg/mL[c]	AB	2 mg/mL[c]	Physically compatible for 4 hr at room temperature	1444	**C**
Anidulafungin	VIC	0.5 mg/mL[a]	AB	5 mg/mL[b]	Physically compatible for 4 hr at 23 °C	2617	**C**
Bivalirudin	TMC	5 mg/mL[a]	AB	5 mg/mL[b]	Physically compatible for 4 hr at 23 °C	2373	**C**
Cefepime HCl	BMS	120 mg/mL[j]		5 mg/mL	Over 10% cefepime loss occurs in 1 hr	2513	**I**
Ceftazidime	SKB	125 mg/mL		50 mg/mL	Precipitates immediately	2434	**I**
	SKB	125 mg/mL		10 mg/mL	Trace precipitation	2434	**I**
	GSK	120 mg/mL[j]		5 mg/mL	Precipitates	2513	**I**
Cyclophosphamide	MJ	20 mg/mL[a]	AB	5 mg/mL[a]	Physically compatible for 4 hr at 25 °C	1194	**C**
Dexmedetomidine HCl	AB	4 mcg/mL[b]	AB	5 mg/mL[b]	Physically compatible for 4 hr at 23 °C	2383	**C**
Diltiazem HCl	MMD	5 mg/mL	ES	5 and 50 mg/mL[b]	Visually compatible	1807	**C**
Doxapram HCl	RB	2 mg/mL[a]	AB	5 mg/mL[a]	Visually compatible for 4 hr at 23 °C	2470	**C**
Enalaprilat	MSD	0.05 mg/mL[b]	AB	5 mg/mL[a]	Physically compatible for 24 hr at room temperature under fluorescent light	1355	**C**
Esmolol HCl	DCC	10 mg/mL[a]	AB	5 mg/mL[a]	Physically compatible for 24 hr at 22 °C	1169	**C**
Famotidine	MSD	0.2 mg/mL[a]	ES	2 mg/mL[b]	Physically compatible for 14 hr	1196	**C**
Fenoldopam mesylate	AB	80 mcg/mL[b]	AB	5 mg/mL[b]	Physically compatible for 4 hr at 23 °C	2467	**C**
Foscarnet sodium	AST	24 mg/mL	AB	20 mg/mL	Physically compatible for 24 hr at room temperature under fluorescent light	1335	**C**
	AST	24 mg/mL	ES	20 mg/mL[c]	Physically compatible for 24 hr at 25 °C under fluorescent light	1393	**C**
Heparin sodium	TR	50 units/mL	AB	3.3 mg/mL[b]	Visually compatible for 4 hr at 25 °C	1793	**C**
Hetastarch in lactated electrolyte	AB	6%	AB	5 mg/mL[b]	Physically compatible for 4 hr at 23 °C	2339	**C**
Hydromorphone HCl	WY	0.2 mg/mL[a]	AB	5 mg/mL[a]	Physically compatible for 4 hr at 25 °C	987	**C**
Idarubicin HCl	AD	1 mg/mL[b]	ES	2 mg/mL[b]	Visually compatible for 24 hr at 25 °C	1525	**C**
Labetalol HCl	SC	1 mg/mL[a]	AB	5 mg/mL[a]	Physically compatible for 24 hr at 18 °C	1171	**C**
Lorazepam	WY	0.33 mg/mL[b]	AB	5 mg/mL	Visually compatible for 24 hr at 22 °C	1855	**C**
Magnesium sulfate	IX	16.7, 33.3, 66.7, 100 mg/mL[a]	AB	5 mg/mL[a]	Physically compatible for at least 4 hr at 32 °C	813	**C**

Y-Site Injection Compatibility (1:1 Mixture) (Cont.)

Erythromycin lactobionate

Drug	Mfr	Conc	Mfr	Conc	Remarks	Ref	C/I
Meperidine HCl	WY	10 mg/mL[a]	AB	5 mg/mL[a]	Physically compatible for 4 hr at 25 °C	987	C
Midazolam HCl	RC	5 mg/mL	AB	5 mg/mL	Visually compatible for 24 hr at 22 °C	1855	C
Morphine sulfate	WI	1 mg/mL[a]	AB	5 mg/mL[a]	Physically compatible for 4 hr at 25 °C	987	C
Multivitamins	USV	5 mL/L[a]	AB	500 mg/250 mL[b]	Physically compatible for 24 hr at room temperature	323	C
Nicardipine HCl	DCC	0.1 mg/mL[a]	AB	5 mg/mL[a]	Visually compatible for 24 hr at room temperature	235	C
Tacrolimus	FUJ	1 mg/mL[b]	AB	20 mg/mL[a]	Visually compatible for 24 hr at 25 °C	1630	C
Theophylline	TR	4 mg/mL	AB	3.3 mg/mL[b]	Visually compatible for 6 hr at 25 °C	1793	C
TNA #73[d]		32.5 mL[e]	AB	20 mg/mL[b]	Visually compatible for 4 hr at 25 °C	1008	C
TPN #61[d]		[f]	AB	50 mg/1 mL[g]	Physically compatible	1012	C
		[h]	AB	300 mg/6 mL[g]	Physically compatible	1012	C
TPN #189[d]			DB	10 mg/mL[a]	Visually compatible for 24 hr at 22 °C	1767	C
Zidovudine	BW	4 mg/mL[a]	AB	20 mg/mL[a,i]	Physically compatible for 4 hr at 25 °C	1193	C

[a]*Tested in dextrose 5%.*
[b]*Tested in sodium chloride 0.9%.*
[c]*Tested in both dextrose 5% and sodium chloride 0.9%.*
[d]*Refer to Appendix I for the composition of parenteral nutrition solutions. TNA indicates a 3-in-1 admixture, and TPN indicates a 2-in-1 admixture.*
[e]*A 32.5-mL sample of parenteral nutrition solution mixed with 50 mL of antibiotic solution.*
[f]*Run at 21 mL/hr.*
[g]*Given over 30 minutes by syringe pump.*
[h]*Run at 94 mL/hr.*
[i]*Sodium bicarbonate 2.5 mEq added to adjust pH.*
[j]*Tested in sterile water for injection.*

ESMOLOL HYDROCHLORIDE
AHFS 24:24

Products — Ready-to-use esmolol hydrochloride 10 mg/mL is available in 10-mL single-dose vials and 250-mL bags with sodium chloride 5.9 mg/mL. Each milliliter of the ready-to-use products is buffered with sodium acetate 2.8 mg and glacial acetic acid 0.546 mg and may contain sodium hydroxide and/or hydrochloric acid for pH adjustment during manufacturing. (1; 4)

Esmolol hydrochloride is also available as a double-strength ready-to-use 20-mg/mL solution in 10-mL vials and 250-mL bags with sodium chloride 4.1 mg/mL. Each milliliter of the double-strength ready-to-use products is buffered with sodium acetate 2.8 mg and glacial acetic acid 0.546 mg and may contain sodium hydroxide and/or hydrochloric acid for pH.

pH — From 4.5 to 5.5. (1; 4)

Osmolarity — Esmolol hydrochloride 10- and 20-mg/mL ready-to-use solutions are iso-osmotic having an osmolarity of 312 mOsm/L. (1; 4)

Trade Name(s) — Brevibloc.

Administration — Esmolol hydrochloride is administered by intravenous infusion at a concentration of 10 or 20 mg/mL, usually with an infusion control device. Esmolol hydrochloride concentrations greater than 10 mg/mL are associated with more serious venous irritation, including thrombophlebitis, and more serious local reactions, including skin necrosis. The manufacturer recommends not infusing concentrations greater than 10 mg/mL into a small vein or through a butterfly catheter. (1; 4)

Stability — Esmolol hydrochloride is a clear, colorless to light yellow solution. It should be stored at controlled room temperature and protected from elevated temperatures and freezing. (1)

pH Effects — Esmolol hydrochloride is relatively stable at neutral pH; the optimal pH is 4.5 to 5.5. However, ester hydrolysis occurs rapidly in strongly acidic or basic solutions. (1358; 1359)

Compatibility Information

Solution Compatibility

Esmolol HCl

Solution	Mfr	Mfr	Conc/L	Remarks	Ref	C/I
Dextrose 5% in Ringer's injection			10 g	Compatible and stable for 24 hr at 4 and 25 °C	1	**C**
Dextrose 5% in Ringer's injection, lactated	BA[a], MG[b]	ACC	10 g	Visually compatible with little or no drug loss in 7 days at 5 or 27 °C, 48 hr at 40 °C, and 24 hr under intense light	1831	**C**
Dextrose 5% in sodium chloride 0.45%	BA[a], MG[b]	ACC	10 g	Visually compatible with little or no drug loss in 7 days at 5 or 27 °C, 48 hr at 40 °C, and 24 hr under intense light	1831	**C**
Dextrose 5% in sodium chloride 0.9%	BA[a], MG[b]	ACC	10 g	Visually compatible with little or no drug loss in 7 days at 5 or 27 °C, 48 hr at 40 °C, and 24 hr under intense light	1831	**C**
Dextrose 5%	TR[a]	DU	6 g	Physically compatible with no loss in 24 hr at room temperature under fluorescent light	1358	**C**
	BA[a]	DU	10, 20, 30 g	Visually compatible with little or no drug loss in 48 hr at 23 °C	1830	**C**
Dextrose 5%[c]	BA[a], MG[b]	ACC	10 g	Visually compatible with little or no drug loss in 7 days at 5 or 27 °C, 48 hr at 40 °C, and 24 hr under intense light	1831	**C**
Ringer's injection, lactated	BA[a], MG[b]	ACC	10 g	Visually compatible with little or no drug loss in 7 days at 5 or 27 °C, 48 hr at 40 °C, and 24 hr under intense light	1831	**C**
Sodium chloride 0.45%	BA[a], MG[b]	ACC	10 g	Visually compatible with little or no drug loss in 7 days at 5 or 27 °C, 48 hr at 40 °C, and 24 hr under intense light	1831	**C**
Sodium chloride 0.9%	BA[a], MG[b]	ACC	10 g	Visually compatible with little or no drug loss in 7 days at 5 or 27 °C, 48 hr at 40 °C, and 24 hr under intense light	1831	**C**

[a]*Tested in PVC containers.*
[b]*Tested in glass containers.*
[c]*Tested with and without potassium chloride 40 mEq/L.*

Additive Compatibility

Esmolol HCl

Drug	Mfr	Conc/L	Mfr	Conc/L	Test Soln	Remarks	Ref	C/I
Aminophylline	LY	1 g	DU	6 g	D5W	Physically compatible with no loss of either drug in 24 hr at room temperature under fluorescent light	1358	**C**
Atracurium besylate	BW	500 mg		10 g	D5W	Physically compatible and atracurium stable for 24 hr at 5 and 30 °C	1694	**C**
Heparin sodium	LY	50,000 units	DU	6 g	D5W	Physically compatible with no esmolol loss in 24 hr at room temperature under fluorescent light. Heparin not tested	1358	**C**
Procainamide HCl	ES	4 g	DU	6 g	D5W	43% procainamide loss in 24 hr at room temperature under fluorescent light	1358	**I**

Additive Compatibility (Cont.)

Esmolol HCl

Drug	Mfr	Conc/L	Mfr	Conc/L	Test Soln	Remarks	Ref	C/I
Sodium bicarbonate	MG[a]	5%	ACC	10 g		Visually compatible. 5 and 8% esmolol losses in 7 days at 4 and 27 °C, respectively	1831	C

[a]*Tested in glass containers.*

Y-Site Injection Compatibility (1:1 Mixture)

Esmolol HCl

Drug	Mfr	Conc	Mfr	Conc	Remarks	Ref	C/I
Amikacin sulfate	BR	5 mg/mL[a]	DCC	10 mg/mL[a]	Physically compatible for 24 hr at 22 °C	1169	C
Aminophylline	ES	1 mg/mL[a]	DCC	10 mg/mL[a]	Physically compatible for 24 hr at 22 °C	1169	C
Amiodarone HCl	WY	4.8 mg/mL[a]	DU	40 mg/mL[a]	Visually compatible for 24 hr at 23 °C	1877	C
Amphotericin B cholesteryl sulfate complex	SEQ	0.83 mg/mL[a]	OHM	10 mg/mL[a]	Microprecipitate forms in 4 hr at 23 °C	2117	I
Ampicillin sodium	WY	20 mg/mL[b]	DCC	10 mg/mL[a]	Physically compatible for 24 hr at 22 °C	1169	C
Atracurium besylate	BW	0.5 mg/mL[a]	DCC	10 mg/mL[a]	Physically compatible for 24 hr at 28 °C	1337	C
Bivalirudin	TMC	5 mg/mL[a]	BA	10 mg/mL[a]	Physically compatible for 4 hr at 23 °C	2373	C
Butorphanol tartrate	BR	0.04 mg/mL[a]	DCC	10 mg/mL[a]	Physically compatible for 24 hr at 22 °C	1169	C
Calcium chloride	AB	20 mg/mL[a]	DCC	10 mg/mL[a]	Physically compatible for 24 hr at 22 °C	1169	C
Cefazolin sodium	LI	10 mg/mL[a]	DCC	10 mg/mL[a]	Physically compatible for 24 hr at 22 °C	1169	C
Ceftazidime	GL	10 mg/mL[a]	DCC	10 mg/mL[a]	Physically compatible for 24 hr at 22 °C	1169	C
Chloramphenicol sodium succinate	PD	10 mg/mL[a]	DCC	10 mg/mL[a]	Physically compatible for 24 hr at 22 °C	1169	C
Cisatracurium besylate	GW	0.1, 2, 5 mg/mL[a]	OHM	10 mg/mL[a]	Physically compatible for 4 hr at 23 °C	2074	C
Clindamycin phosphate	UP	9 mg/mL[a]	DCC	10 mg/mL[a]	Physically compatible for 24 hr at 22 °C	1169	C
Dexmedetomidine HCl	AB	4 mcg/mL[b]	BA	10 mg/mL[b]	Physically compatible for 4 hr at 23 °C	2383	C
Diltiazem HCl	MMD	1 mg/mL[a]	DU	10 mg/mL[a]	Visually compatible for 24 hr at 25 °C	1530	C
Dopamine HCl	IMS	1.6 mg/mL[a]	DCC	10 mg/mL[a]	Physically compatible for 24 hr at 22 °C	1169	C
Doripenem	JJ	5 mg/mL[a,b]	BED	10 mg/mL[a,b]	Physically compatible for 4 hr at 23 °C	2743	C
Enalaprilat	MSD	0.05 mg/mL[b]	DU	10 mg/mL[a]	Physically compatible for 24 hr at room temperature under fluorescent light	1355	C
Erythromycin lactobionate	AB	5 mg/mL[a]	DCC	10 mg/mL[a]	Physically compatible for 24 hr at 22 °C	1169	C
Famotidine	MSD	0.2 mg/mL[a]	DU	10 mg/mL[b]	Physically compatible for 4 hr at 25 °C	1188	C
Fenoldopam mesylate	AB	80 mcg/mL[b]	BA	10 mg/mL[b]	Physically compatible for 4 hr at 23 °C	2467	C
Fentanyl citrate	JN	0.05 mg/1 mL	DCC	1 g/100 mL[d]	Physically compatible when fentanyl is injected into Y-site of flowing admixture[e]	1168	C
	JN	0.05 mg/mL	DCC	10 mg/mL[d]	Physically compatible. No drug loss in 8 hr at room temperature in light	1168	C
Furosemide	HO	10 mg/mL	ACC	10 mg/mL[f]	Cloudy precipitate forms immediately	1146	I
Gentamicin sulfate	ES	0.8 mg/mL[a]	DCC	10 mg/mL[a]	Physically compatible for 24 hr at 22 °C	1169	C
Heparin sodium	IX	40 units/mL[a]	DCC	10 mg/mL[a]	Physically compatible for 24 hr at 22 °C	1169	C

Y-Site Injection Compatibility (1:1 Mixture) (Cont.)

Esmolol HCl

Drug	Mfr	Conc	Mfr	Conc	Remarks	Ref	C/I
Hetastarch in lactated electrolyte	AB	6%	OHM	10 mg/mL	Physically compatible for 4 hr at 23 °C	2339	**C**
Hydrocortisone sodium succinate	LY	1 mg/mL[a]	DCC	10 mg/mL[a]	Physically compatible for 24 hr at 22 °C	1169	**C**
Hydroxyethyl starch 130/0.4 in sodium chloride 0.9%	FRK	6%	BA	10 mg/mL[a]	Visually compatible for 24 hr at room temperature	2770	**C**
Insulin, regular	LI	1 unit/mL[a]	DU	40 mg/mL[a]	Visually compatible for 24 hr at 23 °C	1877	**C**
Labetalol HCl	GL	5 mg/mL	DU	40 mg/mL[a]	Visually compatible for 24 hr at 23 °C	1877	**C**
Linezolid	PHU	2 mg/mL	OHM	10 mg/mL	Physically compatible for 4 hr at 23 °C	2264	**C**
Magnesium sulfate	LY	10 mg/mL[a]	DCC	10 mg/mL[a]	Physically compatible for 24 hr at 22 °C	1169	**C**
Methyldopate HCl	MSD	5 mg/mL[a]	DCC	10 mg/mL[a]	Physically compatible for 24 hr at 22 °C	1169	**C**
Metronidazole	SE	5 mg/mL	DCC	10 mg/mL[a]	Physically compatible for 24 hr at 22 °C	1169	**C**
Micafungin sodium	ASP	1.5 mg/mL[b]	BA	10 mg/mL[b]	Physically compatible for 4 hr at 23 °C	2683	**C**
Midazolam HCl	RC	1 mg/mL[a]	DU	40 mg/mL[a]	Visually compatible for 24 hr at 23 °C	1877	**C**
Morphine sulfate	ES	15 mg/1 mL	DCC	1 g/100 mL[d]	Physically compatible when morphine is injected in Y-site[d]	1168	**C**
	ES	15 mg/mL	DCC	10 mg/mL[d]	Physically compatible. No drug loss in 8 hr at room temperature in light	1168	**C**
Nafcillin sodium	BR	10 mg/mL[a]	DCC	10 mg/mL[a]	Physically compatible for 24 hr at 22 °C	1169	**C**
Nicardipine HCl	DCC	0.1 mg/mL[a]	DU	10 mg/mL	Visually compatible for 24 hr at room temperature	235	**C**
Nitroglycerin	OM	0.2 mg/mL[a]	DU	40 mg/mL[a]	Visually compatible for 24 hr at 23 °C	1877	**C**
Norepinephrine bitartrate	STR	0.064 mg/mL[a]	DU	40 mg/mL[a]	Visually compatible for 24 hr at 23 °C	1877	**C**
Pancuronium bromide	ES	0.05 mg/mL[a]	DCC	10 mg/mL[a]	Physically compatible for 24 hr at 28 °C	1337	**C**
Pantoprazole sodium	ALT[g]	0.16 to 0.8 mg/mL[b]	BA	10 to 20 mg/mL[a]	Discoloration and reddish-brown precipitate form	2603	**I**
Penicillin G potassium	PF	50,000 units/mL[a]	DCC	10 mg/mL[a]	Physically compatible for 24 hr at 22 °C	1169	**C**
Phenytoin sodium	IX	1 mg/mL[a]	DCC	10 mg/mL[a]	Physically compatible for 24 hr at 22 °C	1169	**C**
Polymyxin B sulfate	PF	0.005 unit/mL[a]	DCC	10 mg/mL[a]	Physically compatible for 24 hr at 22 °C	1169	**C**
Potassium chloride	IX	0.4 mEq/mL[a]	DCC	10 mg/mL[b]	Physically compatible for 24 hr at 22 °C	1169	**C**
Potassium phosphates	LY	0.44 mEq/mL[a]	DCC	10 mg/mL[a]	Physically compatible for 24 hr at 22 °C	1169	**C**
Propofol	ZEN	10 mg/mL	OHM	10 mg/mL	Physically compatible for 1 hr at 23 °C	2066	**C**
Ranitidine HCl	GL	0.5 mg/mL[a]	DCC	10 mg/mL[a]	Physically compatible for 24 hr at 22 °C	1169	**C**
Remifentanil HCl	GW	0.025 and 0.25 mg/mL[b]	OHM	10 mg/mL[a]	Physically compatible for 4 hr at 23 °C	2075	**C**
Sodium acetate	LY	0.4 mEq/mL[a]	DCC	10 mg/mL[a]	Physically compatible for 24 hr at 22 °C	1169	**C**
Sodium nitroprusside	RC	0.2 mg/mL[a]	DU	40 mg/mL[a]	Visually compatible for 24 hr at 23 °C	1877	**C**
Streptomycin sulfate	PF	10 mg/mL[a]	DCC	10 mg/mL[a]	Physically compatible for 24 hr at 22 °C	1169	**C**
Tacrolimus	FUJ	1 mg/mL[b]	DU	10 mg/mL[a]	Visually compatible for 24 hr at 25 °C	1630	**C**
Tobramycin sulfate	LI	0.8 mg/mL[a]	DCC	10 mg/mL[a]	Physically compatible for 24 hr at 22 °C	1169	**C**

Y-Site Injection Compatibility (1:1 Mixture) (Cont.)

Esmolol HCl

Drug	Mfr	Conc	Mfr	Conc	Remarks	Ref	C/I
Trimethoprim–sulfamethoxazole	BW	0.64 + 3.2 mg/mL[a]	DCC	10 mg/mL[a]	Physically compatible for 24 hr at 22 °C	1169	C
Vancomycin HCl	LE	5 mg/mL[a]	DCC	10 mg/mL[a]	Physically compatible for 24 hr at 22 °C	1169	C
Vecuronium bromide	OR	0.1 mg/mL[a]	DCC	10 mg/mL[a]	Physically compatible for 24 hr at 28 °C	1337	C
Warfarin sodium	DU	2 mg/mL[c]	OHM	10 mg/mL[a]	Haze forms immediately	2010	I
	DME	2 mg/mL[c]	OHM	10 mg/mL[a]	Haze forms immediately	2078	I

[a]*Tested in dextrose 5%.*
[b]*Tested in sodium chloride 0.9%.*
[c]*Tested in sterile water for injection.*
[d]*Tested in dextrose 5% in sodium chloride 0.9%.*
[e]*Flowing at 1.6 mL/min.*
[f]*Tested in both dextrose 5% and sodium chloride 0.9%.*
[g]*Test performed using the formulation WITHOUT edetate disodium.*

ESOMEPRAZOLE SODIUM
AHFS 56:28.36

Products — Esomeprazole is available as a lyophilized powder in 20- and 40-mg vials as the sodium salt with edetate disodium 1.5 mg and sodium hydroxide to adjust pH during manufacturing. For direct intravenous injection, reconstitute either size vial with 5 mL of sodium chloride 0.9%. (1)

For intravenous infusion, reconstitute either size vial with 5 mL of sodium chloride 0.9%, Ringer's injection, lactated, or dextrose 5% and dilute the reconstituted solution to 50 mL with additional infusion solution. (1)

pH — From 9 to 11. (1)

Trade Name(s) — Nexium I.V.

Administration — Esomeprazole sodium is administered by direct intravenous injection over at least three minutes or by intravenous infusion over 10 to 30 minutes. (1)

Stability — Intact vials of esomeprazole sodium should be stored at controlled room temperature and protected from light. The drug reconstituted with sodium chloride 0.9% for direct intravenous injection should be administered within 12 hours after reconstitution when stored at room temperature. Esomeprazole sodium reconstituted and diluted for intravenous infusion should be administered with 12 hours at room temperature after reconstitution and dilution if sodium chloride 0.9% or Ringer's injection, lactated, is the reconstitution and dilution solution. If dextrose 5% is used for reconstitution and dilution, the drug should be used within six hours at room temperature. The manufacturer states that refrigeration is not required for esomeprazole sodium solutions. (1)

The manufacturer states that esomeprazole sodium administration requires flushing the administration line with sodium chloride 0.9%, Ringer's injection, lactated, or dextrose 5% both before and after administering the drug, and that esomeprazole sodium should not be administered concomitantly with other drugs. (1)

pH Effects — The stability of esomeprazole sodium in solution is strongly dependent on pH. The stability of the drug decreases with decreasing pH. (1)

Compatibility Information

Solution Compatibility

Esomeprazole sodium

Solution	Mfr	Mfr	Conc/L	Remarks	Ref	C/I
Dextrose 5%	BA[a]	ASZ	4 and 8 g	Physically compatible with less than 7% loss in 48 hr at 25 °C and no loss in 120 hr at 4 °C	2760	C
Ringer's injection, lactated	BA[a]	ASZ	4 and 8 g	Physically compatible with less than 4% loss in 48 hr at 25 °C and little or no loss in 120 hr at 4 °C	2760	C

Solution Compatibility (Cont.)

Esomeprazole sodium

Solution	Mfr	Mfr	Conc/L	Remarks	Ref	C/I
Sodium chloride 0.9%	BA[a]	ASZ	4 and 8 g	Physically compatible with less than 3% loss in 48 hr at 25 °C and about 1% loss in 120 hr at 4 °C	2760	C

[a]Tested in PVC containers.

Y-Site Injection Compatibility (1:1 Mixture)

Esomeprazole sodium

Drug	Mfr	Conc	Mfr	Conc	Remarks	Ref	C/I
Ceftaroline fosamil	FOR	2.22 mg/mL[a,b,c]	ASZ	0.4 mg/mL[a,b,c]	Physically compatible for 4 hr at 23 °C	2826	C
Doripenem	JJ	5 mg/mL[a,b]	ASZ	0.4 mg/mL[b]	Physically compatible for 4 hr at 23 °C	2743	C
Telavancin HCl	ASP	7.5 mg/mL[a,b,c]	ASZ	0.4 mg/mL[a,b,c]	Discoloration and increase in measured turbidity	2830	I

[a]Tested in dextrose 5% in water.
[b]Tested in sodium chloride 0.9%.
[c]Tested in Ringer's injection, lactated.

ESTROGENS, CONJUGATED
AHFS 68:16.04

Products — Estrogens, conjugated is available in packages containing a vial with lyophilized estrogens, conjugated, 25 mg; lactose 200 mg; sodium citrate 12.2 mg; simethicone 0.2 mg; and sodium hydroxide or hydrochloric acid for pH adjustment. Reconstitute the vial with 5 mL of sterile water for injection flowing along the side of the vial and agitate gently – not violently. (1)

Trade Name(s) — Premarin Intravenous.

Administration — Estrogens, conjugated may be administered by deep intramuscular injection or slow direct intravenous injection. Intravenous infusion is not recommended, but injection into the tubing of a running infusion may be performed. (1; 4)

Stability — The manufacturer recommends refrigeration of the intact containers at 2 to 8 °C. (1) Such storage provides a shelflife of up to 60 months. Although refrigerated storage is required, the manufacturer has stated the drug may be stored at room temperature for seven days. (2745) The manufacturer recommends use immediately after reconstitution. (1)

pH Effects — Estrogens, conjugated, has been stated to be incompatible with any solution with an acid pH. (1; 4)

Compatibility Information

Solution Compatibility

Estrogens, conjugated

Solution	Mfr	Mfr	Conc/L	Remarks	Ref	C/I
Dextrose 5%				Compatible	1	C
Sodium chloride 0.9%				Compatible	1	C

Drugs in Syringe Compatibility

Estrogens, conjugated

Drug (in syringe)	Mfr	Amt	Mfr	Amt	Remarks	Ref	C/I
Pantoprazole sodium	a	4 mg/ 1 mL		5 mg/ 1 mL	Possible precipitate within 1 hr	2574	I

[a]Test performed using the formulation WITHOUT edetate disodium.

Y-Site Injection Compatibility (1:1 Mixture)

Estrogens, conjugated

Drug	Mfr	Conc	Mfr	Conc	Remarks	Ref	C/I
Heparin sodium[b]	RI	1000 units/L[a]	AY	5 mg/mL	Physically compatible for 4 hr at room temperature	322	C
Hydrocortisone sodium succinate[c]	UP	100 mg/L[a]	AY	5 mg/mL	Physically compatible for 4 hr at room temperature	322	C
Potassium chloride		40 mEq/L[a]	AY	5 mg/mL	Physically compatible for 4 hr at room temperature	322	C

[a]Tested in dextrose 5%, sodium chloride 0.9%, and Ringer's injection, lactated.
[b]Tested in combination with hydrocortisone sodium succinate (Upjohn) 100 mg/L.
[c]Tested in combination with heparin sodium (Riker) 1000 units/L.

ETHACRYNATE SODIUM
AHFS 40:28.08

Products — Each vial has ethacrynate sodium equivalent to ethacrynic acid 50 mg and mannitol 62.5 mg. Reconstitute with 50 mL of dextrose 5% or sodium chloride 0.9% to yield a 1-mg/mL solution. Some dextrose 5% has a pH below 5 and results in a hazy or opalescent solution, which is not recommended for use. (1; 4)

pH — Reconstitution with dextrose 5% or sodium chloride 0.9% results in a solution having a pH of 6.3 to 7.7. (4)

Sodium Content — Ethacrynate sodium contains 0.165 mEq of sodium per 50 mg of ethacrynic acid equivalent. (846)

Trade Name(s) — Sodium Edecrin.

Administration — Ethacrynate sodium may be given slowly through the tubing of a running intravenous solution or directly into a vein over several minutes. (1; 4) Subcutaneous or intramuscular injection should not be used because of local pain and irritation. (1; 4)

Stability — Solutions of ethacrynate sodium are relatively stable for short periods at pH 7 at room temperature; but as the pH or temperature or both increase, the solutions are less stable. Ethacrynate sodium is incompatible with solutions or drugs with a final pH below 5. The reconstituted solution should be discarded after 24 hours. (1; 4)

Compatibility Information

Solution Compatibility

Ethacrynate sodium

Solution	Mfr	Mfr	Conc/L	Remarks	Ref	C/I
Dextrose 5%				Compatible	4	C
Dextrose 5% in sodium chloride 0.9%				Compatible	4	C
Ringer's injection				Compatible	4	C
Ringer's injection, lactated				Compatible	4	C
Sodium chloride 0.9%				Compatible	4	C

Additive Compatibility

Ethacrynate sodium

Drug	Mfr	Conc/L	Mfr	Conc/L	Test Soln	Remarks	Ref	C/I
Chlorpromazine HCl	SKF	50 mg	MSD	50 mg	NS	Little alteration of UV spectra within 8 hr at room temperature	16	**C**
Hydralazine HCl	CI	20 mg	MSD	50 mg	NS	Altered UV spectra at room temperature	16	**I**
Procainamide HCl	SQ	1 g	MSD	50 mg	NS	Altered UV spectra at room temperature	16	**I**
Prochlorperazine edisylate	SKF	20 mg	MSD	80 mg	NS	Little alteration of UV spectra within 8 hr at room temperature	16	**C**
Ranitidine HCl	GL	50 mg and 2 g		500 mg	D5W	Ranitidine stable for only 6 hr at 25 °C. Ethacrynate not tested	1515	**I**
Triflupromazine HCl	SQ		MSD		NS	Occasional gas bubble formation	16	**I**

Y-Site Injection Compatibility (1:1 Mixture)

Ethacrynate sodium

Drug	Mfr	Conc	Mfr	Conc	Remarks	Ref	C/I
Heparin sodium[d]	RI	1000 units/L[a,b,c]	MSD	1 mg/mL	Physically compatible for 4 hr at room temperature	322	**C**
Hydrocortisone sodium succinate[e]	UP	100 mg/L[a,b,c]	MSD	1 mg/mL	Physically compatible for 4 hr at room temperature	322	**C**
Nesiritide	SCI	50 mcg/mL[a,b]		1 mg/mL	Physically incompatible	2625	**I**
Potassium chloride		40 mEq/L[a,b,c]	MSD	1 mg/mL	Physically compatible for 4 hr at room temperature	322	**C**

[a] Tested in dextrose 5%.
[b] Tested in sodium chloride 0.9%.
[c] Tested in Ringer's injection, lactated.
[d] Tested in combination with hydrocortisone sodium succinate (Upjohn) 100 mg/L.
[e] Tested in combination with heparin sodium (Riker) 1000 units/L.

ETOMIDATE
AHFS 28:04.92

Products — Etomidate is available at a concentration of 2 mg/mL in 10- and 20-mL single-dose vials. Each milliliter also contains propylene glycol 35% (v/v). (1)

pH — From 4 to 7. (1)

Trade Name(s) — Amidate.

Administration — Etomidate is administered by intravenous injection over 30 to 60 seconds. (1)

Stability — Intact containers should be stored at controlled room temperature. Unused portions remaining in vials should be discarded. (1)

Compatibility Information

Drugs in Syringe Compatibility

Etomidate

Drug (in syringe)	Mfr	Amt	Mfr	Amt	Remarks	Ref	C/I
Heparin sodium		2500 units/ 1 mL	JN	20 mg/ 10 mL	Visually compatible for at least 5 min	1053	C

Y-Site Injection Compatibility (1:1 Mixture)

Etomidate

Drug	Mfr	Conc	Mfr	Conc	Remarks	Ref	C/I
Alfentanil HCl	JN	0.5 mg/mL	AB	2 mg/mL	Visually compatible for 7 days at 25 °C	1801	C
Ascorbic acid	AB	500 mg/mL	AB	2 mg/mL	Yellow color and precipitate form in 24 hr	1801	I
Atracurium besylate	BW	10 mg/mL	AB	2 mg/mL	Visually compatible for 7 days at 25 °C	1801	C
Atropine sulfate	GNS	0.4 mg/mL	AB	2 mg/mL	Visually compatible for 7 days at 25 °C	1801	C
Dexmedetomidine HCl	HOS				Stated to be compatible	1	C
Ephedrine sulfate	AB	50 mg/mL	AB	2 mg/mL	Visually compatible for 7 days at 25 °C	1801	C
Fentanyl citrate	ES	0.05 mg/mL	AB	2 mg/mL	Visually compatible for 7 days at 25 °C	1801	C
Lidocaine HCl	AST	20 mg/mL	AB	2 mg/mL	Visually compatible for 7 days at 25 °C	1801	C
Lorazepam	WY	2 mg/mL	AB	2 mg/mL	Visually compatible for 7 days at 25 °C	1801	C
Midazolam HCl	RC	5 mg/mL	AB	2 mg/mL	Visually compatible for 7 days at 25 °C	1801	C
Morphine sulfate	ES	10 mg/mL	AB	2 mg/mL	Visually compatible for 7 days at 25 °C	1801	C
Pancuronium bromide	GNS	2 mg/mL	AB	2 mg/mL	Visually compatible for 7 days at 25 °C	1801	C
Phenylephrine HCl	ES	10 mg/mL	AB	2 mg/mL	Visually compatible for 7 days at 25 °C	1801	C
Succinylcholine chloride	AB	20 mg/mL	AB	2 mg/mL	Visually compatible for 7 days at 25 °C	1801	C
Sufentanil citrate	JN	0.05 mg/mL	AB	2 mg/mL	Visually compatible for 7 days at 25 °C	1801	C
Vecuronium bromide	OR	1 mg/mL	AB	2 mg/mL	Slight turbidity and white particles form	1801	I

ETOPOSIDE
AHFS 10:00

Products — Etoposide 20 mg/mL is available in 5-, 25-, and 50-mL multiple-dose vials. Each milliliter also contains polyethylene glycol 300 650 mg, ethanol 30.5% (v/v), polysorbate 80 80 mg, benzyl alcohol 30 mg, and citric acid 2 mg. (1)

pH — From 3 to 4. (1)

Administration — Etoposide should be diluted for administration and given by slow intravenous infusion; concentrations of 0.2 to 0.4 mg/mL should be given over at least 30 to 60 minutes. (1; 4)

Continuous intravenous infusion has also been used. The drug should not be given by rapid intravenous injection. (4)

The surfactant content of the etoposide formulation decreases surface tension and has been found to produce a 30% reduction in drop size compared to simple aqueous solutions. The altered drop size may interfere with accurate infusion rates if infusion devices that rely on drop counting are used. The use of infusion devices that operate independently of drop size has been recommended. (181)

The manufacturer notes that accidental exposure to this potentially toxic agent may cause skin reactions. Therefore, protective gloves and syringes with Luer-Lok fittings should be used during preparation of solutions. A soap and water wash should be employed after accidental contact with the skin or mucosa. (1; 4)

In the event of spills or leaks, the use of sodium hypochlorite 5% (household bleach) or potassium permanganate 1% to inactivate etoposide has been recommended. (1200)

Stability — Store intact containers at controlled room temperature. (1) Stability is not affected by exposure to normal room fluorescent light. (1374)

Devices composed of hard ABS plastic may be incompatible with undiluted etoposide. In one study, a multiport disposable infusion cassette (Omni-Flow) developed cracks within five minutes after infusion was started and leakage was evident within 15 minutes. This phenomenon did not occur when etoposide was diluted to concentrations up to 1 mg/mL. In addition, a venting pin and a connector on an extension set reportedly cracked. Exposure to the polyethylene glycol 300 content of the etoposide formulation can cause cracks in minutes. However, dehydrated alcohol did not cause any cracks within one hour. (1261)

Immersion of a needle with an aluminum component in etoposide (Bristol) 20 mg/mL resulted in no visually apparent reaction after seven days at 24 °C. (988)

Precipitation — Dextrose 5% and sodium chloride 0.9% have been recommended as diluents for the infusion of etoposide. The aqueous solubility of etoposide is poor (0.03 mg/mL), but the formulation temporarily increases its miscibility in an aqueous medium. Nevertheless, the drug will eventually crystallize in varying time periods, and the crystallization is reported to be exacerbated by peristaltic pumps. (1949) At concentrations of 0.2 and 0.4 mg/mL in dextrose 5% and sodium chloride 0.9%, the solutions are stable for 96 and 24 hours, respectively, at 25 °C under normal fluorescent light in either glass or plastic containers. However, precipitation in shorter time periods has been observed. At concentrations of 0.2 and 0.4 mg/mL in Ringer's injection, lactated, or mannitol 10% in glass containers under the same conditions, the solutions are stable for eight hours. No precipitate formed in 72 hours at 20 °C in solutions of etoposide 0.4 mg/mL in dextrose 5% in sodium chloride 0.45%. (1162) However, at 1 mg/mL, crystallization may occur in 30 minutes in a standing solution or five minutes if the solution is stirred. Occasionally, 1-mg/mL concentrations may remain in solution for extended periods. (1374) Nevertheless, concentrations greater than 0.4 mg/mL are not recommended by the manufacturer. Because of the poor solubility of etoposide in aqueous media, monitor closely for precipitation before and during administration. (1; 4; 915; 916)

The rate of precipitation of a supersaturated etoposide solution depends on the presence of crystalline nuclei, agitation, contact with incompatible surfaces, and possibly other factors. (1374)

Etoposide 1 mg/mL in sodium chloride 0.9% in polypropylene syringes (Braun Omnifix) developed a pure etoposide precipitate in about 10% of the prefilled syringes. It also precipitated at various locations in subclavian lines. (1564)

Precipitation of etoposide from infusion solutions is reportedly exacerbated by the use of peristaltic pumps, especially at concentrations of 0.4 mg/mL or above. Use of volumetric pumps has been recommended to reduce this problem. (1832; 1949)

pH Effects — Etoposide is most stable at a pH of about 3.5 to 6, with a calculated minimum degradation rate occurring at pH 4.8. (1262) Epimerization to the less active *cis*-etoposide may occur at pH values above 6. Hydrolysis may occur in alkaline solutions. (1379)

Syringes — When etoposide 1 mg/mL in sodium chloride 0.9% was stored in plastic syringes (Gillette), seizing of the syringes occurred. (1564)

Ambulatory Pumps — Etoposide (Bristol-Myers Squibb) 0.5 mg/mL in sterile water for injection was evaluated for stability and compatibility in PVC reservoirs of Graseby 9000 ambulatory pumps. Etoposide was chemically stable at 37 °C for seven days with no loss of drug. However, refrigerated storage at 4 °C resulted in precipitation of the etoposide in some samples. In addition, substantial amounts of diethylhexyl phthalate (DEHP) plasticizer (up to 90 mcg/mL) were leached from the PVC reservoirs. The authors concluded that etoposide was unsuitable for use in this pump reservoir and recommended consideration of etoposide phosphate, which should not be subject to precipitation and leaching of plasticizer. (2288)

Sorption — No loss of etoposide because of sorption to PVC containers has been observed. (1374) At a concentration of 0.2 mg/mL in dextrose 5% or sodium chloride 0.9% in PVC containers, no etoposide loss due to sorption was found during 72 hours at 5 and 25 °C. (1369)

In an admixture composed of cytarabine (Upjohn) 0.157 mg/mL, daunorubicin hydrochloride (Bellon) 15.7 mcg/mL, and etoposide (Sandoz) 0.157 mg/mL in dextrose 5%, little or no loss of the drugs due to sorption occurred when delivered through PVC, PVC with polyethylene-lined sets, and silicone central catheter. (1955)

Plasticizer Leaching — The surfactant in the etoposide formulation leaches DEHP plasticizer from PVC containers and tubing. The amount of DEHP leached is variable, depending on surfactant concentration, container size, tubing diameter and length, ambient temperature, DEHP concentration in the plastic, and contact time. The use of non-PVC containers and tubing has been recommended to reduce patient exposure to DEHP. If there is sufficient concern, the use of the water-soluble ester form, etoposide phosphate, which does not leach DEHP plasticizer, could be used.

Etoposide 0.4 mg/mL in PVC bags of dextrose 5% leached relatively minor amounts of DEHP plasticizer from PVC bags. This leaching was due to the surfactant polysorbate 80 (Tween 80) in the formulation. After 24 hours at 24 °C, the DEHP concentration in 50-mL bags of infusion solution was 2.6 mcg/mL. This finding is consistent with the low surfactant concentration (0.16%) in the final admixture solution. The actual amount of DEHP leached from PVC containers and administration sets may vary in clinical situations, depending on surfactant concentration, bag size, and contact time. (1683)

Etoposide (Sandoz) 0.4 mg/mL in sodium chloride 0.9% in PVC containers leached DEHP plasticizer from the container material. This leaching increased with storage time from about 12 mcg/mL in eight hours to over 50 mcg/mL in 96 hours at 24 °C. Refrigeration reduced, but did not eliminate, DEHP leaching. (1833)

Etoposide (Novartis) 0.4 mg/mL in dextrose 5% and sodium chloride 0.9% was evaluated for the leaching of DEHP plasticizer from PVC bags of the infusion solution from four manufacturers (Aguettant, Baxter, Biosedra-Fresenius, and Macopharma) over 24 hours stored at 24 °C. Both solutions from all manufacturers leached DEHP in amounts near 20 mcg/mL. (2447)

The low-density polyethylene inner linings of trilayer Vygon tubing and bilayer Cair tubing have been reported not to act as effective barriers to DEHP leaching from the outer PVC layers. Leached DEHP was nearly identical to plain PVC tubing. (2587; 2605)

Filtration — Etoposide 0.1 to 0.4 mg/mL in dextrose 5% or sodium chloride 0.9% has been filtered through several commercially available filters (such as the 0.22-μm Millex-GS or Millex GV) without filter decomposition. (4)

Etoposide (Sandoz) 0.2 mg/mL in dextrose 5% and sodium chloride 0.9% was filtered through a 0.22-μm cellulose ester membrane filter (Ivex-HP, Millipore) over six hours. No significant drug loss due to binding to the filter was noted. (1034)

Central Venous Catheter — Etoposide infused undiluted at a rate of 30 mL/hr for 24 hours through a polyurethane central catheter caused substantial damage to the catheter. In addition to cracking the catheter, a 36% decrease in elasticity, a 3.7% increase in catheter length, and damage similar to melting on the internal catheter wall were found. The damage also occurred with the etoposide vehicle and ethanol alone. Consequently, the damage was attributed to the ethanol component of the formulation. (2286)

The damage to polyurethane catheters caused by the etoposide formulation did not extend to silicone central catheters. Administration of undiluted etoposide could be performed using silicone catheters. (2286)

Compatibility Information

Solution Compatibility

Etoposide

Solution	Mfr	Mfr	Conc/L	Remarks	Ref	C/I
Dextrose 5%	a	BR	400 mg	Physically compatible. 4% loss in 4 days at 21 °C in dark or fluorescent light	1374	C
		SZ	157 mg	2% or less loss in 48 hr at room temperature, in light and dark, and at 4 °C	1955	C
Ringer's injection, lactated	a	BR	400 mg	Physically compatible. 5% loss in 4 days at 21 °C in fluorescent light	1374	C
Sodium chloride 0.9%	b	BR	400 mg	Physically compatible. 1 to 5% loss in 4 days at 21 °C in dark or in fluorescent light	1374	C
	a	BR	50 to 400 mg	Physically compatible for at least 4 days	1374	C
	a	BR	500 mg	Precipitate forms after 48 hr at 21 °C exposed to fluorescent light	1374	C
	a	BR	600 and 700 mg	Precipitate forms within 24 hr at 21 °C exposed to fluorescent light	1374	I
	c		400 mg	Stable for 24 hr at 4 and 24 °C. Precipitation at varying times after 24 hr	1833	C
		BA	0.2 g	Compatible and stable for 22 days at 24 and 4 °C	2541	C
		BA	0.3 g	Compatible and stable for 2 days at 24 °C and 7 days at 4 °C. Precipitate forms after these times	2541	C
		BA	0.4 g	Compatible and stable for 1 day at 24 °C and 2 days at 4 °C. Precipitate forms after these times	2541	C
		BA	0.5 g	Compatible and stable for 1 day at 24 and 4 °C. Precipitate forms after this time	2541	C
		BA	1 to 8 g	Precipitate forms within a few hours	2541	I
		BA	9.5 g	Compatible and stable for 1 day at 24 °C and 2 days at 4 °C. Precipitate forms after these times	2541	C
		BA	10 g	Compatible and stable for 5 days at 24 °C and 7 days at 4 °C. Precipitate forms after these times	2541	C
		BA	11 g	Compatible and stable for 7 days at 24 °C and 22 days at 4 °C	2541	C
		BA	12 g	Compatible and stable for 7 days at 24 °C and 14 days at 4 °C	2541	C

aTested in glass containers.
bTested in both glass and PVC containers.
cTested in glass, PVC, and polyethylene containers.

Additive Compatibility

Etoposide

Drug	Mfr	Conc/L	Mfr	Conc/L	Test Soln	Remarks	Ref	C/I
Carboplatin		1 g		200 mg	W	Under 10% drug loss in 7 days at 23 °C	1954	C
Cisplatin	BR	200 mg	BR	200 and 400 mg	NS[a]	Physically compatible. Under 10% loss of both drugs in 24 hr at 22 °C	1329	C
	BR	200 mg	BR	200 and 400 mg	D5½S[a]	Physically compatible. Under 10% loss of both drugs in 24 hr at 22 °C	1329	C
		200 mg		200 mg	NS	Both drugs stable for 14 days at room temperature protected from light	1379	C
		200 mg		400 mg	NS	10% etoposide loss and no cisplatin loss in 7 days at room temperature	1388	C
Cisplatin[d]	BR	200 mg	BR	400 mg	D5½S, NS[a]	Physically compatible. Drugs stable for 8 hr at 22 °C. Precipitate within 24 to 48 hr	1329	I
Cisplatin with cyclophosphamide		200 mg 2 g		200 mg	NS	All drugs stable for 7 days at room temperature	1379	C
Cisplatin with floxuridine		200 mg 700 mg		300 mg	NS	All drugs stable for 7 days at room temperature	1379	C
Cisplatin with ifosfamide		200 mg 2 g		200 mg	NS	All drugs stable for 5 days at room temperature	1379	C
Cyclophosphamide with cisplatin		2 g 200 mg		200 mg	NS	All drugs stable for 7 days at room temperature	1379	C
Cytarabine with daunorubicin HCl	UP RP	267 mg 33 mg	BR	400 mg	D5½S	Physically compatible with about 6% cytarabine loss and no loss of other drugs in 72 hr at 20 °C	1162	C
Cytarabine with daunorubicin HCl	UP BEL	157 mg 15.7 mg	SZ	157 mg	D5W[b]	Less than 10% loss of any drug in 48 hr at room temperature, exposed to light and in the dark, and at 4 °C	1955	C
Daunorubicin HCl with cytarabine	RP UP	33 mg 267 mg	BR	400 mg	D5½S	Physically compatible with about 6% cytarabine loss and no loss of other drugs in 72 hr at 20 °C	1162	C
Daunorubicin HCl with cytarabine	BEL UP	15.7 mg 157 mg	SZ	157 mg	D5W[b]	Less than 10% loss of any drug in 48 hr at room temperature, exposed to light and in the dark, and at 4 °C	1955	C
Doxorubicin HCl with vincristine sulfate	PHU LI	40 mg 1.6 mg	BMS	200 mg	NS	Visually compatible. All drugs stable for 72 hr at 30 °C in the dark	2239	C
Doxorubicin HCl with vincristine sulfate	PHU LI	25 mg 1 mg	BMS	125 mg	NS	Visually compatible. All drugs stable for 96 hr at 24 °C in light or dark	2239	C
Doxorubicin HCl with vincristine sulfate	PHU LI	35 mg 1.4 mg	BMS	175 mg	NS	Visually compatible. All drugs stable for 96 hr at 24 °C in light or dark	2239	C
Doxorubicin HCl with vincristine sulfate	PHU LI	50 mg 2 mg	BMS	250 mg	NS	Visually compatible. All drugs stable for 48 hr at 24 °C in light or dark. Etoposide precipitate in 72 hr	2239	C
Doxorubicin HCl with vincristine sulfate	PHU LI	70 mg 2.8 mg	BMS	350 mg	NS	Visually compatible. All drugs stable for 24 hr at 24 °C in light or dark. Etoposide precipitate in 36 hr	2239	C
Doxorubicin HCl with vincristine sulfate	PHU LI	100 mg 4 mg	BMS	500 mg	NS	Etoposide precipitate formed in 12 hr at 24 °C in light or dark	2239	I
Floxuridine		10 g		200 mg	NS	Both drugs stable for 15 days at room temperature	1379	C
Floxuridine with cisplatin		700 mg 200 mg		300 mg	NS	All drugs stable for 7 days at room temperature	1379	C

Additive Compatibility (Cont.)

Etoposide

Drug	Mfr	Conc/L	Mfr	Conc/L	Test Soln	Remarks	Ref	C/I
Fluorouracil		10 g		200 mg	NS	Both drugs stable for 7 days at room temperature and 1 day at 35 °C	1379	C
Hydroxyzine HCl	LY	500 mg	BR	1 g	D5W[c]	Physically compatible for 48 hr	1190	C
Ifosfamide		2 g		200 mg	NS	Both drugs stable for 5 days at room temperature	1379	C
Ifosfamide with cisplatin		2 g 200 mg		200 mg	NS	All drugs stable for 5 days at room temperature	1379	C
Mitoxantrone HCl	LE	50 mg	BR	500 mg	NS	Visually compatible with no loss of either drug in 22 hr at room temperature	2271	C
Ondansetron HCl	GL	30 and 300 mg	BR	100 mg	D5W[b]	Physically compatible. Little or no loss of ondansetron in 48 hr at 23 °C. 4% etoposide loss in 24 hr and 6% loss in 48 hr at 23 °C	1876	C
	GL	30 and 300 mg	BR	400 mg	D5W[b]	Physically compatible with little or no loss of either drug in 48 hr at 23 °C	1876	C
Vincristine sulfate with doxorubicin HCl	LI PHU	1.6 mg 40 mg	BMS	200 mg	NS	Visually compatible. All drugs stable for 72 hr at 30 °C in the dark	2239	C
Vincristine sulfate with doxorubicin HCl	LI PHU	1 mg 25 mg	BMS	125 mg	NS	Visually compatible. All drugs stable for 96 hr at 24 °C in light or dark	2239	C
Vincristine sulfate with doxorubicin HCl	LI PHU	1.4 mg 35 mg	BMS	175 mg	NS	Visually compatible. All drugs stable for 96 hr at 24 °C in light or dark	2239	C
Vincristine sulfate with doxorubicin HCl	LI PHU	2 mg 50 mg	BMS	250 mg	NS	Visually compatible. All drugs stable for 48 hr at 24 °C in light or dark. Etoposide precipitate in 72 hr	2239	C
Vincristine sulfate with doxorubicin HCl	LI PHU	2.8 mg 70 mg	BMS	350 mg	NS	Visually compatible. All drugs stable for 24 hr at 24 °C in light or dark. Etoposide precipitate in 36 hr	2239	C
Vincristine sulfate with doxorubicin HCl	LI PHU	4 mg 100 mg	BMS	500 mg	NS	Etoposide precipitate formed in 12 hr at 24 °C in light or dark	2239	I

[a]*Tested in both glass and PVC containers.*
[b]*Tested in PVC containers.*
[c]*Tested in glass containers.*
[d]*Tested with mannitol 1.875% and potassium chloride 20 mEq/L present.*

Y-Site Injection Compatibility (1:1 Mixture)

Etoposide

Drug	Mfr	Conc	Mfr	Conc	Remarks	Ref	C/I
Allopurinol sodium	BW	3 mg/mL[b]	BR	0.4 mg/mL[b]	Physically compatible for 4 hr at 22 °C	1686	C
Amifostine	USB	10 mg/mL[a]	BR	0.4 mg/mL[a]	Physically compatible for 4 hr at 23 °C	1845	C
Aztreonam	SQ	40 mg/mL[a]	BMS	0.4 mg/mL[a]	Physically compatible for 4 hr at 23 °C	1758	C
Cladribine	ORT	0.015[b] and 0.5[c] mg/mL	BR	0.4 mg/mL[b]	Physically compatible for 4 hr at 23 °C	1969	C
Doxorubicin HCl liposomal	SEQ	0.4 mg/mL[a]	BR	0.4 mg/mL[a]	Physically compatible for 4 hr at 23 °C	2087	C
Filgrastim	AMG	30 mcg/mL[a]	BR	0.4 mg/mL[a]	Particles form immediately. Filaments form in 1 hr	1687	I
Fludarabine phosphate	BX	1 mg/mL[a]	BR	0.4 mg/mL[a]	Visually compatible for 4 hr at 22 °C	1439	C

Y-Site Injection Compatibility (1:1 Mixture) (Cont.)

Etoposide

Drug	Mfr	Conc	Mfr	Conc	Remarks	Ref	C/I
Gallium nitrate	FUJ	1 mg/mL[b]	BR	0.4 mg/mL[b]	Precipitate forms after 60 min	1673	I
Gemcitabine HCl	LI	10 mg/mL[b]	BR	0.4 mg/mL[b]	Physically compatible for 4 hr at 23 °C	2226	C
Granisetron HCl	SKB	1 mg/mL	BMS	0.4 mg/mL[b]	Physically compatible with little or no loss of either drug in 4 hr at 22 °C	1883	C
	SKB	0.05 mg/mL[a]	BR	0.4 mg/mL[a]	Physically compatible for 4 hr at 23 °C	2000	C
Idarubicin HCl	AD	1 mg/mL[b]	BR	0.4 mg/mL[a]	Gas forms immediately	1525	I
Melphalan HCl	BW	0.1 mg/mL[b]	BR	0.4 mg/mL[b]	Physically compatible for 3 hr at 22 °C	1557	C
Methotrexate sodium		30 mg/mL	BR	0.6 mg/mL[b]	Visually compatible for 4 hr at room temperature	1788	C
Micafungin sodium	ASP	1.5 mg/mL[b]	SIC	0.4 mg/mL[b]	Physically compatible for 4 hr at 23 °C	2683	C
Mitoxantrone HCl	LE	2 mg/mL	BR	20 mg/mL	Visually compatible with no loss of either drug in 22 hr at room temperature	2271	C
Ondansetron HCl	GL	1 mg/mL[b]	BR	0.4 mg/mL[a]	Visually compatible for 4 hr at 22 °C	1365	C
	GL	16 to 160 mcg/mL		0.144 to 0.25 mg/mL	Physically compatible when etoposide given over 30 to 60 min via Y-site	1366	C
Paclitaxel	NCI	1.2 mg/mL[a]		0.4 mg/mL[a]	Physically compatible for 4 hr at 22 °C	1528	C
Piperacillin sodium–tazobactam sodium	LE[e]	40 + 5 mg/mL[a]	BR	0.4 mg/mL[a]	Physically compatible for 4 hr at 22 °C	1688	C
Sargramostim	IMM	10 mcg/mL[b]	BR	0.4 mg/mL[b]	Visually compatible for 4 hr at 22 °C	1436	C
Sodium bicarbonate		1.4%	BR	0.6 mg/mL[b]	Visually compatible for 4 hr at room temperature	1788	C
Teniposide	BR	0.1 mg/mL[a]	BR	0.4 mg/mL[a]	Physically compatible for 4 hr at 23 °C	1725	C
Thiotepa	IMM[d]	1 mg/mL[a]	BR	0.4 mg/mL[a]	Physically compatible for 4 hr at 23 °C	1861	C
Topotecan HCl	SKB	56 mcg/mL[a,b]	BR	0.4 mg/mL[a,b]	Visually compatible. Little loss of either drug in 4 hr at 22 °C	2245	C
Vinorelbine tartrate	BW	1 mg/mL[b]	BR	0.4 mg/mL[b]	Physically compatible for 4 hr at 22 °C	1558	C

[a]*Tested in dextrose 5%.*
[b]*Tested in sodium chloride 0.9%.*
[c]*Tested in bacteriostatic sodium chloride 0.9% preserved with benzyl alcohol 0.9%.*
[d]*Lyophilized formulation tested.*
[e]*Test performed using the formulation WITHOUT edetate disodium.*

ETOPOSIDE PHOSPHATE
AHFS 10:00

Products — Etoposide phosphate is available in single-dose vials containing the equivalent of 100 mg of etoposide as the phosphate along with sodium citrate 32.7 mg and 300 mg of dextran 40. Reconstitute with 5 or 10 mL of compatible diluent to yield solutions of 20 or 10 mg/mL, respectively. Sterile water for injection, dextrose 5%, sodium chloride 0.9%, bacteriostatic water for injection preserved with benzyl alcohol, or bacteriostatic sodium chloride 0.9% preserved with benzyl alcohol may be used for reconstitution. (1)

pH — Reconstitution with sterile water for injection to a concentration of 1 mg/mL results in a pH of approximately 2.9. (4)

Trade Name(s) — Etopophos.

Administration — Etoposide phosphate is administered by intravenous infusion from 5 to 210 minutes. The reconstituted drug may be given without further dilution or may be diluted to a concentration as low as 0.1 mg/mL with dextrose 5% or sodium chloride 0.9%. (1; 4)

Stability — Etoposide phosphate is a white to off-white powder. (4) Intact vials should be stored under refrigeration at 2 to 8 °C and protected from light. (1)

The manufacturer states that etoposide phosphate reconstituted with an unpreserved diluent (such as sterile water for injection, dextrose 5%, or sodium chloride 0.9%) is stable for 24 hours at room temperatures of 20 to 25 °C and seven days under refrigeration at 2 to 8 °C. If a diluent containing benzyl alcohol as a preservative (such as bacteriostatic water for injection or bacteriostatic sodium chloride 0.9%) is used to reconstitute etoposide phosphate, the solution is stable for 48 hours at room temperatures of 20 to 25 °C and for seven days under refrigeration at 2 to 8 °C. (1; 4)

Unlike etoposide, the phosphate ester is highly water soluble, having a solubility over 100 mg/mL. (4) Consequently, the potential for precipitation in aqueous media is reduced greatly compared with the older surfactant- and organic solvent-based formulation. (2219)

Etoposide production by hydrolysis from infusion admixtures of etoposide phosphate (Bristol-Myers Squibb) was measured. The admixtures, equivalent to etoposide 1.5 mg/mL in 66.7 mL and 15 mg/mL in 20 mL of sodium chloride 0.9%, were filled into PVC ambulatory infusion pump reservoirs (Pharmacia Deltec) and stored at 20 and 37 °C protected from light. Etoposide levels in the etoposide phosphate admixtures increased at both temperatures; in seven days the increase in concentration was about 2% at 20 °C and about 7% at 37 °C. The authors concluded that etoposide phosphate is suitable for multiple-day ambulatory infusion. (2024)

Doxorubicin hydrochloride, etoposide phosphate, and vincristine sulfate admixtures at a variety of concentrations were unable to pass the USP test for antimicrobial effectiveness. Mixtures of these drugs are not "self-preserving" and permit microbial growth. (2343)

Etoposide phosphate (Bristol Myers Squibb) 0.09 mg/mL in sodium chloride 0.9% did not result in the loss of viability of *Staphylococcus aureus*, *Enterococcus faecium*, *Pseudomonas aeruginosa*, and *Candida albicans* within 120 hours at 22 °C. Diluted solutions should be stored under refrigeration whenever possible, and the potential for microbiological growth should be considered when assigning expiration periods. (2740)

Light Effects — An evaluation of etoposide phosphate (Bristol-Myers Squibb) 2 mg/mL, doxorubicin hydrochloride 0.4 mg/mL, and vincristine sulfate 0.016 mg/mL (16 mcg/mL) in sodium chloride 0.9% in polyolefin plastic bags (McGaw) found little or no effect of constant exposure to normal fluorescent room light for 124 hours. The admixtures were physically compatible, and all three drugs in the admixture remained stable throughout the time stored at an elevated temperature of 35 to 40 °C. (2343)

Syringes — Etoposide phosphate (Bristol Laboratories Oncology Products) 10 and 20 mg/mL was prepared with bacteriostatic water for injection preserved with benzyl alcohol 0.9% (Abbott). The solutions were packaged as 4 mL of solution in 5-mL polypropylene syringes (Becton-Dickinson) and sealed with tip caps (Red Cap, Burron Medical). The syringes were stored at 32 °C for seven days, 23 °C for 31 days, and 4 °C for 31 days. All samples were physically stable, with no visual change and no increase in measured haze or particle content, and little drug loss occurred. At 32 °C, 2 to 4% loss occurred in seven days. At 23 °C, about 6 to 7% loss occurred in 31 days. Losses under refrigeration were 4% or less in 31 days. (2219)

Compatibility Information

Solution Compatibility

Etoposide phosphate

Solution	Mfr	Mfr	Conc/L	Remarks	Ref	C/I
Dextrose 5%	a,b	BMS	100 mg	Compatible and stable for 24 hr at 4 and 25 °C	1	C
	BA[a]	BR	0.1 and 10 g	Physically compatible and little loss in 7 days at 32 °C and in 31 days at 23 and 4 °C	2219	C
Sodium chloride 0.9%	a,b	BMS	100 mg	Compatible and stable for 24 hr at 4 and 25 °C	1	C
	BA[a]	BR	0.1 and 10 g	Physically compatible and little loss in 7 days at 32 °C and in 31 days at 23 and 4 °C	2219	C

[a]Tested in PVC containers.
[b]Tested in glass containers.

Additive Compatibility

Etoposide phosphate

Drug	Mfr	Conc/L	Mfr	Conc/L	Test Soln	Remarks	Ref	C/I
Doxorubicin HCl with vincristine sulfate	PHU LI	120 mg 5 mg	BMS	600 mg	NS[a]	Physically compatible. Little loss of any drug in 124 hr at 4 and 40 °C	2343	C
Doxorubicin HCl with vincristine sulfate	PHU LI	240 mg 10 mg	BMS	1.2 g	NS[a]	Physically compatible. Little loss of any drug in 124 hr at 4 and 40 °C	2343	C
Doxorubicin HCl with vincristine sulfate	PHU LI	400 mg 16 mg	BMS	2 g	NS[a]	Physically compatible. Under 4% loss of any drug in 124 hr at 4 and 40 °C	2343	C

Additive Compatibility (Cont.)

Etoposide phosphate

Drug	Mfr	Conc/L	Mfr	Conc/L	Test Soln	Remarks	Ref	C/I
Vincristine sulfate with doxorubicin HCl	LI PHU	5 mg 120 mg	BMS	600 mg	NS[a]	Physically compatible. Little loss of any drug in 124 hr at 4 and 40 °C	2343	C
Vincristine sulfate with doxorubicin HCl	LI PHU	10 mg 240 mg	BMS	1.2 g	NS[a]	Physically compatible. Little loss of any drug in 124 hr at 4 and 40 °C	2343	C
Vincristine sulfate with doxorubicin HCl	LI PHU	16 mg 400 mg	BMS	2 g	NS[a]	Physically compatible. Under 4% loss of any drug in 124 hr at 4 and 40 °C	2343	C

[a]Tested in polyolefin-lined plastic bags.

Y-Site Injection Compatibility (1:1 Mixture)

Etoposide phosphate

Drug	Mfr	Conc	Mfr	Conc	Remarks	Ref	C/I
Acyclovir sodium	GW	7 mg/mL[a]	BR	5 mg/mL[a]	Physically compatible for 4 hr at 23 °C	2218	C
Amikacin sulfate	APC	5 mg/mL[a]	BR	5 mg/mL[a]	Physically compatible for 4 hr at 23 °C	2218	C
Aminophylline	AB	2.5 mg/mL[a]	BR	5 mg/mL[a]	Physically compatible for 4 hr at 23 °C	2218	C
Amphotericin B	GNS	0.6 mg/mL[a]	BR	5 mg/mL[a]	Yellow-orange precipitate forms immediately	2218	I
Ampicillin sodium	APC	20 mg/mL[b]	BR	5 mg/mL[a]	Physically compatible for 4 hr at 23 °C	2218	C
Ampicillin sodium–sulbactam sodium	RR	20 + 10 mg/mL[b]	BR	5 mg/mL[a]	Physically compatible for 4 hr at 23 °C	2218	C
Anidulafungin	VIC	0.5 mg/mL[a]	BMS	5 mg/mL[a]	Physically compatible for 4 hr at 23 °C	2617	C
Aztreonam	SQ	40 mg/mL[a]	BR	5 mg/mL[a]	Physically compatible for 4 hr at 23 °C	2218	C
Bleomycin sulfate	MJ	1 unit/mL[b]	BR	5 mg/mL[a]	Physically compatible for 4 hr at 23 °C	2218	C
Bumetanide	RC	0.04 mg/mL[a]	BR	5 mg/mL[a]	Physically compatible for 4 hr at 23 °C	2218	C
Buprenorphine HCl	RKC	0.04 mg/mL[a]	BR	5 mg/mL[a]	Physically compatible for 4 hr at 23 °C	2218	C
Butorphanol tartrate	APC	0.04 mg/mL[a]	BR	5 mg/mL[a]	Physically compatible for 4 hr at 23 °C	2218	C
Calcium gluconate	FUJ	40 mg/mL[a]	BR	5 mg/mL[a]	Physically compatible for 4 hr at 23 °C	2218	C
Carboplatin	BR	5 mg/mL[a]	BR	5 mg/mL[a]	Physically compatible for 4 hr at 23 °C	2218	C
Carmustine	BR	1.5 mg/mL[a]	BR	5 mg/mL[a]	Physically compatible for 4 hr at 23 °C	2218	C
Caspofungin acetate	ME	0.7 mg/mL[b]	SIC	5 mg/mL[b]	Physically compatible for 4 hr at room temperature	2758	C
Cefazolin sodium	APC	20 mg/mL[a]	BR	5 mg/mL[a]	Physically compatible for 4 hr at 23 °C	2218	C
Cefepime HCl	BMS	20 mg/mL[a]	BR	5 mg/mL[a]	Increased haze and particulates form within 1 hr	2218	I
Cefotaxime sodium	HO	20 mg/mL[a]	BR	5 mg/mL[a]	Physically compatible for 4 hr at 23 °C	2218	C
Cefotetan disodium	ZEN	20 mg/mL[a]	BR	5 mg/mL[a]	Physically compatible for 4 hr at 23 °C	2218	C
Cefoxitin sodium	ME	20 mg/mL[a]	BR	5 mg/mL[a]	Physically compatible for 4 hr at 23 °C	2218	C
Ceftazidime	SKB	40 mg/mL[a]	BR	5 mg/mL[a]	Physically compatible for 4 hr at 23 °C	2218	C
Ceftriaxone sodium	RC	20 mg/mL[a]	BR	5 mg/mL[a]	Physically compatible for 4 hr at 23 °C	2218	C
Cefuroxime sodium	GW	30 mg/mL[a]	BR	5 mg/mL[a]	Physically compatible for 4 hr at 23 °C	2218	C
Chlorpromazine HCl	ES	2 mg/mL[a]	BR	5 mg/mL[a]	Cloudy solution forms immediately with particulates in 4 hr	2218	I

Y-Site Injection Compatibility (1:1 Mixture) (Cont.)

Etoposide phosphate

Drug	Mfr	Conc	Mfr	Conc	Remarks	Ref	C/I
Ciprofloxacin	BAY	1 mg/mL[a]	BR	5 mg/mL[a]	Physically compatible for 4 hr at 23 °C	2218	C
Cisplatin	BR	1 mg/mL	BR	5 mg/mL[a]	Physically compatible for 4 hr at 23 °C	2218	C
Clindamycin phosphate	AST	10 mg/mL[a]	BR	5 mg/mL[a]	Physically compatible for 4 hr at 23 °C	2218	C
Cyclophosphamide	MJ	10 mg/mL[a]	BR	5 mg/mL[a]	Physically compatible for 4 hr at 23 °C	2218	C
Cytarabine	BED	50 mg/mL	BR	5 mg/mL[a]	Physically compatible for 4 hr at 23 °C	2218	C
Dacarbazine	MI	4 mg/mL[a]	BR	5 mg/mL[a]	Physically compatible for 4 hr at 23 °C	2218	C
Dactinomycin	ME	0.01 mg/mL[a]	BR	5 mg/mL[a]	Physically compatible for 4 hr at 23 °C	2218	C
Daunorubicin HCl	BED	1 mg/mL[b]	BR	5 mg/mL[a]	Physically compatible for 4 hr at 23 °C	2218	C
Dexamethasone sodium phosphate	ES	1 mg/mL[a]	BR	5 mg/mL[a]	Physically compatible for 4 hr at 23 °C	2218	C
Diphenhydramine HCl	ES	2 mg/mL[a]	BR	5 mg/mL[a]	Physically compatible for 4 hr at 23 °C	2218	C
Dobutamine HCl	AST	4 mg/mL[a]	BR	5 mg/mL[a]	Physically compatible for 4 hr at 23 °C	2218	C
Dopamine HCl	AST	3.2 mg/mL[a]	BR	5 mg/mL[a]	Physically compatible for 4 hr at 23 °C	2218	C
Doripenem	JJ	5 mg/mL[a,b]	SIC	5 mg/mL[a,b]	Physically compatible for 4 hr at 23 °C	2743	C
Doxorubicin HCl	GEN	2 mg/mL	BR	5 mg/mL[a]	Physically compatible for 4 hr at 23 °C	2218	C
Doxycycline hyclate	FUJ	1 mg/mL[a]	BR	5 mg/mL[a]	Physically compatible for 4 hr at 23 °C	2218	C
Droperidol	AST	0.4 mg/mL[a]	BR	5 mg/mL[a]	Physically compatible for 4 hr at 23 °C	2218	C
Enalaprilat	ME	0.1 mg/mL[a]	BR	5 mg/mL[a]	Physically compatible for 4 hr at 23 °C	2218	C
Famotidine	ME	2 mg/mL[a]	BR	5 mg/mL[a]	Physically compatible for 4 hr at 23 °C	2218	C
Floxuridine	RC	3 mg/mL[a]	BR	5 mg/mL[a]	Physically compatible for 4 hr at 23 °C	2218	C
Fluconazole	RR	2 mg/mL	BR	5 mg/mL[a]	Physically compatible for 4 hr at 23 °C	2218	C
Fludarabine phosphate	BX	1 mg/mL[a]	BR	5 mg/mL[a]	Physically compatible for 4 hr at 23 °C	2218	C
Fluorouracil	PH	16 mg/mL[a]	BR	5 mg/mL[a]	Physically compatible for 4 hr at 23 °C	2218	C
Furosemide	AMR	3 mg/mL[a]	BR	5 mg/mL[a]	Physically compatible for 4 hr at 23 °C	2218	C
Ganciclovir sodium	RC	20 mg/mL[a]	BR	5 mg/mL[a]	Physically compatible for 4 hr at 23 °C	2218	C
Gemcitabine HCl	LI	10 mg/mL[b]	BR	5 mg/mL[b]	Physically compatible for 4 hr at 23 °C	2226	C
Gentamicin sulfate	AB	5 mg/mL[a]	BR	5 mg/mL[a]	Physically compatible for 4 hr at 23 °C	2218	C
Granisetron HCl	SKB	0.05 mg/mL[a]	BR	5 mg/mL[a]	Physically compatible for 4 hr at 23 °C	2218	C
Haloperidol lactate	MN	0.2 mg/mL[a]	BR	5 mg/mL[a]	Physically compatible for 4 hr at 23 °C	2218	C
Heparin sodium	ES	100 units/mL[a]	BR	5 mg/mL[a]	Physically compatible for 4 hr at 23 °C	2218	C
Hydrocortisone sodium succinate	UP	1 mg/mL[a]	BR	5 mg/mL[a]	Physically compatible for 4 hr at 23 °C	2218	C
Hydromorphone HCl	ES	0.5 mg/mL[a]	BR	5 mg/mL[a]	Physically compatible for 4 hr at 23 °C	2218	C
Hydroxyzine HCl	ES	4 mg/mL[a]	BR	5 mg/mL[a]	Physically compatible for 4 hr at 23 °C	2218	C
Idarubicin HCl	AD	0.5 mg/mL[a]	BR	5 mg/mL[a]	Physically compatible for 4 hr at 23 °C	2218	C
Ifosfamide	MJ	25 mg/mL[a]	BR	5 mg/mL[a]	Physically compatible for 4 hr at 23 °C	2218	C
Imipenem–cilastatin sodium	ME	10 mg/mL[b]	BR	5 mg/mL[a]	Yellow color forms in 4 hr at 23 °C	2218	I
Leucovorin calcium	IMM	2 mg/mL[a]	BR	5 mg/mL[a]	Physically compatible for 4 hr at 23 °C	2218	C
Linezolid	PHU	2 mg/mL	BR	5 mg/mL[a]	Physically compatible for 4 hr at 23 °C	2264	C
Lorazepam	WY	0.5 mg/mL[a]	BR	5 mg/mL[a]	Physically compatible for 4 hr at 23 °C	2218	C

Y-Site Injection Compatibility (1:1 Mixture) (Cont.)

Etoposide phosphate

Drug	Mfr	Conc	Mfr	Conc	Remarks	Ref	C/I
Magnesium sulfate	AST	100 mg/mL[a]	BR	5 mg/mL[a]	Physically compatible for 4 hr at 23 °C	2218	C
Mannitol	BA	15%	BR	5 mg/mL[a]	Physically compatible for 4 hr at 23 °C	2218	C
Meperidine HCl	AST	4 mg/mL[a]	BR	5 mg/mL[a]	Physically compatible for 4 hr at 23 °C	2218	C
Mesna	MJ	10 mg/mL[a]	BR	5 mg/mL[a]	Physically compatible for 4 hr at 23 °C	2218	C
Methotrexate sodium	IMM	15 mg/mL[a]	BR	5 mg/mL[a]	Physically compatible for 4 hr at 23 °C	2218	C
Methylprednisolone sodium succinate	AB	5 mg/mL[a]	BR	5 mg/mL[a]	Haze with subvisible microparticles forms immediately. Particle content increases fivefold over 4 hr at 23 °C	2218	I
Metoclopramide HCl	FAU	5 mg/mL	BR	5 mg/mL[a]	Physically compatible for 4 hr at 23 °C	2218	C
Metronidazole	AB	5 mg/mL	BR	5 mg/mL[a]	Physically compatible for 4 hr at 23 °C	2218	C
Mitomycin	BR	0.5 mg/mL	BR	5 mg/mL[a]	Color changed from light blue to reddish purple in 4 hr at 23 °C	2218	I
Mitoxantrone HCl	IMM	0.5 mg/mL[a]	BR	5 mg/mL[a]	Physically compatible for 4 hr at 23 °C	2218	C
Morphine sulfate	ES	1 mg/mL[a]	BR	5 mg/mL[a]	Physically compatible for 4 hr at 23 °C	2218	C
Nalbuphine HCl	AST	10 mg/mL	BR	5 mg/mL[a]	Physically compatible for 4 hr at 23 °C	2218	C
Ondansetron HCl	GW	1 mg/mL[a]	BR	5 mg/mL[a]	Physically compatible for 4 hr at 23 °C	2218	C
Oxaliplatin	SS	0.5 mg/mL[a]	BR	5 mg/mL[a]	Physically compatible for 4 hr at 23 °C	2566	C
Paclitaxel	MJ	1.2 mg/mL[a]	BR	5 mg/mL[a]	Physically compatible for 4 hr at 23 °C	2218	C
Piperacillin sodium–tazobactam sodium	LE[c]	40 + 5 mg/ mL[b]	BR	5 mg/mL[a]	Physically compatible for 4 hr at 23 °C	2218	C
Potassium chloride	AB	0.1 mEq/mL[a]	BR	5 mg/mL[a]	Physically compatible for 4 hr at 23 °C	2218	C
Prochlorperazine edisylate	ES	0.5 mg/mL[a]	BR	5 mg/mL[a]	White cloudy solution forms immediately with precipitate in 4 hr	2218	I
Promethazine HCl	SCN	2 mg/mL[a]	BR	5 mg/mL[a]	Physically compatible for 4 hr at 23 °C	2218	C
Ranitidine HCl	GL	2 mg/mL[a]	BR	5 mg/mL[a]	Physically compatible for 4 hr at 23 °C	2218	C
Sodium bicarbonate	AB	1 mEq/mL	BR	5 mg/mL[a]	Physically compatible for 4 hr at 23 °C	2218	C
Streptozocin	UP	40 mg/mL[a]	BR	5 mg/mL[a]	Physically compatible for 4 hr at 23 °C	2218	C
Teniposide	BR	0.1 mg/mL[a]	BR	5 mg/mL[a]	Physically compatible for 4 hr at 23 °C	2218	C
Thiotepa	IMM	1 mg/mL[a]	BR	5 mg/mL[a]	Physically compatible for 4 hr at 23 °C	2218	C
Ticarcillin disodium–clavulanate potassium	SKB	31 mg/mL[a]	BR	5 mg/mL[a]	Physically compatible for 4 hr at 23 °C	2218	C
Tobramycin sulfate	LI	5 mg/mL[a]	BR	5 mg/mL[a]	Physically compatible for 4 hr at 23 °C	2218	C
Trimethoprim–sulfamethoxazole	ES	0.8 + 4 mg/ mL[a]	BR	5 mg/mL[a]	Physically compatible for 4 hr at 23 °C	2218	C
Vancomycin HCl	LI	10 mg/mL[a]	BR	5 mg/mL[a]	Physically compatible for 4 hr at 23 °C	2218	C
Vinblastine sulfate	FAU	0.12 mg/mL[a]	BR	5 mg/mL[a]	Physically compatible for 4 hr at 23 °C	2218	C
Vincristine sulfate	FAU	0.05 mg/mL[a]	BR	5 mg/mL[a]	Physically compatible for 4 hr at 23 °C	2218	C
Zidovudine	BW	4 mg/mL[a]	BR	5 mg/mL[a]	Physically compatible for 4 hr at 23 °C	2218	C

[a]Tested in dextrose 5%.
[b]Tested in sodium chloride 0.9%.
[c]Test performed using the formulation WITHOUT edetate disodium.

FAMOTIDINE
AHFS 56:28.12

Products — Famotidine is available as a 10-mg/mL concentrated injection in 2-mL single-dose vials and 4- and 20-mL multiple-dose vials. Each milliliter of the solution also contains l-aspartic acid 4 mg and mannitol 20 mg. Benzyl alcohol 0.9% is present as a preservative in the multiple-dose product. (1)

Famotidine is also available premixed at a concentration of 20 mg/ 50 mL. Each 50 mL of solution also contains l-aspartic acid 6.8 mg and sodium chloride 450 mg in water for injection. Additional l-aspartic acid or sodium hydroxide may be added to adjust the pH. (1)

pH — The injection has a pH from 5 to 5.6. (4) The premixed solution has a pH from 5.7 to 6.4. (1)

Osmolarity — The osmolarities of the single- and multiple-dose products are 217 and 290 mOsm/L, respectively. (4)

Sodium Content — Famotidine premixed infusion solution has 7.8 mEq of sodium per 50 mL. (4)

Trade Name(s) — Pepcid.

Administration — Famotidine is administered by slow intravenous injection or infusion. For injection, 20 mg should be diluted to 5 to 10 mL with a compatible diluent and injected no faster than 10 mg/ min. For infusion, 20 mg should be diluted in 100 mL of dextrose 5% or another compatible diluent and infused over 15 to 30 minutes. Alternatively, famotidine premixed solution may be administered by intravenous infusion over 15 to 30 minutes. (1; 4)

Stability — Famotidine injection is a clear, colorless solution. The vials should be stored under refrigeration and protected from freezing. If freezing occurs, thaw at room temperature; make sure that all components have resolubilized. (1; 4) Use of a microwave oven for thawing is not recommended because of the potential hazard of vapor pressure increases in the vials. (4)

Although refrigeration is recommended, the manufacturer has indicated that the drug may be stored at room temperature for 26 weeks (1239) and for three months (2745) at controlled room temperature in differing statements.

Famotidine premixed infusion solution should be stored at controlled room temperature (25 °C) and protected from excessive heat. Brief exposure to temperatures up to 35 °C does not affect the stability of the product adversely. (1)

Freezing Solutions — Famotidine (MSD) 200 mcg/mL in dextrose 5% or sodium chloride 0.9% in PVC bags showed no loss when frozen at −20 °C for 28 days followed by storage at 4 °C for 14 days. (1271)

Famotidine (MSD) 2 mg/mL in dextrose 5%, sodium chloride 0.9%, or sterile water for injection stored in polypropylene syringes (Becton Dickinson) exhibited a 5 to 8% loss in eight weeks when frozen at −20 °C. (1486)

Syringes — Famotidine (MSD) 2 mg/mL in dextrose 5%, sodium chloride 0.9%, or sterile water for injection stored in plastic syringes (Becton Dickinson) exhibited no loss in 14 days at 4 °C. (1487)

Central Venous Catheter — Famotidine (Merck) 2 mg/mL in dextrose 5% was found to be compatible with the ARROWg+ard Blue Plus (Arrow International) chlorhexidine-bearing triple-lumen central catheter. Essentially complete delivery of the drug was found with little or no drug loss occurring. Furthermore, chlorhexidine delivered from the catheter remained at trace amounts with no substantial increase due to the delivery of the drug through the catheter. (2335)

Compatibility Information

Solution Compatibility

Famotidine

Solution	Mfr	Mfr	Conc/L	Remarks	Ref	C/I
Dextrose 5%				Under 10% loss in 7 days at room temperature	1	**C**
	TR[a]		200 mg	Physically compatible with 6% loss in 15 days at 25 °C and no loss in 63 days at 5 °C	1342	**C**
		MSD	20 mg	No loss in 48 hr at 25 °C in light or dark and at 5 °C	1344	**C**
	AB[a,b]	ME	200 mg	Visually compatible with less than 5% loss in 15 days at 22 °C both in dark and light	1936	**C**
Dextrose 10%				Under 10% loss in 7 days at room temperature	1	**C**
Ringer's injection, lactated				Under 10% loss in 7 days at room temperature	1	**C**
Sodium chloride 0.9%				Under 10% loss in 7 days at room temperature	1	**C**
	TR[a]		200 mg	Physically compatible with little or no loss in 15 days at 25 °C and in 63 days at 5 °C	1342	**C**
		MSD	20 mg	No loss in 48 hr at 25 °C in light or dark and at 5 °C	1344	**C**
	AB[a,b]	ME	200 mg	Visually compatible with less than 5% loss in 15 days at 22 °C both in dark and light	1936	**C**

Solution Compatibility (Cont.)

Famotidine

Solution	Mfr	Mfr	Conc/L	Remarks	Ref	C/I
TNA #111, #112[c]		MSD	20 and 50 mg	Physically compatible. Little loss and no change in fat particle size in 48 hr at 4 and 21 °C	1332	C
TNA #114[c]		MSD	20 and 40 mg	Physically compatible. No loss and no change in fat particle size in 72 hr at 21 °C in light	1333	C
TNA #182[c]		MSD	20 mg	Visually compatible. No loss in 24 hr at 24 °C in light	1576	C
TNA #197 to #200[c]		MSD	20 mg	Physically compatible. No loss in 48 hr at 22 °C in light	1921	C
TPN #109, #110[c]		MSD	20 and 40 mg	Physically compatible with no famotidine loss and little change in amino acids in 48 hr at 21 °C and in 7 days at 4 °C	1331	C
TPN #113[c]		MSD	20 mg	Physically compatible. Little loss in 35 days at 4 °C in light	1334	C
TPN #115, #116[c]		MSD	16.7 and 33.3 mg	No famotidine loss in 7 days at 23 and 4 °C	1352	C
TPN #196[c]		MSD	20 mg	Physically compatible. No loss in 48 hr at 22 °C in light	1921	C

[a]Tested in PVC containers.
[b]Tested in polypropylene syringes.
[c]Refer to Appendix I for the composition of parenteral nutrition solutions. TNA indicates a 3-in-1 admixture, and TPN indicates a 2-in-1 admixture.

Additive Compatibility

Famotidine

Drug	Mfr	Conc/L	Mfr	Conc/L	Test Soln	Remarks	Ref	C/I
Cefazolin sodium	FUJ	10 g	YAM	200 mg	D5W	Visually compatible with 10% cefazolin and 5% famotidine loss in 24 hr at 25 °C. 9% cefazolin and 5% famotidine loss in 48 hr at 4 °C	1763	C
Fat emulsion, intravenous		10%	MSD	200 mg		Little loss in 48 hr at 25 °C in light or dark and at 5 °C	1344	C
Flumazenil	RC	20 mg	MSD	80 mg	D5W[a]	Visually compatible. 3% flumazenil loss in 24 hr at 23 °C in fluorescent light. Famotidine not tested	1710	C
Vancomycin HCl	AB	5 g	YAM	200 mg	D5W[b]	Visually compatible. 9% vancomycin and 6% famotidine loss in 14 days at 25 °C. At 4 °C, 4% loss of both drugs in 14 days	2111	C

[a]Tested in PVC containers.
[b]Tested in methyl-methacrylate-butadiene-styrene plastic containers.

Y-Site Injection Compatibility (1:1 Mixture)

Famotidine

Drug	Mfr	Conc	Mfr	Conc	Remarks	Ref	C/I
Acyclovir sodium		7 mg/mL[a]	ME	2 mg/mL[b]	Visually compatible for 4 hr at 22 °C	1936	C
Allopurinol sodium	BW	3 mg/mL[b]	MSD	2 mg/mL[b]	Physically compatible for 4 hr at 22 °C	1686	C
Amifostine	USB	10 mg/mL[a]	ME	2 mg/mL[a]	Physically compatible for 4 hr at 23 °C	1845	C
Aminophylline	LY	2.5 mg/mL[b]	MSD	0.2 mg/mL[a]	Physically compatible for 14 hr	1196	C
		2.5 mg/mL[a]	ME	2 mg/mL	Visually compatible for 4 hr at 22 °C	1936	C
Amiodarone HCl	WY	6 mg/mL[a]	ME	10 mg/mL	Visually compatible for 24 hr at 22 °C	2352	C
Amphotericin B cholesteryl sulfate complex	SEQ	0.83 mg/mL[a]	ME	2 mg/mL[a]	Microprecipitate and increased turbidity form immediately	2117	I
Ampicillin sodium	ES	20 mg/mL[b]	MSD	0.2 mg/mL[a]	Physically compatible for 14 hr	1196	C
		20 mg/mL[b]	ME	2 mg/mL[b]	Visually compatible for 4 hr at 22 °C	1936	C
Ampicillin sodium–sulbactam sodium	RR	20 + 10 mg/mL[b]	MSD	0.2 mg/mL[a]	Physically compatible for 14 hr	1196	C
Amsacrine	NCI	1 mg/mL[a]	MSD	2 mg/mL[a]	Visually compatible for 4 hr at 22 °C	1381	C
Anakinra	SYN	4 and 36 mg/mL[b]		1 mg/mL[b]	Physically compatible with little or no loss of either drug in 4 hr at 22 °C	2511	C
Anidulafungin	VIC	0.5 mg/mL[a]	BV	2 mg/mL[a]	Physically compatible for 4 hr at 23 °C	2617	C
Atropine sulfate	AST	0.1 mg/mL[a]	MSD	0.2 mg/mL[a]	Physically compatible for 4 hr at 25 °C	1188	C
Azithromycin	PF	2 mg/mL[b]	ME	2 mg/mL[j]	Grayish-white microcrystals found	2368	I
Aztreonam	SQ	40 mg/mL[a]	ME	2 mg/mL[a]	Physically compatible for 4 hr at 23 °C	1758	C
Bivalirudin	TMC	5 mg/mL[a]	ME	2 mg/mL[a]	Physically compatible for 4 hr at 23 °C	2373	C
Calcium gluconate	LY	0.00465 mEq/mL[b]	MSD	0.2 mg/mL[a]	Physically compatible for 14 hr	1196	C
Caspofungin acetate	ME	0.5 mg/mL[b]	BA	2 mg/mL[b]	Physically compatible with famotidine i.v. push over 2 to 5 min	2766	C
Cefazolin sodium	LY	20 mg/mL[b]	MSD	0.2 mg/mL[a]	Physically compatible for 14 hr	1196	C
		20 mg/mL[a]	ME	2 mg/mL[b]	Visually compatible for 4 hr at 22 °C	1936	C
Cefotaxime sodium	HO	20 mg/mL[b]	MSD	0.2 mg/mL[a]	Physically compatible for 14 hr	1196	C
		20 mg/mL[a]	ME	2 mg/mL[b]	Visually compatible for 4 hr at 22 °C	1936	C
Cefotetan disodium	STU	20 mg/mL[b]	MSD	0.2 mg/mL[a]	Physically compatible for 14 hr	1196	C
Cefoxitin sodium	MSD	20 mg/mL[b]	MSD	0.2 mg/mL[a]	Physically compatible for 14 hr	1196	C
		20 mg/mL[a]	ME	2 mg/mL[b]	Visually compatible for 4 hr at 22 °C	1936	C
Ceftaroline fosamil	FOR	2.22 mg/mL[a,b,c]	ABX	2 mg/mL[a,b,c]	Physically compatible for 4 hr at 23 °C	2826	C
Ceftazidime	GL	20 mg/mL[b]	MSD	0.2 mg/mL[a]	Physically compatible for 14 hr	1196	C
		20 mg/mL[a]	ME	2 mg/mL[b]	Visually compatible for 4 hr at 22 °C	1936	C
Ceftriaxone sodium		20 mg/mL[a]	ME	2 mg/mL[b]	Visually compatible for 4 hr at 22 °C	1936	C
Cefuroxime sodium	GL	15 mg/mL[b]	MSD	0.2 mg/mL[a]	Physically compatible for 14 hr	1196	C
		20 mg/mL[a]	ME	2 mg/mL[b]	Visually compatible for 4 hr at 22 °C	1936	C
Chlorpromazine HCl		2 mg/mL[a]	ME	2 mg/mL[b]	Visually compatible for 4 hr at 22 °C	1936	C
Cisatracurium besylate	GW	0.1, 2, 5 mg/mL[a]	ME	2 mg/mL[a]	Physically compatible for 4 hr at 23 °C	2074	C
Cladribine	ORT	0.015[b] and 0.5[d] mg/mL	ME	2 mg/mL[b]	Physically compatible for 4 hr at 23 °C	1969	C

Y-Site Injection Compatibility (1:1 Mixture) (Cont.)

Famotidine

Drug	Mfr	Conc	Mfr	Conc	Remarks	Ref	C/I
Dexamethasone sodium phosphate	ES	10 mg/mL	MSD	0.2 mg/mL[a]	Physically compatible for 14 hr	1196	C
		1 mg/mL[a]	ME	2 mg/mL[b]	Visually compatible for 4 hr at 22 °C	1936	C
Dexmedetomidine HCl	AB	4 mcg/mL[b]	ME	2 mg/mL[b]	Physically compatible for 4 hr at 23 °C	2383	C
Dextran 40	PH	100 mg/mL[a]	MSD	0.2 mg/mL[a]	Physically compatible for 4 hr at 25 °C	1188	C
Digoxin	ES	0.25 mg/mL	MSD	0.2 mg/mL[a]	Physically compatible for 14 hr	1196	C
Diphenhydramine HCl		2 mg/mL[a]	ME	2 mg/mL[b]	Visually compatible for 4 hr at 22 °C	1936	C
Dobutamine HCl	LI	1 mg/mL[a]	MSD	0.2 mg/mL[a]	Physically compatible for 4 hr at 25 °C	1188	C
		4 mg/mL[a]	ME	2 mg/mL[b]	Visually compatible for 4 hr at 22 °C	1936	C
Docetaxel	RPR	0.9 mg/mL[a]	ME	2 mg/mL[a]	Physically compatible for 4 hr at 23 °C	2224	C
Dopamine HCl	TR	1.6 mg/mL[a]	MSD	0.2 mg/mL[a]	Physically compatible for 4 hr at 25 °C	1188	C
		1.6 mg/mL[a]	ME	2 mg/mL[b]	Visually compatible for 4 hr at 22 °C	1936	C
Doripenem	JJ	5 mg/mL[a,b]	BED	2 mg/mL[a,b]	Physically compatible for 4 hr at 23 °C	2743	C
Doxorubicin HCl liposomal	SEQ	0.4 mg/mL[a]	ME	2 mg/mL[a]	Physically compatible for 4 hr at 23 °C	2087	C
Droperidol		0.4 mg/mL[a]	ME	2 mg/mL[b]	Visually compatible for 4 hr at 22 °C	1936	C
Enalaprilat	MSD	0.05 mg/mL[b]	MSD	0.2 mg/mL[a]	Physically compatible for 24 hr at room temperature under fluorescent light	1355	C
Epinephrine HCl	ES	4 mcg/mL[a]	MSD	0.2 mg/mL[a]	Physically compatible for 4 hr at 25 °C	1188	C
Erythromycin lactobionate	ES	2 mg/mL[b]	MSD	0.2 mg/mL[a]	Physically compatible for 14 hr	1196	C
Esmolol HCl	DU	10 mg/mL[b]	MSD	0.2 mg/mL[a]	Physically compatible for 4 hr at 25 °C	1188	C
Etoposide phosphate	BR	5 mg/mL[a]	ME	2 mg/mL[a]	Physically compatible for 4 hr at 23 °C	2218	C
Fenoldopam mesylate	AB	80 mcg/mL[b]	ME	2 mg/mL[b]	Physically compatible for 4 hr at 23 °C	2467	C
Filgrastim	AMG	30 mcg/mL[a]	MSD	2 mg/mL[a]	Physically compatible for 4 hr at 22 °C	1687	C
Fluconazole	RR	2 mg/mL	MSD	10 mg/mL	Physically compatible for 24 hr at 25 °C	1407	C
		2 mg/mL[a]	ME	2 mg/mL[b]	Visually compatible for 4 hr at 22 °C	1936	C
Fludarabine phosphate	BX	1 mg/mL[a]	MSD	2 mg/mL[a]	Visually compatible for 4 hr at 22 °C	1439	C
Folic acid	LE	5 mg/mL	MSD	0.2 mg/mL[a]	Physically compatible for 14 hr	1196	C
Furosemide	ES	10 mg/mL	MSD	0.2 mg/mL[a]	Physically compatible for 14 hr	1196	C
	IMS	0.8 mg/mL[a]	MSD	0.2 mg/mL[a]	Physically compatible for 4 hr at 25 °C	1188	C
		3 mg/mL[a]	ME	2 mg/mL[b]	White precipitate forms immediately	1936	I
Gemcitabine HCl	LI	10 mg/mL[b]	ME	2 mg/mL[b]	Physically compatible for 4 hr at 23 °C	2226	C
Gentamicin sulfate	ES	0.8 mg/mL[b]	MSD	0.2 mg/mL[a]	Physically compatible for 14 hr	1196	C
		5 mg/mL[a]	ME	2 mg/mL[b]	Visually compatible for 4 hr at 22 °C	1936	C
Granisetron HCl	SKB	0.05 mg/mL[a]	ME	2 mg/mL[a]	Physically compatible for 4 hr at 23 °C	2000	C
Haloperidol lactate	MN	0.5[a] and 5 mg/mL	MSD	0.267 mg/mL[a]	Visually compatible for 24 hr at 21 °C	1523	C
		0.2 mg/mL[a]	ME	2 mg/mL[b]	Visually compatible for 4 hr at 22 °C	1936	C
Heparin sodium	ES	40 units/mL[b]	MSD	0.2 mg/mL[a]	Physically compatible for 14 hr	1196	C
	TR	50 units/mL[a]	MSD	0.2 mg/mL[a]	Physically compatible for 4 hr at 25 °C	1188	C
		40 units/mL[a]	ME	2 mg/mL[b]	Visually compatible for 4 hr at 22 °C	1936	C
Hetastarch in lactated electrolyte	AB	6%	ME	2 mg/mL[a]	Physically compatible for 4 hr at 23 °C	2339	C
Hydrocortisone sodium succinate	AB	1 mg/mL[a]	MSD	0.2 mg/mL[a]	Physically compatible for 4 hr at 25 °C	1188	C
	AB	125 mg/mL	MSD	0.2 mg/mL[a]	Physically compatible for 14 hr	1196	C

Y-Site Injection Compatibility (1:1 Mixture) (Cont.)

Famotidine

Drug	Mfr	Conc	Mfr	Conc	Remarks	Ref	C/I
Hydromorphone HCl		0.5 mg/mL[a]	ME	2 mg/mL[b]	Visually compatible for 4 hr at 22 °C	1936	C
Hydroxyzine HCl		4 mg/mL[a]	ME	2 mg/mL[b]	Visually compatible for 4 hr at 22 °C	1936	C
Imipenem–cilastatin sodium	MSD	10 mg/mL[b]	MSD	0.2 mg/mL[a]	Physically compatible for 14 hr	1196	C
		5 mg/mL[b]	ME	2 mg/mL[b]	Visually compatible for 4 hr at 22 °C	1936	C
Insulin, regular	LI	0.03 unit/mL[a]	MSD	0.2 mg/mL[a]	Physically compatible for 4 hr at 25 °C	1188	C
Isoproterenol HCl	ES	0.004 mg/mL[a]	MSD	0.2 mg/mL[a]	Physically compatible for 4 hr at 25 °C	1188	C
Labetalol HCl	SC	1 mg/mL[a]	MSD	0.2 mg/mL[a]	Physically compatible for 4 hr at 25 °C	1188	C
Lidocaine HCl	LY	1 mg/mL[a]	MSD	0.2 mg/mL[a]	Physically compatible for 14 hr	1196	C
	TR	4 mg/mL[a]	MSD	0.2 mg/mL[a]	Physically compatible for 4 hr at 25 °C	1188	C
Linezolid	PHU	2 mg/mL	ME	2 mg/mL[a]	Physically compatible for 4 hr at 23 °C	2264	C
Lorazepam		0.1 mg/mL[a]	ME	2 mg/mL[b]	Visually compatible for 4 hr at 22 °C	1936	C
Magnesium sulfate	SO	100 mg/mL[b]	MSD	0.2 mg/mL[a]	Physically compatible for 14 hr	1196	C
		100 mg/mL[a]	ME	2 mg/mL[b]	Visually compatible for 4 hr at 22 °C	1936	C
Melphalan HCl	BW	0.1 mg/mL[b]	MSD	2 mg/mL[b]	Physically compatible for 3 hr at 22 °C	1557	C
Meperidine HCl	AB	10 mg/mL	MSD	0.2 mg/mL[a]	Physically compatible for 4 hr at 25 °C	1397	C
		4 mg/mL[a]	ME	2 mg/mL[b]	Visually compatible for 4 hr at 22 °C	1936	C
Methylprednisolone sodium succinate	QU	40 mg/mL	MSD	0.2 mg/mL[a]	Physically compatible for 14 hr	1196	C
	AB	1 mg/mL[a]	MSD	0.2 mg/mL[a]	Physically compatible for 4 hr at 25 °C	1188	C
		5 mg/mL[a]	ME	2 mg/mL[b]	Visually compatible for 4 hr at 22 °C	1936	C
Metoclopramide HCl	RB	5 mg/mL	MSD	0.2 mg/mL[a]	Physically compatible for 14 hr	1196	C
		5 mg/mL	ME	2 mg/mL[b]	Visually compatible for 4 hr at 22 °C	1936	C
Midazolam HCl	RC	0.15 mg/mL[a]	MSD	0.2 mg/mL[a]	Physically compatible for 4 hr at 25 °C	1188	C
		1.5 mg/mL[a]	ME	2 mg/mL[b]	Visually compatible for 4 hr at 22 °C	1936	C
Morphine sulfate	ES	0.2 mg/mL[a]	MSD	0.2 mg/mL[a]	Physically compatible for 4 hr at 25 °C	1188	C
	AB	1 mg/mL	MSD	0.2 mg/mL[a]	Physically compatible for 4 hr at 25 °C	1397	C
		1 mg/mL[a]	ME	2 mg/mL[b]	Visually compatible for 4 hr at 22 °C	1936	C
Nafcillin sodium	WY	15 mg/mL[b]	MSD	0.2 mg/mL[a]	Physically compatible for 14 hr	1196	C
Nicardipine HCl	DCC	0.1 mg/mL[a]	MSD	0.2 mg/mL[a]	Visually compatible for 24 hr at room temperature	235	C
Nitroglycerin	PD	85 mcg/mL[b]	MSD	0.2 mg/mL[a]	Physically compatible for 14 hr	1196	C
	IMS	0.8 mg/mL[a]	MSD	0.2 mg/mL[a]	Physically compatible for 4 hr at 25 °C	1188	C
Norepinephrine bitartrate	WI	0.004 mg/mL[a]	MSD	0.2 mg/mL[a]	Physically compatible for 4 hr at 25 °C	1188	C
Ondansetron HCl	GL	1 mg/mL[b]	MSD	2 mg/mL[a]	Visually compatible for 4 hr at 22 °C	1365	C
Oxacillin sodium	BE	20 mg/mL[b]	MSD	0.2 mg/mL[a]	Physically compatible for 14 hr	1196	C
Oxaliplatin	SS	0.5 mg/mL[a]	ESL	2 mg/mL[a]	Physically compatible for 4 hr at 23 °C	2566	C
Paclitaxel	NCI	1.2 mg/mL[a]	MSD	2 mg/mL[a]	Physically compatible for 4 hr at 22 °C	1556	C
Palonosetron HCl	MGI	50 mcg/mL	BED	2 mg/mL[a]	Physically compatible and no loss of either drug in 4 hr at room temperature	2771	C
Pemetrexed disodium	LI	20 mg/mL[b]	ESL	2 mg/mL[a]	Physically compatible for 4 hr at 23 °C	2564	C
Phenylephrine HCl	WI	0.02 mg/mL[a]	MSD	0.2 mg/mL[a]	Physically compatible for 4 hr at 25 °C	1188	C

Y-Site Injection Compatibility (1:1 Mixture) (Cont.)

Famotidine

Drug	Mfr	Conc	Mfr	Conc	Remarks	Ref	C/I
Phenytoin sodium	PD	50 mg/mL	MSD	0.2 mg/mL[a]	Physically compatible for 14 hr	1196	C
Phytonadione	MSD	2 mg/mL	MSD	0.2 mg/mL[a]	Physically compatible for 14 hr	1196	C
Piperacillin sodium–tazobactam sodium	LE[k]	40 + 5 mg/mL[a]	MSD	2 mg/mL[a]	Particles form immediately	1688	I
Potassium chloride	AB	0.04 mEq/mL[a]	MSD	0.2 mg/mL[a]	Physically compatible for 4 hr at 25 °C	1188	C
		0.1 mEq/mL[a]	ME	2 mg/mL[b]	Visually compatible for 4 hr at 22 °C	1936	C
Potassium phosphates	LY	0.03 mmol/mL[b]	MSD	0.2 mg/mL[a]	Physically compatible for 14 hr	1196	C
Procainamide HCl	ASC	5 mg/mL[a]	MSD	0.2 mg/mL[a]	Physically compatible for 4 hr at 25 °C	1188	C
Propofol	ZEN	10 mg/mL	ME	2 mg/mL[a]	Physically compatible for 1 hr at 23 °C	2066	C
Remifentanil HCl	GW	0.025 and 0.25 mg/mL[b]	MSD	2 mg/mL[a]	Physically compatible for 4 hr at 23 °C	2075	C
Sargramostim	IMM	10 mcg/mL[b]	MSD	2 mg/mL[b]	Visually compatible for 4 hr at 22 °C	1436	C
Sodium bicarbonate	AB	1 mEq/mL	MSD	0.2 mg/mL[a]	Physically compatible for 4 hr at 25 °C	1188	C
Sodium nitroprusside	ES	0.2 mg/mL[a]	MSD	0.2 mg/mL[a]	Physically compatible for 4 hr at 25 °C protected from light	1188	C
Telavancin HCl	ASP	7.5 mg/mL[a,b,c]	BED	2 mg/mL[a,b,c]	Physically compatible for 2 hr	2830	C
Teniposide	BR	0.1 mg/mL[a]	MSD	2 mg/mL[a]	Physically compatible for 4 hr at 23 °C	1725	C
Theophylline	TR	1.6 mg/mL[a]	MSD	0.2 mg/mL[a]	Physically compatible for 4 hr at 25 °C	1188	C
Thiamine HCl	ES	100 mg/mL	MSD	0.2 mg/mL[a]	Physically compatible for 14 hr	1196	C
Thiotepa	IMM[g]	1 mg/mL[a]	ME	2 mg/mL[a]	Physically compatible for 4 hr at 23 °C	1861	C
Ticarcillin disodium–clavulanate potassium	BE	31 mg/mL[b]	MSD	0.2 mg/mL[a]	Physically compatible for 14 hr	1196	C
Tirofiban HCl	ME	0.05 mg/mL[b]	ME	2 and 4 mg/mL[a]	Physically compatible. Little loss of either drug in 4 hr at room temperature	2250	C
	ME	0.05 mg/mL[a]	ME	2 and 4 mg/mL[b]	Physically compatible. Little loss of either drug in 4 hr at room temperature	2250	C
TNA #218 to #226[h]			ME	2 mg/mL[a]	Visually compatible for 4 hr at 23 °C	2215	C
TPN #212 to #215[h]			ME	2 mg/mL[a]	Physically compatible for 4 hr at 23 °C	2109	C
Verapamil HCl	KN	0.1 mg/mL[a]	MSD	0.2 mg/mL[a]	Physically compatible for 4 hr at 25 °C	1188	C
Vinorelbine tartrate	BW	1 mg/mL[b]	MSD	2 mg/mL[b]	Physically compatible for 4 hr at 22 °C	1558	C

[a]*Tested in dextrose 5%.*
[b]*Tested in sodium chloride 0.9%.*
[c]*Tested in Ringer's injection, lactated.*
[d]*Tested in bacteriostatic sodium chloride 0.9% preserved with benzyl alcohol 0.9%.*
[e]*Form not specified.*
[f]*Tested in dextrose 5% with sodium bicarbonate 0.05 mEq/mL.*
[g]*Lyophilized formulation tested.*
[h]*Refer to Appendix I for the composition of parenteral nutrition solutions. TNA indicates a 3-in-1 admixture, and TPN indicates a 2-in-1 admixture.*
[i]*Diluent not specified.*
[j]*Injected via Y-site into an administration set running azithromycin.*
[k]*Test performed using the formulation WITHOUT edetate disodium.*

FAT EMULSION, INTRAVENOUS
AHFS 40:20

Products — The compositions and characteristics of the fat emulsion products are listed in Table 1.

The pH of fat emulsion, intravenous, products is adjusted with sodium hydroxide.

Administration — Fat emulsion, intravenous, 10 and 20% may be administered intravenously via a peripheral vein or by central venous infusion.

Fat emulsion, intravenous, may also be administered intravenously in total nutrient admixtures (TNA, 3-in-1) in combination with amino acids, dextrose, and other nutrients. Fat emulsion, intravenous 30% is not for direct intravenous administration; it is intended for use as a component in parenteral nutrition admixtures. (513; 655)

Stability — Fat emulsion, intravenous, products may be stored in the intact containers at controlled room temperature. They should be protected from freezing. (513; 655)

Several factors can influence the stability of fat emulsions. A two-year study of Intralipid 10% found an increase in free fatty acids and a decrease of pH on storage. Gross particles formed and toxicity to rabbits increased with time. These changes were greatest during storage at 40 °C but were measurable at 20 and even 4 °C. The toxicity of the emulsions to rabbits could be correlated to the extent of free fatty acid formation in the emulsions. The formation of free fatty acids, with a consequent lowering of pH, is the major route of degradation of fat emulsions. The rate of degradation is minimized at pH 6 to 7. (889)

The container-closure system is important for long-term stability. Plastic containers are generally permeable to oxygen, which can readily oxidize the lipid emulsions, so glass bottles are used. Furthermore, the stoppers must not be permeable to oxygen and must not soften on contact with the emulsions. Teflon-coated stoppers have been recommended. Finally, the emulsions are packed under an atmosphere of nitrogen. (889)

The long-term room temperature stability of the emulsions is lost when the intact containers are entered. The integrity of the nitrogen layer in the sealed container is essential for room temperature stability. Exposure of Intralipid 10% to the atmosphere results in gradual changes in the emulsion system. No changes in the particle size distribution occurred during the first 36 hours of room temperature storage. After 48 hours at room temperature, globule coalescence was noticeable. By 72 hours, the changes had become significant. However, the visual appearance after 72 hours was unchanged. Long-term storage for 15 months at room temperature resulted in formation of a nonhomogeneous cream layer with oil globules on top. (656; 657) If the pH of the emulsion is optimal and the emulsion is stored under nitrogen and not exposed to direct sunlight, oxidative degradation is not likely to be significant. (889)

The manufacturers recommend that a partly used bottle should not be stored for later use, and no bottle should be used if the emulsion appears to be oiling out. (513; 655)

The emulsions should not be frozen. (513; 655) Freezing may cause physical damage. The emulsions may become coarse and coalesce, and they can undergo irreversible phase separation. If accidental freezing occurs, the products should be discarded. (559)

Fat emulsion, intravenous, based on either soybean oil or safflower oil, has been shown to support the growth of various microbes, including both bacterial and fungal species. No visual changes occurred in the emulsions to suggest contamination. (1102; 1103; 1104; 1216) The potential for microbiological growth should be considered when assigning expiration periods.

The 3-in-1 parenteral nutrition solutions that have a lower pH and higher osmolality due to the presence of amino acids and dextrose do not support microbial growth as well as fat emulsion alone. (1216)

Plasticizer Leaching — Fat emulsion extracts diethylhexyl phthalate (DEHP) plasticizer from PVC in amounts exceeding comparable volumes of whole blood. The amount of plasticizer leached from PVC sets by fat emulsion is directly related to the length of administration time and inversely related to the flow rate; these two factors influence the amount of contact time between the fat emulsion and the PVC tubing. Longer administration times and slower administration rates increase the amount of leached plasticizer. Non-PVC plastic containers, such as an ethylene vinyl acetate bag, may be used to avoid plasticizer exposure. If PVC tubing is used, phthalate leaching can be minimized by not storing primed sets. (658; 661; 673; 893; 1105)

Storage of Intralipid 10 and 20% for 24 hours in PVC sets resulted in phthalate contents of 64 to 70 mcg/mL at 5 °C and 144 to 160 mcg/mL at ambient temperature. When the fat emulsions were simply infused through PVC sets, phthalate content dropped to 3.6 to 8.5 mcg/mL. A patient being administered 500 mL of fat emulsion per day would receive about 1.5 to 2.75 mg/day. Negligible levels of phthalate were delivered from a parenteral nutrition admixture containing fat emulsion. (1264)

Table 1. Composition and Characteristics of Several Intravenous Fat Emulsions (513; 655)

Component or Characteristic	Intralipid (Fresenius Kabi)			Liposyn III (Abbott)		
	10%	20%	30%[a]	10%	20%	30%[a]
Soybean oil	10%	20%	30%[a]	10%	20%	30%[a]
Safflower oil	-	-	-	-	-	-
Egg yolk phospholipids	1.2%	1.2%	1.2%	up to 1.2%	1.2%	1.8%
Glycerin	2.25%	2.25%	1.7%	2.5%	2.5%	2.5%
Water for injection	qs	qs	qs	qs	qs	qs
Osmolarity (mOsm/L)	260	260	310	284	292	293
Approximate pH	6–8.9	6–8.9	6–8.9	6–9	6–9	6–9
Fat particle size (μm)	0.5	0.5	0.5	0.4	0.4	0.4
Caloric value (kcal/mL)	1.1	2	3	1.1	2	2.9

[a]*Not for direct infusion. Must be diluted to 20% or less for administration.*

A parenteral nutrition solution containing an amino acid solution, dextrose, and electrolytes in a PVC bag did not leach measurable quantities of DEHP plasticizer during 21 days of storage at 4 and 25 °C. However, addition of fat emulsion 10 or 20% to the formula caused detectable leaching of DEHP from the PVC containers stored for 48 hours. Higher DEHP levels were found in the 25 °C samples than in the 4 °C samples. The authors recommended limiting the use of lipid-containing parenteral nutrition admixtures to 24 to 36 hours. Use of non-PVC containers and tubing is another option. (1430)

Total nutrient admixtures (TNA) with fat emulsion concentrations ranging from 1 to 3.85% were found to leach DEHP plasticizer even though they were packaged in ethylene vinyl acetate bags. The bags had PVC sites in their composition, which contributed the DEHP.

Use of PVC administration sets added additional DEHP. Leached DEHP ranged from about 200 mcg to 2 mg during simulated infusions conducted immediately after preparation. The authors concluded that children who are treated regularly with TNA are exposed to significant amounts of DEHP. (2588)

Filtration — The use of a 1.2- or 5-μm inline filter to remove particulates, aggregates, precipitates, and large fat globules has been suggested to protect patients during parenteral nutrition administration. (569; 1106; 2135; 2346) The particle size of the fat emulsion products may exceed the porosity of some inline filters. Such small porosity filters should not be used with fat emulsion products. (658; 1106)

Compatibility Information

Solution Compatibility

Fat emulsion, intravenous

Solution	Mfr	Mfr	Conc/L	Remarks	Ref	C/I
Amino acids 8.5%	MG	VT	10%	Mixed in equal parts. Physically compatible for 48 hr at 4 °C and room temperature	32	C
	MG	CU	10%	Mixed in equal parts. Physically compatible for 72 hr at room temperature	656	C
	TR	CU	10%	Mixed in equal parts. Physically compatible for 72 hr at room temperature	656	C
Amino acids 7%	AB	CU	10%	Mixed in equal parts. Physically compatible for 72 hr at room temperature	656	C
Amino acids 10%		VT	10%	Mixed in equal parts. Changes in 20 min. Coalescence and creaming in 8 hr at 8 and 25 °C	825	I
Dextrose 5% in Ringer's injection, lactated	CU	VT	10%	Mixed in equal parts. Physically compatible for 48 hr at 4 °C and room temperature	32	C
Dextrose 10%	MG	CU		Mixed in equal parts. Increased globule association in 8 hr at room temperature, considered significant at 48 hr. Formation of a top cream layer by 72 hr	656	I
Dextrose 25%	MG	CU	10%	Mixed in equal parts. Increased globule association in 8 hr, progressing to globule coalescence at 48 hr at room temperature. Formation of a top cream layer by 72 hr	656	I
Dextrose 50%		VT	10%	Mixed in equal parts. Physically compatible for 48 hr at 4 °C and room temperature	32	C
	AB	VT	10%	Mixed in equal parts. Physically compatible for 24 hr at 8 and 25 °C	825	C
Ringer's injection, lactated	CU	VT	10%	Mixed in equal parts. Physically compatible for 48 hr at 4 °C and room temperature	32	C
Sodium chloride 0.9%	CU	VT	10%	Mixed in equal parts. Physically compatible for 48 hr at 4 °C and room temperature	32	C

Additive Compatibility

Fat emulsion, intravenous

Drug	Mfr	Conc/L	Mfr	Conc/L	Test Soln	Remarks	Ref	C/I
Aminophylline	ES	1 g	VT	10%		Physically compatible for 48 hr at 4 °C and room temperature	32	C
	DB	500 mg	VT	10%		Lipid coalescence in 24 hr at 25 and 8 °C	825	I
Amphotericin B	APC, PHT	0.6 g	CL	10 and 20%		Precipitate forms immediately but is concealed by opaque emulsion	1808	I
		90 mg		20%		Yellow precipitate forms in 2 hr. Cumulative delivery of only 56% of total amphotericin B dose	1872	I
	APC	10, 50, 100, and 500 mg, 1 and 5 g	CL	20%		Emulsion separation occurred rapidly, with visible creaming within 4 hr at 27 and 8 °C	1987	I
	SQ	500 mg, 1 and 2 g	KA	20%		Precipitated amphotericin noted on bottom of containers within 4 hr	1988	I
	BMS	50 and 500 mg	CLᶜ	20%		Fat emulsion separates into two phases within 8 hr. Little loss protected from or exposed to fluorescent light in 24 hr at 24 °C	2093	I
	KP	1 and 3 g	BMS	20%		Precipitate forms immediately	2518	I
	KP	150 mg, 300 mg, 1.5 g	BMS	20%	D5Wᵈ	Precipitate forms immediately	2518	I
Ampicillin sodium		20 g		10%		15% ampicillin loss in 24 hr at 23 °C	37	I
	BE	2 g	VT	10%		Lipid coalescence in 24 hr at 25 and 8 °C	825	I
Ascorbic acid	VI	1 g	VT	10%		Physically compatible for 48 hr at 4 °C and room temperature	32	C
	DB	500 mg	VT	10%		Lipid coalescence in 24 hr at 25 and 8 °C	825	I
Calcium chloride		1 g	CU	10%		Immediate flocculation with visually apparent layer in 2 hr at room temperature	656	I
		500 mg	CU	10%		Flocculation within 4 hr at room temperature	656	I
	DB	1 g	VT	10%		Coalescence and creaming in 8 hr at 8 and 25 °C	825	I
		10 and 20 mEq	KV	10%		Immediate flocculation, aggregation, and creaming	1018	I
Calcium gluconate	PR	2 g	CU	10%		Produced cracked emulsion	32	I
		7.2 and 9.6 mEq	KV	10%		Immediate flocculation, aggregation, and creaming	1018	I
Chloramphenicol sodium succinate	PD	2 g	VT	10%		Physically compatible for 48 hr at 4 °C and room temperature	32	C
	PD	2 g	VT	10%		Physically compatible for 24 hr at 8 and 25 °C	825	C
Cloxacillin sodium		10 g		10%		Aggregation of oil droplets	37	I
Cyclosporine	SZ	400 mg	AB	10%		No cyclosporine loss in 72 hr at 21 °C	1616	C
	SZ	500 mg and 2 g	KA	10 and 20%		Physically compatible with no cyclosporine loss in 48 hr at 24 °C under fluorescent light	1625	C

Additive Compatibility (Cont.)

Fat emulsion, intravenous

Drug	Mfr	Conc/L	Mfr	Conc/L	Test Soln	Remarks	Ref	C/I
Diphenhydramine HCl	PD	200 mg	VT	10%		Physically compatible for 48 hr at 4 °C and room temperature	32	C
Famotidine	MSD	20 mg		10%		Little or no famotidine loss in 48 hr at 25 °C in light or dark and at 5 °C	1344	C
Folic acid	USP	20 and 0.2 mg	KV	10%		Physically compatible for 2 weeks at 4 °C and room temperature in the dark but erratic assays	895	?
Fusidate sodium	LEO	1 g		10%		Physically incompatible	1800	I
Gentamicin sulfate	RS	160 mg	VT	10%		Lipid coalescence in 24 hr at 8 and 25 °C	825	I
Hydrocortisone sodium succinate	GL	200 mg	VT	10%		Physically compatible for 24 hr at 8 and 25 °C	825	C
Multivitamins	USV	4 mL	VT	10%		Physically compatible for 48 hr at 4 °C and room temperature	32	C
	KA		KA	10%		Physically compatible for 24 hr at 26 °C. Little loss of most vitamins; up to 52% ascorbate loss	2050	C
Octreotide acetate	SZ	1.5 mg	KV	10%		Octreotide content unstable	1373	I
Phenytoin sodium	PD	1 g	VT	10%		Phenytoin crystal precipitation	32	I
Potassium chloride		100 mEq	VT	10%		Physically compatible for 48 hr at 4 °C and room temperature	32	C
		100 mEq	CU	10%		No change in 24 hr at room temperature, but lipid coalescence in 48 hr	656	C
		200 mEq	CU	10%		Coalescence with surface creaming in 4 hr at room temperature. Oil globules on surface at 48 hr	656	I
	DB	4 g	VT	10%		Lipid coalescence in 24 hr at 8 and 25 °C	825	I
Ranitidine HCl	GL	50 and 100 mg	KV	10%		Physically compatible. 4% or less ranitidine loss in 48 hr at 25 °C in light or dark	1360	C
Sodium bicarbonate	BR	7.5 g	VT	10%		Physically compatible for 48 hr at 4 °C and room temperature	32	C
		3.4 g	VT	10%		Lipid coalescence in 24 hr at 8 and 25 °C	825	I
Sodium chloride		100 mEq	CU	10%		No change for 24 hr at room temperature, but lipid coalescence in 48 hr	656	C
		200 mEq	CU	10%		Lipid coalescence with surface creaming in 4 hr at room temperature. Oil globules on surface at 48 hr	656	I

[a] Refer to Appendix I for the composition of parenteral nutrition solutions. TNA indicates a 3-in-1 admixture.
[b] Tested in ethylene vinyl acetate (EVA) containers.
[c] Tested in glass containers.
[d] Diluted in dextrose 5% before adding to the fat emulsion.

Y-Site Injection Compatibility (1:1 Mixture)

Fat emulsion, intravenous

Drug	Mfr	Conc	Mfr	Conc	Remarks	Ref	C/I
Albumin human		20%		20%	Immediate emulsion destabilization	2267	I

Additional Compatibility Information

Calcium and Phosphate — UNRECOGNIZED CALCIUM PHOS-PHATE PRECIPITATION IN A 3-IN-1 PARENTERAL NU-TRITION MIXTURE RESULTED IN PATIENT DEATH.

The potential for the formation of a calcium phosphate precipitate in parenteral nutrition solutions is well studied and documented (1771; 1777), but the information is complex and difficult to apply to the clinical situation. (1770; 1772; 1777) The incorporation of fat emulsion in 3-in-1 parenteral nutrition solutions obscures any precipitate that is present, which has led to substantial debate on the dangers associated with 3-in-1 parenteral nutrition mixtures and when or if the danger to the patient is warranted therapeutically. (1770; 1771; 1772; 2031; 2032; 2033; 2034; 2035; 2036) Because such precipitation may be life-threatening to patients (2037; 2291), the Food and Drug Administration issued a Safety Alert containing the following recommendations (1769):

1. "The amounts of phosphorus and of calcium added to the admixture are critical. The solubility of the added calcium should be calculated from the volume at the time the calcium is added. It should not be based upon the final volume.

   Some amino acid injections for TPN admixtures contain phosphate ions (as a phosphoric acid buffer). These phosphate ions and the volume at the time the phosphate is added should be considered when calculating the concentration of phosphate additives. Also, when adding calcium and phosphate to an admixture, the phosphate should be added first.

   The line should be flushed between the addition of any potentially incompatible components.
2. A lipid emulsion in a three-in-one admixture obscures the presence of a precipitate. Therefore, if a lipid emulsion is needed, either (1) use a two-in-one admixture with the lipid infused separately, or (2) if a three-in-one admixture is medically necessary, then add the calcium before the lipid emulsion and according to the recommendations in number 1 above.

   If the amount of calcium or phosphate which must be added is likely to cause a precipitate, some or all of the calcium should be administered separately. Such separate infusions must be properly diluted and slowly infused to avoid serious adverse events related to the calcium.
3. When using an automated compounding device, the above steps should be considered when programming the device. In addition, automated compounders should be maintained and operated according to the manufacturer's recommendations.

   Any printout should be checked against the programmed admixture and weight of components.
4. During the mixing process, pharmacists who mix parenteral nutrition admixtures should periodically agitate the admixture and check for precipitates. Medical or home care personnel who start and monitor these infusions should carefully inspect for the presence of precipitates both before and during infusion. Patients and care givers should be trained to visually inspect for signs of precipitation. They also should be advised to stop the infusion and seek medical assistance if precipitates are noted.
5. A filter should be used when infusing either central or peripheral parenteral nutrition admixtures. At this time, data have not been submitted to document which size filter is most effective in trapping precipitates.

Standards of practice vary, but the following is suggested: a 1.2-mcm air-eliminating filter for lipid-containing admixtures and a 0.22-mcm air-eliminating filter for non-lipid-containing admixtures.
6. Parenteral nutrition admixtures should be administered within the following time frames: if stored at room temperature, the infusion should be started within 24 hours after mixing; if stored at refrigerated temperatures, the infusion should be started within 24 hours of rewarming. Because warming parenteral nutrition admixtures may contribute to the formation of precipitates, once administration begins, care should be taken to avoid excessive warming of the admixture.

   Persons administering home care parenteral nutrition admixtures may need to deviate from these time frames. Pharmacists who initially prepare these admixtures should check a reserve sample for precipitates over the duration and under the conditions of storage.
7. If symptoms of acute respiratory distress, pulmonary emboli, or interstitial pneumonitis develop, the infusion should be stopped immediately and thoroughly checked for precipitates. Appropriate medical interventions should be instituted. Home care personnel and patients should immediately seek medical assistance."

Calcium Phosphate Precipitation Fatalities — Fatal cases of paroxysmal respiratory failure in two previously healthy women receiving peripheral vein parenteral nutrition were reported. The patients experienced sudden cardiopulmonary arrest consistent with pulmonary emboli. The authors used in vitro simulations and an animal model to conclude that unrecognized calcium phosphate precipitation in a 3-in-1 total nutrition admixture caused the fatalities. The precipitation resulted during compounding by introducing calcium and phosphate near to one another in the compounding sequence and prior to complete fluid addition. This resulted in a temporarily high concentration of the drugs and precipitation of calcium phosphate. Observation of the precipitate was obscured by the incorporation of 20% fat emulsion, intravenous, into the nutrition mixture. No filter was used during infusion of the fatal nutrition admixtures. (2037)

In a follow-up retrospective review, five patients were identified who had respiratory distress associated with the infusion of the 3-in-1 admixtures at around the same time. Four of these five patients died, although the cause of death could be definitively determined for only two. (2291)

Calcium and Phosphate Conditional Compatibility — Calcium salts are conditionally compatible with phosphates in parenteral nutrition mixtures. The incompatibility is dependent on a solubility and concentration phenomenon and is not entirely predictable. Precipitation may occur during compounding or at some time after compounding is completed.

NOTE: Some amino acid solutions inherently contain calcium and phosphate, which must be considered in any projection of compatibility.

Dextrose — Dextrose in final concentrations of 5 to 12.5% has been shown to cause a progressive coalescence of the globules in Intralipid 10% due to its alteration of pH from about 7 down to about 3.5 in 48 hours. (656)

Monovalent Cations — Monovalent cations such as potassium and sodium also cause progressive globule coalescence in Intralipid 10 and 20%, leading to surface creaming. (480; 490; 656; 890) The degree and rate of this effect are dependent on the concentration of the ions.

A decreasing degree and rate of coalescence were noted as concentrations of sodium chloride or potassium chloride decreased. At 200 mEq/L, the rate is rapid and the effect is severe. In the range of 100 mEq/L or less, significant effects may not occur for over 24 hours. (490; 656)

Divalent Cations — Divalent cations such as calcium and magnesium cause immediate flocculation, with a nonhomogeneous white granular layer forming at the surface of the Intralipid 10%. This is followed by a substantial, visibly distinct layer, which does not redisperse on shaking. (480; 490; 656)

The creaming of Intralipid 20% when calcium chloride was admixed in concentrations from 0.25 to 5% was found to be concentration dependent, with maximum creaming occurring with the 5% additive in 30 minutes. (890)

Multicomponent ("3-in-1") Admixtures — Because of the potential benefits in terms of simplicity, efficiency, time, and cost savings, the concept of mixing amino acids, carbohydrates, electrolytes, fat emulsion, and other nutritional components together in the same container has been explored. Within limits, the feasibility of preparing such "3-in-1" parenteral nutrition admixtures has been demonstrated as long as a careful examination of the emulsion mixtures for signs of instability is performed prior to administration. (1813)

However, these 3-in-1 mixtures are very complex and inherently unstable. Emulsion stability is dependent on both zeta potential and van der Waals forces, influenced by the presence of dextrose. (2029) Because the ultimate stability of each mixture is the result of various complicated factors, a definitive prediction of stability is impossible. Death and injury resulted from administration of unrecognized precipitation in 3-in-1 parenteral nutrition admixtures. In addition, the use of 3-in-1 admixtures is associated with a higher rate of catheter occlusion and reduced catheter life compared with giving the fat emulsion separately from the parenteral nutrition solution. (705; 1518; 2194)

Intravenous administration of unstable fat emulsion with a large amount of large fat globules greater than 5 μm is potentially embolic and has been demonstrated to result in liver toxicity. (2690)

The use of a 5-μm inline filter for a 3-in-1 admixture (containing Travasol 8.5%, Dextrose, Intralipid 10%, various electrolytes, vitamins, and trace elements) showed that fat, in the form of large globules or aggregates, comprised 99.4% of the filter contents. These authors recommend the use of an appropriate filter (≤5 μm) for preventing catheter occlusion with 3-in-1 admixtures. (742)

The presence of glass particles, talc, and plastic has been observed in administration line samples drawn from 20 adults receiving 3-in-1 parenteral nutrition admixtures and in 20 children receiving 2-in-1 admixtures with separate fat emulsion infusions. Particles ranged from 3 to 5 μm to greater than 40 μm and were more consistently seen in the pediatric admixtures. The authors suggest the use of inline filters given that particulate contamination is present, has no therapeutic value, and can be harmful. (2458)

Combining an amino acids–dextrose parenteral nutrition solution containing various electrolytes with fat emulsion 20%, intravenous (Intralipid, Vitrum), resulted in a mixture that was apparently stable for a limited time. However, it ultimately exhibited a creaming phenomenon. Within 12 hours, a distinct 2-cm layer separated on the upper surface. Aggregates believed to be clumps of fat droplets were found. Fewer and smaller aggregates were noted in the lower layer. (560; 561)

Amino acids have been reported to have no adverse effect on the emulsion stability of Intralipid 10%. In addition, the amino acids appeared to prevent the adverse impact of dextrose and to slow the coalescence and flocculation resulting from mono- and divalent cations. However, significant coalescence did result after a somewhat longer time. Therefore, it was recommended that such cations not be mixed with fat emulsion, intravenous. (656)

Three-in-one TNA admixtures prepared with Intralipid 20% and containing mono- and divalent ions as well as heparin sodium 5 units/mL were found to undergo changes consistent with instability including fat particle shape and diameter changes as well as creaming and layering. The changes were evident within 48 hours at room temperature but were delayed to between one and two months when refrigerated. (58)

Travenol has stated that 1:1:1 mixtures of amino acids 5.5, 8.5, or 10% (Travenol), fat emulsion 10 or 20% (Travenol), and dextrose 10 to 70% are physically stable but recommends administration within 24 hours. M.V.I.-12 3.3 mL/L and electrolytes may also be added to the admixtures up to the maximum amounts listed below (850):

Calcium	8.3 mEq/L
Magnesium	3.3 mEq/L
Sodium	23.3 mEq/L
Potassium	20 mEq/L
Chloride	23.3 mEq/L
Phosphate	20 mEq/L
Zinc	3.33 mg/L
Copper	1.33 mg/L
Manganese	0.33 mg/L
Chromium	13.33 mcg/L

The stability of mixtures of Intralipid 20% 1 L, Vamin glucose (amino acids with dextrose 10%) 1.5 L, and dextrose 10% 0.5 L with various electrolytes and vitamins was evaluated. Initial emulsion particle size was around 1 μm. The mixture containing only monovalent cations was stable for at least nine days at 4 °C, with little change in particle size. The mixtures containing the divalent cations, such as calcium and magnesium, demonstrated much greater particle size increases, with mean diameters of around 3.3 to 3.5 μm after nine days at 4 °C. After 48 hours of storage, however, these increases were more modest, around 1.5 to 1.85 μm. After storage at 4 °C for 48 hours followed by 24 hours at room temperature, very few particles exceeded 5 μm. It was found that the effect of particle aggregation caused by electrolytes demonstrates a critical concentration before the effect begins. For calcium and magnesium chlorides, the critical concentrations were 2.4 and 2.6 mmol/L, respectively. Sodium and potassium chloride had critical concentrations of 110 and 150 mmol/L, respectively. The rate of particle aggregation increased linearly with increasing electrolyte concentration. Heparin 667 units/L had no effect on emulsion stability. The quantity of emulsion in the mixture had a relatively small influence on stability, but higher concentrations exhibited a somewhat greater coalescence. (892)

Instability of the emulsion systems is manifested by (1) flocculation of oil droplets to form aggregates that produce a cream-like layer on top or (2) coalescence of oil droplets leading to an increase in the average droplet size and eventually to a separation of free oil. The lowering of pH and adding of electrolytes can adversely affect the mechanical and electrical properties at the oil–water interface, eventually leading to flocculation and coalescence. Amino acids act as buffering agents and provide a protective effect on emulsion stability. Addition of electrolytes, especially the divalent ions Mg^{++} and Ca^{++} in excess of 2.5 mmol/L, to simple fat emulsions causes flocculation. But in mixed parenteral nutrition solutions, the stability of the emulsion is enhanced, depending on the quantity and nature of the amino acids present. The authors recommended a careful examination of emulsion mixtures for instability prior to administration. (849)

The stability of an amino acid 4% (Travenol), dextrose 14%, fat emulsion 4% (Pharmacia) parenteral nutrition solution was reported to be quite good. The solution also contained electrolytes, vitamins, and heparin sodium 4000 units/L. The aqueous solution was prepared first, with the fat emulsion added subsequently. This procedure allowed visual inspection of the aqueous phase and reduced the risk of emulsion breakdown by the divalent cations. Sample mixtures were stored at 18 to 25 and 3 to 8 °C for up to five days. They were evaluated visually and with a Coulter counter for particle size measurements. Both room temperature and refrigerated mixtures were stable for 48 hours. A marked increase in particle size was noted in the room temperature sample after 72 hours, but refrigeration delayed the changes. The authors' experience with over 1400 mixtures for administration to patients resulted in one emulsion creaming and another cracking. The authors had no explanation for the failure of these particular emulsions. (848)

Six parenteral nutrition solutions having various concentrations of amino acids, dextrose, soybean oil emulsion (Kabi-Vitrum), electrolytes, and multivitamins were reported. All of the admixtures were stable for one week under refrigeration followed by 24 hours at room temperature, with no visible changes, pH changes, or significant particle size changes. (1013) However, other researchers questioned this interpretation of the results. (1014; 1015)

The stability of 3-in-1 parenteral nutrition solutions prepared with 500 mL of Intralipid 20% compared to Soyacal 20%, along with 500 or 1000 mL of FreAmine III 8.5% and 500 mL of dextrose 70% was reported. Also present were relatively large amounts of electrolytes and other additives. All mixtures were similarly stable for 28 days at 4 °C followed by five days at 21 to 25 °C, with little change in the emulsion. A slight white cream layer appeared after five days at 4 °C, but it was easily dispersed with gentle agitation. The appearance of this cream layer did not statistically affect particle size distribution. The authors concluded that the emulsion mixture remained suitable for clinical use throughout the study period. The stability of other components was not evaluated. (1019)

The stability of 3-in-1 parenteral nutrition admixtures prepared with Liposyn II 10 and 20%, Aminosyn pH 6, and dextrose along with electrolytes, trace metals, and vitamins was reported. Thirty-one different combinations were evaluated. Samples were stored under the following conditions: (1) 25 °C for one day, (2) 5 °C for two days followed by 30 °C for one day, or (3) 5 °C for nine days followed by 25 °C for one day. In all cases, there was no visual evidence of creaming, free oil droplets, and other signs of emulsion instability. Furthermore, little or no change in the particle size or zeta potential (electrostatic surface charge of lipid particles) was found, indicating emulsion stability. The dextrose and amino acids remained stable over the 10-day storage period. The greatest change of an amino acid occurred with tryptophan, which lost 6% in 10 days. Vitamin stability was not tested. (1025)

The stability of four parenteral nutrition admixtures, ranging from 1 L each of amino acids 5.5% (Travenol), dextrose 10%, and fat emulsion 10% (Travenol) up to a "worst case" of 1 L each of amino acids 10% with electrolytes (Travenol), dextrose 70%, and fat emulsion 10% (Travenol) was reported. The admixtures were stored for 48 hours at 5 to 9 °C followed by 24 hours at room temperature. There were no visible signs of creaming, flocculation, or free oil. The mean emulsion particle size remained within acceptable limits for all admixtures, and there were no significant changes in glucose, soybean oil, and amino acid concentrations. The authors noted that two factors were predominant in determining the stability of such admixtures: electrolyte concentrations and pH. (1065)

Several parenteral nutrition solutions containing amino acids (Travenol), glucose, and lipid, with and without electrolytes and trace elements, produced no visible flocculation or any significant change in mean emulsion particle size during 24 hours at room temperature. (1066)

The compatibility of 10 parenteral nutrition admixtures, evaluated over 96 hours while stored at 20 to 25 °C in both glass bottles and ethylene vinyl acetate bags, was reported. A slight creaming occurred in all admixtures, but this cream layer was easily dispersed by gentle shaking. No fat globules were visually apparent. The mean drop size was larger in the cream layer, but no globules were larger than 5 μm. Analyses of the concentrations of amino acids, dextrose, and electrolytes showed no changes over the study period. The authors concluded that such parenteral nutrition admixtures can be prepared safely as long as the component concentrations are within the following ranges (1067):

Vamin glucose or Vamin N (amino acids 7%)	1000 to 2000 mL
Dextrose 10 to 30%	100 to 550 mL
Intralipid 10 or 20%	500 to 1000 mL
Electrolytes (mmol/L)	
Sodium	20 to 70
Potassium	20 to 55
Calcium	2.3 to 2.9
Magnesium	1.1 to 3.1
Phosphorus	0 to 9.2
Chloride	27 to 71
Zinc	0.005 to 0.03

The stability of eight parenteral nutrition admixtures with various ratios of amino acids, carbohydrates, and fat. FreAmine III 8.5%, dextrose 70%, and Soyacal 10 and 20% (mixed in ratios of 2:1:1, 1:1:1, 1:1:½, and 1:1:¼, where 1 = 500 mL) was evaluated. Additive concentrations were high to stress the admixtures and represent maximum doses likely to be encountered clinically:

Sodium acetate	150 mEq
Sodium chloride	210 mEq
Potassium acetate	45 mEq
Potassium chloride	90 mEq
Potassium phosphate	15 mM
Calcium gluconate	20 mEq
Magnesium sulfate	36 mEq
Trace elements	present
Folic acid	5 mg
M.V.I.-12	10 mL

The admixtures were stored at 4 °C for 14 days followed by four days at 22 to 25 °C. After 24 hours, all admixtures developed a thin white cream layer, which was readily dispersed by gentle agitation. No free oil droplets were observed. The mean particle diameter remained near the original size of the Soyacal throughout the study. Few particles were larger than 3 μm. Osmolality and pH also remained relatively unchanged. (1068)

Parenteral nutrition 3-in-1 admixtures with Aminosyn and Liposyn can be a problem. Standard admixtures were prepared using Aminosyn 7% 1000 mL, dextrose 50% 1000 mL, and Liposyn 10% 500 mL. Concentrated admixtures were prepared using Aminosyn 10% 500 mL, dextrose 70% 500 mL, and Liposyn 20% 500 mL. Vitamins and trace elements were added to the admixtures along with the following electrolytes:

Electrolyte	Standard Admixture	Concentrated Admixture
Sodium	125 mEq	75 mEq
Potassium	95 mEq	74 mEq
Magnesium	25 mEq	25 mEq
Calcium	28 mEq	28 mEq
Phosphate	37 mmol	36 mmol
Chloride	83 mEq	50 mEq

Samples of each admixture were (1) stored at 4 °C, (2) adjusted to pH 6.6 with sodium bicarbonate and stored at 4 °C, or (3) adjusted to pH 6.6 and stored at room temperature. Compatibility was evaluated for three weeks.

Signs of emulsion deterioration were visible by 96 hours in the standard admixture and by 48 hours in the concentrated admixture. Clear rings formed at the meniscus, becoming thicker, yellow, and oily over time. Free-floating oil was obvious in three weeks in the standard admixture and in one week in the concentrated admixture. The samples adjusted to pH 6.6 developed visible deterioration later than the others. The authors indicated that pH may play a greater role than temperature in emulsion stability. However, precipitation (probably calcium phosphate and possibly carbonate) occurred in 36 hours in the pH 6.6 concentrated admixture but not the unadjusted (pH 5.5) samples. Mean particle counts increased for all samples over time but were greatest in the concentrated admixtures. The concentrated admixtures were unsatisfactory for clinical use because of the early increase in particles and precipitation. Furthermore, the standard admixtures should be prepared immediately prior to use. (1069)

The physical stability of 10 parenteral nutrition admixtures with different amino acid sources was studied. The admixtures contained 500 mL each of dextrose 70%, fat emulsion 20% (Alpha Therapeutics), and amino acids in various concentrations from each manufacturer. Also present were standard electrolytes, trace elements, and vitamins. The admixtures were stored for 14 days at 4 °C, followed by four days at 22 to 25 °C. Slight creaming was evident in all admixtures but redispersed easily with agitation. Emulsion particles were uniform in size, showing no tendency to aggregate. No cracked emulsions occurred. (1217)

The stability of parenteral nutrition solutions containing amino acids, dextrose, and fat emulsion along with electrolytes, trace elements, and vitamins has been described. In one study the admixtures were stable for 24 hours at room temperature and for eight days at 4 °C. The visual appearance and particle size of the fat emulsion showed little change over the observation periods. (1218) In another study variable stability periods were found, depending on electrolyte concentrations. Stability ranged from four to 25 days at room temperature. (1219)

The effects of dilution, dextrose concentration, amino acids, and electrolytes on the physical stability of 3-in-1 parenteral nutrition admixtures prepared with Intralipid 10% or Travamulsion 10% was studied. Travamulsion was affected by dilution up to 1:14, exhibiting an increase in mean particle size, while Intralipid remained virtually unchanged for 24 hours at 25 °C and for 72 hours at 4 °C. At dextrose concentrations above 15%, fat droplets larger than 5 mcm formed during storage for 24 hours at either 4 °C or room temperature. The presence of amino acids increased the stability of the fat emulsions in the presence of dextrose. Fat droplets larger than 5 mcm formed at a total electrolyte concentration above approximately 240 mmol/L (monovalent cation equivalent) for Travamulsion 10% and 156 mmol/L for Intralipid 10% in 24 hours at room temperature, although creaming or breaking of the emulsion was not observed visually. (1221)

The stability of 43 parenteral nutrition admixtures composed of various ratios of amino acid products, dextrose 10 to 70%, and four lipid emulsions 10 and 20% with electrolytes, trace elements, and vitamins was studied. One group of admixtures included Travasol 5.5, 8.5, and 10%, FreAmine III 8.5 and 10%, Novamine 8.5 and 11.4%, Nephramine 5.4%, and RenAmine 6.5% with Liposyn II 10 and 20%. In another group, Aminosyn II 7, 8.5, and 10% was combined with Intralipid, Travamulsion, and Soyacal 10 and 20%. A third group was comprised of Aminosyn II 7, 8.5, and 10% with electrolytes combined with the latter three lipid emulsions. The admixtures were stored for 24 hours at 25 °C and for nine days at 5 °C followed by 24 hours at 25 °C. A few admixtures containing FreAmine III and Novamine with Liposyn II developed faint yellow streaks after 10 days of storage. The streaks readily dispersed with gentle shaking, as did the creaming present in most admixtures. Other properties such as pH, zeta-potential, and osmolality underwent little change in all of the admixtures. Particle size increased fourfold in one admixture (Novamine 8.5%, dextrose 50%, and Liposyn II in a 1:1:1 ratio), which the authors noted signaled the onset of particle coalescence. Nevertheless, the authors concluded that all of the admixtures were stable for the storage conditions and time periods tested. (1222)

The stability of 24 parenteral nutrition admixtures composed of various ratios of Aminosyn II 7, 8.5, or 10%, dextrose, and Liposyn II 10 and 20% with electrolytes, trace elements, and vitamins was also studied. Four admixtures were stored for 24 hours at 25 °C, six admixtures were stored for two days at 5 °C followed by one day at 30 °C, and 14 admixtures were stored for nine days at 5 °C followed by one day at 25 °C. No visible instability was evident. Creaming was present in most admixtures but disappeared with gentle shaking. Other properties such as pH, zeta-potential, particle size, and concentrations of the amino acids and dextrose showed little or no change during storage. (1223)

The emulsion stability of five parenteral nutrition formulas (TNA #126 through #130 in Appendix I) containing Liposyn II in concentrations ranging from 1.2 to 7.1% were reported. The parenteral nutrition solutions were prepared using simultaneous pumping of the components into empty containers (as with the Nutrimix compounder) and sequential pumping of the components (as with Automix compounders). The solutions were stored for two days at 5 °C followed by 24 hours at 25 °C. Similar results were obtained for both methods of preparation using visual assessment and oil globule size distribution. (1426)

The stability of 24 parenteral nutrition admixtures containing various concentrations of Aminosyn II, dextrose, and Liposyn II with a variety of electrolytes, trace elements, and multivitamins in dual-chamber, flexible, Nutrimix containers was studied as well. No instability was visible in the admixtures stored at 25 °C for 24 hours or in those stored for nine days at 5 °C followed by 24 hours at 25 °C. Creaming was observed, but neither particle coalescence nor free oil was noted. The pH, particle size distribution, and amino acid and dextrose concentrations remained acceptable during the observation period. (1432)

The physical stability of 10 parenteral nutrition formulas (TNA #149 through #158 in Appendix I) containing TrophAmine and Intralipid 20%, Liposyn II 20%, and Nutrilipid 20% in varying concentrations with low and high electrolyte concentrations was studied. All test formulas were prepared with an automatic compounder and protected from light. TNA #149 through #156 were stored for 48 hours at 4 °C followed by 24 hours at 21 °C; TNA #157 and #158 were stored for 24 hours at 4 °C followed by 24 hours at 21 °C. Although some minor creaming occurred in all formulas, it was completely reversible with agitation. No other changes were visible, and particle size analysis indicated little variation during the study period. The addition of cysteine hydrochloride 1 g/25 g of amino acids, alone or with l-carnitine 16 mg/g fat, to TNA #157 and #158 did not adversely affect the physical stability of 3-in-1 admixtures within the study period. (1620)

The physical stability of five 3-in-1 parenteral nutrition admixtures (TNA #167 through #171 in Appendix I) was evaluated by visual observation, pH and osmolality determinations, and particle size distribution analysis. All five admixtures were physically stable for 90 days at 4 °C. However, some irreversible flocculation occurred in all combinations after 180 days. (1651)

The stability of several parenteral nutrition formulas (TNA #159 through #166 in Appendix I), with and without iron dextran 2 mg/L was studied. All formulas were physically compatible both visually and microscopically for 48 hours at 4 and 25 °C, and particle size distribution remained unchanged. The order of mixing and deliberate agitation had no effect on physical compatibility. (1648)

The maximum allowable concentrations of calcium and phosphate in a 3-in-1 parenteral nutrition mixture for children (TNA #192 in Appendix I) was reported. Added calcium varied from 1.5 to 150 mmol/L, while added phosphate varied from 21 to 300 mmol/L. The mixtures were stable for 48 hours at 22 and 37 °C as long as the pH was not greater than 5.7, the calcium concentration was below 16 mmol/L, the phosphate concentration was below 52 mM/L, and the product of the calcium and phosphate concentrations was below 250 mmol^2/L^2. (1773)

The influence of six factors on the stability of fat emulsion in 45 different 3-in-1 parenteral nutrition mixtures was evaluated. The factors were amino acid concentration (2.5 to 7%); dextrose (5 to 20%); fat emulsion, intravenous (2 to 5%); monovalent cations (0 to 150 mEq/L); divalent cations (4 to 20 mEq/L); and trivalent cations from iron dextran (0 to 10 mg elemental iron/L). Although many formulations were unstable, visual examination could identify instability in only 65% of the samples. Electronic evaluation of particle size identified the remaining unstable mixtures. Furthermore, only the concentration of trivalent ferric ions significantly and consistently affected the emulsion stability during the 30-hour test period. Of the parenteral nutrition mixtures containing iron dextran, 16% were unstable, exhibiting emulsion cracking. The authors suggested that iron dextran should not be incorporated into 3-in-1 mixtures. (1814)

The compatibility of eight parenteral nutrition admixtures, four with and four without electrolytes, comparing Liposyn II and Intralipid (TNA #250 through #257 in Appendix I) was reported. The 3-in-1 admixtures were evaluated over two to nine days at 4 °C and then 24 hours at 25 °C in ethylene vinyl acetate (EVA) bags. No substantial changes were noted in the fat particle sizes and no visual changes of emulsion breakage were observed. All admixtures tested had particle sizes in the 2- to 40-μm range. (2465)

The stability of 3-in-1 parenteral nutrition admixtures prepared with Vamin 14 with electrolytes and containing either Lipofundin MCT/LCT 20% or Intralipid 20% was evaluated. The admixtures contained 66.7 mmol/L of monovalent and 6.7 mmol/L of divalent cations. Stability of the fat emulsion was evaluated after 2, 7, and 21 days at 4 °C in EVA bags followed by 24 hours of room temperature to simulate infusion. Microscopy, Coulter counter, photon correlation spectroscopy, and laser diffractometry techniques were used to determine stability. Droplet size by microscopy was noted to increase to 18 to 20 μm after 21 days in both of the admixtures with the Intralipid-containing admixture showing particles this large as early as day 2 and with Lipofundin MCT/LCT at day 7. The Coulter counter assessed particles greater than 2 μm to be approximately 1300 to 1500 with Lipofundin MCT/LCT and 37,000 in the Intralipid-containing admixtures immediately after their preparation. Heavy creaming with a thick firm layer was noted after 2 days with the Intralipid-containing admixture, making particle assessment difficult. The authors concluded that storage limitation of two days for the Intralipid-containing admixture and not more than seven days for the Lipofundin-containing admixture appeared justified. They also noted that calcium and magnesium behaved identically in destabilizing fat emulsion with greater concentrations of divalent cations. (867)

The physical instability of 3-in-1 total nutrient admixtures stored for 24 hours at room temperature was reported. The admixtures intended for use in neonates and infants were compounded with TrophAmine 2 to 3%, dextrose 18 to 24%, Liposyn II (Abbott) 2 to 3%, l-cysteine hydrochloride, and the following electrolytes:

Sodium	20 to 50 mEq/L
Potassium	13.3 to 40 mEq/L
Calcium chloride	20 to 26.6 mEq/L
Magnesium	3.4 to 5 mEq/L
Phosphates	6.7 to 15 mmol/L

The emulsion in the admixtures cracked and developed visible free oil within 24 hours after compounding. The incompatibility was considered to create a clinically significant risk of complications if the admixture was administered. The authors determined that these 3-in-1 total nutrient admixtures containing these concentrations of electrolytes were unacceptable and should not be used. (2619)

Another evaluation of 3-in-1 total nutrient admixtures reported physical instabilities of several formulations evaluated over seven days. The parenteral nutrition admixtures were prepared with dextrose 15%, and Intralipos 4% (Fresenius Kabi) along with FreAmine 4.3%, NephrAmine 2.1%, TrophAmine 2.7%, Topanusol 5%, or Hepat-Amine 4%. Various electrolytes and other components were also present including sodium, potassium, calcium (salt form unspecified), magnesium, trace elements, vitamin K, and heparin. The admixtures were stored at 4 °C and evaluated at zero, three, and seven days. After removal from refrigeration, the samples were subjected to additional exposure to room temperature and temperatures exceeding 28 °C for 24 to 48 hours. Flocculation was found in the admixtures prepared with FreAmine and with TrophAmine after 24 hours of storage at room temperature and after three days under refrigeration followed by 24 hours at room temperature. All of the admixtures developed coalescence after seven days under refrigeration followed by 24 hours at greater than 28 °C. (2621)

The physical stability of five highly concentrated 3-in-1 parenteral nutrition admixtures for fluid-restricted adults was evaluated. The admixtures were composed of Aminoplasmal (B. Braun) at concentrations over 7% as the amino acids source, dextrose concentrations of about 20%, and a 50:50 mixture of medium-chain triglycerides and long-chain triglycerides (Lipofundin MCT, B. Braun) at concentrations of about 2.5 to 2.7% as the lipid component with electrolytes and vitamins (TNA #269 through #273 in Appendix I). The parenteral nutrition admixtures were prepared in ethylene vinyl acetate bags and stored at room temperature for 30 hours. Electronic evaluation of mean fat particle sizes and globule size distribution found little change over the 30-hour test period. (2721)

The drop size of 3-in-1 parenteral nutrition solutions in drip chambers is variable, being altered by the constituents of the mixture. In one study, multivitamins (Multibionta, E. Merck) caused the greatest reductions in drop size, up to 37%. This change may affect the rate of delivery if flow is estimated from drops per minute. (1016) Similarly, flow rates delivered by infusion controllers dependent on predictable drop size may be inaccurate. Flow rates up to 29% less than expected have been reported. Therefore, variable-pressure volumetric pumps, which are independent of drop size, should be used rather than infusion controllers. (1215)

When using multicomponent, 3-in-1, parenteral nutrition admixtures, the following points should be considered (490; 703; 892; 893; 1025; 1064; 1070; 1214; 1324; 1406; 1670; 2215; 2282; 2308):

1. The order of mixing is important. The amino acid solution should be added to either the fat emulsion or the dextrose before final mixing. This practice ensures that the protective effect of the amino acids to emulsion disruption by changes in pH and the presence of electrolytes is realized.

2. Electrolytes should not be added directly to the fat emulsion. Instead, they should be added to the amino acids or dextrose before the final mixing.

3. Such 3-in-1 admixtures containing electrolytes (especially divalent cations) are unstable and will eventually aggregate. The mixed systems should be carefully examined visually before use to ensure that a uniform emulsion still exists.

4. Avoid contact of 3-in-1 parenteral nutrition admixtures with heparin, which destabilizes and damages the fat emulsion upon contact.

5. The admixtures should be stored under refrigeration if not used immediately.

6. The ultimate stability of the admixtures will be the result of a complex interaction of pH, component concentrations, electrolyte concentrations, and, probably, storage temperature.

Furthermore, the use of a 1.2-μm filter to remove large lipid particles, electrolyte precipitates, other solid particulates, aggregates, and *Candida albicans* contaminants has been recommended (1106; 1657; 1769; 2061; 2135; 2346), although others recommend a 5-μm filter to minimize the frequency of occlusion alarms. (569; 1951)

Heparin — Heparin sodium has been stated to be compatible in fat emulsion. (480; 660) The addition of heparin sodium (Abbott) 1 and 2 units/mL to Liposyn 10% and Intralipid 10% did not break the emulsion and effectively reversed the blood hypercoagulability associated with intravenous fat emulsion administration. (568)

However, flocculation of fat emulsion (Kabi-Vitrum) has been reported during Y-site administration into a line used to infuse a parenteral nutrition solution containing both calcium gluconate and heparin sodium. Subsequent evaluation indicated that the combination of calcium gluconate (0.46 and 1.8 mmol/125 mL) and heparin sodium (25 and 100 units/125 mL) in amino acids plus dextrose induced flocculation of the fat emulsion within two to four minutes at concentrations that resulted in no visually apparent flocculation in 30 minutes with either agent alone. (1214)

Calcium chloride quantities of 1 to 20 mmol normally result in slow flocculation of fat emulsion 20% over several hours. When heparin sodium 5 units/mL was added, the flocculation rate was accelerated greatly and a cream layer was observed visually in a few minutes. This effect was not observed when sodium ion was substituted for the divalent calcium. (1406)

Similar results were observed during simulated Y-site administration of heparin sodium into nine 3-in-1 nutrient admixtures having different compositions. Damage to the fat emulsion component was found to occur immediately, with the possible formation of free oil over time. (2215)

The destabilization of fat emulsion (Intralipid 20%) when administered simultaneously with a TPN admixture and heparin was ob-

served. The damage, detected by viscosity measurement, occurred immediately upon contact at the Y-site. The extent of the destabilization was dependent on the concentration of heparin and the presence of MVI Pediatric with its surfactant content. Additionally, phase separation was observed in two hours. The authors noted that TPN admixtures containing heparin should never be premixed with fat emulsion as a 3-in-1 total nutrient admixture because of this emulsion destabilization. The authors indicated their belief that the damage could be minimized during Y-site co-administration as long as the heparin was kept at a sufficiently low concentration (no visible separation occurred at a heparin concentration of 0.5 unit/mL) and the length of tubing between the Y-site and the patient was minimized. (2282)

However, because the damage to emulsion integrity has been found to occur immediately upon mixing with heparin in the presence of the calcium ions in TPN admixtures (1214; 2215; 2282) and no evaluation and documentation of the clinical safety of using such destabilized emulsions has been performed, use of such damaged emulsions in patients is suspect.

Amphotericin B — In an effort to reduce toxicity, amphotericin B has been admixed in Intralipid instead of the more usual dextrose 5%. (1809; 1810; 1811; 2178) However, amphotericin B 0.75 mg/kg/day administered using this approach in 250 mL of Intralipid 20% has been associated with acute pulmonary toxicities, including sudden onset of coughing, tachypnea, agitation, cyanosis, and deterioration of oxygen saturation. The temporal relationship between the drug administration and respiratory symptoms suggested a causal relationship. Furthermore, no reduction in renal toxicity or other side effects associated with amphotericin B was observed. The authors concluded amphotericin B should not be administered to patients in Intralipid. (2177)

At a concentration of 0.6 mg/mL in Intralipid 10 or 20%, amphotericin B precipitated immediately or almost immediately. The precipitate was not visible to the unaided eye because of the emulsion's dense opacity. Particle size evaluation found thousands of particles larger than 10 μm per milliliter. In dextrose 5%, very few particles were larger than 10 μm. Centrifuging the Intralipid admixtures resulted in rapid visualization of the precipitate as a mass at the bottom of the test tubes. (1808)

However, amphotericin B precipitation is observed in fat emulsion within two to four hours without centrifuging. In concentrations ranging from 90 mg/L to 2 g/L in Intralipid 20%, amphotericin precipitate is easily seen as yellow particulate matter on the bottom of the lipid emulsion containers. (1872; 1988) Damage to the emulsion integrity with creaming has also been reported. (1987)

In other reports, the appearance of problems was observed in as little as 15 minutes, and actual amphotericin B precipitate formed within 20 minutes of mixing. Analysis of the precipitate confirmed its identity as amphotericin B. The authors hypothesized that amphotericin B precipitates because the excipient deoxycholic acid, an anion, attracts oppositely charged choline groups from the egg yolk components of the fat emulsion and forms a precipitate with phosphatidylcholine, leaving insufficient surfactant to keep the amphotericin B dispersed. (2204; 2205)

Plasma Expanders — Fat emulsion (Abbott) 10 and 20% were combined with the plasma expanders Macrodex 6% in sodium chloride 0.9% (Schiwa), Gelafundin (Braun), Haes Steril 10% (Fresenius), and Expafusin Sine (Pfrimmer); fat particles exceeding 5 μm resulted, as observed by microscopic examination. These combinations were incompatible. (1668)

FENOLDOPAM MESYLATE
AHFS 24:08.20

Products — Fenoldopam mesylate is available as a concentrated solution in 1- and 2-mL sizes; each milliliter contains fenoldopam 10 mg (as mesylate), propylene glycol 518 mg, citric acid 3.44 mg, sodium citrate dihydrate 0.61 mg, and sodium metabisulfite. The contents must be diluted for use. (1)

Trade Name(s) — Corlopam.

Administration — Fenoldopam mesylate is administered by continuous intravenous infusion only after dilution in dextrose 5% or sodium chloride 0.9% and preferably using a controlled delivery infusion pump capable of delivering the desired infusion rate. A concentration of 40 mcg/mL is recommended for administration. Bolus doses should not be given. (1)

Stability — Intact ampuls should be stored between 2 and 30 °C (refrigerated or at room temperature). After dilution in dextrose 5% or sodium chloride 0.9%, fenoldopam mesylate is stated to be stable for at least 24 hours under normal ambient light and temperature. Unused solutions should be discarded after 24 hours. (1)

Compatibility Information

Solution Compatibility

Fenoldopam mesylate

Solution	Mfr	Mfr	Conc/L	Remarks	Ref	C/I
Dextrose 5%	AB[a]	AB	4, 8, 40, 80, 200, 300 mg	Physically compatible. Little loss in 72 hr at 4 °C in dark and at 23 °C in light	2369	C
Sodium chloride 0.9%	AB[a]	AB	4, 8, 40, 80, 200, 300 mg	Physically compatible. Little loss in 72 hr at 4 °C in dark and at 23 °C in light	2369	C

[a]*Tested in PVC containers.*

Y-Site Injection Compatibility (1:1 Mixture)

Fenoldopam mesylate

Drug	Mfr	Conc	Mfr	Conc	Remarks	Ref	C/I
Alfentanil HCl	TAY	0.5 mg/mL	AB	80 mcg/mL[b]	Physically compatible for 4 hr at 23 °C	2467	C
Amikacin sulfate	APO	5 mg/mL[b]	AB	80 mcg/mL[b]	Physically compatible for 4 hr at 23 °C	2467	C
Aminocaproic acid	AMR	50 mg/mL[b]	AB	80 mcg/mL[b]	Physically compatible for 4 hr at 23 °C	2467	C
Aminophylline	AB	2.5 mg/mL[b]	AB	80 mcg/mL[b]	Haze and microparticulates form immediately. Yellow turbidity in 4 hr	2467	I
Amiodarone HCl	WAY	4 mg/mL[b]	AB	80 mcg/mL[b]	Physically compatible for 4 hr at 23 °C	2467	C
Amphotericin B	APO	0.6 mg/mL[b]	AB	80 mcg/mL[b]	Yellow precipitate forms immediately	2467	I
Ampicillin sodium	APO	20 mg/mL[b]	AB	80 mcg/mL[b]	Yellow color forms in 4 hr	2467	I
Ampicillin sodium–sulbactam sodium	PF	20 + 10 mg/mL[b]	AB	80 mcg/mL[b]	Physically compatible for 4 hr at 23 °C	2467	C
Argatroban	SKB	1 mg/mL[a]	AB	0.1 mg/mL[a]	Physically compatible for 24 hr at 23 °C	2572	C
Atracurium besylate	BA	0.5 mg/mL[b]	AB	80 mcg/mL[b]	Physically compatible for 4 hr at 23 °C	2467	C
Atropine sulfate	APP	0.1 mg/mL[b]	AB	80 mcg/mL[b]	Physically compatible for 4 hr at 23 °C	2467	C
Aztreonam	BMS	40 mg/mL[b]	AB	80 mcg/mL[b]	Physically compatible for 4 hr at 23 °C	2467	C
Bumetanide	BA	40 mcg/mL[b]	AB	80 mcg/mL[b]	Trace haze forms immediately	2467	I
Butorphanol tartrate	APO	40 mcg/mL[b]	AB	80 mcg/mL[b]	Physically compatible for 4 hr at 23 °C	2467	C
Calcium gluconate	APP	40 mg/mL[b]	AB	80 mcg/mL[b]	Physically compatible for 4 hr at 23 °C	2467	C

Y-Site Injection Compatibility (1:1 Mixture) (Cont.)

Fenoldopam mesylate

Drug	Mfr	Conc	Mfr	Conc	Remarks	Ref	C/I
Cefazolin sodium	APO	20 mg/mL[b]	AB	80 mcg/mL[b]	Physically compatible for 4 hr at 23 °C	2467	C
Cefepime HCl	BMS	20 mg/mL[b]	AB	80 mcg/mL[b]	Physically compatible for 4 hr at 23 °C	2467	C
Cefotaxime sodium	HO	20 mg/mL[b]	AB	80 mcg/mL[b]	Physically compatible for 4 hr at 23 °C	2467	C
Cefotetan disodium	ZEN	20 mg/mL[b]	AB	80 mcg/mL[b]	Physically compatible for 4 hr at 23 °C	2467	C
Cefoxitin sodium	ME	20 mg/mL[b]	AB	80 mcg/mL[b]	Microparticulates form immediately	2467	I
Ceftazidime	GW	40 mg/mL[b]	AB	80 mcg/mL[b]	Physically compatible for 4 hr at 23 °C	2467	C
Ceftriaxone sodium	RC	20 mg/mL[b]	AB	80 mcg/mL[b]	Physically compatible for 4 hr at 23 °C	2467	C
Cefuroxime sodium	GW	30 mg/mL[b]	AB	80 mcg/mL[b]	Physically compatible for 4 hr at 23 °C	2467	C
Chlorpromazine HCl	ES	2 mg/mL[b]	AB	80 mcg/mL[b]	Physically compatible for 4 hr at 23 °C	2467	C
Ciprofloxacin	BAY	2 mg/mL[b]	AB	80 mcg/mL[b]	Physically compatible for 4 hr at 23 °C	2467	C
Cisatracurium besylate	AB	0.5 mg/mL[b]	AB	80 mcg/mL[b]	Physically compatible for 4 hr at 23 °C	2467	C
Clindamycin phosphate	AB	10 mg/mL[b]	AB	80 mcg/mL[b]	Physically compatible for 4 hr at 23 °C	2467	C
Dexamethasone sodium phosphate	AMR	1 mg/mL[b]	AB	80 mcg/mL[b]	Trace haze forms immediately	2467	I
Dexmedetomidine HCl	AB	4 mcg/mL[b]	AB	80 mcg/mL[b]	Physically compatible for 4 hr at 23 °C	2383	C
Diazepam	AB	5 mg/mL	AB	80 mcg/mL[b]	Gross white turbidity forms immediately	2467	I
Digoxin	ES	0.25 mg/mL	AB	80 mcg/mL[b]	Physically compatible for 4 hr at 23 °C	2467	C
Diltiazem HCl	BA	5 mg/mL	AB	80 mcg/mL[b]	Physically compatible for 4 hr at 23 °C	2467	C
Diphenhydramine HCl	ES	2 mg/mL[b]	AB	80 mcg/mL[b]	Physically compatible for 4 hr at 23 °C	2467	C
Dobutamine HCl	BED	4 mg/mL[b]	AB	80 mcg/mL[b]	Physically compatible for 4 hr at 23 °C	2467	C
Dolasetron mesylate	AVE	2 mg/mL[b]	AB	80 mcg/mL[b]	Physically compatible for 4 hr at 23 °C	2467	C
Dopamine HCl	AB	3.2 mg/mL[b]	AB	80 mcg/mL[b]	Physically compatible for 4 hr at 23 °C	2467	C
Doxycycline hyclate	APP	1 mg/mL[b]	AB	80 mcg/mL[b]	Physically compatible for 4 hr at 23 °C	2467	C
Droperidol	AB	2.5 mg/mL	AB	80 mcg/mL[b]	Physically compatible for 4 hr at 23 °C	2467	C
Enalaprilat	BA	0.1 mg/mL[b]	AB	80 mcg/mL[b]	Physically compatible for 4 hr at 23 °C	2467	C
Ephedrine sulfate	BED	5 mg/mL[b]	AB	80 mcg/mL[b]	Physically compatible for 4 hr at 23 °C	2467	C
Epinephrine HCl	AMR	50 mcg/mL[b]	AB	80 mcg/mL[b]	Physically compatible for 4 hr at 23 °C	2467	C
Erythromycin lactobionate	AB	5 mg/mL[b]	AB	80 mcg/mL[b]	Physically compatible for 4 hr at 23 °C	2467	C
Esmolol HCl	BA	10 mg/mL[b]	AB	80 mcg/mL[b]	Physically compatible for 4 hr at 23 °C	2467	C
Famotidine	ME	2 mg/mL[b]	AB	80 mcg/mL[b]	Physically compatible for 4 hr at 23 °C	2467	C
Fentanyl citrate	AB	12.5 mcg/mL[b]	AB	80 mcg/mL[b]	Physically compatible for 4 hr at 23 °C	2467	C
Fluconazole	PF	2 mg/mL	AB	80 mcg/mL[b]	Physically compatible for 4 hr at 23 °C	2467	C
Fosphenytoin sodium	PD	20 mg PE/mL[b,c]	AB	80 mcg/mL[b]	Trace haze and microparticulates form in 4 hr	2467	I
Furosemide	AMR	3 mg/mL[b]	AB	80 mcg/mL[b]	Trace haze forms immediately	2467	I
Gentamicin sulfate	APP	5 mg/mL[b]	AB	80 mcg/mL[b]	Physically compatible for 4 hr at 23 °C	2467	C
Granisetron HCl	SKB	50 mcg/mL[b]	AB	80 mcg/mL[b]	Physically compatible for 4 hr at 23 °C	2467	C
Haloperidol lactate	APP	0.2 mg/mL[b]	AB	80 mcg/mL[b]	Physically compatible for 4 hr at 23 °C	2467	C
Heparin sodium	AB	100 units/mL	AB	80 mcg/mL[b]	Physically compatible for 4 hr at 23 °C	2467	C

Y-Site Injection Compatibility (1:1 Mixture) (Cont.)

Fenoldopam mesylate

Drug	Mfr	Conc	Mfr	Conc	Remarks	Ref	C/I
Hetastarch in lactated electrolyte	AB	6%	AB	80 mcg/mL[b]	Physically compatible for 4 hr at 23 °C	2467	C
Hydrocortisone sodium succinate	PHU	1 mg/mL[b]	AB	80 mcg/mL[b]	Physically compatible for 4 hr at 23 °C	2467	C
Hydromorphone HCl	ES	0.5 mg/mL[b]	AB	80 mcg/mL[b]	Physically compatible for 4 hr at 23 °C	2467	C
Hydroxyzine HCl	ES	2 mg/mL[b]	AB	80 mcg/mL[b]	Physically compatible for 4 hr at 23 °C	2467	C
Iodixanol	NYC	55%	AB	80 mcg/mL[b]	Physically compatible for 4 hr at 23 and 37 °C	2467	C
Iohexol	NYC	51.8%	AB	80 mcg/mL[b]	Physically compatible for 4 hr at 23 and 37 °C	2467	C
Iopamidol	BRD	51%	AB	80 mcg/mL[b]	Physically compatible for 4 hr at 23 and 37 °C	2467	C
Ioxaglate meglumine–ioxaglate sodium	MA	39.3% + 19.6%	AB	80 mcg/mL[b]	Physically compatible for 4 hr at 23 and 37 °C	2467	C
Isoproterenol HCl	AB	20 mcg/mL[b]	AB	80 mcg/mL[b]	Physically compatible for 4 hr at 23 °C	2467	C
Ketorolac tromethamine	AB	15 mg/mL[b]	AB	80 mcg/mL[b]	Trace haze forms immediately	2467	I
Labetalol HCl	AB	2 mg/mL[b]	AB	80 mcg/mL[b]	Physically compatible for 4 hr at 23 °C	2467	C
Levofloxacin	OMN	5 mg/mL[b]	AB	80 mcg/mL[b]	Physically compatible for 4 hr at 23 °C	2467	C
Lidocaine HCl	AST	10 mg/mL[b]	AB	80 mcg/mL[b]	Physically compatible for 4 hr at 23 °C	2467	C
Linezolid	PHU	2 mg/mL	AB	80 mcg/mL[b]	Physically compatible for 4 hr at 23 °C	2467	C
Lorazepam	ES	0.5 mg/mL[b]	AB	80 mcg/mL[b]	Physically compatible for 4 hr at 23 °C	2467	C
Magnesium sulfate	APP	100 mg/mL[b]	AB	80 mcg/mL[b]	Physically compatible for 4 hr at 23 °C	2467	C
Mannitol	BA	15%	AB	80 mcg/mL[b]	Physically compatible for 4 hr at 23 °C	2467	C
Meperidine HCl	AB	4 mg/mL[b]	AB	80 mcg/mL[b]	Physically compatible for 4 hr at 23 °C	2467	C
Methohexital sodium	JP	10 mg/mL[b]	AB	80 mcg/mL[b]	Microparticulates and yellow color form immediately	2467	I
Methylprednisolone sodium succinate	PHU	5 mg/mL[b]	AB	80 mcg/mL[b]	Microparticulates form immediately	2467	I
Metoclopramide HCl	RB	5 mg/mL	AB	80 mcg/mL[b]	Physically compatible for 4 hr at 23 °C	2467	C
Metronidazole	BA	5 mg/mL	AB	80 mcg/mL[b]	Physically compatible for 4 hr at 23 °C	2467	C
Micafungin sodium	ASP	1.5 mg/mL[b]	BA	80 mcg/mL[b]	Physically compatible for 4 hr at 23 °C	2683	C
Midazolam HCl	APP	1 mg/mL[b]	AB	80 mcg/mL[b]	Physically compatible for 4 hr at 23 °C	2467	C
Milrinone lactate	SAN	0.2 mg/mL[b]	AB	80 mcg/mL[b]	Physically compatible for 4 hr at 23 °C	2467	C
Morphine sulfate	ES	1 mg/mL[b]	AB	80 mcg/mL[b]	Physically compatible for 4 hr at 23 °C	2467	C
Nalbuphine HCl	EN	10 mg/mL	AB	80 mcg/mL[b]	Physically compatible for 4 hr at 23 °C	2467	C
Naloxone HCl	AB	0.4 mg/mL[b]	AB	80 mcg/mL[b]	Physically compatible for 4 hr at 23 °C	2467	C
Nicardipine HCl	WAY	1 mg/mL[b]	AB	80 mcg/mL[b]	Physically compatible for 4 hr at 23 °C	2467	C
Nitroglycerin	AMR	0.4 mg/mL[b]	AB	80 mcg/mL[b]	Physically compatible for 4 hr at 23 °C	2467	C
Norepinephrine bitartrate	AB	0.12 mg/mL[b]	AB	80 mcg/mL[b]	Physically compatible for 4 hr at 23 °C	2467	C
Ondansetron HCl	GW	1 mg/mL[b]	AB	80 mcg/mL[b]	Physically compatible for 4 hr at 23 °C	2467	C
Pancuronium bromide	BA	0.1 mg/mL[b]	AB	80 mcg/mL[b]	Physically compatible for 4 hr at 23 °C	2467	C
Pentobarbital sodium	AB	5 mg/mL[b]	AB	80 mcg/mL[b]	Trace haze and microparticulates form immediately	2467	I

Y-Site Injection Compatibility (1:1 Mixture) (Cont.)

Fenoldopam mesylate

Drug	Mfr	Conc	Mfr	Conc	Remarks	Ref	C/I
Phenylephrine HCl	AMR	1 mg/mL[b]	AB	80 mcg/mL[b]	Physically compatible for 4 hr at 23 °C	2467	C
Phenytoin sodium	ES	50 mg/mL	AB	80 mcg/mL[b]	Microcrystals and yellowish darkening form immediately	2467	I
Piperacillin sodium–tazobactam sodium	LE[d]	40 + 5 mg/mL[b]	AB	80 mcg/mL[b]	Physically compatible for 4 hr at 23 °C	2467	C
Potassium chloride	APP	0.1 mEq/mL[b]	AB	80 mcg/mL[b]	Physically compatible for 4 hr at 23 °C	2467	C
Procainamide HCl	ES	10 mg/mL[b]	AB	80 mcg/mL[b]	Physically compatible for 4 hr at 23 °C	2467	C
Prochlorperazine edisylate	SKB	0.5 mg/mL[b]	AB	80 mcg/mL[b]	Trace haze forms in 4 hr	2467	I
Promethazine HCl	ES	2 mg/mL[b]	AB	80 mcg/mL[b]	Physically compatible for 4 hr at 23 °C	2467	C
Propofol	ASZ	10 mg/mL	AB	80 mcg/mL[b]	Physically compatible for 4 hr at 23 °C	2467	C
Propranolol HCl	WAY	1 mg/mL	AB	80 mcg/mL[b]	Physically compatible for 4 hr at 23 °C	2467	C
Quinupristin–dalfopristin	AVE	5 mg/mL[b]	AB	80 mcg/mL[b]	Physically compatible for 4 hr at 23 °C	2467	C
Ranitidine HCl	GW	2 mg/mL[b]	AB	80 mcg/mL[b]	Physically compatible for 4 hr at 23 °C	2467	C
Remifentanil HCl	AB	0.2 mg/mL[b]	AB	80 mcg/mL[b]	Physically compatible for 4 hr at 23 °C	2467	C
Rocuronium bromide	OR	1 mg/mL[b]	AB	80 mcg/mL[b]	Physically compatible for 4 hr at 23 °C	2467	C
Sodium bicarbonate	APP	1 mEq/mL	AB	80 mcg/mL[b]	Trace haze and microparticulates form immediately with turbidity in 4 hr	2467	I
Sufentanil citrate	BA	12.5 mcg/mL[b]	AB	80 mcg/mL[b]	Physically compatible for 4 hr at 23 °C	2467	C
Theophylline	BA	4 mg/mL[a]	AB	80 mcg/mL[b]	Physically compatible for 4 hr at 23 °C	2467	C
Ticarcillin disodium–clavulanate potassium	SKB	31 mg/mL[b]	AB	80 mcg/mL[b]	Physically compatible for 4 hr at 23 °C	2467	C
Tobramycin sulfate	LI	5 mg/mL[b]	AB	80 mcg/mL[b]	Physically compatible for 4 hr at 23 °C	2467	C
Trimethoprim–sulfamethoxazole	ES	0.8 + 4 mg/mL[b]	AB	80 mcg/mL[b]	Physically compatible for 4 hr at 23 °C	2467	C
Vancomycin HCl	APP	10 mg/mL[b]	AB	80 mcg/mL[b]	Physically compatible for 4 hr at 23 °C	2467	C
Vecuronium bromide	ES	0.2 mg/mL[b]	AB	80 mcg/mL[b]	Physically compatible for 4 hr at 23 °C	2467	C
Verapamil HCl	AB	1.25 mg/mL[b]	AB	80 mcg/mL[b]	Physically compatible for 4 hr at 23 °C	2467	C

[a]Tested in dextrose 5%.
[b]Tested in sodium chloride 0.9%.
[c]Concentration expressed in milligrams of phenytoin sodium equivalents (PE) per milliliter.
[d]Test performed using the formulation WITHOUT edetate disodium.

FENTANYL CITRATE
AHFS 28:08.08

Products — Fentanyl citrate is available in 2-, 5-, 10-, and 20-mL ampuls, 2- and 5-mL syringe cartridges, and 30- and 50-mL vials. Each milliliter contains fentanyl (as the citrate) 50 mcg (0.05 mg) with hydrochloric acid and/or sodium hydroxide for pH adjustment. (1; 4)

pH — From 4 to 7.5. (1; 4)

Osmolality — The product osmolality was determined to be essentially 0 mOsm/kg. (1233)

Trade Name(s) — Sublimaze.

Administration — Fentanyl citrate is administered by intramuscular or intravenous injection. (1)

Stability — Intact containers should be stored at controlled room temperature and protected from light. Brief exposure to temperatures up to 40 °C does not affect concentration. (1; 4)

pH Effects — Fentanyl citrate is most stable at pH 3.5 to 7.5. (1638) Fentanyl is hydrolyzed in acidic solutions. (4)

Syringes — Undiluted fentanyl citrate 50 mcg/mL was tested for stability in polypropylene syringes. The fentanyl citrate injection was filled into polypropylene syringes that were then capped off. The samples were stored for 28 days under refrigeration at 5 °C and at room temperature of 22 °C exposed to light. No change in color or clarity occurred. No loss of fentanyl citrate at either set of storage conditions occurred. (2648)

Fentanyl citrate (Elkins Sinn) 0.0167 mg/mL in sodium chloride 0.9% packaged in polypropylene syringes (Sherwood) was physically stable and exhibited little or no loss in 24 hours stored at 4 or 23 °C in the dark. (2199)

Fentanyl citrate (David Bull) 12.5 mcg/mL in sodium chloride 0.9% was packaged as 8 mL in 10-mL polypropylene syringes (Terumo) with attached needles. Fentanyl citrate (David Bull) 33.3 mcg/mL in sodium chloride 0.9% was packaged as 18 mL in 20-mL polypropylene syringes (Terumo) with attached needles. The syringes were stored at 5, 22, and 38 °C for seven days. The solutions were visually unchanged with no loss of drug at 5 and 22 °C. At 38 °C, the 12.5-mcg/mL solution had under 7% loss and the 33.3-mcg/mL solution had no loss. (2202)

Fentanyl citrate (Janssen) 35 mcg/mL in sodium chloride 0.9% was packaged in two types of polypropylene syringes. The Omnifix (B. Braun) syringes had polyisoprene piston tips while the Terumo syringes had no natural or synthetic rubber in the product. Stored at 4, 21, and 35 °C for 30 days, the test solutions exhibited no visible or pH changes. Although the pH remained within the stability range for the drug, this does not demonstrate stability. (2387)

Ambulatory Pumps — Fentanyl citrate (Merck) 50 and 30 mcg/mL in sodium chloride 0.9% was evaluated in CADD-1 and CADD-PRIZM medication cassettes. About 4% drug loss occurred in 14 days at room and refrigeration temperatures. (2717)

Sorption — Fentanyl citrate 2 mcg/mL in various buffer solutions ranging from pH 5.5 to pH 6.7 packaged in PVC containers (Baxter) was shown to undergo slow sorption to the PVC in amounts dependent on the pH of the solution. The lower pH solutions exhibited less loss with increasing loss as the pH increased. At the highest pH tested of 6.7, 17% fentanyl loss occurred in one day. Refrigeration decreased the extent of loss but did not eliminate it. See Table 1. Little or no fentanyl loss was found in identical fentanyl citrate 2-mcg/mL solutions packaged in glass containers. (2305)

Undiluted fentanyl citrate 50 mcg/mL was tested for stability in PVC bags. The fentanyl citrate injection was filled into PVC bags that were stored for 28 days under refrigeration at 5 °C and at room temperature of 22 °C exposed to light. No change in color or clarity occurred. No loss of fentanyl citrate at either set of storage conditions occurred. (2648)

Filtration — Fentanyl citrate (Janssen) 2.5 mcg/mL in dextrose 5% or sodium chloride 0.9% was delivered over four hours through three kinds of 0.2-μm membrane filters varying in size and composition. No fentanyl loss occurred due to sorption to the filter. (1399)

Central Venous Catheter — Fentanyl citrate (Abbott) 10 mcg/mL in dextrose 5% was found to be compatible with the ARROWg+ard Blue Plus (Arrow International) chlorhexidine-bearing triple-lumen central catheter. Essentially complete delivery of the drug was found with little or no drug loss occurring. Furthermore, chlorhexidine delivered from the catheter remained at trace amounts with no substantial increase due to the delivery of the drug through the catheter. (2335)

Table 1. Percentage of Fentanyl Citrate 2 mcg/mL Remaining After Storage for 30 Days at 23 °C in PVC Containers (2305)

Buffer pH	Fentanyl Remaining (%)
5.5	85
5.8	77
6.3	56
6.7	27

Compatibility Information

Solution Compatibility

Fentanyl citrate

Solution	Mfr	Mfr	Conc/L	Remarks	Ref	C/I
Dextrose 5%	DB,[a] TR[b]	JN	5 mg	Physically compatible. No loss in 48 hr at 22 °C in light	1357	C
	AB	JN	20 and 40 mg	Visually compatible. 3% or less loss in 3 hr at 24 °C	1852	C
Sodium chloride 0.9%	TR[b]	JN	20 mg	Physically compatible. Little loss in 30 days at 3 and 23 °C	1356	C
	DB,[a] TR[b]	JN	5 mg	Physically compatible. No loss in 48 hr at 22 °C in light	1357	C

[a]Tested in glass containers.
[b]Tested in PVC containers.

Additive Compatibility

Fentanyl citrate

Drug	Mfr	Conc/L	Mfr	Conc/L	Test Soln	Remarks	Ref	C/I
Bupivacaine HCl	WI	1.25 g	JN	20 mg	NS[a]	Physically compatible with little or no loss of either drug in 30 days at 3 and 23 °C	1396	C
		1.25 g		2 mg	NS[a]	Physically compatible with no bupivacaine loss and about 6 to 7% fentanyl loss in 30 days at 4 and 23 °C	2305	C
		600 mg		2 mg	NS[a]	Physically compatible with no bupivacaine loss and about 2 to 4% fentanyl loss in 30 days at 4 and 23 °C	2305	C
Bupivacaine HCl with clonidine HCl	AST BI	1 g 9 mg	JN	35 mg	NS[a]	Visually compatible with less than 10% change of any drug in 28 days at 4 °C and 24 days at 25 °C in the dark	2437	C
Bupivacaine HCl with epinephrine bitartrate	WI AB	440 mg 0.69 mg	JN	1.25 mg	e	No bupivacaine and fentanyl loss and 10% epinephrine loss in 30 days at 3 and 23 °C then 48 hr at 30 °C	1627	C
Bupivacaine HCl with epinephrine bitartrate	IVX	1 g 2 mg	IVX	2 mg		Visually compatible with less than 10% loss of epinephrine and no loss of other drugs in 182 days at 4 and 22 °C	2613	C
Clonidine HCl with bupivacaine HCl	BI AST	9 mg 1 g	JN	35 mg	NS[a]	Visually compatible with less than 10% change of any drug in 28 days at 4 °C and 24 days at 25 °C in the dark	2437	C
Droperidol with ketamine HCl	JN JN	50 mg 1 g	DB	10 mg	NS[a]	Visually compatible. 5% increase in all drugs in 30 days at 4 and 25 °C due to water loss	2653	C
Droperidol with ketamine HCl	JN JN	50 mg 1 g	DB	10 mg	NS[d]	Visually compatible with little loss of the drugs in 30 days at 25 °C	2653	C
Epinephrine bitartrate with bupivacaine HCl	AB WI	0.69 mg 440 mg	JN	1.25 mg	e	No bupivacaine and fentanyl loss and 10% epinephrine loss in 30 days at 3 and 23 °C then 48 hr at 30 °C	1627	C
Epinephrine bitartrate with bupivacaine HCl	IVX	2 mg 1 g	IVX	2 mg		Visually compatible with less than 10% loss of epinephrine and no loss of other drugs in 182 days at 4 and 22 °C	2613	C
Fluorouracil	AB	1 and 16 g	AB	12.5 mg	D5W, NS[a]	25% fentanyl loss in 15 min due to sorption to PVC	2064	I
Ketamine HCl with droperidol	JN JN	1 g 50 mg	DB	10 mg	NS[a]	Visually compatible. 5% increase in all drugs in 30 days at 4 and 25 °C due to water loss	2653	C
Ketamine HCl with droperidol	JN JN	1 g 50 mg	DB	10 mg	NS[d]	Visually compatible with little loss of the drugs in 30 days at 25 °C	2653	C
Lidocaine HCl	AST	2.5 g		2 mg	NS[a]	Physically compatible with no loss of lidocaine or fentanyl at pH 5.8 in 30 days at 4 and 23 °C	2305	C
	BRN	2.5 g		2 mg	NS[a]	Physically compatible with little lidocaine loss but 18% fentanyl loss at 23 °C and 10% loss at 4 °C in 2 days due to sorption at pH 6.7 from higher pH lidocaine product	2305	I
Ropivacaine HCl	ASZ	1 g	JN	1 mg	NS[b]	Physically compatible. No loss of either drug in 30 days at 30 °C in the dark	2433	C
	ASZ	2 g	JN	1 and 10 mg	b	Physically compatible. No loss of either drug in 30 days at 30 °C in the dark	2433	C

Additive Compatibility (Cont.)

Fentanyl citrate

Drug	Mfr	Conc/L	Mfr	Conc/L	Test Soln	Remarks	Ref	C/I
	ASZ	1.5 g	CUR	3 mg	NS[c]	Physically compatible. No loss of either drug in 51 days at 20 and 4 °C	2498	C
	ASZ	1.5 g	CUR	3 mg	NS[a]	Physically compatible. No loss of either drug in 7 days at 20 and 4 °C	2498	C
Ziconotide acetate	ELN	25 mg[b]	BB	1 g[f]		10% ziconotide loss in 26 days. No fentanyl loss in 40 days at 37 °C	2772	C

[a]Tested in PVC containers.
[b]Tested in polypropylene bags (Mark II Polybags).
[c]Tested in glass and ethylene vinyl acetate containers.
[d]Tested in glass containers.
[e]Tested in portable infusion pump reservoirs (Pharmacia Deltec).
[f]Fentanyl citrate powder dissolved in ziconotide acetate injection.

Drugs in Syringe Compatibility

Fentanyl citrate

Drug (in syringe)	Mfr	Amt	Mfr	Amt	Remarks	Ref	C/I
Atracurium besylate	BW	10 mg/mL		50 mcg/mL	Physically compatible and atracurium stable for 24 hr at 5 and 30 °C	1694	C
Atropine sulfate		0.6 mg/1.5 mL	MN	100 mcg/1 mL	Physically compatible for at least 15 min	14	C
	ST	0.4 mg/1 mL	MN	0.05 mg/1 mL	Physically compatible for at least 15 min	326	C
Bupivacaine HCl with clonidine HCl	AST BI	50 mg 0.45 mg	JN	1.75 mg	Diluted to 50 mL with NS. Visually compatible with less than 10% loss of any drug in 25 days at 4 and 25 °C in the dark	2437	C
Bupivacaine HCl with ketamine HCl	SW PD	1.5 mg/mL 2 mg/mL	JN	0.01 mg/mL	Diluted to 5 mL with NS. Visually compatible with no new GC/MS peaks in 1 hr at room temperature	1956	C
Butorphanol tartrate	BR	4 mg/2 mL	MN	0.1 mg/2 mL	Physically compatible for 30 min at room temperature	566	C
Caffeine citrate		20 mg/1 mL	ES	50 mcg/1 mL	Visually compatible for 4 hr at 25 °C	2440	C
Chlorpromazine HCl	PO	50 mg/2 mL	MN	0.05 mg/1 mL	Physically compatible for at least 15 min	326	C
Clonidine HCl with bupivacaine HCl	BI AST	0.45 mg 50 mg	JN	1.75 mg	Diluted to 50 mL with NS. Visually compatible with less than 10% loss of any drug in 25 days at 4 and 25 °C in the dark	2437	C
Clonidine HCl with lidocaine HCl	BI AST	0.03 mg/mL 2 mg/mL	JN	0.01 mg/mL	Diluted to 5 mL with NS. Visually compatible with no new GC/MS peaks in 1 hr at room temperature	1956	C
Dimenhydrinate	HR	50 mg/1 mL	MN	0.05 mg/1 mL	Physically compatible for at least 15 min	326	C

Drugs in Syringe Compatibility (Cont.)

Fentanyl citrate

Drug (in syringe)	Mfr	Amt	Mfr	Amt	Remarks	Ref	C/I
Diphenhydramine HCl	PD	50 mg/ 1 mL	MN	0.05 mg/ 1 mL	Physically compatible for at least 15 min	326	C
Droperidol	MN	2.5 mg/ 1 mL	MN	0.05 mg/ 1 mL	Physically compatible for at least 15 min	326	C
Heparin sodium		2500 units/ 1 mL	JN	0.1 mg/ 2 mL	Physically compatible for at least 5 min	1053	C
Hydromorphone HCl	KN	4 mg/ 2 mL	MN	0.05 mg/ 1 mL	Physically compatible for 30 min	517	C
Hydroxyzine HCl	PF	50 mg/ 1 mL	MN	0.05 mg/ 1 mL	Physically compatible for at least 15 min	326	C
	PF	50 mg/ 1 mL	CR	0.05 mg/ 1 mL	Physically compatible	771	C
	PF	100 mg/ 2 mL	CR	0.05 mg/ 1 mL	Physically compatible	771	C
Ketamine HCl	PF	1 mg/mL		40 mcg/ mL	Diluted in sodium chloride 0.9%. Physically compatible for 96 hr at 25 °C	2563	C
Ketamine HCl with bupivacaine HCl	PD SW	2 mg/mL 1.5 mg/ mL	JN	0.01 mg/ mL	Diluted to 5 mL with NS. Visually compatible with no new GC/MS peaks in 1 hr at room temperature	1956	C
Lidocaine HCl with clonidine HCl	AST BI	2 mg/mL 0.03 mg/ mL	JN	0.01 mg/ mL	Diluted to 5 mL with NS. Visually compatible with no new GC/MS peaks in 1 hr at room temperature	1956	C
Meperidine HCl	WI	50 mg/ 1 mL	MN	0.05 mg/ 1 mL	Physically compatible for at least 15 min	326	C
Metoclopramide HCl	NO	10 mg/ 2 mL	MN	0.05 mg/ 1 mL	Physically compatible for 15 min at room temperature	565	C
Metoclopramide HCl with midazolam HCl	AST RC	20 mg/ 4 mL 15 mg/ 3 mL	DB	1 mg/ 20 mL	Visually compatible with 7% or less loss of each drug in 10 days at 32 °C	2268	C
Midazolam HCl	RC	5 mg/ 1 mL	ES	0.1 mg/ 2 mL	Physically compatible for 4 hr at 25 °C	1145	C
	RC	0.625 and 0.938 mg/mL[a]	DB	12.5 mcg/mL[a]	Visually compatible. Little fentanyl loss. 7 and 9% midazolam loss in 7 days at 5 and 22 °C, respectively	2202	C
	RC	0.625 mg/mL[a]	DB	37.5 mcg/mL[a]	Visually compatible. No fentanyl loss. 5 and 8% midazolam loss in 7 days at 5 and 22 °C, respectively	2202	C
	RC	0.938 mg/mL[a]	DB	37.5 mcg/mL[a]	Visually compatible. Little fentanyl loss. 7 and 9% midazolam loss in 7 days at 5 and 22 °C, respectively	2202	C
	RC	0.278 and 0.833 mg/mL[a]	DB	33.3 mcg/mL[a]	Visually compatible. No fentanyl loss. 5 and 7% midazolam loss in 7 days at 5 and 22 °C, respectively	2202	C

Drugs in Syringe Compatibility (Cont.)

Fentanyl citrate

Drug (in syringe)	Mfr	Amt	Mfr	Amt	Remarks	Ref	C/I
Midazolam HCl with metoclopramide HCl	RC AST	15 mg/ 3 mL 20 mg/ 4 mL	DB	1 mg/ 20 mL	Visually compatible with 7% or less loss of each drug in 10 days at 32 °C	2268	C
Morphine sulfate	ST	15 mg/ 1 mL	MN	0.05 mg/ 1 mL	Physically compatible for at least 15 min	326	C
Ondansetron HCl	GW	1.33 mg/ mL[a]	ES	16.7 mcg/mL[a]	Physically compatible. Little loss of either drug in 24 hr at 4 or 23 °C	2199	C
Pantoprazole sodium	[b]	4 mg/ 1 mL		50 mcg/ 1 mL	Possible precipitate within 15 min	2574	I
Pentazocine lactate	WI	30 mg/ 1 mL	MN	0.05 mg/ 1 mL	Physically compatible for at least 15 min	326	C
Pentobarbital sodium	AB	50 mg/ 1 mL	MN	0.05 mg/ 1 mL	Physically incompatible within 15 min	326	I
Prochlorperazine edisylate	PO	5 mg/ 1 mL	MN	0.05 mg/ 1 mL	Physically compatible for at least 15 min	326	C
Promethazine HCl	PO	50 mg/ 2 mL	MN	0.05 mg/ 1 mL	Physically compatible for at least 15 min	326	C
Ranitidine HCl	GL	50 mg/ 2 mL	JN	0.1 mg/ 2 mL	Physically compatible for 1 hr at 25 °C	978	C
Scopolamine HBr		0.6 mg/ 1.5 mL	MN	100 mcg/ 1 mL	Physically compatible for at least 15 min	14	C
	ST	0.4 mg/ 1 mL	MN	0.05 mg/ 1 mL	Physically compatible for at least 15 min	326	C

[a]Tested in sodium chloride 0.9%.
[b]Test performed using the formulation WITHOUT edetate disodium.

Y-Site Injection Compatibility (1:1 Mixture)

Fentanyl citrate

Drug	Mfr	Conc	Mfr	Conc	Remarks	Ref	C/I
Abciximab	LI	36 mcg/mL[a]	AB	50 mcg/mL	Visually compatible for 12 hr at 23 °C	2374	C
Acyclovir sodium	BV	5 mg/mL[b]	HOS	50 mcg/mL	Physically compatible	2794	C
Alprostadil	BED	7.5 mcg/mL[k,l]	JN	10 mcg/mL[j]	Visually compatible for 1 hr	2746	C
Amiodarone HCl	WY	6 mg/mL[a]	BA	50 mcg/mL	Visually compatible for 24 hr at 22 °C	2352	C
Amphotericin B cholesteryl sulfate complex	SEQ	0.83 mg/mL[a]	AB	0.05 mg/mL	Physically compatible for 4 hr at 23 °C	2117	C
Anidulafungin	VIC	0.5 mg/mL[a]	AB	50 mcg/mL	Physically compatible for 4 hr at 23 °C	2617	C
Argatroban	GSK	1 mg/mL[b]	ES	50 mcg/mL	Visually compatible for 24 hr at 23 °C	2391	C
Atracurium besylate	BW	0.5 mg/mL[a]	ES	10 mcg/mL[a]	Physically compatible for 24 hr at 28 °C	1337	C
Atropine sulfate	LY	0.4 mg/mL	JN	25 mcg/mL[a]	Physically compatible for 48 hr at 22 °C	1706	C
Azithromycin	PF	2 mg/mL[b]	AB	50 mcg/mL[j]	Whitish-yellow microcrystals found	2368	I
Bivalirudin	TMC	5 mg/mL[a]	AB	50 mcg/mL	Physically compatible for 4 hr at 23 °C	2373	C
	TMC	5 mg/mL[a,b]	TAY	50 mcg/mL	Visually compatible for 6 hr at 23 °C	2680	C

Y-Site Injection Compatibility (1:1 Mixture) (Cont.)

Fentanyl citrate

Drug	Mfr	Conc	Mfr	Conc	Remarks	Ref	C/I
Caffeine citrate		20 mg/mL		10 mcg/mL[a]	Compatible and stable for 24 hr at room temperature	1	C
Caspofungin acetate	ME	0.7 mg/mL[b]	HOS	0.05 mg/mL	Physically compatible for 4 hr at room temperature	2758	C
	ME	0.5 mg/mL[b]	HOS	0.05 mg/mL	Physically compatible with fentanyl citrate i.v. push over 2 to 5 min	2766	C
Ceftaroline fosamil	FOR	2.22 mg/mL[a,b,m]	HOS	50 mcg/mL	Physically compatible for 4 hr at 23 °C	2826	C
Cisatracurium besylate	GW	0.1, 2, 5 mg/mL[a]	AB	12.5 mcg/mL[a]	Physically compatible for 4 hr at 23 °C	2074	C
Clonidine HCl	BI	18 mcg/mL[b]	ALP	50 mcg/mL	Visually compatible	2642	C
Dexamethasone sodium phosphate	AMR	1 mg/mL[a]	JN	0.025 mg/mL[a]	Physically compatible for 48 hr at 22 °C	1706	C
Dexmedetomidine HCl	HOS				Stated to be compatible	1	C
Diazepam	ES	0.5 mg/mL[a]	JN	0.025 mg/mL[a]	Physically compatible for 48 hr at 22 °C	1706	C
Diltiazem HCl	MMD	1 mg/mL[a]	ES	0.05 mg/mL	Visually compatible for 4 hr at 27 °C	2062	C
Diphenhydramine HCl	SCN	2 mg/mL[a]	JN	0.025 mg/mL[a]	Physically compatible for 48 hr at 22 °C	1706	C
Dobutamine HCl	LI	4 mg/mL[a]	ES	0.05 mg/mL	Visually compatible for 4 hr at 27 °C	2062	C
Dopamine HCl	AB	3.2 mg/mL[a]	ES	0.05 mg/mL	Visually compatible for 4 hr at 27 °C	2062	C
Doripenem	JJ	5 mg/mL[a,b]	HOS	0.05 mg/mL	Physically compatible for 4 hr at 23 °C	2743	C
Doxapram HCl	RB	2 mg/mL[a]	ESL	25 mcg/mL[a]	Visually compatible for 4 hr at 23 °C	2470	C
Enalaprilat	MSD	0.05 mg/mL[b]	ES	2 mcg/mL[a]	Physically compatible for 24 hr at room temperature under fluorescent light	1355	C
Epinephrine HCl	AB	0.02 mg/mL[a]	ES	0.05 mg/mL	Visually compatible for 4 hr at 27 °C	2062	C
Esmolol HCl	DCC	1 g/100 mL[c]	JN	0.05 mg/1 mL	Physically compatible when fentanyl is injected into Y-site of flowing admixture[d]	1168	C
	DCC	10 mg/mL[c]	JN	0.05 mg/mL	Physically compatible. No drug loss in 8 hr at room temperature in light	1168	C
Etomidate	AB	2 mg/mL	ES	0.05 mg/mL	Visually compatible for 7 days at 25 °C	1801	C
Fenoldopam mesylate	AB	80 mcg/mL[b]	AB	12.5 mcg/mL[b]	Physically compatible for 4 hr at 23 °C	2467	C
Furosemide	AMR	10 mg/mL	ES	0.05 mg/mL	Visually compatible for 4 hr at 27 °C	2062	C
Haloperidol lactate	MN	0.2 mg/mL[a]	JN	0.025 mg/mL[a]	Physically compatible for 48 hr at 22 °C	1706	C
Heparin sodium	UP	1000 units/L[e]	MN	0.05 mg/mL	Physically compatible for 4 hr at room temperature	534	C
	ES	100 units/mL[a]	ES	0.05 mg/mL	Visually compatible for 4 hr at 27 °C	2062	C
Hetastarch in lactated electrolyte	AB	6%	ES	12.5 mcg/mL[a]	Physically compatible for 4 hr at 23 °C	2339	C
Hydrocortisone sodium succinate	UP	10 mg/L[e]	MN	0.05 mg/mL	Physically compatible for 4 hr at room temperature	534	C
Hydromorphone HCl	KN	1 mg/mL	ES	0.05 mg/mL	Visually compatible for 4 hr at 27 °C	2062	C

Y-Site Injection Compatibility (1:1 Mixture) (Cont.)

Fentanyl citrate

Drug	Mfr	Conc	Mfr	Conc	Remarks	Ref	C/I
Hydroxyethyl starch 130/0.4 in sodium chloride 0.9%	FRK	6%	SZ	20[a], 35[a], 50 mcg/mL	Visually compatible for 24 hr at room temperature	2770	C
Hydroxyzine HCl	WI	4 mg/mL[a]	JN	0.025 mg/mL[a]	Physically compatible for 48 hr at 22 °C	1706	C
Ketorolac tromethamine	WY	1 mg/mL[a]	JN	0.025 mg/mL[a]	Physically compatible for 48 hr at 22 °C	1706	C
Labetalol HCl	SC	1 mg/mL[a]	JN	10 mcg/mL[a]	Physically compatible for 24 hr at 18 °C	1171	C
	AH	2 mg/mL[a]	ES	0.05 mg/mL	Visually compatible for 4 hr at 27 °C	2062	C
Levofloxacin	OMN	5 mg/mL[a]	AB	0.05 mg/mL	Visually compatible for 4 hr at 24 °C	2233	C
Linezolid	PHU	2 mg/mL	AB	0.05 mg/mL	Physically compatible for 4 hr at 23 °C	2264	C
Lorazepam	WY	0.33 mg/mL[b]		0.05 mg/mL	Visually compatible for 24 hr at 22 °C	1855	C
	WY	0.5 mg/mL[a]	ES	0.05 mg/mL	Visually compatible for 4 hr at 27 °C	2062	C
	WY	0.1 mg/mL[a]	JN	0.025 mg/mL[a]	Physically compatible for 48 hr at 22 °C	1706	C
Methotrimeprazine HCl	LE	0.2 mg/mL[a]	JN	0.025 mg/mL[a]	Physically compatible for 48 hr at 22 °C	1706	C
Metoclopramide HCl	DU	5 mg/mL	JN	0.025 mg/mL[a]	Physically compatible for 48 hr at 22 °C	1706	C
Midazolam HCl	RC	1 mg/mL[a]	ES	0.05 mg/mL	Visually compatible for 24 hr at 23 °C	1847	C
	RC	0.1 and 0.5 mg/mL[a]	JN	0.02 mg/mL[a]	Visually compatible. No midazolam and 4% fentanyl loss in 3 hr at 24 °C	1852	C
	RC	0.1 and 0.5 mg/mL[a]	JN	0.04 mg/mL[a]	Visually compatible with no loss of either drug in 3 hr at 24 °C	1852	C
	RC	5 mg/mL		0.05 mg/mL	Visually compatible for 24 hr at 22 °C	1855	C
	RC	2 mg/mL[a]	ES	0.05 mg/mL	Visually compatible for 4 hr at 27 °C	2062	C
	RC	0.2 mg/mL[a]	JN	0.025 mg/mL[a]	Physically compatible for 48 hr at 22 °C	1706	C
Milrinone lactate	SW	0.2 mg/mL[a]	ES	0.05 mg/mL	Visually compatible for 4 hr at 27 °C	2062	C
	SW	0.4 mg/mL[a]	ES	50 mcg/mL	Visually compatible. Little loss of either drug in 4 hr at 23 °C	2214	C
Morphine sulfate	SCN	2 mg/mL[a]	ES	0.05 mg/mL	Visually compatible for 4 hr at 27 °C	2062	C
Nafcillin sodium	WY	33 mg/mL[b]		0.05 mg/mL	No precipitation	547	C
Nesiritide	SCI	50 mcg/mL[a,b]		0.05 mg/mL	Physically compatible for 4 hr	2625	C
Nicardipine HCl	WY	1 mg/mL[a]	ES	0.05 mg/mL	Visually compatible for 4 hr at 27 °C	2062	C
	DCC	0.1 mg/mL[a]	ES	2 mcg/mL[a]	Visually compatible for 24 hr at room temperature	235	C
Nitroglycerin	AB	0.4 mg/mL[a]	ES	0.05 mg/mL	Visually compatible for 4 hr at 27 °C	2062	C
Norepinephrine bitartrate	AB	0.128 mg/mL[a]	ES	0.05 mg/mL	Visually compatible for 4 hr at 27 °C	2062	C
Oxaliplatin	SS	0.5 mg/mL[a]	AB	0.05 mg/mL[a]	Physically compatible for 4 hr at 23 °C	2566	C
Palonosetron HCl	MGI	50 mcg/mL	AB	50 mcg/mL	Physically compatible and no loss of either drug in 4 hr	2720	C
Pancuronium bromide	ES	0.05 mg/mL[a]	ES	10 mcg/mL[a]	Physically compatible for 24 hr at 28 °C	1337	C
Phenobarbital sodium	WY	2 mg/mL[a]	JN	0.025 mg/mL[a]	Physically compatible for 48 hr at 22 °C	1706	C
Phenytoin sodium	ES	2 mg/mL[a,b]	JN	0.025 mg/mL[a]	Precipitate forms within 1 hr	1706	I

Y-Site Injection Compatibility (1:1 Mixture) (Cont.)

Fentanyl citrate

Drug	Mfr	Conc	Mfr	Conc	Remarks	Ref	C/I
Potassium chloride	AB	40 mEq/L[e]	MN	0.05 mg/mL	Physically compatible for 4 hr at room temperature	534	**C**
Propofol	ZEN	10 mg/mL	AB	0.05 mg/mL	Physically compatible for 1 hr at 23 °C	2066	**C**
Ranitidine HCl	GL	1 mg/mL[a]	ES	0.05 mg/mL	Visually compatible for 4 hr at 27 °C	2062	**C**
Remifentanil HCl	GW	0.025 and 0.25 mg/mL[b]	ES	12.5 mcg/mL[a]	Physically compatible for 4 hr at 23 °C	2075	**C**
Sargramostim	IMM	6[f] and 15 mcg/mL[b]	ES	50 mcg/mL	Visually compatible for 2 hr	1618	**C**
Scopolamine HBr	LY	0.05 mg/mL[a]	JN	0.025 mg/mL[a]	Physically compatible for 48 hr at 22 °C	1706	**C**
TNA #218 to #226[h]			AB	12.5[a] and 50 mcg/mL	Visually compatible for 4 hr at 23 °C	2215	**C**
TPN #203, #204[h]			ES	0.05 mg/mL	Visually compatible for 4 hr at 23 °C	1974	**C**
TPN #212 to #215[h]			AB	0.0125[a]and 0.05 mg/mL	Physically compatible for 4 hr at 23 °C	2109	**C**
TPN #216[h]			ES	0.01 mg/mL[g]	Mixed 1 mL of fentanyl with 9 mL of TPN. Visually compatible for 24 hr	2104	**C**
Vecuronium bromide	OR	0.1 mg/mL[a]	ES	10 mcg/mL[a]	Physically compatible for 24 hr at 28 °C	1337	**C**
	OR	1 mg/mL	ES	0.05 mg/mL	Visually compatible for 4 hr at 27 °C	2062	**C**

[a]*Tested in dextrose 5%.*
[b]*Tested in sodium chloride 0.9%.*
[c]*Tested in dextrose 5% in sodium chloride 0.9%.*
[d]*Flowing at 1.6 mL/min.*
[e]*Tested in dextrose 5% in Ringer's injection, dextrose 5% in Ringer's injection, lactated, dextrose 5%, Ringer's injection, lactated, and sodium chloride 0.9%.*
[f]*Tested with albumin human 0.1%.*
[g]*Tested in sterile water for injection.*
[h]*Refer to Appendix I for the composition of parenteral nutrition solutions. TNA indicates a 3-in-1 admixture, and TPN indicates a 2-in-1 admixture.*
[i]*Injected via Y-site into an administration set running azithromycin.*
[j]*Tested in either dextrose 5% or in sodium chloride 0.9%, but the report did not specify which solution.*
[k]*Tested in a 1:1 mixture of (1) dextrose 5% and dextrose 5% in sodium chloride 0.45% with and without potassium chloride 20 mEq/L and also in (2) dextrose 10% in sodium chloride 0.45% with and without potassium chloride 20 mEq/L.*
[l]*Tested in a 1:1 mixture of dextrose 5% and TPN #274 (see Appendix I).*
[m]*Tested in Ringer's injection, lactated.*

FILGRASTIM
AHFS 20:16

Products — Filgrastim is available in 300-mcg and 480-mcg sizes with the product compositions and package configurations shown in Table 1. (1)

pH — 4. (4)

Trade Name(s) — Neupogen.

Administration — Filgrastim is administered by subcutaneous injection undiluted or by intravenous or subcutaneous infusion. For intravenous infusion, it is diluted in 50 to 100 mL of dextrose 5% and

Table 1. Filgrastim Products and Compositions (1)

	300 mcg/ 1-mL Vial	480 mcg/ 1.6-mL Vial	300 mcg/ 0.5-mL Syringe	480 mcg/ 0.8-mL Syringe
Filgrastim	300 mcg	480 mcg	300 mcg	480 mcg
Acetate	0.59 mg	0.94 mg	0.295 mg	0.472 mg
Sorbitol	50 mg	80 mg	25 mg	40 mg
Polysorbate 80	0.004%	0.004%	0.004%	0.004%
Sodium	0.035 mg	0.056 mg	0.0175 mg	0.028 mg
Water for injection qs	1 mL	1.6 mL	0.5 mL	0.8 mL

given over 15 to 30 or 60 minutes or over 24 hours by continuous infusion. It may also be given over 24 hours by continuous subcutaneous infusion after diluting the dose in 10 to 50 mL of dextrose 5% and infusing at a rate not exceeding 10 mL/24 hours. For extended infusions by either route, a controlled-infusion device is used. For filgrastim concentrations of 5 to 15 mcg/mL albumin human should be added to the solution at a final concentration of 0.2% (2 mg/mL) before the filgrastim is added. The drug should not be diluted to concentrations less than 5 mcg/mL. (1; 4)

Stability — Filgrastim injection is a clear, colorless solution. Intact containers should be refrigerated at 2 to 8 °C and protected from direct sunlight. The product also should be protected from freezing and temperatures above 30 °C to avoid aggregation. The solution should not be shaken since bubbles and/or foam may form. If foaming occurs, the solution should be left undisturbed for a few minutes until bubbles dissipate. (1; 4)

Although refrigerated storage is required, the manufacturer has stated that filgrastim may be stored at room temperature for 24 hours (1; 4), while others have stated that the drug is stable for seven days at room temperature. (2745) The product is packaged in single-use containers with no antibacterial preservative. The manufacturer recommends that vials not be reentered and that unused portions be discarded. (1)

Filgrastim dilutions in dextrose 5% prepared for infusion should be stored under refrigeration and used within 24 hours of preparation because of concern about possible bacterial contamination. (1; 4)

pH Effects — Filgrastim is stable at pH 3.8 to 4.2, but stability is limited at neutral pH. (4)

Syringes — Undiluted filgrastim is stable for 24 hours at 15 to 30 °C and for seven days refrigerated at 2 to 8 °C repackaged in tuberculin syringes (Becton-Dickinson). However, refrigeration and use within 24 hours are recommended because of concern about bacterial contamination. (4)

Although studies have found filgrastim in syringes remained sterile stored under refrigeration, (1764; 2186) the sterility of repackaged injections is a function of the quality of the specific aseptic process of packaging, the quality of the environment in which the sterile product is packaged, and the capability of the personnel involved rather than a property of this unpreserved injection. Consequently, sterility is only valid for the specific facilities and operators for that specific test. The adequacy and safety of repackaging in another location or with other individuals or on another occasion should be verified independently for each institution and batch of repackaged filgrastim injection. Each institution needs to establish specific validation testing results for its own aseptic processing facilities, equipment, procedures, and personnel. (1765; 2187) The potential for microbiological growth should be considered when assigning expiration periods.

The sterility of filgrastim 0.2 mL (60 mcg) extemporaneously drawn aseptically into tuberculin syringes and kept under "patient use" storage conditions was evaluated. The syringes were sent home with patients to be stored in their home refrigerators for seven days and then were returned for sterility testing. A contamination rate as high as 1.25% was reported. The authors expressed the opinion and hope that the high rate of contamination was an artifact of the sterility testing itself. However, contamination during storage in the patients' refrigerators may have occurred. (2294)

Sorption — Filgrastim in dextrose 5% at concentrations above 15 mcg/mL and between 2 and 15 mcg/mL with added albumin human 0.2% is compatible with common plastics used in syringes, administration sets, solution containers, and pump cassettes including PVC, polyolefin, and polypropylene. (4)

Filgrastim sorption occurs to a greater extent with lower concentrations and with longer infusion tubing. (2601) For filgrastim concentrations between 5 and 15 mcg/mL, albumin human should be added before adding the filgrastim to make a final albumin human concentration of 0.2% (2 mg/mL) to minimize filgrastim adsorption to infusion containers and equipment. At filgrastim concentrations above 15 mcg/mL, albumin human is unnecessary. The product should not be diluted to a final concentration of less than 5 mcg/mL. (1; 4)

The amount of loss of filgrastim (Amgen) from the undiluted injection at a concentration of 300 mcg/mL when delivered through 6.6-French, single-lumen, silicone rubber, Broviac catheters (Bard) was evaluated. The catheters were filled with dextrose 5% (about 0.45 mL) and flushed before and after introduction of the filgrastim. Injected amounts of filgrastim 300 mcg/mL ranged from 0.17 to 1 mL. The delivered flush solution was collected and analyzed for filgrastim content and activity. The lowest volume (0.17 mL) incurred about 32% loss of filgrastim upon delivery. The other volumes incurred lower losses, ranging from 12% to none. A second repeat filgrastim injection incurred similar losses. The filgrastim that was delivered through the catheters remained active. (2017)

Compatibility Information

Solution Compatibility

	Filgrastim					
Solution	*Mfr*	*Mfr*	*Conc/L*	*Remarks*	*Ref*	*C/I*
Dextrose 5%		AMG	5 mcg/mL or more[a]	Use within 24 hours	1	**C**
		AMG	2 mcg/mL or more[a]	Stable for 7 days at 4 °C	4	**C**
Sodium chloride 0.9%		AMG		Physically incompatible	1	**I**

[a]*Concentrations between 5 and 15 mcg/mL require human albumin 2 mg/mL.*

Y-Site Injection Compatibility (1:1 Mixture)

Filgrastim

Drug	Mfr	Conc	Mfr	Conc	Remarks	Ref	C/I
Acyclovir sodium	BW	7 mg/mL[a]	AMG	30 mcg/mL[a]	Physically compatible for 4 hr at 22 °C	1687	C
Allopurinol sodium	BW	3 mg/mL[a]	AMG	30 mcg/mL[a]	Physically compatible for 4 hr at 22 °C	1687	C
Amikacin sulfate	ES	5 mg/mL[a]	AMG	30 mcg/mL[a]	Physically compatible for 4 hr at 22 °C	1687	C
	BMS	5 mg/mL[a]	AMG	10[d] and 40[a] mcg/mL	Visually compatible. Little loss of filgrastim and fluconazole in 4 hr at 25 °C	2060	C
Aminophylline	AB	2.5 mg/mL[a]	AMG	30 mcg/mL[a]	Physically compatible for 4 hr at 22 °C	1687	C
Amphotericin B	SQ	0.6 mg/mL[a]	AMG	30 mcg/mL[a]	Yellow turbidity and precipitate form	1687	I
Ampicillin sodium	WY	20 mg/mL[a]	AMG	30 mcg/mL[a]	Physically compatible for 4 hr at 22 °C	1687	C
Ampicillin sodium–sulbactam sodium	RR	20 + 10 mg/mL[a]	AMG	30 mcg/mL[a]	Physically compatible for 4 hr at 22 °C	1687	C
Aztreonam	SQ	40 mg/mL[a]	AMG	30 mcg/mL[a]	Physically compatible for 4 hr at 22 °C	1687	C
	SQ	40 mg/mL[a]	AMG	30 mcg/mL[a]	Physically compatible for 4 hr at 23 °C	1758	C
Bleomycin sulfate	BR	1 unit/mL[a]	AMG	30 mcg/mL[a]	Physically compatible for 4 hr at 22 °C	1687	C
Bumetanide	RC	0.04 mg/mL[a]	AMG	30 mcg/mL[a]	Physically compatible for 4 hr at 22 °C	1687	C
Buprenorphine HCl	RKC	0.04 mg/mL[a]	AMG	30 mcg/mL[a]	Physically compatible for 4 hr at 22 °C	1687	C
Butorphanol tartrate	BR	0.04 mg/mL[a]	AMG	30 mcg/mL[a]	Physically compatible for 4 hr at 22 °C	1687	C
Calcium gluconate	AST	40 mg/mL[a]	AMG	30 mcg/mL[a]	Physically compatible for 4 hr at 22 °C	1687	C
Carboplatin	BR	5 mg/mL[a]	AMG	30 mcg/mL[a]	Physically compatible for 4 hr at 22 °C	1687	C
Carmustine	BR	1.5 mg/mL[a]	AMG	30 mcg/mL[a]	Physically compatible for 4 hr at 22 °C	1687	C
Cefazolin sodium	LI	20 mg/mL[a]	AMG	30 mcg/mL[a]	Physically compatible for 4 hr at 22 °C	1687	C
Cefotaxime sodium	HO	20 mg/mL[a]	AMG	30 mcg/mL[a]	Particles form in 4 hr	1687	I
Cefotetan disodium	STU	20 mg/mL[a]	AMG	30 mcg/mL[a]	Physically compatible for 4 hr at 22 °C	1687	C
Cefoxitin sodium	MSD	20 mg/mL[a]	AMG	30 mcg/mL[a]	Haze, particles, and filaments form immediately	1687	I
Ceftaroline fosamil	FOR	2.22 mg/mL[a,b,c]	AMG	30 mcg/mL[a]	Microparticulates formed	2826	I
Ceftazidime	LI	40 mg/mL[a]	AMG	30 mcg/mL[a]	Physically compatible for 4 hr at 22 °C	1687	C
	LI	10 mg/mL[a]	AMG	10[d] and 40[a] mcg/mL	Visually compatible. Little loss of filgrastim and fluconazole in 4 hr at 25 °C	2060	C
Ceftriaxone sodium	RC	20 mg/mL[a]	AMG	30 mcg/mL[a]	Particles and filaments form in 1 hr	1687	I
Cefuroxime sodium	GL	20 mg/mL[a]	AMG	30 mcg/mL[a]	Haze, particles, and filaments form immediately	1687	I
Chlorpromazine HCl	RU	2 mg/mL[a]	AMG	30 mcg/mL[a]	Physically compatible for 4 hr at 22 °C	1687	C
Cisplatin	BR	1 mg/mL	AMG	30 mcg/mL[a]	Physically compatible for 4 hr at 22 °C	1687	C
Clindamycin phosphate	AB	10 mg/mL[a]	AMG	30 mcg/mL[a]	Particles and filaments form immediately	1687	I
Cyclophosphamide	MJ	10 mg/mL[a]	AMG	30 mcg/mL[a]	Physically compatible for 4 hr at 22 °C	1687	C
Cytarabine	CET	50 mg/mL	AMG	30 mcg/mL[a]	Physically compatible for 4 hr at 22 °C	1687	C
Dacarbazine	MI	4 mg/mL[a]	AMG	30 mcg/mL[a]	Physically compatible for 4 hr at 22 °C	1687	C
Dactinomycin	MSD	0.01 mg/mL[a]	AMG	30 mcg/mL[a]	Particles and filaments form immediately	1687	I
Daunorubicin HCl	WY	1 mg/mL[a]	AMG	30 mcg/mL[a]	Physically compatible for 4 hr at 22 °C	1687	C
Dexamethasone sodium phosphate	LY	1 mg/mL[a]	AMG	30 mcg/mL[a]	Physically compatible for 4 hr at 22 °C	1687	C

Y-Site Injection Compatibility (1:1 Mixture) (Cont.)

Filgrastim

Drug	Mfr	Conc	Mfr	Conc	Remarks	Ref	C/I
Diphenhydramine HCl	ES	2 mg/mL[a]	AMG	30 mcg/mL[a]	Physically compatible for 4 hr at 22 °C	1687	**C**
Doxorubicin HCl	CET	2 mg/mL	AMG	30 mcg/mL[a]	Physically compatible for 4 hr at 22 °C	1687	**C**
Doxycycline hyclate	ES	1 mg/mL[a]	AMG	30 mcg/mL[a]	Physically compatible for 4 hr at 22 °C	1687	**C**
Droperidol	JN	0.4 mg/mL[a]	AMG	30 mcg/mL[a]	Physically compatible for 4 hr at 22 °C	1687	**C**
Enalaprilat	MSD	0.1 mg/mL[a]	AMG	30 mcg/mL[a]	Physically compatible for 4 hr at 22 °C	1687	**C**
Etoposide	BR	0.4 mg/mL[a]	AMG	30 mcg/mL[a]	Particles form immediately. Filaments form in 1 hr	1687	**I**
Famotidine	MSD	2 mg/mL[a]	AMG	30 mcg/mL[a]	Physically compatible for 4 hr at 22 °C	1687	**C**
Floxuridine	RC	3 mg/mL[a]	AMG	30 mcg/mL[a]	Physically compatible for 4 hr at 22 °C	1687	**C**
Fluconazole	RR	2 mg/mL	AMG	30 mcg/mL[a]	Physically compatible for 4 hr at 22 °C	1687	**C**
	RR	2 mg/mL[a]	AMG	10[d] and 40[a] mcg/mL	Visually compatible. Little loss of filgrastim and fluconazole in 4 hr at 25 °C	2060	**C**
Fludarabine phosphate	BX	1 mg/mL[a]	AMG	30 mcg/mL[a]	Physically compatible for 4 hr at 22 °C	1687	**C**
Fluorouracil	RC	16 mg/mL[a]	AMG	30 mcg/mL[a]	Particles and long filaments form in 1 hr	1687	**I**
Furosemide	AB	3 mg/mL[a]	AMG	30 mcg/mL[a]	Turbidity forms immediately. Filaments and particles form in 1 hr	1687	**I**
Gallium nitrate	FUJ	0.4 mg/mL[a]	AMG	30 mcg/mL[a]	Physically compatible for 4 hr at 22 °C	1687	**C**
Ganciclovir sodium	SY	20 mg/mL[a]	AMG	30 mcg/mL[a]	Physically compatible for 4 hr at 22 °C	1687	**C**
Gentamicin sulfate	LY	5 mg/mL[a]	AMG	30 mcg/mL[a]	Physically compatible for 4 hr at 22 °C	1687	**C**
	GNS	1.6 mg/mL[a]	AMG	40 mcg/mL[a]	Visually compatible. Little loss of filgrastim and gentamicin in 4 hr at 25 °C	2060	**C**
	GNS	1.6 mg/mL[a]	AMG	10 mcg/mL[d]	23% loss of filgrastim in 4 hr at 25 °C. Little gentamicin loss	2060	**I**
Granisetron HCl	SKB	0.05 mg/mL[a]	AMG	30 mcg/mL[a]	Physically compatible for 4 hr at 23 °C	2000	**C**
Haloperidol lactate	MN	0.2 mg/mL[a]	AMG	30 mcg/mL[a]	Physically compatible for 4 hr at 22 °C	1687	**C**
Heparin sodium	ES	100 units/mL[a]	AMG	30 mcg/mL[a]	Particles and filaments form immediately	1687	**I**
Hydrocortisone sodium succinate	UP	1 mg/mL[a]	AMG	30 mcg/mL[a]	Physically compatible for 4 hr at 22 °C	1687	**C**
Hydromorphone HCl	KN	0.5 mg/mL[a]	AMG	30 mcg/mL[a]	Physically compatible for 4 hr at 22 °C	1687	**C**
Hydroxyzine HCl	ES	4 mg/mL[a]	AMG	30 mcg/mL[a]	Physically compatible for 4 hr at 22 °C	1687	**C**
Idarubicin HCl	AD	0.5 mg/mL[a]	AMG	30 mcg/mL[a]	Physically compatible for 4 hr at 22 °C	1687	**C**
Ifosfamide	MJ	25 mg/mL[a]	AMG	30 mcg/mL[a]	Physically compatible for 4 hr at 22 °C	1687	**C**
Imipenem–cilastatin sodium	MSD	10 mg/mL[a]	AMG	30 mcg/mL[a]	Physically compatible for 4 hr at 22 °C	1687	**C**
	ME	5 mg/mL[a]	AMG	40 mcg/mL[a]	16% loss of filgrastim in 4 hr at 25 °C. Little imipenem–cilastatin loss	2060	**I**
	ME	5 mg/mL[a]	AMG	10 mcg/mL[d]	Visually compatible. Little loss of filgrastim and imipenem–cilastatin in 4 hr at 25 °C	2060	**C**
Leucovorin calcium	LE	2 mg/mL[a]	AMG	30 mcg/mL[a]	Physically compatible for 4 hr at 22 °C	1687	**C**
Lorazepam	WY	0.1 mg/mL[a]	AMG	30 mcg/mL[a]	Physically compatible for 4 hr at 22 °C	1687	**C**
Mannitol	BA	15%	AMG	30 mcg/mL[a]	Filaments form immediately	1687	**I**
Mechlorethamine HCl	MSD	1 mg/mL	AMG	30 mcg/mL[a]	Physically compatible for 4 hr at 22 °C	1687	**C**
Melphalan HCl	BW	0.1 mg/mL[a]	AMG	30 mcg/mL[a]	Physically compatible for 4 hr at 22 °C	1687	**C**

Y-Site Injection Compatibility (1:1 Mixture) (Cont.)

Filgrastim

Drug	Mfr	Conc	Mfr	Conc	Remarks	Ref	C/I
Meperidine HCl	WY	4 mg/mL[a]	AMG	30 mcg/mL[a]	Physically compatible for 4 hr at 22 °C	1687	C
Mesna	MJ	10 mg/mL[a]	AMG	30 mcg/mL[a]	Physically compatible for 4 hr at 22 °C	1687	C
Methotrexate sodium	LE	15 mg/mL[a]	AMG	30 mcg/mL[a]	Physically compatible for 4 hr at 22 °C	1687	C
Methylprednisolone sodium succinate	AB	5 mg/mL[a]	AMG	30 mcg/mL[a]	Haze, particles, and filaments form immediately	1687	I
Metoclopramide HCl	ES	5 mg/mL	AMG	30 mcg/mL[a]	Physically compatible for 4 hr at 22 °C	1687	C
Metronidazole	BA	5 mg/mL	AMG	30 mcg/mL[a]	Particles form immediately. Filaments form in 1 hr	1687	I
Mitomycin	BR	0.5 mg/mL	AMG	30 mcg/mL[a]	Color changes to reddish purple in 1 hr	1687	I
Mitoxantrone HCl	LE	0.5 mg/mL[a]	AMG	30 mcg/mL[a]	Physically compatible for 4 hr at 22 °C	1687	C
Morphine sulfate	WY	1 mg/mL[a]	AMG	30 mcg/mL[a]	Physically compatible for 4 hr at 22 °C	1687	C
Nalbuphine HCl	DU	10 mg/mL	AMG	30 mcg/mL[a]	Physically compatible for 4 hr at 22 °C	1687	C
Ondansetron HCl	GL	1 mg/mL[a]	AMG	30 mcg/mL[a]	Physically compatible for 4 hr at 22 °C	1687	C
Potassium chloride	AB	0.1 mEq/mL[a]	AMG	30 mcg/mL[a]	Physically compatible for 4 hr at 22 °C	1687	C
Prochlorperazine edisylate	SCN	0.5 mg/mL[a]	AMG	30 mcg/mL[a]	Particles form immediately. Filaments form in 1 hr	1687	I
Promethazine HCl	SCN	2 mg/mL[a]	AMG	30 mcg/mL[a]	Physically compatible for 4 hr at 22 °C	1687	C
Ranitidine HCl	GL	2 mg/mL[a]	AMG	30 mcg/mL[a]	Physically compatible for 4 hr at 22 °C	1687	C
Sodium bicarbonate	AB	1 mEq/mL	AMG	30 mcg/mL[a]	Physically compatible for 4 hr at 22 °C	1687	C
Streptozocin	UP	40 mg/mL[a]	AMG	30 mcg/mL[a]	Physically compatible for 4 hr at 22 °C	1687	C
Thiotepa	LE	1 mg/mL[a]	AMG	30 mcg/mL[a]	Particles and filaments form immediately	1687	I
Ticarcillin disodium–clavulanate potassium	SKB	31 mg/mL[a]	AMG	30 mcg/mL[a]	Physically compatible for 4 hr at 22 °C	1687	C
Tobramycin sulfate	LI	5 mg/mL[a]	AMG	30 mcg/mL[a]	Physically compatible for 4 hr at 22 °C	1687	C
	LI	1.6 mg/mL[a]	AMG	10[d] and 40[a] mcg/mL	Visually compatible. Little loss of filgrastim and tobramycin in 4 hr at 25 °C	2060	C
Trimethoprim–sulfamethoxazole	ES	0.8 + 4 mg/mL[a]	AMG	30 mcg/mL[a]	Physically compatible for 4 hr at 22 °C	1687	C
Vancomycin HCl	AB	10 mg/mL[a]	AMG	30 mcg/mL[a]	Physically compatible for 4 hr at 22 °C	1687	C
Vinblastine sulfate	LI	0.12 mg/mL[a]	AMG	30 mcg/mL[a]	Physically compatible for 4 hr at 22 °C	1687	C
Vincristine sulfate	LI	0.05 mg/mL[a]	AMG	30 mcg/mL[a]	Physically compatible for 4 hr at 22 °C	1687	C
Vinorelbine tartrate	BW	1 mg/mL[a]	AMG	30 mcg/mL[a]	Physically compatible for 4 hr at 22 °C	1687	C
Zidovudine	BW	4 mg/mL[a]	AMG	30 mcg/mL[a]	Physically compatible for 4 hr at 22 °C	1687	C

[a]*Tested in dextrose 5%.*
[b]*Tested in sodium chloride 0.9%.*
[c]*Tested in Ringer's injection, lactated.*
[d]*Tested in dextrose 5% with albumin human 2 mg/mL.*

FLOXACILLIN SODIUM
(FLUCLOXACILLIN SODIUM)
AHFS 8:12.16.12

Products — Floxacillin sodium is available in vials containing 250 mg, 500 mg, and 1 g of floxacillin as the sodium salt. To reconstitute for intramuscular use, add 1.5 mL of sterile water for injection to the 250-mg vial, 2 mL to the 500-mg vial, or 2.5 mL to the 1-g vial. (38; 115)

For intravenous use, reconstitute the 250- or 500-mg vial with 5 to 10 mL and the 1-g vial with 15 to 20 mL of sterile water for injection. For intravenous infusion, the solution may be diluted further in a compatible infusion fluid. (38; 115)

For intrapleural use, reconstitute the 250-mg vial with 5 to 10 mL of sterile water for injection. For intra-articular use, reconstitute the 250- or 500-mg vial with up to 5 mL of sterile water for injection or lidocaine hydrochloride 0.5% injection. (38; 115)

For smaller doses, the reconstitution volumes in Table 1 will yield the indicated concentrations.

Sodium and Magnesium Content — Each gram of drug contains 2.2 mmol (51 mg) of sodium and 1 mmol of magnesium. (38; 89; 115)

Trade Name(s) — Floxapen, Ladropen.

Administration — Floxacillin sodium may be administered by intramuscular injection, direct intravenous injection slowly over three to four minutes, continuous intravenous infusion, and intrapleural and intra-articular injection. (38)

Stability — Floxacillin sodium in intact vials should be stored below 25 °C. The injection reconstituted for intramuscular or direct intravenous injection should be freshly prepared and administered within

Table 1. Floxacillin Reconstitution Volumes for Smaller Doses (38; 115)

Vial Size	Concentration (mg/1 mL)					
	50	100	125	200	250	500
250 mg	4.8 mL	2.3 mL	1.8 mL	1.05 mL		
500 mg		4.7 mL	3.7 mL	2.2 mL	1.7 mL	
1 g		9.3 mL			3.3 mL	1.3 mL

30 minutes. However, reconstituted floxacillin sodium injection is stated to be stable for 24 hours when stored under refrigeration. (38; 115)

Losses of 8% in three days were reported for reconstituted solutions containing floxacillin sodium (Beecham) 100 mg/mL stored at 20 to 25 °C. (89)

Freezing Solutions — Floxacillin sodium (Beecham) 20 mg/mL in sodium chloride 0.9% or dextrose 5% in PVC bags (Travenol) retained greater than 90% after being frozen and stored at −27 °C for up to 270 days. Thawing by microwave radiation and subsequent storage for 24 hours at 4 °C did not cause drug loss below 90% of the stated concentration. However, a distinct yellow discoloration was produced after 90 days of storage, rendering the solutions unacceptable. (1176)

Floxacillin sodium (Beecham) 1 g in 50 mL of sodium chloride 0.9% or dextrose 5% in PVC bags (Travenol) was stored at −20 °C for 30 days, followed by natural thawing and storage at 5 °C for 21 hours. The drug was stable under these conditions for the duration of the study. (299)

Sorption — Floxacillin sodium was shown not to exhibit sorption to PVC bags and tubing, polyethylene tubing, Silastic tubing, and polypropylene syringes. (536; 606)

Compatibility Information

Solution Compatibility

Floxacillin sodium

Solution	Mfr	Mfr	Conc/L	Remarks	Ref	C/I
Dextrose 2.5% in sodium chloride 0.45%		BE	1 g	6% loss in 24 hr at 20 to 25 °C	89	C
Dextrose 5%				Under 10% loss in 24 hr at room temperature	1475	C
		BE	1 g	1% loss in 24 hr at 20 to 25 °C	89	C
Ringer's injection, lactated				Under 10% loss in 24 hr at room temperature	1475	C
Sodium chloride 0.9%				Under 10% loss in 24 hr at room temperature	1475	C
		BE	1 g	3% loss in 24 hr at 20 to 25 °C	89	C
	BA	BE	5, 10, 20 g	Visually compatible. 2 to 3% loss in 14 days and 7 to 9% loss in 28 days at 5 °C	1844	C
	BA[a]		120 g	Stable for 6 days at 4 °C. 28% loss in 24 hr at 37 °C	2206	C
	[b]		50 g	2% loss in 6 days at 4 °C, 6% loss in 24 hr at 31 °C, and 13% in 7 hr at 37 °C	2715	C
Sodium lactate ⅙ M				Under 10% loss in 24 hr at room temperature	1475	C
		BE	1 g	4% loss in 24 hr at 20 to 25 °C	89	C

[a]*Tested in PVC containers.*
[b]*Tested in Infusor LV reservoirs.*

Additive Compatibility

Floxacillin sodium

Drug	Mfr	Conc/L	Mfr	Conc/L	Test Soln	Remarks	Ref	C/I
Aminophylline	ANT	1 g	BE	20 g	NS	Physically compatible for 72 hr at 15 and 30 °C	1479	**C**
Amiodarone HCl	LZ	4 g	BE	20 g	D5W	Precipitates immediately	1479	**I**
Ampicillin sodium	BE	20 g	BE	20 g	NS	Physically compatible for 72 hr at 15 and 30 °C	1479	**C**
Atropine sulfate	ANT	60 mg	BE	20 g	W	Haze forms in 24 hr and precipitate forms in 48 hr at 30 °C. No change at 15 °C	1479	**I**
Bumetanide	LEO	6 mg	BE	20 g	NS	Physically compatible for 72 hr at 15 and 30 °C	1479	**C**
Buprenorphine HCl		75 mg	BE	20 g	W	Thick haze forms in 24 hr and precipitate forms in 47 hr at 30 °C. No change at 15 °C	1479	**I**
Calcium gluconate	ANT	2 g	BE	20 g	NS	White precipitate forms immediately	1479	**I**
Ceftazidime	GSK	40 g	GSK	40 g	NS, W	Physically compatible. Under 10% loss in 24 hr at room temperature and 4 °C	2658	**C**
	GSK	60 g	GSK	120 g	NS, W	Physically compatible. Under 10% loss in 24 hr at room temperature and 4 °C	2658	**C**
	GSK	180 g	GSK	240 g	NS, W	Physically compatible. Under 10% loss in 24 hr at room temperature and 4 °C	2658	**C**
Cefuroxime sodium	GL	37.5 g	BE	20 g	W	Physically compatible for 72 hr at 15 and 30 °C	1479	**C**
	GL	7.5 g	BE	10 g	D5W, NS	Physically compatible for 48 hr. Both drugs stable for 1 hr at room temperature	1036	**C**
Chlorpromazine HCl	ANT	5 g	BE	20 g	W	Yellow precipitate forms immediately	1479	**I**
Ciprofloxacin		2 g		10 g	a	Precipitates immediately	1473	**I**
Cloxacillin sodium	BE	20 g	BE	20 g	NS	Physically compatible for 24 hr at 15 and 30 °C. Haze forms in 48 hr at 30 °C. No change at 15 °C	1479	**C**
Dexamethasone sodium phosphate	MSD	4 g	BE	20 g	NS	Physically compatible for 72 hr at 15 and 30 °C	1479	**C**
Dextran 40		10%			D5W, NS	Under 10% loss in 24 hr at room temperature	1475	**C**
Diamorphine HCl	EV	500 mg	BE	20 g	W	Physically compatible for 24 hr at 15 and 30 °C. Haze forms in 48 hr at 30 °C. No change at 15 °C	1479	**C**
Diazepam	PHX	1 g	BE	20 g	D5W	Haze forms in 7 hr at 30 °C and 48 hr at 15 °C	1479	**I**
Digoxin	BW	25 mg	BE	20 g	NS	Physically compatible for 72 hr at 15 and 30 °C	1479	**C**
Dobutamine HCl	LI	500 mg	BE	20 g	NS	Haze forms immediately and precipitate forms in 24 to 48 hr at 15 and 30 °C	1479	**I**
Epinephrine HCl	ANT	8 mg	BE	20 g	W	Physically compatible for 72 hr at 15 and 30 °C	1479	**C**
Erythromycin lactobionate	AB	5 g	BE	20 g	NS	Precipitates immediately. Crystals form in 5 hr at 15 °C	1479	**I**

Additive Compatibility (Cont.)

Floxacillin sodium

Drug	Mfr	Conc/L	Mfr	Conc/L	Test Soln	Remarks	Ref	C/I
Fusidate sodium	LEO	500 mg		2.5 g	D–S	Physically compatible and chemically stable for 48 hr at room temperature	1800	C
Gentamicin sulfate	RS	8 g	BE	20 g	NS	Haze forms immediately and precipitate forms in 2 hr	1479	I
	EX	8 g	BE	10 g	NS	Physically compatible for 48 hr. Both drugs stable for 1 hr at room temperature	1036	C
	EX	8 g	BE	10 g	D5W	Precipitates immediately	1036	I
Heparin sodium	WED	20,000 units	BE	20 g	NS	Physically compatible for 24 hr at 15 and 30 °C. Haze forms in 48 hr at 30 °C. No change at 15 °C	1479	C
Hydrocortisone sodium succinate	UP	50 g	BE	20 g	NS	Physically compatible for 72 hr at 15 and 30 °C	1479	C
Isoproterenol HCl	PX	4 mg	BE	20 g	D5W	Physically compatible for 24 hr at 15 and 30 °C. Haze forms in 48 hr and precipitate forms in 72 hr	1479	C
Isosorbide dinitrate		1 g	BE	20 g		Physically compatible for 24 hr at 15 and 30 °C. Haze forms in 48 hr and precipitate forms in 72 hr at 30 °C. No change at 15 °C	1479	C
Lidocaine HCl	ANT	2 g	BE	20 g	NS	Physically compatible for 72 hr at 15 and 30 °C	1479	C
Meperidine HCl	RC	5 g	BE	20 g	W	Haze forms immediately and precipitate forms in 5 to 24 hr	1479	I
Metoclopramide HCl	ANT	1 g	BE	20 g	NS	White precipitate forms immediately	1479	I
Metronidazole		5 g	BE	10 g		Physically compatible for 48 hr. Both drugs stable for 1 hr at room temperature	1036	C
Morphine sulfate	EV	1 g	BE	20 g	W	Haze forms in 24 hr and precipitate forms in 48 hr at 30 °C. No change at 15 °C	1479	I
Pefloxacin		4 g	BE	10 g	D5W, NS	Precipitates immediately	1473	I
Potassium chloride	ANT	40 mM	BE	20 g	W	Physically compatible for 72 hr at 15 and 30 °C	1479	C
Prochlorperazine edisylate	MB	1.25 g	BE	20 g	W	Precipitates immediately	1479	I
Promethazine HCl	MB	5 g	BE	20 g	W	White precipitate forms immediately	1479	I
Ranitidine HCl	GL	500 mg	BE	20 g	NS	Physically compatible for 72 hr at 15 and 30 °C	1479	C
Scopolamine butylbromide	BI	2 g	BE	20 g	W	Physically compatible for 24 hr at 15 and 30 °C. Precipitate forms in 48 hr at 30 °C. No change in 48 hr at 15 °C	1479	C
Tobramycin sulfate	LI	8 g	BE	20 g	NS	White precipitate forms in 7 hr	1479	I
Verapamil HCl	AB	500 mg	BE	20 g	NS	Haze and precipitate form in 24 hr at 30 °C. No change at 15 °C	1479	I

[a] *Floxacillin sodium added to ciprofloxacin solvent.*

Drugs in Syringe Compatibility

Floxacillin sodium

Drug (in syringe)	Mfr	Amt	Mfr	Amt	Remarks	Ref	C/I
Heparin sodium		2500 units/ 1 mL	BE	1 g	Visually compatible for at least 5 min	1053	C

Y-Site Injection Compatibility (1:1 Mixture)

Floxacillin sodium

Drug	Mfr	Conc	Mfr	Conc	Remarks	Ref	C/I
Clarithromycin	AB	4 mg/mL[a]	BE	40 mg/mL[a]	Translucent precipitate in 1 to 2 hr becoming a gel in 3 hr at 30 and 17 °C	2174	I
Lorazepam	WY	0.33 mg/mL[b]	SKB	50 mg/mL	White opalescence forms in 4 hr	1855	I
Midazolam HCl	RC	5 mg/mL	SKB	50 mg/mL	White precipitate forms immediately	1855	I
TPN #189[c]			BE	50 mg/mL[b]	Visually compatible for 24 hr at 22 °C	1767	C

[a]Tested in dextrose 5%.
[b]Tested in sodium chloride 0.9%.
[c]Refer to Appendix I for the composition of parenteral nutrition solutions. TPN indicates a 2-in-1 admixture.

FLOXURIDINE
AHFS 10:00

Products — Floxuridine is supplied in 5-mL vials containing 500 mg of drug. Reconstitute with 5 mL of sterile water for injection to yield a 100-mg/mL concentration. (1; 4)

pH — From 4 to 5.5. (1; 4)

Administration — Floxuridine is administered by continuous arterial infusion using an infusion device after dilution in dextrose 5% or sodium chloride 0.9%. (1; 4) Floxuridine has also been administered investigationally by intravenous injection or infusion. (4)

Stability — The reconstituted solution should be stored under refrigeration at 2 to 8 °C and used within two weeks. (1; 4)

The pH of optimum stability is 4 to 7. Extreme acidity or alkalinity may result in hydrolysis. (1379)

At a concentration of 5 mg/mL in sodium chloride 0.9%, floxuridine supported the growth of several microorganisms commonly implicated in nosocomial infections, including *Escherichia coli*, *Pseudomonas aeruginosa*, and *Candida albicans*. The arbitrary application of an extended expiration date to floxuridine solutions is, therefore, highly questionable. (827)

Syringes — Floxuridine (Roche) 50 mg/mL and 1 mg/mL in sodium chloride 0.9% was packaged as 3 mL in 10-mL polypropylene infusion pump syringes (Pharmacia Deltec). Little or no loss occurred during 21 days of storage at 30 °C. (1967)

Implantable Pumps — Floxuridine 10 mg/mL was filled into an implantable infusion pump (Fresenius VIP 30) and associated capillary tubing and stored at 37 °C. No floxuridine loss and no contamination from components of pump materials occurred during six weeks of storage. However, an unidentified substance appeared in seven weeks, and 22% loss of floxuridine occurred by eight weeks. (1903)

Floxuridine (Roche), at concentrations ranging from about 2.5 to 12 mg/mL with heparin sodium 200 units/mL in bacteriostatic sodium chloride 0.9%, was evaluated for stability in an implantable infusion pump (Infusaid model 400). In this in vivo assessment, the floxuridine concentrations were determined prior to implantation in patients and again at the time of pump refills. No appreciable floxuridine loss occurred during eight courses of therapy, from 4 to 12 days in duration, in five patients. (767)

Compatibility Information

Solution Compatibility

Floxuridine

Solution	Mfr	Mfr	Conc/L	Remarks	Ref	C/I
Dextrose 5%			5 to 10 g	Under 10% loss in 14 days at room temperature	1379	C
Sodium chloride 0.9%			5 to 10 g	Under 10% loss in 14 days at room temperature	1379	C

Additive Compatibility

Floxuridine

Drug	Mfr	Conc/L	Mfr	Conc/L	Test Soln	Remarks	Ref	C/I
Carboplatin		1 g		10 g	W	Under 10% drug loss in 7 days at 23 °C	1954	C
Cisplatin	BR	500 mg	RC	10 g	NS	13% floxuridine loss in 7 days at room temperature in dark	1386	C
Cisplatin with etoposide		200 mg 300 mg		700 mg	NS	All drugs stable for 7 days at room temperature	1379	C
Cisplatin with leucovorin calcium		200 mg 140 mg		700 mg	NS	All drugs stable for 7 days at room temperature	1379	C
Etoposide		200 mg		10 g	NS	Both drugs stable for 15 days at room temperature	1379	C
Etoposide with cisplatin		300 mg 200 mg		700 mg	NS	All drugs stable for 7 days at room temperature	1379	C
Fluorouracil		10 g		10 g	NS	Both drugs stable for 15 days at room temperature	1390	C
Leucovorin calcium	QU	30 mg	QU	1 g	NS	Physically compatible. Stable for 48 hr at 4 and 20 °C. No floxuridine and 10% leucovorin loss in 48 hr at 40 °C	1317	C
	QU	240 mg	QU	2 g	NS	Physically compatible. Stable for 48 hr at 4 and 20 °C. No floxuridine and 7% leucovorin loss in 48 hr at 40 °C	1317	C
	QU	960 mg	QU	4 g	NS	Physically compatible. Stable for 48 hr at 4, 20, and 40 °C	1317	C
		200 mg		10 g	NS	Both drugs stable for 15 days at room temperature protected from light	1387	C
Leucovorin calcium with cisplatin		140 mg 200 mg		700 mg	NS	All drugs stable for 7 days at room temperature	1379	C

Y-Site Injection Compatibility (1:1 Mixture)

Floxuridine

Drug	Mfr	Conc	Mfr	Conc	Remarks	Ref	C/I
Allopurinol sodium	BW	3 mg/mL[b]	RC	3 mg/mL[b]	Tiny particles form in 1 to 4 hr	1686	**I**
Amifostine	USB	10 mg/mL[a]	RC	3 mg/mL[a]	Physically compatible for 4 hr at 23 °C	1845	**C**
Aztreonam	SQ	40 mg/mL[a]	RC	3 mg/mL[a]	Physically compatible for 4 hr at 23 °C	1758	**C**
Etoposide phosphate	BR	5 mg/mL[a]	RC	3 mg/mL[a]	Physically compatible for 4 hr at 23 °C	2218	**C**
Filgrastim	AMG	30 mcg/mL[a]	RC	3 mg/mL[a]	Physically compatible for 4 hr at 22 °C	1687	**C**
Fludarabine phosphate	BX	1 mg/mL[a]	RC	3 mg/mL[a]	Visually compatible for 4 hr at 22 °C	1439	**C**
Gemcitabine HCl	LI	10 mg/mL[b]	RC	3 mg/mL[b]	Physically compatible for 4 hr at 23 °C	2226	**C**
Granisetron HCl	SKB	0.05 mg/mL[a]	RC	3 mg/mL[a]	Physically compatible for 4 hr at 23 °C	2000	**C**
Melphalan HCl	BW	0.1 mg/mL[b]	RC	3 mg/mL[b]	Physically compatible for 3 hr at 22 °C	1557	**C**
Ondansetron HCl	GL	1 mg/mL[b]	RC	3 mg/mL[a]	Visually compatible for 4 hr at 22 °C	1365	**C**
Paclitaxel	NCI	1.2 mg/mL[a]	RC	3 mg/mL[a]	Physically compatible for 4 hr at 22 °C	1556	**C**
Piperacillin sodium–tazobactam sodium	LE[d]	40 + 5 mg/mL[a]	RC	3 mg/mL[a]	Physically compatible for 4 hr at 22 °C	1688	**C**
Sargramostim	IMM	10 mcg/mL[b]	RC	3 mg/mL[b]	Visually compatible for 4 hr at 22 °C	1436	**C**
Teniposide	BR	0.1 mg/mL[a]	RC	3 mg/mL[a]	Physically compatible for 4 hr at 23 °C	1725	**C**
Thiotepa	IMM[c]	1 mg/mL[a]	RC	3 mg/mL[a]	Physically compatible for 4 hr at 23 °C	1861	**C**
Vinorelbine tartrate	BW	1 mg/mL[b]	RC	3 mg/mL[b]	Physically compatible for 4 hr at 22 °C	1558	**C**

[a] Tested in dextrose 5%.
[b] Tested in sodium chloride 0.9%.
[c] Lyophilized formulation tested.
[d] Test performed using the formulation WITHOUT edetate disodium.

FLUCONAZOLE
AHFS 8:14.08

Products — Fluconazole is available for intravenous infusion in 100- and 200-mL glass bottles and PVC bags in sodium chloride or dextrose diluents. Each milliliter of solution contains fluconazole 2 mg and either sodium chloride 9 mg or dextrose 56 mg. (1)

pH — From 4 to 8 in the sodium chloride diluent and from 3.5 to 6.5 in the dextrose diluent. (1)

Osmolarity — The infusion solution is iso-osmotic (1), having an osmolarity of 300 to 315 mOsm/L. (4)

Trade Name(s) — Diflucan.

Administration — Fluconazole is administered by intravenous infusion at a rate not exceeding 200 mg/hr. (1; 4)

Stability — Fluconazole injection in glass bottles or PVC bags should be stored between 5 and 30 °C or between 5 and 25 °C, respectively, and protected from freezing. Brief exposure to temperatures up to 40 °C does not adversely affect the product in PVC bags. The overwrap moisture barrier should not be removed from the PVC bags until ready for use. The solution should not be used if it is cloudy or precipitated. (1; 4)

Elastomeric Reservoir Pumps — Fluconazole (Pfizer) 2 mg/mL in sodium chloride 0.9% was evaluated for binding to natural rubber elastomeric reservoirs (Baxter). Less than 2% binding was found after storage for two weeks at 35 °C with gentle agitation. (2014)

Central Venous Catheter — Fluconazole (Roerig) 2 mg/mL in dextrose 5% was found to be compatible with the ARROWg+ard Blue Plus (Arrow International) chlorhexidine-bearing triple-lumen central catheter. Essentially complete delivery of the drug was found with little or no drug loss occurring. Furthermore, chlorhexidine delivered from the catheter remained at trace amounts with no substantial increase due to the delivery of the drug through the catheter. (2335)

Compatibility Information

Solution Compatibility

Fluconazole

Solution	Mfr	Mfr	Conc/L	Remarks	Ref	C/I
Dextrose 5%	BA[a]	PF	1 g	Stable for 24 hr at 25 °C in fluorescent light	1676	C
Ringer's injection, lactated	BA[a]	PF	1 g	Stable for 24 hr at 25 °C in fluorescent light	1676	C

[a]Tested in PVC containers.

Additive Compatibility

Fluconazole

Drug	Mfr	Conc/L	Mfr	Conc/L	Test Soln	Remarks	Ref	C/I
Acyclovir sodium	BW	5 g	PF	1 g	D5W	Visually compatible with no fluconazole loss in 72 hr at 25 °C under fluorescent light. Acyclovir not tested	1677	C
Amikacin sulfate	BR	2.5 g	PF	1 g	D5W	Visually compatible with no fluconazole loss in 72 hr at 25 °C under fluorescent light. Amikacin not tested	1677	C
Amphotericin B	LY	50 mg	PF	1 g	D5W	Visually compatible with no fluconazole loss in 72 hr at 25 °C. Amphotericin B not tested	1677	C
Cefazolin sodium	SM	10 g	PF	1 g	D5W	Visually compatible with no fluconazole loss in 72 hr at 25 °C under fluorescent light. Cefazolin not tested	1677	C
Ceftazidime	GL	20 g	PF	1 g	D5W	Visually compatible with no fluconazole loss in 72 hr at 25 °C under fluorescent light. Ceftazidime not tested	1677	C
Ciprofloxacin	BAY	1 g	RR	1 g		Visually compatible with no loss of ciprofloxacin in 24 hr at 22 °C under fluorescent light. Fluconazole not tested	2413	C
Clindamycin phosphate	AST	6 g	PF	1 g	D5W	Visually compatible with no fluconazole loss in 72 hr at 25 °C under fluorescent light. Clindamycin not tested	1677	C
Gentamicin sulfate	SO	0.5 g	PF	1 g	D5W	Visually compatible with no fluconazole loss in 72 hr at 25 °C under fluorescent light. Gentamicin not tested	1677	C
Heparin sodium	BA	50,000 units	PF	1 g	D5W[a]	Fluconazole stable for 24 hr at 25 °C in fluorescent light. Heparin not tested	1676	C
Meropenem	ZEN	1 and 20 g	RR	2 g	NS	Visually compatible for 4 hr at room temperature	1994	C
Metronidazole	AB	2.5 g	PF	1 g		Visually compatible with no fluconazole loss in 72 hr at 25 °C under fluorescent light. Metronidazole not tested	1677	C
Morphine sulfate	ES	0.25 g	PF	1 g	D5W[a]	Fluconazole stable for 24 hr at 25 °C in fluorescent light. Morphine not tested	1676	C
Ondansetron HCl with ranitidine HCl	GL GL	100 mg 500 mg	RR	2 g	[a]	Visually compatible with no loss of any drug in 4 hr	1730	C
Potassium chloride	AB	10 mEq	PF	1 g	D5W[a]	Fluconazole stable for 24 hr at 25 °C in fluorescent light	1676	C

Additive Compatibility (Cont.)

Fluconazole

Drug	Mfr	Conc/L	Mfr	Conc/L	Test Soln	Remarks	Ref	C/I
Ranitidine HCl with ondansetron HCl	GL GL	500 mg 100 mg	RR	2 g	a	Visually compatible with no loss of any drug in 4 hr	1730	**C**
Theophylline	BA	0.4 g	PF	1 g	D5W[a]	Fluconazole stable for 72 hr at 25 °C in fluorescent light. Theophylline not tested	1676	**C**
Trimethoprim–sulfamethoxazole	ES	0.4 + 2 g	PF	1 g	D5W	Delayed cloudiness and precipitation. No fluconazole loss in 72 hr at 25 °C under fluorescent light	1677	**I**

[a]Tested in PVC containers.

Drugs in Syringe Compatibility

Fluconazole

Drug (in syringe)	Mfr	Amt	Mfr	Amt	Remarks	Ref	C/I
Pantoprazole sodium	a	4 mg/ 1 mL		2 mg/ 1 mL	Possible precipitate within 4 hr	2574	**I**

[a]Test performed using the formulation WITHOUT edetate disodium.

Y-Site Injection Compatibility (1:1 Mixture)

Fluconazole

Drug	Mfr	Conc	Mfr	Conc	Remarks	Ref	C/I
Acyclovir sodium	BW	10 mg/mL	RR	2 mg/mL	Physically compatible for 24 hr at 25 °C	1407	**C**
Aldesleukin	CHI	33,800 I.U./ mL[a]	RR	2 mg/mL[a]	Visually compatible with little or no loss of aldesleukin activity	1857	**C**
Allopurinol sodium	BW	3 mg/mL[b]	RR	2 mg/mL	Physically compatible for 4 hr at 22 °C	1686	**C**
Amifostine	USB	10 mg/mL[a]	RR	2 mg/mL	Physically compatible for 4 hr at 23 °C	1845	**C**
Amikacin sulfate	BR	20 mg/mL	RR	2 mg/mL	Physically compatible for 24 hr at 25 °C	1407	**C**
Aminophylline	ES AMR	25 mg/mL 0.8 and 1.5 mg/mL[a,b]	RR PF	2 mg/mL 0.5 and 1.5 mg/mL[a,b]	Physically compatible for 24 hr at 25 °C Visually compatible with no loss of either drug in 3 hr at 24 °C	1407 1626	**C** **C**
Amiodarone HCl	WY	6 mg/mL[a]	PF	2 mg/mL[b]	Visually compatible for 24 hr at 22 °C	2352	**C**
Amphotericin B	SQ	5 mg/mL	RR	2 mg/mL	Cloudiness and yellow precipitate	1407	**I**
Amphotericin B cholesteryl sulfate complex	SEQ	0.83 mg/mL[a]	RR	2 mg/mL	Gross precipitate forms	2117	**I**
Ampicillin sodium	WY	20 mg/mL	RR	2 mg/mL	Cloudiness develops	1407	**I**
Ampicillin sodium–sulbactam sodium	PF	40 + 20 mg/ mL	RR	2 mg/mL	Physically compatible for 24 hr at 25 °C	1407	**C**
Anakinra	SYN	4 and 36 mg/ mL[b]	PF	2 mg/mL[b]	Physically compatible. No fluconazole loss in 4 hr at 25 °C. Anakinra uncertain	2508	**?**
Anidulafungin	VIC	0.5 mg/mL[a]	PF	2 mg/mL	Physically compatible for 4 hr at 23 °C	2617	**C**
Aztreonam	SQ SQ	40 mg/mL 40 mg/mL[a]	RR RR	2 mg/mL 2 mg/mL	Visually compatible for 24 hr at 25 °C Physically compatible for 4 hr at 23 °C	1407 1758	**C** **C**
Benztropine mesylate	MSD	1 mg/mL	RR	2 mg/mL	Physically compatible for 24 hr at 25 °C	1407	**C**

Y-Site Injection Compatibility (1:1 Mixture) (Cont.)

Fluconazole

Drug	Mfr	Conc	Mfr	Conc	Remarks	Ref	C/I
Bivalirudin	TMC	5 mg/mL[a]	PF	2 mg/mL	Physically compatible for 4 hr at 23 °C	2373	C
Calcium gluconate	ES	100 mg/mL	RR	2 mg/mL	Cloudiness develops	1407	I
Caspofungin acetate	ME	0.5 mg/mL[b]	HOS	2 mg/mL	Physically compatible over 60 min	2766	C
Cefazolin sodium	LY	40 mg/mL	RR	2 mg/mL	Physically compatible for 24 hr at 25 °C	1407	C
Cefepime HCl	BMS	120 mg/mL[k]		2 mg/mL	Physically compatible with less than 10% cefepime loss. Fluconazole not tested	2513	C
Cefotaxime sodium	HO	20 mg/mL	RR	2 mg/mL	Cloudiness and amber color develop	1407	I
Cefotetan disodium	STU	40 mg/mL	RR	2 mg/mL	Physically compatible for 24 hr at 25 °C	1407	C
Cefoxitin sodium	MSD	40 mg/mL	RR	2 mg/mL	Physically compatible for 24 hr at 25 °C	1407	C
Ceftaroline fosamil	FOR	2.22 mg/mL[a,b,j]	BED	2 mg/mL	Physically compatible for 4 hr at 23 °C	2826	C
Ceftazidime	GL	20 mg/mL	RR	2 mg/mL	Precipitates immediately	1407	I
	SKB	125 mg/mL		2 mg/mL	Visually compatible with less than 10% loss of ceftazidime in 30 min. Fluconazole not tested	2434	C
	GSK	120 mg/mL[k]		2 mg/mL	Physically compatible with less than 10% ceftazidime loss. Fluconazole not tested	2513	C
Ceftriaxone sodium	RC	40 mg/mL	RR	2 mg/mL	Precipitates immediately	1407	I
Cefuroxime sodium	GL	30 mg/mL	RR	2 mg/mL	Precipitates immediately	1407	I
Chloramphenicol sodium succinate	PD	20 mg/mL	RR	2 mg/mL	Gas production	1407	I
Chlorpromazine HCl	ES	25 mg/mL	RR	2 mg/mL	Physically compatible for 24 hr at 25 °C	1407	C
Cisatracurium besylate	GW	0.1, 2, 5 mg/mL[a]	RR	2 mg/mL	Physically compatible for 4 hr at 23 °C	2074	C
Clindamycin phosphate	AB	24 mg/mL	RR	2 mg/mL	Precipitates immediately	1407	I
Daptomycin	CUB	6.3 mg/mL[b,c]	PF	1.3 mg/mL[c]	Physically compatible. No daptomycin loss and 4% fluconazole loss in 2 hr at 25 °C	2553	C
Dexamethasone sodium phosphate	ES	4 mg/mL	RR	2 mg/mL	Physically compatible for 24 hr at 25 °C	1407	C
Dexmedetomidine HCl	AB	4 mcg/mL[b]	PF	2 mg/mL	Physically compatible for 4 hr at 23 °C	2383	C
Diazepam	ES	5 mg/mL	RR	2 mg/mL	Precipitates immediately	1407	I
Digoxin	BW	0.25 mg/mL	RR	2 mg/mL	Gas production	1407	I
Diltiazem HCl	MMD	5 mg/mL	RR	2 mg/mL	Visually compatible	1807	C
Dimenhydrinate		10 mg/mL		2 mg/mL	Clear solution	2569	C
Diphenhydramine HCl	ES	50 mg/mL	RR	2 mg/mL	Physically compatible for 24 hr at 25 °C	1407	C
Dobutamine HCl	LI	2 mg/mL[a]	RR	2 mg/mL	Visually compatible for 24 hr at 28 °C under fluorescent light	1760	C
Docetaxel	RPR	0.9 mg/mL[a]	RR	2 mg/mL	Physically compatible for 4 hr at 23 °C	2224	C
Dopamine HCl	AMR	1.6 mg/mL[a]	RR	2 mg/mL	Visually compatible for 24 hr at 28 °C under fluorescent light	1760	C
Doripenem	JJ	5 mg/mL[a,b]	HAE	2 mg/mL	Physically compatible for 4 hr at 23 °C	2743	C
Doxorubicin HCl liposomal	SEQ	0.4 mg/mL[a]	RR	2 mg/mL	Physically compatible for 4 hr at 23 °C	2087	C
Droperidol	DU	2.5 mg/mL	RR	2 mg/mL	Physically compatible for 24 hr at 25 °C	1407	C

Y-Site Injection Compatibility (1:1 Mixture) (Cont.)

Fluconazole

Drug	Mfr	Conc	Mfr	Conc	Remarks	Ref	C/I
Etoposide phosphate	BR	5 mg/mL[a]	RR	2 mg/mL	Physically compatible for 4 hr at 23 °C	2218	**C**
Famotidine	MSD	10 mg/mL	RR	2 mg/mL	Physically compatible for 24 hr at 25 °C	1407	**C**
	ME	2 mg/mL[b]		2 mg/mL[a]	Visually compatible for 4 hr at 22 °C	1936	**C**
Fenoldopam mesylate	AB	80 mcg/mL[b]	PF	2 mg/mL	Physically compatible for 4 hr at 23 °C	2467	**C**
Filgrastim	AMG	30 mcg/mL[a]	RR	2 mg/mL	Physically compatible for 4 hr at 22 °C	1687	**C**
	AMG	10[e] and 40[a] mcg/mL	RR	2 mg/mL[a]	Visually compatible. Little loss of filgrastim and fluconazole in 4 hr at 25 °C	2060	**C**
Fludarabine phosphate	BX	1 mg/mL[a]	RR	2 mg/mL	Visually compatible for 4 hr at 22 °C	1439	**C**
Foscarnet sodium	AST	24 mg/mL	RR	2 mg/mL	Physically compatible for 24 hr at 25 °C	1407	**C**
Furosemide	ES	10 mg/mL	RR	2 mg/mL	Precipitate forms	1407	**I**
Gallium nitrate	FUJ	1 mg/mL[b]	PF	2 mg/mL	Visually compatible for 24 hr at 25 °C	1673	**C**
Ganciclovir sodium	SY	50 mg/mL	RR	2 mg/mL	Physically compatible for 24 hr at 25 °C	1407	**C**
Gemcitabine HCl	LI	10 mg/mL[b]	RR	2 mg/mL	Physically compatible for 4 hr at 23 °C	2226	**C**
Gentamicin sulfate	ES	4 mg/mL	RR	2 mg/mL	Physically compatible for 24 hr at 25 °C	1407	**C**
Granisetron HCl	SKB	0.05 mg/mL[a]	PF	2 mg/mL	Physically compatible for 4 hr at 23 °C	2000	**C**
Haloperidol lactate	MN	5 mg/mL	RR	2 mg/mL	Precipitate forms	1407	**I**
Heparin sodium	LY	1000 units/mL	RR	2 mg/mL	Physically compatible for 24 hr at 25 °C	1407	**C**
	TR	50 units/mL	PF	2 mg/mL	Visually compatible for 4 hr at 25 °C	1793	**C**
Hetastarch in lactated electrolyte	AB	6%	PF	2 mg/mL	Physically compatible for 4 hr at 23 °C	2339	**C**
Hydroxyzine HCl	ES	50 mg/mL	RR	2 mg/mL	Cloudiness develops	1407	**I**
Imipenem–cilastatin sodium	MSD	10 mg/mL	RR	2 mg/mL	Precipitates immediately	1407	**I**
Immune globulin intravenous	CU	50 mg/mL	RR	2 mg/mL	Physically compatible for 24 hr at 25 °C	1407	**C**
Leucovorin calcium	LE	10 mg/mL	RR	2 mg/mL	Physically compatible for 24 hr at 25 °C	1407	**C**
Linezolid	PHU	2 mg/mL	RR	2 mg/mL	Physically compatible for 4 hr at 23 °C	2264	**C**
Lorazepam	WY	0.33 mg/mL[b]	PF	2 mg/mL	Visually compatible for 24 hr at 22 °C	1855	**C**
Melphalan HCl	BW	0.1 mg/mL[b]	RR	2 mg/mL	Physically compatible for 3 hr at 22 °C	1557	**C**
Meperidine HCl	AB	10 mg/mL	RR	2 mg/mL	Physically compatible for 4 hr at 25 °C	1397	**C**
Meropenem	ZEN	1 and 50 mg/mL[b]	RR	2 mg/mL	Visually compatible for 4 hr at room temperature	1994	**C**
Metoclopramide HCl	RB	5 mg/mL	RR	2 mg/mL	Physically compatible for 24 hr at 25 °C	1407	**C**
Metronidazole	AB	5 mg/mL	RR	2 mg/mL	Physically compatible for 24 hr at 25 °C	1407	**C**
Midazolam HCl	RC	5 mg/mL	RR	2 mg/mL	Physically compatible for 24 hr at 25 °C	1407	**C**
	RC	5 mg/mL	PF	2 mg/mL	Visually compatible for 24 hr at 22 °C	1855	**C**
Morphine sulfate	IMS	25 mg/mL	RR	2 mg/mL	Physically compatible for 24 hr at 25 °C	1407	**C**
	AB	1 mg/mL	RR	2 mg/mL	Physically compatible for 4 hr at 25 °C	1397	**C**
Nafcillin sodium	BR	20 mg/mL	RR	2 mg/mL	Physically compatible for 24 hr at 25 °C	1407	**C**
Nitroglycerin	AMR	0.2 mg/mL[a]	RR	2 mg/mL	Visually compatible for 24 hr at 28 °C under fluorescent light	1760	**C**
Ondansetron HCl	GL	1 mg/mL[b]	PF	2 mg/mL	Visually compatible for 4 hr at 22 °C	1365	**C**
	GL	0.03 and 0.3 mg/mL[a]	RR	2 mg/mL[b]	Visually compatible. Little loss of either drug in 4 hr at 25 °C in light	1732	**C**

Y-Site Injection Compatibility (1:1 Mixture) (Cont.)

Fluconazole

Drug	Mfr	Conc	Mfr	Conc	Remarks	Ref	C/I
	GL	0.03, 0.1, 0.3 mg/mL[a,b]	RR	2 mg/mL	Visually compatible. Little loss of both drugs in 4 hr. 5% or less loss of both in 12 hr at room temperature	2168	C
Oxacillin sodium	BE	40 mg/mL	RR	2 mg/mL	Physically compatible for 24 hr at 25 °C	1407	C
Paclitaxel	NCI	1.2 mg/mL[a]	RR	2 mg/mL	Physically compatible for 4 hr at 22 °C	1556	C
	BR	0.3 and 1.2 mg/mL[a]	PF	2 mg/mL	Visually compatible. No loss of either drug in 4 hr at 23 °C	1790	C
Pancuronium bromide	GNS	0.5 mg/mL[b]	RR	2 mg/mL	Visually compatible for 24 hr at 28 °C under fluorescent light	1760	C
Pemetrexed disodium	LI	20 mg/mL[b]	PF	2 mg/mL	Physically compatible for 4 hr at 23 °C	2564	C
Penicillin G potassium	RR	100,000 units/mL	RR	2 mg/mL	Physically compatible for 24 hr at 25 °C	1407	C
Pentamidine isethionate	LY	6 mg/mL	RR	2 mg/mL	Cloudiness develops	1407	I
Phenytoin sodium	PD	50 mg/mL	RR	2 mg/mL	Physically compatible for 24 hr at 25 °C	1407	C
Piperacillin sodium–tazobactam sodium	LE[l]	40 + 5 mg/mL[a]	RR	2 mg/mL	Physically compatible for 4 hr at 22 °C	1688	C
Prochlorperazine edisylate	SKF	5 mg/mL	RR	2 mg/mL	Physically compatible for 24 hr at 25 °C	1407	C
Promethazine HCl	ES	50 mg/mL	RR	2 mg/mL	Physically compatible for 24 hr at 25 °C	1407	C
Propofol	ZEN	10 mg/mL	PF	2 mg/mL[a]	Physically compatible for 1 hr at 23 °C	2066	C
Quinupristin–dalfopristin	AVE	2 mg/mL[a]		2 mg/mL	Physically compatible	1	C
Ranitidine HCl	GL	0.5 and 2 mg/mL[a]	RR	2 mg/mL[b]	Visually compatible. No loss of either drug in 4 hr	1730	C
Remifentanil HCl	GW	0.025 and 0.25 mg/mL[b]	RR	2 mg/mL	Physically compatible for 4 hr at 23 °C	2075	C
Sargramostim	IMM	10 mcg/mL[b]	RR	2 mg/mL	Visually compatible for 4 hr at 22 °C	1436	C
Tacrolimus	FUJ	1 mg/mL[b]	RR	2 mg/mL[a]	Visually compatible for 24 hr at 25 °C	1630	C
	FUJ	5 and 20 mcg/mL[b]	PF	0.5 and 1.5 mg/mL[b]	Visually compatible. No loss of either drug in 3 hr at 24 °C	2236	C
Telavancin HCl	ASP	7.5 mg/mL[b]	SAG	2 mg/mL[b]	Physically compatible for 2 hr	2830	C
Teniposide	BR	0.1 mg/mL[a]	RR	2 mg/mL	Physically compatible for 4 hr at 23 °C	1725	C
Theophylline	AMR	1.6 mg/mL[a]	RR	2 mg/mL	Visually compatible for 24 hr at 28 °C under fluorescent light	1760	C
	TR	4 mg/mL	PF	2 mg/mL	Visually compatible for 6 hr at 25 °C	1793	C
Thiotepa	IMM[f]	1 mg/mL[a]	RR	2 mg/mL	Physically compatible for 4 hr at 23 °C	1861	C
Ticarcillin disodium–clavulanate potassium	BE	60 mg/mL	RR	2 mg/mL	Physically compatible for 24 hr at 25 °C	1407	C
Tigecycline	WY	1 mg/mL[b]		2 mg/mL	Physically compatible for 4 hr	2714	C
Tobramycin sulfate	LI	40 mg/mL	RR	2 mg/mL	Physically compatible for 24 hr at 25 °C	1407	C
TNA #218 to #226[g]			PF	2 mg/mL	Visually compatible for 4 hr at 23 °C	2215	C
TPN #146[g]		[h]	PF	0.5 and 1.75 mg/mL[h]	Visually compatible with no fluconazole loss in 2 hr at 24 °C in fluorescent light. Amino acids greater than 93%	1554	C

Y-Site Injection Compatibility (1:1 Mixture) (Cont.)

Fluconazole

Drug	Mfr	Conc	Mfr	Conc	Remarks	Ref	C/I
TPN #147, #148[g]	[h]		PF	0.5 and 1.75 mg/mL[h]	Visually compatible with no fluconazole loss in 2 hr at 24 °C in fluorescent light. Amino acids not analyzed	1554	**C**
TPN #212 to #215[g]			RR	2 mg/mL	Physically compatible for 4 hr at 23 °C	2109	**C**
Trimethoprim–sulfamethoxazole	BW	16 + 80 mg/mL	RR	2 mg/mL	Viscous gel-like substance forms	1407	**I**
Vancomycin HCl	LY	20 mg/mL	RR	2 mg/mL	Physically compatible for 24 hr at 25 °C	1407	**C**
Vasopressin	APP	0.2 unit/mL[b]	PF	2 mg/mL	Physically compatible	2641	**C**
Vecuronium bromide	OR	1 mg/mL[a]	RR	2 mg/mL	Visually compatible for 24 hr at 28 °C under fluorescent light	1760	**C**
Vinorelbine tartrate	BW	1 mg/mL[b]	RR	2 mg/mL	Physically compatible for 4 hr at 22 °C	1558	**C**
Zidovudine	BW	10 mg/mL	RR	2 mg/mL	Physically compatible for 24 hr at 25 °C	1407	**C**

[a]*Tested in dextrose 5%.*
[b]*Tested in sodium chloride 0.9%.*
[c]*Final concentration after mixing.*
[d]*Tested in dextrose 5%, Ringer's injection, lactated, sodium chloride 0.45%, and sodium chloride 0.9%.*
[e]*Tested in dextrose 5% with albumin human 2 mg/mL.*
[f]*Lyophilized formulation tested.*
[g]*Refer to Appendix I for the composition of parenteral nutrition solutions. TNA indicates a 3-in-1 admixture, and TPN indicates a 2-in-1 admixture.*
[h]*Varying volumes to simulate varying administration rates.*
[i]*Final concentrations were 1.5 mg/mL of fluconazole and 5 and 20 mcg/mL of tacrolimus.*
[j]*Tested in Ringer's injection, lactated.*
[k]*Tested in sterile water for injection.*
[l]*Test performed using the formulation WITHOUT edetate disodium.*

FLUDARABINE PHOSPHATE
AHFS 10:00

Products — Fludarabine phosphate is supplied as a lyophilized product in 6-mL vials containing 50 mg of drug with mannitol 50 mg and sodium hydroxide for pH adjustment. Reconstitute with 2 mL of sterile water for injection to yield a 25-mg/mL concentration. (1)

Fludarabine phosphate is also available as a 50-mg/2 mL solution with disodium phosphate dihydrate and sodium hydroxide for pH adjustment. (1)

pH — From pH 7.2 to 8.2 for the reconstituted powder. From pH 7.3 to 7.7 for the liquid. (1)

Trade Name(s) — Fludara.

Administration — Fludarabine phosphate is administered by intravenous infusion over 30 minutes in 100 or 125 mL of dextrose 5% or sodium chloride 0.9%. (1; 4) The drug also has been administered by rapid intravenous injection and continuous infusion, although the risk of toxicity may be increased. (4)

Stability — Intact vials should be stored under refrigeration. The manufacturer recommends use of the reconstituted solution within eight hours because it does not contain an antibacterial preservative. (1) Nevertheless, the drug is chemically stable in solution, exhibiting less than 2% decomposition in 16 days when stored at room temperature and exposed to normal laboratory light. (234)

Fludarabine phosphate (Berlex) 0.2 mg/mL diluted in sodium chloride 0.9% and stored at 22 °C did not exhibit an antimicrobial effect on the growth of *Enterococcus faecium, Staphylococcus aureus, Pseudomonas aeruginosa,* and *Candida albicans* inoculated into the solution. Diluted solutions should be stored under refrigeration whenever possible, and the potential for microbiological growth should be considered when assigning expiration dates. (2160)

pH Effects — Fludarabine phosphate is stable in aqueous solution at pH 4.5 to 8. The pH of optimum stability is approximately 7.6. (234)

Sorption — Fludarabine phosphate 0.04 mg/mL in dextrose 5% or sodium chloride 0.9% was equally stable in either glass or PVC containers, exhibiting no loss due to sorption during 48 hours at room temperature or under refrigeration. (234)

Compatibility Information

Solution Compatibility

Fludarabine phosphate

Solution	Mfr	Mfr	Conc/L	Remarks	Ref	C/I
Dextrose 5%			1 g	Under 3% loss in 16 days at room temperature in light	234	C
			40 mg	No loss in 48 hr at room temperature or refrigerated	234	C
Sodium chloride 0.9%			1 g	Under 3% loss in 16 days at room temperature in light	234	C

Y-Site Injection Compatibility (1:1 Mixture)

Fludarabine phosphate

Drug	Mfr	Conc	Mfr	Conc	Remarks	Ref	C/I
Acyclovir sodium	BW	7 mg/mL[a]	BX	1 mg/mL[a]	Color darkens within 4 hr	1439	I
Allopurinol sodium	BW	3 mg/mL[b]	BX	1 mg/mL[b]	Physically compatible for 4 hr at 22 °C	1686	C
Amifostine	USB	10 mg/mL[a]	BX	1 mg/mL[a]	Physically compatible for 4 hr at 23 °C	1845	C
Amikacin sulfate	BR	5 mg/mL[a]	BX	1 mg/mL[a]	Visually compatible for 4 hr at 22 °C	1439	C
Aminophylline	ES	2.5 mg/mL[a]	BX	1 mg/mL[a]	Visually compatible for 4 hr at 22 °C	1439	C
Amphotericin B	SQ	0.6 mg/mL[a]	BX	1 mg/mL[a]	Precipitate forms in 4 hr at 22 °C	1439	I
Ampicillin sodium	BR	20 mg/mL[b]	BX	1 mg/mL[a]	Visually compatible for 4 hr at 22 °C	1439	C
Ampicillin sodium–sulbactam sodium	RR	20 + 10 mg/mL[b]	BX	1 mg/mL[a]	Visually compatible for 4 hr at 22 °C	1439	C
Amsacrine	NCI	1 mg/mL[a]	BX	1 mg/mL[a]	Visually compatible for 4 hr at 22 °C	1439	C
Aztreonam	SQ	40 mg/mL[a]	BX	1 mg/mL[a]	Visually compatible for 4 hr at 22 °C	1439	C
	SQ	40 mg/mL[a]	BX	1 mg/mL[a]	Physically compatible for 4 hr at 23 °C	1758	C
Bleomycin sulfate	BR	1 unit/mL[b]	BX	1 mg/mL[a]	Visually compatible for 4 hr at 22 °C	1439	C
Butorphanol tartrate	BR	0.04 mg/mL[a]	BX	1 mg/mL[a]	Visually compatible for 4 hr at 22 °C	1439	C
Carboplatin	BR	5 mg/mL[a]	BX	1 mg/mL[a]	Visually compatible for 4 hr at 22 °C	1439	C
Carmustine	BR	1.5 mg/mL[a]	BX	1 mg/mL[a]	Visually compatible for 4 hr at 22 °C	1439	C
Cefazolin sodium	LEM	20 mg/mL[a]	BX	1 mg/mL[a]	Visually compatible for 4 hr at 22 °C	1439	C
Cefotaxime sodium	HO	20 mg/mL[a]	BX	1 mg/mL[a]	Visually compatible for 4 hr at 22 °C	1439	C
Cefotetan disodium	STU	20 mg/mL[a]	BX	1 mg/mL[a]	Visually compatible for 4 hr at 22 °C	1439	C
Ceftazidime	GL	40 mg/mL[a]	BX	1 mg/mL[a]	Visually compatible for 4 hr at 22 °C	1439	C
Ceftriaxone sodium	RC	20 mg/mL[a]	BX	1 mg/mL[a]	Visually compatible for 4 hr at 22 °C	1439	C
Cefuroxime sodium	GL	30 mg/mL[a]	BX	1 mg/mL[a]	Visually compatible for 4 hr at 22 °C	1439	C
Chlorpromazine HCl	ES	2 mg/mL[a]	BX	1 mg/mL[a]	Initial light haze intensifies within 30 min	1439	I
Cisplatin	BR	1 mg/mL	BX	1 mg/mL[a]	Visually compatible for 4 hr at 22 °C	1439	C
Clindamycin phosphate	LY	10 mg/mL[a]	BX	1 mg/mL[a]	Visually compatible for 4 hr at 22 °C	1439	C
Cyclophosphamide	MJ	10 mg/mL[a]	BX	1 mg/mL[a]	Visually compatible for 4 hr at 22 °C	1439	C
Cytarabine	UP	50 mg/mL	BX	1 mg/mL[a]	Visually compatible for 4 hr at 22 °C	1439	C
Dacarbazine	MI	4 mg/mL[a]	BX	1 mg/mL[a]	Visually compatible for 4 hr at 22 °C	1439	C
Dactinomycin	MSD	0.01 mg/mL[a]	BX	1 mg/mL[a]	Visually compatible for 4 hr at 22 °C	1439	C

Y-Site Injection Compatibility (1:1 Mixture) (Cont.)

Fludarabine phosphate

Drug	Mfr	Conc	Mfr	Conc	Remarks	Ref	C/I
Daunorubicin HCl	WY	2 mg/mL[a]	BX	1 mg/mL[a]	Slight haze forms in 4 hr at 22 °C	1439	I
Dexamethasone sodium phosphate	MSD	1 mg/mL[a]	BX	1 mg/mL[a]	Visually compatible for 4 hr at 22 °C	1439	C
Diphenhydramine HCl	WY	2 mg/mL[a]	BX	1 mg/mL[a]	Visually compatible for 4 hr at 22 °C	1439	C
Doxorubicin HCl	CET	2 mg/mL	BX	1 mg/mL[a]	Visually compatible for 4 hr at 22 °C	1439	C
Doxycycline hyclate	ES	1 mg/mL[a]	BX	1 mg/mL[a]	Visually compatible for 4 hr at 22 °C	1439	C
Droperidol	JN	0.4 mg/mL[a]	BX	1 mg/mL[a]	Visually compatible for 4 hr at 22 °C	1439	C
Etoposide	BR	0.4 mg/mL[a]	BX	1 mg/mL[a]	Visually compatible for 4 hr at 22 °C	1439	C
Etoposide phosphate	BR	5 mg/mL[a]	BX	1 mg/mL[a]	Physically compatible for 4 hr at 23 °C	2218	C
Famotidine	MSD	2 mg/mL[a]	BX	1 mg/mL[a]	Visually compatible for 4 hr at 22 °C	1439	C
Filgrastim	AMG	30 mcg/mL[a]	BX	1 mg/mL[a]	Physically compatible for 4 hr at 22 °C	1687	C
Floxuridine	RC	3 mg/mL[a]	BX	1 mg/mL[a]	Visually compatible for 4 hr at 22 °C	1439	C
Fluconazole	RR	2 mg/mL	BX	1 mg/mL[a]	Visually compatible for 4 hr at 22 °C	1439	C
Fluorouracil	LY	16 mg/mL[a]	BX	1 mg/mL[a]	Visually compatible for 4 hr at 22 °C	1439	C
Furosemide	AB	3 mg/mL[a]	BX	1 mg/mL[a]	Visually compatible for 4 hr at 22 °C	1439	C
Ganciclovir sodium	SY	20 mg/mL[a]	BX	1 mg/mL[a]	Darker color forms within 4 hr	1439	I
Gemcitabine HCl	LI	10 mg/mL[b]	BX	1 mg/mL[b]	Physically compatible for 4 hr at 23 °C	2226	C
Gentamicin sulfate	ES	5 mg/mL[a]	BX	1 mg/mL[a]	Visually compatible for 4 hr at 22 °C	1439	C
Granisetron HCl	SKB	0.05 mg/mL[a]	BX	1 mg/mL[a]	Physically compatible for 4 hr at 23 °C	2000	C
Haloperidol lactate	MN	0.2 mg/mL[a]	BX	1 mg/mL[a]	Visually compatible for 4 hr at 22 °C	1439	C
Heparin sodium	SO, WY	40[a], 100, 1000 units/ mL	BX	1 mg/mL[a]	Visually compatible for 4 hr at 22 °C	1439	C
Hydrocortisone sodium succinate	UP	1 mg/mL[a]	BX	1 mg/mL[a]	Visually compatible for 4 hr at 22 °C	1439	C
Hydromorphone HCl	KN	0.5 mg/mL[a]	BX	1 mg/mL[a]	Visually compatible for 4 hr at 22 °C	1439	C
Hydroxyzine HCl	WI	4 mg/mL[a]	BX	1 mg/mL[a]	Slight haze forms immediately	1439	I
Ifosfamide	MJ	25 mg/mL[a]	BX	1 mg/mL[a]	Visually compatible for 4 hr at 22 °C	1439	C
Imipenem–cilastatin sodium	MSD	5 mg/mL[b]	BX	1 mg/mL[a]	Visually compatible for 4 hr at 22 °C	1439	C
Lorazepam	WY	0.1 mg/mL[a]	BX	1 mg/mL[a]	Visually compatible for 4 hr at 22 °C	1439	C
Magnesium sulfate	SO	100 mg/mL[a]	BX	1 mg/mL[a]	Visually compatible for 4 hr at 22 °C	1439	C
Mannitol	BA	15%	BX	1 mg/mL[a]	Visually compatible for 4 hr at 22 °C	1439	C
Mechlorethamine HCl	MSD	1 mg/mL	BX	1 mg/mL[a]	Visually compatible for 4 hr at 22 °C	1439	C
Melphalan HCl	BW	0.1 mg/mL[b]	BX	1 mg/mL[b]	Physically compatible for 3 hr at 22 °C	1557	C
Meperidine HCl	WI	4 mg/mL[a]	BX	1 mg/mL[a]	Visually compatible for 4 hr at 22 °C	1439	C
Mesna	BR	10 mg/mL[a]	BX	1 mg/mL[a]	Visually compatible for 4 hr at 22 °C	1439	C
Methotrexate sodium	CET	15 mg/mL[a]	BX	1 mg/mL[a]	Visually compatible for 4 hr at 22 °C	1439	C
Methylprednisolone sodium succinate	UP	5 mg/mL[a]	BX	1 mg/mL[a]	Visually compatible for 4 hr at 22 °C	1439	C
Metoclopramide HCl	DU	5 mg/mL	BX	1 mg/mL[a]	Visually compatible for 4 hr at 22 °C	1439	C
Mitoxantrone HCl	LE	0.5 mg/mL[a]	BX	1 mg/mL[a]	Visually compatible for 4 hr at 22 °C	1439	C

Y-Site Injection Compatibility (1:1 Mixture) (Cont.)

Fludarabine phosphate

Drug	Mfr	Conc	Mfr	Conc	Remarks	Ref	C/I
Morphine sulfate	WI	1 mg/mL[a]	BX	1 mg/mL[a]	Visually compatible for 4 hr at 22 °C	1439	C
Multivitamins	ROR	0.01 mL/mL[a]	BX	1 mg/mL[a]	Visually compatible for 4 hr at 22 °C	1439	C
Nalbuphine HCl	DU	10 mg/mL	BX	1 mg/mL[a]	Visually compatible for 4 hr at 22 °C	1439	C
Ondansetron HCl	GL	0.5 mg/mL[a]	BX	1 mg/mL[a]	Visually compatible for 4 hr at 22 °C	1439	C
Pentostatin	NCI	0.4 mg/mL[b]	BX	1 mg/mL[a]	Visually compatible for 4 hr at 22 °C	1439	C
Piperacillin sodium–tazobactam sodium	LE[d]	40 + 5 mg/mL[a]	BX	1 mg/mL[a]	Physically compatible for 4 hr at 22 °C	1688	C
Potassium chloride	AB	0.1 mEq/mL[a]	BX	1 mg/mL[a]	Visually compatible for 4 hr at 22 °C	1439	C
Prochlorperazine edisylate	WY	0.5 mg/mL[a]	BX	1 mg/mL[a]	Slight haze forms within 30 min	1439	I
Promethazine HCl	WY	2 mg/mL[a]	BX	1 mg/mL[a]	Visually compatible for 4 hr at 22 °C	1439	C
Ranitidine HCl	GL	2 mg/mL[a]	BX	1 mg/mL[a]	Visually compatible for 4 hr at 22 °C	1439	C
Sodium bicarbonate	AB	1 mEq/mL	BX	1 mg/mL[a]	Visually compatible for 4 hr at 22 °C	1439	C
Teniposide	BR	0.1 mg/mL[a]	BX	1 mg/mL[a]	Physically compatible for 4 hr at 23 °C	1725	C
Thiotepa	IMM[c]	1 mg/mL[a]	BX	1 mg/mL[a]	Physically compatible for 4 hr at 23 °C	1861	C
Ticarcillin disodium–clavulanate potassium	BE	31 mg/mL[a]	BX	1 mg/mL[a]	Visually compatible for 4 hr at 22 °C	1439	C
Tobramycin sulfate	LI	5 mg/mL[a]	BX	1 mg/mL[a]	Visually compatible for 4 hr at 22 °C	1439	C
Trimethoprim–sulfamethoxazole	ES	0.8 + 4 mg/mL[a]	BX	1 mg/mL[a]	Visually compatible for 4 hr at 22 °C	1439	C
Vancomycin HCl	LI	10 mg/mL[a]	BX	1 mg/mL[a]	Visually compatible for 4 hr at 22 °C	1439	C
Vinblastine sulfate	LY	0.12 mg/mL[a]	BX	1 mg/mL[a]	Visually compatible for 4 hr at 22 °C	1439	C
Vincristine sulfate	LY	1 mg/mL	BX	1 mg/mL[a]	Visually compatible for 4 hr at 22 °C	1439	C
Vinorelbine tartrate	BW	1 mg/mL[b]	BX	1 mg/mL[b]	Physically compatible for 4 hr at 22 °C	1558	C
Zidovudine	BW	4 mg/mL[a]	BX	1 mg/mL[a]	Visually compatible for 4 hr at 22 °C	1439	C

[a]Tested in dextrose 5%.
[b]Tested in sodium chloride 0.9%.
[c]Lyophilized formulation tested.
[d]Test performed using the formulation WITHOUT edetate disodium.

FLUMAZENIL
AHFS 28:92

Products — Flumazenil is available as a 0.1-mg/mL solution in 5- and 10-mL multiple-dose vials. In addition to flumazenil, each milliliter also contains methylparaben 1.8 mg, propylparaben 0.2 mg, sodium chloride 0.9%, edetate disodium 0.01%, and acetic acid 0.01%. The pH is adjusted with hydrochloric acid and, if necessary, sodium hydroxide. (1)

pH — The injection has a pH of approximately 4. (1)

Trade Name(s) — Romazicon.

Administration — Flumazenil is administered intravenously over 15 to 30 seconds. To minimize pain at the injection site, flumazenil should be administered through a freely running intravenous infusion line into a large vein. Extravasation should be avoided. (1; 4)

Stability — Flumazenil injection is a stable aqueous solution; it should be stored at controlled room temperature. Discard the product 24 hours after removal from its original vial, whether admixed in an infusion solution or simply drawn into a syringe. (1)

Compatibility Information

Solution Compatibility

Flumazenil

Solution	Mfr	Mfr	Conc/L	Remarks	Ref	C/I
Dextrose 5%				Compatible	1	C
	BA[a]	RC	20 mg	Visually compatible. No loss in 24 hr at 23 °C in fluorescent light	1710	C
Ringer's injection, lactated				Compatible	1	C
Sodium chloride 0.9%				Compatible	1	C

[a]Tested in PVC containers.

Additive Compatibility

Flumazenil

Drug	Mfr	Conc/L	Mfr	Conc/L	Test Soln	Remarks	Ref	C/I
Aminophylline	AMR	2 g	RC	20 mg	D5W[a]	Visually compatible. No flumazenil loss in 24 hr at 23 °C in fluorescent light. Aminophylline not tested	1710	C
Dobutamine HCl	LI	2 g	RC	20 mg	D5W[a]	Visually compatible. No flumazenil loss in 24 hr at 23 °C in fluorescent light. Dobutamine not tested	1710	C
Dopamine HCl	AB	3.2 g	RC	20 mg	D5W[a]	Visually compatible. 7% flumazenil loss in 24 hr at 23 °C in fluorescent light. Dopamine not tested	1710	C
Famotidine	MSD	80 mg	RC	20 mg	D5W[a]	Visually compatible. 3% flumazenil loss in 24 hr at 23 °C in fluorescent light. Famotidine not tested	1710	C
Heparin sodium	ES	50,000 units	RC	20 mg	D5W[a]	Visually compatible. 4% flumazenil loss in 24 hr at 23 °C in fluorescent light. Heparin not tested	1710	C
Lidocaine HCl	AB	4 g	RC	20 mg	D5W[a]	Visually compatible. 4% flumazenil loss in 24 hr at 23 °C in fluorescent light. Lidocaine not tested	1710	C
Procainamide HCl	ES	4 g	RC	20 mg	D5W[a]	Visually compatible. No flumazenil loss in 24 hr at 23 °C in fluorescent light. Procainamide not tested	1710	C
Ranitidine HCl	GL	300 mg	RC	20 mg	D5W[a]	Visually compatible. 3% flumazenil loss in 24 hr at 23 °C in light. Ranitidine not tested	1710	C

[a]Tested in PVC containers.

FLUOROURACIL
(5-FLUOROURACIL)
AHFS 10:00

Products — Fluorouracil injection is available in 10- and 20-mL single-use vials and in 50- and 100-mL bulk pharmacy vials for preparation of individual doses. (4) Each milliliter contains fluorouracil 50 mg with sodium hydroxide and/or hydrochloric acid for pH adjustment. (1)

pH — The pH is adjusted to approximately 9.2 with a range of 8.6 to 9.4. (1; 4)

Administration — Fluorouracil is administered intravenously. Care should be taken to avoid extravasation. Dilution of the injection is not required for administration. (1; 4) Fluorouracil has also been given by portal vein or hepatic artery infusion. (4)

In the event of spills or leaks, the use of sodium hypochlorite 5% (household bleach) to inactivate fluorouracil is recommended. (1200)

Stability — Fluorouracil is normally colorless to faint yellow. Its stability and safety are not affected by slight discoloration during storage. It should be stored at controlled room temperature and protected from light (1; 4) and freezing (4). Storing the vials in the original cartons until the time of use is recommended. (1) The color of the solution results from the presence of free fluorine. A dark yellow indicates greater decomposition. Such decomposition may result from storage for several months at temperatures above room temperature. It is suggested that solutions having a darker yellow color be discarded. (398) Exposure to sunlight or intense incandescent light has also caused degradation. The solutions changed to dark amber to brown. (760) A precipitate may form from exposure to low temperatures and may be resolubilized by heating to 60 °C with vigorous shaking. (1; 4) (Note: Allow the solution to cool to body temperature before administration.)

Microwave radiation also has been used to resolubilize the precipitate. Ampuls of fluorouracil containing a precipitate were exposed to microwave radiation and shaken until clear. These ampuls were then compared to ampuls that were heated to 60 °C and shaken until clear and also to unheated controls. The precipitate was redissolved by microwave radiation without significantly affecting the drug. No significant decrease in concentration was observed. There was a slight change in pH. The authors concluded that microwave radiation was a suitable method for solubilizing the precipitate that may form in fluorouracil ampuls. However, they warned that extreme care should be taken to avoid overheating and the resulting explosions from excessive pressure in the ampuls. (662)

Fluorouracil (Roche) 1 mg/mL in dextrose 5% was evaluated for stability in translucent containers (Perfupack Y, Baxter) and five opaque containers [green PVC Opafuseur (Bruneau), white EVA Perfu-opaque (Baxter), orange PVC PF170 (Cair), white PVC V86 (Codan), and white EVA Perfecran (Fandre)] when exposed to sunlight for 28 days. No photodegradation or sorption was found. However, an increase in concentration due to moisture permeation was detected after two weeks. (1750)

Immersion of a needle with an aluminum component in fluorouracil (Adria) 50 mg/mL resulted in no visually apparent reaction after seven days at 24 °C. (988)

Fluorouracil (Adria) 500 mg/10 mL did not support the growth of several microorganisms commonly implicated in nosocomial infections. The bacteriostatic properties were observed against *Escherichia coli*, *Klebsiella pneumoniae*, *Staphylococcus epidermidis*, *Pseudomonas aeruginosa*, *Candida albicans*, and *Clostridium perfringens*. (828)

In another study, fluorouracil (Adria) 1 g/20 mL transferred to PVC containers did not support the growth of several microorganisms and may have imparted an antimicrobial effect at this concentration. Loss of viability was observed for *Staphylococcus aureus*, *Escherichia coli*, *Pseudomonas aeruginosa*, *Pseudomonas cepacia*, *Candida albicans*, and *Aspergillus niger*. (1187)

Fluorouracil eliminated the viability of *Staphylococcus epidermidis* (10^6 to 10^7 CFU/mL) in varying time periods, depending on concentration and diluent, when stored at near-body temperature (35 °C). At 50 mg/mL, no viability was found after five days of incubation. At 10 mg/mL in sodium chloride 0.9% and dextrose 5%, no viability was found after seven and five days, respectively. Following dilution to 10 mg/mL with bacteriostatic sodium chloride 0.9%, no viability was found after two days. (1659)

pH Effects — At a pH greater than 11, slow hydrolysis of fluorouracil occurs. At a pH less than 8, solubility is reduced and precipitation may or may not occur, depending on the concentration. (1369; 1379)

Fluorouracil 50 mg/mL (Lyphomed, Roche, and SoloPak) exhibited precipitation in two to four hours at pH 8.6 to 8.68; precipitation occurred immediately at pH 8.52 or less. The precipitate consisted of needle-shaped crystals at pH 8.26 to 8.68. Cluster-shaped crystals formed at pH 8.18 and below. (1489)

Admixture with acidic drugs or drugs that decompose in an alkaline environment should be avoided. (524)

A color change to deep purple was reported for the mixtures of doxorubicin hydrochloride (Adria) 10 mg/L with fluorouracil (Roche) 250 mg/L in dextrose 5%. (296) This color change is indicative of decomposition occurring in solutions with an alkaline pH. It also occurs with other anthracyclines. (394)

Freezing Solutions — Fluorouracil (Abic) 5 mg/0.5 mL in sodium chloride 0.9% in polypropylene syringes (Plastipak, Becton Dickinson) was stored frozen at −20 °C. No fluorouracil loss occurred in eight weeks. Refreezing and further storage at −20 °C for another two weeks also did not result in a fluorouracil loss. (1666)

Fluorouracil (Teva) near 6.8 mg/mL in sodium chloride 0.9% in PVC bags was stored frozen at −20 °C for 79 days, thawed in a microwave oven, and stored for an additional 28 days under refrigeration. No precipitation or crystallization occurred. No fluorouracil loss occurred after frozen storage and about 6% loss occurred after the subsequent refrigerated storage. (2807)

Syringes — Fluorouracil 25 mg/mL in polypropylene syringes (Braun Omnifix) was stable for 28 days at 4 and 20 °C. (1564)

Fluorouracil (Roche) 50 mg/mL was packaged as 3 mL in 10-mL polypropylene infusion pump syringes (Pharmacia Deltec). Little or no loss occurred during 21 days of storage at 30 °C. (1967)

Fluorouracil (Roche) 12 and 40 mg/mL diluted with sodium chloride 0.9% and dextrose 5% was packaged in 60-mL polypropylene syringes and stored at 25 °C protected from light. Losses of 5% or less occurred in the solutions after storage for 72 hours. Furthermore, the solutions had no visually apparent precipitate or discoloration. (1983)

Ambulatory Pumps — The stability of undiluted fluorouracil 50 mg/mL from three manufacturers (Lyphomed, Roche, and SoloPak) in the reservoirs of four portable infusion pumps (Pharmacia Deltec CADD-

1, Model 5100; Cormed II, Model 10500; Medfusion Infumed 200; and Pancretec Provider I.V., Model 2000) was evaluated. The fluorouracil was delivered by the pumps at a rate of 10 mL/day over a seven-day cycle at 25 and 37 °C. All fluorouracil samples in all pump reservoirs were stable over the seven-day study period, exhibiting little or no drug loss and only minimal leached plasticizer (DEHP) at either temperature. (1489)

However, precipitation of the Roche fluorouracil was observed with all pumps; a fine white precipitate originated close to the connection junction and migrated in both directions until it occupied most of the tubing and was in the drug reservoir. In some cases, the pumps stopped due to the extent of precipitation. The authors noted that various factors, including solution pH, temperature, drug concentration and solubility, and the manipulative techniques used could contribute to precipitate formation. (1489)

Undiluted fluorouracil (Roche) 50 mg/mL in ethylene vinyl acetate (EVA) bags for use with portable infusion pumps remained stable, with little or no loss after 28 days at 4, 22, and 35 °C. The containers at 35 °C did sustain approximately a 3% water loss due to evaporation during storage, increasing the fluorouracil concentration slightly. (1548)

Fluorouracil (David Bull Laboratories) 25 mg/mL was stable in PVC reservoirs (Parker Micropump) for 14 days at 4 and 37 °C, exhibiting no loss. (1696)

The stability of undiluted fluorouracil injection (Roche) 50 mg/mL in EVA reservoirs (Celsa) and PVC reservoirs (Pharmacia) for use with ambulatory infusion pumps was evaluated. The filled reservoirs were stored for 14 days at 4 °C and at 33 °C to simulate the conditions of prolonged infusion from the reservoirs kept under patients' clothing. No loss of fluorouracil due to decomposition was found. However, the refrigerated samples exhibited substantial (up to 15%) loss of drug content from solution due to gross precipitation. Flocculent precipitation was observed in as little as three days. (Subvisible precipitation may occur earlier.) At the elevated temperature, substantial increases in concentration of fluorouracil occurred in the EVA reservoirs due to water loss from permeation through the plastic reservoir. Approximately 5% increase in drug concentration occurred in

14 days. No change in concentration occurred in the PVC reservoirs during this time frame. (2004)

Implantable Pumps — Fluorouracil 50 mg/mL was filled into an implantable infusion pump (Fresenius VIP 30) and associated capillary tubing and stored at 37 °C. No fluorouracil loss and no contamination from components of pump materials occurred during eight weeks of storage. (1903)

Fluorouracil combined with leucovorin calcium for repeated administration using a Fresenius implanted port resulted in blockage of the pump catheter and necessitated surgical removal of the port. The blockage was caused by precipitation of calcium carbonate in the catheter. (2504)

Sorption — Fluorouracil was shown not to exhibit sorption to PVC bags and tubing, polyethylene bags or tubing, Silastic tubing, and polypropylene and polyethylene syringes. (536; 606; 760; 2420; 2430)

Fluorouracil may be more extensively adsorbed to glass surfaces than to plastic. In one report, significant loss occurred from solutions in glass vials, but almost quantitative recovery was obtained from polyethylene and polypropylene plastic vials. The loss was ascribed to adsorption to the glass surface. (663) This difference was also observed in dextrose 5% in glass and PVC infusion containers. A 10% loss of fluorouracil occurred in 43 hours in the PVC containers but in only seven hours in the glass containers. (519)

Filtration — Fluorouracil 10 to 75 mcg/mL exhibited little or no loss due to sorption to either cellulose nitrate/cellulose acetate ester (Millex OR) or Teflon (Millex FG) filters. (1415; 1416)

Central Venous Catheter — Fluorouracil (Roche) 5 mg/mL in dextrose 5% was found to be compatible with the ARROWg+ard Blue Plus (Arrow International) chlorhexidine-bearing triple-lumen central catheter. Essentially complete delivery of the drug was found with little or no drug loss occurring. Furthermore, chlorhexidine delivered from the catheter remained at trace amounts with no substantial increase due to the delivery of the drug through the catheter. (2335)

Compatibility Information

Solution Compatibility

Fluorouracil

Solution	Mfr	Mfr	Conc/L	Remarks	Ref	C/I
Amino acids 4.25%, dextrose 25%	MG	RC	500 mg	No increase in particulate matter in 24 hr at 5 °C	349	C
Dextrose 5% in Ringer's injection, lactated	MG[a]		500 mg	No decomposition in 24 hr	399	C
Dextrose 5%	[d]	RC	10 g	No loss in 16 weeks at 5 °C. Little change in 7 days at 25 °C	894	C
	[h]	RC	10 g	No loss in 16 weeks at 5 °C	894	C
	TR[b]	RC	1.5 g	Physically compatible. Stable for 8 weeks at ambient temperature both in dark and light	1153	C
			1 and 2 g	Physically compatible and no loss in 48 hr at room temperature and 7 °C	1152	C
	[c]	RC	10 g	Visually compatible with little loss in 28 days at 4, 22, and 35 °C in dark. At 35 °C, concentration increased due to water evaporation	1548	C
	MG[a]		8.3 g	Less than 10% loss in 48 hr at room temperature exposed to light	1658	C

Solution Compatibility (Cont.)

Fluorouracil

Solution	Mfr	Mfr	Conc/L	Remarks	Ref	C/I
	BA[d]	RC	1 and 10 g	Visually compatible with less than 3% loss in 14 days at 4 and 21 °C	2004	C
	BA[d]	RC[e]	0.5 and 5 g	Little or no loss in 13 days at 4 and 25 °C	2175	C
	BA[g]	ICN	25 g	Physically compatible. Little loss in 14 days at 4 °C, 21 days at 25 and 31 °C	2483	C
Sodium chloride 0.9%	TR[b]	RC	1.5 g	Physically compatible and chemically stable for 8 weeks at ambient temperature both in the dark and exposed to fluorescent light	1153	C
			1 and 2 g	Physically compatible and no loss in 48 hr at room temperature and 7 °C	1152	C
	[c]	RC	10 g	Visually compatible with little loss in 28 days at 4, 22, and 35 °C in dark. At 35 °C, concentration increased due to water evaporation	1548	C
	[b]	FA, RC	5 and 50 g	Visually compatible. Little loss in 91 days at 4 °C followed by 7 days at 25 °C in the dark	1567	C
	[c]	RC	15 and 45 g	Visually compatible with little or no loss in 72 hr at 25 °C protected from light	1983	C
	BA[d]	RC	1 and 10 g	Visually compatible with less than 3% loss in 14 days at 4 and 21 °C	2004	C
	BA[d]	RC[e]	0.5 and 5 g	Little or no loss in 13 days at 4 and 25 °C	2175	C
	BA[g]	ICN	25 g	Physically compatible. Little loss in 14 days at 4 °C, 21 days at 25 and 31 °C	2483	C
TPN #23[f]		RC	1 and 4 g	Physically compatible for 42 hr at room temperature in light. Erratic assay results	562	?
		RC	1 g	Physically compatible and fluorouracil stable for 48 hr at room temperature in ambient light	826	C

[a]*Tested in both glass and polyolefin containers.*
[b]*Tested in both glass and PVC containers.*
[c]*Tested in ethylene vinyl acetate (EVA) containers.*
[d]*Tested in PVC containers.*
[e]*A modified fluorouracil formulation containing tromethamine (TRIS, THAM, trometamol) instead of sodium hydroxide.*
[f]*Refer to Appendix I for the composition of parenteral nutrition solutions. TPN indicates a 2-in-1 admixture.*
[g]*Tested in Easypump (Braun) elastomeric reservoir pumps.*
[h]*Tested in Infusor (Travenol) elastomeric reservoir pumps.*

Additive Compatibility

Fluorouracil

Drug	Mfr	Conc/L	Mfr	Conc/L	Test Soln	Remarks	Ref	C/I
Bleomycin sulfate	BR	20 and 30 units	RC	1 g	NS	Physically compatible and bleomycin activity retained for 1 week at 4 °C. Fluorouracil not tested	763	C
Carboplatin		1 g		10 g	W	Greater than 20% carboplatin loss in 24 hr at room temperature	1379	I
	BR	100 mg	DB	1 g	D5W	9% carboplatin loss in 5 hr at 25 °C	2415	I
Ciprofloxacin						Physically incompatible with loss of ciprofloxacin reported due to pH over 6.0	1924	I
Cisplatin	BR	200 mg	SO	1 g	NS[a]	10% cisplatin loss in 1.5 hr and 25% loss in 4 hr at 25 °C	1339	I

Additive Compatibility (Cont.)

Fluorouracil

Drug	Mfr	Conc/L	Mfr	Conc/L	Test Soln	Remarks	Ref	C/I
	BR	500 mg	SO	10 g	NS[a]	10% cisplatin loss in 1.2 hr and 25% loss in 3 hr at 25 °C	1339	I
	BR	500 mg	AD	10 g	NS	80% cisplatin loss in 24 hr at room temperature due to low pH	1386	I
Cyclophosphamide		1.67 g		8.3 g	NS	Both drugs stable for 14 days at room temperature	1389	C
Cyclophosphamide with methotrexate sodium		1.67 g 25 mg		8.3 g	NS	9.3% cyclophosphamide loss in 7 days at room temperature. No loss of other drugs observed	1389	C
Cytarabine	UP	400 mg	RC	250 mg	D5W	Altered UV spectra for cytarabine within 1 hr at room temperature	207	I
Diazepam	RC					Precipitates immediately	524	I
Doxorubicin HCl	AD					Discolors from red to blue-purple	524	I
	AD	10 mg	RC	250 mg	D5W	Color changes to deep purple	296	I
Epirubicin HCl		0.5 to 1 g		10 g	NS	Greater than 10% epirubicin loss in 1 day	1379	I
Etoposide		200 mg		10 g	NS	Both drugs stable for 7 days at room temperature and 1 day at 35 °C	1379	C
Fentanyl citrate	AB	12.5 mg	AB	1 and 16 g	D5W, NS[a]	25% fentanyl loss in 15 min due to sorption to PVC	2064	I
Floxuridine		10 g		10 g	NS	Both drugs stable for 15 days at room temperature	1390	C
Hydromorphone HCl	AST	500 mg	AB	1 g	D5W, NS[a]	Physically compatible. Little loss of either drug in 7 days at 32 °C and 35 days at 23, 4, and −20 °C	1977	C
	AST	500 mg	AB	16 g	D5W, NS[a]	Physically compatible. Little loss of either drug in 3 days at 32 °C, 7 days at 23 °C, and 35 days at 4 and −20 °C	1977	C
Ifosfamide		2 g		10 g	NS	Both drugs stable for 5 days at room temperature	1379	C
Leucovorin calcium	LE	1.5 to 13.3 g	AD	16.7 to 46.2 g	[b]	Subvisible particulates form in all combinations in variable periods from 1 to 4 days at 4, 23, and 32 °C	1816	I
Methotrexate sodium		30 mg		10 g	NS	Both drugs stable for 15 days at room temperature	1379	C
Methotrexate sodium with cyclophosphamide		25 mg 1.67 g		8.3 g	NS	9.3% cyclophosphamide loss in 7 days at room temperature. No loss of other drugs observed	1389	C
Metoclopramide HCl	FUJ	100 mg	RC	2.5 g	D5W	10% metoclopramide loss in 6 hr and 27% loss in 24 hr at 25 °C. 5% metoclopramide loss in 120 hr at 4 °C. 5 and 7% fluorouracil losses in 120 hr at 4 and 25 °C, respectively	1780	I
Mitoxantrone HCl	LE	500 mg		25 g	D5W	Visually compatible. Mitoxantrone stable for 24 hr at room temperature. Fluorouracil not tested	1531	C

Additive Compatibility (Cont.)

Fluorouracil

Drug	Mfr	Conc/L	Mfr	Conc/L	Test Soln	Remarks	Ref	C/I
Morphine sulfate	AST	1 g	AB	1 and 16 g	D5W, NS[a]	Subvisible morphine precipitate forms immediately, becoming grossly visible within 24 hr. Morphine losses of 60 to 80% occur within 1 day	1977	I
Vincristine sulfate	LI	4 mg	RC	10 mg	D5W	Physically compatible. No alteration in UV spectra in 8 hr at room temperature	207	C

[a]Tested in PVC containers.
[b]Tested with both drugs undiluted and diluted by 25% with dextrose 5%.

Drugs in Syringe Compatibility

Fluorouracil

Drug (in syringe)	Mfr	Amt	Mfr	Amt	Remarks	Ref	C/I
Bleomycin sulfate		1.5 units/ 0.5 mL		25 mg/ 0.5 mL	Physically compatible for 5 min at room temperature followed by 8 min of centrifugation	980	C
Cisplatin		0.5 mg/ 0.5 mL		25 mg/ 0.5 mL	Physically compatible for 5 min at room temperature followed by 8 min of centrifugation	980	C
Cyclophosphamide		10 mg/ 0.5 mL		25 mg/ 0.5 mL	Physically compatible for 5 min at room temperature followed by 8 min of centrifugation	980	C
Doxorubicin HCl		1 mg/ 0.5 mL		25 mg/ 0.5 mL	Physically compatible for 5 min at room temperature followed by 8 min of centrifugation	980	C
		5 and 10 mg/ 10 mL[a]		500 mg/ 10 mL	Precipitate forms within several hours of mixing	1564	I
Droperidol		1.25 mg/ 0.5 mL		25 mg/ 0.5 mL	Precipitates immediately	980	I
Epirubicin HCl		5 and 10 mg/ 10 mL[a]		500 mg/ 10 mL	Precipitate forms within several hours of mixing	1564	I
Furosemide		5 mg/ 0.5 mL		25 mg/ 0.5 mL	Physically compatible for 5 min at room temperature followed by 8 min of centrifugation	980	C
Heparin sodium		500 units/ 0.5 mL		25 mg/ 0.5 mL	Physically compatible for 5 min at room temperature followed by 8 min of centrifugation	980	C
	LEO	20,000 units/ 0.8 mL	DB	500 mg/ 20 mL	Visually compatible with no loss of either drug in 7 days at 25 °C and 14 days at 4 °C in the dark	2415	C
Leucovorin calcium		5 mg/ 0.5 mL		25 mg/ 0.5 mL	Physically compatible for 5 min at room temperature followed by 8 min of centrifugation	980	C
Methotrexate sodium		12.5 mg/ 0.5 mL		25 mg/ 0.5 mL	Physically compatible for 5 min at room temperature followed by 8 min of centrifugation	980	C
Metoclopramide HCl		2.5 mg/ 0.5 mL		25 mg/ 0.5 mL	Physically compatible for 5 min at room temperature followed by 8 min of centrifugation	980	C
Mitomycin		0.25 mg/ 0.5 mL		25 mg/ 0.5 mL	Physically compatible for 5 min at room temperature followed by 8 min of centrifugation	980	C

Drugs in Syringe Compatibility (Cont.)

Fluorouracil

Drug (in syringe)	Mfr	Amt	Mfr	Amt	Remarks	Ref	C/I
Vinblastine sulfate		0.5 mg/ 0.5 mL		25 mg/ 0.5 mL	Physically compatible for 5 min at room temperature followed by 8 min of centrifugation	980	C
Vincristine sulfate		0.5 mg/ 0.5 mL		25 mg/ 0.5 mL	Physically compatible for 5 min at room temperature followed by 8 min of centrifugation	980	C

ªDiluted in sodium chloride 0.9%.

Y-Site Injection Compatibility (1:1 Mixture)

Fluorouracil

Drug	Mfr	Conc	Mfr	Conc	Remarks	Ref	C/I
Aldesleukin	CHIª	ª			Unacceptable loss of aldesleukin activity	1890	I
Allopurinol sodium	BW	3 mg/mLᵇ	RC	16 mg/mLᵇ	Physically compatible for 4 hr at 22 °C	1686	C
Amifostine	USB	10 mg/mLª	AD	16 mg/mLᵇ	Physically compatible for 4 hr at 23 °C	1845	C
Amphotericin B cholesteryl sulfate complex	SEQ	0.83 mg/mLª	PH	16 mg/mLª	Microprecipitate forms immediately	2117	I
Anidulafungin	VIC	0.5 mg/mLª	APP	16 mg/mLª	Physically compatible for 4 hr at 23 °C	2617	C
Aztreonam	SQ	40 mg/mLª	AD	16 mg/mLª	Physically compatible for 4 hr at 23 °C	1758	C
Bleomycin sulfate		3 units/mL		50 mg/mL	Drugs injected sequentially in Y-site with no flush. No precipitate seen	980	C
Cisplatin		1 mg/mL		50 mg/mL	Drugs injected sequentially in Y-site with no flush. No precipitate seen	980	C
Cyclophosphamide		20 mg/mL		50 mg/mL	Drugs injected sequentially in Y-site with no flush. No precipitate seen	980	C
Doripenem	JJ	5 mg/mLªᵇ	ABX	16 mg/mLªᵇ	Physically compatible for 4 hr at 23 °C	2743	C
Doxorubicin HCl		2 mg/mL		50 mg/mL	Drugs injected sequentially in Y-site with no flush. No precipitate seen	980	C
Doxorubicin HCl liposomal	SEQ	0.4 mg/mLª	PH	16 mg/mLª	Physically compatible for 4 hr at 23 °C	2087	C
Droperidol		2.5 mg/mL		50 mg/mL	Drugs injected sequentially in Y-site with no flush. Precipitates immediately	980	I
Etoposide phosphate	BR	5 mg/mLª	PH	16 mg/mLª	Physically compatible for 4 hr at 23 °C	2218	C
Filgrastim	AMG	30 mcg/mLª	RC	16 mg/mLª	Particles and long filaments form in 1 hr	1687	I
Fludarabine phosphate	BX	1 mg/mLª	LY	16 mg/mLª	Visually compatible for 4 hr at 22 °C	1439	C
Furosemide		10 mg/mL		50 mg/mL	Drugs injected sequentially in Y-site with no flush. No precipitate seen	980	C
Gallium nitrate	FUJ	1 mg/mLᵇ	RC	50 mg/mL	Precipitate forms immediately but clears after 60 min	1673	I
Gemcitabine HCl	LI	10 mg/mLᵇ	PH	16 mg/mLᵇ	Physically compatible for 4 hr at 23 °C	2226	C
Granisetron HCl	SKB	0.05 mg/mLᵇ	AD	16 mg/mLᵇ	Physically compatible for 4 hr at 23 °C	1804	C
	SKB	1 mg/mL	RC	2 mg/mLᵇ	Physically compatible with little or no loss of either drug in 4 hr at 22 °C	1883	C
	SKB	0.05 mg/mLª	AD	16 mg/mLª	Physically compatible for 4 hr at 23 °C	2000	C

Y-Site Injection Compatibility (1:1 Mixture) (Cont.)

Fluorouracil

Drug	Mfr	Conc	Mfr	Conc	Remarks	Ref	C/I
Heparin sodium		1000 units/mL		50 mg/mL	Drugs injected sequentially in Y-site with no flush. No precipitate seen	980	C
	UP	1000 units/L[c]	RC	50 mg/mL	Physically compatible for 4 hr at room temperature	534	C
Hydrocortisone sodium succinate	UP	10 mg/L[c]	RC	50 mg/mL	Physically compatible for 4 hr at room temperature	534	C
Leucovorin calcium		10 mg/mL		50 mg/mL	Drugs injected sequentially in Y-site with no flush. No precipitate seen	980	C
Linezolid	PHU	2 mg/mL	PH	16 mg/mL[a]	Physically compatible for 4 hr at 23 °C	2264	C
Mannitol		20%	SO	1 and 2 mg/mL[d]	Physically compatible and fluorouracil stable for 24 hr. Mannitol not tested	1526	C
Melphalan HCl	BW	0.1 mg/mL[b]	LY	16 mg/mL[b]	Physically compatible for 3 hr at 22 °C	1557	C
Methotrexate sodium		25 mg/mL		50 mg/mL	Drugs injected sequentially in Y-site with no flush. No precipitate seen	980	C
Metoclopramide HCl		5 mg/mL		50 mg/mL	Drugs injected sequentially in Y-site with no flush. No precipitate seen	980	C
Mitomycin		0.5 mg/mL		50 mg/mL	Drugs injected sequentially in Y-site with no flush. No precipitate seen	980	C
Ondansetron HCl	GL	1 mg/mL[b]	SO	16 mg/mL[a]	Precipitates immediately	1365	I
	GL	16 to 160 mcg/mL		≤0.8 mg/mL	Physically compatible when fluorouracil given at 20 mL/hr via Y-site	1366	C
Paclitaxel	NCI	1.2 mg/mL[a]		16 mg/mL[a]	Physically compatible for 4 hr at 22 °C	1528	C
Palonosetron HCl	MGI	50 mcg/mL	APP	16 mg/mL[a]	Physically compatible and no loss of either drug in 4 hr	2627	C
Pemetrexed disodium	LI	20 mg/mL[b]	APP	16 mg/mL[a]	Physically compatible for 4 hr at 23 °C	2564	C
Piperacillin sodium–tazobactam sodium	LE[h]	40 + 5 mg/mL[a]	LY	16 mg/mL[a]	Physically compatible for 4 hr at 22 °C	1688	C
Potassium chloride	AB	40 mEq/L[c]	RC	50 mg/mL	Physically compatible for 4 hr at room temperature	534	C
Propofol	ZEN	10 mg/mL	AD	16 mg/mL[a]	Physically compatible for 1 hr at 23 °C	2066	C
Sargramostim	IMM	10 mcg/mL[b]	SO	16 mg/mL[b]	Visually compatible for 4 hr at 22 °C	1436	C
Teniposide	BR	0.1 mg/mL[a]	AD	16 mg/mL[b]	Physically compatible for 4 hr at 23 °C	1725	C
Thiotepa	IMM[e]	1 mg/mL[a]	AD	16 mg/mL[a]	Physically compatible for 4 hr at 23 °C	1861	C
TNA #218, #219, #221, #222, #224 to #226[f]			PH	16 mg/mL[a]	Visually compatible for 4 hr at 23 °C	2215	C
TNA #220, #223[f]			PH	16 mg/mL[a]	Small amount of white precipitate forms immediately	2215	I
Topotecan HCl	SKB	56 mcg/mL[b]	RC	50 mg/mL	Immediate haze and yellow color	2245	I
TPN #212, #213[f]			PH	16 mg/mL[a]	Slight subvisible haze, crystals, and amber discoloration form in 1 to 4 hr	2109	I
TPN #214, #215[f]			PH	16 mg/mL[a]	Turbidity forms immediately	2109	I
Vinblastine sulfate		1 mg/mL		50 mg/mL	Drugs injected sequentially in Y-site with no flush. No precipitate seen	980	C

Y-Site Injection Compatibility (1:1 Mixture) (Cont.)

Fluorouracil

Drug	Mfr	Conc	Mfr	Conc	Remarks	Ref	C/I
Vincristine sulfate		1 mg/mL		50 mg/mL	Drugs injected sequentially in Y-site with no flush. No precipitate seen	980	C
Vinorelbine tartrate	BW	1 mg/mL[b]	RC	16 mg/mL[b]	Heavy white precipitate forms immediately	1558	I

[a]Tested in dextrose 5%.
[b]Tested in sodium chloride 0.9%.
[c]Tested in dextrose 5% in Ringer's injection, dextrose 5% in Ringer's injection, lactated, dextrose 5%, Ringer's injection, lactated, and sodium chloride 0.9%.
[d]Tested in dextrose 5% in sodium chloride 0.45%, dextrose 5%, and sodium chloride 0.9%.
[e]Lyophilized formulation tested.
[f]Refer to Appendix I for the composition of parenteral nutrition solutions. TNA indicates a 3-in-1 admixture, and TPN indicates a 2-in-1 admixture.
[g]Tested with albumin human 0.1%.
[h]Test performed using the formulation WITHOUT edetate disodium.

FLUPHENAZINE HYDROCHLORIDE
AHFS 28:16.08.24

Products — Fluphenazine hydrochloride is available in 10-mL multiple-dose vials. Each milliliter contains fluphenazine hydrochloride 2.5 mg with sodium chloride for isotonicity, sodium hydroxide or hydrochloric acid to adjust the pH, and methylparaben 0.1% and propylparaben 0.01% as preservatives. (1)

pH — From 4.8 to 5.2. (1; 4)

Administration — Fluphenazine hydrochloride is administered by intramuscular injection. (1; 4)

Stability — Intact vials should be stored at controlled room temperature and protected from freezing and light. Parenteral solutions of fluphenazine hydrochloride vary from colorless to light amber. Solutions that are darker than light amber, are discolored in some other way, or contain a precipitate should not be used. (1; 4)

Compatibility Information

Drugs in Syringe Compatibility

Fluphenazine HCl

Drug (in syringe)	Mfr	Amt	Mfr	Amt	Remarks	Ref	C/I
Benztropine mesylate	MSD	2 mg/ 2 mL	LY	5 mg/ 2 mL	Visually compatible for 60 min	1784	C
Diphenhydramine HCl	ES	100 mg/ 2 mL	LY	5 mg/ 2 mL	Visually compatible for 60 min	1784	C
Hydroxyzine HCl	ES	100 mg/ 2 mL	LY	5 mg/ 2 mL	Visually compatible for 60 min	1784	C

FOLIC ACID
AHFS 88:08

Products — Folic acid 5 mg/mL injection is available in 10-mL vials. Each milliliter of solution also contains edetate sodium 5 mg, benzyl alcohol 2 mg, and hydrochloric acid and/or sodium hydroxide to adjust pH in water for injection. (1)

pH — From 8 to 11. (1; 4)

Administration — Folic acid injection is administered by deep intramuscular, intravenous, or subcutaneous injection. (1; 4)

Stability — Intact vials should be stored at controlled room temperature and protected from light. (1) The yellow to orange-yellow solutions are heat sensitive and should be protected from light (4) for long-term storage. However, exposure of folic acid in parenteral nutrition solutions to fluorescent light for 48 hours did not cause any significant loss of folic acid. (896)

pH Effects — Folic acid is soluble in solutions of pH 5.6 or above at room temperature to a concentration of 1 g/L. However, below about pH 4.5 to 5, folic acid may precipitate in varying time periods, depending on the acidity of the solution. In the small concentrations used for parenteral nutrition, a pH of above 5 ensures that folic acid will remain in solution. Most parenteral nutrition solutions are buffered by the amino acids to pH 5 to 6. (895)

The rate of folic acid photodegradation is higher in an acidic medium compared to the rate in an alkaline medium. (2496)

Sorption — A parenteral nutrition solution containing 13 mcg/L of folic acid injection in a 3-L PVC bag and run through an administration set delivered the full amount of folic acid, with no loss. (895)

Filtration — Folic acid (Lederle) 0.5 mg/L in dextrose 5% and sodium chloride 0.9% was filtered at 120 mL/hr for six hours through a 0.22-μm cellulose ester membrane filter (Ivex-2). No significant reduction due to binding to the filter was noted. (533)

Compatibility Information

Solution Compatibility

Folic acid

Solution	Mfr	Mfr	Conc/L	Remarks	Ref	C/I
Amino acids 4.25%, dextrose 25%	MG	USP	0.2 and 10 mg	Physically compatible. Stable for 7 days at 4 °C and room temperature in dark	895	C
Dextrose 20%		USP	0.2 and 20 mg	Physically compatible. Stable for 7 days at 4 °C and room temperature in dark	895	C
Dextrose 40%		USP	0.2 and 20 mg	17 to 25% loss in 24 hr at 4 °C and room temperature in dark, with precipitation at the higher concentration after 48 hr	895	I
Dextrose 50%		USP	20 mg	Precipitate forms within 24 hr at 4 °C and room temperature protected from light	895	I
TPN #69[a]		USP	0.4 mg	Physically compatible and folic acid stable for at least 7 days at 4 and 25 °C protected from light	895	C
TPN #70[a]		LE	0.25 to 1 mg	Folic acid stable for at least 48 hr at 6 and 21 °C in the light or dark	896	C
TPN #74[a]			1 mg	Folic acid stable over 8 hr at room temperature in fluorescent or sunlight	842	C
TPN #189[a]		AB	15 mg/mL	Visually compatible for 24 hr at 22 °C	1767	C

[a]*Refer to Appendix I for the composition of parenteral nutrition solutions. TPN indicates a 2-in-1 admixture.*

Additive Compatibility

Folic acid

Drug	Mfr	Conc/L	Mfr	Conc/L	Test Soln	Remarks	Ref	C/I
Fat emulsion, intravenous	KV	10%	USP	0.2 and 20 mg		Physically compatible for 2 weeks at 4 °C and room temperature in the dark but erratic assays	895	?

Drugs in Syringe Compatibility

Folic acid

Drug (in syringe)	Mfr	Amt	Mfr	Amt	Remarks	Ref	C/I
Doxapram HCl	RB	400 mg/ 20 mL		15 mg/ 1 mL	Immediate turbidity	1177	**I**

Y-Site Injection Compatibility (1:1 Mixture)

Folic acid

Drug	Mfr	Conc	Mfr	Conc	Remarks	Ref	C/I
Famotidine	MSD	0.2 mg/mL[a]	LE	5 mg/mL	Physically compatible for 14 hr	1196	**C**

[a]*Tested in dextrose 5%.*

Additional Compatibility Information

Parenteral Nutrition Solutions — A 40% drop in folic acid concentration occurred immediately after admixture in a parenteral nutrition solution composed of amino acids, dextrose, electrolytes, trace elements, and multivitamins in PVC bags. The folic acid concentration then remained relatively constant for 28 days when stored at both 4 and 25 °C. (1063)

Extensive decomposition of ascorbic acid and folic acid was reported in a parenteral nutrition solution composed of amino acids 3.3%, dextrose 12.5%, electrolytes, trace elements, and M.V.I.-12 (USV) in PVC bags. Half-lives were 1.1, 2.9, and 8.9 hours for ascorbic acid and 2.7, 5.4, and 24 hours for folic acid stored at 24 °C in daylight, 24 °C protected from light, and 4 °C protected from light, respectively. The decomposition was much greater than for solutions not containing catalyzing metal ions. Also, it was greater than for the vitamins singly because of interactions with the other vitamins present. (1059)

Because of these interactions, recommendations to separate the administration of vitamins and trace elements have been made. (1056; 1060; 1061) Other researchers have termed such recommendations premature based on differing reports (895; 896) and the apparent absence of epidemic vitamin deficiency in parenteral nutrition patients. (1062)

The stability of several vitamins from M.V.I.-12 (Armour) admixed in parenteral nutrition solutions composed of different amino acid products, with or without Intralipid 10%, in glass bottles and PVC bags at 25 and 5 °C for 48 hours was reported. Folic acid was stable in all samples. (1431)

In another study, the stability of several vitamins (from M.V.I.-12) following admixture with four different amino acid products (Fre-Amine III, Neopham, Novamine, Travasol) with or without Intralipid when stored in glass bottles or PVC bags at 25 °C for 48 hours was reported. High-intensity phototherapy light did not affect folic acid. When bisulfite was added to the Neopham admixture, folic acid was unaffected. The authors concluded that intravenous multivitamins should be added to parenteral nutrition admixtures immediately prior to administration to reduce losses of vitamins other than folic acid since commercially available amino acid products may contain bisulfites and have varying pH values. (487)

The vitamins in Cernevit (Baxter) diluted in three 2-in-1 parenteral nutrition admixtures were tested for stability over 48 hours. Most of the other vitamins, including folic acid, retained their initial concentrations. (2796)

FOSCARNET SODIUM
AHFS 8:18.92

Products — Foscarnet sodium is available as a 24-mg/mL infusion solution in water for injection in 250- and 500-mL glass bottles. Hydrochloric acid and/or sodium hydroxide may have been added to adjust the pH. (1)

pH — Adjusted to pH 7.4. (1)

Trade Name(s) — Foscavir.

Administration — Foscarnet sodium is administered by intravenous infusion, using an infusion pump. It should not be given by rapid injection. Recommended rates of infusion are a minimum of one hour for doses of 60 mg/kg and up to two hours for doses of 120 mg/kg. Recommended dosage, frequency, and administration rates should not be exceeded. For peripheral administration, foscarnet sodium solution must be diluted to 12 mg/mL with dextrose 5% or sodium chloride 0.9%. The drug may be infused without dilution through a central catheter. (1; 4)

Stability — Foscarnet sodium injection is a clear, colorless solution. It should be stored at controlled room temperature and protected from temperatures above 40 °C and from freezing. The product should be used only if the seal is intact and a vacuum is present. (1)

The manufacturer has stated that foscarnet sodium diluted in dextrose 5% or sodium chloride 0.9% and transferred to PVC containers is stable for 24 hours at room temperature or under refrigeration. (71)

Foscarnet sodium may chelate divalent metal ions and is chemically incompatible with solutions containing calcium such as Ringer's injection, lactated, and parenteral nutrition solutions. (1)

Foscarnet sodium (Astra) 13 mg/mL diluted in sodium chloride 0.9% at 22 °C did not exhibit an antibacterial effect on the growth of three organisms (*Enterococcus faecium, Staphylococcus aureus,* and *Pseudomonas aeruginosa*) inoculated into the solution. Foscarnet sodium did exhibit moderate antifungal activity against *Candida albicans.* The authors recommended that ready-to-use solutions be stored under refrigeration whenever possible and that the potential for mi-

crobiological growth should be considered when assigning expiration periods. (2160)

Autoclaving — The concentration of foscarnet sodium (Astra), diluted in sodium chloride 0.9% to 12 mg/mL and packaged in glass infusion bottles with rubber bungs, was compared before and after autoclaving at 30 psi for 15 minutes at 121 °C. The foscarnet sodium concentration did not change after autoclaving. Therefore, the dilution may be autoclaved to avoid limiting its shelf life due to sterility concerns. (1835)

Elastomeric Reservoir Pumps — Foscarnet sodium (Astra) 24 mg/mL was evaluated for binding potential to natural rubber elastomeric reservoirs (Baxter). No binding was found after storage for two weeks at 35 °C with gentle agitation. (2014)

Compatibility Information

Solution Compatibility

Foscarnet sodium

Solution	Mfr	Mfr	Conc/L	Remarks	Ref	C/I
Dextrose 5%	BA[a]	AST	12 g	Visually compatible and chemically stable for 35 days at 5 and 25 °C	1834	**C**
Ringer's injection, lactated				Chemically incompatible	1	**I**
Sodium chloride 0.9%	MG[a]	AST	12 g	Visually compatible. Stable for 30 days at 25 °C in light or dark and at 5 °C in dark	1726	**C**
	BA[a]	AST	12 g	Visually compatible and chemically stable for 35 days at 5 and 25 °C	1834	**C**

[a]*Tested in PVC containers.*

Additive Compatibility

Foscarnet sodium

Drug	Mfr	Conc/L	Mfr	Conc/L	Test Soln	Remarks	Ref	C/I
Potassium chloride		20 to 120 mmol	AST	12 g	NS	Foscarnet concentrations of 93 to 99% were maintained for at least 65 hr	2156	**C**

Y-Site Injection Compatibility (1:1 Mixture)

Foscarnet sodium

Drug	Mfr	Conc	Mfr	Conc	Remarks	Ref	C/I
Acyclovir sodium	BW	10 mg/mL	AST	24 mg/mL	Precipitates immediately	1335	**I**
	BW	7 mg/mL[a,b]	AST	24 mg/mL	Acyclovir crystals form immediately	1393	**I**
Aldesleukin	CHI	33,800 I.U./mL[a]	AST	24 mg/mL	Visually compatible with little or no loss of aldesleukin activity	1857	**C**
Amikacin sulfate	BR	20 mg/mL	AST	24 mg/mL	Physically compatible for 24 hr at room temperature under fluorescent light	1335	**C**
Aminophylline	LY	25 mg/mL	AST	24 mg/mL	Physically compatible for 24 hr at room temperature under fluorescent light	1335	**C**

Y-Site Injection Compatibility (1:1 Mixture) (Cont.)

Foscarnet sodium

Drug	Mfr	Conc	Mfr	Conc	Remarks	Ref	C/I
Amphotericin B	SQ	5 mg/mL	AST	24 mg/mL	Cloudy yellow precipitate forms	1335	**I**
	SQ	0.6 mg/mL[a]	AST	24 mg/mL	Dense haze forms immediately	1393	**I**
Ampicillin sodium	WY	20 mg/mL	AST	24 mg/mL	Physically compatible for 24 hr at room temperature under fluorescent light	1335	**C**
Aztreonam	SQ	40 mg/mL	AST	24 mg/mL	Physically compatible for 24 hr at room temperature under fluorescent light	1335	**C**
	SQ	40 mg/mL[a,b]	AST	24 mg/mL	Physically compatible for 24 hr at 25 °C under fluorescent light	1393	**C**
Cefazolin sodium	SKF	40 mg/mL	AST	24 mg/mL	Physically compatible for 24 hr at room temperature under fluorescent light	1335	**C**
Cefoxitin sodium	MSD	40 mg/mL	AST	24 mg/mL	Physically compatible for 24 hr at room temperature under fluorescent light	1335	**C**
Ceftazidime	GL	20 mg/mL	AST	24 mg/mL	Physically compatible for 24 hr at room temperature under fluorescent light	1335	**C**
	GL	20 mg/mL[a,b]	AST	24 mg/mL	Physically compatible for 24 hr at 25 °C under fluorescent light	1393	**C**
Ceftriaxone sodium	RC	20 mg/mL[a,b]	AST	24 mg/mL	Physically compatible for 24 hr at 25 °C under fluorescent light	1393	**C**
Cefuroxime sodium	GL	30 mg/mL	AST	24 mg/mL	Physically compatible for 24 hr at room temperature under fluorescent light	1335	**C**
Chloramphenicol sodium succinate	PD	20 mg/mL	AST	24 mg/mL	Physically compatible for 24 hr at room temperature under fluorescent light	1335	**C**
Clindamycin phosphate	AB	24 mg/mL	AST	24 mg/mL	Physically compatible for 24 hr at room temperature under fluorescent light	1335	**C**
	UP	12 mg/mL[a,b]	AST	24 mg/mL	Physically compatible for 24 hr at 25 °C under fluorescent light	1393	**C**
Dexamethasone sodium phosphate	OR	10 mg/mL	AST	24 mg/mL	Physically compatible for 24 hr at room temperature under fluorescent light	1335	**C**
Diazepam	ES	5 mg/mL	AST	24 mg/mL	Gas production	1335	**I**
Digoxin	WY	0.25 mg/mL	AST	24 mg/mL	Gas production	1335	**I**
Diphenhydramine HCl	PD	50 mg/mL	AST	24 mg/mL	Cloudy solution	1335	**I**
Dobutamine HCl	LI	12.5 mg/mL	AST	24 mg/mL	Delayed formation of muddy precipitate	1335	**I**
Dopamine HCl	DU	80 mg/mL	AST	24 mg/mL	Physically compatible for 24 hr at room temperature under fluorescent light	1335	**C**
Doripenem	JJ	5 mg/mL[a,b]	HOS	24 mg/mL	Physically compatible for 4 hr at 23 °C	2743	**C**
Droperidol	QU	2.5 mg/mL	AST	24 mg/mL	Delayed formation of yellow precipitate	1335	**I**
Erythromycin lactobionate	AB	20 mg/mL	AST	24 mg/mL	Physically compatible for 24 hr at room temperature under fluorescent light	1335	**C**
	ES	20 mg/mL[a,b]	AST	24 mg/mL	Physically compatible for 24 hr at 25 °C under fluorescent light	1393	**C**
Fluconazole	RR	2 mg/mL	AST	24 mg/mL	Physically compatible for 24 hr at 25 °C	1407	**C**
Furosemide	AB	10 mg/mL	AST	24 mg/mL	Physically compatible for 24 hr at room temperature under fluorescent light	1335	**C**
Ganciclovir sodium		50 mg/mL	AST	24 mg/mL	Precipitates immediately	1335	**I**
Gentamicin sulfate	ES	4 mg/mL	AST	24 mg/mL	Physically compatible for 24 hr at room temperature under fluorescent light	1335	**C**

Y-Site Injection Compatibility (1:1 Mixture) (Cont.)

Foscarnet sodium

Drug	Mfr	Conc	Mfr	Conc	Remarks	Ref	C/I
	ES	2 mg/mL[a,b]	AST	24 mg/mL	Physically compatible for 24 hr at 25 °C under fluorescent light	1393	C
Haloperidol lactate	LY	5 mg/mL	AST	24 mg/mL	Delayed formation of fine white precipitate	1335	I
Heparin sodium	ES	1000 units/mL	AST	24 mg/mL	Physically compatible for 24 hr at room temperature under fluorescent light	1335	C
	LY	100 units/mL[a,b]	AST	24 mg/mL	Physically compatible for 24 hr at 25 °C under fluorescent light	1393	C
Hydrocortisone sodium succinate	UP	50 mg/mL	AST	24 mg/mL	Physically compatible for 24 hr at room temperature under fluorescent light	1335	C
Hydromorphone HCl	KN	10 mg/mL	AST	24 mg/mL	Physically compatible for 24 hr at room temperature under fluorescent light	1335	C
Hydroxyzine HCl	LY	50 mg/mL	AST	24 mg/mL	Physically compatible for 24 hr at room temperature under fluorescent light	1335	C
Imipenem–cilastatin sodium	MSD	10 mg/mL	AST	24 mg/mL	Physically compatible for 24 hr at room temperature under fluorescent light	1335	C
	MSD	5 mg/mL[a]	AST	24 mg/mL	Physically compatible for 24 hr at 25 °C under fluorescent light	1393	C
Leucovorin calcium	QU	10 mg/mL	AST	24 mg/mL	Cloudy yellow solution	1335	I
Lorazepam	WY	4 mg/mL	AST	24 mg/mL	Gas production	1335	I
	WY	0.08 mg/mL[a,b]	AST	24 mg/mL	Physically compatible for 24 hr at 25 °C under fluorescent light	1393	C
Metoclopramide HCl	RB	4 mg/mL	AST	24 mg/mL	Physically compatible for 24 hr at room temperature under fluorescent light	1335	C
	RB	2 mg/mL[a,b]	AST	24 mg/mL	Physically compatible for 24 hr at 25 °C under fluorescent light	1393	C
Metronidazole	AB	5 mg/mL	AST	24 mg/mL	Physically compatible for 24 hr at room temperature under fluorescent light	1335	C
	SE	5 mg/mL	AST	24 mg/mL	Physically compatible for 24 hr at 25 °C under fluorescent light	1393	C
Midazolam HCl	RC	5 mg/mL	AST	24 mg/mL	Gas production	1335	I
Morphine sulfate	IMS	1 mg/mL	AST	24 mg/mL	Physically compatible for 24 hr at room temperature under fluorescent light	1335	C
	ES	1 mg/mL[a,b]	AST	24 mg/mL	Physically compatible for 24 hr at 25 °C under fluorescent light	1393	C
	ES	5[b] and 15 mg/mL	AST	24 mg/mL	Visually compatible for 24 hr at 23 °C under fluorescent light	1529	C
Nafcillin sodium	BR	20 mg/mL[a,b]	AST	24 mg/mL	Physically compatible for 24 hr at 25 °C under fluorescent light	1393	C
Oxacillin sodium	BR	40 mg/mL	AST	24 mg/mL	Physically compatible for 24 hr at room temperature under fluorescent light	1335	C
	BE	20 mg/mL[a,b]	AST	24 mg/mL	Physically compatible for 24 hr at 25 °C under fluorescent light	1393	C
Penicillin G potassium	SQ	100,000 units/mL	AST	24 mg/mL	Physically compatible for 24 hr at room temperature under fluorescent light	1335	C
Pentamidine isethionate	LY	6 mg/mL	AST	24 mg/mL	Precipitates immediately	1335	I
	LY	6 mg/mL[a,b]	AST	24 mg/mL	Pentamidine crystals form immediately	1393	I

Y-Site Injection Compatibility (1:1 Mixture) (Cont.)

Foscarnet sodium

Drug	Mfr	Conc	Mfr	Conc	Remarks	Ref	C/I
Prochlorperazine edisylate	SKF	5 mg/mL	AST	24 mg/mL	Cloudy brown solution	1335	I
Promethazine HCl	ES	50 mg/mL	AST	24 mg/mL	Gas production	1335	I
Ranitidine HCl	GL	2 mg/mL[a,b]	AST	24 mg/mL	Physically compatible for 24 hr at 25 °C under fluorescent light	1393	C
Ticarcillin disodium–clavulanate potassium	BE	100 mg/mL[a,b]	AST	24 mg/mL	Physically compatible for 24 hr at 25 °C under fluorescent light	1393	C
Tobramycin sulfate	LI	40 mg/mL	AST	24 mg/mL	Physically compatible for 24 hr at room temperature under fluorescent light	1335	C
TPN #121[d]		[c]	AST	24 mg/mL	Physically compatible for 24 hr at 25 °C	1393	C
Trimethoprim–sulfamethoxazole	RC	16 + 80 mg/mL	AST	24 mg/mL	Precipitates immediately and gas production	1335	I
	BW	0.53 + 2.6 mg/mL[a]	AST	24 mg/mL	Physically compatible for 24 hr at 25 °C under fluorescent light	1393	C
Vancomycin HCl	LE	20 mg/mL	AST	24 mg/mL	Precipitates immediately	1335	I
	LE	15 mg/mL[a,b]	AST	24 mg/mL	Physically compatible for 24 hr at 25 °C under fluorescent light	1393	C
	LE	10 mg/mL[b]	AST	24 mg/mL	Visually compatible for 24 hr at room temperature. No precipitate found	2063	C

[a]*Tested in dextrose 5%.*
[b]*Tested in sodium chloride 0.9%.*
[c]*Tested in equal quantities.*
[d]*Refer to Appendix I for the composition of parenteral nutrition solutions. TPN indicates a 2-in-1 admixture.*

FOSPHENYTOIN SODIUM
AHFS 28:12.12

Products — Fosphenytoin is the prodrug for its metabolite, phenytoin. Fosphenytoin sodium is available in 2- and 10-mL vials as a 75-mg/mL solution, which is the equivalent of phenytoin sodium 50 mg/mL after administration. Each milliliter also contains tromethamine (TRIS) buffer along with hydrochloric acid or sodium hydroxide to adjust pH in water for injection. (1) CAUTION: Care should be taken to avoid confusion between the two different forms (fosphenytoin sodium and phenytoin sodium) to prevent dosing errors.

Units — Each 75 mg of fosphenytoin sodium is metabolically converted to 50 mg of phenytoin after administration. NOTE: The amount and concentration of fosphenytoin sodium are expressed in terms of the equivalent mass of phenytoin sodium, called phenytoin sodium equivalents (PE). The manufacturer indicates that this avoids the need to perform conversions based on molecular weight between the two forms. (1) However, it creates the need to express all prescribing, dispensing, and dosing consistently in PE to avoid dosing errors that could result from confusion between the two forms.

pH — From 8.6 to 9.0. (1)

Trade Name(s) — Cerebyx.

Administration — Fosphenytoin sodium is dosed in terms of phenytoin sodium equivalents (PE). CAUTION: Care should be taken to ensure that all prescribing, preparation, and dosing is performed using the correct units and that any confusion between the two forms (fosphenytoin sodium and phenytoin sodium) is avoided.

Fosphenytoin sodium is administered intravenously at a rate no greater than 150 mg PE/min. The drug may be diluted in dextrose 5% or sodium chloride 0.9% to a concentration of 1.5 to 25 mg PE/mL. It has also been given intramuscularly. (1)

Stability — Fosphenytoin sodium injection is a clear, colorless to pale yellow solution. Intact vials should be stored under refrigeration at 2 to 8 °C. Storage at controlled room temperature should not exceed 48 hours. Any vials that develop particulate matter should not be used. (1)

Freezing Solutions — Fosphenytoin sodium (Parke-Davis) 1, 8, and 20 PE (phenytoin sodium equivalents) per milliliter in dextrose 5% (Baxter) and sodium chloride 0.9% (Baxter) in PVC containers and undiluted fosphenytoin sodium 50 mg PE per milliliter were packaged in 3-mL polypropylene syringes sealed with tip caps (Becton Dickinson). The samples were frozen at −20 °C. Little or no loss occurred after 30 days of frozen storage followed by seven days at 4 or 25 °C. Stability was also maintained if the thawed samples that had been stored at 25 °C were returned to the freezer for an additional seven days. (2083)

Syringes — Fosphenytoin sodium (Parke-Davis) 50 mg PE (phenytoin sodium equivalents) per milliliter was packaged in 3-mL polypropylene syringes with syringe caps (Becton Dickinson) and stored at −20, 4, and 25 °C. The samples stored at 4 and 25 °C exhibited little or no loss of fosphenytoin sodium in 30 days. The samples stored at −20 °C also showed little or no loss of fosphenytoin sodium after 30 days' storage followed by seven days at 4 °C or at 25 °C. Also, stability was maintained if the thawed samples that had been stored at 25 °C were returned to the freezer for an additional seven days. (2083)

Compatibility Information

Solution Compatibility

Fosphenytoin sodium

Solution	Mfr	Mfr	Conc/L	Remarks	Ref	C/I
Dextrose 5% in Ringer's injection, lactated	BA[a]	PD	1, 8, 20 mg PE/mL	Visually compatible with little or no loss in 7 days at 25 °C under fluorescent light	2083	C
Dextrose 5% in sodium chloride 0.45%	BA[a]	PD	1, 8, 20 mg PE/mL	Visually compatible with little or no loss in 7 days at 25 °C under fluorescent light	2083	C
Dextrose 5%	BA[a,b]	PD	1, 8, 20 mg PE/mL	Visually compatible with little or no loss in 7 days at 25 °C under fluorescent light	2083	C
Dextrose 10%	BA[a]	PD	1, 8, 20 mg PE/mL	Visually compatible with little or no loss in 7 days at 25 °C under fluorescent light	2083	C
Plasma-Lyte A, pH 7.4	BA[a]	PD	1, 8, 20 mg PE/mL	Visually compatible with little or no loss in 7 days at 25 °C under fluorescent light	2083	C
Ringer's injection, lactated	BA[a]	PD	1, 8, 20 mg PE/mL	Visually compatible with little or no loss in 7 days at 25 °C under fluorescent light	2083	C
Sodium chloride 0.9%	BA[a,b]	PD	1, 8, 20 mg PE/mL	Visually compatible with little or no loss in 7 days at 25 °C under fluorescent light	2083	C

[a]Tested in PVC containers.
[b]Tested in glass containers.

Additive Compatibility

Fosphenytoin sodium

Drug	Mfr	Conc/L	Mfr	Conc/L	Test Soln	Remarks	Ref	C/I
Hetastarch in sodium chloride 0.9%	MG	6%	PD	1, 8, 20 mg PE/mL	NS	Visually compatible with little or no loss in 7 days at 25 °C under fluorescent light	2083	C
Mannitol	BA[a]	20%	PD	2, 8, 20 mg PE/mL		Visually compatible with little or no loss in 7 days at 25 °C under fluorescent light	2083	C
Potassium chloride	BA	20 and 40 mEq	PD	1, 8, 20 mg PE/mL	D5½S[a]	Visually compatible with little or no loss in 7 days at 25 °C under fluorescent light	2083	C

[a]Tested in PVC containers.

Y-Site Injection Compatibility (1:1 Mixture)

Fosphenytoin sodium

Drug	Mfr	Conc	Mfr	Conc	Remarks	Ref	C/I
Fenoldopam mesylate	AB	80 mcg/mL[a]	PD	20 mg PE/mL[a]	Trace haze and microparticulates form in 4 hr	2467	I
Lorazepam	WY	2 mg/mL	PD	1 mg PE/mL[a]	Samples remained clear with no loss of either drug in 8 hr	2223	C
Midazolam HCl	RC	2 mg/mL[a]	PD	1 mg PE/mL[a]	Midazolam base precipitates immediately	2223	I
Phenobarbital sodium		130 mg/mL	PD	10 mg PE/mL[a]	Visually compatible with no loss of either drug in 8 hr at room temperature	2212	C

[a]Tested in sodium chloride 0.9%.

FUROSEMIDE
(FRUSEMIDE)
AHFS 40:28.08

Products — Furosemide is available in 2-, 4-, and 10-mL amber ampuls, single-use vials, prefilled syringes, and syringe cartridges. Each milliliter of solution contains furosemide 10 mg, water for injection, with sodium chloride for isotonicity, sodium hydroxide, and, if necessary, hydrochloric acid to adjust pH. (1; 4)

pH — From 8 to 9.3. (1; 4)

Osmolality — Furosemide (Hoechst-Roussel) 10 mg/mL has an osmolality of 287 mOsm/kg. (50) The osmolality of the Elkins-Sinn product has been determined to be 289 mOsm/kg by freezing-point depression. (1071)

In another study, the osmolality of furosemide injection (manufacturer unspecified) was determined to be 291 mOsm/kg. (1233)

Sodium Content — The injection contains 0.162 mEq of sodium per milliliter. (4)

Administration — Furosemide may be administered by intramuscular injection, by direct intravenous injection over one to two minutes, and by intravenous infusion at a rate not exceeding 4 mg/min. (1; 4)

Stability — Exposure to light may cause discoloration; protection from light for the syringes once they are removed from the package is recommended. Do not use furosemide solutions if they have a yellow color. Furosemide products should be stored at controlled room temperature. (1; 4) Refrigeration may result in precipitation or crystallization. However, resolubilization at room temperature or on warming may be performed without affecting the drug's stability. (593)

Furosemide under simulated summer conditions in paramedic vehicles was exposed to temperatures from 26 to 38 °C over 4 weeks. Analysis found no loss of drug under these conditions. (2562)

pH Effects — Furosemide is soluble in alkaline solutions and is prepared as a mildly buffered alkaline product. (1; 4) It can usually be mixed with infusion solutions that are neutral or weakly basic (pH 7 to 10) and with some weakly acidic solutions that have a low buffer capacity. (4) It should not be mixed with acidic solutions having a pH below 5.5. Solutions such as sodium chloride 0.9%, Ringer's injection, lactated, and dextrose 5% have been recommended. If the solution pH is below 5.5, pH adjustment has been recommended. (1; 4) In addition, furosemide has been found to be unstable in acidic media (96; 664) but very stable in basic media. (664)

A 2-mL fluid barrier of dextrose 5% in a microbore retrograde infusion set failed to prevent precipitation when used between gentamicin sulfate 5 mg/0.5 mL and furosemide 2 mg/0.2 mL. (1385)

Autoclaving — Autoclaving of furosemide 1 mg/mL in sodium chloride 0.9% in glass bottles at 115 °C for 34 minutes resulted in no loss of furosemide. Storage of the solution for 70 days at room temperature with protection from light also showed no detectable change in furosemide content. However, storage at room temperature with exposure to light for 70 days resulted in about a 60% loss of furosemide and the formation of a yellow-orange precipitate. (1108)

Light Effects — Furosemide is subject to photodegradation by several mechanisms. (358; 400; 2067) Photodegradation is minimized at pH 7; rates of decomposition increase as the pH becomes more acidic or basic. (400; 2067) Photodegradation is unaffected by ionic strength and initial concentration (in the range of 10 mcg/mL to 1 mg/mL), but the rate of loss may decrease at the higher concentration due to a light-filtering effect of the yellow discoloration. In pH 7 phosphate buffer, more than 60% furosemide loss occurred in transparent glass vials exposed to fluorescent light for 90 hours; little or no loss occurred if the transparent vials were covered with aluminum foil or if amber glass containers were used. (2067)

Syringes — Furosemide (Hoechst) 10 mg/mL was filled into 25-mL polypropylene syringes (Becton Dickinson) and stored at 25 °C while exposed to normal room light or in the dark for 24 hours. There was no detectable change in furosemide content in either light-exposed or light-protected syringes. (1108)

Furosemide (Abbott) 1, 2, 4, and 8 mg/mL diluted in sodium chloride 0.9% was packaged in polypropylene syringes. Samples were stored for 84 days at 22 °C and also at 4 °C protected from light for 84 days. This was followed by an additional 7 days of storage at 22 °C exposed to fluorescent light. No visible changes occurred and little or no loss of furosemide occurred in any of the samples. (2389)

Filtration — Furosemide (Hoechst) 0.04 mg/mL in dextrose 5% and sodium chloride 0.9% was filtered through a 0.22-μm cellulose ester membrane filter (Ivex-HP, Millipore) over six hours. No significant drug loss due to binding to the filter was noted. (1034)

Central Venous Catheter — Furosemide (American Regent) 1 mg/mL in dextrose 5% was found to be compatible with the ARROWg+ard Blue Plus (Arrow International) chlorhexidine-bearing triple-lumen central catheter. Essentially complete delivery of the drug was found with little or no drug loss occurring. Furthermore, chlorhexidine delivered from the catheter remained at trace amounts with no substantial increase due to the delivery of the drug through the catheter. (2335)

Compatibility Information

Solution Compatibility

Furosemide

Solution	Mfr	Mfr	Conc/L	Remarks	Ref	C/I
Amino acids 4.25%, dextrose 25%	MG	HO	40 mg	No increase in particulate matter in 24 hr at 25 °C	349	C
Dextrose 5% in Ringer's injection, lactated	BA	HO	600 mg	Physically compatible for 24 hr	315	C
Dextrose 5% in sodium chloride 0.9%	BA	HO	600 mg	Physically compatible for 24 hr	315	C
Dextrose 5%	BA	HO	600 mg	Physically compatible for 24 hr	315	C
			200 and 400 mg	4 to 5% loss in 24 hr at 25 °C	1348	C
Dextrose 10%	BA	HO	600 mg	Physically compatible for 24 hr	315	C
Dextrose 20%	BA	HO	600 mg	Physically compatible for 24 hr	315	C
Ringer's injection, lactated	BA	HO	600 mg	Physically compatible for 24 hr	315	C
	TR[a]	HO	1 g	No furosemide loss in 24 hr at 25 °C exposed to light or in the dark	1108	C
Sodium chloride 0.9%	BA	HO	600 mg	Physically compatible for 24 hr	315	C
	TR[a]	HO	1 g	No furosemide loss in 24 hr at 25 °C exposed to light or in the dark. 10% loss in 26 days at 6 °C	1108	C
			200 and 400 mg	5 to 7% loss in 24 hr at 25 °C	1348	C
	BA[a]	AB	1.2, 2.4, 3.2 g	Visually compatible. Little loss in 84 days at 4 and 22 °C in dark then 7 days at 22 °C in fluorescent light	2389	C
Sodium lactate ⅙ M	BA	HO	600 mg	Physically compatible for 24 hr	315	C

[a]Tested in PVC containers.

Additive Compatibility

Furosemide

Drug	Mfr	Conc/L	Mfr	Conc/L	Test Soln	Remarks	Ref	C/I
Amikacin sulfate	BR	2 g	HO	160 mg	D5W, NS	Transient cloudiness, then visually compatible for 24 hr at 21 °C	876	?
Aminophylline	ANT	1 g	HO	1 g	NS	Physically compatible for 72 hr at 15 and 30 °C	1479	C
Amiodarone HCl	LZ	1.8 g	ES	200 mg	D5W, NS[a]	Physically compatible. 8% or less amiodarone loss in 24 hr at 24 °C in light	1031	C
	LZ	4 g	HO	1 g	D5W	Haze in 5 hr and precipitate in 24 to 72 hr at 30 °C. No changes at 15 °C	1479	I

Additive Compatibility (Cont.)

Furosemide

Drug	Mfr	Conc/L	Mfr	Conc/L	Test Soln	Remarks	Ref	C/I
Ampicillin sodium	BE	20 g	HO	1 g	NS	Physically compatible for 72 hr at 15 and 30 °C	1479	C
Atropine sulfate	ANT	60 mg	HO	1 g	W	Physically compatible for 72 hr at 15 and 30 °C	1479	C
Bumetanide	LEO	6 mg	HO	1 g	NS	Physically compatible for 72 hr at 15 and 30 °C	1479	C
Buprenorphine HCl		75 mg	HO	1 g	W	Haze for 6 hr at 30 °C. No change at 15 °C	1479	I
Calcium gluconate	ANT	2 g	HO	1 g	NS	Physically compatible for 72 hr at 15 and 30 °C	1479	C
Cefuroxime sodium	GL	37.5 g	HO	1 g	W	Physically compatible for 72 hr at 15 and 30 °C	1479	C
Chlorpromazine HCl	ANT	5 g	HO	1 g	W	Precipitates immediately	1479	I
Cloxacillin sodium	BE	20 g	HO	1 g	NS	Physically compatible for 72 hr at 15 and 30 °C	1479	C
Dexamethasone sodium phosphate	MSD	4 g	HO	1 g	NS	Physically compatible for 72 hr at 15 and 30 °C	1479	C
Diamorphine HCl	EV	500 mg	HO	1 g	W	Physically compatible for 72 hr at 15 and 30 °C	1479	C
Diazepam	PHX	1 g	HO	1 g	D5W	Precipitates immediately	1479	I
Digoxin	BW	25 mg	HO	1 g	NS	Physically compatible for 72 hr at 15 and 30 °C	1479	C
Dobutamine HCl	LI	1 g	HO	1 g	D5W, NS	Cloudy in 1 hr at 25 °C	789	I
	LI	1 g	WY	5 g	D5W, NS	Immediate white precipitate	812	I
	LI	500 mg	HO	1 g	NS	Haze forms immediately	1479	I
Epinephrine HCl	ANT	8 mg	HO	1 g	W	Physically compatible for 72 hr at 15 and 30 °C	1479	C
Erythromycin lactobionate	AB	5 g	HO	1 g	NS	Precipitates immediately. Crystals form in 12 to 24 hr at 15 and 30 °C	1479	I
Gentamicin sulfate	SC	1.6 g	HO	800 mg	D5W, NS	Furosemide precipitates immediately	876	I
	RS	8 g	HO	1 g	NS	Physically compatible for 24 hr at 15 and 30 °C. Precipitate forms in 48 to 72 hr	1479	C
Heparin sodium	WED	20,000 units	HO	1 g	NS	Physically compatible for 72 hr at 15 and 30 °C	1479	C
Hydrocortisone sodium succinate		1 g		200 and 400 mg	D5W, NS	6 to 8% hydrocortisone loss and 5 to 6% furosemide loss in 24 hr at 25 °C	1348	C
		300 mg		200 and 400 mg	D5W, NS	6 to 8% hydrocortisone loss in 6 hr and 10 to 14% loss in 24 hr at 25 °C. 5 to 6% furosemide loss in 24 hr	1348	I
	UP	50 g	HO	1 g	NS	Physically compatible for 72 hr at 15 and 30 °C	1479	C
Isoproterenol HCl	PX	4 mg	HO	1 g	D5W	Precipitates immediately	1479	I
Isosorbide dinitrate		1 g	HO	1 g		Physically compatible for 72 hr at 15 and 30 °C	1479	C
Lidocaine HCl	ANT	2 g	HO	1 g	NS	Physically compatible for 72 hr at 15 and 30 °C	1479	C

Additive Compatibility (Cont.)

Furosemide

Drug	Mfr	Conc/L	Mfr	Conc/L	Test Soln	Remarks	Ref	C/I
Mannitol	BA[c]	20%	AB	200, 400, 800 mg		Visually compatible for 72 hr at 22 °C	1803	C
Meperidine HCl	RC	5 g	HO	1 g	W	Fine precipitate forms immediately	1479	I
Meropenem	ZEN	1 and 20 g	HO	1 g	NS	Visually compatible for 4 hr at room temperature	1994	C
Metoclopramide HCl	ANT	1 g	HO	1 g	NS	Precipitates immediately	1479	I
Midazolam HCl	RC	50 and 250 mg		80 mg	NS	Visually compatible for 4 hr	355	C
Morphine sulfate	EV	1 g	HO	1 g	W	Physically compatible for 72 hr at 15 and 30 °C	1479	C
Nitroglycerin	ACC	400 mg	HO	1 g	D5W[b]	Physically compatible with no nitroglycerin loss in 48 hr at 23 °C. Furosemide not tested	929	C
	ACC	400 mg	HO	1 g	NS[b]	Physically compatible with 3% nitroglycerin loss in 48 hr at 23 °C. Furosemide not tested	929	C
Potassium chloride	ANT	40 mmol	HO	1 g	W	Physically compatible for 72 hr at 15 and 30 °C	1479	C
Prochlorperazine edisylate	MB	1.25 g	HO	1 g	W	Yellow precipitate forms immediately	1479	I
Promethazine HCl	MB	5 g	HO	1 g	W	White precipitate forms immediately	1479	I
Ranitidine HCl	GL	500 mg	HO	1 g	NS	Physically compatible for 72 hr at 15 and 30 °C	1479	C
	GL	50 mg and 2 g		400 mg	D5W	Physically compatible. Ranitidine stable for 24 hr at 25 °C. Furosemide not tested	1515	C
Scopolamine butylbromide	BI	2 g	HO	1 g	W	Physically compatible for 72 hr at 15 and 30 °C	1479	C
Sodium bicarbonate	IMS	8.4%	HO	1 g		Physically compatible for 72 hr at 15 and 30 °C	1479	C
Theophylline		2 g		330 mg	D5W	Visually compatible. Little theophylline and 10% furosemide loss in 48 hr	1909	C
Tobramycin sulfate	DI	1.6 g	HO	800 mg	D5W, NS	Transient cloudiness then physically compatible for 24 hr at 21 °C	876	?
	LI	8 g	HO	1 g	NS	Physically compatible for 72 hr at 15 and 30 °C	1479	C
Verapamil HCl	KN	80 mg	HO	200 mg	D5W, NS	Physically compatible for 24 hr	764	C
	AB	500 mg	HO	1 g	NS	Slight precipitate forms but dissipates	1479	?

[a]*Tested in both polyolefin and PVC containers.*
[b]*Tested in glass containers.*
[c]*Tested in PVC containers.*

Drugs in Syringe Compatibility

Furosemide

Drug (in syringe)	Mfr	Amt	Mfr	Amt	Remarks	Ref	C/I
Bleomycin sulfate		1.5 units/ 0.5 mL		5 mg/ 0.5 mL	Physically compatible for 5 min at room temperature followed by 8 min of centrifugation	980	C
Caffeine citrate		20 mg/ 1 mL	AST	10 mg/ 1 mL	Precipitates immediately	2440	I
Cisplatin		0.5 mg/ 0.5 mL		5 mg/ 0.5 mL	Physically compatible for 5 min at room temperature followed by 8 min of centrifugation	980	C
Cyclophosphamide		10 mg/ 0.5 mL		5 mg/ 0.5 mL	Physically compatible for 5 min at room temperature followed by 8 min of centrifugation	980	C
Dexamethasone sodium phosphate	ME	0.33 to 3.33 mg/ mL	HO	3.33 to 10 mg/ mL	Tested in NS. No visible precipitation with under 10% loss of either drug in 5 days at 4 and 25 °C. Precipitation with over 10% drug loss in 15 days	2711	C
Dimenhydrinate		10 mg/ 1 mL		10 mg/ 1 mL	Precipitate forms	2569	I
Doxapram HCl	RB	400 mg/ 20 mL	HO	100 mg/ 10 mL	Immediate turbidity	1177	I
Doxorubicin HCl		1 mg/ 0.5 mL		5 mg/ 0.5 mL	Precipitates immediately	980	I
Droperidol		1.25 mg/ 0.5 mL		5 mg/ 0.5 mL	Precipitates immediately	980	I
Fluorouracil		25 mg/ 0.5 mL		5 mg/ 0.5 mL	Physically compatible for 5 min at room temperature followed by 8 min of centrifugation	980	C
Heparin sodium		500 units/ 0.5 mL		5 mg/ 0.5 mL	Physically compatible for 5 min at room temperature followed by 8 min of centrifugation	980	C
		2500 units/ 1 mL		20 mg/ 2 mL	Physically compatible for at least 5 min	1053	C
Leucovorin calcium		5 mg/ 0.5 mL		5 mg/ 0.5 mL	Physically compatible for 5 min at room temperature followed by 8 min of centrifugation	980	C
Methotrexate sodium		12.5 mg/ 0.5 mL		5 mg/ 0.5 mL	Physically compatible for 5 min at room temperature followed by 8 min of centrifugation	980	C
Metoclopramide HCl		2.5 mg/ 0.5 mL		5 mg/ 0.5 mL	Precipitates immediately	980	I
Milrinone lactate	WI	3.5 mg/ 3.5 mL	LY	40 mg/ 4 mL	Brought to 10-mL total volume with D5W. Precipitates immediately	1191	I
Mitomycin		0.25 mg/ 0.5 mL		5 mg/ 0.5 mL	Physically compatible for 5 min at room temperature followed by 8 min of centrifugation	980	C
Pantoprazole sodium	[a]	4 mg/ 1 mL		10 mg/ 1 mL	Possible precipitate within 15 min	2574	I
Vinblastine sulfate		0.5 mg/ 0.5 mL		5 mg/ 0.5 mL	Precipitates immediately	980	I
Vincristine sulfate		0.5 mg/ 0.5 mL		5 mg/ 0.5 mL	Precipitates immediately	980	I

[a]*Test performed using the formulation WITHOUT edetate disodium.*

Y-Site Injection Compatibility (1:1 Mixture)

Furosemide

Drug	Mfr	Conc	Mfr	Conc	Remarks	Ref	C/I
Allopurinol sodium	BW	3 mg/mL[b]	ES	3 mg/mL[b]	Physically compatible for 4 hr at 22 °C	1686	C
Amifostine	USB	10 mg/mL[a]	AB	3 mg/mL[a]	Physically compatible for 4 hr at 23 °C	1845	C
Amikacin sulfate	BR	2 mg/mL[c]	HO	10 mg/mL	Physically compatible for 24 hr at 21 °C	876	C
Amiodarone HCl	WY	6 mg/mL[a]	AMR	1 mg/mL[a]	Visually compatible for 24 hr at 22 °C	2352	C
	WY	6 mg/mL[a]	AMR	10 mg/mL	Immediate opaque white turbidity	2352	I
Amphotericin B cholesteryl sulfate complex	SEQ	0.83 mg/mL[a]	AMR	3 mg/mL[a]	Physically compatible for 4 hr at 23 °C	2117	C
Amsacrine	NCI	1 mg/mL[a]	ES	3 mg/mL[a]	Yellow turbidity becoming colorless liquid with yellow precipitate	1381	I
Anidulafungin	VIC	0.5 mg/mL[a]	AB	3 mg/mL[a]	Physically compatible for 4 hr at 23 °C	2617	C
Argatroban	SKB	1 mg/mL[a]	AB	10 mg/mL	Physically compatible for 24 hr at 23 °C	2572	C
Azithromycin	PF	2 mg/mL[b]	AMR	10 mg/mL[l]	White microcrystals found	2368	I
Aztreonam	SQ	40 mg/mL[a]	AB	3 mg/mL[a]	Physically compatible for 4 hr at 23 °C	1758	C
Bivalirudin	TMC	5 mg/mL[a]	AMR	3 mg/mL[a]	Physically compatible for 4 hr at 23 °C	2373	C
Bleomycin sulfate		3 units/mL		10 mg/mL	Drugs injected sequentially in Y-site with no flush. No precipitate seen	980	C
Caspofungin acetate	ME	0.7 mg/mL[b]	AMR	3 mg/mL[b]	Immediate white turbid precipitate forms	2758	I
	ME	0.5 mg/mL[b]	HOS	10 mg/mL	Gelatinous material reported	2766	I
Cefepime HCl	BMS	120 mg/mL[c]		10 mg/mL[a]	Physically compatible with less than 10% cefepime loss. Furosemide not tested	2513	C
Ceftaroline fosamil	FOR	2.22 mg/mL[a,b,m]	HOS	3 mg/mL[a,b,m]	Physically compatible for 4 hr at 23 °C	2826	C
Ceftazidime	SKB	125 mg/mL		10 mg/mL	Visually compatible with less than 10% loss of ceftazidime in 30 min. Furosemide not tested	2434	C
	GSK	120 mg/mL[d]		10 mg/mL	Physically compatible with less than 10% ceftazidime loss. Furosemide not tested	2513	C
Chlorpromazine HCl	RPR	0.13 mg/mL[a]	HMR	2.6 mg/mL[a]	Precipitate forms immediately	2244	I
Ciprofloxacin	MI	2 mg/mL[c]	AB	10 mg/mL	Precipitates immediately	1655	I
	BAY	2 mg/mL[b]	DMX	5 mg/mL	White precipitate forms immediately	1934	I
Cisatracurium besylate	GW	0.1 mg/mL[a]	AB	3 mg/mL[a]	Physically compatible for 4 hr at 23 °C	2074	C
	GW	2 and 5 mg/mL[a]	AB	3 mg/mL[a]	White cloudiness forms immediately	2074	I
Cisplatin		1 mg/mL		10 mg/mL	Drugs injected sequentially in Y-site with no flush. No precipitate seen	980	C
Cladribine	ORT	0.015[b] and 0.5[e] mg/mL	AB	3 mg/mL[b]	Physically compatible for 4 hr at 23 °C	1969	C
Clarithromycin	AB	4 mg/mL[a]	ANT	10 mg/mL	White cloudiness forms immediately, becoming an obvious precipitate in 15 min	2174	I
Cyclophosphamide		20 mg/mL		10 mg/mL	Drugs injected sequentially in Y-site with no flush. No precipitate seen	980	C
Dexmedetomidine HCl	AB	4 mcg/mL[b]	AMR	3 mg/mL[b]	Physically compatible for 4 hr at 23 °C	2383	C
Diltiazem HCl	MMD	1[b] and 5 mg/mL	AMR	10 mg/mL	Heavy precipitate forms	1807	I
	MMD	1 mg/mL[a]	AMR	10 mg/mL	Precipitate forms immediately	2062	I

Y-Site Injection Compatibility (1:1 Mixture) (Cont.)

Drug	Mfr	Conc	Mfr	Conc	Remarks	Ref	C/I
				Furosemide			
Dobutamine HCl	LI	4 mg/mL[b]	ES	1 mg/mL[b]	Physically compatible for 3 hr	1316	C
	LI	4 mg/mL[a]	ES	1 mg/mL[a]	Slight precipitate in 1 hr	1316	I
	LI	4 mg/mL[a]	AMR	10 mg/mL	Precipitate forms immediately	2062	I
Docetaxel	RPR	0.9 mg/mL[a]	AMR	3 mg/mL[a]	Physically compatible for 4 hr at 23 °C	2224	C
Dopamine HCl	AST, DU	12.8 mg/mL	AB, AMR	5 mg/mL	Physically compatible for 3 hr at room temperature	1978	C
	AB, AMR	12.8 mg/mL	AB, AMR	5 mg/mL	White precipitate forms immediately	1978	I
	AB	3.2 mg/mL[a]	AMR	10 mg/mL	Precipitate forms in 4 hr at 27 °C	2062	I
Doripenem	JJ	5 mg/mL[a,b]	AMR	3 mg/mL[a,b]	Physically compatible for 4 hr at 23 °C	2743	C
Doxorubicin HCl		2 mg/mL		10 mg/mL	Drugs injected sequentially in Y-site with no flush. Precipitates immediately	980	I
Doxorubicin HCl liposomal	SEQ	0.4 mg/mL[a]	AMR	3 mg/mL[a]	Physically compatible for 4 hr at 23 °C	2087	C
Droperidol		2.5 mg/mL		10 mg/mL	Drugs injected sequentially in Y-site with no flush. Precipitates immediately	980	I
		2.5 mg/mL		10 mg/mL	Precipitate forms	977	I
Epinephrine HCl	AB	0.02 mg/mL[a]	AMR	10 mg/mL	Visually compatible for 4 hr at 27 °C	2062	C
Esmolol HCl	ACC	10 mg/mL[c]	HO	10 mg/mL	Cloudy precipitate forms immediately	1146	I
Etoposide phosphate	BR	5 mg/mL[a]	AMR	3 mg/mL[a]	Physically compatible for 4 hr at 23 °C	2218	C
Famotidine	MSD	0.2 mg/mL[a]	IMS	0.8 mg/mL[a]	Physically compatible for 4 hr at 25 °C	1188	C
	MSD	0.2 mg/mL[a]	ES	10 mg/mL	Physically compatible for 14 hr	1196	C
	ME	2 mg/mL[b]		3 mg/mL[a]	White precipitate forms immediately	1936	I
Fenoldopam mesylate	AB	80 mcg/mL[b]	AMR	3 mg/mL[b]	Trace haze forms immediately	2467	I
Fentanyl citrate	ES	0.05 mg/mL	AMR	10 mg/mL	Visually compatible for 4 hr at 27 °C	2062	C
Filgrastim	AMG	30 mcg/mL[a]	AB	3 mg/mL[a]	Turbidity forms immediately. Filaments and particles form in 1 hr	1687	I
Fluconazole	RR	2 mg/mL	ES	10 mg/mL	Precipitate forms	1407	I
Fludarabine phosphate	BX	1 mg/mL[a]	AB	3 mg/mL[a]	Visually compatible for 4 hr at 22 °C	1439	C
Fluorouracil		50 mg/mL		10 mg/mL	Drugs injected sequentially in Y-site with no flush. No precipitate seen	980	C
Foscarnet sodium	AST	24 mg/mL	AB	10 mg/mL	Physically compatible for 24 hr at room temperature under fluorescent light	1335	C
Gallium nitrate	FUJ	1 mg/mL[b]	AB	10 mg/mL	Visually compatible for 24 hr at 25 °C	1673	C
Gemcitabine HCl	LI	10 mg/mL[b]	AMR	3 mg/mL[b]	Gross precipitation occurs immediately	2226	I
Gentamicin sulfate	SC	1.6 mg/mL[c]	HO	10 mg/mL	Furosemide precipitates immediately	876	I
Granisetron HCl	SKB	0.05 mg/mL[a]	AB	3 mg/mL[a]	Physically compatible for 4 hr at 23 °C	1804	C
	SKB	1 mg/mL	HO	0.4 mg/mL[b]	Physically compatible with little or no loss of either drug in 4 hr at 22 °C	1883	C
Heparin sodium		1000 units/mL		10 mg/mL	Drugs injected sequentially in Y-site with no flush. No precipitate seen	980	C
	UP	1000 units/L[f]	HO	10 mg/mL	Physically compatible for 4 hr at room temperature	534	C
	ES	100 units/mL[a]	AMR	10 mg/mL	Visually compatible for 4 hr at 27 °C	2062	C
	NOV	29.2 units/mL[a]	HMR	2.6 mg/mL[a]	Visually compatible for 150 min	2244	C

Y-Site Injection Compatibility (1:1 Mixture) (Cont.)

Furosemide

Drug	Mfr	Conc	Mfr	Conc	Remarks	Ref	C/I
Hetastarch in lactated electrolyte	AB	6%	AMR	3 mg/mL[a]	Physically compatible for 4 hr at 23 °C	2339	C
Hydralazine HCl	SO	1 mg/mL[c]	ES	1 mg/mL[c]	Slight color change in 3 hr	1316	I
Hydrocortisone sodium succinate	UP	10 mg/L[f]	HO	10 mg/mL	Physically compatible for 4 hr at room temperature	534	C
Hydromorphone HCl	KN	1 mg/mL	AMR	10 mg/mL	Visually compatible for 4 hr at 27 °C	2062	C
Hydroxyethyl starch 130/0.4 in sodium chloride 0.9%	FRK	6%	SZ	1, 1.5, 2 mg/mL[a]	Visually compatible for 24 hr at room temperature	2770	C
Idarubicin HCl	AD	1 mg/mL[b]	AB	10 mg/mL	Precipitate forms immediately	1525	I
	AD	1 mg/mL[b]	AB	0.8 mg/mL[b]	Haze forms immediately	1525	I
Indomethacin sodium trihydrate	MSD	1 mg/mL[b]	AB	10 mg/mL	Visually compatible for 24 hr at 28 °C	1527	C
Labetalol HCl	SC	1.6 mg/mL[g]	ES	10 mg/mL[g]	White precipitate forms immediately	1715	I
	AH	2 mg/mL[a]	AMR	10 mg/mL	Precipitate forms immediately	2062	I
Leucovorin calcium		10 mg/mL		10 mg/mL	Drugs injected sequentially in Y-site with no flush. No precipitate seen	980	C
Levofloxacin	OMN	5 mg/mL[a]	AST	10 mg/mL	Cloudy precipitate forms	2233	I
Linezolid	PHU	2 mg/mL	AMR	3 mg/mL[a]	Physically compatible for 4 hr at 23 °C	2264	C
Lorazepam	WY	0.33 mg/mL[b]	CNF	10 mg/mL	Visually compatible for 24 hr at 22 °C	1855	C
	WY	0.5 mg/mL[a]	AMR	10 mg/mL	Visually compatible for 4 hr at 27 °C	2062	C
Melphalan HCl	BW	0.1 mg/mL[b]	AB	3 mg/mL[b]	Physically compatible for 3 hr at 22 °C	1557	C
Meperidine HCl	AB	10 mg/mL	ES	0.8 mg/mL[a]	Physically compatible for 4 hr at 25 °C	1397	C
	AB	10 mg/mL	ES	2.4 mg/mL[a]	White cloudiness forms immediately	1397	I
	AB	10 mg/mL	ES	10 mg/mL	White precipitate forms immediately	1397	I
Meropenem	ZEN	1 and 50 mg/mL[b]	HO	10 mg/mL	Visually compatible for 4 hr at room temperature	1994	C
Methotrexate sodium		25 mg/mL		10 mg/mL	Drugs injected sequentially in Y-site with no flush. No precipitate seen	980	C
Metoclopramide HCl		5 mg/mL		10 mg/mL	Drugs injected sequentially in Y-site with no flush. Precipitates immediately	980	I
Metoprolol tartrate	BED	1 mg/mL	HOS	10 mg/mL	Visually compatible for 24 hr at 19 °C	2795	C
Micafungin sodium	ASP	1.5 mg/mL[b]	AMR	3 mg/mL[b]	Physically compatible for 4 hr at 23 °C	2683	C
Midazolam HCl	RC	1 mg/mL[a]	AST	10 mg/mL	Immediate haze. Precipitate in 2 hr	1847	I
	RC	5 mg/mL	CNF	10 mg/mL	White precipitate forms immediately	1855	I
	RC	2 mg/mL[a]	AMR	10 mg/mL	Precipitate forms immediately	2062	I
Milrinone lactate	WI	200 mcg/mL[a]	LY	10 mg/mL	Precipitates immediately	1191	I
	SW	0.2 mg/mL[a]	AMR	10 mg/mL	Precipitate forms in 4 hr at 27 °C	2062	I
Mitomycin		0.5 mg/mL		10 mg/mL	Drugs injected sequentially in Y-site with no flush. No precipitate seen	980	C
Morphine sulfate	AB	1 mg/mL	ES	0.8[a], 2.4[a], 10 mg/mL	White precipitate in 1 hr at 25 °C	1397	I
	SCN	2 mg/mL[a]	AMR	10 mg/mL	Visually compatible for 4 hr at 27 °C	2062	C
Nesiritide	SCI	50 mcg/mL[a,b]		10 mg/mL	Physically incompatible	2625	I
Nicardipine HCl	WY	1 mg/mL[a]	AMR	10 mg/mL	Precipitate forms immediately	2062	I
Nitroglycerin	AB	0.4 mg/mL[a]	AMR	10 mg/mL	Visually compatible for 4 hr at 27 °C	2062	C
	BA	0.1 mg/mL[o]	AMR	10 mg/mL	Precipitation occurs immediately	2725	I

Y-Site Injection Compatibility (1:1 Mixture) (Cont.)

Furosemide

Drug	Mfr	Conc	Mfr	Conc	Remarks	Ref	C/I
	AMR	0.1 mg/mL[a]	AMR	10 mg/mL	Physically compatible for 48 hr at room temperature	2725	C
Norepinephrine bitartrate	AB	0.128 mg/mL[a]	AMR	10 mg/mL	Visually compatible for 4 hr at 27 °C	2062	C
Ondansetron HCl	GL	1 mg/mL[b]	AB	3 mg/mL[a]	Immediate turbidity and precipitation	1365	I
Oxaliplatin	SS	0.5 mg/mL[a]	AMR	3 mg/mL[a]	Physically compatible for 4 hr at 23 °C	2566	C
Paclitaxel	NCI	1.2 mg/mL[a]	AST	3 mg/mL[a]	Physically compatible for 4 hr at 22 °C	1556	C
Pantoprazole sodium	ALT[n]	0.16 to 0.8 mg/mL[b]	SX	1 to 2 mg/mL[a]	Visually compatible for 12 hr at 23 °C	2603	C
Phenylephrine HCl	BA	0.64 mg/mL[a,b]	AB	4 mg/mL[a,b]	Precipitates in 5 to 15 min	2687	I
Piperacillin sodium–tazobactam sodium	LE[n]	40 + 5 mg/mL[a]	AB	3 mg/mL[a]	Physically compatible for 4 hr at 22 °C	1688	C
Potassium chloride	AB	40 mEq/L[f]	HO	10 mg/mL	Physically compatible for 4 hr at room temperature	534	C
	BRN	0.625 mEq/mL[a]	HMR	2.6 mg/mL[a]	Visually compatible for 150 min	2244	C
Propofol	ZEN	10 mg/mL	AB	3 mg/mL[a]	Physically compatible for 1 hr at 23 °C	2066	C
Quinidine gluconate	LI	6 mg/mL[c]	ES	4 mg/mL[c]	Immediate gross precipitation	1316	I
Ranitidine HCl	GL	1 mg/mL[a]	AMR	10 mg/mL	Visually compatible for 4 hr at 27 °C	2062	C
Remifentanil HCl	GW	0.025 and 0.25 mg/mL[b]	AMR	3 mg/mL[a]	Physically compatible for 4 hr at 23 °C	2075	C
Sargramostim	IMM	10 mcg/mL[b]	AB	3 mg/mL[b]	Visually compatible for 4 hr at 22 °C	1436	C
Sodium nitroprusside	RC	0.3, 1.2, 3 mg/mL[a]	SX	1.2[k] and 10 mg/mL	Visually compatible for 48 hr at 24 °C protected from light	2357	C
	RC	1.2 and 3 mg/mL[a]	SX	5 mg/mL[a]	Visually compatible for 48 hr at 24 °C protected from light	2357	C
Tacrolimus	FUJ	1 mg/mL[b]	ES	10 mg/mL	Visually compatible for 24 hr at 25 °C	1630	C
Telavancin HCl	ASP	7.5 mg/mL[a,b,m]	HOS	3 mg/mL[a,b,m]	Immediate precipitation	2830	I
Teniposide	BR	0.1 mg/mL[a]	AB	3 mg/mL[a]	Physically compatible for 4 hr at 23 °C	1725	C
Thiotepa	IMM[i]	1 mg/mL[a]	AMR	3 mg/mL[a]	Physically compatible for 4 hr at 23 °C	1861	C
Tirofiban HCl	ME	50 mcg/mL[a,b]	AB	0.5[a,b] and 10 mg/mL	Physically compatible with no loss of either drug in 4 hr at 23 °C	2356	C
TNA #73[j]			ES	3.3 mg/mL[c]	Visually compatible for 4 hr	1009	C
TNA #218 to #226[j]			AB	3 mg/mL[a]	Visually compatible for 4 hr at 23 °C	2215	C
Tobramycin sulfate	DI	1.6 mg/mL[c]	HO	10 mg/mL	Physically compatible for 24 hr at 21 °C	876	C
TPN #189[j]				10 mg/mL[b]	Visually compatible for 24 hr at 22 °C	1767	C
TPN #203, #204[j]			AMR	10 mg/mL	Visually compatible for 2 hr at 23 °C	1974	C
TPN #212 to #215[j]			AB	3 mg/mL[a]	Small amount of subvisible precipitate forms immediately	2109	I
Vasopressin	APP	0.4 unit/mL[a,b]	AB	4 mg/mL[a,b]	Precipitates in 5 to 15 min	2687	I
Vecuronium bromide	OR	1 mg/mL	AMR	10 mg/mL	Precipitate forms immediately	2062	I

Y-Site Injection Compatibility (1:1 Mixture) (Cont.)

Furosemide

Drug	Mfr	Conc	Mfr	Conc	Remarks	Ref	C/I
Vinblastine sulfate		1 mg/mL		10 mg/mL	Drugs injected sequentially in Y-site with no flush. Precipitates immediately	980	I
Vincristine sulfate		1 mg/mL		10 mg/mL	Drugs injected sequentially in Y-site with no flush. Precipitates immediately	980	I
Vinorelbine tartrate	BW	1 mg/mL[b]	ES	3 mg/mL[b]	Heavy white precipitate forms immediately	1558	I

[a]*Tested in dextrose 5%.*
[b]*Tested in sodium chloride 0.9%.*
[c]*Tested in both dextrose 5% and sodium chloride 0.9%.*
[d]*Tested in sterile water for injection.*
[e]*Tested in bacteriostatic sodium chloride 0.9% preserved with benzyl alcohol 0.9%.*
[f]*Tested in dextrose 5% in Ringer's injection, dextrose 5% in Ringer's injection, lactated, dextrose 5%, Ringer's injection, lactated, and sodium chloride 0.9%.*
[g]*Furosemide 0.5 mL injected in the Y-site port of a running infusion of labetalol hydrochloride in dextrose 5%.*
[h]*Tested in dextrose 5% with sodium bicarbonate 0.05 mEq/mL.*
[i]*Lyophilized formulation tested.*
[j]*Refer to Appendix I for the composition of parenteral nutrition solutions. TNA indicates a 3-in-1 admixture, and TPN indicates a 2-in-1 admixture.*
[k]*Tested in dextrose 5% in sodium chloride 0.2%.*
[l]*Injected via Y-site into an administration set running azithromycin.*
[m]*Tested in Ringer's injection, lactated.*
[n]*Test performed using the formulation WITHOUT edetate disodium.*
[o]*Tested using premixed nitroglycerin infusion in dextrose 5% with citrate buffer (Baxter Healthcare).*

FUSIDATE SODIUM
AHFS 8:12.28.92

Products — Fusidate sodium is available as a dry powder in vials containing 500 mg (equivalent to 480 mg of fusidic acid). It is packaged with a diluent vial containing 10 mL of phosphate–citrate buffer (pH 7.4 to 7.6). The drug should be reconstituted with the diluent and diluted further with sodium chloride 0.9% or other compatible diluent for administration. (38)

Sodium and Phosphate Content — Each vial of fusidate sodium contains 3.1 mmol of sodium and 1.1 mmol of phosphate. (38)

Trade Name(s) — Fucidin.

Administration — Fusidate sodium is administered by slow intravenous infusion over not less than six hours if a superficial vein is employed. If a central venous line is used, the infusion should be given over two to four hours. The reconstituted fusidate sodium in 10 mL of buffer solution is diluted in 500 mL of sodium chloride 0.9% or other compatible infusion solution for administration. The drug must not be given by other routes. (38)

Stability — Fusidate sodium should be stored below 25 °C and protected from light. Reconstituted solutions that are added to 500 mL of compatible infusion solutions are stable for 24 hours at room temperature. Unused portions of the reconstituted solution should be discarded. (38)

Fusidate sodium reconstituted with the buffer solution to 50 mg/mL is physically incompatible with infusion solutions containing amino acids solutions, dextrose 20% or greater, and lipid infusions. (38)

Fusidate sodium (Leo) at a concentration of 0.125 mg/mL is stated to be physically incompatible with the following peritoneal dialysis solutions (1800):

Dianeal PD2 with dextrose 1.36%
Dianeal PD3 with dextrose 1.36%
Dianeal with dextrose 3.86%
Peritoneal Dialysis Solution 6.36%
Peritoneal Dialysis Solution 6.36% + acetate
Peritoneal Dialysis Solution with dextrose 2.27%

pH Effects — Precipitation may occur upon dilution if the resulting pH is less than 7.4. (38)

Freezing Solutions — Fusidate sodium (Leo) 1 mg/mL in sodium chloride 0.9% and dextrose 5% is stated to be stable frozen at −20 °C for 24 hours followed by thawing in a microwave oven. (1800)

Fusidic acid (Leo) 500 mg, reconstituted in buffer and diluted to 550 mL in sodium chloride 0.9% in PVC bags, was stored frozen at −20 °C. No loss was found after 12 months of storage followed by microwave thawing. Furthermore, the solution was physically compatible, with no increase in subvisible particles. In addition, there was no loss of fusidate sodium after six months of storage at −20 °C followed by three freeze–thaw cycles. (1612)

Compatibility Information

Solution Compatibility

Fusidate sodium

Solution	Mfr	Mfr	Conc/L	Remarks	Ref	C/I
Dextrose 5%	BA[a]	LEO	1.16 and 2.32 g	Physically compatible. Under 10% loss in 162 days at 4 °C. 10% loss in 10.4 days at 25 °C or 2.1 days at 37 °C	1709	C
Dextrose 5%[b]	BP	LEO	1 or 2 g	Physically compatible and chemically stable for 48 hr at room temperature	1800	C
Sodium chloride 0.9%[b]	BP	LEO	1 and 2 g	Physically compatible and chemically stable for 48 hr at room temperature	1800	C
Sodium chloride 0.18% and dextrose 4%	BP	LEO	1 g	Physically compatible and chemically stable for 48 hr at room temperature	1800	C
Sodium lactate ⅙ M	BP	LEO	1 g	Physically compatible and chemically stable for 48 hr at room temperature	1800	C

[a]Tested in PVC containers.
[b]Tested both with and without potassium chloride 0.3%.

Additive Compatibility

Fusidate sodium

Drug	Mfr	Conc/L	Mfr	Conc/L	Test Soln	Remarks	Ref	C/I
Cefotaxime sodium		2.5 g	LEO	500 mg	D–S	Physically compatible and chemically stable for 48 hr at room temperature	1800	C
Erythromycin lactobionate		5 g	LEO	1 g	D–S	Physically compatible and chemically stable for 48 hr at room temperature	1800	C
Fat emulsion, intravenous		10%	LEO	1 g		Physically incompatible	1800	I
Floxacillin sodium		2.5 g	LEO	500 mg	D–S	Physically compatible and chemically stable for 48 hr at room temperature	1800	C
Gentamicin sulfate		160 mg	LEO	1 g	D–S	Physically compatible and chemically stable for 48 hr at room temperature	1800	C
		1.5 g	LEO	1 g	D–S	Physically incompatible	1800	I
Vancomycin HCl		25 g	LEO	500 mg	D–S	Physically incompatible	1800	I

GALLIUM NITRATE
AHFS 92:24

Products — Gallium nitrate is available in 20-mL vials. Each milliliter of solution contains gallium nitrate 25 mg, sodium citrate dihydrate 28.75 mg, and sodium hydroxide or hydrochloric acid for pH adjustment during manufacturing in water for injection. (1)

pH — 6 to 7. (1)

Trade Name(s) — Ganite.

Administration — Gallium nitrate is administered by intravenous infusion over 24 hours after dilution in 1000 mL of dextrose 5% or sodium chloride 0.9%. (1)

Stability — Gallium nitrate in intact vials should be stored at controlled room temperature. The manufacturer states that unused portions of the vials should be discarded because no preservative is present. (1)

Gallium nitrate diluted in 1000 mL of dextrose 5% or sodium chloride 0.9% is stable for 48 hours at room temperature and for seven days stored under refrigeration. (1)

Compatibility Information

Y-Site Injection Compatibility (1:1 Mixture)

Gallium nitrate

Drug	Mfr	Conc	Mfr	Conc	Remarks	Ref	C/I
Acyclovir sodium	BW	7 mg/mL[b]	FUJ	1 mg/mL[b]	Visually compatible for 24 hr at 25 °C	1673	C
Allopurinol sodium	BW	3 mg/mL[b]	FUJ	0.4 mg/mL[b]	Physically compatible for 4 hr at 22 °C	1686	C
Amifostine	USB	10 mg/mL[a]	FUJ	0.4 mg/mL[a]	Physically compatible for 4 hr at 23 °C	1845	C
Aminophylline	AMR	25 mg/mL	FUJ	1 mg/mL[b]	Visually compatible for 24 hr at 25 °C	1673	C
Ampicillin sodium–sulbactam sodium	RR	45 + 22.5 mg/mL[b]	FUJ	1 mg/mL[b]	Visually compatible for 24 hr at 25 °C	1673	C
Aztreonam	SQ	40 mg/mL[a]	FUJ	0.4 mg/mL[a]	Physically compatible for 4 hr at 23 °C	1758	C
Cefazolin sodium	GEM	100 mg/mL[b]	FUJ	1 mg/mL[b]	Visually compatible for 24 hr at 25 °C	1673	C
Ceftazidime	LI	100 mg/mL[b]	FUJ	1 mg/mL[b]	Visually compatible for 24 hr at 25 °C	1673	C
Ceftriaxone sodium	RC	40 mg/mL[b]	FUJ	1 mg/mL[b]	Visually compatible for 24 hr at 25 °C	1673	C
Ciprofloxacin	MI	2 mg/mL[b]	FUJ	1 mg/mL[b]	Visually compatible for 24 hr at 25 °C	1673	C
Cisplatin	BR	1 mg/mL	FUJ	1 mg/mL[b]	Precipitates immediately	1673	I
Cladribine	ORT	0.015[b] and 0.5[c] mg/mL	FUJ	0.4 mg/mL[b]	Physically compatible for 4 hr at 23 °C	1969	C
Cyclophosphamide	MJ	20 mg/mL	FUJ	1 mg/mL[b]	Visually compatible for 24 hr at 25 °C	1673	C
Cytarabine	CET	50 mg/mL	FUJ	1 mg/mL[b]	Precipitates immediately	1673	I
Dexamethasone sodium phosphate	AMR	4 mg/mL	FUJ	1 mg/mL[b]	Visually compatible for 24 hr at 25 °C	1673	C
Diphenhydramine HCl	ES	50 mg/mL	FUJ	1 mg/mL[b]	Visually compatible for 24 hr at 25 °C	1673	C
Doxorubicin HCl	CET	2 mg/mL	FUJ	1 mg/mL[b]	Precipitates immediately	1673	I
Etoposide	BR	0.4 mg/mL[b]	FUJ	1 mg/mL[b]	Precipitate forms after 60 min	1673	I
Filgrastim	AMG	30 mcg/mL[a]	FUJ	0.4 mg/mL[a]	Physically compatible for 4 hr at 22 °C	1687	C
Fluconazole	PF	2 mg/mL	FUJ	1 mg/mL[b]	Visually compatible for 24 hr at 25 °C	1673	C
Fluorouracil	RC	50 mg/mL	FUJ	1 mg/mL[b]	Precipitate forms immediately but clears after 60 min	1673	I
Furosemide	AB	10 mg/mL	FUJ	1 mg/mL[b]	Visually compatible for 24 hr at 25 °C	1673	C
Granisetron HCl	SKB	0.05 mg/mL[a]	FUJ	0.4 mg/mL[a]	Physically compatible for 4 hr at 23 °C	2000	C
Haloperidol lactate	MN	5 mg/mL	FUJ	1 mg/mL[b]	Immediate white cloudiness	1673	I
Heparin sodium	ES	40 units/mL[b]	FUJ	1 mg/mL[b]	Visually compatible for 24 hr at 25 °C	1673	C
Hydrocortisone sodium succinate	AB	50 mg/mL	FUJ	1 mg/mL[b]	Visually compatible for 24 hr at 25 °C	1673	C

Y-Site Injection Compatibility (1:1 Mixture) (Cont.)

Gallium nitrate

Drug	Mfr	Conc	Mfr	Conc	Remarks	Ref	C/I
Hydromorphone HCl	WY	4 mg/mL	FUJ	1 mg/mL[b]	Precipitate forms in 24 hr at 25 °C	1673	I
Ifosfamide	MJ	20 mg/mL[b]	FUJ	1 mg/mL[b]	Visually compatible for 24 hr at 25 °C	1673	C
Imipenem–cilastatin sodium	MSD	5 mg/mL[b]	FUJ	1 mg/mL[b]	Precipitates immediately	1673	I
Lorazepam	WY	1 mg/mL[b]	FUJ	1 mg/mL[b]	White haze and precipitate form immediately but clear in 30 min	1673	I
Magnesium sulfate	AMR	200 mg/mL[b]	FUJ	1 mg/mL[b]	Visually compatible for 24 hr at 25 °C	1673	C
Mannitol	AB	250 mg/mL	FUJ	1 mg/mL[b]	Visually compatible for 24 hr at 25 °C	1673	C
Melphalan HCl	BW	0.1 mg/mL[b]	FUJ	0.4 mg/mL[b]	Physically compatible for 3 hr at 22 °C	1557	C
Meperidine HCl	WY	50 mg/mL	FUJ	1 mg/mL[b]	Visually compatible for 24 hr at 25 °C	1673	C
Mesna	MJ	20 mg/mL	FUJ	1 mg/mL[b]	Visually compatible for 24 hr at 25 °C	1673	C
Methotrexate sodium	LE	25 mg/mL[b]	FUJ	1 mg/mL[b]	Visually compatible for 24 hr at 25 °C	1673	C
Metoclopramide HCl	SO	5 mg/mL	FUJ	1 mg/mL[b]	Visually compatible for 24 hr at 25 °C	1673	C
Morphine sulfate	SCN	1 mg/mL[b]	FUJ	1 mg/mL[b]	Precipitate forms in 24 hr at 25 °C	1673	I
Ondansetron HCl	GL	0.3 mg/mL[b]	FUJ	1 mg/mL[b]	Visually compatible for 24 hr at 25 °C	1673	C
Piperacillin sodium–tazobactam sodium	LE[e]	40 + 5 mg/mL[a]	FUJ	0.4 mg/mL[a]	Physically compatible for 4 hr at 22 °C	1688	C
Potassium chloride	AB	0.3 mEq/mL[b]	FUJ	1 mg/mL[b]	Visually compatible for 24 hr at 25 °C	1673	C
Prochlorperazine edisylate	SCN	5 mg/mL	FUJ	1 mg/mL[b]	Precipitates immediately	1673	I
Ranitidine HCl	GL	2.5 mg/mL[b]	FUJ	1 mg/mL[b]	Visually compatible for 24 hr at 25 °C	1673	C
Sodium bicarbonate	AB	1 mEq/mL	FUJ	1 mg/mL[b]	Visually compatible for 24 hr at 25 °C	1673	C
Teniposide	BR	0.1 mg/mL[a]	FUJ	0.4 mg/mL[a]	Physically compatible for 4 hr at 23 °C	1725	C
Thiotepa	IMM[d]	1 mg/mL[a]	FUJ	0.4 mg/mL[a]	Physically compatible for 4 hr at 23 °C	1861	C
Ticarcillin disodium–clavulanate potassium	SKB	103.3 mg/mL[b]	FUJ	1 mg/mL[b]	Visually compatible for 24 hr at 25 °C	1673	C
Trimethoprim–sulfamethoxazole	ES	0.8 + 4 mg/mL[b]	FUJ	1 mg/mL[b]	Visually compatible for 24 hr at 25 °C	1673	C
Vancomycin HCl	AB	5 mg/mL[b]	FUJ	1 mg/mL[b]	Visually compatible for 24 hr at 25 °C	1673	C
Vinorelbine tartrate	BW	1 mg/mL[b]	FUJ	0.4 mg/mL[b]	Physically compatible for 4 hr at 22 °C	1558	C

[a]*Tested in dextrose 5%.*
[b]*Tested in sodium chloride 0.9%.*
[c]*Tested in bacteriostatic water for injection preserved with benzyl alcohol 0.9%.*
[d]*Lyophilized formulation tested.*
[e]*Test performed using the formulation WITHOUT edetate disodium.*

GANCICLOVIR SODIUM
AHFS 8:18.32

Products — Ganciclovir sodium is available in vials containing, in dry form, the equivalent of ganciclovir 500 mg. Reconstitute with 10 mL of sterile water for injection and shake to dissolve the drug to yield a solution containing ganciclovir 50 mg/mL. Do not use paraben-containing diluents to reconstitute ganciclovir sodium because precipitation may result. (1)

pH — Approximately 11. (1)

Sodium Content — Each 500-mg vial contains 46 mg of sodium. (1)

Trade Name(s) — Cytovene-IV.

Administration — Ganciclovir sodium is administered by intravenous infusion. After reconstitution, the dose may be diluted in 50 to 250 mL (usually 100 mL) of compatible infusion solution and given over one hour. Concentrations over 10 mg/mL are not recommended. Ganciclovir sodium should not be administered by intramuscular, subcutaneous, or rapid intravenous injection or infusion. (1; 4)

Stability — Intact vials should be stored at controlled room temperature and protected from temperatures above 40 °C. The reconstituted solution is stable for 12 hours at room temperature. Refrigeration of the reconstituted solution is not recommended because of possible precipitation. (1; 4) However, ganciclovir sodium 500 mg/10 mL in sterile water for injection had no significant loss in 60 days when stored at 4 °C. (1637)

Ganciclovir sodium (Syntex) 0.35 mg/mL diluted in sodium chloride 0.9% and stored at 22 °C did not exhibit a substantial antimicrobial effect on the growth of four organisms (*Enterococcus faecium, Staphylococcus aureus, Pseudomonas aeruginosa,* and *Candida albicans*) inoculated into the solution. *S. aureus* and *C. albicans* remained viable for 24 hours, and the others remained viable to the end of the study at 120 hours. The author recommended that diluted solutions of ganciclovir sodium be stored under refrigeration whenever possible and that the potential for microbiological growth should be considered when assigning expiration periods. (2160)

Freezing Solutions — The manufacturer does not recommend freezing ganciclovir sodium solutions. (1) However, ganciclovir sodium (Syntex) 1.4, 4, and 7 mg/mL in sodium chloride 0.9% packaged in polypropylene syringes and 0.28 and 1.4 mg/mL in sodium chloride 0.9% packaged in PVC containers was evaluated. All samples exhibited 4% or less drug loss after 364 days at −20 °C. (1836)

No ganciclovir sodium loss occurred in a 10-mg/mL solution in sodium chloride 0.9% in 48 weeks when stored frozen at –8 °C. (2595)

Syringes — Ganciclovir sodium (Syntex) 5.8 mg/mL in sodium chloride 0.9%, packaged in polypropylene infusion-pump syringes (Healthtek), exhibited 3% or less drug loss in 10 days at 4 °C and no loss in 12 hours at 25 °C. (1742)

Ganciclovir sodium (Syntex) 1.4, 4, and 7 mg/mL in sodium chloride 0.9% was packaged in polypropylene syringes and stored at 20, 4, and −20 °C. Drug loss occurred of 4% or less in seven days at 20 °C, in 80 days at 4 °C, and in 364 days at −20 °C. (1836)

Central Venous Catheter — Ganciclovir sodium (Roche) 5 mg/mL in dextrose 5% was found to be compatible with the ARROWg+ard Blue Plus (Arrow International) chlorhexidine-bearing triple-lumen central catheter. Essentially complete delivery of the drug was found with little or no drug loss occurring. Furthermore, chlorhexidine delivered from the catheter remained at trace amounts with no substantial increase due to the delivery of the drug through the catheter. (2335)

Compatibility Information

Solution Compatibility

Ganciclovir sodium

Solution	Mfr	Mfr	Conc/L	Remarks	Ref	C/I
Dextrose 5%				Physically and chemically compatible	1	C
	TR[a]	SY	2.44 g	Physically compatible with no loss in 5 days at 25 °C in light or dark and at 4 °C	1288	C
	BA[a]	SY	1, 5, 10 g	Visually compatible with 3 to 7% loss in 35 days at 4 to 8 °C in the dark	1545	C
	AB[a]	SY	1 and 5 g	Visually compatible with 1% or less loss in 35 days at 5 and 25 °C	1643	C
Ringer's injection				Physically and chemically compatible	1	C
Ringer's injection, lactated				Physically and chemically compatible	1	C
Sodium chloride 0.9%	[a]			Physically compatible and stable for 14 days refrigerated but use within 24 hr recommended	1	C
	TR[a]	SY	2.59 g	Physically compatible with no loss in 5 days at 25 °C in light or dark and at 4 °C	1288	C
	AB[a]	SY	1 and 5 g	Visually compatible with 1% or less loss in 35 days at 5 and 25 °C	1643	C
		SY	2.2 g	Little or no loss in 14 days at 4 °C	1637	C
	[a]	SY	0.28 and 1.4 g	4% or less loss in 7 days at 20 °C, 80 days at 4 °C, and 364 days at −20 °C	1836	C
	BA[a]	RC	1 and 5 g	No ganciclovir loss in 35 days at 4 °C in the dark. No visible particles but an increase in microparticulates under 10 μm in size	2251	C
	BA[b]	RC	1 and 5 g	Physically compatible with no loss in 35 days at 4 °C protected from light	2251	C

Solution Compatibility (Cont.)

Ganciclovir sodium

Solution	Mfr	Mfr	Conc/L	Remarks	Ref	C/I
TPN #183[c]		SY	2 g	Precipitate forms	1744	I
TPN #183 to #185[c]		SY	3 and 5 g	Precipitate forms	1744	I

[a]Tested in PVC containers.
[b]Tested in latex elastomeric pump reservoirs (Baxter Intermate).
[c]Refer to Appendix I for the composition of parenteral nutrition solutions. TPN indicates a 2-in-1 admixture.

Y-Site Injection Compatibility (1:1 Mixture)

Ganciclovir sodium

Drug	Mfr	Conc	Mfr	Conc	Remarks	Ref	C/I
Aldesleukin	CHI	33,800 I.U./mL[a]	SY	10 mg/mL[a]	Aldesleukin bioactivity inhibited	1857	I
Allopurinol sodium	BW	3 mg/mL[b]	SY	20 mg/mL[b]	Physically compatible for 4 hr at 22 °C	1686	C
Amifostine	USB	10 mg/mL[a]	SY	20 mg/mL[a]	Crystalline needles form immediately. Dense precipitate in 1 hr	1845	I
Amphotericin B cholesteryl sulfate complex	SEQ	0.83 mg/mL[a]	RC	20 mg/mL[a]	Physically compatible for 4 hr at 23 °C	2117	C
Amsacrine	NCI	1 mg/mL[a]	SY	20 mg/mL[a]	Immediate dark orange turbidity	1381	I
Anidulafungin	VIC	0.5 mg/mL[a]	RC	20 mg/mL[a]	Physically compatible for 4 hr at 23 °C	2617	C
Aztreonam	SQ	40 mg/mL[a]	SY	20 mg/mL[a]	White needles form immediately. Dense precipitate in 1 hr	1758	I
Caspofungin acetate	ME	0.7 mg/mL[b]	RC	20 mg/mL[b]	Physically compatible for 4 hr at room temperature	2758	C
Cisatracurium besylate	GW	0.1 and 2 mg/mL[a]	SY	20 mg/mL[a]	Physically compatible for 4 hr at 23 °C	2074	C
	GW	5 mg/mL[a]	SY	20 mg/mL[a]	White cloudiness forms immediately	2074	I
Docetaxel	RPR	0.9 mg/mL[a]	RC	20 mg/mL[a]	Physically compatible for 4 hr at 23 °C	2224	C
Doxorubicin HCl liposomal	SEQ	0.4 mg/mL[a]	RC	20 mg/mL[a]	Physically compatible for 4 hr at 23 °C	2087	C
Enalaprilat	MSD	1.25 mg/mL	SY	5 mg/mL[c]	Physically compatible for 4 hr at 21 °C	1409	C
Etoposide phosphate	BR	5 mg/mL[a]	RC	20 mg/mL[a]	Physically compatible for 4 hr at 23 °C	2218	C
Filgrastim	AMG	30 mcg/mL[a]	SY	20 mg/mL[a]	Physically compatible for 4 hr at 22 °C	1687	C
Fluconazole	RR	2 mg/mL	SY	50 mg/mL	Physically compatible for 24 hr at 25 °C	1407	C
Fludarabine phosphate	BX	1 mg/mL[a]	SY	20 mg/mL[a]	Darker color forms within 4 hr	1439	I
Foscarnet sodium	AST	24 mg/mL		50 mg/mL	Precipitates immediately	1335	I
Gemcitabine HCl	LI	10 mg/mL[b]	RC	20 mg/mL[b]	Subvisible crystals form immediately. Gross precipitate in 1 hr	2226	I
Granisetron HCl	SKB	0.05 mg/mL[a]	SY	20 mg/mL[a]	Physically compatible for 4 hr at 23 °C	2000	C
Linezolid	PHU	2 mg/mL	RC	20 mg/mL[a]	Physically compatible for 4 hr at 23 °C	2264	C
Melphalan HCl	BW	0.1 mg/mL[b]	SY	20 mg/mL[b]	Physically compatible for 3 hr at 22 °C	1557	C
Ondansetron HCl	GL	1 mg/mL[b]	SY	20 mg/mL[a]	Immediate turbidity and precipitation	1365	I
Paclitaxel	NCI	1.2 mg/mL[a]	SY	20 mg/mL[a]	Physically compatible for 4 hr at 22 °C	1556	C
Pemetrexed disodium	LI	20 mg/mL[b]	RC	20 mg/mL[a]	Physically compatible for 4 hr at 23 °C	2564	C

Y-Site Injection Compatibility (1:1 Mixture) (Cont.)

Ganciclovir sodium

Drug	Mfr	Conc	Mfr	Conc	Remarks	Ref	C/I
Piperacillin sodium–tazobactam sodium	LE[d]	40 + 5 mg/mL[a]	SY	20 mg/mL[a]	Large crystals form in 1 hr and become heavy white precipitate in 4 hr	1688	I
Propofol	ZEN	10 mg/mL	SY	20 mg/mL[a]	Physically compatible for 1 hr at 23 °C	2066	C
Remifentanil HCl	GW	0.025 and 0.25 mg/mL[b]	SY	20 mg/mL[a]	Physically compatible for 4 hr at 23 °C	2075	C
Sargramostim	IMM	10 mcg/mL[b]	SY	20 mg/mL[b]	Small particles form in 4 hr	1436	I
Tacrolimus	FUJ				Significant tacrolimus loss within 15 min	191	I
Teniposide	BR	0.1 mg/mL[a]	SY	20 mg/mL[a]	Physically compatible for 4 hr at 23 °C	1725	C
Thiotepa	IMM[e]	1 mg/mL[a]	SY	20 mg/mL[a]	Physically compatible for 4 hr at 23 °C	1861	C
TNA #218 to #226[f]			RC	20 mg/mL[a]	White precipitate forms immediately	2215	I
TPN #144[f]			SY	1 and 5 mg/mL[a]	Visually compatible for 2 hr at 20 °C	1522	C
			SY	10 mg/mL[a]	Heavy precipitate forms within 30 min	1522	I
TPN #183[f]			SY	2 mg/mL	Precipitate forms	1744	I
			SY	1 mg/mL[g]	Visually compatible with no ganciclovir loss in 3 hr at 24 °C. Less than 10% amino acids loss in 2 hr	1744	C
TPN #183 to #185[f]			SY	3 and 5 mg/mL	Precipitate forms	1744	I
TPN #184, #185[f]			SY	2 mg/mL[h]	Visually compatible with no ganciclovir loss in 3 hr at 24 °C. Less than 10% amino acid loss in 3 hr	1744	C
TPN #212 to #215[f]			SY	20 mg/mL[a]	Gross white precipitate forms immediately	2109	I
Vinorelbine tartrate	BW	1 mg/mL[b]	SY	20 mg/mL[b]	Turbid precipitate forms immediately	1558	I

[a]*Tested in dextrose 5%.*
[b]*Tested in sodium chloride 0.9%.*
[c]*Tested in both dextrose 5% and sodium chloride 0.9%.*
[d]*Test performed using the formulation WITHOUT edetate disodium.*
[e]*Lyophilized formulation tested.*
[f]*Refer to Appendix I for the composition of parenteral nutrition solutions. TNA indicates a 3-in-1 admixture, and TPN indicates a 2-in-1 admixture.*
[g]*Ganciclovir sodium concentration after mixing was 0.83 mg/mL.*
[h]*Ganciclovir sodium concentration after mixing was 1.4 mg/mL.*

GEMCITABINE HYDROCHLORIDE
AHFS 10:00

Products — Gemcitabine hydrochloride is available as a lyophilized powder in vials containing 200 mg of drug (as the base) with mannitol 200 mg and sodium acetate 12.5 mg. Reconstitute the 200-mg vial with 5 mL of sodium chloride 0.9% (without preservatives) and shake to dissolve the powder. (1)

Gemcitabine hydrochloride is also available as a lyophilized powder in vials containing 1 g of drug (as the base) with mannitol 1 g and sodium acetate 62.5 mg. Reconstitute the 1-g vial with 25 mL of sodium chloride 0.9% (without preservatives) and shake to dissolve the powder. (1)

When reconstituted as directed, the resulting solution from either size vial has a gemcitabine concentration of 38 mg/mL, which accounts for the displacement volume of the powder. The total volumes after reconstitution will be 5.26 mL for the 200-mg vial and 26.3 mL for the 1-g vial. (1)

Because of the drug's aqueous solubility, reconstitution to concentrations higher than 40 mg/mL may result in incomplete dissolution and should be avoided. (1)

The pH of the products may have been adjusted by the manufacturer with sodium hydroxide and/or hydrochloric acid. (1)

pH — The reconstituted solution has a pH in the range of 2.7 to 3.3. (1)

Trade Name(s) — Gemzar.

Administration — Gemcitabine hydrochloride is administered weekly by intravenous infusion over 30 minutes. It may be administered as reconstituted or diluted further in additional sodium chloride 0.9% to a concentration as low as 0.1 mg/mL. (1)

Stability — Gemcitabine hydrochloride in intact vials should be stored at controlled room temperature. The white lyophilized powder becomes a colorless to light straw-colored solution on reconstitution. The manufacturer states that the reconstituted solution is stable for 24 hours at controlled room temperature. Unused solution should be discarded. (1) However, other information indicates the reconstituted solution may be stable for longer periods. (2227) See Reconstituted Solutions below. The reconstituted solution should not be refrigerated because crystallization may occur. (1)

Gemcitabine hydrochloride (Lilly) 2.4 mg/mL diluted in sodium chloride 0.9% and stored at 22 °C did not exhibit a substantial antimicrobial effect on the growth of four organisms (*Enterococcus faecium, Staphylococcus aureus, Pseudomonas aeruginosa,* and *Candida albicans*) inoculated into the solution. *C. albicans* maintained viability for 120 hours, and the others were viable for 24 hours. The author recommended that diluted solutions of gemcitabine hydrochloride be stored under refrigeration whenever possible and that the potential for microbiological growth should be considered when assigning expiration periods. (2160)

Reconstituted Solutions — Gemcitabine hydrochloride (Lilly) 200-mg and 1-g vials reconstituted to 38 mg/mL with sterile water for injection and also sodium chloride 0.9% were evaluated over periods of 35 days at 23 °C exposed to and protected from fluorescent light and at 4 °C protected from light. The samples stored at 23 °C were physically stable throughout the study period. Under 4% loss occurred in 35 days at 23 °C. When refrigerated, the solutions remained physically and chemically stable for at least seven days, but large colorless crystals formed in some samples after that time. The crystals did not redissolve on warming to room temperature. No loss occurred in the refrigerated solutions unless crystals formed; gemcitabine losses of 20 to 35% were determined in samples containing crystals. Exposure to or protection from fluorescent light did not affect gemcitabine stability. (2227)

Syringes — Gemcitabine hydrochloride (Lilly) 38 mg/mL in sodium chloride 0.9% was repackaged as 10 mL of solution in 20-mL polypropylene plastic syringes (Becton Dickinson) and sealed with tip caps (Red Cap, Burron). Sample syringes were stored at 23 °C both exposed to and protected from fluorescent light and at 4 °C protected from light for 35 days. All samples were physically stable throughout the study period. Although not observed in these solutions packaged in plastic syringes, reconstituted solutions stored under refrigeration are subject to possible crystal formation. No loss occurred in 35 days under any of the conditions. (2227)

Sorption — Gemcitabine hydrochloride has not exhibited any incompatibilities with bottles or PVC bags and administration sets. (1)

Gemcitabine hydrochloride (Lilly) 5.12 mg/mL in sodium chloride 0.9% exhibited no loss due to sorption in polyethylene and PVC containers compared to glass containers over 48 hours at room temperature. (2420; 2430)

Compatibility Information

Solution Compatibility

Gemcitabine HCl

Solution	Mfr	Mfr	Conc/L	Remarks	Ref	C/I
Dextrose 5%	BA[a]	LI	0.1 and 10 g	Physically compatible and chemically stable with no loss in 35 days at 23 °C in light and dark and at 4 and 32 °C in the dark	2227	C
Sodium chloride 0.9%	BA[a]	LI	0.1 and 10 g	Physically compatible and chemically stable with no loss in 35 days at 23 °C in light and dark and at 4 and 32 °C in the dark	2227	C
	GRI[a,b]	LI	7.5 and 25 g	Visually compatible. Under 4% loss in 27 days at 25 °C in light and dark	2741	C

[a]*Tested in PVC containers.*
[b]*Tested in glass containers.*

Y-Site Injection Compatibility (1:1 Mixture)

Gemcitabine HCl

Drug	Mfr	Conc	Mfr	Conc	Remarks	Ref	C/I
Acyclovir sodium	GW	7 mg/mL[b]	LI	10 mg/mL[b]	Gross precipitation occurs immediately	2226	I
Amifostine	USB	10 mg/mL[b]	LI	10 mg/mL[b]	Physically compatible for 4 hr at 23 °C	2226	C
Amikacin sulfate	APC	5 mg/mL[b]	LI	10 mg/mL[b]	Physically compatible for 4 hr at 23 °C	2226	C

Y-Site Injection Compatibility (1:1 Mixture) (Cont.)

Gemcitabine HCl

Drug	Mfr	Conc	Mfr	Conc	Remarks	Ref	C/I
Aminophylline	AB	2.5 mg/mL[b]	LI	10 mg/mL[b]	Physically compatible for 4 hr at 23 °C	2226	C
Amphotericin B	PH	0.6 mg/mL[a]	LI	10 mg/mL[b]	Gross precipitation occurs immediately	2226	I
Ampicillin sodium	SKB	20 mg/mL[b]	LI	10 mg/mL[b]	Physically compatible for 4 hr at 23 °C	2226	C
Ampicillin sodium–sulbactam sodium	RR	20 + 10 mg/mL[b]	LI	10 mg/mL[b]	Physically compatible for 4 hr at 23 °C	2226	C
Anidulafungin	VIC	0.5 mg/mL[a]	LI	10 mg/mL[a]	Physically compatible for 4 hr at 23 °C	2617	C
Aztreonam	SQ	40 mg/mL[b]	LI	10 mg/mL[b]	Physically compatible for 4 hr at 23 °C	2226	C
Bleomycin sulfate	MJ	1 unit/mL[b]	LI	10 mg/mL[b]	Physically compatible for 4 hr at 23 °C	2226	C
Bumetanide	RC	0.04 mg/mL[b]	LI	10 mg/mL[b]	Physically compatible for 4 hr at 23 °C	2226	C
Buprenorphine HCl	RKC	0.04 mg/mL[b]	LI	10 mg/mL[b]	Physically compatible for 4 hr at 23 °C	2226	C
Butorphanol tartrate	APC	0.04 mg/mL[b]	LI	10 mg/mL[b]	Physically compatible for 4 hr at 23 °C	2226	C
Calcium gluconate	FUJ	40 mg/mL[b]	LI	10 mg/mL[b]	Physically compatible for 4 hr at 23 °C	2226	C
Carboplatin	BR	5 mg/mL[b]	LI	10 mg/mL[b]	Physically compatible for 4 hr at 23 °C	2226	C
Carmustine	BR	1.5 mg/mL[b]	LI	10 mg/mL[b]	Physically compatible for 4 hr at 23 °C	2226	C
Cefazolin sodium	APC	20 mg/mL[b]	LI	10 mg/mL[b]	Physically compatible for 4 hr at 23 °C	2226	C
Cefotaxime sodium	HO	20 mg/mL[b]	LI	10 mg/mL[b]	Subvisible haze forms in 1 hr. Increased haze and a microprecipitate in 4 hr	2226	I
Cefotetan disodium	ZEN	20 mg/mL[b]	LI	10 mg/mL[b]	Physically compatible for 4 hr at 23 °C	2226	C
Cefoxitin sodium	ME	20 mg/mL[b]	LI	10 mg/mL[b]	Physically compatible for 4 hr at 23 °C	2226	C
Ceftazidime	SKB	40 mg/mL[b]	LI	10 mg/mL[b]	Physically compatible for 4 hr at 23 °C	2226	C
Ceftriaxone sodium	RC	20 mg/mL[b]	LI	10 mg/mL[b]	Physically compatible for 4 hr at 23 °C	2226	C
Cefuroxime sodium	GW	30 mg/mL[b]	LI	10 mg/mL[b]	Physically compatible for 4 hr at 23 °C	2226	C
Chlorpromazine HCl	ES	2 mg/mL[b]	LI	10 mg/mL[b]	Physically compatible for 4 hr at 23 °C	2226	C
Ciprofloxacin	BAY	1 mg/mL[b]	LI	10 mg/mL[b]	Physically compatible for 4 hr at 23 °C	2226	C
Cisplatin	BR	1 mg/mL	LI	10 mg/mL[b]	Physically compatible for 4 hr at 23 °C	2226	C
Clindamycin phosphate	AST	10 mg/mL[b]	LI	10 mg/mL[b]	Physically compatible for 4 hr at 23 °C	2226	C
Cyclophosphamide	BR	10 mg/mL[b]	LI	10 mg/mL[b]	Physically compatible for 4 hr at 23 °C	2226	C
Cytarabine	BED	50 mg/mL	LI	10 mg/mL[b]	Physically compatible for 4 hr at 23 °C	2226	C
Dactinomycin	ME	0.01 mg/mL[b]	LI	10 mg/mL[b]	Physically compatible for 4 hr at 23 °C	2226	C
Daunorubicin HCl	BED	1 mg/mL[b]	LI	10 mg/mL[b]	Physically compatible for 4 hr at 23 °C	2226	C
Dexamethasone sodium phosphate	ES	1 mg/mL[b]	LI	10 mg/mL[b]	Physically compatible for 4 hr at 23 °C	2226	C
Dexrazoxane	PH	5 mg/mL[b]	LI	10 mg/mL[b]	Physically compatible for 4 hr at 23 °C	2226	C
Diphenhydramine HCl	SCN	2 mg/mL[b]	LI	10 mg/mL[b]	Physically compatible for 4 hr at 23 °C	2226	C
Dobutamine HCl	AST	4 mg/mL[b]	LI	10 mg/mL[b]	Physically compatible for 4 hr at 23 °C	2226	C
Docetaxel	RPR	2 mg/mL[a]	LI	10 mg/mL[b]	Physically compatible for 4 hr at 23 °C	2226	C
Dopamine HCl	AB	3.2 mg/mL[b]	LI	10 mg/mL[b]	Physically compatible for 4 hr at 23 °C	2226	C
Doripenem	JJ	5 mg/mL[a,b]	LI	10 mg/mL[b]	Physically compatible for 4 hr at 23 °C	2743	C
Doxorubicin HCl	PH	2 mg/mL	LI	10 mg/mL[b]	Physically compatible for 4 hr at 23 °C	2226	C
Doxycycline hyclate	FUJ	1 mg/mL[b]	LI	10 mg/mL[b]	Physically compatible for 4 hr at 23 °C	2226	C

Y-Site Injection Compatibility (1:1 Mixture) (Cont.)

Gemcitabine HCl

Drug	Mfr	Conc	Mfr	Conc	Remarks	Ref	C/I
Droperidol	AST	0.4 mg/mL[b]	LI	10 mg/mL[b]	Physically compatible for 4 hr at 23 °C	2226	**C**
Enalaprilat	ME	0.1 mg/mL[b]	LI	10 mg/mL[b]	Physically compatible for 4 hr at 23 °C	2226	**C**
Etoposide	BR	0.4 mg/mL[b]	LI	10 mg/mL[b]	Physically compatible for 4 hr at 23 °C	2226	**C**
Etoposide phosphate	BR	5 mg/mL[b]	LI	10 mg/mL[b]	Physically compatible for 4 hr at 23 °C	2226	**C**
Famotidine	ME	2 mg/mL[b]	LI	10 mg/mL[b]	Physically compatible for 4 hr at 23 °C	2226	**C**
Floxuridine	RC	3 mg/mL[b]	LI	10 mg/mL[b]	Physically compatible for 4 hr at 23 °C	2226	**C**
Fluconazole	RR	2 mg/mL	LI	10 mg/mL[b]	Physically compatible for 4 hr at 23 °C	2226	**C**
Fludarabine phosphate	BX	1 mg/mL[b]	LI	10 mg/mL[b]	Physically compatible for 4 hr at 23 °C	2226	**C**
Fluorouracil	PH	16 mg/mL[b]	LI	10 mg/mL[b]	Physically compatible for 4 hr at 23 °C	2226	**C**
Furosemide	AMR	3 mg/mL[b]	LI	10 mg/mL[b]	Gross precipitation occurs immediately	2226	**I**
Ganciclovir sodium	RC	20 mg/mL[b]	LI	10 mg/mL[b]	Subvisible crystals form immediately. Gross precipitate in 1 hr	2226	**I**
Gentamicin sulfate	AB	5 mg/mL[b]	LI	10 mg/mL[b]	Physically compatible for 4 hr at 23 °C	2226	**C**
Granisetron HCl	SKB	0.05 mg/mL[b]	LI	10 mg/mL[b]	Physically compatible for 4 hr at 23 °C	2226	**C**
Haloperidol lactate	MN	0.2 mg/mL[b]	LI	10 mg/mL[b]	Physically compatible for 4 hr at 23 °C	2226	**C**
Heparin sodium	ES	100 units/mL[b]	LI	10 mg/mL[b]	Physically compatible for 4 hr at 23 °C	2226	**C**
Hydrocortisone sodium succinate	UP	1 mg/mL[b]	LI	10 mg/mL[b]	Physically compatible for 4 hr at 23 °C	2226	**C**
Hydromorphone HCl	AST	0.5 mg/mL[b]	LI	10 mg/mL[b]	Physically compatible for 4 hr at 23 °C	2226	**C**
Hydroxyzine HCl	ES	2 mg/mL[b]	LI	10 mg/mL[b]	Physically compatible for 4 hr at 23 °C	2226	**C**
Idarubicin HCl	AD	0.5 mg/mL[b]	LI	10 mg/mL[b]	Physically compatible for 4 hr at 23 °C	2226	**C**
Ifosfamide	MJ	25 mg/mL[b]	LI	10 mg/mL[b]	Physically compatible for 4 hr at 23 °C	2226	**C**
Imipenem–cilastatin sodium	ME	10 mg/mL[b]	LI	10 mg/mL[b]	Yellow-green discoloration forms in 1 hr	2226	**I**
Irinotecan HCl	PHU	5 mg/mL[b]	LI	10 mg/mL[b]	Subvisible haze with green discoloration forms immediately	2226	**I**
Leucovorin calcium	IMM	2 mg/mL[b]	LI	10 mg/mL[b]	Physically compatible for 4 hr at 23 °C	2226	**C**
Linezolid	PHU	2 mg/mL	LI	10 mg/mL[a]	Physically compatible for 4 hr at 23 °C	2264	**C**
Lorazepam	WY	0.5 mg/mL[a]	LI	10 mg/mL[b]	Physically compatible for 4 hr at 23 °C	2226	**C**
Mannitol	BA	15%	LI	10 mg/mL[b]	Physically compatible for 4 hr at 23 °C	2226	**C**
Meperidine HCl	AST	4 mg/mL[b]	LI	10 mg/mL[b]	Physically compatible for 4 hr at 23 °C	2226	**C**
Mesna	MJ	10 mg/mL[b]	LI	10 mg/mL[b]	Physically compatible for 4 hr at 23 °C	2226	**C**
Methotrexate sodium	IMM	15 mg/mL[b]	LI	10 mg/mL[b]	Precipitate forms immediately, redissolves, but reprecipitates in 15 to 20 min	2226	**I**
Methylprednisolone sodium succinate	AB	5 mg/mL[b]	LI	10 mg/mL[b]	Gross precipitation occurs immediately	2226	**I**
Metoclopramide HCl	FAU	5 mg/mL	LI	10 mg/mL[b]	Physically compatible for 4 hr at 23 °C	2226	**C**
Metronidazole	AB	5 mg/mL	LI	10 mg/mL[b]	Physically compatible for 4 hr at 23 °C	2226	**C**
Mitomycin	BR	0.5 mg/mL	LI	10 mg/mL[b]	Reddish-purple color forms in 1 hr	2226	**I**
Mitoxantrone HCl	IMM	0.5 mg/mL[b]	LI	10 mg/mL[b]	Physically compatible for 4 hr at 23 °C	2226	**C**
Morphine sulfate	ES	1 mg/mL[b]	LI	10 mg/mL[b]	Physically compatible for 4 hr at 23 °C	2226	**C**
Nalbuphine HCl	AST	10 mg/mL	LI	10 mg/mL[b]	Physically compatible for 4 hr at 23 °C	2226	**C**

Y-Site Injection Compatibility (1:1 Mixture) (Cont.)

Gemcitabine HCl

Drug	Mfr	Conc	Mfr	Conc	Remarks	Ref	C/I
Ondansetron HCl	GW	1 mg/mL[b]	LI	10 mg/mL[b]	Physically compatible for 4 hr at 23 °C	2226	C
Oxaliplatin	SS	0.5 mg/mL[a]	LI	10 mg/mL[a]	Physically compatible for 4 hr at 23 °C	2566	C
Paclitaxel	MJ	1.2 mg/mL[a]	LI	10 mg/mL[b]	Physically compatible for 4 hr at 23 °C	2226	C
Palonosetron HCl	MGI	50 mcg/mL	LI	10 mg/mL[a]	Physically compatible and no loss of either drug in 4 hr	2627	C
Pemetrexed disodium	LI	20 mg/mL[b]	LI	10 mg/mL[a]	Cloudy precipitate forms immediately	2564	I
Piperacillin sodium–tazobactam sodium	LE[c]	40 + 5 mg/mL[b]	LI	10 mg/mL[b]	Cloudiness forms immediately, becoming flocculent precipitate in 1 hr	2226	I
Potassium chloride	AB	0.1 mEq/mL[b]	LI	10 mg/mL[b]	Physically compatible for 4 hr at 23 °C	2226	C
Prochlorperazine edisylate	SCN	0.5 mg/mL[b]	LI	10 mg/mL[b]	Subvisible haze forms immediately	2226	I
Promethazine HCl	SCN	2 mg/mL[b]	LI	10 mg/mL[b]	Physically compatible for 4 hr at 23 °C	2226	C
Ranitidine HCl	GL	2 mg/mL[b]	LI	10 mg/mL[b]	Physically compatible for 4 hr at 23 °C	2226	C
Sodium bicarbonate	AB	1 mEq/mL	LI	10 mg/mL[b]	Physically compatible for 4 hr at 23 °C	2226	C
Streptozocin	UP	40 mg/mL[b]	LI	10 mg/mL[b]	Physically compatible for 4 hr at 23 °C	2226	C
Teniposide	BR	0.1 mg/mL[a]	LI	10 mg/mL[b]	Physically compatible for 4 hr at 23 °C	2226	C
Thiotepa	IMM	1 mg/mL[b]	LI	10 mg/mL[b]	Physically compatible for 4 hr at 23 °C	2226	C
Ticarcillin disodium–clavulanate potassium	SKB	31 mg/mL[b]	LI	10 mg/mL[b]	Physically compatible for 4 hr at 23 °C	2226	C
Tobramycin sulfate	LI	5 mg/mL[b]	LI	10 mg/mL[b]	Physically compatible for 4 hr at 23 °C	2226	C
Topotecan HCl	SKB	0.1 mg/mL[b]	LI	10 mg/mL[b]	Physically compatible for 4 hr at 23 °C	2226	C
Trimethoprim–sulfamethoxazole	ES	0.8 + 4 mg/mL[b]	LI	10 mg/mL[b]	Physically compatible for 4 hr at 23 °C	2226	C
Vancomycin HCl	LI	10 mg/mL[b]	LI	10 mg/mL[b]	Physically compatible for 4 hr at 23 °C	2226	C
Vinblastine sulfate	FAU	0.12 mg/mL[b]	LI	10 mg/mL[b]	Physically compatible for 4 hr at 23 °C	2226	C
Vincristine sulfate	FAU	0.05 mg/mL[b]	LI	10 mg/mL[b]	Physically compatible for 4 hr at 23 °C	2226	C
Vinorelbine tartrate	GW	1 mg/mL[b]	LI	10 mg/mL[b]	Physically compatible for 4 hr at 23 °C	2226	C
Zidovudine	GW	4 mg/mL[b]	LI	10 mg/mL[b]	Physically compatible for 4 hr at 23 °C	2226	C

[a]Tested in dextrose 5%.
[b]Tested in sodium chloride 0.9%.
[c]Test performed using the formulation WITHOUT edetate disodium.

GENTAMICIN SULFATE
AHFS 8:12.02

Products — Gentamicin (as the sulfate) is available at a concentration of 40 mg/mL in 2- and 20-mL vials. The drug is also available at a concentration of 10 mg/mL for pediatric use. The products may also contain edetate disodium, sodium bisulfite, and parabens. (1; 4)

Gentamicin sulfate is also available from several manufacturers premixed in various concentrations in sodium chloride 0.9%. (4)

pH — The injection for intravenous or intramuscular administration has a pH of 3 to 5.5. Premixed infusions of gentamicin sulfate in sodium chloride 0.9% have a pH of around 4 to 4.5. (4)

Osmolality — Gentamicin sulfate (Wyeth) 40 mg/mL has an osmolality of 160 mOsm/kg. (50) Gentamicin sulfate pediatric injection (Elkins-Sinn) 10 mg/mL has an osmolality of 116 mOsm/kg by freezing-point depression or 212 mOsm/kg by vapor pressure. (1071)

The osmolality of gentamicin sulfate 1 mg/mL was 262 mOsm/kg in dextrose 5% and 278 mOsm/kg in sodium chloride 0.9%. At a 2.5-mg/mL concentration, the osmolality was 278 mOsm/kg in dextrose 5% and 293 mOsm/kg in sodium chloride 0.9%. (1375)

The osmolality of gentamicin sulfate 80 mg was calculated for the following dilutions (1054):

	Osmolality (mOsm/kg)	
Diluent	50 mL	100 mL
Dextrose 5%	293	285
Sodium chloride 0.9%	320	315

The osmolarity of the premixed infusions in sodium chloride 0.9% is approximately 284 to 308 mOsm/L. (4)

Administration — Gentamicin sulfate is administered by intramuscular injection or intermittent intravenous infusion over 0.5 to two hours. For adults, intravenous administration in 50 to 200 mL of sodium chloride 0.9% or dextrose 5% is recommended, while the volume for pediatric patients should be reduced to meet patient's needs. (1; 4)

Stability — Gentamicin sulfate injection is colorless to slightly yellow. (4) Intact containers should be stored at controlled room temperature and protected from freezing. (1; 4) Drug concentration is unrelated to color intensity of gentamicin sulfate solutions. (2139)

Freezing Solutions — Gentamicin sulfate (Schering) 50 mg in 50 mL of dextrose 5% and also sodium chloride 0.9% in PVC containers frozen at −20 °C was stable for 30 days. (299)

Gentamicin sulfate (Schering) 80 mg/100 mL of dextrose 5% in PVC bags was frozen at −20 °C for 30 days and then thawed by exposure to ambient temperature or microwave radiation. No precipitation or color change was observed, and no drug loss occurred. Subsequent storage of the admixture at room temperature for 24 hours also yielded a physically compatible solution, exhibiting little or no drug loss. (554)

Gentamicin sulfate (Elkins-Sinn) 120 mg/50 mL lost 6% in dextrose 5% and 2% in sodium chloride 0.9% in 28 days when frozen at −20 °C. (981)

The stability of gentamicin sulfate (Schering) 5.45 mg/mL in dextrose 5% frozen in an ambulatory pump reservoir was studied. The drug-filled reservoirs were stored at −20 °C for 30 days and then thawed at 5 °C for four days. This thawing was then followed by two days of drug delivery through the pump at 37 °C. No visible changes and no loss occurred during storage and delivery. Furthermore, plasticizer (DEHP) levels were insignificant. (1490)

Syringes — The stability of gentamicin sulfate (Schering) repackaged in plastic syringes (Monoject) was significantly less than in glass syringes (Glaspak, Becton Dickinson) at both 4 and 25 °C. The commercial concentrations were tested in the following amounts: 40 mg/mL—1, 0.75, 0.5, and 0.25 mL; and 10 mg/mL—1.5, 1, and 0.5 mL. Storage in plastic syringes resulted in an average loss of 16% in 30 days and in the formation of a brown precipitate. In glass syringes, the average loss was 7% at 30 days. The brown precipitate did not appear after 30 days but was present at 60 days. It appeared in the cannula of the needle in both glass and plastic syringes. For the 40-mg/mL concentration, the volume of the sample also affected stability. Significantly less loss was noted in the smaller volumes (0.25 and 0.5 mL) than in the larger volumes (0.5 and 1 mL). This volume-related phenomenon

was not demonstrated in the 10-mg/mL pediatric concentration. Storage temperature had no effect on stability over 90 days. (297)

The manufacturer also expressed concern about plastic packaging of gentamicin, noting a possibly inadequate oxygen and moisture barrier both through the tip and the walls of the syringe. It was indicated that gentamicin is oxygen sensitive and that depletion of the antioxidant present could result in instability. Further, loss of moisture at the tip could result in occlusion by the dried product. (403)

Gentamicin sulfate 40 mg/1 mL was packaged in polypropylene syringes (Plastipak, Becton Dickinson). No significant change in concentration occurred over 30 days at 4 or 25 °C. (401)

Gentamicin sulfate (Elkins-Sinn) 120 mg, diluted with 1 mL of sodium chloride 0.9% to a final volume of 4 mL, was stable (less than 10% loss) when stored in polypropylene syringes (Becton Dickinson) for 48 hours at 23 °C under fluorescent light. (1159)

The stability of gentamicin sulfate (Elkins-Sinn) diluted to 10 mg/mL with sodium chloride 0.9% and stored in glass syringes (Becton Dickinson) at 4 °C was studied. No loss of gentamicin sulfate was found during 12 weeks of storage. (1265)

Sorption — Gentamicin sulfate was shown not to exhibit sorption to PVC bags and tubing, polyethylene bags and tubing, multilayer bags of polyethylene, polyamide, and polypropylene, Silastic tubing, polypropylene syringes, and elastomeric reservoirs. (536; 606; 2014; 2269)

Filtration — The effect of several filters on the delivered concentration of gentamicin sulfate (Roussel) from simulated pediatric infusions was studied. A syringe containing dextrose 10% on a syringe pump set at 8.26 mL/hr was connected by intravenous tubing to a 0.5-μm air-blocking filter set (Travenol), a 0.22-μm air-eliminating filter set (Travenol), and a 0.2-μm air-eliminating filter set (Pall). Gentamicin doses of 2.5 and 7.5 mg were injected antegrade to the filter. The effluents were sampled at 1, 1.5, 2, and 4 hours. No significant drug sorption to the plastic tubing or inline filters occurred. However, because of the difference in specific gravity of the drug (1.010) and intravenous solution (1.032), variations in delivered gentamicin did occur due to filter design and position. With the Travenol filters, gentamicin delivery was more rapid with ascending flow in both horizontal and vertical positions. Drug delivery was significantly delayed with descending flow in both positions. The Pall filter delivered gentamicin more rapidly in the horizontal position with either ascending or descending flow. The vertical filter position significantly delayed drug delivery in both flow directions. (804)

However, in another study, gentamicin sulfate 60 mg/15 mL was injected as a bolus through a 0.2-μm nylon air-eliminating filter (Ultipor, Pall) to evaluate the effect of filtration on simulated intravenous push delivery. About 38% of the drug was delivered through the filter after flushing with 10 mL of sodium chloride 0.9%. (809)

Gentamicin sulfate 5 and 10 mg/55 mL of dextrose 5% and sodium chloride 0.9% was filtered over 20 minutes through a 0.22-μm cellulose ester filter set (Ivex-2, Millipore). Virtually all of the drug was delivered through the filter. (1003)

The binding of gentamicin sulfate to the filter of a set used for continuous ambulatory peritoneal dialysis (CAPD) was studied. Gentamicin sulfate 60 mg/2 L in Dianeal 137 with dextrose 4.25 and 1.5% was filtered through a Peridex CAPD filter set (Millipore); this set has a surface area 27 times larger than an inline intravenous filter. About 25% binding occurred from the solution containing dextrose 4.25%, but only 7.5% was bound with the 1.5% solution. (1112)

Gentamicin sulfate (Unicet-Unilabo) 0.32 mg/mL in dextrose 5% and sodium chloride 0.9% was filtered through a 0.22-μm cellulose ester membrane filter (Ivex-HP, Millipore) over six hours. No significant drug loss due to binding to the filter was noted. (1034)

Central Venous Catheter — Gentamicin sulfate (Fujisawa) 1 mg/mL in dextrose 5% was found to be compatible with the ARROWg+ard Blue Plus (Arrow International) chlorhexidine-bearing triple-lumen central catheter. Essentially complete delivery of the drug was found with little or no drug loss occurring. Furthermore, chlorhexidine delivered from the catheter remained at trace amounts with no substantial increase due to the delivery of the drug through the catheter. (2335)

Compatibility Information

Solution Compatibility

Gentamicin sulfate

Solution	Mfr	Mfr	Conc/L	Remarks	Ref	C/I
Amino acids 4.25%, dextrose 25%	MG	SC	80 mg	No increase in particulate matter in 24 hr at 5 °C	349	C
Dextrose 5%		RS	160 mg	Stable for 48 hr at room temperature	157	C
	AB	SC	160 mg	Stable for 24 hr at 5 and 25 °C	88	C
	BA[a], TR	SC	1 g	Stable for 24 hr at 5 and 22 °C	298	C
	TR[b]	SC	800 mg	Physically compatible with little loss in 24 hr at room temperature	554	C
			120 mg	Physically compatible. Stable for 24 hr at 25 °C	897	C
	AB[b]	LY	1.2 g	Visually compatible. Stable for 48 hr at 25 °C in light and 4 °C	1541	C
			600 mg	Decomposition products in 48 hr at room temperature. Gentamicin not quantified	2139	?
Dextrose 10%	SO	SC	60 mg/ 21.5 mL[c]	Visually compatible with no loss in 30 days at 5 °C in the dark	1731	C
	SO	SC	120 mg/ 23 mL[c]	Visually compatible with no loss in 30 days at 5 °C in the dark	1731	C
Isolyte M in dextrose 5%				Stable for 24 hr at room temperature	227	C
Isolyte P in dextrose 5%				Stable for 24 hr at room temperature	227	C
Normosol M in dextrose 5%				Stable for 24 hr at room temperature	227	C
Normosol R				Stable for 24 hr at room temperature	227	C
Normosol R in dextrose 5%				Stable for 24 hr at room temperature	227	C
Ringer's injection			120 mg	Physically compatible and stable for 24 hr at 25 °C	897	C
Ringer's injection, lactated				Stable for 24 hr at room temperature	227	C
Sodium chloride 0.9%			120 mg	Physically compatible and stable for 24 hr at 25 °C	897	C
		RS	160 mg	Stable for 48 hr at room temperature	157	C
	BA[a], TR	SC	1 g	Stable for 24 hr at 5 and 22 °C	298	C
	AB[b]	LY	1.2 g	Visually compatible and stable for 48 hr at 25 °C in light and 4 °C	1541	C
TPN #22[d]		SC	800 mg	Physically compatible. No loss in 24 hr at 22 °C in the dark	837	C
TPN #52 and TPN #53[d]		SC	50 mg	Physically compatible. No loss in 24 hr at 29 °C	440	C
TPN #107[d]			75 mg	Physically compatible and stable for 24 hr at 21 °C	1326	C

[a]Tested in both glass and PVC containers.
[b]Tested in PVC containers.
[c]Tested in glass vials as a concentrate.
[d]Refer to Appendix I for the composition of parenteral nutrition solutions. TPN indicates a 2-in-1 admixture.

Additive Compatibility

Gentamicin sulfate

Drug	Mfr	Conc/L	Mfr	Conc/L	Test Soln	Remarks	Ref	C/I
Amphotericin B		200 mg		320 mg	D5W	Haze develops over 3 hr	26	**I**
Ampicillin sodium	BE	8 g	RS	160 mg	D5¼S, D5W, NS	50% gentamicin loss in 2 hr at room temperature	157	**I**
		1 g		100 mg	TPN #107[a]	42% gentamicin loss and 25% ampicillin loss in 24 hr at 21 °C	1326	**I**
Atracurium besylate	BW	500 mg		2 g	D5W	Physically compatible and atracurium stable for 24 hr at 5 and 30 °C	1694	**C**
Aztreonam	SQ	10 and 20 g	SC	200 and 800 mg	D5W, NS[b]	Little aztreonam loss in 48 hr at 25 °C and 7 days at 4 °C. Gentamicin stable for 12 hr at 25 °C and 24 hr at 4 °C. Up to 10% loss in 48 hr at 25 °C and 7 days at 4 °C	1023	**C**
Bleomycin sulfate	BR	20 and 30 units	SC	50, 100, 300, 600 mg	NS	Physically compatible and bleomycin activity retained for 1 week at 4 °C. Gentamicin not tested	763	**C**
Cefazolin sodium[f]	SKF	10 g	ES	800 mg	D5W, NS[c]	10% cefazolin loss in 4 hr in D5W and 12 hr in NS at 25 °C. No clindamycin and gentamicin loss in 24 hr	1328	**I**
Cefepime HCl	BR	40 g	ES	1.2 g	D5W, NS	Cloudy in 18 hr at room temperature	1681	**I**
Cefotaxime sodium	RS	50 mg	SC	9 mg	D5W	30% loss of gentamicin in 2 hr at 22 °C	504	**I**
	RS	50 mg	SC	6 mg	D5W	4% loss of gentamicin in 24 hr at 22 °C	504	**C**
Cefoxitin sodium	MSD	5 g	SC	400 mg	D5S	4% cefoxitin loss in 24 hr and 11% in 48 hr at 25 °C. 2% in 48 hr at 5 °C. 9% gentamicin loss in 24 hr and 23% in 48 hr at 25 °C. 2% in 48 hr at 5 °C	308	**C**
Ceftazidime	GL	50 mg	SC	6 and 9 mg	D5W	10 to 20% gentamicin loss in 2 hr at 22 °C	504	**I**
Ceftriaxone sodium	RC	100 mg	SC	9 mg	D5W	13% loss of gentamicin in 8 hr at 22 °C	504	**I**
	RC	100 mg	SC	6 mg	D5W	5% loss of gentamicin in 24 hr at 22 °C	504	**C**
Cefuroxime sodium	GL	7.5 g	EX	800 mg	D5W, NS[b]	Physically compatible with no loss of either drug in 1 hr	1036	**C**
		1 g		100 mg	TPN #107[a]	32% gentamicin loss in 24 hr at 21 °C	1326	**I**
Ciprofloxacin	MI	1.6 g	LY	1 g	D5W, NS	Visually compatible and both drugs stable for 48 hr at 25 °C under fluorescent light and 4 °C in the dark	1541	**C**
	BAY	2 g	SC	10 g	NS	Visually compatible. Little ciprofloxacin loss in 24 hr at 25 °C. Gentamicin not tested	1934	**C**
	BAY	2 g	SC	1.6 g	D5W	Visually compatible with no loss of ciprofloxacin in 24 hr at 22 °C under fluorescent light. Gentamicin not tested	2413	**C**
Clindamycin phosphate	UP	2.4 g		120 mg	D5W	Physically compatible. Clindamycin stable for 24 hr at room temperature	104	**C**
	UP	1.2 g		60 mg	D5W	Physically compatible. Clindamycin stable for 24 hr at room temperature	104	**C**
	UP	12 g		600 mg	D5W	Physically compatible	101	**C**
	UP	9 g		800 mg	D5W	Clindamycin stable for 24 hr	101	**C**

Additive Compatibility (Cont.)

Gentamicin sulfate

Drug	Mfr	Conc/L	Mfr	Conc/L	Test Soln	Remarks	Ref	C/I
	UP	9 g	AB	1 g	D5W, NS[d]	Physically compatible and both drugs stable for 48 hr at room temperature exposed to light and 1 week frozen	174	C
	UP	9 g	LY	1.2 g	D5W[c]	Physically compatible and both drugs stable for 7 days at 4 and 25 °C	174	C
	UP	9 g	LY	1.2 g	NS[c]	Physically compatible and both drugs stable for 14 days at 4 and 25 °C	174	C
	UP	18 g	LY	2.4 g	D5W, NS[b]	Physically compatible and both drugs stable for 14 days at 4 and 25 °C	174	C
	UP	9 g	ES	1.2 g	D5W, NS[c]	Physically compatible and both drugs stable for 28 days frozen at −20 °C	174	C
	UP	18 g	ES	2.4 g	D5W, NS[b]	Both drugs stable for 28 days frozen at −20 °C	981	C
	UP	6 g	ES	667 mg	D5W[b]	Physically compatible with no clindamycin loss and 9% gentamicin loss in 24 hr at room temperature	995	C
		400 mg		75 mg	TPN #107[a]	19% gentamicin loss and 15% clindamycin loss in 24 hr at 21 °C	1326	I
Clindamycin phosphate[g]	UP	9 g	ES	800 mg	D5W, NS[c]	10% cefazolin loss in 4 hr in D5W and 12 hr in NS at 25 °C. No clindamycin and gentamicin loss in 24 hr	1328	I
Cloxacillin sodium	BE	4 g	RS	160 mg	D5¼S, D5W, NS	Precipitate forms	157	I
Cytarabine	UP	100 mg		80 mg	D5W	Physically compatible for 24 hr	174	C
	UP	300 mg		240 mg	D5W	Physically incompatible	174	I
Dextran 40		10%			D5W	Gentamicin stable for 24 hr at room temperature	227	C
Dopamine HCl	AS	800 mg	SC	2 g	D5W	No dopamine and 7% gentamicin loss in 24 hr at 25 °C	312	C
	AS	800 mg	SC	320 mg	D5W	Gentamicin stable through 6 hr. 80% gentamicin loss in 24 hr at 25 °C. Dopamine stable for 24 hr	78	I
Fat emulsion, intravenous	VT	10%	RS	160 mg		Lipid coalescence in 24 hr at 8 and 25 °C	825	I
Floxacillin sodium	BE	20 g	RS	8 g	NS	Haze forms immediately and precipitate forms in 2 hr	1479	I
	BE	10 g	EX	8 g	NS	Physically compatible for 48 hr. Both drugs stable for 1 hr at room temperature	1036	C
	BE	10 g	EX	8 g	D5W	Precipitates immediately	1036	I
Fluconazole	PF	1 g	SO	0.5 g	D5W	Visually compatible with no fluconazole loss in 72 hr at 25 °C under fluorescent light. Gentamicin not tested	1677	C
Furosemide	HO	800 mg	SC	1.6 g	D5W, NS	Furosemide precipitates immediately	876	I
	HO	1 g	RS	8 g	NS	Physically compatible for 24 hr at 15 and 30 °C. Precipitate forms in 48 to 72 hr	1479	C
Fusidate sodium	LEO	1 g		160 mg	D–S	Physically compatible and chemically stable for 48 hr at room temperature	1800	C
	LEO	1 g		1.5 g	D–S	Physically incompatible	1800	I
Heparin sodium	BP	20,000 units		320 mg	D5W, NS	Precipitates immediately	26	I

Additive Compatibility (Cont.)

Gentamicin sulfate

Drug	Mfr	Conc/L	Mfr	Conc/L	Test Soln	Remarks	Ref	C/I
	OR	20,000 units	SC	1 g	D5W, NS	Opalescence	113	I
	BRN	1000 to 6000 units	ME	88 mg	D10W, NS	Activity of both drugs greatly reduced	1570	I
Linezolid	PHU	2 g	AB	800 mg	e	Physically compatible. Little linezolid loss in 7 days at 4 and 23 °C in dark. Gentamicin losses of 5 to 7% in 7 days at 4 °C and 8% in 5 days at 23 °C	2332	C
Mannitol		20%		120 mg		Physically compatible and gentamicin stable for 24 hr at 25 °C	897	C
Meropenem	ZEN	1 and 20 g	SC	800 mg	NS	Visually compatible for 4 hr at room temperature	1994	C
Metronidazole	SE	5 g	SC	800 mg and 1.2 g		Physically compatible with no loss of either drug in 2 days at 18 °C. At 4 °C, no metronidazole loss but up to 10% gentamicin loss in 7 days	1242	C
	RP	5 g		800 mg		Visually compatible with no loss of metronidazole in 15 days at 5 and 25 °C. 10% gentamicin loss in 63 hr at 25 °C and 10.6 days at 5 °C	1931	C
Midazolam HCl	RC	50, 250, 400 mg	EX	800 mg	NS	Visually compatible for 4 hr	355	C
Nafcillin sodium		1 g		75 mg	TPN #107[a]	10% gentamicin loss in 24 hr at 21 °C	1326	I
Penicillin G sodium	GL	13 and 40 million units	RS	160 mg	D5¼S, D5W, NS	Gentamicin stable for 24 hr at room temperature	157	C
Ranitidine HCl	GL	100 mg		160 mg	D5W	Physically compatible for 24 hr at ambient temperature in light	1151	C
	GL	50 mg and 2 g		80 mg	D5W, NS	Physically compatible. Ranitidine stable for 24 hr at 25 °C. Gentamicin not tested	1515	C
Verapamil HCl	KN	80 mg	SC	160 mg	D5W, NS	Physically compatible for 24 hr	764	C

[a]*Refer to Appendix I for the composition of parenteral nutrition solutions. TPN indicates a 2-in-1 admixture.*
[b]*Tested in PVC containers.*
[c]*Tested in glass containers.*
[d]*Tested in both glass and PVC containers.*
[e]*Admixed in the linezolid infusion container.*
[f]*Tested in combination with clindamycin phosphate 9 g/L.*
[g]*Tested in combination with cefazolin sodium 10 g/L.*

Drugs in Syringe Compatibility

Gentamicin sulfate

Drug (in syringe)	Mfr	Amt	Mfr	Amt	Remarks	Ref	C/I
Ampicillin sodium	AY	500 mg		80 mg/ 2 mL	Physically incompatible within 1 hr at room temperature	99	I
Caffeine citrate		20 mg/ 1 mL	ES	10 mg/ 1 mL	Visually compatible for 4 hr at 25 °C	2440	C
Clindamycin phosphate	UP	900 mg/ 6 mL	ES	120 mg/ 4 mL[a]	Physically compatible with little loss of either drug for 48 hr at 25 °C	1159	C
Cloxacillin sodium	BE	250 mg		80 mg/ 2 mL	Physically incompatible within 1 hr at room temperature	99	I
Dimenhydrinate		10 mg/ 1 mL		10 mg/ 1 mL	Clear solution	2569	C
		10 mg/ 1 mL		40 mg/ 1 mL	Clear solution	2569	C
Heparin sodium		2500 units/ 1 mL		40 mg	Turbidity or precipitate forms within 5 min	1053	I
Iohexol	WI	64.7%, 5 mL	SC	0.8 mg/ 1 mL	Physically compatible for at least 2 hr	1438	C
Iopamidol	SQ	61%, 5 mL	SC	0.8 mg/ 1 mL	Physically compatible for at least 2 hr	1438	C
Iothalamate meglumine	MA	60%, 5 mL	SC	0.8 mg/ 1 mL	Physically compatible for at least 2 hr	1438	C
Ioxaglate meglumine–ioxaglate sodium	MA	5 mL	SC	0.8 mg/ 1 mL	Transient precipitate clears within 5 min	1438	?
Pantoprazole sodium	[b]	4 mg/ 1 mL		40 mg/ 1 mL	Whitish precipitate	2574	I
Penicillin G sodium		1 million units		80 mg/ 2 mL	No precipitate or color change within 1 hr at room temperature	99	C

[a]Diluted to 4 mL with 1 mL of sodium chloride 0.9%.
[b]Test performed using the formulation WITHOUT edetate disodium.

Y-Site Injection Compatibility (1:1 Mixture)

Gentamicin sulfate

Drug	Mfr	Conc	Mfr	Conc	Remarks	Ref	C/I
Acyclovir sodium	BW	5 mg/mL[a]	TR	1.6 mg/mL[a]	Physically compatible for 4 hr at 25 °C	1157	C
	BV	5 mg/mL[b]	AMS	30 mg/mL[e]	White paste-like precipitate	2794	I
Allopurinol sodium	BW	3 mg/mL[b]	ES	5 mg/mL[b]	Hazy solution with crystals forms in 1 hr	1686	I
Alprostadil	BED	7.5 mcg/mL[t,u]	ES	1 mg/mL[s]	Visually compatible for 1 hr	2746	C
Amifostine	USB	10 mg/mL[a]	ES	5 mg/mL[a]	Physically compatible for 4 hr at 23 °C	1845	C
Amiodarone HCl	LZ	4 mg/mL[c]	LY	0.8 mg/mL[c]	Physically compatible for 4 hr at room temperature	1444	C
	WY	6 mg/mL[a]	APP	5 mg/mL[a]	Visually compatible for 24 hr at 22 °C	2352	C
Amphotericin B cholesteryl sulfate complex	SEQ	0.83 mg/mL[a]	FUJ	5 mg/mL[a]	Gross precipitate forms	2117	I
Amsacrine	NCI	1 mg/mL[a]	SO	5 mg/mL[a]	Visually compatible for 4 hr at 22 °C	1381	C
Anidulafungin	VIC	0.5 mg/mL[a]	AB	5 mg/mL[a]	Physically compatible for 4 hr at 23 °C	2617	C

Y-Site Injection Compatibility (1:1 Mixture) (Cont.)

Gentamicin sulfate

Drug	Mfr	Conc	Mfr	Conc	Remarks	Ref	C/I
Atracurium besylate	BW	0.5 mg/mL[a]	ES	2 mg/mL[a]	Physically compatible for 24 hr at 28 °C	1337	C
Azithromycin	PF	2 mg/mL[b]	AMR	21 mg/mL[e,p]	Whitish-yellow microcrystals found	2368	I
Aztreonam	SQ	40 mg/mL[a]	ES	5 mg/mL[a]	Physically compatible for 4 hr at 23 °C	1758	C
Bivalirudin	TMC	5 mg/mL[a]	AB	5 mg/mL[a]	Physically compatible for 4 hr at 23 °C	2373	C
Caspofungin acetate	ME	0.7 mg/mL[b]	HOS	5 mg/mL[b]	Physically compatible for 4 hr at room temperature	2758	C
Cefepime HCl	BMS	120 mg/mL[c]		6 mg/mL	Physically compatible with less than 10% cefepime loss. Gentamicin not tested	2513	C
Ceftaroline fosamil	FOR	2.22 mg/mL[a,b,q]	HOS	5 mg/mL[a,b,q]	Physically compatible for 4 hr at 23 °C	2826	C
Ceftazidime	SKB	125 mg/mL		0.6 mg/mL	Visually compatible with less than 10% loss of both drugs in 1 hr	2434	C
	GSK	120 mg/mL[g]		6 mg/mL	Physically compatible with less than 10% ceftazidime loss. Gentamicin not tested	2513	C
Ciprofloxacin	MI	2 mg/mL[c]	LY	1.6 mg/mL[c]	Visually compatible for 24 hr at 24 °C	1655	C
Cisatracurium besylate	GW	0.1, 2, 5 mg/mL[a]	ES	5 mg/mL[a]	Physically compatible for 4 hr at 23 °C	2074	C
Clarithromycin	AB	4 mg/mL[a]	RS	40 mg/mL	Visually compatible for 72 hr at both 30 and 17 °C	2174	C
Cyclophosphamide	MJ	20 mg/mL[a]	TR	1.6 mg/mL[a]	Physically compatible for 4 hr at 25 °C	1194	C
Cytarabine	UP	16 mg/mL[b]	GNS	15 mg/mL[e]	Visually compatible for 24 hr at room temperature in test tubes. No precipitate found on filter from Y-site delivery	2063	C
Daptomycin	CUB	19.2 mg/mL[b,r]	AB	1.5 mg/mL[r]	Physically compatible with no loss of either drug in 2 hr at 25 °C	2553	C
Dexmedetomidine HCl	AB	4 mcg/mL[b]	APP	5 mg/mL[b]	Physically compatible for 4 hr at 23 °C	2383	C
Diltiazem HCl	MMD	1[b] and 5 mg/mL	SC	2.4[b] and 40 mg/mL	Visually compatible	1807	C
Docetaxel	RPR	0.9 mg/mL[a]	AB	5 mg/mL[a]	Physically compatible for 4 hr at 23 °C	2224	C
Doripenem	JJ	5 mg/mL[a,b]	HOS	5 mg/mL[a,b]	Physically compatible for 4 hr at 23 °C	2743	C
Doxapram HCl	RB	2 mg/mL[a]	APP	10 mg/mL[a]	Visually compatible for 4 hr at 23 °C	2470	C
Doxorubicin HCl liposomal	SEQ	0.4 mg/mL[a]	ES	5 mg/mL[a]	Physically compatible for 4 hr at 23 °C	2087	C
Enalaprilat	MSD	0.05 mg/mL[b]	ES	0.8 mg/mL[a]	Physically compatible for 24 hr at room temperature under fluorescent light	1355	C
Esmolol HCl	DCC	10 mg/mL[a]	ES	0.8 mg/mL[a]	Physically compatible for 24 hr at 22 °C	1169	C
Etoposide phosphate	BR	5 mg/mL[a]	AB	5 mg/mL[a]	Physically compatible for 4 hr at 23 °C	2218	C
Famotidine	MSD	0.2 mg/mL[a]	ES	0.8 mg/mL[b]	Physically compatible for 14 hr	1196	C
	ME	2 mg/mL[b]		5 mg/mL[a]	Visually compatible for 4 hr at 22 °C	1936	C
Fenoldopam mesylate	AB	80 mcg/mL[b]	APP	5 mg/mL[b]	Physically compatible for 4 hr at 23 °C	2467	C
Filgrastim	AMG	30 mcg/mL[a]	LY	5 mg/mL[a]	Physically compatible for 4 hr at 22 °C	1687	C
	AMG	40 mcg/mL[a]	GNS	1.6 mg/mL[a]	Visually compatible. Little loss of filgrastim and gentamicin in 4 hr at 25 °C	2060	C
	AMG	10 mcg/mL[f]	GNS	1.6 mg/mL[a]	23% loss of filgrastim in 4 hr at 25 °C. Little gentamicin loss	2060	I

Y-Site Injection Compatibility (1:1 Mixture) (Cont.)

Gentamicin sulfate

Drug	Mfr	Conc	Mfr	Conc	Remarks	Ref	C/I
Fluconazole	RR	2 mg/mL	ES	4 mg/mL	Physically compatible for 24 hr at 25 °C	1407	C
Fludarabine phosphate	BX	1 mg/mL[a]	ES	5 mg/mL[a]	Visually compatible for 4 hr at 22 °C	1439	C
Foscarnet sodium	AST	24 mg/mL	ES	4 mg/mL	Physically compatible for 24 hr at room temperature under fluorescent light	1335	C
	AST	24 mg/mL	ES	2 mg/mL[c]	Physically compatible for 24 hr at 25 °C under fluorescent light	1393	C
Furosemide	HO	10 mg/mL	SC	1.6 mg/mL[c]	Furosemide precipitates immediately	876	I
Gemcitabine HCl	LI	10 mg/mL[b]	AB	5 mg/mL[b]	Physically compatible for 4 hr at 23 °C	2226	C
Granisetron HCl	SKB	1 mg/mL	ES	1.5 mg/mL[b]	Physically compatible with little loss of either drug in 4 hr at 22 °C	1883	C
Heparin sodium		[b]	RS	80 mg	Precipitates immediately	528	I
	ES	50 units/mL[c]	ES	3.2 mg/mL[c]	Immediate gross haze	1316	I
	TR	50 units/mL	TR	2 mg/mL	Visually incompatible within 4 hr at 25 °C	1793	I
Hetastarch in lactated electrolyte	AB	6%	SC	5 mg/mL[a]	Physically compatible for 4 hr at 23 °C	2339	C
Hetastarch in sodium chloride 0.9%	DCC	6%	TR	0.8 mg/mL[b]	Precipitates immediately but disappears after 1 hr at room temperature	1313	I
Hydromorphone HCl	WY	0.2 mg/mL[a]	TR	0.8 mg/mL[a]	Physically compatible for 4 hr at 25 °C	987	C
Hydroxyethyl starch 130/0.4 in sodium chloride 0.9%	FRK	6%	SX	1, 3, 5 mg/mL[a]	Visually compatible for 24 hr at room temperature	2770	C
Indomethacin sodium trihydrate	MSD	0.5 and 1 mg/mL[a]		1 mg/mL[a]	White turbidity forms immediately and becomes white flakes in 1 hr	1550	I
Insulin	LI	0.2 unit/mL[b]	TR	1.2 mg/mL[b]	Physically compatible for 2 hr at 25 °C	1395	C
Iodipamide meglumine	SQ				White precipitate forms immediately downstream to Y-site when given into a set through which gentamicin was administered previously	324	I
Labetalol HCl	SC	1 mg/mL[a]	ES	0.8 mg/mL[a]	Physically compatible for 24 hr at 18 °C	1171	C
Levofloxacin	OMN	5 mg/mL[a]	ES	10 mg/mL	Visually compatible for 4 hr at 24 °C	2233	C
Linezolid	PHU	2 mg/mL	FUJ	5 mg/mL[a]	Physically compatible for 4 hr at 23 °C	2264	C
Lorazepam	WY	0.33 mg/mL[b]	CNF	3 mg/mL	Visually compatible for 24 hr at 22 °C	1855	C
Magnesium sulfate	IX	16.7, 33.3, 66.7, 100 mg/mL[a]	SC	0.8 mg/mL[a]	Physically compatible for at least 4 hr at 32 °C	813	C
Melphalan HCl	BW	0.1 mg/mL[b]	LY	5 mg/mL[b]	Physically compatible for 3 hr at 22 °C	1557	C
Meperidine HCl	WY	10 mg/mL[a]	TR	0.8 mg/mL[a]	Physically compatible for 4 hr at 25 °C	987	C
	WY	10 mg/mL[b]	ES	1.2 and 2 mg/mL[b]	Physically compatible for 1 hr at 25 °C	1338	C
Meropenem	ZEN	1 and 50 mg/mL[b]	SC	4 mg/mL[g]	Visually compatible for 4 hr at room temperature	1994	C
	ASZ	10 mg/mL[b]	AMS	30 mg/mL[e]	Physically compatible	2794	C
Midazolam HCl	RC	1 mg/mL[a]	ES	10 mg/mL	Visually compatible for 24 hr at 23 °C	1847	C
	RC	5 mg/mL	CNF	3 mg/mL	Visually compatible for 24 hr at 22 °C	1855	C

Y-Site Injection Compatibility (1:1 Mixture) (Cont.)

Gentamicin sulfate

Drug	Mfr	Conc	Mfr	Conc	Remarks	Ref	C/I
Milrinone lactate	SS	0.2 mg/mL[a]	APP	10 mg/mL[a]	Visually compatible for 4 hr at 25 °C	2381	C
Morphine sulfate	WI	1 mg/mL[a]	TR	0.8 mg/mL[a]	Physically compatible for 4 hr at 25 °C	987	C
	ES	1 mg/mL[b]	ES	1.2 and 2 mg/mL[b]	Physically compatible for 1 hr at 25 °C	1338	C
Multivitamins	USV	5 mL/L[a]	SC	80 mg/100 mL[a]	Physically compatible for 24 hr at room temperature	323	C
Nicardipine HCl	DCC	0.1 mg/mL[a]	ES	0.8 mg/mL[a]	Visually compatible for 24 hr at room temperature	235	C
Ondansetron HCl	GL	1 mg/mL[b]	ES	5 mg/mL[a]	Visually compatible for 4 hr at 22 °C	1365	C
Paclitaxel	NCI	1.2 mg/mL[a]	ES	5 mg/mL[a]	Physically compatible for 4 hr at 22 °C	1556	C
Palonosetron HCl	MGI	50 mcg/mL	APP	5 mg/mL[a]	Physically compatible. No loss of either drug in 4 hr at room temperature	2765	C
Pancuronium bromide	ES	0.05 mg/mL[a]	ES	2 mg/mL[a]	Physically compatible for 24 hr at 28 °C	1337	C
Pemetrexed disodium	LI	20 mg/mL[b]	AB	5 mg/mL[a]	Gross white precipitate forms immediately	2564	I
Potassium chloride	BA	0.02 mEq/mL[v]	AMS	30 mg/mL[e]	Physically compatible	2794	C
Propofol	ZEN	10 mg/mL	ES	5 mg/mL[a]	White precipitate forms immediately	2066	I
Remifentanil HCl	GW	0.025 and 0.25 mg/mL[b]	ES	5 mg/mL[a]	Physically compatible for 4 hr at 23 °C	2075	C
Sargramostim	IMM	10 mcg/mL[b]	SO	5 mg/mL[a]	Visually compatible for 4 hr at 22 °C	1436	C
Tacrolimus	FUJ	1 mg/mL[b]	SCN	4 mg/mL[a]	Visually compatible for 24 hr at 25 °C	1630	C
Telavancin HCl	ASP	7.5 mg/mL[a,b,q]	HOS	5 mg/mL[a,b,q]	Physically compatible for 2 hr	2830	C
Teniposide	BR	0.1 mg/mL[a]	LY	5 mg/mL[a]	Physically compatible for 4 hr at 23 °C	1725	C
Theophylline	TR	4 mg/mL	TR	2 mg/mL	Visually compatible for 6 hr at 25 °C	1793	C
Thiotepa	IMM[h]	1 mg/mL[a]	ES	5 mg/mL[a]	Physically compatible for 4 hr at 23 °C	1861	C
Tigecycline	WY	1 mg/mL[b]		1.4 mg/mL[b]	Physically compatible for 4 hr	2714	C
TNA #73[i]		32.5 mL[j]	SC	1.6 mg/mL[a]	Visually compatible for 4 hr at 25 °C	1008	C
TNA #97 to #104[i]			ES	40 mg/mL	Physically compatible and gentamicin content retained for 6 hr at 21 °C	1324	C
TNA #218 to #226[i]			AB, FUJ	5 mg/mL[a]	Visually compatible for 4 hr at 23 °C	2215	C
TPN #54[i]				13 and 20 mg/mL	Physically compatible and gentamicin activity retained over 6 hr at 22 °C	1045	C
TPN #61[i]		[k]	IX	12.5 mg/1.25 mL[l]	Physically compatible	1012	C
		[m]	IX	75 mg/1.9 mL[l]	Physically compatible	1012	C
TPN #91[i]		[n]	IX	5 mg[o]	Physically compatible	1170	C
TPN #189[i]			DB	1 mg/mL[b]	Visually compatible for 24 hr at 22 °C	1767	C
TPN #203, #204[i]			ES	10 mg/mL	Visually compatible for 2 hr at 23 °C	1974	C
TPN #212 to #215[i]			AB	5 mg/mL[a]	Physically compatible for 4 hr at 23 °C	2109	C
Vasopressin	APP	0.2 unit/mL[b]	APP	1.2 mg/mL[e]	Physically compatible	2641	C

Y-Site Injection Compatibility (1:1 Mixture) (Cont.)

Gentamicin sulfate

Drug	Mfr	Conc	Mfr	Conc	Remarks	Ref	C/I
Vecuronium bromide	OR	0.1 mg/mL[a]	ES	2 mg/mL[a]	Physically compatible for 24 hr at 28 °C	1337	**C**
Vinorelbine tartrate	BW	1 mg/mL[b]	ES	5 mg/mL[b]	Physically compatible for 4 hr at 22 °C	1558	**C**
Warfarin sodium	DU	2 mg/mL[g]	SC	1.6 mg/mL[a]	Haze forms immediately	2010	**I**
	DME	2 mg/mL[g]	SC	1.6 mg/mL[a]	Haze forms immediately	2078	**I**
Zidovudine	BW	4 mg/mL[a]	IMS	2 mg/mL[a]	Physically compatible for 4 hr at 25 °C	1193	**C**

[a]*Tested in dextrose 5%.*
[b]*Tested in sodium chloride 0.9%.*
[c]*Tested in both dextrose 5% and sodium chloride 0.9%.*
[d]*Tested in dextrose 5%, Ringer's injection, lactated, sodium chloride 0.45%, and sodium chloride 0.9%.*
[e]*Tested in sodium chloride 0.45%.*
[f]*Tested in dextrose 5% with albumin human 2 mg/mL.*
[g]*Tested in sterile water for injection.*
[h]*Lyophilized formulation tested.*
[i]*Refer to Appendix I for the composition of parenteral nutrition solutions. TNA indicates a 3-in-1 admixture, and TPN indicates a 2-in-1 admixture.*
[j]*A 32.5-mL sample of parenteral nutrition solution mixed with 50 mL of antibiotic solution.*
[k]*Run at 21 mL/hr.*
[l]*Given over 30 minutes by syringe pump.*
[m]*Run at 94 mL/hr.*
[n]*Run at 10 mL/hr.*
[o]*Given over one hour by syringe pump.*
[p]*Injected via Y-site into an administration set running azithromycin.*
[q]*Tested in Ringer's injection, lactated.*
[r]*Final concentration after mixing.*
[s]*Tested in either dextrose 5% or in sodium chloride 0.9%, but the report did not specify which solution.*
[t]*Tested in a 1:1 mixture of (1) dextrose 5% and dextrose 5% in sodium chloride 0.45% with and without potassium chloride 20 mEq/L and also in (2) dextrose 10% in sodium chloride 0.45% with and without potassium chloride 20 mEq/L.*
[u]*Tested in a 1:1 mixture of dextrose 5% and TPN #274 (see Appendix I).*
[v]*Tested in dextrose 5% in sodium chloride 0.45%.*

Additional Compatibility Information

Peritoneal Dialysis Solutions — The activity of gentamicin 10 mg/L was evaluated in peritoneal dialysis fluids containing 1.5 or 4.25% dextrose (Dianeal 137, Travenol). Storage at 25 °C resulted in no loss of antimicrobial activity in 24 hours. (515)

Gentamicin sulfate (Schering) 3 and 10 mg/L in peritoneal dialysis concentrate with 50% dextrose retained about 90% of initial activity in seven hours and about 50 to 70% in 24 hours at room temperature. (1044)

The stability of gentamicin sulfate 8 mg/L, alone and with cefazolin sodium 75 and 150 mg/L, was evaluated in a peritoneal dialysis solution of dextrose 1.5% with heparin sodium 1000 units/L. Gentamicin activity was retained for 48 hours at both 4 and 26 °C, alone and with both concentrations of cefazolin. Cefazolin activity was also retained over the study period. At 37 °C, gentamicin losses ranged from 4 to 8% and cefazolin losses ranged from 10 to 12% in 48 hours. (1029)

In another study, the stability of gentamicin sulfate (Schering) was evaluated in peritoneal dialysate concentrates containing dextrose 30 and 50% (Dianeal) as well as in a diluted solution containing dextrose 2.5%. The gentamicin sulfate concentrations were 100 and 160 mg/L in the peritoneal dialysate concentrates and 5 and 8 mg/L in the diluted solutions. Gentamicin sulfate was found to be stable in all of these solutions for at least 24 hours at 23 °C. (1229)

Gentamicin 4 mcg/mL was evaluated in Dianeal PDS with dextrose 1.5 and 4.25% (Travenol) with cefazolin 125 mcg/mL, heparin 500 units, and albumin human 80 mg in 2-L bags. The gentamicin content was retained for 72 hours. (1413)

The retention of antimicrobial activity of gentamicin sulfate (SoloPak) 120 mg/L alone and with vancomycin hydrochloride (Lilly) 1 g/L was evaluated in Dianeal PD-2 (Travenol) with dextrose 1.5%. Little or no loss of either antibiotic occurred in eight hours at 37 °C. Gentamicin sulfate alone retained activity for at least 48 hours at 4 and 25 °C. In combination with vancomycin hydrochloride, antimicrobial activity of both antibiotics was retained for up to 48 hours. However, the authors recommended refrigeration at 4 °C for storage periods greater than 24 hours. (1414)

Gentamicin sulfate (Schering) 25 mcg/mL combined separately with the cephalosporins cefazolin sodium (Lilly) and cefoxitin (MSD) at a concentration of 125 mcg/mL in peritoneal dialysis solution (Dianeal 1.5%) exhibited enhanced rates of lethality to *Staphylococcus aureus*, *Escherichia coli*, and *Pseudomonas aeruginosa* compared to any of the drugs alone. (1623)

Gentamicin sulfate (American Pharmaceutical Partners) 8 mcg/mL in Delflex peritoneal dialysis solution bags with 2.5% dextrose (Fresenius) is stable with little or no loss occurring in 14 days refrigerated and at room temperature. (2573)

Gentamicin sulfate (American Pharmaceutical Partners) 8 mcg/mL with vancomycin hydrochloride (Lederle) 25 mcg/mL in Delflex peritoneal dialysis solution bags with 2.5% dextrose (Fresenius) is stable with little or no loss of either drug occurring in 14 days refrigerated and at room temperature. (2573)

β-Lactam Antibiotics — In common with other aminoglycoside antibiotics, gentamicin activity may be impaired by β-lactam antibiotics. The inactivation is dependent on concentration, temperature, and time of exposure. (68; 219; 504; 574; 575; 654; 667; 740; 792; 816; 824; 973; 1052; 1382)

The clinical significance of these interactions in patients appears to be primarily confined to those with renal failure. (218; 334; 361; 364; 616; 737; 816; 847) Literature reports of greatly reduced aminoglycoside levels in such patients have appeared frequently. (363; 365; 366; 367; 614; 666; 962) In addition, the interaction may be clinically important if assays for aminoglycoside levels in serum are sufficiently delayed. (576; 618; 735; 832; 847; 1052; 1382)

Most authors believe that in vitro mixing of penicillins with aminoglycoside antibiotics should be avoided but that clinical use of the drugs in combination can be of great value. It is generally recommended that the drugs be given separately in such combined therapy. (157; 218; 222; 224; 361; 364; 368; 369; 370)

Local Anesthetics — Gentamicin sulfate 80 mg (2 mL) was physically compatible with 1 mL of each of the following local anesthetics and did not show significant loss in 24 hours at room temperature or under refrigeration (227):

Lidocaine hydrochloride 1 and 2% (Astra)
Lidocaine hydrochloride 1 and 2% with epinephrine 1:100,000 (Astra)
Mepivacaine hydrochloride 1 and 2% (Winthrop)

Heparin — Addition of gentamicin sulfate (Roussel) 80 mg to the tubing of an infusion solution of sodium chloride 0.9% containing heparin resulted in immediate precipitation. (528)

Gentamicin sulfate 10 mg/L with heparin sodium 1000 units/L in Dianeal with dextrose 5% peritoneal dialysis solution was reported to be conditionally compatible. No significant reduction in gentamicin sulfate concentration occurred in four to six hours. (228) However, a marked reduction in the anticoagulant activity of heparin sodium occurred if opalescence or a precipitate formed (which results if the undiluted drugs are combined), even if the precipitate redissolved. Heparin activity was retained if one drug was added to a dilute solution of the other and no precipitate formed. (295)

The incompatibility of heparin sodium with gentamicin sulfate is said to result from coprecipitation. (230)

A white precipitate may result from the administration of gentamicin sulfate through a heparinized intravenous cannula. (976) Flushing heparin locks with sodium chloride 0.9% before and after administering drugs incompatible with heparin has been recommended. (4)

Sodium Citrate — The physical stability of gentamicin sulfate (Schering) 1, 2, and 5 mg/mL in sodium citrate 4% anticoagulant solution (Baxter) was evaluated. The combination has been used in preventing hemodialysis catheter-related infections. The gentamicin dilutions were packaged in 3-mL syringes and were stored at 4 and 23 °C. The solutions remained clear and colorless for 35 days at both temperatures. The pH was found to be near 5.1 initially and did not change throughout the study. Although the gentamicin content was not measured, the authors pointed out that other studies had reported that the drug in solutions within the pH range of 4 to 7 was stable for up to 90 days. Furthermore, in another study, sodium citrate had also been documented to be stable for 28 days at room temperature. (2631)

Gentamicin sulfate (Sandoz) 2.5 mg/mL in sodium citrate 4% (Cytasol) was found to be physically and chemically stable for 112 days at 24 °C packaged in polyethylene plastic syringes sealed with tip caps. (2824)

GLYCOPYRROLATE
AHFS 12:08.08

Products — Glycopyrrolate is available in 1- and 2-mL single-dose vials and 5- and 20-mL multiple-dose vials. Each milliliter contains glycopyrrolate 0.2 mg, sodium hydroxide and/or hydrochloric acid to adjust the pH, and benzyl alcohol 0.9% in water for injection. (1)

pH — From 2 to 3. (1)

Trade Name(s) — Robinul.

Administration — Glycopyrrolate may be administered by intravenous or intramuscular injection without dilution. The drug may also be given via the tubing of a running intravenous infusion. (1; 4)

Stability — Glycopyrrolate is a clear, colorless solution; intact vials should be stored at controlled room temperature. (1)

pH Effects — The stability of glycopyrrolate in solution is pH dependent. At pH 2 to 3, the drug is very stable. Above pH 6, the stability becomes questionable because of ester hydrolysis. The speed of this hydrolysis is increased with increasing pH. A significant decline in glycopyrrolate stability as the pH is increased above 6 can be seen in Table 1. (331)

Glycopyrrolate 0.8 mg/L in Ringer's injection, lactated, is physically compatible for 48 hours at 25 °C. The pH of the solution (6.1) is slightly higher than the pH range yielding acceptable glycopyrrolate stability (2 to 6). However, the drug can be administered via the tubing of a running intravenous infusion of Ringer's injection, lactated. (1; 4)

Because of the low pH of glycopyrrolate, mixtures with alkaline drugs such as barbiturates result in precipitation of the free acid. If

Table 1. Stability of Glycopyrrolate 0.8 mg/L in Dextrose 5% Adjusted to Various pH Values (25 °C)

Admixture pH	Approximate Time for 5% Decomposition (hr)
4.0	>48
5.0	>48
6.0	30
6.5	7
7.0	4
8.0	2

the pH of the admixture is increased above 6 by an alkaline additive or solution, rapid ester hydrolysis of the glycopyrrolate results. (331)

Syringes — Glycopyrrolate (American Regent) 0.1 mg/mL in sodium chloride 0.9% in polypropylene syringes (Sherwood) was physically stable and exhibited little loss in 24 hours stored at 4 and 23 °C. (2199)

Glycopyrrolate (Robins) 0.2 mg/mL packaged as 4 mL of undiluted injection in 6-mL polypropylene syringes (Becton Dickinson) was stored at 4 and 25 °C exposed to fluorescent light. The injection remained visually clear, and little loss of glycopyrrolate occurred in 90 days at both storage conditions. (2439)

Compatibility Information

Solution Compatibility

Glycopyrrolate

Solution	Mfr	Mfr	Conc/L	Remarks	Ref	C/I
Dextrose 5% in sodium chloride 0.45%	MG	RB	0.8 mg	Physically compatible. pH in glycopyrrolate stability range for 48 hr at 25 °C	331	C
Dextrose 5%	AB	RB	0.8 mg	Physically compatible. pH in glycopyrrolate stability range for 48 hr at 25 °C	331	C
Dextrose 10%			0.8 mg	Physically compatible	1	C
Ringer's injection	AB	RB	0.8 mg	Physically compatible. pH in glycopyrrolate stability range for 48 hr at 25 °C	331	C
Ringer's injection, lactated			0.8 mg	Physically compatible for 48 hr at 25 °C but pH outside stability range	1	I
Sodium chloride 0.9%	CU	RB	0.8 mg	Physically compatible. pH in glycopyrrolate stability range for 48 hr at 25 °C	331	C

Additive Compatibility

Glycopyrrolate

Drug	Mfr	Conc/L	Mfr	Conc/L	Test Soln	Remarks	Ref	C/I
Buprenorphine HCl with haloperidol lactate	RKC	84 mg 104 mg		25 mg	NS[a]	Visually compatible with less than 10% loss of any drug in 30 days at 4 and 25 °C in the dark	2436	C
Haloperidol lactate with buprenorphine HCl	RKC	104 mg 84 mg		25 mg	NS[a]	Visually compatible with less than 10% loss of any drug in 30 days at 4 and 25 °C in the dark	2436	C
Methylprednisolone sodium succinate	UP	250 mg	RB	1.33 mg	D5½S	Physically incompatible	329	I

[a]*Tested in PVC containers.*

Drugs in Syringe Compatibility

Glycopyrrolate

Drug (in syringe)	Mfr	Amt	Mfr	Amt	Remarks	Ref	C/I
Atropine sulfate	ES	0.4 mg/ 1 mL	RB	0.2 mg/ 1 mL	Physically compatible. pH in glycopyrrolate stability range for 48 hr at 25 °C	331	C
	ES	0.8 mg/ 2 mL	RB	0.2 mg/ 1 mL	Physically compatible. pH in glycopyrrolate stability range for 48 hr at 25 °C	331	C
	ES	0.4 mg/ 1 mL	RB	0.4 mg/ 2 mL	Physically compatible. pH in glycopyrrolate stability range for 48 hr at 25 °C	331	C

Drugs in Syringe Compatibility (Cont.)

Glycopyrrolate

Drug (in syringe)	Mfr	Amt	Mfr	Amt	Remarks	Ref	C/I
Buprenorphine HCl with haloperidol lactate	RKC ON	4 mg 5 mg		1.2 mg	Diluted to 48 mL with NS. Visually compatible with less than 10% loss of any drug in 30 days at 4 and 25 °C in the dark	2436	**C**
Chloramphenicol sodium succinate	PD	100 mg/ 1 mL	RB	0.2 mg/ 1 mL	Gas evolves	331	**I**
	PD	200 mg/ 2 mL	RB	0.2 mg/ 1 mL	Gas evolves	331	**I**
	PD	100 mg/ 1 mL	RB	0.4 mg/ 2 mL	Gas evolves	331	**I**
Chlorpromazine HCl	SKF	25 mg/ 1 mL	RB	0.2 mg/ 1 mL	Physically compatible. pH in glycopyrrolate stability range for 48 hr at 25 °C	331	**C**
	SKF	50 mg/ 2 mL	RB	0.2 mg/ 1 mL	Physically compatible. pH in glycopyrrolate stability range for 48 hr at 25 °C	331	**C**
	SKF	25 mg/ 1 mL	RB	0.4 mg/ 2 mL	Physically compatible. pH in glycopyrrolate stability range for 48 hr at 25 °C	331	**C**
Dexamethasone sodium phosphate	MSD	4 mg/ 1 mL	RB	0.2 mg/ 1 mL	Physically compatible for 48 hr at 25 °C. pH >6.0. 5% glycopyrrolate loss may occur in 4 to 7 hr	331	**I**
	MSD	8 mg/ 2 mL	RB	0.2 mg/ 1 mL	Physically compatible for 48 hr at 25 °C. pH >6.0. 5% glycopyrrolate loss may occur in 4 to 7 hr	331	**I**
	MSD	4 mg/ 1 mL	RB	0.4 mg/ 2 mL	Physically compatible for 48 hr at 25 °C. pH >6.0. 5% glycopyrrolate loss may occur in 4 to 7 hr	331	**I**
	MSD	24 mg/ 1 mL	RB	0.2 mg/ 1 mL	Physically compatible for 48 hr at 25 °C. pH >6.0. 5% glycopyrrolate loss may occur in 4 to 7 hr	331	**I**
	MSD	48 mg/ 2 mL	RB	0.2 mg/ 1 mL	Physically compatible for 48 hr at 25 °C. pH >6.0. 5% glycopyrrolate loss may occur in 4 to 7 hr	331	**I**
	MSD	24 mg/ 1 mL	RB	0.4 mg/ 2 mL	Physically compatible for 48 hr at 25 °C. pH >6.0. 5% glycopyrrolate loss may occur in 4 to 7 hr	331	**I**
Diazepam	RC	5 mg/ 1 mL	RB	0.2 mg/ 1 mL	Precipitates immediately	331	**I**
	RC	10 mg/ 2 mL	RB	0.2 mg/ 1 mL	Precipitates immediately	331	**I**
	RC	5 mg/ 1 mL	RB	0.4 mg/ 2 mL	Precipitates immediately	331	**I**
Dimenhydrinate	SE	50 mg/ 1 mL	RB	0.2 mg/ 1 mL	Precipitates immediately	331	**I**
	SE	100 mg/ 2 mL	RB	0.2 mg/ 1 mL	Precipitates immediately	331	**I**
	SE	50 mg/ 1 mL	RB	0.4 mg/ 2 mL	Precipitates immediately	331	**I**
Diphenhydramine HCl	PD	10 mg/ 1 mL	RB	0.2 mg/ 1 mL	Physically compatible. pH in glycopyrrolate stability range for 48 hr at 25 °C	331	**C**
	PD	20 mg/ 2 mL	RB	0.2 mg/ 1 mL	Physically compatible. pH in glycopyrrolate stability range for 48 hr at 25 °C	331	**C**
	PD	10 mg/ 1 mL	RB	0.4 mg/ 2 mL	Physically compatible. pH in glycopyrrolate stability range for 48 hr at 25 °C	331	**C**
	PD	50 mg/ 1 mL	RB	0.2 mg/ 1 mL	Physically compatible. pH in glycopyrrolate stability range for 48 hr at 25 °C	331	**C**

Drugs in Syringe Compatibility (Cont.)

Glycopyrrolate

Drug (in syringe)	Mfr	Amt	Mfr	Amt	Remarks	Ref	C/I
	PD	100 mg/ 2 mL	RB	0.2 mg/ 1 mL	Physically compatible. pH in glycopyrrolate stability range for 48 hr at 25 °C	331	**C**
	PD	50 mg/ 1 mL	RB	0.4 mg/ 2 mL	Physically compatible. pH in glycopyrrolate stability range for 48 hr at 25 °C	331	**C**
Droperidol	MN	2.5 mg/ 1 mL	RB	0.2 mg/ 1 mL	Physically compatible. pH in glycopyrrolate stability range for 48 hr at 25 °C	331	**C**
	MN	5 mg/ 2 mL	RB	0.2 mg/ 1 mL	Physically compatible. pH in glycopyrrolate stability range for 48 hr at 25 °C	331	**C**
	MN	2.5 mg/ 1 mL	RB	0.4 mg/ 2 mL	Physically compatible. pH in glycopyrrolate stability range for 48 hr at 25 °C	331	**C**
Haloperidol lactate with buprenorphine HCl	ON RKC	5 mg 4 mg		1.2 mg	Diluted to 48 mL with NS. Visually compatible with less than 10% loss of any drug in 30 days at 4 and 25 °C in the dark	2436	**C**
Hydromorphone HCl	KN	2 mg/ 1 mL	RB	0.2 mg/ 1 mL	Physically compatible. pH in glycopyrrolate stability range for 48 hr at 25 °C	331	**C**
	KN	4 mg/ 2 mL	RB	0.2 mg/ 1 mL	Physically compatible. pH in glycopyrrolate stability range for 48 hr at 25 °C	331	**C**
	KN	2 mg/ 1 mL	RB	0.4 mg/ 2 mL	Physically compatible. pH in glycopyrrolate stability range for 48 hr at 25 °C	331	**C**
Hydroxyzine HCl	PF	25 mg/ 1 mL	RB	0.2 mg/ 1 mL	Physically compatible. pH in glycopyrrolate stability range for 48 hr at 25 °C	331	**C**
	PF	50 mg/ 2 mL	RB	0.2 mg/ 1 mL	Physically compatible. pH in glycopyrrolate stability range for 48 hr at 25 °C	331	**C**
	PF	25 mg/ 1 mL	RB	0.4 mg/ 2 mL	Physically compatible. pH in glycopyrrolate stability range for 48 hr at 25 °C	331	**C**
Lidocaine HCl	ES	10 mg/ 1 mL	RB	0.2 mg/ 1 mL	Physically compatible. pH in glycopyrrolate stability range for 48 hr at 25 °C	331	**C**
	ES	20 mg/ 2 mL	RB	0.2 mg/ 1 mL	Physically compatible. pH in glycopyrrolate stability range for 48 hr at 25 °C	331	**C**
	ES	10 mg/ 1 mL	RB	0.4 mg/ 2 mL	Physically compatible. pH in glycopyrrolate stability range for 48 hr at 25 °C	331	**C**
	ES	20 mg/ 1 mL	RB	0.2 mg/ 1 mL	Physically compatible. pH in glycopyrrolate stability range for 48 hr at 25 °C	331	**C**
	ES	40 mg/ 2 mL	RB	0.2 mg/ 1 mL	Physically compatible. pH in glycopyrrolate stability range for 48 hr at 25 °C	331	**C**
	ES	20 mg/ 1 mL	RB	0.4 mg/ 2 mL	Physically compatible. pH in glycopyrrolate stability range for 48 hr at 25 °C	331	**C**
Meperidine HCl	WI	50 mg/ 1 mL	RB	0.2 mg/ 1 mL	Physically compatible. pH in glycopyrrolate stability range for 48 hr at 25 °C	331	**C**
	WI	100 mg/ 2 mL	RB	0.2 mg/ 1 mL	Physically compatible. pH in glycopyrrolate stability range for 48 hr at 25 °C	331	**C**
	WI	50 mg/ 1 mL	RB	0.4 mg/ 2 mL	Physically compatible. pH in glycopyrrolate stability range for 48 hr at 25 °C	331	**C**
Methohexital sodium	LI	10 mg/ 1 mL	RB	0.2 mg/ 1 mL	Precipitates immediately	331	**I**
	LI	20 mg/ 2 mL	RB	0.2 mg/ 1 mL	Precipitates immediately	331	**I**
	LI	10 mg/ 1 mL	RB	0.4 mg/ 2 mL	Precipitates immediately	331	**I**
Midazolam HCl	RC	5 mg/ 1 mL	RB	0.2 mg/ 1 mL	Physically compatible for 4 hr at 25 °C	1145	**C**

Drugs in Syringe Compatibility (Cont.)

Glycopyrrolate

Drug (in syringe)	Mfr	Amt	Mfr	Amt	Remarks	Ref	C/I
Morphine sulfate	LI	15 mg/ 1 mL	RB	0.2 mg/ 1 mL	Physically compatible. pH in glycopyrrolate stability range for 48 hr at 25 °C	331	**C**
	LI	30 mg/ 2 mL	RB	0.2 mg/ 1 mL	Physically compatible. pH in glycopyrrolate stability range for 48 hr at 25 °C	331	**C**
	LI	15 mg/ 1 mL	RB	0.4 mg/ 2 mL	Physically compatible. pH in glycopyrrolate stability range for 48 hr at 25 °C	331	**C**
Nalbuphine HCl	DU	10 mg/ 1 mL	RB	0.2 mg/ 1 mL	Physically compatible for 48 hr	128	**C**
	DU	20 mg/ 1 mL	RB	0.2 mg/ 1 mL	Physically compatible for 48 hr	128	**C**
Neostigmine methylsulfate	RC	0.5 mg/ 1 mL	RB	0.2 mg/ 1 mL	Physically compatible. pH in glycopyrrolate stability range for 48 hr at 25 °C	331	**C**
	RC	1 mg/ 2 mL	RB	0.2 mg/ 1 mL	Physically compatible. pH in glycopyrrolate stability range for 48 hr at 25 °C	331	**C**
	RC	0.5 mg/ 1 mL	RB	0.4 mg/ 2 mL	Physically compatible. pH in glycopyrrolate stability range for 48 hr at 25 °C	331	**C**
Ondansetron HCl	GW	1 mg/mL[a]	AMR	0.1 mg/ mL[a]	Physically compatible. Little loss of either drug in 24 hr at 4 or 23 °C	2199	**C**
Pentazocine lactate	WI	30 mg/ 1 mL	RB	0.2 mg/ 1 mL	Precipitates immediately	331	**I**
	WI	60 mg/ 2 mL	RB	0.2 mg/ 1 mL	Precipitates immediately	331	**I**
	WI	30 mg/ 1 mL	RB	0.4 mg/ 2 mL	Precipitates immediately	331	**I**
Pentobarbital sodium	AB	50 mg/ 1 mL	RB	0.2 mg/ 1 mL	Precipitates immediately	331	**I**
	AB	100 mg/ 2 mL	RB	0.2 mg/ 1 mL	Precipitates immediately	331	**I**
	AB	50 mg/ 1 mL	RB	0.4 mg/ 2 mL	Precipitates immediately	331	**I**
Prochlorperazine edisylate	SKF	5 mg/ 1 mL	RB	0.2 mg/ 1 mL	Physically compatible. pH in glycopyrrolate stability range for 48 hr at 25 °C	331	**C**
	SKF	10 mg/ 2 mL	RB	0.2 mg/ 1 mL	Physically compatible. pH in glycopyrrolate stability range for 48 hr at 25 °C	331	**C**
	SKF	5 mg/ 1 mL	RB	0.4 mg/ 2 mL	Physically compatible. pH in glycopyrrolate stability range for 48 hr at 25 °C	331	**C**
Promethazine HCl	WY	25 mg/ 1 mL	RB	0.2 mg/ 1 mL	Physically compatible. pH in glycopyrrolate stability range for 48 hr at 25 °C	331	**C**
	WY	50 mg/ 2 mL	RB	0.2 mg/ 1 mL	Physically compatible. pH in glycopyrrolate stability range for 48 hr at 25 °C	331	**C**
	WY	25 mg/ 1 mL	RB	0.4 mg/ 2 mL	Physically compatible. pH in glycopyrrolate stability range for 48 hr at 25 °C	331	**C**
Ranitidine HCl	GL	50 mg/ 2 mL	RB	0.2 mg/ 1 mL	Physically compatible for 1 hr at 25 °C	978	**C**
Scopolamine HBr	ES	0.4 mg/ 1 mL	RB	0.2 mg/ 1 mL	Physically compatible. pH in glycopyrrolate stability range for 48 hr at 25 °C	331	**C**
	ES	0.8 mg/ 2 mL	RB	0.2 mg/ 1 mL	Physically compatible. pH in glycopyrrolate stability range for 48 hr at 25 °C	331	**C**
	ES	0.4 mg/ 1 mL	RB	0.4 mg/ 2 mL	Physically compatible. pH in glycopyrrolate stability range for 48 hr at 25 °C	331	**C**

Drugs in Syringe Compatibility (Cont.)

Glycopyrrolate

Drug (in syringe)	Mfr	Amt	Mfr	Amt	Remarks	Ref	C/I
Sodium bicarbonate	AB	75 mg/ 1 mL	RB	0.2 mg/ 1 mL	Gas evolves	331	I
	AB	150 mg/ 2 mL	RB	0.2 mg/ 1 mL	Gas evolves	331	I
	AB	75 mg/ 1 mL	RB	0.4 mg/ 2 mL	Gas evolves	331	I
Trimethobenzamide HCl	BE	100 mg/ 1 mL	RB	0.2 mg/ 1 mL	Physically compatible. pH in glycopyrrolate stability range for 48 hr at 25 °C	331	C
	BE	200 mg/ 2 mL	RB	0.2 mg/ 1 mL	Physically compatible. pH in glycopyrrolate stability range for 48 hr at 25 °C	331	C
	BE	100 mg/ 1 mL	RB	0.4 mg/ 2 mL	Physically compatible. pH in glycopyrrolate stability range for 48 hr at 25 °C	331	C

^aTested in sodium chloride 0.9%.

Y-Site Injection Compatibility (1:1 Mixture)

Glycopyrrolate

Drug	Mfr	Conc	Mfr	Conc	Remarks	Ref	C/I
Dexmedetomidine HCl	HOS				Stated to be compatible	1	C
Palonosetron HCl	MGI	50 mcg/mL	BA	0.2 mg/mL	Physically compatible. No loss of either drug in 4 hr at room temperature	2773	C
Propofol	ZEN	10 mg/mL	RB	0.2 mg/mL	Physically compatible for 1 hr at 23 °C	2066	C

GRANISETRON HYDROCHLORIDE
AHFS 56:22.20

Products — Granisetron hydrochloride is available in 1-mL single-use and 4-mL multiple-use vials containing in each milliliter the equivalent of granisetron 1 mg, sodium chloride 0.9%, citric acid 2 mg, and benzyl alcohol 10 mg as a preservative. (1)

Granisetron hydrochloride is also available in 1-mL single-use vials containing the equivalent of granisetron 0.1 mg, sodium chloride 9 mg, and citric acid 2 mg. (1)

pH — From 4.0 to 6.0. (1)

Equivalency — Granisetron hydrochloride 1.12 mg provides 1 mg of granisetron. (1)

Administration — Granisetron hydrochloride may be administered intravenously undiluted over 30 seconds or by intravenous infusion over five minutes after dilution to 20 to 50 mL with dextrose 5% or sodium chloride 0.9%. (1; 4)

Stability — Granisetron hydrochloride is a clear, colorless injection. Intact vials should be stored at controlled room temperature and pro-

tected from freezing and light. The drug is stable for at least 24 hours when diluted as directed in dextrose 5% or sodium chloride 0.9% and stored at room temperature under normal lighting conditions. (1)

Syringes — Granisetron hydrochloride (SmithKline Beecham) 0.05, 0.07, and 0.1 mg/mL (as granisetron) in sodium chloride 0.9% and in dextrose 5% was repackaged in polypropylene syringes (Sherwood Medical) (closure used not cited). Little or no granisetron hydrochloride loss occurred after 14 days at 5 and 24 °C. (1968)

Granisetron hydrochloride (SmithKline Beecham) 1 mg/mL was repackaged into Plastipak (Becton Dickinson) polypropylene syringes and stored at room temperature exposed to or protected from light and refrigerated at 4 °C. Little granisetron hydrochloride loss occurred in 15 days under any of these storage conditions. (2149)

Central Venous Catheter — Granisetron hydrochloride (SmithKline Beecham) 10 mcg/mL in dextrose 5% was found to be compatible with the ARROWg+ard Blue Plus (Arrow International) chlorhexidine-bearing triple-lumen central catheter. Essentially complete delivery of the drug was found with little or no drug loss occurring. Furthermore, chlorhexidine delivered from the catheter remained at trace amounts with no substantial increase due to the delivery of the drug through the catheter. (2335)

Compatibility Information

Solution Compatibility

Granisetron HCl

Solution	Mfr	Mfr	Conc/L	Remarks	Ref	C/I
Dextrose 5% in sodium chloride 0.45%	BA[b]	SKB	20 mg	Physically compatible. Little loss in 24 hr at 20 °C under fluorescent light	1883	C
Dextrose 5% in sodium chloride 0.9%	BA[b]	SKB	20 mg	Physically compatible. Little loss in 24 hr at 20 °C under fluorescent light	1883	C
Dextrose 5%	BA[b]	SKB	20 mg	Physically compatible. Little loss in 24 hr at 20 °C under fluorescent light	1883	C
	BA[a]	SKB	200 mg	Physically compatible. Little loss in 24 hr at 20 °C under fluorescent light	1883	C
		BE	56[b] and 150[a] mg	Visually compatible. Little loss in 30 days at −20 °C then 7 days at 4 °C then 3 days at 20 °C	1884	C
	MG[c]	SKB	20 mg	5% or less loss in 14 days at 4 °C	1837	C
Sodium chloride 0.9%	BA[b]	SKB	20 mg	Physically compatible. Little loss in 24 hr at 20 °C under fluorescent light	1883	C
	BA[a]	SKB	200 mg	Physically compatible. Little loss in 24 hr at 20 °C under fluorescent light	1883	C
		BE	56[b] and 150[a] mg	Visually compatible. Little loss in 30 days at −20 °C then 7 days at 4 °C then 3 days at 20 °C	1884	C
	MG[c]	SKB	20 mg	5% or less drug loss in 7 days at 4 °C, but 13% loss in 14 days	1837	C

[a]Tested in polypropylene syringes.
[b]Tested in PVC containers.
[c]Tested in Homepump (Block Medical) elastomeric reservoir pumps.

Additive Compatibility

Granisetron HCl

Drug	Mfr	Conc/L	Mfr	Conc/L	Test Soln	Remarks	Ref	C/I
Dexamethasone sodium phosphate	AMR	92 mg	SKB	10 and 40 mg	D5W, NS[a]	Visually compatible. Little loss of either drug in 14 days at 4 and 24 °C in dark	1875	C
	AMR	660 mg	SKB	10 and 40 mg	D5W, NS[a]	Visually compatible. Little dexamethasone and 8% granisetron loss in 14 days at 4 and 24 °C in dark	1875	C
	MSD	75 and 345 mg	BE	55 and 51 mg	D5W, NS[a]	Visually compatible. Little loss of either drug in 72 hr at room temperature	1884	C
Methylprednisolone sodium succinate	DAK	2.26 g	BE	56 mg	D5W, NS[a]	Visually compatible. Little loss of either drug in 72 hr at room temperature	1884	C

[a]Tested in PVC containers.

Drugs in Syringe Compatibility

Granisetron HCl

Drug (in syringe)	Mfr	Amt	Mfr	Amt	Remarks	Ref	C/I
Dexamethasone sodium phosphate	MSD	0.2 and 1 mg/mL[a]	BE	0.15 mg/mL[a]	Visually compatible. Little loss of either drug in 72 hr at room temperature	1884	**C**
Methylprednisolone sodium succinate	DAK	6 mg/mL[a]	BE	0.15 mg/mL[a]	Visually compatible. Little loss of either drug in 72 hr at room temperature	1884	**C**

[a]Diluted with water.

Y-Site Injection Compatibility (1:1 Mixture)

Granisetron HCl

Drug	Mfr	Conc	Mfr	Conc	Remarks	Ref	C/I
Acyclovir sodium	BW	7 mg/mL[a]	SKB	0.05 mg/mL[a]	Physically compatible for 4 hr at 23 °C	2000	**C**
	BV	5 mg/mL[b]	RC	1 mg/mL	Crystals form	2794	**I**
Allopurinol sodium	BW	3 mg/mL[a]	SKB	0.05 mg/mL[a]	Physically compatible for 4 hr at 23 °C	2000	**C**
Amifostine	USB	10 mg/mL[a]	SKB	0.05 mg/mL[a]	Physically compatible for 4 hr at 23 °C	2000	**C**
Amikacin sulfate	AB	5 mg/mL[a]	SKB	0.05 mg/mL[a]	Physically compatible for 4 hr at 23 °C	2000	**C**
Aminophylline	AB	2.5 mg/mL[a]	SKB	0.05 mg/mL[a]	Physically compatible for 4 hr at 23 °C	2000	**C**
Amphotericin B	PH	0.6 mg/mL[a]	SKB	0.05 mg/mL[a]	Large increase in measured turbidity occurs immediately	2000	**I**
Amphotericin B cholesteryl sulfate complex	SEQ	0.83 mg/mL[a]	SKB	0.05 mg/mL[a]	Physically compatible for 4 hr at 23 °C	2117	**C**
Ampicillin sodium	MAR	20 mg/mL[b]	SKB	0.05 mg/mL[a]	Physically compatible for 4 hr at 23 °C	2000	**C**
Ampicillin sodium–sulbactam sodium	RR	20 + 10 mg/mL[b]	SKB	0.05 mg/mL[a]	Physically compatible for 4 hr at 23 °C	2000	**C**
Amsacrine	NCI	1 mg/mL[a]	SKB	0.05 mg/mL[a]	Physically compatible for 4 hr at 23 °C. Precipitate forms in 24 hr	2000	**C**
Aztreonam	SQ	40 mg/mL[a]	SKB	0.05 mg/mL[a]	Physically compatible for 4 hr at 23 °C	2000	**C**
Bleomycin sulfate	MJ	1 unit/mL[b]	SKB	0.05 mg/mL[a]	Physically compatible for 4 hr at 23 °C	2000	**C**
Bumetanide	RC	0.04 mg/mL[a]	SKB	0.05 mg/mL[a]	Physically compatible for 4 hr at 23 °C	2000	**C**
Buprenorphine HCl	RKC	0.04 mg/mL[a]	SKB	0.05 mg/mL[a]	Physically compatible for 4 hr at 23 °C	2000	**C**
Butorphanol tartrate	APC	0.04 mg/mL[a]	SKB	0.05 mg/mL[a]	Physically compatible for 4 hr at 23 °C	2000	**C**
Calcium gluconate	AB	40 mg/mL[a]	SKB	0.05 mg/mL[a]	Physically compatible for 4 hr at 23 °C	2000	**C**
Carboplatin	BR	1 mg/mL[b]	SKB	1 mg/mL	Physically compatible with little or no loss of either drug in 4 hr at 22 °C	1883	**C**
Carmustine	BMS	1.5 mg/mL[a]	SKB	0.05 mg/mL[a]	Physically compatible for 4 hr at 23 °C	2000	**C**
Cefazolin sodium	SKB	20 mg/mL[a]	SKB	0.05 mg/mL[a]	Physically compatible for 4 hr at 23 °C	2000	**C**
Cefepime HCl	BMS	20 mg/mL[a]	SKB	0.05 mg/mL[a]	Physically compatible for 4 hr at 23 °C	2000	**C**
Cefotaxime sodium	HO	20 mg/mL[a]	SKB	0.05 mg/mL[a]	Physically compatible for 4 hr at 23 °C	2000	**C**
Cefotetan disodium	STU	20 mg/mL[a]	SKB	0.05 mg/mL[a]	Physically compatible for 4 hr at 23 °C	2000	**C**
Cefoxitin sodium	ME	20 mg/mL[a]	SKB	0.05 mg/mL[a]	Physically compatible for 4 hr at 23 °C	2000	**C**
Ceftaroline fosamil	FOR	2.22 mg/mL[a,b,c]	CUP	50 mcg/mL[a,b,c]	Physically compatible for 4 hr at 23 °C	2826	**C**
Ceftazidime	SKB	16.7 mg/mL[b]	SKB	1 mg/mL	Physically compatible with little or no loss of either drug in 4 hr at 22 °C	1883	**C**

Y-Site Injection Compatibility (1:1 Mixture) (Cont.)

Granisetron HCl

Drug	Mfr	Conc	Mfr	Conc	Remarks	Ref	C/I
Ceftriaxone sodium	RC	20 mg/mL[a]	SKB	0.05 mg/mL[a]	Physically compatible for 4 hr at 23 °C	2000	C
Cefuroxime sodium	LI	30 mg/mL[a]	SKB	0.05 mg/mL[a]	Physically compatible for 4 hr at 23 °C	2000	C
Chlorpromazine HCl	SCN	2 mg/mL[a]	SKB	0.05 mg/mL[a]	Physically compatible for 4 hr at 23 °C	2000	C
Ciprofloxacin	MI	1 mg/mL[a]	SKB	0.05 mg/mL[a]	Physically compatible for 4 hr at 23 °C	2000	C
Cisplatin	BR	0.05 mg/mL[b]	SKB	1 mg/mL	Physically compatible with little or no granisetron loss in 4 hr at 22 °C	1883	C
	BR	1 mg/mL	SKB	1 mg/mL	Physically compatible with little or no loss of either drug in 4 hr at 22 °C	1883	C
Cladribine	ORT	0.015[b] and 0.5[d] mg/mL	SKB	0.05 mg/mL[b]	Physically compatible for 4 hr at 23 °C	1969	C
Clindamycin phosphate	AB	10 mg/mL[a]	SKB	0.05 mg/mL[a]	Physically compatible for 4 hr at 23 °C	2000	C
Cyclophosphamide	MJ	2 mg/mL[b]	SKB	1 mg/mL	Physically compatible with little loss of either drug in 4 hr at 22 °C	1883	C
Cytarabine	UP	2 mg/mL[b]	SKB	1 mg/mL	Physically compatible with little loss of either drug in 4 hr at 22 °C	1883	C
	UP	50 mg/mL	SKB	0.05 mg/mL[a]	Physically compatible for 4 hr at 23 °C	2000	C
Dacarbazine	MI	1.7 mg/mL[b]	SKB	1 mg/mL	Physically compatible with little loss of either drug in 4 hr at 22 °C	1883	C
Dactinomycin	ME	0.01 mg/mL[a]	SKB	0.05 mg/mL[a]	Physically compatible for 4 hr at 23 °C	2000	C
Daunorubicin HCl	CHI	1 mg/mL[a]	SKB	0.05 mg/mL[a]	Physically compatible for 4 hr at 23 °C	2000	C
Dexamethasone sodium phosphate	ME	0.24 mg/mL[b]	SKB	1 mg/mL	Physically compatible with little or no loss of either drug in 4 hr at 22 °C	1883	C
Dexmedetomidine HCl	AB	4 mcg/mL[b]	SKB	50 mcg/mL[b]	Physically compatible for 4 hr at 23 °C	2383	C
Diphenhydramine HCl	PD	1 mg/mL[b]	SKB	1 mg/mL	Physically compatible with little loss of either drug in 4 hr at 22 °C	1883	C
	SCN	2 mg/mL[a]	SKB	0.05 mg/mL[a]	Physically compatible for 4 hr at 23 °C	2000	C
Dobutamine HCl	BA	4 mg/mL[a]	SKB	0.05 mg/mL[a]	Physically compatible for 4 hr at 23 °C	2000	C
Docetaxel	RPR	0.9 mg/mL[a]	SKB	0.05 mg/mL[a]	Physically compatible for 4 hr at 23 °C	2224	C
Dopamine HCl	AB	3.2 mg/mL[a]	SKB	0.05 mg/mL[a]	Physically compatible for 4 hr at 23 °C	2000	C
Doripenem	JJ	5 mg/mL[a,b]	RC	0.05 mg/mL[a,b]	Physically compatible for 4 hr at 23 °C	2743	C
Doxorubicin HCl	AD	0.2 mg/mL[b]	SKB	1 mg/mL	Physically compatible with little loss of either drug in 4 hr at 22 °C	1883	C
Doxorubicin HCl liposomal	SEQ	0.4 mg/mL[a]	SKB	0.05 mg/mL[a]	Physically compatible for 4 hr at 23 °C	2087	C
Doxycycline hyclate	LY	1 mg/mL[a]	SKB	0.05 mg/mL[a]	Physically compatible for 4 hr at 23 °C	2000	C
Droperidol	AB	0.4 mg/mL[a]	SKB	0.05 mg/mL[a]	Physically compatible for 4 hr at 23 °C	2000	C
Enalaprilat	MSD	0.1 mg/mL[a]	SKB	0.05 mg/mL[a]	Physically compatible for 4 hr at 23 °C	2000	C
Etoposide	BMS	0.4 mg/mL[b]	SKB	1 mg/mL	Physically compatible with little or no loss of either drug in 4 hr at 22 °C	1883	C
	BR	0.4 mg/mL[a]	SKB	0.05 mg/mL[a]	Physically compatible for 4 hr at 23 °C	2000	C
Etoposide phosphate	BR	5 mg/mL[a]	SKB	0.05 mg/mL[a]	Physically compatible for 4 hr at 23 °C	2218	C
Famotidine	ME	2 mg/mL[a]	SKB	0.05 mg/mL[a]	Physically compatible for 4 hr at 23 °C	2000	C
Fenoldopam mesylate	AB	80 mcg/mL[b]	SKB	50 mcg/mL[b]	Physically compatible for 4 hr at 23 °C	2467	C
Filgrastim	AMG	30 mcg/mL[a]	SKB	0.05 mg/mL[a]	Physically compatible for 4 hr at 23 °C	2000	C

Y-Site Injection Compatibility (1:1 Mixture) (Cont.)

Granisetron HCl

Drug	Mfr	Conc	Mfr	Conc	Remarks	Ref	C/I
Floxuridine	RC	3 mg/mL[a]	SKB	0.05 mg/mL[a]	Physically compatible for 4 hr at 23 °C	2000	C
Fluconazole	PF	2 mg/mL	SKB	0.05 mg/mL[a]	Physically compatible for 4 hr at 23 °C	2000	C
Fludarabine phosphate	BX	1 mg/mL[a]	SKB	0.05 mg/mL[a]	Physically compatible for 4 hr at 23 °C	2000	C
Fluorouracil	AD	16 mg/mL[a]	SKB	0.05 mg/mL[a]	Physically compatible for 4 hr at 23 °C	1804	C
	RC	2 mg/mL[b]	SKB	1 mg/mL	Physically compatible with little or no loss of either drug in 4 hr at 22 °C	1883	C
	AD	16 mg/mL[a]	SKB	0.05 mg/mL[a]	Physically compatible for 4 hr at 23 °C	2000	C
Furosemide	AB	3 mg/mL[a]	SKB	0.05 mg/mL[a]	Physically compatible for 4 hr at 23 °C	1804	C
	HO	0.4 mg/mL[b]	SKB	1 mg/mL	Physically compatible with little or no loss of either drug in 4 hr at 22 °C	1883	C
Gallium nitrate	FUJ	0.4 mg/mL[a]	SKB	0.05 mg/mL[a]	Physically compatible for 4 hr at 23 °C	2000	C
Ganciclovir sodium	SY	20 mg/mL[a]	SKB	0.05 mg/mL[a]	Physically compatible for 4 hr at 23 °C	2000	C
Gemcitabine HCl	LI	10 mg/mL[b]	SKB	0.05 mg/mL[b]	Physically compatible for 4 hr at 23 °C	2226	C
Gentamicin sulfate	ES	1.5 mg/mL[b]	SKB	1 mg/mL	Physically compatible with little loss of either drug in 4 hr at 22 °C	1883	C
Haloperidol lactate	MN	0.2 mg/mL[a]	SKB	0.05 mg/mL[a]	Physically compatible for 4 hr at 23 °C	2000	C
Heparin sodium	AB	100 units/mL[a]	SKB	0.05 mg/mL[a]	Physically compatible for 4 hr at 23 °C	2000	C
Hetastarch in lactated electrolyte	AB	6%	SKB	0.05 mg/mL[a]	Physically compatible for 4 hr at 23 °C	2339	C
Hydrocortisone sodium succinate	AB	1 mg/mL[a]	SKB	0.05 mg/mL[a]	Physically compatible for 4 hr at 23 °C	2000	C
Hydromorphone HCl	KN	0.5 mg/mL[b]	SKB	1 mg/mL	Physically compatible with little or no loss of either drug in 4 hr at 22 °C	1883	C
	ES	0.5 mg/mL[a]	SKB	0.05 mg/mL[a]	Physically compatible for 4 hr at 23 °C	2000	C
Hydroxyzine HCl	ES	2 mg/mL[a]	SKB	0.05 mg/mL[a]	Physically compatible for 4 hr at 23 °C	2000	C
Idarubicin HCl	AD	0.5 mg/mL[a]	SKB	0.05 mg/mL[a]	Physically compatible for 4 hr at 23 °C	2000	C
Ifosfamide	MJ	4 mg/mL[b]	SKB	1 mg/mL	Physically compatible with little or no loss of either drug in 4 hr at 22 °C	1883	C
Imipenem–cilastatin sodium	ME	10 mg/mL[a]	SKB	0.05 mg/mL[a]	Physically compatible for 4 hr at 23 °C	2000	C
Leucovorin calcium	IMM	2 mg/mL[a]	SKB	0.05 mg/mL[a]	Physically compatible for 4 hr at 23 °C	2000	C
Linezolid	PHU	2 mg/mL	SKB	0.05 mg/mL[a]	Physically compatible for 4 hr at 23 °C	2264	C
Lorazepam	WY	0.1 mg/mL[b]	SKB	1 mg/mL	Physically compatible with little or no loss of either drug in 4 hr at 22 °C	1883	C
	WY	0.1 mg/mL[a]	SKB	0.05 mg/mL[a]	Physically compatible for 4 hr at 23 °C	2000	C
Magnesium sulfate	AB	16 mg/mL[b]	SKB	1 mg/mL	Physically compatible with little or no loss of granisetron in 4 hr at 22 °C	1883	C
	AB	100 mg/mL[a]	SKB	0.05 mg/mL[a]	Physically compatible for 4 hr at 23 °C	2000	C
Mechlorethamine HCl	MSD	0.5 mg/mL[b]	SKB	1 mg/mL	Physically compatible with little or no loss of either drug in 4 hr at 22 °C	1883	C
Melphalan HCl	BW	0.1 mg/mL[b]	SKB	0.05 mg/mL[a]	Physically compatible for 4 hr at 23 °C	2000	C
Meperidine HCl	WY	4 mg/mL[a]	SKB	0.05 mg/mL[a]	Physically compatible for 4 hr at 23 °C	2000	C
Mesna	MJ	4 mg/mL[b]	SKB	1 mg/mL	Physically compatible with little or no loss of either drug in 4 hr at 22 °C	1883	C
Methotrexate sodium	CET	12.5 mg/mL[b]	SKB	1 mg/mL	Physically compatible with little or no loss of either drug in 4 hr at 22 °C	1883	C

Y-Site Injection Compatibility (1:1 Mixture) (Cont.)

Granisetron HCl

Drug	Mfr	Conc	Mfr	Conc	Remarks	Ref	C/I
Methylprednisolone sodium succinate	WY	5 mg/mL[a]	SKB	0.05 mg/mL[a]	Physically compatible for 4 hr at 23 °C	2000	C
Metoclopramide HCl	AB	5 mg/mL	SKB	0.05 mg/mL[a]	Physically compatible for 4 hr at 23 °C	2000	C
Metronidazole	BA	5 mg/mL	SKB	0.05 mg/mL[a]	Physically compatible for 4 hr at 23 °C	2000	C
Mitomycin	BMS	0.5 mg/mL	SKB	0.05 mg/mL[a]	Physically compatible for 4 hr at 23 °C	2000	C
Mitoxantrone HCl	IMM	0.5 mg/mL[a]	SKB	0.05 mg/mL[a]	Physically compatible for 4 hr at 23 °C	2000	C
Morphine sulfate	AST	1 mg/mL[b]	SKB	1 mg/mL	Physically compatible with little or no loss of either drug in 4 hr at 22 °C	1883	C
	AST	1 mg/mL[a]	SKB	0.05 mg/mL[a]	Physically compatible for 4 hr at 23 °C	2000	C
Nalbuphine HCl	AB	10 mg/mL	SKB	0.05 mg/mL[a]	Physically compatible for 4 hr at 23 °C	2000	C
Oxaliplatin	SS	0.5 mg/mL[a]	SKB	0.05 mg/mL[a]	Physically compatible for 4 hr at 23 °C	2566	C
Paclitaxel	MJ	0.3 mg/mL[b]	SKB	1 mg/mL	Physically compatible with little or no loss of either drug in 4 hr at 22 °C	1883	C
	MJ	1.2 mg/mL[a]	SKB	0.05 mg/mL[a]	Physically compatible for 4 hr at 23 °C	2000	C
Pemetrexed disodium	LI	20 mg/mL[b]	RC	0.05 mg/mL[a]	Physically compatible for 4 hr at 23 °C	2564	C
Piperacillin sodium–tazobactam sodium	CY[h]	40 + 5 mg/mL[a]	SKB	0.05 mg/mL[a]	Physically compatible for 4 hr at 23 °C	2000	C
Potassium chloride	LY	0.04 mEq/mL[b]	SKB	1 mg/mL	Physically compatible with little or no loss of granisetron in 4 hr at 22 °C	1883	C
Prochlorperazine edisylate	SCN	0.5 mg/mL[a]	SKB	0.05 mg/mL[a]	Physically compatible for 4 hr at 23 °C	2000	C
Promethazine HCl	WY	2 mg/mL[a]	SKB	0.05 mg/mL[a]	Physically compatible for 4 hr at 23 °C	2000	C
Propofol	ZEN	10 mg/mL	SKB	0.05 mg/mL[a]	Physically compatible for 1 hr at 23 °C	2066	C
Ranitidine HCl	GL	2 mg/mL[a]	SKB	0.05 mg/mL[a]	Physically compatible for 4 hr at 23 °C	2000	C
Sargramostim	IMM	10 mcg/mL[b]	SKB	0.05 mg/mL[a]	Physically compatible for 4 hr at 23 °C	2000	C
Sodium bicarbonate	AB	1 mEq/mL	SKB	0.05 mg/mL[a]	Physically compatible for 4 hr at 23 °C	1804	C
	AB	0.33 mEq/mL[b]	SKB	1 mg/mL	Physically compatible with 8% loss of granisetron in 4 hr at 22 °C	1883	C
	AB	1 mEq/mL	SKB	0.05 mg/mL[a]	Physically compatible for 4 hr at 23 °C	2000	C
Streptozocin	UP	9.1 mg/mL[b]	SKB	1 mg/mL	Physically compatible with little or no loss of either drug in 4 hr at 22 °C	1883	C
Teniposide	BMS	0.1 mg/mL[a]	SKB	0.05 mg/mL[a]	Physically compatible for 4 hr at 23 °C	2000	C
Thiotepa	IMM[f]	1 mg/mL[a]	SKB	0.05 mg/mL[a]	Physically compatible for 4 hr at 23 °C	1861	C
Ticarcillin disodium–clavulanate potassium	SKB	27 mg/mL[b]	SKB	1 mg/mL	Physically compatible with little or no loss of either drug in 4 hr at 22 °C	1883	C
	SKB	31 mg/mL[a]	SKB	0.05 mg/mL[a]	Physically compatible for 4 hr at 23 °C	2000	C
TNA #218 to #226[g]			SKB	0.05 mg/mL[a]	Visually compatible for 4 hr at 23 °C	2215	C
Tobramycin sulfate	AB	5 mg/mL[a]	SKB	0.05 mg/mL[a]	Physically compatible for 4 hr at 23 °C	2000	C
Topotecan HCl	SKB	56 mcg/mL[a,b]	SKB	20 mcg/mL[a,b]	Visually compatible. Little loss of either drug in 4 hr at 22 °C	2245	C
TPN #212 to #215[g]			SKB	0.05 mg/mL[a]	Physically compatible for 4 hr at 23 °C	2109	C
Trimethoprim–sulfamethoxazole	ES	0.8 + 4 mg/mL[a]	SKB	0.05 mg/mL[a]	Physically compatible for 4 hr at 23 °C	2000	C
Vancomycin HCl	AB	10 mg/mL[a]	SKB	0.05 mg/mL[a]	Physically compatible for 4 hr at 23 °C	2000	C
Vinblastine sulfate	LI	0.12 mg/mL[a]	SKB	0.05 mg/mL[a]	Physically compatible for 4 hr at 23 °C	2000	C

Y-Site Injection Compatibility (1:1 Mixture) (Cont.)

Granisetron HCl

Drug	Mfr	Conc	Mfr	Conc	Remarks	Ref	C/I
Vincristine sulfate	LI	0.01 and 0.34 mg/mL[b]	SKB	1 mg/mL	Physically compatible with little or no loss of either drug in 4 hr at 22 °C	1883	C
Vinorelbine tartrate	BW	1 mg/mL[a]	SKB	0.05 mg/mL[a]	Physically compatible for 4 hr at 23 °C	2000	C
Zidovudine	BW	4 mg/mL[a]	SKB	0.05 mg/mL[a]	Physically compatible for 4 hr at 23 °C	2000	C

[a]*Tested in dextrose 5%.*
[b]*Tested in sodium chloride 0.9%.*
[c]*Tested in Ringer's injection, lactated.*
[d]*Tested in bacteriostatic sodium chloride 0.9% preserved with benzyl alcohol 0.9%.*
[e]*Granisetron HCl tested in both sodium chloride 0.9% and dextrose 5%.*
[f]*Lyophilized formulation tested.*
[g]*Refer to Appendix I for the composition of parenteral nutrition solutions. TNA indicates a 3-in-1 admixture, and TPN indicates a 2-in-1 admixture.*
[h]*Test performed using the formulation WITHOUT edetate disodium.*

HALOPERIDOL LACTATE
AHFS 28:16.08.08

Products — Haloperidol lactate is available in 1-mL ampuls and vials and 10-mL multiple-dose vials. Each milliliter of solution contains haloperidol 5 mg (as the lactate) and lactic acid for pH adjustment. (1)

pH — From 3 to 3.6 (1) or 3.8. (17)

Trade Name(s) — Haldol.

Administration — Haloperidol lactate should be administered intramuscularly (1; 4), although intravenous administration has been performed. (4; 571; 1258)

Stability — Haloperidol lactate should be stored at controlled room temperature and protected from light; freezing and temperatures above 40 °C should be avoided. (1; 4)

Central Venous Catheter — Haloperidol lactate (McNeil) 0.2 mg/mL in dextrose 5% was found to be compatible with the ARROWg+ard Blue Plus (Arrow International) chlorhexidine-bearing triple-lumen central catheter. Essentially complete delivery of the drug was found with little or no drug loss occurring. Furthermore, chlorhexidine delivered from the catheter remained at trace amounts with no substantial increase due to the delivery of the drug through the catheter. (2335)

Compatibility Information

Solution Compatibility

Haloperidol lactate

Solution	Mfr	Mfr	Conc/L	Remarks	Ref	C/I
Dextrose 5% in sodium chloride 0.2%	AB	MN	0.1 to 1 g	Visually compatible for 7 days at 21 °C	1740	C
	AB	MN	2 and 3 g	Precipitate forms in 30 to 60 min	1740	I
Dextrose 5%	TR[a]	MN	100 mg	Physically compatible and stable for 38 days at 24 °C	571	C
	AB	MN	0.1 to 3 g	Visually compatible for 7 days at 21 °C	1740	C
Ringer's injection, lactated	AB	MN	0.1 to 1 g	Visually compatible for 7 days at 21 °C	1740	C
	AB	MN	2 g	Precipitate forms within 15 min	1740	I
	AB	MN	3 g	Precipitate forms immediately	1740	I

Solution Compatibility (Cont.)

Haloperidol lactate

Solution	Mfr	Mfr	Conc/L	Remarks	Ref	C/I
Sodium chloride 0.45%	AB	MN	0.1 to 1 g	Visually compatible for 7 days at 21 °C	1740	C
	AB	MN	2 g	Precipitate forms within 15 min	1740	I
	AB	MN	3 g	Precipitate forms immediately	1740	I
Sodium chloride 0.9%	AB[b]	MN	2 and 3 g	Slight precipitate forms immediately and becomes much heavier within 15 to 30 min	1523	I
	AB[b]	MN	1 g	Slight precipitate forms immediately and persists through 8 hr	1523	I
	AB[b]	MN	100 and 500 mg	Visually compatible for 8 hr at 21 °C under fluorescent light	1523	C
	AB	MN	0.1 to 0.75 g	Visually compatible for 7 days at 21 °C	1740	C
	AB	MN	1 to 3 g	Precipitate forms immediately	1740	I

[a]Tested in both glass and PVC containers.
[b]Tested in glass containers.

Additive Compatibility

Haloperidol lactate

Drug	Mfr	Conc/L	Mfr	Conc/L	Test Soln	Remarks	Ref	C/I
Buprenorphine HCl with glycopyrrolate	RKC	84 mg 25 mg	ON	104 mg	NS[a]	Visually compatible with less than 10% loss of any drug in 30 days at 4 and 25 °C in the dark	2436	C
Glycopyrrolate with buprenorphine HCl	RKC	25 mg 84 mg	ON	104 mg	NS[a]	Visually compatible with less than 10% loss of any drug in 30 days at 4 and 25 °C in the dark	2436	C
Oxycodone HCl	NAP	1 g	JC	125 mg	NS, W	Visually compatible. Under 4% concentration change in 24 hr at 25 °C	2600	C
Tramadol HCl	AND	11.18 g	EST	210 mg	NS[b]	Visually compatible for 7 days at 25 °C protected from light	2701	C
	AND	33.3 g	EST	620 mg	NS[b]	Visually compatible for 7 days at 25 °C protected from light	2701	C

[a]Tested in PVC containers.
[b]Tested in elastomeric pump reservoirs (Baxter).

Drugs in Syringe Compatibility

Haloperidol lactate

Drug (in syringe)	Mfr	Amt	Mfr	Amt	Remarks	Ref	C/I
Benztropine mesylate	MSD	2 mg	MN	0.25, 0.5, 1 mg	Visually compatible for 24 hr at 21 °C	1781	C
	MSD	2 mg	MN	2 mg	Precipitate forms within 4 hr at 21 °C	1781	I
	MSD	2 mg	MN	3, 4, 5 mg	Precipitate forms within 15 min at 21 °C	1781	I
	MSD	1 mg	MN	0.25 and 0.5 mg	Visually compatible for 24 hr at 21 °C	1781	C
	MSD	1 mg	MN	1 to 5 mg	Precipitate forms within 15 min at 21 °C	1781	I
	MSD	0.5 mg	MN	0.25 to 5 mg	Precipitate forms within 15 min at 21 °C	1781	I

Drugs in Syringe Compatibility (Cont.)

Haloperidol lactate

Drug (in syringe)	Mfr	Amt	Mfr	Amt	Remarks	Ref	C/I
	MSD	2 mg/ 2 mL	MN	10 mg/ 2 mL	White precipitate forms within 5 min	1784	I
Buprenorphine HCl with glycopyrrolate	RKC	4 mg 1.2 mg	ON	5 mg	Diluted to 48 mL with NS. Visually compatible with less than 10% loss of any drug in 30 days at 4 and 25 °C in the dark	2436	C
Cyclizine lactate	WEL	150 mg/ 3 mL	SE	1.5 mg/ 0.3 mL	Diluted with 17 mL of NS. Crystals of cyclizine form within 24 hr at 25 °C	1761	I
	WEL	150 mg/ 3 mL	SE	1.5 mg/ 0.3 mL	Diluted with 17 mL of D5W or W. Visually compatible for 24 hr at 25 °C	1761	C
Cyclizine lactate with diamorphine HCl	WEL BP	16 mg/ mL 11 mg/ mL	JC	2.2 mg/ mL	Physically compatible with less than 10% loss of any drug in 7 days at 23 °C	2071	C
Cyclizine lactate with diamorphine HCl	WEL BP	16 mg/ mL 25 mg/ mL	JC	2.2 mg/ mL	Physically compatible with less than 10% loss of any drug in 7 days at 23 °C	2071	C
Cyclizine lactate with diamorphine HCl	WEL BP	11 mg/ mL 40 mg/ mL	JC	2.2 mg/ mL	Physically compatible with less than 10% loss of any drug in 7 days at 23 °C	2071	C
Cyclizine lactate with diamorphine HCl	WEL BP	13 mg/ mL 42 mg/ mL	JC	2.1 mg/ mL	Physically compatible with less than 10% loss of any drug in 7 days at 23 °C	2071	C
Cyclizine lactate with diamorphine HCl	WEL BP	9 mg/mL 55 mg/ mL	JC	2.1 mg/ mL	Physically compatible with less than 10% loss of any drug in 7 days at 23 °C	2071	C
Cyclizine lactate with diamorphine HCl	WEL BP	13 mg/ mL 56 mg/ mL	JC	2.1 mg/ mL	Physically compatible with less than 10% loss of any drug in 7 days at 23 °C	2071	C
Diamorphine HCl	MB	10, 25, 50 mg/ 1 mL	SE	1.5 mg/ 1 mL[a]	Physically compatible and diamorphine content retained for 24 hr at room temperature	1454	C
	EV	20 mg/ 1 mL	SE	2 mg/ 1 mL	Crystallization with 58% haloperidol loss in 7 days at room temperature	1455	I
	EV	50 and 150 mg/ 1 mL	SE	5 mg/ 1 mL	Precipitates immediately	1455	I
	EV	100 mg/ 8 mL	SE	2.5 mg/ 8 mL	Physically compatible for 24 hr at room temperature and 7 days at 6 °C	1456	C
	HC	20 to 100 mg/ mL	SE	0.75 mg/ mL	Visually compatible for 48 hr at 5 and 20 °C	1672	C
	HC	2 mg/mL	SE	0.75 mg/ mL	5% diamorphine loss in 14.8 days at 20 °C. Haloperidol stable for 45 days	1672	C
	HC	20 mg/ mL	SE	0.75 mg/ mL	5% diamorphine loss in 20.7 days at 20 °C. Haloperidol stable for 45 days	1672	C
	BP	20, 50, 100 mg/ mL	JC	2 and 3 mg/mL	Physically compatible with less than 10% loss of either drug in 7 days at 23 °C	2071	C

Drugs in Syringe Compatibility (Cont.)

Haloperidol lactate

Drug (in syringe)	Mfr	Amt	Mfr	Amt	Remarks	Ref	C/I
	BP	20 and 50 mg/mL	JC	4 mg/mL	Physically compatible with less than 10% loss of either drug in 7 days at 23 °C	2071	C
Diamorphine HCl with cyclizine lactate	BP WEL	11 mg/mL 16 mg/mL	JC	2.2 mg/mL	Physically compatible with less than 10% loss of any drug in 7 days at 23 °C	2071	C
Diamorphine HCl with cyclizine lactate	BP WEL	25 mg/mL 16 mg/mL	JC	2.2 mg/mL	Physically compatible with less than 10% loss of any drug in 7 days at 23 °C	2071	C
Diamorphine HCl with cyclizine lactate	BP WEL	40 mg/mL 11 mg/mL	JC	2.2 mg/mL	Physically compatible with less than 10% loss of any drug in 7 days at 23 °C	2071	C
Diamorphine HCl with cyclizine lactate	BP WEL	42 mg/mL 13 mg/mL	JC	2.1 mg/mL	Physically compatible with less than 10% loss of any drug in 7 days at 23 °C	2071	C
Diamorphine HCl with cyclizine lactate	BP WEL	55 mg/mL 9 mg/mL	JC	2.1 mg/mL	Physically compatible with less than 10% loss of any drug in 7 days at 23 °C	2071	C
Diamorphine HCl with cyclizine lactate	BP WEL	56 mg/mL 13 mg/mL	JC	2.1 mg/mL	Physically compatible with less than 10% loss of any drug in 7 days at 23 °C	2071	C
Diphenhydramine HCl	ES	100 mg/2 mL	MN	10 mg/2 mL	White precipitate forms within 5 min	1784	I
	ES	50 mg/1 mL	MN	5 mg/1 mL	White cloudy precipitate forms in 2 hr at room temperature	1886	I
Glycopyrrolate with buprenorphine HCl	RKC	1.2 mg 4 mg	ON	5 mg	Diluted to 48 mL with NS. Visually compatible with less than 10% loss of any drug in 30 days at 4 and 25 °C in the dark	2436	C
Heparin sodium		2500 units/1 mL	JN	5 mg/1 mL	Turbidity or precipitate forms within 5 min	1053	I
Hydromorphone HCl	KN	1[a] and 10 mg/1 mL	MN	1[a], 2[a], 5 mg/1 mL	Visually compatible for 24 hr at 25 °C under fluorescent light	1785	C
	KN	10 and 15 mg/mL	MN	2 mg/mL	White precipitate of haloperidol forms immediately	668	I
Hydroxyzine HCl	ES	100 mg/2 mL	MN	10 mg/2 mL	White precipitate forms within 5 min	1784	I
Ketorolac tromethamine	SY	30 mg/1 mL	SO	5 mg/1 mL	White crystalline precipitate forms immediately	1786	I
Lorazepam	WY	2 mg/1 mL	MN	5 mg/1 mL	Physically compatible and chemically stable for 16 hr at room temperature	1838	C
	WY	4 mg/1 mL	MN	5 mg/1 mL	Visually compatible with no loss of either drug in 24 hr at 4 and 25 °C	260	C
	WY	2 mg/1 mL	MN	5 mg/1 mL	Visually compatible for 4 hr at room temperature	260	C

Drugs in Syringe Compatibility (Cont.)

Haloperidol lactate

Drug (in syringe)	Mfr	Amt	Mfr	Amt	Remarks	Ref	C/I
Morphine sulfate		5 and 10 mg/ 1 mL[c]	MN	5 mg/ 1 mL	Cloudiness forms immediately, becoming a crystalline precipitate of haloperidol and parabens	1901	I
	ME	20 mg/ mL[a]	MN	2 mg/mL	White precipitate of haloperidol forms on mixing	668	I
Oxycodone HCl	NAP	200 mg/ 20 mL	JC	15 mg/ 3 mL	Visually compatible. Under 4% concentration change in 24 hr at 25 °C	2600	C
Scopolamine butylbromide	BI	2.5, 5, 10 mg/ mL		0.3125 mg/mL	Physically compatible. Less than 10% loss of both drugs in 15 days at 4 and 25 °C	2521	C
	BI	2.5, 5, 10 mg/ mL		0.625 mg/mL	Physically compatible. Less than 10% loss of both drugs in 7 days at 4 and 25 °C. Over 10% loss of scopolamine in 15 days at both temperatures	2521	C
	BI	2.5, 5, 10 mg/ mL		1.25 mg/ mL	Physically incompatible. Haloperidol precipitates in 15 days at 25 °C and 7 days at 4 °C	2521	I
Tramadol HCl	GRU	8.33, 16.67, 33.33 mg/mL[d]	EST	0.208 mg/mL[d]	Physically compatible with no loss of either drug in 15 days at 4 and 25 °C protected from light	2672	C

[a] Diluted with sterile water for injection.
[b] Morphine sulfate powder dissolved in dextrose 5%.
[c] Morphine sulfate powder dissolved in water.
[d] Diluted with sodium chloride 0.9%.

Y-Site Injection Compatibility (1:1 Mixture)

Haloperidol lactate

Drug	Mfr	Conc	Mfr	Conc	Remarks	Ref	C/I
Allopurinol sodium	BW	3 mg/mL[b]	MN	0.2 mg/mL[b]	Immediate turbidity. Crystals in 1 hr	1686	I
Amifostine	USB	10 mg/mL[a]	MN	0.2 mg/mL[a]	Physically compatible for 4 hr at 23 °C	1845	C
Amphotericin B cholesteryl sulfate complex	SEQ	0.83 mg/mL[a]	MN	0.2 mg/mL[a]	Gross precipitate forms	2117	I
Amsacrine	NCI	1 mg/mL[a]	MN	0.2 mg/mL[a]	Visually compatible for 4 hr at 22 °C	1381	C
Aztreonam	SQ	40 mg/mL[a]	MN	0.2 mg/mL[a]	Physically compatible for 4 hr at 23 °C	1758	C
Bivalirudin	TMC	5 mg/mL[a]	MN	0.2 mg/mL[a]	Physically compatible for 4 hr at 23 °C	2373	C
Ceftaroline fosamil	FOR	2.22 mg/ mL[a,b,f]	BED	0.2 mg/mL[a,b,f]	Physically compatible for 4 hr at 23 °C	2826	C
Cisatracurium besylate	GW	0.1, 2, 5 mg/ mL[a]	MN	0.2 mg/mL[a]	Physically compatible for 4 hr at 23 °C	2074	C
Cladribine	ORT	0.015[b] and 0.5[c] mg/mL	MN	0.2 mg/mL[b]	Physically compatible for 4 hr at 23 °C	1969	C
Dexmedetomidine HCl	AB	4 mcg/mL[b]	MN	0.2 mg/mL[b]	Physically compatible for 4 hr at 23 °C	2383	C
Dobutamine HCl	LI	4 mg/mL[a]	MN	0.5[a] and 5 mg/mL	Visually compatible for 24 hr at 21 °C	1523	C

Y-Site Injection Compatibility (1:1 Mixture) (Cont.)

Haloperidol lactate

Drug	Mfr	Conc	Mfr	Conc	Remarks	Ref	C/I
Docetaxel	RPR	0.9 mg/mL[a]	MN	0.2 mg/mL[a]	Physically compatible for 4 hr at 23 °C	2224	C
Dopamine HCl	DU	1.6 mg/mL[a]	MN	0.5[a] and 5 mg/mL	Visually compatible for 24 hr at 21 °C	1523	C
Doxorubicin HCl liposomal	SEQ	0.4 mg/mL[a]	MN	0.2 mg/mL[a]	Physically compatible for 4 hr at 23 °C	2087	C
Etoposide phosphate	BR	5 mg/mL[a]	MN	0.2 mg/mL[a]	Physically compatible for 4 hr at 23 °C	2218	C
Famotidine	MSD	0.267 mg/mL[a]	MN	0.5[a] and 5 mg/mL	Visually compatible for 24 hr at 21 °C	1523	C
	ME	2 mg/mL[b]		0.2 mg/mL[a]	Visually compatible for 4 hr at 22 °C	1936	C
Fenoldopam mesylate	AB	80 mcg/mL[b]	APP	0.2 mg/mL[b]	Physically compatible for 4 hr at 23 °C	2467	C
Fentanyl citrate	JN	0.025 mg/mL[a]	MN	0.2 mg/mL[a]	Physically compatible for 48 hr at 22 °C	1706	C
Filgrastim	AMG	30 mcg/mL[a]	MN	0.2 mg/mL[a]	Physically compatible for 4 hr at 22 °C	1687	C
Fluconazole	RR	2 mg/mL	MN	5 mg/mL	Precipitate forms	1407	I
Fludarabine phosphate	BX	1 mg/mL[a]	MN	0.2 mg/mL[a]	Visually compatible for 4 hr at 22 °C	1439	C
Foscarnet sodium	AST	24 mg/mL	LY	5 mg/mL	Delayed formation of fine white precipitate	1335	I
Gallium nitrate	FUJ	1 mg/mL[b]	MN	5 mg/mL	Immediate white cloudiness	1673	I
Gemcitabine HCl	LI	10 mg/mL[b]	MN	0.2 mg/mL[b]	Physically compatible for 4 hr at 23 °C	2226	C
Granisetron HCl	SKB	0.05 mg/mL[a]	MN	0.2 mg/mL[a]	Physically compatible for 4 hr at 23 °C	2000	C
Heparin sodium	OR	25,000 and 50,000 units/250 mL[e]	MN	5 mg/1 mL[d]	White precipitate forms immediately	779	I
Hetastarch in lactated electrolyte	AB	6%	MN	0.2 mg/mL[a]	Physically compatible for 4 hr at 23 °C	2339	C
Hydromorphone HCl	AST	0.5 mg/mL[a]	MN	0.2 mg/mL[a]	Physically compatible for 48 hr at 22 °C	1706	C
Lidocaine HCl	AB	4 mg/mL[a]	MN	0.5[a] and 5 mg/mL	Visually compatible for 24 hr at 21 °C	1523	C
Linezolid	PHU	2 mg/mL	MN	0.2 mg/mL[a]	Physically compatible for 4 hr at 23 °C	2264	C
Lorazepam	WY	0.33 mg/mL[b]	JN	0.5 and 5 mg/mL	Visually compatible for 24 hr at 22 °C	1855	C
Melphalan HCl	BW	0.1 mg/mL[b]	MN	0.2 mg/mL[b]	Physically compatible for 3 hr at 22 °C	1557	C
Methadone HCl	LI	1 mg/mL[a]	MN	0.2 mg/mL[a]	Physically compatible for 48 hr at 22 °C	1706	C
Midazolam HCl	RC	5 mg/mL	JN	0.5 and 5 mg/mL	Visually compatible for 24 hr at 22 °C	1855	C
Morphine sulfate	AST	1 mg/mL[a]	MN	0.2 mg/mL[a]	Physically compatible for 48 hr at 22 °C	1706	C
Nitroglycerin	DU	0.4 mg/mL[a]	MN	0.5[a] and 5 mg/mL	Visually compatible for 24 hr at 21 °C	1523	C
Norepinephrine bitartrate	WI	0.032 mg/mL[a]	MN	0.5[a] and 5 mg/mL	Visually compatible for 24 hr at 21 °C	1523	C
Ondansetron HCl	GL	1 mg/mL[b]	LY	0.2 mg/mL[a]	Visually compatible for 4 hr at 22 °C	1365	C
Oxaliplatin	SS	0.5 mg/mL[a]	APP	0.2 mg/mL[a]	Physically compatible for 4 hr at 23 °C	2566	C
Paclitaxel	NCI	1.2 mg/mL[a]		0.2 mg/mL[a]	Physically compatible for 4 hr at 22 °C	1528	C
Pemetrexed disodium	LI	20 mg/mL[b]	APP	0.2 mg/mL[a]	Physically compatible for 4 hr at 23 °C	2564	C
Phenylephrine HCl	WB	0.02 mg/mL[a]	MN	0.5[a] and 5 mg/mL	Visually compatible for 24 hr at 21 °C	1523	C

Y-Site Injection Compatibility (1:1 Mixture) (Cont.)

Haloperidol lactate

Drug	Mfr	Conc	Mfr	Conc	Remarks	Ref	C/I
Piperacillin sodium–tazobactam sodium	LE[h]	40 + 5 mg/mL[a]	MN	0.2 mg/mL[a]	White turbidity and particles form immediately	1688	I
Propofol	ZEN	10 mg/mL	MN	0.2 mg/mL[a]	Physically compatible for 1 hr at 23 °C	2066	C
Quinupristin–dalfopristin	AVE	2 mg/mL[a]		0.2 mg/mL[a]	Physically compatible	1	C
Remifentanil HCl	GW	0.025 and 0.25 mg/mL[b]	MN	0.2 mg/mL[a]	Physically compatible for 4 hr at 23 °C	2075	C
Sargramostim	IMM	10 mcg/mL[b]	LY	0.2 mg/mL[b]	Small particles form in 4 hr	1436	I
Sodium nitroprusside	AB	0.2 mg/mL[a]	MN	5 mg/mL	Immediate turbidity. Precipitate in 24 hr at 21 °C in fluorescent light	1523	I
	AB	0.2 mg/mL[a]	MN	0.5 mg/mL[a]	Visually compatible for 24 hr at 21 °C	1523	C
Tacrolimus	FUJ	1 mg/mL[b]	SO	2.5 mg/mL[a]	Visually compatible for 24 hr at 25 °C	1630	C
Teniposide	BR	0.1 mg/mL[a]	MN	0.2 mg/mL[a]	Physically compatible for 4 hr at 23 °C	1725	C
Theophylline	TR	1.6 mg/mL[a]	MN	0.5[a] and 5 mg/mL	Visually compatible for 24 hr at 21 °C	1523	C
Thiotepa	IMM[i]	1 mg/mL[b]	MN	0.2 mg/mL[b]	Physically compatible for 4 hr at 23 °C	1861	C
Tigecycline	WY	1 mg/mL[b]	MN	0.2 mg/mL[b]	Physically compatible for 4 hr	2714	C
TNA #218 to #226[g]			MN	0.2 mg/mL[a]	Damage to emulsion occurs immediately with free oil possible	2215	I
TPN #189[g]			SE	10 mg/mL	Visually compatible for 24 hr at 22 °C	1767	C
TPN #212 to #215[g]			MN	0.2 mg/mL[a]	Physically compatible for 4 hr at 23 °C	2109	C
Vinorelbine tartrate	BW	1 mg/mL[b]	MN	0.2 mg/mL[b]	Physically compatible for 4 hr at 22 °C	1558	C

[a]Tested in dextrose 5%.
[b]Tested in sodium chloride 0.9%.
[c]Tested in bacteriostatic sodium chloride 0.9% preserved with benzyl alcohol 0.9%.
[d]Injected over one minute.
[e]Tested in both dextrose 5% and sodium chloride 0.9%. Run at 1000 units/hr.
[f]Tested in Ringer's injection, lactated.
[g]Refer to Appendix I for the composition of parenteral nutrition solutions. TNA indicates a 3-in-1 admixture, and TPN indicates a 2-in-1 admixture.
[h]Test performed using the formulation WITHOUT edetate disodium.
[i]Lyophilized formulation tested.

HEPARIN SODIUM
AHFS 20:12.04.16

Products — Heparin sodium is available from various manufacturers in concentrations ranging from 1000 to 20,000 units/mL, packaged in sizes ranging from 0.5- to 1-mL ampuls, vials, or prefilled syringes to 30-mL multiple-dose vials. Benzyl alcohol or parabens may also be present as preservatives, and hydrochloric acid and/or sodium hydroxide may have been added to adjust pH. Sodium chloride may have been added to some products for isotonicity. In addition, dilute solutions of 10 and 100 units/mL in 1- to 5-mL disposable syringes and 1- to 30-mL vials are available for use in flushing heparin locks. (4)

Heparin sodium is also available premixed in various concentrations in sodium chloride 0.45 and 0.9% and dextrose 5%. (4)

pH — Heparin sodium injection and heparin lock flush solution are adjusted to pH 5 to 7.5 during manufacturing. (1; 17)

Osmolality — The osmolality of heparin sodium (Elkins-Sinn) 1000 units/mL was determined to be 384 mOsm/kg by freezing-point depression and 283 mOsm/kg by vapor pressure. (1071)

One heparin lock flush solution is reported to have an osmolarity of 392 mOsm/L. (4)

Commercial heparin sodium infusion solutions in sodium chloride 0.9% and dextrose 5% have osmolalities of 322 and 270 mOsm/kg, respectively. (4)

Administration — Heparin sodium may be administered by deep subcutaneous injection, by intermittent intravenous injection undiluted or diluted in 50 to 100 mL of dextrose 5% or sodium chloride 0.9%, or by continuous intravenous infusion in a liter of compatible solution, preferably using an electronic rate-control device. The container should be inverted at least six times after heparin sodium addition to prevent pooling of the heparin. Intramuscular injection should not be used because of pain and hematoma formation. (4)

Care is required when adding heparin sodium to infusion solutions, especially in flexible containers. When heparin sodium was added to a flexible PVC container of sodium chloride 0.9% hanging in the use position, pooling of the heparin resulted; 97% of the heparin was delivered in the first 30% of the solution. Repeated inversion and agitation of the containers to effect thorough mixing eliminates this pooling (and the danger of overdosage), yielding an even distribution and a constant delivery concentration. (85)

Stability — Heparin sodium solutions are colorless to slightly yellow. (4) Heparin sodium solution should not be used if it is discolored or contains a precipitate. Heparin sodium should be stored at controlled room temperature (1; 4) and protected from freezing and temperatures exceeding 40 °C. (4; 21) In a study of hospital-manufactured heparin sodium 1 unit/mL in sodium chloride 0.9%, full anticoagulant activity was retained for at least 12 months after sterilization by autoclaving and subsequent storage at room temperature exposed to daylight. (675)

pH Effects — A pH profile of heparin sodium 20,000 units/L in dextrose 5% over a pH range of 3.8 to 7.6 did not reveal a loss during the 24-hour study. (21) In another report, heparin sodium in sodium chloride 0.9% was tested at pH 3.2 (adjusted with hydrochloric acid) and 9.2 (adjusted with sodium hydroxide). No loss was noted in 24 hours. (57) However, a pH profile of heparin sodium 660 units/mL, when autoclaved for 10 minutes at 10 pounds/inch^2 at 115 °C, showed loss of activity at pH values above 8.5 and especially below 5. (243)

Syringes — The stability of 50 mL of a 500-unit/mL heparin sodium solution in sodium chloride 0.9% packaged in 50-mL polypropylene syringes was studied. Storage both at room temperature and at 0 to 4 °C showed an overall trend to lower activity by about 8% after three weeks.

When glass containers were compared to plastic syringes, the glass containers consistently showed lower retained activity in as little as two hours after preparation. The possibility of adsorption to glass surfaces was noted (676) but has not been demonstrated.

Heparin sodium 1 unit/mL, prefilled into Injekt (Braun) all-plastic syringes having polyethylene barrels and polypropylene plungers, showed no significant activity loss over 52 weeks at 37 °C due to decomposition or sorption. However, plastic syringes with rubber-tipped plungers, such as Plastipak (Becton Dickinson) and Perfusor (Braun), exhibited extra ultraviolet peaks, presumably due to leaching of rubber components. (1491)

Heparin sodium (Leo) 300 units/mL in dextrose 5% or water for injection was drawn into 50-mL polypropylene syringes (Plastipak, Becton Dickinson) and stored for eight hours at room temperature and 4 °C. No loss in either solvent occurred. (1799)

The stability of heparin sodium repackaged in 10-mL polypropylene syringes for use in CADD-Micro syringe pumps was evaluated. Ten milliliters of heparin sodium 1000 units/mL (Elkins-Sinn) and 40,000 units/mL (Schein) were packaged in the test syringes and capped. Syringes were stored at a near-body temperature of 30 °C for 30 days. Little or no loss of heparin sodium content occurred; actual activity in prolonging blood clotting was not evaluated. (2275)

Sorption — Heparin sodium, BP, 2000 units/2 mL was stored for 18 hours at room temperature in plastic syringes: Brunswick (Sherwood Medical), Plastipak (Becton Dickinson), Steriseal (Needle Industries), and Sabre (Gillette U.K.). The first three syringes have polypropylene barrels; the Sabre has a combination polypropylene–polystyrene barrel. No significant loss of heparin occurred due to sorption. (784)

Heparin sodium (Leo) 300 units/mL in dextrose 5% or water for injection was delivered at 4 mL/hr by syringe pump through PVC and polyethylene-lined PVC infusion tubing for 12 hours at room temperature. No loss occurred due to sorption to the polyethylene-lined tubing. However, losses of about 15 to 25% occurred with the PVC tubing and were especially high during the first 15 minutes of infusion. (1799)

Filtration — Heparin sodium (Abbott) 10,000 units/L in dextrose 5% and sodium chloride 0.9% was filtered at 120 mL/hr for six hours through a 0.22-μm cellulose ester membrane filter (Ivex-2). No significant loss due to binding to the filter was noted. (533)

Central Venous Catheter — Heparin sodium (Elkins-Sinn) 100 units/mL in dextrose 5% was found to be compatible with the AR-ROWg+ard Blue Plus (Arrow International) chlorhexidine-bearing triple-lumen central catheter. Essentially complete delivery of the drug was found with little or no drug loss occurring. Furthermore, chlorhexidine delivered from the catheter remained at trace amounts with no substantial increase due to the delivery of the drug through the catheter. (2335)

Compatibility Information

Solution Compatibility

Heparin sodium

Solution	Mfr	Mfr	Conc/L	Remarks	Ref	C/I
Amino acids 4.25%, dextrose 25%	MG	RI	20,000 units	No increase in particulate matter in 24 hr at 5 °C	349	C
Dextrose–Ringer's injection combinations	AB	AB	1000 and 4000 units	Physically compatible	3	C

Solution Compatibility (Cont.)

Heparin sodium

Solution	Mfr	Mfr	Conc/L	Remarks	Ref	C/I
Dextrose–Ringer's injection, lactated, combinations	AB	AB	1000 and 4000 units	Physically compatible	3	C
Dextrose 5% in Ringer's injection, lactated	TR[a]	UP	10,000 units	Stable for 24 hr at 5 °C	282	C
Dextrose–saline combinations	AB	AB	1000 and 4000 units	Physically compatible	3	C
Dextrose 2.5% in sodium chloride 0.45%	BA	DB	1000 units	Heparin activity retained for 12 months at 4 °C	1914	C
Dextrose 5% in sodium chloride 0.45%	TR	AB	20,000 units	No decrease in activity in 24 hr at room temperature	407	C
Dextrose 5% in sodium chloride 0.9%			12,000 units	Physically compatible	74	C
			32,000 units	Stable for 24 hr	57	C
	AB	AB	20,000 units	Stable for 24 hr	21	C
	AB		20,000 units	Stable for 72 hr	46	C
	TR[a]	UP	10,000 units	Stable for 24 hr at 5 °C	282	C
	BA		30,000 units	40% loss in 5 hr at 15, 25, and 35 °C. Activity recovered 5 to 7 hr later	674	I
Dextrose 2.5%	AB	AB	1000 and 4000 units	Physically compatible	3	C
Dextrose 5%			12,000 units	Physically compatible	74	C
	AB	AB	1000 and 4000 units	Physically compatible	3	C
	BP		40,000 units	Stable for 24 hr at 23 °C	252	C
			32,000 units	Stable for 24 hr	57	C
	AB	AB	20,000 units	Stable for 24 hr	21	C
	AB[a]		20,000 units	Stable for 72 hr	46	C
	TR[b]	OR	20,000 and 40,000 units	Stable for 48 hr at 27 °C	254	C
	TR[a]	UP	10,000 units	Stable for 24 hr at 5 °C	282	C
	TR	AS	20,000 units	No decrease in activity in 24 hr at room temperature	407	C

Solution Compatibility (Cont.)

Heparin sodium

Solution	Mfr	Mfr	Conc/L	Remarks	Ref	C/I
		OR	20,000 units	50% loss within 1 hr at 23 °C	113	**I**
	MG	UP	10,000 units	30 to 50% activity loss in 6 hr at room temperature. Partial rebound in 24 hr	406	**I**
	BA		30,000 units	65% loss in 5 hr at 15, 25, and 35 °C. Activity recovered in 24 to 48 hr	674	**I**
		AH	35,000 units	Apparent temporary 50% loss of heparin activity in 4 hr with recovery in 6 hr at 25 °C. Heparin activity then maintained for 14 days at 4 °C	900	**?**
	BA	DB	1000 units	Heparin activity retained for 7 days at 22 °C	1914	**C**
	BA	DB	10,000 units	Heparin activity retained for 12 months at 22 °C	1914	**C**
	BA[b]	BRN	7000 units	Visually compatible with about 5% loss in 24 hr at 22 °C but little or no loss at 4 °C	2289	**C**
	BRN[d]	BRN	7000 units	Visually compatible with little or no loss in 24 hr at 4 and 22 °C	2289	**C**
Dextrose 10%	AB	AB	1000 and 4000 units	Physically compatible	3	**C**
	MG	UP	10,000 units	40% activity loss in 6 hr at room temperature. Partial rebound at 24 hr	406	**I**
Dextrose 25%		LY	5000 units	About 6% heparin activity loss in 21 days and 11% loss in 28 days at 4 °C	2025	**C**
Ionosol products	AB	AB	1000 and 4000 units	Physically compatible	3	**C**
Normosol R	AB	AB	20,000 units	Stable for 24 hr	21	**C**
Ringer's injection	AB	AB	1000 and 4000 units	Physically compatible	3	**C**
Ringer's injection, lactated	AB	AB	1000 and 4000 units	Physically compatible	3	**C**
			12,000 units	Physically compatible	74	**C**
	TR[a]	UP	10,000 units	Stable for 24 hr at 5 °C	282	**C**
		OR	20,000 units	40% loss within 1 hr at 23 °C	113	**I**
	MG	UP	10,000 units	50 to 60% activity loss in 6 hr at room temperature. Partial rebound at 24 hr	406	**I**
		AH	35,000 units	Apparent temporary 50% loss of heparin activity in 4 hr with recovery in 6 hr at 25 °C. Heparin activity gradually lost over 14 days	900	**?**

Solution Compatibility (Cont.)

Heparin sodium

Solution	Mfr	Mfr	Conc/L	Remarks	Ref	C/I
Sodium chloride 0.45%	AB	AB	1000 and 4000 units	Physically compatible	3	C
Sodium chloride 0.9%			12,000 units	Physically compatible	74	C
	AB	AB	1000 and 4000 units	Physically compatible	3	C
			32,000 units	Stable for 24 hr	57	C
	AB	AB	20,000 units	Stable for 24 hr	21	C
	AB		20,000 units	Stable for 72 hr	46	C
	TR[a]	UP	10,000 units	Stable for 24 hr at 5 °C	282	C
	TR[b]	OR	20,000 and 40,000 units	Stable for 48 hr at 27 °C	254	C
		AH	35,000 units	Heparin activity stable for 24 hr at 25 °C followed by 14 days at 4 °C	900	C
	MG	UP	10,000 units	30 to 50% activity loss in 6 hr at room temperature. Partial rebound at 24 hr	406	I
	BA	DB	1000 units	Heparin activity retained for 12 months at 22 °C	1914	C
	BA	DB	10,000 units	Heparin activity retained for 12 months at 4 and 22 °C	1914	C
		LY	5000 units	Heparin activity retained for 28 days at 4 °C	2025	C
	BA[b]	BRN	7000 units	Visually compatible with about 5% loss in 24 hr at 22 °C but little or no loss at 4 °C	2289	C
	BRN[d]	BRN	7000 units	Visually compatible with little or no loss in 24 hr at 4 and 22 °C	2289	C
Sodium lactate ⅙ M		OR	20,000 units	50% loss within 1 hr at 23 °C	113	I
TPN #48 to #51[c]		AH	35,000 units	Heparin activity retained for 24 hr at 25 °C but significantly decreased after 24 hr	900	C
TPN #205[c]		LY	3000 to 20,000 units	Heparin activity retained for 28 days at 4 °C	2025	C

[a]Tested in both glass and PVC containers.
[b]Tested in PVC containers.
[c]Refer to Appendix I for the composition of parenteral nutrition solutions. TPN indicates a 2-in-1 admixture.
[d]Tested in polyethylene and glass containers.

Additive Compatibility

Heparin sodium

Drug	Mfr	Conc/L	Mfr	Conc/L	Test Soln	Remarks	Ref	C/I
Alteplase	GEN	0.5 g	ES	40,000 units	NS	Heparin interacts with alteplase. Opalescence forms within 5 min with peak intensity at 4 hr at 25 °C. Alteplase clot-lysis activity reduced slightly	1856	I
Amikacin sulfate	BR	5 g	AB	30,000 units	D5LR, D5R, D5S, D5W, D10W, LR, NS, R, SL	Precipitates immediately	294	I
Aminophylline		250 mg		12,000 units	D5W	Physically compatible	74	C
	SE	1 g	UP	4000 units	D5W	Physically compatible	15	C
Amphotericin B	SQ	100 mg	AB	4000 units	D	Physically compatible	21	C
	SQ	100 mg	UP	4000 units	D5W	Physically compatible	15	C
	SQ	70 and 140 mg		2000 units	D5W	Bioactivity not affected over 24 hr at 25 °C	335	C
Ampicillin sodium		2 g		32,000 units	NS	Physically compatible and heparin activity retained for 24 hr	57	C
	BE	10 g	OR	20,000 units	NS	Both stable for 24 hr at 25 °C	113	C
	BR	1 g		12,000 units	D10W, LR, NS	Ampicillin stable for 24 hr at 4 °C	87	C
	BR	1 g		12,000 units	D5S	15% ampicillin decomposition in 24 hr at 4 °C	87	I
	BR	1 g		12,000 units	D5S, D10W, LR	20 to 25% ampicillin decomposition in 24 hr at 25 °C	87	I
Antithymocyte globulin (rabbit)[d]	SGS	200 and 300 mg	ES	2000 units	D5W	Immediate haze and precipitation	2488	I
	SGS	200 and 300 mg	ES	2000 units	NS	Physically compatible for 24 hr at 23 °C	2488	C
Ascorbic acid	UP	500 mg	UP	4000 units	D5W	Physically compatible	15	C
Atracurium besylate	BW	500 mg		40,000 units	D5W	Particles form at 5 and 30 °C	1694	I
Bleomycin sulfate	BR	20 and 30 units	RI	10,000 to 200,000 units	NS	Physically compatible and bleomycin activity retained for 1 week at 4 °C. Heparin not tested	763	C
Calcium gluconate		1 g		12,000 units	D5W	Physically compatible	74	C
	UP	1 g	UP	4000 units	D5W	Physically compatible	15	C
	UP	1 g	AB	20,000 units		Physically compatible	21	C

Additive Compatibility (Cont.)

Heparin sodium

Drug	Mfr	Conc/L	Mfr	Conc/L	Test Soln	Remarks	Ref	C/I
Cefepime HCl	BR	4 g	MG	10,000 and 50,000 units	D5W, NS	Visually compatible with 4% cefepime loss in 24 hr at room temperature and 3% in 7 days at 5 °C. No heparin loss	1681	C
Ceftazidime		4 g		10,000 and 50,000 units	D5W, NS	Ceftazidime stable for 24 hr at room temperature and 7 days refrigerated	4	C
Chloramphenicol sodium succinate	PD	500 mg		12,000 units	D5W	Physically compatible	74	C
	PD	10 g	UP	4000 units	D5W	Physically compatible	15	C
	PD	1 g	AB	20,000 units		Physically compatible	6; 21	C
Ciprofloxacin	BAY	2 g	CP	10,000, 100,000, 1 million units	NS	White precipitate forms immediately	1934	I
	MI	2 g		4100 units	NS	Physically incompatible	888	I
	MI	2 g		8300 units	NS	Physically incompatible	888	I
Clindamycin phosphate	UP	9 g		100,000 units	D5W	Clindamycin stable for 24 hr	101	C
Cloxacillin sodium		2 g		32,000 units	NS	Physically compatible and heparin stable for 24 hr	57	C
Colistimethate sodium	WC	500 mg	AB	20,000 units	D	Physically compatible	21	C
	WC	500 mg	UP	4000 units	D5W	Physically compatible	15	C
Cytarabine	UP	500 mg		10,000 units	NS	Haze formation	174	I
	UP	100 mg		20,000 units	D5W	Haze formation	174	I
Daunorubicin HCl	FA	200 mg	UP	4000 units	D5W	Physically incompatible	15	I
Dimenhydrinate	SE	50 mg		12,000 units	D5W	Physically compatible	74	C
	SE	500 mg	UP	4000 units	D5W	Physically compatible	15	C
	SE	50 mg	AB	20,000 units	D	Physically compatible	21	C
Dobutamine HCl	LI	1 g	ES	40,000 units	D5W, NS	Physically compatible with no color change in 24 hr at 25 °C	789	C
	LI	1 g	LY	50,000 units	D5W, NS	Physically compatible for 24 hr at 21 °C	812	C
	LI	1 g	ES	5 million units	D5W, NS	Pink discoloration within 6 hr at 21 °C	812	I
	LI	1 g	ES	50,000 units	D5W	Precipitate forms within 3 min	841	I

Additive Compatibility (Cont.)

Heparin sodium

Drug	Mfr	Conc/L	Mfr	Conc/L	Test Soln	Remarks	Ref	C/I
	LI	1.5 g	LY	50,000 units	D5W, NS	Obvious precipitation	1318	I
	LI	900 mg	LY	50,000 units	D5W, W	Physically compatible for 4 hr, but heat of reaction detected by microcalorimetry	1318	I
	LI	900 mg	LY	50,000 units	NS	Physically compatible for 4 hr with no heat of reaction detected by microcalorimetry	1318	C
Dopamine HCl	AS	800 mg	AB	200,000 units	D5W	No dopamine or heparin loss in 24 hr at 25 °C	312	C
Enalaprilat	MSD	12 mg	ES	50,000 units	D5Wa	Visually compatible. Little enalaprilat loss in 24 hr at room temperature under fluorescent light. Heparin not tested	1572	C
Epirubicin HCl						Potential precipitation	1	I
Erythromycin lactobionate	AB	1 g	AB	1500 units		Precipitate forms within 1 hr	20	I
	AB	5 g	UP	4000 units	D5W	Physically incompatible	15	I
	AB	1.5 g	OR	20,000 units	D5W, NS	Precipitate forms	113	I
	AB	1 g	AB	20,000 units		Precipitate forms within 1 hr	21	I
Esmolol HCl	DU	6 g	LY	50,000 units	D5W	Physically compatible with no esmolol loss in 24 hr at room temperature under fluorescent light. Heparin not tested	1358	C
Floxacillin sodium	BE	20 g	WED	20,000 units	NS	Physically compatible for 24 hr at 15 and 30 °C. Haze forms in 48 hr at 30 °C. No change at 15 °C	1479	C
Fluconazole	PF	1 g	BA	50,000 units	D5W	Fluconazole stable for 24 hr at 25 °C in fluorescent light. Heparin not tested	1676	C
Flumazenil	RC	20 mg	ES	50,000 units	D5Wa	Visually compatible. 4% flumazenil loss in 24 hr at 23 °C in fluorescent light. Heparin not tested	1710	C
Furosemide	HO	1 g	WED	20,000 units	NS	Physically compatible for 72 hr at 15 and 30 °C	1479	C
Gentamicin sulfate		320 mg	BP	20,000 units	D5W, NS	Precipitates immediately	26	I
	SC	1 g	OR	20,000 units	D5W, NS	Opalescence	113	I
	ME	88 mg	BRN	1000 to 6000 units	D10W, NS	Activity of both drugs greatly reduced	1570	I
Hydrocortisone sodium succinate		800 mg		32,000 units	NS	Physically compatible and heparin activity retained for 24 hr	57	C
	UP	500 mg	UP	4000 units	D5W	Physically incompatible	15	I
	UP	100 mg		12,000 units	D5W	Precipitates immediately	74	I
Hydromorphone HCl	KN	20 g	OR	1000 units	D5Wa	Visually compatible with no loss of hydromorphone in 18 days at 4 and 23 °C. Heparin not tested	2410	C

Additive Compatibility (Cont.)

Heparin sodium

Drug	Mfr	Conc/L	Mfr	Conc/L	Test Soln	Remarks	Ref	C/I
	KN	5 g	OR	500 units	D5W[a]	Visually compatible with no loss of hydromorphone in 18 days at 4 and 23 °C. Heparin not tested	2410	C
	KN	5 g	OR	8000 units	D5W[a]	Visually compatible with no loss of hydromorphone in 18 days at 4 and 23 °C. Heparin not tested	2410	C
Isoproterenol HCl		2 mg		32,000 units	NS	Physically compatible and heparin activity retained for 24 hr	57	C
	WI	4 mg	AB	20,000 units		Physically compatible	59	C
Lidocaine HCl		4 g		32,000 units	NS	Physically compatible and heparin activity retained for 24 hr	57	C
	AST	2 g	AB	20,000 units		Physically compatible	24	C
Lincomycin HCl	UP	600 mg	AB	20,000 units		Physically compatible	21	C
Magnesium sulfate		130 mEq		50,000 units	NS[b]	Visually compatible with heparin activity retained for 14 days at 24 °C under fluorescent light	1908	C
Meropenem	ZEN	1 and 20 g	ES	20,000 units	NS	Visually compatible for 4 hr at room temperature	1994	C
Methyldopate HCl	MSD	1 g	AB	20,000 units	D, D–S, S	Physically compatible	23	C
Methylprednisolone sodium succinate	UP	40 mg		10,000 units	D5S	Clear solution for 24 hr	329	C
	UP	125 mg		5000 units	D5S, D5W, LR, R	Clear solution for 24 hr	329	C
	UP	25 g		40,000 units	NS	Clear solution for 24 hr	329	C
Mitomycin	BR	167 mg	ES	33,300 units	NS[b]	Visually compatible. 10% mitomycin calculated loss in 21 hr and no decrease in heparin bioactivity at 25 °C	1866	I
	BR	167 mg	ES	33,300 units	NS[a]	Visually compatible. 10% mitomycin calculated loss in 25 hr and no decrease in heparin bioactivity at 25 °C	1866	C
	BR	500 mg	ES	33,300 units	NS[b]	Visually compatible. 10% mitomycin calculated loss in 42 hr and no decrease in heparin bioactivity at 25 °C	1866	C
	BR	500 mg	ES	33,300 units	NS[a]	Visually compatible. 10% mitomycin calculated loss in 61 hr and no decrease in heparin bioactivity at 25 °C	1866	C
Nafcillin sodium	WY	500 mg	AB, WY	20,000 units		Physically compatible	27	C
	WY	500 mg	AB	20,000 units		Physically compatible	21	C
Norepinephrine bitartrate	WI	8 mg		12,000 units	D5W	Physically compatible	74	C
	WI	8 mg	AB	20,000 units	D, D–S, S	Physically compatible	77	C

Additive Compatibility (Cont.)

Heparin sodium

Drug	Mfr	Conc/L	Mfr	Conc/L	Test Soln	Remarks	Ref	C/I
Octreotide acetate	SZ	1.5 mg	ES	1000 units	TPN #120[c]	Little octreotide loss over 48 hr at room temperature in ambient light	1373	**C**
Penicillin G potassium		1 million units		12,000 units	D5W	Physically compatible	74	**C**
	SQ	1 million units	AB	20,000 units	D5W	Penicillin stable for 24 hr at 25 °C	47	**C**
	SQ	20 million units	UP	4000 units	D5W	Physically incompatible	15	**I**
Penicillin G sodium	BE	20 million units	OR	20,000 units	NS	Both stable for 24 hr at 25 °C	113	**C**
	UP	20 million units	UP	4000 units	D5W	Physically incompatible	15	**I**
Polymyxin B sulfate	BP	20 mg	BP	20,000 units	D5W	Precipitates immediately	26	**I**
	BP	20 mg	BP	20,000 units	NS	Haze develops over 3 hr	26	**I**
Potassium chloride		3 g		12,000 units	D5W	Physically compatible	74	**C**
	AB	40 mEq	AB	20,000 units		Physically compatible	21	**C**
		80 mEq		32,000 units	NS	Physically compatible and heparin activity retained for 24 hr	57	**C**
Promethazine HCl	WY	250 mg	UP	4000 units	D5W	Physically incompatible	15	**I**
Ranitidine HCl	GL	2 g	ES	10,000 and 40,000 units	D5W, NS[a]	Physically compatible. 2% ranitidine loss in 48 hr at room temperature in light. Heparin not tested	1361	**C**
	GL	50 mg	ES	10,000 and 40,000 units	NS[a]	Physically compatible. No ranitidine loss in 48 hr at room temperature in light. Heparin not tested	1361	**C**
	GL	50 mg	ES	10,000 and 40,000 units	D5W[a]	Physically compatible. 7% ranitidine loss in 24 hr and 12% loss in 48 hr at room temperature in light. Heparin not tested	1361	**C**
Sodium bicarbonate	AB	2.4 mEq[e]	AB	20,000 units	D5W	Physically compatible for 24 hr	772	**C**

Additive Compatibility (Cont.)

Heparin sodium

Drug	Mfr	Conc/L	Mfr	Conc/L	Test Soln	Remarks	Ref	C/I
Streptomycin sulfate		1 g	AB	20,000 units		Precipitate forms within 1 hr	21	I
	BP	4 g	BP	20,000 units	D5W, NS	Precipitates immediately	26	I
Teicoplanin	HO	2 g	CPP	20,000 and 40,000 units	D5W, NS	Visually compatible. No loss of teicoplanin and heparin in 24 hr at 25 °C	2165	C
Vancomycin HCl	LI	1 g		12,000 units	D5W	Precipitates immediately	74	I
	LE	400 mg	IX	1000 units	TPN #95ᶜ	Physically compatible and vancomycin stable for 8 days at room temperature and under refrigeration	1321	C
	LI	25 mg	ES	100,000 units	NS	Physically compatible. Under 10% vancomycin loss and no heparin loss in 30 days at 28 °C and 63 days at 4 °C	2542	C
Verapamil HCl	KN	80 mg	ES	20,000 units	D5W, NS	Physically compatible for 24 hr	764	C

ᵃ*Tested in PVC containers.*
ᵇ*Tested in glass containers.*
ᶜ*Refer to Appendix I for the composition of parenteral nutrition solutions. TPN indicates a 2-in-1 admixture.*
ᵈ*Hydrocortisone sodium succinate (Pharmacia Upjohn) 50 mg/L was also present.*
ᵉ*One vial of Neut added to a liter of admixture.*

Drugs in Syringe Compatibility

Heparin sodium

Drug (in syringe)	Mfr	Amt	Mfr	Amt	Remarks	Ref	C/I
Amikacin sulfate		100 mg		2500 units/1 mL	Turbidity or precipitate forms within 5 min	1053	I
Aminophylline		240 mg/10 mL		2500 units/1 mL	Physically compatible for at least 5 min	1053	C
Amiodarone HCl	LZ	150 mg/3 mL		2500 units/1 mL	Turbidity or precipitate forms within 5 min	1053	I
Amphotericin B		50 mg		2500 units/1 mL	Physically compatible for at least 5 min	1053	C
Ampicillin sodium		2 g		2500 units/1 mL	Physically compatible for at least 5 min	1053	C
Atropine sulfate		0.5 mg/1 mL		2500 units/1 mL	Physically compatible for at least 5 min	1053	C

Drugs in Syringe Compatibility (Cont.)

Heparin sodium

Drug (in syringe)	Mfr	Amt	Mfr	Amt	Remarks	Ref	C/I
Bleomycin sulfate		1.5 units/ 0.5 mL		500 units/ 0.5 mL	Physically compatible for 5 min at room temperature followed by 8 min of centrifugation	980	**C**
Buprenorphine HCl	BM	300 mg/ 1 mL		2500 units/ 1 mL	Visually compatible for at least 5 min	1053	**C**
Caffeine citrate		20 mg/ 1 mL	AB	10 units/ 1 mL	Visually compatible for 4 hr at 25 °C	2440	**C**
Cefazolin sodium		2 g		2500 units/ 1 mL	Physically compatible for at least 5 min	1053	**C**
Cefotaxime sodium	HO	2 g		2500 units/ 1 mL	Physically compatible for at least 5 min	1053	**C**
	WW	10 mg/ mL	HOS	5000 units/mL	Physically compatible. No cefotaxime loss in 3 days at 4 °C. Losses of 7 and 14% in 1 and 2 days at 27 °C	2820	**C**
Cefoxitin sodium	MSD	2 g		2500 units/ 1 mL	Physically compatible for at least 5 min	1053	**C**
Chloramphenicol sodium succinate	PD	1 g	AB	20,000 units/ 1 mL	Physically compatible for at least 30 min	21	**C**
		1 g		2500 units/ 1 mL	Physically compatible for at least 5 min	1053	**C**
Chlorpromazine HCl		50 mg/ 2 mL		2500 units/ 1 mL	Turbidity or precipitate forms within 5 min	1053	**I**
Cisplatin		0.5 mg/ 0.5 mL		500 units/ 0.5 mL	Physically compatible for 5 min at room temperature followed by 8 min of centrifugation	980	**C**
Clindamycin phosphate	UP	300 mg		2500 units/ 1 mL	Physically compatible for at least 5 min	1053	**C**
Clonazepam	RC	1 mg/ 2 mL		2500 units/ 1 mL	Visually compatible for at least 5 min	1053	**C**
Clonidine HCl	BI	0.15 mg/ 1 mL		2500 units/ 1 mL	Visually compatible for at least 5 min	1053	**C**
Cyclophosphamide		10 mg/ 0.5 mL		500 units/ 0.5 mL	Physically compatible for 5 min at room temperature followed by 8 min of centrifugation	980	**C**
Diazepam		10 mg/ 2 mL		2500 units/ 1 mL	Turbidity or precipitate forms within 5 min	1053	**I**

Drugs in Syringe Compatibility (Cont.)

Heparin sodium

Drug (in syringe)	Mfr	Amt	Mfr	Amt	Remarks	Ref	C/I
Digoxin		0.25 mg/ 1 mL		2500 units/ 1 mL	Physically compatible for at least 5 min	1053	C
Dimenhydrinate		65 mg/ 10 mL		2500 units/ 1 mL	Physically compatible for at least 5 min	1053	C
		10 mg/ 1 mL		25,000 units/ 1 mL	Precipitate forms	2569	I
Dobutamine HCl	LI	250 mg/ 10 mL		2500 units/ 1 mL	Physically compatible for at least 5 min	1053	C
Dopamine HCl		50 mg/ 5 mL		2500 units/ 1 mL	Physically compatible for at least 5 min	1053	C
Doxorubicin HCl		1 mg/ 0.5 mL		500 units/ 0.5 mL	Precipitates immediately	980	I
Droperidol		1.25 mg/ 0.5 mL		500 units/ 0.5 mL	Precipitates immediately	980	I
	JN	5 mg/ 2 mL		2500 units/ 1 mL	Turbidity or precipitate forms within 5 min	1053	I
Epinephrine HCl		1 mg/ 1 mL		2500 units/ 1 mL	Physically compatible for at least 5 min	1053	C
Erythromycin lactobionate	AB	1 g	AB	20,000 units/ 1 mL	Physically incompatible	21	I
Etomidate	JN	20 mg/ 10 mL		2500 units/ 1 mL	Visually compatible for at least 5 min	1053	C
Fentanyl citrate	JN	0.1 mg/ 2 mL		2500 units/ 1 mL	Physically compatible for at least 5 min	1053	C
Floxacillin sodium	BE	1 g		2500 units/ 1 mL	Visually compatible for at least 5 min	1053	C
Fluorouracil		25 mg/ 0.5 mL		500 units/ 0.5 mL	Physically compatible for 5 min at room temperature followed by 8 min of centrifugation	980	C
	DB	500 mg/ 20 mL	LEO	20,000 units/ 0.8 mL	Visually compatible with no loss of either drug in 7 days at 25 °C and 14 days at 4 °C in the dark	2415	C

Drugs in Syringe Compatibility (Cont.)

Heparin sodium

Drug (in syringe)	Mfr	Amt	Mfr	Amt	Remarks	Ref	C/I
Furosemide		5 mg/ 0.5 mL		500 units/ 0.5 mL	Physically compatible for 5 min at room temperature followed by 8 min of centrifugation	980	**C**
		20 mg/ 2 mL		2500 units/ 1 mL	Physically compatible for at least 5 min	1053	**C**
Gentamicin sulfate		40 mg		2500 units/ 1 mL	Turbidity or precipitate forms within 5 min	1053	**I**
Haloperidol lactate	JN	5 mg/ 1 mL		2500 units/ 1 mL	Turbidity or precipitate forms within 5 min	1053	**I**
Hydromorphone HCl	KN	50 mg/ 1 mL	OR	10 units/ 1 mL	White cloudy precipitate	2410	**I**
	KN	50 mg/ 1 mL	LEO	100 units/ 1 mL	White cloudy precipitate	2410	**I**
	KN	50 mg/ 1 mL	OR	25,000 units/ 1 mL	White cloudy precipitate	2410	**I**
Iohexol	WI	64.7%, 5 mL	OR	5000 units/ 0.5 mL	Physically compatible for at least 2 hr	1438	**C**
Iopamidol	SQ	61%, 5 mL	OR	5000 units/ 0.5 mL	Physically compatible for at least 2 hr	1438	**C**
Iothalamate meglumine	MA	60%, 5 mL	OR	5000 units/ 0.5 mL	Physically compatible for at least 2 hr	1438	**C**
Ioxaglate meglumine–ioxaglate sodium	MA	5 mL	OR	5000 units/ 0.5 mL	Physically compatible for at least 2 hr	1438	**C**
Leucovorin calcium		5 mg/ 0.5 mL		500 units/ 0.5 mL	Physically compatible for 5 min at room temperature followed by 8 min of centrifugation	980	**C**
Lidocaine HCl	AST	100 mg/ 5 mL		2500 units/ 1 mL	Physically compatible for at least 5 min	1053	**C**
Lincomycin HCl	UP	600 mg/ 2 mL	AB	20,000 units/ 1 mL	Physically compatible for at least 30 min	21	**C**
Meperidine HCl	HO	100 mg/ 2 mL		2500 units/ 1 mL	Turbidity or precipitate forms within 5 min	1053	**I**
Methotrexate sodium		12.5 mg/ 0.5 mL		500 units/ 0.5 mL	Physically compatible for 5 min at room temperature followed by 8 min of centrifugation	980	**C**

Drugs in Syringe Compatibility (Cont.)

Heparin sodium

Drug (in syringe)	Mfr	Amt	Mfr	Amt	Remarks	Ref	C/I
Methotrimeprazine HCl		25 mg/ 1 mL		2500 units/ 1 mL	Turbidity or precipitate forms within 5 min	1053	I
Metoclopramide HCl		2.5 mg/ 0.5 mL		500 units/ 0.5 mL	Physically compatible for 5 min at room temperature followed by 8 min of centrifugation	980	C
		10 mg/ 2 mL		2500 units/ 1 mL	Physically compatible for at least 5 min	1053	C
	RB	10 mg/ 2 mL	ES	2000 units/ 2 mL	Physically compatible for 48 hr at 25 °C	1167	C
	RB	10 mg/ 2 mL	ES	4000 units/ 4 mL	Physically compatible for 48 hr at 25 °C	1167	C
	RB	160 mg/ 32 mL	ES	16,000 units/ 16 mL	Physically compatible for 48 hr at 25 °C	1167	C
Mexiletine HCl	BI	250 mg/ 10 mL		2500 units/ 1 mL	Turbidity or precipitate forms within 5 min	1053	I
Midazolam HCl	RC	15 mg/ 3 mL		2500 units/ 1 mL	Turbidity or precipitate forms within 5 min	1053	I
Mitomycin		0.25 mg/ 0.5 mL		500 units/ 0.5 mL	Physically compatible for 5 min at room temperature followed by 8 min of centrifugation	980	C
Morphine sulfate		1, 2, 5, 10 mg	WY	100 and 200 units	Brought to 5 mL with NS. Physically compatible with no morphine loss in 24 hr at 23 °C	985	C
		1, 2, 5 mg	WY	100 and 200 units	Brought to 5 mL with W. Physically compatible with no morphine loss in 24 hr at 23 °C	985	C
		10 mg	WY	100 and 200 units	Brought to 5 mL with W. Immediate haze with precipitate and 5 to 7% morphine loss	985	I
Nafcillin sodium	WY	500 mg	AB	20,000 units/ 1 mL	Physically compatible for at least 30 min	21	C
Naloxone HCl	DU	0.4 mg/ 1 mL		2500 units/ 1 mL	Physically compatible for at least 5 min	1053	C
Neostigmine methylsulfate	RC	0.5 mg/ 1 mL		2500 units/ 1 mL	Physically compatible for at least 5 min	1053	C
Nitroglycerin		25 mg/ 25 mL		2500 units/ 1 mL	Physically compatible for at least 5 min	1053	C

Drugs in Syringe Compatibility (Cont.)

Heparin sodium

Drug (in syringe)	Mfr	Amt	Mfr	Amt	Remarks	Ref	C/I
Pancuronium bromide		4 mg/ 2 mL		2500 units/ 1 mL	Physically compatible for at least 5 min	1053	C
Pantoprazole sodium	c	4 mg/ 1 mL		25,000 units/ 1 mL	Precipitates within 1 hr	2574	I
Pentazocine lactate	WI	30 mg/ 1 mL		2500 units/ 1 mL	Turbidity or precipitate forms within 5 min	1053	I
Phenobarbital sodium		200 mg/ 1 mL		2500 units/ 1 mL	Physically compatible for at least 5 min	1053	C
Promethazine HCl		50 mg/ 2 mL		2500 units/ 1 mL	Turbidity or precipitate forms within 5 min	1053	I
Ranitidine HCl	GL	50 mg/ 5 mL		2500 units/ 1 mL	Visually compatible for at least 5 min	1053	C
Sodium nitroprusside		60 mg/ 5 mL		2500 units/ 1 mL	Physically compatible for at least 5 min	1053	C
Streptomycin sulfate		1 g	AB	20,000 units/ 1 mL	Physically incompatible	21	I
Succinylcholine chloride		100 mg/ 5 mL		2500 units/ 1 mL	Physically compatible for at least 5 min	1053	C
Tobramycin sulfate		80 mg/ 2 mL		10 units/ 1 mL	Turbidity or fine white precipitate due to formation of an insoluble salt	845	I
	LI	40 mg		2500 units/ 1 mL	Turbidity or precipitate forms within 5 min	1053	I
Tramadol HCl	GRU	100 mg/ 2 mL		2500 units/ 1 mL	Visually compatible for at least 5 min	1053	C
Trimethoprim–sulfamethoxazole		80 + 400 mg/ 5 mL		2500 units/ 1 mL	Physically compatible for at least 5 min	1053	C
Vancomycin HCl	LI	500 mg		2500 units/ 1 mL	Turbidity or precipitate forms within 5 min	1053	I
Verapamil HCl	KN	5 mg/ 2 mL		2500 units/ 1 mL	Physically compatible for at least 5 min	1053	C
Vinblastine sulfate		0.5 mg/ 0.5 mL		500 units/ 0.5 mL	Physically compatible for 5 min at room temperature followed by 8 min of centrifugation	980	C
	LI	1 mg/ 1 mL		200 units/ 1 mL[a]	Turbidity appears in 2 to 3 min	767	I

Drugs in Syringe Compatibility (Cont.)

Heparin sodium

Drug (in syringe)	Mfr	Amt	Mfr	Amt	Remarks	Ref	C/I
Vincristine sulfate		0.5 mg/ 0.5 mL		500 units/ 0.5 mL	Physically compatible for 5 min at room temperature followed by 8 min of centrifugation	980	C
Warfarin sodium	DU	2 mg/ 1 mL[b]	ES	5000 units/ 1 mL	Low-level haze forms immediately and becomes visible in ambient light in 1 hr	2010	I

[a]Tested in bacteriostatic sodium chloride 0.9%.
[b]Tested in sterile water for injection.
[c]Test performed using the formulation WITHOUT edetate disodium.

Y-Site Injection Compatibility (1:1 Mixture)

Heparin sodium

Drug	Mfr	Conc	Mfr	Conc	Remarks	Ref	C/I
Acyclovir sodium	BW	5 mg/mL[a]	ES	50 units/mL[a]	Physically compatible for 4 hr at 25 °C	1157	C
	BV	5 mg/mL[b]	BD	100 units/mL	Physically compatible	2794	C
Aldesleukin	CHI	33,800 I.U./ mL[a]	BA	100 units/mL	Visually compatible with little or no loss of aldesleukin activity	1857	C
	CHI[r]	[a]			Visually compatible but aldesleukin activity was variable depending on rate of delivery. Heparin not tested	1890	?
Allopurinol sodium	BW	3 mg/mL[b]	ES	100 units/ mL[b]	Physically compatible for 4 hr at 22 °C	1686	C
Alteplase	GEN	1 mg/mL	ES	100 units/ mL[a]	Haze noted in 24 hr	1340	I
Amifostine	USB	10 mg/mL[a]	ES	100 units/ mL[a]	Physically compatible for 4 hr at 23 °C	1845	C
Aminophylline	SE	25 mg/mL	RI	1000 units/L[c]	Physically compatible for 4 hr at room temperature	322	C
Amiodarone HCl				300 units/ mL[b]	White precipitate forms upon sequential administration	791	I
Amphotericin B	SQ	0.1 mg/mL[a]	SO	100 units/ mL[b]	Turbidity forms in 45 min	1435	I
Amphotericin B cholesteryl sulfate complex	SEQ	0.83 mg/mL[a]	WY	1000 units/ mL[a]	Gross precipitate forms	2117	I
Ampicillin sodium	BR	25, 50, 100, 125 mg/mL	RI	1000 units/L[c]	Physically compatible for 4 hr at room temperature	322	C
	WY	20 mg/mL[b]	TR	50 units/mL	Visually compatible for 4 hr at 25 °C	1793	C
	NOP	10 mg/mL[b]	LEO	10 and 5000 units/mL[b]	Physically compatible with little change in heparin activity in 14 days at 4 and 37 °C. Antibiotic not tested	2684	C
Ampicillin sodium–sulbactam sodium	PF	20 + 10 mg/ mL[b]	TR	50 units/mL	Visually compatible for 4 hr at 25 °C	1793	C
Amsacrine	NCI	1 mg/mL[a]	SO	40 units/mL[a]	Orange precipitate forms immediately	1381	I
Anidulafungin	VIC	0.5 mg/mL[a]	AB	100 units/mL	Physically compatible for 4 hr at 23 °C	2617	C
Antithymocyte globulin (rabbit)	SGS	0.2 mg/mL[a]	ES	2 units/mL[a]	Haze and precipitate form immediately	2488	I
	SGS	0.3 mg/mL[a]	ES	2 units/mL[a]	Haze and precipitate form immediately	2488	I

Y-Site Injection Compatibility (1:1 Mixture) (Cont.)

Heparin sodium

Drug	Mfr	Conc	Mfr	Conc	Remarks	Ref	C/I
	SGS	0.2 mg/mL[b]	ES	2 units/mL[b]	Physically compatible for 4 hr at 23 °C	2488	C
	SGS	0.3 mg/mL[b]	ES	2 units/mL[b]	Physically compatible for 4 hr at 23 °C	2488	C
	SGS	0.2 mg/mL[a,b]	ES	100 units/mL	Physically compatible for 4 hr at 23 °C	2488	C
	SGS	0.3 mg/mL[a,b]	ES	100 units/mL	Physically compatible for 4 hr at 23 °C	2488	C
Atracurium besylate	BW	0.5 mg/mL[a]	SO	40 units/mL[a]	Physically compatible for 24 hr at 28 °C	1337	C
Atropine sulfate	BW	0.5 mg/mL	UP	1000 units/L[e]	Physically compatible for 4 hr at room temperature	534	C
Aztreonam	SQ	40 mg/mL[a]	ES	100 units/mL[a]	Physically compatible for 4 hr at 23 °C	1758	C
	BV	20 mg/mL[a]	TR	50 units/mL	Visually compatible for 4 hr at 25 °C	1793	C
Bivalirudin	TMC	5 mg/mL[a]	AB	100 units/mL	Physically compatible for 4 hr at 23 °C	2373	C
Bleomycin sulfate		3 units/mL		1000 units/mL	Drugs injected sequentially in Y-site with no flush. No precipitate seen	980	C
Caffeine citrate		20 mg/mL		1 unit/mL[a]	Compatible and stable for 24 hr at room temperature	1	C
Calcium gluconate	ES	100 mg/mL	RI	1000 units/L[c]	Physically compatible for 4 hr at room temperature	322	C
Caspofungin acetate	ME	0.7 mg/mL[b]	HOS	100 units/mL	Immediate white turbid precipitate forms	2758	I
	ME	0.5 mg/mL[b]	BA	100 units/mL	Fine white crystalline material reported	2766	I
Cefazolin sodium	SKB	20 mg/mL	TR	50 units/mL	Visually compatible for 4 hr at 25 °C	1793	C
	NOP	10 mg/mL[b]	LEO	10 and 5000 units/mL[b]	Physically compatible with little change in heparin activity in 14 days at 4 and 37 °C. Antibiotic not tested	2684	C
Cefotetan disodium	STU	40 mg/mL[a]	TR	50 units/mL	Visually compatible for 4 hr at 25 °C	1793	C
Ceftaroline fosamil	FOR	2.22 mg/mL[a,b,k]	HOS	100 units/mL	Physically compatible for 4 hr at 23 °C	2826	C
Ceftazidime	LI	20 mg/mL	TR	50 units/mL	Visually compatible for 4 hr at 25 °C	1793	C
Ceftriaxone sodium	RC	20 mg/mL	TR	50 units/mL	Visually compatible for 4 hr at 25 °C	1793	C
Chlorpromazine HCl	SKF	25 mg/mL	UP	1000 units/L[e]	Physically compatible for 4 hr at room temperature	534	C
	RPR	0.13 mg/mL[a]	NOV	29.2 units/mL[a]	Visually compatible for 150 min	2244	C
Ciprofloxacin		2 mg/mL		10 units/mL	Turbidity forms rapidly with subsequent white precipitate	1483	I
	MI	2 mg/mL[f]	LY	100 units/mL	Crystals form immediately	1655	I
	BAY	2 mg/mL[b]	CP	10, 100, 1000 units/mL[b]	White precipitate forms immediately	1934	I
Cisatracurium besylate	GW	0.1 and 2 mg/mL[a]	AB	100 units/mL	Physically compatible for 4 hr at 23 °C	2074	C
	GW	5 mg/mL[a]	AB	100 units/mL	White cloudiness forms immediately	2074	I
Cisplatin		1 mg/mL		1000 units/mL	Drugs injected sequentially in Y-site with no flush. No precipitate seen	980	C
Cladribine	ORT	0.015[b] and 0.5[g] mg/mL	WY	100 units/mL[b]	Physically compatible for 4 hr at 23 °C	1969	C
Clarithromycin	AB	4 mg/mL[a]	CPP	1000 units/mL[a]	White cloudiness forms immediately	2174	I
Clindamycin phosphate	UP	12 mg/mL[a]	TR	50 units/mL	Visually compatible for 4 hr at 25 °C	1793	C

Y-Site Injection Compatibility (1:1 Mixture) (Cont.)

Heparin sodium

Drug	Mfr	Conc	Mfr	Conc	Remarks	Ref	C/I
Cyanocobalamin	PD	0.1 mg/mL	UP	1000 units/L[e]	Physically compatible for 4 hr at room temperature	534	C
Cyclophosphamide		20 mg/mL		1000 units/mL	Drugs injected sequentially in Y-site with no flush. No precipitate seen	980	C
Dacarbazine	MI	25 mg/mL[b]	WY	100 units/mL	White precipitate forms immediately[h]	1158	I
	MI	10 mg/mL[b]	WY	100 units/mL	No observable precipitation[h]	1158	C
Daptomycin	CUB	19.6 mg/mL[b,l]	ES	98 units/mL[b,l]	Physically compatible with no loss of either drug in 2 hr at 25 °C	2553	C
Dexamethasone sodium phosphate	ES	0.08 mg/mL[a]	TR	50 units/mL	Visually compatible for 4 hr at 25 °C	1793	C
	MSD	4 mg/mL	RI	1000 units/L[c]	Physically compatible for 4 hr at room temperature	322	C
Dexmedetomidine HCl	AB	4 mcg/mL[b]	AB	100 units/mL	Physically compatible for 4 hr at 23 °C	2383	C
Diazepam	RC	5 mg/mL	RI	1000 units/L[c]	Immediate haziness and globule formation	322	I
Digoxin	BW	0.25 mg/mL	RI	1000 units/L[c]	Physically compatible for 4 hr at room temperature	322	C
Diltiazem HCl	MMD	5 mg/mL	LY	20,000 units/mL	Precipitate forms	1807	I
	MMD	1 mg/mL[b]	LY	20,000 units/mL	Visually compatible	1807	C
	MMD	1[b] and 5 mg/mL	SCN	5000 and 10,000 units/mL	Visually compatible	1807	C
	MMD	5 mg/mL	LY, SCN	80 units/mL[f]	Visually compatible	1807	C
	MMD	1 mg/mL[a]	ES	100 units/mL[a]	Visually compatible for 4 hr at 27 °C	2062	C
Diphenhydramine HCl	PD	50 mg/mL	UP	1000 units/L[e]	Physically compatible for 4 hr at room temperature	534	C
Dobutamine HCl	LI	4 mg/mL[b]	ES	50 units/mL[b]	Physically compatible for 3 hr	1316	C
	LI	4 mg/mL[a]	ES	50 units/mL[a]	Immediate gross precipitation	1316	I
	LI	1 mg/mL[a]	TR	50 units/mL	Visually compatible for 4 hr at 25 °C	1793	C
	LI	4 mg/mL[a]	OR	100 units/mL[a]	Haze and white precipitate form	1877	I
	LI	4 mg/mL[a]	ES	100 units/mL[a]	Precipitate forms in 4 hr at 27 °C	2062	I
Docetaxel	RPR	0.9 mg/mL[a]	ES	100 units/mL	Physically compatible for 4 hr at 23 °C	2224	C
Dopamine HCl	ACC	40 mg/mL	UP	1000 units/L[e]	Physically compatible for 4 hr at room temperature	534	C
	BA	1.6 mg/mL	TR	50 units/mL	Visually compatible for 4 hr at 25 °C	1793	C
	AB	3.2 mg/mL[a]	ES	100 units/mL[a]	Visually compatible for 4 hr at 27 °C	2062	C
Doripenem	JJ	5 mg/mL[a,b]	HOS	100 units/mL	Physically compatible for 4 hr at 23 °C	2743	C
Doxapram HCl	RB	2 mg/mL[a]	APP	1 unit/mL[t]	Visually compatible for 4 hr at 23 °C	2470	C
Doxorubicin HCl		2 mg/mL		1000 units/mL	Drugs injected sequentially in Y-site with no flush. Precipitates immediately	980	I
Doxorubicin HCl liposomal	SEQ	0.4 mg/mL[a]	ES	1000 units/mL[a]	Physically compatible for 4 hr at 23 °C	2087	C

Y-Site Injection Compatibility (1:1 Mixture) (Cont.)

Heparin sodium

Drug	Mfr	Conc	Mfr	Conc	Remarks	Ref	C/I
Doxycycline hyclate	ES	1 mg/mL[a]	TR	50 units/mL	Visually incompatible within 4 hr at 25 °C	1793	**I**
Droperidol		2.5 mg/mL		1000 units/mL	Drugs injected sequentially in Y-site with no flush. Precipitates immediately	980	**I**
	CR	1.25 mg/mL	UP	1000 units/L[e]	Physically compatible for 4 hr at room temperature	534	**C**
Edrophonium chloride	RC	10 mg/mL	UP	1000 units/L[e]	Physically compatible for 4 hr at room temperature	534	**C**
Enalaprilat	MSD	0.05 mg/mL[a,b,k]	IX	40 units/mL[a]	Physically compatible for 24 hr at room temperature under fluorescent light	1355	**C**
Epinephrine HCl	AB	0.1 mg/mL	UP	1000 units/L[e]	Physically compatible for 4 hr at room temperature	534	**C**
	AB	0.02 mg/mL[a]	ES	100 units/mL[a]	Visually compatible for 4 hr at 27 °C	2062	**C**
Ertapenem sodium	ME	10 mg/mL[b]	APP	40 and 100 units/mL[a]	Visually compatible with about 4% ertapenem loss in 4 hr	2487	**C**
	ME	10 mg/mL[b]	APP	50 and 100 units/mL[b]	Visually compatible with about 3% ertapenem loss in 4 hr	2487	**C**
Erythromycin lactobionate	AB	3.3 mg/mL[b]	TR	50 units/mL	Visually compatible for 4 hr at 25 °C	1793	**C**
Esmolol HCl	DCC	10 mg/mL[a]	IX	40 units/mL[a]	Physically compatible for 24 hr at 22 °C	1169	**C**
Estrogens, conjugated	AY	5 mg/mL	RI	1000 units/L[c]	Physically compatible for 4 hr at room temperature	322	**C**
Ethacrynate sodium	MSD	1 mg/mL	RI	1000 units/L[c]	Physically compatible for 4 hr at room temperature	322	**C**
Etoposide phosphate	BR	5 mg/mL[a]	ES	100 units/mL[a]	Physically compatible for 4 hr at 23 °C	2218	**C**
Famotidine	MSD	0.2 mg/mL[a]	ES	40 units/mL[b]	Physically compatible for 14 hr	1196	**C**
	MSD	0.2 mg/mL[a]	TR	50 units/mL[a]	Physically compatible for 4 hr at 25 °C	1188	**C**
	ME	2 mg/mL[b]		40 units/mL[a]	Visually compatible for 4 hr at 22 °C	1936	**C**
Fenoldopam mesylate	AB	80 mcg/mL[b]	AB	100 units/mL	Physically compatible for 4 hr at 23 °C	2467	**C**
Fentanyl citrate	MN	0.05 mg/mL	UP	1000 units/L[e]	Physically compatible for 4 hr at room temperature	534	**C**
	ES	0.05 mg/mL	ES	100 units/mL[a]	Visually compatible for 4 hr at 27 °C	2062	**C**
Filgrastim	AMG	30 mcg/mL[a]	ES	100 units/mL[a]	Particles and filaments form immediately	1687	**I**
Fluconazole	RR	2 mg/mL	LY	1000 units/mL	Physically compatible for 24 hr at 25 °C	1407	**C**
	PF	2 mg/mL	TR	50 units/mL	Visually compatible for 4 hr at 25 °C	1793	**C**
Fludarabine phosphate	BX	1 mg/mL[a]	SO, WY	40[a], 100, 1000 units/mL	Visually compatible for 4 hr at 22 °C	1439	**C**
Fluorouracil	RC	50 mg/mL	UP	1000 units/L[e]	Physically compatible for 4 hr at room temperature	534	**C**
		50 mg/mL		1000 units/mL	Drugs injected sequentially in Y-site with no flush. No precipitate seen	980	**C**
Foscarnet sodium	AST	24 mg/mL	ES	1000 units/mL	Physically compatible for 24 hr at room temperature under fluorescent light	1335	**C**

Y-Site Injection Compatibility (1:1 Mixture) (Cont.)

Heparin sodium

Drug	Mfr	Conc	Mfr	Conc	Remarks	Ref	C/I
	AST	24 mg/mL	LY	100 units/mL[f]	Physically compatible for 24 hr at 25 °C under fluorescent light	1393	C
Furosemide		10 mg/mL		1000 units/mL	Drugs injected sequentially in Y-site with no flush. No precipitate seen	980	C
	HO	10 mg/mL	UP	1000 units/L[e]	Physically compatible for 4 hr at room temperature	534	C
	AMR	10 mg/mL	ES	100 units/mL[a]	Visually compatible for 4 hr at 27 °C	2062	C
	HMR	2.6 mg/mL[a]	NOV	29.2 units/mL[a]	Visually compatible for 150 min	2244	C
Gallium nitrate	FUJ	1 mg/mL[b]	ES	40 units/mL[b]	Visually compatible for 24 hr at 25 °C	1673	C
Gemcitabine HCl	LI	10 mg/mL[b]	ES	100 units/mL[b]	Physically compatible for 4 hr at 23 °C	2226	C
Gentamicin sulfate	RS	80 mg		[b]	Precipitates immediately	528	I
	ES	3.2 mg/mL[f]	ES	50 units/mL[f]	Immediate gross haze	1316	I
	TR	2 mg/mL	TR	50 units/mL	Visually incompatible within 4 hr at 25 °C	1793	I
Granisetron HCl	SKB	0.05 mg/mL[a]	AB	100 units/mL[a]	Physically compatible for 4 hr at 23 °C	2000	C
Haloperidol lactate	MN	5 mg/1 mL[i]	OR	25,000 and 50,000 units/250 mL[f]	White precipitate forms immediately	779	I
Hetastarch in lactated electrolyte	AB	6%	ES	100 units/mL	Physically compatible for 4 hr at 23 °C	2339	C
Hydralazine HCl	CI	20 mg/mL	UP	1000 units/L[e]	Physically compatible for 4 hr at room temperature	534	C
Hydrocortisone sodium succinate	UP	2 mg/mL[a]	TR	50 units/mL	Visually compatible for 4 hr at 25 °C	1793	C
	UP	125 mg/mL	ES	100 units/mL[f]	Visually compatible for 24 hr at room temperature in test tubes. No precipitate found on filter from Y-site delivery	2063	C
Hydromorphone HCl	KN	1 mg/mL	ES	100 units/mL[a]	Visually compatible for 4 hr at 27 °C	2062	C
Hydroxyethyl starch 130/0.4 in sodium chloride 0.9%	FRK	6%	HOS	10 units/mL	Visually compatible for 24 hr at room temperature	2770	C
	FRK	6%	PP	1000, 10,000 units/mL	Visually compatible for 24 hr at room temperature	2770	C
Idarubicin HCl	AD	1 mg/mL[b]	ES, SO	100 and 1000 units/mL	Haze forms immediately and precipitate forms in 12 to 20 min	1525	I
Insulin, regular	LI	0.2 unit/mL[b]	ES	60 units/mL[a]	Physically compatible for 2 hr at 25 °C	1395	C
Isoproterenol HCl	WI	0.2 mg/mL	UP	1000 units/L[e]	Physically compatible for 4 hr at room temperature	534	C
Isosorbide dinitrate	RP	10 mg/mL	LEO	300 units/mL[a]	Erratic availability of both drugs delivered through PVC tubing	1799	I
Labetalol HCl	SC	1 mg/mL[a]	IX	40 units/mL[a]	Physically compatible for 24 hr at 18 °C	1171	C
	GL	5 mg/mL	OR	100 units/mL[a]	Cloudiness with particles forms immediately	1877	I
	AH	2 mg/mL[a]	ES	100 units/mL[a]	Visually compatible for 4 hr at 27 °C	2062	C
Leucovorin calcium		10 mg/mL		1000 units/mL	Drugs injected sequentially in Y-site with no flush. No precipitate seen	980	C

Y-Site Injection Compatibility (1:1 Mixture) (Cont.)

Heparin sodium

Drug	Mfr	Conc	Mfr	Conc	Remarks	Ref	C/I
Levofloxacin	OMN	5 mg/mL[a]	ES	10 units/mL	Cloudy precipitate forms	2233	**I**
Lidocaine HCl	AST	20 mg/mL	RI	1000 units/L[c]	Physically compatible for 4 hr at room temperature	322	C
	TR	4 mg/mL	TR	50 units/mL	Visually compatible for 4 hr at 25 °C	1793	C
Linezolid	PHU	2 mg/mL	ES	1000 units/mL[a]	Physically compatible for 4 hr at 23 °C	2264	C
Lorazepam	WY	0.33 mg/mL[b]		417 units/mL	Visually compatible for 24 hr at 22 °C	1855	C
	WY	0.5 mg/mL[a]	ES	100 units/mL[a]	Visually compatible for 4 hr at 27 °C	2062	C
Magnesium sulfate	AB	500 mg/mL	UP	1000 units/L	Physically compatible for 4 hr at room temperature	534	C
Melphalan HCl	BW	0.1 mg/mL[b]	WY	100 units/mL[b]	Physically compatible for 3 hr at 22 °C	1557	C
Meperidine HCl	WY	10 mg/mL[b]	ES	60 units/mL[a]	Physically compatible for 1 hr at 25 °C	1338	C
Meropenem	ZEN	1 and 50 mg/mL[b]	ES	1 unit/mL[j]	Visually compatible for 4 hr at room temperature	1994	C
Methotrexate sodium		25 mg/mL		1000 units/mL	Drugs injected sequentially in Y-site with no flush. No precipitate seen	980	C
Methyldopate HCl	ES	5 mg/mL[a]	TR	50 units/mL	Visually compatible for 4 hr at 25 °C	1793	C
Methylergonovine maleate	SZ	0.2 mg/mL	UP	1000 units/L[e]	Physically compatible for 4 hr at room temperature	534	C
Methylprednisolone sodium succinate	UP	2.5 mg/mL[a]	TR	50 units/mL	Visually compatible for 4 hr at 25 °C	1793	C
	UP	5 mg/mL[b]	ES	100 units/mL[f]	Visually compatible for 24 hr at room temperature in test tubes. No precipitate found on filter from Y-site delivery	2063	C
Metoclopramide HCl		5 mg/mL		1000 units/mL	Drugs injected sequentially in Y-site with no flush. No precipitate seen	980	C
Metoprolol tartrate	BED	1 mg/mL	BA	1000 units/mL[a]	Visually compatible for 24 hr at 19 °C	2795	C
Metronidazole	MG	5 mg/mL	TR	50 units/mL	Visually compatible for 4 hr at 25 °C	1793	C
Micafungin sodium	ASP	1.5 mg/mL[b]	AB	100 units/mL	Physically compatible for 4 hr at 23 °C	2683	C
Midazolam HCl	RC	5 mg/mL		417 units/mL	Visually compatible for 24 hr at 22 °C	1855	C
	RC	2 mg/mL[a]	ES	100 units/mL[a]	Visually compatible for 4 hr at 27 °C	2062	C
	RC[d]	15 mg/3 mL		50 units/mL[b]	Clear solution	1053	C
Milrinone lactate	SW	0.2 mg/mL[a]	ES	100 units/mL[a]	Visually compatible for 4 hr at 27 °C	2062	C
	SW	0.4 mg/mL[a]	ES	100 units/mL[a]	Visually compatible. Little loss of milrinone and heparin in 4 hr at 23 °C	2214	C
Mitomycin		0.5 mg/mL		1000 units/mL	Drugs injected sequentially in Y-site with no flush. No precipitate seen	980	C
Morphine sulfate	WY	15 mg/mL	UP	1000 units/L[e]	Physically compatible for 4 hr at room temperature	534	C
	WY	0.2 mg/mL[f]	ES	50 units/mL[f]	Physically compatible for 3 hr	1316	C
	ES	1 mg/mL[b]	ES	60 units/mL[a]	Physically compatible for 1 hr at 25 °C	1338	C

Y-Site Injection Compatibility (1:1 Mixture) (Cont.)

Heparin sodium

Drug	Mfr	Conc	Mfr	Conc	Remarks	Ref	C/I
	SCN	2 mg/mL[a]	ES	100 units/mL[a]	Visually compatible for 4 hr at 27 °C	2062	C
Nafcillin sodium	WY	20 mg/mL[a]	TR	50 units/mL	Visually compatible for 4 hr at 25 °C	1793	C
Neostigmine methylsulfate	RC	0.5 mg/mL	UP	1000 units/L[e]	Physically compatible for 4 hr at room temperature	534	C
Nesiritide	SCI	50 mcg/mL[a,b]		0.1, 1, 10 units/mL	Physically incompatible	2625	I
Nicardipine HCl	WY	1 mg/mL[a]	ES	100 units/mL[a]	Precipitate forms immediately	2062	I
	DCC	0.1 mg/mL[a]	IX	40 units/mL[a]	Visually compatible for 24 hr at room temperature	235	C
Nitroglycerin	BA	0.2 mg/mL	ES	50 units/mL	Visually compatible for 24 hr at 23 °C	1794	C
	OM	0.2 mg/mL[a]	OR	100 units/mL[a]	Visually compatible for 24 hr at 23 °C	1877	C
	AB	0.4 mg/mL[a]	ES	100 units/mL[a]	Visually compatible for 4 hr at 27 °C	2062	C
Norepinephrine bitartrate	WI	1 mg/mL	UP	1000 units/L[e]	Physically compatible for 4 hr at room temperature	534	C
	AB	0.128 mg/mL[a]	ES	100 units/mL[a]	Visually compatible for 4 hr at 27 °C	2062	C
Ondansetron HCl	GL	1 mg/mL[b]	SO	40 units/mL[a]	Visually compatible for 4 hr at 22 °C	1365	C
Oxacillin sodium	BR	100 mg/mL	UP	1000 units/L[e]	Physically compatible for 4 hr at room temperature	534	C
Oxaliplatin	SS	0.5 mg/mL[a]	AB	100 units/mL	Physically compatible for 4 hr at 23 °C	2566	C
Oxytocin	SZ	1 unit/mL	UP	1000 units/L[e]	Physically compatible for 4 hr at room temperature	534	C
Paclitaxel	NCI	1.2 mg/mL[a]	WY	100 units/mL[a]	Physically compatible for 4 hr at 22 °C	1556	C
Palonosetron HCl	MGI	50 mcg/mL	HOS	100 units/mL	Physically compatible. No loss of either drug in 4 hr at room temperature	2771	C
Pancuronium bromide	ES	0.05 mg/mL[a]	SO	40 units/mL[a]	Physically compatible for 24 hr at 28 °C	1337	C
Pemetrexed disodium	LI	20 mg/mL[b]	AB	100 units/mL	Physically compatible for 4 hr at 23 °C	2564	C
Penicillin G potassium	LI	200,000 units/mL	RI	1000 units/L[c]	Physically compatible for 4 hr at room temperature	322	C
	RR	40,000 units/mL[a]	TR	50 units/mL	Visually compatible for 4 hr at 25 °C	1793	C
Pentazocine lactate	WI	30 mg/mL	UP	1000 units/L[e]	Physically compatible for 4 hr at room temperature	534	C
Phenytoin sodium	PD	50 mg/mL	RI	1000 units/L[c]	Immediate crystal formation	322	I
	ES	2 mg/mL[b]	TR	50 units/mL	Cloudy immediately and becomes white precipitate in 4 hr at 25 °C	1793	I
Phytonadione	RC	10 mg/mL	UP	1000 units/L[e]	Physically compatible for 4 hr at room temperature	534	C
Piperacillin sodium–tazobactam sodium	LE[q]	40 + 5 mg/mL[a]	ES	100 units/mL[a]	Physically compatible for 4 hr at 22 °C	1688	C
Potassium chloride	AB	0.2 mEq/mL[a]	TR	50 units/mL	Visually compatible for 4 hr at 25 °C	1793	C

Y-Site Injection Compatibility (1:1 Mixture) (Cont.)

Heparin sodium

Drug	Mfr	Conc	Mfr	Conc	Remarks	Ref	C/I
	BRN	0.625 mEq/mL[a]	NOV	29.2 units/mL[a]	Visually compatible for 150 min	2244	C
Procainamide HCl	SQ	100 mg/mL	UP	1000 units/L[e]	Physically compatible for 4 hr at room temperature	534	C
Prochlorperazine edisylate	SKF	5 mg/mL	UP	1000 units/L[e]	Physically compatible for 4 hr at room temperature	534	C
Promethazine HCl	SV	50 mg/mL	UP	1000 units/L[m]	Physically compatible for 4 hr at room temperature	534	C
	SV	50 mg/mL	UP	1000 units/L[p]	Clear initially, but cloudiness develops in 4 hr at room temperature	534	I
Propofol	ZEN	10 mg/mL	ES	100 units/mL[a]	Physically compatible for 1 hr at 23 °C	2066	C
Propranolol HCl	AY	1 mg/mL	UP	1000 units/L[e]	Physically compatible for 4 hr at room temperature	534	C
Quinidine gluconate	LI	6 mg/mL[b]	ES	50 units/mL[b]	Physically compatible for 3 hr	1316	C
	LI	6 mg/mL[a]	ES	50 units/mL[a]	Immediate gross haze	1316	I
Ranitidine HCl	GL	0.5 mg/mL	LY	50 units/mL[a]	Physically compatible for 24 hr	1323	C
	GL	1 mg/mL	TR	50 units/mL	Visually compatible for 4 hr at 25 °C	1793	C
	GL	1 mg/mL[a]	ES	100 units/mL[a]	Visually compatible for 4 hr at 27 °C	2062	C
Remifentanil HCl	GW	0.025 and 0.25 mg/mL[b]	AB	100 units/mL	Physically compatible for 4 hr at 23 °C	2075	C
Sargramostim	IMM	10 mcg/mL[b]	WY	100 units/mL	Visually compatible for 4 hr at 22 °C	1436	C
	IMM	6[b,r] and 15[b] mcg/mL	ES	100 units/mL[f]	Visually compatible for 2 hr	1618	C
Scopolamine HBr	BW	0.86 mg/mL	UP	1000 units/L[e]	Physically compatible for 4 hr at room temperature	534	C
Sodium bicarbonate	BR	75 mg/mL	RI	1000 units/L[c]	Physically compatible for 4 hr at room temperature	322	C
		1.4%	CH	500 units/mL[b]	Visually compatible for 4 hr at room temperature	1788	C
Sodium nitroprusside	ES	0.2 mg/mL[a]	TR	50 units/mL	Visually compatible for 4 hr at 25 °C protected from light	1793	C
	RC	0.2 mg/mL[a]	OR	100 units/mL[a]	Visually compatible for 24 hr at 23 °C	1877	C
	RC	1.2 and 3 mg/mL[a]	OR	48, 200, 480 units/mL[s]	Visually compatible for 48 hr at 24 °C protected from light	2357	C
	RC	0.3 mg/mL[a]	OR	480 units/mL[s]	Visually compatible for 48 hr at 24 °C protected from light	2357	C
Succinylcholine chloride	BW	20 mg/mL	RI	1000 units/L[c]	Physically compatible for 4 hr at room temperature	322	C
Tacrolimus	FUJ	1 mg/mL[b]	ES	10 units/mL[a]	Visually compatible for 24 hr at 25 °C	1630	C
Telavancin HCl	ASP	7.5 mg/mL[a,b]	APP	1000 units/mL[a,b]	Measured turbidity increased	2830	I
	ASP	7.5 mg/mL[k]	APP	1000 units/mL[k]	Physically compatible for 2 hr	2830	C
Theophylline	TR	4 mg/mL	TR	50 units/mL	Visually compatible for 4 hr at 25 °C	1793	C

Y-Site Injection Compatibility (1:1 Mixture) (Cont.)

Heparin sodium

Drug	Mfr	Conc	Mfr	Conc	Remarks	Ref	C/I
Thiotepa	IMM[n]	1 mg/mL[a]	ES	100 units/mL[a]	Physically compatible for 4 hr at 23 °C	1861	C
Ticarcillin disodium–clavulanate potassium	BE	31 mg/mL[a]	TR	50 units/mL	Visually compatible for 4 hr at 25 °C	1793	C
Tigecycline	WY	1 mg/mL[b]		10 units/mL	Physically compatible for 4 hr	2714	C
	WY	1 mg/mL[b]		100 units/mL[b]	Physically compatible for 4 hr	2714	C
Tirofiban HCl	ME	0.05 mg/mL[a,b]	AB	40 units/mL[a]	Physically compatible. No tirofiban or heparin loss in 4 hr at room temperature	2250	C
	ME	0.05 mg/mL[b]	AB	50 units/mL[b]	Physically compatible. No tirofiban or heparin loss in 4 hr at room temperature	2250	C
	ME	0.05 mg/mL[a,b]	AB	100 units/mL[a,b]	Physically compatible. No tirofiban or heparin loss in 4 hr at room temperature	2250	C
TNA #218 to #226[o]			AB	100 units/mL	Damage to emulsion occurs immediately with free oil possible	2215[o]	I
Tobramycin sulfate	LI	3.2 mg/mL[f]	ES	50 units/mL[f]	Immediate gross haze	1316	I
	LI	0.8 mg/mL[a]	TR	50 units/mL	Visually incompatible within 4 hr at 25 °C	1793	I
TPN #189[o]			DB	500 units/mL[b]	Visually compatible for 24 hr at 22 °C	1767	C
TPN #212 to #215[o]			AB	100 units/mL	Physically compatible for 4 hr at 23 °C	2109	C
Trimethobenzamide HCl	RC	100 mg/mL	UP	1000 units/L[e]	Physically compatible for 4 hr at room temperature	534	C
Vancomycin HCl	LI	6.6 mg/mL[a]	TR	50 units/mL	Visually incompatible within 4 hr at 25 °C	1793	I
	LE	10 mg/mL[b]	ES	100 units/mL[f]	Precipitate forms	2063	I
	PHS	2.5 mg/mL[b]	LEO	10 and 5000 units/mL[b]	Physically compatible with little change in heparin activity in 14 days at 4 and 37 °C. Antibiotic not tested	2684	C
	PHS	2 mg/mL[b]	LEO	10 units/mL[b]	Physically compatible with little change in heparin activity in 14 days at 4 and 37 °C. Antibiotic not tested	2684	C
Vasopressin	AMR	2 and 4 units/mL[b]	BA	100 units/mL[a]	Physically compatible with vasopressin pushed through a Y-site over 5 sec	2478	C
Vecuronium bromide	OR	0.1 mg/mL[a]	SO	40 units/mL[a]	Physically compatible for 24 hr at 28 °C	1337	C
	OR	1 mg/mL	ES	100 units/mL[a]	Visually compatible for 4 hr at 27 °C	2062	C
Vinblastine sulfate		1 mg/mL		1000 units/mL	Drugs injected sequentially in Y-site with no flush. No precipitate seen	980	C
Vincristine sulfate		1 mg/mL		1000 units/mL	Drugs injected sequentially in Y-site with no flush. No precipitate seen	980	C
Vinorelbine tartrate	BW	1 mg/mL[b]	ES	100 units/mL[b]	Physically compatible for 4 hr at 22 °C	1558	C
	GW	3 mg/mL[b]		100 units/mL[b]	A fine haze forms immediately, becoming cloudy in 15 min	2238	I
	GW	2 mg/mL[b]		100 units/mL[b]	Visually compatible for at least 15 min	2238	C
	GW	1 mg/mL[b]		100 units/mL[b]	Visually compatible for at least 15 min	2238	C
	GW	4 mg/4 mL[b]		100 units/1 mL[b]	Volumes mixed as cited. Visually compatible for at least 15 min	2238	C

Y-Site Injection Compatibility (1:1 Mixture) (Cont.)

Heparin sodium

Drug	Mfr	Conc	Mfr	Conc	Remarks	Ref	C/I
	GW	8 mg/4 mL[b]		100 units/ 1 mL[b]	Volumes mixed as cited. Precipitate forms	2238	**I**
	GW	12 mg/4 mL[b]		100 units/ 1 mL[b]	Volumes mixed as cited. Precipitate forms	2238	**I**
Warfarin sodium	DU	2 mg/mL[j]	AB	100 units/ mL[a]	Visually compatible with no warfarin loss in 30 min	2010	**C**
	DME	2 mg/mL[j]	AB	100 units/ mL[a]	Visually compatible for 24 hr at 24 °C	2078	**C**
Zidovudine	BW	4 mg/mL[a]	LY	100 units/ mL[a]	Physically compatible for 4 hr at 25 °C	1193	**C**

[a]*Tested in dextrose 5%.*
[b]*Tested in sodium chloride 0.9%.*
[c]*Tested in combination with hydrocortisone sodium succinate (Upjohn) 100 mg/L in dextrose 5%, sodium chloride 0.9%, and Ringer's injection, lactated.*
[d]*Given over three minutes into a heparin infusion run at 1 mL/min.*
[e]*Tested in dextrose 5% in Ringer's injection, dextrose 5% in Ringer's injection, lactated, dextrose 5%, Ringer's injection, lactated, and sodium chloride 0.9%.*
[f]*Tested in both dextrose 5% and sodium chloride 0.9%.*
[g]*Tested in bacteriostatic sodium chloride 0.9% preserved with benzyl alcohol 0.9%.*
[h]*Dacarbazine in intravenous tubing flushed with heparin sodium.*
[i]*Injected over one minute.*
[j]*Tested in sterile water for injection.*
[k]*Tested in Ringer's injection, lactated.*
[l]*Final concentration after mixing.*
[m]*Tested in dextrose 5% in Ringer's injection, lactated, dextrose 5%, Ringer's injection, lactated, and sodium chloride 0.9%.*
[n]*Lyophilized formulation tested.*
[o]*Refer to Appendix I for the composition of parenteral nutrition solutions. TNA indicates a 3-in-1 admixture, and TPN indicates a 2-in-1 admixture.*
[p]*Tested in dextrose 5% in Ringer's injection.*
[q]*Test performed using the formulation WITHOUT edetate disodium.*
[r]*Tested with albumin human 0.1%.*
[s]*Tested in dextrose 5% in sodium chloride 0.2%.*
[t]*Tested in sodium chloride 0.45%.*

Additional Compatibility Information

Parenteral Nutrition Admixtures — In solutions of amino acids 5% and dextrose 5 or 25% with vitamins or trace elements, heparin activity was retained for 24 hours at 25 °C. However, the activity fell significantly after 24 hours. (900)

However, flocculation of fat emulsion (Kabi-Vitrum) was reported during Y-site administration into a line being used to infuse a parenteral nutrition solution containing both calcium gluconate and heparin sodium. Subsequent evaluation indicated that the combination of calcium gluconate (0.46 and 1.8 mM/125 mL) plus heparin sodium (25 and 100 units/125 mL) in amino acids plus dextrose would induce flocculation of the fat emulsion within two to four minutes at concentrations that resulted in no visually apparent flocculation in 30 minutes with either agent alone. (1214)

Calcium chloride concentrations of 1 to 20 mM normally result in slow flocculation of fat emulsion 20%, intravenous, over a period of hours. When heparin sodium 5 units/mL was added, the flocculation rate accelerated greatly; a cream layer was observed visually in a few minutes. This effect was not observed when sodium ion was substituted for the divalent calcium. (1406)

Destabilization of fat emulsion (Intralipid 20%) was observed when administered simultaneously with a parenteral nutrition admixture. The damage, detected by viscosity measurement, occurred immediately upon contact at the Y-site. The extent of the destabilization was dependent on the concentration of the heparin and the presence of MVI Pediatric with its surfactant content. In addition to the viscosity changes, phase separation was observed in two hours. Parenteral nutrition admixtures containing heparin should never be premixed with fat emulsion as a 3-in-1 total nutrient admixture because of this emulsion destabilization. The damage might be minimized during Y-site co-administration as long as the heparin was kept at a sufficiently low concentration (no visible separation occurred at a heparin concentration of 0.5 unit/mL) and the length of tubing between the Y-site and the patient was minimized. (2282)

However, because the damage to emulsion integrity has been found to occur immediately upon mixing with heparin in the presence of the calcium ions in parenteral nutrition admixtures (1214; 2215; 2282) and no evaluation and documentation of the clinical safety of using such destabilized emulsions has been performed, use of such damaged emulsions in patients is suspect.

Peritoneal Dialysis Solutions — The activity of heparin 35,000 units/ L was evaluated in peritoneal dialysis fluids containing 1.5 and 2.5% dextrose (Dianeal, Travenol). Storage at 25 °C resulted in an apparent temporary 50% loss of heparin activity in four hours with recovery in six hours. Heparin activity was then retained for 14 days at 4 °C. (900)

Gentamicin sulfate 10 mg/L with heparin sodium 1000 units/L in Dianeal with dextrose 5% had no significant reduction in gentamicin sulfate concentration or of heparin sodium in four to six hours. (228)

However, a marked reduction in the anticoagulant activity of heparin sodium occurred if opalescence or a precipitate is formed, which results if the undiluted drugs are combined, even if the precipitate redissolves. Heparin activity was retained if one drug was added to a dilute solution of the other and no precipitate formed. (295)

Vancomycin hydrochloride (Lilly) 15 mg/L to 5.3 g/L in Dianeal with dextrose 2.5 or 4.25% was physically compatible with heparin sodium (Organon) 500 to 14,300 units/L for 24 hours at 25 °C under fluorescent light. However, a white precipitate formed immediately in combinations of heparin sodium with vancomycin hydrochloride 6.9 to 14.3 g/L. (1322)

Heparin Locks — Heparin locks, weak heparin solutions instilled or "locked" into infusion ports or sets through a resealing latex diaphragm, are useful in providing an established intravenous route for intermittent intravenous injections. To maintain patency, a weak heparin solution is left in the tubing. Concentrations of heparin sodium used have varied from about 10 to 1000 units/mL of sodium chloride 0.9%, with 10 and 100 units/mL being the most common. The volume of dilute heparin sodium in sodium chloride 0.9% usually used to flush the set is 0.2 to 1 mL. (255; 256; 257; 258; 405; 677; 678; 901; 2119) However, the use of sodium chloride 0.9% instead of a solution containing heparin has been suggested to maintain patency. Studies have found sodium chloride 0.9% to be as effective in maintaining patency as 10- and 100-unit/mL solutions of heparin. (902; 903; 1109; 1266; 1267; 1268; 1269; 1639; 1640; 1641; 1656; 1839; 1959; 2003; 2119) Other investigators reported that even small amounts of heparin solution are more effective than sodium chloride 0.9% alone. (678; 1270; 2120; 2121)

Evaluations of the use of heparinized solutions as locks or continuous flow solutions to help maintain patency in central venous catheters and arterial catheters have resulted in similarly variable results and recommendations. (2122; 2123; 2124; 2125; 2126) Although use of such heparinized solutions has been generally considered a benign technique causing minimal problems, a number of adverse effects have been reported, especially from solutions with a high heparin concentration and/or numerous heparin flushes. (2127; 2128; 2129; 2130; 2131; 2132)

Vancomycin hydrochloride (Lilly) 25 mcg/mL and heparin sodium (Elkins-Sinn) 100 units/mL in 0.9% sodium chloride injection as a catheter flush solution was evaluated for stability when stored at 4 °C for 14 days. The flush solution was visually clear, and vancomycin activity and heparin activity were retained throughout the storage period. However, an additional 24 hours at 37 °C to simulate use conditions resulted in losses of both agents ranging from 20 to 37%. (1933)

Vancomycin hydrochloride 25 mcg/mL combined with heparin sodium (Hospira) 10 units/mL in sterile water for injection for use as a lock solution was found to be physically compatible. Little or no vancomycin loss occurred in 3 days at 4 °C. However, losses of 8% occurred in 3 days at 27 °C and 1 day at 40 °C. (2820)

If ciprofloxacin (Sicor) 2 mg/mL was added to this flush solution, a white precipitate appeared within 1 day. Losses of both ciprofloxacin and vancomycin occurred as well. (2820)

Methylprednisolone — The compatibility of methylprednisolone sodium succinate (Upjohn) with heparin sodium added to an auxiliary medication infusion unit has been studied. Primary admixtures were prepared by adding heparin sodium 10,000 units/L to dextrose 5%, dextrose 5% in sodium chloride 0.9%, and Ringer's injection, lactated. Up to 100 mL of the primary admixture was added along with methylprednisolone sodium succinate (Upjohn) to the auxiliary medication infusion unit with the following results (329):

Methylprednisolone Sodium Succinate	Heparin Sodium 10,000 units/L of Primary Solution	Results
500 mg	D5S, D5W qs 100 mL	Clear solution for 24 hr
500 mg	LR qs 100 mL or added to 100 mL LR	Clear solution for 6 hr
1000 mg	D5S, D5W qs 100 mL	Clear solution for 6 hr
1000 mg	Added to 100 mL D5W	Clear solution for 24 hr
1000 mg	LR qs 100 mL or added to 100 mL LR	Clear solution for 4 to 6 hr
2000 mg	D5W qs 100 mL	Clear solution for 6 hr
2000 mg	D5S, LR qs 100 mL	Clear solution for 24 hr

HETASTARCH IN LACTATED ELECTROLYTE
AHFS 40:12

Products — Hetastarch 6% in lactated electrolyte is available in 500- and 1000-mL flexible plastic infusion containers. Each 100 milliliters of solution contains hetastarch 6 g, sodium chloride 672 mg, sodium lactate anhydrous 317 mg, dextrose hydrous 99 mg, calcium chloride dihydrate 37 mg, potassium chloride 22 mg, and magnesium chloride hexahydrate 9 mg in water for injection. The concentrations of electrolytes are shown in Table 1. (1)

Table 1. Electrolyte Composition (1)

Electrolyte	mEq/L
Sodium	143
Calcium	5
Potassium	3
Magnesium	0.9
Chloride	124
Lactate	28

pH — Approximately pH 5.9 with negligible buffering capacity. (1)

Osmolarity — Approximately 307 mOsm/L. (1)

Trade Name(s) — Hextend.

Administration — Hetastarch 6% in lactated electrolyte is administered by intravenous infusion. The amount of solution and rate of administration depend on the clinical condition and needs of the patient. The product should be inspected for cloudiness, haze, and particulate matter prior to use. Solutions such as this product that contain calcium should not be administered simultaneously with blood through the same set because of the likelihood of coagulation. (1)

Stability — Intact containers of hetastarch 6% in lactated electrolyte should be stored at controlled room temperature and protected from freezing and excessive heat. Brief exposure at temperatures up to 40 °C does not adversely affect the product. (1)

The product is a clear, pale yellow to amber solution. Prolonged exposure to adverse conditions may result in the formation of a turbid deep brown appearance or crystalline precipitate; such solutions should not be used. (1)

Compatibility Information

Y-Site Injection Compatibility (1:1 Mixture)

Hetastarch in lactated electrolyte

Drug	Mfr	Conc	Mfr	Conc	Remarks	Ref	C/I
Alfentanil HCl	TAY	0.125 mg/mL[a]	AB	6%	Physically compatible for 4 hr at 23 °C	2339	C
Amikacin sulfate	APC	5 mg/mL[a]	AB	6%	Physically compatible for 4 hr at 23 °C	2339	C
Aminophylline	AMR	2.5 mg/mL[a]	AB	6%	Physically compatible for 4 hr at 23 °C	2339	C
Amiodarone HCl	WAY	4 mg/mL[a]	AB	6%	Physically compatible for 4 hr at 23 °C	2339	C
Amphotericin B	APC	0.6 mg/mL[a]	AB	6%	Immediate gross precipitation	2339	I
Ampicillin sodium	APC	20 mg/mL[b]	AB	6%	Physically compatible for 4 hr at 23 °C	2339	C
Ampicillin sodium–sulbactam sodium	PF	20 + 10 mg/mL[b]	AB	6%	Physically compatible for 4 hr at 23 °C	2339	C
Atracurium besylate	GW	0.5 mg/mL[a]	AB	6%	Physically compatible for 4 hr at 23 °C	2339	C
Azithromycin	PF	2 mg/mL[a]	AB	6%	Physically compatible for 4 hr at 23 °C	2339	C
Aztreonam	BMS	40 mg/mL[a]	AB	6%	Physically compatible for 4 hr at 23 °C	2339	C
Bumetanide	OHM	0.04 mg/mL[a]	AB	6%	Physically compatible for 4 hr at 23 °C	2339	C
Butorphanol tartrate	APC	0.04 mg/mL[a]	AB	6%	Physically compatible for 4 hr at 23 °C	2339	C
Calcium gluconate	FUJ	40 mg/mL[a]	AB	6%	Physically compatible for 4 hr at 23 °C	2339	C
Cefazolin sodium	LI	20 mg/mL[a]	AB	6%	Physically compatible for 4 hr at 23 °C	2339	C
Cefepime HCl	BMS	20 mg/mL[a]	AB	6%	Physically compatible for 4 hr at 23 °C	2339	C
Cefotaxime sodium	HO	20 mg/mL[a]	AB	6%	Physically compatible for 4 hr at 23 °C	2339	C
Cefotetan disodium	ZEN	20 mg/mL[a]	AB	6%	Physically compatible for 4 hr at 23 °C	2339	C
Cefoxitin sodium	ME	20 mg/mL[a]	AB	6%	Physically compatible for 4 hr at 23 °C	2339	C
Ceftazidime	GW	40 mg/mL[a]	AB	6%	Physically compatible for 4 hr at 23 °C	2339	C
Cefuroxime sodium	LI	30 mg/mL[a]	AB	6%	Physically compatible for 4 hr at 23 °C	2339	C
Chlorpromazine HCl	ES	2 mg/mL[a]	AB	6%	Physically compatible for 4 hr at 23 °C	2339	C
Ciprofloxacin	BAY	2 mg/mL[a]	AB	6%	Physically compatible for 4 hr at 23 °C	2339	C
Cisatracurium besylate	GW	0.5 mg/mL[a]	AB	6%	Physically compatible for 4 hr at 23 °C	2339	C
Clindamycin phosphate	PHU	10 mg/mL[a]	AB	6%	Physically compatible for 4 hr at 23 °C	2339	C
Dexamethasone sodium phosphate	APP	1 mg/mL[a]	AB	6%	Physically compatible for 4 hr at 23 °C	2339	C
Diazepam	AB	5 mg/mL	AB	6%	White turbidity forms immediately	2339	I
Digoxin	ES	0.25 mg/mL	AB	6%	Physically compatible for 4 hr at 23 °C	2339	C

Y-Site Injection Compatibility (1:1 Mixture) (Cont.)

Hetastarch in lactated electrolyte

Drug	Mfr	Conc	Mfr	Conc	Remarks	Ref	C/I
Diltiazem HCl	BA	5 mg/mL	AB	6%	Physically compatible for 4 hr at 23 °C	2339	C
Diphenhydramine HCl	SCN	2 mg/mL[a]	AB	6%	Physically compatible for 4 hr at 23 °C	2339	C
Dobutamine HCl	AST	4 mg/mL[a]	AB	6%	Physically compatible for 4 hr at 23 °C	2339	C
Dolasetron mesylate	HO	2 mg/mL[a]	AB	6%	Physically compatible for 4 hr at 23 °C	2339	C
Dopamine HCl	AB	3.2 mg/mL[a]	AB	6%	Physically compatible for 4 hr at 23 °C	2339	C
Doxycycline hyclate	APP	1 mg/mL[a]	AB	6%	Physically compatible for 4 hr at 23 °C	2339	C
Droperidol	AMR	2.5 mg/mL	AB	6%	Physically compatible for 4 hr at 23 °C	2339	C
Enalaprilat	ME	0.1 mg/mL[a]	AB	6%	Physically compatible for 4 hr at 23 °C	2339	C
Ephedrine sulfate	TAY	5 mg/mL[a]	AB	6%	Physically compatible for 4 hr at 23 °C	2339	C
Epinephrine HCl	AB	0.05 mg/mL[a]	AB	6%	Physically compatible for 4 hr at 23 °C	2339	C
Erythromycin lactobionate	AB	5 mg/mL[b]	AB	6%	Physically compatible for 4 hr at 23 °C	2339	C
Esmolol HCl	OHM	10 mg/mL	AB	6%	Physically compatible for 4 hr at 23 °C	2339	C
Famotidine	ME	2 mg/mL[a]	AB	6%	Physically compatible for 4 hr at 23 °C	2339	C
Fenoldopam mesylate	AB	80 mcg/mL[b]	AB	6%	Physically compatible for 4 hr at 23 °C	2467	C
Fentanyl citrate	ES	12.5 mcg/mL[a]	AB	6%	Physically compatible for 4 hr at 23 °C	2339	C
Fluconazole	PF	2 mg/mL	AB	6%	Physically compatible for 4 hr at 23 °C	2339	C
Furosemide	AMR	3 mg/mL[a]	AB	6%	Physically compatible for 4 hr at 23 °C	2339	C
Gentamicin sulfate	SC	5 mg/mL[a]	AB	6%	Physically compatible for 4 hr at 23 °C	2339	C
Granisetron HCl	SKB	0.05 mg/mL[a]	AB	6%	Physically compatible for 4 hr at 23 °C	2339	C
Haloperidol lactate	MN	0.2 mg/mL[a]	AB	6%	Physically compatible for 4 hr at 23 °C	2339	C
Heparin sodium	ES	100 units/mL	AB	6%	Physically compatible for 4 hr at 23 °C	2339	C
Hydrocortisone sodium succinate	PHU	1 mg/mL[a]	AB	6%	Physically compatible for 4 hr at 23 °C	2339	C
Hydromorphone HCl	AST	0.5 mg/mL[a]	AB	6%	Physically compatible for 4 hr at 23 °C	2339	C
Hydroxyzine HCl	ES	2 mg/mL[a]	AB	6%	Physically compatible for 4 hr at 23 °C	2339	C
Isoproterenol HCl	AB	0.02 mg/mL[a]	AB	6%	Physically compatible for 4 hr at 23 °C	2339	C
Ketorolac tromethamine	AB	15 mg/mL	AB	6%	Physically compatible for 4 hr at 23 °C	2339	C
Labetalol HCl	GW	2 mg/mL[a]	AB	6%	Physically compatible for 4 hr at 23 °C	2339	C
Levofloxacin	OMN	5 mg/mL[a]	AB	6%	Physically compatible for 4 hr at 23 °C	2339	C
Lidocaine HCl	AB	8 mg/mL[a]	AB	6%	Physically compatible for 4 hr at 23 °C	2339	C
Lorazepam	OHM	0.5 mg/mL[a]	AB	6%	Physically compatible for 4 hr at 23 °C	2339	C
Magnesium sulfate	AST	100 mg/mL[a]	AB	6%	Physically compatible for 4 hr at 23 °C	2339	C
Mannitol	BA	15%	AB	6%	Physically compatible for 4 hr at 23 °C	2339	C
Meperidine HCl	OHM	4 mg/mL[a]	AB	6%	Physically compatible for 4 hr at 23 °C	2339	C
Methylprednisolone sodium succinate	PHU	5 mg/mL[a]	AB	6%	Physically compatible for 4 hr at 23 °C	2339	C
Metoclopramide HCl	FAU	5 mg/mL	AB	6%	Physically compatible for 4 hr at 23 °C	2339	C
Metronidazole	AB	5 mg/mL	AB	6%	Physically compatible for 4 hr at 23 °C	2339	C
Midazolam HCl	RC	1 mg/mL[a]	AB	6%	Physically compatible for 4 hr at 23 °C	2339	C
Milrinone lactate	SAN	0.2 mg/mL[a]	AB	6%	Physically compatible for 4 hr at 23 °C	2339	C

Y-Site Injection Compatibility (1:1 Mixture) (Cont.)

Hetastarch in lactated electrolyte

Drug	Mfr	Conc	Mfr	Conc	Remarks	Ref	C/I
Morphine sulfate	AST	1 mg/mL[a]	AB	6%	Physically compatible for 4 hr at 23 °C	2339	C
Nalbuphine HCl	AST	10 mg/mL	AB	6%	Physically compatible for 4 hr at 23 °C	2339	C
Nitroglycerin	AMR	0.4 mg/mL[a]	AB	6%	Physically compatible for 4 hr at 23 °C	2339	C
Norepinephrine bitartrate	AB	0.12 mg/mL[a]	AB	6%	Physically compatible for 4 hr at 23 °C	2339	C
Ondansetron HCl	GW	1 mg/mL[a]	AB	6%	Physically compatible for 4 hr at 23 °C	2339	C
Palonosetron HCl	MGI	50 mcg/mL	HOS	6%	Physically compatible. No palonosetron loss in 4 hr at room temperature	2775	C
Pancuronium bromide	ES	0.1 mg/mL[a]	AB	6%	Physically compatible for 4 hr at 23 °C	2339	C
Phenylephrine HCl	OHM	1 mg/mL[a]	AB	6%	Physically compatible for 4 hr at 23 °C	2339	C
Piperacillin sodium–tazobactam sodium	LE[c]	40 + 5 mg/mL[a]	AB	6%	Physically compatible for 4 hr at 23 °C	2339	C
Potassium chloride	AB	0.1 mEq/mL[a]	AB	6%	Physically compatible for 4 hr at 23 °C	2339	C
Procainamide HCl	ES	10 mg/mL[a]	AB	6%	Physically compatible for 4 hr at 23 °C	2339	C
Prochlorperazine edisylate	SO	0.5 mg/mL[a]	AB	6%	Physically compatible for 4 hr at 23 °C	2339	C
Promethazine HCl	SCN	2 mg/mL[a]	AB	6%	Physically compatible for 4 hr at 23 °C	2339	C
Ranitidine HCl	GW	2 mg/mL[a]	AB	6%	Physically compatible for 4 hr at 23 °C	2339	C
Rocuronium bromide	OR	1 mg/mL[a]	AB	6%	Physically compatible for 4 hr at 23 °C	2339	C
Sodium bicarbonate	AB	1 mEq/mL	AB	6%	Microprecipitate develops rapidly	2339	I
Sodium nitroprusside	OHM	2 mg/mL[a]	AB	6%	Physically compatible for 4 hr at 23 °C protected from light	2339	C
Succinylcholine chloride	AB	2 mg/mL[a]	AB	6%	Physically compatible for 4 hr at 23 °C	2339	C
Sufentanil citrate	BA	12.5 mcg/mL[a]	AB	6%	Physically compatible for 4 hr at 23 °C	2339	C
Theophylline	BA	4 mg/mL[a]	AB	6%	Physically compatible for 4 hr at 23 °C	2339	C
Ticarcillin disodium–clavulanate potassium	SKB	31 mg/mL[a]	AB	6%	Physically compatible for 4 hr at 23 °C	2339	C
Tobramycin sulfate	GNS	5 mg/mL[a]	AB	6%	Physically compatible for 4 hr at 23 °C	2339	C
Trimethoprim–sulfamethoxazole	ES	0.8 + 4 mg/mL[a]	AB	6%	Physically compatible for 4 hr at 23 °C	2339	C
Vancomycin HCl	LI	10 mg/mL[a]	AB	6%	Physically compatible for 4 hr at 23 °C	2339	C
Vecuronium bromide	OR	0.2 mg/mL[a]	AB	6%	Physically compatible for 4 hr at 23 °C	2339	C
Verapamil HCl	AMR	1.25 mg/mL[a]	AB	6%	Physically compatible for 4 hr at 23 °C	2339	C

[a]Tested in dextrose 5%.
[b]Tested in sodium chloride 0.9%.
[c]Test performed using the formulation WITHOUT edetate disodium.

HETASTARCH IN SODIUM CHLORIDE 0.9%
AHFS 40:12

Products — Hetastarch is available as a 6% (6 g/100 mL) injection in sodium chloride 0.9% in 500-mL plastic containers. The solution also contains sodium hydroxide for pH adjustment during manufacturing. (1)

pH — Approximately pH 5.5. (1)

Osmolarity — The product has an osmolarity of 309 mOsm/L. (1; 4)

Sodium Content — Hetastarch 6% in sodium chloride 0.9% provides 77 mEq of sodium per 500-mL container. (4)

Trade Name(s) — Hespan.

Administration — Hetastarch is given only by intravenous infusion; discard any remaining solution in partially used containers. The dosage and rate of infusion must be individualized to the patient's condition and response. (1; 4)

Stability — Hetastarch injection is a clear, pale yellow to amber colloidal solution. The product should be stored at controlled room temperature and protected from freezing and excessive heat. Brief exposure to temperatures up to 40 °C does not affect stability. However, prolonged storage under adverse conditions may result in a crystalline precipitate or a deep brown turbid appearance. Such solutions should not be administered. (1; 4)

Amylose starch has been shown to associate and precipitate over time in solution. (2296) Before hetastarch is used, the colloidal solution should be checked for clarity and particulates and the flexible plastic containers should be squeezed to check for small leaks. (1)

Compatibility Information

Additive Compatibility

Hetastarch in sodium chloride 0.9%

Drug	Mfr	Conc/L	Mfr	Conc/L	Test Soln	Remarks	Ref	C/I
Ampicillin sodium		4 g		6%	NS	18% loss in 6 hr and 35% in 24 hr at 20 °C	834	I
Enalaprilat	MSD	25 mg	DU	6%		Physically compatible for 24 hr at room temperature under fluorescent light	1355	C
Fosphenytoin sodium	PD	1, 8, 20 mg PE/mL[a]	MG	6%	NS	Visually compatible with little or no loss in 7 days at 25 °C under fluorescent light	2083	C
Oxacillin sodium		4 g		6%		1% oxacillin loss in 24 hr at 20 °C	834	C

[a]Concentration expressed in milligrams of phenytoin sodium equivalents (PE) per milliliter.

Y-Site Injection Compatibility (1:1 Mixture)

Hetastarch in sodium chloride 0.9%

Drug	Mfr	Conc	Mfr	Conc	Remarks	Ref	C/I
Amikacin sulfate	BR	5 mg/mL[a]	DCC	6%	Small crystals form immediately after mixing and persist for 4 hr	1313	I
Ampicillin sodium	BR	20 mg/mL[a]	DCC	6%	Visually compatible for 4 hr at room temperature	1313	C
	BR	20 mg/mL[a]	DCC	6%	One or two particles in one of five vials. Fine white strands appeared immediately during Y-site infusion	1315	I
Cefazolin sodium	SKF	20 mg/mL[a]	DCC	6%	Visually compatible for 4 hr at room temperature	1313	C
	SKF	20 mg/mL[a]	DCC	6%	Simulation in vials showed no incompatibility, but white precipitate formed in Y-site during infusion	1315	I
Cefotaxime sodium	HO	20 mg/mL[a]	DCC	6%	Small crystals form immediately after mixing and persist for 4 hr	1313	I
Cefoxitin sodium	MSD	20 mg/mL[a]	DCC	6%	Precipitate in 1 hr at room temperature	1313	I
Diltiazem HCl	MMD	5 mg/mL	DU	6%	Visually compatible	1807	C

Y-Site Injection Compatibility (1:1 Mixture) (Cont.)

Hetastarch in sodium chloride 0.9%

Drug	Mfr	Conc	Mfr	Conc	Remarks	Ref	C/I
Doxycycline hyclate	LY	1 mg/mL[a]	DCC	6%	Visually compatible for 4 hr at room temperature	1313	C
	LY	1 mg/mL[a]	DCC	6%	White particle in one of five tests. No incompatibility during Y-site infusion	1315	?
Enalaprilat	MSD	0.05 mg/mL[b]	DCC	6%	Physically compatible for 24 hr at room temperature under fluorescent light	1355	C
Ertapenem sodium	ME	10 mg/mL[b]	AB	6%	Visually compatible with about 3% ertapenem loss in 8 hr	2487	C
Gentamicin sulfate	TR	0.8 mg/mL	DCC	6%	Precipitates immediately but disappears after 1 hr at room temperature	1313	I
Nicardipine HCl	DCC	0.1 mg/mL[a]	DU	6%	Visually compatible for 24 hr at room temperature	235	C
Ranitidine HCl	GL	0.5 mg/mL	DCC	6%	Barely visible single particle appeared after 1 hr but disappeared	1313	?
	GL	0.5 mg/mL	DCC	6%	Barely visible particles appeared and disappeared	1314	I
	GL	0.5 mg/mL	DCC	6%	Small white particles and white fiber	1315	I
Theophylline	TR	4 mg/mL	DCC	6%	Precipitates after 2 hr at room temperature	1313	I
Tobramycin sulfate	LI	0.8 mg/mL	DCC	6%	Small crystals form immediately after mixing and persist for 4 hr	1313	I

[a]Tested in dextrose 5%.
[b]Tested in sodium chloride 0.9%.

HYALURONIDASE
AHFS 44:00

Products — Hyaluronidase is supplied as a 150-unit/mL solution in 1-mL fill vials. Each milliliter also contains sodium chloride 8.5 mg, edetate disodium 1 mg, calcium chloride 0.4 mg, and thimerosal not more than 0.1 mg in sodium phosphate buffer. (1)

pH — From 6.4 to 7.4. (4)

Osmolality — From 295 to 355 mOsm/kg. (1)

Trade Name(s) — Amphadase.

Administration — Hyaluronidase is administered subcutaneously, intradermally, or intramuscularly along with other drugs or solutions. The solutions should be isotonic for subcutaneous administration. It should not be administered intravenously. (1; 4)

Stability — Hyaluronidase injection in intact vials should be stored under refrigeration at 2 to 8 °C. It should not be used if it is discolored or contains a precipitate. (4)

Hyaluronidase (Wyeth) 75 units/mL in citric acid/sodium citrate buffer (pH 4.5) was found to lose about 7 to 8% activity in 24 hours at 4 and 23 °C. Hyaluronidase activity decreased by 25 to 33% in 48 hours. (1907)

Compatibility Information

Solution Compatibility

Hyaluronidase

Solution	Mfr	Mfr	Conc/L	Remarks	Ref	C/I
Dextrose–Ringer's injection combinations	AB	AB	150 units	Physically compatible	3	C

Solution Compatibility (Cont.)

Hyaluronidase

Solution	Mfr	Mfr	Conc/L	Remarks	Ref	C/I
Dextrose–Ringer's injection, lactated, combinations	AB	AB	150 units	Physically compatible	3	**C**
Dextrose–saline combinations	AB	AB	150 units	Physically compatible	3	**C**
Dextrose 2.5%	AB	AB	150 units	Physically compatible	3	**C**
Dextrose 5%	AB	AB	150 units	Physically compatible	3	**C**
Dextrose 10%	AB	AB	150 units	Physically compatible	3	**C**
Ionosol products	AB	AB	150 units	Physically compatible	3	**C**
Ringer's injection	AB	AB	150 units	Physically compatible	3	**C**
Ringer's injection, lactated	AB	AB	150 units	Physically compatible	3	**C**
Sodium chloride 0.45%	AB	AB	150 units	Physically compatible	3	**C**
Sodium chloride 0.9%	AB	AB	150 units	Physically compatible	3	**C**
Sodium lactate ⅙ M	AB	AB	150 units	Physically compatible	3	**C**

Additive Compatibility

Hyaluronidase

Drug	Mfr	Conc/L	Mfr	Conc/L	Test Soln	Remarks	Ref	C/I
Amikacin sulfate	BR	5 g	SE	150 units	D5LR, D5R, D5S, D5W, D10W, LR, NS, R, SL	Physically compatible and amikacin stable for 24 hr at 25 °C. Hyaluronidase not analyzed	294	**C**
Sodium bicarbonate	AB	2.4 mEq[a]	WY	150 units	D5W	Physically compatible for 24 hr	772	**C**

[a] *One vial of Neut added to a liter of admixture.*

Drugs in Syringe Compatibility

Hyaluronidase

Drug (in syringe)	Mfr	Amt	Mfr	Amt	Remarks	Ref	C/I
Hydromorphone HCl	KN	2 mg/mL[a]	WY	150 units/mL[a]	43 and 56% hyaluronidase loss in 24 hr at 4 and 23 °C, respectively	1907	**I**
	KN	10 and 40 mg/mL[a]	WY	150 units/mL[a]	70 to 82% hyaluronidase loss in 24 hr at 4 and 23 °C	1907	**I**

Drugs in Syringe Compatibility (Cont.)

Hyaluronidase

Drug (in syringe)	Mfr	Amt	Mfr	Amt	Remarks	Ref	C/I
Iodipamide meglumine	SQ	52%, 40 to 2 mL	WY	150 units/ 1 mL	Physically compatible for 48 hr	530	C
	SQ	52%, 1 mL	WY	150 units/ 1 mL	Physically compatible for at least 1 hr but a precipitate forms within 48 hr	530	I
Iothalamate meglumine	MA	60%, 40 to 1 mL	WY	150 units/ 1 mL	Physically compatible for 48 hr	530	C
Pentobarbital sodium	AB	500 mg/ 10 mL	AB	150 units	Physically compatible	55	C

ᵃMixed in equal quantities.

HYDRALAZINE HYDROCHLORIDE
AHFS 24:08.20

Products — Hydralazine hydrochloride is available in 1-mL vials. Each milliliter of solution contains hydralazine hydrochloride 20 mg, methylparaben 0.65 mg, propylparaben 0.35 mg, and propylene glycol 103.6 mg in water for injection. The pH may have been adjusted with hydrochloric acid and/or sodium hydroxide. (1)

pH — From 3.4 to 4.4. (1)

Administration — Hydralazine hydrochloride may be administered intramuscularly or as a rapid direct intravenous injection; the manufacturer does not recommend adding the drug to infusion solutions. (1; 4)

Stability — Hydralazine hydrochloride in intact vials should be stored at controlled room temperature and protected from freezing. (1; 4) Refrigeration of the intact containers may result in precipitation or crystallization. (593)

Hydralazine hydrochloride undergoes color changes in most infusion solutions. However, it has been stated that color changes within eight to 12 hours of admixture preparation in solutions stored at 30 °C are not indicative of drug losses. (4) The manufacturer does not recommend admixture in infusion solutions. (1)

Hydralazine hydrochloride may react with various metals (1) to yield discolored solutions, often yellow or pink. One report indicated a pink discoloration in prefilled syringes when the hydralazine hydrochloride had been drawn up through filter needles (Monoject) with a stainless steel filter and stored for up to 12 hours. The reaction is not specific to any one metal. Consequently, contact with metal parts should be minimized, and hydralazine hydrochloride should be prepared just prior to use. (906)

pH Effects — Hydralazine hydrochloride exhibits maximum stability at pH 3.5 and is stable over the pH range of 3 to 5. It undergoes more rapid decomposition as the pH becomes alkaline. (106; 466)

Light Effects — Exposure to light increases the rate of hydralazine hydrochloride decomposition during long-term storage. At a concentration of 0.35 mg/mL in sodium chloride 0.9% in glass bottles, 10% decomposition was calculated to occur in 14.4 weeks in the dark and 12.3 weeks under fluorescent light. In PVC containers, decomposition occurs more rapidly; a 10% loss was calculated to occur in 12.8 weeks in the dark and 9.9 weeks under fluorescent light. (1561)

Sorption — Hydralazine hydrochloride 27 mg/L in sodium chloride 0.9% in PVC bags exhibited approximately 10% loss in one week at 15 to 20 °C due to sorption. (536) However, no loss due to sorption occurred during a seven-hour simulated infusion through an infusion set consisting of a cellulose propionate burette chamber and 170 cm of PVC tubing. (606)

Hydralazine hydrochloride was shown not to exhibit sorption to polyethylene tubing, Silastic tubing, and polypropylene syringes. (606)

Compatibility Information

Solution Compatibility

Hydralazine HCl

Solution	Mfr	Mfr	Conc/L	Remarks	Ref	C/I
Dextrose–Ringer's injection combinations	AB	CI	400 mg	Physically compatible	3	C
Dextrose 5% in Ringer's injection, lactated	AB	CI	400 mg	Physically compatible	3	C
Dextrose 2.5% in half-strength Ringer's injection, lactated	AB	CI	400 mg	Physically compatible	3	C
Dextrose–saline combinations	AB	CI	400 mg	Physically compatible	3	C
Dextrose 2.5%	AB	CI	400 mg	Physically compatible	3	C
Dextrose 5%		CI	40 mg	Yellow color within 1 hr. 4% decomposition in 2 hr and 8% in 3.5 hr	466	I
			200 to 400 mg	Progressive yellow discoloration due to hydralazine reaction with dextrose	845	I
	TR[a]		350 mg	10% loss in 1 hr at 21 °C under fluorescent light. Approximately 11 to 12% loss in 1.5 hr at 21 °C in the dark	1561	I
	BA	AMR	200 mg	41% loss in 24 hr at 25 °C	2644	I
Dextrose 10%	AB	CI	400 mg	Physically compatible	3	C
Dextrose 10% in Ringer's injection, lactated	AB	CI	400 mg	Color change	3	I
Ionosol products	AB	CI	400 mg	Physically compatible	3	C
Ringer's injection	AB	CI	400 mg	Physically compatible	3	C
Ringer's injection, lactated	AB	CI	400 mg	Physically compatible	3	C
		CI	40 mg	No decomposition in 2.5 hr	466	C
Sodium chloride 0.45%	AB	CI	400 mg	Physically compatible	3	C
Sodium chloride 0.9%	AB	CI	400 mg	Physically compatible	3	C
		CI	40 mg	No decomposition in 4 days	466	C
		CI	200 to 400 mg	Physically compatible	845	C
	TR[a]		350 mg	6 to 8% loss in 52 days at 21 °C under fluorescent light	1561	C
	BA	AMR	200 mg	8% loss in 2 days and 13% loss in 3 days at 25 °C	2644	C
Sodium lactate ⅙ M	AB	CI	400 mg	Physically compatible	3	C

[a]*Tested in both glass and PVC containers.*

Additive Compatibility

Hydralazine HCl

Drug	Mfr	Conc/L	Mfr	Conc/L	Test Soln	Remarks	Ref	C/I
Aminophylline	BP	1 g	BP	80 mg	D5W	Yellow color produced	26	I
Ampicillin sodium	BP	2 g	BP	80 mg	D5W	Yellow color produced	26	I
Chlorothiazide sodium	BP	2 g	BP	80 mg	D5W, NS	Yellow color with precipitate in 3 hr	26	I
Dobutamine HCl	LI	200 mg	CI	200 mg	NS	Physically compatible for 24 hr	552	C
Edetate calcium disodium	RI	4 g	BP	80 mg	D5W	Yellow color produced	26	I
Ethacrynate sodium	MSD	50 mg	CI	20 mg	NS	Altered UV spectra at room temperature	16	I
Hydrocortisone sodium succinate	BP	400 mg	BP	80 mg	D5W	Yellow color produced	26	I

Additive Compatibility (Cont.)

Hydralazine HCl

Drug	Mfr	Conc/L	Mfr	Conc/L	Test Soln	Remarks	Ref	C/I
Methohexital sodium	BP	2 g	BP	80 mg	D5W, NS	Yellow color with precipitate in 3 hr	26	I
Nitroglycerin	ACC	400 mg	CI	1 g	D5W[a]	Yellow color. 4% nitroglycerin loss in 48 hr at 23 °C. Hydralazine not tested	929	I
	ACC	400 mg	CI	1 g	NS[a]	Yellow color. No nitroglycerin loss in 48 hr at 23 °C. Hydralazine not tested	929	I
Phenobarbital sodium	BP	800 mg	BP	80 mg	D5W	Yellow color and precipitate in 3 hr	26	I
Verapamil HCl	KN	80 mg	CI	40 mg	D5W, NS	Yellow discoloration	764	I

[a]Tested in glass containers.

Drugs in Syringe Compatibility

Hydralazine HCl

Drug (in syringe)	Mfr	Amt	Mfr	Amt	Remarks	Ref	C/I
Pantoprazole sodium	a	4 mg/1 mL		20 mg/1 mL	Precipitates within 4 hr	2574	I

[a]Test performed using the formulation WITHOUT edetate disodium.

Y-Site Injection Compatibility (1:1 Mixture)

Hydralazine HCl

Drug	Mfr	Conc	Mfr	Conc	Remarks	Ref	C/I
Aminophylline	ES	4 mg/mL[a]	SO	1 mg/mL[a]	Gross color change in 1 hr	1316	I
	ES	4 mg/mL[b]	SO	1 mg/mL[b]	Color change in 1 hr and haze in 3 hr	1316	I
Ampicillin sodium	WY	40 mg/mL[b]	SO	1 mg/mL[a]	Moderate color change in 1 hr	1316	I
	WY	40 mg/mL[b]	SO	1 mg/mL[b]	Moderate color change in 3 hr	1316	I
Caspofungin acetate	ME	0.5 mg/mL[b]	APP	20 mg/mL	Physically compatible with hydralazine HCl i.v. push over 2 to 5 min	2766	C
Furosemide	ES	1 mg/mL[c]	SO	1 mg/mL[c]	Slight color change in 3 hr	1316	I
Heparin sodium	UP	1000 units/L[d]	CI	20 mg/mL	Physically compatible for 4 hr at room temperature	534	C
Hydrocortisone sodium succinate	UP	10 mg/L[d]	CI	20 mg/mL	Physically compatible for 4 hr at room temperature	534	C
Nesiritide	SCI	50 mcg/mL[a,b]		20 mg/mL	Physically incompatible	2625	I
Nitroglycerin	LY	0.4 mg/mL[a]	SO	1 mg/mL[a]	Physically compatible for 3 hr	1316	C
	LY	0.4 mg/mL[b]	SO	1 mg/mL[b]	Slight precipitate in 3 hr	1316	I
Potassium chloride	AB	40 mEq/L[d]	CI	20 mg/mL	Physically compatible for 4 hr at room temperature	534	C
Verapamil HCl	LY	0.2 mg/mL[c]	SO	1 mg/mL[c]	Physically compatible for 3 hr	1316	C

[a]Tested in dextrose 5%.
[b]Tested in sodium chloride 0.9%.
[c]Tested in both dextrose 5% and sodium chloride 0.9%.
[d]Tested in dextrose 5% in Ringer's injection, dextrose 5% in Ringer's injection, lactated, dextrose 5%, Ringer's injection, lactated, and sodium chloride 0.9%.

HYDROCORTISONE SODIUM SUCCINATE
AHFS 68:04

Products — Hydrocortisone sodium succinate is available in a variety of sizes and containers (4), including 100-mg conventional vials containing hydrocortisone sodium succinate equivalent to hydrocortisone 100 mg with monobasic sodium phosphate anhydrous 0.8 mg and dibasic sodium phosphate dried 8.73 mg. Reconstitute the vial by adding not more than 2 mL of bacteriostatic water for injection or bacteriostatic sodium chloride injection. (1)

Hydrocortisone sodium succinate is also supplied in "Act-O-Vial" containers of 100, 250, 500, and 1000 mg. For the "Act-O-Vial" containers, press the plastic activator down to force the diluent into the lower chamber. Agitate gently to dissolve the drug. When reconstituted, each milliliter of solution contains (1):

Component	100 mg	250, 500, 1000 mg
Hydrocortisone equivalent (as sodium succinate)	50 mg	125 mg
Monobasic sodium phosphate anhydrous	0.4 mg	1 mg
Dibasic sodium phosphate dried	4.38 mg	11 mg
Benzyl alcohol	~9 mg	~8.3 mg
Water for injection	qs	qs

The pH has been adjusted when necessary with sodium hydroxide.

pH — From 7 to 8. (1; 4)

Osmolality — The osmolality of hydrocortisone sodium succinate (Abbott) 50 mg/mL was determined to be 292 mOsm/kg by freezing-point depression and 260 mOsm/kg by vapor pressure. (1071)

Sodium Content — Hydrocortisone sodium succinate contains 2.066 mEq of sodium per gram of drug. (846)

Trade Name(s) — Solu-Cortef.

Administration — Hydrocortisone sodium succinate may be administered by intramuscular injection, direct intravenous injection over 30 seconds to several minutes, or continuous or intermittent intravenous infusion at a concentration of 0.1 to 1 mg/mL in a compatible infusion solution. Benzyl alcohol-containing products should not be used in premature infants. (1; 4)

Stability — Hydrocortisone sodium succinate in intact containers should be stored at controlled room temperatures of 20 to 25 °C. (1) After reconstitution, solutions are stable at controlled room temperature or below if protected from light. The solution should only be used if it is clear. Unused solutions should be discarded after three days. Hydrocortisone sodium succinate is heat labile and must not be autoclaved. (1; 4)

pH Effects — Hydrocortisone sodium succinate is optimally stable at pH 7 to 8. It is stable for 72 hours at pH 6 and for 12 hours at pH 5. More acidic solutions cause precipitation. (41)

Solutions of hydrocortisone buffered to pH 9.1 showed oxidation to 21-dehydrocortisone at rates of 1.6 to 2.8%/hr at 26 °C. This rate is four or five times greater than that observed at pH 6.9 to 7.9. (531)

Freezing Solutions — Hydrocortisone sodium succinate (Upjohn) 500-mg/4 mL reconstituted solution exhibited no loss over four weeks when stored frozen. (69)

Intrathecal Injections — In a study of solutions for intrathecal injection, hydrocortisone sodium succinate (Upjohn) was reconstituted to a concentration of 1 mg/mL with Elliott's B solution (295 mOsm/kg, pH 7.3), sodium chloride 0.9% (296 mOsm/kg, pH 7), and Ringer's injection, lactated (258 mOsm/kg, pH 7). In Ringer's injection, lactated, and sodium chloride 0.9%, no decomposition was observed in 24 hours at room temperature under fluorescent light or at 30 °C. However, in seven days, approximately 10% decomposition occurred at room temperature and about 15% at 30 °C. In Elliott's B solution, hydrocortisone sodium succinate is much less stable. In 24 hours, a 7% loss occurred at room temperature and a 12% loss occurred at 30 °C, increasing to 21 and 32%, respectively, at 72 hours. Less than 10% decomposition of this combination occurred in four to eight hours. (327)

In another study, the stability and compatibility of cytarabine (Upjohn), methotrexate (NCI), and hydrocortisone (Upjohn), mixed together in intrathecal injections, were evaluated. Two combinations were tested: (1) cytarabine 50 mg, methotrexate 12 mg (as the sodium salt), and hydrocortisone 25 mg (as the sodium succinate salt); and (2) cytarabine 30 mg, methotrexate 12 mg (as the sodium salt), and hydrocortisone 15 mg (as the sodium succinate salt). Each drug combination was added to 12 mL of Elliott's B solution (NCI), sodium chloride 0.9% (Abbott), dextrose 5% (Abbott), and Ringer's injection, lactated (Abbott), and stored for 24 hours at 25 °C. Cytarabine and methotrexate were both chemically stable, with no drug loss after the full 24 hours in all solutions. Hydrocortisone was also stable in the sodium chloride 0.9%, dextrose 5%, and Ringer's injection, lactated, with about a 2% drug loss. However, in Elliott's B solution, hydrocortisone was significantly less stable, with a 6% loss in the 25-mg concentration over 24 hours. The 15-mg concentration was worse, with a 5% loss in 10 hours and a 13% loss in 24 hours. The higher pH of Elliott's B solution and the lower concentration of hydrocortisone may have been factors in this increased decomposition. All mixtures were physically compatible for 24 hours, but a precipitate formed after several days of storage. (819)

Hydrocortisone sodium succinate (Upjohn) 2 mg/mL diluted in Elliott's B solution (Orphan Medical) was packaged as 20 mL in 30-mL glass vials and 20-mL plastic syringes (Becton Dickinson) with Red Cap (Burron) Luer-lok syringe tip caps. The solution was physically compatible and chemically stable exhibiting about 9% or less loss in 24 hours at 23 °C and 7% or less loss in 48 hours at 4 °C. (1976)

Bacterially contaminated intrathecal solutions could pose grave risks and, consequently, such solutions should be administered as soon as possible after preparation. (328)

Syringes — Hydrocortisone sodium succinate (Upjohn) 10 mg/mL in sodium chloride 0.9% was packaged in polypropylene syringes (Becton Dickinson) and stored under refrigeration at 5 °C and at room temperature of 25 °C. The drug solution remained clear throughout the study, and about 2% hydrocortisone loss occurred after 21 days under refrigeration. At room temperature, about 5% loss occurred in three days and 10% loss occurred in seven days. Stability in glass containers was found to be comparable. (2331)

Hydrocortisone sodium succinate (Pharmacia) 50 mg/mL in sterile water for injection packaged in polypropylene syringes (Braun) was visually compatible with calculated shelf lives of 6.8 days at room temperature and 81 days under refrigeration. (2654)

Sorption — Hydrocortisone sodium succinate was shown not to exhibit sorption to PVC bags and tubing, polyethylene tubing, Silastic tubing, and polypropylene syringes. (12; 536; 606)

Filtration — Hydrocortisone sodium succinate (Upjohn) 10 mg/L in dextrose 5% and sodium chloride 0.9% did not display significant sorption to a 0.45-μm cellulose membrane filter (Abbott S-A-I-F) during an eight-hour simulated infusion. (567)

Central Venous Catheter — Hydrocortisone sodium succinate (Abbott) 1 mg/mL in dextrose 5% was found to be compatible with the AR-ROWg+ard Blue Plus (Arrow International) chlorhexidine-bearing triple-lumen central catheter. Essentially complete delivery of the drug was found with little or no drug loss occurring. Furthermore, chlorhexidine delivered from the catheter remained at trace amounts with no substantial increase due to the delivery of the drug through the catheter. (2335)

Compatibility Information

Solution Compatibility

Hydrocortisone sodium succinate

Solution	Mfr	Mfr	Conc/L	Remarks	Ref	C/I
Dextrose–Ringer's injection combinations	AB	UP	250 mg	Physically compatible	3	C
Dextrose–Ringer's injection, lactated, combinations	AB	UP	250 mg	Physically compatible	3	C
Dextrose 5% in Ringer's injection, lactated	TR[a]	UP	500 mg	Stable for 24 hr at 5 °C	282	C
	BA	UP	600 mg	Physically compatible for 24 hr	315	C
Dextrose–saline combinations	AB	UP	250 mg	Physically compatible	3	C
Dextrose 5% in sodium chloride 0.9%		UP	100, 200, 300 mg	Stable for 48 hr	43	C
	AB	UP	250 mg	Stable for 48 hr	46	C
		UP	100 mg	Physically compatible	74	C
	TR[a]	UP	500 mg	Stable for 24 hr at 5 °C	282	C
	BA	UP	600 mg	Physically compatible for 24 hr	315	C
Dextrose 2.5%	AB	UP	250 mg	Physically compatible	3	C
Dextrose 5%	AB	UP	250 mg	Physically compatible	3	C
	AB	UP	250 mg	Stable for 48 hr	46	C
		UP	100 mg	Physically compatible	74	C
	TR[a]	UP	500 mg	Stable for 24 hr at 5 °C	282	C
	BA	UP	600 mg	Physically compatible for 24 hr	315	C
Dextrose 10%	AB	UP	250 mg	Physically compatible	3	C
	BA	UP	600 mg	Physically compatible for 24 hr	315	C
Dextrose 20%	BA	UP	600 mg	Physically compatible for 24 hr	315	C
Ionosol products	AB	UP	250 mg	Physically compatible	3	C
Ringer's injection	AB	UP	250 mg	Physically compatible	3	C
Ringer's injection, lactated	AB	UP	250 mg	Physically compatible	3	C
		UP	100 mg	Physically compatible	74	C
	TR[a]	UP	500 mg	Stable for 24 hr at 5 °C	282	C
	BA	UP	600 mg	Physically compatible for 24 hr	315	C
Sodium chloride 0.45%	AB	UP	250 mg	Physically compatible	74	C
Sodium chloride 0.9%	AB	UP	250 mg	Physically compatible	3	C
	AB	UP	250 mg	Stable for 48 hr	46	C
		UP	100 mg	Physically compatible	74	C
	TR[a]	UP	500 mg	Stable for 24 hr at 5 °C	282	C
	BA	UP	600 mg	Physically compatible for 24 hr	315	C
	[b]	PH	1 g	Visually compatible. Calculated shelf lives of 7 days at room temperature and 41 days (PVC) and 48 days (polyolefin) under refrigeration	2654	C

Solution Compatibility (Cont.)

Hydrocortisone sodium succinate

Solution	Mfr	Mfr	Conc/L	Remarks	Ref	C/I
Sodium lactate ⅙ M	AB	UP	250 mg	Physically compatible	3	C
	BA	UP	600 mg	Physically compatible for 24 hr	315	C

[a]Tested in both glass and PVC containers.
[b]Tested in PVC (Baxter) and polyolefin (Fresenius Kabi) containers.

Additive Compatibility

Hydrocortisone sodium succinate

Drug	Mfr	Conc/L	Mfr	Conc/L	Test Soln	Remarks	Ref	C/I
Amikacin sulfate	BR	5 g	UP	200 mg	D5LR, D5R, D5S, D5W, D10W, LR, NS, R, SL	Physically compatible and both stable for 24 hr at 25 °C	294	C
Aminophylline		250 mg	UP	100 mg	D5W	Physically compatible	74	C
	SE	1 g	UP	500 mg	D5W	Physically compatible	15	C
	SE	500 mg	UP	100 mg		Physically compatible	6	C
		625 mg		250 mg	D5W	Physically compatible and aminophylline stable for 24 hr at 4 and 30 °C. Total hydrocortisone content changed little but substantial ester hydrolysis	521	C
Amphotericin B	SQ	100 mg	UP	500 mg	D5W	Physically compatible	15	C
	SQ	70 and 140 mg		50 mg	D5W	Bioactivity not significantly affected over 24 hr at 25 °C	335	C
Ampicillin sodium	BR	1 g		200 and 400 mg	LR	Ampicillin stable for 24 hr at 25 °C	87	C
	BR	1 g		1.8 g	D5S, D5W, D10W, IM, IP, LR, NS	Ampicillin stable for 24 hr at 4 °C	87	C
	BR	1 g		50 and 100 mg	LR	14% ampicillin loss in 12 hr at 25 °C	87	I
	BR	1 g		1.8 g	D5S, D10W, IM, IP, LR	11 to 28% ampicillin loss in 24 hr at 25 °C	87	I
	BE	20 g		200 mg	NS	18% ampicillin loss in 6 hr at 25 °C	89	I
	BE	20 g		200 mg	D5W	23% ampicillin loss in 6 hr at 25 °C	89	I
	BE	20 g		200 mg	D–S	32% ampicillin loss in 6 hr at 25 °C	89	I
Antithymocyte globulin (rabbit)[c]	SGS	200 and 300 mg	PHU	50 mg	D5W	Immediate haze and precipitation	2488	I
	SGS	200 and 300 mg	PHU	50 mg	NS	Physically compatible for 24 hr at 23 °C	2488	C
Ascorbic acid	UP		UP			Concentration-dependent incompatibility	15	I
Bleomycin sulfate	BR	20 and 30 units	AB	300 mg, 750 mg, 1 g, 2.5 g	NS	60 to 100% loss of bleomycin activity in 1 week at 4 °C	763	I

Additive Compatibility (Cont.)

Hydrocortisone sodium succinate

Drug	Mfr	Conc/L	Mfr	Conc/L	Test Soln	Remarks	Ref	C/I
Calcium chloride	UP	1 g	UP	500 mg	D5W	Physically compatible	15	**C**
Calcium gluconate		1 g	UP	100 mg	D5W	Physically compatible	74	**C**
	UP	1 g	UP	500 mg	D5W	Physically compatible	15	**C**
Chloramphenicol sodium succinate	PD	500 mg	UP	100 mg	D5W	Physically compatible	74	**C**
	PD	10 g	UP	500 mg	D5W	Physically compatible	15	**C**
	PD	1 g	UP	500 mg		Physically compatible	6	**C**
Clindamycin phosphate	UP	1.2 g	UP	1 g	W	Clindamycin stable for 24 hr	101	**C**
Cloxacillin sodium	BE	20 g	GL	200 mg	D5S, D5W, NS	Physically compatible and cloxacillin stable for 24 hr at 25 °C	89	**C**
Colistimethate sodium	WC	500 mg	UP	500 mg	D5W	Physically incompatible	15	**I**
Cytarabine	UP	360 mg	UP	500 mg	D5S, D10S	Physically compatible for 40 hr	174	**C**
	UP	360 mg	UP	500 mg	R, SL	Physically incompatible	174	**I**
Daunorubicin HCl	FA	200 mg	UP	500 mg	D5W	Physically compatible	15	**C**
Dimenhydrinate	SE	50 mg	UP	100 mg	D5W	Physically compatible	74	**C**
	SE	500 mg	UP	500 mg	D5W	Physically incompatible	15	**I**
Dopamine HCl	AS	800 mg	UP	1 g	D5W	No dopamine loss in 18 hr at 25 °C	312	**C**
Erythromycin lactobionate	AB	5 g	UP	500 mg	D5W	Physically compatible	15	**C**
	AB	1 g	UP	250 mg		Physically compatible	20	**C**
Fat emulsion, intravenous	VT	10%	RS	160 mg		Physically compatible for 24 hr at 8 and 25 °C	825	**C**
Floxacillin sodium	BE	20 g	UP	50 g	NS	Physically compatible for 72 hr at 15 and 30 °C	1479	**C**
Furosemide		200 and 400 mg		1 g	D5W, NS	6 to 8% hydrocortisone loss and 5 to 6% furosemide loss in 24 hr at 25 °C	1348	**C**
		200 and 400 mg		300 mg	D5W, NS	6 to 8% hydrocortisone loss in 6 hr and 10 to 14% loss in 24 hr at 25 °C. 5 to 6% furosemide loss in 24 hr	1348	**I**
	HO	1 g	UP	50 g	NS	Physically compatible for 72 hr at 15 and 30 °C	1479	**C**
Heparin sodium		32,000 units		800 mg	NS	Physically compatible and heparin activity retained for 24 hr	57	**C**
	UP	4000 units	UP	500 mg	D5W	Physically incompatible	15	**I**
		12,000 units	UP	100 mg	D5W	Precipitates immediately	74	**I**
Hydralazine HCl	BP	80 mg	BP	400 mg	D5W	Yellow color produced	26	**I**
Lidocaine HCl	AST	2 g	UP	250 mg		Physically compatible	24	**C**
Magnesium sulfate	ES	750 mg	UP	100 mg	AA 3.5%, D 25%	Physically compatible	302	**C**
Metronidazole	SE	5 g	ES	10 g		No loss of either drug in 7 days at 25 °C and 12 days at 5 °C	993	**C**
Mitomycin	BR	1 g	AB	33.3 g	W[b]	Visually compatible. 10% calculated loss of mitomycin in 172 hr and hydrocortisone in 212 hr at 25 °C	1866	**C**

Additive Compatibility (Cont.)

Hydrocortisone sodium succinate

Drug	Mfr	Conc/L	Mfr	Conc/L	Test Soln	Remarks	Ref	C/I
	BR	1 g	AB	33.3 g	W[a]	Visually compatible. 10% calculated loss of mitomycin in 206 hr and hydrocortisone in 218 hr at 25 °C	1866	C
	BR	1 g	AB	33.3 g	W[b]	Visually compatible. 10% calculated loss of mitomycin in 1423 hr and hydrocortisone in 176 hr at 4 °C	1866	C
	BR	1 g	AB	33.3 g	W[a]	Visually compatible. 10% calculated loss of mitomycin in 820 hr and hydrocortisone in 807 hr at 4 °C	1866	C
Mitoxantrone HCl	LE	50 to 200 mg		100 mg to 2 g	D5W, NS[a]	Physically compatible and both drugs stable for 24 hr at room temperature	1293	C
Nafcillin sodium	WY	500 mg	UP	250 mg		Precipitate forms within 1 hr	27	I
Norepinephrine bitartrate	WI	8 mg	UP	100 mg	D5W	Physically compatible	74	C
Penicillin G potassium		1 million units	UP	100 mg	D5W	Physically compatible	74	C
	SQ	20 million units	UP	500 mg	D5W	Physically compatible	15	C
	SQ	5 million units	UP	250 mg	D	Physically compatible	47	C
Penicillin G sodium	UP	20 million units	UP	500 mg	D5W	Physically compatible	15	C
Pentobarbital sodium	AB	1 g	UP	500 mg	D5W	Physically incompatible	15	I
Phenobarbital sodium	WI	200 mg	UP	500 mg	D5W	Physically incompatible	15	I
Polymyxin B sulfate	BW	200 mg	UP	500 mg	D5W	Physically compatible	15	C
Potassium chloride		3 g	UP	100 mg	D5W	Physically compatible	74	C
Promethazine HCl	WY	250 mg	UP	500 mg	D5W	Physically incompatible	15	I
Vancomycin HCl	LI	1 g	UP	100 mg	D5W	Physically compatible	74	C
Verapamil HCl	KN	80 mg	UP	200 mg	D5W, NS	Physically compatible for 24 hr	764	C

[a]Tested in PVC containers.
[b]Tested in glass containers.
[c]Heparin sodium (Elkins-Sinn) 2000 units/L was also present.

Drugs in Syringe Compatibility

Hydrocortisone sodium succinate

Drug (in syringe)	Mfr	Amt	Mfr	Amt	Remarks	Ref	C/I
Dimenhydrinate		10 mg/ 1 mL		125 mg/ 1 mL	Clear solution	2569	C
Doxapram HCl	RB	400 mg/ 20 mL	UP	500 mg/ 2 mL	Immediate turbidity and precipitation	1177	I
Iohexol	WI	64.7%, 5 mL	UP	10 mg/ 1 mL	Physically compatible for at least 2 hr	1438	C

Drugs in Syringe Compatibility (Cont.)

Hydrocortisone sodium succinate

Drug (in syringe)	Mfr	Amt	Mfr	Amt	Remarks	Ref	C/I
Iopamidol	SQ	61%, 5 mL	UP	10 mg/ 1 mL	Physically compatible for at least 2 hr	1438	**C**
Iothalamate meglumine	MA	60%, 5 mL	UP	10 mg/ 1 mL	Physically compatible for at least 2 hr	1438	**C**
Ioxaglate meglumine–ioxaglate sodium	MA	5 mL	UP	10 mg/ 1 mL	Physically compatible for at least 2 hr	1438	**C**
Magnesium sulfate	ES	500 mg/ mL	UP	100 mg/ 2 mL	White precipitate formed	302	**I**
Pantoprazole sodium	[a]	4 mg/ 1 mL		125 mg/ 1 mL	Possible precipitate within 15 min	2574	**I**

[a]Test performed using the formulation WITHOUT edetate disodium.

Y-Site Injection Compatibility (1:1 Mixture)

Hydrocortisone sodium succinate

Drug	Mfr	Conc	Mfr	Conc	Remarks	Ref	C/I
Acyclovir sodium	BW	5 mg/mL[a]	LY	1 mg/mL[a]	Physically compatible for 4 hr at 25 °C	1157	**C**
Allopurinol sodium	BW	3 mg/mL[b]	UP	1 mg/mL[b]	Physically compatible for 4 hr at 22 °C	1686	**C**
Amifostine	USB	10 mg/mL[a]	UP	1 mg/mL[a]	Physically compatible for 4 hr at 23 °C	1845	**C**
Aminophylline	SE	25 mg/mL	UP	100 mg/L[c]	Physically compatible for 4 hr at room temperature	322	**C**
Amphotericin B cholesteryl sulfate complex	SEQ	0.83 mg/mL[a]	AB	1 mg/mL[a]	Physically compatible for 4 hr at 23 °C	2117	**C**
Ampicillin sodium	BR	25, 50, 100, 125 mg/mL	UP	100 mg/L[c]	Physically compatible for 4 hr at room temperature	322	**C**
Amsacrine	NCI	1 mg/mL[a]	UP	1 mg/mL[a]	Visually compatible for 4 hr at 22 °C	1381	**C**
Anidulafungin	VIC	0.5 mg/mL[a]	PHU	1 mg/mL[a]	Physically compatible for 4 hr at 23 °C	2617	**C**
Antithymocyte globulin (rabbit)	SGS	0.2 and 0.3 mg/mL[a,b]	PHU	0.5 mg/mL[a,b]	Physically compatible for 4 hr at 23 °C	2488	**C**
	SGS	0.2 and 0.3 mg/mL[a,b]	PHU	1 mg/mL[a,b]	Physically compatible for 4 hr at 23 °C	2488	**C**
Argatroban	GSK	1 mg/mL[b]	PHU	50 mg/mL	Visually compatible for 24 hr at 23 °C	2391	**C**
Atracurium besylate	BW	0.5 mg/mL[a]	AB	1 mg/mL[a]	Physically compatible for 24 hr at 28 °C	1337	**C**
Atropine sulfate	BW	0.5 mg/mL	UP	10 mg/L[d]	Physically compatible for 4 hr at room temperature	534	**C**
Aztreonam	SQ	40 mg/mL[a]	UP	1 mg/mL[a]	Physically compatible for 4 hr at 23 °C	1758	**C**
Bivalirudin	TMC	5 mg/mL[a]	PHU	1 mg/mL[a]	Physically compatible for 4 hr at 23 °C	2373	**C**
	TMC	5 mg/mL[a,b]	PHU	50 mg/mL	Visually compatible for 6 hr at 23 °C	2680	**C**
Calcium gluconate	ES	100 mg/mL	UP	100 mg/L[c]	Physically compatible for 4 hr at room temperature	322	**C**
Caspofungin acetate	ME	0.7 mg/mL[b]	HOS	1 mg/mL[b]	Physically compatible for 4 hr at room temperature	2758	**C**
Ceftaroline fosamil	FOR	2.22 mg/ mL[a,b,h]	PF	1 mg/mL[a,b,h]	Physically compatible for 4 hr at 23 °C	2826	**C**

Y-Site Injection Compatibility (1:1 Mixture) (Cont.)

Hydrocortisone sodium succinate

Drug	Mfr	Conc	Mfr	Conc	Remarks	Ref	C/I
Chlorpromazine HCl	SKF	25 mg/mL	UP	10 mg/L[d]	Physically compatible for 4 hr at room temperature	534	C
Ciprofloxacin	MI	2 mg/mL[e]	UP	50 mg/mL	Transient cloudiness rapidly dissipates. Crystals form in 1 hr at 24 °C	1655	I
Cisatracurium besylate	GW	0.1, 2, 5 mg/mL[a]	AB	1 mg/mL[a]	Physically compatible for 4 hr at 23 °C	2074	C
Cladribine	ORT	0.015[b] and 0.5[f] mg/mL	UP	1 mg/mL[b]	Physically compatible for 4 hr at 23 °C	1969	C
Cyanocobalamin	PD	0.1 mg/mL	UP	10 mg/L[d]	Physically compatible for 4 hr at room temperature	534	C
Cytarabine	UP	16 mg/mL[b]	UP	125 mg/mL	Visually compatible for 24 hr at room temperature in test tubes. No precipitate found on filter from Y-site delivery	2063	C
Dacarbazine					Pink precipitate forms immediately	524	I
Dexamethasone sodium phosphate	MSD	4 mg/mL	UP	100 mg/L[c]	Physically compatible for 4 hr at room temperature	322	C
Diazepam	RC	5 mg/mL	UP	100 mg/L[c]	Immediate haziness and globule formation	322	I
Digoxin	BW	0.25 mg/mL	UP	100 mg/L[c]	Physically compatible for 4 hr at room temperature	322	C
Diltiazem HCl	MMD	5 mg/mL	UP	50 and 125 mg/mL	Precipitate forms but clears with swirling	1807	?
	MMD	1 mg/mL[b]	UP	50 and 125 mg/mL	Visually compatible	1807	C
	MMD	5 mg/mL	UP	1[b] and 2[a] mg/mL	Visually compatible	1807	C
Diphenhydramine HCl	PD	50 mg/mL	UP	10 mg/L[d]	Physically compatible for 4 hr at room temperature	534	C
Docetaxel	RPR	0.9 mg/mL[a]	AB	1 mg/mL[a]	Physically compatible for 4 hr at 23 °C	2224	C
Dopamine HCl	ACC	40 mg/mL	UP	10 mg/L[d]	Physically compatible for 4 hr at room temperature	534	C
Doripenem	JJ	5 mg/mL[a,b]	PHU	1 mg/mL[a,b]	Physically compatible for 4 hr at 23 °C	2743	C
Doxorubicin HCl liposomal	SEQ	0.4 mg/mL[a]	AB	1 mg/mL[a]	Physically compatible for 4 hr at 23 °C	2087	C
Droperidol	CR	1.25 mg/mL	UP	10 mg/L[d]	Physically compatible for 4 hr at room temperature	534	C
Edrophonium chloride	RC	10 mg/mL	UP	10 mg/L[d]	Physically compatible for 4 hr at room temperature	534	C
Enalaprilat	MSD	0.05 mg/mL[b]	UP	2 mg/mL[a]	Physically compatible for 24 hr at room temperature under fluorescent light	1355	C
Epinephrine HCl	AB	0.1 mg/mL	UP	10 mg/L[d]	Physically compatible for 4 hr at room temperature	534	C
Esmolol HCl	DCC	10 mg/mL[a]	LY	1 mg/mL[a]	Physically compatible for 24 hr at 22 °C	1169	C
Estrogens, conjugated	AY	5 mg/mL	UP	100 mg/L[c]	Physically compatible for 4 hr at room temperature	322	C
Ethacrynate sodium	MSD	1 mg/mL	UP	100 mg/L[c]	Physically compatible for 4 hr at room temperature	322	C
Etoposide phosphate	BR	5 mg/mL[a]	UP	1 mg/mL[a]	Physically compatible for 4 hr at 23 °C	2218	C

Y-Site Injection Compatibility (1:1 Mixture) (Cont.)

Hydrocortisone sodium succinate

Drug	Mfr	Conc	Mfr	Conc	Remarks	Ref	C/I
Famotidine	MSD	0.2 mg/mL[a]	AB	1 mg/mL[a]	Physically compatible for 4 hr at 25 °C	1188	**C**
	MSD	0.2 mg/mL[a]	AB	125 mg/mL	Physically compatible for 14 hr	1196	**C**
Fenoldopam mesylate	AB	80 mcg/mL[b]	PHU	1 mg/mL[b]	Physically compatible for 4 hr at 23 °C	2467	**C**
Fentanyl citrate	MN	0.05 mg/mL	UP	10 mg/L[d]	Physically compatible for 4 hr at room temperature	534	**C**
Filgrastim	AMG	30 mcg/mL[a]	UP	1 mg/mL[a]	Physically compatible for 4 hr at 22 °C	1687	**C**
Fludarabine phosphate	BX	1 mg/mL[a]	UP	1 mg/mL[a]	Visually compatible for 4 hr at 22 °C	1439	**C**
Fluorouracil	RC	50 mg/mL	UP	10 mg/L[d]	Physically compatible for 4 hr at room temperature	534	**C**
Foscarnet sodium	AST	24 mg/mL	UP	50 mg/mL	Physically compatible for 24 hr at room temperature under fluorescent light	1335	**C**
Furosemide	HO	10 mg/mL	UP	10 mg/L[d]	Physically compatible for 4 hr at room temperature	534	**C**
Gallium nitrate	FUJ	1 mg/mL[b]	AB	50 mg/mL	Visually compatible for 24 hr at 25 °C	1673	**C**
Gemcitabine HCl	LI	10 mg/mL[b]	UP	1 mg/mL[b]	Physically compatible for 4 hr at 23 °C	2226	**C**
Granisetron HCl	SKB	0.05 mg/mL[a]	AB	1 mg/mL[a]	Physically compatible for 4 hr at 23 °C	2000	**C**
Heparin sodium	TR	50 units/mL	UP	2 mg/mL[b]	Visually compatible for 4 hr at 25 °C	1793	**C**
	ES	100 units/mL[e]	UP	125 mg/mL	Visually compatible for 24 hr at room temperature in test tubes. No precipitate found on filter from Y-site delivery	2063	**C**
Hetastarch in lactated electrolyte	AB	6%	PHU	1 mg/mL[a]	Physically compatible for 4 hr at 23 °C	2339	**C**
Hydralazine HCl	CI	20 mg/mL	UP	10 mg/L[d]	Physically compatible for 4 hr at room temperature	534	**C**
Idarubicin HCl	AD	1 mg/mL[b]	UP	2[a] and 50 mg/mL	Haze forms immediately and precipitate forms in 20 min	1525	**I**
Isoproterenol HCl	WI	0.2 mg/mL	UP	10 mg/L[d]	Physically compatible for 4 hr at room temperature	534	**C**
Lidocaine HCl	AST	20 mg/mL	UP	100 mg/L[c]	Physically compatible for 4 hr at room temperature	322	**C**
Linezolid	PHU	2 mg/mL	UP	1 mg/mL[a]	Physically compatible for 4 hr at 23 °C	2264	**C**
Lorazepam	WY	0.33 mg/mL[b]	UP	50 mg/mL	Visually compatible for 24 hr at 22 °C	1855	**C**
Magnesium sulfate	AB	500 mg/mL	UP	10 mg/L[d]	Physically compatible for 4 hr at room temperature	534	**C**
Melphalan HCl	BW	0.1 mg/mL[b]	UP	1 mg/mL[b]	Physically compatible for 3 hr at 22 °C	1557	**C**
Meperidine HCl	AB	10 mg/mL	AB	2 mg/mL[a]	Physically compatible for 4 hr at 25 °C	1397	**C**
Methylergonovine maleate	SZ	0.2 mg/mL	UP	10 mg/L[d]	Physically compatible for 4 hr at room temperature	534	**C**
Midazolam HCl	RC	5 mg/mL	UP	50 mg/mL	White precipitate forms immediately	1855	**I**
Morphine sulfate	WY	15 mg/mL	UP	10 mg/L[d]	Physically compatible for 4 hr at room temperature	534	**C**
Neostigmine methylsulfate	RC	0.5 mg/mL	UP	10 mg/L[d]	Physically compatible for 4 hr at room temperature	534	**C**
Nicardipine HCl	DCC	0.1 mg/mL[a]	UP	2 mg/mL[a]	Visually compatible for 24 hr at room temperature	235	**C**

Y-Site Injection Compatibility (1:1 Mixture) (Cont.)

Hydrocortisone sodium succinate

Drug	Mfr	Conc	Mfr	Conc	Remarks	Ref	C/I
Norepinephrine bitartrate	WI	1 mg/mL	UP	10 mg/L[d]	Physically compatible for 4 hr at room temperature	534	C
Ondansetron HCl	GL	1 mg/mL[b]	UP	1 mg/mL[a]	Visually compatible for 4 hr at 22 °C	1365	C
Oxacillin sodium	BR	100 mg/mL	UP	10 mg/L[d]	Physically compatible for 4 hr at room temperature	534	C
Oxaliplatin	SS	0.5 mg/mL[a]	PHU	1 mg/mL[a]	Physically compatible for 4 hr at 23 °C	2566	C
Oxytocin	SZ	1 unit/mL	UP	10 mg/L[d]	Physically compatible for 4 hr at room temperature	534	C
Paclitaxel	NCI	1.2 mg/mL[a]	AB	1 mg/mL[a]	Physically compatible for 4 hr at 22 °C	1556	C
Pancuronium bromide	ES	0.05 mg/mL[a]	AB	1 mg/mL[a]	Physically compatible for 24 hr at 28 °C	1337	C
Penicillin G potassium	LI	200,000 units/mL	UP	100 mg/L[c]	Physically compatible for 4 hr at room temperature	322	C
Pentazocine lactate	WI	30 mg/mL	UP	10 mg/L[d]	Physically compatible for 4 hr at room temperature	534	C
Phenytoin sodium	PD	50 mg/mL	UP	100 mg/L[c]	Immediate crystal formation	322	I
Phytonadione	RC	10 mg/mL	UP	10 mg/L[d]	Physically compatible for 4 hr at room temperature	534	C
Piperacillin sodium–tazobactam sodium	LE[k]	40 + 5 mg/mL[a]	UP	1 mg/mL[a]	Physically compatible for 4 hr at 22 °C	1688	C
Procainamide HCl	SQ	100 mg/mL	UP	10 mg/L[d]	Physically compatible for 4 hr at room temperature	534	C
Prochlorperazine edisylate	SKF	5 mg/mL	UP	10 mg/L[d]	Physically compatible for 4 hr at room temperature	534	C
Promethazine HCl	SV	50 mg/mL	UP	10 mg/L[l]	Physically compatible for 4 hr at room temperature	534	C
	SV	50 mg/mL	UP	10 mg/L[g]	Clear initially, but cloudiness develops in 4 hr at room temperature	534	I
Propofol	ZEN	10 mg/mL	UP	1 mg/mL[a]	Physically compatible for 1 hr at 23 °C	2066	C
Propranolol HCl	AY	1 mg/mL	UP	10 mg/L[d]	Physically compatible for 4 hr at room temperature	534	C
Remifentanil HCl	GW	0.025 and 0.25 mg/mL[b]	AB	1 mg/mL[a]	Physically compatible for 4 hr at 23 °C	2075	C
Sargramostim	IMM	10 mcg/mL[b]	UP	1 mg/mL[b]	Few small particles in 1 hr	1436	I
Scopolamine HBr	BW	0.86 mg/mL	UP	10 mg/L[d]	Physically compatible for 4 hr at room temperature	534	C
Sodium bicarbonate	BR	75 mg/mL	UP	100 mg/L[c]	Physically compatible for 4 hr at room temperature	322	C
Succinylcholine chloride	BW	20 mg/mL	UP	100 mg/L[c]	Physically compatible for 4 hr at room temperature	322	C
Tacrolimus	FUJ	1 mg/mL[b]	AB	50 mg/mL[a]	Visually compatible for 24 hr at 25 °C	1630	C
Telavancin HCl	ASP	7.5 mg/mL[a,b,h]	PF	1 mg/mL[a,b,h]	Physically compatible for 2 hr	2830	C
Teniposide	BR	0.1 mg/mL[a]	UP	1 mg/mL[a]	Physically compatible for 4 hr at 23 °C	1725	C
Theophylline	TR	4 mg/mL	UP	2 mg/mL[a]	Visually compatible for 6 hr at 25 °C	1793	C

Y-Site Injection Compatibility (1:1 Mixture) (Cont.)

Hydrocortisone sodium succinate

Drug	Mfr	Conc	Mfr	Conc	Remarks	Ref	C/I
Thiotepa	IMM[i]	1 mg/mL[a]	UP	1 mg/mL[a]	Physically compatible for 4 hr at 23 °C	1861	C
TNA #218 to #226[j]			AB	1 mg/mL[a]	Visually compatible for 4 hr at 23 °C	2215	C
TPN #189[j]			UP	50 mg/mL[b]	Visually compatible for 24 hr at 22 °C	1767	C
TPN #212 to #215[j]			AB	1 mg/mL[a]	Physically compatible for 4 hr at 23 °C	2109	C
Trimethobenzamide HCl	RC	100 mg/mL	UP	10 mg/L[d]	Physically compatible for 4 hr at room temperature	534	C
Vecuronium bromide	OR	0.1 mg/mL[a]	AB	1 mg/mL[a]	Physically compatible for 24 hr at 28 °C	1337	C
Vinorelbine tartrate	BW	1 mg/mL[b]	UP	1 mg/mL[b]	Physically compatible for 4 hr at 22 °C	1558	C

[a]*Tested in dextrose 5%.*
[b]*Tested in sodium chloride 0.9%.*
[c]*Tested in combination with heparin sodium (Riker) 1000 units/L in dextrose 5%, sodium chloride 0.9%, and Ringer's injection, lactated.*
[d]*Tested in dextrose 5% in Ringer's injection, dextrose 5% in Ringer's injection, lactated, dextrose 5%, Ringer's injection, lactated, and sodium chloride 0.9%.*
[e]*Tested in both dextrose 5% and sodium chloride 0.9%.*
[f]*Tested in bacteriostatic sodium chloride 0.9% preserved with benzyl alcohol 0.9%.*
[g]*Tested in dextrose 5% in Ringer's injection.*
[h]*Tested in Ringer's injection, lactated.*
[i]*Lyophilized formulation tested.*
[j]*Refer to Appendix I for the composition of parenteral nutrition solutions. TNA indicates a 3-in-1 admixture, and TPN indicates a 2-in-1 admixture.*
[k]*Test performed using the formulation WITHOUT edetate disodium.*
[l]*Tested in dextrose 5% in Ringer's injection, lactated, dextrose 5%, Ringer's injection, lactated, and sodium chloride 0.9%.*

HYDROMORPHONE HYDROCHLORIDE
AHFS 28:08.08

Products — Hydromorphone hydrochloride is available in 1-mL ampuls and 20-mL multiple-dose vials. In ampuls, each milliliter of the solution contains hydromorphone hydrochloride 1, 2, or 4 mg with sodium citrate 0.2% and citric acid 0.2%. In vials, each milliliter of the solution contains hydromorphone hydrochloride 2 mg, edetate disodium 0.5 mg, methylparaben 1.8 mg, and propylparaben 0.2 mg. Sodium hydroxide or hydrochloric acid may have been used to adjust the pH of the solutions in vials. (1)

Hydromorphone hydrochloride is also available in 1- and 5-mL amber ampuls and 50-mL single-dose vials as a high potency form (Dilaudid-HP). Each milliliter of the solution contains 10 mg of hydromorphone hydrochloride with citric acid 0.2% and sodium citrate 0.2%. (1)

In addition to the liquid dosage forms, high potency hydromorphone hydrochloride (Dilaudid-HP) is available as a 250-mg single-dose vial as a lyophilized powder. Reconstitute with 25 mL of sterile water for injection to yield a 10-mg/mL solution. (1)

pH — From 4 to 5.5. (4)

Trade Name(s) — Dilaudid, Dilaudid-HP.

Administration — Hydromorphone hydrochloride may be administered by subcutaneous, intramuscular, or slow direct intravenous injection over at least two to three minutes. (1; 4)

Stability — Hydromorphone hydrochloride products should be stored at controlled room temperature and protected from light. (1) The liquid dosage forms in intact ampuls or vials should not be stored under refrigeration because of possible precipitation or crystallization. Resolubilization at room temperature or on warming may be performed without affecting the stability of the drug. (593) The manufacturer recommends inspecting for particulate matter or discoloration. A slight yellowish discoloration may develop in both the ampuls and vials, but it has not been associated with drug loss. (1; 4)

Extemporaneously prepared hydromorphone hydrochloride 10 and 50 mg/mL, stored in 100-mL glass vials or PVC bags, exhibited no loss in 42 days at 4 and 23 °C. (1394)

Syringes — Hydromorphone hydrochloride (Knoll) 10 mg/mL undiluted and diluted to 0.1 mg/mL in sodium chloride 0.9% was packaged as 3 mL in 10-mL polypropylene infusion pump syringes (Pharmacia Deltec). No loss occurred over 30 days at 30 °C. (1967)

Hydromorphone hydrochloride 1.5 and 80 mg/mL in sodium chloride 0.9% packaged as 20 mL in 30-mL polypropylene syringes was evaluated for physical and chemical stability. Sample solutions were stored for 60 days at 4 °C protected from light and 23 °C exposed to normal fluorescent light. Other sample solutions were stored frozen at −20 °C and at elevated temperature of 37 °C for two days to simulate more extreme conditions during express shipping. About 2 to 5% loss occurred in 60 days at 4 and 23 °C. The frozen and 37 °C samples exhibited little change in concentration in two days. However, samples stored frozen at −20 °C exhibited the formation of microparticulates in the thousands per milliliter, possibly shed by the syringe components. (2377)

Implantable Pumps — The stability of hydromorphone hydrochloride 2 (Dilaudid) and 10 (Dilaudid-HP) mg/mL was evaluated in

SynchroMed implantable pumps over 16 weeks at 37 °C. Little or no drug loss and no adverse effects on the pumps occurred. (2584)

Central Venous Catheter — Hydromorphone hydrochloride (Knoll) 0.5 mg/mL in dextrose 5% was found to be compatible with the ARROWg+ard Blue Plus (Arrow International) chlorhexidine-bearing triple-lumen central catheter. Essentially complete delivery of the drug was found with little or no drug loss occurring. Furthermore, chlorhexidine delivered from the catheter remained at trace amounts with no substantial increase due to the delivery of the drug through the catheter. (2335)

Compatibility Information

Solution Compatibility

Hydromorphone HCl

Solution	Mfr	Mfr	Conc/L	Remarks	Ref	C/I
Dextrose 5% in Ringer's injection	CU	KN[a]	80 mg	Physically compatible. No loss in 24 hr at 25 °C	572	C
Dextrose 5% in Ringer's injection, lactated	MG	KN[a]	80 mg	Physically compatible. No loss in 24 hr at 25 °C	572	C
Dextrose 5%	TR[b]	KN[a]	80 mg	Physically compatible. No loss in 24 hr at 25 °C	572	C
	MG[c]	KN[a]	80 mg	Physically compatible. No loss in 24 hr at 25 °C	572	C
	[b]	KN	1 and 5 g	No loss in 42 days at 4 and 23 °C	1394	C
Dextrose 5% in sodium chloride 0.45%	MG	KN[a]	80 mg	Physically compatible. No loss in 24 hr at 25 °C	572	C
Dextrose 5% in sodium chloride 0.9%	MG	KN[a]	80 mg	Physically compatible. No loss in 24 hr at 25 °C	572	C
Ringer's injection	MG	KN[a]	80 mg	Physically compatible. No loss in 24 hr at 25 °C	572	C
Ringer's injection, lactated	MG	KN[a]	80 mg	Physically compatible. No loss in 24 hr at 25 °C	572	C
Sodium chloride 0.45%	MG	KN[a]	80 mg	Physically compatible. No loss in 24 hr at 25 °C	572	C
Sodium chloride 0.9%	TR[b]	KN[a]	80 mg	Physically compatible. No loss in 24 hr at 25 °C	572	C
	MG[c]	KN[a]	80 mg	Physically compatible. No loss in 24 hr at 25 °C	572	C
	[b]	KN	1 and 5 g	No loss in 42 days at 4 and 23 °C	1394	C
	AB[b]	KN	20 and 100 mg	Visually compatible. Little or no loss in 72 hr at 24 °C under fluorescent light	1870	C
	BA[d]	[e]	1.5 to 80 g	Physically compatible. 2 to 5% hydromorphone loss in 60 days at 4 °C protected from light and 23 °C under fluorescent light	2377	C
	[f]	BA	200 mg	Under 8% loss in 112 days at 4 and 20 °C	2818	C
Sodium lactate ⅙ M	CU	KN[a]	80 mg	Physically compatible. No loss in 24 hr at 25 °C	572	C

[a] *Both ampul and vial formulations tested.*
[b] *Tested in PVC containers.*
[c] *Tested in polyolefin containers.*
[d] *Tested in polypropylene syringes.*
[e] *Extemporaneously compounded from hydromorphone hydrochloride powder.*
[f] *Tested in PCA injectors.*

Additive Compatibility

Hydromorphone HCl

Drug	Mfr	Conc/L	Mfr	Conc/L	Test Soln	Remarks	Ref	C/I
Bupivacaine HCl	AB	625 mg and 1.25 g	KN	20 mg	NS[a]	Visually compatible with little or no loss of either drug in 72 hr at 24 °C under fluorescent light	1870	C
	AB	625 mg and 1.25 g	KN	100 mg	NS[a]	Visually compatible with little or no loss of either drug in 72 hr at 24 °C under fluorescent light	1870	C
Clonidine HCl	BI	150 mg		25 mg	[b]	No clonidine loss in 35 days at 37 °C	2593	C
Fluorouracil	AB	1 g	AST	500 mg	D5W, NS[a]	Physically compatible. Little loss of either drug in 7 days at 32 °C and 35 days at 23, 4, and −20 °C	1977	C
	AB	16 g	AST	500 mg	D5W, NS[a]	Physically compatible. Little loss of either drug in 3 days at 32 °C, 7 days at 23 °C, and 35 days at 4 and −20 °C	1977	C
Heparin sodium	OR	1000 units	KN	20 g	D5W[a]	Visually compatible with no loss of hydromorphone in 18 days at 4 and 23 °C. Heparin not tested	2410	C
	OR	500 units	KN	5 g	D5W[a]	Visually compatible with no loss of hydromorphone in 18 days at 4 and 23 °C. Heparin not tested	2410	C
	OR	8000 units	KN	5 g	D5W[a]	Visually compatible with no loss of hydromorphone in 18 days at 4 and 23 °C. Heparin not tested	2410	C
Ketamine HCl	SZ	200 mg, 600 mg, 1 g	SZ	200 mg	NS[d]	Visually compatible. Under 10% loss of both drugs in 7 days at 25 °C	2799	C
Midazolam HCl	RC	0.1 to 4.5 g	KN	0.5 to 45 g	D5W, NS	Visually compatible for 24 hr at room temperature	2086	C
	RC	100 and 500 mg	KN	2 and 20 g	D5W, NS	Visually compatible. Under 7% hydromorphone and midazolam loss in 23 days at 4 and 23 °C	2086	C
Ondansetron HCl	GL	100 mg and 1 g	ES	500 mg	NS	Physically compatible. No loss of either drug in 7 days at 32 °C or 31 days at 4 and 22 °C protected from light	1690	C
Potassium chloride	AST	0.5 and 1 mEq/mL	KN	2 and 20 mg/mL	D5W[a]	Visually compatible with no loss of hydromorphone in 18 days at 4 and 23 °C. Potassium chloride not tested	2410	C
Promethazine HCl	ES	300 mg	KN	1 g	NS[a]	Visually compatible for 21 days at 4 and 25 °C	1992	C
Verapamil HCl	KN	80 mg	KN	16 mg	D5W, NS	Physically compatible for 24 hr	764	C
Ziconotide acetate	ELN	25 mg[b]	BB	35 g[c]		90% ziconotide retained for 19 days at 37 °C. No hydromorphone loss in 25 days	2702	C

[a]*Tested in PVC containers.*
[b]*Tested in SynchroMed implantable pumps.*
[c]*Hydromorphone HCl powder dissolved in ziconotide acetate injection.*
[d]*Tested in amber glass and PVC containers.*

Drugs in Syringe Compatibility

Hydromorphone HCl

Drug (in syringe)	Mfr	Amt	Mfr	Amt	Remarks	Ref	C/I
Ampicillin sodium	AY	250 mg/ 1 mL	KN	2, 10, 40 mg/ 1 mL	Visually compatible but 10% loss of ampicillin in 5 hr at room temperature	2082	I
Atropine sulfate	ES	0.4 mg/ 0.5 mL	KN	4 mg/ 2 mL[a]	Physically compatible for 30 min	517	C
Bupivacaine HCl	AST	7.5 mg/ mL	KN	65 mg/ mL	Visually compatible for 30 days at 25 °C	1660	C
Cefazolin sodium	SKF	>200 mg/1 mL	KN	2, 10, 40 mg/ 1 mL	Precipitate forms	2082	I
	SKF	150 mg/ 1 mL	KN	2, 10, 40 mg/ 1 mL	Visually compatible with less than 10% loss of each drug in 24 hr at room temperature	2082	C
Ceftazidime	GL	180 mg/ 1 mL	KN	2, 10, 40 mg/ 1 mL	Visually compatible with less than 10% loss of either drug in 24 hr at room temperature	2082	C
Chlorpromazine HCl	ES	25 mg/ 1 mL	KN	4 mg/ 2 mL[a]	Physically compatible for 30 min	517	C
Cloxacillin sodium	AY	250 mg/ 1 mL	KN	2, 10, 40 mg/ 1 mL	Precipitate forms but dissipates with shaking. Under 10% loss of both drugs in 24 hr at room temperature	2082	?
Dexamethasone sodium phosphate	SX	4 mg/ mL[b]	KN	2, 10, 40 mg/ mL[b]	Visually compatible and both drugs stable for 24 hr at 24 °C	1542	C
	DB	10 mg/ mL[b]	KN	2 and 10 mg/ mL[b]	Visually compatible and both drugs stable for 24 hr at 24 °C	1542	C
	DB	10 mg/ mL[b]	KN	40 mg/ mL[b]	White turbidity forms immediately	1542	I
	DB	7.1 mg/ mL[c]	KN	11.6 mg/ mL[c]	Visually compatible for 24 hr at 24 °C	1542	C
	DB	5.5 to 6.6 mg/ mL[c]	KN	13.3 to 17.5 mg/ mL[c]	Precipitate forms	1542	I
	DB	4.75 mg/ mL[c]	KN	10.5 mg/ mL[c]	Visually compatible for 24 hr at 24 °C	1542	C
	DB	3 to 4.1 mg/ mL[c]	KN	14.75 to 25 mg/ mL[c]	Precipitate forms	1542	I
	SX	3.34 mg/ mL[c]	KN	26.66 mg/mL[c]	Visually compatible for 24 hr at 24 °C	1542	C

Drugs in Syringe Compatibility (Cont.)

Hydromorphone HCl

Drug (in syringe)	Mfr	Amt	Mfr	Amt	Remarks	Ref	C/I
Diazepam	SX	5 mg/ 1 mL	KN	2, 10, 40 mg/ 1 mL	Diazepam precipitate forms immediately due to aqueous dilution	2082	I
Dimenhydrinate	SQ	50 mg/ 1 mL	KN	2, 10, 40 mg/ 1 mL	Visually compatible with both drugs stable for 24 hr at 4, 23, and 37 °C. Precipitate forms after 24 hr	1776	C
		10 mg/ 1 mL		50 mg/ 1 mL	Precipitate forms in about 2 hr	2569	I
Diphenhydramine HCl	PD	50 mg/ 1 mL	KN	4 mg/ 2 mL[a]	Physically compatible for 30 min	517	C
Fentanyl citrate	MN	0.05 mg/ 1 mL	KN	4 mg/ 2 mL[a]	Physically compatible for 30 min	517	C
Glycopyrrolate	RB	0.2 mg/ 1 mL	KN	2 mg/ 1 mL	Physically compatible. pH in glycopyrrolate stability range for 48 hr at 25 °C	331	C
	RB	0.2 mg/ 1 mL	KN	4 mg/ 2 mL	Physically compatible. pH in glycopyrrolate stability range for 48 hr at 25 °C	331	C
	RB	0.4 mg/ 2 mL	KN	2 mg/ 1 mL	Physically compatible. pH in glycopyrrolate stability range for 48 hr at 25 °C	331	C
Haloperidol lactate	MN	1[d], 2[d], 5 mg/ 1 mL	KN	1[d] and 10 mg/ 1 mL	Visually compatible for 24 hr at 25 °C under fluorescent light	1785	C
	MN	2 mg/mL	KN	10 and 15 mg/ mL	White precipitate of haloperidol forms immediately	668	I
Heparin sodium	OR	10 units/ 1 mL	KN	50 mg/ 1 mL	White cloudy precipitate	2410	I
	LEO	100 units/ 1 mL	KN	50 mg/ 1 mL	White cloudy precipitate	2410	I
	OR	25,000 units/ 1 mL	KN	50 mg/ 1 mL	White cloudy precipitate	2410	I
Hyaluronidase	WY	150 units/mL[e]	KN	2 mg/mL[e]	43 and 56% hyaluronidase loss in 24 hr at 4 and 23 °C, respectively	1907	I
	WY	150 units/mL[e]	KN	10 and 40 mg/ mL[e]	70 to 82% hyaluronidase loss in 24 hr at 4 and 23 °C	1907	I
Hydroxyzine HCl	PF	50 mg/ 1 mL	KN	4 mg/ 2 mL[a]	Physically compatible for 30 min	517	C
	PF	100 mg/ 2 mL	KN	0.75 mg/ 0.8 mL	Physically compatible	771	C
Ketamine HCl	SZ	0.2, 0.6, 1 mg/mL[j]	SZ	0.2 mg/ mL[j]	Visually compatible. Under 10% loss of both drugs in 7 days at 25 °C	2799	C
Ketorolac tromethamine	SY	30 mg/ 1 mL	KN	10 mg/ 1 mL	Cloudiness forms immediately but clears with swirling	1785	?
	SY	30 mg/ 1 mL	KN	1 mg/ 1 mL[d]	Visually compatible for 24 hr at 25 °C under fluorescent light	1785	C
	SY	15 mg/ 1 mL[d]	KN	1[d] and 10 mg/ 1 mL	Visually compatible for 24 hr at 25 °C under fluorescent light	1785	C

Drugs in Syringe Compatibility (Cont.)

Hydromorphone HCl

Drug (in syringe)	Mfr	Amt	Mfr	Amt	Remarks	Ref	C/I
Lorazepam	WY	4 mg/ 1 mL	KN	2, 10, 40 mg/ 1 mL	Visually compatible. 10% lorazepam loss in 6 days at 4 °C, 4 days at 23 °C, and 24 hr at 37 °C. Little hydromorphone loss in 7 days at all temperatures	1776	C
Methotrimeprazine HCl	LE	10 mg/ mL	KN	10 mg/ mL	Visually compatible with less than 10% loss of either drug in 7 days at 8 °C	668	C
Metoclopramide HCl	RB	5 mg/mL	KN	10 and 20 mg/ mL	Visually compatible with less than 10% loss of either drug in 7 days at 8 °C	668	C
Midazolam HCl	RC	5 mg/ 1 mL	WB	2 mg/ 0.5 mL	Physically compatible for 4 hr at 25 °C	1145	C
Pantoprazole sodium	i	4 mg/ 1 mL		10 mg/ 1 mL	Whitish precipitate forms within 4 hr	2574	I
Pentazocine lactate	WI	30 mg/ 1 mL	KN	4 mg/ 2 mL[a]	Physically compatible for 30 min	517	C
Pentobarbital sodium	AB	50 mg/ 1 mL	KN	4 mg/ 2 mL[f]	Physically compatible for 30 min	517	C
	AB	50 mg/ 1 mL	KN	4 mg/ 2 mL[g]	Transient precipitate that dissipates after mixing and stays clear for 30 min	517	?
Phenobarbital sodium	AB	120 mg/ 1 mL	KN	2, 10, 40 mg/ 1 mL	Precipitate forms immediately but dissipates with shaking. Phenobarbital precipitates after 6 hr at room temperature	2082	I
Phenytoin sodium	AB	50 mg/ 1 mL	KN	2, 10, 40 mg/ 1 mL	White precipitate of phenytoin forms immediately	2082	I
Potassium chloride	AST	2 mEq/ 1 mL	KN	50 mg/ 1 mL	Visually compatible for 24 hr at room temperature	2410	C
Prochlorperazine edisylate	SKF	5 mg/ 1 mL	KN	4 mg/ 2 mL[f]	Precipitates immediately	517	I
	SKF	5 mg/ 1 mL	KN	4 mg/ 2 mL[g]	Physically compatible for 30 min	517	C
Prochlorperazine mesylate	RP	5 mg/ 1 mL	KN	2, 10, 40 mg/ 1 mL	Visually compatible. Little or no loss of either drug in 7 days at 4, 23, and 37 °C	1776	C
	RP	1.5 mg/ mL[j]	SX	0.5 mg/ mL[j]	Physically compatible for 96 hr at room temperature exposed to light	2171	C
Promethazine HCl	WY	50 mg/ 1 mL	KN	4 mg/ 2 mL[a]	Physically compatible for 30 min	517	C
	WY	25 mg/ 1 mL	KN	4 mg/ 2 mL[a]	Physically compatible for 30 min	517	C
Ranitidine HCl	GL	50 mg/ 2 mL	PE	2 mg/ 1 mL	Physically compatible for 1 hr at 25 °C	978	C
Salbutamol	GL	2.5 mg/ 2.5 mL[b]	KN	1 mg/ 0.5 mL	Physically compatible for 1 hr	1904	C
Scopolamine HBr	BW	0.43 mg/ 0.5 mL	KN	4 mg/ 2 mL[a]	Physically compatible for 30 min	517	C

Drugs in Syringe Compatibility (Cont.)

Hydromorphone HCl

Drug (in syringe)	Mfr	Amt	Mfr	Amt	Remarks	Ref	C/I
Trimethobenzamide HCl	BE	100 mg/ 1 mL	KN	4 mg/ 2 mL[a]	Physically compatible for 30 min	517	**C**
Ziconotide acetate	ELN	25 mcg/ mL	BB	35 mg/ mL[k]	No loss of either drug in 25 days at 5 °C	2702	**C**

[a] Both ampul and vial formulations tested.
[b] Mixed in equal quantities. Final concentration is one-half the indicated concentration.
[c] Mixed in varying quantities to yield the final concentrations noted.
[d] Dilution prepared in sterile water for injection.
[e] Mixed in equal quantities for testing.
[f] Vial formulation tested.
[g] Ampul formulation tested.
[h] Both preserved (benzyl alcohol 0.9%; benzalkonium chloride 0.01%) and unpreserved sodium chloride 0.9% were used as a diluent.
[i] Test performed using the formulation WITHOUT edetate disodium.
[j] Diluted in sodium chloride 0.9%.
[k] Hydromorphone HCl powder dissolved in ziconotide acetate injection.

Y-Site Injection Compatibility (1:1 Mixture)

Hydromorphone HCl

Drug	Mfr	Conc	Mfr	Conc	Remarks	Ref	C/I
Acyclovir sodium	BW	5 mg/mL[a]	WB	0.04 mg/mL[a]	Physically compatible for 4 hr at 25 °C	1157	**C**
Allopurinol sodium	BW	3 mg/mL[b]	KN	0.5 mg/mL[b]	Physically compatible for 4 hr at 22 °C	1686	**C**
Amifostine	USB	10 mg/mL[a]	AST	0.5 mg/mL[a]	Physically compatible for 4 hr at 23 °C	1845	**C**
Amikacin sulfate	BR	5 mg/mL[a]	WY	0.2 mg/mL[a]	Physically compatible for 4 hr at 25 °C	987	**C**
Amphotericin B cholesteryl sulfate complex	SEQ	0.83 mg/mL[a]	ES	0.5 mg/mL[a]	Decreased natural turbidity occurs	2117	**I**
Ampicillin sodium	BR	20 mg/mL[b]	WY	0.2 mg/mL[a]	Physically compatible for 4 hr at 25 °C	987	**C**
	AY	20[a] and 250 mg/mL	KN	2, 10, 40 mg/ mL	Visually compatible. Hydromorphone stable for 24 hr. 10% ampicillin loss in 5 hr	1532	**I**
Amsacrine	NCI	1 mg/mL[a]	AST	0.5 mg/mL[a]	Visually compatible for 4 hr at 22 °C	1381	**C**
Atropine sulfate	LY	0.4 mg/mL	AST	0.5 mg/mL[a]	Physically compatible for 48 hr at 22 °C	1706	**C**
Aztreonam	SQ	40 mg/mL[a]	KN	0.5 mg/mL[a]	Physically compatible for 4 hr at 23 °C	1758	**C**
Bivalirudin	TMC	5 mg/mL[a]	AST	0.5 mg/mL[a]	Physically compatible for 4 hr at 23 °C	2373	**C**
Caspofungin acetate	ME	0.7 mg/mL[b]	BA	1 mg/mL[b]	Physically compatible for 4 hr at room temperature	2758	**C**
	ME	0.5 mg/mL[b]	HOS	1 mg/mL	Physically compatible with hydromorphone HCl i.v. push over 2 to 5 min	2766	**C**
Cefazolin sodium	SKF	20 mg/mL[a]	WY	0.2 mg/mL[a]	Physically compatible for 4 hr at 25 °C	987	**C**
	SKF	20[a] and 150 mg/mL	KN	2, 10, 40 mg/ mL	Visually compatible and both drugs stable for 24 hr	1532	**C**
	SKF	>200 mg/mL	KN	2, 10, 40 mg/ mL	Precipitate forms immediately	1532	**I**
Cefotaxime sodium	HO	20 mg/mL[a]	WY	0.2 mg/mL[a]	Physically compatible for 4 hr at 25 °C	987	**C**
Cefoxitin sodium	MSD	20 mg/mL[a]	WY	0.2 mg/mL[a]	Physically compatible for 4 hr at 25 °C	987	**C**
Ceftaroline fosamil	FOR	2.22 mg/ mL[a,b,f]	HOS	0.5 mg/mL[a,b,f]	Physically compatible for 4 hr at 23 °C	2826	**C**

Y-Site Injection Compatibility (1:1 Mixture) (Cont.)

Hydromorphone HCl

Drug	Mfr	Conc	Mfr	Conc	Remarks	Ref	C/I
Ceftazidime	GL	40[a] and 180 mg/mL	KN	2, 10, 40 mg/mL	Visually compatible and both drugs stable for 24 hr	1532	C
Cefuroxime sodium	GL	30 mg/mL[a]	WY	0.2 mg/mL[a]	Physically compatible for 4 hr at 25 °C	987	C
Chloramphenicol sodium succinate	LY	20 mg/mL[a]	WY	0.2 mg/mL[a]	Physically compatible for 4 hr at 25 °C	987	C
Cisatracurium besylate	GW	0.1, 2, 5 mg/mL[a]	ES	0.5 mg/mL[a]	Physically compatible for 4 hr at 23 °C	2074	C
Cladribine	ORT	0.015[b] and 0.5[d] mg/mL	KN	0.5 mg/mL[b]	Physically compatible for 4 hr at 23 °C	1969	C
Clindamycin phosphate	UP	12 mg/mL[a]	WY	0.2 mg/mL[a]	Physically compatible for 4 hr at 25 °C	987	C
Cloxacillin sodium	AY	250 mg/mL	KN	2, 10, 40 mg/mL	Turbidity forms but dissipates with shaking and solution remains clear. Both drugs stable for 24 hr	1532	?
	AY	40 mg/mL[a]	KN	2, 10, 40 mg/mL	Turbidity forms immediately and cloxacillin precipitate develops	1532	I
	AY	27 mg/mL[a]	KN	2, 10, 40 mg/mL	Turbidity forms immediately	1532	I
	AY	12 mg/mL[a]	KN	2, 10, 40 mg/mL	Visually compatible for 24 hr; precipitate forms in 96 hr	1532	C
Dexamethasone sodium phosphate	AMR	1 mg/mL[a]	AST	0.5 mg/mL[a]	Physically compatible for 48 hr at 22 °C	1706	C
Dexmedetomidine HCl	AB	4 mcg/mL[b]	AST	0.5 mg/mL[b]	Physically compatible for 4 hr at 23 °C	2383	C
Diazepam	SX	5 mg/mL	KN	2, 10, 40 mg/mL	Turbidity forms immediately and diazepam precipitate develops	1532	I
	ES	0.5 mg/mL[a]	AST	0.5 mg/mL[a]	Physically compatible for 48 hr at 22 °C	1706	C
Diltiazem HCl	MMD	1 mg/mL[a]	KN	1 mg/mL	Visually compatible for 4 hr at 27 °C	2062	C
Diphenhydramine HCl	SCN	2 mg/mL[a]	AST	0.5 mg/mL[a]	Physically compatible for 48 hr at 22 °C	1706	C
Dobutamine HCl	LI	4 mg/mL[a]	KN	1 mg/mL	Visually compatible for 4 hr at 27 °C	2062	C
Docetaxel	RPR	0.9 mg/mL[a]	AST	0.5 mg/mL[a]	Physically compatible for 4 hr at 23 °C	2224	C
Dopamine HCl	AB	3.2 mg/mL[a]	KN	1 mg/mL	Visually compatible for 4 hr at 27 °C	2062	C
Doripenem	JJ	5 mg/mL[a,b]	BA	1 mg/mL[a,b]	Physically compatible for 4 hr at 23 °C	2743	C
Doxorubicin HCl liposomal	SEQ	0.4 mg/mL[a]	ES	0.5 mg/mL[a]	Physically compatible for 4 hr at 23 °C	2087	C
Doxycycline hyclate	ES	1 mg/mL[a]	WY	0.2 mg/mL[a]	Physically compatible for 4 hr at 25 °C	987	C
Epinephrine HCl	AB	0.02 mg/mL[a]	KN	1 mg/mL	Visually compatible for 4 hr at 27 °C	2062	C
Erythromycin lactobionate	AB	5 mg/mL[a]	WY	0.2 mg/mL[a]	Physically compatible for 4 hr at 25 °C	987	C
Etoposide phosphate	BR	5 mg/mL[a]	ES	0.5 mg/mL[a]	Physically compatible for 4 hr at 23 °C	2218	C
Famotidine	ME	2 mg/mL[b]		0.5 mg/mL[a]	Visually compatible for 4 hr at 22 °C	1936	C
Fenoldopam mesylate	AB	80 mcg/mL[b]	ES	0.5 mg/mL[b]	Physically compatible for 4 hr at 23 °C	2467	C
Fentanyl citrate	ES	0.05 mg/mL	KN	1 mg/mL	Visually compatible for 4 hr at 27 °C	2062	C
Filgrastim	AMG	30 mcg/mL[a]	KN	0.5 mg/mL[a]	Physically compatible for 4 hr at 22 °C	1687	C
Fludarabine phosphate	BX	1 mg/mL[a]	KN	0.5 mg/mL[a]	Visually compatible for 4 hr at 22 °C	1439	C
Foscarnet sodium	AST	24 mg/mL	KN	10 mg/mL	Physically compatible for 24 hr at room temperature under fluorescent light	1335	C
Furosemide	AMR	10 mg/mL	KN	1 mg/mL	Visually compatible for 4 hr at 27 °C	2062	C

Y-Site Injection Compatibility (1:1 Mixture) (Cont.)

Hydromorphone HCl

Drug	Mfr	Conc	Mfr	Conc	Remarks	Ref	C/I
Gallium nitrate	FUJ	1 mg/mL[b]	WY	4 mg/mL	Precipitate forms in 24 hr at 25 °C	1673	I
Gemcitabine HCl	LI	10 mg/mL[b]	AST	0.5 mg/mL[b]	Physically compatible for 4 hr at 23 °C	2226	C
Gentamicin sulfate	TR	0.8 mg/mL[a]	WY	0.2 mg/mL[a]	Physically compatible for 4 hr at 25 °C	987	C
Granisetron HCl	SKB	1 mg/mL	KN	0.5 mg/mL[b]	Physically compatible with little or no loss of either drug in 4 hr at 22 °C	1883	C
	SKB	0.05 mg/mL[a]	ES	0.5 mg/mL[a]	Physically compatible for 4 hr at 23 °C	2000	C
Haloperidol lactate	MN	0.2 mg/mL[a]	AST	0.5 mg/mL[a]	Physically compatible for 48 hr at 22 °C	1706	C
Heparin sodium	ES	100 units/mL[a]	KN	1 mg/mL	Visually compatible for 4 hr at 27 °C	2062	C
Hetastarch in lactated electrolyte	AB	6%	AST	0.5 mg/mL[a]	Physically compatible for 4 hr at 23 °C	2339	C
Hydroxyethyl starch 130/0.4 in sodium chloride 0.9%	FRK	6%	SZ	0.4[a], 1.2[a], 2 mg/mL	Visually compatible for 24 hr at room temperature	2770	C
Hydroxyzine HCl	WI	4 mg/mL[a]	AST	0.5 mg/mL[a]	Physically compatible for 48 hr at 22 °C	1706	C
Ketorolac tromethamine	WY	1 mg/mL[a]	AST	0.5 mg/mL[a]	Physically compatible for 48 hr at 22 °C	1706	C
Labetalol HCl	AH	2 mg/mL[a]	KN	1 mg/mL	Visually compatible for 4 hr at 27 °C	2062	C
Levofloxacin	OMN	5 mg/mL[a]	HOS	2 mg/mL	Physically compatible	2794	C
Linezolid	PHU	2 mg/mL	AST	0.5 mg/mL[a]	Physically compatible for 4 hr at 23 °C	2264	C
Lorazepam	WY	0.5 mg/mL[a]	KN	1 mg/mL	Visually compatible for 4 hr at 27 °C	2062	C
	WY	0.1 mg/mL[a]	AST	0.5 mg/mL[a]	Physically compatible for 48 hr at 22 °C	1706	C
Magnesium sulfate	LY	16.7, 33.3, 50, 100 mg/mL[a]	KN	2 mg/mL[a]	Visually compatible for 4 hr at 25 °C	1549	C
Melphalan HCl	BW	0.1 mg/mL[b]	KN	0.5 mg/mL[b]	Physically compatible for 3 hr at 22 °C	1557	C
Methotrimeprazine HCl	LE	0.2 mg/mL[a]	AST	0.5 mg/mL[a]	Physically compatible for 48 hr at 22 °C	1706	C
Metoclopramide HCl	DU	5 mg/mL	AST	0.5 mg/mL[a]	Physically compatible for 48 hr at 22 °C	1706	C
Metronidazole	SE	5 mg/mL	WY	0.2 mg/mL[a]	Physically compatible for 4 hr at 25 °C	987	C
Micafungin sodium	ASP	1.5 mg/mL[b]	BA	0.5 mg/mL[b]	Physically compatible for 4 hr at 23 °C	2683	C
Midazolam HCl	RC	2 mg/mL[a]	KN	1 mg/mL	Visually compatible for 4 hr at 27 °C	2062	C
	RC	0.2 mg/mL[a]	AST	0.5 mg/mL[a]	Physically compatible for 48 hr at 22 °C	1706	C
Milrinone lactate	SW	0.2 mg/mL[a]	KN	1 mg/mL	Visually compatible for 4 hr at 27 °C	2062	C
Morphine sulfate	SCN	2 mg/mL[a]	KN	1 mg/mL	Visually compatible for 4 hr at 27 °C	2062	C
Nafcillin sodium	WY	20 mg/mL[a]	WY	0.2 mg/mL[a]	Physically compatible for 4 hr at 25 °C	987	C
Nicardipine HCl	WY	1 mg/mL[a]	KN	1 mg/mL	Visually compatible for 4 hr at 27 °C	2062	C
Nitroglycerin	AB	0.4 mg/mL[a]	KN	1 mg/mL	Visually compatible for 4 hr at 27 °C	2062	C
Norepinephrine bitartrate	AB	0.128 mg/mL[a]	KN	1 mg/mL	Visually compatible for 4 hr at 27 °C	2062	C
Ondansetron HCl	GL	1 mg/mL[b]	KN	0.5 mg/mL[a]	Visually compatible for 4 hr at 22 °C	1365	C
Oxacillin sodium	BE	20 mg/mL[a]	WY	0.2 mg/mL[a]	Physically compatible for 4 hr at 25 °C	987	C
Oxaliplatin	SS	0.5 mg/mL[a]	ES	0.5 mg/mL[a]	Physically compatible for 4 hr at 23 °C	2566	C
Paclitaxel	NCI	1.2 mg/mL[a]	KN	0.5 mg/mL[a]	Physically compatible for 4 hr at 22 °C	1556	C

Y-Site Injection Compatibility (1:1 Mixture) (Cont.)

Hydromorphone HCl

Drug	Mfr	Conc	Mfr	Conc	Remarks	Ref	C/I
Palonosetron HCl	MGI	50 mcg/mL	BA	0.5 mg/mL[a]	Physically compatible and no loss of either drug in 4 hr	2720	C
Pemetrexed disodium	LI	20 mg/mL[b]	ES	0.5 mg/mL[a]	Physically compatible for 4 hr at 23 °C	2564	C
Penicillin G potassium	PF	100,000 units/mL[a]	WY	0.2 mg/mL[a]	Physically compatible for 4 hr at 25 °C	987	C
Phenobarbital sodium	AB	120 mg/mL	KN	2, 10, 40 mg/mL	Turbidity forms but dissipates; phenobarbital precipitates in 6 hr	1532	I
	WY	2 mg/mL[a]	AST	0.5 mg/mL[a]	Physically compatible for 48 hr at 22 °C	1706	C
Phenytoin sodium	AB	50 mg/mL	KN	2, 10, 40 mg/mL	Turbidity forms immediately and phenytoin precipitate develops	1532	I
	ES	2 mg/mL[a,b]	AST	0.5 mg/mL[a]	Precipitate forms within 1 hr	1706	I
Piperacillin sodium–tazobactam sodium	LE[e]	40 + 5 mg/mL[a]	ES	0.5 mg/mL[a]	Physically compatible for 4 hr at 22 °C	1688	C
Propofol	ZEN	10 mg/mL	AST	0.5 mg/mL[a]	Physically compatible for 1 hr at 23 °C	2066	C
Ranitidine HCl	GL	1 mg/mL[a]	KN	1 mg/mL	Visually compatible for 4 hr at 27 °C	2062	C
Remifentanil HCl	GW	0.025 and 0.25 mg/mL[b]	ES	0.5 mg/mL[a]	Physically compatible for 4 hr at 23 °C	2075	C
Sargramostim	IMM	10 mcg/mL[b]	WI	0.5 mg/mL[b]	Few small particles in 30 min	1436	I
Scopolamine HBr	LY	0.05 mg/mL[a]	AST	0.5 mg/mL[a]	Physically compatible for 48 hr at 22 °C	1706	C
Tacrolimus	FUJ	10 and 40 mcg/mL[a]	KN	2 and 0.2 mg/mL[a]	Visually compatible. No loss of either drug in 4 hr at 24 °C	2216	C
Teniposide	BR	0.1 mg/mL[a]	KN	0.5 mg/mL[a]	Physically compatible for 4 hr at 23 °C	1725	C
Thiotepa	IMM[g]	1 mg/mL[a]	AST	0.5 mg/mL[a]	Physically compatible for 4 hr at 23 °C	1861	C
TNA #218, #220, #221, #223[h]			ES	0.5 mg/mL[a]	Visually compatible for 4 hr at 23 °C	2215	C
TNA #219, #222, #224 to #226[h]			ES	0.5 mg/mL[a]	Damage to emulsion occurs immediately with free oil formation possible	2215	I
Tobramycin sulfate	DI	0.8 mg/mL[a]	WY	0.2 mg/mL[a]	Physically compatible for 4 hr at 25 °C	987	C
TPN #212 to #215[h]			ES	0.5 mg/mL[a]	Physically compatible for 4 hr at 23 °C	2109	C
Trimethoprim–sulfamethoxazole	BW	0.8 + 4 mg/mL[a]	WY	0.2 mg/mL[a]	Physically compatible for 4 hr at 25 °C	987	C
Vancomycin HCl	LI	5 mg/mL[a]	WY	0.2 mg/mL[a]	Physically compatible for 4 hr at 25 °C	987	C
	HOS	4 mg/mL[b]	HOS	2 mg/mL	Physically compatible	2794	C
Vecuronium bromide	OR	1 mg/mL	KN	1 mg/mL	Visually compatible for 4 hr at 27 °C	2062	C
Vinorelbine tartrate	BW	1 mg/mL[b]	KN	0.5 mg/mL[b]	Physically compatible for 4 hr at 22 °C	1558	C

[a]*Tested in dextrose 5%.*
[b]*Tested in sodium chloride 0.9%.*
[c]*Tested in sterile water for injection.*
[d]*Tested in bacteriostatic sodium chloride 0.9% preserved with benzyl alcohol 0.9%.*
[e]*Test performed using the formulation WITHOUT edetate disodium.*
[f]*Tested in Ringer's injection, lactated.*
[g]*Lyophilized formulation tested.*
[h]*Refer to Appendix I for the composition of parenteral nutrition solutions. TNA indicates a 3-in-1 admixture, and TPN indicates a 2-in-1 admixture.*

HYDROXYETHYL STARCH 130/0.4 6% IN SODIUM CHLORIDE 0.9%
AHFS 40:12

Products — Hydroxyethyl starch 130/0.4 is available as a 6% (6 g/ 100 mL) in sodium chloride 0.9% in 500-mL plastic containers. The solution also contains sodium hydroxide or hydrochloric acid for pH adjustment during manufacturing. (1)

pH — From 4.0 to 5.5. (1)

Osmolarity — The calculated osmolarity is 308 mOsm/L. (1)

Sodium Content — The product provides 77 mEq of sodium per 500-mL container. (1)

Trade Name(s) — Voluven.

Administration — Hydroxyethyl starch 130/0.4 6% in sodium chloride 0.9% is given by intravenous infusion only. Any remaining solution in partially used containers should be discarded. The dosage and rate of infusion should be individualized to the patient's condition and response. The container is made of non-DEHP plastic and is latex free. The container does not require a vented set. If using pressure infusion, withdraw or expel air from the container through the medication/administration port prior to infusion. (1)

Stability — Hydroxyethyl starch 130/0.4 6% in sodium chloride 0.9% is a clear to slightly opalescent colorless to slightly yellow colloidal solution. The product should be stored at controlled room temperature and protected from freezing. The bag of solution should not be removed from the overwrap until immediately before use. It should only be administered if the solution is clear and free from particles. The solution should be administered immediately after insertion of the administration set. (1)

Compatibility Information

Y-Site Injection Compatibility (1:1 Mixture)

Hydroxyethyl starch 130/0.4 6% in sodium chloride 0.9%

Drug	Mfr	Conc	Mfr	Conc	Remarks	Ref	C/I
Ampicillin sodium	NOP	10, 25, 40 mg/mL[a]	FRK	6%	Visually compatible for 24 hr at room temperature	2770	C
Calcium chloride	HOS	20, 40, 80 mg/mL[a]	FRK	6%	Visually compatible for 24 hr at room temperature	2770	C
Calcium gluconate	PP	20, 30, 40 mg/mL[a]	FRK	6%	Visually compatible for 24 hr at room temperature	2770	C
Cefazolin sodium	NOP	20, 30, 40 mg/mL[a]	FRK	6%	Visually compatible for 24 hr at room temperature	2770	C
Ceftriaxone sodium	RC	20, 30, 40 mg/mL[a]	FRK	6%	Visually compatible for 24 hr at room temperature	2770	C
Ciprofloxacin	AB	0.5, 1, 2 mg/mL[a]	FRK	6%	Visually compatible for 24 hr at room temperature	2770	C
Clindamycin phosphate	SZ	6, 12, 24 mg/mL[a]	FRK	6%	Visually compatible for 24 hr at room temperature	2770	C
Dimenhydrinate	SZ	0.5, 0.75, 1 mg/mL[a]	FRK	6%	Visually compatible for 24 hr at room temperature	2770	C
Dobutamine HCl	SZ	1, 2, 4 mg/mL[a]	FRK	6%	Visually compatible for 24 hr at room temperature	2770	C
Dopamine HCl	BMS	0.8, 3.2, 6.4 mg/mL[a]	FRK	6%	Visually compatible for 24 hr at room temperature	2770	C
Epinephrine HCl	BIO	16, 24, 32 mcg/mL[a]	FRK	6%	Color change within 4 hr	2770	I
Esmolol HCl	BA	10 mg/mL[a]	FRK	6%	Visually compatible for 24 hr at room temperature	2770	C
Fentanyl citrate	SZ	20[a], 35[a], 50 mcg/mL	FRK	6%	Visually compatible for 24 hr at room temperature	2770	C
Furosemide	SZ	1, 1.5, 2 mg/mL[a]	FRK	6%	Visually compatible for 24 hr at room temperature	2770	C
Gentamicin sulfate	SX	1, 3, 5 mg/mL[a]	FRK	6%	Visually compatible for 24 hr at room temperature	2770	C

Y-Site Injection Compatibility (1:1 Mixture) (Cont.)

Hydroxyethyl starch 130/0.4 6% in sodium chloride 0.9%

Drug	Mfr	Conc	Mfr	Conc	Remarks	Ref	C/I
Heparin sodium	HOS	10 units/mL	FRK	6%	Visually compatible for 24 hr at room temperature	2770	C
	PP	1000, 10,000 units/mL	FRK	6%	Visually compatible for 24 hr at room temperature	2770	C
Hydromorphone HCl	SZ	0.4[a], 1.2[a], 2 mg/mL	FRK	6%	Visually compatible for 24 hr at room temperature	2770	C
Insulin, regular	NOV	5, 27.5, 50 units/mL[a]	FRK	6%	Visually compatible for 24 hr at room temperature	2770	C
Labetalol HCl	SZ	1.25[a], 2.5[a], 5 mg/mL	FRK	6%	Visually compatible for 24 hr at room temperature	2770	C
Levofloxacin	OMN	1, 2.5, 5 mg/mL[a]	FRK	6%	Visually compatible for 24 hr at room temperature	2770	C
Magnesium sulfate	SZ	125[a], 250[a], 500 mg/mL	FRK	6%	Visually compatible for 24 hr at room temperature	2770	C
Meperidine HCl	SZ	1, 5, 10 mg/mL[a]	FRK	6%	Visually compatible for 24 hr at room temperature	2770	C
Methylprednisolone sodium succinate	NOP	0.25[a], 5[a], 62.5 mg/mL	FRK	6%	Visually compatible for 24 hr at room temperature	2770	C
Metronidazole	HOS	1[a], 2.5[a], 5 mg/mL	FRK	6%	Visually compatible for 24 hr at room temperature	2770	C
Midazolam HCl	SZ	1, 1.5, 2 mg/mL[a]	FRK	6%	Visually compatible for 24 hr at room temperature	2770	C
Morphine sulfate	SZ	1, 5, 10 mg/mL[a]	FRK	6%	Visually compatible for 24 hr at room temperature	2770	C
Moxifloxacin HCl	BAY	0.4[a], 0.8[a], 1.6 mg/mL	FRK	6%	Visually compatible for 24 hr at room temperature	2770	C
Multivitamins	SX	2.5, 5, 10 mL/L[a]	FRK	6%	Visually compatible for 24 hr at room temperature	2770	C
Nitroglycerin	SZ	0.1, 0.25, 0.4 mg/mL[a]	FRK	6%	Visually compatible for 24 hr at room temperature	2770	C
Norepinephrine bitartrate	SZ	6, 8, 64 mcg/mL[a]	FRK	6%	Visually compatible for 24 hr at room temperature	2770	C
Octreotide acetate	NVA	5, 7.5, 10 mcg/mL[a]	FRK	6%	Visually compatible for 24 hr at room temperature	2770	C
Phenytoin sodium	SZ	6, 7.5, 9 mg/mL[a]	FRK	6%	White precipitate forms immediately	2770	I
Potassium chloride	HOS	0.02, 0.4, 0.8 mEq/mL[a]	FRK	6%	Visually compatible for 24 hr at room temperature	2770	C
Potassium phosphates	SX	0.003, 0.0765, 0.15 mmol/mL[a]	FRK	6%	Visually compatible for 24 hr at room temperature	2770	C
Propofol	NOP	2.5[a], 5[a], 10 mg/mL	FRK	6%	Visually compatible for 24 hr at room temperature	2770	C
Sodium bicarbonate	HOS	0.25[a], 0.5[a], 1 mmol/mL	FRK	6%	Visually compatible for 24 hr at room temperature	2770	C
Vasopressin	SZ	0.4, 0.7, 1 unit/mL[a]	FRK	6%	Visually compatible for 24 hr at room temperature	2770	C

[a]Tested in dextrose 5%.

HYDROXYZINE HYDROCHLORIDE
AHFS 28:24.92

Products — Hydroxyzine hydrochloride is available as a 25-mg/mL solution in 1-mL vials and 10-mL multiple-dose vials. It is also available as a 50-mg/mL solution in 1- and 2-mL single-dose vials and 10-mL multiple-dose vials. Also present in the solutions are benzyl alcohol 0.9% and sodium hydroxide and/or hydrochloric acid to adjust the pH. (1; 4)

pH — From 3.5 to 6. (17)

Administration — Hydroxyzine hydrochloride may be administered undiluted by intramuscular injection only, preferably into the upper outer quadrant of the buttock or the midlateral thigh muscles in adults. In children, the midlateral muscles of the thigh are preferred. (1; 4)

Stability — Hydroxyzine should be stored at controlled room temperature and protected from freezing and excessive temperatures. (1; 4)

Compatibility Information

Additive Compatibility

Hydroxyzine HCl

Drug	Mfr	Conc/L	Mfr	Conc/L	Test Soln	Remarks	Ref	C/I
Aminophylline	SE	1 g	RR	250 mg	D5W	Physically incompatible	15	I
Chloramphenicol sodium succinate	PD	10 g	RR	250 mg	D5W	Physically incompatible	15	I
Cisplatin	BR	200 mg	LY	500 mg	NS[a]	Physically compatible for 48 hr	1190	C
Cyclophosphamide	AD	1 g	LY	500 mg	D5W[a]	Physically compatible for 48 hr	1190	C
Cytarabine	UP	1 g	LY	500 mg	D5W[a]	Physically compatible for 48 hr	1190	C
Dimenhydrinate	SE	500 mg	RR	250 mg	D5W	Physically compatible	15	C
Etoposide	BR	1 g	LY	500 mg	D5W[a]	Physically compatible for 48 hr	1190	C
Lidocaine HCl	AST	2 g	PF	100 mg		Physically compatible	24	C
Mesna	AW	3 g	LY	500 mg	D5W[a]	Physically compatible for 48 hr	1190	C
Methotrexate sodium	BV	1 and 3 g	LY	500 mg	D5W[a]	Physically compatible for 48 hr	1190	C
Nafcillin sodium	WY	500 mg	PF	100 mg		Physically compatible	27	C
Penicillin G potassium	SQ	20 million units	RR	250 mg	D5W	Physically incompatible	15	I
Penicillin G sodium	UP	20 million units	RR	250 mg	D5W	Physically incompatible	15	I
Pentobarbital sodium	AB	1 g	RR	250 mg	D5W	Physically incompatible	15	I
Phenobarbital sodium	WI	200 mg	RR	250 mg	D5W	Physically incompatible	15	I

[a]*Tested in glass containers.*

Drugs in Syringe Compatibility

Hydroxyzine HCl

Drug (in syringe)	Mfr	Amt	Mfr	Amt	Remarks	Ref	C/I
Atropine sulfate		0.4 mg/ 1 mL	PF	100 mg/ 2 mL	Physically compatible	771	C
		0.4 mg/ 1 mL	PF	50 mg/ 1 mL	Physically compatible	771	C
		0.6 mg/ 1.5 mL	PF	100 mg/ 4 mL	Physically compatible for at least 15 min	14	C

Drugs in Syringe Compatibility (Cont.)

Hydroxyzine HCl

Drug (in syringe)	Mfr	Amt	Mfr	Amt	Remarks	Ref	C/I
	USP	0.4 mg/ 0.4 mL	NF	50 mg/ 1 mL	Hydroxyzine stable for at least 10 days at 3 and 25 °C	49	C
	ST	0.4 mg/ 1 mL	PF	50 mg/ 1 mL	Physically compatible for at least 15 min	326	C
Buprenorphine HCl					Physically and chemically compatible	4	C
Butorphanol tartrate	BR	2 mg/ 1 mL	PF	50 mg/ 1 mL	Physically compatible	771	C
	BR	1 mg/ 1 mL	PF	100 mg/ 2 mL	Physically compatible	771	C
Chlorpromazine HCl	PO	50 mg/ 2 mL	PF	50 mg/ 1 mL	Physically compatible for at least 15 min	326	C
	STS	50 mg/ 2 mL	ES	100 mg/ 2 mL	Visually compatible for 60 min	1784	C
Dimenhydrinate	HR	50 mg/ 1 mL	PF	50 mg/ 1 mL	Physically incompatible within 15 min	326	I
Diphenhydramine HCl	PD	50 mg/ 1 mL	PF	50 mg/ 1 mL	Physically compatible for at least 15 min	326	C
Doxapram HCl	RB	400 mg/ 20 mL		25 mg/ 1 mL	Physically compatible with no doxapram loss in 24 hr	1177	C
Droperidol	MN	2.5 mg/ 1 mL	PF	50 mg/ 1 mL	Physically compatible for at least 15 min	326	C
Fentanyl citrate	MN	0.05 mg/ 1 mL	PF	50 mg/ 1 mL	Physically compatible for at least 15 min	326	C
	CR	0.05 mg/ 1 mL	PF	50 mg/ 1 mL	Physically compatible	771	C
	CR	0.05 mg/ 1 mL	PF	100 mg/ 2 mL	Physically compatible	771	C
Fluphenazine HCl	LY	5 mg/ 2 mL	ES	100 mg/ 2 mL	Visually compatible for 60 min	1784	C
Glycopyrrolate	RB	0.2 mg/ 1 mL	PF	25 mg/ 1 mL	Physically compatible. pH in glycopyrrolate stability range for 48 hr at 25 °C	331	C
	RB	0.2 mg/ 1 mL	PF	50 mg/ 2 mL	Physically compatible. pH in glycopyrrolate stability range for 48 hr at 25 °C	331	C
	RB	0.4 mg/ 2 mL	PF	25 mg/ 1 mL	Physically compatible. pH in glycopyrrolate stability range for 48 hr at 25 °C	331	C
Haloperidol lactate	MN	10 mg/ 2 mL	ES	100 mg/ 2 mL	White precipitate forms within 5 min	1784	I
Hydromorphone HCl	KN	4 mg/ 2 mL	PF	50 mg/ 1 mL	Physically compatible for 30 min	517	C
	KN	0.75 mg/ 0.8 mL	PF	100 mg/ 2 mL	Physically compatible	771	C
Ketorolac tromethamine	SY	180 mg/ 6 mL	SO	150 mg/ 3 mL	Heavy white precipitate forms immediately, separating into two layers over time	1703	I
Lidocaine HCl	AST	2%/2 mL	PF	50 mg/ 2 mL	Physically compatible	771	C
	AST	2%/2 mL	PF	100 mg/ 2 mL	Physically compatible	771	C
Meperidine HCl	WI	100 mg/ 2 mL	PF	50 mg/ 1 mL	Physically compatible	771	C

Drugs in Syringe Compatibility (Cont.)

Hydroxyzine HCl

Drug (in syringe)	Mfr	Amt	Mfr	Amt	Remarks	Ref	C/I
	WI	50 mg/ 1 mL	PF	100 mg/ 2 mL	Physically compatible	771	**C**
	WY	100 mg/ 1 mL	PF	100 mg/ 4 mL	Physically compatible for at least 15 min	14	**C**
	WI	50 mg/ 1 mL	PF	50 mg/ 1 mL	Physically compatible for at least 15 min	326	**C**
Methotrimeprazine HCl	LE	20 mg/ 1 mL	PF	50 mg/ 1 mL	Physically compatible	771	**C**
	LE	10 mg/ 0.5 mL	PF	100 mg/ 2 mL	Physically compatible	771	**C**
Metoclopramide HCl	NO	10 mg/ 2 mL	PF	50 mg/ 1 mL	Physically compatible for 15 min at room temperature	565	**C**
Midazolam HCl	RC	5 mg/ 1 mL	ES	100 mg/ 2 mL	Physically compatible for 4 hr at 25 °C	1145	**C**
Morphine sulfate	WY	15 mg/ 1 mL	PF	100 mg/ 4 mL	Physically compatible for at least 15 min	14	**C**
	ST	15 mg/ 1 mL	PF	50 mg/ 1 mL	Physically compatible for at least 15 min	326	**C**
		10 mg/ 0.7 mL	PF	50 mg/ 1 mL	Physically compatible	771	**C**
		5 mg/ 0.3 mL	PF	100 mg/ 2 mL	Physically compatible	771	**C**
Nalbuphine HCl	EN	10 mg/ 1 mL	PF	50 mg	Physically compatible for 36 hr at 27 °C	762	**C**
	EN	5 mg/ 0.5 mL	PF	50 mg	Physically compatible for 36 hr at 27 °C	762	**C**
	EN	2.5 mg/ 0.25 mL	PF	50 mg	Physically compatible for 36 hr at 27 °C	762	**C**
	DU	10 mg/ 1 mL	PF	25 mg/ 1 mL	Physically compatible for 48 hr	128	**C**
	DU	20 mg/ 1 mL	PF	25 mg/ 1 mL	Physically compatible for 48 hr	128	**C**
Pentazocine lactate	WI	60 mg/ 2 mL	PF	50 mg/ 1 mL	Physically compatible	771	**C**
	WI	30 mg/ 1 mL	PF	100 mg/ 2 mL	Physically compatible	771	**C**
	WI	30 mg/ 1 mL	PF	100 mg/ 4 mL	Physically compatible for at least 15 min	14	**C**
	WI	30 mg/ 1 mL	PF	50 mg/ 1 mL	Physically compatible for at least 15 min	326	**C**
Pentobarbital sodium	WY	100 mg/ 2 mL	PF	100 mg/ 4 mL	Precipitate forms within 15 min	14	**I**
	AB	50 mg/ 1 mL	PF	50 mg/ 1 mL	Physically incompatible within 15 min	326	**I**
Prochlorperazine edisylate	PO	5 mg/ 1 mL	PF	50 mg/ 1 mL	Physically compatible for at least 15 min	326	**C**
Promethazine HCl	WY	50 mg/ 2 mL	PF	100 mg/ 4 mL	Physically compatible for at least 15 min	14	**C**
	PO	50 mg/ 2 mL	PF	50 mg/ 1 mL	Physically compatible for at least 15 min	326	**C**

Drugs in Syringe Compatibility (Cont.)

Hydroxyzine HCl

Drug (in syringe)	Mfr	Amt	Mfr	Amt	Remarks	Ref	C/I
Ranitidine HCl	GL	50 mg/ 2 mL	PF	50 mg/ 1 mL	Immediate white haze that disappears following vortex mixing	978	I
Scopolamine HBr		0.6 mg/ 1.5 mL	PF	100 mg/ 4 mL	Physically compatible for at least 15 min	14	C
	ST	0.4 mg/ 1 mL	PF	50 mg/ 1 mL	Physically compatible for at least 15 min	326	C
		0.65 mg/ 1 mL	PF	100 mg/ 2 mL	Physically compatible	771	C
		0.65 mg/ 1 mL	PF	50 mg/ 1 mL	Physically compatible	771	C

Y-Site Injection Compatibility (1:1 Mixture)

Hydroxyzine HCl

Drug	Mfr	Conc	Mfr	Conc	Remarks	Ref	C/I
Allopurinol sodium	BW	3 mg/mL[b]	ES	4 mg/mL[b]	Immediate turbidity and precipitate	1686	I
Amifostine	USB	10 mg/mL[a]	WI	4 mg/mL[a]	Subvisible haze forms immediately	1845	I
Amphotericin B cholesteryl sulfate complex	SEQ	0.83 mg/mL[a]	ES	2 mg/mL[a]	Gross precipitate forms	2117	I
Aztreonam	SQ	40 mg/mL[a]	WI	4 mg/mL[a]	Physically compatible for 4 hr at 23 °C	1758	C
Ceftaroline fosamil	FOR	2.22 mg/ mL[a,b,h]	ABX	2 mg/mL[a,b,h]	Physically compatible for 4 hr at 23 °C	2826	C
Ciprofloxacin	MI	2 mg/mL[c]	ES	50 mg/mL	Visually compatible for 24 hr at 24 °C	1655	C
Cisatracurium besylate	GW	0.1, 2, 5 mg/ mL[a]	ES	2 mg/mL[a]	Physically compatible for 4 hr at 23 °C	2074	C
Cladribine	ORT	0.015[b] and 0.5[d] mg/mL	ES	4 mg/mL[b]	Physically compatible for 4 hr at 23 °C	1969	C
Dexmedetomidine HCl	AB	4 mcg/mL[b]	ES	2 mg/mL[b]	Physically compatible for 4 hr at 23 °C	2383	C
Docetaxel	RPR	0.9 mg/mL[a]	ES	2 mg/mL[a]	Physically compatible for 4 hr at 23 °C	2224	C
Doxorubicin HCl liposomal	SEQ	0.4 mg/mL[a]	ES	2 mg/mL[a]	10-fold increase in particles $\geq$10 μm in 4 hr	2087	I
Etoposide phosphate	BR	5 mg/mL[a]	ES	4 mg/mL[a]	Physically compatible for 4 hr at 23 °C	2218	C
Famotidine	ME	2 mg/mL[b]		4 mg/mL[a]	Visually compatible for 4 hr at 22 °C	1936	C
Fenoldopam mesylate	AB	80 mcg/mL[b]	ES	2 mg/mL[b]	Physically compatible for 4 hr at 23 °C	2467	C
Fentanyl citrate	JN	0.025 mg/ mL[a]	WI	4 mg/mL[a]	Physically compatible for 48 hr at 22 °C	1706	C
Filgrastim	AMG	30 mcg/mL[a]	ES	4 mg/mL[a]	Physically compatible for 4 hr at 22 °C	1687	C
Fluconazole	RR	2 mg/mL	ES	50 mg/mL	Cloudiness develops	1407	I
Fludarabine phosphate	BX	1 mg/mL[a]	WI	4 mg/mL[a]	Slight haze forms immediately	1439	I
Foscarnet sodium	AST	24 mg/mL	LY	50 mg/mL	Physically compatible for 24 hr at room temperature under fluorescent light	1335	C
Gemcitabine HCl	LI	10 mg/mL[b]	ES	2 mg/mL[b]	Physically compatible for 4 hr at 23 °C	2226	C
Granisetron HCl	SKB	0.05 mg/mL[a]	ES	2 mg/mL[a]	Physically compatible for 4 hr at 23 °C	2000	C
Hetastarch in lactated electrolyte	AB	6%	ES	2 mg/mL[a]	Physically compatible for 4 hr at 23 °C	2339	C

Y-Site Injection Compatibility (1:1 Mixture) (Cont.)

Hydroxyzine HCl

Drug	Mfr	Conc	Mfr	Conc	Remarks	Ref	C/I
Hydromorphone HCl	AST	0.5 mg/mL[a]	WI	4 mg/mL[a]	Physically compatible for 48 hr at 22 °C	1706	**C**
Linezolid	PHU	2 mg/mL	ES	2 mg/mL[a]	Physically compatible for 4 hr at 23 °C	2264	**C**
Melphalan HCl	BW	0.1 mg/mL[b]	WI	4 mg/mL[b]	Physically compatible for 3 hr at 22 °C	1557	**C**
Methadone HCl	LI	1 mg/mL[a]	WI	4 mg/mL[a]	Physically compatible for 48 hr at 22 °C	1706	**C**
Morphine sulfate	AST	1 mg/mL[a]	WI	4 mg/mL[a]	Physically compatible for 48 hr at 22 °C	1706	**C**
Ondansetron HCl	GL	1 mg/mL[b]	WI	4 mg/mL[a]	Visually compatible for 4 hr at 22 °C	1365	**C**
Oxaliplatin	SS	0.5 mg/mL[a]	ES	2 mg/mL[a]	Physically compatible for 4 hr at 23 °C	2566	**C**
Paclitaxel	NCI	1.2 mg/mL[a]	ES	4 mg/mL[a]	Normal inherent haze from paclitaxel decreases immediately	1556	**I**
Pemetrexed disodium	LI	20 mg/mL[b]	APP	2 mg/mL[a]	Physically compatible for 4 hr at 23 °C	2564	**C**
Piperacillin sodium–tazobactam sodium	LE[g]	40 + 5 mg/mL[a]	WI	4 mg/mL[a]	Haze and particles form immediately	1688	**I**
Propofol	ZEN	10 mg/mL	ES	2 mg/mL[a]	Physically compatible for 1 hr at 23 °C	2066	**C**
Remifentanil HCl	GW	0.025 and 0.25 mg/mL[b]	ES	2 mg/mL[a]	Physically compatible for 4 hr at 23 °C	2075	**C**
Sargramostim	IMM	10 mcg/mL[b]	ES	4 mg/mL[b]	Slight haze and particles form in 4 hr	1436	**I**
Teniposide	BR	0.1 mg/mL[a]	WI	4 mg/mL[a]	Physically compatible for 4 hr at 23 °C	1725	**C**
Thiotepa	IMM[e]	1 mg/mL[a]	ES	4 mg/mL[a]	Physically compatible for 4 hr at 23 °C	1861	**C**
TNA #218 to #226[f]			ES	2 mg/mL[a]	Visually compatible for 4 hr at 23 °C	2215	**C**
TPN #212 to #215[f]			ES	2 mg/mL[a]	Physically compatible for 4 hr at 23 °C	2109	**C**
Vinorelbine tartrate	BW	1 mg/mL[b]	ES	4 mg/mL[b]	Physically compatible for 4 hr at 22 °C	1558	**C**

[a]*Tested in dextrose 5%.*
[b]*Tested in sodium chloride 0.9%.*
[c]*Tested in both dextrose 5% and sodium chloride 0.9%.*
[d]*Tested in bacteriostatic sodium chloride 0.9% preserved with benzyl alcohol 0.9%.*
[e]*Lyophilized formulation tested.*
[f]*Refer to Appendix I for the composition of parenteral nutrition solutions. TNA indicates a 3-in-1 admixture, and TPN indicates a 2-in-1 admixture.*
[g]*Test performed using the formulation WITHOUT edetate disodium.*
[h]*Tested in Ringer's injection, lactated.*

Additional Compatibility Information

Chlorpromazine and Meperidine — Chlorpromazine hydrochloride (Elkins-Sinn) 6.25 mg/mL, hydroxyzine hydrochloride (Pfizer) 12.5 mg/mL, and meperidine hydrochloride (Winthrop) 25 mg/mL, in both glass and plastic syringes, were reported to be physically compatible and chemically stable for at least one year at 4 and 25 °C when protected from light. (989)

IBUPROFEN LYSINATE
AHFS 28:08.04.92

Products — Ibuprofen lysinate is available as a preservative-free injection containing in each milliliter the L-lysine salt of (±) ibuprofen 17.1 mg (equivalent to ibuprofen 10 mg) with sodium hydroxide and/or hydrochloric acid to adjust pH during manufacturing in water for injection. The injection is packaged in single-use 2-mL vials. (1)

pH — About 7.0. (1)

Trade Name(s) — NeoProfen.

Administration — Ibuprofen lysinate is administered intravenously after dilution in a suitable volume of dextrose or saline infusion solution. The drug should be prepared and administered within 30 minutes of preparation by intravenous infusion over 15 minutes taking care to avoid extravasation. (1)

Stability — Intact vials of ibuprofen lysinate should be stored at controlled room temperature protected from light. The manufacturer recommends retaining the vials in their carton until use. (1)

After dilution in an appropriate volume of dextrose or saline intravenous infusion solution, ibuprofen lysinate should be administered within 30 minutes over a period of 15 minutes. Any remaining solution in the single-use vials should be discarded because no antimicrobial preservative is present. The manufacturer recommends not administering ibuprofen lysinate into a line running a TPN admixture; the TPN should be interrupted if necessary for 15 minutes both before and after administering ibuprofen lysinate maintaining line patency using dextrose or saline infusion solution. (1)

Compatibility Information

Solution Compatibility

Ibuprofen lysinate

Solution	Mfr	Mfr	Conc/L	Remarks	Ref	C/I
Dextrose 5%			1 and 4 g	6 to 7% loss occurred in 15 days at 25 °C	2610	C
Sodium chloride 0.9%			1 and 4 g	4 to 7% loss occurred in 15 days at 25 °C	2610	C

IDARUBICIN HYDROCHLORIDE
AHFS 10:00

Products — Idarubicin hydrochloride is available as a 1-mg/mL orange-red solution in single-use vials containing 5, 10, and 20 mL. In addition to the drug, each milliliter also contains glycerin 25 mg and hydrochloric acid to adjust pH in water for injection. (1)

pH — The idarubicin hydrochloride has been adjusted with hydrochloric acid to a target pH of 3.5. (1)

Trade Name(s) — Idamycin PFS.

Administration — Idarubicin hydrochloride should be administered by slow intravenous injection over 10 to 15 minutes into the tubing of a running infusion of sodium chloride 0.9% or dextrose 5%. The drug should not be given subcutaneously or intramuscularly, and extravasation should be avoided to prevent severe tissue necrosis. Care should be exercised during dose preparation to avoid inadvertent skin contact with the drug. (1)

Stability — Idarubicin hydrochloride in intact vials should be stored under refrigeration at 2 to 8 °C and protected from light. Leaving the vials in the carton until the time of use is recommended. (1)

Idarubicin hydrochloride (Farmitalia) 0.07 mg/mL diluted in sodium chloride 0.9% and stored at 22 °C did not exhibit an antimicrobial effect on the growth of four organisms (*Enterococcus faecium, Staphylococcus aureus, Pseudomonas aeruginosa,* and *Candida albicans*) inoculated into the solution. Viability was maintained for periods of 48 to 120 hours. The author recommended that diluted solutions of idarubicin hydrochloride be stored under refrigeration whenever possible and that the potential for microbiological growth should be considered when assigning expiration periods. (2160)

pH Effects — Idarubicin hydrochloride in prolonged contact with alkaline solutions will undergo decomposition. (1; 1368)

Light Effects — Dilute solutions (0.01 mg/mL) of idarubicin hydrochloride are light sensitive, undergoing some degradation with exposure to light over periods greater than six hours. (1368) However, the manufacturer indicates that no special precautions are necessary to protect freshly prepared solutions for administration. (1369)

Sorption — Idarubicin hydrochloride is compatible with PVC, glass, and polypropylene. (1369)

Compatibility Information

Solution Compatibility

Idarubicin HCl

Solution	Mfr	Mfr	Conc/L	Remarks	Ref	C/I
Dextrose 5% in sodium chloride 0.9%		FA	10 mg	No loss in 72 hr at room temperature protected from light. Less than 10% loss in 6 hr at room temperature exposed to light	1493	**C**
Dextrose 5%		FA	100 mg	Up to 5% loss in 4 weeks at 25 °C in the dark	1007	**C**
		FA	10 mg	No loss in 72 hr at room temperature protected from light. Less than 10% loss in 6 hr at room temperature exposed to light	1493	**C**
Ringer's injection, lactated		FA	100 mg	Up to 5% loss in 4 weeks at 25 °C in the dark	1007	**C**
Sodium chloride 0.9%		FA	100 mg	Up to 5% loss in 4 weeks at 25 °C in the dark	1007	**C**
		FA	10 mg	No loss in 72 hr at room temperature protected from light. Less than 10% loss in 6 hr at room temperature exposed to light	1493	**C**

Y-Site Injection Compatibility (1:1 Mixture)

Idarubicin HCl

Drug	Mfr	Conc	Mfr	Conc	Remarks	Ref	C/I
Acyclovir sodium	BW	5 mg/mL[b]	AD	1 mg/mL[b]	Haze forms and color changes immediately. Precipitate forms in 12 min	1525	**I**
Allopurinol sodium	BW	3 mg/mL[b]	AD	0.5 mg/mL[b]	Immediate reddish-purple color. Particles in 1 hr. Total color loss in 24 hr	1686	**I**
Amifostine	USB	10 mg/mL[a]	AD	0.5 mg/mL[a]	Physically compatible for 4 hr at 23 °C	1845	**C**
Amikacin sulfate	BR	5 mg/mL[a]	AD	1 mg/mL[b]	Visually compatible for 24 hr at 25 °C	1525	**C**
Ampicillin sodium–sulbactam sodium	RR	20 + 10 mg/mL[b]	AD	1 mg/mL[b]	Haze forms and color changes immediately. Precipitate forms in 20 min	1525	**I**
Aztreonam	SQ	40 mg/mL[a]	AD	0.5 mg/mL[a]	Physically compatible for 4 hr at 23 °C	1758	**C**
Cefazolin sodium	LI	20 mg/mL[a]	AD	1 mg/mL[b]	Precipitate forms in 1 hr	1525	**I**
Ceftazidime	LI	20 mg/mL[a]	AD	1 mg/mL[b]	Haze forms in 1 hr	1525	**I**
Cladribine	ORT	0.015[b] and 0.5[c] mg/mL	AD	0.5 mg/mL[b]	Physically compatible for 4 hr at 23 °C	1969	**C**
Clindamycin phosphate	AST	12 mg/mL[a]	AD	1 mg/mL[b]	Haze and precipitate form immediately	1525	**I**
Cyclophosphamide	AD	4 mg/mL[a]	AD	1 mg/mL[b]	Visually compatible for 24 hr at 25 °C	1525	**C**
Cytarabine	CET	6 mg/mL[a]	AD	1 mg/mL[b]	Visually compatible for 24 hr at 25 °C	1525	**C**
Dexamethasone sodium phosphate	OR	10 mg/mL	AD	1 mg/mL[b]	Haze forms immediately and precipitate forms in 20 min	1525	**I**
	AMR	0.2 mg/mL[b]	AD	1 mg/mL[b]	Haze forms in 20 min	1525	**I**
Diphenhydramine HCl	ES	1[a] and 50 mg/mL	AD	1 mg/mL[b]	Visually compatible for 24 hr at 25 °C	1525	**C**
Droperidol	AMR	0.04[a] and 2.5 mg/mL	AD	1 mg/mL[b]	Visually compatible for 24 hr at 25 °C	1525	**C**
Erythromycin lactobionate	ES	2 mg/mL[b]	AD	1 mg/mL[b]	Visually compatible for 24 hr at 25 °C	1525	**C**
Etoposide	BR	0.4 mg/mL[a]	AD	1 mg/mL[b]	Gas forms immediately	1525	**I**
Etoposide phosphate	BR	5 mg/mL[a]	AD	0.5 mg/mL[a]	Physically compatible for 4 hr at 23 °C	2218	**C**

Y-Site Injection Compatibility (1:1 Mixture) (Cont.)

Idarubicin HCl

Drug	Mfr	Conc	Mfr	Conc	Remarks	Ref	C/I
Filgrastim	AMG	30 mcg/mL[a]	AD	0.5 mg/mL[a]	Physically compatible for 4 hr at 22 °C	1687	C
Furosemide	AB	10 mg/mL	AD	1 mg/mL[b]	Precipitate forms immediately	1525	I
	AB	0.8 mg/mL[b]	AD	1 mg/mL[b]	Haze forms immediately	1525	I
Gemcitabine HCl	LI	10 mg/mL[b]	AD	0.5 mg/mL[b]	Physically compatible for 4 hr at 23 °C	2226	C
Granisetron HCl	SKB	0.05 mg/mL[a]	AD	0.5 mg/mL[a]	Physically compatible for 4 hr at 23 °C	2000	C
Heparin sodium	ES, SO	100 and 1000 units/mL	AD	1 mg/mL[b]	Haze forms immediately and precipitate forms in 12 to 20 min	1525	I
Hydrocortisone sodium succinate	UP	2[a] and 50 mg/mL	AD	1 mg/mL[b]	Haze forms immediately and precipitate forms in 20 min	1525	I
Imipenem–cilastatin sodium	MSD	5 mg/mL[b]	AD	1 mg/mL[b]	Visually compatible for 12 hr at 25 °C in light. Precipitate in 24 hr	1525	C
Lorazepam	WY	2 mg/mL	AD	1 mg/mL[b]	Color changes immediately	1525	I
Magnesium sulfate	SO	2 mg/mL[b]	AD	1 mg/mL[b]	Visually compatible for 24 hr at 25 °C	1525	C
Mannitol	AB	12.5 mg/mL[a]	AD	1 mg/mL[b]	Visually compatible for 24 hr at 25 °C	1525	C
Melphalan HCl	BW	0.1 mg/mL[b]	AD	0.5 mg/mL[b]	Physically compatible for 3 hr at 22 °C	1557; 1675	C
Meperidine HCl	WY	1[a] and 50 mg/mL	AD	1 mg/mL[b]	Color changes immediately	1525	I
Methotrexate sodium	LE	25 mg/mL	AD	1 mg/mL[b]	Color changes immediately	1525	I
Metoclopramide HCl	SO	5 mg/mL	AD	1 mg/mL[b]	Visually compatible for 24 hr at 25 °C	1525	C
Piperacillin sodium–tazobactam sodium	LE[f]	40 + 5 mg/mL[a]	AD	0.5 mg/mL[a]	Immediate increase in haze	1688	I
Potassium chloride	AB	0.03 mEq/mL[b]	AD	1 mg/mL[b]	Visually compatible for 24 hr at 25 °C	1525	C
Ranitidine HCl	GL	1 mg/mL[a]	AD	1 mg/mL[b]	Visually compatible for 24 hr at 25 °C	1525	C
Sargramostim	IMM	10 mcg/mL[b]	AD	0.5 mg/mL[b]	Physically compatible	1675	C
Sodium bicarbonate	AB	0.09 mEq/mL[a]	AD	1 mg/mL[b]	Haze forms and color changes immediately. Precipitate forms in 20 min	1525	I
Teniposide	BR	0.1 mg/mL[a]	AD	0.5 mg/mL[a]	Unacceptable increase in turbidity	1725	I
Thiotepa	IMM[d]	1 mg/mL[a]	AD	0.5 mg/mL[a]	Physically compatible for 4 hr at 23 °C	1861	C
TPN #140[e]			AD	1 mg/mL[b]	Visually compatible for 24 hr at 25 °C	1525	C
Vancomycin HCl	AD	4 mg/mL[a]	AD	1 mg/mL[b]	Color changes immediately	1525	I
Vincristine sulfate	AD	1 mg/mL	AD	1 mg/mL[b]	Color changes immediately	1525	I
Vinorelbine tartrate	BW	1 mg/mL[b]	AD	0.5 mg/mL[b]	Physically compatible for 4 hr at 22 °C	1558; 1675	C

[a]Tested in dextrose 5%.
[b]Tested in sodium chloride 0.9%.
[c]Tested in bacteriostatic sodium chloride 0.9% preserved with benzyl alcohol 0.9%.
[d]Lyophilized formulation tested.
[e]Refer to Appendix I for the composition of parenteral nutrition solutions. TPN indicates a 2-in-1 admixture.
[f]Test performed using the formulation WITHOUT edetate disodium.

IFOSFAMIDE
AHFS 10:00

Products — Ifosfamide is available in vials containing 1 or 3 g of drug. Reconstitute the ifosfamide with 20 or 60 mL of sterile water for injection or bacteriostatic water for injection (parabens or benzyl alcohol), respectively, to yield a 50-mg/mL solution. (1)

pH — Approximately 6. (72)

Trade Name(s) — Ifex.

Administration — Ifosfamide is administered by slow intravenous infusion over a minimum of 30 minutes diluted to a concentration between 0.6 and 20 mg/mL. (1; 4) Ifosfamide has also been administered by continuous intravenous infusion. (4) To prevent bladder toxicity, mesna and at least 2 L/day of fluid should be given. (1; 4)

Stability — Intact vials of ifosfamide should be stored at controlled room temperature and protected from temperatures above 30 °C. (1) Ifosfamide may liquify at temperatures above 35 °C. (72)

The reconstituted solution is stated to be chemically and physically stable for seven days at 30 °C and for up to six weeks under refrigeration. (4; 72) Because of microbiological concerns, the manufacturer recommends storage under refrigeration and use in 24 hours for reconstituted or diluted ifosfamide solutions. (1)

Ifosfamide (Boehringer-Ingelheim) 80 mg/mL in sodium chloride 0.9% exhibited about 7% loss in nine days at 37 °C in the dark. (1494)

Reconstitution to an ifosfamide concentration of 100 mg/mL with benzyl alcohol-preserved bacteriostatic water for injection resulted in a turbid mixture, separating into two distinct liquid phases. The separate phases dissolved completely, with no loss of drug or preservative, when diluted to about 60 mg/mL or less. (1289)

pH Effects — Ifosfamide exhibits maximum solution stability in the pH range of 4 to 10; the rate of decomposition is essentially the same over this pH range. At pH values less than 4 and above 10, increased rates of decomposition have been observed. (2002; 2401)

Syringes — Ifosfamide 0.6 and 20 mg/mL in dextrose 5%, lactated Ringer's injection, sodium chloride 0.9%, and sterile water for injection in polypropylene syringes (Becton Dickinson) is physically and chemically stable for at least 24 hours at 30 °C. (1496)

Ambulatory Pumps — Ifosfamide (Asta Medica) 20 mg/mL and mesna (Asta Medica) 20 mg/mL in water for injection were evaluated for stability and compatibility in PVC reservoirs for Graseby 9000 ambulatory pumps. The solutions were physically compatible and analysis found about 3% ifosfamide and 9% mesna loss in 7 days at 37 °C. About 2% or less loss of both drugs was found after 14 days at 4 °C. Furthermore, weight losses due to moisture loss were minimal. (2288)

Compatibility Information

Solution Compatibility

Ifosfamide

Solution	Mfr	Mfr	Conc/L	Remarks	Ref	C/I
Dextrose 5% in Ringer's injection			600 mg and 16 g	Physically compatible. Under 5% loss in 7 days at 30 °C and no loss in 6 weeks at 5 °C	72	C
Dextrose 5% in sodium chloride 0.9%	b		0.6 to 20 g	Physically compatible and stable for 7 days at 30 °C and 6 weeks at 5 °C	4	C
			600 mg and 16 g	Physically compatible. Under 5% loss in 7 days at 30 °C and no loss in 6 weeks at 5 °C	72	C
Dextrose 5%	b		0.6 to 20 g	Physically compatible and stable for 7 days at 30 °C and 6 weeks at 5 °C	4	C
			600 mg and 16 g	Physically compatible. Under 5% loss in 7 days at 30 °C and no loss in 6 weeks at 5 °C	72	C
Ringer's injection, lactated	b		0.6 to 20 g	Physically compatible and stable for 7 days at 30 °C and 6 weeks at 5 °C	4	C
			600 mg and 16 g	Physically compatible. Under 5% loss in 7 days at 30 °C and no loss in 6 weeks at 5 °C	72	C
Sodium chloride 0.45%			600 mg and 16 g	Physically compatible. Under 5% loss in 7 days at 30 °C and no loss in 6 weeks at 5 °C	72	C
Sodium chloride 0.9%	b		0.6 to 20 g	Physically compatible and stable for 7 days at 30 °C and 6 weeks at 5 °C	4	C
			600 mg and 16 g	Physically compatible. Under 5% loss in 7 days at 30 °C and no loss in 6 weeks at 5 °C	72	C
		BI	80 g	7% loss in 9 days at 37 °C in dark	1494	C
	a		10 g	No loss in 8 days at 4 and 25 °C protected from light and at 25 °C in light	1551	C

Solution Compatibility (Cont.)

Ifosfamide

Solution	Mfr	Mfr	Conc/L	Remarks	Ref	C/I
a			20, 40, 80 g	No loss in 8 days at 35 °C	1551	C
Sodium lactate ⅙ M			600 mg and 16 g	Physically compatible. Under 5% loss in 7 days at 30 °C and no loss in 6 weeks at 5 °C	72	C

[a]Tested in PVC containers.
[b]Tested in glass, PVC, and polyolefin containers.

Additive Compatibility

Ifosfamide

Drug	Mfr	Conc/L	Mfr	Conc/L	Test Soln	Remarks	Ref	C/I
Carboplatin		1 g		1 g	W	Both drugs stable for 5 days at room temperature	1379	C
Cisplatin		200 mg		2 g	NS	Both drugs stable for 7 days at room temperature	1379	C
Cisplatin with etoposide		200 mg 200 mg		2 g	NS	All drugs stable for 5 days at room temperature	1379	C
Epirubicin HCl		1 g		2.5 g	NS	Under 10% loss of either drug in 14 days	1379	C
Etoposide		200 mg		2 g	NS	Both drugs stable for 5 days at room temperature	1379	C
Etoposide with cisplatin		200 mg 200 mg		2 g	NS	All drugs stable for 5 days at room temperature	1379	C
Fluorouracil		10 g		2 g	NS	Both drugs stable for 5 days at room temperature	1379	C
Mesna	AW	3.3 g	MJ	3.3 g	D5W, LR	Physically compatible. No ifosfamide loss and about 5% mesna loss in 24 hr at 21 °C exposed to light	72	C
	AW	5 g	MJ	5 g	D5W, LR	Physically compatible. No ifosfamide loss and about 5% mesna loss in 24 hr at 21 °C exposed to light	72	C
	BI	79 g	BI	83.3 g	NS	Little or no ifosfamide loss in 9 days at room temperature and 7% ifosfamide loss in 9 days at 37 °C. Mesna not tested	1494	C
		1.6 g		2.6 g	D5S[a]	No increase in decomposition products in 8 hr at room temperature	1495	C
	BR	600 mg	BR	600 mg	D5½S, D5W, LR, NS[b]	Both drugs chemically stable for at least 24 hr at room temperature	1496	C
	AM	20 g	AM	20 g	W[c]	Physically compatible with about 3% ifosfamide loss and 9% mesna loss in 7 days at 37 °C. About 2% or less loss of both drugs in 14 days at 4 °C	2288	C

[a]Tested in polyethylene containers.
[b]Tested in PVC containers.
[c]Tested in PVC reservoirs for Graseby 9000 ambulatory pumps.

Drugs in Syringe Compatibility

Ifosfamide

Drug (in syringe)	Mfr	Amt	Mfr	Amt	Remarks	Ref	C/I
Epirubicin HCl		1 mg/mL[a]		50 mg/mL[a]	Little or no loss of either drug in 28 days at 4 and 20 °C	1564	C
Epirubicin HCl with mesna		1 mg/mL 40 mg/mL[a]		50 mg/mL[a]	50% epirubicin loss in 7 days at 4 and 20 °C. No loss of other drugs in 7 days	1564	I
Mesna		200 mg/5 mL		250 mg/5 mL	3% ifosfamide loss in 7 days and 12% in 4 weeks at 4 °C and room temperature. No mesna loss	1290	C
		40 mg/mL[a]		50 mg/mL[a]	Little or no loss of either drug in 28 days at 4 and 20 °C	1564	C
Mesna with epirubicin HCl		40 mg/mL[a] 1 mg/mL		50 mg/mL[a]	50% epirubicin loss in 7 days at 4 and 20 °C. No loss of other drugs in 7 days	1564	I

[a]Diluted in sodium chloride 0.9%.

Y-Site Injection Compatibility (1:1 Mixture)

Ifosfamide

Drug	Mfr	Conc	Mfr	Conc	Remarks	Ref	C/I
Allopurinol sodium	BW	3 mg/mL[b]	MJ	25 mg/mL[b]	Physically compatible for 4 hr at 22 °C	1686	C
Amifostine	USB	10 mg/mL[a]	MJ	25 mg/mL[a]	Physically compatible for 4 hr at 23 °C	1845	C
Amphotericin B cholesteryl sulfate complex	SEQ	0.83 mg/mL[a]	MJ	25 mg/mL[a]	Physically compatible for 4 hr at 23 °C	2117	C
Anidulafungin	VIC	0.5 mg/mL[a]	BMS	25 mg/mL[a]	Physically compatible for 4 hr at 23 °C	2617	C
Aztreonam	SQ	40 mg/mL[a]	MJ	25 mg/mL[a]	Physically compatible for 4 hr at 23 °C	1758	C
Caspofungin acetate	ME	0.7 mg/mL[b]	BA	20 mg/mL[b]	Physically compatible for 4 hr at room temperature	2758	C
Doripenem	JJ	5 mg/mL[a,b]	BMS	20 mg/mL[a,b]	Physically compatible for 4 hr at 23 °C	2743	C
Doxorubicin HCl liposomal	SEQ	0.4 mg/mL[a]	MJ	25 mg/mL[a]	Physically compatible for 4 hr at 23 °C	2087	C
Etoposide phosphate	BR	5 mg/mL[a]	MJ	25 mg/mL[a]	Physically compatible for 4 hr at 23 °C	2218	C
Filgrastim	AMG	30 mcg/mL[a]	MJ	25 mg/mL[a]	Physically compatible for 4 hr at 22 °C	1687	C
Fludarabine phosphate	BX	1 mg/mL[a]	MJ	25 mg/mL[a]	Visually compatible for 4 hr at 22 °C	1439	C
Gallium nitrate	FUJ	1 mg/mL[b]	MJ	20 mg/mL[b]	Visually compatible for 24 hr at 25 °C	1673	C
Gemcitabine HCl	LI	10 mg/mL[b]	MJ	25 mg/mL[b]	Physically compatible for 4 hr at 23 °C	2226	C
Granisetron HCl	SKB	1 mg/mL	MJ	4 mg/mL[b]	Physically compatible with little or no loss of either drug in 4 hr at 22 °C	1883	C
Linezolid	PHU	2 mg/mL	MJ	25 mg/mL[a]	Physically compatible for 4 hr at 23 °C	2264	C
Melphalan HCl	BW	0.1 mg/mL[b]	BR	25 mg/mL[b]	Physically compatible for 3 hr at 22 °C	1557	C
Methotrexate sodium		30 mg/mL		36 mg/mL[a]	Visually compatible for 2 hr at room temperature. Yellow precipitate in 4 hr	1788	I
Ondansetron HCl	GL	1 mg/mL[b]	MJ	25 mg/mL[a]	Visually compatible for 4 hr at 22 °C	1365	C
Oxaliplatin	SS	0.5 mg/mL[a]	MJ	20 mg/mL[a]	Physically compatible for 4 hr at 23 °C	2566	C
Paclitaxel	NCI	1.2 mg/mL[a]	BR	25 mg/mL[a]	Physically compatible for 4 hr at 22 °C	1556	C

Y-Site Injection Compatibility (1:1 Mixture) (Cont.)

Ifosfamide

Drug	Mfr	Conc	Mfr	Conc	Remarks	Ref	C/I
Palonosetron HCl	MGI	50 mcg/mL	MJ	10 mg/mL[a]	Physically compatible and no loss of either drug in 4 hr	2640	C
Pemetrexed disodium	LI	20 mg/mL[b]	MJ	20 mg/mL[a]	Physically compatible for 4 hr at 23 °C	2564	C
Piperacillin sodium–tazobactam sodium	LE[e]	40 + 5 mg/mL[a]	MJ	25 mg/mL[a]	Physically compatible for 4 hr at 22 °C	1688	C
Propofol	ZEN	10 mg/mL	MJ	25 mg/mL[a]	Physically compatible for 1 hr at 23 °C	2066	C
Sargramostim	IMM	10 mcg/mL[b]	MJ	25 mg/mL[b]	Visually compatible for 4 hr at 22 °C	1436	C
Sodium bicarbonate		1.4%		36 mg/mL[a]	Visually compatible for 4 hr at room temperature	1788	C
Teniposide	BR	0.1 mg/mL[a]	MJ	25 mg/mL[a]	Physically compatible for 4 hr at 23 °C	1725	C
Thiotepa	IMM[c]	1 mg/mL[a]	MJ	25 mg/mL[a]	Physically compatible for 4 hr at 23 °C	1861	C
TNA #218 to #226[d]			MJ	25 mg/mL[a]	Visually compatible for 4 hr at 23 °C	2215	C
Topotecan HCl	SKB	56 mcg/mL[a,b]	MJ	14.28 mg/mL[a,b]	Visually compatible. Little loss of either drug in 4 hr at 22 °C	2245	C
TPN #212 to #215[d]			MJ	25 mg/mL[a]	Physically compatible for 4 hr at 23 °C	2109	C
Vinorelbine tartrate	BW	1 mg/mL[b]	MJ	25 mg/mL[b]	Physically compatible for 4 hr at 22 °C	1558	C

[a]*Tested in dextrose 5%.*
[b]*Tested in sodium chloride 0.9%.*
[c]*Lyophilized formulation tested.*
[d]*Refer to Appendix I for the composition of parenteral nutrition solutions. TNA indicates a 3-in-1 admixture, and TPN indicates a 2-in-1 admixture.*
[e]*Test performed using the formulation WITHOUT edetate disodium.*

IMIPENEM–CILASTATIN SODIUM
AHFS 8:12.07.08

Products — Imipenem–cilastatin sodium for intravenous use is available as a fixed combination of equal quantities of both drugs. The combination is provided in vials and infusion bottles containing 250 and 500 mg of each drug with sodium bicarbonate 10 and 20 mg, respectively. (1)

The vials should be reconstituted with about 10 mL of a compatible diluent from a 100-mL infusion container and shaken well to form a suspension. Diluents containing benzyl alcohol should not be used to reconstitute the drug for use in neonates and small pediatric patients. The suspension must be transferred to the remaining solution in the infusion container for dilution. The suspension is *not* for direct injection. The procedure is then repeated: a 10-mL aliquot from the admixture is added to the vial and, once again, returned to the infusion admixture. This procedure ensures that all of the vial contents are transferred. The admixture should be agitated until it is clear to yield either a 2.5- or 5-mg/mL concentration, depending on the vial content. The admixture should *not* be heated to aid dissolution. (1; 4)

ADD-Vantage vials of imipenem–cilastatin sodium should be prepared with 100 mL of dextrose 5% or sodium chloride 0.9% in ADD-Vantage diluent bags. (1; 4)

The 250- and 500-mg piggyback infusion bottles should be reconstituted with 100 mL of compatible diluent and shaken until clear to yield 2.5- and 5-mg/mL concentrations, respectively. (1; 4)

Imipenem–cilastatin sodium for intramuscular use is available in vials containing 500 or 750 mg of each component. The vials should be reconstituted with 2 or 3 mL, respectively, of lidocaine hydrochloride 1% (without epinephrine) and agitated to form a suspension. This intramuscular formulation is not for intravenous use. (1; 4)

pH — The intravenous product is buffered to pH 6.5 to 8.5. (1)

Osmolarity — When reconstituted and diluted as directed by the manufacturer, the osmolarity of the intravenous admixture approximates that of the diluent. (4)

Sodium Content — The 250- and 500-mg intravenous vials contain 0.8 mEq (18.8 mg) and 1.6 mEq (37.5 mg) of sodium, respectively. The 500- and 750-mg intramuscular vials contain 1.4 mEq (32 mg) and 2.1 mEq (48 mg) of sodium, respectively. (1; 4)

Trade Name(s) — Primaxin I.V., Primaxin I.M.

Administration — Imipenem–cilastatin sodium for intravenous use is given by intermittent intravenous infusion at a concentration not exceeding 5 mg/mL. Infusion periods vary from 20 to 60 minutes, depending on the dose. The intramuscular formulation should be injected deeply into a large muscle mass. Suspensions of either formulation should not be given intravenously. (1; 4)

Stability — The product should be stored below 25 °C. (1; 4)

Reconstituted as directed, intravenous solutions are colorless to yellow but may become a deeper yellow over time. Intramuscular suspensions are white to light tan. The manufacturer indicates that stability is not affected by color variations within this range (1), but the solutions should be discarded if they darken to brown. (4) Intramuscular suspensions prepared with lidocaine hydrochloride (without epinephrine) should be used within one hour. (1; 4)

In solution, imipenem is substantially less stable than cilastatin and is the determining factor in the overall stability of the combination product. Reconstitution results in solutions that are stable for four hours at room temperature or 24 hours under refrigeration at 4 °C. (1)

Imipenem degradation kinetics were determined for a 2.5-mg/mL solution in sodium chloride 0.9%. The degradation rates were temperature dependent, with a half-life of over 44 hours at 2 °C dropping to six hours at 25 °C and to two hours at 37 °C. The decomposition was consistent with hydrolysis, and the loss of antimicrobial activity suggests cleavage of the β-lactam ring. (1272)

pH Effects — Imipenem is inactivated at acidic or alkaline pH but is more stable at neutral pH. (4) The pH range of maximum stability appears to be 6.5 to 7.5, with increasing rates of decomposition occurring as the pH moves away from this range. (1273) At a pH of about 4, the half-life of imipenem is about 35 minutes. (2166)

Freezing Solutions — The manufacturer recommends that imipenem–cilastatin solutions not be frozen. (1) At concentrations of 250 and 500 mg/100 mL in sodium chloride 0.9%, imipenem losses of around 15% occurred in one week when frozen at −20 and −10 °C. (1141) Freezing solutions at temperatures above −70 °C offers no stability advantage over refrigerated storage (1141) and results in decomposition of imipenem in a manner similar to ampicillin. (4)

Effects of Solution Components — Dextrose exerts an adverse effect on the stability of imipenem. Dextrose 5 and 10% reduced the time to 10% decomposition by about one-half compared to sterile water. Sodium chloride content increases imipenem stability because of a positive kinetic salt effect similar to other β-lactam antibiotics. Both lactate and bicarbonate anions attack the β-lactam ring and decrease imipenem stability. (1141)

Elastomeric Reservoir Pumps — Imipenem–cilastatin sodium (Merck) 5 mg/mL in both dextrose 5% and sodium chloride 0.9% was evaluated for binding potential to natural rubber elastomeric reservoirs (Baxter). Less than 1% binding was found after storage for two weeks at 35 °C with gentle agitation. (2014)

Central Venous Catheter — Imipenem–cilastatin (MSD) 2 mg/mL in sodium chloride 0.9% was found to be compatible with the ARROWg+ard Blue Plus (Arrow International) chlorhexidine-bearing triple-lumen central catheter. Essentially complete delivery of the drug was found with little or no drug loss occurring. Furthermore, chlorhexidine delivered from the catheter remained at trace amounts with no substantial increase due to the delivery of the drug through the catheter. (2335)

Compatibility Information

Solution Compatibility

Imipenem–cilastatin sodium

Solution	Mfr	Mfr	Conc/L	Remarks	Ref	C/I
Dextrose 5% in Ringer's injection, lactated	AB[a]	MSD	2.5 g	8% imipenem loss in 3 hr, 15% in 6 hr at 25 °C. 9% loss in 24 hr, 15% in 48 hr at 4 °C	1141	**I**
	AB[a]	MSD	5 g	14% imipenem loss in 3 hr at 25 °C and 13% in 24 hr at 4 °C	1141	**I**
Dextrose 5% in sodium chloride 0.225%	AB[a]	MSD	2.5 g	8% imipenem loss in 6 hr and 12% in 9 hr at 25 °C. 10% loss in 48 hr at 4 °C	1141	**I**[b]
	AB[a]	MSD	5 g	5% imipenem loss in 3 hr, 13% in 6 hr at 25 °C. 7% loss in 24 hr, 13% in 48 hr at 4 °C	1141	**I**[b]
Dextrose 5% in sodium chloride 0.45%	AB[a]	MSD	2.5 g	8% imipenem loss in 6 hr, 11% in 9 hr at 25 °C. 9% loss in 48 hr, 13% in 72 hr at 4 °C	1141	**I**[b]
	AB[a]	MSD	5 g	5% imipenem loss in 3 hr, 11% in 6 hr at 25 °C. 6% loss in 24 hr, 13% in 48 hr at 4 °C	1141	**I**[b]
Dextrose 5% in sodium chloride 0.9%	AB[a]	MSD	2.5 g	6% imipenem loss in 6 hr, 10% in 9 hr at 25 °C. 6% loss in 24 hr, 11% in 48 hr at 4 °C	1141	**I**[b]
	AB[a]	MSD	5 g	6% imipenem loss in 3 hr, 11% in 6 hr at 25 °C. 6% loss in 24 hr, 13% in 48 hr at 4 °C	1141	**I**[b]
Dextrose 5%	AB[a]	MSD	2.5 g	5% imipenem loss in 3 hr, 10% in 6 hr at 25 °C. 8% loss in 24 hr, 14% in 48 hr at 4 °C	1141	**I**[b]

Solution Compatibility (Cont.)

Imipenem–cilastatin sodium

Solution	Mfr	Mfr	Conc/L	Remarks	Ref	C/I
	AB[a]	MSD	5 g	6% imipenem loss in 3 hr, 15% in 6 hr at 25 °C. 8% loss in 24 hr, 14% in 48 hr at 4 °C	1141	I[b]
	BA	MSD	5 g	Visually compatible. 10% imipenem loss in about 6 hr at 23 °C and in 48 hr at 4 °C	2166	I[b]
	BA[e], BRN[d]	MSD	2.5 g	Visually compatible. Little or no loss in 24 hr at 4 and 22 °C	2289	C
Dextrose 10%	AB[a]	MSD	2.5 g	6% imipenem loss in 3 hr, 10% in 6 hr at 25 °C. 8% loss in 24 hr, 13% in 48 hr at 4 °C	1141	I[b]
	AB[a]	MSD	5 g	8% imipenem loss in 3 hr and 13% in 6 hr at 25 °C. 10% loss in 24 hr at 4 °C	1141	I[b]
Normosol M in dextrose 5%	AB[a]	MSD	2.5 g	7% imipenem loss in 3 hr, 11% in 6 hr at 25 °C. 9% loss in 24 hr, 19% in 48 hr at 4 °C	1141	I[b]
	AB[a]	MSD	5 g	8% imipenem loss in 3 hr and 14% in 6 hr at 25 °C. 10% loss in 24 hr at 4 °C	1141	I[b]
Ringer's injection, lactated	AB[a]	MSD	2.5 g	9% imipenem loss in 6 hr, 12% in 9 hr at 25 °C. 4% loss in 24 hr, 10% in 48 hr at 4 °C	1141	I
	AB[a]	MSD	5 g	6% imipenem loss in 3 hr, 12% in 6 hr at 25 °C. 7% loss in 24 hr, 12% in 48 hr at 4 °C	1141	I
Sodium chloride 0.9%	AB[a]	MSD	2.5 g	6% imipenem loss in 9 hr at 25 °C. 7% loss in 72 hr at 4 °C	1141	I[b]
	AB[a]	MSD	5 g	8% imipenem loss in 9 hr at 25 °C. 7% loss in 48 hr and 11% in 72 hr at 4 °C	1141	I[b]
	BA[e], BRN[d]	MSD	2.5 g	Visually compatible. Little or no loss in 24 hr at 4 and 22 °C	2289	C
Sodium lactate ⅙ M	AB[a]	MSD	2.5 g	13% imipenem loss in 3 hr at 25 °C. 8% loss in 24 hr and 15% in 48 hr at 4 °C	1141	I
	AB[a]	MSD	5 g	18% imipenem loss in 3 hr at 25 °C. 14% loss in 24 hr at 4 °C	1141	I
TPN #107[c]			500 mg	57% imipenem loss in 24 hr at 21 °C	1326	I
TPN #241, #242[c]		MSD	5 g	8 to 10% imipenem loss within 30 min at 25 °C under fluorescent light	493	I

[a]Tested in glass containers.
[b]Incompatible by conventional standards but recommended for dilution of imipenem–cilastatin with use in shorter periods of time.
[c]Refer to Appendix I for the composition of parenteral nutrition solutions. TPN indicates a 2-in-1 admixture.
[d]Tested in polyethylene and glass containers.
[e]Tested in PVC containers.

Additive Compatibility

Imipenem–cilastatin sodium

Drug	Mfr	Conc/L	Mfr	Conc/L	Test Soln	Remarks	Ref	C/I
Amoxicillin sodium	MSD	8 g	GSK	4 g	NS	Blue discoloration formed in 2 hr. Amoxicillin and imipenem losses of 40 and 72%, respectively, in 12 hr	2800	I
Mannitol	AB[a]	2.5%	MSD	2.5 g		9% imipenem loss in 9 hr at 25 °C. 7% loss in 48 hr and 11% in 72 hr at 4 °C	1141	I[b]
	AB[a]	2.5%	MSD	5 g		6% imipenem loss in 3 hr and 12% in 6 hr at 25 °C. 7% loss in 24 hr and 10% in 48 hr at 4 °C	1141	I[b]

Additive Compatibility (Cont.)

Imipenem–cilastatin sodium

Drug	Mfr	Conc/L	Mfr	Conc/L	Test Soln	Remarks	Ref	C/I
	AB[a]	5%	MSD	2.5 g		6% imipenem loss in 3 hr and 10% in 6 hr at 25 °C. 9% loss in 48 hr and 13% in 72 hr at 4 °C	1141	I[b]
	AB[a]	5%	MSD	5 g		7% imipenem loss in 3 hr and 12% in 6 hr at 25 °C. 12% loss in 48 hr at 4 °C	1141	I[b]
	AB[a]	10%	MSD	2.5 g		6% imipenem loss in 3 hr and 10% in 6 hr at 25 °C. 7% loss in 24 hr and 12% in 48 hr at 4 °C	1141	I[b]
	AB[a]	10%	MSD	5 g		12% imipenem loss in 3 hr at 25 °C. 13% loss in 48 hr at 4 °C	1141	I[b]
Sodium bicarbonate	AB	5%	MSD	2.5 g		43% imipenem loss in 3 hr at 25 °C and 52% in 24 hr at 4 °C	1141	I
	AB	5%	MSD	5 g		45% imipenem loss in 3 hr at 25 °C and 50% in 24 hr at 4 °C	1141	I
Tobramycin sulfate		10 mg		100 mg	W	Little or no loss of antibiotic activity in 24 hr at 37 °C	498	C

[a]*Tested in glass containers.*
[b]*Incompatible by conventional standards but may be used in shorter periods of time.*

Y-Site Injection Compatibility (1:1 Mixture)

Imipenem–cilastatin sodium

Drug	Mfr	Conc	Mfr	Conc	Remarks	Ref	C/I
Acyclovir sodium	BW	5 mg/mL[a]	MSD	5 mg/mL[b]	Physically compatible for 4 hr at 25 °C	1157	C
Allopurinol sodium	BW	3 mg/mL[b]	MSD	10 mg/mL[b]	Haze and particles form in 1 hr	1686	I
Amifostine	USB	10 mg/mL[a]	MSD	10 mg/mL[a]	Physically compatible for 4 hr at 23 °C	1845	C
Amiodarone HCl	WY	6 mg/mL[a]	ME	5 mg/mL[a]	Immediate haze. Becomes yellow in 24 hr	2352	I
Amphotericin B cholesteryl sulfate complex	SEQ	0.83 mg/mL[a]	ME	10 mg/mL[b]	Gross precipitate forms	2117	I
Anidulafungin	VIC	0.5 mg/mL[a]	ME	5 mg/mL[b]	Physically compatible for 4 hr at 23 °C	2617	C
Azithromycin	PF	2 mg/mL[b]	ME	5 mg/mL[b,g]	Whitish-yellow microcrystals found	2368	I
Aztreonam	SQ	40 mg/mL[a]	MSD	10 mg/mL[a]	Physically compatible for 4 hr at 23 °C	1758	C
Caspofungin acetate	ME	0.7 mg/mL[b]	ME	5 mg/mL[b]	Physically compatible for 4 hr at room temperature	2758	C
Cisatracurium besylate	GW	0.1, 2, 5 mg/mL[a]	ME	10 mg/mL[b]	Physically compatible for 4 hr at 23 °C	2074	C
Diltiazem HCl	MMD	5 mg/mL	MSD	5 mg/mL[c]	Visually compatible	1807	C
Docetaxel	RPR	0.9 mg/mL[a]	ME	10 mg/mL[b]	Physically compatible for 4 hr at 23 °C	2224	C
Etoposide phosphate	BR	5 mg/mL[a]	ME	10 mg/mL[b]	Yellow color forms in 4 hr at 23 °C	2218	I
Famotidine	MSD	0.2 mg/mL[a]	MSD	10 mg/mL[b]	Physically compatible for 14 hr	1196	C
	ME	2 mg/mL[b]		5 mg/mL[b]	Visually compatible for 4 hr at 22 °C	1936	C
Filgrastim	AMG	30 mcg/mL[a]	MSD	10 mg/mL[a]	Physically compatible for 4 hr at 22 °C	1687	C
	AMG	40 mcg/mL[a]	ME	5 mg/mL[a]	16% loss of filgrastim in 4 hr at 25 °C. Little imipenem–cilastatin loss	2060	I

Y-Site Injection Compatibility (1:1 Mixture) (Cont.)

Imipenem–cilastatin sodium

Drug	Mfr	Conc	Mfr	Conc	Remarks	Ref	C/I
	AMG	10 mcg/mL[d]	ME	5 mg/mL[a]	Visually compatible. Little loss of filgrastim and imipenem–cilastatin in 4 hr at 25 °C	2060	C
Fluconazole	RR	2 mg/mL	MSD	10 mg/mL	Precipitates immediately	1407	I
Fludarabine phosphate	BX	1 mg/mL[a]	MSD	5 mg/mL[a]	Visually compatible for 4 hr at 22 °C	1439	C
Foscarnet sodium	AST	24 mg/mL	MSD	10 mg/mL	Physically compatible for 24 hr at room temperature under fluorescent light	1335	C
	AST	24 mg/mL	MSD	5 mg/mL[a]	Physically compatible for 24 hr at 25 °C under fluorescent light	1393	C
Gallium nitrate	FUJ	1 mg/mL[b]	MSD	5 mg/mL[b]	Precipitates immediately	1673	I
Gemcitabine HCl	LI	10 mg/mL[b]	ME	10 mg/mL[b]	Yellow-green discoloration forms in 1 hr	2226	I
Granisetron HCl	SKB	0.05 mg/mL[a]	ME	10 mg/mL[a]	Physically compatible for 4 hr at 23 °C	2000	C
Idarubicin HCl	AD	1 mg/mL[b]	MSD	5 mg/mL[b]	Visually compatible for 12 hr at 25 °C in light. Precipitate in 24 hr	1525	C
Insulin, regular	LI	0.2 unit/mL[b]	MSD	4 and 5 mg/mL[b]	Physically compatible for 2 hr at 25 °C	1395	C
Linezolid	PHU	2 mg/mL	ME	10 mg/mL[b]	Physically compatible for 4 hr at 23 °C	2264	C
Lorazepam	WY	0.33 mg/mL[b]	MSD	5 mg/mL	Yellow precipitate forms in 24 hr	1855	I
Melphalan HCl	BW	0.1 mg/mL[b]	MSD	10 mg/mL[b]	Physically compatible for 3 hr at 22 °C	1557	C
Meperidine HCl	AB	10 mg/mL	MSD	5 mg/mL[a]	Yellow color forms in 2 hr at 25 °C	1397	I
Methotrexate sodium		30 mg/mL	MSD	5 mg/mL	Visually compatible for 4 hr at room temperature	1788	C
Midazolam HCl	RC	5 mg/mL	MSD	5 mg/mL	Haze forms in 24 hr	1855	I
Milrinone lactate	SS	0.2 mg/mL[a]	ME	5 mg/mL[b]	Yellow color darkening in 4 hr at 25 °C	2381	I
Ondansetron HCl	GL	1 mg/mL[b]	MSD	5 mg/mL[b]	Visually compatible for 4 hr at 22 °C	1365	C
Propofol	ZEN	10 mg/mL	ME	10 mg/mL[b]	Physically compatible for 1 hr at 23 °C	2066	C
Remifentanil HCl	GW	0.025 and 0.25 mg/mL[b]	ME	10 mg/mL[a]	Physically compatible for 4 hr at 23 °C	2075	C
Sargramostim	IMM	10 mcg/mL[b]	MSD	5 mg/mL[b]	Large particle and clump form in 4 hr	1436	I
Sodium bicarbonate		1.4%	MSD	5 mg/mL[a]	Pale yellow precipitate forms in 1 hr at room temperature	1788	I
Tacrolimus	FUJ	1 mg/mL[b]	MSD	10 mg/mL[b]	Visually compatible for 24 hr at 25 °C	1630	C
Telavancin HCl	ASP	7.5 mg/mL[a]	ME	5 mg/mL[a]	Slight measured turbidity increase	2830	I
	ASP	7.5 mg/mL[b]	ME	5 mg/mL[b]	Physically compatible for 2 hr	2830	C
Teniposide	BR	0.1 mg/mL[a]	MSD	10 mg/mL[b]	Physically compatible for 4 hr at 23 °C	1725	C
Thiotepa	IMM[e]	1 mg/mL[a]	ME	10 mg/mL[a]	Physically compatible for 4 hr at 23 °C	1861	C
Tigecycline	WY	1 mg/mL[b]		5 mg/mL[b]	Physically compatible for 4 hr	2714	C
TNA #218 to #226[f]			ME	10 mg/mL[b]	Visually compatible for 4 hr at 23 °C	2215	C
TPN #212 to #215[f]			ME	10 mg/mL[b]	Physically compatible for 4 hr at 23 °C	2109	C
Vasopressin	APP	0.2 unit/mL[b]	ME	5 mg/mL[a]	Physically compatible	2641	C

Y-Site Injection Compatibility (1:1 Mixture) (Cont.)

Imipenem–cilastatin sodium

Drug	Mfr	Conc	Mfr	Conc	Remarks	Ref	C/I
Vinorelbine tartrate	BW	1 mg/mL[b]	MSD	10 mg/mL[b]	Physically compatible for 4 hr at 22 °C	1558	C
Zidovudine	BW	4 mg/mL[a]	MSD	5 mg/mL[a]	Physically compatible for 4 hr at 25 °C	1193	C

[a]*Tested in dextrose 5%.*
[b]*Tested in sodium chloride 0.9%.*
[c]*Tested in both dextrose 5% and sodium chloride 0.9%.*
[d]*Tested in dextrose 5% with albumin human 2 mg/mL.*
[e]*Lyophilized formulation tested.*
[f]*Refer to Appendix I for the composition of parenteral nutrition solutions. TNA indicates a 3-in-1 admixture, and TPN indicates a 2-in-1 admixture.*
[g]*Injected via Y-site into an administration set running azithromycin.*

IMMUNE GLOBULIN INTRAVENOUS
AHFS 80:04

Products — Immune globulin intravenous is available from a number of manufacturers in both liquid and dry powder forms. Protein concentrations of 5 and 10% are available in liquid forms. Dry powder product sizes vary by product but range from 1 to 12 g of protein. The dry powder products require reconstitution in the volumes specified by the manufacturers for the individual sizes and typically result in protein concentrations of 5 or 10%.

Do not shake the reconstituted product. Rotate or swirl the vial to dissolve particles. (4) Foaming results from shaking and should be avoided (1) because it may impede dissolution. (1499)

Reconstitution of Sandoglobulin with dextrose 5% has resulted in extended dissolution times of 75 and 135 minutes for the 3 and 6% solutions, respectively. With sodium chloride 0.9%, dissolution occurs over a few minutes; exceptional cases take up to 20 minutes. (1498)

pH — The pH of the various immune globulin products varies but is typically within the range of 5 to 7 for the dry powder products and within the range of 4 to 6 for the liquid forms. (1; 4)

Trade Name(s) — Carimune NF, Flebogamma, Gamimune N, Gammagard S/D, Gammar-P IV, Gamunex, Iveegam EN, Octagam, Panglobulin, Polygam S/D, Sandoglobulin, Venoglobulin-S.

Administration — Immune globulin intravenous is administered initially by slow intravenous infusion; the rate is gradually increased after 15 to 30 minutes according to patient tolerance. (1; 4)

Stability — Recommended storage conditions vary among the different immune globulin products. Typically the products are stored either at room temperature or under refrigeration with protection from freezing. The proper storage conditions for each specific product should be verified as it is received. Solutions that have been frozen should not be used. (1; 4)

Partially used immune globulin containers should be discarded. (4)

Immune globulin intravenous (Gammagard S/D, Baxter and Polygam S/D, American Red Cross) was reconstituted with sterile water for injection to concentrations of 50 mg/mL (5%) and 100 mg/mL (10%). Stability of the reconstituted product was evaluated in the original glass vials and also after transfer to PVC bags at 4 °C for 48 hours and at 25 °C for 12 hours. The visual appearance of the solutions remained acceptable, extremely low amounts of diethylhexyl phthalate (DEHP) plasticizer were leached from the PVC bags, and all tests for protein content and antibody activity indicated that stability was maintained throughout the study under both storage conditions. (2435)

Sorption — A stability evaluation of immune globulin intravenous in PVC bags found no loss of activity due to sorption when compared to glass containers. (2435)

Plasticizer Leaching — Storage of reconstituted immune globulin intravenous in PVC containers for 48 hours at 4 °C and 12 hours at 25 °C resulted in very low amounts of leached DEHP plasticizer from undetectable amounts up to a maximum of 86 ng/mL. (2435)

Compatibility Information

Solution Compatibility

Immune globulin intravenous

Solution	Mfr	Mfr	Conc/L	Remarks	Ref	C/I
Dextrose 5%	[a]	HY	2.5%	Visually compatible with no alteration of IgG concentration or functional activity	1885	C

Solution Compatibility (Cont.)

Immune globulin intravenous

Solution	Mfr	Mfr	Conc/L	Remarks	Ref	C/I
Dextrose 15%	a	HY	2.5%	Visually compatible with no alteration of IgG concentration or functional activity	1885	**C**
Dextrose 5% in sodium chloride 0.225%	a	HY	2.5%	Visually compatible with no alteration of IgG concentration or functional activity	1885	**C**
TPN #194 and TPN #195[b]	a	HY	2.5%	Visually compatible with no alteration of IgG concentration or functional activity	1885	**C**

[a]Tested in PVC containers.
[b]Refer to Appendix I for the composition of parenteral nutrition solutions. TPN indicates a 2-in-1 admixture.

Y-Site Injection Compatibility (1:1 Mixture)

Immune globulin intravenous

Drug	Mfr	Conc	Mfr	Conc	Remarks	Ref	C/I
Fluconazole	RR	2 mg/mL	CU	50 mg/mL	Physically compatible for 24 hr at 25 °C	1407	**C**
Sargramostim	IMM	6[a,b] and 15 mcg/mL[b]	CU	50 mg/mL	Visually compatible for 2 hr	1618	**C**

[a]With albumin human 0.1%.
[b]Tested in sodium chloride 0.9%.

Additional Compatibility Information

Immune globulin products may be manufactured using differing procedures and may exhibit differing compatibility characteristics. All manufacturers recommend not mixing other drugs with the immune globulin. In addition, different brands of immune globulin cannot be safely mixed because of possible aggregate formation. The manufacturers make the recommendations cited in Table 1 regarding compatibility with infusion solutions. (1; 1135)

Table 1. Immune Globulin Products: Compatibility with Infusion Solutions

Product	Remarks
Carimune NF	May be reconstituted with sodium chloride 0.9%, dextrose 5%, or sterile water for injection.
Flebogamma	Mixing with infusion solutions is not recommended by the manufacturer.
Gamimune N	Incompatible with sodium chloride 0.9%. Dextrose 5% is recommended for dilution if needed.
Gammagard S/D	Packaged with sterile water for injection for use as a diluent. No other diluents or solutions are recommended.
Gammar-P	Reconstitute with sterile water for injection. May be administered sequentially with dextrose 5% or sodium chloride 0.9%.
Gamunex	May be diluted with dextrose 5%. Incompatible with sodium chloride 0.9%.
Iveegam EN	Reconstitute with sterile water for injection. May be diluted in dextrose 5% or sodium chloride 0.9%.
Panglobulin	May be reconstituted with sodium chloride 0.9%, dextrose 5%, or sterile water for injection.
Venoglobulin-S	May be administered sequentially or flushed with dextrose 5% or sodium chloride 0.9%. Do not add infusion solutions to the immune globulin container.

INDOMETHACIN SODIUM TRIHYDRATE
AHFS 28:08.04.92

Products — Indomethacin sodium trihydrate is supplied as a lyophilized product in vials containing the equivalent of 1 mg of indomethacin. Reconstitute with 1 or 2 mL of preservative-free sterile water for injection or sodium chloride 0.9% to yield a 1- or 0.5-mg/mL solution, respectively. (1)

pH — From 6 to 7.5. (4)

Trade Name(s) — Indocin I.V.

Administration — Indomethacin sodium trihydrate is usually administered by intravenous injection over 20 to 30 minutes, although dilution after reconstitution is not recommended. Extravasation should be avoided. (1; 4)

Stability — Indomethacin sodium trihydrate is supplied as a white to yellow powder. Color variations have no relationship to indomethacin content. The vials should be stored below 30 °C and protected from light. (1)

The manufacturer recommends discarding any unused solution because of the absence of an antibacterial preservative. (1) However, at 1 mg/mL in sodium chloride 0.9%, the drug is stated to be chemically stable for 16 days at room temperature. (4)

Solutions of indomethacin sodium trihydrate (Abbott and Fujisawa) diluted in sodium chloride 0.9% to a concentration of 0.1 mg/mL were evaluated for visual and chemical stability stored in the original vials. Little or no loss was found after storage for 10 days at 25 °C. (2105)

The stability of indomethacin sodium trihydrate (Merck Sharp & Dohme) 0.5 mg/mL reconstituted with sterile water for injection in the original vials and repackaged into 1-mL polypropylene syringes (Sherwood) was reported. The reconstituted solutions were stored at room temperature (about 23 °C) exposed to fluorescent light for 12 hours daily and under refrigeration (about 4 °C) in the dark. Little or no loss of indomethacin in the refrigerated solutions occurred after 14 days of storage. The solutions stored at room temperature exhibited 9% loss in 10 days. The solutions at both temperatures remained visually clear and colorless throughout the study. (2228)

pH Effects — Reconstitution of indomethacin sodium trihydrate with solutions having pH values below 6 may result in precipitation of free indomethacin. (1; 4)

Compatibility Information

Drugs in Syringe Compatibility

Indomethacin sodium trihydrate

Drug (in syringe)	Mfr	Amt	Mfr	Amt	Remarks	Ref	C/I
Pantoprazole sodium	a	4 mg/1 mL		0.5 mg/1 mL	Precipitates within 1 hr	2574	**I**

[a]Test performed using the formulation WITHOUT edetate disodium.

Y-Site Injection Compatibility (1:1 Mixture)

Indomethacin sodium trihydrate

Drug	Mfr	Conc	Mfr	Conc	Remarks	Ref	C/I
Amino acids	MG	1 and 2%[c]	MSD	1 mg/mL[b]	Haze forms in 2 hr and white precipitate forms in 4 hr	1527	**I**
	MG	1 and 2%[d]	MSD	1 mg/mL[b]	Haze forms in 30 min and white precipitate forms in 1 hr	1527	**I**
Calcium gluconate	AMR	100 mg/mL	MSD	1 mg/mL[b]	Fine yellow precipitate forms within 1 hr	1527	**I**
Dextrose injection	BA	2.5%	MSD	1 mg/mL[b]	Visually compatible for 24 hr at 28 °C	1527	**C**
	BA	5%	MSD	1 mg/mL[b]	Visually compatible for 24 hr at 28 °C	1527	**C**
	BA	7.5%	MSD	1 mg/mL[b]	Haze forms in 2 hr, precipitate in 4 hr	1527	**I**
	BA	10%	MSD	1 mg/mL[b]	Haze forms in 2 hr, precipitate in 4 hr	1527	**I**
Dobutamine HCl	LI	1.2 mg/mL[a]	MSD	1 mg/mL[b]	Hazy precipitate forms immediately	1527	**I**
Dopamine HCl	AB	1.2 mg/mL[a]	MSD	1 mg/mL[b]	Hazy precipitate forms immediately	1527	**I**
Furosemide	AB	10 mg/mL	MSD	1 mg/mL[b]	Visually compatible for 24 hr at 28 °C	1527	**C**
Gentamicin sulfate		1 mg/mL[a]	MSD	0.5 and 1 mg/mL[a]	White turbidity forms immediately and becomes white flakes in 1 hr	1550	**I**
Insulin, regular	NOV	1 unit/mL[b]	MSD	1 mg/mL[b]	Visually compatible for 24 hr at 28 °C	1527	**C**

Y-Site Injection Compatibility (1:1 Mixture) (Cont.)

Indomethacin sodium trihydrate

Drug	Mfr	Conc	Mfr	Conc	Remarks	Ref	C/I
Levofloxacin	OMN	5 mg/mL[a]	ME	1 mg/mL	Cloudy precipitate forms	2233	I
Potassium chloride	AB	0.2 mEq/mL[a]	MSD	1 mg/mL[b]	Visually compatible for 24 hr at 28 °C	1527	C
Sodium bicarbonate	AB	0.5 mEq/mL[a]	MSD	1 mg/mL[b]	Visually compatible for 24 hr at 28 °C	1527	C
Sodium nitroprusside	AB	0.2 mg/mL[a]	MSD	1 mg/mL[b]	Visually compatible for 24 hr at 28 °C	1527	C
Tobramycin sulfate		1 mg/mL[a]	MSD	0.5 and 1 mg/mL[a]	White turbidity forms immediately and becomes white flakes in 1 hr	1550	I

[a]*Tested in dextrose 5%.*
[b]*Tested in sodium chloride 0.9%.*
[c]*TrophAmine in dextrose 10%.*
[d]*TrophAmine in sterile water for injection.*

INSULIN
AHFS 68:20.08

Products — Regular insulin is available in 10-mL vials and 1.5-mL prefilled syringes and syringe cartridges at a concentration of 100 units/mL. Human insulin is produced using recombinant DNA technology. Regular concentrated insulin (Lilly) also is available in 20-mL vials containing 500 units/mL. Glycerin 1.4 to 1.8% and phenol or cresol 0.1 to 0.25% may also be present. (1; 4)

Several modified forms of insulin (Isophane, Lente, etc.) are available, each having a characteristic onset of action, time to peak effect, and duration of action. (4)

Adequately mixing these products is necessary prior to use, but vigorous shaking may entrain air bubbles that could interfere with accurate dosing. Gentle shaking of the vial combined with end-over-end inversion and rolling in the palms has been suggested. (2270)

pH — All regular insulin products have a neutral pH of approximately 7 to 7.8. (4; 261)

Trade Name(s) — Humulin R.

Administration — Regular insulin is usually administered by subcutaneous injection into the thighs, arms, buttocks, or abdomen, with sites rotated. Syringes calibrated for the particular concentration of insulin to be given must be used. Regular insulin may also be administered intramuscularly or by intravenous infusion, usually diluted in sodium chloride 0.9%. Regular insulin is the only form of insulin that can be given intravenously. (4)

Care is required when adding insulin to infusion solutions, especially in flexible containers. Adding insulin to a plasma expander carrier solution hanging in the use position resulted in stratification, with the insulin floating to the top. Little insulin was delivered initially, and 87% of the insulin appeared in the last 28% of the solution. Repeated inversion and agitation of the container to effect thorough mixture eliminates this stratification, yielding an even distribution and a constant delivery concentration. (85)

Reuse of disposable insulin syringes has been suggested to reduce cost to patients. However, disposable insulin syringes are usually siliconized. Reuse of disposable plastic insulin syringes (Plastipak Microfine II, Becton Dickinson) has resulted in contamination of vials of insulin with silicone oil, causing a white precipitate and impairment of biological effects. In a test of insulin from several sources, repeated drawing of the insulin into the disposable syringes and then expulsion of it back into the vials introduced substantial amounts of silicone oil; a white precipitate formed within 12 hours at 8 °C. (1110)

Stability — Regular insulin should be stored under refrigeration and protected from freezing. (1; 4) Although refrigerated storage is required, some manufacturers have stated the drug may be stored at room temperature for 28 to 30 days. (2745; 2769) Freezing of insulin products may alter the protein structure, decreasing concentration. (559) In one study of several insulin products, one cycle of freezing for 45 hours followed by slow thawing at 21 °C or rapid thawing in a water bath at 37 °C did not result in a loss of bioactivity. However, microscopic examination revealed particle aggregation, and some crystal damage had occurred. (680)

The stability of regular insulin (Novo Nordisk) was evaluated under simulated shipping conditions. Sample vials were packaged in both insulated and non-insulated mailers and packaged with either two 12-oz. frozen gel packs for simulated summer mailing or one 12-oz. frozen gel pack for simulated winter shipping. The evaluation was conducted for simulated transit periods ranging from 24 hours to 120 hours (overnight air delivery to ground delivery). Visual inspection found no change in appearance in any of the samples tested. Microscopy found no formation of aggregates. No loss of insulin content occurred in any of the samples with any of the shipping methods and conditions. Size exclusion chromatography found little or no change in high-molecular-weight protein content. The regular insulin remained within USP specifications with all of the shipping methods and time periods studied. (2769)

As with other protein and peptide products, insulin aggregation with possible reduced bioactivity can be a problem. Aggregates have been found to form in a variety of infusion devices and under various storage conditions, including static storage and continuous rotational or reciprocating motion. (1948; 1995; 2406) Aggregation may occur at air-water interfaces. Such interfaces have been generated by turbulence, such as shaking and repeatedly passing insulin through a syringe and needle. With sufficient vigor, both actions can turn the insulin turbid from insoluble aggregates. (1948) In addition, contact with silicone rubber appears to promote insulin aggregation. (1995)

Factors that increase the formation rate of insulin transformation products (such as deamidated insulin, covalent dimers, and higher oligamers) in beef and human insulin products were evaluated during six months of storage. A low rate of transformation product appeared at 4 °C. Higher temperatures, as might occur when insulin is carried in a shirt pocket or car glove compartment, accelerated this production (especially for human insulin) and also fibril formation. Exposure to light increased the dimer and higher oligomer content. Insulin should not be exposed to direct sunlight or subjected to vibration or extremes of temperature. (1663)

The appearance of transformation products was found to be two- to three-fold greater when using PVC administration sets compared to polyethylene and polypropylene infusion equipment. Furthermore, use of the PVC sets resulted in up to 30% reduction in the concentration of methylparaben, phenol, and m-cresol preservatives in insulin products. (311)

Regular insulin, containing 100 units/mL, is clear and colorless or almost colorless. The concentrated injection containing 500 units/mL may be straw colored. Discoloration, turbidity, or unusual viscosity indicates deterioration or contamination. (4)

Insulin 4, 10, 20, and 40 units/L was evaluated in the following Baxter peritoneal dialysis solutions in PVC and Clear-Flex polyolefin containers:

> Dianeal PD4 with 1.36% dextrose in PVC containers
> Physioneal 40 with 1.36% dextrose in PVC containers
> Physioneal 40 Clear-Flex with 1.36% dextrose in Clear-Flex

In Dianeal PD4, more than 90% of the insulin concentration remained over 24 hours. The insulin 10, 20, and 40 units/L in Physioneal 40 retained more than 90% of the insulin concentration over six hours and more than 80% over 24 hours. The insulin 4 units/L in Physioneal 40 retained more than 90% of the insulin concentration over three hours and more than 70% over 24 hours. No difference was found between the results in PVC and Clear-Flex containers. (2647)

Syringes — It has been stated that neutral regular insulin (and also NPH and Lente insulin) can be stored for five to seven days under refrigeration in either glass or plastic syringes. Mixtures of these insulins can also be stored similarly. (679)

Insulin soluble, BP, 1.6 units/2 mL diluted in sodium chloride 0.9% was stored for 18 hours at room temperature in the following plastic syringes: Brunswick (Sherwood Medical), Plastipak (Becton Dickinson), and Sabre (Gillette U.K.). The first two syringes have polypropylene barrels; the Sabre has a combination polypropylene–polystyrene barrel. No significant loss of insulin occurred due to sorption. Significant (but unspecified) losses did occur when the concentration was reduced to 0.2 unit/mL, but the make of syringe did not influence this adsorption. (784)

No apparent degradation or binding occurred for at least 14 days when insulin, USP (Lilly), 100 units/mL was stored under refrigeration in 1-mL polypropylene syringes (Becton Dickinson). (805)

The soluble insulins Velosulin (Nordisk), Actrapid and Human Actrapid (Novo), Humulin S (Lilly), Neusulin (Wellcome), and

Quicksol (Boots) in 1-mL 100-unit Plastipak syringes (Becton Dickinson) exhibited no loss in 29 days when stored at 4 and 20 °C. (1275)

Regular insulin human (Humulin R, 100 units/mL, Lilly), isophane insulin human (Humulin N, 100 units/mL, Lilly), and the combination product (Humulin N/R 70/30, Lilly) were evaluated for stability packaged in plastic syringes. Test samples of 0.4 mL of each insulin product were drawn into 1-mL polypropylene syringes (Plastipak, Becton Dickinson) and 1-mL polypropylene–ethylene copolymer syringes (Terumo) and stored for 28 days at 4 and 23 °C. No loss of insulin from any insulin product occurred in either syringe type. However, the antibacterial preservatives present in the insulin formulations were lost, especially in the polypropylene syringes at room temperature. Storage under refrigeration to slow the loss of preservative as much as possible was recommended. (1124)

Infusion Pumps — Insulin solutions may form highly insoluble polymers. In areas having high shear rates such as the tubing, cannula, and needle, aggregation can lead to blockage. In low shear areas such as the insulin reservoir of implantable pumps, gentle agitation can lead to the formation of a cross-linked gel. (1112)

Sorption — The adsorption of insulin to the surfaces of intravenous infusion solution containers, glass and plastic (including PVC, ethylene vinyl acetate, polyethylene, and other polyolefins), tubing, and filters has been demonstrated. Estimates of the loss range up to about 80% for the entire infusion apparatus, although varying results using differing test methods, equipment, and procedures have been reported. Estimates of adsorption of around 20 to 30% are common. The percent adsorbed is inversely proportional to the concentration of insulin. Other important factors are the amount of container surface area and the fill volume of the solution. The amount of insulin adsorbed varies directly with the available surface area and indirectly with the ratio of fluid volume to container capacity. The container material is a factor, with glass possibly adsorbing insulin more extensively than some plastics. Other factors influencing the extent of insulin adsorption include the type of solution, type and length of administration set, rate of infusion, temperature, previous exposure of tubing to insulin, and presence of albumin human, whole blood, electrolytes, and other drugs. (266; 267; 268; 269; 420; 422; 423; 424; 425; 426; 428; 533; 681; 682; 683; 684; 685; 686; 687; 688; 689; 690; 854; 908; 909; 910; 911; 912; 913; 1111; 1112; 1274; 1282; 1408; 1497; 1664; 1665; 2079; 2301)

The adsorption of insulin to container surfaces is an instantaneous process. (267; 425; 911; 912; 913) However, the effect of adsorption on the deliverable amount of insulin appears to vary with time. Several investigators reported a dramatic initial drop in delivered insulin followed by a return to higher (although variable) levels. The bulk of the insulin adsorption apparently occurs in the first 30 to 60 minutes. Although flow rate does not influence total insulin binding, the plateau phase of delivered insulin may be reached more quickly at faster infusion rates. (422; 424; 425; 426; 428; 687; 688; 689; 854; 2301)

In a study of insulin loss during simulated delivery to low-birth-weight infants, insulin 0.2 unit/mL was delivered at rates of 0.05 and 0.2 mL/hr through microbore PVC tubing and polyethylene-lined PVC tubing. During the early hours, the amount of insulin delivered through both types of tubing was much reduced, especially at the slower delivery rate. The authors indicated that this loss might contribute to the 14- to 24-hour delays in blood glucose normalization in these infants. The priming of microbore tubing with 5 units/mL of insulin for 20 minutes was suggested to accelerate the achievement of steady-state insulin delivery. The time courses of insulin delivery observed for representative unprimed and primed sets are presented in Table 1. (2301)

Regular human insulin 0.1 unit/mL in sodium chloride 0.9% in VISIV polyolefin bags was tested for 24 hours at room temperature near 23 °C. About 35% loss occurred, which is consistent with the drug's potential for adsorption to surfaces. (2660; 2792)

The addition of albumin human to infusion solutions helps to reduce the adsorption of insulin. The degree to which albumin human prevents adsorption is uncertain. Reported losses of insulin in albumin-containing solutions have varied from about zero to approximately 30%. However, most work indicates a substantial reduction in insulin adsorption. (266; 267; 268; 269; 418; 428; 683; 684; 685; 908; 909) Other additives such as vitamins, electrolytes, and drugs may also have a similar effect. (425; 909; 914)

Other recommended approaches to avoiding or minimizing adsorption include adding a small amount of the patient's blood to the insulin solution (689; 690; 691) and storing or flushing the administration apparatus with the insulin solution to saturate the set prior to administration. (428; 1111; 2301) Addition of extra insulin to compensate for the losses has also been suggested. (1112) As an alternative, administration of insulin using a syringe pump with a short cannula has been recommended. This procedure will reduce the surface area in relation to the amount of insulin present. (1033)

The clinical significance of this adsorption is uncertain. Some clinical studies indicated no relevant effect on the success of therapy. (415; 427; 685) Some in vestigators felt that the importance of insulin adsorption to the surfaces of the infusion container and tubing may be a moot point since the dosage is individualized on the basis of blood and urine glucose determinations. Simply adding more insulin may saturate binding sites and yield the desired response. (270; 271; 854; 909)

Still others indicated that the adsorption may indeed be relevant for solutions with an insulin content of less than 100 or 200 units/L. (424; 426; 428; 908; 2301)

If the apparent dose of intravenous insulin is used as the basis for determining the subsequent dose upon discontinuing the intravenous one, then a potential for dosing error exists. The actual amount of insulin being administered could be substantially less than the apparent amount. (533)

Table 1. Approximate Amount of Insulin Delivered through Unprimed and Primed[a] Administration Sets (2301)

Set Type	Delivered Insulin (%)				
	1 hr	2 hr	4 hr	8 hr	24 hr
Unprimed	17	11	27	55	100
Primed	70	70	70	100	100

[a]Primed with insulin 5 units/mL for 20 minutes.

Whether one attempts to prevent insulin adsorption or not, it does not appear to be possible to add an amount of insulin to an infusion solution and know precisely what portion of that amount will actually be given to the patient. Monitoring the patient's response to therapy and making the appropriate adjustments on the basis of that response are, therefore, of prime importance. (690; 854; 1664)

Implantable Pumps — Insulin, regular human (Genapol, Hoeschst-Roussel) 400 units/mL with heparin sodium 500 units/mL was evaluated in MIP 2001 implantable pumps (MiniMed) at 37 °C for three months. The drug solution remained visually clear, but the insulin content dropped to 65% of the initial amount. The activity of heparin declined by even more. Only 45% remained after three months. The losses were attributed to the shaking that occurred during use rather than temperature, interaction with pump materials, or interaction of the two drugs with each other. (239)

Filtration — A filter material specially treated with a proprietary agent was evaluated for a reduction in insulin binding. Insulin, regular (Lilly), 40 units/L in dextrose 5% and sodium chloride 0.9% was run through an administration set with a treated 0.22-μm cellulose ester inline filter at a rate of 2 mL/min. Cumulative insulin losses from the first 150 mL of solution were about 12% from dextrose 5% and 4% from sodium chloride 0.9%, compared to much higher losses previously reported for untreated cellulose ester filter material. Furthermore, equilibrium binding studies showed a reduction to 5% of the binding to untreated filter material from either solution. (904) All Abbott Ivex integral filter and extension sets currently use this treated filter material. (1074)

Compatibility Information

Solution Compatibility

Insulin, regular

Solution	Mfr	Mfr	Conc/L	Remarks	Ref	C/I
Sodium chloride 0.9%	HOS[b]	NOV	100 units	35 to 45% loss in 24 hr due to adsorption	2660; 2792	?
	BA[a]	LI	1000 units	10% loss in 1 hr in 50-mL bag and in 4 hr in 250-mL bag	2079	I
TNA #267[c]	[d]	NOV	10 units	40 to 60% loss likely due to sorption	2599	I

[a]Tested in PVC containers.
[b]Tested in VISIV polyolefin containers.
[c]Refer to Appendix I for the composition of parenteral nutrition solutions. TPN indicates a 2-in-1 admixture.
[d]Tested in EVA containers.

Additive Compatibility

Insulin, regular

Drug	Mfr	Conc/L	Mfr	Conc/L	Test Soln	Remarks	Ref	C/I
Cytarabine	UP	100 and 500 mg		40 units	D5W	Fine precipitate forms	174	**I**
Meropenem	ZEN	1 and 20 g	LI	1000 units	NS	Visually compatible for 4 hr at room temperature	1994	**C**
Octreotide acetate		50 mcg		5 units	TPN	Substantial insulin loss	1377	**I**
Ranitidine HCl	GL	600 mg	LI	1000 units	NS[a]	Visually compatible. Little ranitidine loss in 24 hr at ambient temperature but insulin losses of 9% in 4 hr and 14% in 24 hr, presumably due to sorption	2079	**I**

[a]*Tested in PVC containers.*

Drugs in Syringe Compatibility

Insulin, regular

Drug (in syringe)	Mfr	Amt	Mfr	Amt	Remarks	Ref	C/I
Pantoprazole sodium	[a]	4 mg/ 1 mL		100 units/ 1 mL	Precipitates within 1 hr	2574	**I**

[a]*Test performed using the formulation WITHOUT edetate disodium.*

Y-Site Injection Compatibility (1:1 Mixture)

Insulin, regular

Drug	Mfr	Conc	Mfr	Conc	Remarks	Ref	C/I
Amiodarone HCl	WY	4.8 mg/mL[a]	LI	1 unit/mL[a]	Visually compatible for 24 hr at 23 °C	1877	**C**
Ampicillin sodium	WY	20 mg/mL[b]	LI	0.2 unit/mL[b]	Physically compatible for 2 hr at 25 °C	1395	**C**
Ampicillin sodium–sulbactam sodium	RR	20 + 10 mg/ mL[b]	LI	0.2 unit/mL[b]	Physically compatible for 2 hr at 25 °C	1395	**C**
Aztreonam	SQ	20 mg/mL	LI	0.2 unit/mL[b]	Physically compatible for 2 hr at 25 °C	1395	**C**
Caspofungin acetate	ME	0.7 mg/mL[b]	NOV	1 unit/mL[b]	Physically compatible for 4 hr at room temperature	2758	**C**
	ME	0.5 mg/mL[b]	NOV	1 unit/mL[b]	Physically compatible over 60 min	2766	**C**
Cefazolin sodium	LI	20 mg/mL[a]	LI	0.2 unit/mL[b]	Physically compatible for 2 hr at 25 °C	1395	**C**
Cefepime HCl	BMS	120 mg/mL[c]		100 units/mL	Physically compatible with less than 10% cefepime loss. Insulin not tested	2513	**C**
Cefotetan disodium	STU	20 and 40 mg/mL[a]	LI	0.2 unit/mL[b]	Physically compatible for 2 hr at 25 °C	1395	**C**
Ceftaroline fosamil	FOR	2.22 mg/mL[f]	NOV	1 unit/mL[f]	Physically compatible for 4 hr at 23 °C	2826	**C**
Ceftazidime	GSK	120 mg/mL[h]		100 units/mL	Physically compatible with less than 10% ceftazidime loss. Insulin not tested	2513	**C**
Clarithromycin	AB	4 mg/mL[a]	NOV	4 units/mL[a]	Visually compatible for 72 hr at both 30 and 17 °C	2174	**C**
Digoxin	ES	0.005 mg/ mL[b]	LI	1 unit/mL[b]	Physically compatible for 3 hr	1316	**C**

Y-Site Injection Compatibility (1:1 Mixture) (Cont.)

Insulin, regular

Drug	Mfr	Conc	Mfr	Conc	Remarks	Ref	C/I
	ES	0.005 mg/mL[a]	LI	1 unit/mL[a]	Slight haze in 1 hr	1316	I
Dobutamine HCl	LI	4 mg/mL[e]	LI	1 unit/mL[e]	Physically compatible for 3 hr	1316	C
Dopamine HCl	DU	3.2 mg/mL[a]	LI	1 unit/mL[a]	White precipitate forms immediately, dissolves quickly, and reforms in 24 hr at 23 °C	1877	I
Doripenem	JJ	5 mg/mL[a,b]	NOV	1 unit/mL[a,b]	Physically compatible for 4 hr at 23 °C	2743	C
Doxapram HCl	RB	2 mg/mL[a]	NOV	1 unit/mL[d]	Visually compatible for 4 hr at 23 °C	2470	C
Esmolol HCl	DU	40 mg/mL[a]	LI	1 unit/mL[a]	Visually compatible for 24 hr at 23 °C	1877	C
Famotidine	MSD	0.2 mg/mL[a]	LI	0.03 unit/mL[a]	Physically compatible for 4 hr at 25 °C	1188	C
Gentamicin sulfate	TR	1.2 mg/mL[b]	LI	0.2 unit/mL[b]	Physically compatible for 2 hr at 25 °C	1395	C
Heparin sodium	ES	60 units/mL[a]	LI	0.2 unit/mL[b]	Physically compatible for 2 hr at 25 °C	1395	C
Hydroxyethyl starch 130/0.4 in sodium chloride 0.9%	FRK	6%	NOV	5, 27.5, 50 units/mL[a]	Visually compatible for 24 hr at room temperature	2770	C
Imipenem–cilastatin sodium	MSD	4 and 5 mg/mL[b]	LI	0.2 unit/mL[b]	Physically compatible for 2 hr at 25 °C	1395	C
Indomethacin sodium trihydrate	MSD	1 mg/mL[b]	NOV	1 unit/mL[b]	Visually compatible for 24 hr at 28 °C	1527	C
Labetalol HCl	GL	5 mg/mL	LI	1 unit/mL[a]	Visually compatible for 4 hr. White precipitate forms in 24 hr at 23 °C	1877	?
Levofloxacin	OMN	5 mg/mL[a]	LI	100 units/mL	Cloudy precipitate forms	2233	I
	OMN	5 mg/mL[a]	LI	1 unit/mL	Visually compatible for 4 hr at 24 °C	2233	C
Magnesium sulfate	LY	40 mg/mL[g]	LI	0.2 unit/mL[b]	Physically compatible for 2 hr at 25 °C	1395	C
Meperidine HCl	WY	10 mg/mL[b]	LI	0.2 unit/mL[b]	Physically compatible for 1 hr at 25 °C	1338	C
	AST	50 mg/mL[a]	LI	0.2 unit/mL[b]	Physically compatible for 2 hr at 25 °C	1395	C
Meropenem	ZEN	1 and 50 mg/mL[b]	LI	0.2 unit/mL[h]	Visually compatible for 4 hr at room temperature	1994	C
Micafungin sodium	ASP	1.5 mg/mL[b]	NOV	1 unit/mL[b]	Increase in haze and microparticulates form in 4 hr	2683	I
Midazolam HCl	RC	1 mg/mL[a]	LI	1 unit/mL[a]	Visually compatible for 24 hr at 23 °C	1877	C
Milrinone lactate	SW	0.4 mg/mL[a]	NOV	1 unit/mL[b]	Visually compatible. Little loss of either drug in 4 hr at 23 °C	2214	C
Morphine sulfate	ES	1 mg/mL[b]	LI	0.2 unit/mL[b]	Physically compatible for 1 hr at 25 °C	1338	C
	ES	5 mg/mL[a]	LI	0.2 unit/mL[b]	Physically compatible for 2 hr at 25 °C	1395	C
	SX	1 mg/mL[a]	LI	1 unit/mL[a]	Visually compatible for 24 hr at 23 °C	1877	C
Nafcillin sodium	BA	20 and 40 mg/mL[a]	LI	0.2 unit/mL[b]	Precipitates immediately	1395	I
Nesiritide	SCI	50 mcg/mL[a,b]		Up to 100 units/mL	Physically incompatible	2625	I
Nitroglycerin	OM	0.2 mg/mL[a]	LI	1 unit/mL[a]	Visually compatible for 24 hr at 23 °C	1877	C
Norepinephrine bitartrate	STR	0.064 mg/mL[a]	LI	1 unit/mL[a]	White precipitate forms immediately	1877	I
Oxytocin	PD	0.02 unit/mL[i]	LI	0.2 unit/mL[b]	Physically compatible for 2 hr at 25 °C	1395	C
Pantoprazole sodium	ALT[c]	0.16 to 0.8 mg/mL[b]	LI	5 to 50 units/mL[a]	Visually compatible for 12 hr at 23 °C	2603	C

Y-Site Injection Compatibility (1:1 Mixture) (Cont.)

Insulin, regular

Drug	Mfr	Conc	Mfr	Conc	Remarks	Ref	C/I
Pentobarbital sodium	WY	2 mg/mL[e]	LI	1 unit/mL[e]	Physically compatible for 3 hr	1316	**C**
Propofol	ZEN	10 mg/mL	NOV	1 unit/mL[a]	Physically compatible for 1 hr at 23 °C	2066	**C**
Ranitidine HCl	GL	1 mg/mL[b]	LI	1 unit/mL[b]	Visually compatible. Little loss of ranitidine in 4 hr but insulin losses of 9% in 1 hr and 20% in 4 hr, presumably due to sorption	2079	**I**
Sodium bicarbonate	AB	1 mEq/mL	LI	1 unit/mL	Physically compatible for 3 hr	1316	**C**
Sodium nitroprusside	RC	0.2 mg/mL[a]	LI	1 unit/mL[a]	Visually compatible for 24 hr at 23 °C	1877	**C**
	RC	1.2 and 3 mg/mL[a]	LI	1 and 2 units/mL[b]	Visually compatible for 48 hr at 24 °C protected from light	2357	**C**
Tacrolimus	FUJ	1 mg/mL[b]	LI	0.1 unit/mL[a]	Visually compatible for 24 hr at 25 °C	1630	**C**
Terbutaline sulfate	CI	0.02 mg/mL[a]	LI	0.2 unit/mL[b]	Physically compatible for 2 hr at 25 °C	1395	**C**
Ticarcillin disodium–clavulanate potassium	BE	31 mg/mL[b]	LI	0.2 unit/mL[b]	Physically compatible for 2 hr at 25 °C	1395	**C**
Tobramycin sulfate	LI	1.6 and 2 mg/mL[a]	LI	0.2 unit/mL[b]	Physically compatible for 2 hr at 25 °C	1395	**C**
TNA #218 to #226[j]			NOV	1 unit/mL[a]	Visually compatible for 4 hr at 23 °C	2215	**C**
TPN #189[j]			NOV	2 units/mL[k]	Visually compatible for 24 hr at 22 °C	1767	**C**
TPN #212 to #215[j]			NOV	1 unit/mL[b]	Physically compatible for 4 hr at 23 °C	2109	**C**
Vancomycin HCl	LI	4 mg/mL[a]	LI	0.2 unit/mL[b]	Physically compatible for 2 hr at 25 °C	1395	**C**
Vasopressin	APP	0.2 unit/mL[b]	NOV	1 unit/mL[b]	Physically compatible	2641	**C**

[a]*Tested in dextrose 5%.*
[b]*Tested in sodium chloride 0.9%.*
[c]*Test performed using the formulation WITHOUT edetate disodium.*
[d]*Tested in sodium chloride 0.45%.*
[e]*Tested in both dextrose 5% and sodium chloride 0.9%.*
[f]*Tested in dextrose 5%, sodium chloride 0.9%, and Ringer's injection, lactated.*
[g]*Tested in Ringer's injection, lactated.*
[h]*Tested in sterile water for injection.*
[i]*Tested in dextrose 5% in Ringer's injection, lactated.*
[j]*Refer to Appendix I for the composition of parenteral nutrition solutions. TNA indicates a 3-in-1 admixture, and TPN indicates a 2-in-1 admixture.*
[k]*Tested in Haemaccel (Behring).*

Additional Compatibility Information

Mixing Insulin Products — Mixing of the various types of insulin has been utilized. The following compatibility results have been cited (1076):

Insulin Types	Compatibility
Regular with NPH	Mixtures are stable in all ratios
Regular with protamine zinc	Stability is unpredictable
Regular with Lente	Reduces activity of regular due to binding to excess zinc
Lente, Semilente, Ultralente	Mixtures are stable in all ratios
Lente, Semilente, Ultralente with phosphate-buffered insulins[a]	Should not be mixed due to precipitation

[a]*Includes Humulin BR, NPH, protamine zinc, Velosulin insulins.*

It has been stated that neutral regular insulin may be combined with modified insulin in any proportions. (263; 264) However, losses of soluble insulins when mixed with zinc and isophane insulins were reported. These losses generally ranged from about 20 to 50% but were as high as 99%, depending on the ratio and sources of the two insulins in the mixture. The reaction occurred within the first 90 to 120 seconds after mixing, with no further losses occurring after this time. This phenomenon could explain clinical reports of failure to control postprandial blood sugar levels. (1275)

The loss of solubility when short-acting insulins were mixed in ratios of 1:1, 1:2, 1:3, and 1:5 with long-acting insulins was reported. Iletin II Regular (Lilly) was mixed with Iletin II Lente, NPH, or Ultralente (Lilly). Actrapid (Novo) was mixed with Monotard (Novo). Velosulin (Nordisk) was mixed with Insulatard (Nordisk). The mixtures were centrifuged after storage times of approximately 20 minutes and 75 seconds. The level of soluble short-acting insulin in the supernatant was determined. In a 1:1 ratio, no significant loss of solubility occurred with the Iletin II Lente combination within 20 minutes and with the Actrapid–Monotard combination in 75 seconds. All other combinations, ratios, and time periods had losses ranging from 10 to 75%. The worst losses were experienced with the highest ratios of long-acting insulins and with the longer time period. The method used to prolong insulin action (precipitation) might affect the solubility of the short-acting insulin when admixed. (1156)

The loss of initial hypoglycemic effect when Actrapid HM (Novo) was mixed with Ultratard HM (Novo), an ultralente insulin, for five minutes before injection was noted. The authors recommended not mixing the two types of insulin to preserve the rapid hypoglycemic effect of regular insulin. (73)

Octreotide — Insulin levels in a 3-L bag of parenteral nutrition solution showed a marked reduction when octreotide 150 mcg was added to the container. Sample parenteral nutrition solutions, with and without octreotide, were prepared with regular insulin 15 units/3-L bag. Subsequent analysis found an insulin level of 3.5 units/L in the plain parenteral nutrition solution, an amount consistent with the losses occurring due to surface adsorption. However, in the parenteral nutrition solution containing octreotide, the insulin level was only 0.6 unit/L. The reason for this potential incompatibility is not known. (1377)

INSULIN LISPRO
AHFS 68:20.08

Products — Insulin lispro is available in vials, cartridges, and pens as a suspension containing in each milliliter insulin lispro 100 units with glycerin 16 mg, dibasic sodium phosphate 1.88 mg, metacresol 3.15 mg, zinc ion 0.0197 mg (as oxide), a trace of phenol, and sodium hydroxide and/or hydrochloric acid to adjust pH during manufacturing in water for injection. (1)

pH — From 7.0 to 7.8. (1)

Trade Name(s) — Humalog.

Administration — Insulin lispro is an injectable suspension intended for subcutaneous injection including using some external insulin pumps. (1)

Stability — Intact vials of insulin lispro should be stored under refrigeration and protected from freezing, excessive heat, and light. (1)

Although refrigerated storage is required, the manufacturer has stated the drug may be stored at room temperature for 28 days. Visually inspect insulin lispro before use. Discard if it is cloudy, contains a precipitate, has thickened, or is discolored. (1; 2745)

Insulin lispro diluted with Sterile Diluent for Humalog to 10 or 50 units/mL can be used for 28 days refrigerated and for 14 days at room temperatures up to 30 °C. If diluting insulin lispro, great care is essential to avoid concentration errors. Insulin lispro in a cartridge or used in an external insulin pump must not be diluted. (1)

Insulin lispro cartridges used in D-TRON and D-TRON Plus external pumps should be discarded after seven days and the cartridge adapters and external pump reservoir should be discarded every 48 hours. (1)

The physical and chemical stability of insulin lispro 100 units/mL in MiniMed507c, H-TRONplus, and D-TRON CSII insulin infusion devices stored at 37 °C and subjected to mechanical shaking at 100 strokes/min was evaluated over 7 days. The insulin lispro solution remained clear and free of aggregation and precipitation, and concentrations remained at 95%. (2638)

INTERFERON ALFA-2B
AHFS 10:00

Products — Interferon alfa-2b is available as a dry powder in vials containing 10, 18, and 50 million International Units (I.U.) packaged with bacteriostatic water for injection containing benzyl alcohol 0.9% diluent. Only the 10-million I.U. vial is recommended for intralesional use. The 50-million I.U. vials are used in malignant melanoma and AIDS-related Kaposi's sarcoma only. (1)

For intramuscular, subcutaneous, or intralesional use, reconstitute the appropriate-size vial contents with the bacteriostatic water for injection diluent using the requisite volume noted in Table 1. Direct

Table 1. Reconstitution of Interferon Alfa-2b Powder for Injection Vials (1)

Vial Size (million I.U.)	Diluent Volume (mL)	Concentration (I.U./mL)
10	2	5
10	1	10 (for intralesional use only)
18	1	18
50	1	50 (for malignant melanoma and AIDS-related Kaposi's sarcoma only)

the stream at the vial wall and not at the powder in the bottom of the vial. Swirl gently to dissolve the powder; do not shake. (1)

In addition to the drug, the reconstituted solutions also contain in each milliliter glycine 20 mg, sodium phosphate dibasic 2.3 mg, sodium phosphate monobasic 0.55 mg, and albumin human 1 mg. (1)

For intravenous infusion, reconstitute the appropriate-size vial contents with the diluent provided. Swirl gently to dissolve the powder; do not shake. Withdraw the appropriate dose and add it to 100 mL of sodium chloride 0.9%, ensuring that the final concentration is not less than 10 million I.U./100 mL. (1)

Interferon alfa-2b is also available for intramuscular or subcutaneous use as solutions in multidose vials, which contain 22.8 million I.U./3.8 mL (6 million I.U./mL), and 25 million I.U., which contain 32 million I.U./3.2 mL (10 million I.U./mL). Multidose injection "pens" are also available containing 3, 5, and 10 million I.U. per 0.2 mL injection with a total of 1.5 mL per pen for subcutaneous injection. (1)

Each milliliter of solution also contains sodium chloride 7.5 mg, sodium phosphate dibasic 1.8 mg, sodium phosphate monobasic 1.3 mg, edetate disodium 0.1 mg, polysorbate 80 0.1 mg, and metacresol 1.5 mg. The solution products are albumin-free. (1)

Vial size to be used and appropriate concentration are dependent on the intended use of the product. In addition to intramuscular and subcutaneous use, the 10-million I.U. vials are also for intralesional use. Interferon alfa-2b solution products are not recommended for intravenous administration in the United States labeling. (1)

In the Canadian labeling, intravenous infusion of the solution products is permitted with dilution in sodium chloride 0.9% immediately before administration to a concentration no lower than 0.3 million I.U./mL. These albumin-free dosage forms require this higher minimum concentration to avoid loss due to sorption to plastic bags. (1)

Specific Activity — Approximately 2×10^8 I.U./mg of protein. (1)

pH — The reconstituted powder for injection has a pH in the range of 6.9 to 7.5. (4)

Tonicity — Reconstitution of the 10-million I.U. vial with 1 mL of water for injection results in an isotonic solution. (1369)

Trade Name(s) — Intron A.

Administration — The administration of interferon alfa-2b is dependent on the intended use and specific dosage form. The dry powder products, reconstituted as directed, may be administered by intramuscular and subcutaneous injection or intravenous infusion. The contents of the 10-million I.U. vial, reconstituted as directed, may also be given intralesionally. For intravenous infusions, interferon alfa-2b may be diluted further to a concentration of not less than 10 million I.U./100 mL of sodium chloride 0.9% for intravenous infusion over 20 minutes. (1)

The solution products are administered by intramuscular or subcutaneous injection. The 5-million I.U. and 10-million I.U. vials and the 25-million I.U. multidose vials may also be used for intralesional injection. The solution products are not for use in malignant melanoma or AIDS-related Kaposi's sarcoma. In addition, the Canadian product labeling permits intravenous infusion in sodium chloride 0.9% at concentrations no lower than 0.3 million units/mL. (1)

Stability — Interferon alfa-2b dry powder in vials is a white to cream color. (1; 4) It is not photosensitive. (1369) The reconstituted solution

is clear and colorless to light yellow. Intact vials should be stored under refrigeration at 2 to 8 °C but are stable for up to seven days at 45 °C (4) or 28 days at room temperature. (1369) The reconstituted solution should be stored under refrigeration. In concentrations between 3 and 50 million I.U./mL, reconstituted solutions are stable for up to one month under refrigeration and up to two days at ambient temperatures up to 40 °C. (1)

Interferon alfa-2b solution in vials is colorless. Intact vials of solution should be stored under refrigeration at 2 to 8 °C. The solution products are stable for up to seven days at 35 °C and up to 14 days at 30 °C. Interferon alfa-2b in multidose pens is stable for up to two days at 30 °C. (1)

Interferon alfa-2b (Schering) containing albumin human in the formulation reconstituted with the accompanying diluent and diluted further to 2 million I.U./mL with sterile water for injection was stored at 4 °C for 21 days in polypropylene centrifuge tubes. Biological activity was retained throughout the study period. (2022)

In another study, the retention of bioactivity by albumin-free interferon alfa-2b 6 million units/mL stability was compared to samples of that product to which albumin human 1 mg/mL was added and also to the reconstituted product containing albumin human in the formulation. The solutions were packaged as 0.5 mL in polypropylene syringes and stored at 4 °C for 42 days. In addition, the albumin-free product was diluted to 2 million units/mL with sterile water for injection and stored in a 60-mL polypropylene syringe under the same conditions. No substantial loss of biological activity was found in any of the samples. (2188)

Sodium chloride 0.9% is recommended for preparation of intravenous infusion admixtures. (1)

Interferon alfa-2b is stated to be compatible with sodium chloride 0.9%, Ringer's injection, and Ringer's injection, lactated. It is stated to be incompatible with dextrose solutions. (1369)

pH Effects — Reconstituted interferon alfa-2b is stable over a pH range of 6.5 to 8 (4), with greatest stability between pH 6.9 and 7.5. (1369)

Freezing Solutions — Reconstituted interferon alfa-2b 10 million I.U./mL packaged in plastic syringes is stated to be stable for up to four weeks when frozen at −10 °C or colder. (4) Solutions frozen at −20 °C are stated to be stable for 56 days including four freeze-thaw cycles. Frozen solutions stored at −80 °C are stable for one year. (1369)

Syringes — Interferon alfa-2b (Intron A, Kirby-Warwick) 3 million units was diluted in 6 mL of sterile water for injection and packaged in 10-mL polypropylene syringes. The samples were stored for 14 days under refrigeration and for 24 hours at 37 °C. Analysis found changes indicating interconversion between interferon monomers and possibly oligomer formation. Dilution and packaging in polypropylene syringes was considered to be unsuitable. (744)

Sorption — Like other interferons, interferon alfa-2b can bind to surfaces, including glass and plastics. Consequently, albumin human is incorporated into the dry powder dosage forms to minimize adsorption and permit the use of glass or plastic syringes for administration without substantial loss at concentrations not less than 0.1 million I.U./mL. (1; 4) The solution dosage forms are albumin-free. Consequently, the Canadian product labeling recommends dilution of the solution products in sodium chloride 0.9% to a concentration not lower than 0.3 million I.U./mL to prevent losses. (1)

IODIPAMIDE MEGLUMINE
AHFS 36:68

Products — Iodipamide meglumine is available in 20-mL vials containing an aqueous solution composed of 52% iodipamide meglumine (5.2 g bound iodine/20 mL) with 0.32% sodium citrate buffer and 0.04% edetate disodium. (1; 4)

pH — From 6.5 to 7.7. (1; 4)

Sodium Content — The 52% solution contains approximately 18.2 mg of sodium per 20 mL. (1)

Trade Name(s) — Cholografin Meglumine.

Administration — Iodipamide meglumine is administered slowly intravenously only. After warming to body temperature, the 52% injection is injected over 10 minutes. (1; 4)

Stability — The solutions may vary from colorless to pale yellow or light amber. Darker solutions should not be used. Crystallization may occur in the 52% solution. To redissolve it, place the vial in hot water and shake gently for several minutes. If cloudiness does not disappear, the solution should not be used. (1; 4)

Plastic syringes have been stated to be unsuitable for accommodating radiopaque solutions for any length of time. The plastic is attacked, and the plunger tends to freeze on prolonged storage. (40) However, when iodipamide meglumine (Squibb) 52% was stored in polystyrene syringes (Pharmaseal) at 25 and 37 °C, no apparent changes were noted visually or spectrophotometrically over five days. (530)

Iodipamide meglumine solutions should be protected from light and excessive heat. (1)

Compatibility Information

Additive Compatibility

Iodipamide meglumine

Drug	Mfr	Conc/L	Mfr	Conc/L	Test Soln	Remarks	Ref	C/I
Diphenhydramine HCl	PD	20 to 200 mg	SQ		NS	Dense putty-like white precipitate forms immediately	309	I

Drugs in Syringe Compatibility

Iodipamide meglumine

Drug (in syringe)	Mfr	Amt	Mfr	Amt	Remarks	Ref	C/I
Dimenhydrinate	SE	50 mg/ 1 mL	SQ	52%, 40 mL	Forms a precipitate initially but clears within 1 hr and remains clear for 48 hr	530	?
	SE	50 mg/ 1 mL	SQ	52%, 20 to 1 mL	Forms a precipitate initially but clears within 1 hr. Precipitate reforms on standing	530	I
Diphenhydramine HCl	PD	5 mg/ 0.1 mL to 50 mg/ 1 mL	SQ		Dense putty-like white precipitate forms immediately	309	I
	PD	1 mL[a]	SQ	52%, 40 to 1 mL	Forms a precipitate initially but clears within 1 hr and remains clear for 48 hr	530	?
Hyaluronidase	WY	150 units/ 1 mL	SQ	52%, 40 to 2 mL	Physically compatible for 48 hr	530	C
	WY	150 units/ 1 mL	SQ	52%, 1 mL	Physically compatible for at least 1 hr but a precipitate forms within 48 hr	530	I
Promethazine HCl	WY	1 mL[a]	SQ	52%, 40 and 20 mL	Forms a precipitate initially but clears within 1 hr and remains clear for 48 hr	530	?
	WY	1 mL[a]	SQ	52%, 10 to 1 mL	Precipitates immediately	530	I

[a]*Concentration unspecified.*

Y-Site Injection Compatibility (1:1 Mixture)

Iodipamide meglumine

Drug	Mfr	Conc	Mfr	Conc	Remarks	Ref	C/I
Gentamicin sulfate			SQ		White precipitate forms immediately downstream to Y-site when given into a set through which gentamicin was administered previously	324	I

IODIXANOL
AHFS 36:68

Products — Iodixanol is available at 270 mg/mL of organically bound iodine (as 550 mg/mL of iodixanol) with calcium chloride dihydrate 0.074 mg/mL and sodium chloride 1.87 mg/mL. It is also available at 320 mg/mL of organically bound iodine (as 652 mg/mL of iodixanol) with calcium chloride dihydrate 0.044 mg/mL and sodium chloride 1.11 mg/mL. Each milliliter of the solutions also contains tromethamine 1.2 mg, edetate calcium disodium 0.1 mg, and hydrochloric acid and/or sodium hydroxide to adjust pH. The products are packaged from 50 to 200 mL. (1)

pH — Adjusted during manufacturing to pH 7.4 with a range from 6.8 to 7.7 at 22 °C. (1)

Osmolarity — Both concentrations have an osmolality of 290 mOsm/kg. (1)

Density — The 270-mg I/mL product has a density of 1.314 g/mL at 20 °C and 1.303 g/mL at 37 °C. The 320-mg I/mL product has a density of 1.369 g/mL at 20 °C and 1.356 g/mL at 37 °C. (1)

Trade Name(s) — Vispaque.

Administration — Iodixanol is administered intravenously and intra-arterially. It is not intended for intrathecal use. The drug may be administered at either body or room temperature. (1)

Stability — Intact containers of clear, colorless to pale yellow iodixanol injection should be stored at controlled room temperature and protected from exposure to direct sunlight and from freezing. Discard the product if inadvertently frozen because of possible damage to closure integrity. The foil overwrap on the flexible plastic containers serves as both a moisture and light barrier and should not be removed until immediately before use. Vials and bottles of iodixanol may be stored for up to one month at 37 °C in a contrast agent warmer using circulating warm air. (1)

Compatibility Information

Y-Site Injection Compatibility (1:1 Mixture)

Iodixanol

Drug	Mfr	Conc	Mfr	Conc	Remarks	Ref	C/I
Fenoldopam mesylate	AB	80 mcg/mL[a]	NYC	55%	Physically compatible for 4 hr at 23 and 37 °C	2467	C

[a]*Tested in sodium chloride 0.9%.*

IOHEXOL
AHFS 36:68

Products — Iohexol is available in concentrations ranging from 30.2% (140 mg/mL organically bound iodine) to 75.5% (350 mg/mL organically bound iodine) in numerous vial and bottle sizes from 10 to 250 mL; not all concentrations are available in all sizes. Also present in each milliliter are tromethamine 1.21 mg, edetate calcium disodium 0.1 mg, and hydrochloric acid or sodium hydroxide to adjust the pH. (1) Table 1 presents the characteristics of iohexol products.

pH — From 6.8 to 7.7. (1)

Trade Name(s) — Omnipaque.

Table 1. Iohexol Product Characteristics (1)

Iohexol Concentration (%)	Iodine Concentration (mg/mL)	Osmolality (mOsm/kg)	Specific Gravity (37 °C)
30.2	140	322	1.164
38.8	180	408	1.209
51.8	240	520	1.280
64.7	300	672	1.349
75.5	350	844	1.406

Administration — Iohexol at appropriate concentrations may be administered intravenously, intra-arterially, intrathecally (except for Omnipaque 350) slowly over one to two minutes, intra-articularly, or directly into selected areas for visualization. Solutions should be warmed to body temperature prior to administration. (1)

Stability — Iohexol is colorless to pale yellow. Intact vials should be stored at controlled room temperature and protected from direct exposure to sunlight and freezing. The product should not be used if particulate matter is present. Do not remove the iohexol containers from the moisture- and light-protective foil overwrap until immediately before use. (1)

Compatibility Information

Drugs in Syringe Compatibility

Iohexol

Drug (in syringe)	Mfr	Amt	Mfr	Amt	Remarks	Ref	C/I
Ampicillin sodium	BR	30 mg/ 1 mL	WI	64.7%, 5 mL	Physically compatible for at least 2 hr	1438	C
Bupivacaine HCl	AST	0.25 and 0.125%[b], 4 mL		1 mL[a]	Visually compatible with no bupivacaine loss in 24 hr at room temperature. Iohexol not tested	1611	C
Chloramphenicol sodium succinate	PD	33 mg/ 1 mL	WI	64.7%, 5 mL	Physically compatible for at least 2 hr	1438	C
Diphenhydramine HCl	PD	12.5 mg/ 0.25 mL	WI	64.7%, 5 mL	Physically compatible for at least 2 hr	1438	C
Epinephrine HCl	PD	1 mg/ 1 mL	WI	64.7%, 5 mL	Physically compatible for at least 2 hr	1438	C
Gentamicin sulfate	SC	0.8 mg/ 1 mL	WI	64.7%, 5 mL	Physically compatible for at least 2 hr	1438	C
Heparin sodium	OR	5000 units/ 0.5 mL	WI	64.7%, 5 mL	Physically compatible for at least 2 hr	1438	C
Hydrocortisone sodium succinate	UP	10 mg/ 1 mL	WI	64.7%, 5 mL	Physically compatible for at least 2 hr	1438	C
Methylprednisolone sodium succinate	UP	10 mg/ 1 mL	WI	64.7%, 5 mL	Physically compatible for at least 2 hr	1438	C
Papaverine HCl	LI	30 mg/ 1 mL	WI	64.7%, 5 mL	Physically compatible for at least 2 hr	1438	C
Protamine sulfate	LI	10 mg/ 1 mL	WI	64.7%, 5 mL	Physically compatible for at least 2 hr	1438	C

[a]Concentration unspecified.
[b]Diluted 1:1 in sodium chloride 0.9%.

Y-Site Injection Compatibility (1:1 Mixture)

Iohexol

Drug	Mfr	Conc	Mfr	Conc	Remarks	Ref	C/I
Fenoldopam mesylate	AB	80 mcg/mL[a]	NYC	51.8%	Physically compatible for 4 hr at 23 and 37 °C	2467	C

[a]Tested in sodium chloride 0.9%.

IOPAMIDOL
AHFS 36:68

Products — Iopamidol products are available in concentrations ranging from 41% (200 mg/mL organically bound iodine) to 76% (370 mg/mL organically bound iodine) in numerous vial and bottle sizes from 20 to 200 mL; not all concentrations are available in all sizes. Also present in each milliliter are tromethamine 1 mg, edetate calcium disodium, with hydrochloric acid and/or sodium hydroxide to adjust the pH. (1) Table 1 presents the characteristics of iopamidol products.

Table 1. Iopamidol Product Characteristics (1)

Iopamidol Concentration (%)	Iodine Concentration (mg/mL)	Osmolality (mOsm/kg)	Specific Gravity (37 °C)
41	200	413	1.227
51	250	524	1.281
61	300	616	1.339
76	370	796	1.405

pH — From 6.5 to 7.5. (1)

Trade Name(s) — Isovue.

Administration — Iopamidol may be administered intravenously or intra-arterially. Solutions should be warmed to body temperature prior to administration. (1)

Stability — Iopamidol injection is colorless to pale yellow. Intact vials should be stored at controlled room temperature and protected from light. If crystals form, they should be dissolved by warming of the vial in hot (60 to 100 °C) water for about five minutes and gentle shaking. The vials should cool to body temperature before use. If crystals fail to dissolve, the vials should be discarded. (1)

Compatibility Information

Drugs in Syringe Compatibility

Iopamidol

Drug (in syringe)	Mfr	Amt	Mfr	Amt	Remarks	Ref	C/I
Ampicillin sodium	BR	30 mg/ 1 mL	SQ	61%, 5 mL	Physically compatible for at least 2 hr	1438	C
Chloramphenicol sodium succinate	PD	33 mg/ 1 mL	SQ	61%, 5 mL	Physically compatible for at least 2 hr	1438	C
Diphenhydramine HCl	PD	12.5 mg/ 0.25 mL	SQ	61%, 5 mL	Physically compatible for at least 2 hr	1438	C
Epinephrine HCl	PD	1 mg/ 1 mL	SQ	61%, 5 mL	Physically compatible for at least 2 hr	1438	C
Gentamicin sulfate	SC	0.8 mg/ 1 mL	SQ	61%, 5 mL	Physically compatible for at least 2 hr	1438	C
Heparin sodium	OR	5000 units/ 0.5 mL	SQ	61%, 5 mL	Physically compatible for at least 2 hr	1438	C
Hydrocortisone sodium succinate	UP	10 mg/ 1 mL	SQ	61%, 5 mL	Physically compatible for at least 2 hr	1438	C
Methylprednisolone sodium succinate	UP	10 mg/ 1 mL	SQ	61%, 5 mL	Physically compatible for at least 2 hr	1438	C
Papaverine HCl	LI	30 mg/ 1 mL	SQ	61%, 5 mL	Physically compatible for at least 2 hr	1438	C
Protamine sulfate	LI	10 mg/ 1 mL	SQ	61%, 5 mL	Physically compatible for at least 2 hr	1438	C

Y-Site Injection Compatibility (1:1 Mixture)

Iopamidol

Drug	Mfr	Conc	Mfr	Conc	Remarks	Ref	C/I
Fenoldopam mesylate	AB	80 mcg/mL[a]	BRD	51%	Physically compatible for 4 hr at 23 and 37 °C	2467	C

[a]*Tested in sodium chloride 0.9%.*

IOTHALAMATE MEGLUMINE
AHFS 36:68

Products — Iothalamate meglumine is available in concentrations ranging from 17.2 to 60. The formulations may also contain edetate and phosphate buffers. Some examples of single-agent products are listed in Table 1. (1; 4)

pH — From 6.5 to 7.7. (1)

Osmolarity — The injections are hypertonic having osmolalities of 600 to 1400 mOsm/kg. (1)

Administration — Iothalamate meglumine solutions may be administered intravenously, intra-arterially, by injection into pancreatic and biliary ducts, and by bladder, ureter, or renal pelvis instillation. Solutions should be warmed to body temperature before administration. (4)

Stability — Iothalamate meglumine solutions are colorless to pale yellow. They should be stored below 30 °C. Crystallization does not occur at room temperature, but exposure to cold temperatures may result in crystallization. Should crystallization occur, the solution should be brought to room temperature, with shaking of the container if necessary to redissolve the crystals. The speed of dissolution may be increased by heating the vials in warm air. (1; 4)

Table 1. Some Representative Iothalamate Meglumine Products

Iothalamate Meglumine Content (%)	Bound Iodine (mg/mL)	Representative Trade Names
Urogenital solutions (not for intravascular use)		
17.2	81	Cysto-Conray II
Parenteral solutions		
30	141	Conray 30
43	202	Conray 43
60	282	Conray

pH Effects — Iothalamate meglumine is sensitive to low pH values. At pH values reported as about 2.4 to 2.7 (479) and below 3 (4), turbidity or frank precipitation may appear in the 60% product. (479)

Light Effects — Iothalamate meglumine is light sensitive and should be protected from strong daylight and direct sunlight. (4)

Syringes — Iothalamate meglumine 60% (Conray) was stored in polystyrene syringes (Pharmaseal) at 25 and 37 °C. No apparent changes were noted over five days. (530)

Compatibility Information

Drugs in Syringe Compatibility

Iothalamate meglumine

Drug (in syringe)	Mfr	Amt	Mfr	Amt	Remarks	Ref	C/I
Ampicillin sodium	BR	30 mg/1 mL	MA	60%, 5 mL	Physically compatible for at least 2 hr	1438	C
Chloramphenicol sodium succinate	PD	33 mg/1 mL	MA	60%, 5 mL	Physically compatible for at least 2 hr	1438	C
Dimenhydrinate	SE	50 mg/1 mL	MA	60%, 40 to 1 mL	Physically compatible for 48 hr	530	C
Diphenhydramine HCl	PD	1 mL[a]	MA	60%, 40 to 1 mL	Physically compatible for 48 hr	530	C
	PD	50 mg/1 mL	MA	5 mL[a]	No precipitate observed	309	C

Drugs in Syringe Compatibility (Cont.)

Iothalamate meglumine

Drug (in syringe)	Mfr	Amt	Mfr	Amt	Remarks	Ref	C/I
	PD	12.5 mg/ 0.25 mL	MA	60%, 5 mL	Physically compatible for at least 2 hr	1438	C
Epinephrine HCl	PD	1 mg/ 1 mL	MA	60%, 5 mL	Physically compatible for at least 2 hr	1438	C
Gentamicin sulfate	SC	0.8 mg/ 1 mL	MA	60%, 5 mL	Physically compatible for at least 2 hr	1438	C
Heparin sodium	OR	5000 units/ 0.5 mL	MA	60%, 5 mL	Physically compatible for at least 2 hr	1438	C
Hyaluronidase	WY	150 units/ 1 mL	MA	60%, 40 to 1 mL	Physically compatible for 48 hr	530	C
Hydrocortisone sodium succinate	UP	10 mg/ 1 mL	MA	60%, 5 mL	Physically compatible for at least 2 hr	1438	C
Methylprednisolone sodium succinate	UP	10 mg/ 1 mL	MA	60%, 5 mL	Physically compatible for at least 2 hr	1438	C
Papaverine HCl	LI	30 mg/ 1 mL	MA	60%, 5 mL	Physically compatible for at least 2 hr	1438	C
Promethazine HCl	WY	1 mL[a]	MA	60%, 40 to 1 mL	Precipitates immediately	530	I
Protamine sulfate	LI	10 mg/ 1 mL	MA	60%, 5 mL	Physically compatible for at least 2 hr	1438	C

[a]*Concentration unspecified.*

IOXAGLATE MEGLUMINE AND IOXAGLATE SODIUM
AHFS 36:68

Products — Ioxaglate meglumine 39.3% and ioxaglate sodium 19.6% (Mallinckrodt) is available in containers ranging in size from 20 to 200 mL. Each milliliter contains ioxaglate meglumine 393 mg, ioxaglate sodium 196 mg, and edetate calcium disodium 0.1 mg. The product provides 32% organically bound iodine. (1)

pH — From 6 to 7.6. (1)

Osmolality — The osmolality of the product is 600 mOsm/kg. (1)

Sodium Content — Each milliliter provides 0.15 mEq (3.48 mg) of sodium. (1)

Trade Name(s) — Hexabrix.

Administration — The product may be administered intravenously, intra-arterially, or intra-articularly. It also may be injected or instilled directly into selected areas to be visualized. The solutions should be warmed to body temperature before administration. (1)

Stability — The product should be stored below 30 °C and protected from freezing and direct exposure to sun or strong daylight. The solution is colorless to pale yellow. Crystallization does not occur at normal room temperatures. If the product is frozen or crystallization occurs, bring it to room temperature and shake vigorously to dissolve all crystals. Warming with circulating warm air is recommended to speed dissolution. Submersion in water is not recommended. (1)

Compatibility Information

Drugs in Syringe Compatibility

Ioxaglate meglumine + Ioxaglate sodium

Drug (in syringe)	Mfr	Amt	Mfr	Amt	Remarks	Ref	C/I
Ampicillin sodium	BR	30 mg/ 1 mL	MA	5 mL	Physically compatible for at least 2 hr	1438	C
Chloramphenicol sodium succinate	PD	33 mg/ 1 mL	MA	5 mL	Physically compatible for at least 2 hr	1438	C
Diphenhydramine HCl	PD	12.5 mg/ 0.25 mL	MA	5 mL	Precipitate forms immediately and persists for at least 2 hr	1438	I
Epinephrine HCl	PD	1 mg/ 1 mL	MA	5 mL	Physically compatible for at least 2 hr	1438	C
Gentamicin sulfate	SC	0.8 mg/ 1 mL	MA	5 mL	Transient precipitate clears within 5 min	1438	?
Heparin sodium	OR	5000 units/ 0.5 mL	MA	5 mL	Physically compatible for at least 2 hr	1438	C
Hydrocortisone sodium succinate	UP	10 mg/ 1 mL	MA	5 mL	Physically compatible for at least 2 hr	1438	C
Methylprednisolone sodium succinate	UP	10 mg/ 1 mL	MA	5 mL	Physically compatible for at least 2 hr	1438	C
Papaverine HCl	ME	32 mg/ 1 mL	MA	5 mL	Precipitate forms immediately and persists for at least 2 hr	1438	I
	LI	30 mg/ 1 mL	MA	3 and 5 mL	White amorphous precipitate forms immediately and persists for 24 hr. If shaken, it dissolves in 20 to 30 min	1437	I
	LI	30 mg/2 to 6 mL[a]	MA	5 mL	Precipitate forms	1437	I
	LI	30 mg/11 and 16 mL[a]	MA	5 mL	Precipitate forms and then redissolves	1437	?
	LI	30 mg/ 21 mL[a]	MA	5 mL	Physically compatible	1437	C
	LI	30 mg/ 11 mL[a]	MA	15 and 30 mL	Physically compatible	1437	C
	LI	60 mg/12 and 17 mL[a]	MA	5 mL	Precipitate forms	1437	I
	LI	60 mg/ 22 mL[a]	MA	5 mL	Precipitate forms	1437	I
Protamine sulfate	LI	10 mg/ 1 mL	MA	5 mL	Precipitate forms immediately and persists for at least 2 hr	1438	I

[a]Diluted in sodium chloride 0.9%.

Y-Site Injection Compatibility (1:1 Mixture)

Ioxaglate meglumine–ioxaglate sodium

Drug	Mfr	Conc	Mfr	Conc	Remarks	Ref	C/I
Fenoldopam mesylate	AB	80 mcg/mL[a]	MA	39.3% + 19.6%	Physically compatible for 4 hr at 23 and 37 °C	2467	C

[a]Tested in sodium chloride 0.9%.

IRINOTECAN HYDROCHLORIDE
AHFS 10:00

Products — Irinotecan hydrochloride is available in 2- and 5-mL single-use vials containing 40 and 100 mg of drug, respectively, on the basis of the trihydrate. Each milliliter of solution contains irinotecan hydrochloride trihydrate 20 mg, sorbitol 45 mg, lactic acid 0.9 mg, and hydrochloric acid or sodium hydroxide to adjust the pH. The product must be diluted prior to use. (1)

pH — From 3 to 3.8. (1)

Trade Name(s) — Camptosar.

Administration — Irinotecan hydrochloride is administered by intravenous infusion over 90 minutes after dilution to a final concentration in the range of 0.12 to 2.8 mg/mL in dextrose 5% or sodium chloride 0.9%. In most clinical trials, the doses were given in 500 mL of dextrose 5%. (1)

Stability — Irinotecan hydrochloride injection is supplied as a pale yellow solution. Intact vials should be stored at controlled room temperature and protected from light. Freezing of irinotecan hydrochloride solutions may result in precipitation and should be avoided. Upon dilution in dextrose 5%, the manufacturer recommends use periods of 6 hours at room temperature and 24 hours refrigerated. (1)

Irinotecan hydrochloride (Aventis Pharma) 0.35 mg/mL in sodium chloride 0.9% did not result in the loss of viability of *Staphylococcus aureus, Enterococcus faecium, Pseudomonas aeruginosa,* and *Candida albicans* within 120 hours at room temperature of 22 °C. Diluted solutions should be stored under refrigeration whenever possible, and the potential for microbiological growth should be considered when assigning expiration periods. (2740)

pH Effects — Irinotecan hydrochloride stability is pH dependent. In solution at acidic pH the drug is stable, but neutral and alkaline solutions are problematic. Maximum stability is demonstrated at pH 6 or lower. Increasing solution pH to more than pH 6.5 has resulted in 10% loss in as little as three hours. At pH 7.4, decomposition is rapid. Mixing irinotecan hydrochloride with neutral or alkaline drugs and solutions should be avoided. (1881; 2274; 2375)

Light Effects — Irinotecan hydrochloride is subject to photodegradation, including the formation of a precipitate. The structural changes exhibited by the decomposition products would indicate that they are unlikely to be active antineoplastic compounds. (1997; 1998; 2137) Exposure to ultraviolet light for three days produced a darkening in the solution color and the formation of a yellow precipitate composed of several decomposition products. (1997) Photodegradation of irinotecan hydrochloride occurs under any pH condition but is accelerated in neutral and alkaline solutions compared with acidic solutions. At pH 10, photodegradation is very rapid; at pH 3 it is much slower. At pH 7, irinotecan 0.34 mg/mL lost 32% in six hours exposed to a daylight lamp and 19% exposed to a white fluorescent light. In infusion solutions having neutral pH, irinotecan hydrochloride exposed to lighting (such as that of a medical facility) may have rapid decomposition. Protection from light exposure has been recommended to maintain product quality during administration. (1998) Other researchers have found that unacceptable losses occur within seven days when exposed to fluorescent light but that light protection during administration is not needed. (2419)

Compatibility Information

Solution Compatibility

Irinotecan HCl

Solution	Mfr	Mfr	Conc/L	Remarks	Ref	C/I
Dextrose 5%			0.12 to 2.8 g	Physically compatible. Stable for 24 hr at room temperature in fluorescent light and 48 hr refrigerated	1	**C**
	AB[a]	PH	20 mg	About 9% loss occurred in 24 hr at 25 °C	2375	**C**
	LME[a], BA[b]	RPR	2 g	Visually compatible with little or no loss in 2 hr at room temperature and in 4 days refrigerated	2396	**C**
	BA[a,b]	RPR	2.8 g	Visually compatible with little or no loss in 24 hr at room temperature in light or dark	2397	**C**
	BA[b]	RPR	0.4, 1, 2.8 g	Visually compatible with no loss in 28 days at both 4 and 25 ° protected from light	2419	**C**
Sodium chloride 0.9%			0.12 to 2.8 g	Physically compatible. Stable for 24 hr at room temperature in fluorescent light. May precipitate if refrigerated	1	**C**
	AB[a]	PH	20 mg	About 11% loss occurred in 2 hr at 25 °C	2375	**I**
	LME[a], BA[b]	RPR	2 g	Visually compatible with little or no loss in 2 hr at room temperature and in 4 days refrigerated	2396	**C**
	BA[a,b]	RPR	2.8 g	Visually compatible with little or no loss in 24 hr at room temperature in light or dark	2397	**C**
	BA[b]	RPR	0.4, 1, 2.8 g	Visually compatible with no loss in 28 days at both 4 and 25 °C protected from light	2419	**C**

Solution Compatibility (Cont.)

Irinotecan HCl

Solution	Mfr	Mfr	Conc/L	Remarks	Ref	C/I
	BA[b]	RPR	0.4 and 1 g	8 to 10% loss in 7 days and 13 to 17% loss in 14 days at 25 °C exposed to light. Color darkens and a precipitate may appear within 4 weeks	2419	C
	BA[b]	RPR	2.8 g	9% loss in 14 days and 15% loss in 21 days at 25 °C exposed to light. Color darkens and a precipitate may appear within 4 weeks	2419	C

[a] Tested in glass containers.
[b] Tested in PVC containers.

Additive Compatibility

Irinotecan HCl

Drug	Mfr	Conc/L	Mfr	Conc/L	Test Soln	Remarks	Ref	C/I
Epirubicin HCl	CE	560 mg	RPR	640 mg	NS	UV spectrum changes immediately upon mixing	2670	I

Y-Site Injection Compatibility (1:1 Mixture)

Irinotecan HCl

Drug	Mfr	Conc	Mfr	Conc	Remarks	Ref	C/I
Gemcitabine HCl	LI	10 mg/mL[b]	PHU	5 mg/mL[b]	Subvisible haze with green discoloration forms immediately	2226	I
Oxaliplatin	SS	0.5 mg/mL[a]	PHU	1 mg/mL[a]	Physically compatible for 4 hr at 23 °C	2566	C
Palonosetron HCl	MGI	50 mcg/mL	PHU	1 mg/mL[a]	Physically compatible. No palonosetron and 5% irinotecan loss in 4 hr	2609	C
Pemetrexed disodium	LI	20 mg/mL[b]	PHU	1 mg/mL[a]	Color darkening occurs over 4 hr	2564	I

[a] Tested in dextrose 5%.
[b] Tested in sodium chloride 0.9%.

IRON DEXTRAN
AHFS 20:04.04

Products — Iron dextran is available in 1- and 2-mL vials for intravenous or intramuscular use. It is composed of a dark brown liquid complex of ferric hydroxide and dextran in sodium chloride 0.9%, providing 50 mg of elemental iron per milliliter. (1)

pH — From 5.2 to 6.5. (1)

Trade Name(s) — INFeD.

Administration — Iron dextran (INFeD) may be administered by slow intravenous injection at a rate of no more than 1 mL/min or by deep intramuscular injection into the upper outer quadrant of the buttock. Subsequent injections should be made into alternate buttocks. Staining of the skin can be minimized by using a separate needle to withdraw the drug from the container and by displacing the skin laterally prior to injection. (1; 4) Iron dextran also has been administered by intravenous infusion over one to six hours after dilution in sodium chloride 0.9%. (4) Dilution in dextrose 5% results in a greater incidence of pain and phlebitis. (75) The manufacturer recommends not adding iron dextran injection to parenteral nutrition solutions, (1) especially 3-in-1 mixtures. (1814) In adults, a test dose of 25 mg should be given over five minutes (4), with the remainder given after at least one hour has elapsed if no hypersensitivity reaction occurs. (1; 4)

Stability — The commercial injection should be stored at controlled room temperature. (1; 4)

Filtration — Iron dextran adsorbs to sterilizing membrane filters composed of cellulose nitrate and acetate combined. An iron dextran solution containing 5 mcg/mL in water was estimated to lose 93% of the iron from the first milliliter passed through the filter. As more solution was passed through the filter, a decreasing proportion of the iron was adsorbed, indicating that the filter was approaching satura-tion. The extent of iron adsorption increased in the presence of elec-trolytes and trace elements. Adsorption can be substantial, especially when small amounts of iron dextran are involved. (918)

Compatibility Information

Solution Compatibility

Iron dextran

Solution	Mfr	Mfr	Conc/L	Remarks	Ref	C/I
TNA #122[a]		FI	50 mg	Lipid oiling out in 18 to 19 hr with formation of yellow-brown layer	1383	**I**
TNA #159 to #166[a]		FI	2 mg	Physically compatible with no change in particle size distribution in 48 hr at 4 and 25 °C	1648	**C**
TPN #31 to #33[a]		FI	100 mg	Physically compatible with minimal changes to iron dextran and amino acids for 18 hr at room temperature	692	**C**
TPN #207, #208[a]		SCN	10 mg	Rust-colored precipitate forms in 12 hr at 19 °C protected from sunlight	2103	**I**
TPN #209[a]		SCN	10 mg	Rust-colored precipitate forms in 18 to 24 hr at 19 °C protected from sunlight	2103	**I**
TPN #210[a]		SCN	10 mg	Visually compatible for 48 hr at 19 °C protected from sunlight. Trace iron precipitation found after 48 hr	2103	**?**
TPN #211[a]		SCN	10 mg	Visually compatible for 48 hr at 19 °C protected from sunlight. No iron precipitation found after 48 hr	2103	**C**

[a]Refer to Appendix I for the composition of parenteral nutrition solutions. TNA indicates a 3-in-1 admixture, and TPN indicates a 2-in-1 admixture.

ISOPROTERENOL HYDROCHLORIDE (ISOPRENALINE HYDROCHLORIDE)
AHFS 12:12.08.04

Products — Isoproterenol hydrochloride is available at a concentration of 0.2 mg/mL in 1- and 5-mL ampuls. In addition to the drug, each milliliter contains sodium chloride 7 mg, sodium lactate 1.8 mg, lactic acid 0.12 mg, sodium metabisulfite 1 mg, and hydrochloric acid to adjust pH in water for injection. (1)

pH — From 2.5 to 4.5. (1)

Osmolality — The osmolality of isoproterenol hydrochloride 0.2 mg/mL was determined to be 277 mOsm/kg by freezing-point depression and 293 mOsm/kg by vapor pressure. (1071)

Trade Name(s) — Isuprel HCl.

Administration — Isoproterenol hydrochloride may be administered by intravenous infusion; by direct intravenous, intramuscular, or sub-cutaneous injection; and, in extreme emergencies, by intracardiac in-jection. For direct intravenous injection, 1 mL of the 1:5000 injection should be diluted to 10 mL with sodium chloride 0.9% or dextrose 5% to provide a 20-mcg/mL solution. Intravenous infusions are pre-pared by adding 1 to 10 mL of the 1:5000 injection to 500 mL of compatible diluent. (1; 4)

Stability — Isoproterenol hydrochloride injection in intact containers should be stored at controlled room temperature and protected from light. Ampuls should be kept in opaque containers until used. The drug should not be used if a color or precipitate is present. Exposure to air, light, or increased temperature may cause a pink to brownish pink color to develop. (1; 4; 975)

Isoproterenol hydrochloride under simulated summer conditions in paramedic vehicles was exposed to temperatures ranging from 26 to 38 °C over four weeks. Analysis found about 4% loss of the drug in seven days and 11% loss in four weeks. (2562)

pH Effects — The pH of a solution is the primary determinant of cate-cholamine stability in intravenous admixtures. (527) Isoproterenol hy-drochloride 5 mg/L in dextrose 5% was stable for more than 24 hours at 25 °C over a pH range of 3.7 to 5.7. (59) However, isoproterenol hydrochloride displayed significant decomposition at a pH value above approximately 6. (48; 59; 430) If drugs that may raise the pH above 6 are mixed, they should be administered immediately after preparation (59), or, preferably, administered separately. (24)

Visual inspection for color changes related to decomposition may be inadequate to assess the compatibility of admixtures. In one evaluation with aminophylline stored at 25 °C, a color change was not noted until 24 hours had elapsed. However, no intact isoproterenol hydrochloride was present in the admixture at 24 hours. (527)

Filtration — Isoproterenol hydrochloride (Winthrop) 2 mg/L in dextrose 5%, sodium chloride 0.9%, and Ringer's injection, lactated, filtered over 12 hours through a 5-μm stainless steel depth filter (Argyle Filter Connector), a 0.22-μm cellulose ester membrane filter (Ivex-2 Filter Set), and a 0.22-μm polycarbonate membrane filter (In-Sure Filter Set), showed no significant reduction due to binding to the filters. (320)

In another study, isoproterenol hydrochloride (Winthrop) 4 mg/L in dextrose 5% and sodium chloride 0.9% did not display significant sorption to a 0.45-μm cellulose membrane filter (Abbott S-A-I-F) during an eight-hour simulated infusion. (567)

Central Venous Catheter — Isoproterenol hydrochloride (Abbott) 0.02 mg/mL in dextrose 5% was found to be compatible with the ARROWg+ard Blue Plus (Arrow International) chlorhexidine-bearing triple-lumen central catheter. Essentially complete delivery of the drug was found with little or no drug loss occurring. Furthermore, chlorhexidine delivered from the catheter remained at trace amounts with no substantial increase due to the delivery of the drug through the catheter. (2335)

Compatibility Information

Solution Compatibility

Isoproterenol HCl

Solution	Mfr	Mfr	Conc/L	Remarks	Ref	C/I
Amino acids 4.25%, dextrose 25%	MG	WI	2 mg	No increase in particulate matter in 24 hr at 5 °C	349	C
Dextrose 5% in Ringer's injection, lactated	TR[a]	WI	2 mg	Stable for 24 hr at 5 °C	282	C
Dextrose 5% in sodium chloride 0.9%	TR[a]	WI	2 mg	Stable for 24 hr at 5 °C	282	C
Dextrose 5%	TR[a]	WI	2 mg	Stable for 24 hr at 5 °C	282	C
	AB	BN	2 mg	Physically compatible and chemically stable. 10% decomposition is calculated to occur in 24 hr in the light and 250 hr in the dark at 25 °C	527	C
Ringer's injection, lactated	TR[a]	WI	2 mg	Stable for 24 hr at 5 °C	282	C
Sodium chloride 0.9%	TR[a]	WI	2 mg	Stable for 24 hr at 5 °C	282	C

[a]*Tested in both glass and PVC containers.*

Additive Compatibility

Isoproterenol HCl

Drug	Mfr	Conc/L	Mfr	Conc/L	Test Soln	Remarks	Ref	C/I
Aminophylline	SE	500 mg	BN	2 mg	D5W	At 25 °C, 10% isoproterenol decomposition in 2.2 to 2.5 hr in light and dark	527	I
Atracurium besylate	BW	500 mg		4 mg	D5W	Physically compatible and atracurium stable for 24 hr at 5 and 30 °C	1694	C
Calcium chloride	UP	1 g	WI	4 mg		Physically compatible	59	C
Dobutamine HCl	LI	1 g	ES	2 mg	D5W, NS	Physically compatible for 24 hr at 21 °C	812	C
Floxacillin sodium	BE	20 g	PX	4 mg	D5W	Physically compatible for 24 hr at 15 and 30 °C. Haze forms in 48 hr and precipitate forms in 72 hr	1479	C
Furosemide	HO	1 g	PX	4 mg	D5W	Precipitates immediately	1479	I
Heparin sodium		32,000 units		2 mg	NS	Physically compatible and heparin activity retained for 24 hr	57	C
	AB	20,000 units	WI	4 mg		Physically compatible	59	C
Magnesium sulfate		1 g	WI	4 mg		Physically compatible	59	C
Multivitamins	USV	10 mL	WI	4 mg		Physically compatible	59	C

Additive Compatibility (Cont.)

Isoproterenol HCl

Drug	Mfr	Conc/L	Mfr	Conc/L	Test Soln	Remarks	Ref	C/I
Potassium chloride	AB	40 mEq	WI	4 mg		Physically compatible	59	C
Ranitidine HCl	GL	50 mg and 2 g		20 mg	D5W	Physically compatible. Ranitidine stable for 24 hr at 25 °C. Isoproterenol not tested	1515	C
Sodium bicarbonate	AB	2.4 mEq[a]	BN	1 mg	D5W	Isoproterenol decomposition	772	I
		5%	WI	5 mg		Isoproterenol decomposition	48	I
Succinylcholine chloride	AB	2 g	WI	4 mg		Physically compatible	59	C
Verapamil HCl	KN	80 mg	BN	10 mg	D5W, NS	Physically compatible for 24 hr	764	C

[a]One vial of Neut added to a liter of admixture.

Drugs in Syringe Compatibility

Isoproterenol HCl

Drug (in syringe)	Mfr	Amt	Mfr	Amt	Remarks	Ref	C/I
Caffeine citrate		20 mg/ 1 mL	SW	0.2 mg/ 1 mL	Visually compatible for 4 hr at 25 °C	2440	C
Pantoprazole sodium	[a]	4 mg/ 1 mL		0.2 mg/ 1 mL	Whitish precipitate	2574	I

[a]Test performed using the formulation WITHOUT edetate disodium.

Y-Site Injection Compatibility (1:1 Mixture)

Isoproterenol HCl

Drug	Mfr	Conc	Mfr	Conc	Remarks	Ref	C/I
Amiodarone HCl	LZ	4 mg/mL[c]	ES	4 mcg/mL[c]	Physically compatible for 24 hr at 21 °C	1032	C
Atracurium besylate	BW	0.5 mg/mL[a]	ES	4 mcg/mL[a]	Physically compatible for 24 hr at 28 °C	1337	C
Bivalirudin	TMC	5 mg/mL[a]	AB	20 mcg/mL[a]	Physically compatible for 4 hr at 23 °C	2373	C
Cisatracurium besylate	GW	0.1, 2, 5 mg/ mL[a]	AB	0.02 mg/mL[a]	Physically compatible for 4 hr at 23 °C	2074	C
Dexmedetomidine HCl	AB	4 mcg/mL[b]	AB	20 mcg/mL[b]	Physically compatible for 4 hr at 23 °C	2383	C
Famotidine	MSD	0.2 mg/mL[a]	ES	0.004 mg/ mL[a]	Physically compatible for 4 hr at 25 °C	1188	C
Fenoldopam mesylate	AB	80 mcg/mL[b]	AB	20 mcg/mL[b]	Physically compatible for 4 hr at 23 °C	2467	C
Heparin sodium	UP	1000 units/L[d]	WI	0.2 mg/mL	Physically compatible for 4 hr at room temperature	534	C
Hetastarch in lactated electrolyte	AB	6%	AB	0.02 mg/mL[a]	Physically compatible for 4 hr at 23 °C	2339	C
Hydrocortisone sodium succinate	UP	10 mg/L[d]	WI	0.2 mg/mL	Physically compatible for 4 hr at room temperature	534	C
Levofloxacin	OMN	5 mg/mL[a]	ES	0.2 mg/mL	Visually compatible for 4 hr at 24 °C	2233	C
Milrinone lactate	SW	0.4 mg/mL[a]	ES	8 mcg/mL[a]	Visually compatible. Little loss of either drug in 4 hr at 23 °C	2214	C
Pancuronium bromide	ES	0.05 mg/mL[a]	ES	4 mcg/mL[a]	Physically compatible for 24 hr at 28 °C	1337	C

Y-Site Injection Compatibility (1:1 Mixture) (Cont.)

Isoproterenol HCl

Drug	Mfr	Conc	Mfr	Conc	Remarks	Ref	C/I
Potassium chloride	AB	40 mEq/L[d]	WI	0.2 mg/mL	Physically compatible for 4 hr at room temperature	534	C
Propofol	ZEN	10 mg/mL	AB	0.004 mg/mL[a]	Physically compatible for 1 hr at 23 °C	2066	C
Remifentanil HCl	GW	0.025 and 0.25 mg/mL[b]	SW	0.02 mg/mL[a]	Physically compatible for 4 hr at 23 °C	2075	C
Sodium nitroprusside	RC	0.3, 1.2, 3 mg/mL[a]	SX	20 mcg/mL[f]	Visually compatible for 48 hr at 24 °C protected from light	2357	C
	RC	1.2 and 3 mg/mL[a]	SX	80 mcg/mL[f]	Visually compatible for 48 hr at 24 °C protected from light	2357	C
Tacrolimus	FUJ	1 mg/mL[b]	ES	0.04 mg/mL[a]	Visually compatible for 24 hr at 25 °C	1630	C
TNA #73[e]			BR	4 mcg/mL[c]	Visually compatible for 4 hr	1009	C
Vecuronium bromide	OR	0.1 mg/mL[a]	ES	4 mcg/mL[a]	Physically compatible for 24 hr at 28 °C	1337	C

[a]*Tested in dextrose 5%.*
[b]*Tested in sodium chloride 0.9%.*
[c]*Tested in both dextrose 5% and sodium chloride 0.9%.*
[d]*Tested in dextrose 5% in Ringer's injection, dextrose 5% in Ringer's injection, lactated, dextrose 5%, Ringer's injection, lactated, and sodium chloride 0.9%.*
[e]*Refer to Appendix I for the composition of parenteral nutrition solutions. TNA indicates a 3-in-1 admixture.*
[f]*Tested in dextrose 5% in sodium chloride 0.2%.*

ISOSORBIDE DINITRATE
AHFS 24:12.08

Products — Isosorbide dinitrate is available as a 0.1% solution in 10-mL ampuls and 50- and 100-mL vials. Each milliliter contains isosorbide dinitrate 1 mg. It also is available as a 0.05% solution in 50-mL vials and 10-mL prefilled syringes. Each milliliter contains isosorbide dinitrate 0.5 mg. (38)

Trade Name(s) — Isoket, Risordan.

Administration — Isosorbide dinitrate is administered by intravenous infusion when diluted to a maximum concentration of 0.05% in sodium chloride 0.9% or dextrose 5%. The delivery rate should be controlled using an infusion or syringe pump. (38)

Isosorbide dinitrate is also administered as an intracoronary bolus injection during percutaneous transluminal coronary angioplasty. (38)

Stability — Isosorbide dinitrate injections are colorless and stable in the intact ampuls or vials when stored at room temperature. Once opened, ampuls and vials should be used immediately, and any remainder should be discarded. (38)

Syringes — Isosorbide dinitrate (Rhone-Poulenc) 1 mg/mL was repackaged in polypropylene syringes (Plastipak, Becton Dickinson) and stored for eight hours at room temperature and 4 °C. No loss of drug was found. (1799)

Sorption — Several studies have described or evaluated isosorbide dinitrate sorption characteristics. The drug undergoes rapid and extensive sorption to PVC and polyamide containers and PVC administration tubing. Studies have reported isosorbide dinitrate losses ranging from about 15 to 50%, depending on concentration, flow rate, contact time, length of tubing, and temperature. The majority of loss occurs at the beginning of contact with the plastic and then declines as saturation occurs. Isosorbide dinitrate also undergoes sorption of about 16 to 26% to cellulose propionate and butadiene styrene burette chambers but only 2% to methacrylate butadiene styrene burette chambers. However, little or no sorption occurs to glass, polyethylene, polybutadiene, nylon, and polypropylene containers and administration equipment. Consequently, glass, polyethylene, polypropylene, polybutadiene, and polyethylene containers and equipment are recommended while PVC and polyamide are not. (769; 782; 795; 1027; 1392; 1464; 1465; 1466; 1467; 1619; 2143; 2289)

Filtration — Losses due to sorption of isosorbide dinitrate 250 mg/L in sodium chloride 0.9% delivered at 20 mL/hr through cellulose acetate filters (Sterifix, Ivex HP) were 15 to 26%. Losses to polyamide filters (Pall) were 9 to 13% under the same conditions. (1465)

The loss of isosorbide dinitrate due to sorption to filters extends to filters used in hemodialysis. Isosorbide dinitrate 0.1 mg/mL in sodium chloride 0.9% during simulated hemodialysis using five different filter media underwent substantial drug losses from the solution and binding to some of the filters. Losses of approximately 86% with polysulfone (Fresenius), 72% with cellulose acetate (Baxter), 43% with polyacrylonitrile (Hospal), and 12% cuprophan (Gambro) were found. However, with hemophan filters (Gambro), no loss of drug due to sorption occurred. (2138)

Compatibility Information

Solution Compatibility

Isosorbide dinitrate

Solution	Mfr	Mfr	Conc/L	Remarks	Ref	C/I
Dextrose 5%	BA[a]	BRN	20 mg	Visually compatible but 43% loss of drug due to sorption to the PVC container at 22 °C and 17% loss at 4 °C in 24 hr	2289	I
	BRN[b,c]	BRN	20 mg	Visually compatible with 2 to 3% loss in 24 hr at 4 and 22 °C	2289	C
Sodium chloride 0.9%	TR[a], BT[a]		80 mg	38% loss in 24 hr at room temperature	1464	I
	TR[b], BT[c]		80 mg	Physically compatible with little or no loss in 6 hr at room temperature	1464	C
	TR[a]		100 mg	9% loss in 2 hr and 23% loss in 24 hr at 21 °C in the dark	1392	I
	[b,d]		100 mg	Physically compatible with little or no loss in 24 hr at 21 °C in the dark	1392	C
	BA[a]	BRN	20 mg	Visually compatible but 43% loss of drug due to sorption to the PVC container at 22 °C and 17% loss at 4 °C in 24 hr	2289	I
	BRN[b,c]	BRN	20 mg	Visually compatible with 2 to 3% loss in 24 hr at 4 and 22 °C	2289	C

[a]Tested in PVC containers.
[b]Tested in glass containers.
[c]Tested in polypropylene containers.
[d]Tested in Clear-Flex polyethylene-lined laminated containers.

Additive Compatibility

Isosorbide dinitrate

Drug	Mfr	Conc/L	Mfr	Conc/L	Test Soln	Remarks	Ref	C/I
Floxacillin sodium	BE	20 g		1 g		Physically compatible for 24 hr at 15 and 30 °C. Haze forms in 48 hr and precipitate forms in 72 hr at 30 °C. No change at 15 °C	1479	C
Furosemide	HO	1 g		1 g		Physically compatible for 72 hr at 15 and 30 °C	1479	C

Y-Site Injection Compatibility (1:1 Mixture)

Isosorbide dinitrate

Drug	Mfr	Conc	Mfr	Conc	Remarks	Ref	C/I
Cefepime HCl	BMS	120 mg/mL[b]		0.2 mg/mL	Physically compatible with less than 10% cefepime loss. Isosorbide not tested	2513	C
Ceftazidime	GSK	120 mg/mL[b]		0.2 mg/mL	Physically compatible with less than 10% ceftazidime loss. Isosorbide not tested	2513	C
Heparin sodium	LEO	300 units/mL[a]	RP	10 mg/mL	Erratic availability of both drugs delivered through PVC tubing	1799	I

[a]Tested in dextrose 5%.
[b]Tested in sterile water for injection.

KETAMINE HYDROCHLORIDE
AHFS 28:04.92

Products — Ketamine hydrochloride is available in concentrations equivalent to 10, 50, or 100 mg/mL of ketamine base. The injections also contain 0.1 mg/mL of benzethonium chloride. The 10-mg/mL concentration is made isotonic with sodium chloride and is available in 20-mL vials. The 50-mg/mL concentration is available in 10-mL vials, and the 100-mg/mL concentration is available in 5-mL vials. (1)

The 100-mg/mL concentration must be diluted before intravenous use. Dilution of the dose with an equal volume of sterile water for injection, dextrose 5%, or sodium chloride 0.9% is recommended. (1)

pH — From 3.5 to 5.5. (1)

Osmolality — The osmolalities of ketamine hydrochloride products were determined to be 300 mOsm/kg for the 10-mg/mL concentration and 387 mOsm/kg for the 50-mg/mL concentration. (1233)

Trade Name(s) — Ketalar.

Administration — Ketamine hydrochloride may be administered intramuscularly or by slow intravenous injection over at least 60 seconds.

The 100-mg/mL preparation should not be given undiluted. For intravenous infusion, a 1- or 2-mg/mL solution may be prepared by adding 500 mg of ketamine to 500 mL or to 250 mL, respectively, of dextrose 5% or sodium chloride 0.9%. Diazepam and barbiturates must be given separately from ketamine hydrochloride and not be mixed in the same container. (1)

Stability — Intact vials of ketamine hydrochloride should be stored at controlled room temperature and protected from light. Ketamine hydrochloride injection is a colorless to slightly yellow solution. The drug may darken upon prolonged exposure to light, but this darkening does not affect concentration. Do not use the product if a precipitate is present. (1)

Syringes — Ketamine hydrochloride (Abbott) 10 mg/mL diluted in sterile water for injection was packaged in 1-mL polypropylene tuberculin syringes (Becton Dickinson) and was stored at 25 °C. The drug solution remained clear and no loss occurred in 30 days. (2431)

Ketamine hydrochloride diluted in sodium chloride 0.9% to 1 mg/mL was packaged in polypropylene syringes with tip caps and stored at 4, 25, and 40 °C for 12 months. No visible changes occurred, and drug concentrations remained above 95% at all temperatures. (2779)

Compatibility Information

Additive Compatibility

Ketamine HCl

Drug	Mfr	Conc/L	Mfr	Conc/L	Test Soln	Remarks	Ref	C/I
Droperidol with fentanyl citrate	JN DB	50 mg 10 mg	JN	1 g	NS[a]	Visually compatible. 5% increase in all drugs in 30 days at 4 and 25 °C due to water loss	2653	C
Droperidol with fentanyl citrate	JN DB	50 mg 10 mg	JN	1 g	NS[c]	Visually compatible with little loss of the drugs in 30 days at 25 °C	2653	C
Fentanyl citrate with droperidol	DB JN	10 mg 50 mg	JN	1 g	NS[a]	Visually compatible. 5% increase in all drugs in 30 days at 4 and 25 °C due to water loss	2653	C
Fentanyl citrate with droperidol	DB JN	10 mg 50 mg	JN	1 g	NS[c]	Visually compatible with little loss of the drugs in 30 days at 25 °C	2653	C
Hydromorphone HCl	SZ	200 mg	SZ	200 mg, 600 mg, 1 g	NS[a,c]	Visually compatible. Under 10% loss of both drugs in 7 days at 25 °C	2799	C
Morphine sulfate	SX	1 g	PD	1 g	NS[a]	At least 90% of both drugs retained for 6 days at room temperature	2260	C
	SX	25 g	PD	25 g	NS[a]	At least 90% of both drugs retained for 6 days at room temperature	2260	C
	SX	25 g	PD	25 g	NS[b]	At least 90% of both drugs retained for 6 days at room temperature	2260	C
	AB	2 g	PD	1.33 g	NS	Little loss of either drug in 4 days at room temperature	2786	C

[a] Tested in PVC containers.
[b] Tested in plastic medication cassette reservoirs (Deltec).
[c] Tested in glass containers.

Drugs in Syringe Compatibility

Ketamine HCl

Drug (in syringe)	Mfr	Amt	Mfr	Amt	Remarks	Ref	C/I
Bupivacaine HCl with fentanyl citrate	SW JN	1.5 mg/mL 0.01 mg/mL	PD	2 mg/mL	Diluted to 5 mL with NS. Visually compatible with no new GC/MS peaks in 1 hr at room temperature	1956	C
Clonidine HCl with tetracaine HCl	BI SW	0.03 mg/mL 2 mg/mL	PD	2 mg/mL	Diluted to 5 mL with NS. Visually compatible with no new GC/MS peaks in 1 hr at room temperature	1956	C
Dexamethasone sodium phosphate	OR	50 and 600 mg	PF	1 mg	Diluted to 14 mL with NS. Physically compatible with no loss of either drug in 8 days at 4 and 23 °C	2677	C
Doxapram HCl	RB	400 mg/20 mL	PD	200 mg/20 mL	Physically compatible with no doxapram loss in 9 hr but 12% loss in 24 hr	1177	I
Fentanyl citrate		40 mcg/mL	PF	1 mg/mL	Diluted in sodium chloride 0.9%. Physically compatible for 96 hr at 25 °C	2563	C
Fentanyl citrate with bupivacaine HCl	JN SW	0.01 mg/mL 1.5 mg/mL	PD	2 mg/mL	Diluted to 5 mL with NS. Visually compatible with no new GC/MS peaks in 1 hr at room temperature	1956	C
Hydromorphone HCl	SZ	0.2 mg/mL[a]	SZ	0.2, 0.6, 1 mg/mL[a]	Visually compatible. Under 10% loss of both drugs in 7 days at 25 °C	2799	C
Lidocaine HCl with morphine sulfate	AST ES	2 mg/mL 0.2 mg/mL	PD	2 mg/mL	Diluted to 5 mL with NS. Visually compatible with no new GC/MS peaks in 1 hr at room temperature	1956	C
Meperidine HCl	DB	12 mg/mL	PD	2 mg/mL	Diluted to 50 mL with NS. Visually compatible for 48 hr at 25 °C	2059	C
Morphine sulfate	SX	1 mg/mL[a], 10 mg/mL[a]	PD	1 mg/mL[a]	At least 90% of both drugs retained for 6 days at room temperature	2260	C
	SX	25 mg/mL[a]	PD	1 mg/mL[a]	5% morphine loss in 6 days at room temperature. Up to 15% ketamine loss in 2 to 6 days	2260	C
	SX	1, 10, 25 mg/mL[a]	PD[a]	10, 25 mg/mL	At least 90% of both drugs retained for 6 days at room temperature	2260	C
		1 mg/1 mL		5, 10, 20 mg/1 mL	No substantial change in the concentration of either drug over 4 days	669	C
	SZ	2, 5, 10 mg/mL[a]	SZ	2 mg/mL[a]	Physically compatible. Little loss of either drug at 23 and 5 °C in 91 days	2797	C
Morphine sulfate with lidocaine HCl	ES AST	0.2 mg/mL 2 mg/mL	PD	2 mg/mL	Diluted to 5 mL with NS. Visually compatible with no new GC/MS peaks in 1 hr at room temperature	1956	C
Propofol	NOP	50 mg/5 mL	SZ	50 mg/5 mL	Physically compatible. Little loss of either drug in 3 hr at room temperature	2790	C
	NOP	70 mg/7 mL	SZ	30 mg/3 mL	Physically compatible. Little loss of either drug in 3 hr at room temperature	2790	C
Tetracaine HCl with clonidine HCl	SW BI	2 mg/mL 0.03 mg/mL	PD	2 mg/mL	Diluted to 5 mL with NS. Visually compatible with no new GC/MS peaks in 1 hr at room temperature	1956	C

[a]Diluted in sodium chloride 0.9%.

Y-Site Injection Compatibility (1:1 Mixture)

Ketamine HCl

Drug	Mfr	Conc	Mfr	Conc	Remarks	Ref	C/I
Cefepime HCl	BMS	120 mg/mL[a]		10 mg/mL	Physically compatible with less than 10% cefepime loss. Ketamine not tested	2513	C
Ceftazidime	SKB	125 mg/mL		10 mg/mL	Visually compatible with less than 10% loss of ceftazidime in 24 hr. Ketamine not tested	2434	C
	GSK	120 mg/mL[a]		10 mg/mL	Physically compatible with less than 10% ceftazidime loss. Ketamine not tested	2513	C
Propofol	ZEN	10 mg/mL	PD	10 mg/mL	Physically compatible for 1 hr at 23 °C	2066	C

[a]*Tested in sterile water for injection.*

KETOROLAC TROMETHAMINE
AHFS 28:08.04.92

Products — Ketorolac tromethamine is available as a 15-mg/mL solution in 1-mL vials and also as a 30-mg/mL solution in 1-mL vials. Ketorolac tromethamine 30 mg/mL is also available in 2-mL vials for intramuscular use. In addition to ketorolac tromethamine, the formulations contain ethanol, sodium chloride, and citric acid in water for injection. The product also contains sodium hydroxide or hydrochloric acid to adjust the pH. (1)

pH — From 6.9 to 7.9. (1; 4)

Tonicity — Both ketorolac tromethamine concentrations are isotonic. (4)

Administration — Ketorolac tromethamine is administered slowly by deep intramuscular injection or by intravenous injection over no less than 15 seconds. (1; 4) The 60 mg/2 mL injection is for intramuscular use only. (1)

Stability — Ketorolac tromethamine injection should be stored at controlled room temperature and protected from light. The injection is clear and has a slight yellow color. (1; 4) Prolonged exposure to light may result in discoloration of the solution and precipitation. (4) Ketorolac tromethamine is chemically stable over a wide pH range from about pH 3 to 11 (499), but precipitation may occur in solutions and with drugs having a relatively low pH. (4)

Compatibility Information

Solution Compatibility

Ketorolac tromethamine

Solution	Mfr	Mfr	Conc/L	Remarks	Ref	C/I
Dextrose 5% in sodium chloride 0.9%	TR[a]	SY	600 mg	Physically compatible. No loss in 48 hr at room temperature	1646	C
Dextrose 5%	TR[b]	SY	600 mg	Physically compatible. No loss in 48 hr at room temperature	1646	C
	BA[a]	RC	600 mg	Visually compatible. Little loss in 7 days and 14% loss in 14 days at 25 °C. Less than 2% loss in 50 days at 5 °C	2095	C
	[a]	RC	300 and 600 mg	Visually compatible. Little loss in 21 days at 4 and 23 °C	2442	C
	[c]	RC	200 mg	Visually compatible. Less than 10% loss after −20 °C storage for 90 days, microwave thawing, and storage at 4 °C for 60 days	2645	C
	BA[c]	RC	100 and 300 mg	Visually compatible. Less than 3% drug loss after 15 days at −20 °C then 35 days at 4 °C	2707	C

Solution Compatibility (Cont.)

Ketorolac tromethamine

Solution	Mfr	Mfr	Conc/L	Remarks	Ref	C/I
Plasma-Lyte A, pH 7.4	TR[a]	SY	600 mg	Physically compatible. No loss in 48 hr at room temperature	1646	C
	TR[b]	SY	60 mg	Physically compatible. No loss in 48 hr at room temperature	1646	C
Ringer's injection	TR[a]	SY	600 mg	Physically compatible. No loss in 48 hr at room temperature	1646	C
	TR[b]	SY	60 mg	Physically compatible. No loss in 48 hr at room temperature	1646	C
Ringer's injection, lactated	TR[a]	SY	600 mg	Physically compatible. No loss in 48 hr at room temperature	1646	C
Sodium chloride 0.9%	TR[b]	SY	600 mg	Physically compatible. No loss in 48 hr at room temperature	1646	C
	BA[a]	RC	600 mg	Visually compatible. No loss in 35 days at 25 °C and in 50 days at 5 °C	2095	C

[a]Tested in PVC containers.
[b]Tested in both glass and PVC containers.
[c]Tested in polyolefin containers.

Drugs in Syringe Compatibility

Ketorolac tromethamine

Drug (in syringe)	Mfr	Amt	Mfr	Amt	Remarks	Ref	C/I
Cyclizine lactate	WEL	50 mg/mL	RC	30 mg/mL	White precipitate forms	2495	I
Diazepam	ES	15 mg/3 mL	SY	180 mg/6 mL	Visually compatible for 4 hr at 24 °C. Increase in absorbance occurs immediately, persists for 30 min, and dissipates by 1 hr	1703	?
Haloperidol lactate	SO	5 mg/1 mL	SY	30 mg/1 mL	White crystalline precipitate forms immediately	1786	I
Hydromorphone HCl	KN	10 mg/1 mL	SY	30 mg/1 mL	Cloudiness forms immediately but clears with swirling	1785	?
	KN	1 mg/1 mL[a]	SY	30 mg/1 mL	Visually compatible for 24 hr at 25 °C under fluorescent light	1785	C
	KN	1[a] and 10 mg/1 mL	SY	15 mg/1 mL[a]	Visually compatible for 24 hr at 25 °C under fluorescent light	1785	C
Hydroxyzine HCl	SO	150 mg/3 mL	SY	180 mg/6 mL	Heavy white precipitate forms immediately, separating into two layers over time	1703	I
Nalbuphine HCl	DU	30 mg/3 mL	SY	180 mg/6 mL	Solid white precipitate forms immediately and settles to bottom	1703	I
Prochlorperazine edisylate	STS	15 mg/3 mL	SY	180 mg/6 mL	Heavy white precipitate forms immediately, separating into two layers over time	1703	I
Promethazine HCl	ES	75 mg/3 mL	SY	180 mg/6 mL	Heavy white precipitate forms immediately, separating into two layers over time	1703	I

[a]Dilutions prepared with sterile water for injection.

Y-Site Injection Compatibility (1:1 Mixture)

Ketorolac tromethamine

Drug	Mfr	Conc	Mfr	Conc	Remarks	Ref	C/I
Azithromycin	PF	2 mg/mL[b]	AB	15 mg/mL[c]	Amber microcrystals found	2368	I
Cisatracurium besylate	GW	0.1, 2, 5 mg/mL[a]	RC	15 mg/mL[a]	Physically compatible for 4 hr at 23 °C	2074	C
Dexmedetomidine HCl	AB	4 mcg/mL[b]	AB	15 mg/mL	Physically compatible for 4 hr at 23 °C	2383	C
Fenoldopam mesylate	AB	80 mcg/mL[b]	AB	15 mg/mL[b]	Trace haze forms immediately	2467	I
Fentanyl citrate	JN	0.025 mg/mL[a]	WY	1 mg/mL[a]	Physically compatible for 48 hr at 22 °C	1706	C
Hetastarch in lactated electrolyte	AB	6%	AB	15 mg/mL	Physically compatible for 4 hr at 23 °C	2339	C
Hydromorphone HCl	AST	0.5 mg/mL[a]	WY	1 mg/mL[a]	Physically compatible for 48 hr at 22 °C	1706	C
Methadone HCl	LI	1 mg/mL[a]	WY	1 mg/mL[a]	Physically compatible for 48 hr at 22 °C	1706	C
Morphine sulfate	AST	1 mg/mL[a]	WY	1 mg/mL[a]	Physically compatible for 48 hr at 22 °C	1706	C
Remifentanil HCl	GW	0.025 and 0.25 mg/mL[b]	RC	15 mg/mL[a]	Physically compatible for 4 hr at 23 °C	2075	C

[a] *Tested in dextrose 5%.*
[b] *Tested in sodium chloride 0.9%.*
[c] *Injected via Y-site into an administration set running azithromycin.*

LABETALOL HYDROCHLORIDE
AHFS 24:24

Products — Labetalol hydrochloride is available in 20- and 40-mL multiple-dose vials and 4- and 8-mL vials and disposable syringes. Each milliliter of solution contains labetalol hydrochloride 5 mg, dextrose, anhydrous 45 mg, edetate disodium 0.1 mg, methylparaben 0.8 mg, propylparaben 0.1 mg, and citric acid anhydrous and sodium hydroxide as necessary to adjust pH in water for injection. (1)

pH — From 3 to 4.5. (17)

Administration — Labetalol hydrochloride is administered by slow direct intravenous injection, over two minutes, or by continuous intravenous infusion at an initial rate of 2 mg/min with subsequent adjustments based on blood pressure response. For continuous infusion, concentrations of 1 mg/mL or 2 mg/3 mL can be made by adding 200 mg (40 mL) to 160 or 250 mL of compatible infusion solution. To facilitate the infusion of labetalol hydrochloride at an accurate rate of administration, a controlled-infusion device, such as a pump, may be used. (1; 4)

Stability — Labetalol hydrochloride may be stored at room temperature or under refrigeration and should be protected from light and freezing. The solution is clear and colorless to slightly yellow. (1)

pH Effects — Labetalol hydrochloride has optimal stability at pH 3 to 4. Addition to an alkaline drug or solution has resulted in precipitate formation. (757; 1715; 2062)

Compatibility Information

Solution Compatibility

Labetalol HCl

Solution	Mfr	Mfr	Conc/L	Remarks	Ref	C/I
Dextrose 5% in Ringer's injection	TR	SC	1.25 and 3.75 g	Physically compatible and chemically stable for 72 hr at 4 and 25 °C	757	C
Dextrose 5% in Ringer's injection, lactated	TR	SC	1.25 and 3.75 g	Physically compatible and chemically stable for 72 hr at 4 and 25 °C	757	C

Solution Compatibility (Cont.)

Labetalol HCl

Solution	Mfr	Mfr	Conc/L	Remarks	Ref	C/I
Dextrose 2.5% in sodium chloride 0.45%	TR	SC	1.25 and 3.75 g	Physically compatible and chemically stable for 72 hr at 4 and 25 °C	757	**C**
Dextrose 5% in sodium chloride 0.2%	TR	SC	1.25 and 3.75 g	Physically compatible and chemically stable for 72 hr at 4 and 25 °C	757	**C**
Dextrose 5% in sodium chloride 0.33%	TR	SC	1.25 and 3.75 g	Physically compatible and chemically stable for 72 hr at 4 and 25 °C	757	**C**
Dextrose 5% in sodium chloride 0.9%	TR	SC	1.25 and 3.75 g	Physically compatible and chemically stable for 72 hr at 4 and 25 °C	757	**C**
Dextrose 5%	TR	SC	1.25 and 3.75 g	Physically compatible and chemically stable for 72 hr at 4 and 25 °C	757	**C**
Ringer's injection	TR	SC	1.25 and 3.75 g	Physically compatible and chemically stable for 72 hr at 4 and 25 °C	757	**C**
Ringer's injection, lactated	TR	SC	1.25 and 3.75 g	Physically compatible and chemically stable for 72 hr at 4 and 25 °C	757	**C**
Sodium chloride 0.9%				Physically compatible and stable for 24 hr at room temperature or refrigerated	1	**C**

Additive Compatibility

Labetalol HCl

Drug	Mfr	Conc/L	Mfr	Conc/L	Test Soln	Remarks	Ref	C/I
Sodium bicarbonate	TR	5%	SC	1.25, 2.5, 3.75 g		White precipitate forms within 6 hr after mixing at 4 and 25 °C	757	**I**

Drugs in Syringe Compatibility

Labetalol HCl

Drug (in syringe)	Mfr	Amt	Mfr	Amt	Remarks	Ref	C/I
Pantoprazole sodium	a	4 mg/ 1 mL		5 mg/ 1 mL	Whitish precipitate	2574	**I**

[a]Test performed using the formulation WITHOUT edetate disodium.

Y-Site Injection Compatibility (1:1 Mixture)

Labetalol HCl

Drug	Mfr	Conc	Mfr	Conc	Remarks	Ref	C/I
Amikacin sulfate	BR	5 mg/mL[a]	SC	1 mg/mL[a]	Physically compatible for 24 hr at 18 °C	1171	**C**
Aminophylline	ES	1 mg/mL[a]	SC	1 mg/mL[a]	Physically compatible for 24 hr at 18 °C	1171	**C**
Amiodarone HCl	WY	4.8 mg/mL[a]	GL	5 mg/mL	Visually compatible for 24 hr at 23 °C	1877	**C**
	WY	6 mg/mL[a]	BED	5 mg/mL	Visually compatible for 24 hr at 22 °C	2352	**C**
Amphotericin B cholesteryl sulfate complex	SEQ	0.83 mg/mL[a]	AH	5 mg/mL	Gross precipitate forms	2117	**I**
Ampicillin sodium	WY	10 mg/mL[b]	SC	1 mg/mL[a]	Physically compatible for 24 hr at 18 °C	1171	**C**

Y-Site Injection Compatibility (1:1 Mixture) (Cont.)

Labetalol HCl

Drug	Mfr	Conc	Mfr	Conc	Remarks	Ref	C/I
Bivalirudin	TMC	5 mg/mL[a]	FP	2 mg/mL[a]	Physically compatible for 4 hr at 23 °C	2373	C
Butorphanol tartrate	BR	0.04 mg/mL[a]	SC	1 mg/mL[a]	Physically compatible for 24 hr at 18 °C	1171	C
Calcium gluconate	AMR	0.23 mEq/mL[a]	SC	1 mg/mL[a]	Physically compatible for 24 hr at 18 °C	1171	C
Cefazolin sodium	LI	10 mg/mL[a]	SC	1 mg/mL[a]	Physically compatible for 24 hr at 18 °C	1171	C
Ceftaroline fosamil	FOR	2.22 mg/mL[a]	HOS	5 mg/mL	Increase in measured haze and microparticulates	2826	I
	FOR	2.22 mg/mL[b,e]	HOS	5 mg/mL	Increase in measured haze	2826	I
Ceftazidime	GL	10 mg/mL[a]	SC	1 mg/mL[a]	Physically compatible for 24 hr at 18 °C	1171	C
Ceftriaxone sodium	RC	20[a,b] and 100[c] mg/mL	GL	2.5[c] and 5 mg/mL	Fluffy white precipitate forms immediately	1964	I
Chloramphenicol sodium succinate	PD	10 mg/mL[a]	SC	1 mg/mL[a]	Physically compatible for 24 hr at 18 °C	1171	C
Clindamycin phosphate	UP	9 mg/mL[a]	SC	1 mg/mL[a]	Physically compatible for 24 hr at 18 °C	1171	C
Clonidine HCl	BI	18 mcg/mL[b]	GSK	1 mg/mL[a,b]	Visually compatible	2642	C
Dexmedetomidine HCl	AB	4 mcg/mL[b]	AB	2 mg/mL[b]	Physically compatible for 4 hr at 23 °C	2383	C
Diltiazem HCl	MMD	1 mg/mL[a]	AH	2 mg/mL[a]	Visually compatible for 4 hr at 27 °C	2062	C
Dobutamine HCl	LI	2.5 mg/mL[a]	GL	1 mg/mL[a]	Visually compatible. Little loss of either drug in 4 hr at room temperature	1762	C
	LI	4 mg/mL[a]	GL	5 mg/mL	Visually compatible for 24 hr at 23 °C	1877	C
	LI	4 mg/mL[a]	AH	2 mg/mL[a]	Visually compatible for 4 hr at 27 °C	2062	C
Dopamine HCl	IMS	1.6 mg/mL[a]	SC	1 mg/mL[a]	Physically compatible for 24 hr at 18 °C	1171	C
	ES	1.6 mg/mL[a]	GL	1 mg/mL[a]	Visually compatible. Little loss of either drug in 4 hr at room temperature	1762	C
	AB	3.2 mg/mL[a]	AH	2 mg/mL[a]	Visually compatible for 4 hr at 27 °C	2062	C
Doripenem	JJ	5 mg/mL[a,b]	HOS	2 mg/mL[a,b]	Physically compatible for 4 hr at 23 °C	2743	C
Enalaprilat	MSD	0.05 mg/mL[b]	GL	1 mg/mL[a]	Physically compatible for 24 hr at room temperature under fluorescent light	1355	C
Epinephrine HCl	AB	0.02 mg/mL[a]	AH	2 mg/mL[a]	Visually compatible for 4 hr at 27 °C	2062	C
Erythromycin lactobionate	AB	5 mg/mL[a]	SC	1 mg/mL[a]	Physically compatible for 24 hr at 18 °C	1171	C
Esmolol HCl	DU	40 mg/mL[a]	GL	5 mg/mL	Visually compatible for 24 hr at 23 °C	1877	C
Famotidine	MSD	0.2 mg/mL[a]	SC	1 mg/mL[a]	Physically compatible for 4 hr at 25 °C	1188	C
Fenoldopam mesylate	AB	80 mcg/mL[b]	AB	2 mg/mL[b]	Physically compatible for 4 hr at 23 °C	2467	C
Fentanyl citrate	JN	10 mcg/mL[a]	SC	1 mg/mL[a]	Physically compatible for 24 hr at 18 °C	1171	C
	ES	0.05 mg/mL	AH	2 mg/mL[a]	Visually compatible for 4 hr at 27 °C	2062	C
Furosemide	ES	10 mg/mL[d]	SC	1.6 mg/mL[d]	White precipitate forms immediately	1715	I
	AMR	10 mg/mL	AH	2 mg/mL[a]	Precipitate forms immediately	2062	I
Gentamicin sulfate	ES	0.8 mg/mL[a]	SC	1 mg/mL[a]	Physically compatible for 24 hr at 18 °C	1171	C
Heparin sodium	IX	40 units/mL[a]	SC	1 mg/mL[a]	Physically compatible for 24 hr at 18 °C	1171	C
	OR	100 units/mL[a]	GL	5 mg/mL	Cloudiness with particles forms immediately	1877	I
	ES	100 units/mL[a]	AH	2 mg/mL[a]	Visually compatible for 4 hr at 27 °C	2062	C
Hetastarch in lactated electrolyte	AB	6%	GW	2 mg/mL[a]	Physically compatible for 4 hr at 23 °C	2339	C

Y-Site Injection Compatibility (1:1 Mixture) (Cont.)

Labetalol HCl

Drug	Mfr	Conc	Mfr	Conc	Remarks	Ref	C/I
Hydromorphone HCl	KN	1 mg/mL	AH	2 mg/mL[a]	Visually compatible for 4 hr at 27 °C	2062	C
Hydroxyethyl starch 130/0.4 in sodium chloride 0.9%	FRK	6%	SZ	1.25[a], 2.5[a], 5 mg/mL	Visually compatible for 24 hr at room temperature	2770	C
Insulin, regular	LI	1 unit/mL[a]	GL	5 mg/mL	Visually compatible for 4 hr. White precipitate forms in 24 hr at 23 °C	1877	?
Lidocaine HCl	AST	20 mg/mL[a]	SC	1 mg/mL[a]	Physically compatible for 24 hr at 18 °C	1171	C
Linezolid	PHU	2 mg/mL	GW	5 mg/mL	Physically compatible for 4 hr at 23 °C	2264	C
Lorazepam	WY	0.5 mg/mL[a]	AH	2 mg/mL[a]	Visually compatible for 4 hr at 27 °C	2062	C
Magnesium sulfate	LY	10 mg/mL[a]	SC	1 mg/mL[a]	Physically compatible for 24 hr at 18 °C	1171	C
Meperidine HCl	AB	10 mg/mL	GL	5 mg/mL	Physically compatible for 4 hr at 25 °C	1397	C
Metronidazole	SE	5 mg/mL	SC	1 mg/mL[a]	Physically compatible for 24 hr at 18 °C	1171	C
Micafungin sodium	ASP	1.5 mg/mL[b]	AB	2 mg/mL[b]	White cloudiness forms immediately	2683	I
Midazolam HCl	RC	1 mg/mL[a]	GL	5 mg/mL	Visually compatible for 24 hr at 23 °C	1877	C
	RC	2 mg/mL[a]	AH	2 mg/mL[a]	Visually compatible for 4 hr at 27 °C	2062	C
Milrinone lactate	SW	0.2 mg/mL[a]	AH	2 mg/mL[a]	Visually compatible for 4 hr at 27 °C	2062	C
Morphine sulfate	WY	1 mg/mL[a]	SC	1 mg/mL[a]	Physically compatible for 24 hr at 18 °C	1171	C
	AB	1 mg/mL	GL	5 mg/mL	Physically compatible for 4 hr at 25 °C	1397	C
	ES	0.5 mg/mL[a]	GL	1 mg/mL[a]	Visually compatible. Little loss of either drug in 4 hr at room temperature	1762	C
	SCN	2 mg/mL[a]	AH	2 mg/mL[a]	Visually compatible for 4 hr at 27 °C	2062	C
Nafcillin sodium	BR	10 mg/mL[a]	SC	1 mg/mL[a]	Cloudy precipitate forms immediately	1171	I
Nicardipine HCl	WY	1 mg/mL[a]	AH	2 mg/mL[a]	Visually compatible for 4 hr at 27 °C	2062	C
	DCC	0.1 mg/mL[a]	GL	1 mg/mL[a]	Visually compatible for 24 hr at room temperature	235	C
Nitroglycerin	DU	0.2 mg/mL[a]	GL	1 mg/mL[a]	Visually compatible. No labetalol loss and 6% nitroglycerin loss in 4 hr at room temperature	1762	C
	OM	0.2 mg/mL[a]	GL	5 mg/mL	Visually compatible for 24 hr at 23 °C	1877	C
	AB	0.4 mg/mL[a]	AH	2 mg/mL[a]	Visually compatible for 4 hr at 27 °C	2062	C
Norepinephrine bitartrate	STR	64 mcg/mL[a]	GL	5 mg/mL	Visually compatible for 24 hr at 23 °C	1877	C
	AB	0.128 mg/mL[a]	AH	2 mg/mL[a]	Visually compatible for 4 hr at 27 °C	2062	C
Oxacillin sodium	BR	10 mg/mL[a]	SC	1 mg/mL[a]	Physically compatible for 24 hr at 18 °C	1171	C
Penicillin G potassium	PF	50,000 units/mL[a]	SC	1 mg/mL[a]	Physically compatible for 24 hr at 18 °C	1171	C
Potassium chloride	IX	0.4 mEq/mL[a]	SC	1 mg/mL[a]	Physically compatible for 24 hr at 18 °C	1171	C
Potassium phosphates	LY	0.44 mEq/mL[a]	SC	1 mg/mL[a]	Physically compatible for 24 hr at 18 °C	1171	C
Propofol	ZEN	10 mg/mL	AH	5 mg/mL	Physically compatible for 1 hr at 23 °C	2066	C
Ranitidine HCl	GL	0.5 mg/mL[a]	SC	1 mg/mL[a]	Physically compatible for 24 hr at 18 °C	1171	C
	GL	0.6 mg/mL[a]	GL	1 mg/mL[a]	Visually compatible. Little ranitidine and 5% labetalol loss in 4 hr at room temperature	1762	C
	GL	1 mg/mL[a]	AH	2 mg/mL[a]	Visually compatible for 4 hr at 27 °C	2062	C
Sodium acetate	LY	0.4 mEq/mL[a]	SC	1 mg/mL[a]	Physically compatible for 24 hr at 18 °C	1171	C

Y-Site Injection Compatibility (1:1 Mixture) (Cont.)

Labetalol HCl

Drug	Mfr	Conc	Mfr	Conc	Remarks	Ref	C/I
Sodium nitroprusside	RC	0.2 mg/mL[a]	GL	5 mg/mL	Visually compatible for 24 hr at 23 °C	1877	C
Telavancin HCl	ASP	7.5 mg/mL[a,b,e]	BED	5 mg/mL	Physically compatible for 2 hr	2830	C
Tobramycin sulfate	LI	0.8 mg/mL[a]	SC	1 mg/mL[a]	Physically compatible for 24 hr at 18 °C	1171	C
Trimethoprim–sulfamethoxazole	BW	0.8 + 4 mg/mL[a]	SC	1 mg/mL[a]	Physically compatible for 24 hr at 18 °C	1171	C
Vancomycin HCl	LE	5 mg/mL[a]	SC	1 mg/mL[a]	Physically compatible for 24 hr at 18 °C	1171	C
Vecuronium bromide	OR	1 mg/mL	AH	2 mg/mL[a]	Visually compatible for 4 hr at 27 °C	2062	C
Warfarin sodium	DU	2 mg/mL[c]	SC	0.8 mg/mL[a]	Haze forms immediately	2010	I
	DME	2 mg/mL[c]	SC	0.8 mg/mL[a]	Haze forms immediately	2078	I

[a]*Tested in dextrose 5%.*
[b]*Tested in sodium chloride 0.9%.*
[c]*Tested in sterile water for injection.*
[d]*Furosemide 0.5 mL injected in the Y-site port of a running infusion of labetalol hydrochloride in dextrose 5%.*
[e]*Tested in Ringer's injection, lactated.*

LENOGRASTIM
AHFS 20:16

Products — Lenograstim (rHuG-CSF) is available as a lyophilized powder in single-use vials containing 13.4 million I.U. (Granocyte-13) or 33.6 million I.U. (Granocyte-34). In addition to lenograstim, each vial of the product contains mannitol 2.5%, arginine 1%, phenylalanine 1%, methionine 0.1%, polysorbate 20 0.01%, and hydrochloric acid to adjust pH. (38)

Lenograstim vials of either strength should be reconstituted with 1.05 mL of the accompanying water for injection diluent. Gently mix to effect dissolution, usually about 5 seconds. Do not shake the vials vigorously. Both the lenograstim vials and the diluent are overfilled by 5% to permit withdrawal of a full 1 mL of the reconstituted product containing 13.4 or 33.6 million I.U. (38)

Units — Each 13.4-million I.U. vial contains 105 mcg of lenograstim. Each 33.6-million I.U. vial contains 263 mcg of lenograstim. (38)

pH — The reconstituted solution has a pH buffered to 6.5. (38)

Trade Name(s) — Granocyte-13, Granocyte-34.

Administration — Lenograstim is administered by subcutaneous injection and intravenous infusion after dilution in sodium chloride 0.9% in glass or PVC containers or dextrose 5% in glass containers. Granocyte 13 should not be diluted to a concentration lower than 0.26 million I.U. per milliliter (2 mcg/mL); Granocyte-34 should not be diluted to a concentration lower than 0.32 million I.U. per milliliter (2.5 mcg/mL). The dilution volume should not exceed 50 mL for each vial of Granocyte-13 and 100 mL for each vial of Granocyte-34. (38)

Stability — Intact vials of lenograstim should be stored at 30 °C or below and protected from freezing. When reconstituted as directed, lenograstim is stable for 24 hours under refrigeration. Diluted for administration to concentrations not less than 0.26 million I.U. (Granocyte-13) or 0.32 million I.U. (Granocyte-34) per milliliter, lenograstim is stable for up to 24 hours at 5 or 25 °C. (38)

At concentrations not less than 0.26 million I.U. (Granocyte-13) or 0.32 million I.U. (Granocyte-34) per milliliter, lenograstim is stable for up to 24 hours at 5 or 25 °C in sodium chloride 0.9% in both PVC and glass containers and in dextrose 5% in glass containers. (38)

Ambulatory Pumps — The stability of lenograstim (Rhône-Poulenc Rorer) 33.6 million I.U. (263 mcg) and 67.2 million I.U. (526 mcg) each in 100 mL of sodium chloride 0.9% filled into Intermate elastomeric infusion devices (Baxter) was evaluated stored at 4 °C for 14 days. No loss of lenograstim was found. (2048)

Sorption — Lenograstim prepared in sodium chloride 0.9% is compatible with PVC containers and common administration sets. (38)

LEPIRUDIN
AHFS 20:12.04.92

Products — Lepirudin is available as a lyophilized powder in vials containing 50 mg of drug along with 40 mg of mannitol and sodium hydroxide for pH adjustment. Reconstitute the vials with 1 mL of sterile water for injection or sodium chloride 0.9% and shake gently to yield a 50-mg/mL solution. Dissolution usually occurs within a few seconds but definitely in less than three minutes. The reconstituted solution must be diluted for use. (1)

pH — Approximately 7. (1)

Units — Lepirudin activity is measured in antithrombin units (ATU). One ATU is the amount of lepirudin that neutralizes one unit of World Health Organization preparation 89/588 thrombin. (1)

Specific Activity — Lepirudin has a specific activity of 16,000 ATU per milligram of drug. (1)

Trade Name(s) — Refludan.

Administration — Lepirudin is administered slowly intravenously over 15 to 20 seconds initially and is followed by continuous intravenous infusion. For the initial intravenous bolus dose, the reconstituted solution is diluted to a concentration of 5 mg/mL. One milliliter of the reconstituted solution is diluted with 9 mL of sodium chloride 0.9%, dextrose 5%, or sterile water for injection in a sterile 10-mL or larger syringe. For intravenous infusion, lepirudin concentrations of 0.2 or 0.4 mg/mL are prepared by adding the reconstituted contents of two vials to 500 or 250 mL, respectively, of sodium chloride 0.9% or dextrose 5%. (1)

Stability — Intact vials of lepirudin should be stored between 2 and 25 °C. The manufacturer recommends use of the reconstituted solution immediately after preparation. The clear, colorless reconstituted solution is stable 24 hours at room temperature. Diluted for administration to a concentration between 0.2 and 5 mg/mL, lepirudin is also stable for 24 hours at room temperature. (1; 4)

Compatibility Information

Y-Site Injection Compatibility (1:1 Mixture)

			Lepirudin				
Drug	Mfr	Conc	Mfr	Conc	Remarks	Ref	C/I
Amiodarone HCl	WY	6 mg/mL[a]	HMR	0.4 mg/mL[a]	Visually compatible for 24 hr at 22 °C	2352	C
Metoprolol tartrate	BED	1 mg/mL	BX	0.4 mg/mL[a]	Trace precipitate in 5 hr at 19 °C	2795	I

[a]*Tested in dextrose 5%.*

LEUCOVORIN CALCIUM
AHFS 92:12

Products — Leucovorin calcium is available in lyophilized form in vials containing leucovorin 50, 100, 200, 350, and 500 mg as the calcium salt with sodium chloride and sodium hydroxide or hydrochloric acid to adjust the pH. Reconstitute the vials with bacteriostatic water for injection containing benzyl alcohol or sterile water for injection with the volumes indicated in Table 1. (1; 4)

Leucovorin calcium is also available at a concentration of 10 mg/mL containing no preservative in vials of 10, 25, and 30 mL. (4)

pH — From 6.5 to 8.5. (17)

Administration — Leucovorin calcium is administered by intramuscular or intravenous injection or infusion at a rate not exceeding 160 mg/min. When doses greater than 10 mg/m² are required, diluents containing benzyl alcohol should not be used for reconstitution. (1; 4)

Stability — Leucovorin calcium injection should be stored at room temperature and protected from light. (1; 4)

The reconstituted solution of leucovorin calcium is stated to be stable for seven days. When reconstituted with diluents that contain no preservatives, immediate use is recommended. (1)

Table 1. Recommended Reconstitution of Leucovorin Calcium (1; 4)

Vial Size (mg)	Volume of Diluent (mL)	Concentration (mg/mL)
50	5	10
100	10	10
200	20	10
350	17.5	20
500	50	10

pH Effects — Leucovorin calcium solutions exhibit good stability at pH 6.5 to 10. The pH of maximum stability was determined to be 7.1 to 7.4. Below pH 6, increased decomposition occurs. (1276)

Central Venous Catheter — Leucovorin calcium (Gensia) 2 mg/mL in dextrose 5% was found to be compatible with the ARROWg+ard Blue Plus (Arrow International) chlorhexidine-bearing triple-lumen central catheter. Essentially complete delivery of the drug was found with little or no drug loss occurring. Furthermore, chlorhexidine delivered from the catheter remained at trace amounts with no substantial increase due to the delivery of the drug through the catheter. (2335)

Compatibility Information

Solution Compatibility

Leucovorin calcium

Solution	Mfr	Mfr	Conc/L	Remarks	Ref	C/I
Dextrose 10% in sodium chloride 0.9%		LE	50 mg	Under 10% loss in 24 hr at room temperature in dark	488	C
Dextrose 5%	TR[a]	LE	910 mg	Under 10% loss in 24 hr at room temperature	519	C
	[a]	LE	0.1, 0.5, 1, 1.5 g	Little loss in 4 days at 4 and 23 °C in dark	1596	C
	MG[b]		910 mg	Under 10% loss in 24 hr at room temperature in light	1658	C
Dextrose 10%		LE	50 mg	Under 10% loss in 24 hr at room temperature in dark	488	C
Ringer's injection		LE	50 mg	Under 10% loss in 24 hr at room temperature in dark	488	C
Ringer's injection, lactated		LE	50 mg	Under 10% loss in 24 hr at room temperature in dark	488	C
Sodium chloride 0.9%	[a]	LE	1 and 1.5 g	Little loss in 4 days at 4 and 23 °C in dark	1596	C
	[c]	LE	0.5 g	Little loss in 4 days at 4 and 23 °C in dark	1596	C
	[c]	LE	0.1 g	9% loss in 4 days at 4 and 23 °C in dark	1596	C
	[d]	LE	0.1 and 0.5 g	Variable losses, up to 24%, in 4 days at 4 and 23 °C in dark	1596	I
	[b]	LE	1 g	Stable for 7 days at 4 and 25 °C in dark	1669	C

[a]Tested in both glass and PVC containers.
[b]Tested in both glass and polyolefin containers.
[c]Tested in glass containers.
[d]Tested in PVC containers.

Additive Compatibility

Leucovorin calcium

Drug	Mfr	Conc/L	Mfr	Conc/L	Test Soln	Remarks	Ref	C/I
Cisplatin		200 mg		140 mg	NS	Both drugs stable for 15 days at room temperature protected from light	1379	C
Cisplatin with floxuridine		200 mg 700 mg		140 mg	NS	All drugs stable for 7 days at room temperature	1379	C
Floxuridine	QU	1 g	QU	30 mg	NS	Physically compatible. Stable for 48 hr at 4 and 20 °C. No floxuridine and 10% leucovorin loss in 48 hr at 40 °C	1317	C
	QU	2 g	QU	240 mg	NS	Physically compatible. Stable for 48 hr at 4 and 20 °C. No floxuridine and 7% leucovorin loss in 48 hr at 40 °C	1317	C
	QU	4 g	QU	960 mg	NS	Physically compatible. Stable for 48 hr at 4, 20, and 40 °C	1317	C
		10 g		200 mg	NS	Both drugs stable for 15 days at room temperature protected from light	1387	C
Floxuridine with cisplatin		700 mg 200 mg		140 mg	NS	All drugs stable for 7 days at room temperature	1379	C

Additive Compatibility (Cont.)

Leucovorin calcium

Drug	Mfr	Conc/L	Mfr	Conc/L	Test Soln	Remarks	Ref	C/I
Fluorouracil	AD	16.7 to 46.2 g	LE	1.5 to 13.3 g	a	Subvisible particulates form in all combinations in variable periods from 1 to 4 days at 4, 23, and 32 °C	1816	I

[a]Tested with both drugs undiluted and diluted by 25% with dextrose 5%.

Drugs in Syringe Compatibility

Leucovorin calcium

Drug (in syringe)	Mfr	Amt	Mfr	Amt	Remarks	Ref	C/I
Bleomycin sulfate		1.5 units/ 0.5 mL		5 mg/ 0.5 mL	Physically compatible for 5 min at room temperature followed by 8 min of centrifugation	980	C
Cisplatin		0.5 mg/ 0.5 mL		5 mg/ 0.5 mL	Physically compatible for 5 min at room temperature followed by 8 min of centrifugation	980	C
Cyclophosphamide		10 mg/ 0.5 mL		5 mg/ 0.5 mL	Physically compatible for 5 min at room temperature followed by 8 min of centrifugation	980	C
Doxorubicin HCl		1 mg/ 0.5 mL		5 mg/ 0.5 mL	Physically compatible for 5 min at room temperature followed by 8 min of centrifugation	980	C
Droperidol		1.25 mg/ 0.5 mL		5 mg/ 0.5 mL	Precipitates immediately	980	I
Fluorouracil		25 mg/ 0.5 mL		5 mg/ 0.5 mL	Physically compatible for 5 min at room temperature followed by 8 min of centrifugation	980	C
Furosemide		5 mg/ 0.5 mL		5 mg/ 0.5 mL	Physically compatible for 5 min at room temperature followed by 8 min of centrifugation	980	C
Heparin sodium		500 units/ 0.5 mL		5 mg/ 0.5 mL	Physically compatible for 5 min at room temperature followed by 8 min of centrifugation	980	C
Methotrexate sodium		12.5 mg/ 0.5 mL		5 mg/ 0.5 mL	Physically compatible for 5 min at room temperature followed by 8 min of centrifugation	980	C
Metoclopramide HCl		2.5 mg/ 0.5 mL		5 mg/ 0.5 mL	Physically compatible for 5 min at room temperature followed by 8 min of centrifugation	980	C
Mitomycin		0.25 mg/ 0.5 mL		5 mg/ 0.5 mL	Physically compatible for 5 min at room temperature followed by 8 min of centrifugation	980	C
Vinblastine sulfate		0.5 mg/ 0.5 mL		5 mg/ 0.5 mL	Physically compatible for 5 min at room temperature followed by 8 min of centrifugation	980	C
Vincristine sulfate		0.5 mg/ 0.5 mL		5 mg/ 0.5 mL	Physically compatible for 5 min at room temperature followed by 8 min of centrifugation	980	C

Y-Site Injection Compatibility (1:1 Mixture)

Leucovorin calcium

Drug	Mfr	Conc	Mfr	Conc	Remarks	Ref	C/I
Amifostine	USB	10 mg/mL[a]	LE	2 mg/mL[a]	Physically compatible for 4 hr at 23 °C	1845	C
Amphotericin B cholesteryl sulfate complex	SEQ	0.83 mg/mL[a]	IMM	2 mg/mL[a]	Gross precipitate forms	2117	I

Y-Site Injection Compatibility (1:1 Mixture) (Cont.)

Leucovorin calcium

Drug	Mfr	Conc	Mfr	Conc	Remarks	Ref	C/I
Anidulafungin	VIC	0.5 mg/mL[a]	BED	2 mg/mL[a]	Physically compatible for 4 hr at 23 °C	2617	C
Aztreonam	SQ	40 mg/mL[a]	LE	2 mg/mL[a]	Physically compatible for 4 hr at 23 °C	1758	C
Bleomycin sulfate		3 units/mL		10 mg/mL	Drugs injected sequentially in Y-site with no flush. No precipitate seen	980	C
Cisplatin		1 mg/mL		10 mg/mL	Drugs injected sequentially in Y-site with no flush. No precipitate seen	980	C
Cladribine	ORT	0.015[b] and 0.5[c] mg/mL	IMM	2 mg/mL[b]	Physically compatible for 4 hr at 23 °C	1969	C
Cyclophosphamide		20 mg/mL		10 mg/mL	Drugs injected sequentially in Y-site with no flush. No precipitate seen	980	C
Docetaxel	RPR	0.9 mg/mL[a]	ES	2 mg/mL[a]	Physically compatible for 4 hr at 23 °C	2224	C
Doxorubicin HCl		2 mg/mL		10 mg/mL	Drugs injected sequentially in Y-site with no flush. No precipitate seen	980	C
Doxorubicin HCl liposomal	SEQ	0.4 mg/mL[a]	IMM	2 mg/mL[a]	Physically compatible for 4 hr at 23 °C	2087	C
Droperidol		2.5 mg/mL		10 mg/mL	Drugs injected sequentially in Y-site with no flush. Precipitates immediately	980	I
Etoposide phosphate	BR	5 mg/mL[a]	IMM	2 mg/mL[a]	Physically compatible for 4 hr at 23 °C	2218	C
Filgrastim	AMG	30 mcg/mL[a]	LE	2 mg/mL[a]	Physically compatible for 4 hr at 22 °C	1687	C
Fluconazole	RR	2 mg/mL	LE	10 mg/mL	Physically compatible for 24 hr at 25 °C	1407	C
Fluorouracil		50 mg/mL		10 mg/mL	Drugs injected sequentially in Y-site with no flush. No precipitate seen	980	C
Foscarnet sodium	AST	24 mg/mL	QU	10 mg/mL	Cloudy yellow solution	1335	I
Furosemide		10 mg/mL		10 mg/mL	Drugs injected sequentially in Y-site with no flush. No precipitate seen	980	C
Gemcitabine HCl	LI	10 mg/mL[b]	IMM	2 mg/mL[b]	Physically compatible for 4 hr at 23 °C	2226	C
Granisetron HCl	SKB	0.05 mg/mL[a]	IMM	2 mg/mL[a]	Physically compatible for 4 hr at 23 °C	2000	C
Heparin sodium		1000 units/mL		10 mg/mL	Drugs injected sequentially in Y-site with no flush. No precipitate seen	980	C
Linezolid	PHU	2 mg/mL	GNS	2 mg/mL[a]	Physically compatible for 4 hr at 23 °C	2264	C
Methotrexate sodium		25 mg/mL		10 mg/mL	Drugs injected sequentially in Y-site with no flush. No precipitate seen	980	C
		30 mg/mL	LE	10 mg/mL	Visually compatible for 4 hr at room temperature	1788	C
Metoclopramide HCl		5 mg/mL		10 mg/mL	Drugs injected sequentially in Y-site with no flush. No precipitate seen	980	C
Mitomycin		0.5 mg/mL		10 mg/mL	Drugs injected sequentially in Y-site with no flush. No precipitate seen	980	C
Oxaliplatin	SS	0.5 mg/mL[a]	BED	2 mg/mL[a]	Physically compatible for 4 hr at 23 °C	2566	C
Pemetrexed disodium	LI	20 mg/mL[b]	SIC	2 mg/mL[a]	Physically compatible for 4 hr at 23 °C	2564	C
Piperacillin sodium–tazobactam sodium	LE[f]	40 + 5 mg/mL[a]	LE	2 mg/mL[a]	Physically compatible for 4 hr at 22 °C	1688	C
Sodium bicarbonate		1.4%	LE	10 mg/mL	Yellow precipitate forms in 0.5 hr at room temperature	1788	I
Tacrolimus	FUJ	1 mg/mL[b]	ES	10 mg/mL[a]	Visually compatible for 24 hr at 25 °C	1630	C

Y-Site Injection Compatibility (1:1 Mixture) (Cont.)

Leucovorin calcium

Drug	Mfr	Conc	Mfr	Conc	Remarks	Ref	C/I
Teniposide	BR	0.1 mg/mL[a]	LE	2 mg/mL[a]	Physically compatible for 4 hr at 23 °C	1725	**C**
Thiotepa	IMM[d]	1 mg/mL[a]	LE	2 mg/mL[a]	Physically compatible for 4 hr at 23 °C	1861	**C**
TNA #218 to #226[e]			IMM	2 mg/mL[a]	Visually compatible for 4 hr at 23 °C	2215	**C**
TPN #212 to #215[e]			IMM	2 mg/mL[a]	Physically compatible for 4 hr at 23 °C	2109	**C**
Vinblastine sulfate		1 mg/mL		10 mg/mL	Drugs injected sequentially in Y-site with no flush. No precipitate seen	980	**C**
Vincristine sulfate		1 mg/mL		10 mg/mL	Drugs injected sequentially in Y-site with no flush. No precipitate seen	980	**C**

[a]Tested in dextrose 5%.
[b]Tested in sodium chloride 0.9%.
[c]Tested in bacteriostatic sodium chloride 0.9% preserved with benzyl alcohol 0.9%.
[d]Lyophilized formulation tested.
[e]Refer to Appendix I for the composition of parenteral nutrition solutions. TNA indicates a 3-in-1 admixture, and TPN indicates a 2-in-1 admixture.
[f]Test performed using the formulation WITHOUT edetate disodium.

Additional Compatibility Information

Fluorouracil — Several articles reported the chemical stability and physical compatibility of fluorouracil with leucovorin calcium. (505; 980; 1309; 1387; 1817) However, more recent work found substantial amounts of subvisual particles in this drug combination over numerous concentrations when stored at 4, 23, and 32 °C. Particulate formation sometimes clogged filters and disrupted multiple-day treatment. Particulate formation began in about 24 hours in most samples, and particles were found in all samples within seven days. Fluorouracil and leucovorin calcium in the same container can no longer be considered a compatible combination. (1816)

Fluorouracil combined with leucovorin calcium for repeated administration using a Fresenius implanted port resulted in blockage of the pump catheter and necessitated surgical removal of the port. The blockage was caused by precipitation of calcium carbonate in the catheter. (2504)

LEVOFLOXACIN
AHFS 8:12.18

Products — Levofloxacin is available as a 25-mg/mL preservative-free aqueous solution in 20-mL (500-mg) and 30-mL (750-mg) single-use vials. This concentration must be diluted to a 5-mg/mL concentration for administration. Adding 250 mg (10 mL) to 40 mL of diluent, 500 mg (20 mL) to 80 mL of diluent, or 750 mg (30 mL) to 120 mL of diluent will result in a 5-mg/mL concentration. (1)

The drug is also available as premixed infusion solutions of 5 mg/mL in dextrose 5% in 50-mL (250-mg), 100-mL (500-mg), and 150-mL (750-mg) flexible plastic bags. The solutions in plastic bags are ready to use and require no dilution. Sodium hydroxide and hydrochloric acid may have been added to adjust the pH. (1)

pH — From 3.8 to 5.8. (1)

The pH of a 5-mg/mL concentration in dextrose or sodium chloride solutions is about 4.6 to 4.7. In solutions with a greater buffering capacity, pH values are higher. A 5-mg/mL concentration had a pH of 4.9 in dextrose 5% in Ringer's injection, lactated, a pH of 5.0 in Plasma-Lyte 56/5% dextrose, and a pH of 5.5 in sodium lactate ⅙ M. (1)

Tonicity — The premixed infusion solutions are nearly isotonic. (1)

Trade Name(s) — Levaquin.

Administration — Levofloxacin is administered only at 5-mg/mL by slow intravenous infusion over at least 60 minutes. Doses of 750 mg should be administered over 90 minutes. No other route is recommended. Rapid infusion or bolus administration must not be used because of the potential for hypotension. The 25-mg/mL concentrate must be diluted to 5 mg/mL for administration. (1; 4)

Stability — Intact vials should be stored at controlled room temperature and protected from light. The premixed infusion solutions should be stored at or below 25 °C and protected from light, freezing, and excessive heat. A brief exposure to temperatures up to 40 °C does not adversely affect concentration. (1) The injection and infusion admixtures are clear and yellow to greenish yellow in appearance. This color does not adversely affect the product. (1; 1986) Discard any remaining unused portion of the injection because no preservatives are present. (1)

Levofloxacin diluted in a compatible diluent to 5 mg/mL is stated to be stable for 72 hours stored at or below 25 °C and for 14 days stored at 5 °C. (1)

Levofloxacin may form stable coordination compounds with metal ions. The chelation potential is greatest with Al^{3+} and declines from Cu^{2+} to Zn^{2+} to Mg^{2+} to Ca^{2+}. (1)

pH Effects — Levofloxacin has a solubility of 100 mg/mL at pH values ranging from 0.6 to 5.8. The solubility increases as pH increases up to 6.7, with a maximum solubility of 272 mg/mL. Above pH 6.7, solubility decreases to a minimum of 50 mg/mL at pH 6.9. (1)

Freezing Solutions — Levofloxacin 5 mg/mL diluted in a compatible diluent in glass bottles or plastic infusion containers is stable for six months frozen at −20 °C. Frozen solutions should be thawed at room temperature or in the refrigerator. Accelerated thawing using microwaves or hot water immersion is not recommended. Thawed solutions should not be refrozen. (1)

Light Effects — Levofloxacin undergoes slow degradation when exposed to ultraviolet light. (2399) Losses have been reported upon long-term light exposure. (2636)

Central Venous Catheter — Levofloxacin (McNeil) 1 mg/mL in dextrose 5% was found to be compatible with the ARROWg+ard Blue Plus (Arrow International) chlorhexidine-bearing triple-lumen central catheter. Essentially complete delivery of the drug was found with little or no drug loss occurring. Furthermore, chlorhexidine delivered from the catheter remained at trace amounts with no substantial increase due to the delivery of the drug through the catheter. (2335)

Compatibility Information

Solution Compatibility

Levofloxacin

Solution	Mfr	Mfr	Conc/L	Remarks	Ref	C/I
Dextrose 5% in Ringer's injection, lactated	BA[a]	OMJ	0.5 and 5 g	Physically compatible. No loss in 3 days at 25 °C, 14 days at 5 °C, 26 weeks at −20 °C, in dark	1986	C
Dextrose 5% in sodium chloride 0.9%	BA[a]	OMJ	0.5 and 5 g	Physically compatible. No loss in 3 days at 25 °C, 14 days at 5 °C, 26 weeks at −20 °C, in dark	1986	C
Dextrose 5%	BA[a]	OMJ	0.5 and 5 g	Physically compatible. No loss in 3 days at 25 °C, 14 days at 5 °C, 26 weeks at −20 °C, in dark	1986	C
Plasma-Lyte 56 in dextrose 5%	BA[a]	OMJ	0.5 and 5 g	Physically compatible. No loss in 3 days at 25 °C, 14 days at 5 °C, 26 weeks at −20 °C, in dark	1986	C
Sodium chloride 0.9%	BA[a]	OMJ	0.5 and 5 g	Physically compatible. No loss in 3 days at 25 °C, 14 days at 5 °C, 26 weeks at −20 °C, in dark	1986	C
Sodium lactate ⅙ M	BA[a]	OMJ	0.5 and 5 g	Physically compatible. <4% loss in 3 days at 25 °C, 14 days at 5 °C, 26 weeks at −20 °C, in dark	1986	C

[a]Tested in PVC containers.

Additive Compatibility

Levofloxacin

Drug	Mfr	Conc/L	Mfr	Conc/L	Test Soln	Remarks	Ref	C/I
Linezolid	PHU	2 g	OMN	5 g	[a]	Physically compatible. Little drug loss in 7 days at 4 and 23 °C in dark	2334	C
Mannitol	BA	20%	OMJ	0.5 g		Precipitate forms within a few hours	1986	I
	BA	20%	OMJ	5 g		Precipitate forms within 13 weeks at −20 °C	1986	I
	BA	20%	OMJ	5 g		Physically compatible. <4% loss in 3 days at 25 °C, 14 days at 5 °C, in dark	1986	C
Sodium bicarbonate	BA[b]	5%	OMJ	0.5 g		Physically compatible. No loss in 3 days at 25 °C, 14 days at 5 °C, in dark	1986	C
	BA[b]	5%	OMJ	0.5 g		Precipitate forms within 13 weeks at −20 °C	1986	I

Additive Compatibility (Cont.)

Levofloxacin

Drug	Mfr	Conc/L	Mfr	Conc/L	Test Soln	Remarks	Ref	C/I
	BA[b]	5%	OMJ	5 g		Physically compatible. No loss in 3 days at 25 °C, 14 days at 5 °C, 26 weeks at −20 °C, in dark	1986	C

[a]Admixed in the linezolid infusion container.
[b]Tested in PVC containers.

Y-Site Injection Compatibility (1:1 Mixture)

Levofloxacin

Drug	Mfr	Conc	Mfr	Conc	Remarks	Ref	C/I
Acyclovir sodium	BW	50 mg/mL	OMN	5 mg/mL[a]	Cloudy precipitate forms	2233	I
Alprostadil	UP	0.5 mg/mL	OMN	5 mg/mL[a]	Precipitate forms	2233	I
Amikacin sulfate	BED	50 mg/mL	OMN	5 mg/mL[a]	Visually compatible for 4 hr at 24 °C	2233	C
Aminophylline	AMR	25 mg/mL	OMN	5 mg/mL[a]	Visually compatible for 4 hr at 24 °C	2233	C
Ampicillin sodium	MAR	50 mg/mL	OMN	5 mg/mL[a]	Visually compatible for 4 hr at 24 °C	2233	C
Anidulafungin	VIC	0.5 mg/mL[a]	OMN	5 mg/mL[a]	Physically compatible for 4 hr at 23 °C	2617	C
Azithromycin	PF	2 mg/mL[b]	ORT	5 mg/mL[e]	White and amber microcrystals found	2368	I
Bivalirudin	TMC	5 mg/mL[a]	ORT	5 mg/mL[a]	Physically compatible for 4 hr at 23 °C	2373	C
Caffeine citrate		5 mg/mL	OMN	5 mg/mL[a]	Visually compatible for 4 hr at 24 °C	2233	C
Caspofungin acetate	ME	0.7 mg/mL[b]	JN	5 mg/mL[b]	Physically compatible for 4 hr at room temperature	2758	C
	ME	0.5 mg/mL[b]	HOS	5 mg/mL[a]	Physically compatible over 60 min	2766	C
Cefotaxime sodium	HO	200 mg/mL	OMN	5 mg/mL[a]	Visually compatible for 4 hr at 24 °C	2233	C
Ceftaroline fosamil	FOR	2.22 mg/mL[a,b,c]	OMN	5 mg/mL[a,b,c]	Physically compatible for 4 hr at 23 °C	2826	C
Clindamycin phosphate	UP	150 mg/mL	OMN	5 mg/mL[a]	Visually compatible for 4 hr at 24 °C	2233	C
Daptomycin	CUB	14.3 mg/mL[b,f]	OMN	7.1 mg/mL[b,f]	Physically compatible with no loss of either drug in 2 hr at 25 °C	2553	C
Dexamethasone sodium phosphate	ES	4 mg/mL	OMN	5 mg/mL[a]	Visually compatible for 4 hr at 24 °C	2233	C
Dexmedetomidine HCl	AB	4 mcg/mL[b]	ORT	5 mg/mL[b]	Physically compatible for 4 hr at 23 °C	2383	C
Dobutamine HCl	AB	12.5 mg/mL	OMN	5 mg/mL[a]	Visually compatible for 4 hr at 24 °C	2233	C
Dopamine HCl	AMR	80 mg/mL	OMN	5 mg/mL[a]	Visually compatible for 4 hr at 24 °C	2233	C
Doripenem	JJ	5 mg/mL[a,b]	OMN	5 mg/mL[a,b]	Physically compatible for 4 hr at 23 °C	2743	C
Epinephrine HCl	AB	1 mg/mL	OMN	5 mg/mL[a]	Visually compatible for 4 hr at 24 °C	2233	C
Fenoldopam mesylate	AB	80 mcg/mL[b]	OMN	5 mg/mL[b]	Physically compatible for 4 hr at 23 °C	2467	C
Fentanyl citrate	AB	0.05 mg/mL	OMN	5 mg/mL[a]	Visually compatible for 4 hr at 24 °C	2233	C
Furosemide	AST	10 mg/mL	OMN	5 mg/mL[a]	Cloudy precipitate forms	2233	I
Gentamicin sulfate	ES	10 mg/mL	OMN	5 mg/mL[a]	Visually compatible for 4 hr at 24 °C	2233	C
Heparin sodium	ES	10 units/mL	OMN	5 mg/mL[a]	Cloudy precipitate forms	2233	I
Hetastarch in lactated electrolyte	AB	6%	OMN	5 mg/mL[a]	Physically compatible for 4 hr at 23 °C	2339	C

Y-Site Injection Compatibility (1:1 Mixture) (Cont.)

Levofloxacin

Drug	Mfr	Conc	Mfr	Conc	Remarks	Ref	C/I
Hydromorphone HCl	HOS	2 mg/mL	OMN	5 mg/mL[a]	Physically compatible	2794	C
Hydroxyethyl starch 130/0.4 in sodium chloride 0.9%	FRK	6%	OMN	1, 2.5, 5 mg/ mL[a]	Visually compatible for 24 hr at room temperature	2770	C
Indomethacin sodium trihydrate	ME	1 mg/mL	OMN	5 mg/mL[a]	Cloudy precipitate forms	2233	I
Insulin, regular	LI	1 unit/mL	OMN	5 mg/mL[a]	Visually compatible for 4 hr at 24 °C	2233	C
	LI	100 units/mL	OMN	5 mg/mL[a]	Cloudy precipitate forms	2233	I
Isoproterenol HCl	ES	0.2 mg/mL	OMN	5 mg/mL[a]	Visually compatible for 4 hr at 24 °C	2233	C
Lidocaine HCl	AB	10 mg/mL[d]	OMN	5 mg/mL[a]	Visually compatible for 4 hr at 24 °C	2233	C
Linezolid	PHU	2 mg/mL	ORT	5 mg/mL[a]	Physically compatible for 4 hr at 23 °C	2264	C
Lorazepam		2 mg/mL	OMN	5 mg/mL[a]	Visually compatible for 4 hr at 24 °C	2233	C
Magnesium sulfate	AMR	20 mg/mL[b]	OMN	5 mg/mL[a]	Physically compatible	2794	C
Metoclopramide HCl	ES	5 mg/mL	OMN	5 mg/mL[a]	Visually compatible for 4 hr at 24 °C	2233	C
Morphine sulfate	SW	4 mg/mL	OMN	5 mg/mL[a]	Visually compatible for 4 hr at 24 °C	2233	C
Nitroglycerin	AMR	5 mg/mL	OMN	5 mg/mL[a]	Cloudy precipitate forms	2233	I
Oxacillin sodium	APC	167 mg/mL	OMN	5 mg/mL[a]	Visually compatible for 4 hr at 24 °C	2233	C
Pancuronium bromide	ES	1 mg/mL	OMN	5 mg/mL[a]	Visually compatible for 4 hr at 24 °C	2233	C
Penicillin G sodium	MAR	500,000 units/mL	OMN	5 mg/mL[a]	Visually compatible for 4 hr at 24 °C	2233	C
Phenobarbital sodium	ES	130 mg/mL	OMN	5 mg/mL[a]	Visually compatible for 4 hr at 24 °C	2233	C
Phenylephrine HCl	AMR	10 mg/mL	OMN	5 mg/mL[a]	Visually compatible for 4 hr at 24 °C	2233	C
Potassium chloride	HOS	0.04 mEq/ mL[a]	OMN	5 mg/mL[a]	Physically compatible	2794	C
Sodium bicarbonate	AB	0.5 mEq/mL	OMN	5 mg/mL[a]	Visually compatible for 4 hr at 24 °C	2233	C
Sodium nitroprusside	ES	10 mg/mL[b]	OMN	5 mg/mL[a]	Fluffy precipitate forms	2233	I
Telavancin HCl	ASP	7.5 mg/mL[a,b,c]	OMN	5 mg/mL[a,b,c]	Discoloration and measured haze increase	2830	I
Vancomycin HCl	LI	50 mg/mL	OMN	5 mg/mL[a]	Visually compatible for 4 hr at 24 °C	2233	C

[a]*Tested in dextrose 5%.*
[b]*Tested in sodium chloride 0.9%.*
[c]*Tested in Ringer's injection, lactated.*
[d]*Preservative free.*
[e]*Injected via Y-site into an administration set running azithromycin.*
[f]*Final concentration after mixing.*

LEVOTHYROXINE SODIUM
AHFS 68:36.04

Products — Levothyroxine sodium is available in 200- and 500-mcg vials. Also present in the vials are mannitol 10 mg, tribasic sodium phosphate anhydrous 0.7 mg, and sodium hydroxide to adjust pH during manufacturing. Reconstitute the 200-mcg vials by adding 2 or 5 mL of sodium chloride 0.9%, resulting in solutions containing 40 or 100 mcg/mL, respectively. Reconstitute the 500-mcg vials by adding 5 mL of sodium chloride 0.9% or bacteriostatic sodium chloride 0.9% preserved with benzyl alcohol, resulting in a solution containing 100 mcg/mL. Shake well to ensure complete dissolution. (1; 4)

Trade Name(s) — Synthroid.

Administration — Levothyroxine sodium injection may be administered by intravenous or intramuscular injection. (1)

Stability — Intact vials should be stored at controlled room temperature and protected from light. The manufacturer states that the reconstituted levothyroxine sodium should be used immediately after reconstitution. Any remaining solution should be discarded. The manufacturer also states levothyroxine sodium injection should not be added to intravenous solutions. (1)

Syringes — Levothyroxine sodium 0.1 mg/mL in sodium chloride 0.9% was packaged as 5 mL in 6-mL polypropylene syringes (Monoject). No loss of drug was found after seven days at 5 °C. (2354)

Compatibility Information

Solution Compatibility

Levothyroxine sodium

Solution	Mfr	Mfr	Conc/L	Remarks	Ref	C/I
Sodium chloride 0.9%	BAª	PP	0.4 and 2 mg	Physically compatible. <10% loss in 8 hr at 25 °C	2823	C

ª*Tested in PVC containers.*

LIDOCAINE HYDROCHLORIDE
(LIGNOCAINE HYDROCHLORIDE)
AHFS 24:04.04.08

Products — Lidocaine hydrochloride for direct intravenous use is available in concentrations of 10 and 20 mg/mL in ampuls and vials from 5 to 50 mL and in 5-mL prefilled syringes. The drug is also available as 40-, 100-, and 200-mg/mL concentrates for intravenous admixture preparation. The pH of these solutions is adjusted with sodium hydroxide and/or hydrochloric acid. Multiple-dose vials and automatic injection devices may also have methylparaben and EDTA or sulfites. (4)

Lidocaine hydrochloride is also available premixed in dextrose 5% in concentrations of 0.2, 0.4, and 0.8% (2, 4, and 8 mg/mL, respectively). The solutions come in container sizes ranging from 250 to 1000 mL. (4)

pH — The pH of the injection is about 6.5 but may range from 5 to 7. (1; 4) The premixed infusion solutions in dextrose 5% have a pH of 3 to 7. (4; 17)

Osmolality — The osmolalities of lidocaine hydrochloride products were determined to be 296 mOsm/kg for the 10-mg/mL concentration and 352 mOsm/kg for the 20-mg/mL concentration. (1233)

The commercially available lidocaine hydrochloride 0.2, 0.4, and 0.8% premixed solutions have osmolarities of approximately 266, 281, and 308 mOsm/L, respectively. (4)

Trade Name(s) — Xylocaine.

Administration — Lidocaine hydrochloride is administered by direct intravenous injection and continuous intravenous infusion. (4) It may also be administered by intramuscular injection. (4; 118; 119; 120) Products containing 40, 100, or 200 mg/mL should not be administered by direct intravenous injection without prior dilution to 1- or 2-mg/mL (0.1 or 0.2%) solution. Lidocaine hydrochloride products containing preservatives should not be given intravenously. Products containing epinephrine should not be used to treat arrhythmias. (4)

Stability — Lidocaine hydrochloride injection and premixed infusion solutions should be stored at controlled room temperature and protected from excessive heat and freezing. (4)

pH Effects — Although lidocaine hydrochloride is stable across a broad pH range, its pH of maximum stability is 3 to 6. (1277)

Buffering lidocaine hydrochloride injection with sodium bicarbonate has been used to reduce pain on injection. Increasing the pH results in an increased percentage of the drug being present as the unionized base, which is less stable and soluble. Lidocaine base precipitation has been shown to occur at a pH around 7.5 to 7.6. (2409)

The stability of lidocaine hydrochloride 2%, with and without epinephrine hydrochloride, was studied after alkalinization with sodium bicarbonate. Lidocaine hydrochloride alone was alkalinized to pH 7.2, while the lidocaine–epinephrine combination was adjusted to pH 6.5 and also 7.05. The combinations were compatible, and no loss of lidocaine or epinephrine occurred over six hours. (1401)

The stability of lidocaine hydrochloride 1% (Elkins-Sinn) buffered with sodium bicarbonate to pH 6.8, 7.2, and 7.4 was evaluated. No loss occurred in 27 days at pH 6.8. At pH 7.2, adequate concentrations were retained for 19 days but by 27 days concentrations had fallen to about 88% and a crystalline precipitate formed. At pH 7.4, losses of up to 23% were accompanied by crystalline precipitation between 5 and 15 days. (2407)

Lidocaine hydrochloride is stable when mixed with certain acid-stable drugs such as epinephrine hydrochloride, norepinephrine bitartrate, and isoproterenol hydrochloride. However, its buffering action may raise the pH of intravenous admixtures above 5.5, the maximum pH for stability of the other drugs. The final pH is usually about 6. These drugs begin to deteriorate within several hours. Note: This does not apply to commercial lidocaine–epinephrine combinations, which have the pH adjusted to retain epinephrine. (24)

Syringes — Lidocaine hydrochloride (Abbott) 20 mg/mL was packaged as 10 mL of undiluted injection in 12-mL polypropylene syringes (Becton Dickinson) and stored at 23 °C under fluorescent light and 4 °C. No lidocaine loss was found after 90 days of storage. (2428)

Lidocaine hydrochloride 2% (20 mg/mL) in autoinjector syringes (Abbott) was evaluated for stability over 45 days under use conditions in paramedic vehicles. Temperatures fluctuated with locations and conditions and ranged from 6.5 °C (43.7 °F) to 52 °C (125.6 °F) in high desert conditions. No visually apparent changes occurred, and no loss was found. (2548)

Lidocaine hydrochloride under simulated summer conditions in paramedic vehicles was exposed to temperatures ranging from 26 to 38 °C over four weeks. No loss of the drug occurred. (2562)

Sorption — Lidocaine hydrochloride in solutions with acidic pH was shown not to exhibit sorption to PVC bags and tubing, elastomeric pump reservoirs, polyethylene tubing, Silastic tubing, and polypropylene syringes. (12; 536; 606; 2014)

However, in a slightly alkaline (pH 8) cardioplegia solution, the percentage of unionized lidocaine base increased to 58%. This compares to 3% in dextrose 5% and sodium chloride 0.9% at around pH 6. The unionized form is highly lipid soluble and may interact with PVC bags. Storage of the cardioplegia solutions in PVC bags at 22 °C resulted in a 12 to 19% lidocaine loss in two days and a 65 to 75% loss in 21 days. Degradation was not likely because storage in glass bottles did not result in any lidocaine loss after 21 days at 22 °C. Refrigeration of the PVC bags at 4 °C slowed the lidocaine loss to 9% or less in 21 days. (776)

Filtration — Lidocaine hydrochloride (Astra) 200 mg/L in dextrose 5% and sodium chloride 0.9% did not display significant sorption to a 0.45-μm cellulose membrane filter (Abbott S-A-I-F) during an eight-hour simulated infusion. (567)

Central Venous Catheter — Lidocaine hydrochloride (Astra) 2 mg/mL in dextrose 5% was found to be compatible with the ARROWg+ard Blue Plus (Arrow International) chlorhexidine-bearing triple-lumen central catheter. Essentially complete delivery of the drug was found with little or no drug loss occurring. Furthermore, chlorhexidine delivered from the catheter remained at trace amounts with no substantial increase due to the delivery of the drug through the catheter. (2335)

Compatibility Information

Solution Compatibility

Lidocaine HCl

Solution	Mfr	Mfr	Conc/L	Remarks	Ref	C/I
Amino acids 4.25%, dextrose 25%	MG	AST	1 g	No increase in particulate matter in 24 hr at 5 °C	349	C
Dextrose 5% in Ringer's injection, lactated	TR[a]	AST	1 g	Stable for 24 hr at 5 °C	282	C
	TR[a]	AST	2 g	Physically compatible. Little loss in 14 days at 25 °C	775	C
Dextrose 5% in sodium chloride 0.45%	CU, AB[a]	AST	2 g	Physically compatible. Little loss in 14 days at 25 °C	775	C
Dextrose 5% in sodium chloride 0.9%	TR[a]	AST	1 g	Stable for 24 hr at 5 °C	282	C
Dextrose 5%	TR[a]	AST	2 g	Physically compatible. No loss in 14 days at 25 °C	775	C
	AB[a]	ES	515 mg	No loss over 21 days at 20 to 24 °C	776	C
	TR[a]	AST	1 g	Stable for 24 hr at 5 °C	282	C
	TR[b]	ES	4 g	Stable for 120 days at 4 and 30 °C	543	C
	TR[b]	AST	1 and 8 g	Visually compatible. No loss in 48 hr at room temperature	1802	C
Ringer's injection, lactated	TR[a]	AST	1 g	Stable for 24 hr at 5 °C	282	C
	TR[a]	AST	2 g	Physically compatible. No loss in 14 days at 25 °C	775	C
Sodium chloride 0.45%	AB[a]	AST	2 g	Physically compatible. No loss in 14 days at 25 °C	775	C
Sodium chloride 0.9%	TR[a]	AST	2 g	Physically compatible. No loss in 14 days at 25 °C	775	C
	AB[a]	ES	515 mg	No loss over 21 days at 20 to 24 °C	776	C
	BA[c]	AST		Stable for 24 hr	45	C
	TR[a]	AST	1 g	Stable for 24 hr at 5 °C	282	C
	TR[b]	AST	1 g	Stable for 24 hr	45	C
	TR[b]	AST	1 and 8 g	Visually compatible. Little loss in 48 hr at room temperature	1802	C

[a]*Tested in both glass and PVC containers.*
[b]*Tested in PVC containers.*
[c]*Tested in glass containers.*

Additive Compatibility

Lidocaine HCl

Drug	Mfr	Conc/L	Mfr	Conc/L	Test Soln	Remarks	Ref	C/I
Alteplase	GEN	0.5 g	AST	4 g	D5W	Visually compatible with no alteplase clot-lysis activity loss in 24 hr at 25 °C	1856	C
	GEN	0.5 g	AST	4 g	NS	Visually compatible with 7% alteplase clot-lysis activity loss in 24 hr at 25 °C	1856	C
Aminophylline	SE	500 mg	AST	2 g		Physically compatible	24	C
	AQ	1 g	AST	2 g	D5W, LR, NS	Physically compatible for 24 hr at 25 °C	775	C
Amiodarone HCl	LZ	1.8 g	AB	4 g	D5W, NS[a,d]	Physically compatible. 9% or less amiodarone loss in 24 hr at 24 °C in light	1031	C
Atracurium besylate	BW	500 mg		2 g	D5W	Physically compatible and atracurium stable for 24 hr at 5 and 30 °C	1694	C
Calcium chloride	UP	1 g	AST	2 g		Physically compatible	24	C
Calcium gluconate	ES	2 g	AST	2 g	D5W, LR, NS	Physically compatible for 24 hr at 25 °C	775	C
Chloramphenicol sodium succinate	PD	1 g	AST	2 g		Physically compatible	24	C
Chlorothiazide sodium	MSD	500 mg	AST	2 g		Physically compatible	24	C
Ciprofloxacin	MI	2 g		1 g	NS	Compatible for 24 hr at 25 °C	888	C
	MI	2 g		1.5 g	NS	Compatible for 24 hr at 25 °C	888	C
Dexamethasone sodium phosphate	MSD	4 mg	AST	2 g		Physically compatible	24	C
Digoxin	ES	1 mg	AST	2 g	D5W, LR, NS	Physically compatible for 24 hr at 25 °C	775	C
Diphenhydramine HCl	PD	50 mg	AST	2 g		Physically compatible	24	C
Dobutamine HCl	LI	1 g	ES	4 g	D5W, NS	Visually compatible for 24 hr at 25 °C	789	C
	LI	1 g	AST	4 and 10 g	D5W, NS	Physically compatible for 24 hr at 21 °C	812	C
Dopamine HCl	AS	800 mg	AST	4 g	D5W[a]	No dopamine or lidocaine loss in 24 hr at 25 °C	312	C
	ACC	800 mg	AST	2 g	D5W, LR, NS	Physically compatible for 24 hr at 25 °C	775	C
Ephedrine sulfate		50 mg	AST	2 g		Physically compatible	24	C
Erythromycin lactobionate	AB	1 g	AST	2 g		Physically compatible	24	C
Fentanyl citrate		2 mg	AST	2.5 g	NS[a]	Physically compatible with no loss of lidocaine or fentanyl at pH 5.8 in 30 days at 4 and 23 °C	2305	C
		2 mg	BRN	2.5 g	NS[a]	Physically compatible with little lidocaine loss but 18% fentanyl loss at 23 °C and 10% loss at 4 °C in 2 days due to sorption at pH 6.7 from higher pH lidocaine product	2305	I
Floxacillin sodium	BE	20 g	ANT	2 g	NS	Physically compatible for 72 hr at 15 and 30 °C	1479	C
Flumazenil	RC	20 mg	AB	4 g	D5W[a]	Visually compatible. 4% flumazenil loss in 24 hr at 23 °C in fluorescent light. Lidocaine not tested	1710	C

Additive Compatibility (Cont.)

Lidocaine HCl

Drug	Mfr	Conc/L	Mfr	Conc/L	Test Soln	Remarks	Ref	C/I
Furosemide	HO	1 g	ANT	2 g	NS	Physically compatible for 72 hr at 15 and 30 °C	1479	C
Heparin sodium		32,000 units		4 g	NS	Physically compatible and heparin activity retained for 24 hr	57	C
	AB	20,000 units	AST	2 g		Physically compatible	24	C
Hydrocortisone sodium succinate	UP	250 mg	AST	2 g		Physically compatible	24	C
Hydroxyzine HCl	PF	100 mg	AST	2 g		Physically compatible	24	C
Methohexital sodium	BP	2 g	BP	2 g	D5W	Precipitates immediately	26	I
Nafcillin sodium	AP	20 g	AST	0.6 g	D5W[a], NS[d]	Visually compatible. Little nafcillin loss in 48 hr at 23 °C. Lidocaine not tested	1806	C
Nitroglycerin	ACC	400 mg	IMS	4 g	D5W, NS[e]	Physically compatible. No nitroglycerin loss in 48 hr at 23 °C. Lidocaine not tested	929	C
Penicillin G potassium	SQ	1 million units	AST	2 g		Physically compatible	24	C
Pentobarbital sodium	AB	500 mg	AST	2 g		Physically compatible	24	C
Phenylephrine HCl	WI	20 mg	AST	2 g		Physically compatible	24	C
Phenytoin sodium	ES	1 g	AST	2 g	D5W, LR, NS	Immediate formation of a white cloudy precipitate	775	I
Potassium chloride	AB	40 mEq	AST	2 g		Physically compatible	24	C
Procainamide HCl	SQ	1 g	AST	2 g	D5W, LR, NS	Physically compatible for 24 hr at 25 °C	775	C
Prochlorperazine edisylate	SKF	10 mg	AST	2 g		Physically compatible	24	C
Ranitidine HCl	GL	50 mg and 2 g	AST	1 and 8 g	D5W, NS[a]	Physically compatible. 3% ranitidine loss in 24 hr at room temperature in light. Lidocaine not tested	1361	C
	GL	50 mg and 2 g		2.5 g	D5W	Physically compatible. Ranitidine stable for 24 hr at 25 °C. Lidocaine not tested	1515	C
	GL	50 mg and 2 g	AST	1 and 8 g	D5W, NS[a]	Visually compatible. Little loss of either drug in 48 hr at room temperature	1802	C
Sodium bicarbonate	AB	40 mEq	AST	2 g		Physically compatible	24	C
	AB	2.4 mEq[c]		1 g	D5W	Physically compatible for 24 hr	772	C
Sodium lactate	AB	50 mEq	AST	2 g		Physically compatible	24	C
Theophylline		2 g		380 mg	D5W	Visually compatible with little or no loss of either drug in 48 hr	1909	C
Verapamil HCl	KN	80 mg	IMS	2 g	D5W, NS	Physically compatible for 48 hr	739	C

[a]*Tested in PVC containers.*
[b]*Tested in both glass and PVC containers.*
[c]*One vial of Neut added to a liter of admixture.*
[d]*Tested in polyolefin containers.*
[e]*Tested in glass containers.*

Drugs in Syringe Compatibility

Lidocaine HCl

Drug (in syringe)	Mfr	Amt	Mfr	Amt	Remarks	Ref	C/I
Ampicillin sodium	BE	500 mg		0.5 and 2.5% in 1.5 mL	Physically compatible	89	C
	BE	250 mg		0.5 and 2.5% in 1.5 mL	Occasional turbidity	89	I
Caffeine citrate		20 mg/ 1 mL	AB	1%, 1 mL	Visually compatible for 4 hr at 25 °C	2440	C
Cefazolin sodium	SKF	1 g	AST	0.5%, 3 mL	Precipitate forms within 3 to 4 hr at 4 °C	532	I
Ceftriaxone sodium	RC	450 mg/ mL	LY	1%	5% ceftriaxone loss in 8 weeks at −15 °C but solution failed the particulate matter test	1824	I
	RC	250 and 450 mg/ mL	DW	1%	10% ceftriaxone loss in 3 days at 20 °C, 7 to 8% loss in 35 days at 4 °C, and 4 to 6% loss in 168 days at −20 °C. Lidocaine not tested	1991	C
Clonidine HCl with fentanyl citrate	BI JN	0.03 mg/ mL 0.01 mg/ mL	AST	2 mg/mL	Diluted to 5 mL with NS. Visually compatible with no new GC/MS peaks in 1 hr at room temperature	1956	C
Cloxacillin sodium	BE				Physically compatible	89	C
Fentanyl citrate with clonidine HCl	JN BI	0.01 mg/ mL 0.03 mg/ mL	AST	2 mg/mL	Diluted to 5 mL with NS. Visually compatible with no new GC/MS peaks in 1 hr at room temperature	1956	C
Glycopyrrolate	RB	0.2 mg/ 1 mL	ES	10 mg/ 1 mL	Physically compatible. pH in glycopyrrolate stability range for 48 hr at 25 °C	331	C
	RB	0.2 mg/ 1 mL	ES	20 mg/ 2 mL	Physically compatible. pH in glycopyrrolate stability range for 48 hr at 25 °C	331	C
	RB	0.4 mg/ 2 mL	ES	10 mg/ 1 mL	Physically compatible. pH in glycopyrrolate stability range for 48 hr at 25 °C	331	C
	RB	0.2 mg/ 1 mL	ES	20 mg/ 1 mL	Physically compatible. pH in glycopyrrolate stability range for 48 hr at 25 °C	331	C
	RB	0.2 mg/ 1 mL	ES	40 mg/ 2 mL	Physically compatible. pH in glycopyrrolate stability range for 48 hr at 25 °C	331	C
	RB	0.4 mg/ 2 mL	ES	20 mg/ 1 mL	Physically compatible. pH in glycopyrrolate stability range for 48 hr at 25 °C	331	C
Heparin sodium		2500 units/ 1 mL	AST	100 mg/ 5 mL	Physically compatible for at least 5 min	1053	C
Hydroxyzine HCl	PF	50 mg/ 2 mL	AST	2%/2 mL	Physically compatible	771	C
	PF	100 mg/ 2 mL	AST	2%/2 mL	Physically compatible	771	C
Ketamine HCl with morphine sulfate	PD ES	2 mg/mL 0.2 mg/ mL	AST	2 mg/mL	Diluted to 5 mL with NS. Visually compatible with no new GC/MS peaks in 1 hr at room temperature	1956	C
Metoclopramide HCl	RB	10 mg/ 2 mL	ES	50 mg/ 5 mL	Physically compatible for 48 hr at 25 °C	1167	C
	RB	10 mg/ 2 mL	ES	100 mg/ 10 mL	Physically compatible for 48 hr at 25 °C	1167	C

Drugs in Syringe Compatibility (Cont.)

Lidocaine HCl

Drug (in syringe)	Mfr	Amt	Mfr	Amt	Remarks	Ref	C/I
	RB	160 mg/32 mL	ES	50 mg/5 mL	Physically compatible for 48 hr at 25 °C	1167	C
	RB	160 mg/32 mL	ES	100 mg/10 mL	Physically compatible for 48 hr at 25 °C	1167	C
Milrinone lactate	STR	5.25 mg/5.25 mL	AB	100 mg/10 mL	Physically compatible. No loss of either drug in 20 min at 23 °C	1410	C
Morphine sulfate with ketamine HCl	ES / PD	0.2 mg/mL / 2 mg/mL	AST	2 mg/mL	Diluted to 5 mL with NS. Visually compatible with no new GC/MS peaks in 1 hr at room temperature	1956	C
Nalbuphine HCl	DU	10 mg/1 mL		40 mg	Physically compatible for 48 hr	128	C
	DU	20 mg/1 mL		40 mg	Physically compatible for 48 hr	128	C
Pantoprazole sodium	d	4 mg/1 mL		200 mg/1 mL	Precipitates within 4 hr	2574	I
Phenylephrine HCl		0.25%		2%	No loss of either drug in 66 days at 25 °C	1278	C
Propofol		1%		5 and 10 mg	Physically compatible for 24 hr	2490	C
		1%		20 and 40 mg	Physically incompatible. Increased fat droplet size and layering in 3 hr	2490	I
	ZEN	1%, 20 mL		10 mg	Physically compatible for 6 hr	2543	C
	ZEN	1%, 20 mL		30 to 50 mg	Increased fat droplet size	2543	I
Sodium bicarbonate	AB	3 mEq/3 mL	ES	2%[a], 30 mL	11% lidocaine and 28% epinephrine loss in 1 week at 25 °C	1712	I
	AB	3 mEq/3 mL	ES	2%[a], 30 mL	6% lidocaine loss in 4 weeks at 4 °C. 12% epinephrine loss in 3 weeks at 4 °C	1712	C
	LY	0.1 mEq/mL	AST	1%[a]	25% epinephrine loss in 1 week at room temperature. Lidocaine not tested	1713	I
		0.088 mEq/mL		0.9%	11% lidocaine loss in 7 days at room temperature	1723	C
	AST	8.4%/2 mL	AST	1 and 1.5%[b], 20 mL	Visually compatible for up to 5 hr at room temperature	1724	C
	AST	8.4%/2 mL	AST	2%[b], 20 mL	Haze forms but dissipates with gentle agitation	1724	?
	AB	4%/4 mL	AST	1 and 1.5%[b], 20 mL	Visually compatible for up to 5 hr at room temperature	1724	C
	AB	4%/4 mL	AST	2%[b], 20 mL	Haze forms but dissipates with gentle agitation	1724	?
		1.4 and 8.4%/1.5 mL	BEL	2%[c], 20 mL	8% epinephrine loss in 7 days at room temperature. Lidocaine not tested	1743	C
		8.4%/1 mL		2%/10 mL	Physically compatible. No loss of lidocaine in 6 hr	1401	C
		8.4%/1.5 mL		2%[a], 10 mL	Physically compatible. No loss of lidocaine or epinephrine in 6 hr	1401	C
		1.4%/1.5 mL		2%[a], 10 mL	Physically compatible. No loss of lidocaine or epinephrine in 6 hr	1401	C

Drugs in Syringe Compatibility (Cont.)

Lidocaine HCl

Drug (in syringe)	Mfr	Amt	Mfr	Amt	Remarks	Ref	C/I
		8.4%/ 1 mL		1%[a], 10 mL	Cloudiness in some samples with no epinephrine loss for 72 hr in the dark. Exposed to light and air, precipitation and 20% epinephrine loss in 24 hr. Lidocaine not tested	2408	?
	HOS	8.4%/ 0.3 mL	ASZ	1 and 2%,[a] 2.7 mL	Physically compatible. 10% epinephrine loss in 7 days and 5% lidocaine loss in 28 days at 5 °C in dark	2815	C

[a]*Tested with epinephrine hydrochloride 1:100,000 added.*
[b]*Tested with epinephrine hydrochloride 1:200,000 added.*
[c]*Tested with epinephrine hydrochloride 1:80,000 added.*
[d]*Test performed using the formulation WITHOUT edetate disodium.*

Y-Site Injection Compatibility (1:1 Mixture)

Lidocaine HCl

Drug	Mfr	Conc	Mfr	Conc	Remarks	Ref	C/I
Alteplase	GEN	1 mg/mL	AB	8 mg/mL[a]	Physically compatible for 6 days	1340	C
Amiodarone HCl	LZ	4 mg/mL[c]	AST	8 mg/mL[c]	Physically compatible for 24 hr at 21 °C	1032	C
Amphotericin B cholesteryl sulfate complex	SEQ	0.83 mg/mL[a]	AST	10 mg/mL	Gross precipitate forms	2117	I
Argatroban	SKB	1 mg/mL[a]	BA	8 mg/mL[a]	Physically compatible for 24 hr at 23 °C	2572	C
Bivalirudin	TMC	5 mg/mL[a]	AST	10 mg/mL[a]	Physically compatible for 4 hr at 23 °C	2373	C
Cefazolin sodium	LI	40 mg/mL[c]	AB	8 mg/mL[c]	Physically compatible for 3 hr	1316	C
Ceftaroline fosamil	FOR	2.22 mg/mL[d]	HOS	10 mg/mL	Physically compatible for 4 hr at 23 °C	2826	C
Ciprofloxacin	MI	2 mg/mL[c]	AB	4[a] and 20 mg/mL	Visually compatible for 24 hr at 24 °C	1655	C
Cisatracurium besylate	GW	0.1, 2, 5 mg/mL[a]	AST	8 mg/mL[a]	Physically compatible for 4 hr at 23 °C	2074	C
Clarithromycin	AB	4 mg/mL[a]	ANT	4 mg/mL[a]	Visually compatible for 72 hr at both 30 and 17 °C	2174	C
Daptomycin	CUB	16.7 mg/mL[b,i]	ASZ	3.3 mg/mL[b,i]	Physically compatible with no loss of either drug in 2 hr at 25 °C	2553	C
Dexmedetomidine HCl	AB	4 mcg/mL[b]	AST	10 mg/mL[b]	Physically compatible for 4 hr at 23 °C	2383	C
Diltiazem HCl	MMD	1 mg/mL[a]	AST	8 mg/mL[a]	Visually compatible for 24 hr at 25 °C	1530	C
	MMD	1[b] and 5 mg/mL	AB	10 mg/mL[b]	Visually compatible	1807	C
	MMD	5 mg/mL	AB, SCN	4 and 8 mg/mL[a]	Visually compatible	1807	C
Dobutamine HCl	LI	4 mg/mL[c]	AB	8 mg/mL[c]	Physically compatible for 3 hr	1316	C
Dobutamine HCl with dopamine HCl	LI DCC	4 mg/mL[c] 3.2 mg/mL[c]	AB	8 mg/mL[c]	Physically compatible for 3 hr	1316	C
Dobutamine HCl with nitroglycerin	LI LY	4 mg/mL[c] 0.4 mg/mL[c]	AB	8 mg/mL[c]	Physically compatible for 3 hr	1316	C
Dobutamine HCl with sodium nitroprusside	LI ES	4 mg/mL[c] 0.4 mg/mL[c]	AB	8 mg/mL[c]	Physically compatible for 3 hr	1316	C
Dopamine HCl	DCC	3.2 mg/mL[c]	AB	8 mg/mL[c]	Physically compatible for 3 hr	1316	C

Y-Site Injection Compatibility (1:1 Mixture) (Cont.)

Lidocaine HCl

Drug	Mfr	Conc	Mfr	Conc	Remarks	Ref	C/I
Dopamine HCl with dobutamine HCl	DCC LI	3.2 mg/mL[c] 4 mg/mL[c]	AB	8 mg/mL[c]	Physically compatible for 3 hr	1316	C
Dopamine HCl with nitroglycerin	DCC LY	3.2 mg/mL[c] 0.4 mg/mL[c]	AB	8 mg/mL[c]	Physically compatible for 3 hr	1316	C
Dopamine HCl with sodium nitroprusside	DCC ES	3.2 mg/mL[c] 0.4 mg/mL[c]	AB	8 mg/mL[c]	Physically compatible for 3 hr	1316	C
Enalaprilat	MSD	0.05 mg/mL[b]	AST	4 mg/mL[a]	Physically compatible for 24 hr at room temperature under fluorescent light	1355	C
Etomidate	AB	2 mg/mL	AST	20 mg/mL	Visually compatible for 7 days at 25 °C	1801	C
Famotidine	MSD MSD	0.2 mg/mL[a] 0.2 mg/mL[a]	TR LY	4 mg/mL[a] 1 mg/mL[a]	Physically compatible for 4 hr at 25 °C Physically compatible for 14 hr	1188 1196	C C
Fenoldopam mesylate	AB	80 mcg/mL[b]	AST	10 mg/mL[b]	Physically compatible for 4 hr at 23 °C	2467	C
Haloperidol lactate	MN	0.5[a] and 5 mg/mL	AB	4 mg/mL[a]	Visually compatible for 24 hr at 21 °C	1523	C
Heparin sodium	TR	50 units/mL	TR	4 mg/mL	Visually compatible for 4 hr at 25 °C	1793	C
Heparin sodium[k]	RI	1000 units/L[d]	AST	20 mg/mL	Physically compatible for 4 hr at room temperature	322	C
Hetastarch in lactated electrolyte	AB	6%	AB	8 mg/mL[a]	Physically compatible for 4 hr at 23 °C	2339	C
Hydrocortisone sodium succinate[l]	UP	100 mg/L[d]	AST	20 mg/mL	Physically compatible for 4 hr at room temperature	322	C
Labetalol HCl	SC	1 mg/mL[a]	AST	20 mg/mL[a]	Physically compatible for 24 hr at 18 °C	1171	C
Levofloxacin	OMN	5 mg/mL[a]	AB	10 mg/mL[g]	Visually compatible for 4 hr at 24 °C	2233	C
Linezolid	PHU	2 mg/mL	AB	10 mg/mL[a]	Physically compatible for 4 hr at 23 °C	2264	C
Meperidine HCl	AB	10 mg/mL	AB	1 mg/mL[a]	Physically compatible for 4 hr at 25 °C	1397	C
Metoprolol tartrate	BED	1 mg/mL	BA	8 mg/mL[a]	Trace precipitate in 8 hr at 19 °C	2795	I
Micafungin sodium	ASP	1.5 mg/mL[b]	AB	10 mg/mL[b]	Physically compatible for 4 hr at 23 °C	2683	C
Morphine sulfate	AB	1 mg/mL	AB	1 mg/mL[a]	Physically compatible for 4 hr at 25 °C	1397	C
Nesiritide	SCI	50 mcg/mL[a,b]		20 mg/mL	Physically compatible for 4 hr. May be chemically incompatible with nesiritide[j]	2625	?
Nicardipine HCl	DCC	0.1 mg/mL[a]	AST	4 mg/mL[a]	Visually compatible for 24 hr at room temperature	235	C
Nitroglycerin	LY	0.4 mg/mL[c]	AB	8 mg/mL[c]	Physically compatible for 3 hr	1316	C
Nitroglycerin with dobutamine HCl	LY LI	0.4 mg/mL[c] 4 mg/mL[c]	AB	8 mg/mL[c]	Physically compatible for 3 hr	1316	C
Nitroglycerin with dopamine HCl	LY DCC	0.4 mg/mL[c] 3.2 mg/mL[c]	AB	8 mg/mL[c]	Physically compatible for 3 hr	1316	C
Nitroglycerin with sodium nitroprusside	LY ES	0.4 mg/mL[c] 0.4 mg/mL[c]	AB	8 mg/mL[c]	Physically compatible for 3 hr	1316	C
Palonosetron HCl	MGI	50 mcg/mL	AB	10 mg/mL[a]	Physically compatible. No loss of either drug in 4 hr at room temperature	2771	C
Potassium chloride		40 mEq/L[d]	AST	20 mg/mL	Physically compatible for 4 hr at room temperature	322	C
Propofol	ZEN	10 mg/mL	AST	10 mg/mL	Physically compatible for 1 hr at 23 °C	2066	C

Y-Site Injection Compatibility (1:1 Mixture) (Cont.)

Lidocaine HCl

Drug	Mfr	Conc	Mfr	Conc	Remarks	Ref	C/I
Remifentanil HCl	GW	0.025 and 0.25 mg/mL[b]	AST	8 mg/mL[a]	Physically compatible for 4 hr at 23 °C	2075	C
Sodium nitroprusside	ES	0.4 mg/mL[c]	AB	8 mg/mL[c]	Physically compatible for 3 hr	1316	C
	RC	1.2 and 3 mg/mL[a]	AST	6 mg/mL[h]	Visually compatible for 48 hr at 24 °C protected from light	2357	C
	RC	0.3, 1.2, 3 mg/mL[a]	AST	20 and 40 mg/mL[h]	Visually compatible for 48 hr at 24 °C protected from light	2357	C
Sodium nitroprusside with dobutamine HCl	ES LI	0.4 mg/mL[c] 4 mg/mL[c]	AB	8 mg/mL[c]	Physically compatible for 3 hr	1316	C
Sodium nitroprusside with dopamine HCl	ES DCC	0.4 mg/mL[c] 3.2 mg/mL[c]	AB	8 mg/mL[c]	Physically compatible for 3 hr	1316	C
Sodium nitroprusside with nitroglycerin	ES LY	0.4 mg/mL[c] 0.4 mg/mL[c]	AB	8 mg/mL[c]	Physically compatible for 3 hr	1316	C
Theophylline	TR	4 mg/mL	TR	4 mg/mL	Visually compatible for 6 hr at 25 °C	1793	C
Tigecycline	WY	1 mg/mL[b]		200 mg/mL	Physically compatible for 4 hr	2714	C
Tirofiban HCl	ME	0.05 mg/mL[a,b]	AB	1 and 20 mg/mL[a,b]	Physically compatible. Little loss of either drug in 4 hr at room temperature	2250	C
TNA #73[e]			ES	4 mg/mL[c]	Visually compatible for 4 hr	1009	C
Vasopressin	AMR	2 and 4 units/mL[b]	BA	4 mg/mL[a]	Physically compatible with vasopressin pushed into a Y-site over 5 sec	2478	C
Warfarin sodium	DU	2 mg/mL[f]	AST	2 mg/mL[a]	Visually compatible with no warfarin loss in 30 min	2010	C
	DME	2 mg/mL[f]	AST	2 mg/mL[a]	Visually compatible for 24 hr at 24 °C	2078	C

[a]*Tested in dextrose 5%.*
[b]*Tested in sodium chloride 0.9%.*
[c]*Tested in both dextrose 5% and sodium chloride 0.9%.*
[d]*Tested in dextrose 5%, sodium chloride 0.9%, and Ringer's injection, lactated.*
[e]*Refer to Appendix I for the composition of parenteral nutrition solutions. TNA indicates a 3-in-1 admixture.*
[f]*Tested in sterile water for injection.*
[g]*Preservative free.*
[h]*Tested in dextrose 5% in sodium chloride 0.2%.*
[i]*Final concentration after mixing.*
[j]*Nesiritide is incompatible with bisulfite antioxidants used in some drug formulations. The specific formulation of the product to be used should be checked to ensure that no sulfite antioxidants are present.*
[k]*Tested in combination with hydrocortisone sodium succinate (Upjohn) 100 mg/L*
[l]*Tested in combination with heparin sodium (Riker) 1000 units/L.*

LINCOMYCIN HYDROCHLORIDE
AHFS 8:12.28.20

Products — Lincomycin hydrochloride is available in 2- and 10-mL vials. Each milliliter contains lincomycin hydrochloride equivalent to lincomycin base 300 mg and benzyl alcohol 9.45 mg in water for injection. (1; 4)

pH — From 3 to 5.5. (17)

Trade Name(s) — Lincocin.

Administration — Lincomycin hydrochloride may be administered by deep intramuscular injection, slow intravenous infusion, or subconjunctival injection. (1; 4) For intravenous administration, each gram of lincomycin should be diluted in 100 mL or more of compatible infusion solution and infused over at least one hour. (4)

Stability — Lincomycin hydrochloride injection should be stored at controlled room temperature and protected from freezing. (1; 4)

Compatibility Information

Solution Compatibility

Lincomycin HCl

Solution	Mfr	Mfr	Conc/L	Remarks	Ref	C/I
Dextrose 5% in sodium chloride 0.9%		UP	1.2 g	Stable for 24 hr	109	**C**
Dextrose 5%		UP	1.2 g	Stable for 24 hr	109	**C**
Dextrose 10%		UP	1.2 g	Stable for 24 hr	109	**C**
Dextrose 10% in sodium chloride 0.9%				Physically compatible for 24 hr at room temperature	1	**C**
Ringer's injection				Physically compatible for 24 hr at room temperature	1	**C**
Sodium chloride 0.9%		UP	1.2 g	Stable for 24 hr	109	**C**
Sodium lactate ⅙ M				Physically compatible for 24 hr at room temperature	1	**C**

Additive Compatibility

Lincomycin HCl

Drug	Mfr	Conc/L	Mfr	Conc/L	Test Soln	Remarks	Ref	C/I
Amikacin sulfate	BR	5 g	UP	10 g	D5LR, D5R, D5S, D5W, D10W, LR, NS, R, SL	Physically compatible and both stable for 24 hr at 25 °C	293	**C**
Ampicillin sodium						Physically compatible for 24 hr at room temperature	1	**C**
Chloramphenicol sodium succinate						Physically compatible for 24 hr at room temperature	1	**C**
Cytarabine	UP	500 mg		1, 1.5, 2, 2.4, 3 g		Physically compatible for 48 hr	174	**C**
Heparin sodium	AB	20,000 units	UP	600 mg		Physically compatible	21	**C**
Penicillin G potassium	SQ	20 million units	UP	6 g	D5W	Physically compatible	15	**C**
	SQ	5 million units	UP	600 mg	D	Physically compatible	47	**C**
Penicillin G sodium	UP	20 million units	UP	6 g	D5W	Physically compatible	15	**C**
Polymyxin B sulfate						Physically compatible for 24 hr at room temperature	1	**C**
Ranitidine HCl	GL	50 mg and 2 g		2.4 g	D5W	Physically compatible. Ranitidine stable for 24 hr at 25 °C. Lincomycin not tested	1515	**C**

Drugs in Syringe Compatibility

Lincomycin HCl

Drug (in syringe)	Mfr	Amt	Mfr	Amt	Remarks	Ref	C/I
Ampicillin sodium	AY	500 mg	UP	600 mg/ 2 mL	Physically incompatible within 1 hr at room temperature	99	**I**
	AY	500 mg	UP	600 mg/ 2 mL	Precipitate forms within 1 hr at room temperature	300	**I**
Cloxacillin sodium	AY	250 mg	UP	600 mg/ 2 mL	Physically compatible for 1 hr at room temperature	300	**C**
	BE	250 mg	UP	600 mg/ 2 mL	No precipitate or color change within 1 hr at room temperature	99	**C**
Doxapram HCl	RB	400 mg/ 20 mL		300 mg/ 1 mL	Physically compatible with no doxapram loss in 24 hr	1177	**C**
Heparin sodium	AB	20,000 units/ 1 mL	UP	600 mg/ 2 mL	Physically compatible for at least 30 min	21	**C**
Penicillin G sodium		1 million units	UP	600 mg/ 2 mL	No precipitate or color change within 1 hr at room temperature	99	**C**

LINEZOLID
AHFS 8:12.28.24

Products — Linezolid is available as a single-use, ready-to-use solution for infusion in 100-, 200-, and 300-mL plastic (Excel) containers. Each milliliter of the ready-to-use infusion provides linezolid 2 mg along with dextrose 50.24 mg, sodium citrate 1.64 mg, and citric acid 0.85 mg in water for injection. (1)

pH — Adjusted to pH 4.8. (1)

Sodium Content — The sodium concentration is 0.38 mg/mL. The sodium content in a 100-mL bag is 1.7 mEq, in a 200-mL bag is 3.3 mEq, and in a 300-mL bag is 5 mEq. (1)

Trade Name(s) — Zyvox.

Administration — Linezolid ready-to-use solution is administered only by intravenous infusion over a period of 30 to 120 minutes. (1)

Stability — Linezolid ready-to-use solutions may exhibit a yellow color that can intensify over time without affecting the stability of the drug. Intact containers should be kept in their protective overwrap until ready to use, and should be stored at controlled room temperature and protected from light and freezing. (1)

Linezolid 150, 300, and 600 mg/L in Dianeal PD-2 with 1.5 or 4.25% dextrose stored at 37, 25, and 4 °C protected from light was physically compatible and exhibited no loss. (2500)

Sorption — Linezolid was found to be compatible with common types of intravenous administration sets including diethylhexyl phthalate (DEHP) plasticized PVC, trioctyl trimellitate (TOTM) plasticized PVC, and polyolefin sets. The total dose of linezolid was fully delivered with the delivered concentration remaining constant throughout. In addition, no detectable levels of plasticizer were found in the delivered solutions. (2338)

Compatibility Information

Solution Compatibility

Linezolid

Solution	Mfr	Mfr	Conc/L	Remarks	Ref	C/I
Dextrose 5%		PF		Compatible	1	**C**
Ringer's injection, lactated		PF		Compatible	1	**C**
Sodium chloride 0.9%		PF		Compatible	1	**C**

Additive Compatibility

Linezolid

Drug	Mfr	Conc/L	Mfr	Conc/L	Test Soln	Remarks	Ref	C/I
Aztreonam	SQ	20 g	PHU	2 g	a	Physically compatible with no linezolid loss in 7 days at 4 and 23 °C protected from light. About 9% aztreonam loss at 23 °C and less than 4% loss at 4 °C in 7 days	2263	C
Cefazolin sodium	APC	10 g	PHU	2 g	a	Physically compatible with 5% or less loss of each drug in 3 days at 23 °C and 7 days at 4 °C protected from light	2262	C
Ceftazidime	GW	20 g	PHU	2 g	a	Physically compatible with no linezolid loss in 7 days at 4 and 23 °C protected from light. Ceftazidime losses of 5% in 24 hr and 12% in 3 days at 23 °C and about 3% in 7 days at 4 °C	2262	C
Ceftriaxone sodium	RC	10 g	PHU	2 g	a	Physically compatible, but up to 37% ceftriaxone loss in 24 hr at 23 °C and 10% loss in 3 days at 4 °C	2262	I
Ciprofloxacin	BAY	4 g	PHU	2 g	a	Physically compatible with little or no loss of either drug in 7 days at 23 °C protected from light. Refrigeration results in precipitation after 1 day	2334	C
Erythromycin lactobionate	AB	5 g	PHU	2 g	a	Erythromycin loss of 15% in 1 hr and 30% in 4 hr at 23 °C. Loss of 45% in 1 day at 4 °C	2333	I
Gentamicin sulfate	AB	800 mg	PHU	2 g	a	Physically compatible. Little linezolid loss in 7 days at 4 and 23 °C in dark. Gentamicin losses of 5 to 7% in 7 days at 4 °C and 8% in 5 days at 23 °C	2332	C
Levofloxacin	OMN	5 g	PHU	2 g	a	Physically compatible. Little drug loss in 7 days at 4 and 23 °C in dark	2334	C
Tobramycin sulfate	GNS	800 mg	PHU	2 g	a	Physically compatible. Little linezolid loss in 7 days at 4 and 23 °C in dark. No tobramycin loss in 7 days at 4 °C but losses of 4% in 1 day and 12% in 3 days at 23 °C	2332	C
Trimethoprim–sulfamethoxazole	ES	800 mg + 4 g	PHU	2 g	a	A large amount of white needle-like crystals forms immediately	2333	I

[a]Admixed in the linezolid infusion container.

Y-Site Injection Compatibility (1:1 Mixture)

Linezolid

Drug	Mfr	Conc	Mfr	Conc	Remarks	Ref	C/I
Acyclovir sodium	APP	7 mg/mL[a]	PHU	2 mg/mL	Physically compatible for 4 hr at 23 °C	2264	C
Alfentanil HCl	TAY	0.5 mg/mL	PHU	2 mg/mL	Physically compatible for 4 hr at 23 °C	2264	C
Amikacin sulfate	AB	5 mg/mL[a]	PHU	2 mg/mL	Physically compatible for 4 hr at 23 °C	2264	C
Aminophylline	AB	2.5 mg/mL[a]	PHU	2 mg/mL	Physically compatible for 4 hr at 23 °C	2264	C
Amphotericin B	AB	0.6 mg/mL[a]	PHU	2 mg/mL	Yellow precipitate forms within 5 min	2264	I

Y-Site Injection Compatibility (1:1 Mixture) (Cont.)

Linezolid

Drug	Mfr	Conc	Mfr	Conc	Remarks	Ref	C/I
Ampicillin sodium	APC	20 mg/mL[b]	PHU	2 mg/mL	Physically compatible for 4 hr at 23 °C	2264	C
Ampicillin sodium–sulbactam sodium	PF	20 + 10 mg/mL[b]	PHU	2 mg/mL	Physically compatible for 4 hr at 23 °C	2264	C
Anidulafungin	VIC	0.5 mg/mL[a]	PH	2 mg/mL	Physically compatible for 4 hr at 23 °C	2617	C
Aztreonam	SQ	40 mg/mL[a]	PHU	2 mg/mL	Physically compatible for 4 hr at 23 °C	2264	C
Buprenorphine HCl	RKC	0.04 mg/mL[a]	PHU	2 mg/mL	Physically compatible for 4 hr at 23 °C	2264	C
Butorphanol tartrate	APC	0.04 mg/mL[a]	PHU	2 mg/mL	Physically compatible for 4 hr at 23 °C	2264	C
Calcium gluconate	AMR	40 mg/mL[a]	PHU	2 mg/mL	Physically compatible for 4 hr at 23 °C	2264	C
Carboplatin	BR	5 mg/mL[a]	PHU	2 mg/mL	Physically compatible for 4 hr at 23 °C	2264	C
Caspofungin acetate	ME	0.7 mg/mL[b]	PHU	2 mg/mL[b]	Physically compatible for 4 hr at room temperature	2758	C
	ME	0.5 mg/mL[b]	PF	2 mg/mL	Physically compatible over 60 min	2766	C
Cefazolin sodium	SKB	20 mg/mL[a]	PHU	2 mg/mL	Physically compatible for 4 hr at 23 °C	2264	C
Cefotetan disodium	ZEN	20 mg/mL[a]	PHU	2 mg/mL	Physically compatible for 4 hr at 23 °C	2264	C
Cefoxitin sodium	ME	20 mg/mL[a]	PHU	2 mg/mL	Physically compatible for 4 hr at 23 °C	2264	C
Ceftazidime	SKB	40 mg/mL[a]	PHU	2 mg/mL	Physically compatible for 4 hr at 23 °C	2264	C
Ceftriaxone sodium	RC	20 mg/mL[a]	PHU	2 mg/mL	Physically compatible for 4 hr at 23 °C	2264	C
Cefuroxime sodium	GL	30 mg/mL[a]	PHU	2 mg/mL	Physically compatible for 4 hr at 23 °C	2264	C
Chlorpromazine HCl	ES	2 mg/mL[a]	PHU	2 mg/mL	Measured haze level increases immediately	2264	I
Ciprofloxacin	BAY	1 mg/mL[a]	PHU	2 mg/mL	Physically compatible for 4 hr at 23 °C	2264	C
Cisatracurium besylate	GW	2 mg/mL	PHU	2 mg/mL	Physically compatible for 4 hr at 23 °C	2264	C
Cisplatin	BR	1 mg/mL	PHU	2 mg/mL	Physically compatible for 4 hr at 23 °C	2264	C
Clindamycin phosphate	UP	10 mg/mL[a]	PHU	2 mg/mL	Physically compatible for 4 hr at 23 °C	2264	C
Cyclophosphamide	MJ	10 mg/mL[a]	PHU	2 mg/mL	Physically compatible for 4 hr at 23 °C	2264	C
Cyclosporine	SZ	5 mg/mL[a]	PHU	2 mg/mL	Physically compatible for 4 hr at 23 °C	2264	C
Cytarabine	BED	50 mg/mL	PHU	2 mg/mL	Physically compatible for 4 hr at 23 °C	2264	C
Dexamethasone sodium phosphate	FUJ	1 mg/mL[a]	PHU	2 mg/mL	Physically compatible for 4 hr at 23 °C	2264	C
Dexmedetomidine HCl	AB	4 mcg/mL[b]	PHU	2 mg/mL	Physically compatible for 4 hr at 23 °C	2383	C
Diazepam	AB	5 mg/mL	PHU	2 mg/mL	Turbid precipitate forms immediately	2264	I
Digoxin	ES	0.25 mg/mL	PHU	2 mg/mL	Physically compatible for 4 hr at 23 °C	2264	C
Diphenhydramine HCl	ES	2 mg/mL[a]	PHU	2 mg/mL	Physically compatible for 4 hr at 23 °C	2264	C
Dobutamine HCl	AST	4 mg/mL[a]	PHU	2 mg/mL	Physically compatible for 4 hr at 23 °C	2264	C
Dopamine HCl	AB	3.2 mg/mL[a]	PHU	2 mg/mL	Physically compatible for 4 hr at 23 °C	2264	C
Doripenem	JJ	5 mg/mL[a,b]	PHU	2 mg/mL	Physically compatible for 4 hr at 23 °C	2743	C
Doxorubicin HCl	FUJ	2 mg/mL	PHU	2 mg/mL	Physically compatible for 4 hr at 23 °C	2264	C
Doxycycline hyclate	FUJ	1 mg/mL[a]	PHU	2 mg/mL	Physically compatible for 4 hr at 23 °C	2264	C
Droperidol	AMR	0.4 mg/mL[a]	PHU	2 mg/mL	Physically compatible for 4 hr at 23 °C	2264	C
Enalaprilat	ME	0.1 mg/mL[a]	PHU	2 mg/mL	Physically compatible for 4 hr at 23 °C	2264	C
Esmolol HCl	OHM	10 mg/mL	PHU	2 mg/mL	Physically compatible for 4 hr at 23 °C	2264	C

Y-Site Injection Compatibility (1:1 Mixture) (Cont.)

Linezolid

Drug	Mfr	Conc	Mfr	Conc	Remarks	Ref	C/I
Etoposide phosphate	BR	5 mg/mL[a]	PHU	2 mg/mL	Physically compatible for 4 hr at 23 °C	2264	C
Famotidine	ME	2 mg/mL[a]	PHU	2 mg/mL	Physically compatible for 4 hr at 23 °C	2264	C
Fenoldopam mesylate	AB	80 mcg/mL[b]	PHU	2 mg/mL	Physically compatible for 4 hr at 23 °C	2467	C
Fentanyl citrate	AB	0.05 mg/mL	PHU	2 mg/mL	Physically compatible for 4 hr at 23 °C	2264	C
Fluconazole	RR	2 mg/mL	PHU	2 mg/mL	Physically compatible for 4 hr at 23 °C	2264	C
Fluorouracil	PH	16 mg/mL[a]	PHU	2 mg/mL	Physically compatible for 4 hr at 23 °C	2264	C
Furosemide	AMR	3 mg/mL[a]	PHU	2 mg/mL	Physically compatible for 4 hr at 23 °C	2264	C
Ganciclovir sodium	RC	20 mg/mL[a]	PHU	2 mg/mL	Physically compatible for 4 hr at 23 °C	2264	C
Gemcitabine HCl	LI	10 mg/mL[a]	PHU	2 mg/mL	Physically compatible for 4 hr at 23 °C	2264	C
Gentamicin sulfate	FUJ	5 mg/mL[a]	PHU	2 mg/mL	Physically compatible for 4 hr at 23 °C	2264	C
Granisetron HCl	SKB	0.05 mg/mL[a]	PHU	2 mg/mL	Physically compatible for 4 hr at 23 °C	2264	C
Haloperidol lactate	MN	0.2 mg/mL[a]	PHU	2 mg/mL	Physically compatible for 4 hr at 23 °C	2264	C
Heparin sodium	ES	1000 units/mL[a]	PHU	2 mg/mL	Physically compatible for 4 hr at 23 °C	2264	C
Hydrocortisone sodium succinate	UP	1 mg/mL[a]	PHU	2 mg/mL	Physically compatible for 4 hr at 23 °C	2264	C
Hydromorphone HCl	AST	0.5 mg/mL[a]	PHU	2 mg/mL	Physically compatible for 4 hr at 23 °C	2264	C
Hydroxyzine HCl	ES	2 mg/mL[a]	PHU	2 mg/mL	Physically compatible for 4 hr at 23 °C	2264	C
Ifosfamide	MJ	25 mg/mL[a]	PHU	2 mg/mL	Physically compatible for 4 hr at 23 °C	2264	C
Imipenem–cilastatin sodium	ME	10 mg/mL[b]	PHU	2 mg/mL	Physically compatible for 4 hr at 23 °C	2264	C
Labetalol HCl	GW	5 mg/mL	PHU	2 mg/mL	Physically compatible for 4 hr at 23 °C	2264	C
Leucovorin calcium	GNS	2 mg/mL[a]	PHU	2 mg/mL	Physically compatible for 4 hr at 23 °C	2264	C
Levofloxacin	ORT	5 mg/mL[a]	PHU	2 mg/mL	Physically compatible for 4 hr at 23 °C	2264	C
Lidocaine HCl	AB	10 mg/mL[a]	PHU	2 mg/mL	Physically compatible for 4 hr at 23 °C	2264	C
Lorazepam	WY	0.1 mg/mL[a]	PHU	2 mg/mL	Physically compatible for 4 hr at 23 °C	2264	C
Magnesium sulfate	AST	100 mg/mL[a]	PHU	2 mg/mL	Physically compatible for 4 hr at 23 °C	2264	C
Mannitol	BA	15%	PHU	2 mg/mL	Physically compatible for 4 hr at 23 °C	2264	C
Meperidine HCl	AST	4 mg/mL[a]	PHU	2 mg/mL	Physically compatible for 4 hr at 23 °C	2264	C
Meropenem	ZEN	2.5 mg/mL[b]	PHU	2 mg/mL	Physically compatible for 4 hr at 23 °C	2264	C
Mesna	MJ	10 mg/mL[a]	PHU	2 mg/mL	Physically compatible for 4 hr at 23 °C	2264	C
Methotrexate sodium	IMM	15 mg/mL[a]	PHU	2 mg/mL	Physically compatible for 4 hr at 23 °C	2264	C
Methylprednisolone sodium succinate	AB	5 mg/mL[a]	PHU	2 mg/mL	Physically compatible for 4 hr at 23 °C	2264	C
Metoclopramide HCl	FAU	5 mg/mL	PHU	2 mg/mL	Physically compatible for 4 hr at 23 °C	2264	C
Metronidazole	BA	5 mg/mL	PHU	2 mg/mL	Physically compatible for 4 hr at 23 °C	2264	C
Midazolam HCl	RC	2 mg/mL[a]	PHU	2 mg/mL	Physically compatible for 4 hr at 23 °C	2264	C
Mitoxantrone HCl	IMM	0.5 mg/mL[a]	PHU	2 mg/mL	Physically compatible for 4 hr at 23 °C	2264	C
Morphine sulfate	AST	1 mg/mL[a]	PHU	2 mg/mL	Physically compatible for 4 hr at 23 °C	2264	C
Nalbuphine HCl	AST	10 mg/mL	PHU	2 mg/mL	Physically compatible for 4 hr at 23 °C	2264	C
Naloxone HCl	DU	0.4 mg/mL	PHU	2 mg/mL	Physically compatible for 4 hr at 23 °C	2264	C

Y-Site Injection Compatibility (1:1 Mixture) (Cont.)

Linezolid

Drug	Mfr	Conc	Mfr	Conc	Remarks	Ref	C/I
Nicardipine HCl	WAY	1 mg/mL[a]	PHU	2 mg/mL	Physically compatible for 4 hr at 23 °C	2264	**C**
Nitroglycerin	FAU	0.4 mg/mL[a]	PHU	2 mg/mL	Physically compatible for 4 hr at 23 °C	2264	**C**
Ondansetron HCl	GW	1 mg/mL[a]	PHU	2 mg/mL	Physically compatible for 4 hr at 23 °C	2264	**C**
Paclitaxel	MJ	0.6 mg/mL[a]	PHU	2 mg/mL	Physically compatible for 4 hr at 23 °C	2264	**C**
Pentamidine isethionate	FUJ	6 mg/mL[a]	PHU	2 mg/mL	Crystalline precipitate forms in 1 to 4 hr	2264	**I**
Pentobarbital sodium	AB	5 mg/mL[a]	PHU	2 mg/mL	Physically compatible for 4 hr at 23 °C	2264	**C**
Phenobarbital sodium	WY	5 mg/mL[a]	PHU	2 mg/mL	Physically compatible for 4 hr at 23 °C	2264	**C**
Phenytoin sodium	ES	50 mg/mL	PHU	2 mg/mL	Crystalline precipitate forms immediately	2264	**I**
Piperacillin sodium–tazobactam sodium	LE[c]	40 + 5 mg/ mL[a]	PHU	2 mg/mL	Physically compatible for 4 hr at 23 °C	2264	**C**
Potassium chloride	FUJ	0.1 mEq/mL[a]	PHU	2 mg/mL	Physically compatible for 4 hr at 23 °C	2264	**C**
Prochlorperazine edisylate	SO	0.5 mg/mL[a]	PHU	2 mg/mL	Physically compatible for 4 hr at 23 °C	2264	**C**
Promethazine HCl	SCN	2 mg/mL[a]	PHU	2 mg/mL	Physically compatible for 4 hr at 23 °C	2264	**C**
Propranolol HCl	WAY	1 mg/mL	PHU	2 mg/mL	Physically compatible for 4 hr at 23 °C	2264	**C**
Ranitidine HCl	GW	2 mg/mL[a]	PHU	2 mg/mL	Physically compatible for 4 hr at 23 °C	2264	**C**
Remifentanil HCl	GW	0.5 mg/mL[a]	PHU	2 mg/mL	Physically compatible for 4 hr at 23 °C	2264	**C**
Sodium bicarbonate	AB	1 mEq/mL	PHU	2 mg/mL	Physically compatible for 4 hr at 23 °C	2264	**C**
Sufentanil citrate	ES	0.05 mg/mL	PHU	2 mg/mL	Physically compatible for 4 hr at 23 °C	2264	**C**
Theophylline	BA	4 mg/mL[a]	PHU	2 mg/mL	Physically compatible for 4 hr at 23 °C	2264	**C**
Tigecycline	WY	1 mg/mL[b]	PF	2 mg/mL	Physically compatible for 4 hr	2714	**C**
Tobramycin sulfate	AB	5 mg/mL[a]	PHU	2 mg/mL	Physically compatible for 4 hr at 23 °C	2264	**C**
Vancomycin HCl	FUJ	10 mg/mL[a]	PHU	2 mg/mL	Physically compatible for 4 hr at 23 °C	2264	**C**
Vasopressin	APP	0.2 unit/mL[b]	PHU	2 mg/mL	Physically compatible	2641	**C**
Vecuronium bromide	OR	1 mg/mL	PHU	2 mg/mL	Physically compatible for 4 hr at 23 °C	2264	**C**
Verapamil HCl	AB	2.5 mg/mL	PHU	2 mg/mL	Physically compatible for 4 hr at 23 °C	2264	**C**
Vincristine sulfate	LI	0.05 mg/mL[a]	PHU	2 mg/mL	Physically compatible for 4 hr at 23 °C	2264	**C**
Zidovudine	GW	4 mg/mL[a]	PHU	2 mg/mL	Physically compatible for 4 hr at 23 °C	2264	**C**

[a]*Tested in dextrose 5%.*
[b]*Tested in sodium chloride 0.9%.*
[c]*Test performed using the formulation WITHOUT edetate disodium.*

LORAZEPAM
AHFS 28:24.08

Products — Lorazepam is available in 2- and 4-mg/mL concentrations in 1- and 10-mL vials. The 2-mg/mL concentration is also available in 0.5- and 1-mL disposable syringe cartridges, and the 4-mg/mL concentration is available in 1-mL syringe cartridges. Each milliliter also contains 0.18 mL of polyethylene glycol 400 and 2% benzyl alcohol in propylene glycol. (1)

For intramuscular use, lorazepam may be injected as is. For intravenous use, however, lorazepam *must* be diluted immediately prior to injection with an equal volume of compatible diluent. To dilute the dose in a syringe cartridge or when aspirated from a vial into a syringe, first eliminate all air and then aspirate the proper volume of diluent. Pull the plunger back slightly to provide some mixing space and gently invert the syringe cartridge or syringe repeatedly to mix the contents. To avoid air entrapment, do not shake vigorously. (1)

Trade Name(s) — Ativan.

Administration — Lorazepam may be administered by deep intramuscular injection or by intravenous injection when diluted immediately before use with an equal volume of compatible diluent. Intravenous injection is made directly into a vein or into the tubing of a running intravenous infusion at a rate not exceeding 2 mg/min. Care should be taken to ensure that intra-arterial administration and perivascular infiltration will not occur. (1; 4)

Stability — Intact vials of lorazepam should be refrigerated and protected from light and freezing. (1; 4) The manufacturer has stated that the product may be stored for up to two weeks at room temperature. (1181) However, manufacturers have acknowledged that both physical and chemical stability are acceptable for 60 to 90 days at room temperature. (1674; 2829) Lorazepam should be inspected and should not be used if it is discolored or contains a precipitate. (1; 4)

Precipitation — The choice of commercial lorazepam concentration to use in the preparation of dilutions is a critical factor in the physical stability of the dilutions. Both the 2- and 4-mg/mL concentrations utilize the same concentrations of solubilizing solvents. On admixture, the solvents that keep the aqueous insoluble lorazepam in solution are diluted twice as much using the 4-mg/mL concentration than if the 2-mg/mL were used, resulting in different precipitation potentials for the same concentration of lorazepam. Care should be taken to ensure that the compounding procedure that is to be used for lorazepam admixtures has been demonstrated to result in solutions in which the lorazepam remains soluble.

Lorazepam concentrations up to 0.08 mg/mL have been reported to be physically stable, while occasional precipitate formation in admixtures of lorazepam 0.1 to 0.2 mg/mL has been reported. The precipitate has been observed in both containers and in administration set tubing. (1943; 1979; 1980) In one case, a visible precipitate formed in a lorazepam 0.5-mg/mL admixture in sodium chloride 0.9% in a glass bottle. (1945) However, a 0.5-mg/mL concentration may remain in solution longer if prepared from the 2-mg/mL concentration, yielding a higher concentration of organic solvents in the final admixture. (1981; 2207) Concentrations of 1 and 2 mg/mL have been reported to be physically stable for up to 24 hours as well as concentrations below 0.08 mg/mL. (1980; 2208) Concentrations in the middle range of 0.08 to 1 mg/mL may be problematic. (1980) In one report, use of lorazepam 2 mg/mL to prepare lorazepam 1-mg/mL admixtures in dextrose 5% or sodium chloride 0.9% was acceptable but use of the lorazepam 4-mg/mL concentration to prepare the same solutions resulted in almost immediate precipitation. (2207)

Lorazepam solubility in common infusion solutions has been reported (Table 1). Its solubility in sodium chloride 0.9% is approximately half that found in the other tested solutions. This result was attributed to the pH of the sodium chloride 0.9% (pH 6.3) being essentially the same as the isoelectric point of lorazepam (pH 6.4), where aqueous solubility would be the lowest. Dextrose 5% was the best diluent for lorazepam. (787)

Bacteriostatic Water — Dilution of lorazepam (Wyeth) to 1 mg/mL with bacteriostatic water for injection (bacteriostat not noted), packaged in glass vials, resulted in lorazepam losses. Losses of about 10% at 4 °C and 12% at 22 °C occurred in seven days. Drug precipitated in varying periods after the first week of storage. (1840)

Table 1. Lorazepam Equilibrium Solubility (787)

Solution	Lorazepam Solubility (mg/mL)	Solution pH
Deionized water	0.054	7.09
Dextrose 5%	0.062	4.41
Ringer's injection, lactated	0.055	7.21
Sodium chloride 0.9%	0.027	6.30

Syringes — Lorazepam (Wyeth) 2 mg/mL was packaged as 3 mL in 10-mL polypropylene infusion pump syringes (Pharmacia Deltec). About 12 to 14% loss occurred in three days and 25% loss in 10 days at 5 and 30 °C. The authors recommended not storing lorazepam in the syringes for these time periods. (1967)

Lorazepam (Wyeth) 1 mg/mL, prepared from the 2-mg/mL commercial concentration, diluted in dextrose 5% or in sodium chloride 0.9% was filled as 40 mL in 60-mL polypropylene syringes (Becton-Dickinson). The filled syringes were stored at 22 °C for 28 hours. Visual inspection found the solutions remained physically stable, and less than 3% drug loss occurred in this time period. (2208)

The physical and chemical stability of lorazepam (Wyeth-Ayerst) 0.2, 0.5, and 1 mg/mL in dextrose 5% and in sodium chloride 0.9% was evaluated when packaged in polypropylene syringes. When prepared using lorazepam 2 mg/mL, the solutions were found to be physically stable over 24 hours and chemically stable for 48 hours at room temperature. If prepared using lorazepam 4 mg/mL, the solutions consistently precipitated. (2416)

Sorption — Lorazepam (Wyeth) 2- and 4-mg/mL concentrations were diluted 1:1 using dextrose 5%, sodium chloride 0.9%, and water for injection. A 2-mL sample of each dilution was injected into the Y-sites of administration sets from five different manufacturers through which dextrose 5%, sodium chloride 0.9%, Ringer's injection, or Ringer's injection, lactated, was flowing at rates of 30 and 125 mL/hr. No differences were found among the various infusion sets, infusion solutions, or flow rates. All effluent solutions were visually acceptable and had no loss of lorazepam. (786)

In another study, lorazepam (Wyeth) 2 mg/50 mL in dextrose 5% was delivered at rates of 600, 200, and 100 mL/hr using an infusion controller fitted with 180 or 350 cm of PVC tubing. Lorazepam loss due to sorption was greater with the longer tubing and at slower rates. Losses ranged from a high of 5% (350 cm, 100 mL/hr) to a low of 0.7% (180 cm, 600 mL/hr). (787)

In static sorption studies, lorazepam (Wyeth) 2 mg/50 mL in dextrose 5% was filled into PVC containers in the following amounts: 50 mL into 50-mL bags, 100 mL into 50-mL bags, and 100 mL into 250-mL bags. The bags were stored at 23 °C. A rapid initial loss of lorazepam occurred (about 3.9 to 5.8% in the first hour) followed by a slower, approximately constant loss after eight hours. Cumulative losses of 6 to 8% occurred in about five hours in the smaller bags with smaller bag surface area to volume ratios. The solution in the larger bags exhibited over a 10% loss in two hours. (787)

Plasticizer Leaching — Lorazepam (Wyeth-Ayerst) 0.1 mg/mL in dextrose 5% did not leach diethylhexyl phthalate (DEHP) plasticizer from 50-mL PVC bags in 24 hours at 24 °C. (1683)

Compatibility Information

Solution Compatibility

Lorazepam

Solution	Mfr	Mfr	Conc/L	Remarks	Ref	C/I
Dextrose 5%	BA[a]	WY	0.1 g	Sorption losses of 11% in 8 hr and 27% in 24 hr at 37 °C, 8% in 8 hr and 17% in 24 hr at 24 °C, and 3% in 24 hr and 8% in 7 days at 4 °C	1684	I
	MG[b]	WY	0.1 g	3% loss in 24 hr and 9% in 72 hr at 37 °C, little or no loss in 24 hr and 5% in 7 days at 24 °C, and no loss in 7 days at 4 and −20 °C	1684	C
	AB[c]	WY	0.16, 0.24, 0.5 g	About 10 to 20% loss due to sorption throughout 24-hr delivery at 24 °C under fluorescent light	1858	I
	BA[a]	WY	0.08 g	10 to 17% loss due to sorption in 4 hr at 4 °C. 17% loss in 1 hr, increasing to over 30% in 24 hr at 21 °C	1873	I
	BA[a]	WY	0.5 g	About 14% loss due to sorption in 4 hr at 21 °C	1873	I
	BA[a]	WY	1 g	6% sorption loss in 6 hr with no further loss in 24 hr at 25 °C	2203	C
	AB[e]	WY	1 g	Prepared with 4-mg/mL lorazepam. White precipitate forms in 8 hours at 22 °C	2208	I
	AB[e]	WY	1 g	Prepared with 2-mg/mL lorazepam. Visually compatible with little loss in 28 hr at 22 °C under fluorescent light	2208	C
	AB[e]	WY	2 g	Prepared with 4-mg/mL lorazepam. Visually compatible with little loss in 28 hr at 22 °C under fluorescent light	2208	C
	HOS[f]	BA	200 mg	No loss in 24 hr	2660; 2792	C
Ringer's injection, lactated	BA[a]	WY	0.1 g	Sorption losses of 25% in 8 hr at 37 °C, 14% in 8 hr at 24 °C, and 5% in 24 hr and 9% in 72 hr at 4 °C	1684	I
	MG[b]	WY	0.1 g	2% loss in 24 hr and 7% in 72 hr at 37 °C, little or no loss in 24 hr and 4% in 7 days at 24 °C, and no loss in 7 days at 4 °C	1684	C
Sodium chloride 0.9%	[d]		40 mg	Physically compatible with less than 3% loss in 24 hr at 21 °C in the dark	1392	C
	BA[a]	WY	0.1 g	Sorption losses of 13% in 8 hr and 29% in 24 hr at 37 °C, 8% in 8 hr and 17% in 24 hr at 24 °C, and 3% in 24 hr and 8% in 7 days at 4 °C	1684	I
	MG[b]	WY	0.1 g	2% loss in 24 hr and 7% in 72 hr at 37 °C, little or no loss in 24 hr and 4% in 7 days at 24 °C, and no loss in 7 days at 4 °C	1684	C
	AB[c]	WY	0.16, 0.24, 0.5 g	About 10 to 20% loss due to sorption throughout 24-hr delivery at 24 °C under fluorescent light	1858	I
	BA[a]	WY	0.08 g	8 to 10% sorption loss in 4 hr at 4 °C. 17 to 23% loss in 1 hr, increasing to 25 to 30% loss in 4 hr at 21 °C	1873	I
	BA[a]	WY	0.5 g	17% or more sorption loss in 4 hr at 21 °C	1873	I
	BRN[b]	AB	1 g	No loss in 35 days at −20, 4, and 24 °C	2525	C

[a]Tested in PVC containers.
[b]Tested in polyolefin containers.
[c]Tested in PVC and glass containers and delivered through PVC administration sets.
[d]Tested in PVC, glass, and polyethylene-lined laminated containers.
[e]Tested in glass containers.
[f]Tested in VISIV polyolefin containers.

Additive Compatibility

Lorazepam

Drug	Mfr	Conc/L	Mfr	Conc/L	Test Soln	Remarks	Ref	C/I
Dexamethasone sodium phosphate with diphenhydramine HCl and metoclopramide HCl	AMR ES DU	400 mg 2 g 4 g	WY	40 mg	NS[a]	Rapid lorazepam losses of 8, 10, and 15% at 3, 23, and 30 °C, respectively, in 24 hr. Other drugs stable for 14 days at all three storage temperatures	1733	I
Diphenhydramine HCl with dexamethasone sodium phosphate and metoclopramide HCl	ES AMR DU	2 g 400 mg 4 g	WY	40 mg	NS[a]	Rapid lorazepam losses of 8, 10, and 15% at 3, 23, and 30 °C, respectively, in 24 hr. Other drugs stable for 14 days at all three storage temperatures	1733	I
Metoclopramide HCl with dexamethasone sodium phosphate and diphenhydramine HCl	DU AMR ES	4 g 400 mg 2 g	WY	40 mg	NS[a]	Rapid lorazepam losses of 8, 10, and 15% at 3, 23, and 30 °C, respectively, in 24 hr. Other drugs stable for 14 days at all three storage temperatures	1733	I

[a]*Tested in Pharmacia-Deltec PVC pump reservoirs.*

Drugs in Syringe Compatibility

Lorazepam

Drug (in syringe)	Mfr	Amt	Mfr	Amt	Remarks	Ref	C/I
Aripiprazole	BMS	6.75 mg/ 0.9 mL	HOS	0.2 mg/ 0.1 mL	Visually compatible for 30 min	2719	C
	BMS	5.25 mg/ 0.7 mL	HOS	0.6 mg/ 0.3 mL	Visually compatible for 30 min	2719	C
	BMS	3.75 mg/ 0.5 mL	HOS	1 mg/ 0.5 mL	Visually compatible for 30 min	2719	C
	BMS	2.25 mg/ 0.3 mL	HOS	1.4 mg/ 0.7 mL	Visually compatible for 30 min	2719	C
	BMS	0.75 mg/ 0.1 mL	HOS	1.8 mg/ 0.9 mL	Visually compatible for 30 min	2719	C
Buprenorphine HCl					Incompatible	4	I
Caffeine citrate		20 mg/ 1 mL	SW	2 mg/ 1 mL	Haze forms immediately becoming two layers over time	2440	I
Dimenhydrinate		10 mg/ 1 mL		4 mg/ 1 mL	Clear solution	2569	C
Haloperidol lactate	MN	5 mg/ 1 mL	WY	2 mg/ 1 mL	Physically compatible and chemically stable for 16 hr at room temperature	1838	C
	MN	5 mg/ 1 mL	WY	4 mg/ 1 mL	Visually compatible with no loss of either drug in 24 hr at 4 and 25 °C	260	C
	MN	5 mg/ 1 mL	WY	2 mg/ 1 mL	Visually compatible for 4 hr at room temperature	260	C
Hydromorphone HCl	KN	2, 10, 40 mg/ 1 mL	WY	4 mg/ 1 mL	Visually compatible. 10% lorazepam loss in 6 days at 4 °C, 4 days at 23 °C, and 24 hr at 37 °C. Little hydromorphone loss in 7 days at all temperatures	1776	C
Pantoprazole sodium	[a]	4 mg/ 1 mL		4 mg/ 1 mL	Precipitates	2574	I
Ranitidine HCl	GL	50 mg/ 2 mL	WY	4 mg/ 1 mL	Poor mixing and layering, which disappears following vortex mixing	978	?

[a]*Test performed using the formulation WITHOUT edetate disodium.*

Y-Site Injection Compatibility (1:1 Mixture)

Lorazepam

Drug	Mfr	Conc	Mfr	Conc	Remarks	Ref	C/I
Acyclovir sodium	BW	5 mg/mL[a]	WY	0.04 mg/mL[a]	Physically compatible for 4 hr at 25 °C	1157	C
Albumin human		200 mg/mL	WY	0.33 mg/mL[b]	Visually compatible for 24 hr at 22 °C	1855	C
Aldesleukin	CHI	33,800 I.U./mL[a]	WY	2 mg/mL	Globules form immediately	1857	I
Allopurinol sodium	BW	3 mg/mL[b]	WY	0.1 mg/mL[b]	Physically compatible for 4 hr at 22 °C	1686	C
Amifostine	USB	10 mg/mL[a]	WY	0.1 mg/mL[a]	Physically compatible for 4 hr at 23 °C	1845	C
Amikacin sulfate	BMS	5 mg/mL	WY	0.33 mg/mL[b]	Visually compatible for 24 hr at 22 °C	1855	C
Amiodarone HCl	WY	6 mg/mL[a]	WY	1 mg/mL[a]	Visually compatible for 24 hr at 22 °C	2352	C
Amoxicillin sodium	SKB	50 mg/mL	WY	0.33 mg/mL[b]	Visually compatible for 24 hr at 22 °C	1855	C
Amoxicillin sodium–clavulanate potassium	SKB	20 + 2 mg/mL	WY	0.33 mg/mL[b]	Visually compatible for 24 hr at 22 °C	1855	C
Amphotericin B cholesteryl sulfate complex	SEQ	0.83 mg/mL[a]	WY	0.1 mg/mL[a]	Physically compatible for 4 hr at 23 °C	2117	C
Amsacrine	NCI	1 mg/mL[a]	WY	0.1 mg/mL[a]	Visually compatible for 4 hr at 22 °C	1381	C
Anakinra	SYN	4 and 36 mg/mL[b]	WY	0.1 mg/mL[b]	Physically compatible with no loss of either drug in 4 hr at 22 °C	2512	C
Atracurium besylate	BW	0.5 mg/mL[a]	WY	0.5 mg/mL[a]	Physically compatible for 24 hr at 28 °C	1337	C
Aztreonam	SQ	40 mg/mL[a]	WY	0.1 mg/mL[a]	Haze forms within 1 hr	1758	I
Bivalirudin	TMC	5 mg/mL[a]	ESL[a]	0.5 mg/mL	Physically compatible for 4 hr at 23 °C	2373	C
Bumetanide	LEO	0.5 mg/mL	WY	0.33 mg/mL[b]	Visually compatible for 24 hr at 22 °C	1855	C
Caspofungin acetate	ME	0.7 mg/mL[b]	HOS	0.5 mg/mL[b]	Physically compatible for 4 hr at room temperature	2758	C
Cefotaxime sodium	RS	10 mg/mL	WY	0.33 mg/mL[b]	Visually compatible for 24 hr at 22 °C	1855	C
Ceftaroline fosamil	FOR	2.22 mg/mL[a,b,e]	HOS	0.5 mg/mL[a,b,e]	Physically compatible for 4 hr at 23 °C	2826	C
Ciprofloxacin	BAY	2 mg/mL	WY	0.33 mg/mL[b]	Visually compatible for 24 hr at 22 °C	1855	C
Cisatracurium besylate	GW	0.1, 2, 5 mg/mL[a]	WY	0.5 mg/mL[a]	Physically compatible for 4 hr at 23 °C	2074	C
Cladribine	ORT	0.015[b] and 0.5[d] mg/mL	WY	0.1 mg/mL[b]	Physically compatible for 4 hr at 23 °C	1969	C
Clonidine HCl	BI	0.015 mg/mL	WY	0.33 mg/mL[b]	Visually compatible for 24 hr at 22 °C	1855	C
Dexamethasone sodium phosphate		4 mg/mL	WY	0.33 mg/mL[b]	Visually compatible for 24 hr at 22 °C	1855	C
Dexmedetomidine HCl	AB	4 mcg/mL[b]	ESL	0.5 mg/mL[b]	Physically compatible for 4 hr at 23 °C	2383	C
Diltiazem HCl	MMD	5 mg/mL	WY	4 mg/mL	Visually compatible	1807	C
	MMD	1 mg/mL[b]	WY	2 mg/mL[b]	Visually compatible	1807	C
	MMD	1 mg/mL[a]	WY	0.5 mg/mL[a]	Visually compatible for 4 hr at 27 °C	2062	C
Dobutamine HCl	LI	4 mg/mL[a]	WY	0.5 mg/mL[a]	Visually compatible for 4 hr at 27 °C	2062	C
Docetaxel	RPR	0.9 mg/mL[a]	WY	0.5 mg/mL[a]	Physically compatible for 4 hr at 23 °C	2224	C
Dopamine HCl	AB	3.2 mg/mL[a]	WY	0.5 mg/mL[a]	Visually compatible for 4 hr at 27 °C	2062	C
Doripenem	JJ	5 mg/mL[a,b]	BED	0.5 mg/mL[a,b]	Physically compatible for 4 hr at 23 °C	2743	C

Y-Site Injection Compatibility (1:1 Mixture) (Cont.)

Lorazepam

Drug	Mfr	Conc	Mfr	Conc	Remarks	Ref	C/I
Doxorubicin HCl liposomal	SEQ	0.4 mg/mL[a]	WY	0.1 mg/mL[a]	Physically compatible for 4 hr at 23 °C	2087	C
Epinephrine HCl	AB	0.02 mg/mL[a]	WY	0.5 mg/mL[a]	Visually compatible for 4 hr at 27 °C	2062	C
Erythromycin lactobionate	AB	5 mg/mL	WY	0.33 mg/mL[b]	Visually compatible for 24 hr at 22 °C	1855	C
Etomidate	AB	2 mg/mL	WY	2 mg/mL	Visually compatible for 7 days at 25 °C	1801	C
Etoposide phosphate	BR	5 mg/mL[a]	WY	0.5 mg/mL[a]	Physically compatible for 4 hr at 23 °C	2218	C
Famotidine	ME	2 mg/mL[b]		0.1 mg/mL[a]	Visually compatible for 4 hr at 22 °C	1936	C
Fenoldopam mesylate	AB	80 mcg/mL[b]	ES	0.5 mg/mL[b]	Physically compatible for 4 hr at 23 °C	2467	C
Fentanyl citrate	ES	0.05 mg/mL	WY	0.33 mg/mL[b]	Visually compatible for 24 hr at 22 °C	1855	C
		0.05 mg/mL	WY	0.5 mg/mL[a]	Visually compatible for 4 hr at 27 °C	2062	C
	JN	0.025 mg/mL[a]	WY	0.1 mg/mL[a]	Physically compatible for 48 hr at 22 °C	1706	C
Filgrastim	AMG	30 mcg/mL[a]	WY	0.1 mg/mL[a]	Physically compatible for 4 hr at 22 °C	1687	C
Floxacillin sodium	SKB	50 mg/mL	WY	0.33 mg/mL[b]	White opalescence forms in 4 hr	1855	I
Fluconazole	PF	2 mg/mL	WY	0.33 mg/mL[b]	Visually compatible for 24 hr at 22 °C	1855	C
Fludarabine phosphate	BX	1 mg/mL[a]	WY	0.1 mg/mL[a]	Visually compatible for 4 hr at 22 °C	1439	C
Foscarnet sodium	AST	24 mg/mL	WY	4 mg/mL	Gas production	1335	I
	AST	24 mg/mL	WY	0.08 mg/mL[a]	Physically compatible for 24 hr at 25 °C under fluorescent light	1393	C
Fosphenytoin sodium	PD	1 mg PE/mL[b,h]	WY	2 mg/mL	Samples remained clear with no loss of either drug in 8 hr	2223	C
Furosemide	CNF	10 mg/mL	WY	0.33 mg/mL[b]	Visually compatible for 24 hr at 22 °C	1855	C
	AMR	10 mg/mL	WY	0.5 mg/mL[a]	Visually compatible for 4 hr at 27 °C	2062	C
Gallium nitrate	FUJ	1 mg/mL[b]	WY	1 mg/mL[b]	White haze and precipitate form immediately but clear in 30 min	1673	I
Gemcitabine HCl	LI	10 mg/mL[b]	WY	0.5 mg/mL[a]	Physically compatible for 4 hr at 23 °C	2226	C
Gentamicin sulfate	CNF	3 mg/mL	WY	0.33 mg/mL[b]	Visually compatible for 24 hr at 22 °C	1855	C
Granisetron HCl	SKB	1 mg/mL	WY	0.1 mg/mL[b]	Physically compatible with little or no loss of either drug in 4 hr at 22 °C	1883	C
	SKB	0.05 mg/mL[a]	WY	0.1 mg/mL[a]	Physically compatible for 4 hr at 23 °C	2000	C
Haloperidol lactate	JN	0.5 and 5 mg/mL	WY	0.33 mg/mL[b]	Visually compatible for 24 hr at 22 °C	1855	C
Heparin sodium		417 units/mL	WY	0.33 mg/mL[b]	Visually compatible for 24 hr at 22 °C	1855	C
	ES	100 units/mL[a]	WY	0.5 mg/mL[a]	Visually compatible for 4 hr at 27 °C	2062	C
Hetastarch in lactated electrolyte	AB	6%	OHM	0.5 mg/mL[a]	Physically compatible for 4 hr at 23 °C	2339	C
Hydrocortisone sodium succinate	UP	50 mg/mL	WY	0.33 mg/mL[b]	Visually compatible for 24 hr at 22 °C	1855	C
Hydromorphone HCl	KN	1 mg/mL	WY	0.5 mg/mL[a]	Visually compatible for 4 hr at 27 °C	2062	C
	AST	0.5 mg/mL[a]	WY	0.1 mg/mL[a]	Physically compatible for 48 hr at 22 °C	1706	C
Idarubicin HCl	AD	1 mg/mL[b]	WY	2 mg/mL	Color changes immediately	1525	I
Imipenem–cilastatin sodium	MSD	5 mg/mL	WY	0.33 mg/mL[b]	Yellow precipitate forms in 24 hr	1855	I
Labetalol HCl	AH	2 mg/mL[a]	WY	0.5 mg/mL[a]	Visually compatible for 4 hr at 27 °C	2062	C
Levofloxacin	OMN	5 mg/mL[a]		2 mg/mL	Visually compatible for 4 hr at 24 °C	2233	C

Y-Site Injection Compatibility (1:1 Mixture) (Cont.)

Lorazepam

Drug	Mfr	Conc	Mfr	Conc	Remarks	Ref	C/I
Linezolid	PHU	2 mg/mL	WY	0.1 mg/mL[a]	Physically compatible for 4 hr at 23 °C	2264	**C**
Melphalan HCl	BW	0.1 mg/mL[b]	WY	0.1 mg/mL[b]	Physically compatible for 3 hr at 22 °C	1557	**C**
Methadone HCl	LI	1 mg/mL[a]	WY	0.1 mg/mL[a]	Physically compatible for 48 hr at 22 °C	1706	**C**
Metronidazole	BRN	5 mg/mL	WY	0.33 mg/mL[b]	Visually compatible for 24 hr at 22 °C	1855	**C**
Micafungin sodium	ASP	1.5 mg/mL[b]	AB	0.5 mg/mL[b]	Physically compatible for 4 hr at 23 °C	2683	**C**
Midazolam HCl	RC	2 mg/mL[a]	WY	0.5 mg/mL[a]	Visually compatible for 4 hr at 27 °C	2062	**C**
Milrinone lactate	SW	0.2 mg/mL[a]	WY	0.5 mg/mL[a]	Visually compatible for 4 hr at 27 °C	2062	**C**
	SW	0.4 mg/mL[a]	WY	0.2 mg/mL[a]	Visually compatible. Little loss of either drug in 4 hr at 23 °C	2214	**C**
	SS	0.2 mg/mL[a]	WY	1 mg/mL[a]	Visually compatible for 4 hr at 25 °C	2381	**C**
	SS	0.2 mg/mL[a]	WY	2 mg/mL[a]	Visually compatible for 4 hr at 25 °C	2381	**C**
Morphine sulfate	SCN	2 mg/mL[a]	WY	0.5 mg/mL[a]	Visually compatible for 4 hr at 27 °C	2062	**C**
	AST	1 mg/mL[a]	WY	0.1 mg/mL[a]	Physically compatible for 48 hr at 22 °C	1706	**C**
Nicardipine HCl	WY	1 mg/mL[a]	WY	0.5 mg/mL[a]	Visually compatible for 4 hr at 27 °C	2062	**C**
Nitroglycerin	AB	0.4 mg/mL[a]	WY	0.5 mg/mL[a]	Visually compatible for 4 hr at 27 °C	2062	**C**
Norepinephrine bitartrate	AB	0.128 mg/mL[a]	WY	0.5 mg/mL[a]	Visually compatible for 4 hr at 27 °C	2062	**C**
Omeprazole	AST	4 mg/mL	WY	0.33 mg/mL[b]	Yellow discoloration forms	1855	**I**
Ondansetron HCl	GL	1 mg/mL[b]	WY	0.1 mg/mL[a]	Light haze develops immediately	1365	**I**
Oxaliplatin	SS	0.5 mg/mL[a]	ESL	0.5 mg/mL[a]	Physically compatible for 4 hr at 23 °C	2566	**C**
Paclitaxel	NCI	1.2 mg/mL[a]		0.1 mg/mL[a]	Physically compatible for 4 hr at 22 °C	1528	**C**
Palonosetron HCl	MGI	50 mcg/mL	BA	0.5 mg/mL[a]	Physically compatible. No loss of either drug in 4 hr	2608	**C**
Pancuronium bromide	ES	0.05 mg/mL[a]	WY	0.5 mg/mL[a]	Physically compatible for 24 hr at 28 °C	1337	**C**
Pemetrexed disodium	LI	20 mg/mL[b]	ES	0.5 mg/mL[a]	Physically compatible for 4 hr at 23 °C	2564	**C**
Piperacillin sodium–tazobactam sodium	LE[c]	40 + 5 mg/mL[a]	WY	0.1 mg/mL[a]	Physically compatible for 4 hr at 22 °C	1688	**C**
Potassium chloride	BRN	1 mEq/mL	WY	0.33 mg/mL[b]	Visually compatible for 24 hr at 22 °C	1855	**C**
Propofol	ZEN	10 mg/mL	WY	0.1 mg/mL[a]	Physically compatible for 1 hr at 23 °C	2066	**C**
Ranitidine HCl	GL	0.5 mg/mL	WY	0.33 mg/mL[b]	Visually compatible for 24 hr at 22 °C	1855	**C**
	GL	1 mg/mL[a]	WY	0.5 mg/mL[a]	Visually compatible for 4 hr at 27 °C	2062	**C**
Remifentanil HCl	GW	0.025 and 0.25 mg/mL[b]	WY	0.5 mg/mL[a]	Physically compatible for 4 hr at 23 °C	2075	**C**
Sargramostim	IMM	10 mcg/mL[b]	WY	0.1 mg/mL[b]	Slightly bluish haze forms in 1 hr	1436	**I**
Tacrolimus	FUJ	1 mg/mL[b]	WY	1 mg/mL[a]	Visually compatible for 24 hr at 25 °C	1630	**C**
Teniposide	BR	0.1 mg/mL[a]	WY	0.1 mg/mL[a]	Physically compatible for 4 hr at 23 °C	1725	**C**
Thiotepa	IMM[f]	1 mg/mL[a]	WY	0.1 mg/mL[a]	Physically compatible for 4 hr at 23 °C	1861	**C**
TNA #218 to #226[g]			WY	0.1 mg/mL[a]	Damage to emulsion occurs in 1 hr	2215	**I**
TPN #212 to #215[g]			WY	0.1 mg/mL[a]	Physically compatible for 4 hr at 23 °C	2109	**C**
Trimethoprim–sulfamethoxazole	RC	0.8 + 4 mg/mL	WY	0.33 mg/mL[b]	Visually compatible for 24 hr at 22 °C	1855	**C**
Vancomycin HCl	LI	5 mg/mL	WY	0.33 mg/mL[b]	Visually compatible for 24 hr at 22 °C	1855	**C**

Y-Site Injection Compatibility (1:1 Mixture) (Cont.)

Lorazepam

Drug	Mfr	Conc	Mfr	Conc	Remarks	Ref	C/I
Vecuronium bromide	OR	0.1 mg/mL[a]	WY	0.5 mg/mL[a]	Physically compatible for 24 hr at 28 °C	1337	C
	OR	4 mg/mL	WY	0.33 mg/mL[b]	Visually compatible for 24 hr at 22 °C	1855	C
	OR	1 mg/mL	WY	0.5 mg/mL[a]	Visually compatible for 4 hr at 27 °C	2062	C
Vinorelbine tartrate	BW	1 mg/mL[b]	WY	0.1 mg/mL[b]	Physically compatible for 4 hr at 22 °C	1558	C
Zidovudine	BW	4 mg/mL[a]	WY	80 mcg/mL[a]	Physically compatible for 4 hr at 25 °C	1193	C

[a]*Tested in dextrose 5%.*
[b]*Tested in sodium chloride 0.9%.*
[c]*Test performed using the formulation WITHOUT edetate disodium.*
[d]*Tested in bacteriostatic sodium chloride 0.9% preserved with benzyl alcohol 0.9%.*
[e]*Tested in Ringer's injection, lactated.*
[f]*Lyophilized formulation tested.*
[g]*Refer to Appendix I for the composition of parenteral nutrition solutions. TNA indicates a 3-in-1 admixture, and TPN indicates a 2-in-1 admixture.*
[h]*Concentration expressed in milligrams of phenytoin sodium equivalents (PE) per milliliter.*

MAGNESIUM SULFATE
AHFS 28:12.92

Products — Magnesium sulfate is available in concentrations of 50, 8, 4, 2, and 1% in a variety of container sizes. (4) The 50% solution provides 500 mg/mL of magnesium sulfate (magnesium 4.06 mEq/mL). The pH of these concentrations may have been adjusted with sodium hydroxide and/or sulfuric acid. (1; 4)

Magnesium sulfate is available as 4% (40 mg/mL; 0.325 mEq/mL) and 8% (80 mg/mL; 0.65 mEq/mL) solutions in water for injection. Magnesium sulfate in dextrose 5% is available as 1% (10 mg/mL; 0.081 mEq/mL) and 2% (20 mg/mL; 0.162 mEq/mL). (1)

pH — Magnesium sulfate injection has a pH adjusted to 5.5 to 7.0. (1) The premixed infusion solutions have pH values in the range of 3.5 to 6.5. (17)

Osmotic Values — The 50% solution has a calculated osmolarity of 4060 mOsm/L. (1)

Magnesium sulfate 4 and 8% solutions in water for injection have osmolarities of 325 and 649 mOsm/L, respectively. Magnesium sulfate 1 and 2% solutions in dextrose 5% have osmolarities of 333 and 415 mOsm/L. (1)

Administration — Magnesium sulfate may be administered by intramuscular or direct intravenous injection and by continuous or intermittent intravenous infusion. For intravenous injection, a concentration of 20% or less should be used; the rate of injection should not exceed 1.5 mL of a 10% solution (or equivalent) per minute. For intramuscular injection, a 25 or 50% concentration is satisfactory for adults, but dilute to 20% for infants and children. (1; 4)

Stability — Magnesium sulfate 50% injection and magnesium sulfate 4 and 8% in water for injection or 1 and 2% in dextrose 5% should be stored at controlled room temperature and protected from freezing. (1; 4) Refrigeration of intact ampuls may result in precipitation or crystallization. (593)

Compatibility Information

Solution Compatibility

Magnesium sulfate

Solution	Mfr	Mfr	Conc/L	Remarks	Ref	C/I
Dextrose 5%	MG	AB	40 g	Physically compatible. Stable for 60 days at 0 °C	922	C
Ringer's injection, lactated	BA[a,b]	AMR	37 g	Visually compatible. No change in composition in 3 months stored at room temperature	2184	C
Sodium chloride 0.9%	BA[a,b]	AMR	37 g	Visually compatible. No change in composition in 3 months stored at room temperature	2184	C

[a]*Tested in glass containers.*
[b]*Tested in PVC containers.*

Additive Compatibility

Magnesium sulfate

Drug	Mfr	Conc/L	Mfr	Conc/L	Test Soln	Remarks	Ref	C/I
Amphotericin B	SQ	40 and 80 mg	IMS	2 and 4 g	D5W	Physically incompatible in 3 hr at 24 °C with decreased clarity and development of supernatant	1578	**I**
Calcium chloride	DB	20 to 4 g	DB	50 to 10 g	D5W, NS	Visible precipitate or microprecipitate forms at room temperature	2597	**I**
	DB	2 g	DB	4 g	D5W, NS	No visible precipitate. Microscopic examination was inconclusive	2597	**?**
	DB	2 g	DB	2.5 g	TPN #266[c]	No visible precipitate or microprecipitate in 24 hr at room temperature	2597	**C**
Calcium gluconate	DB	60 to 12 g	DB	50 to 10 g	D5W, NS	Visible precipitate or microprecipitate forms at room temperature	2597	**I**
	DB	6 g	DB	5 g	D5W, NS	No visible precipitate or microprecipitate in 24 hr at room temperature	2597	**C**
Chloramphenicol sodium succinate	PD	10 g	LI	16 mEq	D5W	Physically compatible	15	**C**
Cisplatin	BR	50 and 200 mg		1 and 2 g	D5½S[a]	Compatible for 48 hr at 25 °C and 96 hr at 4 °C followed by 48 hr at 25 °C	1088	**C**
Cyclosporine	SZ	2 g	LY	30 g	D5W	Transient turbidity upon preparation. 5% cyclosporine loss in 6 hr and 10% loss in 12 hr at 24 °C under fluorescent light	1629	**I**
Dobutamine HCl	LI	167 mg	ES	83 g	NS	Haze forms between 20 and 24 hr	552	**I**
	LI	1 g	TO	2 g	D5W, NS	Slightly pink in 24 hr at 25 °C	789	**I**
Heparin sodium		50,000 units		130 mEq	NS[b]	Visually compatible with heparin activity retained for 14 days at 24 °C under fluorescent light	1908	**C**
Hydrocortisone sodium succinate	UP	100 mg	ES	750 mg	AA 3.5%, D 25%	Physically compatible	302	**C**
Isoproterenol HCl	WI	4 mg		1 g		Physically compatible	59	**C**
Meropenem	ZEN	1 and 20 g	AST	1 g	NS	Visually compatible for 4 hr at room temperature	1994	**C**
Methyldopa HCl	MSD	1 g		1 g	D, D–S, S	Physically compatible	23	**C**
Norepinephrine bitartrate	WI	8 mg		1 g	D, D–S, S	Physically compatible	77	**C**
Penicillin G potassium	PF	500 mg		1 g	W	5% penicillin loss in 1 day and 13% in 2 days at 24 °C	999	**C**
	PF	500 mg		2 to 8 g	W	7 to 8% penicillin loss in 1 day and 20 to 25% in 2 days at 24 °C	999	**C**
Polymyxin B sulfate	BW	200 mg	LI	16 mEq	D5W	Physically incompatible	15	**I**
Potassium acetate		25 mmol		10 mmol	TPN	Transient precipitate forms	2266	**?**
Potassium chloride	BRN	80 mEq	DB	3.9 g	D5W, NS	Visually compatible. Under 5% loss of ions in 24 hr at 22 °C	2360	**C**

Additive Compatibility (Cont.)

Magnesium sulfate

Drug	Mfr	Conc/L	Mfr	Conc/L	Test Soln	Remarks	Ref	C/I
Sodium bicarbonate	AB	80 mEq	LI	16 mEq	D5W	Physically incompatible	15	I
	BA	50 mEq	HOS	1.5 and 15 mEq	[d]	Physically compatible. No loss of ions for 48 hr at 23 °C	2814	C
Verapamil HCl	KN	80 mg	IX	10 g	D5W, NS	Physically compatible for 24 hr	764	C

[a]Tested in PVC containers.
[b]Tested in glass containers.
[c]Refer to Appendix I for the composition of parenteral nutrition solutions. TPN indicates a 2-in-1 admixture.
[d]Tested in an extemporaneously-compounded hemofiltration solution.

Drugs in Syringe Compatibility

Magnesium sulfate

Drug (in syringe)	Mfr	Amt	Mfr	Amt	Remarks	Ref	C/I
Dimenhydrinate		10 mg/1 mL		500 mg/1 mL	Clear solution	2569	C
Hydrocortisone sodium succinate	UP	100 mg/2 mL	ES	500 mg/mL	White precipitate formed	302	I
Metoclopramide HCl	RB	10 mg/2 mL	ES	500 mg/1 mL	Physically compatible for 48 hr at 25 °C	1167	C
	RB	10 mg/2 mL	ES	1 g/2 mL	Physically compatible for 48 hr at 25 °C	1167	C
	RB	160 mg/32 mL	ES	1 g/2 mL	Physically compatible for 48 hr at 25 °C	1167	C
Pantoprazole sodium	[a]	4 mg/1 mL		500 mg/1 mL	Whitish precipitate	2574	I

[a]Test performed using the formulation WITHOUT edetate disodium.

Y-Site Injection Compatibility (1:1 Mixture)

Magnesium sulfate

Drug	Mfr	Conc	Mfr	Conc	Remarks	Ref	C/I
Acyclovir sodium	BW	5 mg/mL[a]	LY	20 mg/mL[a]	Physically compatible for 4 hr at 25 °C	1157	C
Aldesleukin	CHI	33,800 I.U./mL[a]	LY	20 mg/mL[a]	Visually compatible with little or no loss of aldesleukin activity	1857	C
Amifostine	USB	10 mg/mL[a]	AST	100 mg/mL[a]	Physically compatible for 4 hr at 23 °C	1845	C
Amikacin sulfate	BR	5 mg/mL[a]	IX	16.7, 33.3, 66.7, 100 mg/mL[a]	Physically compatible for at least 4 hr at 32 °C	813	C
Amiodarone HCl	WY	6 mg/mL[a]	APP	500 mg/mL	Immediate opaque white turbidity becoming thick precipitate in 24 hr at 22 °C	2352	I
	WY	6 mg/mL[a]	APP	20 mg/mL[a]	Visually compatible for 24 hr at 22 °C	2352	C
Amphotericin B cholesteryl sulfate complex	SEQ	0.83 mg/mL[a]	AST	100 mg/mL[a]	Gross precipitate forms	2117	I
Ampicillin sodium	WY	20 mg/mL[b]	IX	16.7, 33.3, 66.7, 100 mg/mL[a]	Physically compatible for at least 4 hr at 32 °C	813	C

Y-Site Injection Compatibility (1:1 Mixture) (Cont.)

Magnesium sulfate

Drug	Mfr	Conc	Mfr	Conc	Remarks	Ref	C/I
Aztreonam	SQ	40 mg/mL[a]	AST	100 mg/mL[a]	Physically compatible for 4 hr at 23 °C	1758	C
Bivalirudin	TMC	5 mg/mL[a]	APP	100 mg/mL[a]	Physically compatible for 4 hr at 23 °C	2373	C
Caspofungin acetate	ME	0.7 mg/mL[b]	AMR	100 mg/mL[b]	Physically compatible for 4 hr at room temperature	2758	C
	ME	0.5 mg/mL[b]	HOS	40 mg/mL	Physically compatible over 60 min	2766	C
Cefazolin sodium	LI	20 mg/mL[a]	IX	16.7, 33.3, 66.7, 100 mg/mL[a]	Physically compatible for at least 4 hr at 32 °C	813	C
Cefotaxime sodium	HO	20 mg/mL[a]	IX	16.7, 33.3, 66.7, 100 mg/mL[a]	Physically compatible for at least 4 hr at 32 °C	813	C
Cefoxitin sodium	MSD	20 mg/mL[a]	IX	16.7, 33.3, 66.7, 100 mg/mL[a]	Physically compatible for at least 4 hr at 32 °C	813	C
Ceftaroline fosamil	FOR	2.22 mg/mL[a,b]	AMR	100 mg/mL[a,b]	Physically compatible for 4 hr at 23 °C	2826	C
	FOR	2.22 mg/mL[f]	AMR	100 mg/mL[f]	Increase in measured haze	2826	I
Chloramphenicol sodium succinate	PD	20 mg/mL[a]	IX	16.7, 33.3, 66.7, 100 mg/mL[a]	Physically compatible for at least 4 hr at 32 °C	813	C
Ciprofloxacin	MI	2 mg/mL[a]	LY	50%	Visually compatible for 2 hr at 25 °C	1628	C
	MI	2 mg/mL[d]	AB	4 mEq/mL	Precipitate forms in 4 hr in D5W and 1 hr in NS at 24 °C	1655	I
Cisatracurium besylate	GW	0.1, 2, 5 mg/mL[a]	AB	100 mg/mL[a]	Physically compatible for 4 hr at 23 °C	2074	C
Clindamycin phosphate	UP	12 mg/mL[a]	IX	16.7, 33.3, 66.7, 100 mg/mL[a]	Physically compatible for at least 4 hr at 32 °C	813	C
Clonidine HCl	BI	18 mcg/mL[b]	BRN	9.6 mg/mL[a]	Visually compatible	2642	C
Dexmedetomidine HCl	AB	4 mcg/mL[b]	APP	100 mg/mL[b]	Physically compatible for 4 hr at 23 °C	2383	C
Dobutamine HCl	LI	4 mg/mL[d]	LY	40 mg/mL[d]	Physically compatible for 3 hr	1316	C
Docetaxel	RPR	0.9 mg/mL[a]	AST	100 mg/mL[a]	Physically compatible for 4 hr at 23 °C	2224	C
Doripenem	JJ	5 mg/mL[a,b]	AMR	100 mg/mL[a,b]	Physically compatible for 4 hr at 23 °C	2743	C
Doxorubicin HCl liposomal	SEQ	0.4 mg/mL[a]	AST	100 mg/mL[a]	Physically compatible for 4 hr at 23 °C	2087	C
Doxycycline hyclate	PF	1 mg/mL[a]	IX	16.7, 33.3, 66.7, 100 mg/mL[a]	Physically compatible for at least 4 hr at 32 °C	813	C
Enalaprilat	MSD	0.05 mg/mL[b]	LY	10 mEq/mL[a]	Physically compatible for 24 hr at room temperature under fluorescent light	1355	C
Erythromycin lactobionate	AB	5 mg/mL[a]	IX	16.7, 33.3, 66.7, 100 mg/mL[a]	Physically compatible for at least 4 hr at 32 °C	813	C
Esmolol HCl	DCC	10 mg/mL[a]	LY	10 mg/mL[a]	Physically compatible for 24 hr at 22 °C	1169	C
Etoposide phosphate	BR	5 mg/mL[a]	AST	100 mg/mL[a]	Physically compatible for 4 hr at 23 °C	2218	C
Famotidine	MSD	0.2 mg/mL[a]	SO	100 mg/mL[b]	Physically compatible for 14 hr	1196	C
	ME	2 mg/mL[b]		100 mg/mL[a]	Visually compatible for 4 hr at 22 °C	1936	C

Y-Site Injection Compatibility (1:1 Mixture) (Cont.)

Magnesium sulfate

Drug	Mfr	Conc	Mfr	Conc	Remarks	Ref	C/I
Fenoldopam mesylate	AB	80 mcg/mL[b]	APP	100 mg/mL[b]	Physically compatible for 4 hr at 23 °C	2467	C
Fludarabine phosphate	BX	1 mg/mL[a]	SO	100 mg/mL[a]	Visually compatible for 4 hr at 22 °C	1439	C
Gallium nitrate	FUJ	1 mg/mL[b]	AMR	200 mg/mL[b]	Visually compatible for 24 hr at 25 °C	1673	C
Gentamicin sulfate	SC	0.8 mg/mL[a]	IX	16.7, 33.3, 66.7, 100 mg/mL[a]	Physically compatible for at least 4 hr at 32 °C	813	C
Granisetron HCl	SKB	1 mg/mL	AB	16 mg/mL[b]	Physically compatible with little or no loss of granisetron in 4 hr at 22 °C	1883	C
	SKB	0.05 mg/mL[a]	AB	100 mg/mL[a]	Physically compatible for 4 hr at 23 °C	2000	C
Heparin sodium	UP	1000 units/L[e]	AB	500 mg/mL	Physically compatible for 4 hr at room temperature	534	C
Hetastarch in lactated electrolyte	AB	6%	AST	100 mg/mL[a]	Physically compatible for 4 hr at 23 °C	2339	C
Hydrocortisone sodium succinate	UP	10 mg/L[e]	AB	500 mg/mL	Physically compatible for 4 hr at room temperature	534	C
Hydromorphone HCl	KN	2 mg/mL[a]	LY	16.7, 33.3, 50, 100 mg/mL[a]	Visually compatible for 4 hr at 25 °C	1549	C
Hydroxyethyl starch 130/0.4 in sodium chloride 0.9%	FRK	6%	SZ	125[a], 250[a], 500 mg/mL	Visually compatible for 24 hr at room temperature	2770	C
Idarubicin HCl	AD	1 mg/mL[b]	SO	2 mg/mL[b]	Visually compatible for 24 hr at 25 °C	1525	C
Insulin, regular	LI	0.2 unit/mL[b]	LY	40 mg/mL[f]	Physically compatible for 2 hr at 25 °C	1395	C
Labetalol HCl	SC	1 mg/mL[a]	LY	10 mg/mL[a]	Physically compatible for 24 hr at 18 °C	1171	C
Levofloxacin	OMN	5 mg/mL[a]	AMR	20 mg/mL[b]	Physically compatible	2794	C
Linezolid	PHU	2 mg/mL	AST	100 mg/mL[a]	Physically compatible for 4 hr at 23 °C	2264	C
Meperidine HCl	WI	10 mg/mL[a]	LY	16.7, 33.3, 50, 100 mg/mL[a]	Visually compatible for 4 hr at 25 °C	1549	C
Metronidazole	SE	5 mg/mL	IX	16.7, 33.3, 66.7, 100 mg/mL[a]	Physically compatible for at least 4 hr at 32 °C	813	C
Micafungin sodium	ASP	1.5 mg/mL[b]	AMR	100 mg/mL[b]	Physically compatible for 4 hr at 23 °C	2683	C
Milrinone lactate	SW	0.4 mg/mL[a]	SO	40 mg/mL[a]	Visually compatible. No milrinone loss in 4 hr at 23 °C	2214	C
Morphine sulfate	ES	1 mg/mL[a]	LY	16.7, 33.3, 50, 100 mg/mL[a]	Visually compatible for 4 hr at 25 °C	1549	C
	g	2 mg/mL[b]	AB	2, 4, 8 mg/mL[b]	Visually compatible for 8 hr at room temperature	1719	C
Nafcillin sodium	WY	20 mg/mL[a]	IX	16.7, 33.3, 66.7, 100 mg/mL[a]	Physically compatible for at least 4 hr at 32 °C	813	C
Nicardipine HCl	DCC	0.1 mg/mL[a]	LY	10 mg/mL[a]	Visually compatible for 24 hr at room temperature	235	C
Ondansetron HCl	GL	1 mg/mL[b]	SO	100 mg/mL[a]	Visually compatible for 4 hr at 22 °C	1365	C

Y-Site Injection Compatibility (1:1 Mixture) (Cont.)

Magnesium sulfate

Drug	Mfr	Conc	Mfr	Conc	Remarks	Ref	C/I
Oxacillin sodium	BE	20 mg/mL[a]	IX	16.7, 33.3, 66.7, 100 mg/mL[a]	Physically compatible for at least 4 hr at 32 °C	813	**C**
Oxaliplatin	SS	0.5 mg/mL[a]	APP	100 mg/mL[a]	Physically compatible for 4 hr at 23 °C	2566	**C**
Paclitaxel	NCI	1.2 mg/mL[a]	AST	100 mg/mL[a]	Physically compatible for 4 hr at 22 °C	1556	**C**
Penicillin G potassium	SQ	100,000 units/mL[a]	IX	16.7, 33.3, 66.7, 100 mg/mL[a]	Physically compatible for at least 4 hr at 32 °C	813	**C**
Piperacillin sodium–tazobactam sodium	LE[c]	40 + 5 mg/mL[a]	AST	100 mg/mL[a]	Physically compatible for 4 hr at 22 °C	1688	**C**
Potassium chloride	AB	40 mEq/L[e]	AB	500 mg/mL	Physically compatible for 4 hr at room temperature	534	**C**
Propofol	ZEN	10 mg/mL	AST	100 mg/mL[a]	Physically compatible for 1 hr at 23 °C	2066	**C**
Remifentanil HCl	GW	0.025 and 0.25 mg/mL[b]	AB	100 mg/mL[a]	Physically compatible for 4 hr at 23 °C	2075	**C**
Sargramostim	IMM	10 mcg/mL[b]	LY	100 mg/mL[b]	Visually compatible for 4 hr at 22 °C	1436	**C**
Sodium nitroprusside	RC	0.3, 1.2, 3 mg/mL[a]	SX	0.4 and 0.8 mEq/mL[j]	Visually compatible for 48 hr at 24 °C protected from light	2357	**C**
Telavancin HCl	ASP	7.5 mg/mL[a,b,f]	AMR	100 mg/mL[a,b,f]	Physically compatible for 2 hr	2830	**C**
Thiotepa	IMM[h]	1 mg/mL[a]	AST	100 mg/mL[a]	Physically compatible for 4 hr at 23 °C	1861	**C**
TNA #218 to #226[i]			AB	100 mg/mL[a]	Visually compatible for 4 hr at 23 °C	2215	**C**
Tobramycin sulfate	DI	0.8 mg/mL[a]	IX	16.7, 33.3, 66.7, 100 mg/mL[a]	Physically compatible for at least 4 hr at 32 °C	813	**C**
TPN #212 to #215[i]			AB	100 mg/mL[a]	Physically compatible for 4 hr at 23 °C	2109	**C**
Trimethoprim–sulfamethoxazole	RC	0.8 + 4 mg/mL[a]	IX	16.7, 33.3, 66.7, 100 mg/mL[a]	Physically compatible for at least 4 hr at 32 °C	813	**C**
Vancomycin HCl	LI	5 mg/mL[a]	IX	16.7, 33.3, 66.7, 100 mg/mL[a]	Physically compatible for at least 4 hr at 32 °C	813	**C**

[a]Tested in dextrose 5%.
[b]Tested in sodium chloride 0.9%.
[c]Test performed using the formulation WITHOUT edetate disodium.
[d]Tested in both dextrose 5% and sodium chloride 0.9%.
[e]Tested in dextrose 5% in Ringer's injection, dextrose 5% in Ringer's injection, lactated, dextrose 5%, Ringer's injection, lactated, and sodium chloride 0.9%.
[f]Tested in Ringer's injection, lactated.
[g]Extemporaneously prepared product.
[h]Lyophilized formulation tested.
[i]Refer to Appendix I for the composition of parenteral nutrition solutions. TNA indicates a 3-in-1 admixture, and TPN indicates a 2-in-1 admixture.
[j]Tested in dextrose 5% in sodium chloride 0.2%.

MANNITOL
AHFS 40:28.12

Products — Mannitol is available in concentrations ranging from 5 to 25% (1; 4):

Concentration	Osmolarity	Available Sizes
5%	275 mOsm/L	1000 mL
10%	550 mOsm/L	500 and 1000 mL
15%	825 mOsm/L	500 mL
20%	1100 mOsm/L	250 and 500 mL
25%	1375 mOsm/L	50 mL

pH — From 4.5 to 7. (1; 4)

Trade Name(s) — Osmitrol.

Administration — Mannitol is administered by intravenous infusion. An administration set with a filter should be used for infusion solutions containing mannitol 20% or more. The dosage, concentration, and administration rate are dependent on the patient's condition and response. (1; 4)

Stability — Mannitol solutions should be stored at controlled room temperature and protected from freezing. (1; 4) The solutions are chemically stable. Mannitol 25% was chemically and physically stable after five autoclavings at 250 °F for 15 minutes. In addition, no extracts or visible particles from the rubber closures were found. (83)

Crystallization — In concentrations of 15% or greater, mannitol may crystallize when exposed to low temperatures. (1; 4; 593) Do not use a mannitol solution containing crystals. If such crystallization occurs, the recommended procedure for resolubilization is to heat the mannitol in a dry heat cabinet to 70 °C for flexible plastic containers with the overwrap intact or to 80 °C for glass containers with vigorous shaking. The use of a water bath is not recommended. Mannitol 25% in glass vials may be autoclaved at 121 °C. The solution should cool to body temperature before use. (1; 4)

The use of a microwave oven to resolubilize crystallized mannitol in glass ampuls has been suggested. Exposure to microwave radiation followed by shaking satisfactorily resolubilized the crystals in a shorter total time than the water bath and autoclave methods and resulted in no chemical decomposition. (694)

Unfortunately, the use of microwave radiation to solubilize mannitol crystals is a highly risky undertaking. Explosions of mannitol ampuls during microwave exposure have been reported. (695; 697) Such explosions could injure someone as well as ruin the microwave oven. The explosion results from pressure building during the heating of the solution that occurs from the microwave exposure. (696; 697)

One inventive pharmacist redissolved mannitol crystals using a coffeemaker. (1114)

As an alternative to resolubilizing techniques, the use of warming chambers to maintain the solutions in a crystal-free condition has been recommended. (698; 699; 700) Various chambers have been described including a wooden cabinet (698), a metal kettle (699), and even a bun warmer. (700) Storage temperatures of 35 and 50 °C have been utilized. (698; 699)

A related but differing effect is seen when supersaturated solutions of mannitol are placed in PVC bags. Within a few minutes, a heavy white flocculent precipitate forms. The needle-like crystals in mannitol solutions result from slow undisturbed growth. The white flocculent mannitol precipitate results from contact with the PVC surfaces, which act as nuclei for rapid crystallization of small crystals. Attempts to resolubilize the precipitate with the aid of heat are not fruitful because crystallization may recur in a short time. (432)

Compatibility Information

Additive Compatibility

Mannitol

Drug	Mfr	Conc/L	Mfr	Conc/L	Test Soln	Remarks	Ref	C/I
Amikacin sulfate	BR	250 mg and 5 g	BA	20%		Compatible and stable for 24 hr at 25 °C, 60 days at 4 °C, 30 days at −15 °C	292	C
Aztreonam				5 and 10%		Manufacturer recommended solution	1	C
Cefoxitin sodium	MSD	1, 2, 10, 20 g		10%		4 to 5% cefoxitin loss in 24 hr and 10 to 11% in 48 hr at 25 °C. 2 to 5% cefoxitin loss in 7 days at 5 °C	308	C
Ceftriaxone sodium	RC	10 to 40 g		5 and 10%		Less than 10% loss in 24 hr at 25 °C	1	C
Cisplatin	BR	50 and 200 mg		18.75 g	D5½S[a]	Compatible for 48 hr at 25 °C and 96 hr at 4 °C followed by 48 hr at 25 °C	1088	C
Dopamine HCl	AS	800 mg	MG	20%		Under 5% dopamine loss in 48 hr at 25 °C	79	C
Ertapenem sodium	ME	10 and 20 g	AB	5%		Precipitate in <1 hr. 15% loss in 20 hr at 25 °C. 7% loss in 2 days at 4 °C	2487	I

Additive Compatibility (Cont.)

Mannitol

Drug	Mfr	Conc/L	Mfr	Conc/L	Test Soln	Remarks	Ref	C/I
	ME	10 and 20 g	AB	20%		Precipitate in <1 hr. 13% loss in 6 hr at 25 °C. 8% loss in 1 day at 4 °C	2487	**I**
Fosphenytoin sodium	PD	2, 8, 20 mg PE/mL[b]	BA[a]	20%		Visually compatible with little or no loss in 7 days at 25 °C under fluorescent light	2083	**C**
Furosemide	AB	200, 400, 800 mg	BA[a]	20%		Visually compatible for 72 hr at 22 °C	1803	**C**
Gentamicin sulfate		120 mg		20%		Physically compatible and gentamicin stable for 24 hr at 25 °C	897	**C**
Imipenem–cilastatin sodium	MSD	2.5 g	AB[c]	2.5%		9% imipenem loss in 9 hr at 25 °C. 7% loss in 48 hr and 11% in 72 hr at 4 °C	1141	**I**[d]
	MSD	5 g	AB[c]	2.5%		6% imipenem loss in 3 hr and 12% in 6 hr at 25 °C. 7% loss in 24 hr and 10% in 48 hr at 4 °C	1141	**I**[d]
	MSD	2.5 g	AB[c]	5%		6% imipenem loss in 3 hr and 10% in 6 hr at 25 °C. 9% loss in 48 hr and 13% in 72 hr at 4 °C	1141	**I**[d]
	MSD	5 g	AB[c]	5%		7% imipenem loss in 3 hr and 12% in 6 hr at 25 °C. 12% loss in 48 hr at 4 °C	1141	**I**[d]
	MSD	2.5 g	AB[c]	10%		6% imipenem loss in 3 hr and 10% in 6 hr at 25 °C. 7% loss in 24 hr and 12% in 48 hr at 4 °C	1141	**I**[d]
	MSD	5 g	AB[c]	10%		12% imipenem loss in 3 hr at 25 °C. 13% loss in 48 hr at 4 °C	1141	**I**[d]
Levofloxacin	OMJ	0.5 g	BA	20%		Precipitate forms within a few hours	1986	**I**
	OMJ	5 g	BA	20%		Precipitate forms within 13 weeks at −20 °C	1986	**I**
	OMJ	5 g	BA	20%		Physically compatible. <4% loss in 3 days at 25 °C, 14 days at 5 °C, in dark	1986	**C**
Meropenem	ZEN	1 g	BA[a]	2.5%		7 to 8% meropenem loss in 8 hr at 24 °C and in 24 hr at 4 °C	2089	**I**[d]
	ZEN	20 g	BA[a]	2.5%		7 to 9% meropenem loss in 4 hr at 24 °C and 6% loss in 20 hr at 4 °C	2089	**I**[d]
	ZEN	1 g	BA[a]	10%		10 to 11% meropenem loss in 4 hr at 24 °C and in 20 hr at 4 °C	2089	**I**[d]
	ZEN	20 g	BA[a]	10%		10% meropenem loss in 3 hr at 24 °C and in 20 hr at 4 °C	2089	**I**[d]
Metoclopramide HCl	RB	40 and 100 mg	AB	20%		Physically compatible for 48 hr at room temperature	924	**C**
	RB	40 and 100 mg	AB	20%		Physically compatible for 48 hr at 25 °C	1167	**C**
	RB	640 mg and 1.6 g	AB	20%		Physically compatible for 48 hr at 25 °C	1167	**C**
Ondansetron HCl	GL	16 mg	BP[a]	10%		Physically compatible. Stable for 7 days at room temperature in light and at 4 °C	1366	**C**

Additive Compatibility (Cont.)

Mannitol

Drug	Mfr	Conc/L	Mfr	Conc/L	Test Soln	Remarks	Ref	C/I
Sodium bicarbonate	AB	44.6 mEq	AMR	25 g	D5LR, D5¼S, D5½S, D5S, D5W, D10W, NS, ½S[e]	Visually compatible for 24 hr at 24 °C	1853; 1973	C
Tobramycin sulfate	LI	200 mg and 1 g		20%		Physically compatible and chemically stable for 48 hr at 25 °C	147	C
Tramadol HCl	GRU	0.4 g		20%		Visually compatible with no tramadol loss in 24 hr at room temperature and 4 °C	2652	C
Verapamil HCl	KN	80 mg	IX	25 g	D5W, NS	Physically compatible for 24 hr	764	C

[a]Tested in PVC containers.
[b]Concentration expressed in milligrams of phenytoin sodium equivalents (PE) per milliliter.
[c]Tested in glass containers.
[d]Incompatible by conventional standards but may be used in shorter periods of time.
[e]Tested in polyolefin containers.

Y-Site Injection Compatibility (1:1 Mixture)

Mannitol

Drug	Mfr	Conc	Mfr	Conc	Remarks	Ref	C/I
Allopurinol sodium	BW	3 mg/mL[b]	BA	15%	Physically compatible for 4 hr at 22 °C	1686	C
Amifostine	USB	10 mg/mL[a]	BA	15%	Physically compatible for 4 hr at 23 °C	1845	C
Amphotericin B cholesteryl sulfate complex	SEQ	0.83 mg/mL[a]	BA	15%	Physically compatible for 4 hr at 23 °C	2117	C
Aztreonam	SQ	40 mg/mL[a]	BA	15%	Physically compatible for 4 hr at 23 °C	1758	C
Bivalirudin	TMC	5 mg/mL[a]	BA	15%	Physically compatible for 4 hr at 23 °C	2373	C
Ceftaroline fosamil	FOR	2.22 mg/mL[a,b,h]	HOS	15%	Physically compatible for 4 hr at 23 °C	2826	C
Cisatracurium besylate	GW	0.1, 2, 5 mg/mL[a]	BA	15%	Physically compatible for 4 hr at 23 °C	2074	C
Cladribine	ORT	0.015[b] and 0.5[c] mg/mL	BA	15%	Physically compatible for 4 hr at 23 °C	1969	C
Docetaxel	RPR	0.9 mg/mL[a]	BA	15%	Physically compatible for 4 hr at 23 °C	2224	C
Doripenem	JJ	5 mg/mL[a,b]	HOS	15%	Physically compatible for 4 hr at 23 °C	2743	C
Doxorubicin HCl liposomal	SEQ	0.4 mg/mL[a]	BA	15%	Partial loss of measured natural turbidity	2087	I
Etoposide phosphate	BR	5 mg/mL[a]	BA	15%	Physically compatible for 4 hr at 23 °C	2218	C
Fenoldopam mesylate	AB	80 mcg/mL[b]	BA	15%	Physically compatible for 4 hr at 23 °C	2467	C
Filgrastim	AMG	30 mcg/mL[a]	BA	15%	Filaments form immediately	1687	I
Fludarabine phosphate	BX	1 mg/mL[a]	BA	15%	Visually compatible for 4 hr at 22 °C	1439	C
Fluorouracil	SO	1 and 2 mg/mL[d]		20%	Physically compatible and fluorouracil stable for 24 hr. Mannitol not tested	1526	C

Y-Site Injection Compatibility (1:1 Mixture) (Cont.)

Mannitol

Drug	Mfr	Conc	Mfr	Conc	Remarks	Ref	C/I
Gallium nitrate	FUJ	1 mg/mL[b]	AB	250 mg/mL	Visually compatible for 24 hr at 25 °C	1673	C
Gemcitabine HCl	LI	10 mg/mL[b]	BA	15%	Physically compatible for 4 hr at 23 °C	2226	C
Hetastarch in lactated electrolyte	AB	6%	BA	15%	Physically compatible for 4 hr at 23 °C	2339	C
Idarubicin HCl	AD	1 mg/mL[b]	AB	12.5 mg/mL[b]	Visually compatible for 24 hr at 25 °C	1525	C
Linezolid	PHU	2 mg/mL	BA	15%	Physically compatible for 4 hr at 23 °C	2264	C
Melphalan HCl	BW	0.1 mg/mL[b]	BA	15%	Physically compatible for 3 hr at 22 °C	1557	C
Ondansetron HCl	GL	1 mg/mL[b]	BA	15%	Visually compatible for 4 hr at 22 °C	1365	C
Oxaliplatin	SS	0.5 mg/mL[a]	BA	15%	Physically compatible for 4 hr at 23 °C	2566	C
Paclitaxel	NCI	1.2 mg/mL[a]	BA	15%	Physically compatible for 4 hr at 22 °C	1556	C
Palonosetron HCl	MGI	50 mcg/mL	HOS	15%	Physically compatible. No palonosetron loss in 4 hr at room temperature	2775	C
Pantoprazole sodium	[g]	4 mg/mL		25%	Precipitates	2574	I
Pemetrexed disodium	LI	20 mg/mL[b]	BA	15%	Physically compatible for 4 hr at 23 °C	2564	C
Piperacillin sodium–tazobactam sodium	LE[g]	40 + 5 mg/ mL[a]	BA	15%	Physically compatible for 4 hr at 22 °C	1688	C
Propofol	ZEN	10 mg/mL	BA	15%	Physically compatible for 1 hr at 23 °C	2066	C
Remifentanil HCl	GW	0.025 and 0.25 mg/mL[b]	BA	15%	Physically compatible for 4 hr at 23 °C	2075	C
Sargramostim	IMM	10 mcg/mL[b]	BA	15%	Visually compatible for 4 hr at 22 °C	1436	C
Telavancin HCl	ASP	7.5 mg/ mL[a,b,h]	HOS	20%	Physically compatible for 2 hr	2830	C
Teniposide	BR	0.1 mg/mL[a]	BA	15%	Physically compatible for 4 hr at 23 °C	1725	C
Thiotepa	IMM[e]	1 mg/mL[b]	BA	15%	Physically compatible for 4 hr at 23 °C	1861	C
TNA #218 to #226[f]			BA	15%	Visually compatible for 4 hr at 23 °C	2215	C
TPN #212 to #215[f]			BA	15%	Physically compatible for 4 hr at 23 °C	2109	C
Vinorelbine tartrate	BW	1 mg/mL[b]	BA	15%	Physically compatible for 4 hr at 22 °C	1558	C

[a]*Tested in dextrose 5%.*
[b]*Tested in sodium chloride 0.9%.*
[c]*Tested in bacteriostatic sodium chloride 0.9% preserved with benzyl alcohol 0.9%.*
[d]*Tested in dextrose 5% in sodium chloride 0.45%, dextrose 5%, and sodium chloride 0.9%.*
[e]*Lyophilized formulation tested.*
[f]*Refer to Appendix I for the composition of parenteral nutrition solutions. TNA indicates a 3-in-1 admixture, and TPN indicates a 2-in-1 admixture.*
[g]*Test performed using the formulation WITHOUT edetate disodium.*
[h]*Tested in Ringer's injection, lactated.*

MECHLORETHAMINE HYDROCHLORIDE (MUSTINE HYDROCHLORIDE) AHFS 10:00

Products — Mechlorethamine hydrochloride is available in vials containing 10 mg of drug and sodium chloride qs 100 mg. While taking appropriate protective measures, including wearing protective gloves, reconstitute the vial with 10 mL of water for injection or sodium chloride 0.9%. With the needle in the rubber stopper, shake the vial several times to dissolve the drug. The resultant solution contains mechlorethamine hydrochloride 1 mg/mL. (1)

pH — The reconstituted solution has a pH of 3 to 5. (1; 4)

Trade Name(s) — Mustargen.

Administration — Mechlorethamine hydrochloride is administered intravenously or into body cavities. (1; 4) The drug is extremely irritating to tissues and should not be given intramuscularly or subcutaneously. (4) For intravenous use, the drug may be injected over a few minutes directly into the vein or into the tubing of a running infusion solution. (1; 4) After administration, flushing the vein with about 5 to 10 mL of intravenous solution has been recommended. (4) The drug is a powerful vesicant, and extravasation should be avoided. (1; 4; 377) For intracavitary administration, the drug may be diluted up to 100 mL with sodium chloride 0.9%. (1; 4)

Spillage of the drug on gloves, etc., can be neutralized by soaking in an aqueous solution containing equal amounts of sodium thiosulfate 5% and sodium bicarbonate 5% for 45 minutes. Unused injection solution also may be neutralized by mixing with an equal volume of the sodium thiosulfate–sodium bicarbonate solution for 45 minutes. (1; 1200)

Stability — In dry form, the drug is a light yellow-brown and is stable at temperatures up to 40 °C. (4) Solutions decompose on standing and should be prepared immediately before use. The drug is even less stable in neutral or alkaline solutions than in the acidic reconstituted solution. Do not use if the solution is discolored or if water droplets form within the vial before reconstitution. Discard unused portions after neutralization. (1; 4)

Because of the rapid decomposition of mechlorethamine hydrochloride in solution, administration in intravenous infusion solutions is not recommended. (4) One report indicated a 7% loss of mechlorethamine in one hour at room temperature when diluted to 0.1 mg/mL in sodium chloride 0.9%. (923) Injecting the drug into the tubing of a running intravenous infusion rather than adding it to the entire volume of the solution minimizes the extent of chemical decomposition. (1)

The stability of mechlorethamine hydrochloride (Boots) 1 mg/mL when reconstituted with water for injection or sodium chloride 0.9% in vials and plastic syringes was determined. About an 8 to 10% loss occurred in samples over six hours at 22 °C; losses of 4 to 6% occurred in six hours in samples stored at 4 °C. (1279)

Immersion of a needle with an aluminum component in mechlorethamine (MSD) 1 mg/mL resulted in no visually apparent reaction after seven days at 24 °C. (988)

Freezing Solutions — The stability of mechlorethamine hydrochloride (Boots) 1 mg/mL in water for injection and sodium chloride 0.9% frozen at −20 °C was determined. In water for injection, about a 7% loss occurred after 12 weeks; about a 15% loss occurred in eight weeks with sodium chloride 0.9% as the diluent. At a concentration of 10 mg/500 mL in sodium chloride 0.9% in PVC bags, about a 10% loss occurred in eight weeks frozen at −20 °C. (1279)

Compatibility Information

Solution Compatibility

Mechlorethamine HCl

Solution	Mfr	Mfr	Conc/L	Remarks	Ref	C/I
Dextrose 5%	a	BT	20 mg	10% loss in 5 hr at 22 °C. 4% loss in 6 hr at 4 °C	1279	I
Sodium chloride 0.9%	a	BT	20 mg	10% loss in 3 hr at 22 °C. 10% loss in 4 hr at 4 °C	1279	I

ᵃTested in PVC containers.

Additive Compatibility

Mechlorethamine HCl

Drug	Mfr	Conc/L	Mfr	Conc/L	Test Soln	Remarks	Ref	C/I
Methohexital sodium	BP	2 g	BP	40 mg	D5W, NS	Haze develops over 3 hr	26	I

Y-Site Injection Compatibility (1:1 Mixture)

Mechlorethamine HCl

Drug	Mfr	Conc	Mfr	Conc	Remarks	Ref	C/I
Allopurinol sodium	BW	3 mg/mLᵇ	MSD	1 mg/mL	Haze and small particles form immediately. Numerous large particles in 4 hr	1686	I
Amifostine	USB	10 mg/mLᵃ	MSD	1 mg/mL	Physically compatible for 4 hr at 23 °C	1845	C
Aztreonam	SQ	40 mg/mLᵃ	MSD	1 mg/mL	Physically compatible for 4 hr at 23 °C	1758	C
Filgrastim	AMG	30 mcg/mLᵃ	MSD	1 mg/mL	Physically compatible for 4 hr at 22 °C	1687	C
Fludarabine phosphate	BX	1 mg/mLᵃ	MSD	1 mg/mL	Visually compatible for 4 hr at 22 °C	1439	C

Y-Site Injection Compatibility (1:1 Mixture) (Cont.)

Mechlorethamine HCl

Drug	Mfr	Conc	Mfr	Conc	Remarks	Ref	C/I
Granisetron HCl	SKB	1 mg/mL	MSD	0.5 mg/mL[b]	Physically compatible with little or no loss of either drug in 4 hr at 22 °C	1883	**C**
Melphalan HCl	BW	0.1 mg/mL[b]	MSD	1 mg/mL	Physically compatible for 3 hr at 22 °C	1557	**C**
Ondansetron HCl	GL	1 mg/mL[b]	MSD	1 mg/mL	Visually compatible for 4 hr at 22 °C	1365	**C**
Sargramostim	IMM	10 mcg/mL[b]	MSD	1 mg/mL	Visually compatible for 4 hr at 22 °C	1436	**C**
Teniposide	BR	0.1 mg/mL[a]	MSD	1 mg/mL	Physically compatible for 4 hr at 23 °C	1725	**C**
Vinorelbine tartrate	BW	1 mg/mL[b]	MSD	1 mg/mL	Physically compatible for 4 hr at 22 °C	1558	**C**

[a]Tested in dextrose 5%.
[b]Tested in sodium chloride 0.9%.

MELPHALAN HYDROCHLORIDE
AHFS 10:00

Products — Melphalan hydrochloride is available in 50-mg vials with povidone 20 mg. It is packaged with a vial of special diluent containing sodium citrate 0.2 g, propylene glycol 6 mL, ethanol (96%) 0.52 mL, and sterile water for injection qs to 10 mL. While taking appropriate protective measures, including wearing protective gloves, reconstitute by rapidly injecting 10 mL of special diluent and shake vigorously to yield a 5-mg/mL melphalan concentration. (1)

pH — The reconstituted solution has a pH of about 7. (4)

Trade Name(s) — Alkeran.

Administration — Melphalan is administered intravenously. Immediately after reconstitution, the drug should be diluted in sodium chloride 0.9% to a concentration not greater than 0.45 mg/mL. It should be infused over 15 to 20 minutes. (1; 4)

Stability — Intact vials should be stored at controlled room temperature and protected from light. The reconstituted solution is stable for no more than 90 minutes at room temperature. (4) Refrigeration of the reconstituted solution results in precipitation. (1; 4)

Because of rapid decomposition, the manufacturer recommends that drug administration be completed within 60 minutes of initial reconstitution. Degradation products are detected within 30 minutes. (1); a 10% loss occurs within approximately three hours at 30 °C. (234) After dilution in sodium chloride 0.9%, nearly 1% of the drug is hydrolyzed every 10 minutes. (1)

pH Effects — Melphalan is most stable over a pH range of 3 to 7; decomposition increases at pH 9. (971)

Sorption — Melphalan hydrochloride (GlaxoWellcome) 60 mcg/mL in sodium chloride 0.9% exhibited no loss due to sorption in polyethylene, PVC containers, and glass containers over 24 hours under refrigeration and eight hours at room temperature. (2420; 2430)

Filtration — Melphalan hydrochloride 20 mcg/mL in 1 mL of sodium chloride 0.9% was filtered through the following filters; minimal adsorption occurred in all cases (970):

Filter	Delivered Concentration (% of initial)
Cellulose acetate 0.2 μm (Minisart-N, Sartorius)	99
Polysulfone 0.45 μm (Acrodisc, Gelman)	98
Polytetrafluoroethylene 0.45 μm (Acrodisc-CR, Gelman)	96

Compatibility Information

Solution Compatibility

Melphalan HCl

Solution	Mfr	Mfr	Conc/L	Remarks	Ref	C/I
Dextrose 5%		BW	40 and 400 mg	10% loss in 90 min at 20 °C and 36 min at 25 °C	971	**I**
Ringer's injection, lactated		BW	40 and 400 mg	10% loss in 2.9 hr at 20 °C and 90 min at 25 °C	971	**I**

Solution Compatibility (Cont.)

Melphalan HCl

Solution	Mfr	Mfr	Conc/L	Remarks	Ref	C/I
Sodium chloride 0.9%			20 mg	4% loss in 6 months at −20 °C	970	C
		BW	40 and 400 mg	10% loss in 4.5 hr at 20 °C and 2.4 hr at 25 °C	971	I[a]
		BW	100 and 450 mg	10% loss in 45 min at 30 °C	234	I
		BW	100 mg	10% loss in 3 hr at 20 °C	234	I[a]
	b	WEL	200 mg	Visually compatible. 6% loss in 3 hr and 17% in 6 hr at room temperature. 6% loss in 6 hr and 13% in 24 hr at 4 °C. No loss in 72 hr at −20 °C	1841	I[a]

[a] Incompatible by conventional standards. May be used in shorter time periods.
[b] Tested in PVC containers.

Y-Site Injection Compatibility (1:1 Mixture)

Melphalan HCl

Drug	Mfr	Conc	Mfr	Conc	Remarks	Ref	C/I
Acyclovir sodium	BW	7 mg/mL[b]	BW	0.1 mg/mL[b]	Physically compatible for 3 hr at 22 °C	1557	C
Amikacin sulfate	BR	5 mg/mL[b]	BW	0.1 mg/mL[b]	Physically compatible for 3 hr at 22 °C	1557	C
Aminophylline	AB	2.5 mg/mL[b]	BW	0.1 mg/mL[b]	Physically compatible for 3 hr at 22 °C	1557	C
Amphotericin B	SQ	0.6 mg/mL[a]	BW	0.1 mg/mL[b]	Immediate increase in measured turbidity	1557	I
	SQ	0.6 mg/mL[a]	BW	0.1 mg/mL[a]	Physically compatible but rapid melphalan loss in D5W precludes use	1557	I
Ampicillin sodium	WY	20 mg/mL[b]	BW	0.1 mg/mL[b]	Physically compatible for 3 hr at 22 °C	1557	C
Aztreonam	SQ	40 mg/mL[b]	BW	0.1 mg/mL[b]	Physically compatible for 3 hr at 22 °C	1557	C
Bleomycin sulfate	BR	1 unit/mL[b]	BW	0.1 mg/mL[b]	Physically compatible for 3 hr at 22 °C	1557	C
Bumetanide	RC	0.04 mg/mL[b]	BW	0.1 mg/mL[b]	Physically compatible for 3 hr at 22 °C	1557	C
Buprenorphine HCl	RKC	0.04 mg/mL[b]	BW	0.1 mg/mL[b]	Physically compatible for 3 hr at 22 °C	1557	C
Butorphanol tartrate	BR	0.04 mg/mL[b]	BW	0.1 mg/mL[b]	Physically compatible for 3 hr at 22 °C	1557	C
Calcium gluconate	AST	40 mg/mL[b]	BW	0.1 mg/mL[b]	Physically compatible for 3 hr at 22 °C	1557	C
Carboplatin	BR	5 mg/mL[b]	BW	0.1 mg/mL[b]	Physically compatible for 3 hr at 22 °C	1557	C
Carmustine	BR	1.5 mg/mL[b]	BW	0.1 mg/mL[b]	Physically compatible for 3 hr at 22 °C	1557	C
Caspofungin acetate	ME	0.7 mg/mL[b]	CAR	1 mg/mL[b]	Physically compatible for 4 hr at room temperature	2758	C
Cefazolin sodium	GEM	20 mg/mL[b]	BW	0.1 mg/mL[b]	Physically compatible for 3 hr at 22 °C	1557	C
Cefotaxime sodium	HO	20 mg/mL[b]	BW	0.1 mg/mL[b]	Physically compatible for 3 hr at 22 °C	1557	C
Cefotetan disodium	STU	20 mg/mL[b]	BW	0.1 mg/mL[b]	Physically compatible for 3 hr at 22 °C	1557	C
Ceftazidime	LI	40 mg/mL[b]	BW	0.1 mg/mL[b]	Physically compatible for 3 hr at 22 °C	1557	C
Ceftriaxone sodium	RC	20 mg/mL[b]	BW	0.1 mg/mL[b]	Physically compatible for 3 hr at 22 °C	1557	C
Cefuroxime sodium	GL	20 mg/mL[b]	BW	0.1 mg/mL[b]	Physically compatible for 3 hr at 22 °C	1557	C
Chlorpromazine HCl	ES	2 mg/mL[b]	BW	0.1 mg/mL[b]	Large increase in measured turbidity occurs within 1 hr and grows over 3 hr	1557	I
Cisplatin	BR	1 mg/mL	BW	0.1 mg/mL[b]	Physically compatible for 3 hr at 22 °C	1557	C
Clindamycin phosphate	AB	10 mg/mL[b]	BW	0.1 mg/mL[b]	Physically compatible for 3 hr at 22 °C	1557	C

Y-Site Injection Compatibility (1:1 Mixture) (Cont.)

Melphalan HCl

Drug	Mfr	Conc	Mfr	Conc	Remarks	Ref	C/I
Cyclophosphamide	BR	10 mg/mL[b]	BW	0.1 mg/mL[b]	Physically compatible for 3 hr at 22 °C	1557	C
Cytarabine	UP	50 mg/mL	BW	0.1 mg/mL[b]	Physically compatible for 3 hr at 22 °C	1557	C
Dacarbazine	MI	4 mg/mL[b]	BW	0.1 mg/mL[b]	Physically compatible for 3 hr at 22 °C	1557	C
Dactinomycin	MSD	0.01 mg/mL[b]	BW	0.1 mg/mL[b]	Physically compatible for 3 hr at 22 °C	1557	C
Daunorubicin HCl	WY	1 mg/mL[b]	BW	0.1 mg/mL[b]	Physically compatible for 3 hr at 22 °C	1557	C
Dexamethasone sodium phosphate	LY	1 mg/mL[b]	BW	0.1 mg/mL[b]	Physically compatible for 3 hr at 22 °C	1557	C
Diphenhydramine HCl	WY	2 mg/mL[b]	BW	0.1 mg/mL[b]	Physically compatible for 3 hr at 22 °C	1557	C
Doxorubicin HCl	AD	2 mg/mL	BW	0.1 mg/mL[b]	Physically compatible for 3 hr at 22 °C	1557	C
Doxycycline hyclate	LY	1 mg/mL[b]	BW	0.1 mg/mL[b]	Physically compatible for 3 hr at 22 °C	1557	C
Droperidol	JN	0.4 mg/mL[b]	BW	0.1 mg/mL[b]	Physically compatible for 3 hr at 22 °C	1557	C
Enalaprilat	MSD	0.1 mg/mL[b]	BW	0.1 mg/mL[b]	Physically compatible for 3 hr at 22 °C	1557	C
Etoposide	BR	0.4 mg/mL[b]	BW	0.1 mg/mL[b]	Physically compatible for 3 hr at 22 °C	1557	C
Famotidine	MSD	2 mg/mL[b]	BW	0.1 mg/mL[b]	Physically compatible for 3 hr at 22 °C	1557	C
Filgrastim	AMG	30 mcg/mL[a]	BW	0.1 mg/mL[a]	Physically compatible for 4 hr at 22 °C	1687	C
Floxuridine	RC	3 mg/mL[b]	BW	0.1 mg/mL[b]	Physically compatible for 3 hr at 22 °C	1557	C
Fluconazole	RR	2 mg/mL	BW	0.1 mg/mL[b]	Physically compatible for 3 hr at 22 °C	1557	C
Fludarabine phosphate	BX	1 mg/mL[b]	BW	0.1 mg/mL[b]	Physically compatible for 3 hr at 22 °C	1557	C
Fluorouracil	LY	16 mg/mL[b]	BW	0.1 mg/mL[b]	Physically compatible for 3 hr at 22 °C	1557	C
Furosemide	AB	3 mg/mL[b]	BW	0.1 mg/mL[b]	Physically compatible for 3 hr at 22 °C	1557	C
Gallium nitrate	FUJ	0.4 mg/mL[b]	BW	0.1 mg/mL[b]	Physically compatible for 3 hr at 22 °C	1557	C
Ganciclovir sodium	SY	20 mg/mL[b]	BW	0.1 mg/mL[b]	Physically compatible for 3 hr at 22 °C	1557	C
Gentamicin sulfate	LY	5 mg/mL[b]	BW	0.1 mg/mL[b]	Physically compatible for 3 hr at 22 °C	1557	C
Granisetron HCl	SKB	0.05 mg/mL[a]	BW	0.1 mg/mL[b]	Physically compatible for 4 hr at 23 °C	2000	C
Haloperidol lactate	MN	0.2 mg/mL[b]	BW	0.1 mg/mL[b]	Physically compatible for 3 hr at 22 °C	1557	C
Heparin sodium	WY	100 units/mL[b]	BW	0.1 mg/mL[b]	Physically compatible for 3 hr at 22 °C	1557	C
Hydrocortisone sodium succinate	UP	1 mg/mL[b]	BW	0.1 mg/mL[b]	Physically compatible for 3 hr at 22 °C	1557	C
Hydromorphone HCl	KN	0.5 mg/mL[b]	BW	0.1 mg/mL[b]	Physically compatible for 3 hr at 22 °C	1557	C
Hydroxyzine HCl	WI	4 mg/mL[b]	BW	0.1 mg/mL[b]	Physically compatible for 3 hr at 22 °C	1557	C
Idarubicin HCl	AD	0.5 mg/mL[b]	BW	0.1 mg/mL[b]	Physically compatible for 3 hr at 22 °C	1557; 1675	C
Ifosfamide	BR	25 mg/mL[b]	BW	0.1 mg/mL[b]	Physically compatible for 3 hr at 22 °C	1557	C
Imipenem–cilastatin sodium	MSD	10 mg/mL[b]	BW	0.1 mg/mL[b]	Physically compatible for 3 hr at 22 °C	1557	C
Lorazepam	WY	0.1 mg/mL[b]	BW	0.1 mg/mL[b]	Physically compatible for 3 hr at 22 °C	1557	C
Mannitol	BA	15%	BW	0.1 mg/mL[b]	Physically compatible for 3 hr at 22 °C	1557	C
Mechlorethamine HCl	MSD	1 mg/mL	BW	0.1 mg/mL[b]	Physically compatible for 3 hr at 22 °C	1557	C
Meperidine HCl	WY	4 mg/mL[b]	BW	0.1 mg/mL[b]	Physically compatible for 3 hr at 22 °C	1557	C
Mesna	BR	10 mg/mL[b]	BW	0.1 mg/mL[b]	Physically compatible for 3 hr at 22 °C	1557	C
Methotrexate sodium	LE	15 mg/mL[b]	BW	0.1 mg/mL[b]	Physically compatible for 3 hr at 22 °C	1557	C

Y-Site Injection Compatibility (1:1 Mixture) (Cont.)

Melphalan HCl

Drug	Mfr	Conc	Mfr	Conc	Remarks	Ref	C/I
Methylprednisolone sodium succinate	AB	5 mg/mL[b]	BW	0.1 mg/mL[b]	Physically compatible for 3 hr at 22 °C	1557	C
Metoclopramide HCl	RB	5 mg/mL	BW	0.1 mg/mL[b]	Physically compatible for 3 hr at 22 °C	1557	C
Metronidazole	AB	5 mg/mL	BW	0.1 mg/mL[b]	Physically compatible for 3 hr at 22 °C	1557	C
Mitomycin	BR	0.5 mg/mL	BW	0.1 mg/mL[b]	Physically compatible for 3 hr at 22 °C	1557	C
Mitoxantrone HCl	LE	0.5 mg/mL[b]	BW	0.1 mg/mL[b]	Physically compatible for 3 hr at 22 °C	1557	C
Morphine sulfate	WI	1 mg/mL[b]	BW	0.1 mg/mL[b]	Physically compatible for 3 hr at 22 °C	1557	C
Nalbuphine HCl	AST	10 mg/mL	BW	0.1 mg/mL[b]	Physically compatible for 3 hr at 22 °C	1557	C
Ondansetron HCl	GL	1 mg/mL[b]	BW	0.1 mg/mL[b]	Physically compatible for 3 hr at 22 °C	1557	C
Pentostatin	PD	0.4 mg/mL[b]	BW	0.1 mg/mL[b]	Physically compatible for 3 hr at 22 °C	1557	C
Potassium chloride	AB	0.1 mEq/mL[b]	BW	0.1 mg/mL[b]	Physically compatible for 3 hr at 22 °C	1557	C
Prochlorperazine edisylate	SKB	0.5 mg/mL[b]	BW	0.1 mg/mL[b]	Physically compatible for 3 hr at 22 °C	1557	C
Promethazine HCl	WY	2 mg/mL[b]	BW	0.1 mg/mL[b]	Physically compatible for 3 hr at 22 °C	1557	C
Ranitidine HCl	GL	2 mg/mL[b]	BW	0.1 mg/mL[b]	Physically compatible for 3 hr at 22 °C	1557	C
Sodium bicarbonate	AB	1 mEq/mL	BW	0.1 mg/mL[b]	Physically compatible for 3 hr at 22 °C	1557	C
Streptozocin	UP	40 mg/mL[b]	BW	0.1 mg/mL[b]	Physically compatible for 3 hr at 22 °C	1557	C
Teniposide	BR	0.1 mg/mL[a]	BW	0.1 mg/mL[a]	Physically compatible for 4 hr at 23 °C	1725	C
Thiotepa	LE	10 mg/mL[b]	BW	0.1 mg/mL[b]	Physically compatible for 3 hr at 22 °C	1557	C
Ticarcillin disodium–clavulanate potassium	SKB	31 mg/mL[b]	BW	0.1 mg/mL[b]	Physically compatible for 3 hr at 22 °C	1557	C
Tobramycin sulfate	LI	5 mg/mL[b]	BW	0.1 mg/mL[b]	Physically compatible for 3 hr at 22 °C	1557	C
Trimethoprim–sulfamethoxazole	ES	0.8 + 4 mg/mL[b]	BW	0.1 mg/mL[b]	Physically compatible for 3 hr at 22 °C	1557	C
Vancomycin HCl	LY	10 mg/mL[b]	BW	0.1 mg/mL[b]	Physically compatible for 3 hr at 22 °C	1557	C
Vinblastine sulfate	LI	0.12 mg/mL[b]	BW	0.1 mg/mL[b]	Physically compatible for 3 hr at 22 °C	1557	C
Vincristine sulfate	LI	0.05 mg/mL[b]	BW	0.1 mg/mL[b]	Physically compatible for 3 hr at 22 °C	1557	C
Vinorelbine tartrate	BW	1 mg/mL[b]	BW	0.1 mg/mL[b]	Physically compatible for 4 hr at 22 °C	1558	C
Zidovudine	BW	4 mg/mL[b]	BW	0.1 mg/mL[b]	Physically compatible for 3 hr at 22 °C	1557	C

[a]*Tested in dextrose 5%.*
[b]*Tested in sodium chloride 0.9%.*

MEPERIDINE HYDROCHLORIDE (PETHIDINE HYDROCHLORIDE)
AHFS 28:08.08

Products — Meperidine hydrochloride is available in concentrations of 10, 25, 50, 75, and 100 mg/mL in a variety of packaging sizes and configurations, including ampuls, vials, and disposable cartridge units. (1) Some products also contain an antioxidant such as sodium metabisulfite and antibacterial preservatives such as phenol and metacresol. (4)

pH — The pH is adjusted to 3.5 to 6. (1; 4)

Osmolality — The osmolality of meperidine hydrochloride 50 mg/mL was determined to be 302 mOsm/kg. (1233)

Trade Name(s) — Demerol Hydrochloride.

Administration — Meperidine hydrochloride is administered by intramuscular injection into a large muscle mass. It may also be given subcutaneously or slowly by intravenous injection or infusion in a diluted solution. (1; 4) A 10-mg/mL concentration has been recommended for slow intravenous injection. The 10-mg/mL commercial injection does not require further dilution and is for use with a compatible infusion device. Intravenous infusion of a 1-mg/mL concentration has been used to supplement anesthesia. (4)

Stability — Meperidine hydrochloride should be stored at controlled room temperature and protected from light and freezing. (4)

Syringes — Meperidine hydrochloride (Wyeth) 5 and 10 mg/mL in dextrose 5% and sodium chloride 0.9% was packaged in 30-mL Plastipak (Becton Dickinson) syringes capped with Monoject (Sherwood) tip caps. Syringes were stored at 23 °C exposed to light and protected from light, 4 °C protected from light, and frozen at −20 °C protected from light for 12 weeks. Both concentrations at all storage conditions were stable for at least 12 weeks. (1894)

Preservative-free meperidine hydrochloride (Abbott) was diluted to concentrations of 0.25, 1, 10, 20, and 30 mg/mL with dextrose 5% and with sodium chloride 0.9%. The solutions were packaged in 60-

mL polypropylene syringes (Becton Dickinson), sealed with Luer lock caps, and stored at 22 and 4 °C for 28 days protected from light. The solutions were visually colorless and free of precipitation over the course of the study. Little or no loss of meperidine hydrochloride occurred in either solution at either temperature in 28 days. (2200)

Sorption — Meperidine hydrochloride was shown not to exhibit sorption to PVC bags and tubing, polyethylene tubing, Silastic tubing, and polypropylene syringes. (536; 606)

Central Venous Catheter — Meperidine hydrochloride (Wyeth) 4 mg/mL in dextrose 5% was found to be compatible with the ARROWg+ard Blue Plus (Arrow International) chlorhexidine-bearing triple-lumen central catheter. Essentially complete delivery of the drug was found with little or no drug loss occurring. Furthermore, chlorhexidine delivered from the catheter remained at trace amounts with no substantial increase due to the delivery of the drug through the catheter. (2335)

Compatibility Information

Solution Compatibility

Meperidine HCl

Solution	Mfr	Mfr	Conc/L	Remarks	Ref	C/I
Dextrose–Ringer's injection combinations	AB	WI	100 mg	Physically compatible	3	C
Dextrose–Ringer's injection, lactated, combinations	AB	WI	100 mg	Physically compatible	3	C
Dextrose–saline combinations	AB	WI	100 mg	Physically compatible	3	C
Dextrose 2.5%	AB	WI	100 mg	Physically compatible	3	C
Dextrose 5%	AB	WI	100 mg	Physically compatible	3	C
	TR[a]	WI	1.2 g	Physically compatible. No loss in 36 hr at 22 °C	1000	C
		DB	300 mg	Stable for at least 24 hr at 25 °C	53	C
Dextrose 10%	AB	WI	100 mg	Physically compatible	3	C
Ionosol products	AB	WI	100 mg	Physically compatible	3	C
Ringer's injection	AB	WI	100 mg	Physically compatible	3	C
Ringer's injection, lactated	AB	WI	100 mg	Physically compatible	3	C
Sodium chloride 0.18%		DB	300 mg	Stable for at least 24 hr at 25 °C	53	C
Sodium chloride 0.45%	AB	WI	100 mg	Physically compatible	3	C
Sodium chloride 0.9%	AB	WI	100 mg	Physically compatible	3	C
	FRE[a]		2.5 g	Visually compatible with little or no loss in 24 days at room temperature	1791	C
		DB	300 mg	Stable for at least 24 hr at 25 °C	53	C
	BA	SW	10 g	No loss occurs in 90 days at 37 °C in an implantable pump[c]	2246	C
	MAC	AGT	1 and 40 g[d]	Physically compatible with little or no loss in 30 days at room temperature protected from light	2633	C
Sodium lactate ⅙ M	AB	WI	100 mg	Physically compatible	3	C
TPN #71[b]	[a]	WI	100 mg	Physically compatible. No loss in 36 hr at 22 °C	1000	C

[a]Tested in PVC containers.
[b]Refer to Appendix I for the composition of parenteral nutrition solutions. TPN indicates a 2-in-1 admixture.
[c]Tested in an Infusaid implantable pump.
[d]Tested in Deltec medication cassettes.

Additive Compatibility

Meperidine HCl

Drug	Mfr	Conc/L	Mfr	Conc/L	Test Soln	Remarks	Ref	C/I
Cefazolin sodium	FUJ	10 g		0.5 g	D5W	Visually compatible. 5% loss of each drug in 5 days at 25 °C. 5% cefazolin and 7% meperidine loss in 20 days at 4 °C	1966	C
Clonidine HCl	BI	3 mg		8 g	NS[a]	Visually compatible with no loss of either drug in 21 days at room temperature	2710	C
Dobutamine HCl	LI	1 g	ES	50 g	D5W, NS	Physically compatible for 24 hr at 21 °C	812	C
Floxacillin sodium	BE	20 g	RC	5 g	W	Haze forms immediately and precipitate forms in 5 to 24 hr	1479	I
Furosemide	HO	1 g	RC	5 g	W	Fine precipitate forms immediately	1479	I
Metoclopramide HCl	DW	150 mg	DW	7.35 g	D5W, NS	Visually compatible. Little loss of drugs over 48 hr at 32 °C in light or dark	2253	C
Ondansetron HCl	GL	100 mg and 1 g	WY	4 g	NS[a]	Physically compatible. No loss of either drug in 31 days at 4 and 22 °C and in 7 days at 32 °C	1862	C
Scopolamine HBr		0.43 mg	WI	100 mg		Physically compatible	3	C
Sodium bicarbonate	AB	2.4 mEq[b]	WI	100 mg	D5W	Physically compatible for 24 hr	772	C
Succinylcholine chloride	AB	2 g	WI	100 mg		Physically compatible	3	C
Verapamil HCl	KN	80 mg	WI	150 mg	D5W, NS	Physically compatible for 24 hr	764	C

[a]Tested in PVC containers.
[b]One vial of Neut added to a liter of admixture.

Drugs in Syringe Compatibility

Meperidine HCl

Drug (in syringe)	Mfr	Amt	Mfr	Amt	Remarks	Ref	C/I
Atropine sulfate		0.6 mg/ 1.5 mL	WY	100 mg/ 1 mL	Physically compatible for at least 15 min	14	C
	ST	0.4 mg/ 1 mL	WI	50 mg/ 1 mL	Physically compatible for at least 15 min	326	C
Butorphanol tartrate	BR	4 mg/ 2 mL	WI	50 mg/ 1 mL	Physically compatible for 30 min at room temperature	566	C
Chlorpromazine HCl	SKF	50 mg/ 2 mL	WY	100 mg/ 1 mL	Physically compatible for at least 15 min	14	C
	PO	50 mg/ 2 mL	WI	50 mg/ 1 mL	Physically compatible for at least 15 min	326	C
Dimenhydrinate	HR	50 mg/ 1 mL	WI	50 mg/ 1 mL	Physically compatible for at least 15 min	326	C
Diphenhydramine HCl	PD	50 mg/ 1 mL	WY	100 mg/ 1 mL	Physically compatible for at least 15 min	14	C
	PD	50 mg/ 1 mL	WI	50 mg/ 1 mL	Physically compatible for at least 15 min	326	C
Droperidol	MN	2.5 mg/ 1 mL	WI	50 mg/ 1 mL	Physically compatible for at least 15 min	326	C
Fentanyl citrate	MN	0.05 mg/ 1 mL	WI	50 mg/ 1 mL	Physically compatible for at least 15 min	326	C

Drugs in Syringe Compatibility (Cont.)

Meperidine HCl

Drug (in syringe)	Mfr	Amt	Mfr	Amt	Remarks	Ref	C/I
Glycopyrrolate	RB	0.2 mg/ 1 mL	WI	50 mg/ 1 mL	Physically compatible. pH in glycopyrrolate stability range for 48 hr at 25 °C	331	C
	RB	0.2 mg/ 1 mL	WI	100 mg/ 2 mL	Physically compatible. pH in glycopyrrolate stability range for 48 hr at 25 °C	331	C
	RB	0.4 mg/ 2 mL	WI	50 mg/ 1 mL	Physically compatible. pH in glycopyrrolate stability range for 48 hr at 25 °C	331	C
Heparin sodium		2500 units/ 1 mL	HO	100 mg/ 2 mL	Turbidity or precipitate forms within 5 min	1053	I
Hydroxyzine HCl	PF	100 mg/ 4 mL	WY	100 mg/ 1 mL	Physically compatible for at least 15 min	14	C
	PF	50 mg/ 1 mL	WI	50 mg/ 1 mL	Physically compatible for at least 15 min	326	C
	PF	50 mg/ 1 mL	WI	100 mg/ 2 mL	Physically compatible	771	C
	PF	100 mg/ 2 mL	WI	50 mg/ 1 mL	Physically compatible	771	C
Ketamine HCl	PD	2 mg/mL	DB	12 mg/ mL	Diluted to 50 mL with NS. Visually compatible for 48 hr at 25 °C	2059	C
Metoclopramide HCl	NO	10 mg/ 2 mL	WI	50 mg/ 1 mL	Physically compatible for 15 min at room temperature	565	C
	DW	10 mg/ 2 mL	DW	50 mg/ 1 mL	Visually compatible. Little loss of either drug over 48 hr at 32 °C in light or dark	2253	C
Midazolam HCl	RC	5 mg/ 1 mL	WB	100 mg/ 1 mL	Physically compatible for 4 hr at 25 °C	1145	C
Morphine sulfate	ST	15 mg/ 1 mL	WI	50 mg/ 1 mL	Physically incompatible within 15 min	326	I
Ondansetron HCl	GW	1.33 mg/ mL[a]	ES	8.33 mg/ mL[a]	Physically compatible. Little loss of either drug in 24 hr at 4 or 23 °C	2199	C
Pantoprazole sodium	[b]	4 mg/ 1 mL		100 mg/ 1 mL	Yellowish precipitate within 15 min	2574	I
Pentazocine lactate	WI	30 mg/ 1 mL	WI	50 mg/ 1 mL	Physically compatible for at least 15 min	326	C
Pentobarbital sodium	WY	100 mg/ 2 mL	WY	100 mg/ 1 mL	Precipitate forms within 15 min	14	I
	AB	500 mg/ 10 mL	WI	100 mg/ 2 mL	Physically incompatible	55	I
	AB	50 mg/ 1 mL	WI	50 mg/ 1 mL	Physically incompatible within 15 min	326	I
Prochlorperazine edisylate	SKF		WY	100 mg/ 1 mL	Physically compatible for at least 15 min	14	C
	PO	5 mg/ 1 mL	WI	50 mg/ 1 mL	Physically compatible for at least 15 min	326	C
Promethazine HCl	WY	50 mg/ 2 mL	WY	100 mg/ 1 mL	Physically compatible for at least 15 min	14	C
	PO	50 mg/ 2 mL	WI	50 mg/ 1 mL	Physically compatible for at least 15 min	326	C
Ranitidine HCl	GL	50 mg/ 2 mL	WI	100 mg/ 1 mL	Physically compatible for 1 hr at 25 °C	978	C

Drugs in Syringe Compatibility (Cont.)

Meperidine HCl

Drug (in syringe)	Mfr	Amt	Mfr	Amt	Remarks	Ref	C/I
Scopolamine HBr		0.6 mg/ 1.5 mL	WY	100 mg/ 1 mL	Physically compatible for at least 15 min	14	C
	ST	0.4 mg/ 1 mL	WI	50 mg/ 1 mL	Physically compatible for at least 15 min	326	C

[a] Tested in sodium chloride 0.9%.
[b] Test performed using the formulation WITHOUT edetate disodium.

Y-Site Injection Compatibility (1:1 Mixture)

Meperidine HCl

Drug	Mfr	Conc	Mfr	Conc	Remarks	Ref	C/I
Acyclovir sodium	BW	5 mg/mL[a]	WB	1 mg/mL[a]	Physically compatible for 4 hr at 25 °C	1157	C
	BW	5 mg/mL[a]	AB	10 mg/mL	White crystalline precipitate forms within 1 hr at 25 °C	1397	I
	BW	5 mg/mL[a,b]	WY	100 mg/mL	Visually compatible for 24 hr at room temperature in test tubes. No precipitate found on filter from Y-site delivery	2063	C
Allopurinol sodium	BW	3 mg/mL[b]	WY	4 mg/mL[b]	Tiny particles form immediately and increase in number over 4 hr	1686	I
Amifostine	USB	10 mg/mL[a]	WY	4 mg/mL[a]	Physically compatible for 4 hr at 23 °C	1845	C
Amikacin sulfate	BR	5 mg/mL[a]	WY	10 mg/mL[a]	Physically compatible for 4 hr at 25 °C	987	C
Amphotericin B cholesteryl sulfate complex	SEQ	0.83 mg/mL[a]	AST	4 mg/mL[a]	Increased turbidity forms immediately.	2117	I
Ampicillin sodium	BR	20 mg/mL[b]	WY	10 mg/mL[a]	Physically compatible for 4 hr at 25 °C	987	C
Ampicillin sodium–sulbactam sodium	RR	20 + 10 mg/ mL[b]	WY	10 mg/mL[b]	Physically compatible for 1 hr at 25 °C	1338	C
Anidulafungin	VIC	0.5 mg/mL[a]	AB	10 mg/mL[a]	Physically compatible for 4 hr at 23 °C	2617	C
Aztreonam	SQ	20 mg/mL[a]	AB	10 mg/mL	Physically compatible for 4 hr at 25 °C	1397	C
	SQ	40 mg/mL[a]	WY	4 mg/mL[a]	Physically compatible for 4 hr at 23 °C	1758	C
Bivalirudin	TMC	5 mg/mL[a]	AST	10 mg/mL[a]	Physically compatible for 4 hr at 23 °C	2373	C
Bumetanide	RC	0.25 mg/mL	AB	10 mg/mL	Physically compatible for 4 hr at 25 °C	1397	C
Caspofungin acetate	ME	0.7 mg/mL[b]	HOS	10 mg/mL[b]	Physically compatible for 4 hr at room temperature	2758	C
Cefazolin sodium	SKF	20 mg/mL[a]	WY	10 mg/mL[a]	Physically compatible for 4 hr at 25 °C	987	C
Cefotaxime sodium	HO	20 mg/mL[a]	WY	10 mg/mL[a]	Physically compatible for 4 hr at 25 °C	987	C
Cefotetan disodium	STU	20 and 40 mg/mL[a]	WY	10 mg/mL[b]	Physically compatible for 1 hr at 25 °C	1338	C
Cefoxitin sodium	MSD	20 mg/mL[a]	WY	10 mg/mL[a]	Physically compatible for 4 hr at 25 °C	987	C
	MSD	40 mg/mL[a]	WY	10 mg/mL[b]	Physically compatible for 1 hr at 25 °C	1338	C
Ceftaroline fosamil	FOR	2.22 mg/ mL[a,b,c]	HOS	10 mg/mL[a,b,c]	Physically compatible for 4 hr at 23 °C	2826	C
Ceftazidime	LI	20 and 40 mg/mL[a]	AB	10 mg/mL	Physically compatible for 4 hr at 25 °C	1397	C
Ceftriaxone sodium	RC	20 and 40 mg/mL[a]	AB	10 mg/mL	Physically compatible for 4 hr at 25 °C	1397	C

Y-Site Injection Compatibility (1:1 Mixture) (Cont.)

Meperidine HCl

Drug	Mfr	Conc	Mfr	Conc	Remarks	Ref	C/I
Cefuroxime sodium	GL	30 mg/mL[a]	WY	10 mg/mL[a]	Physically compatible for 4 hr at 25 °C	987	C
Chloramphenicol sodium succinate	LY	20 mg/mL[a]	WY	10 mg/mL[a]	Physically compatible for 4 hr at 25 °C	987	C
Cisatracurium besylate	GW	0.1, 2, 5 mg/mL[a]	AST	4 mg/mL[a]	Physically compatible for 4 hr at 23 °C	2074	C
Cladribine	ORT	0.015[b] and 0.5[e] mg/mL	WY	4 mg/mL[b]	Physically compatible for 4 hr at 23 °C	1969	C
Clindamycin phosphate	UP	12 mg/mL[a]	WY	10 mg/mL[a]	Physically compatible for 4 hr at 25 °C	987	C
Dexamethasone sodium phosphate	LY	0.2 mg/mL[a]	AB	10 mg/mL	Physically compatible for 4 hr at 25 °C	1397	C
Dexmedetomidine HCl	AB	4 mcg/mL[b]	AST	10 mg/mL[b]	Physically compatible for 4 hr at 23 °C	2383	C
Digoxin	BW	0.25 mg/mL	AB	10 mg/mL	Physically compatible for 4 hr at 25 °C	1397	C
Diltiazem HCl	MMD	1[b] and 5 mg/mL	WY	100 mg/mL	Visually compatible	1807	C
	MMD	5 mg/mL	WY	10 mg/mL[b]	Visually compatible	1807	C
Diphenhydramine HCl	ES	1[a] and 50 mg/mL	AB	10 mg/mL	Physically compatible for 4 hr at 25 °C	1397	C
Dobutamine HCl	LI	1 mg/mL	AB	10 mg/mL	Physically compatible for 4 hr at 25 °C	1397	C
Docetaxel	RPR	0.9 mg/mL[a]	AST	4 mg/mL[a]	Physically compatible for 4 hr at 23 °C	2224	C
Dopamine HCl	AB	1.6 mg/mL	AB	10 mg/mL	Physically compatible for 4 hr at 25 °C	1397	C
Doripenem	JJ	5 mg/mL[a,b]	HOS	10 mg/mL[a,b]	Physically compatible for 4 hr at 23 °C	2743	C
Doxorubicin HCl liposomal	SEQ	0.4 mg/mL[a]	AST	4 mg/mL[a]	Increase in measured turbidity	2087	I
Doxycycline hyclate	ES	1 mg/mL[a]	WY	10 mg/mL[a]	Physically compatible for 4 hr at 25 °C	987	C
Droperidol	AMR	2.5 mg/mL[a]	AB	10 mg/mL	Physically compatible for 4 hr at 25 °C	1397	C
Erythromycin lactobionate	AB	5 mg/mL[a]	WY	10 mg/mL[a]	Physically compatible for 4 hr at 25 °C	987	C
Etoposide phosphate	BR	5 mg/mL[a]	AST	4 mg/mL[a]	Physically compatible for 4 hr at 23 °C	2218	C
Famotidine	MSD	0.2 mg/mL[a]	AB	10 mg/mL	Physically compatible for 4 hr at 25 °C	1397	C
	ME	2 mg/mL[b]		4 mg/mL[a]	Visually compatible for 4 hr at 22 °C	1936	C
Fenoldopam mesylate	AB	80 mcg/mL[b]	AB	4 mg/mL[b]	Physically compatible for 4 hr at 23 °C	2467	C
Filgrastim	AMG	30 mcg/mL[a]	WY	4 mg/mL[a]	Physically compatible for 4 hr at 22 °C	1687	C
Fluconazole	RR	2 mg/mL	AB	10 mg/mL	Physically compatible for 4 hr at 25 °C	1397	C
Fludarabine phosphate	BX	1 mg/mL[a]	WI	4 mg/mL[a]	Visually compatible for 4 hr at 22 °C	1439	C
Furosemide	ES	0.8 mg/mL[a]	AB	10 mg/mL	Physically compatible for 4 hr at 25 °C	1397	C
	ES	2.4 mg/mL[a]	AB	10 mg/mL	White cloudiness forms immediately	1397	I
	ES	10 mg/mL	AB	10 mg/mL	White precipitate forms immediately	1397	I
Gallium nitrate	FUJ	1 mg/mL[b]	WY	50 mg/mL	Visually compatible for 24 hr at 25 °C	1673	C
Gemcitabine HCl	LI	10 mg/mL[b]	AST	4 mg/mL[b]	Physically compatible for 4 hr at 23 °C	2226	C
Gentamicin sulfate	TR	0.8 mg/mL[a]	WY	10 mg/mL[a]	Physically compatible for 4 hr at 25 °C	987	C
	ES	1.2 and 2 mg/mL[b]	WY	10 mg/mL[b]	Physically compatible for 1 hr at 25 °C	1338	C
Granisetron HCl	SKB	0.05 mg/mL[a]	WY	4 mg/mL[a]	Physically compatible for 4 hr at 23 °C	2000	C
Heparin sodium	ES	60 units/mL[a]	WY	10 mg/mL[b]	Physically compatible for 1 hr at 25 °C	1338	C
Hetastarch in lactated electrolyte	AB	6%	OHM	4 mg/mL[a]	Physically compatible for 4 hr at 23 °C	2339	C

Y-Site Injection Compatibility (1:1 Mixture) (Cont.)

Meperidine HCl

Drug	Mfr	Conc	Mfr	Conc	Remarks	Ref	C/I
Hydrocortisone sodium succinate	AB	2 mg/mL[a]	AB	10 mg/mL	Physically compatible for 4 hr at 25 °C	1397	C
Hydroxyethyl starch 130/0.4 in sodium chloride 0.9%	FRK	6%	SZ	1, 5, 10 mg/mL[a]	Visually compatible for 24 hr at room temperature	2770	C
Idarubicin HCl	AD	1 mg/mL[b]	WY	1[a] and 50 mg/mL	Color changes immediately	1525	I
Imipenem–cilastatin sodium	MSD	5 mg/mL[a]	AB	10 mg/mL	Yellow color forms in 2 hr at 25 °C	1397	I
Insulin, regular	LI	0.2 unit/mL[b]	WY	10 mg/mL[b]	Physically compatible for 1 hr at 25 °C	1338	C
	LI	0.2 unit/mL[b]	AST	50 mg/mL[a]	Physically compatible for 2 hr at 25 °C	1395	C
Labetalol HCl	GL	5 mg/mL	AB	10 mg/mL	Physically compatible for 4 hr at 25 °C	1397	C
Lidocaine HCl	AB	1 mg/mL[a]	AB	10 mg/mL	Physically compatible for 4 hr at 25 °C	1397	C
Linezolid	PHU	2 mg/mL	AST	4 mg/mL[a]	Physically compatible for 4 hr at 23 °C	2264	C
Magnesium sulfate	LY	16.7, 33.3, 50, 100 mg/mL[a]	WI	10 mg/mL[a]	Visually compatible for 4 hr at 25 °C	1549	C
Melphalan HCl	BW	0.1 mg/mL[b]	WY	4 mg/mL[b]	Physically compatible for 3 hr at 22 °C	1557	C
Methyldopate HCl	AMR	2.5 mg/mL[a]	AB	10 mg/mL	Physically compatible for 4 hr at 25 °C	1397	C
Methylprednisolone sodium succinate	UP	2.5 mg/mL[a]	AB	10 mg/mL	Physically compatible for 4 hr at 25 °C	1397	C
Metoclopramide HCl	SN	0.2 mg/mL[a]	AB	10 mg/mL	Physically compatible for 4 hr at 25 °C	1397	C
Metoprolol tartrate	CI	1 mg/mL	AB	10 mg/mL	Physically compatible for 4 hr at 25 °C	1397	C
Metronidazole	SE	5 mg/mL	WY	10 mg/mL	Physically compatible for 4 hr at 25 °C	987	C
Micafungin sodium	ASP	1.5 mg/mL[b]	AB	10 mg/mL[b]	Milky precipitate forms immediately	2683	I
Nafcillin sodium	WY	20 mg/mL[a]	WY	10 mg/mL[a]	Cloudy haze cleared on mixing and remained clear for 4 hr at 25 °C	987	?
	WY	20 and 30 mg/mL[a]	WY	10 mg/mL[b]	Cloudy solution formed immediately and persisted for at least 1 hr at 25 °C	1338	I
Nesiritide	SCI	50 mcg/mL[a,b]		100 mg/mL	Physically compatible for 4 hr. May be chemically incompatible with nesiritide[f]	2625	?
Ondansetron HCl	GL	1 mg/mL[b]	WI	4 mg/mL[a]	Visually compatible for 4 hr at 22 °C	1365	C
Oxacillin sodium	BE	20 mg/mL[a]	WY	10 mg/mL[a]	Physically compatible for 4 hr at 25 °C	987	C
Oxaliplatin	SS	0.5 mg/mL[a]	AB	10 mg/mL[a]	Physically compatible for 4 hr at 23 °C	2566	C
Oxytocin	PD	0.02 unit/mL[h]	WY	10 mg/mL[b]	Physically compatible for 1 hr at 25 °C	1338	C
Paclitaxel	NCI	1.2 mg/mL[a]	WY	4 mg/mL[a]	Physically compatible for 4 hr at 22 °C	1556	C
Palonosetron HCl	MGI	50 mcg/mL	AB	10 mg/mL[a]	Physically compatible. No loss of either drug in 4 hr	2720	C
Pemetrexed disodium	LI	20 mg/mL[b]	AB	10 mg/mL[a]	Physically compatible for 4 hr at 23 °C	2564	C
Penicillin G potassium	PF	100,000 units/mL[a]	WY	10 mg/mL[a]	Physically compatible for 4 hr at 25 °C	987	C
Piperacillin sodium–tazobactam sodium	LE[d]	40 + 5 mg/mL[a]	WY	4 mg/mL[a]	Physically compatible for 4 hr at 22 °C	1688	C
Potassium chloride	AB	0.4 mEq/mL[a]	AB	10 mg/mL	Physically compatible for 4 hr at 25 °C	1397	C
Propofol	ZEN	10 mg/mL	WY	4 mg/mL[a]	Physically compatible for 1 hr at 23 °C	2066	C
Propranolol HCl	WY	1 mg/mL	AB	10 mg/mL	Physically compatible for 4 hr at 25 °C	1397	C

Y-Site Injection Compatibility (1:1 Mixture) (Cont.)

Meperidine HCl

Drug	Mfr	Conc	Mfr	Conc	Remarks	Ref	C/I
Ranitidine HCl	GL	0.5 mg/mL[i]	WY	10 mg/mL[b]	Physically compatible for 1 hr at 25 °C	1338	C
Remifentanil HCl	GW	0.025 and 0.25 mg/mL[b]	AST	4 mg/mL[a]	Physically compatible for 4 hr at 23 °C	2075	C
Sargramostim	IMM	10 mcg/mL[b]	WI	4 mg/mL[b]	Visually compatible for 4 hr at 22 °C	1436	C
Teniposide	BR	0.1 mg/mL[a]	WY	4 mg/mL[a]	Physically compatible for 4 hr at 23 °C	1725	C
Thiotepa	IMM[j]	1 mg/mL[a]	WY	4 mg/mL[a]	Physically compatible for 4 hr at 23 °C	1861	C
Ticarcillin disodium–clavulanate potassium	BE	31 mg/mL[b]	WY	10 mg/mL[b]	Physically compatible for 1 hr at 25 °C	1338	C
TNA #218 to #226[g]			AST	4 mg/mL[a]	Visually compatible for 4 hr at 23 °C	2215	C
Tobramycin sulfate	DI	0.8 mg/mL[a]	WY	10 mg/mL[a]	Physically compatible for 4 hr at 25 °C	987	C
	LI	1.6, 2, 2.4 mg/mL[a]	WY	10 mg/mL[b]	Physically compatible for 1 hr at 25 °C	1338	C
TPN #131, #132[g]			AB	10 mg/mL	Physically compatible for 4 hr at 25 °C	1397	C
TPN #189[g]			DB	50 mg/mL	Visually compatible for 24 hr at 22 °C	1767	C
TPN #212 to #215[g]			AST	4 mg/mL[a]	Physically compatible for 4 hr at 23 °C	2109	C
Trimethoprim–sulfamethoxazole	BW	0.8 + 4 mg/mL[a]	WY	10 mg/mL[a]	Physically compatible for 4 hr at 25 °C	987	C
Vancomycin HCl	LI	5 mg/mL[a]	WY	10 mg/mL[a]	Physically compatible for 4 hr at 25 °C	987	C
Verapamil HCl	DU	2.5 mg/mL	AB	10 mg/mL	Physically compatible for 4 hr at 25 °C	1397	C
Vinorelbine tartrate	BW	1 mg/mL[b]	WY	4 mg/mL[b]	Physically compatible for 4 hr at 22 °C	1558	C

[a]*Tested in dextrose 5%.*
[b]*Tested in sodium chloride 0.9%.*
[c]*Tested in Ringer's injection, lactated.*
[d]*Test performed using the formulation WITHOUT edetate disodium.*
[e]*Tested in bacteriostatic sodium chloride 0.9% preserved with benzyl alcohol 0.9%.*
[f]*Nesiritide is incompatible with bisulfite antioxidants used in some drug formulations. The specific formulation of the product to be used should be checked to ensure that no sulfite antioxidants are present.*
[g]*Refer to Appendix I for the composition of parenteral nutrition solutions. TNA indicates a 3-in-1 admixture, and TPN indicates a 2-in-1 admixture.*
[h]*Tested in dextrose 5% in Ringer's injection, lactated.*
[i]*Tested in sodium chloride 0.45%.*
[j]*Lyophilized formulation tested.*

Additional Compatibility Information

Chlorpromazine and Hydroxyzine — Chlorpromazine hydrochloride (Elkins-Sinn) 6.25 mg/mL, hydroxyzine hydrochloride (Pfizer) 12.5 mg/mL, and meperidine hydrochloride (Winthrop) 25 mg/mL, in both glass and plastic syringes, have been reported to be physically compatible and chemically stable for at least one year at 4 and 25 °C when protected from light. (989)

Chlorpromazine and Promethazine — Chlorpromazine hydrochloride, meperidine hydrochloride, and promethazine hydrochloride combined as an extemporaneous mixture for preoperative sedation, developed a brownish-yellow color after two weeks of storage with protection from light. The discoloration was attributed to the meta-cresol preservative content of the meperidine hydrochloride product used. Use of meperidine hydrochloride which contains a different preservative resulted in a solution that remained clear and colorless for at least three months when protected from light. (1148)

MEPIVACAINE HYDROCHLORIDE
AHFS 72:00

Products — Mepivacaine hydrochloride is available in concentrations of 1, 1.5, and 2.0%. Methylparaben is incorporated into multiple-dose containers, but single-dose containers may be preservative free. The pH may have been adjusted with sodium hydroxide and/or hydrochloric acid. (1; 4)

pH — From 4.5 to 6.8. (1; 4)

Osmolality — Mepivacaine hydrochloride injections are isotonic. (1)

Trade Name(s) — Carbocaine, Polocaine, Polocaine-MPF.

Administration — Mepivacaine hydrochloride may be administered by infiltration and by peripheral or sympathetic nerve block. Mepivacaine hydrochloride *without* preservatives may be administered by epidural block, including caudal anesthesia; forms containing preservatives should not be administered by this route (4).

Stability — Mepivacaine hydrochloride in intact containers should be stored at controlled room temperature and protected from temperatures above 40 °C and from freezing. Mepivacaine hydrochloride is resistant to hydrolysis and may be autoclaved repeatedly. (1; 4) However, mepivacaine hydrochloride in dental cartridges should not be subjected to autoclaving because of breakdown of the dental cartridge closures. (4)

Syringes — The stability of mepivacaine (salt form unspecified) 10 mg/mL repackaged in polypropylene syringes was evaluated. Little change in concentration was found after four weeks of storage at room temperature not exposed to direct light. (2164)

Compatibility Information

Drugs in Syringe Compatibility

Mepivacaine HCl

Drug (in syringe)	Mfr	Amt	Mfr	Amt	Remarks	Ref	C/I
Sodium bicarbonate	AB	4%; 1, 2, 4 mL	AST, WI	1 and 1.5%/ 20 mL	Precipitate forms within approximately 1 hr	1724	**I**
	AST	8.4%; 0.5, 1, 2 mL	AST, WI	1 and 1.5%/ 20 mL	Precipitate forms within approximately 1 hr	1724	**I**

MEROPENEM
AHFS 8:12.07.08

Products — Meropenem is available in dosage forms containing 500 mg and 1 g of drug along with sodium carbonate. (1)

Reconstitute the 500-mg vials with 10 mL and the 1-g vials with 20 mL of sterile water for injection, shake the vial, and allow it to stand until the solution is clear. Each milliliter of the resultant solution contains 50 mg of meropenem. (1)

pH — The reconstituted solution has a pH from 7.3 to 8.3. (1)

Sodium Content — Each gram of meropenem provides 3.92 mEq (90.2 mg) of sodium from the sodium carbonate present in the formulation. (1)

Trade Name(s) — Merrem.

Administration — Meropenem is administered by direct intravenous injection of 5 to 20 mL over three to five minutes or by intravenous infusion diluted in a compatible infusion solution over 15 to 30 minutes. (1)

Stability — Intact vials should be stored at controlled room temperature between 20 and 25 °C. The drug is a white to pale yellow powder that yields a colorless to yellow solution on reconstitution. (1)

The manufacturer indicates that reconstituted solutions in vials of meropenem up to 50 mg/mL in sterile water for injection are stable for two hours at room temperature and up to 12 hours under refrigeration. The infusion vials diluted in sodium chloride 0.9% to a meropenem concentration of 2.5 to 50 mg/mL are stated to be stable for two hours at room temperature and 18 hours under refrigeration; in dextrose 5% at these concentrations, stability is only one hour at room temperature and eight hours under refrigeration. (1)

Meropenem 50 mg/mL reconstituted with sodium chloride 0.9% is reported to reach 10% loss in 4.8 hours at 25 °C. (2697)

Solutions of meropenem 2.5 to 20 mg/mL in sodium chloride 0.9% in the Minibag Plus (Baxter) are stable for up to four hours at room temperature and up to 24 hours under refrigeration. In dextrose 5% in the same concentration range, the drug is stable for only one hour at room temperature and up to six hours under refrigeration. (1)

In addition, the manufacturer notes that meropenem 1 to 20 mg/mL in sterile water for injection or sodium chloride 0.9% is stable for up to four hours and in dextrose 5% for up to two hours at room temperature in plastic administration set tubing, drip chambers, and volume control devices. (1)

The manufacturer notes that meropenem 1 to 20 mg/mL in sterile water for injection or sodium chloride 0.9% is stable for up to 48 hours and in dextrose 5% for up to six hours in plastic syringes stored under refrigeration. (1)

Central Venous Catheter — Meropenem (Zeneca) 5 mg/mL in sodium chloride 0.9% was found to be compatible with the ARROWg+ard Blue Plus (Arrow International) chlorhexidine-bearing triple-lumen central catheter. Essentially complete delivery of the drug was found with little or no drug loss occurring. Furthermore, chlorhexidine delivered from the catheter remained at trace amounts with no substantial increase due to the delivery of the drug through the catheter. (2335)

Compatibility Information

Solution Compatibility

Meropenem

Solution	Mfr	Mfr	Conc/L	Remarks	Ref	C/I
Dextrose 5% with potassium chloride 0.15%	BA[a]	ZEN	1 g	10 to 11% loss in 4 hr at 24 °C and in 18 hr at 4 °C	2089	I[c]
	BA[a]	ZEN	20 g	8 to 10% loss in 3 hr at 24 °C and in 18 hr at 4 °C	2089	I[c]
Dextrose 5% in Ringer's injection, lactated	BA[a]	ZEN	1 g	11% loss in 8 hr at 24 °C and 4 to 10% loss in 48 hr at 4 °C	2089	I[c]
	BA[a]	ZEN	20 g	15% loss in 4 hr at 24 °C and 10% loss in 18 hr at 4 °C	2089	I[c]
Dextrose 5% with sodium bicarbonate 0.02%	BA[a]	ZEN	1 g	11% loss in 4 hr at 24 °C and 9% in 18 hr at 4 °C	2089	I[c]
	BA[a]	ZEN	20 g	10 to 12% loss in 3 hr at 24 °C and 10% loss in 20 hr at 4 °C	2089	I[c]
Dextrose 2.5% in sodium chloride 0.45%	BA[a]	ZEN	1 g	10% loss in 6 hr at 24 °C and 7% loss in 24 hr at 4 °C	2089	I[c]
	BA[a]	ZEN	20 g	8% loss in 4 hr at 24 °C and 7% loss in 24 hr at 4 °C	2089	I[c]
Dextrose 5% in sodium chloride 0.2%	BA[a]	ZEN	1 g	10 to 11% loss in 4 hr at 24 °C and in 16 hr at 4 °C	2089	I[c]
	BA[a]	ZEN	20 g	Up to 10% loss in 3 hr at 24 °C and 9% loss in 18 hr at 4 °C	2089	I[c]
Dextrose 5% in sodium chloride 0.9%	BA[a]	ZEN	1 g	11 to 13% loss in 4 hr at 24 °C and in 14 hr at 4 °C	2089	I[c]
	BA[a]	ZEN	20 g	9 to 11% loss in 3 hr at 24 °C and in 14 hr at 4 °C	2089	I[c]
Dextrose 5%	BA[a]	ZEN	1 g	9% loss in 4 hr at 24 °C and in 14 hr at 4 °C	2089	I[c]
	BA[b]	ZEN	2.5 g	6 to 7% loss in 4 hr at 24 °C and 8 to 10% in 24 hr at 4 °C	2089	I[c]
	BA[a]	ZEN	20 g	11 to 12% loss in 4 hr at 24 °C and in 18 hr at 4 °C	2089	I[c]
	BA[b]	ZEN	50 g	9 to 10% loss in 3 hr at 24 °C and in 24 hr at 4 °C	2089	I[c]
	[a]	ZEN	1 g	Visually compatible. Calculated time to 10% loss in 4.5 hr at 23 °C, 1.8 days at 4 °C, and 1.2 days at −20 °C	2492	I
	[a]	ZEN	22 g	Visually compatible. Calculated time to 10% loss in 8 hr at 23 °C, 2.1 days at 4 °C, and 7.8 days at −20 °C	2492	I
Dextrose 10%	BA[a]	ZEN	1 g	10 to 12% loss in 3 hr at 24 °C and in 8 hr at 4 °C	2089	I[c]
	BA[a]	ZEN	20 g	9 to 10% loss in 2 hr at 24 °C and in 8 hr at 4 °C	2089	I[c]
Normosol M with dextrose 5%	AB[a]	ZEN	1 g	5% loss in 8 hr at 24 °C and 4% loss in 48 hr at 4 °C	2089	I[c]
	AB[a]	ZEN	20 g	10% loss in 3 hr at 24 °C and 7 to 8% loss in 24 hr at 4 °C	2089	I[c]
Ringer's injection	BA[a]	ZEN	1 g	6% loss in 10 hr at 24 °C and 4 to 5% loss in 48 hr at 4 °C	2089	I[c]

Solution Compatibility (Cont.)

Meropenem

Solution	Mfr	Mfr	Conc/L	Remarks	Ref	C/I
	BA[a]	ZEN	20 g	7% loss in 8 hr at 24 °C and 7% loss in 48 hr at 4 °C	2089	I[c]
Ringer's injection, lactated	BA[a]	ZEN	1 g	10 to 12% loss in 10 hr at 24 °C and 9% loss in 48 hr at 4 °C	2089	I[c]
	BA[a]	ZEN	20 g	9% loss in 8 hr at 24 °C and 7% loss in 48 hr at 4 °C	2089	I[c]
Sodium chloride 0.45%	AB[d]	ZEN	5 g	9 to 10% loss in 22 hr at 24 °C and 3% loss in 48 hr at 4 °C	2089	I[c]
	AB[d]	ZEN	20 g	6 to 8% loss in 10 hr at 24 °C and 5 to 6% loss in 48 hr at 4 °C	2089	I[c]
Sodium chloride 0.9%	BA[a]	ZEN	1 g	8 to 10% loss in 20 hr at 24 °C and 3 to 4% loss in 48 hr at 4 °C	2089	I[c]
	BA[b]	ZEN	2.5 g	10% loss in 24 hr at 24 °C and 2% loss in 48 hr at 4 °C	2089	C
	BA[a]	ZEN	20 g	8% loss in 10 hr at 24 °C and 5 to 7% loss in 48 hr at 4 °C	2089	I[c]
	BA[b]	ZEN	50 g	9 to 10% loss in 8 hr at 24 °C and in 48 hr at 4 °C	2089	I[c]
	[e]	ZEN	20 and 30 g	Less than 3% loss in 24 hr when kept at less than 5 °C	2261	C
	[h]	ZEN	5 g	Visually compatible. Calculated times to 10% loss were 34 hr at 24 °C and 120 hr at 5 °C	2151	C
	[h]	ZEN	10 g	Visually compatible. Calculated times to 10% loss were 20 hr at 24 °C and 120 hr at 5 °C	2151	C
	[a]	ZEN	1 g	Visually compatible. Calculated time to 10% loss in 22 hr at 23 °C, 10.7 days at 4 °C, and 33.4 days at −20 °C	2492	I
	[a]	ZEN	22 g	Visually compatible. Calculated time to 10% loss in 17 hr at 23 °C, 4.9 days at 4 °C, and 11.4 days at −20 °C	2492	I
		ASZ	5 g	6% loss in 8 hr at 20 °C; 12% loss in 8 hr at 37 °C	2532	C
	[f]	ASZ	30 g	No loss in 24 hr kept in a cold pouch with two freezer packs	2568	C
	[a,g]	ZEN	4 g	3 to 4% loss in 168 hr at 5 °C	2554	C
	[a,g]	ZEN	10 g	2 to 5% loss in 120 hr at 5 °C	2554	C
	[a,g]	ZEN	20 g	7% loss in 120 hr at 5 °C	2554	C
Sodium lactate ⅙ M	BA[a]	ZEN	1 g	7% loss in 8 hr at 24 °C and 6 to 7% loss in 48 hr at 4 °C	2089	I[c]
	BA[a]	ZEN	20 g	9% loss in 8 hr at 24 °C and 4 to 5% loss in 24 hr at 4 °C	2089	I[c]

[a]Tested in PVC containers.
[b]Tested in glass containers.
[c]Incompatible by conventional standards but recommended for dilution of meropenem with use in shorter periods of time.
[d]Tested in Abbott ADD-Vantage system.
[e]Tested in CADD-Plus medication cassettes.
[f]Tested in Deltec medication cassettes.
[g]Tested in Homepump Eclipse elastomeric pump reservoirs.
[h]Tested in Intermate SV elastomeric pump reservoirs.

Additive Compatibility

Meropenem

Drug	Mfr	Conc/L	Mfr	Conc/L	Test Soln	Remarks	Ref	C/I
Acyclovir sodium	BW	5 g	ZEN	1 g	NS	Visually compatible for 4 hr at room temperature	1994	C
	BW	5 g	ZEN	20 g	NS	Precipitates immediately	1994	I
Aminophylline	AMR	1 g	ZEN	1 and 20 g	NS	Visually compatible for 4 hr at room temperature	1994	C
Amphotericin B	SQ	200 mg	ZEN	1 and 20 g	NS	Precipitate forms	2068	I
Atropine sulfate	ES	40 mg	ZEN	1 and 20 g	NS	Visually compatible for 4 hr at room temperature	1994	C
Dexamethasone sodium phosphate	MSD	4 g	ZEN	1 and 20 g	NS	Visually compatible for 4 hr at room temperature	1994	C
Dobutamine HCl	LI	1 g	ZEN	1 and 20 g	NS	Visually compatible for 4 hr at room temperature	1994	C
Dopamine HCl	DU	800 mg	ZEN	1 and 20 g	NS	Visually compatible for 4 hr at room temperature	1994	C
Doxycycline hyclate	RR	200 mg	ZEN	1 g	NS	Visually compatible for 4 hr at room temperature	1994	C
	RR	200 mg	ZEN	20 g	NS	Brown discoloration forms in 1 hr at room temperature	1994	I
Enalaprilat	MSD	50 mg	ZEN	1 and 20 g	NS	Visually compatible for 4 hr at room temperature	1994	C
Fluconazole	RR	2 g	ZEN	1 and 20 g	NS	Visually compatible for 4 hr at room temperature	1994	C
Furosemide	HO	1 g	ZEN	1 and 20 g	NS	Visually compatible for 4 hr at room temperature	1994	C
Gentamicin sulfate	SC	800 mg	ZEN	1 and 20 g	NS	Visually compatible for 4 hr at room temperature	1994	C
Heparin sodium	ES	20,000 units	ZEN	1 and 20 g	NS	Visually compatible for 4 hr at room temperature	1994	C
Insulin, regular	LI	1000 units	ZEN	1 and 20 g	NS	Visually compatible for 4 hr at room temperature	1994	C
Magnesium sulfate	AST	1 g	ZEN	1 and 20 g	NS	Visually compatible for 4 hr at room temperature	1994	C
Mannitol	BA[a]	2.5%	ZEN	1 g		7 to 8% meropenem loss in 8 hr at 24 °C and in 24 hr at 4 °C	2089	I[b]
	BA[a]	2.5%	ZEN	20 g		7 to 9% meropenem loss in 4 hr at 24 °C and 6% loss in 20 hr at 4 °C	2089	I[b]
	BA[a]	10%	ZEN	1 g		10 to 11% meropenem loss in 4 hr at 24 °C and in 20 hr at 4 °C	2089	I[b]
	BA[a]	10%	ZEN	20 g		10% meropenem loss in 3 hr at 24 °C and in 20 hr at 4 °C	2089	I[b]
Metoclopramide HCl	RB	100 mg	ZEN	1 and 20 g	NS	Visually compatible for 4 hr at room temperature	1994	C
Morphine sulfate	ES	1 g	ZEN	1 and 20 g	NS	Visually compatible for 4 hr at room temperature	1994	C
Multivitamins	AST	50 mL	ZEN	1 and 20 g	NS	Color darkened in 4 hr at room temperature	1994	I

Additive Compatibility (Cont.)

Meropenem

Drug	Mfr	Conc/L	Mfr	Conc/L	Test Soln	Remarks	Ref	C/I
Norepinephrine bitartrate	WI	8 g	ZEN	1 and 20 g	NS	Visually compatible for 4 hr at room temperature	1994	C
Ondansetron HCl	GL	1 g	ZEN	1 g	NS	Visually compatible for 4 hr at room temperature	1994	C
	GL	1 g	ZEN	20 g	NS	White precipitate forms immediately	1994	I
Phenobarbital sodium	ES	200 mg	ZEN	1 and 20 g	NS	Visually compatible for 4 hr at room temperature	1994	C
Ranitidine HCl	GL	100 mg	ZEN	1 and 20 g	NS	Visually compatible for 4 hr at room temperature	1994	C
Sodium bicarbonate	BA	5%	ZEN	1 g		10% meropenem loss in 4 hr at 24 °C and 18 hr at 4 °C	2089	I[b]
	BA	5%	ZEN	20 g		9 to 10% meropenem loss in 3 hr at 24 °C and 18 hr at 4 °C	2089	I[b]
Vancomycin HCl	LI	1 g	ZEN	1 and 20 g	NS	Visually compatible for 4 hr at room temperature	1994	C
Zidovudine	BW	4 g	ZEN	1 g	NS	Visually compatible for 4 hr at room temperature	1994	C
	BW	4 g	ZEN	20 g	NS	Dark yellow discoloration forms in 4 hr at room temperature	1994	I

[a]*Tested in PVC containers.*
[b]*Incompatible by conventional standards but may be used in shorter periods of time.*

Drugs in Syringe Compatibility

Meropenem

Drug (in syringe)	Mfr	Amt	Mfr	Amt	Remarks	Ref	C/I
Pantoprazole sodium	[a]	4 mg/ 1 mL		50 mg/ 1 mL	Precipitates within 15 min	2574	I

[a]*Test performed using the formulation WITHOUT edetate disodium.*

Y-Site Injection Compatibility (1:1 Mixture)

Meropenem

Drug	Mfr	Conc	Mfr	Conc	Remarks	Ref	C/I
Acyclovir sodium	BW	5 mg/mL[c]	ZEN	1 mg/mL[b]	Visually compatible for 4 hr at room temperature	1994	C
	BW	5 mg/mL[c]	ZEN	50 mg/mL[b]	Precipitate forms	2068	I
Aminophylline	AMR	25 mg/mL	ZEN	1 and 50 mg/mL[b]	Visually compatible for 4 hr at room temperature	1994	C
Amphotericin B	SQ	5 mg/mL	ZEN	1 and 50 mg/mL[b]	Precipitate forms	2068	I
Anidulafungin	VIC	0.5 mg/mL[a]	ASZ	2.5 mg/mL[b]	Physically compatible for 4 hr at 23 °C	2617	C
Atropine sulfate	ES	0.4 mg/mL	ZEN	1 and 50 mg/mL[b]	Visually compatible for 4 hr at room temperature	1994	C
Calcium gluconate	AMR	4 mg/mL[c]	ZEN	1 mg/mL[b]	Visually compatible for 4 hr at room temperature	1994	C

Y-Site Injection Compatibility (1:1 Mixture) (Cont.)

Meropenem

Drug	Mfr	Conc	Mfr	Conc	Remarks	Ref	C/I
	AMR	4 mg/mL[c]	ZEN	50 mg/mL[b]	Yellow discoloration forms in 4 hr at room temperature	1994	I
Caspofungin acetate	ME	0.7 mg/mL[b]	ASZ	2.5 mg/mL[b]	Physically compatible for 4 hr at room temperature	2758	C
	ME	0.5 mg/mL[b]	ASZ	10 mg/mL[b]	Physically compatible over 30 min	2766	C
Cyclosporine	BED	1 mg/mL[a]	ASZ	10 mg/mL[b]	Physically compatible	2794	C
Dexamethasone sodium phosphate	MSD	10 mg/mL[c]	ZEN	1 and 50 mg/mL[b]	Visually compatible for 4 hr at room temperature	1994	C
Diazepam	RC	5 mg/mL	ZEN	1 and 50 mg/mL[b]	White precipitate forms immediately	1994	I
Digoxin	BW	0.25 mg/mL	ZEN	1 and 50 mg/mL[b]	Visually compatible for 4 hr at room temperature	1994	C
Diphenhydramine HCl	PD	50 mg/mL	ZEN	1 and 50 mg/mL[b]	Visually compatible for 4 hr at room temperature	1994	C
Docetaxel	RPR	0.9 mg/mL[a]	ZEN	20 mg/mL[b]	Physically compatible for 4 hr at 23 °C	2224	C
Doxycycline hyclate	RR	1 mg/mL[c]	ZEN	1 mg/mL[b]	Visually compatible for 4 hr at room temperature	1994	C
	RR	1 mg/mL[c]	ZEN	50 mg/mL[b]	Amber discoloration forms within 30 min	1994	I
Enalaprilat	MSD	0.05 mg/mL[c]	ZEN	1 and 50 mg/mL[b]	Visually compatible for 4 hr at room temperature	1994	C
Fluconazole	RR	2 mg/mL	ZEN	1 and 50 mg/mL[b]	Visually compatible for 4 hr at room temperature	1994	C
Furosemide	HO	10 mg/mL	ZEN	1 and 50 mg/mL[b]	Visually compatible for 4 hr at room temperature	1994	C
Gentamicin sulfate	SC	4 mg/mL[c]	ZEN	1 and 50 mg/mL[b]	Visually compatible for 4 hr at room temperature	1994	C
	AMS	30 mg/mL[e]	ASZ	10 mg/mL[b]	Physically compatible	2794	C
Heparin sodium	ES	1 unit/mL[c]	ZEN	1 and 50 mg/mL[b]	Visually compatible for 4 hr at room temperature	1994	C
Insulin, regular	LI	0.2 unit/mL[c]	ZEN	1 and 50 mg/mL[b]	Visually compatible for 4 hr at room temperature	1994	C
Linezolid	PHU	2 mg/mL	ZEN	2.5 mg/mL[b]	Physically compatible for 4 hr at 23 °C	2264	C
Metoclopramide HCl	RB	5 mg/mL	ZEN	1 and 50 mg/mL[b]	Visually compatible for 4 hr at room temperature	1994	C
Milrinone lactate	SS	0.2 mg/mL[a]	ZEN	50 mg/mL[a]	Visually compatible for 4 hr at 25 °C	2381	C
Morphine sulfate	ES	1 mg/mL[c]	ZEN	1 and 50 mg/mL[b]	Visually compatible for 4 hr at room temperature	1994	C
Norepinephrine bitartrate	WI	1 mg/mL	ZEN	1 and 50 mg/mL[b]	Visually compatible for 4 hr at room temperature	1994	C
Ondansetron HCl	GL	1 mg/mL[c]	ZEN	1 mg/mL[b]	Visually compatible for 4 hr at room temperature	1994	C
	GL	1 mg/mL[c]	ZEN	50 mg/mL[b]	White precipitate forms immediately	1994	I
Phenobarbital sodium	ES	0.32 mg/mL[c]	ZEN	1 and 50 mg/mL[b]	Visually compatible for 4 hr at room temperature	1994	C
Potassium chloride		10 and 40 mEq/L[a]	ZEN	1 mg/mL[a]	Visually compatible. Calculated 10% meropenem loss in 3.3 hr at 23 °C	2492	C

Y-Site Injection Compatibility (1:1 Mixture) (Cont.)

Meropenem

Drug	Mfr	Conc	Mfr	Conc	Remarks	Ref	C/I
		10 and 40 mEq/L[b]	ZEN	1 mg/mL[a]	Visually compatible. Calculated 10% meropenem loss in 5 hr at 23 °C	2492	C
		10 and 40 mEq/L[a]	ZEN	1 mg/mL[b]	Visually compatible. Calculated 10% meropenem loss in 5.8 hr at 23 °C	2492	C
		10 and 40 mEq/L[b]	ZEN	1 mg/mL[b]	Visually compatible. Calculated 10% meropenem loss in 22 hr at 23 °C	2492	C
		10 and 40 mEq/L[a]	ZEN	22 mg/mL[a]	Visually compatible. Calculated 10% meropenem loss in 7.7 hr at 23 °C	2492	C
		10 and 40 mEq/L[b]	ZEN	22 mg/mL[a]	Visually compatible. Calculated 10% meropenem loss in 13 hr at 23 °C	2492	C
		10 and 40 mEq/L[a]	ZEN	22 mg/mL[b]	Visually compatible. Calculated 10% meropenem loss in 8 hr at 23 °C	2492	C
		10 and 40 mEq/L[b]	ZEN	22 mg/mL[b]	Visually compatible. Calculated 10% meropenem loss in 20 hr at 23 °C	2492	C
Telavancin HCl	ASP	7.5 mg/mL[a,b,f]	ASZ	10 mg/mL[a,b,f]	Physically compatible for 2 hr	2830	C
TNA #218 to #226[d]			ZEN	20 mg/mL[a]	Visually compatible for 4 hr at 23 °C	2215	C
Vancomycin HCl	LI	5 mg/mL[c]	ZEN	1 and 50 mg/mL[b]	Visually compatible for 4 hr at room temperature	1994	C
Vasopressin	APP	0.2 unit/mL[b]	ASZ	5 mg/mL[a]	Physically compatible	2641	C
Zidovudine	BW	4 mg/mL[c]	ZEN	1 mg/mL[b]	Visually compatible for 4 hr at room temperature	1994	C
	BW	4 mg/mL[c]	ZEN	50 mg/mL[b]	Yellow color in 4 hr at room temperature	1994	I

[a]Tested in dextrose 5%.
[b]Tested in sodium chloride 0.9%.
[c]Tested in sterile water for injection.
[d]Refer to Appendix I for the composition of parenteral nutrition solutions. TNA indicates a 3-in-1 admixture.
[e]Tested in sodium chloride 0.45%.
[f]Tested in Ringer's injection, lactated.

MESNA
AHFS 92:56

Products — Mesna is available as a 100-mg/mL solution in 10-mL multidose vials. Each milliliter of solution also contains edetate disodium 0.25 mg and sodium hydroxide to adjust the pH. In addition, the multidose vials contain benzyl alcohol 10.4 mg/mL. (1)

pH — The pH of mesna injection is stated to be pH 6.5 to 7.3 or pH 7.5 to 8.5, depending on the specific product. (1)

Trade Name(s) — Mesnex.

Administration — Mesna may be administered by intravenous injection or infusion. (1; 4) Infusion is usually performed over 15 to 30 minutes, but continuous infusion has also been utilized. (4) Dilution to a concentration of 20 mg/mL in a compatible solution is recommended for intravenous infusion. (1; 4)

Stability — Intact ampuls of mesna should be stored at controlled room temperature. The solution is clear and colorless (1) and is not light sensitive. (72) When exposed to oxygen, mesna oxidizes to the disulfide form, dimesna. Unused mesna injection in opened ampuls should be discarded after dose preparation. However, the multidose vials may be stored and used for up to eight days after initial entry. (1)

pH Effects — Mesna and ifosfamide have been found to be stable in combined admixtures (72; 1380; 1494; 1495; 1496). However, mesna has been found to undergo more extensive decomposition when mixed with ifosfamide in an infusion solution made alkaline with sodium bicarbonate. At pH 8, mesna was stable for six hours, but lost about 13% in 24 hours and 23% in 48 hours. Ifosfamide underwent only 6% loss in 24 hours, but lost 14% in 48 hours. (2281)

Syringes — The short-term use of plastic syringes for preparing mesna infusions appears to be satisfactory. However, extended storage of mesna in a plastic and a glass syringe resulted in the formation of dark or thread-like particles and a change in viscosity after 12 hours at room temperature. (72)

Mesna (Asta Pharma) 100 mg/mL was packaged as 10 mL in 20-mL polypropylene syringes (Becton-Dickinson). Samples having the air expelled from the syringes were stored at 5, 24, and 35 °C, and samples with air drawn into the syringes were stored at 24 °C. After nine days of storage, little or no change in the mesna concentration was found in all samples with no air present. The maximum loss was less than 4% found in the samples stored at 35 °C. However, the syringes containing air exhibited 10% loss in eight days at 24 °C. Minimizing the exposure of mesna to air during storage was recommended to slow the formation of dimesna. (2181)

Compatibility Information

Solution Compatibility

Mesna

Solution	Mfr	Mfr	Conc/L	Remarks	Ref	C/I
Dextrose 5% in sodium chloride 0.2%			20 g	Physically and chemically stable for 24 hr at 25 °C	1	C
Dextrose 5% in sodium chloride 0.45%			20 g	Physically and chemically stable for 24 hr at 25 °C	1	C
		AW	1 g	4% loss in 72 hr at room temperature	72	C
		AW	20 g	5% loss in 48 hr at room temperature	72	C
Dextrose 5%			20 g	Physically and chemically stable for 24 hr at 25 °C	1	C
		AW	1 g	5% loss in 24 hr and 13% in 48 hr at room temperature	72	C
		AW	20 g	5% loss in 48 hr at room temperature	72	C
	BA[a]	BED	10 g	Under 10% loss in 14 days at 25 °C and 28 days at 5 °C	2810	C
Ringer's injection, lactated			20 g	Physically and chemically stable for 24 hr at 25 °C	1	C
		AW	1 g	4% loss in 24 hr and 11% in 48 hr at room temperature	72	C
Sodium chloride 0.9%			20 g	Physically and chemically stable for 24 hr at 25 °C	1	C
		AW	1 g	10% loss in 48 hr at room temperature	72	C

[a]Tested in ReadyMed elastomeric pump reservoirs.

Additive Compatibility

Mesna

Drug	Mfr	Conc/L	Mfr	Conc/L	Test Soln	Remarks	Ref	C/I
Carboplatin		1 g		1 g	W	More than 10% carboplatin loss in 24 hr at room temperature	1379	I
Cisplatin		67 mg		3.33 g	NS	Cisplatin not detectable after 1 hr	1291	I
		67 mg		110 mg	NS	Cisplatin weakly detected after 1 hr	1291	I
Cyclophosphamide	AM	10.8 g	AM	3.2 g	D5W	Physically compatible with about 5% loss of both drugs in 24 hr at 22 °C. 7% cyclophosphamide loss and 10% mesna loss occurred in 72 hr at 4 °C	2486	C
	AM	1.8 g	AM	540 mg	D5W	Physically compatible with about 10% loss of both drugs in 12 hr at 22 °C	2486	I
	AM	1.8 g	AM	540 mg	D5W	Physically compatible with about 9% loss of both drugs in 72 hr at 4 °C	2486	C
Hydroxyzine HCl	LY	500 mg	AW	3 g	D5W[a]	Physically compatible for 48 hr	1190	C
Ifosfamide	MJ	3.3 g	AW	3.3 g	D5W, LR	Physically compatible. No ifosfamide loss and about 5% mesna loss in 24 hr at 21 °C exposed to light	72	C
	MJ	5 g	AW	5 g	D5W, LR	Physically compatible. No ifosfamide loss and about 5% mesna loss in 24 hr at 21 °C exposed to light	72	C

Additive Compatibility (Cont.)

						Mesna		
Drug	*Mfr*	*Conc/L*	*Mfr*	*Conc/L*	*Test Soln*	*Remarks*	*Ref*	*C/I*
	BI	83.3 g	BI	79 g	NS	Little or no ifosfamide loss in 9 days at room temperature and 7% ifosfamide loss in 9 days at 37 °C. Mesna not tested	1494	**C**
		2.6 g		1.6 g	D5S[b]	No increase in decomposition products in 8 hr at room temperature	1495	**C**
	BR	600 mg	BR	600 mg	D5½S, D5W, LR, NS[c]	Both drugs chemically stable for at least 24 hr at room temperature	1496	**C**
	AM	20 g	AM	20 g	W[d]	Physically compatible with about 3% ifosfamide loss and 9% mesna loss in 7 days at 37 °C. About 2% or less loss of both drugs in 14 days at 4 °C	2288	**C**

[a]*Tested in glass containers.*
[b]*Tested in polyethylene containers.*
[c]*Tested in PVC containers.*
[d]*Tested in PVC reservoirs for the Graseby 9000 ambulatory pump.*

Drugs in Syringe Compatibility

					Mesna		
Drug (in syringe)	*Mfr*	*Amt*	*Mfr*	*Amt*	*Remarks*	*Ref*	*C/I*
Epirubicin HCl with ifosfamide		1 mg/mL[a] 50 mg/mL[a]		40 mg/mL[a]	50% epirubicin loss in 7 days at 4 and 20 °C. No loss of other drugs in 7 days	1564	**I**
Ifosfamide		250 mg/5 mL		200 mg/5 mL	3% ifosfamide loss in 7 days and 12% in 4 weeks at 4 °C and room temperature. No mesna loss	1290	**C**
		50 mg/mL[a]		40 mg/mL[a]	Little or no loss of either drug in 28 days at 4 and 20 °C	1564	**C**
Ifosfamide with epirubicin HCl		50 mg/mL[a] 1 mg/mL[a]		40 mg/mL[a]	50% epirubicin loss in 7 days at 4 and 20 °C. No loss of other drugs in 7 days	1564	**I**

[a]*Diluted with sodium chloride 0.9%.*

Y-Site Injection Compatibility (1:1 Mixture)

					Mesna		
Drug	*Mfr*	*Conc*	*Mfr*	*Conc*	*Remarks*	*Ref*	*C/I*
Allopurinol sodium	BW	3 mg/mL[b]	MJ	10 mg/mL[b]	Physically compatible for 4 hr at 22 °C	1686	**C**
Amifostine	USB	10 mg/mL[a]	MJ	10 mg/mL[a]	Physically compatible for 4 hr at 23 °C	1845	**C**
Amphotericin B cholesteryl sulfate complex	SEQ	0.83 mg/mL[a]	MJ	10 mg/mL[a]	Microprecipitate forms immediately	2117	**I**

Y-Site Injection Compatibility (1:1 Mixture) (Cont.)

Mesna

Drug	Mfr	Conc	Mfr	Conc	Remarks	Ref	C/I
Aztreonam	SQ	40 mg/mL[a]	MJ	10 mg/mL[a]	Physically compatible for 4 hr at 23 °C	1758	C
Cladribine	ORT	0.015[b] and 0.5[c] mg/mL	MJ	10 mg/mL[b]	Physically compatible for 4 hr at 23 °C	1969	C
Docetaxel	RPR	0.9 mg/mL[a]	MJ	10 mg/mL[a]	Physically compatible for 4 hr at 23 °C	2224	C
Doxorubicin HCl liposomal	SEQ	0.4 mg/mL[a]	MJ	10 mg/mL[a]	Physically compatible for 4 hr at 23 °C	2087	C
Etoposide phosphate	BR	5 mg/mL[a]	MJ	10 mg/mL[a]	Physically compatible for 4 hr at 23 °C	2218	C
Filgrastim	AMG	30 mcg/mL[a]	MJ	10 mg/mL[a]	Physically compatible for 4 hr at 22 °C	1687	C
Fludarabine phosphate	BX	1 mg/mL[a]	BR	10 mg/mL[a]	Visually compatible for 4 hr at 22 °C	1439	C
Gallium nitrate	FUJ	1 mg/mL[b]	MJ	20 mg/mL	Visually compatible for 24 hr at 25 °C	1673	C
Gemcitabine HCl	LI	10 mg/mL[b]	MJ	10 mg/mL[b]	Physically compatible for 4 hr at 23 °C	2226	C
Granisetron HCl	SKB	1 mg/mL	MJ	4 mg/mL[b]	Physically compatible with little or no loss of either drug in 4 hr at 22 °C	1883	C
Linezolid	PHU	2 mg/mL	MJ	10 mg/mL[a]	Physically compatible for 4 hr at 23 °C	2264	C
Melphalan HCl	BW	0.1 mg/mL[b]	BR	10 mg/mL[b]	Physically compatible for 3 hr at 22 °C	1557	C
Methotrexate sodium		30 mg/mL		1.8 mg/mL[a]	Visually compatible for 4 hr at room temperature	1788	C
Micafungin sodium	ASP	1.5 mg/mL[b]	APP	20 mg/mL[b]	Physically compatible for 4 hr at 23 °C	2683	C
Ondansetron HCl	GL	1 mg/mL[b]	BR	10 mg/mL[a]	Visually compatible for 4 hr at 22 °C	1365	C
Oxaliplatin	SS	0.5 mg/mL[a]	MJ	10 mg/mL[a]	Physically compatible for 4 hr at 23 °C	2566	C
Paclitaxel	NCI	1.2 mg/mL[a]	MJ	10 mg/mL[a]	Physically compatible for 4 hr at 22 °C	1556	C
Pemetrexed disodium	LI	20 mg/mL[b]	APP	10 mg/mL[a]	Physically compatible for 4 hr at 23 °C	2564	C
Piperacillin sodium–tazobactam sodium	LE[f]	40 + 5 mg/mL[a]	MJ	10 mg/mL[a]	Physically compatible for 4 hr at 22 °C	1688	C
Sargramostim	IMM	10 mcg/mL[b]	MJ	10 mg/mL[b]	Visually compatible for 4 hr at 22 °C	1436	C
Sodium bicarbonate		1.4%		1.8 mg/mL[a]	Visually compatible for 4 hr at room temperature	1788	C
Teniposide	BR	0.1 mg/mL[a]	MJ	10 mg/mL[a]	Physically compatible for 4 hr at 23 °C	1725	C
Thiotepa	IMM[d]	1 mg/mL[a]	MJ	10 mg/mL[a]	Physically compatible for 4 hr at 23 °C	1861	C
TNA #218 to #226[e]			MJ	10 mg/mL[a]	Visually compatible for 4 hr at 23 °C	2215	C
TPN #212 to #215[e]			MJ	10 mg/mL[a]	Physically compatible for 4 hr at 23 °C	2109	C
Vinorelbine tartrate	BW	1 mg/mL[b]	MJ	10 mg/mL[b]	Physically compatible for 4 hr at 22 °C	1558	C

[a]Tested in dextrose 5%.
[b]Tested in sodium chloride 0.9%.
[c]Tested in bacteriostatic sodium chloride 0.9% preserved with benzyl alcohol 0.9%.
[d]Lyophilized formulation tested.
[e]Refer to Appendix I for the composition of parenteral nutrition solutions. TNA indicates a 3-in-1 admixture, and TPN indicates a 2-in-1 admixture.
[f]Test performed using the formulation WITHOUT edetate disodium.

METHADONE HYDROCHLORIDE
AHFS 28:08.08

Products — Methadone hydrochloride is available in 20-mL multidose vials. Each milliliter of solution contains methadone hydrochloride 10 mg and sodium chloride 0.9% with sodium hydroxide and/or hydrochloric acid to adjust the pH. In addition, the 20-mL vials contain chlorobutanol 0.5%. (1)

pH — From 4.5 to 6.5. (1)

Administration — Methadone hydrochloride may be administered by subcutaneous, intramuscular, or intravenous injection. (1; 4)

Stability — Methadone hydrochloride in intact vials should be stored at controlled room temperature and protected from light. (1)

Compatibility Information

Solution Compatibility

Methadone HCl

Solution	Mfr	Mfr	Conc/L	Remarks	Ref	C/I
Sodium chloride 0.9%	TR[a]	LI	1, 2, 5 g	Little or no loss in 28 days at room temperature exposed to light	1500	C

[a]*Tested in PVC containers.*

Y-Site Injection Compatibility (1:1 Mixture)

Methadone HCl

Drug	Mfr	Conc	Mfr	Conc	Remarks	Ref	C/I
Atropine sulfate	LY	0.4 mg/mL	LI	1 mg/mL[a]	Physically compatible for 48 hr at 22 °C	1706	C
Dexamethasone sodium phosphate	AMR	1 mg/mL[a]	LI	1 mg/mL[a]	Physically compatible for 48 hr at 22 °C	1706	C
Diazepam	ES	0.5 mg/mL[a]	LI	1 mg/mL[a]	Physically compatible for 48 hr at 22 °C	1706	C
Diphenhydramine HCl	SCN	2 mg/mL[a]	LI	1 mg/mL[a]	Physically compatible for 48 hr at 22 °C	1706	C
Haloperidol lactate	MN	0.2 mg/mL[a]	LI	1 mg/mL[a]	Physically compatible for 48 hr at 22 °C	1706	C
Hydroxyzine HCl	WI	4 mg/mL[a]	LI	1 mg/mL[a]	Physically compatible for 48 hr at 22 °C	1706	C
Ketorolac tromethamine	WY	1 mg/mL[a]	LI	1 mg/mL[a]	Physically compatible for 48 hr at 22 °C	1706	C
Lorazepam	WY	0.1 mg/mL[a]	LI	1 mg/mL[a]	Physically compatible for 48 hr at 22 °C	1706	C
Methotrimeprazine HCl	LE	0.2 mg/mL[a]	LI	1 mg/mL[a]	Physically compatible for 48 hr at 22 °C	1706	C
Metoclopramide HCl	DU	5 mg/mL	LI	1 mg/mL[a]	Physically compatible for 48 hr at 22 °C	1706	C
Midazolam HCl	RC	0.2 mg/mL[a]	LI	1 mg/mL[a]	Physically compatible for 48 hr at 22 °C	1706	C
Phenobarbital sodium	WY	2 mg/mL[a]	LI	1 mg/mL[a]	Physically compatible for 48 hr at 22 °C	1706	C
Phenytoin sodium	ES	2 mg/mL[a,b]	LI	1 mg/mL[a]	Precipitate forms immediately	1706	I
Scopolamine HBr	LY	0.05 mg/mL[a]	LI	1 mg/mL[a]	Physically compatible for 48 hr at 22 °C	1706	C

[a]*Tested in dextrose 5%.*
[b]*Tested in sodium chloride 0.9%.*

METHOCARBAMOL
AHFS 12:20.04

Products — Methocarbamol 100 mg/mL is available in 10-mL vials. Also present in the formulation is polyethylene glycol 300 50% in water for injection with sodium hydroxide and/or hydrochloric acid to adjust pH during manufacturing. (1)

pH — From 3.5 to 6.0. (1)

Tonicity — Methocarbamol injection is hypertonic. (4)

Trade Name(s) — Robaxin.

Administration — Methocarbamol injection is administered intramuscularly or intravenously. It should not be given subcutaneously. For intramuscular injection, not more than 5 mL (500 mg) should be given into each gluteal region. Direct intravenous injection should be made slowly at a maximum rate of 3 mL (300 mg) per minute. For intravenous infusion, 1 g of methocarbamol may be diluted in 250 mL of dextrose 5% or sodium chloride 0.9%. (1)

Stability — Store at controlled room temperature (1) and protected from freezing. Methocarbamol was stable for up to six days when diluted in sterile water for injection, dextrose 5%, or sodium chloride 0.9% to a concentration of 4 mg/mL. Refrigeration of methocarbamol diluted for intravenous infusion to concentrations of 15.4 mg/mL and greater may result in precipitation. (4)

Compatibility Information

Solution Compatibility

Methocarbamol

Solution	Mfr	Mfr	Conc/L	Remarks	Ref	C/I
Dextrose 5% in sodium chloride 0.45%		RB	≤15.4 g	Physically compatible. Stable for 6 days at room temperature	2449	**C**
		RB	>15.4 g	Methocarbamol precipitates	2449	**I**
Dextrose 5%		RB	≤15.4 g	Physically compatible. Stable for 6 days at room temperature	2449	**C**
		RB	>15.4 g	Methocarbamol precipitates	2449	**I**
Sodium chloride 0.9%		RB	≤15.4 g	Physically compatible. Stable for 6 days at room temperature	2449	**C**
		RB	>15.4 g	Methocarbamol precipitates	2449	**I**

METHOHEXITAL SODIUM
AHFS 28:04.04

Products — Methohexital sodium is available in 50-mL vials (with or without accompanying vials of sterile water for injection) containing methohexital sodium 500 mg with anhydrous sodium carbonate 30 mg and in vials containing methohexital sodium 2.5 g with sodium carbonate 150 mg, and in vials containing methohexital sodium 5 g with sodium carbonate 300 mg. (1)

To prepare a 1% (10 mg/mL) solution of methohexital sodium for intravenous use, reconstitute with sterile water for injection, preferably, or sodium chloride 0.9% 50 mL for the 500-mg vials or 15 mL initially and then bring to 250 mL for the 2.5-g size. Do not use diluents containing bacteriostats. (1)

The initial dilution of the 2.5-g vials results in a yellow solution. When further diluted, the solution must be clear and colorless or it should not be used. (1; 4)

To prepare a 0.2% (2 mg/mL) solution of methohexital sodium for intravenous use, add 500 mg to 250 mL of dextrose 5% or sodium chloride 0.9%. Sterile water for injection should not be used for this concentration to avoid extreme hypotonicity. (1)

To prepare a 5% (50-mg/mL) solution for intramuscular use, the 500-mg and 2.5-g vials should be reconstituted with 10 and 50 mL, respectively, of compatible diluent. (1)

pH — A 0.2% solution in dextrose 5% has a pH of 9.5 to 10.5; a 1% solution in sterile water for injection has a pH of 10 to 11. (1; 4)

Sodium Content — Methohexital sodium contains 4.652 mEq of sodium per gram of drug; the sodium carbonate provides 1.132 mEq while the balance comes from the drug itself. (869)

Trade Name(s) — Brevital Sodium.

Administration — Methohexital sodium is administered intravenously, by injection or continuous infusion, in concentrations no higher than 1%. Intra-arterial injection and extravasation should be avoided. Intramuscular injection of 5% solutions has also been described. (1)

Methohexital sodium is stated to be incompatible with silicone and, as a consequence, should not contact rubber stoppers or parts of disposable syringes that have been treated with silicone. (4)

Stability — Intact vials should be stored at controlled room temperature. (1; 4) Solutions of methohexital sodium in dextrose 5% or sodium chloride 0.9% are stable for about 24 hours. (4) The manufacturer does not recommend the use of Ringer's injection, lactated, as a diluent. The potential for incompatibility exists between the sodium carbonate in the drug formulation and the calcium ions of the infusion solution. (1; 282)

pH Effects — Methohexital sodium is alkaline in solution and is incompatible with acidic solutions and phenol-containing solutions. (4)

Methohexital sodium exhibits poor solubility in an acidic medium and may precipitate in solutions containing acidic drugs. (22)

Since solubility is maintained only at relatively high pH, mixing methohexital sodium with acidic solutions is not recommended. (4) Mixed with methohexital sodium, a haze or precipitate forms in 15 minutes with atropine sulfate and tubocurarine chloride, in 30 minutes with metocurine iodide and succinylcholine chloride, and in 60 minutes with scopolamine HBr. (1)

When barbiturates are mixed with succinylcholine chloride, either free barbiturate precipitates or the succinylcholine chloride is hydrolyzed, depending on the final pH of the admixture. (4; 21) Similarly, atracurium besylate may be inactivated by alkaline solutions, such as barbiturates, and a free acid of the admixed drug may precipitate, depending on the resultant pH of the admixture. (4)

Methohexital sodium may raise the pH of admixture solutions to the alkaline range and, therefore, should not be mixed with drugs that are alkali labile. (4)

Sorption — Methohexital sodium (Lilly) 32 mg/L displayed 7.9% sorption to a PVC plastic test strip in 24 hours. (12) However, another test did not confirm this finding. No significant loss in PVC containers and no difference between glass and PVC containers were found. (282)

Compatibility Information

Solution Compatibility

Methohexital sodium

Solution	Mfr	Mfr	Conc/L	Remarks	Ref	C/I
Dextrose 5% in Ringer's injection, lactated	TR[a]	LI	2 g	Stable for 24 hr at 5 °C	282	**C**
Dextrose 5% in sodium chloride 0.9%	TR[a]	LI	2 g	Stable for 24 hr at 5 °C	282	**C**
Dextrose 5%	TR[a]	LI	2 g	Stable for 24 hr at 5 °C	282	**C**
Ringer's injection, lactated	TR[a]	LI	2 g	Stable for 24 hr at 5 °C	282	**C**
Sodium chloride 0.9%	TR[a]	LI	2 g	Stable for 24 hr at 5 °C	282	**C**

[a]*Tested in both glass and PVC containers.*

Additive Compatibility

Methohexital sodium

Drug	Mfr	Conc/L	Mfr	Conc/L	Test Soln	Remarks	Ref	C/I
Chlorpromazine HCl	BP	200 mg	BP	2 g	D5W, NS	Precipitates immediately	26	**I**
Hydralazine HCl	BP	80 mg	BP	2 g	D5W, NS	Yellow color with precipitate in 3 hr	26	**I**
Lidocaine HCl	BP	2 g	BP	2 g	D5W	Precipitates immediately	26	**I**
Mechlorethamine HCl	BP	40 mg	BP	2 g	D5W, NS	Haze develops over 3 hr	26	**I**
Methyldopate HCl		1 g	BP	2 g	D5W	Haze develops over 3 hr	26	**I**
		1 g	BP	2 g	NS	Crystals produced	26	**I**
Prochlorperazine mesylate	BP	100 mg	BP	2 g	D5W	Haze develops over 3 hr	26	**I**
Promethazine HCl	BP	100 mg	BP	2 g	D5W, NS	Precipitates immediately	26	**I**
Streptomycin sulfate	BP	4 g	BP	2 g	NS	Crystals produced	26	**I**

Drugs in Syringe Compatibility

Methohexital sodium

Drug (in syringe)	Mfr	Amt	Mfr	Amt	Remarks	Ref	C/I
Glycopyrrolate	RB	0.2 mg/ 1 mL	LI	10 mg/ 1 mL	Precipitates immediately	331	I
	RB	0.2 mg/ 1 mL	LI	20 mg/ 2 mL	Precipitates immediately	331	I
	RB	0.4 mg/ 2 mL	LI	10 mg/ 1 mL	Precipitates immediately	331	I
Scopolamine HBr					Haze forms in 1 hr	4	I

Y-Site Injection Compatibility (1:1 Mixture)

Methohexital sodium

Drug	Mfr	Conc	Mfr	Conc	Remarks	Ref	C/I
Fenoldopam mesylate	AB	80 mcg/mL[a]	JP	10 mg/mL[a]	Microparticulates and yellow color form immediately	2467	I

[a]*Tested in sodium chloride 0.9%.*

METHOTREXATE SODIUM
AHFS 10:00

Products — Methotrexate sodium is available in liquid and lyophilized dosage forms.

The liquid dosage forms contain methotrexate sodium 25 mg/mL and are available in vials of various sizes from 2 to 10 mL. The products also contain sodium chloride, and the preserved products contain benzyl alcohol. The pH has been adjusted during manufacturing with sodium hydroxide and, if necessary, hydrochloric acid. (1; 4)

Methotrexate (as the sodium salt) is available in single-use lyophilized vials containing 1 g. The pH has been adjusted during manufacturing with sodium hydroxide. The 1-g vial requires 19.4 mL of sterile, preservative-free diluent for reconstitution to yield a 50-mg/mL concentration. (4)

pH — The pH of the commercially available dosage forms of methotrexate sodium is approximately 8.5 (range 7.5 to 9). (1; 4)

Tonicity — The liquid forms of methotrexate sodium are isotonic. (1; 4)

Sodium Content — Methotrexate sodium liquid injections contain sodium 0.43, 0.86, and 2.15 mEq in the 2-, 4-, and 10-mL sizes, respectively. The lyophilized product contains 7 mEq of sodium in the 1-g vial. (1)

Administration — Methotrexate sodium may be administered by intramuscular, intra-arterial, or intrathecal injection, by direct intravenous injection, or by continuous or intermittent intravenous infusion. (1; 4) For intrathecal injection, a preservative-free form is diluted to a 1-mg/mL concentration in sodium chloride 0.9%, Elliott's B solution, or the patient's own spinal fluid. (4; 435; 830) For high-dose regimens, it is recommended that preservative-free forms of methotrexate sodium be used (241; 242); high doses of methotrexate sodium require leucovorin rescue. (4)

Stability — Store the lyophilized powder and injection at controlled room temperature with protection from light. (1; 4)

For intrathecal injection, the preservative-free dosage forms should be diluted immediately prior to use. (4) Although reconstitution of the lyophilized vials immediately prior to use is also recommended because of the absence of antibacterial preservatives, the reconstituted solution is stable for at least one week at room temperature. (234)

Immersion of a needle with an aluminum component in methotrexate sodium (Lederle) 25 mg/mL resulted in the formation of orange crystals on the aluminum surface after 36 hours at 24 °C with protection from light. (988)

pH Effects — Methotrexate is most stable between pH 6 and 8. Drugs producing extremes of pH should not be added to methotrexate. (1072; 1369; 1379)

Freezing Solutions — Methotrexate sodium (Lederle) 50 mg/100 mL in PVC bags of dextrose 5% (Travenol) was frozen at −20 °C for at least 30 days and thawed by microwave radiation for two minutes with no significant change in concentration. Even after five repetitions of the freeze–thaw treatment, the methotrexate concentration showed no significant change. (818)

The stability of methotrexate 5 mg, 50 mg, and 1 g in 50 mL of sodium chloride 0.9% in PVC bags frozen at −20 °C for up to 12 weeks and thawed in a microwave oven was evaluated. No loss was found in any of the concentrations. (1281)

Light Effects — Photolability, although unrecognized for many years, is a stability problem that is increased by dilution and mixture with sodium bicarbonate. (1202)

In dilute solutions of 0.1 mg/mL, methotrexate is reported to undergo photodegradation on exposure to light. Decomposition of 5 to 8% in 10 days and 11 to 17% in 20 days has been reported. This effect was not observed in the more concentrated solutions of the commercial preparation (25 mg/mL) (433) or in admixtures of methotrexate during short-term light exposure. No significant loss of methotrexate occurred due to light exposure for four hours in solutions composed of 5 mg, 50 mg, or 1 g of methotrexate in 50 mL of sodium chloride 0.9% in PVC containers. (1281)

Little methotrexate loss was found from a 1-mg/mL solution in sodium chloride 0.9% in three burette drip chambers made of cellulose propionate (Avon A200 standard and A2000 Amberset) and methacrylate butadiene styrene (Avon A2001 Sureset) when exposed to normal mixed daylight and fluorescent lighting conditions for 24 hours. However, in 48 hours about 10 and 12% losses were observed in the A200 and A2001, respectively. With exposure to direct sunlight, an 11% loss occurred in the A200 in seven hours. No loss occurred when the Amberset or Sureset was wrapped in foil and exposed to either light condition for 48 hours. (1378)

Exposure of methotrexate 1-mg/mL solution in PVC and polybutadiene tubing to mixed daylight and fluorescent light produced significant losses after eight to 12 hours. The Amberset PVC tubing or foil wrapping for the polybutadiene tubing to protect solutions from light reduced losses to 12 to 16% in 48 hours. (1378)

Methotrexate sodium (R. Bellon), reconstituted to a concentration of 1 mg/mL with sodium chloride 0.9%, was evaluated for stability in translucent containers (Perfupack, Baxter) and five opaque containers [green PVC Opafuseur (Bruneau), white EVA Perfu-opaque (Baxter), orange PVC PF170 (Cair), white PVC V86 (Codan), and white EVA Perfecran (Fandre)] when exposed to sunlight for 28 days. Photodegradation was found after storage in the translucent Perfupack. Losses ranged from 18.5 to 27% after 24 hours at a methotrexate sodium concentration of 5 mg/mL. At 1 mg/mL, losses of 4% or less occurred in 24 hours in the opaque containers. (1750)

Intrathecal Injections — In a study of intrathecal injections, preservative-free methotrexate sodium (Ben Venue) was reconstituted to a concentration of 2.5 mg/mL with Elliott's B solution (305 mOsm/kg, pH 7.2), sodium chloride 0.9% injection (303 mOsm/kg, pH 7.6), or Ringer's injection, lactated (270 mOsm/kg, pH 7.6). In all three solutions, methotrexate exhibited no change in concentration over seven days under fluorescent light at 30 °C. (327)

In another study, the stability and compatibility of cytarabine (Upjohn), methotrexate (National Cancer Institute), and hydrocortisone (Upjohn), mixed together in intrathecal injections, were evaluated. Two combinations were tested: (1) cytarabine 50 mg, methotrexate 12 mg (as the sodium salt), and hydrocortisone 25 mg (as the sodium succinate salt); and (2) cytarabine 30 mg, methotrexate 12 mg (as the sodium salt), and hydrocortisone 15 mg (as the sodium succinate salt). Each drug combination was added to 12 mL of Elliott's B solution (National Cancer Institute), sodium chloride 0.9% (Abbott), dextrose 5% (Abbott), and Ringer's injection, lactated (Abbott), and stored for 24 hours at 25 °C. Cytarabine and methotrexate were both chemically stable, with no drug loss after the full 24 hours in all solutions. Hydrocortisone was also stable in the sodium chloride 0.9%, dextrose 5%, and Ringer's injection, lactated, with about a 2% drug loss. However, in Elliott's B solution, hydrocortisone was significantly less stable, with a 6% loss in the 25-mg concentration over 24 hours. The 15-mg concentration was worse, with a 5% loss in 10 hours and a 13% loss in 24 hours. The higher pH of Elliott's B solution and the lower concentration of hydrocortisone may have been factors in this increased decomposition. All mixtures were physically compatible during this study, but a precipitate formed after several days of storage. (819)

Methotrexate sodium (Lederle) 2 mg/mL diluted in Elliott's B solution (Orphan Medical) was packaged as 20 mL in 30-mL glass vials and 20-mL plastic syringes (Becton Dickinson) with Red Cap (Burron) Luer-Lok syringe tip caps. The solution was physically compatible and chemically stable exhibiting little loss during storage for 48 hours at 4 and 23 °C. (1976)

Bacterially contaminated intrathecal solutions can pose very grave risks. Consequently, intrathecal solutions should be administered as soon as possible after preparation. (328)

Syringes — Methotrexate (Lederle) 50 mg/mL was stable for up to eight months when stored in Monoject or Plastipak plastic syringes at 25 °C. Because of possible alteration in water vapor permeability, use of Sabre and Steriseal plastic syringes is limited to 70 days at 25 °C. (1280)

Methotrexate sodium (Lederle) 2.5 mg/mL was repackaged into 10-mL plastic syringes (Becton Dickinson) and stored at 4 and 25 °C for seven days. No loss of methotrexate was found. Furthermore, no contaminants from the syringes were observed. (1913)

Sorption — Methotrexate sodium 22.5 mg/100 mL and 12 g/500 mL in both dextrose 5% and sodium chloride 0.9% in PVC containers (Macroflex, Macopharma) exhibited no sorption loss during 30 days of storage at 4 °C protected from light. Simulated infusion of methotrexate sodium 2.25 g/500 mL in dextrose 5% and sodium chloride 0.9% over 24 hours through opaque PVC infusion sets (Perfecran, Fandre) also showed no sorption loss to the PVC tubing. (1867)

Methotrexate sodium (Medac) 0.36 mg/mL in dextrose 5% and in sodium chloride 0.9% exhibited little or no loss due to sorption in polyethylene, PVC, and glass containers over 72 hours at room and refrigeration temperatures. (2420; 2430)

Central Venous Catheter — Methotrexate sodium (Immunex) 2.5 mg/mL in dextrose 5% was found to be compatible with the ARROWg+ard Blue Plus (Arrow International) chlorhexidine-bearing triple-lumen central catheter. Essentially complete delivery of the drug was found with little or no drug loss occurring. Furthermore, chlorhexidine delivered from the catheter remained at trace amounts with no substantial increase due to the delivery of the drug through the catheter. (2335)

Compatibility Information

Solution Compatibility

Methotrexate sodium

Solution	Mfr	Mfr	Conc/L	Remarks	Ref	C/I
Amino acids 4.25%, dextrose 25%	MG	LE	50 mg	No increase in particulate matter in 24 hr at 5 °C	349	C
Dextrose 5%	TR[a]	LE	960 mg	Under 10% loss in 24 hr at room temperature	519	C
	[b]		225 mg and 24 g	Visually compatible with no loss in 30 days at 4 °C protected from light	1867	C
Sodium chloride 0.9%	[a]	FA	1.25 and 12.5 g	Visually compatible with little or no loss in 105 days at 4 °C followed by 7 days at 25 °C in the dark	1567	C
	[b]		225 mg and 24 g	Visually compatible with no loss in 30 days at 4 °C protected from light	1867	C

[a]Tested in both glass and PVC containers.
[b]Tested in PVC containers.

Additive Compatibility

Methotrexate sodium

Drug	Mfr	Conc/L	Mfr	Conc/L	Test Soln	Remarks	Ref	C/I
Bleomycin sulfate	BR	20 and 30 units	LE	250 and 500 mg	NS	About 60% loss of bleomycin activity in 1 week at 4 °C	763	I
Cyclophosphamide		1.67 g		25 mg	NS	6.6% cyclophosphamide loss in 14 days at room temperature	1379; 1389	C
Cyclophosphamide with fluorouracil		1.67 g 8.3 g		25 mg	NS	9.3% cyclophosphamide loss in 7 days at room temperature. No loss of other drugs observed	1389	C
Cytarabine	UP	400 mg	LE	200 mg	D5W	Physically compatible. Very little change in UV spectra in 8 hr at room temperature	207	C
Fluorouracil		10 g		30 mg	NS	Both drugs stable for 15 days at room temperature	1379	C
Fluorouracil with cyclophosphamide		8.3 g 1.67 g		25 mg	NS	9.3% cyclophosphamide loss in 7 days at room temperature. No loss of other drugs observed	1389	C
Hydroxyzine HCl	LY	500 mg	BV	1 and 3 g	D5W[a]	Physically compatible for 48 hr	1190	C
Mercaptopurine sodium	BW	1 g	LE	100 mg	D5W	Physically compatible	15	C
Ondansetron HCl	GL	30 and 300 mg	LE	0.5 and 6 g	D5W[b]	Physically compatible with little or no loss of either drug in 48 hr at 23 °C	1876	C
Sodium bicarbonate		50 mEq	LE	750 mg	D5W	6% methotrexate loss in 1 week at 5 °C in dark. At 23 °C in light, 6% loss in 72 hr and 15% in 1 week	465	C
		50 mEq		2 g		No photodegradation products in 12 hr in room light	433	C
Vincristine sulfate	LI	10 mg	LE	100 mg	D5W	Physically compatible	15	C
	LI	4 mg	LE	8 mg	D5W	Physically compatible. No change in UV spectra in 8 hr at room temperature	207	C

[a]Tested in glass containers.
[b]Tested in PVC containers.

Drugs in Syringe Compatibility

Methotrexate sodium

Drug (in syringe)	Mfr	Amt	Mfr	Amt	Remarks	Ref	C/I
Bleomycin sulfate		1.5 units/ 0.5 mL		12.5 mg/ 0.5 mL	Physically compatible for 5 min at room temperature followed by 8 min of centrifugation	980	C
Cisplatin		0.5 mg/ 0.5 mL		12.5 mg/ 0.5 mL	Physically compatible for 5 min at room temperature followed by 8 min of centrifugation	980	C
Cyclophosphamide		10 mg/ 0.5 mL		12.5 mg/ 0.5 mL	Physically compatible for 5 min at room temperature followed by 8 min of centrifugation	980	C
Doxapram HCl	RB	400 mg/ 20 mL		50 mg/ 20 mL	Physically compatible with 4% doxapram loss in 24 hr	1177	C
Doxorubicin HCl		1 mg/ 0.5 mL		12.5 mg/ 0.5 mL	Physically compatible for 5 min at room temperature followed by 8 min of centrifugation	980	C
Droperidol		1.25 mg/ 0.5 mL		12.5 mg/ 0.5 mL	Precipitates immediately	980	I
Fluorouracil		25 mg/ 0.5 mL		12.5 mg/ 0.5 mL	Physically compatible for 5 min at room temperature followed by 8 min of centrifugation	980	C
Furosemide		5 mg/ 0.5 mL		12.5 mg/ 0.5 mL	Physically compatible for 5 min at room temperature followed by 8 min of centrifugation	980	C
Heparin sodium		500 units/ 0.5 mL		12.5 mg/ 0.5 mL	Physically compatible for 5 min at room temperature followed by 8 min of centrifugation	980	C
Leucovorin calcium		5 mg/ 0.5 mL		12.5 mg/ 0.5 mL	Physically compatible for 5 min at room temperature followed by 8 min of centrifugation	980	C
Metoclopramide HCl		2.5 mg/ 0.5 mL		12.5 mg/ 0.5 mL	Physically compatible for 5 min at room temperature followed by 8 min of centrifugation	980	C
	RB	10 mg/ 2 mL	LE	50 mg/ 2 mL	Incompatible. If mixed, use immediately	1167	I
	RB	160 mg/ 32 mL	LE	200 mg/ 8 mL	Incompatible. If mixed, use immediately	1167	I
Mitomycin		0.25 mg/ 0.5 mL		12.5 mg/ 0.5 mL	Physically compatible for 5 min at room temperature followed by 8 min of centrifugation	980	C
Vinblastine sulfate		0.5 mg/ 0.5 mL		12.5 mg/ 0.5 mL	Physically compatible for 5 min at room temperature followed by 8 min of centrifugation	980	C
Vincristine sulfate		0.5 mg/ 0.5 mL		12.5 mg/ 0.5 mL	Physically compatible for 5 min at room temperature followed by 8 min of centrifugation	980	C

Y-Site Injection Compatibility (1:1 Mixture)

Methotrexate sodium

Drug	Mfr	Conc	Mfr	Conc	Remarks	Ref	C/I
Allopurinol sodium	BW	3 mg/mL[b]	LE	15 mg/mL[b]	Physically compatible for 4 hr at 22 °C	1686	C
Amifostine	USB	10 mg/mL[a]	LE	15 mg/mL[a]	Physically compatible for 4 hr at 23 °C	1845	C
Amphotericin B cholesteryl sulfate complex	SEQ	0.83 mg/mL[a]	IMM	15 mg/mL[a]	Physically compatible for 4 hr at 23 °C	2117	C
Asparaginase	BEL	120 I.U./mL[a]		30 mg/mL	Visually compatible for 4 hr at room temperature	1788	C

Y-Site Injection Compatibility (1:1 Mixture) (Cont.)

Methotrexate sodium

Drug	Mfr	Conc	Mfr	Conc	Remarks	Ref	C/I
Aztreonam	SQ	40 mg/mL[a]	LE	15 mg/mL[a]	Physically compatible for 4 hr at 23 °C	1758	C
Bleomycin sulfate		3 units/mL		25 mg/mL	Drugs injected sequentially in Y-site with no flush. No precipitate seen	980	C
Ceftriaxone sodium	RC	100 mg/mL		30 mg/mL	Visually compatible for 4 hr at room temperature	1788	C
Cisplatin		1 mg/mL		25 mg/mL	Drugs injected sequentially in Y-site with no flush. No precipitate seen	980	C
Cyclophosphamide		20 mg/mL		25 mg/mL	Drugs injected sequentially in Y-site with no flush. No precipitate seen	980	C
		20 mg/mL[a]		30 mg/mL	Visually compatible for 4 hr at room temperature	1788	C
Cytarabine	UP	0.6 mg/mL[a]		30 mg/mL	Visually compatible for 4 hr at room temperature	1788	C
Daunorubicin HCl	BEL	0.52 mg/mL[a]		30 mg/mL	Visually compatible for 4 hr at room temperature	1788	C
Dexamethasone sodium phosphate	MSD	4 mg/mL		30 mg/mL	Visually compatible for 2 hr at room temperature. Precipitate forms in 4 hr	1788	I
Doripenem	JJ	5 mg/mL[a,b]	BED	12.5 mg/mL[a,b]	Physically compatible for 4 hr at 23 °C	2743	C
Doxorubicin HCl		2 mg/mL		25 mg/mL	Drugs injected sequentially in Y-site with no flush. No precipitate seen	980	C
	FA	0.4 mg/mL[a]		30 mg/mL	Visually compatible for 4 hr at room temperature	1788	C
Doxorubicin HCl liposomal	SEQ	0.4 mg/mL[a]	IMM	15 mg/mL[a]	Physically compatible for 4 hr at 23 °C	2087	C
Droperidol		2.5 mg/mL		25 mg/mL	Precipitate forms	977	I
		2.5 mg/mL		25 mg/mL	Drugs injected sequentially in Y-site with no flush. Precipitates immediately	980	I
Etoposide	BR	0.6 mg/mL[b]		30 mg/mL	Visually compatible for 4 hr at room temperature	1788	C
Etoposide phosphate	BR	5 mg/mL[a]	IMM	15 mg/mL[a]	Physically compatible for 4 hr at 23 °C	2218	C
Filgrastim	AMG	30 mcg/mL[a]	LE	15 mg/mL[a]	Physically compatible for 4 hr at 22 °C	1687	C
Fludarabine phosphate	BX	1 mg/mL[a]	CET	15 mg/mL[a]	Visually compatible for 4 hr at 22 °C	1439	C
Fluorouracil		50 mg/mL		25 mg/mL	Drugs injected sequentially in Y-site with no flush. No precipitate seen	980	C
Furosemide		10 mg/mL		25 mg/mL	Drugs injected sequentially in Y-site with no flush. No precipitate seen	980	C
Gallium nitrate	FUJ	1 mg/mL[b]	LE	25 mg/mL[b]	Visually compatible for 24 hr at 25 °C	1673	C
Gemcitabine HCl	LI	10 mg/mL[b]	IMM	15 mg/mL[b]	Precipitate forms immediately, redissolves, but reprecipitates in 15 to 20 min	2226	I
Granisetron HCl	SKB	1 mg/mL	CET	12.5 mg/mL[b]	Physically compatible with little or no loss of either drug in 4 hr at 22 °C	1883	C
Heparin sodium		1000 units/mL		25 mg/mL	Drugs injected sequentially in Y-site with no flush. No precipitate seen	980	C

Y-Site Injection Compatibility (1:1 Mixture) (Cont.)

Methotrexate sodium

Drug	Mfr	Conc	Mfr	Conc	Remarks	Ref	C/I
Idarubicin HCl	AD	1 mg/mL[b]	LE	25 mg/mL	Color changes immediately	1525	I
Ifosfamide		36 mg/mL[a]		30 mg/mL	Visually compatible for 2 hr at room temperature. Yellow precipitate in 4 hr	1788	I
Imipenem–cilastatin sodium	MSD	5 mg/mL		30 mg/mL	Visually compatible for 4 hr at room temperature	1788	C
Leucovorin calcium		10 mg/mL		25 mg/mL	Drugs injected sequentially in Y-site with no flush. No precipitate seen	980	C
	LE	10 mg/mL		30 mg/mL	Visually compatible for 4 hr at room temperature	1788	C
Linezolid	PHU	2 mg/mL	IMM	15 mg/mL[a]	Physically compatible for 4 hr at 23 °C	2264	C
Melphalan HCl	BW	0.1 mg/mL[b]	LE	15 mg/mL[b]	Physically compatible for 3 hr at 22 °C	1557	C
Mesna		1.8 mg/mL[a]		30 mg/mL	Visually compatible for 4 hr at room temperature	1788	C
Methylprednisolone sodium succinate	UP	20 mg/mL		30 mg/mL	Visually compatible for 4 hr at room temperature	1788	C
Metoclopramide HCl		5 mg/mL		25 mg/mL	Drugs injected sequentially in Y-site with no flush. No precipitate seen	980	C
Midazolam HCl	RC	5 mg/mL		30 mg/mL	Yellow precipitate forms immediately	1788	I
Mitomycin		0.5 mg/mL		25 mg/mL	Drugs injected sequentially in Y-site with no flush. No precipitate seen	980	C
Nalbuphine HCl	DU	10 mg/mL		30 mg/mL	Yellow precipitate forms immediately	1788	I
Ondansetron HCl	GL	1 mg/mL[b]	CET	15 mg/mL[a]	Visually compatible for 4 hr at 22 °C	1365	C
	GL	2 mg/mL		30 mg/mL	Visually compatible for 4 hr at room temperature	1788	C
Oxacillin sodium	BR	250 mg/mL		30 mg/mL	Visually compatible for 4 hr at room temperature	1788	C
Oxaliplatin	SS	0.5 mg/mL[a]	BED	12.5 mg/mL[a]	Physically compatible for 4 hr at 23 °C	2566	C
Paclitaxel	NCI	1.2 mg/mL[a]		15 mg/mL[a]	Physically compatible for 4 hr at 22 °C	1528	C
Piperacillin sodium–tazobactam sodium	LE[c]	40 + 5 mg/mL[a]	LE	15 mg/mL[a]	Physically compatible for 4 hr at 22 °C	1688	C
Propofol	ZEN	10 mg/mL	LE	15 mg/mL[a]	White precipitate forms in 1 hr	2066	I
Sargramostim	IMM	10 mcg/mL[b]	CET	15 mg/mL[b]	Visually compatible for 4 hr at 22 °C	1436	C
Teniposide	BR	0.1 mg/mL[a]	LE	15 mg/mL[a]	Physically compatible for 4 hr at 23 °C	1725	C
Thiotepa	IMM[e]	1 mg/mL[a]	LE	15 mg/mL[a]	Physically compatible for 4 hr at 23 °C	1861	C
TNA #218 to #226[d]			IMM	15 mg/mL[a]	Visually compatible for 4 hr at 23 °C	2215[d]	C
TPN #212 to #215[d]			LE	15 mg/mL[a]	Substantial loss of natural haze with a microprecipitate	2109[d]	I
Vancomycin HCl	AB	510 mg[f]	LE	[g]	Physically compatible during 1-hr simultaneous infusion	1405	C
		5 mg/mL[a]		30 mg/mL	Visually compatible for 2 hr at room temperature. Yellow precipitate in 4 hr	1788	I
Vinblastine sulfate		1 mg/mL		25 mg/mL	Drugs injected sequentially in Y-site with no flush. No precipitate seen	980	C
Vincristine sulfate		1 mg/mL		25 mg/mL	Drugs injected sequentially in Y-site with no flush. No precipitate seen	980	C

Y-Site Injection Compatibility (1:1 Mixture) (Cont.)

Methotrexate sodium

Drug	Mfr	Conc	Mfr	Conc	Remarks	Ref	C/I
	LI	0.1 mg/mL		30 mg/mL	Visually compatible for 4 hr at room temperature	1788	C
Vinorelbine tartrate	BW	1 mg/mL[b]	LE	15 mg/mL[b]	Physically compatible for 4 hr at 22 °C	1558	C

[a]Tested in dextrose 5%.
[b]Tested in sodium chloride 0.9%.
[c]Test performed using the formulation WITHOUT edetate disodium.
[d]Refer to Appendix I for the composition of parenteral nutrition solutions. TNA indicates a 3-in-1 admixture, and TPN indicates a 2-in-1 admixture.
[e]Lyophilized formulation tested.
[f]Infused over one hour simultaneously with methotrexate.
[g]Diluted in dextrose 5%; concentration not cited.

METHOTRIMEPRAZINE HYDROCHLORIDE
(LEVOMEPROMAZINE HYDROCHLORIDE)
AHFS 28:24.92

Products — Methotrimeprazine hydrochloride is available in 1-mL ampuls as a 25-mg/mL (2.5% w/v) solution. The injection also contains ascorbic acid, sodium sulfite, and sodium chloride in water for injection. (38; 115)

pH — From 3 to 5. (17)

Osmolality — Methotrimeprazine hydrochloride injection is an isotonic solution. (38; 115)

Trade Name(s) — Nozinan.

Administration — Methotrimeprazine hydrochloride is administered by intramuscular injection or intravenously after dilution with an equal volume of sodium chloride 0.9% immediately before use. It may also be given by continuous subcutaneous infusion diluted with the appropriate volume of sodium chloride 0.9%. (38; 115)

Stability — Methotrimeprazine hydrochloride injection is a clear, colorless solution. It should be stored at controlled room temperature and protected from light. On exposure to light, methotrimeprazine hydrochloride rapidly develops a pink or yellow discoloration; discolored solutions should be discarded. The drug is incompatible with alkaline solutions. (38; 115)

Compatibility Information

Additive Compatibility

Methotrimeprazine HCl

Drug	Mfr	Conc/L	Mfr	Conc/L	Test Soln	Remarks	Ref	C/I
Oxycodone HCl	NAP	1 g		250 mg	NS, W	Visually compatible. Under 4% concentration change in 24 hr at 25 °C	2600	C

Drugs in Syringe Compatibility

Methotrimeprazine HCl

Drug (in syringe)	Mfr	Amt	Mfr	Amt	Remarks	Ref	C/I
Butorphanol tartrate	BR	4 mg/ 2 mL		25 mg/ 1 mL	Physically compatible for 30 min at room temperature	566	C
Diamorphine HCl	MB	50 mg/ 1 mL	MB	1.25 and 2.5 mg/ 1 mL[a]	Physically compatible and diamorphine stable for 24 hr at room temperature	1454	C

Drugs in Syringe Compatibility (Cont.)

Methotrimeprazine HCl

Drug (in syringe)	Mfr	Amt	Mfr	Amt	Remarks	Ref	C/I
Heparin sodium		2500 units/ 1 mL		25 mg/ 1 mL	Turbidity or precipitate forms within 5 min	1053	I
Hydromorphone HCl	KN	10 mg/ mL	LE	10 mg/ mL	Visually compatible with less than 10% loss of either drug in 7 days at 8 °C	668	C
Hydroxyzine HCl	PF	50 mg/ 1 mL	LE	20 mg/ 1 mL	Physically compatible	771	C
	PF	100 mg/ 2 mL	LE	10 mg/ 0.5 mL	Physically compatible	771	C
Metoclopramide HCl	NO	10 mg/ 2 mL	RP	10 mg/ 2 mL	Physically compatible for 15 min at room temperature	565	C
Oxycodone HCl	NAP	200 mg/ 20 mL		200 mg/ 8 mL	Visually compatible. Under 4% concentration change in 24 hr at 25 °C	2600	C
Ranitidine HCl	GL	50 mg/ 2 mL	RP	25 mg/ 1 mL	Immediate white turbidity	978	I

[a]Diluted with sterile water for injection.

Y-Site Injection Compatibility (1:1 Mixture)

Methotrimeprazine HCl

Drug	Mfr	Conc	Mfr	Conc	Remarks	Ref	C/I
Fentanyl citrate	JN	0.025 mg/ mL[a]	LE	0.2 mg/mL[a]	Physically compatible for 48 hr at 22 °C	1706	C
Hydromorphone HCl	AST	0.5 mg/mL[a]	LE	0.2 mg/mL[a]	Physically compatible for 48 hr at 22 °C	1706	C
Methadone HCl	LI	1 mg/mL[a]	LE	0.2 mg/mL[a]	Physically compatible for 48 hr at 22 °C	1706	C
Morphine sulfate	AST	1 mg/mL[a]	LE	0.2 mg/mL[a]	Physically compatible for 48 hr at 22 °C	1706	C

[a]Tested in dextrose 5%.

METHYLDOPATE HYDROCHLORIDE
AHFS 24:08.16

Products — Methyldopate hydrochloride 50 mg/mL is available in 5- and 10-mL vials. Each milliliter of solution also contains citric acid, anhydrous 5 mg, sodium bisulfite 3.2 mg, monothioglycerol 2 mg, methylparaben 1.5 mg, sodium edetate 0.5 mg, propylparaben 0.2 mg, and sodium hydroxide and/or hydrochloric acid to adjust pH in water for injection. (1)

pH — From 3 to 4.2. (17)

Administration — Methyldopate hydrochloride is administered by intravenous infusion. Intramuscular and subcutaneous injections are not recommended due to erratic absorption. It is recommended that the desired dose be added to 100 mL of dextrose 5%. Alternatively, the dose may be administered at 100 mg/10 mL in dextrose 5%. The dose should be infused slowly over 30 to 60 minutes. (1; 4)

Stability — Intact vials should be stored at controlled room temperature and protected from freezing. (1; 4) In aqueous solutions, the drug is most stable at acid to neutral pH. Oxidation of the catechol ring is the most important degradation process. The rate of such oxidation increases with increasing oxygen supply, increasing pH, and decreasing drug concentration. (1072)

The pH of infusion solutions containing methyldopate hydrochloride tends to be 7 or less, even when alkaline intravenous infusion solutions are used. (4) It has been suggested that drugs poorly soluble in acidic media, such as barbiturate salts, be mixed cautiously with methyldopate hydrochloride since its acidity imparts some buffer capacity to intravenous admixtures. Furthermore, it should not be used with drugs known to be acid labile. (23)

Methyldopate hydrochloride oxidation is facilitated in alkaline solutions, yielding inactive dark-colored compounds. (23; 436) At pH 7.8, more than a 5% loss occurred over 24 hours. (437)

Compatibility Information

Solution Compatibility

Methyldopate HCl

Solution	Mfr	Mfr	Conc/L	Remarks	Ref	C/I
Amino acids 4.25%, dextrose 25%	MG	MSD	500 mg	No increase in particulate matter in 24 hr at 5 °C	349	C
Dextrose 5% in sodium chloride 0.9%	AB	MSD	1 g	Stable for 24 hr	23	C
Dextrose 5%	AB	MSD	1 g	Stable for 24 hr	23	C
	AB	MSD	1 g	Physically compatible. 10% calculated loss in 125 hr at 25 °C	527	C
Normosol M in dextrose 5%	AB	MSD	1 g	Stable for 24 hr	23	C
Normosol R	AB	MSD	1 g	Stable for 24 hr	23	C
Ringer's injection	AB	MSD	1 g	Stable for 24 hr	23	C
Sodium chloride 0.9%	AB	MSD	1 g	Stable for 24 hr	23	C

Additive Compatibility

Methyldopate HCl

Drug	Mfr	Conc/L	Mfr	Conc/L	Test Soln	Remarks	Ref	C/I
Aminophylline	SE	500 mg	MSD	1 g	D, D–S, S	Physically compatible	23	C
	SE	500 mg	MSD	1 g	D5W	Physically compatible. At 25 °C, 10% methyldopate decomposition in 90 hr	527	C
Amphotericin B		200 mg		1 g	D5W	Haze develops over 3 hr	26	I
Ascorbic acid	AB	1 g	MSD	1 g	D, D–S, S	Physically compatible	23	C
Chloramphenicol sodium succinate	PD	1 g	MSD	1 g	D, D–S, S	Physically compatible	23	C
Diphenhydramine HCl	PD	50 mg	MSD	1 g	D, D–S, S	Physically compatible	23	C
Heparin sodium	AB	20,000 units	MSD	1 g	D, D–S, S	Physically compatible	23	C
Magnesium sulfate		1 g	MSD	1 g	D, D–S, S	Physically compatible	23	C
Methohexital sodium	BP	2 g		1 g	D5W	Haze develops over 3 hr	26	I
	BP	2 g		1 g	NS	Crystals produced	26	I
Multivitamins	USV	10 mL	MSD	1 g	D, D–S, S	Physically compatible	23	C
Potassium chloride		40 mEq	MSD	1 g	D, D–S, S	Physically compatible	23	C
Sodium bicarbonate		50 mEq	MSD	1 g	D, D–S, S	Physically compatible	23	C
	AB	5%	MSD	1 g		Stable for 24 hr	23	C
Succinylcholine chloride	AB	2 g	MSD	1 g	D, D–S, S	Physically compatible	23	C
Verapamil HCl	KN	80 mg	MSD	500 mg	D5W, NS	Physically compatible for 24 hr	764	C

Y-Site Injection Compatibility (1:1 Mixture)

Methyldopate HCl

Drug	Mfr	Conc	Mfr	Conc	Remarks	Ref	C/I
Esmolol HCl	DCC	10 mg/mL[a]	MSD	5 mg/mL[a]	Physically compatible for 24 hr at 22 °C	1169	C
Heparin sodium	TR	50 units/mL	ES	5 mg/mL[a]	Visually compatible for 4 hr at 25 °C	1793	C
Meperidine HCl	AB	10 mg/mL	AMR	2.5 mg/mL[a]	Physically compatible for 4 hr at 25 °C	1397	C
Morphine sulfate	AB	1 mg/mL	AMR	2.5 mg/mL[a]	Physically compatible for 4 hr at 25 °C	1397	C
Theophylline	TR	4 mg/mL	ES	5 mg/mL[a]	Visually compatible for 6 hr at 25 °C	1793	C
TNA #73[c]			MSD	5 mg/mL[a]	Cracked the lipid emulsion	1009	I
			MSD	5 mg/mL[b]	Visually compatible for 4 hr	1009	C

[a]*Tested in dextrose 5%.*
[b]*Tested in sodium chloride 0.9%.*
[c]*Refer to Appendix I for the composition of parenteral nutrition solutions. TNA indicates a 3-in-1 admixture.*

METHYLERGONOVINE MALEATE
AHFS 76:00

Products — Methylergonovine maleate 0.2 mg/mL is available in 1-mL ampuls. Each milliliter of solution also contains maleic acid 0.1 mg and sodium chloride 7 mg in water for injection. (1)

pH — From 2.7 to 3.5. (17)

Trade Name(s) — Methergine.

Administration — Methylergonovine maleate may be administered intramuscularly or, in severe or life-threatening situations, intravenously slowly over no less than one minute. (1; 4) Dilution of the dose to 5 mL with sodium chloride 0.9% has also been recommended for intravenous injection. (4)

Stability — Methylergonovine maleate injection is a clear, colorless solution. If the product becomes discolored, it should not be used. (1; 4) The drug darkens with age and exposure to light. (4) The manufacturer recommends storage of intact ampuls below 25 °C and protection from light. (1)

Compatibility Information

Y-Site Injection Compatibility (1:1 Mixture)

Methylergonovine maleate

Drug	Mfr	Conc	Mfr	Conc	Remarks	Ref	C/I
Heparin sodium	UP	1000 units/L[a]	SZ	0.2 mg/mL	Physically compatible for 4 hr at room temperature	534	C
Hydrocortisone sodium succinate	UP	10 mg/L[a]	SZ	0.2 mg/mL	Physically compatible for 4 hr at room temperature	534	C

[a]*Tested in dextrose 5% in Ringer's injection, dextrose 5% in Ringer's injection, lactated, dextrose 5%, Ringer's injection, lactated, and sodium chloride 0.9%.*

METHYLPREDNISOLONE ACETATE
AHFS 68:04

Products — Methylprednisolone acetate is an injectable suspension that is available in 20-, 40-, and 80-mg/mL concentrations in 5- and 10-mL multiple-dose vials. Each milliliter contains (1):

Component	Concentration/mL		
Methylprednisolone acetate	20 mg	40 mg	80 mg
Polyethylene glycol 3350	29.5 mg	29.1 mg	28.2 mg
Polysorbate 80	1.97 mg	1.94 mg	1.88 mg
Monobasic sodium phosphate	6.9 mg	6.8 mg	6.59 mg
Dibasic sodium phosphate	1.44 mg	1.42 mg	1.37 mg
Benzyl alcohol	9.3 mg	9.16 mg	8.88 mg
Sodium chloride	to adjust tonicity	to adjust tonicity	to adjust tonicity
Sodium hydroxide and/or hydrochloric acid	qs	qs	qs

Methylprednisolone acetate is also available at concentrations of 40- and 80-mg/mL in 1-mL single-dose vials. Each milliliter contains (1):

Component	Concentration/mL	
Methylprednisolone acetate	40 mg	80 mg
Polyethylene glycol 3350	29 mg	28 mg
Myristyl-gamma-picolinium chloride	0.195 mg	0.189 mg
Sodium chloride	to adjust tonicity	to adjust tonicity
Sodium hydroxide and/or hydrochloric acid	qs	qs

pH — From 3.5 to 7.0. (1)

Trade Name(s) — Depo-Medrol.

Administration — Methylprednisolone acetate is administered by intramuscular, intra-articular, intrasynovial, soft tissue, and intralesional injection without dilution. The drug is a suspension that must not be administered intravenously. (1)

Stability — The intact vials should be stored at controlled room temperature. (1)

Compatibility Information

Drugs in Syringe Compatibility

Methylprednisolone acetate

Drug (in syringe)	Mfr	Amt	Mfr	Amt	Remarks	Ref	C/I
Ropivacaine HCl	AST	6 mg/ 3 mL	PHU	80 mg/ 2 mL	Little loss of either drug in 30 days at 4 and 24 °C in light or dark	2367	C

METHYLPREDNISOLONE SODIUM SUCCINATE
AHFS 68:04

Products — Methylprednisolone sodium succinate is available in 40-mg (1 mL), 125-mg (2 mL), 500-mg (4 mL), and 1-g (8 mL) dual-chamber containers and 500-mg (8 mL), 1-g (16 mL), and 2-g (30.6 mL) vials with and without diluent. Monobasic sodium phosphate anhydrous, dibasic sodium phosphate dried, and lactose in the 40-mg size are also present. Use only the special diluent or bacteriostatic water for injection with benzyl alcohol to reconstitute the vials. The reconstituted solutions contain the methylprednisolone equivalent (as sodium succinate) of 40, 62.5, 125, or 65.4 mg/mL depending on the vial size and reconstitution volume used. (1)

pH — The pH is adjusted to 7 to 8. (1; 4)

Osmolarity — The osmolarities of the 40-, 62.5-, 125-, and 65.4-mg/mL concentrations are 500, 400, 440, and 420 mOsm/L, respectively. (1) The osmolality of methylprednisolone sodium succinate was calculated for the following dilutions (1054):

Diluent	Osmolality (mOsm/kg)	
	50 mL	100 mL
500 mg		
Dextrose 5%	291	275
Sodium chloride 0.9%	317	301
1 g		
Dextrose 5%	318	292
Sodium chloride 0.9%	345	319

Sodium Content — Each gram of methylprednisolone sodium succinate contains 2.01 mEq of sodium. (846)

Trade Name(s) — A-MethaPred, Solu-Medrol.

Administration — Methylprednisolone sodium succinate may be administered by intramuscular and direct intravenous injection and by intermittent or continuous intravenous infusion. (1; 4) Direct intravenous injection should be performed over at least one minute (4) or over several minutes. High-dose therapy is given intravenously over at least 30 minutes. (1)

Stability — Intact vials should be stored at controlled room temperature between 20 and 25 °C and protected from light. Reconstituted solutions also should be stored between 20 and 25 °C and should used within 48 hours. (1)

The drug is subject to both ester hydrolysis and acyl migration. Degradation products include free methylprednisolone, succinate, and methylprednisolone-17-succinate. (1072) Gross decomposition may result in insoluble free methylprednisolone. (2426) The solution should not be used unless it is clear and free of particulate matter. (4)

Methylprednisolone sodium succinate (Upjohn) diluted to a concentration of 4 mg/mL with sterile water for injection and packaged in glass vials was evaluated for stability. The samples stored at 22 °C lost 10% in 24 hours while those stored at 4 °C lost 6% in seven days and 17% in 14 days. (1938)

pH Effects — The minimum rate of hydrolysis occurs at pH 3.5. Between pH 3.4 and 7.4, acyl migration is the dominant effect. (1501)

Freezing Solutions — Reconstituted methylprednisolone sodium succinate (Upjohn) 125 mg/2 mL, when stored frozen, exhibited no loss over four weeks. (69)

When stored frozen at −20 °C, methylprednisolone sodium succinate (Upjohn) 500 mg/108 mL in sodium chloride 0.9% in PVC bags exhibited no loss after 12 months followed by microwave thawing. Furthermore, the solution was physically compatible. (1612)

Syringes — Methylprednisolone sodium succinate (Pharmacia & Upjohn) 10 mg/mL in sodium chloride 0.9% was packaged in 10-mL polypropylene syringes (Becton Dickinson) and 12-mL polypropylene syringes (Monoject) and stored at 5 and 25 °C. The drug solutions remained clear, and about 10% loss occurred in seven days at 25 °C and about 4% loss in 21 days at 5 °C. The losses were comparable to the drug solution stored in a glass flask, indicating sorption to syringe components did not occur. (2340)

Central Venous Catheter — Methylprednisolone sodium succinate (Abbott) 5 mg/mL in dextrose 5% was found to be compatible with the ARROWg+ard Blue Plus (Arrow International) chlorhexidine-bearing triple-lumen central catheter. Essentially complete delivery of the drug was found with little or no drug loss occurring. Furthermore, chlorhexidine delivered from the catheter remained at trace amounts with no substantial increase due to the delivery of the drug through the catheter. (2335)

Compatibility Information

Solution Compatibility

Methylprednisolone sodium succinate

Solution	Mfr	Mfr	Conc/L	Remarks	Ref	C/I
Amino acids 4.25%, dextrose 25%	MG	UP	250 mg	No increase in particulate matter in 24 hr at 5 °C	349	**C**
Dextrose 5% in sodium chloride 0.45%		UP	5 to 10 g	Physically compatible for at least 4 hr	329	**C**
Dextrose 5% in sodium chloride 0.9%		UP	80 mg	Physically compatible for 24 hr	329	**C**
Dextrose 5%	AB	AB	500 mg to 1 g	Physically compatible and chemically stable for 24 hr at 25 °C	758	**C**
	AB	AB	1.25 g	Physically compatible for 12 hr at 25 °C. Haze from free methylprednisolone possible after 12 hr	758	**I**
	AB	AB	2 to 20 g	Physically compatible for 8 hr at 25 °C. Haze from free methylprednisolone possible after 8 hr	758	**I**
	AB	AB	30 g	Physically compatible and chemically stable for 24 hr at 25 °C	758	**C**
	TR[a]	UP	400 mg and 1.25 g	Physically compatible with 6 to 8% methylprednisolone 21-succinate ester loss in 24 hr at 24 °C	1418	**C**
	TR[a]	UP	40 mg and 2 g	Visually compatible with 4% or less loss in 48 hr at room temperature	1802	**C**
	BA[a], BRN[b]	HO	125 mg	Visually compatible with little or no loss in 24 hr at 4 and 22 °C	2289	**C**
Ringer's injection, lactated		UP	80 mg	Physically compatible for 24 hr	329	**C**
Sodium chloride 0.9%	AB	AB	500 mg to 30 g	Physically compatible and chemically stable for 24 hr at 25 °C	758	**C**
	TR[a]	UP	40 mg	Visually compatible with 6% loss in 48 hr at room temperature	1802	**C**

Solution Compatibility (Cont.)

Methylprednisolone sodium succinate

Solution	Mfr	Mfr	Conc/L	Remarks	Ref	C/I
	TRᵃ	UP	2 g	Visually compatible with 9% loss in 24 hr and 12% loss in 48 hr at room temperature	1802	C
	BAᵃ, BRNᵇ	HO	125 mg	Visually compatible with little or no loss in 24 hr at 4 and 22 °C	2289	C
TNA #237ᶜ		PHU	25, 63, 125 mg	Physically compatible with no substantial change in lipid particle size. Variable assay results, but less than 10% change in drug concentration and less than 8% change in TNA components after 7 days at 4 °C, followed by 24 hr at ambient temperature and light	2347	C
TPN #236ᶜ		PHU	25, 63, 125 mg	Variable assay results, but less than 10% change in drug concentration and less than 12% change in TPN components after 7 days at 4 °C, followed by 24 hr at ambient temperature and light	2347	C

ᵃTested in PVC containers.
ᵇTested in polyethylene and glass containers.
ᶜRefer to Appendix I for the composition of parenteral nutrition solutions. TNA indicates a 3-in-1 admixture, and TPN indicates a 2-in-1 admixture.

Additive Compatibility

Methylprednisolone sodium succinate

Drug	Mfr	Conc/L	Mfr	Conc/L	Test Soln	Remarks	Ref	C/I
Aminophylline		500 mg	UP	40 to 250 mg	D5W, NS	Clear solution for 24 hr	329	C
		1 g	UP	80 mg	D5W	Clear solution for 24 hr	329	C
	SE	500 mg	UP	125 mg		Precipitate forms after 6 hr but within 24 hr	6	I
		1 g	UP	250 mg to 1 g	D5W	Precipitate forms	329	I
		~400 mg	UP	10 to 20 g	D5S, D5W, LR	Yellow color forms	329	I
	SE	1 g	UP	500 mg and 2 g	D5W	Physically compatible. No aminophylline or methylprednisolone alcohol loss in 3 hr at room temperature, but 7 to 10% ester hydrolysis	1022	C
	SE	1 g	UP	500 mg and 2 g	NS	Physically compatible. No aminophylline or methylprednisolone alcohol loss in 3 hr at room temperature, but 12 to 18% ester hydrolysis	1022	C
Calcium gluconate		1 g	UP	40 mg	D5S	Physically incompatible	329	I
Chloramphenicol sodium succinate	PD	1 g	UP	40 mg	D5W	Clear solution for 20 hr	329	C
	PD	2 g	UP	80 mg	D5W	Clear solution for 20 hr	329	C
Clindamycin phosphate	UP	1.2 g	UP	500 mg	D5W, W	Clindamycin stable for 24 hr	101	C
Cytarabine	UP	360 mg	UP	250 mg	D5S, D10S, NS	Clear solution for 24 hr	329	C
	UP	360 mg	UP	250 mg	R, SL	Physically incompatible	329	I
Dopamine HCl	AS	800 mg	UP	500 mg	D5W	No dopamine loss in 18 hr at 25 °C	312	C
	AS	800 mg	UP	500 mg	D5W	Clear solution for 24 hr	329	C
Glycopyrrolate	RB	1.33 mg	UP	250 mg	D5½S	Physically incompatible	329	I

Additive Compatibility (Cont.)

Methylprednisolone sodium succinate

Drug	Mfr	Conc/L	Mfr	Conc/L	Test Soln	Remarks	Ref	C/I
Granisetron HCl	BE	56 mg	DAK	2.26 g	D5W, NS[a]	Visually compatible. Little loss of either drug in 72 hr at room temperature	1884	C
Heparin sodium		5000 units	UP	125 mg	D5S, D5W, LR, R	Clear solution for 24 hr	329	C
		10,000 units	UP	40 mg	D5S	Clear solution for 24 hr	329	C
		40,000 units	UP	25 g	NS	Clear solution for 24 hr	329	C
Nafcillin sodium	WY	500 mg	UP	125 mg	D5W	Precipitate forms	329	I
Norepinephrine bitartrate	WI	8 mg	UP	40 mg	D5S	Physically compatible	329	C
Ondansetron HCl	GSK	160 mg	PH	2.4 g	D5W, NS	Transient turbidity forms then clears. 5% or less loss of either drug in 24 hr at 23 °C and 48 hr at 6 °C	2643	?
Penicillin G potassium		2 to 10 million units	UP	80 mg	D5S, D5W, LR	Clear solution for 24 hr	329	C
Penicillin G sodium		5 million units	UP	125 mg	D5W, LR	Precipitate forms	329	I
Ranitidine HCl	GL	50 mg	UP	40 mg	D5W[a]	Visually compatible with 7% ranitidine loss and no methylprednisolone loss in 48 hr at room temperature	1802	C
	GL	50 mg	UP	2 g	D5W[a]	Visually compatible with 6% ranitidine loss and 10% methylprednisolone loss in 48 hr at room temperature	1802	C
	GL	2 g	UP	40 mg and 2 g	D5W[a]	Visually compatible with no loss of either drug in 48 hr at room temperature	1802	C
	GL	50 mg and 2 g	UP	40 mg and 2 g	NS[a]	Visually compatible with no ranitidine loss and about 10% methylprednisolone loss in 48 hr at room temperature	1802	C
Theophylline	AB[b]	4 g	UP	500 mg and 2 g	D5W	Physically compatible. Little theophylline or methylprednisolone alcohol loss in 24 hr at room temperature, but 8% ester hydrolysis	1150	C
	AB[b]	400 mg	UP	500 mg and 2 g	D5W	Physically compatible. Little theophylline or methylprednisolone alcohol loss in 24 hr at room temperature, but 11% ester hydrolysis	1150	C
Verapamil HCl	KN	80 mg	UP	250 mg	D5W, NS	Physically compatible for 24 hr	764	C

[a]*Tested in PVC containers.*
[b]*Tested in premixed infusion solution.*

Drugs in Syringe Compatibility

Methylprednisolone sodium succinate

Drug (in syringe)	Mfr	Amt	Mfr	Amt	Remarks	Ref	C/I
Doxapram HCl	RB	400 mg/ 20 mL	UP	40 mg/ 2 mL	Immediate turbidity and precipitation	1177	**I**
Granisetron HCl	BE	0.15 mg/ mL[a]	DAK	6 mg/mL[a]	Visually compatible. Little loss of either drug in 72 hr at room temperature	1884	**C**
Iohexol	WI	64.7%, 5 mL	UP	10 mg/ 1 mL	Physically compatible for at least 2 hr	1438	**C**
Iopamidol	SQ	61%, 5 mL	UP	10 mg/ 1 mL	Physically compatible for at least 2 hr	1438	**C**
Iothalamate meglumine	MA	60%, 5 mL	UP	10 mg/ 1 mL	Physically compatible for at least 2 hr	1438	**C**
Ioxaglate meglumine–ioxaglate sodium	MA	5 mL	UP	10 mg/ 1 mL	Physically compatible for at least 2 hr	1438	**C**
Metoclopramide HCl	RB	10 mg/ 2 mL	ES	62.5 mg/ 1 mL	Physically compatible for 24 hr at 25 °C	1167	**C**
	RB	10 mg/ 2 mL	ES	250 mg/ 4 mL	Physically compatible for 24 hr at 25 °C	1167	**C**
	RB	160 mg/ 32 mL	ES	250 mg/ 4 mL	Physically compatible for 24 hr at 25 °C	1167	**C**
Pantoprazole sodium	[b]	4 mg/ 1 mL		62.5 mg/ 1 mL	Precipitates within 15 min	2574	**I**

[a] Diluted with water.
[b] Test performed using the formulation WITHOUT edetate disodium.

Y-Site Injection Compatibility (1:1 Mixture)

Methylprednisolone sodium succinate

Drug	Mfr	Conc	Mfr	Conc	Remarks	Ref	C/I
Acyclovir sodium	BW	5 mg/mL[a]	LY	0.8 mg/mL[a]	Physically compatible for 4 hr at 25 °C	1157	**C**
Allopurinol sodium	BW	3 mg/mL[b]	AB	5 mg/mL[b]	Haze forms in 1 hr with white precipitate in 24 hr	1686	**I**
Alprostadil	BED	7.5 mcg/mL[f]	PH	40 mg/mL[e]	Visually compatible for 1 hr	2746	**C**
Amifostine	USB	10 mg/mL[a]	AB	5 mg/mL[a]	Physically compatible for 4 hr at 23 °C	1845	**C**
Amiodarone HCl	WY	6 mg/mL[a]	PHU	125 mg/mL	Visually compatible for 24 hr at 22 °C	2352	**C**
Amphotericin B cholesteryl sulfate complex	SEQ	0.83 mg/mL[a]	PHU	5 mg/mL[a]	Physically compatible for 4 hr at 23 °C	2117	**C**
Amsacrine	NCI	1 mg/mL[a]	UP	5 mg/mL[a]	Immediate orange turbidity and precipitate in 4 hr	1381	**I**
Anidulafungin	VIC	0.5 mg/mL[a]	PH	5 mg/mL[a]	Physically compatible for 4 hr at 23 °C	2617	**C**
Aztreonam	SQ	40 mg/mL[a]	AB	5 mg/mL[a]	Physically compatible for 4 hr at 23 °C	1758	**C**
Bivalirudin	TMC	5 mg/mL[a]	PHU	5 mg/mL[a]	Physically compatible for 4 hr at 23 °C	2373	**C**
Caspofungin acetate	ME	0.7 mg/mL[b]	PHU	5 mg/mL[b]	Immediate white turbid precipitate forms	2758	**I**
Cefepime HCl	BMS	120 mg/mL[j]		50 mg/mL	Physically compatible with less than 10% cefepime loss. Methylprednisolone not tested	2513	**C**

Y-Site Injection Compatibility (1:1 Mixture) (Cont.)

Methylprednisolone sodium succinate

Drug	*Mfr*	*Conc*	*Mfr*	*Conc*	*Remarks*	*Ref*	*C/I*
Ceftaroline fosamil	FOR	2.22 mg/mL[a,b,g]	PHU	5 mg/mL[a,b,g]	Physically compatible for 4 hr at 23 °C	2826	C
Ceftazidime	GSK	120 mg/mL[j]		50 mg/mL	Physically compatible. Less than 10% ceftazidime loss. Methylprednisolone not tested	2513	C
Ciprofloxacin	MI	2 mg/mL[c]	UP	62.5 mg/mL	Transient cloudiness rapidly dissipates. Crystals form in 2 hr at 24 °C	1655	I
Cisatracurium besylate	GW	0.1 mg/mL[a]	AB	5 mg/mL[a]	Physically compatible for 4 hr at 23 °C	2074	C
	GW	2 mg/mL[a]	AB	5 mg/mL[a]	Subvisible haze forms immediately	2074	I
	GW	5 mg/mL[a]	AB	5 mg/mL[a]	Haze forms immediately	2074	I
Cladribine	ORT	0.015[b] and 0.5[d] mg/mL	AB	5 mg/mL[b]	Physically compatible for 4 hr at 23 °C	1969	C
Cytarabine	UP	16 mg/mL[b]	UP	5 mg/mL[a]	Visually compatible for 24 hr at room temperature in test tubes. No precipitate found on filter from Y-site delivery	2063	C
Dexmedetomidine HCl	AB	4 mcg/mL[b]	PHU	5 mg/mL[b]	Physically compatible for 4 hr at 23 °C	2383	C
Diltiazem HCl	MMD	5 mg/mL	UP	2.5 mg/mL[a]	Cloudiness forms	1807	I
	MMD	5 mg/mL	UP	20 mg/mL[b]	Precipitate forms	1807	I
	MMD	5 mg/mL	UP	62.5 mg/mL	Cloudiness forms but clears with swirling	1807	?
	MMD	1 mg/mL[b]	UP	2.5[a], 20[b], 62.5 mg/mL	Visually compatible	1807	C
Docetaxel	RPR	0.9 mg/mL[a]	PHU	5 mg/mL[a]	Partial loss of measured natural turbidity occurs immediately	2224	I
Dopamine HCl	AB	0.8 mg/mL[a]	UP	5 mg/mL[a]	Visually compatible for 24 hr at room temperature in test tubes. No precipitate found on filter from Y-site delivery	2063	C
Doripenem	JJ	5 mg/mL[a,b]	PHU	5 mg/mL[a,b]	Physically compatible for 4 hr at 23 °C	2743	C
Doxorubicin HCl liposomal	SEQ	0.4 mg/mL[a]	UP	5 mg/mL[a]	Physically compatible for 4 hr at 23 °C	2087	C
Enalaprilat	MSD	0.05 mg/mL[b]	UP	0.8 mg/mL[a]	Physically compatible for 24 hr at room temperature under fluorescent light	1355	C
Etoposide phosphate	BR	5 mg/mL[a]	AB	5 mg/mL[a]	Haze with subvisible microparticles forms immediately. Particle content increases fivefold over 4 hr at 23 °C	2218	I
Famotidine	MSD	0.2 mg/mL[a]	AB	1 mg/mL[a]	Physically compatible for 4 hr at 25 °C	1188	C
	MSD	0.2 mg/mL[a]	QU	40 mg/mL	Physically compatible for 14 hr	1196	C
	ME	2 mg/mL[b]		5 mg/mL[a]	Visually compatible for 4 hr at 22 °C	1936	C
Fenoldopam mesylate	AB	80 mcg/mL[b]	PHU	5 mg/mL[b]	Microparticulates form immediately	2467	I
Filgrastim	AMG	30 mcg/mL[a]	AB	5 mg/mL[a]	Haze, particles, and filaments form immediately	1687	I
Fludarabine phosphate	BX	1 mg/mL[a]	UP	5 mg/mL[a]	Visually compatible for 4 hr at 22 °C	1439	C
Gemcitabine HCl	LI	10 mg/mL[b]	AB	5 mg/mL[b]	Gross precipitation occurs immediately	2226	I
Granisetron HCl	SKB	0.05 mg/mL[a]	WY	5 mg/mL[a]	Physically compatible for 4 hr at 23 °C	2000	C

Y-Site Injection Compatibility (1:1 Mixture) (Cont.)

Methylprednisolone sodium succinate

Drug	Mfr	Conc	Mfr	Conc	Remarks	Ref	C/I
Heparin sodium	TR	50 units/mL	UP	2.5 mg/mL[a]	Visually compatible for 4 hr at 25 °C	1793	C
	ES	100 units/mL[c]	UP	5 mg/mL[a]	Visually compatible for 24 hr at room temperature in test tubes. No precipitate found on filter from Y-site delivery	2063	C
Hetastarch in lactated electrolyte	AB	6%	PHU	5 mg/mL[a]	Physically compatible for 4 hr at 23 °C	2339	C
Hydroxyethyl starch 130/0.4 in sodium chloride 0.9%	FRK	6%	NOP	0.25[a], 5[a], 62.5 mg/mL	Visually compatible for 24 hr at room temperature	2770	C
Linezolid	PHU	2 mg/mL	AB	5 mg/mL[a]	Physically compatible for 4 hr at 23 °C	2264	C
Melphalan HCl	BW	0.1 mg/mL[b]	AB	5 mg/mL[b]	Physically compatible for 3 hr at 22 °C	1557	C
Meperidine HCl	AB	10 mg/mL	UP	2.5 mg/mL[a]	Physically compatible for 4 hr at 25 °C	1397	C
Methotrexate sodium		30 mg/mL	UP	20 mg/mL	Visually compatible for 4 hr at room temperature	1788	C
Metronidazole	MG	5 mg/mL	UP	5 mg/mL[a]	Visually compatible for 24 hr at room temperature in test tubes. No precipitate found on filter from Y-site delivery	2063	C
Midazolam HCl	RC	1 mg/mL[a]	UP	40 mg/mL	Visually compatible for 24 hr at 23 °C	1847	C
Milrinone lactate	SS	0.2 mg/mL[a]	PHU	125 mg/mL	Visually compatible for 4 hr at 25 °C	2381	C
Morphine sulfate	AB	1 mg/mL	UP	2.5 mg/mL[a]	Physically compatible for 4 hr at 25 °C	1397	C
Nicardipine HCl	DCC	0.1 mg/mL[a]	UP	0.8 mg/mL[a]	Visually compatible for 24 hr at room temperature	235	C
Ondansetron HCl	GL	1 mg/mL[b]	UP	5 mg/mL[a]	Light haze develops in 30 min	1365	I
Oxaliplatin	SS	0.5 mg/mL[a]	PHU	5 mg/mL[a]	Physically compatible for 4 hr at 23 °C	2566	C
Paclitaxel	NCI	1.2 mg/mL[a]	UP	5 mg/mL[a]	Normal inherent haze from paclitaxel decreases immediately	1556	I
Palonosetron HCl	MGI	50 mcg/mL	PHU	5 mg/mL[a]	Microprecipitate begins to form immediately and becomes visible within 4 hr	2681	I
Pemetrexed disodium	LI	20 mg/mL[b]	PHU	5 mg/mL[a]	Physically compatible for 4 hr at 23 °C	2564	C
Piperacillin sodium–tazobactam sodium	LE[k]	40 + 5 mg/mL[a]	AB	5 mg/mL[a]	Physically compatible for 4 hr at 22 °C	1688	C
Potassium chloride		40 mEq/L[a]	UP	40 mg/mL	Physically compatible for 4 hr at room temperature	322	C
		40 mEq/L[b]	UP	40 mg/mL	Physically compatible initially but haze forms in 4 hr at room temperature	322	I
		40 mEq/L[g]	UP	40 mg/mL	Immediate haze formation	322	I
Propofol	ZEN	10 mg/mL	AB	5 mg/mL[a]	White precipitate forms immediately	2066	I
Remifentanil HCl	GW	0.025 and 0.25 mg/mL[b]	AB	5 mg/mL[a]	Physically compatible for 4 hr at 23 °C	2075	C
Sargramostim	IMM	10 mcg/mL[b]	UP	5 mg/mL[b]	Small amounts of particles and filaments form in 4 hr	1436	I

Y-Site Injection Compatibility (1:1 Mixture) (Cont.)

Methylprednisolone sodium succinate

Drug	Mfr	Conc	Mfr	Conc	Remarks	Ref	C/I
Sodium bicarbonate		1.4%	UP	20 mg/mL	Visually compatible for 4 hr at room temperature	1788	C
Tacrolimus	FUJ	1 mg/mL[b]	UP	0.8 mg/mL[a]	Visually compatible for 24 hr at 25 °C	1630	C
Telavancin HCl	ASP	7.5 mg/mL[a]	PF	5 mg/mL[a]	Slight measured turbidity increase	2830	I
	ASP	7.5 mg/mL[b,g]	PF	5 mg/mL[b,g]	Physically compatible for 2 hr	2830	C
Teniposide	BR	0.1 mg/mL[a]	AB	5 mg/mL[a]	Physically compatible for 4 hr at 23 °C	1725	C
Theophylline	TR	4 mg/mL	UP	2.5 mg/mL[a]	Visually compatible for 6 hr at 25 °C	1793	C
Thiotepa	IMM[h]	1 mg/mL[a]	AB	5 mg/mL[a]	Physically compatible for 4 hr at 23 °C	1861	C
Tigecycline	WY	1 mg/mL[b]		20 mg/mL[b]	Microparticulates form	2714	I
TNA #218 to #226[i]			AB	5 mg/mL[a]	Visually compatible for 4 hr at 23 °C	2215	C
Topotecan HCl	SKB	56 mcg/mL[a,b]	UP	2.4 mg/mL[a,b]	Yellow color forms. Little loss of either drug in 4 hr at 22 °C	2245	C
TPN #212 to #215[i]			AB	5 mg/mL[a]	Physically compatible for 4 hr at 23 °C	2109	C
Vinorelbine tartrate	BW	1 mg/mL[b]	AB	5 mg/mL[b]	Heavy white precipitate forms immediately	1558	I

[a]*Tested in dextrose 5%.*
[b]*Tested in sodium chloride 0.9%.*
[c]*Tested in both dextrose 5% and sodium chloride 0.9%.*
[d]*Tested in bacteriostatic sodium chloride 0.9% preserved with benzyl alcohol 0.9%.*
[e]*Tested in either dextrose 5% or in sodium chloride 0.9%, but the report did not specify which solution.*
[f]*Tested in a 1:1 mixture of (1) dextrose 5% and dextrose 5% in sodium chloride 0.45% with and without potassium chloride 20 mEq/L, and also (2) dextrose 10% in sodium chloride 0.45% with and without potassium chloride 20 mEq/L, and also (3) dextrose 5% and TPN #274 (see Appendix I).*
[g]*Tested in Ringer's injection, lactated.*
[h]*Lyophilized formulation tested.*
[i]*Refer to Appendix I for the composition of parenteral nutrition solutions. TNA indicates a 3-in-1 admixture, and TPN indicates a 2-in-1 admixture.*
[j]*Tested in sterile water for injection.*
[k]*Test performed using the formulation WITHOUT edetate disodium.*

Additional Compatibility Information

Infusion Solutions — Solution haziness was reported for methylprednisolone sodium succinate admixtures in intravenous fluids. (702; 758) Changes in the manufacturing process for bulk methylprednisolone sodium succinate powder have resulted in substantial improvements in admixture clarity and absence of the haze formation that developed previously in solutions of Solu-Medrol. (670; 702)

In a study of the turbidity produced by methylprednisolone sodium succinate (Abbott) 500 mg to 30 g/L, turbidity was substantially higher in dextrose 5% than in sodium chloride 0.9%. (758) Another important factor was the concentration of methylprednisolone sodium succinate. Turbidity was generally higher at intermediate concentrations (2 to 15 g/L) than at low (300 mg/L) or high (20 g/L) concentrations. (758)

These differences in the development of turbidity cannot be explained by simple increased ester hydrolysis due to differing pH values and drug concentrations. Rather, the solubility of free methylprednisolone in various concentrations of methylprednisolone sodium succinate has been suggested as the primary factor. The solubility of free methylprednisolone is increased as the concentration of the sodium succinate ester increases. The increased solubilization is believed to overshadow increased formation of free methylprednisolone in concentrations over 10 g/L, preventing or minimizing precipitation and turbidity. Differences in turbidity between the drug in dextrose 5% and sodium chloride 0.9% are believed to result primarily from the electrolyte content of sodium chloride 0.9% and, to a much lesser extent, the pH of the dextrose admixtures. These differences are presumed to affect the solubilizing capacity and reactivity of the ester. (758)

Other Drugs — The compatibility of methylprednisolone sodium succinate (Upjohn) with several drugs added to auxiliary medication infusion units has been studied. Primary admixtures were prepared by adding various drugs to dextrose 5%, dextrose 5% in sodium chloride 0.9%, and Ringer's injection, lactated. Up to 100 mL of the primary admixture was added along with methylprednisolone sodium succinate (Upjohn) to the auxiliary medication infusion unit with the following results (329):

Methylprednisolone Sodium Succinate	Primary Solution	Result
	Aminophylline 500 mg/L	
500 mg	D5S, D5W qs 100 mL	Clear solution for 24 hr
500 mg	LR qs 100 mL	Clear solution for 24 hr
500 mg	Added to 100 mL LR	Clear solution for 1 hr
1000 mg	D5W qs 100 mL	Yellow solution, clear for 24 hr
1000 mg	D5S qs 100 mL	Yellow solution, clear for 6 hr
1000 mg	Added to 100 mL D5S	Yellow solution, clear for 24 hr
1000 mg	LR qs 100 mL or added to 100 mL LR	Yellow solution, clear for 4 hr
2000 mg	D5S, D5W, LR qs 100 mL	Yellow solution, clear for 24 hr
	Heparin Sodium 10,000 units/L	
500 mg	D5S, D5W qs 100 mL	Clear solution for 24 hr
500 mg	LR qs 100 mL or added to 100 mL LR	Clear solution for 6 hr
1000 mg	D5S, D5W qs 100 mL	Clear solution for 6 hr
1000 mg	Added to 100 mL D5W	Clear solution for 24 hr
1000 mg	LR qs 100 mL or added to 100 mL LR	Clear solution for 4 to 6 hr
2000 mg	D5W qs 100 mL	Clear solution for 6 hr
2000 mg	D5S, LR qs 100 mL	Clear solution for 24 hr
	Potassium Chloride 40 mEq/L	
500 mg	D5S, D5W, LR qs 100 mL	Clear solution for 24 hr
1000 mg	D5W qs 100 mL	Clear solution for 24 hr
1000 mg	D5S, LR qs 100 mL or added to 100 mL D5S, LR	Clear solution for 6 hr
2000 mg	D5S, D5W, LR qs 100 mL	Clear solution for 24 hr
	Sodium Bicarbonate 44.6 mEq/L	
500 mg	D5S, D5W qs 100 mL	Clear solution for 24 hr
500 mg	LR qs 100 mL or added to 100 mL LR	Clear solution for 1 hr
1000 mg	D5W qs 100 mL	Clear solution for 24 hr
1000 mg	D5S qs 100 mL or added to 100 mL D5S	Clear solution for 24 hr
1000 mg	LR qs 100 mL	Clear solution for 1 hr
1000 mg	Added to 100 mL LR	Clear solution for 4 hr
2000 mg	D5S, D5W qs 100 mL	Clear solution for 24 hr
2000 mg	LR qs 100 mL	Clear solution for 30 min
2000 mg	Added to 100 mL LR	Clear solution for 4 hr

METOCLOPRAMIDE HYDROCHLORIDE
AHFS 56:32

Products — Metoclopramide hydrochloride is available in 2-mL ampuls and 2-, 10-, and 30-mL vials. Each milliliter of solution contains metoclopramide (as the hydrochloride) 5 mg with sodium chloride 8.5 mg and hydrochloric acid and/or sodium hydroxide, if necessary, in water for injection. (1)

pH — From 4.5 to 6.5. (1) Metoclopramide hydrochloride 1.25, 2.22, and 3.75 mg/mL in sodium chloride 0.9% had pH values of 4.4, 4.1, and 4.0, respectively. (2161)

Osmolality — The osmolality of metoclopramide hydrochloride 5 mg/mL was determined to be 280 mOsm/kg. (1233) Metoclopramide hydrochloride 1.25, 2.22, and 3.75 mg/mL in sodium chloride 0.9% had osmolalities of 285, 286, and 294 mOsm/kg, respectively. (2161)

Trade Name(s) — Reglan.

Administration — Metoclopramide hydrochloride is administered by intramuscular injection, by direct intravenous injection undiluted slowly over one or two minutes for 10 mg doses of drug, or by intermittent intravenous infusion over 15 minutes diluted in 50 mL of compatible diluent for larger doses. (1; 4)

Stability — Metoclopramide hydrochloride injection is a clear, colorless solution; it should be stored at controlled room temperature and protected from freezing. The drug is stable over a pH range of 2 to 9. Metoclopramide hydrochloride is photosensitive; protection from light for the product during storage has been recommended. (4) However, the manufacturer no longer recommends light protection for dilutions under normal lighting conditions, stating that they may be stored up to 24 hours. (1)

Freezing Solutions — Undiluted metoclopramide hydrochloride (Robins) 5 mg/mL packaged as 3 mL in plastic infusion-pump syringes (MiniMed) fitted with Luer-Lok tip caps (Burron) exhibited microprecipitation that did not redissolve upon warming to room temperature when stored frozen at −20 °C for as little as one day. The precipitate was not visible with the unaided eye. Freezing is not an acceptable storage method for undiluted metoclopramide hydrochloride injection. (2001)

Syringes — Undiluted metoclopramide hydrochloride (Robins) 5 mg/mL was packaged as 3 mL in plastic infusion-pump syringes (MiniMed) fitted with Luer-Lok tip caps (Burron). Stored for seven days at 32 °C to simulate wearing a portable infusion pump close to the body, metoclopramide hydrochloride was physically stable and little loss occurred. At 23 °C, metoclopramide hydrochloride was physically and chemically stable for up to 60 days with little loss occurring. However, large quantities of subvisible particulates formed after that time, making the drug unsuitable for use. Stored under refrigeration at 4 °C, metoclopramide hydrochloride remained both physically and chemically stable for up to 90 days. (2001)

Metoclopramide hydrochloride (Solopak) 2.5 mg/mL in sodium chloride 0.9% packaged in polypropylene syringes (Sherwood) was physically stable and exhibited little or no loss in 24 hours stored at 4 and 23 °C. (2199)

Central Venous Catheter — Metoclopramide hydrochloride (Abbott) 0.5 mg/mL in dextrose 5% was found to be compatible with the AR-ROWg+ard Blue Plus (Arrow International) chlorhexidine-bearing triple-lumen central catheter. Essentially complete delivery of the drug was found with little or no drug loss occurring. Furthermore, chlorhexidine delivered from the catheter remained at trace amounts with no substantial increase due to the delivery of the drug through the catheter. (2335)

Compatibility Information

Solution Compatibility

Metoclopramide HCl

Solution	Mfr	Mfr	Conc/L	Remarks	Ref	C/I
Amino acids 2.75%, dextrose 25%, electrolytes	TR	RB	5 and 20 mg	Metoclopramide chemically stable for 72 hr at room temperature	854	C
Dextrose 5% in sodium chloride 0.45%				Compatible for 48 hr at room temperature	1	C
	TR[a]	RB	200 mg	Physically compatible with 2% loss in 24 hr at 25 °C exposed to normal room light	1167	C
	TR[a]	RB	3.2 g	Physically compatible with 4 to 5% loss in 24 hr at 25 °C exposed to normal room light	1167	C
Dextrose 5%				Compatible for 24 hr at room temperature	1	C
	TR[a]	RB	200 mg	Physically compatible with no loss in 24 hr at 25 °C exposed to normal room light	1167	C
	TR[a]	RB	200 mg	9% loss after 2 weeks and 14% loss after 4 weeks frozen at −20 °C followed by 24 hr at room temperature	1167	C
	TR[a]	RB	3.2 g	Physically compatible with 5% loss in 24 hr at 25 °C exposed to normal room light	1167	C
	TR[a]	RB	3.2 g	11% loss after 1 week and 37% loss after 4 weeks frozen at −20 °C followed by 24 hr at room temperature	1167	I
Ringer's injection				Compatible for 48 hr at room temperature	1	C
Ringer's injection, lactated				Compatible for 48 hr at room temperature	1	C
Sodium chloride 0.9%				Compatible for 48 hr at room temperature	1	C
	TR[a]	RB	200 mg and 3.2 g	No loss after 4 weeks frozen at −20 °C followed by 24 hr at room temperature	1167	C
	TR[a]	RB	200 mg and 3.2 g	Physically compatible with no loss in 24 hr at 25 °C exposed to normal room light	1167	C
	BA	BA	500 mg	Physically compatible with no drug loss in 21 days at 25 °C	2586	C
TPN #89[b]		RB	5 mg	Physically compatible with no metoclopramide loss in 24 hr and 10% loss in 48 hr at 25 °C	1167	C
		RB	20 mg	Physically compatible with no metoclopramide loss in 72 hr at 25 °C	1167	C

Solution Compatibility (Cont.)

Metoclopramide HCl

Solution	Mfr	Mfr	Conc/L	Remarks	Ref	C/I
TPN #90[b]		RB	5 mg	Physically compatible with no metoclopramide loss in 72 hr at 25 °C	1167	**C**
		RB	20 mg	Physically compatible with 3% metoclopramide loss in 72 hr at 25 °C	1167	**C**

[a]Tested in PVC containers.
[b]Refer to Appendix I for the composition of parenteral nutrition solutions. TPN indicates a 2-in-1 admixture.

Additive Compatibility

Metoclopramide HCl

Drug	Mfr	Conc/L	Mfr	Conc/L	Test Soln	Remarks	Ref	C/I
Clindamycin phosphate	UP	6 g	RB	100 and 200 mg		Physically compatible for 24 hr at 25 °C	1167	**C**
	UP	3.5 g	RB	1.9 g		Physically compatible for 24 hr at 25 °C	1167	**C**
	UP	4.4 g	RB	1.2 g		Physically compatible for 24 hr at 25 °C	1167	**C**
Dexamethasone sodium phosphate with lorazepam and diphenhydramine HCl	AMR WY ES	400 mg 40 mg 2 g	DU	4 g	NS[a]	Rapid lorazepam losses of 8, 10, and 15% at 3, 23, and 30 °C, respectively, in 24 hr. Other drugs stable for 14 days at all three storage temperatures	1733	**I**
Diphenhydramine HCl with dexamethasone sodium phosphate and lorazepam	ES AMR WY	2 g 400 mg 40 mg	DU	4 g	NS[a]	Rapid lorazepam losses of 8, 10, and 15% at 3, 23, and 30 °C, respectively, in 24 hr. Other drugs stable for 14 days at all three storage temperatures	1733	**I**
Erythromycin lactobionate	AB	4 g	RB	400 mg	NS	Incompatible. If mixed, use immediately	924	**I**
	AB	4.1 g	RB	416 mg		Incompatible. If mixed, use immediately	1167	**I**
	AB	5 g	RB	100 mg	NS	Incompatible. If mixed, use immediately	924	**I**
	AB	3.5 g	RB	1.1 g		Incompatible. If mixed, use immediately	1167	**I**
Floxacillin sodium	BE	20 g	ANT	1 g	NS	White precipitate forms immediately	1479	**I**
Fluorouracil	RC	2.5 g	FUJ	100 mg	D5W	10% metoclopramide loss in 6 hr and 27% loss in 24 hr at 25 °C. 5% metoclopramide loss in 120 hr at 4 °C. 5 and 7% fluorouracil losses in 120 hr at 4 and 25 °C, respectively	1780	**I**
Furosemide	HO	1 g	ANT	1 g	NS	Precipitates immediately	1479	**I**
Lorazepam with dexamethasone sodium phosphate and diphenhydramine HCl	WY AMR ES	40 mg 400 mg 2 g	DU	4 g	NS[a]	Rapid lorazepam losses of 8, 10, and 15% at 3, 23, and 30 °C, respectively, in 24 hr. Other drugs stable for 14 days at all three storage temperatures	1733	**I**
Mannitol	AB	20%	RB	40 and 100 mg		Physically compatible for 48 hr at room temperature	924	**C**
	AB	20%	RB	40 and 100 mg		Physically compatible for 48 hr at 25 °C	1167	**C**
	AB	20%	RB	640 mg and 1.6 g		Physically compatible for 48 hr at 25 °C	1167	**C**
Meperidine HCl	DW	7.35 g	DW	150 mg	D5W, NS	Visually compatible. Little loss of drugs over 48 hr at 32 °C in light or dark	2253	**C**
Meropenem	ZEN	1 and 20 g	RB	100 mg	NS	Visually compatible for 4 hr at room temperature	1994	**C**

Additive Compatibility (Cont.)

Metoclopramide HCl

Drug	Mfr	Conc/L	Mfr	Conc/L	Test Soln	Remarks	Ref	C/I
Morphine sulfate	EV	1 g	SKB	500 mg	NS[b]	Visually compatible. Little loss of either drug in 35 days at 22 °C and 182 days at 4 °C followed by 7 days at 32 °C	1939	C
	EV	1 g	SKB	500 mg	D5W[c]	Visually compatible. 8% metoclopramide loss in 14 days at 22 °C and 98 days at 4 °C. No morphine loss	1939	C
Multivitamins	USV	20 mL	RB	20 and 320 mg	NS	Physically compatible for 48 hr at room temperature	924	C
	USV	20 mL	RB	20 and 320 mg	NS	Physically compatible for 48 hr at room temperature	924	C
Oxycodone HCl	NAP	770 mg		1.2 g	NS, W	Visually compatible. Under 4% concentration change in 24 hr at 25 °C	2600	C
Potassium acetate	IX	20 mEq	RB	10 and 160 mg	NS	Physically compatible for 48 hr at room temperature	924	C
Potassium chloride	ES	30 mEq	RB	10 and 160 mg	NS	Physically compatible for 48 hr at room temperature	924	C
Potassium phosphates	IX	15 mmol	RB	10 and 160 mg	NS	Physically compatible for 48 hr at room temperature	924	C
Tramadol HCl	AND	1.118 g	SYO	1.11 g	NS[d]	Visually compatible for 7 days at 25 °C protected from light	2701	C
	AND	3.33 g	SYO	3.33 g	NS[d]	Visually compatible for 7 days at 25 °C protected from light	2701	C
Verapamil HCl	KN	80 mg	RB	20 mg	D5W, NS	Physically compatible for 24 hr	764	C

[a]Tested in Pharmacia-Deltec PVC pump reservoirs.
[b]Tested in PVC containers.
[c]Tested in PCA Infusors (Baxter).
[d]Tested in elastomeric pump reservoirs (Baxter).

Drugs in Syringe Compatibility

Metoclopramide HCl

Drug (in syringe)	Mfr	Amt	Mfr	Amt	Remarks	Ref	C/I
Aminophylline	ES	500 mg/ 20 mL	RB	160 mg/ 32 mL	Physically compatible for 24 hr at 25 °C	1167	C
	ES	80 mg/ 3.2 mL	RB	10 mg/ 2 mL	Physically compatible for 24 hr at 25 °C	1167	C
	ES	500 mg/ 20 mL	RB	10 mg/ 2 mL	Physically compatible for 24 hr at 25 °C	1167	C
Ampicillin sodium	BR	250 mg/ 2.5 mL	RB	10 mg/ 2 mL	Incompatible. If mixed, use immediately	1167	I
	BR	1 g/ 10 mL	RB	10 mg/ 2 mL	Incompatible. If mixed, use immediately	1167	I
	BR	1 g/ 10 mL	RB	160 mg/ 32 mL	Incompatible. If mixed, use immediately	1167	I
Ascorbic acid	AB	250 mg/ 0.5 mL	RB	160 mg/ 32 mL	Physically compatible for 48 hr at 25 °C	1167	C
	AB	250 mg/ 0.5 mL	RB	10 mg/ 2 mL	Physically compatible for 48 hr at 25 °C	1167	C

Drugs in Syringe Compatibility (Cont.)

Metoclopramide HCl

Drug (in syringe)	Mfr	Amt	Mfr	Amt	Remarks	Ref	C/I
Atropine sulfate	GL	0.4 mg/ 1 mL	NO	10 mg/ 2 mL	Physically compatible for 15 min at room temperature	565	**C**
Benztropine mesylate	MSD	2 mg/ 2 mL	RB	160 mg/ 32 mL	Physically compatible for 48 hr at 25 °C	1167	**C**
	MSD	2 mg/ 2 mL	RB	10 mg/ 2 mL	Physically compatible for 48 hr at 25 °C	1167	**C**
Bleomycin sulfate		1.5 units/ 0.5 mL		2.5 mg/ 0.5 mL	Physically compatible for 5 min at room temperature followed by 8 min of centrifugation	980	**C**
Butorphanol tartrate	BR	4 mg/ 2 mL	NO	10 mg/ 2 mL	Physically compatible for 30 min at room temperature	566	**C**
Caffeine citrate		20 mg/ 1 mL	ES	5 mg/ 1 mL	Visually compatible for 4 hr at 25 °C	2440	**C**
Calcium gluconate	ES	1 g/ 10 mL	RB	10 mg/ 2 mL	Possible precipitate formation	924	**I**
	ES	1 g/ 10 mL	RB	160 mg/ 32 mL	Incompatible. If mixed, use immediately	1167	**I**
Chloramphenicol sodium succinate	PD	250 mg/ 2.5 mL	RB	10 mg/ 2 mL	White precipitate forms immediately at 25 °C	1167	**I**
	PD	2 g/ 20 mL	RB	10 mg/ 2 mL	White precipitate forms immediately at 25 °C	1167	**I**
	PD	2 g/ 20 mL	RB	160 mg/ 32 mL	White precipitate forms immediately at 25 °C	1167	**I**
Chlorpromazine HCl	MB	25 mg/ 1 mL	NO	10 mg/ 2 mL	Physically compatible for 15 min at room temperature	565	**C**
Cisplatin		0.5 mg/ 0.5 mL		2.5 mg/ 0.5 mL	Physically compatible for 5 min at room temperature followed by 8 min of centrifugation	980	**C**
Cyclophosphamide		10 mg/ 0.5 mL		2.5 mg/ 0.5 mL	Physically compatible for 5 min at room temperature followed by 8 min of centrifugation	980	**C**
	MJ	1 g/ 50 mL	RB	10 mg/ 2 mL	Physically compatible for 24 hr at 25 °C	1167	**C**
	MJ	1 g/ 50 mL	RB	160 mg/ 32 mL	Physically compatible for 24 hr at 25 °C	1167	**C**
	MJ	40 mg/ 2 mL	RB	10 mg/ 2 mL	Physically compatible for 24 hr at 25 °C	1167	**C**
Cytarabine	UP	500 mg/ 10 mL	RB	160 mg/ 32 mL	Physically compatible for 48 hr at 25 °C	1167	**C**
	UP	50 mg/ 1 mL	RB	10 mg/ 2 mL	Physically compatible for 48 hr at 25 °C	1167	**C**
Dexamethasone sodium phosphate	ES, MSD	8 mg/ 2 mL	RB	160 mg/ 32 mL	Physically compatible for 48 hr at 25 °C	1167	**C**
	ES, MSD	8 mg/ 2 mL	RB	10 mg/ 2 mL	Physically compatible for 48 hr at 25 °C	1167	**C**
Diamorphine HCl	MB	10, 25, 50 mg/ 1 mL	BK	5 mg/ 1 mL	Physically compatible and diamorphine stable for 24 hr at room temperature	1454	**C**
	EV	50 and 150 mg/ 1 mL	LA	5 mg/ 1 mL	Slight discoloration with 8% metoclopramide loss and 9% diamorphine loss in 7 days at room temperature	1455	**C**
Dimenhydrinate	HR	50 mg/ 1 mL	NO	10 mg/ 2 mL	Physically compatible for 15 min at room temperature	565	**C**

Drugs in Syringe Compatibility (Cont.)

Metoclopramide HCl

Drug (in syringe)	Mfr	Amt	Mfr	Amt	Remarks	Ref	C/I
Diphenhydramine HCl	PD	50 mg/ 1 mL	NO	10 mg/ 2 mL	Physically compatible for 15 min at room temperature	565	C
	PD	40 mg/ 4 mL	RB	160 mg/ 32 mL	Physically compatible for 48 hr at 25 °C	1167	C
	PD	200 mg/ 20 mL	RB	160 mg/ 32 mL	Physically compatible for 48 hr at 25 °C	1167	C
	PD	50 mg/ 5 mL	RB	10 mg/ 2 mL	Physically compatible for 48 hr at 25 °C	1167	C
	PD	250 mg/ 25 mL	RB	10 mg/ 2 mL	Physically compatible for 48 hr at 25 °C	1167	C
Doxorubicin HCl		1 mg/ 0.5 mL		2.5 mg/ 0.5 mL	Physically compatible for 5 min at room temperature followed by 8 min of centrifugation	980	C
	AD	90 mg/ 45 mL	RB	160 mg/ 32 mL	Physically compatible for 48 hr at 25 °C	1167	C
	AD	40 mg/ 20 mL	RB	10 mg/ 2 mL	Physically compatible for 48 hr at 25 °C	1167	C
Droperidol	MN	2.5 mg/ 1 mL	NO	10 mg/ 2 mL	Physically compatible for 15 min at room temperature	565	C
		1.25 mg/ 0.5 mL		2.5 mg/ 0.5 mL	Physically compatible for 5 min at room temperature followed by 8 min of centrifugation	980	C
Fentanyl citrate	MN	0.05 mg/ 1 mL	NO	10 mg/ 2 mL	Physically compatible for 15 min at room temperature	565	C
Fentanyl citrate with midazolam HCl	DB RC	1 mg/ 20 mL 15 mg/ 3 mL	AST	20 mg/ 4 mL	Visually compatible with 7% or less loss of each drug in 10 days at 32 °C	2268	C
Fluorouracil		25 mg/ 0.5 mL		2.5 mg/ 0.5 mL	Physically compatible for 5 min at room temperature followed by 8 min of centrifugation	980	C
Furosemide		5 mg/ 0.5 mL		2.5 mg/ 0.5 mL	Precipitates immediately	980	I
Heparin sodium		500 units/ 0.5 mL		2.5 mg/ 0.5 mL	Physically compatible for 5 min at room temperature followed by 8 min of centrifugation	980	C
		2500 units/ 1 mL		10 mg/ 2 mL	Physically compatible for at least 5 min	1053	C
	ES	16,000 units/ 16 mL	RB	160 mg/ 32 mL	Physically compatible for 48 hr at 25 °C	1167	C
	ES	2000 units/ 2 mL	RB	10 mg/ 2 mL	Physically compatible for 48 hr at 25 °C	1167	C
	ES	4000 units/ 4 mL	RB	10 mg/ 2 mL	Physically compatible for 48 hr at 25 °C	1167	C
Hydromorphone HCl	KN	10 and 20 mg/ mL	RB	5 mg/mL	Visually compatible with less than 10% loss of either drug in 7 days at 8 °C	668	C
Hydroxyzine HCl	PF	50 mg/ 1 mL	NO	10 mg/ 2 mL	Physically compatible for 15 min at room temperature	565	C

Drugs in Syringe Compatibility (Cont.)

Metoclopramide HCl

Drug (in syringe)	Mfr	Amt	Mfr	Amt	Remarks	Ref	C/I
Leucovorin calcium		5 mg/ 0.5 mL		2.5 mg/ 0.5 mL	Physically compatible for 5 min at room temperature followed by 8 min of centrifugation	980	**C**
Lidocaine HCl	ES	50 mg/ 5 mL	RB	160 mg/ 32 mL	Physically compatible for 48 hr at 25 °C	1167	**C**
	ES	100 mg/ 10 mL	RB	160 mg/ 32 mL	Physically compatible for 48 hr at 25 °C	1167	**C**
	ES	50 mg/ 5 mL	RB	10 mg/ 2 mL	Physically compatible for 48 hr at 25 °C	1167	**C**
	ES	100 mg/ 10 mL	RB	10 mg/ 2 mL	Physically compatible for 48 hr at 25 °C	1167	**C**
Magnesium sulfate	ES	1 g/2 mL	RB	160 mg/ 32 mL	Physically compatible for 48 hr at 25 °C	1167	**C**
	ES	500 mg/ 1 mL	RB	10 mg/ 2 mL	Physically compatible for 48 hr at 25 °C	1167	**C**
	ES	1 g/2 mL	RB	10 mg/ 2 mL	Physically compatible for 48 hr at 25 °C	1167	**C**
Meperidine HCl	WI	50 mg/ 1 mL	NO	10 mg/ 2 mL	Physically compatible for 15 min at room temperature	565	**C**
	DW	50 mg/ 1 mL	DW	10 mg/ 2 mL	Visually compatible. Little loss of either drug over 48 hr at 32 °C in light or dark	2253	**C**
Methotrexate sodium		12.5 mg/ 0.5 mL		2.5 mg/ 0.5 mL	Physically compatible for 5 min at room temperature followed by 8 min of centrifugation	980	**C**
	LE	200 mg/ 8 mL	RB	160 mg/ 32 mL	Incompatible. If mixed, use immediately	1167	**I**
	LE	50 mg/ 2 mL	RB	10 mg/ 2 mL	Incompatible. If mixed, use immediately	1167	**I**
Methotrimeprazine HCl	RP	10 mg/ 2 mL	NO	10 mg/ 2 mL	Physically compatible for 15 min at room temperature	565	**C**
Methylprednisolone sodium succinate	ES	250 mg/ 4 mL	RB	160 mg/ 32 mL	Physically compatible for 24 hr at 25 °C	1167	**C**
	ES	62.5 mg/ 1 mL	RB	10 mg/ 2 mL	Physically compatible for 24 hr at 25 °C	1167	**C**
	ES	250 mg/ 4 mL	RB	10 mg/ 2 mL	Physically compatible for 24 hr at 25 °C	1167	**C**
Midazolam HCl	RC	5 mg/ 1 mL	RB	10 mg/ 2 mL	Physically compatible for 4 hr at 25 °C	1145	**C**
Midazolam HCl with fentanyl citrate	RC DB	15 mg/ 3 mL 1 mg/ 20 mL	AST	20 mg/ 4 mL	Visually compatible with 7% or less loss of each drug in 10 days at 32 °C	2268	**C**
Mitomycin		0.25 mg/ 0.5 mL		2.5 mg/ 0.5 mL	Physically compatible for 5 min at room temperature followed by 8 min of centrifugation	980	**C**
Morphine sulfate	AH	10 mg/ 1 mL	NO	10 mg/ 2 mL	Physically compatible for 15 min at room temperature	565	**C**
	EV	1 mg/mL	SKB	0.5 mg/ mL	Diluted with NS. 5% or less loss of both drugs in 35 days at 22 °C and 182 days at 4 °C followed by 7 days at 32 °C	1939	**C**
	ME	25 mg/ mL[b]	RB	5 mg/mL	Visually compatible with less than 10% drug loss in 7 days at 8 °C	668	**C**

Drugs in Syringe Compatibility (Cont.)

Metoclopramide HCl

Drug (in syringe)	Mfr	Amt	Mfr	Amt	Remarks	Ref	C/I
Ondansetron HCl	GW	1 mg/mL[c]	SO	2.5 mg/mL[c]	Physically compatible. Under 6% ondansetron and under 5% metoclopramide losses in 24 hr at 4 or 23 °C	2199	C
Oxycodone HCl	NAP	200 mg/20 mL		100 mg/20 mL	Visually compatible. Under 4% concentration change in 24 hr at 25 °C	2600	C
Pantoprazole sodium	[a]	4 mg/1 mL		5 mg/1 mL	Precipitates within 15 min	2574	I
Penicillin G potassium	SQ	250,000 units/1 mL	RB	10 mg/2 mL	Incompatible. If mixed, use immediately	924; 1167	I
	SQ	1 million units/4 mL	RB	10 mg/2 mL	Incompatible. If mixed, use immediately	924; 1167	I
Pentazocine lactate	WI	30 mg/1 mL	NO	10 mg/2 mL	Physically compatible for 15 min at room temperature	565	C
Prochlorperazine edisylate	MB	10 mg/2 mL	NO	10 mg/2 mL	Physically compatible for 15 min at room temperature	565	C
Promethazine HCl	WY	25 mg/1 mL	NO	10 mg/2 mL	Physically compatible for 15 min at room temperature	565	C
Ranitidine HCl	GL	50 mg/2 mL	RB	10 mg/1 mL	Physically compatible for 1 hr at 25 °C	978	C
Scopolamine HBr	ST	0.4 mg/1 mL	NO	10 mg/2 mL	Physically compatible for 15 min at room temperature	565	C
Sodium bicarbonate	AB	100 mEq/100 mL	RB	10 mg/2 mL	Gas evolves	1167	I
	AB	100 mEq/100 mL	RB	160 mg/32 mL	Gas evolves	1167	I
Vinblastine sulfate		0.5 mg/0.5 mL		2.5 mg/0.5 mL	Physically compatible for 5 min at room temperature followed by 8 min of centrifugation	980	C
Vincristine sulfate		0.5 mg/0.5 mL		2.5 mg/0.5 mL	Physically compatible for 5 min at room temperature followed by 8 min of centrifugation	980	C

[a]*Test performed using the formulation WITHOUT edetate disodium.*
[b]*Tested in sterile water for injection.*
[c]*Tested in sodium chloride 0.9%.*

Y-Site Injection Compatibility (1:1 Mixture)

Metoclopramide HCl

Drug	Mfr	Conc	Mfr	Conc	Remarks	Ref	C/I
Acyclovir sodium	BW	5 mg/mL[a]	ES	0.2 mg/mL[a]	Physically compatible for 4 hr at 25 °C	1157	C
	BV	5 mg/mL[b]	SIC	5 mg/mL	Crystals form	2794	I
Aldesleukin	CHI	33,800 I.U./mL[a]	DU	5 mg/mL	Visually compatible with little or no loss of aldesleukin activity	1857	C
Allopurinol sodium	BW	3 mg/mL[b]	DU	5 mg/mL	Heavy white precipitate forms immediately	1686	I
Amifostine	USB	10 mg/mL[a]	ES	5 mg/mL	Physically compatible for 4 hr at 23 °C	1845	C
Amphotericin B cholesteryl sulfate complex	SEQ	0.83 mg/mL[a]	FAU	5 mg/mL	Gross precipitate forms	2117	I

Y-Site Injection Compatibility (1:1 Mixture) (Cont.)

Metoclopramide HCl

Drug	Mfr	Conc	Mfr	Conc	Remarks	Ref	C/I
Amsacrine	NCI	1 mg/mL[a]	RB	2.5 mg/mL[a]	Orange turbidity becomes orange precipitate in 1 hr	1381	I
Aztreonam	SQ	40 mg/mL[a]	ES	5 mg/mL	Physically compatible for 4 hr at 23 °C	1758	C
Bivalirudin	TMC	5 mg/mL[a]	FAU	5 mg/mL	Physically compatible for 4 hr at 23 °C	2373	C
Bleomycin sulfate		3 units/mL		5 mg/mL	Drugs injected sequentially in Y-site with no flush. No precipitate seen	980	C
Ceftaroline fosamil	FOR	2.22 mg/mL[a,b,e]	HOS	5 mg/mL	Physically compatible for 4 hr at 23 °C	2826	C
Ciprofloxacin	MI	2 mg/mL[c]	DU	5 mg/mL	Visually compatible for 24 hr at 24 °C	1655	C
	BAY	2 mg/mL[b]		5 mg/mL	Visually compatible. No ciprofloxacin loss in 15 min. Metoclopramide not tested	1934	C
Cisatracurium besylate	GW	0.1, 2, 5 mg/mL[a]	AB	5 mg/mL	Physically compatible for 4 hr at 23 °C	2074	C
Cisplatin		1 mg/mL		5 mg/mL	Drugs injected sequentially in Y-site with no flush. No precipitate seen	980	C
Cladribine	ORT	0.015[b] and 0.5[d] mg/mL	RB	5 mg/mL	Physically compatible for 4 hr at 23 °C	1969	C
Clarithromycin	AB	4 mg/mL[a]	ANT	5 mg/mL	Visually compatible for 72 hr at both 30 and 17 °C	2174	C
Cyclophosphamide		20 mg/mL		5 mg/mL	Drugs injected sequentially in Y-site with no flush. No precipitate seen	980	C
Dexmedetomidine HCl	AB	4 mcg/mL[b]	FAU	5 mg/mL	Physically compatible for 4 hr at 23 °C	2383	C
Diltiazem HCl	MMD	1[b] and 5 mg/mL	RB	5 mg/mL	Visually compatible	1807	C
	MMD	5 mg/mL	RB	0.2 mg/mL[b]	Visually compatible	1807	C
Docetaxel	RPR	0.9 mg/mL[a]	AB	5 mg/mL	Physically compatible for 4 hr at 23 °C	2224	C
Doripenem	JJ	5 mg/mL[a,b]	HOS	5 mg/mL	Physically compatible for 4 hr at 23 °C	2743	C
Doxapram HCl	RB	2 mg/mL[a]	AB	1 mg/mL	Visually compatible for 4 hr at 23 °C	2470	C
Doxorubicin HCl		2 mg/mL		5 mg/mL	Drugs injected sequentially in Y-site with no flush. No precipitate seen	980	C
Doxorubicin HCl liposomal	SEQ	0.4 mg/mL[a]	GNS	5 mg/mL	Increase in measured turbidity	2087	I
Droperidol		2.5 mg/mL		5 mg/mL	Drugs injected sequentially in Y-site with no flush. No precipitate seen	980	C
Etoposide phosphate	BR	5 mg/mL[a]	FAU	5 mg/mL	Physically compatible for 4 hr at 23 °C	2218	C
Famotidine	MSD	0.2 mg/mL[a]	RB	5 mg/mL	Physically compatible for 14 hr	1196	C
	ME	2 mg/mL[b]		5 mg/mL	Visually compatible for 4 hr at 22 °C	1936	C
Fenoldopam mesylate	AB	80 mcg/mL[b]	RB	5 mg/mL	Physically compatible for 4 hr at 23 °C	2467	C
Fentanyl citrate	JN	0.025 mg/mL[a]	DU	5 mg/mL	Physically compatible for 48 hr at 22 °C	1706	C
Filgrastim	AMG	30 mcg/mL[a]	ES	5 mg/mL	Physically compatible for 4 hr at 22 °C	1687	C
Fluconazole	RR	2 mg/mL	RB	5 mg/mL	Physically compatible for 24 hr at 25 °C	1407	C
Fludarabine phosphate	BX	1 mg/mL[a]	DU	5 mg/mL	Visually compatible for 4 hr at 22 °C	1439	C
Fluorouracil		50 mg/mL		5 mg/mL	Drugs injected sequentially in Y-site with no flush. No precipitate seen	980	C

Y-Site Injection Compatibility (1:1 Mixture) (Cont.)

Metoclopramide HCl

Drug	Mfr	Conc	Mfr	Conc	Remarks	Ref	C/I
Foscarnet sodium	AST	24 mg/mL	RB	4 mg/mL	Physically compatible for 24 hr at room temperature under fluorescent light	1335	C
	AST	24 mg/mL	RB	2 mg/mL[c]	Physically compatible for 24 hr at 25 °C under fluorescent light	1393	C
Furosemide		10 mg/mL		5 mg/mL	Drugs injected sequentially in Y-site with no flush. Precipitates immediately	980	I
Gallium nitrate	FUJ	1 mg/mL[b]	SO	5 mg/mL	Visually compatible for 24 hr at 25 °C	1673	C
Gemcitabine HCl	LI	10 mg/mL[b]	FAU	5 mg/mL	Physically compatible for 4 hr at 23 °C	2226	C
Granisetron HCl	SKB	0.05 mg/mL[a]	AB	5 mg/mL	Physically compatible for 4 hr at 23 °C	2000	C
Heparin sodium		1000 units/mL		5 mg/mL	Drugs injected sequentially in Y-site with no flush. No precipitate seen	980	C
Hetastarch in lactated electrolyte	AB	6%	FAU	5 mg/mL	Physically compatible for 4 hr at 23 °C	2339	C
Hydromorphone HCl	AST	0.5 mg/mL[a]	DU	5 mg/mL	Physically compatible for 48 hr at 22 °C	1706	C
Idarubicin HCl	AD	1 mg/mL[b]	SO	5 mg/mL	Visually compatible for 24 hr at 25 °C	1525	C
Leucovorin calcium		10 mg/mL		5 mg/mL	Drugs injected sequentially in Y-site with no flush. No precipitate seen	980	C
Levofloxacin	OMN	5 mg/mL[a]	ES	5 mg/mL	Visually compatible for 4 hr at 24 °C	2233	C
Linezolid	PHU	2 mg/mL	FAU	5 mg/mL	Physically compatible for 4 hr at 23 °C	2264	C
Melphalan HCl	BW	0.1 mg/mL[b]	RB	5 mg/mL	Physically compatible for 3 hr at 22 °C	1557	C
Meperidine HCl	AB	10 mg/mL	SN	0.2 mg/mL[a]	Physically compatible for 4 hr at 25 °C	1397	C
Meropenem	ZEN	1 and 50 mg/mL[b]	RB	5 mg/mL	Visually compatible for 4 hr at room temperature	1994	C
Methadone HCl	LI	1 mg/mL[a]	DU	5 mg/mL	Physically compatible for 48 hr at 22 °C	1706	C
Methotrexate sodium		25 mg/mL		5 mg/mL	Drugs injected sequentially in Y-site with no flush. No precipitate seen	980	C
Mitomycin		0.5 mg/mL		5 mg/mL	Drugs injected sequentially in Y-site with no flush. No precipitate seen	980	C
Morphine sulfate	AB	1 mg/mL	SN	0.2 mg/mL[a]	Physically compatible for 4 hr at 25 °C	1397	C
	AST	1 mg/mL[a]	DU	5 mg/mL	Physically compatible for 48 hr at 22 °C	1706	C
Ondansetron HCl	GL	1 mg/mL[b]	DU	5 mg/mL	Visually compatible for 4 hr at 22 °C	1365	C
Oxaliplatin	SS	0.5 mg/mL[a]	RB	5 mg/mL	Physically compatible for 4 hr at 23 °C	2566	C
Paclitaxel	NCI	1.2 mg/mL[a]		5 mg/mL	Physically compatible for 4 hr at 22 °C	1528	C
Palonosetron HCl	MGI	50 mcg/mL	BA	5 mg/mL	Physically compatible. No loss of either drug in 4 hr	2716	C
Pemetrexed disodium	LI	20 mg/mL[b]	RB	5 mg/mL	Physically compatible for 4 hr at 23 °C	2564	C
Piperacillin sodium–tazobactam sodium	LE[h]	40 + 5 mg/mL[a]	RB	5 mg/mL	Physically compatible for 4 hr at 22 °C	1688	C
Quinupristin–dalfopristin	AVE	2 mg/mL[a]		5 mg/mL	Physically compatible	1	C
Remifentanil HCl	GW	0.025 and 0.25 mg/mL[b]	AB	5 mg/mL	Physically compatible for 4 hr at 23 °C	2075	C
Sargramostim	IMM	10 mcg/mL[b]	DU	5 mg/mL	Visually compatible for 4 hr at 22 °C	1436	C
Tacrolimus	FUJ	1 mg/mL[b]	DU	0.2 mg/mL[a]	Visually compatible for 24 hr at 25 °C	1630	C
Telavancin HCl	ASP	7.5 mg/mL[a,b,e]	HOS	1 mg/mL[a,b,e]	Physically compatible for 2 hr	2830	C

Y-Site Injection Compatibility (1:1 Mixture) (Cont.)

Metoclopramide HCl

Drug	Mfr	Conc	Mfr	Conc	Remarks	Ref	C/I
Teniposide	BR	0.1 mg/mL[a]	ES	5 mg/mL	Physically compatible for 4 hr at 23 °C	1725	C
Thiotepa	IMM[f]	1 mg/mL[a]	RB	5 mg/mL	Physically compatible for 4 hr at 23 °C	1861	C
Tigecycline	WY	1 mg/mL[b]		5 mg/mL	Physically compatible for 4 hr	2714	C
TNA #218 to #226[g]			AB	5 mg/mL	Visually compatible for 4 hr at 23 °C	2215	C
Topotecan HCl	SKB	56 mcg/mL[a,b]	RB	1.72 mg/mL[a,b]	Visually compatible. Little loss of either drug in 4 hr at 22 °C	2245	C
TPN #212 to #215[g]			AB	5 mg/mL	Substantial loss of natural haze occurs immediately	2109	I
Vinblastine sulfate		1 mg/mL		5 mg/mL	Drugs injected sequentially in Y-site with no flush. No precipitate seen	980	C
Vincristine sulfate		1 mg/mL		5 mg/mL	Drugs injected sequentially in Y-site with no flush. No precipitate seen	980	C
Vinorelbine tartrate	BW	1 mg/mL[b]	RB	5 mg/mL	Physically compatible for 4 hr at 22 °C	1558	C
Zidovudine	BW	4 mg/mL[a]	RB	2 mg/mL[a]	Physically compatible for 4 hr at 25 °C	1193	C

[a]*Tested in dextrose 5%.*
[b]*Tested in sodium chloride 0.9%.*
[c]*Tested in both dextrose 5% and sodium chloride 0.9%.*
[d]*Tested in bacteriostatic sodium chloride 0.9% preserved with benzyl alcohol 0.9%.*
[e]*Tested in Ringer's injection, lactated.*
[f]*Lyophilized formulation tested.*
[g]*Refer to Appendix I for the composition of parenteral nutrition solutions. TNA indicates a 3-in-1 admixture, and TPN indicates a 2-in-1 admixture.*
[h]*Test performed using the formulation WITHOUT edetate disodium.*

METOPROLOL TARTRATE
AHFS 24:24

Products — Metoprolol tartrate is available in 5-mL ampuls, vials, and syringe cartridges. Each milliliter of solution contains 1 mg of metoprolol tartrate and 9 mg of sodium chloride. (1)

pH — From 5 to 8. (17)

Trade Name(s) — Lopressor.

Administration — Metoprolol tartrate is administered intravenously. (1)

Stability — Metoprolol tartrate injection should be stored at controlled room temperature and protected from light and freezing. (1; 4)

Metoprolol tartrate under simulated summer conditions in paramedic vehicles was exposed to temperatures ranging from 26 to 38 °C over 4 weeks. Analysis found no loss of the drug under these conditions. (2562)

Compatibility Information

Solution Compatibility

Metoprolol tartrate

Solution	Mfr	Mfr	Conc/L	Remarks	Ref	C/I
Dextrose 5%	BA[a]	CI	300 mg	Visually compatible. Little loss in 36 hr at 24 °C in light	1679	C
			0.5 g	Physically compatible. No loss in 30 hr at room temperature	2728	C

Solution Compatibility (Cont.)

Metoprolol tartrate

Solution	Mfr	Mfr	Conc/L	Remarks	Ref	C/I
Sodium chloride 0.9%	BA[a]	CI	300 mg	Visually compatible. Little loss in 36 hr at 24 °C in light	1679	C
			0.5 g	Physically compatible. No loss in 30 hr at room temperature	2728	C

[a]Tested in PVC containers.

Y-Site Injection Compatibility (1:1 Mixture)

Metoprolol tartrate

Drug	Mfr	Conc	Mfr	Conc	Remarks	Ref	C/I
Abciximab	LI	36 mcg/mL[a]	AB	1 mg/mL	Visually compatible for 12 hr at 23 °C	2374	C
Alteplase	GEN	1 mg/mL	CI	1 mg/mL	Visually compatible with no alteplase clot-lysis activity loss in 24 hr at 25 °C	1856	C
Amiodarone HCl	BIO	1.8 mg/mL[a]	BED	1 mg/mL	Visually compatible for 24 hr at 19 °C	2795	C
Amphotericin B cholesteryl sulfate complex	SEQ	0.83 mg/mL[a]	GEM	1 mg/mL	Gross precipitate forms	2117	I
Argatroban	GSK	1 mg/mL[b]	AB	1 mg/mL	Visually compatible for 24 hr at 23 °C	2391	C
Bivalirudin	TMC	5 mg/mL[a,b]	AB	1 mg/mL	Visually compatible for 6 hr at 23 °C	2680	C
Ceftaroline fosamil	FOR	2.22 mg/mL[a,b,c]	HOS	1 mg/mL	Physically compatible for 4 hr at 23 °C	2826	C
Diltiazem HCl	NVP[a]	1 mg/mL	BED	1 mg/mL	Visually compatible for 24 hr at 19 °C	2795	C
Eptifibatide	SC	0.75 mg/mL	BED	1 mg/mL	Visually compatible for 24 hr at 19 °C	2795	C
Furosemide	HOS	10 mg/mL	BED	1 mg/mL	Visually compatible for 24 hr at 19 °C	2795	C
Heparin sodium	BA	1000 units/mL[a]	BED	1 mg/mL	Visually compatible for 24 hr at 19 °C	2795	C
Lepirudin	BX	0.4 mg/mL[a]	BED	1 mg/mL	Trace precipitate in 5 hr at 19 °C	2795	I
Lidocaine HCl	BA	8 mg/mL[a]	BED	1 mg/mL	Trace precipitate in 8 hr at 19 °C	2795	I
Meperidine HCl	AB	10 mg/mL	CI	1 mg/mL	Physically compatible for 4 hr at 25 °C	1397	C
Milrinone lactate	NVP	0.2 mg/mL[a]	BED	1 mg/mL	Visually compatible for 24 hr at 19 °C	2795	C
Morphine sulfate	AB	1 mg/mL	CI	1 mg/mL	Physically compatible for 4 hr at 25 °C	1397	C
Nesiritide	SCI	50 mcg/mL[a,b]		1 mg/mL	Physically compatible for 4 hr	2625	C
	SCI	6 mcg/mL[a]	BED	1 mg/mL	Trace precipitate in 24 hr at 19 °C	2795	I
Nitroglycerin	BA	0.2 mg/mL[a]	BED	1 mg/mL	Trace precipitate in 8 hr at 19 °C	2795	I
Procainamide HCl	HOS	8 mg/mL[b]	BED	1 mg/mL	Visually compatible for 24 hr at 19 °C	2795	C
Sodium nitroprusside	HOS	0.4 mg/mL[a]	BED	1 mg/mL	Visually compatible for 24 hr at 19 °C	2795	C

[a]Tested in dextrose 5%.
[b]Tested in sodium chloride 0.9%.
[c]Tested in Ringer's injection, lactated.

METRONIDAZOLE
AHFS 8:30.92

Products — Metronidazole 5 mg/mL is available as a ready-to-use solution in 100-mL (500-mg) single-dose PVC plastic bags. No dilution or buffering is required. Each bag also contains dibasic sodium phosphate 48 mg, citric acid anhydrous 23 mg, and sodium chloride 790 mg in water for injection. (1)

pH — Metronidazole has a pH of 5.5 (range 4.5 to 7). (1; 17)

Osmolarity — Metronidazole has an osmolarity of 310 mOsm/L. (1)

Sodium Content — Metronidazole contains 14 mEq of sodium from the excipients per 500 mg of metronidazole. (1; 4)

Administration — Metronidazole is administered by continuous intravenous infusion or by intermittent intravenous infusion over one hour. (1; 4)

Stability — Metronidazole ready-to-use is a clear, colorless solution which should be stored at controlled room temperature and protected from light. It should not be stored under refrigeration. (1; 4) Refrigeration may result in crystal formation. However, the crystals redissolve on warming to room temperature. (1115)

Light Effects — Prolonged exposure to light will cause a darkening of the product. (4) However, most manufacturers indicate that short-term exposure to normal room light does not adversely affect metronidazole stability. Direct sunlight should be avoided. (1115)

Sorption — Metronidazole was shown not to exhibit sorption to PVC bags and tubing, polyethylene tubing, Silastic tubing, and polypropylene syringes. (536; 606)

Central Venous Catheter — Metronidazole (Baxter) 5 mg/mL in dextrose 5% was found to be compatible with the ARROWg+ard Blue Plus (Arrow International) chlorhexidine-bearing triple-lumen central catheter. Essentially complete delivery of the drug was found with little or no drug loss occurring. Furthermore, chlorhexidine delivered from the catheter remained at trace amounts with no substantial increase due to the delivery of the drug through the catheter. (2335)

Compatibility Information

Additive Compatibility

Metronidazole

Drug	Mfr	Conc/L	Mfr	Conc/L	Test Soln	Remarks	Ref	C/I
Amoxicillin sodium–clavulanate potassium	BE	20 + 2 g	BAY	5 g		Physically compatible with 8% clavulanate loss in 2 hr and 25% loss in 6 hr at 21 °C. 7 to 8% amoxicillin and no metronidazole loss in 6 hr at 21 °C	1920	**I**
Ampicillin sodium	BR	20 g	SE	5 g		9% ampicillin loss in 22 hr at 25 °C and in 12 days at 5 °C. No metronidazole loss	993	**C**
Aztreonam	SQ	10 and 20 g	MG	5 g		Pink color develops in 12 hr, becoming cherry red in 48 hr at 25 °C. Pink color develops in 3 days at 4 °C. No loss of either drug detected	1023	**I**
Cefazolin sodium	LI	10 g	SE	5 g		5% cefazolin loss and no metronidazole loss in 7 days at 25 °C. No loss of either drug in 12 days at 5 °C	993	**C**
	LI	10 g	AB	5 g		Visually compatible with no loss of either drug in 72 hr at 8 °C	1649	**C**
Cefepime HCl	BR	4 and 40 g	AB, ES, SE	5 g		4 to 5% cefepime loss in 24 hr at room temperature exposed to light and up to 10% loss in 7 days at 5 °C. No metronidazole loss. Orange color develops in 18 hr at room temperature and 24 hr at 5 °C	1682	**?**
	BMS	2.5, 5, 10, and 20 g	SCS	5 g	a	Visually compatible. 7 to 9% cefepime loss in 48 hr at 23 °C; 2 to 8% cefepime loss in 7 days at 4 °C. 7% or less metronidazole loss in 7 days at 4 and 23 °C	2324	**C**

Additive Compatibility (Cont.)

Metronidazole

Drug	Mfr	Conc/L	Mfr	Conc/L	Test Soln	Remarks	Ref	C/I
	ELN	3.3, 6.6, 10, 20 g	AB	5 g	[a]	Physically compatible and less than 6% metronidazole loss at 4 and 23 °C in 14 days. 2 to 5% cefepime loss in 14 days at 4 °C. At 23 °C, 10 to 12% cefepime loss in 72 hr	2726	C
Cefotaxime sodium	HO	10 g	AB	5 g		Both drugs stable for 72 hr at 8 °C	1547	C
	HO	10 g	AB	5 g		Visually compatible with 10% cefotaxime loss in 19 hr at 28 °C and 8% loss in 96 hr at 5 °C. No metronidazole loss in 96 hr at 5 or 28 °C	1754	C
Cefoxitin sodium	MSD	30 g	SE	5 g		9% cefoxitin loss in 48 hr at 25 °C and 3% in 12 days at 5 °C. No metronidazole loss	993	C
Ceftazidime	GL	20 g		5 g		No loss of either drug in 4 hr	1345	C
	LI	10 g	AB	5 g		Visually compatible with little or no loss of either drug in 72 hr at 8 °C	1849	C
Ceftriaxone sodium	RC	10 g	AB	5 g		Visually compatible with little or no loss of either drug in 72 hr at 8 °C	1849	C
	RC	10 g	BA	5 g		Visually compatible with no metronidazole loss and with 6% ceftriaxone loss in 3 days and 8% in 4 days at 25 °C	2101	C
Cefuroxime sodium	GL	7.5 g		5 g		Physically compatible with no loss of either drug in 1 hr	1036	C
	GL	15 g		5 g		No loss of either drug in 4 hr at 24 °C	1376	C
	GL	7.5 g		5 g		10% cefuroxime loss in 16 days at 4 °C and 35 hr at 25 °C. No metronidazole loss in 15 days at 4 and 25 °C	1565	C
	GL	7.5 and 15 g	IVX	5 g		Physically compatible. No loss of metronidazole and about 6% cefuroxime loss in 49 days at 5 °C	2192	C
Ciprofloxacin		2 g		5 g		No loss of either drug in 4 hr at 24 °C	1346	C
	MI	1.6 g	SE	4.2 g		Visually compatible. Both drugs stable for 48 hr at 25 °C in light and 4 °C in dark	1541	C
		1 g	RPR	2.5 g		Under 3% metronidazole loss in 24 hr at 25 °C in light or dark. Ciprofloxacin not tested	2361	C
	BAY	1 g	SCS	2.5 g		Visually compatible. No ciprofloxacin loss in 24 hr at 22 °C in light. Metronidazole not tested	2413	C
Floxacillin sodium	BE	10 g		5 g		Physically compatible for 48 hr. Both drugs stable for 1 hr at room temperature	1036	C
Fluconazole	PF	1 g	AB	2.5 g		Visually compatible with no fluconazole loss in 72 hr at 25 °C under fluorescent light. Metronidazole not tested	1677	C
Gentamicin sulfate	SC	800 mg and 1.2 g	SE	5 g		Physically compatible with no loss of either drug in 2 days at 18 °C. At 4 °C, no metronidazole loss but up to 10% gentamicin loss in 7 days	1242	C

Additive Compatibility (Cont.)

Metronidazole

Drug	Mfr	Conc/L	Mfr	Conc/L	Test Soln	Remarks	Ref	C/I
		800 mg	RP	5 g		Visually compatible with no loss of metronidazole in 15 days at 5 and 25 °C. 10% gentamicin loss in 63 hr at 25 °C and 10.6 days at 5 °C	1931	C
Hydrocortisone sodium succinate	ES	10 g	SE	5 g		No loss of either drug in 7 days at 25 °C and 12 days at 5 °C	993	C
Midazolam HCl	RC	50, 250, 400 mg		5 g	NS	Visually compatible for 4 hr	355	C
Penicillin G potassium	PF	200 million units	SE	5 g		5% penicillin loss in 22 hr and 8% in 72 hr at 25 °C. 2% penicillin loss in 12 days at 5 °C. No metronidazole loss	993	C
Tobramycin sulfate	LI	1 g	RP	5 g		Visually compatible with no loss of metronidazole in 15 days at 5 and 25 °C. 10% tobramycin loss in 73 hr at 25 °C and 12.1 days at 5 °C	1931	C

[a]Tested in PVC containers.

Y-Site Injection Compatibility (1:1 Mixture)

Metronidazole

Drug	Mfr	Conc	Mfr	Conc	Remarks	Ref	C/I
Acyclovir sodium	BW	5 mg/mL[a]	SE	5 mg/mL	Physically compatible for 4 hr at 25 °C	1157	C
Allopurinol sodium	BW	3 mg/mL[b]	BA	5 mg/mL	Physically compatible for 4 hr at 22 °C	1686	C
Amifostine	USB	10 mg/mL[a]	BA	5 mg/mL	Physically compatible for 4 hr at 23 °C	1845	C
Amphotericin B cholesteryl sulfate complex	SEQ	0.83 mg/mL[a]	AB	5 mg/mL	Gross precipitate forms	2117	I
Anidulafungin	VIC	0.5 mg/mL[a]	BA	5 mg/mL	Physically compatible for 4 hr at 23 °C	2617	C
Aztreonam	SQ	40 mg/mL[a]	BA	5 mg/mL	Orange color forms in 4 hr	1758	I
Bivalirudin	TMC	5 mg/mL[a]	BA	5 mg/mL	Physically compatible for 4 hr at 23 °C	2373	C
Caspofungin acetate	ME	0.7 mg/mL[b]	BA	5 mg/mL	Physically compatible for 4 hr at room temperature	2758	C
	ME	0.5 mg/mL[b]	BA	5 mg/mL	Physically compatible over 60 min	2766	C
Ceftaroline fosamil	FOR	2.22 mg/mL[a,b,e]	BA	5 mg/mL	Physically compatible for 4 hr at 23 °C	2826	C
Cisatracurium besylate	GW	0.1, 2, 5 mg/mL[a]	AB	5 mg/mL	Physically compatible for 4 hr at 23 °C	2074	C
Clarithromycin	AB	4 mg/mL[a]	PRK	5 mg/mL	Visually compatible for 72 hr at both 30 and 17 °C	2174	C
Cyclophosphamide	MJ	20 mg/mL[a]	SE	5 mg/mL	Physically compatible for 4 hr at 25 °C	1194	C
Dexmedetomidine HCl	AB	4 mcg/mL[b]	BA	5 mg/mL	Physically compatible for 4 hr at 23 °C	2383	C
Diltiazem HCl	MMD	5 mg/mL	SE	5 mg/mL	Visually compatible	1807	C
Dimenhydrinate		10 mg/mL		5 mg/mL	Clear solution	2569	C
Docetaxel	RPR	0.9 mg/mL[a]	BA	5 mg/mL	Physically compatible for 4 hr at 23 °C	2224	C

Y-Site Injection Compatibility (1:1 Mixture) (Cont.)

Metronidazole

Drug	Mfr	Conc	Mfr	Conc	Remarks	Ref	C/I
Dopamine HCl	AB	0.8 mg/mL[a]	MG	5 mg/mL	Visually compatible for 24 hr at room temperature in test tubes. No precipitate found on filter from Y-site delivery	2063	C
Doripenem	JJ	5 mg/mL[a,b]	BA	5 mg/mL	Physically compatible for 4 hr at 23 °C	2743	C
Doxapram HCl	RB	2 mg/mL[a]	AB	5 mg/mL	Visually compatible for 4 hr at 23 °C	2470	C
Doxorubicin HCl liposomal	SEQ	0.4 mg/mL[a]	AB	5 mg/mL	Physically compatible for 4 hr at 23 °C	2087	C
Enalaprilat	MSD	0.05 mg/mL[b]	SE	5 mg/mL	Physically compatible for 24 hr at room temperature under fluorescent light	1355	C
Esmolol HCl	DCC	10 mg/mL[a]	SE	5 mg/mL	Physically compatible for 24 hr at 22 °C	1169	C
Etoposide phosphate	BR	5 mg/mL[a]	AB	5 mg/mL	Physically compatible for 4 hr at 23 °C	2218	C
Fenoldopam mesylate	AB	80 mcg/mL[b]	BA	5 mg/mL	Physically compatible for 4 hr at 23 °C	2467	C
Filgrastim	AMG	30 mcg/mL[a]	BA	5 mg/mL	Particles form immediately. Filaments form in 1 hr	1687	I
Fluconazole	RR	2 mg/mL	AB	5 mg/mL	Physically compatible for 24 hr at 25 °C	1407	C
Foscarnet sodium	AST	24 mg/mL	AB	5 mg/mL	Physically compatible for 24 hr at room temperature under fluorescent light	1335	C
	AST	24 mg/mL	SE	5 mg/mL	Physically compatible for 24 hr at 25 °C under fluorescent light	1393	C
Gemcitabine HCl	LI	10 mg/mL[b]	AB	5 mg/mL	Physically compatible for 4 hr at 23 °C	2226	C
Granisetron HCl	SKB	0.05 mg/mL[a]	BA	5 mg/mL	Physically compatible for 4 hr at 23 °C	2000	C
Heparin sodium	TR	50 units/mL	MG	5 mg/mL	Visually compatible for 4 hr at 25 °C	1793	C
Hetastarch in lactated electrolyte	AB	6%	AB	5 mg/mL	Physically compatible for 4 hr at 23 °C	2339	C
Hydromorphone HCl	WY	0.2 mg/mL[a]	SE	5 mg/mL	Physically compatible for 4 hr at 25 °C	987	C
Hydroxyethyl starch 130/0.4 in sodium chloride 0.9%	FRK	6%	HOS	1[a], 2.5[a], 5 mg/mL	Visually compatible for 24 hr at room temperature	2770	C
Labetalol HCl	SC	1 mg/mL[a]	SE	5 mg/mL	Physically compatible for 24 hr at 18 °C	1171	C
Linezolid	PHU	2 mg/mL	BA	5 mg/mL	Physically compatible for 4 hr at 23 °C	2264	C
Lorazepam	WY	0.33 mg/mL[b]	BRN	5 mg/mL	Visually compatible for 24 hr at 22 °C	1855	C
Magnesium sulfate	IX	16.7, 33.3, 66.7, 100 mg/mL[a]	SE	5 mg/mL	Physically compatible for at least 4 hr at 32 °C	813	C
Melphalan HCl	BW	0.1 mg/mL[b]	AB	5 mg/mL	Physically compatible for 3 hr at 22 °C	1557	C
Meperidine HCl	WY	10 mg/mL[a]	SE	5 mg/mL	Physically compatible for 4 hr at 25 °C	987	C
Methylprednisolone sodium succinate	UP	5 mg/mL[a]	MG	5 mg/mL	Visually compatible for 24 hr at room temperature in test tubes. No precipitate found on filter from Y-site delivery	2063	C
Midazolam HCl	RC	1 mg/mL[a]	BA	5 mg/mL	Visually compatible for 24 hr at 23 °C	1847	C
	RC	5 mg/mL	BRN	5 mg/mL	Visually compatible for 24 hr at 22 °C	1855	C
Milrinone lactate	SS	0.2 mg/mL[a]	AB	5 mg/mL	Visually compatible for 4 hr at 25 °C	2381	C
Morphine sulfate	WI	1 mg/mL[a]	SE	5 mg/mL	Physically compatible for 4 hr at 25 °C	987	C

Y-Site Injection Compatibility (1:1 Mixture) (Cont.)

Metronidazole

Drug	Mfr	Conc	Mfr	Conc	Remarks	Ref	C/I
Nicardipine HCl	DCC	0.1 mg/mL[a]	SE	5 mg/mL	Visually compatible for 24 hr at room temperature	235	C
Palonosetron HCl	MGI	50 mcg/mL	BA	5 mg/mL	Physically compatible. No loss of either drug in 4 hr at room temperature	2765	C
Pemetrexed disodium	LI	20 mg/mL[b]	BA	5 mg/mL	Color darkening and brownish discoloration occur immediately	2564	I
Piperacillin sodium–tazobactam sodium	LE[f]	40 + 5 mg/mL[a]	BA	5 mg/mL	Physically compatible for 4 hr at 22 °C	1688	C
Remifentanil HCl	GW	0.025 and 0.25 mg/mL[b]	AB	5 mg/mL	Physically compatible for 4 hr at 23 °C	2075	C
Sargramostim	IMM	10 mcg/mL[b]	MG	5 mg/mL	Visually compatible for 4 hr at 22 °C	1436	C
Tacrolimus	FUJ	1 mg/mL[b]	AB	5 mg/mL	Visually compatible for 24 hr at 25 °C	1630	C
Teniposide	BR	0.1 mg/mL[a]	BA	5 mg/mL	Physically compatible for 4 hr at 23 °C	1725	C
Theophylline	TR	4 mg/mL	MG	5 mg/mL	Visually compatible for 6 hr at 25 °C	1793	C
Thiotepa	IMM[c]	1 mg/mL[a]	BA	5 mg/mL	Physically compatible for 4 hr at 23 °C	1861	C
TNA #218 to #226[d]			AB	5 mg/mL	Visually compatible for 4 hr at 23 °C	2215	C
TPN #189[d]			DB	5 mg/mL	Visually compatible for 24 hr at 22 °C	1767	C
TPN #203, #204[d]			AB	5 mg/mL	Visually compatible for 2 hr at 23 °C	1974	C
TPN #212 to #215[d]			SCS	5 mg/mL	Physically compatible for 4 hr at 23 °C	2109	C
Vasopressin	APP	0.2 unit/mL[b]	AB	5 mg/mL	Physically compatible	2641	C
Vinorelbine tartrate	BW	1 mg/mL[b]	BA	5 mg/mL	Physically compatible for 4 hr at 22 °C	1558	C

[a]*Tested in dextrose 5%.*
[b]*Tested in sodium chloride 0.9%.*
[c]*Lyophilized formulation tested.*
[d]*Refer to Appendix I for the composition of parenteral nutrition solutions. TNA indicates a 3-in-1 admixture, and TPN indicates a 2-in-1 admixture.*
[e]*Tested in Ringer's injection, lactated.*
[f]*Test performed using the formulation WITHOUT edetate disodium*

MEXILETINE HYDROCHLORIDE
AHFS 24:04.04.08

Products — Mexiletine hydrochloride is available as a 25-mg/mL solution in 10-mL (250-mg) ampuls. The product also contains sodium chloride and water for injection. (38)

Trade Name(s) — Mexitil.

Administration — Mexiletine hydrochloride is administered intravenously. It should never be given as a bolus. A loading dose is given by intravenous injection at a rate of 1 mL (25 mg) per minute. This is followed by intravenous infusion of a 500-mg/500 mL (1-mg/mL) dilution in a suitable infusion solution. The initial infusion rate of the first 250 mL of the admixture is 4 mL/min over the first hour followed by infusion of the next 250 mL at 2 mL/min over the next two hours. Maintenance is performed using a 250-mg/500 mL (0.5-mg/mL) dilution administered at a rate of 1 mL/min. (38)

Stability — Mexiletine hydrochloride injection is a clear, colorless solution that should be stored below 25 °C and protected from light. Dilutions for infusion are stable for up to eight hours. (38)

Compatibility Information

Solution Compatibility

Mexiletine HCl

Solution	Mfr	Mfr	Conc/L	Remarks	Ref	C/I
Dextrose 5%				Compatible for 8 hr	38	C
Sodium chloride 0.9%[a]				Compatible for 8 hr	38	C
Sodium lactate ⅙ M				Compatible for 8 hr	38	C

[a]Tested with and without potassium chloride 0.3 and 0.6% present.

Drugs in Syringe Compatibility

Mexiletine HCl

Drug (in syringe)	Mfr	Amt	Mfr	Amt	Remarks	Ref	C/I
Heparin sodium		2500 units/ 1 mL	BI	250 mg/ 10 mL	Turbidity or precipitate forms within 5 min	1053	I

MICAFUNGIN SODIUM
AHFS 8:14.16

Products — Micafungin sodium is available in vials containing 50 and 100 mg of drug with lactose 200 mg and citric acid and/or sodium hydroxide added during manufacturing to adjust pH. Reconstitute the 50- or 100-mg vials with 5 mL of sodium chloride 0.9%, resulting in solutions containing micafungin 10 or 20 mg/mL, respectively. As an alternative, dextrose 5% may used for reconstitution. However, diluents containing a bacteriostatic agent should not be used for reconstitution. To minimize foaming, gently swirl the vials to dissolve the contents. Do not shake vigorously. (1)

pH — From 5.0 to 7.0. (1)

Trade Name(s) — Mycamine.

Administration — Micafungin sodium is administered by intravenous infusion in 100 mL of sodium chloride 0.9% or dextrose 5% over one hour. Existing infusion lines should be flushed with sodium chloride 0.9% prior to starting the micafungin sodium infusion. (1)

Stability — Store intact vials at controlled room temperature. When reconstituted as directed, the manufacturer indicates micafungin sodium is stable for up to 24 hours at room temperature. However, the drug does not contain a preservative, and the manufacturer recommends discarding partially used vials. Micafungin sodium diluted for administration is also stable for up to 24 hours at room temperature when protected from light. (1)

Light Effects — The manufacturer states that micafungin sodium dilutions should be protected from light but that covering tubing and drip chambers is not necessary. (1)

Compatibility Information

Y-Site Injection Compatibility (1:1 Mixture)

Micafungin sodium

Drug	Mfr	Conc	Mfr	Conc	Remarks	Ref	C/I
Albumin human	ZLB	25%	ASP	1.5 mg/mL[b]	Immediate increase in measured haze	2683	I
Aminophylline	AMR	2.5 mg/mL[b]	ASP	1.5 mg/mL[b]	Physically compatible for 4 hr at 23 °C	2683	C
Amiodarone HCl	BA	4 mg/mL[b]	ASP	1.5 mg/mL[b]	Gross milky white precipitate forms	2683	I
Bumetanide	BED	40 mcg/mL[b]	ASP	1.5 mg/mL[b]	Physically compatible for 4 hr at 23 °C	2683	C
Calcium chloride	AB	40 mg/mL[b]	ASP	1.5 mg/mL[b]	Physically compatible for 4 hr at 23 °C	2683	C
Calcium gluconate	AMR	40 mg/mL[b]	ASP	1.5 mg/mL[b]	Physically compatible for 4 hr at 23 °C	2683	C

Y-Site Injection Compatibility (1:1 Mixture) (Cont.)

Micafungin sodium

Drug	Mfr	Conc	Mfr	Conc	Remarks	Ref	C/I
Carboplatin	BA	5 mg/mL[b]	ASP	1.5 mg/mL[b]	Physically compatible for 4 hr at 23 °C	2683	**C**
Cisatracurium besylate	AB	0.5 mg/mL[b]	ASP	1.5 mg/mL[b]	Gross precipitate forms immediately	2683	**I**
Cyclosporine	BED	5 mg/mL[b]	ASP	1.5 mg/mL[b]	Physically compatible for 4 hr at 23 °C	2683	**C**
Diltiazem HCl	BA	5 mg/mL	ASP	1.5 mg/mL[b]	Gross precipitate forms immediately	2683	**I**
Dobutamine HCl	AB	4 mg/mL[b]	ASP	1.5 mg/mL[b]	Gross precipitate forms immediately	2683	**I**
Dopamine HCl	AMR	3.2 mg/mL[b]	ASP	1.5 mg/mL[b]	Physically compatible for 4 hr at 23 °C	2683	**C**
Doripenem	JJ	5 mg/mL[a,b]	ASP	1.5 mg/mL[a,b]	Physically compatible for 4 hr at 23 °C	2743	**C**
Epinephrine HCl	AB	50 mcg/mL[b]	ASP	1.5 mg/mL[b]	Microparticulates form in 4 hr	2683	**I**
Eptifibatide	SC	0.75 mg/mL	ASP	1.5 mg/mL[b]	Physically compatible for 4 hr at 23 °C	2683	**C**
Esmolol HCl	BA	10 mg/mL[b]	ASP	1.5 mg/mL[b]	Physically compatible for 4 hr at 23 °C	2683	**C**
Etoposide	SIC	0.4 mg/mL[b]	ASP	1.5 mg/mL[b]	Physically compatible for 4 hr at 23 °C	2683	**C**
Fenoldopam mesylate	BA	80 mcg/mL[b]	ASP	1.5 mg/mL[b]	Physically compatible for 4 hr at 23 °C	2683	**C**
Furosemide	AMR	3 mg/mL[b]	ASP	1.5 mg/mL[b]	Physically compatible for 4 hr at 23 °C	2683	**C**
Heparin sodium	AB	100 units/mL	ASP	1.5 mg/mL[b]	Physically compatible for 4 hr at 23 °C	2683	**C**
Hydromorphone HCl	BA	0.5 mg/mL[b]	ASP	1.5 mg/mL[b]	Physically compatible for 4 hr at 23 °C	2683	**C**
Insulin, regular	NOV	1 unit/mL[b]	ASP	1.5 mg/mL[b]	Increase in haze and microparticulates form in 4 hr	2683	**I**
Labetalol HCl	AB	2 mg/mL[b]	ASP	1.5 mg/mL[b]	White cloudiness forms immediately	2683	**I**
Lidocaine HCl	AB	10 mg/mL[b]	ASP	1.5 mg/mL[b]	Physically compatible for 4 hr at 23 °C	2683	**C**
Lorazepam	AB	0.5 mg/mL[b]	ASP	1.5 mg/mL[b]	Physically compatible for 4 hr at 23 °C	2683	**C**
Magnesium sulfate	AMR	100 mg/mL[b]	ASP	1.5 mg/mL[b]	Physically compatible for 4 hr at 23 °C	2683	**C**
Meperidine HCl	AB	10 mg/mL[b]	ASP	1.5 mg/mL[b]	Milky precipitate forms immediately	2683	**I**
Mesna	APP	20 mg/mL[b]	ASP	1.5 mg/mL[b]	Physically compatible for 4 hr at 23 °C	2683	**C**
Midazolam HCl	APP	2 mg/mL[b]	ASP	1.5 mg/mL[b]	Gross precipitate forms immediately	2683	**I**
Milrinone lactate	BED	0.2 mg/mL[b]	ASP	1.5 mg/mL[b]	Physically compatible for 4 hr at 23 °C	2683	**C**
Morphine sulfate	APP	15 mg/mL	ASP	1.5 mg/mL[b]	White precipitate forms immediately	2683	**I**
Mycophenolate mofetil HCl	RC	6 mg/mL[a]	ASP	1.5 mg/mL[b]	White precipitate forms immediately	2683	**I**
Nesiritide	SCI	6 mcg/mL[a]	ASP	1.5 mg/mL[b]	Microparticulates form immediately	2683	**I**
Nicardipine HCl	ESP	1 mg/mL[b]	ASP	1.5 mg/mL[b]	Precipitate forms immediately	2683	**I**
Nitroglycerin	AMR	0.4 mg/mL[b]	ASP	1.5 mg/mL[b]	Physically compatible for 4 hr at 23 °C	2683	**C**
Norepinephrine bitartrate	BED	0.128 mg/mL[b]	ASP	1.5 mg/mL[b]	Physically compatible for 4 hr at 23 °C	2683	**C**
Octreotide acetate	NVA	5 mcg/mL[b]	ASP	1.5 mg/mL[b]	Microparticulates form in 4 hr	2683	**I**
Ondansetron HCl	GSK	1 mg/mL[b]	ASP	1.5 mg/mL[b]	White precipitate forms immediately	2683	**I**
Phenylephrine HCl	BA	1 mg/mL[b]	ASP	1.5 mg/mL[b]	Physically compatible for 4 hr at 23 °C	2683	**C**
Phenytoin sodium	HOS	50 mg/mL	ASP	1.5 mg/mL[b]	Measured haze increases within 1 hr	2683	**I**
Potassium chloride	AB	0.1 mEq/mL[b]	ASP	1.5 mg/mL[b]	Physically compatible for 4 hr at 23 °C	2683	**C**
Potassium phosphates	APP	0.5 mmol/mL[b]	ASP	1.5 mg/mL[b]	Physically compatible for 4 hr at 23 °C	2683	**C**
Rocuronium bromide	OR	1 mg/mL[b]	ASP	1.5 mg/mL[b]	White precipitate forms immediately	2683	**I**

Y-Site Injection Compatibility (1:1 Mixture) (Cont.)

Micafungin sodium

Drug	Mfr	Conc	Mfr	Conc	Remarks	Ref	C/I
Sodium nitroprusside	AB	2 mg/mL[b]	ASP	1.5 mg/mL[b]	Physically compatible for 4 hr at 23 °C protected from light	2683	C
Sodium phosphates	AMR	0.5 mmol/mL[b]	ASP	1.5 mg/mL[b]	Physically compatible for 4 hr at 23 °C	2683	C
Tacrolimus	FUJ	20 mcg/mL[b]	ASP	1.5 mg/mL[b]	Physically compatible for 4 hr at 23 °C	2683	C
Telavancin HCl	ASP	7.5 mg/mL[a,b]	ASP	5 mg/mL[a,b]	Visible haze forms	2830	I
Theophylline	AB	4 mg/mL	ASP	1.5 mg/mL[b]	Physically compatible for 4 hr at 23 °C	2683	C
TPN #268[c]			ASP	1.5 mg/mL[b]	Physically compatible for 4 hr at 23 °C	2683	C
Vasopressin	AMR	1 unit/mL	ASP	1.5 mg/mL[b]	Physically compatible for 4 hr at 23 °C	2683	C
Vecuronium bromide	BED	1 mg/mL	ASP	1.5 mg/mL[b]	White precipitate forms immediately	2683	I

[a]*Tested in dextrose 5%.*
[b]*Tested in sodium chloride 0.9%.*
[c]*Refer to Appendix I for the composition of parenteral nutrition solutions. TPN indicates a 2-in-1 admixture.*

MIDAZOLAM HYDROCHLORIDE
AHFS 28:24.08

Products — Midazolam hydrochloride is available at a concentration equivalent to midazolam 5 mg/mL in vials containing 1, 2, 5, or 10 mL. It also is available at a concentration equivalent to midazolam 1 mg/mL in vials containing 2, 5, or 10 mL. Each milliliter also contains sodium chloride 0.8%, disodium edetate 0.01%, and benzyl alcohol 1%, with hydrochloric acid and, if necessary, sodium hydroxide to adjust the pH. Preservative-free midazolam hydrochloride 1 and 5 mg/mL is also available. (1; 4)

pH — The pH of the injection is 2.9 to 3.7. (1; 4) Midazolam (Roche) 0.625, 1.25, and 1.67 mg/mL in sodium chloride 0.9% had pH values of 3.6, 3.4, and 3.4, respectively. (2161)

Osmolality — The 5-mg/mL concentration has an osmolality of 385 mOsm/kg. (4) Midazolam (Roche) 0.625, 1.25, and 1.67 mg/mL in sodium chloride 0.9% had osmolalities of 274, 262, and 259 mOsm/kg, respectively. (2161)

Sodium Content — Each milliliter of the available products contains about 0.14 mEq of sodium. (4)

Administration — Midazolam hydrochloride is administered by intramuscular injection deep into a large muscle mass or by slow intravenous injection in incremental doses (1; 4) or intravenous infusion. (4) Use of the 1-mg/mL concentration is recommended to facilitate slower injection and dosage titration. Both concentrations may be diluted with sodium chloride 0.9% or dextrose 5%. (1; 4)

Stability — Midazolam hydrochloride (Roche) is a colorless to light yellow solution. It should be stored at controlled room temperature and protected from light. (1; 4)

pH Effects — Midazolam hydrochloride is stable at pH 3 to 3.6. (4) It is highly water soluble at pH 4 or less; at higher pH values, increased lipid solubility occurs. (1145) The rate of photodecomposition increases with increasing pH from 1.3 to 6.4. (1944)

Light Effects — Midazolam hydrochloride in intact containers should be stored protected from light for long-term stability of the drug. (1; 4) Exposure of the commercial injection (Roche) to sunlight for four months resulted in the yellowing of the solution in one month and a midazolam loss of about 8% in four months. (1944) However, admixtures in compatible infusion solutions do not require protection from light for short-term storage and administration. (4)

Freezing Solutions — The injection was physically stable when frozen for three days followed by room temperature thawing. (4)

Syringes — Midazolam hydrochloride (Roche) 2 mg/mL in sodium chloride 0.9% was packaged as 3 mL in 10-mL polypropylene infusion pump syringes (Pharmacia Deltec). Little or no loss occurred during 10 days of storage at 5 and 30 °C. (1967)

Midazolam hydrochloride (Roche) 3 mg/mL in sodium chloride 0.9% exhibited no visual changes and had losses of 6.5% at 20 °C and 8.7% at 32 °C in polypropylene syringes (Terumo) and of 8.9% at 32 °C in glass vials after 13 days. (1595)

The stability of midazolam (salt form unspecified) 1 mg/mL repackaged in polypropylene syringes was evaluated. Little change in concentration was found after four weeks of storage at room temperature not exposed to direct light. (2164)

Midazolam hydrochloride (Roche) 5 mg/mL was packaged as 10 mL in 12-mL polypropylene syringes (Sherwood). No loss occurred in 36 days stored at 25 °C protected from light. (2088)

Compatibility Information

Solution Compatibility

Midazolam HCl

Solution	Mfr	Mfr	Conc/L	Remarks	Ref	C/I
Dextrose 5% with potassium chloride 0.15%	BA[a]	RC	0.1 and 0.5 g	13% loss in 24 hr at ambient temperature. 10% calculated loss in 20 hr	1868	I
	BA[a]	RC	1 g	7% loss in 24 hr at ambient temperature. 10% calculated loss in 35 hr	1868	C
Dextrose 5% in sodium chloride 0.9%	GRI	RC	0.1 and 0.5 g	8 to 10% loss in 24 hr at ambient temperature	1868	C
	GRI	RC	1 g	4% loss in 24 hr at ambient temperature. 10% calculated loss in 54 hr	1868	C
Dextrose 5%	MG[b]	RC	0.5 g	Visually compatible. No loss in 30 days at 23 °C in the dark or at 4 °C	1717	C
	c	RC	30 mg	No loss in 72 hr at 20 °C	1798	C
	AB	RC	0.1 and 0.5 g	Visually compatible. No loss in 3 hr at 24 °C	1852	C
	GRI	RC	0.1, 0.5, 1 g	3 to 5% loss in 24 hr at ambient temperature. 10% calculated loss in 63 to 112 hr	1868	C
	BA[g]	RC	500 mg	Visually compatible. No loss in 36 days at 4, 25, and 40 °C protected from light	2088	C
	BA[a], BRN[g,h]	RC	35 mg	Visually compatible. 4 to 6% loss in 24 hr at 4 and 22 °C	2289	C
	g	RC	100 and 500 mg	Visually compatible for 4 hr	355	C
Ringer's injection, lactated	GRI	RC	0.1 g	10% calculated loss in 2 hr at ambient temperature	1868	I
	GRI	RC	0.5 g	10% calculated loss in 6 hr at ambient temperature	1868	I
	GRI	RC	1 g	10% calculated loss in 10 hr at ambient temperature	1868	I
	g	RC	100 and 500 mg	Visually compatible for 4 hr	355	C
Sodium chloride 0.9%	d	RC	40 mg	Physically compatible. No loss in 24 hr at 21 °C in the dark	1392	C
	MG[b]	RC	0.5 g	Visually compatible. No loss in 30 days at 23 °C in the dark or at 4 °C	1717	C
	c	RC	30 mg	No loss in 72 hr at 20 °C	1798	C
	BA[a]	RC	1 g[e]	Visually compatible. 5% or less loss in 10 days at 23 °C both in light and dark	1859	C
	BA[a]	RC	1 g	Visually compatible. 4 to 6% loss in 49 days at 4 and 20 °C in light and at 20 °C in dark	1863	C
	GRI	RC	0.1, 0.5, 1 g	8 to 10% loss in 24 hr at ambient temperature	1868	C
	BA[g]	RC	500 mg	Visually compatible. No loss in 36 days at 4, 25, and 40 °C protected from light	2088	C
	BA[a], BRN[g,h]	RC	35 mg	Visually compatible. 4 to 6% loss in 24 hr at 4 and 22 °C	2289	C
	g	RC	100 and 500 mg	Visually compatible for 4 hr	355	C
	BA	RC	300, 600, 900 mg	Visually compatible. No loss in 48 hr at room temperature	2531	C

Solution Compatibility (Cont.)

Midazolam HCl

Solution	Mfr	Mfr	Conc/L	Remarks	Ref	C/I
TPN #174 to #176[f]		RC	600 mg to 1 g	Precipitates immediately	1624	I
		RC	100 and 500 mg	Visually compatible with no midazolam loss and less than 10% loss of any amino acid in 5 hr at 22 °C	1624	C

[a]Tested in PVC containers.
[b]Tested in polyolefin containers.
[c]Tested in both glass and PVC containers.
[d]Tested in PVC, glass, and polyethylene-lined laminated containers.
[e]Also contained benzyl alcohol 1%.
[f]Refer to Appendix I for the composition of parenteral nutrition solutions. TPN indicates a 2-in-1 admixture.
[g]Tested in glass containers.
[h]Tested in polyethylene containers.

Additive Compatibility

Midazolam HCl

Drug	Mfr	Conc/L	Mfr	Conc/L	Test Soln	Remarks	Ref	C/I
Aminophylline		720 mg	RC	50 mg	NS	Visually compatible for 4 hr	355	C
		720 mg	RC	250 mg	NS	Transient precipitate that dissipates	355	?
		720 mg	RC	400 mg	NS	Precipitate forms immediately	355	I
Amoxicillin sodium	BE	10 g	RC	50 and 250 mg	NS	Transient precipitate	355	?
	BE	10 g	RC	400 mg	NS	Precipitate forms immediately	355	I
Cefuroxime sodium	GL	7.5 g	RC	50, 250, 400 mg	NS	Visually compatible for 4 hr	355	C
Ciprofloxacin	BAY	2 g	RC	200 mg	D5W	Visually compatible. No ciprofloxacin loss in 24 hr at 22 °C in light. Midazolam not tested	2413	C
Furosemide		80 mg	RC	50 and 250 mg	NS	Visually compatible for 4 hr	355	C
Gentamicin sulfate	EX	800 mg	RC	50, 250, 400 mg	NS	Visually compatible for 4 hr	355	C
Hydromorphone HCl	KN	0.5 to 45 g	RC	0.1 to 4.5 g	D5W, NS	Visually compatible for 24 hr at room temperature	2086	C
	KN	2 and 20 g	RC	100 and 500 mg	D5W, NS	Visually compatible. Under 7% hydromorphone and midazolam loss in 23 days at 4 and 23 °C	2086	C
Metronidazole		5 g	RC	50, 250, 400 mg	NS	Visually compatible for 4 hr	355	C
Oxycodone HCl	NAP	830 mg	RC	830 mg	NS, W	Visually compatible. Under 4% concentration change in 24 hr at 25 °C	2600	C
Ranitidine HCl	GL	400 mg	RC	50 and 250 mg	NS	Visually compatible for 4 hr	355	C
Sodium bicarbonate	[b]	5%	RC	100 mg		Transient precipitation upon mixing	355	?
	[b]	5%	RC	500 mg		Precipitation upon mixing	355	I

Additive Compatibility (Cont.)

Midazolam HCl

Drug	Mfr	Conc/L	Mfr	Conc/L	Test Soln	Remarks	Ref	C/I
Tramadol HCl	AND	11.18 g	RC	500 mg	NS[a]	Visually compatible for 7 days at 25 °C protected from light	2701	**C**
	AND	33.3 g	RC	1.5 g	NS[a]	Visually compatible for 7 days at 25 °C protected from light	2701	**C**

[a]*Tested in elastomeric pump reservoirs (Baxter).*
[b]*Tested in glass containers.*

Drugs in Syringe Compatibility

Midazolam HCl

Drug (in syringe)	Mfr	Amt	Mfr	Amt	Remarks	Ref	C/I
Alfentanil HCl	JN	0.5 mg/mL	RC	0.2 mg/mL[a]	Visually compatible. 8% midazolam and 2% alfentanil loss in 3 weeks at 20 °C in light. No alfentanil loss and 7% midazolam loss in 4 weeks at 6 °C in dark	2133	**C**
Atracurium besylate	BW	10 mg/mL		5 mg/mL	Physically compatible and atracurium stable for 24 hr at 5 and 30 °C	1694	**C**
Atropine sulfate	IX	0.4 mg/1 mL	RC	5 mg/1 mL	Physically compatible for 4 hr at 25 °C	1145	**C**
Buprenorphine HCl	NE	0.3 mg/1 mL	RC	5 mg/1 mL	Physically compatible for 4 hr at 25 °C	1145	**C**
Butorphanol tartrate	BR	2 mg/1 mL	RC	5 mg/1 mL	Physically compatible for 4 hr at 25 °C	1145	**C**
Chlorpromazine HCl	SKF	50 mg/2 mL	RC	5 mg/1 mL	Physically compatible for 4 hr at 25 °C	1145	**C**
Dexamethasone sodium phosphate	DB	2 mg/8 mL	RC	2.5 mg/8 mL	Diluted in NS. Visually clear. No dexamethasone loss in 48 hr. Midazolam losses over 10% beyond 24 hr at room temperature	2531	**C**
	DB	2 mg/8 mL	RC	5 mg/8 mL	Diluted in NS. Visually clear. No dexamethasone loss in 48 hr. Midazolam losses were 7% in 48 hr at room temperature	2531	**C**
	DB	4 mg/8 mL	RC	5 mg/8 mL	Diluted in NS. Cloudiness forms immediately	2531	**I**
	DB	4 mg/8 mL	RC	7.5 mg/8 mL	Diluted in NS. Cloudiness forms immediately	2531	**I**
	DB	2 mg/8 mL	RC	7.5 mg/8 mL	Diluted in NS. Crystals form in some samples within 24 hr	2531	**I**
Diamorphine HCl	EV	10 mg	RC	10[b] and 75[c] mg	Visually compatible. 10% diamorphine and no midazolam loss in 15.9 days at 22 °C	1792	**C**
	EV	500 mg	RC	10[b] and 75[c] mg	Visually compatible. 10% diamorphine and no midazolam loss in 22.2 days at 22 °C	1792	**C**
Dimenhydrinate	SE	50 mg/1 mL	RC	5 mg/1 mL	White precipitate forms immediately	1145	**I**
Diphenhydramine HCl	ES	50 mg/1 mL	RC	5 mg/1 mL	Physically compatible for 4 hr at 25 °C	1145	**C**

Drugs in Syringe Compatibility (Cont.)

Midazolam HCl

Drug (in syringe)	Mfr	Amt	Mfr	Amt	Remarks	Ref	C/I
Droperidol	JN	2.5 mg/ 1 mL	RC	5 mg/ 1 mL	Physically compatible for 4 hr at 25 °C	1145	C
Fentanyl citrate	ES	0.1 mg/ 2 mL	RC	5 mg/ 1 mL	Physically compatible for 4 hr at 25 °C	1145	C
	DB	12.5 mcg/mL[a]	RC	0.625 and 0.938 mg/mL[a]	Visually compatible. Little fentanyl loss. 7 and 9% midazolam loss in 7 days at 5 and 22 °C, respectively	2202	C
	DB	37.5 mcg/mL[a]	RC	0.625 mg/mL[a]	Visually compatible. No fentanyl loss. 5 and 8% midazolam loss in 7 days at 5 and 22 °C, respectively	2202	C
	DB	37.5 mcg/mL[a]	RC	0.938 mg/mL[a]	Visually compatible. Little fentanyl loss. 7 and 9% midazolam loss in 7 days at 5 and 22 °C, respectively	2202	C
	DB	33.3 mcg/mL[a]	RC	0.278 and 0.833 mg/mL[a]	Visually compatible. No fentanyl loss. 5 and 7% midazolam loss in 7 days at 5 and 22 °C, respectively	2202	C
Fentanyl citrate with metoclopramide HCl	DB AST	1 mg/ 20 mL 20 mg/ 4 mL	RC	15 mg/ 3 mL	Visually compatible with 7% or less loss of each drug in 10 days at 32 °C	2268	C
Glycopyrrolate	RB	0.2 mg/ 1 mL	RC	5 mg/ 1 mL	Physically compatible for 4 hr at 25 °C	1145	C
Heparin sodium		2500 units/ 1 mL	RC	15 mg/ 3 mL	Turbidity or precipitate forms within 5 min	1053	I
Hydromorphone HCl	WB	2 mg/ 0.5 mL	RC	5 mg/ 1 mL	Physically compatible for 4 hr at 25 °C	1145	C
Hydroxyzine HCl	ES	100 mg/ 2 mL	RC	5 mg/ 1 mL	Physically compatible for 4 hr at 25 °C	1145	C
Meperidine HCl	WB	100 mg/ 1 mL	RC	5 mg/ 1 mL	Physically compatible for 4 hr at 25 °C	1145	C
Metoclopramide HCl	RB	10 mg/ 2 mL	RC	5 mg/ 1 mL	Physically compatible for 4 hr at 25 °C	1145	C
Metoclopramide HCl with fentanyl citrate	AST DB	20 mg/ 4 mL 1 mg/ 20 mL	RC	15 mg/ 3 mL	Visually compatible with 7% or less loss of each drug in 10 days at 32 °C	2268	C
Morphine sulfate	WB	10 mg/ 1 mL	RC	5 mg/ 1 mL	Physically compatible for 4 hr at 25 °C	1145	C
		5 and 10 mg/ 1 mL[d]	RC	5 mg/ 1 mL	Visually compatible. 9% or less morphine and 8% or less midazolam loss in 14 days at 22 °C in dark. Microprecipitate may form, requiring filtration	1901	C
		5 and 10 mg/ 1 mL[e]	RC	5 mg/ 1 mL	Visually compatible. 8% or less morphine and 3% or less midazolam loss in 14 days at 22 °C protected from light. Microprecipitate may form, requiring filtration	1901	C
Nalbuphine HCl	DU	10 mg/ 1 mL	RC	5 mg/ 1 mL	Physically compatible for 4 hr at 25 °C	1145	C

Drugs in Syringe Compatibility (Cont.)

Midazolam HCl

Drug (in syringe)	Mfr	Amt	Mfr	Amt	Remarks	Ref	C/I
Ondansetron HCl	GW	1.33 mg/mL[a]	RC	1.66 mg/mL[a]	Physically compatible. Under 4% ondansetron and under 7% midazolam losses in 24 hr at 4 or 23 °C	2199	**C**
Oxycodone HCl	NAP	200 mg/20 mL	RC	100 mg/20 mL	Visually compatible. Under 4% concentration change in 24 hr at 25 °C	2600	**C**
Pantoprazole sodium	f	4 mg/1 mL		5 mg/1 mL	Precipitates immediately	2574	**I**
Pentobarbital sodium	WY	100 mg/2 mL	RC	5 mg/1 mL	White precipitate forms immediately	1145	**I**
Prochlorperazine edisylate	SKF	10 mg/2 mL	RC	5 mg/1 mL	White precipitate forms immediately	1145	**I**
Promethazine HCl	WY	25 mg/1 mL	RC	5 mg/1 mL	Physically compatible for 4 hr at 25 °C	1145	**C**
Ranitidine HCl	GL	50 mg/2 mL	RC	5 mg/1 mL	White precipitate forms immediately	1145	**I**
Scopolamine HBr	BW	0.43 mg/0.5 mL	RC	5 mg/1 mL	Physically compatible for 4 hr at 25 °C	1145	**C**
Trimethobenzamide HCl	BE	200 mg/2 mL	RC	5 mg/1 mL	Physically compatible for 4 hr at 25 °C	1145	**C**

[a] Diluted with sodium chloride 0.9%.
[b] Diluted with sterile water to 15 mL.
[c] Diamorphine hydrochloride constituted with midazolam injection.
[d] Morphine sulfate powder dissolved in dextrose 5%.
[e] Morphine sulfate powder dissolved in water and sodium chloride 0.9%.
[f] Test performed using the formulation WITHOUT edetate disodium.

Y-Site Injection Compatibility (1:1 Mixture)

Midazolam HCl

Drug	Mfr	Conc	Mfr	Conc	Remarks	Ref	C/I
Abciximab	LI	36 mcg/mL[a]	BED	2 mg/mL	Visually compatible for 12 hr at 23 °C	2374	**C**
Albumin human		200 mg/mL	RC	5 mg/mL	White precipitate forms immediately	1855	**I**
Amikacin sulfate	BMS	5 mg/mL	RC	5 mg/mL	Visually compatible for 24 hr at 22 °C	1855	**C**
Amiodarone HCl	WY	4.8 mg/mL[a]	RC	1 mg/mL[a]	Visually compatible for 24 hr at 23 °C	1877	**C**
	WY	6 mg/mL[a]	RC	1 mg/mL[a]	Visually compatible for 24 hr at 22 °C	2352	**C**
Amoxicillin sodium	SKB	50 mg/mL	RC	5 mg/mL	White precipitate forms immediately	1855	**I**
Amoxicillin sodium–clavulanate potassium	SKB	20 + 2 mg/mL	RC	5 mg/mL	White precipitate forms immediately	1855	**I**
Amphotericin B cholesteryl sulfate complex	SEQ	0.83 mg/mL[a]	RC	2 mg/mL[a]	Gross precipitate forms	2117	**I**
Ampicillin sodium	WY	20 mg/mL[b]	RC	1 mg/mL[a]	Haze forms immediately	1847	**I**
Anidulafungin	VIC	0.5 mg/mL[a]	BA	1 mg/mL[a]	Physically compatible for 4 hr at 23 °C	2617	**C**
Argatroban	GSK	1 mg/mL[b]	AB	2 mg/mL	Visually compatible for 24 hr at 23 °C	2391	**C**
Atracurium besylate	BW	0.5 mg/mL[a]	RC	0.05 mg/mL[a]	Physically compatible for 24 hr at 28 °C	1337	**C**
	GW	1 and 5 mg/mL[a]	RC	0.1 mg/mL[a]	Visually compatible with no loss of either drug in 3 hr at 25 °C	2112	**C**

Y-Site Injection Compatibility (1:1 Mixture) (Cont.)

Midazolam HCl

Drug	Mfr	Conc	Mfr	Conc	Remarks	Ref	C/I
	GW	5 mg/mL[a]	RC	0.5 mg/mL[a]	Visually compatible with no loss of either drug in 3 hr at 25 °C	2112	C
	GW	1 mg/mL[a]	RC	0.5 mg/mL[a]	Visually compatible with no loss of midazolam and 4% loss of atracurium in 3 hr at 25 °C	2112	C
Bivalirudin	TMC	5 mg/mL[a]	BA	1 mg/mL[a]	Physically compatible for 4 hr at 23 °C	2373	C
	TMC	5 mg/mL[a,b]	AB	2 mg/mL	Visually compatible for 6 hr at 23 °C	2680	C
Bumetanide	LEO	0.5 mg/mL	RC	5 mg/mL	White precipitate forms immediately	1855	I
Butorphanol tartrate	BR	f	RC	f	Crystalline midazolam precipitate forms	2144	I
Calcium gluconate	FUJ	100 mg/mL	RC	1 mg/mL[a]	Visually compatible for 24 hr at 23 °C	1847	C
Caspofungin acetate	ME	0.7 mg/mL[b]	APP	2 mg/mL[b]	Physically compatible for 4 hr at room temperature	2758	C
Cefazolin sodium	MAR	20 mg/mL[a]	RC	1 mg/mL[a]	Visually compatible for 24 hr at 23 °C	1847	C
Cefepime HCl	BMS	120 mg/mL[c]		5 mg/mL	Over 10% cefepime loss occurs in 1 hr	2513	I
Cefotaxime sodium	HO	20 mg/mL[a]	RC	1 mg/mL[a]	Visually compatible for 24 hr at 23 °C	1847	C
	RS	10 mg/mL	RC	5 mg/mL	Visually compatible for 24 hr at 22 °C	1855	C
Ceftaroline fosamil	FOR	2.22 mg/mL[a,b,d]	BV	2 mg/mL[a,b,d]	Physically compatible for 4 hr at 23 °C	2826	C
Ceftazidime	LI	20 mg/mL[a]	RC	1 mg/mL[a]	Haze forms in 1 hr	1847	I
	SKB	125 mg/mL		5 mg/mL	Precipitates immediately	2434	I
	GSK	120 mg/mL[c]		5 mg/mL	Precipitates	2513	I
Cefuroxime sodium	LI	15 mg/mL[a]	RC	1 mg/mL[a]	Particles form in 8 hr	1847	I
Ciprofloxacin	BAY	2 mg/mL	RC	5 mg/mL	Visually compatible for 24 hr at 22 °C	1855	C
Cisatracurium besylate	GW	0.1, 2, 5 mg/mL[a]	RC	1 mg/mL[a]	Physically compatible for 4 hr at 23 °C	2074	C
Clindamycin phosphate	UP	9 mg/mL[a]	RC	1 mg/mL[a]	Visually compatible for 24 hr at 23 °C	1847	C
Clonidine HCl	BI	0.015 mg/mL	RC	5 mg/mL	Orange color in 24 hr at 22 °C	1855	I
	BI	18 mcg/mL[b]	ALP	1 mg/mL	Visually compatible	2642	C
Dexamethasone sodium phosphate	ES	4 mg/mL	RC	1 mg/mL[a]	Immediate haze. Precipitate in 8 hr	1847	I
		4 mg/mL	RC	5 mg/mL	White precipitate forms immediately	1855	I
Dexmedetomidine HCl	HOS				Stated to be compatible	1	C
Digoxin	BW	0.1 mg/mL	RC	1 mg/mL[a]	Visually compatible for 24 hr at 23 °C	1847	C
Diltiazem HCl	MMD	1 mg/mL[a]	RC	2 mg/mL[a]	Visually compatible for 4 hr at 27 °C	2062	C
Dobutamine HCl	GNS	2 mg/mL[a]	RC	1 mg/mL[a]	Particles form in 8 hr	1847	I
	LI	4 mg/mL[a]	RC	1 mg/mL[a]	Visually compatible for 24 hr at 23 °C	1877	C
	LI	4 mg/mL[a]	RC	2 mg/mL[a]	Visually compatible for 4 hr at 27 °C	2062	C
Dopamine HCl	AB	1.6 mg/mL[a]	RC	1 mg/mL[a]	Visually compatible for 24 hr at 23 °C	1847	C
	DU	3.2 mg/mL[a]	RC	1 mg/mL[a]	Visually compatible for 24 hr at 23 °C	1877	C
	AB	3.2 mg/mL[a]	RC	2 mg/mL[a]	Visually compatible for 4 hr at 27 °C	2062	C
Doripenem	JJ	5 mg/mL[a,b]	BED	2 mg/mL[a,b]	Physically compatible for 4 hr at 23 °C	2743	C
Epinephrine HCl	AB	0.02 mg/mL[a]	RC	2 mg/mL[a]	Visually compatible for 4 hr at 27 °C	2062	C
Erythromycin lactobionate	AB	5 mg/mL	RC	5 mg/mL	Visually compatible for 24 hr at 22 °C	1855	C
Esmolol HCl	DU	40 mg/mL[a]	RC	1 mg/mL[a]	Visually compatible for 24 hr at 23 °C	1877	C

Y-Site Injection Compatibility (1:1 Mixture) (Cont.)

Midazolam HCl

Drug	Mfr	Conc	Mfr	Conc	Remarks	Ref	C/I
Etomidate	AB	2 mg/mL	RC	5 mg/mL	Visually compatible for 7 days at 25 °C	1801	**C**
Famotidine	MSD	0.2 mg/mL[a]	RC	0.15 mg/mL[a]	Physically compatible for 4 hr at 25 °C	1188	**C**
	ME	2 mg/mL[b]		1.5 mg/mL[a]	Visually compatible for 4 hr at 22 °C	1936	**C**
Fenoldopam mesylate	AB	80 mcg/mL[b]	APP	1 mg/mL[b]	Physically compatible for 4 hr at 23 °C	2467	**C**
Fentanyl citrate	ES	0.05 mg/mL	RC	1 mg/mL[a]	Visually compatible for 24 hr at 23 °C	1847	**C**
	JN	0.02 mg/mL[a]	RC	0.1 and 0.5 mg/mL[a]	Visually compatible. No midazolam and 4% fentanyl loss in 3 hr at 24 °C	1852	**C**
	JN	0.04 mg/mL[a]	RC	0.1 and 0.5 mg/mL[a]	Visually compatible with no loss of either drug in 3 hr at 24 °C	1852	**C**
		0.05 mg/mL	RC	5 mg/mL	Visually compatible for 24 hr at 22 °C	1855	**C**
	ES	0.05 mg/mL	RC	2 mg/mL[a]	Visually compatible for 4 hr at 27 °C	2062	**C**
	JN	0.025 mg/mL[a]	RC	0.2 mg/mL[a]	Physically compatible for 48 hr at 22 °C	1706	**C**
Floxacillin sodium	SKB	50 mg/mL	RC	5 mg/mL	White precipitate forms immediately	1855	**I**
Fluconazole	RR	2 mg/mL	RC	5 mg/mL	Physically compatible for 24 hr at 25 °C	1407	**C**
	PF	2 mg/mL	RC	5 mg/mL	Visually compatible for 24 hr at 22 °C	1855	**C**
Foscarnet sodium	AST	24 mg/mL	RC	5 mg/mL	Gas production	1335	**I**
Fosphenytoin sodium	PD	1 mg PE/mL[b,g]	RC	2 mg/mL[b]	Midazolam base precipitates immediately	2223	**I**
Furosemide	AST	10 mg/mL	RC	1 mg/mL[a]	Immediate haze. Precipitate in 2 hr	1847	**I**
	CNF	10 mg/mL	RC	5 mg/mL	White precipitate forms immediately	1855	**I**
	AMR	10 mg/mL	RC	2 mg/mL[a]	Precipitate forms immediately	2062	**I**
Gentamicin sulfate	ES	10 mg/mL	RC	1 mg/mL[a]	Visually compatible for 24 hr at 23 °C	1847	**C**
	CNF	3 mg/mL	RC	5 mg/mL	Visually compatible for 24 hr at 22 °C	1855	**C**
Haloperidol lactate	JN	0.5 and 5 mg/mL	RC	5 mg/mL	Visually compatible for 24 hr at 22 °C	1855	**C**
Heparin sodium		417 units/mL	RC	5 mg/mL	Visually compatible for 24 hr at 22 °C	1855	**C**
	ES	100 units/mL[a]	RC	2 mg/mL[a]	Visually compatible for 4 hr at 27 °C	2062	**C**
		50 units/mL[b]	RC[h]	15 mg/3 mL	Clear solution	1053	**C**
Hetastarch in lactated electrolyte	AB	6%	RC	1 mg/mL[a]	Physically compatible for 4 hr at 23 °C	2339	**C**
Hydrocortisone sodium succinate	UP	50 mg/mL	RC	5 mg/mL	White precipitate forms immediately	1855	**I**
Hydromorphone HCl	KN	1 mg/mL	RC	2 mg/mL[a]	Visually compatible for 4 hr at 27 °C	2062	**C**
	AST	0.5 mg/mL[a]	RC	0.2 mg/mL[a]	Physically compatible for 48 hr at 22 °C	1706	**C**
Hydroxyethyl starch 130/0.4 in sodium chloride 0.9%	FRK	6%	SZ	1, 1.5, 2 mg/mL[a]	Visually compatible for 24 hr at room temperature	2770	**C**
Imipenem–cilastatin sodium	MSD	5 mg/mL	RC	5 mg/mL	Haze forms in 24 hr	1855	**I**
Insulin, regular	LI	1 unit/mL[a]	RC	1 mg/mL[b]	Visually compatible for 24 hr at 23 °C	1877	**C**
Labetalol HCl	GL	5 mg/mL	RC	1 mg/mL[a]	Visually compatible for 24 hr at 23 °C	1877	**C**
	AH	2 mg/mL[a]	RC	2 mg/mL[a]	Visually compatible for 4 hr at 27 °C	2062	**C**
Linezolid	PHU	2 mg/mL	RC	2 mg/mL[a]	Physically compatible for 4 hr at 23 °C	2264	**C**
Lorazepam	WY	0.5 mg/mL[a]	RC	2 mg/mL[a]	Visually compatible for 4 hr at 27 °C	2062	**C**
Methadone HCl	LI	1 mg/mL[a]	RC	0.2 mg/mL[a]	Physically compatible for 48 hr at 22 °C	1706	**C**
Methotrexate sodium		30 mg/mL	RC	5 mg/mL	Yellow precipitate forms immediately	1788	**I**

Y-Site Injection Compatibility (1:1 Mixture) (Cont.)

Midazolam HCl

Drug	Mfr	Conc	Mfr	Conc	Remarks	Ref	C/I
Methylprednisolone sodium succinate	UP	40 mg/mL	RC	1 mg/mL[a]	Visually compatible for 24 hr at 23 °C	1847	C
Metronidazole	BA	5 mg/mL	RC	1 mg/mL[a]	Visually compatible for 24 hr at 23 °C	1847	C
	BRN	5 mg/mL	RC	5 mg/mL	Visually compatible for 24 hr at 22 °C	1855	C
Micafungin sodium	ASP	1.5 mg/mL[b]	APP	2 mg/mL[b]	Gross precipitate forms immediately	2683	I
Milrinone lactate	SW	0.2 mg/mL[a]	RC	2 mg/mL	Visually compatible for 4 hr at 27 °C	2062	C
	SW	0.4 mg/mL[a]	RC	1 mg/mL	Visually compatible. Little loss of either drug in 4 hr at 23 °C	2214	C
Morphine sulfate	AST	1 mg/mL[a]	RC	0.2 mg/mL[a]	Physically compatible for 48 hr at 22 °C	1706	C
	ES	0.25 mg/mL[a]	RC	0.1 and 0.5 mg/mL[a]	Visually compatible with no loss of either drug in 3 hr at 24 °C	1789	C
	ES	1 mg/mL[a]	RC	0.1 and 0.5 mg/mL[a]	Visually compatible with no loss of either drug in 3 hr at 24 °C	1789	C
	SX	1 mg/mL[a]	RC	1 mg/mL[a]	Visually compatible for 24 hr at 23 °C	1877	C
	SCN	2 mg/mL[a]	RC	2 mg/mL[a]	Visually compatible for 4 hr at 27 °C	2062	C
Nafcillin sodium	WY	20 mg/mL[a]	RC	1 mg/mL[a]	Immediate haze. Particles in 4 hr	1847	I
Nicardipine HCl	WY	1 mg/mL[a]	RC	2 mg/mL[a]	Visually compatible for 4 hr at 27 °C	2062	C
Nitroglycerin	SO	0.2 mg/mL[a]	RC	1 mg/mL[a]	Visually compatible for 24 hr at 23 °C	1847	C
	OM	0.2 mg/mL[a]	RC	1 mg/mL[a]	Visually compatible for 24 hr at 23 °C	1877	C
	AB	0.4 mg/mL[a]	RC	2 mg/mL[a]	Visually compatible for 4 hr at 27 °C	2062	C
Norepinephrine bitartrate	STR	0.064 mg/mL[a]	RC	1 mg/mL[a]	Visually compatible for 24 hr at 23 °C	1877	C
	AB	0.128 mg/mL[a]	RC	2 mg/mL[a]	Visually compatible for 4 hr at 27 °C	2062	C
Omeprazole	AST	4 mg/mL	RC	5 mg/mL	Brown color then precipitate	1855	I
Palonosetron HCl	MGI	50 mcg/mL	BA	2 mg/mL[a]	Physically compatible. No loss of either drug in 4 hr	2608	C
Pancuronium bromide	ES	0.05 mg/mL[a]	RC	0.05 mg/mL[a]	Physically compatible for 24 hr at 28 °C	1337	C
Pantoprazole sodium	ALT[j]	0.16 to 0.8 mg/mL[b]	SX	1 to 2 mg/mL[a]	Discoloration and reddish-brown precipitate form	2603	I
	ALT[j]	8 mg/mL	RC	0.1 mg/mL	Yellow color forms immediately	2727	I
Potassium chloride	BRN	1 mEq/mL	RC	5 mg/mL	Visually compatible for 24 hr at 22 °C	1855	C
Propofol	STU	2 mg/mL	RC	5 mg/mL	Oil droplets form within 7 days at 25 °C. No visible change in 24 hr	1801	?
	ZEN	10 mg/mL	RC	2 mg/mL[a]	Physically compatible for 1 hr at 23 °C	2066	C
Ranitidine HCl	GL	0.5 mg/mL	RC	5 mg/mL	Visually compatible for 24 hr at 22 °C	1855	C
	GL	1 mg/mL[a]	RC	2 mg/mL[a]	Visually compatible for 4 hr at 27 °C	2062	C
Remifentanil HCl	GW	0.025 and 0.25 mg/mL[b]	RC	1 mg/mL[a]	Physically compatible for 4 hr at 23 °C	2075	C
Sodium bicarbonate		1.4%	RC	5 mg/mL	White precipitate forms immediately	1788	I
	IMS	1 mEq/mL	RC	1 mg/mL[a]	Immediate haze. Precipitate in 2 hr	1847	I
Sodium nitroprusside	ES	0.2 mg/mL[a]	RC	1 mg/mL[a]	Visually compatible for 24 hr at 23 °C	1847	C
	RC	0.2 mg/mL[a]	RC	1 mg/mL[a]	Visually compatible for 24 hr at 23 °C	1877	C
	RC	1.2 and 3 mg/mL[a]	RC	1.2 and 2.4 mg/mL[i]	Visually compatible for 48 hr at 24 °C protected from light	2357	C
	RC	0.3, 1.2, 3 mg/mL[a]	RC	5 mg/mL[i]	Visually compatible for 48 hr at 24 °C protected from light	2357	C

Y-Site Injection Compatibility (1:1 Mixture) (Cont.)

Midazolam HCl

Drug	Mfr	Conc	Mfr	Conc	Remarks	Ref	C/I
Theophylline	BA	1.6 mg/mL[a]	RC	1 mg/mL[a]	Visually compatible for 24 hr at 23 °C	1847	C
Tirofiban HCl	ME	50 mcg/mL[a,b]	RC	5 and 0.05[a,b] mg/mL	Physically compatible. No loss of either drug in 4 hr at 23 °C	2356	C
TNA #218 to #226[e]			RC	2 mg/mL[a]	Damage to emulsion occurs immediately with free oil formation possible	2215	I
Tobramycin sulfate	LI	10 mg/mL	RC	1 mg/mL[a]	Visually compatible for 24 hr at 23 °C	1847	C
TPN #189[e]			RC	5 mg/mL	White haze and precipitate form immediately. Crystals form in 24 hr	1767	I
TPN #212 to #215[e]			RC	2 mg/mL[a]	White cloudiness forms rapidly	2109	I
Trimethoprim–sulfamethoxazole	RC	0.8 + 4 mg/mL	RC	5 mg/mL	White precipitate forms immediately	1855	I
Vancomycin HCl	LI	5 mg/mL[a]	RC	1 mg/mL[a]	Visually compatible for 24 hr at 23 °C	1847	C
	LI	5 mg/mL	RC	5 mg/mL	Visually compatible for 24 hr at 22 °C	1855	C
Vecuronium bromide	OR	0.1 mg/mL[a]	RC	0.05 mg/mL[a]	Physically compatible for 24 hr at 28 °C	1337	C
	OR	4 mg/mL	RC	5 mg/mL	Visually compatible for 24 hr at 22 °C	1855	C
	OR	1 mg/mL	RC	2 mg/mL[a]	Visually compatible for 4 hr at 27 °C	2062	C

[a]*Tested in dextrose 5%.*
[b]*Tested in sodium chloride 0.9%.*
[c]*Tested in sterile water for injection.*
[d]*Tested in Ringer's injection, lactated.*
[e]*Refer to Appendix I for the composition of parenteral nutrition solutions. TNA indicates a 3-in-1 admixture, and TPN indicates a 2-in-1 admixture.*
[f]*Concentration unspecified.*
[g]*Concentration expressed in milligrams of phenytoin sodium equivalents (PE) per milliliter.*
[h]*Given over three minutes into a heparin infusion run at 1 mL/min.*
[i]*Tested in dextrose 5% in sodium chloride 0.2%.*
[j]*Test performed using the formulation WITHOUT edetate disodium.*

MILRINONE LACTATE
AHFS 24:04.08

Products — Milrinone lactate is available as a solution containing the equivalent of milrinone 1 mg/mL in 10-, 20-, and 50-mL single-dose vials. Each milliliter also contains dextrose, anhydrous, 47 mg in water for injection. Lactic acid or sodium hydroxide may have been used to adjust the pH. The total lactic acid concentration may vary between 0.95 and 1.29 mg/mL. The 1-mg/mL concentration must be diluted for use. (1)

Milrinone lactate is also available as a ready-to-use solution in 100- and 200-mL flexible PVC plastic containers at a concentration equivalent to milrinone 0.2 mg/mL (200 mcg/mL). The solution has a nominal lactic acid concentration of 0.282 mg/mL and also contains dextrose, anhydrous 49.4 mg/mL. (1)

pH — From 3.2 to 4. (1)

Administration — Milrinone lactate is administered intravenously. For maintenance administration by continuous intravenous infusion, milrinone lactate in vials is diluted in a compatible diluent, usually to 200 mcg/mL. The premixed 200-mcg/mL infusion in flexible plastic containers need not be diluted for use. When milrinone lactate is administered by continuous infusion, the use of a calibrated electronic infusion device is recommended. (1)

Stability — Milrinone lactate solutions are colorless to pale yellow. The 1-mg/mL concentration should be stored at controlled room temperature and protected from freezing. The 0.2-mg/mL concentration in PVC containers should be stored at room temperature of 25 °C and should be protected from freezing and exposure to excessive heat. Brief exposure to temperatures up to 40 °C does not adversely affect the product. (1)

Compatibility Information

Solution Compatibility

Milrinone lactate

Solution	Mfr	Mfr	Conc/L	Remarks	Ref	C/I
Dextrose 5%	c	WI	200 mg	Physically compatible. Stable for 72 hr at room temperature in light or dark	1468	C
	a	SW	0.2 g	Visually compatible. Little loss after 14 days at 23 °C in light and at 4 °C	2106	C
	BAa	SW	0.4, 0.6, 0.8 g	Visually compatible. Little loss after 14 days at 23 °C and at 4 °C	2107	C
	BAa	SW	0.4 g	Visually compatible. No loss after 7 days at 23 °C under fluorescent light	2214	C
Ringer's injection, lactated	BAa	SW	0.4 g	Visually compatible. 3% loss after 7 days at 23 °C under fluorescent light	2214	C
Sodium chloride 0.45%	c	WI	200 mg	Physically compatible. Stable for 72 hr at room temperature in light or dark	1468	C
	BAa	SW	0.4 g	Visually compatible. No loss after 7 days at 23 °C under fluorescent light	2214	C
Sodium chloride 0.9%	c	WI	200 mg	Physically compatible. Stable for 72 hr at room temperature in light or dark	1468	C
	a	SW	0.2 g	Visually compatible. Little loss after 14 days at 23 °C in light and at 4 °C	2106	C
	MGb	SW	0.4, 0.6, 0.8 g	Visually compatible. Little loss after 14 days at 23 and 4 °C	2107	C
	BAa	SW	0.4 g	Visually compatible. No loss after 7 days at 23 °C under fluorescent light	2214	C

[a]Tested in PVC containers.
[b]Tested in polyolefin containers.
[c]Tested in glass (Abbott), Accumed (McGaw), and PVC (Travenol) containers.

Additive Compatibility

Milrinone lactate

Drug	Mfr	Conc/L	Mfr	Conc/L	Test Soln	Remarks	Ref	C/I
Procainamide HCl	SQ	2 and 4 g	WI	200 mg	D5W	3% procainamide loss in 1 hr and 11% in 4 hr at 23 °C. No milrinone loss	1191	I
Quinidine gluconate	LI	16 g	WI	200 mg	D5W	Physically compatible with no loss of either drug in 4 hr at 23 °C	1191	C

Drugs in Syringe Compatibility

Milrinone lactate

Drug (in syringe)	Mfr	Amt	Mfr	Amt	Remarks	Ref	C/I
Atropine sulfate	IX	2 mg/ 2 mL	STR	5.25 mg/ 5.25 mL	Physically compatible. No loss of either drug in 20 min at 23 °C	1410	C
Calcium chloride	AB	3 g/ 30 mL	STR	5.25 mg/ 5.25 mL	Physically compatible. No milrinone loss in 20 min at 23 °C	1410	C
Digoxin	BW	0.5 mg/ 2 mL	WI	3.5 mg/ 3.5 mL	Brought to 10-mL total volume with D5W. Physically compatible with no loss of either drug in 4 hr at 23 °C	1191	C

Drugs in Syringe Compatibility (Cont.)

Milrinone lactate

Drug (in syringe)	Mfr	Amt	Mfr	Amt	Remarks	Ref	C/I
Epinephrine HCl	AB	0.5 mg/ 0.5 mL	STR	5.25 mg/ 5.25 mL	Physically compatible. No loss of either drug in 20 min at 23 °C	1410	C
Furosemide	LY	40 mg/ 4 mL	WI	3.5 mg/ 3.5 mL	Brought to 10-mL total volume with D5W. Precipitates immediately	1191	I
Lidocaine HCl	AB	100 mg/ 10 mL	STR	5.25 mg/ 5.25 mL	Physically compatible. No loss of either drug in 20 min at 23 °C	1410	C
Morphine sulfate	WI	40 mg/ 5 mL	STR	5.25 mg/ 5.25 mL	Physically compatible. No loss of either drug in 20 min at 23 °C	1410	C
Propranolol HCl	AY	3 mg/ 3 mL	WI	3.5 mg/ 3.5 mL	Brought to 10-mL total volume with D5W. Physically compatible with no loss of either drug in 4 hr at 23 °C	1191	C
Sodium bicarbonate	AB	3.75 g/ 50 mL	STR	5.25 mg/ 5.25 mL	Physically compatible. No milrinone loss in 20 min at 23 °C	1410	C
Verapamil HCl	KN	10 mg/ 4 mL	WI	3.5 mg/ 3.5 mL	Brought to 10-mL total volume with D5W. Physically compatible with no loss of either drug in 4 hr at 23 °C	1191	C

Y-Site Injection Compatibility (1:1 Mixture)

Milrinone lactate

Drug	Mfr	Conc	Mfr	Conc	Remarks	Ref	C/I
Acyclovir sodium	APP	7 mg/mL[a]	SS	0.2 mg/mL[a]	Visually compatible for 4 hr at 25 °C	2381	C
Amikacin sulfate	AB	5 mg/mL[a]	SS	0.2 mg/mL[a]	Visually compatible for 4 hr at 25 °C	2381	C
Amiodarone HCl	WY	6 mg/mL[a]	SAN	0.4 mg/mL[a]	Visually compatible for 24 hr at 22 °C	2352	C
Ampicillin sodium	APO	100 mg/mL[b]	SS	0.2 mg/mL[a]	Visually compatible for 4 hr at 25 °C	2381	C
Argatroban	SKB	1 mg/mL[a]	NVP	0.4 mg/mL[a]	Physically compatible for 24 hr at 23 °C	2572	C
Atracurium besylate	BW	1 mg/mL[a]	SW	0.4 mg/mL[a]	Visually compatible with little or no loss of either drug in 4 hr at 23 °C	2214	C
Bivalirudin	TMC	5 mg/mL[a]	SAN	0.2 mg/mL[a]	Physically compatible for 4 hr at 23 °C	2373	C
Bumetanide	RC	0.25 mg/mL	SW	0.4 mg/mL[a]	Visually compatible with little or no loss of either drug in 4 hr at 23 °C	2214	C
Calcium chloride	AMR	20 mg/mL[a]	SS	0.2 mg/mL[a]	Visually compatible for 4 hr at 25 °C	2381	C
Calcium gluconate	LY	0.465 mEq/ mL	SW	0.4 mg/mL[a]	Visually compatible with no loss of milrinone in 4 hr at 23 °C	2214	C
	AMR	50 mg/mL[a]	SS	0.2 mg/mL[a]	Visually compatible for 4 hr at 25 °C	2381	C
Caspofungin acetate	ME	0.7 mg/mL[b]	BA	0.2 mg/mL[b]	Physically compatible for 4 hr at room temperature	2758	C
Cefazolin sodium	APO	100 mg/mL[a]	SS	0.2 mg/mL[a]	Visually compatible for 4 hr at 25 °C	2381	C
Cefepime HCl	BMS	100 mg/mL	SS	0.2 mg/mL[a]	Visually compatible for 4 hr at 25 °C	2381	C
Cefotaxime sodium	HO	150 mg/mL[a]	SS	0.2 mg/mL[a]	Visually compatible for 4 hr at 25 °C	2381	C
Ceftaroline fosamil	FOR	2.22 mg/ mL[a,b,e]	BED	0.2 mg/mL[a,b,e]	Physically compatible for 4 hr at 23 °C	2826	C
Ceftazidime	GW	100 mg/mL[a]	SS	0.2 mg/mL[a]	Visually compatible for 4 hr at 25 °C	2381	C
Cefuroxime sodium	LI	100 mg/mL[a]	SS	0.2 mg/mL[a]	Visually compatible for 4 hr at 25 °C	2381	C

Y-Site Injection Compatibility (1:1 Mixture) (Cont.)

Milrinone lactate

Drug	Mfr	Conc	Mfr	Conc	Remarks	Ref	C/I
Ciprofloxacin	BAY	2 mg/mL	SS	0.2 mg/mL[a]	Visually compatible for 4 hr at 25 °C	2381	C
Clindamycin phosphate	PHU	18 mg/mL[a]	SS	0.2 mg/mL[a]	Visually compatible for 4 hr at 25 °C	2381	C
Dexamethasone sodium phosphate	ES	10 mg/mL[a]	SS	0.2 mg/mL[a]	Visually compatible for 4 hr at 25 °C	2381	C
Dexmedetomidine HCl	AB	4 mcg/mL[b]	SAN	0.2 mg/mL[b]	Physically compatible for 4 hr at 23 °C	2383	C
Digoxin	BW	0.25 mg/mL	WI	200 mcg/mL[a]	Physically compatible with no loss of either drug in 4 hr at 23 °C	1191	C
Diltiazem HCl	MMD	1 mg/mL[a]	SW	0.2 mg/mL[a]	Visually compatible for 4 hr at 27 °C	2062	C
	MMD	1 mg/mL[a]	SW	0.4 mg/mL[a]	Visually compatible with little loss of either drug in 4 hr at 23 °C	2214	C
Dobutamine HCl	LI	4 mg/mL[a]	SW	0.2 mg/mL[a]	Visually compatible for 4 hr at 27 °C	2062	C
	GEN	8 mg/mL[a]	SW	0.4 mg/mL[a]	Visually compatible. Little loss of either drug in 4 hr at 23 °C	2214	C
Dopamine HCl	AB	3.2 mg/mL[a]	SW	0.2 mg/mL[a]	Visually compatible for 4 hr at 27 °C	2062	C
	SO	6.4 mg/mL[a]	SW	0.4 mg/mL[a]	Visually compatible. Little loss of either drug in 4 hr at 23 °C	2214	C
Doripenem	JJ	5 mg/mL[a,b]	BA	0.2 mg/mL[a,b]	Physically compatible for 4 hr at 23 °C	2743	C
Epinephrine HCl	AB	0.02 mg/mL[a]	SW	0.2 mg/mL[a]	Visually compatible for 4 hr at 27 °C	2062	C
	AB	0.064 mg/mL[a]	SW	0.4 mg/mL[a]	Visually compatible. Little loss of either drug in 4 hr at 23 °C	2214	C
Fenoldopam mesylate	AB	80 mcg/mL[b]	SAN	0.2 mg/mL[b]	Physically compatible for 4 hr at 23 °C	2467	C
Fentanyl citrate	ES	0.05 mg/mL	SW	0.2 mg/mL[a]	Visually compatible for 4 hr at 27 °C	2062	C
	ES	50 mcg/mL	SW	0.4 mg/mL[a]	Visually compatible. Little loss of either drug in 4 hr at 23 °C	2214	C
Furosemide	LY	10 mg/mL	WI	200 mcg/mL[a]	Precipitates immediately	1191	I
	AMR	10 mg/mL	SW	0.2 mg/mL[a]	Precipitate forms in 4 hr at 27 °C	2062	I
Gentamicin sulfate	APP	10 mg/mL[a]	SS	0.2 mg/mL[a]	Visually compatible for 4 hr at 25 °C	2381	C
Heparin sodium	ES	100 units/mL[a]	SW	0.2 mg/mL[a]	Visually compatible for 4 hr at 27 °C	2062	C
	ES	100 units/mL[a]	SW	0.4 mg/mL[a]	Visually compatible. Little loss of milrinone and heparin in 4 hr at 23 °C	2214	C
Hetastarch in lactated electrolyte	AB	6%	SAN	0.2 mg/mL[a]	Physically compatible for 4 hr at 23 °C	2339	C
Hydromorphone HCl	KN	1 mg/mL	SW	0.2 mg/mL[a]	Visually compatible for 4 hr at 27 °C	2062	C
Imipenem–cilastatin sodium	ME	5 mg/mL[b]	SS	0.2 mg/mL[a]	Yellow color darkening in 4 hr at 25 °C	2381	I
Insulin, regular human	NOV	1 unit/mL[b]	SW	0.4 mg/mL[a]	Visually compatible. Little loss of either drug in 4 hr at 23 °C	2214	C
Isoproterenol HCl	ES	8 mcg/mL[a]	SW	0.4 mg/mL[a]	Visually compatible. Little loss of either drug in 4 hr at 23 °C	2214	C
Labetalol HCl	AH	2 mg/mL[a]	SW	0.2 mg/mL[a]	Visually compatible for 4 hr at 27 °C	2062	C
Lorazepam	WY	0.5 mg/mL[a]	SW	0.2 mg/mL[a]	Visually compatible for 4 hr at 27 °C	2062	C
	WY	0.2 mg/mL[a]	SW	0.4 mg/mL[a]	Visually compatible. Little loss of either drug in 4 hr at 23 °C	2214	C
	WY	1 mg/mL[a]	SS	0.2 mg/mL[a]	Visually compatible for 4 hr at 25 °C	2381	C
	WY	2 mg/mL[a]	SS	0.2 mg/mL[a]	Visually compatible for 4 hr at 25 °C	2381	C
Magnesium sulfate	SO	40 mg/mL[a]	SW	0.4 mg/mL[a]	Visually compatible. No milrinone loss in 4 hr at 23 °C	2214	C

Y-Site Injection Compatibility (1:1 Mixture) (Cont.)

Milrinone lactate

Drug	Mfr	Conc	Mfr	Conc	Remarks	Ref	C/I
Meropenem	ZEN	50 mg/mL[a]	SS	0.2 mg/mL[a]	Visually compatible for 4 hr at 25 °C	2381	C
Methylprednisolone sodium succinate	PHU	125 mg/mL	SS	0.2 mg/mL[a]	Visually compatible for 4 hr at 25 °C	2381	C
Metoprolol tartrate	BED	1 mg/mL	NVP	0.2 mg/mL[a]	Visually compatible for 24 hr at 19 °C	2795	C
Metronidazole	AB	5 mg/mL	SS	0.2 mg/mL[a]	Visually compatible for 4 hr at 25 °C	2381	C
Micafungin sodium	ASP	1.5 mg/mL[b]	BED	0.2 mg/mL[b]	Physically compatible for 4 hr at 23 °C	2683	C
Midazolam HCl	RC	2 mg/mL	SW	0.2 mg/mL[a]	Visually compatible for 4 hr at 27 °C	2062	C
	RC	1 mg/mL	SW	0.4 mg/mL[a]	Visually compatible. Little loss of either drug in 4 hr at 23 °C	2214	C
Morphine sulfate	SCN	2 mg/mL[a]	SW	0.2 mg/mL[a]	Visually compatible for 4 hr at 27 °C	2062	C
	AST	1 mg/mL[a]	SW	0.4 mg/mL[a]	Visually compatible. Little loss of either drug in 4 hr at 23 °C	2214	C
	FAU	25 mg/mL[a]	SS	0.2 mg/mL[a]	Visually compatible for 4 hr at 25 °C	2381	C
Nesiritide	SCI	50 mcg/mL[a,b]		1 mg/mL	Physically compatible for 4 hr	2625	C
Nicardipine HCl	WY	1 mg/mL[a]	SW	0.2 mg/mL[a]	Visually compatible for 4 hr at 27 °C	2062	C
Nitroglycerin	AB	0.4 mg/mL[a]	SW	0.2 mg/mL[a]	Visually compatible for 4 hr at 27 °C	2062	C
	SO	0.8 mg/mL[a]	SW	0.4 mg/mL[a]	Visually compatible. Little loss of either drug in 4 hr at 23 °C	2214	C
Norepinephrine bitartrate	AB	0.128 mg/mL[a]	SW	0.2 mg/mL[a]	Visually compatible for 4 hr at 27 °C	2062	C
	SW	0.064 mg/mL[a]	SW	0.4 mg/mL[a]	Visually compatible. Little loss of either drug in 4 hr at 23 °C	2214	C
Oxacillin sodium	APO	100 mg/mL[a]	SS	0.2 mg/mL[a]	Visually compatible for 4 hr at 25 °C	2381	C
Pancuronium bromide	GNS	1 mg/mL	SW	0.4 mg/mL[a]	Visually compatible. Little loss of either drug in 4 hr at 23 °C	2214	C
Piperacillin sodium–tazobactam sodium	LE[c]	200 + 25 mg/mL	SS	0.2 mg/mL[a]	Visually compatible for 4 hr at 25 °C	2381	C
Potassium chloride	AB	1 mEq/mL[a]	SW	0.4 mg/mL[a]	Visually compatible. No milrinone loss in 4 hr at 23 °C	2214	C
Procainamide HCl	SQ	2 and 4 mg/mL[a]	WI	350 mcg/mL[a]	3 to 6% procainamide loss in 1 hr and 10 to 13% in 4 hr at 23 °C. No milrinone loss	1191	I
Propofol	ZEN	10 mg/mL	SW	0.4 mg/mL[a]	Little loss of either drug in 4 hr at 23 °C	2214	C
Propranolol HCl	AY	1 mg/mL[a]	WI	200 mcg/mL[a]	Physically compatible with no loss of either drug in 4 hr at 23 °C	1191	C
Quinidine gluconate	LI	16 mg/mL[a]	WI	350 mcg/mL[a]	Physically compatible with no loss of either drug in 4 hr at 23 °C	1191	C
Ranitidine HCl	GL	1 mg/mL[a]	SW	0.2 mg/mL[a]	Visually compatible for 4 hr at 27 °C	2062	C
	GL	2 mg/mL[a]	SW	0.4 mg/mL[a]	Visually compatible. Little loss of either drug in 4 hr at 23 °C	2214	C
Rocuronium bromide	OR	2 mg/mL[a]	SW	0.4 mg/mL[a]	Visually compatible. Little loss of either drug in 4 hr at 23 °C	2214	C
Sodium bicarbonate	AB	1 mEq/mL	SW	0.4 mg/mL[a]	Visually compatible with 4% loss of milrinone in 4 hr at 23 °C	2214	C

Y-Site Injection Compatibility (1:1 Mixture) (Cont.)

Milrinone lactate

Drug	Mfr	Conc	Mfr	Conc	Remarks	Ref	C/I
Sodium nitroprusside	AB	0.8 mg/mL[a]	SW	0.4 mg/mL[a]	Visually compatible. Little loss of either drug in 4 hr at 23 °C protected from light	2214	C
	RC	0.3, 1.2, 3 mg/mL[a]	SW	0.1[f], 0.4[f], 1 mg/mL	Visually compatible for 48 hr at 24 °C protected from light	2357	C
Telavancin HCl	ASP	7.5 mg/mL[a,b,e]	BED	0.2 mg/mL[a,b,e]	Physically compatible for 2 hr	2830	C
Theophylline	AB	1.6 mg/mL[a]	SW	0.4 mg/mL[a]	Visually compatible. Little loss of either drug in 4 hr at 23 °C	2214	C
Ticarcillin disodium–clavulanate potassium	SKB	100 mg/mL[a]	SS	0.2 mg/mL[a]	Visually compatible for 4 hr at 25 °C	2381	C
Tobramycin sulfate	LI	10 mg/mL[a]	SS	0.2 mg/mL[a]	Visually compatible for 4 hr at 25 °C	2381	C
Torsemide	BM	10 mg/mL	SW	0.4 mg/mL[a]	Visually compatible. Little loss of either drug in 4 hr at 23 °C	2214	C
TPN #217[d]			SW	0.4 mg/mL[a]	Visually compatible with no loss of milrinone in 4 hr at 23 °C	2214	C
TPN #243, #244[d]			SS	0.2 mg/mL[a]	Visually compatible for 4 hr at 25 °C	2381	C
Vancomycin HCl	OR	5 mg/mL[a]	SS	0.2 mg/mL[a]	Visually compatible for 4 hr at 25 °C	2381	C
Vasopressin	AMR	2 and 4 units/mL[b]	AB	0.2 mg/mL[a]	Physically compatible with vasopressin pushed through a Y-site over 5 sec	2478	C
Vecuronium bromide	OR	1 mg/mL	SW	0.2 mg/mL[a]	Visually compatible for 4 hr at 27 °C	2062	C
	OR	1 mg/mL	SW	0.4 mg/mL[a]	Visually compatible. Little loss of either drug in 4 hr at 23 °C	2214	C
Verapamil HCl	KN	2.5 mg/mL[a]	WI	200 mcg/mL[a]	Physically compatible with no loss of either drug in 4 hr at 23 °C	1191	C

[a]Tested in dextrose 5%.
[b]Tested in sodium chloride 0.9%.
[c]Test performed using the formulation WITHOUT edetate disodium.
[d]Refer to Appendix I for the composition of parenteral nutrition solutions. TPN indicates a 2-in-1 admixture.
[e]Tested in Ringer's injection, lactated.
[f]Tested in dextrose 5% in sodium chloride 0.2%.

MITOMYCIN
AHFS 10:00

Products — Mitomycin is available in 5-, 20-, and 40-mg vials with mannitol 10, 40, and 80 mg, respectively. Reconstitute the 5-mg vials with 10 mL, the 20-mg vials with 40 mL, and the 40-mg vials with 80 mL of sterile water for injection and shake to aid dissolution. Allow to stand at room temperature if dissolution does not take place immediately. The reconstituted solution contains 500 mcg/mL of mitomycin. (1; 4)

pH — From 6 to 8. (4)

Administration — Mitomycin is administered intravenously through a functioning intravenous catheter. Extravasation should be avoided because cellulitis, ulceration, and sloughing may occur. It has been recommended that mitomycin be administered through the tubing of a running infusion solution to avoid this problem. (1; 4)

In the event of spills or leaks, Bristol-Myers Squibb recommends the use of sodium hypochlorite 5% (household bleach) or potassium permanganate 1% to inactivate mitomycin. (1200)

Stability — Intact vials should be stored at controlled room temperature and protected from light. Temperatures exceeding 40 °C should be avoided. Reconstituted solutions are stable for two weeks stored under refrigeration or for one week at room temperature. (1; 4)

Mitomycin (Kyowa) 0.6 and 0.8 mg/mL in water for injection exhibited 10% loss in seven days at 21 °C in the dark. When stored at 4 °C in the dark, the 0.6-mg/mL concentration lost 7% in seven days. Although exhibiting no loss in 24 hours when stored at 4 °C in the dark, the 0.8-mg/mL concentration developed a fine, pink, needle-like precipitate in three days. At a higher concentration of 1 mg/mL in water for injection similar results were obtained. Refrigeration resulted in fine, pink, needle-like precipitate formation in 24 hours. The 1-mg/mL concentration stored at 21 °C exposed to fluorescent light exhibited 6% loss in 24 hours and developed the fine, pink, needle-like precipitate in four days. Stored at a higher temperature of 25 °C in the dark, losses of 6% in 24 hours and 10% in seven days were found with no precipitate forming. (1503)

pH Effects — Mitomycin is very stable in solution at a neutral pH but undergoes more rapid decomposition at acidic and basic pH. (1119; 1203; 1204; 1866) The decomposition is complex and pH dependent, producing different decomposition products in acidic and basic solutions. (1119; 1283; 1284) The pH of maximum stability is approximately pH 7. (1072; 1203; 1204; 1379) At pH 7, a 10% mitomycin loss occurs in seven days at room temperature. (1072) At a concentration of 0.05 mg/mL in dextrose 5% buffered to pH 7.8 with a mixture of phosphates, mitomycin was stable for 15 days at room temperature and over 120 days when refrigerated. (1118)

Both pH and storage temperature are important to mitomycin stability. Mitomycin (150 to 600 mcg/mL) stability was tested in pH 6, 7, and 8 buffer solutions. The drug was less stable at pH 6 than at pH 7 and especially pH 8. At pH 6, drug losses of around 96 and 41% occurred at room temperature and under refrigeration, respectively, over 28 days. However, mitomycin was more stable at pH 7 and 8. Drug losses when stored under refrigeration for 28 days were about 10 to 20% in this pH range. (2651)

Temperature Effects — Heating mitomycin 0.6 mg/mL in sodium chloride 0.9% to 100 °C resulted in a 24% drug loss in 30 minutes and a 58% loss in one hour. (1285)

Freezing Solutions — Mitomycin 0.6 mg/mL in sodium chloride 0.9% crystallized out of solution when frozen at −20 °C. The particles did not redissolve after thawing in a microwave oven. Freezing to −30 °C, below the eutectic temperature, resulted in no loss of mitomycin during four weeks of storage, microwave thawing, and refreezing at −30 °C for another four weeks. (1285)

Light Effects — The stability of mitomycin is not adversely affected by the presence or absence of normal fluorescent light. (1503)

Syringes — Mitomycin (Bristol-Myers Squibb) reconstituted to a concentration of 0.5 mg/mL with sterile water was repackaged in 1-mL polypropylene tuberculin syringes (Sherwood). Syringes were stored at both 5 and 25 °C protected from light. About 7% mitomycin loss occurred in 11 days at 25 °C and about 8% loss in 42 days at 5 °C. (2179)

Filtration — Mitomycin 10 to 75 mcg/mL exhibited little or no loss due to sorption to either cellulose nitrate/cellulose acetate ester (Millex OR) or Teflon (Millex FG) filters. (1415; 1416)

Compatibility Information

Solution Compatibility

Mitomycin

Solution	Mfr	Mfr	Conc/L	Remarks	Ref	C/I
Dextrose 3.3% in sodium chloride 0.3%		BR	50 mg	10% loss in 1.6 hr at 25 °C	1205	I
Dextrose 5%			20 and 40 mg	Stable for 3 hr at room temperature	1	C
	TRa	BR	400 mg	10% loss in 1 or 2 hr at room temperature	519	I
	TRb	CH	50 mg	Violet color appeared in 4 hr and intensified over 12 hr. 74% loss in 12 hr at 28 °C in light and 33% in 12 hr at 5 °C in dark	1118	I
		BR	50 mg	10% loss in 2.6 hr at 25 °C	1205	I
	MGc	BR	20 mg	10% loss in 3 hr at 25 °C	1866	I
	MGc	BR	40 mg	10% loss in 24 hr at 4 °C	1866	C
	TRb	BR	20 mg	10% loss in 7 hr at 25 °C	1866	I
	TRb	BR	40 mg	10% loss in 23 hr at 4 °C	1866	C
Ringer's injection, lactated		BR	50 mg	10% loss in 43 hr at 25 °C	1205	C
	MGc	BR	20 mg	10% loss in 143 hr at 25 °C	1866	C
	MGc	BR	40 mg	10% loss in 480 hr at 4 °C	1866	C
	TRb	BR	20 mg	10% loss in 142 hr at 25 °C	1866	C
	TRb	BR	40 mg	10% loss in 370 hr at 4 °C	1866	C
Sodium chloride 0.4%	a,d	KY	600 mg	6 to 8% loss in 7 days at 4 °C in the dark	1503	C
Sodium chloride 0.6%	b,d	KY	400 mg	9% loss in 7 days at 4 °C in the dark	1503	C
Sodium chloride 0.9%			20 and 40 mg	Stable for 12 hr at room temperature	1	C
	TRa	BR	400 mg	Under 10% loss in 24 hr at room temperature	519	C
	TRb	CH	50 mg	Violet color appeared in 4 hr and intensified over 12 hr. 10% loss in 12 hr at 5 °C in dark	1118	I

Solution Compatibility (Cont.)

Mitomycin

Solution	Mfr	Mfr	Conc/L	Remarks	Ref	C/I
		BR	50 mg	10% loss in 5 days at 25 °C	1205	C
	[a]	KY	600 mg	5% loss in 24 hr and 9% in 4 days at 4 °C in dark	1503	C
	MG[c]	BR	40 mg	10% loss in 128 hr at 4 °C	1866	C
	TR[b]	BR	40 mg	10% loss in 126 hr at 4 °C	1866	C
Sodium lactate ⅙ M			20 and 40 mg	Stable for 24 hr at room temperature	1	C

[a]Tested in both glass and PVC containers.
[b]Tested in PVC containers.
[c]Tested in glass containers.
[d]Prepared from sodium chloride 0.9% and water for injection.

Additive Compatibility

Mitomycin

Drug	Mfr	Conc/L	Mfr	Conc/L	Test Soln	Remarks	Ref	C/I
Bleomycin sulfate	BR	20 and 30 units	BR	10 mg	NS	20% loss of bleomycin activity in 1 week at 4 °C	763	I
	BR	20 and 30 units	BR	50 mg	NS	52% loss of bleomycin activity in 1 week at 4 °C	763	I
Dexamethasone sodium phosphate	LY	5 g	BR	100 mg	NS[a]	Visually compatible. 10% calculated loss of mitomycin in 68 hr and dexamethasone in 250 hr at 25 °C	1866	C
	LY	5 g	BR	100 mg	NS[b]	Visually compatible. 10% calculated loss of mitomycin in 91 hr and dexamethasone in 154 hr at 25 °C	1866	C
	LY	5 g	BR	100 mg	NS[a]	Visually compatible. 10% calculated loss of mitomycin in 211 hr and dexamethasone in 98 hr at 4 °C	1866	C
	LY	5 g	BR	100 mg	NS[b]	Visually compatible. 10% calculated loss of mitomycin in 238 hr and dexamethasone in 355 hr at 4 °C	1866	C
Heparin sodium	ES	33,300 units	BR	167 mg	NS[a]	Visually compatible. 10% mitomycin calculated loss in 21 hr and no decrease in heparin bioactivity at 25 °C	1866	I
	ES	33,300 units	BR	167 mg	NS[b]	Visually compatible. 10% mitomycin calculated loss in 25 hr and no decrease in heparin bioactivity at 25 °C	1866	C
	ES	33,300 units	BR	500 mg	NS[a]	Visually compatible. 10% mitomycin calculated loss in 42 hr and no decrease in heparin bioactivity at 25 °C	1866	C
	ES	33,300 units	BR	500 mg	NS[b]	Visually compatible. 10% mitomycin calculated loss in 61 hr and no decrease in heparin bioactivity at 25 °C	1866	C
Hydrocortisone sodium succinate	AB	33.3 g	BR	1 g	W[a]	Visually compatible. 10% calculated loss of mitomycin in 172 hr and hydrocortisone in 212 hr at 25 °C	1866	C
	AB	33.3 g	BR	1 g	W[b]	Visually compatible. 10% calculated loss of mitomycin in 206 hr and hydrocortisone in 218 hr at 25 °C	1866	C

Additive Compatibility (Cont.)

Mitomycin

Drug	Mfr	Conc/L	Mfr	Conc/L	Test Soln	Remarks	Ref	C/I
	AB	33.3 g	BR	1 g	W[a]	Visually compatible. 10% calculated loss of mitomycin in 1423 hr and hydrocortisone in 176 hr at 4 °C	1866	**C**
	AB	33.3 g	BR	1 g	W[b]	Visually compatible. 10% calculated loss of mitomycin in 820 hr and hydrocortisone in 807 hr at 4 °C	1866	**C**

[a]Tested in glass containers.
[b]Tested in PVC containers.

Drugs in Syringe Compatibility

Mitomycin

Drug (in syringe)	Mfr	Amt	Mfr	Amt	Remarks	Ref	C/I
Bleomycin sulfate		1.5 units/ 0.5 mL		0.25 mg/ 0.5 mL	Physically compatible for 5 min at room temperature followed by 8 min of centrifugation	980	**C**
Cisplatin		0.5 mg/ 0.5 mL		0.25 mg/ 0.5 mL	Physically compatible for 5 min at room temperature followed by 8 min of centrifugation	980	**C**
Cisplatin with doxorubicin HCl	BMS BED	50 mg 25 mg	BMS	5 mg	Brought to a 5-mL final volume with NS. Visually compatible but more than 10% loss of mitomycin in 4 hr at 25 °C. At 4 °C, less than 10% loss of all three drugs in 12 hr, but about 16% mitomycin loss in 24 hr	2423	**I**
Cyclophosphamide		10 mg/ 0.5 mL		0.25 mg/ 0.5 mL	Physically compatible for 5 min at room temperature followed by 8 min of centrifugation	980	**C**
Doxorubicin HCl		1 mg/ 0.5 mL		0.25 mg/ 0.5 mL	Physically compatible for 5 min at room temperature followed by 8 min of centrifugation	980	**C**
Doxorubicin HCl with cisplatin	BED BMS	25 mg 50 mg	BMS	5 mg	Brought to a 5-mL final volume with NS. Visually compatible but more than 10% loss of mitomycin in 4 hr at 25 °C. At 4 °C, less than 10% loss of all three drugs in 12 hr, but about 16% mitomycin loss in 24 hr	2423	**I**
Droperidol		1.25 mg/ 0.5 mL		0.25 mg/ 0.5 mL	Physically compatible for 5 min at room temperature followed by 8 min of centrifugation	980	**C**
Fluorouracil		25 mg/ 0.5 mL		0.25 mg/ 0.5 mL	Physically compatible for 5 min at room temperature followed by 8 min of centrifugation	980	**C**
Furosemide		5 mg/ 0.5 mL		0.25 mg/ 0.5 mL	Physically compatible for 5 min at room temperature followed by 8 min of centrifugation	980	**C**
Heparin sodium		500 units/ 0.5 mL		0.25 mg/ 0.5 mL	Physically compatible for 5 min at room temperature followed by 8 min of centrifugation	980	**C**
Leucovorin calcium		5 mg/ 0.5 mL		0.25 mg/ 0.5 mL	Physically compatible for 5 min at room temperature followed by 8 min of centrifugation	980	**C**
Methotrexate sodium		12.5 mg/ 0.5 mL		0.25 mg/ 0.5 mL	Physically compatible for 5 min at room temperature followed by 8 min of centrifugation	980	**C**
Metoclopramide HCl		2.5 mg/ 0.5 mL		0.25 mg/ 0.5 mL	Physically compatible for 5 min at room temperature followed by 8 min of centrifugation	980	**C**

Drugs in Syringe Compatibility (Cont.)

Mitomycin

Drug (in syringe)	Mfr	Amt	Mfr	Amt	Remarks	Ref	C/I
Vinblastine sulfate		0.5 mg/ 0.5 mL		0.25 mg/ 0.5 mL	Physically compatible for 5 min at room temperature followed by 8 min of centrifugation	980	C
Vincristine sulfate		0.5 mg/ 0.5 mL		0.25 mg/ 0.5 mL	Physically compatible for 5 min at room temperature followed by 8 min of centrifugation	980	C

Y-Site Injection Compatibility (1:1 Mixture)

Mitomycin

Drug	Mfr	Conc	Mfr	Conc	Remarks	Ref	C/I
Amifostine	USB	10 mg/mL[a]	BR	0.5 mg/mL	Physically compatible for 4 hr at 23 °C	1845	C
Aztreonam	SQ	40 mg/mL[a]	BMS	0.5 mg/mL	Reddish-purple color forms in 4 hr	1758	I
Bleomycin sulfate		3 units/mL		0.5 mg/mL	Drugs injected sequentially in Y-site with no flush. No precipitate seen	980	C
Caspofungin acetate	ME	0.7 mg/mL[b]	BED	0.5 mg/mL[b]	Physically compatible for 4 hr at room temperature	2758	C
Cisplatin		1 mg/mL		0.5 mg/mL	Drugs injected sequentially in Y-site with no flush. No precipitate seen	980	C
Cyclophosphamide		20 mg/mL		0.5 mg/mL	Drugs injected sequentially in Y-site with no flush. No precipitate seen	980	C
Doxorubicin HCl		2 mg/mL		0.5 mg/mL	Drugs injected sequentially in Y-site with no flush. No precipitate seen	980	C
Droperidol		2.5 mg/mL		0.5 mg/mL	Drugs injected sequentially in Y-site with no flush. No precipitate seen	980	C
Etoposide phosphate	BR	5 mg/mL[a]	BR	0.5 mg/mL	Color changed from light blue to reddish purple in 4 hr at 23 °C	2218	I
Filgrastim	AMG	30 mcg/mL[a]	BR	0.5 mg/mL	Color changes to reddish purple in 1 hr	1687	I
Fluorouracil		50 mg/mL		0.5 mg/mL	Drugs injected sequentially in Y-site with no flush. No precipitate seen	980	C
Furosemide		10 mg/mL		0.5 mg/mL	Drugs injected sequentially in Y-site with no flush. No precipitate seen	980	C
Gemcitabine HCl	LI	10 mg/mL[b]	BR	0.5 mg/mL	Reddish-purple color forms in 1 hr	2226	I
Granisetron HCl	SKB	0.05 mg/mL[a]	BMS	0.5 mg/mL	Physically compatible for 4 hr at 23 °C	2000	C
Heparin sodium		1000 units/ mL		0.5 mg/mL	Drugs injected sequentially in Y-site with no flush. No precipitate seen	980	C
Leucovorin calcium		10 mg/mL		0.5 mg/mL	Drugs injected sequentially in Y-site with no flush. No precipitate seen	980	C
Melphalan HCl	BW	0.1 mg/mL[b]	BR	0.5 mg/mL	Physically compatible for 3 hr at 22 °C	1557	C
Methotrexate sodium		25 mg/mL		0.5 mg/mL	Drugs injected sequentially in Y-site with no flush. No precipitate seen	980	C
Metoclopramide HCl		5 mg/mL		0.5 mg/mL	Drugs injected sequentially in Y-site with no flush. No precipitate seen	980	C
Ondansetron HCl	GL	1 mg/mL[b]	BR	0.5 mg/mL	Visually compatible for 4 hr at 22 °C	1365	C
Piperacillin sodium–tazobactam sodium	LE[d]	40 + 5 mg/ mL[a]	BR	0.5 mg/mL	Blue color darkens in 4 hr, becoming reddish purple in 24 hr	1688	I

Y-Site Injection Compatibility (1:1 Mixture) (Cont.)

Mitomycin

Drug	Mfr	Conc	Mfr	Conc	Remarks	Ref	C/I
Sargramostim	IMM	10 mcg/mL[b]	BR	0.5 mg/mL	Slight haze in 30 min	1436	I
Teniposide	BR	0.1 mg/mL[a]	BR	0.5 mg/mL	Physically compatible for 4 hr at 23 °C	1725	C
Thiotepa	IMM[c]	1 mg/mL[a]	BMS	0.5 mg/mL	Physically compatible for 4 hr at 23 °C	1861	C
Topotecan HCl	SKB	56 mcg/mL[a,b]	BR	84 mcg/mL[a,b]	Pale purple color forms immediately becoming a dark pinkish-lavender in 4 hr. 15 to 20% mitomycin loss in 4 hr at 22 °C	2245	I
Vinblastine sulfate		1 mg/mL		0.5 mg/mL	Drugs injected sequentially in Y-site with no flush. No precipitate seen	980	C
Vincristine sulfate		1 mg/mL		0.5 mg/mL	Drugs injected sequentially in Y-site with no flush. No precipitate seen	980	C
Vinorelbine tartrate	BW	1 mg/mL[b]	BR	0.5 mg/mL	Reddish-purple color in 1 hr	1558	I

[a]*Tested in dextrose 5%.*
[b]*Tested in sodium chloride 0.9%.*
[c]*Lyophilized formulation tested.*
[d]*Test performed using the formulation WITHOUT edetate disodium.*

MITOXANTRONE HYDROCHLORIDE
AHFS 10:00

Products — Mitoxantrone hydrochloride is supplied as a concentrate for further dilution in 10-mL multidose vials. Each milliliter of the dark blue aqueous solution contains mitoxantrone 2 mg (as the hydrochloride salt), sodium chloride 0.8%, sodium acetate 0.005%, and acetic acid 0.046%. (1)

pH — From 3 to 4.5. (1)

Sodium Content — Each milliliter contains sodium 0.14 mEq. (1)

Trade Name(s) — Novantrone.

Administration — Mitoxantrone hydrochloride must be diluted for use. The drug is administered by slow intravenous infusion after dilution to at least 50 mL in dextrose 5% or sodium chloride 0.9%. Mitoxantrone hydrochloride is usually administered over 15 to 30 minutes through the tubing of a freely running intravenous solution (1; 4) or by continuous intravenous infusion over 24 hours. (4) It should not be given over less than three minutes. (1; 4)

Stability — Intact vials of the dark blue concentrate should be stored at controlled room temperature and protected from freezing. (1) Refrigeration of the concentrate may cause a precipitate, which redissolves upon warming to room temperature. (72; 1369)

The manufacturer indicates that mitoxantrone hydrochloride concentrate remaining in partially used vials may be stored for up to seven days at 15 to 25 °C and up to 14 days under refrigeration but should not be stored frozen. (4)

Combining heparin with mitoxantrone hydrochloride may result in precipitate formation. (1293)

pH Effects — The pH range of maximum stability is 2 to 4.5 but was unstable when the pH was increased to 7.4. (1379)

Light Effects — Mitoxantrone hydrochloride is not photolabile. Exposure of the product to direct sunlight for one month caused no change in its appearance or concentration. (72; 1293)

Syringes — Mitoxantrone hydrochloride 0.2 mg/mL in sodium chloride 0.9% in polypropylene syringes (Braun Omnifix) is reported to be stable for 28 days at 4 and 20 °C (1564) and for 24 hours at 37 °C. (1369)

Mitoxantrone hydrochloride (Lederle) 2 mg/mL in glass vials and drawn into 12-mL plastic syringes (Monoject) exhibited no visual changes and little or no loss when stored for 42 days at 4 and 23 °C. Potential extractable materials from the syringes were not detectable during the study period. (1593)

Sorption — Mitoxantrone hydrochloride (Lederle) 1 mg/mL in sodium chloride 0.9% exhibited no loss due to sorption to PVC and polyethylene administration lines during simulated infusion at 0.875 mL/hr for 2.5 hours via a syringe pump. (1795)

Filtration — Although binding of mitoxantrone hydrochloride to filters has been reported (1249; 1415; 1416), the manufacturer states that filtration of mitoxantrone hydrochloride through a 0.22-μm filter (Millipore) results in no loss. (1293)

Mitoxantrone hydrochloride (Lederle) 1 mg/mL in sodium chloride 0.9%, during simulated infusion at 0.875 mL/hr for 2.5 hours via a syringe pump, exhibited no loss due to sorption to cellulose acetate (Minisart 45, Sartorius), polysulfone (Acrodisc 45, Gelman), and nylon (Posidyne ELD96, Pall) filters. (1795)

Compatibility Information

Solution Compatibility

Mitoxantrone HCl

Solution	Mfr	Mfr	Conc/L	Remarks	Ref	C/I
Dextrose 5% in sodium chloride 0.9%	a	LE	20 to 500 mg	Physically compatible. At least 90% retained for 48 hr at room temperature	1293	C
Dextrose 5%	a	LE	20 to 500 mg	Physically compatible. At least 90% retained for 7 days at room temperature and under refrigeration	72; 1293	C
		LE	5 mg	Physically compatible. No loss in 48 hr	72	C
Sodium chloride 0.9%	a	LE	20 to 500 mg	Physically compatible. At least 90% retained for 7 days at room temperature and under refrigeration	72; 1293	C
	b	LE	20 to 500 mg	Physically compatible. At least 90% retained for 48 hr at room temperature	1293	C
		LE	5 mg	Physically compatible. No loss in 48 hr	72	C

[a]Tested in PVC containers.
[b]Tested in glass containers.

Additive Compatibility

Mitoxantrone HCl

Drug	Mfr	Conc/L	Mfr	Conc/L	Test Soln	Remarks	Ref	C/I
Cyclophosphamide	AD	10 g	LE	500 mg	D5W	Visually compatible. Mitoxantrone stable for 24 hr at room temperature. Cyclophosphamide not tested	1531	C
Cytarabine	UP	500 mg	LE	500 mg	D5W	Visually compatible. Mitoxantrone stable for 24 hr at room temperature. Cytarabine not tested	1531	C
Etoposide	BR	500 mg	LE	50 mg	NS	Visually compatible with no loss of either drug in 22 hr at room temperature	2271	C
Fluorouracil		25 g	LE	500 mg	D5W	Visually compatible. Mitoxantrone stable for 24 hr at room temperature. Fluorouracil not tested	1531	C
Hydrocortisone sodium succinate		100 mg to 2 g	LE	50 to 200 mg	D5W, NS[a]	Physically compatible and both drugs stable for 24 hr at room temperature	1293	C
Potassium chloride		50 mEq	LE	500 mg	D5W	Visually compatible. Mitoxantrone stable for 24 hr at room temperature	1531	C

[a]Tested in PVC containers.

Y-Site Injection Compatibility (1:1 Mixture)

Mitoxantrone HCl

Drug	Mfr	Conc	Mfr	Conc	Remarks	Ref	C/I
Allopurinol sodium	BW	3 mg/mL[b]	LE	0.5 mg/mL[b]	Physically compatible for 4 hr at 22 °C	1686	C
Amifostine	USB	10 mg/mL[a]	LE	0.5 mg/mL[a]	Physically compatible for 4 hr at 23 °C	1845	C
Amphotericin B cholesteryl sulfate complex	SEQ	0.83 mg/mL[a]	IMM	0.5 mg/mL[a]	Gross precipitate forms	2117	I

Y-Site Injection Compatibility (1:1 Mixture) (Cont.)

Mitoxantrone HCl

Drug	Mfr	Conc	Mfr	Conc	Remarks	Ref	C/I
Aztreonam	SQ	40 mg/mL[a]	LE	0.5 mg/mL[a]	Heavy precipitate forms in 1 hr	1758	I
Cladribine	ORT	0.015[b] and 0.5[c] mg/mL	LE	0.5 mg/mL[b]	Physically compatible for 4 hr at 23 °C	1969	C
Doxorubicin HCl liposomal	SEQ	0.4 mg/mL[a]	IMM	0.5 mg/mL[a]	Partial loss of measured natural turbidity	2087	I
Etoposide	BR	20 mg/mL	LE	2 mg/mL	Visually compatible with no loss of either drug in 22 hr at room temperature	2271	C
Etoposide phosphate	BR	5 mg/mL[a]	IMM	0.5 mg/mL[a]	Physically compatible for 4 hr at 23 °C	2218	C
Filgrastim	AMG	30 mcg/mL[a]	LE	0.5 mg/mL[a]	Physically compatible for 4 hr at 22 °C	1687	C
Fludarabine phosphate	BX	1 mg/mL[a]	LE	0.5 mg/mL[a]	Visually compatible for 4 hr at 22 °C	1439	C
Gemcitabine HCl	LI	10 mg/mL[b]	IMM	0.5 mg/mL[b]	Physically compatible for 4 hr at 23 °C	2226	C
Granisetron HCl	SKB	0.05 mg/mL[a]	IMM	0.5 mg/mL[a]	Physically compatible for 4 hr at 23 °C	2000	C
Linezolid	PHU	2 mg/mL	IMM	0.5 mg/mL[a]	Physically compatible for 4 hr at 23 °C	2264	C
Melphalan HCl	BW	0.1 mg/mL[b]	LE	0.5 mg/mL[b]	Physically compatible for 3 hr at 22 °C	1557	C
Ondansetron HCl	GL	1 mg/mL[b]	LE	0.5 mg/mL[a]	Visually compatible for 4 hr at 22 °C	1365	C
Oxaliplatin	SS	0.5 mg/mL[a]	IMM	0.5 mg/mL[a]	Physically compatible for 4 hr at 23 °C	2566	C
Paclitaxel	NCI	1.2 mg/mL[a]	LE	0.5 mg/mL[a]	Normal inherent haze from paclitaxel decreases immediately	1556	I
Pemetrexed disodium	LI	20 mg/mL[b]	IMM	0.5 mg/mL[a]	Dark-blue precipitate forms immediately	2564	I
Piperacillin sodium–tazobactam sodium	LE[f]	40 + 5 mg/mL[a]	LE	0.5 mg/mL[a]	Haze and particles form immediately. Large particles form in 4 hr	1688	I
Propofol	ZEN	10 mg/mL	IMM	0.5 mg/mL[a]	Particles form immediately	2066	I
Sargramostim	IMM	10 mcg/mL[b]	LE	0.5 mg/mL[b]	Visually compatible for 4 hr at 22 °C	1436	C
Teniposide	BR	0.1 mg/mL[a]	LE	0.5 mg/mL[a]	Physically compatible for 4 hr at 23 °C	1725	C
Thiotepa	IMM[d]	1 mg/mL[a]	IMM	0.5 mg/mL[a]	Physically compatible for 4 hr at 23 °C	1861	C
TNA #218 to #226[e]			IMM	0.5 mg/mL[a]	Visually compatible for 4 hr at 23 °C	2215	C
TPN #212 to #215[e]			IMM	0.5 mg/mL[a]	Substantial loss of natural haze occurs immediately	2109	I
Vinorelbine tartrate	BW	1 mg/mL[b]	LE	0.5 mg/mL[b]	Physically compatible for 4 hr at 22 °C	1558	C

[a]Tested in dextrose 5%.
[b]Tested in sodium chloride 0.9%.
[c]Tested in bacteriostatic sodium chloride 0.9% preserved with benzyl alcohol 0.9%.
[d]Lyophilized formulation tested.
[e]Refer to Appendix I for the composition of parenteral nutrition solutions. TNA indicates a 3-in-1 admixture, and TPN indicates a 2-in-1 admixture.
[f]Test performed using the formulation WITHOUT edetate disodium.

MORPHINE SULFATE
AHFS 28:08.08

Products — Morphine sulfate is available in a variety of concentrations and sizes ranging from 0.5 to 50 mg/mL. The Astramorph PF and Duramorph 0.5- and 1-mg/mL concentrations and the Infumorph 200- (10 mg/mL) and Infumorph 500- (25 mg/mL) formulations are preservative free. Morphine hydrochloride and morphine tartrate injections are also available in some countries. Other morphine products may contain various preservatives, antioxidants, and buffers, including chlorobutanol, phenol, sodium bisulfite, sodium phosphates, and sodium formaldehyde sulfoxylate. (4; 38)

pH — From 2.5 to 6.5 for most products. Duramorph has a pH of 3.5 to 7, and Infumorph has a pH of about 4.5. (4; 17) Morphine sulfate 7.5 mg/mL in sodium chloride 0.9% had a pH of 3.5. (2161)

Osmolality — Morphine sulfate 7.5 mg/mL in sodium chloride 0.9% had an osmolality of 236 mOsm/kg. (2161)

Trade Name(s) — Astramorph PF, Duramorph, Infumorph.

Administration — Morphine sulfate is usually administered subcutaneously but may be administered by intramuscular or slow intravenous injection and by slow continuous subcutaneous or intravenous infusion. For continuous intravenous infusion, a concentration of 0.1 to 1 mg/mL in dextrose 5% may be infused using an infusion control device; more concentrated solutions also have been used. Duramorph, Infumorph, and Astramorph PF contain no preservatives and may be administered intrathecally or epidurally. (1; 4)

High-concentration morphine sulfate is not recommended for subcutaneous, intramuscular, or intravenous injection of individual doses or for intrathecal or epidural administration. The products are intended for continuous intravenous infusion using a suitable microinfusion control device. (4)

Stability — Morphine sulfate injections are clear, colorless solutions. Intact containers should be stored at controlled room temperature and protected from freezing and light. The manufacturers state that the products should not be heat sterilized. (1) Morphine sulfate darkens upon prolonged exposure to light. (4)

Undiluted morphine sulfate 10 mg/mL, stored in 100-mL glass vials and PVC bags, exhibited no loss in 30 days at 23 °C. (1394)

Morphine sulfate (Wyeth) 1 mg/mL in bacteriostatic sodium chloride 0.9% containing benzyl alcohol 0.9%, when stored in glass vials with protection from light, exhibited no loss at 4 °C and a 4% loss at 22 °C after 91 days. (1583)

Morphine sulfate 15 and 2 mg/mL diluted with sterile water for injection at 4 and 24 °C in 200-mL PVC bags (Baxter) was stable at both temperatures with little loss in 15 days. (1504)

Morphine sulfate under simulated summer conditions in paramedic vehicles was exposed to 26 to 38 °C over four weeks. No drug loss occurred under these conditions. (2562)

Morphine sulfate 1 mg/mL compounded in sodium chloride 0.9% was packaged in 100-mL polypropylene infusion bags and was autoclaved at 121 °C for 20 minutes for sterilization. No visible precipitation appeared and microparticulate levels remained acceptable in all samples when stored at 25 °C for three years and at 30 and 40 °C for six months. No evidence of evaporation was found in the samples, and no loss of morphine sulfate occurred in any of the solutions throughout the study. While PVC bags cannot be autoclaved and ex-

hibit excessive loss of water through evaporation upon storage, polypropylene bags can be successfully used for compounding bags of morphine sulfate solutions with three-year stability for use in patient-controlled analgesia. (2665)

pH Effects — Morphine sulfate is relatively stable at acidic pH, especially below pH 4, but degradation increases greatly at neutral or basic pH. Degradation is often accompanied by a yellow to brown discoloration in the normally colorless solution. (1072; 2170)

Morphine sulfate stability at a low concentration of 2 mg/mL in an admixture with ketamine hydrochloride in sodium chloride 0.9% with the pH adjusted over a range of pH 5.5 to 7.5 was stored at room temperature over 4 days. No difference in physical or chemical drug stability was observed among the samples. (2786)

However, at higher concentrations precipitation of morphine at pH values of pH 6.4 and above precipitation may occur. Morphine sulfate at about 18 mg/mL mixed with ketamine hydrochloride exhibited a pH near 4.85. Adjusting the pH higher with sodium bicarbonate injection up to pH 5.9 resulted in mixtures that were clear over 24 hours at 21 °C. However, adjusting to pH 6.2 resulted in precipitation within 2 hours. Adjusting to pH 6.4 and above resulted in immediate precipitation. (2787)

Freezing Solutions — Morphine sulfate (Lilly) 1 and 2 mg/mL in dextrose 5% and sodium chloride 0.9% in PVC bags exhibited no loss during 14 weeks of frozen storage at −20 °C. (1286)

Syringes — Prefilled into plastic syringes with syringe caps (Braun), morphine sulfate is stated to remain within acceptable limits of degradation for at least 69 days at room temperature. (982)

In another study, less than a 3% loss of morphine sulfate occurred in 12 weeks when stored in plastic syringes at 22 °C and exposed to light. A smaller loss occurred when the morphine sulfate was stored at 3 °C with light protection. (1287)

Morphine sulfate (Lilly) 1 and 5 mg/mL in dextrose 5% and sodium chloride 0.9% was packaged in 30-mL Plastipak (Becton Dickinson) syringes capped with Monoject (Sherwood) tip caps. Syringes were stored at 23 °C in light and dark, 4 °C protected from light, and frozen at −20 °C protected from light for 12 weeks. Both concentrations at all three temperatures were stable for at least six weeks when protected from light. However, the samples at 23 °C exposed to light were stable for a week, but developed unacceptable losses after that. (1894)

Morphine sulfate 2 mg/mL in sodium chloride 0.9% was packaged in 50-mL (Becton Dickinson) and 30-mL (Becton Dickinson and Sherwood) polypropylene syringes for use in patient-controlled analgesia and in stoppered glass vials. The samples were stored at room temperature in the dark for six weeks. Little loss of morphine sulfate occurred in the 50-mL syringes and the glass vials in six weeks. About 5% loss occurred when packaged in both brands of 30-mL syringes. Addition of sodium metabisulfite 0.1% as an antioxidant increased the rate of drug loss up to 10% in two weeks. (2040)

Morphine sulfate 5 mg/mL in sodium chloride 0.9% and 50 mg/mL in sterile water for injection and also in sodium chloride 0.9% packaged as 20 mL in 30-mL polypropylene syringes were stored for 60 days at 4 °C protected from light and 23 °C exposed to normal fluorescent light. Other solutions were stored frozen at −20 °C and at elevated temperature of 37 °C for two days to simulate more extreme conditions during express shipping. Little or no morphine sulfate loss occurred in the 50-mg/mL samples stored for 60 days at 4 and 23 °C even though slight yellow discoloration appeared after 30 days. The 5-mg/mL samples stored at 4 and 23 °C exhibited about 4 to 5% loss in 60 days. The frozen and 37 °C samples exhibited little or no change in morphine sulfate concentration in two days. However, samples of the 50-mg/mL concentration stored at −20 and 4 °C and samples of the 5-mg/mL concentration stored frozen at −20 °C precipitated upon low temperature storage. Although the precipitate redissolved upon warming at 37 °C for several hours, large amounts of microparticulates in the tens of thousands per milliliter remained, possibly shed by the syringe components. (2376)

Elastomeric Reservoir Pumps — Morphine sulfate 15 and 2 mg/mL was diluted with sterile water for injection at 4 and 24 °C in Intermate 200 (Infusion Systems) and Infusor (Baxter) disposable elastomeric infusion devices. In the Intermate 200 with 100 mL of morphine sulfate solution, little or no loss occurred in 15 days at either 4 or 24 °C and even at 31 °C (simulating use next to a patient's skin or clothing). In the Infusor, with 50 mL, losses of 5% or more were observed in 12 days in some containers. (1504)

Morphine sulfate 0.5 mg/mL in both dextrose 5% and sodium chloride 0.9% was evaluated for binding potential to natural rubber elastomeric reservoirs (Baxter). No binding was found after storage for two weeks at 35 °C with gentle agitation. (2014)

Morphine sulfate 2 and 10 mg/mL is reported to be physically and chemically stable in Accufuser Plus silicone balloon infusers when stored at room temperature and refrigerated. Little or no loss of morphine sulfate occurred in 40 days. (2678)

Implantable Pumps — Morphine sulfate 10 mg/mL was filled into a VIP 30 implantable infusion pump (Fresenius) and associated capillary tubing and stored at 37 °C. No morphine loss and no contamination from components of pump materials occurred during eight weeks of storage. (1903)

Morphine sulfate (Infumorph) 20 mg/mL with clonidine hydrochloride (Boehringer Ingelheim) 50 mcg/mL and morphine sulfate 2 mg/mL with clonidine hydrochloride 1.84 mg/mL were evaluated in SynchroMed EL (Medtronic) implantable pumps with silicone elastomer intrathecal catheters at 37 °C for three months. No visible incompatibilities were observed; delivered concentrations of both drugs were in the range of 94.0 to 99.6% throughout the study. Furthermore, no impairment of mechanical performance of the pump or any of its components was found. (2477)

An admixture of bupivacaine hydrochloride 25 mg/mL, clonidine hydrochloride 2 mg/mL, and morphine sulfate 50 mg/mL in sterile water for injection was reported to be physically and chemically stable for 90 days at 37 °C in SynchroMed implantable pumps. Little or no loss of any of the drugs was found. (2585)

Clonidine hydrochloride and morphine sulfate powders were dissolved in ziconotide acetate (Elan) injection to yield concentrations of 2 and 35 mg/mL and 25 mcg/mL, respectively. Stored at 37 °C, 11% ziconotide loss in 7 days, 4% clonidine loss in 20 days, and no morphine loss in 28 days occurred. (2752)

Other Devices — The stability of two intrathecal solutions of morphine sulfate 10 mg/mL in sodium chloride 0.9% (isobaric) and 5 mg/mL in dextrose 7% in water (hyperbaric) was evaluated. The solutions were stored at 4 and 37 °C in glass ampuls and pump reservoirs composed of silicone rubber reinforced with polyester (Cordis Europa). No precipitation or discoloration and no loss of morphine sulfate or increase in degradation products occurred in the solutions in glass ampuls after two months at either temperature. However, in the pump reservoirs, the isobaric solution in sodium chloride 0.9% developed a yellow color. Furthermore, a decomposition product, pseudomorphine, was detectable in three days and increased to 1% in one month at 37 °C. This level was 20 times that of the pseudomorphine found in the hyperbaric dextrose 7% in water solution under the same conditions. The decomposition was attributed to dissolved oxygen, ethylene oxide sterilant, and silicone rubber. (1508)

Central Venous Catheter — Morphine sulfate (Astra) 1 mg/mL in dextrose 5% was found to be compatible with the ARROWg+ard Blue Plus (Arrow International) chlorhexidine-bearing triple-lumen central catheter. Essentially complete delivery of the drug was found with little or no drug loss occurring. Furthermore, chlorhexidine delivered from the catheter remained at trace amounts with no substantial increase due to the delivery of the drug through the catheter. (2335)

Compatibility Information

Solution Compatibility

Morphine sulfate

Solution	Mfr	Mfr	Conc/L	Remarks	Ref	C/I
Dextrose–Ringer's injection combinations	AB		16.2 mg	Physically compatible	3	C
Dextrose–Ringer's injection, lactated, combinations	AB		16.2 mg	Physically compatible	3	C
Dextrose–saline combinations	AB		16.2 mg	Physically compatible	3	C
Dextrose 2.5%	AB		16.2 mg	Physically compatible	3	C
Dextrose 5%	AB		16.2 mg	Physically compatible	3	C
	TR[a]	LI	1.2 g	Physically compatible. No loss in 36 hr at 22 °C	1000	C
	TR[b]	AB, AH	40 and 400 mg	Physically compatible with little or no loss in 7 days at 23 and 4 °C	1349	C
	[a]	AH	5 g	No loss in 30 days at 23 °C	1394	C
	[g]	SX	10 g	Visually compatible. Losses of 5 to 8% in 31 days at 4 and 23 °C	1505	C

Solution Compatibility (Cont.)

Morphine sulfate

Solution	Mfr	Mfr	Conc/L	Remarks	Ref	C/I
Dextrose 10%	AB		16.2 mg	Physically compatible	3	**C**
Ionosol products	AB		16.2 mg	Physically compatible	3	**C**
Ringer's injection	AB		16.2 mg	Physically compatible	3	**C**
Ringer's injection, lactated	AB		16.2 mg	Physically compatible	3	**C**
Sodium chloride 0.45%	AB		16.2 mg	Physically compatible	3	**C**
Sodium chloride 0.9%	AB		16.2 mg	Physically compatible	3	**C**
	TR[b]	AB, AH	40 and 400 mg	Physically compatible with little or no loss in 7 days at 23 and 4 °C	1349	**C**
	[a]	AH	5 g	No loss in 30 days at 23 °C	1394	**C**
	AB[a]	SCN	100 and 500 mg	Visually compatible with no loss in 72 hr at 24 °C under fluorescent light	2058	**C**
	[e]	PHS	1 and 10 g	Visually compatible. No loss in 16 days at 32 °C in the dark. 4% concentration increase consistent with slight evaporation	2254	**C**
	[f]	CNF	0.5, 1.5, 2.5 g	Visually compatible. No loss in 60 days at 32 °C. 8% concentration increase was due to evaporation	1312	**C**
	[g]	SX	10 g	Visually compatible. Losses of 5 to 8% at 4 and 23 °C	1505	**C**
	[h]		0.5, 15, 30 g[i]	No loss in 14 days at 5 °C. Slight concentration increase at 37 °C due to evaporation. Light brown color after 5 days at 37 °C	1506	**C**
	[h]		60 g[i]	At 37 °C, slight concentration increase in 14 days due to evaporation. Light brown color in 5 days	1506	**C**
	[h]		60 g[i]	At 5 °C, morphine precipitates in 4 days with over 40% loss	1506	**I**
	[e]	ES	1 and 5 g	Visually compatible for 30 days at 5 and 25 °C. Increased concentration due to evaporation. Maximum storage of 30 days at 5 °C and 14 days at 25 °C	1507	**C**
	BA[j]	[i]	5 g	Physically compatible. 4 to 5% loss in 60 days at 23 °C in light and at 4 °C in dark	2376	**C**
	BA[j]	[i]	50 g	Physically compatible. Little loss in 60 days at 23 °C in light. Yellow color not indicative of decomposition	2376	**C**
	BA[j]	[i]	50 g	At 4 °C, morphine sulfate precipitates but redissolves on warming leaving tens of thousands of microparticulates. Little loss in 60 days at 4 °C	2376	**?**
	MAC[e]	AGT	1 and 40 g	Physically compatible. No loss in 30 days at room temperature protected from light. Concentration increase due to water loss	2633	**C**
	BA[k]	ANT	2 and 3 g	Physically compatible. Little drug loss in 60 days at 4 and 25 °C. Less than 2.5% loss of moisture during storage	2628	**C**
Sodium lactate ⅙ M	AB		16.2 mg	Physically compatible	3	**C**
Sterile water for injection	BA[c]	[i]	50 g	Physically compatible. Little loss in 60 days at 23 °C in light. Yellow color not indicative of decomposition	2376	**C**
	BA[c]	[i]	50 g	At 4 °C, morphine sulfate precipitates but redissolves on warming leaving tens of thousands of microparticulates. Little loss in 60 days at 4 °C	2376	**?**

Solution Compatibility (Cont.)

Morphine sulfate

Solution	Mfr	Mfr	Conc/L	Remarks	Ref	C/I
TPN #71[d]	[a]	LI	100 mg	Physically compatible and no morphine loss in 36 hr at 22 °C	1000	**C**

[a]Tested in PVC containers.
[b]Tested in both glass and PVC containers.
[c]Note: Not suitable for large-volume infusion.
[d]Refer to Appendix I for the composition of parenteral nutrition solutions. TPN indicates a 2-in-1 admixture.
[e]Tested in Pharmacia or SIMS Deltec medication cassette reservoirs.
[f]Tested in Pharmacia Deltec PVC/Kalex phthalate ester medication cassette reservoirs.
[g]Tested in Pharmacia cassette reservoirs.
[h]Tested in Cormed III Kalex reservoirs.
[i]Prepared from morphine sulfate powder.
[j]Tested in polypropylene syringes.
[k]Tested in ANAPA Plus (E-WHA International) ambulatory infusion device and PEGA (Pegasus) sets.

Additive Compatibility

Morphine sulfate

Drug	Mfr	Conc/L	Mfr	Conc/L	Test Soln	Remarks	Ref	C/I
Alteplase	GEN	0.5 g	WY	1 g	NS	Visually compatible with 5 to 8% alteplase clot-lysis activity loss in 24 hr at 25 °C	1856	**C**
Atracurium besylate	BW	500 mg		1 g	D5W	Physically compatible and atracurium stable for 24 hr at 5 and 30 °C	1694	**C**
Baclofen	CI	200 mg	DB	1 and 1.5 g	NS[d]	Physically compatible. Little loss of either drug in 30 days at 37 °C	1911	**C**
	CI	800 mg	DB	1 g	NS[d]	Physically compatible. Little baclofen loss and less than 7% morphine loss in 29 days at 37 °C	1911	**C**
	CI	800 mg	DB	1.5 g	NS[d]	Physically compatible. Little loss of either drug in 30 days at 37 °C	1911	**C**
	CI	1.5 g	DB	7.5 g	NS[d]	Physically compatible. Little loss of either drug in 30 days at 37 °C	2170	**C**
	CI	1 g	DB	15 g	NS[d]	Physically compatible. Little loss of either drug in 30 days at 37 °C	2170	**C**
	CI	200 mg	DB	21 g	NS[d]	Physically compatible. 7% baclofen loss and little morphine loss in 30 days at 37 °C	2170	**C**
Bupivacaine HCl	AST	3 g		1 g	[b]	Little loss of either drug in 30 days at 18 °C	1932	**C**
	AB	625 mg and 1.25 g	SCN	100 mg	NS[b]	Visually compatible. No loss of either drug in 72 hr at 24 °C in light	2058	**C**
	AB	625 mg and 1.25 g	SCN	500 mg	NS[b]	Visually compatible. No loss of either drug in 72 hr at 24 °C in light	2058	**C**
Dobutamine HCl	LI	1 g	ES	5 g	D5W, NS	Physically compatible for 24 hr at 21 °C	812	**C**
Floxacillin sodium	BE	20 g	EV	1 g	W	Haze forms in 24 hr and precipitate forms in 48 hr at 30 °C. No change at 15 °C	1479	**I**
Fluconazole	PF	1 g	ES	0.25 g	D5W[b]	Fluconazole stable for 24 hr at 25 °C in fluorescent light. Morphine not tested	1676	**C**

Additive Compatibility (Cont.)

Morphine sulfate

Drug	Mfr	Conc/L	Mfr	Conc/L	Test Soln	Remarks	Ref	C/I
Fluorouracil	AB	1 and 16 g	AST	1 g	D5W, NS[b]	Subvisible morphine precipitate forms immediately, becoming grossly visible within 24 hr. Morphine losses of 60 to 80% occur within 1 day	1977	I
Furosemide	HO	1 g	EV	1 g	W	Physically compatible for 72 hr at 15 and 30 °C	1479	C
Ketamine HCl	PD	1 g	SX	1 g	NS[b]	At least 90% of both drugs retained for 6 days at room temperature	2260	C
	PD	25 g	SX	25 g	NS[b]	At least 90% of both drugs retained for 6 days at room temperature	2260	C
	PD	25 g	SX	25 g	NS[e]	At least 90% of both drugs retained for 6 days at room temperature	2260	C
	PD	1.33 g	AB	2 g	NS	Little loss of either drug in 4 days at room temperature	2786	C
Meropenem	ZEN	1 and 20 g	ES	1 g	NS	Visually compatible for 4 hr at room temperature	1994	C
Metoclopramide HCl	SKB	500 mg	EV	1 g	NS[b]	Visually compatible. Little loss of either drug in 35 days at 22 °C and 182 days at 4 °C followed by 7 days at 32 °C	1939	C
	SKB	500 mg	EV	1 g	D5W[c]	Visually compatible. 8% metoclopramide loss in 14 days at 22 °C and 98 days at 4 °C. No morphine loss	1939	C
Ondansetron HCl	GL	100 mg and 1 g	AST	1 g	NS[b]	Physically compatible. No ondansetron loss and 5% or less morphine loss in 7 days at 32 °C or 31 days at 4 and 22 °C protected from light	1690	C
Ropivacaine HCl	ASZ	1 g	AST	20 mg	NS[f]	Physically compatible. Little loss of either drug in 30 days at 30 °C in the dark	2433	C
	ASZ	2 g	AST	20 and 100 mg	[f]	Physically compatible. Little loss of either drug in 30 days at 30 °C in the dark	2433	C
Succinylcholine chloride	AB	2 g		16.2 mg		Physically compatible	3	C
Verapamil HCl	KN	80 mg	KN	30 mg	D5W, NS	Physically compatible for 24 hr	764	C
Ziconotide acetate	ELN	25 mg[a]	BB	35 g[g]		90% ziconotide retained for 8 days at 37 °C. No morphine loss in 17 days	2702	C
	ELN	25 mg[a]	BB	20 g[g]		90% ziconotide retained for 19 days at 37 °C. No morphine loss in 28 days	2713	C
	ELN	25 mg[a]	BB	10 g[g]		10% ziconotide loss in 34 days. No morphine loss in 60 days at 37 °C	2780	C
	ELN	25 mg[a]	BB	20 g[g]		10% ziconotide loss in 19 days. No morphine loss in 28 days at 37 °C	2780	C

[a]*Tested in SynchroMed II implantable pumps.*
[b]*Tested in PVC containers.*
[c]*Tested in PCA Infusors (Baxter).*
[d]*Tested in glass containers.*
[e]*Tested in Deltec plastic medication cassette reservoirs.*
[f]*Tested in polypropylene bags (Mark II Polybags).*
[g]*Morphine sulfate powder dissolved in ziconotide acetate injection.*

Drugs in Syringe Compatibility

Morphine sulfate

Drug (in syringe)	Mfr	Amt	Mfr	Amt	Remarks	Ref	C/I
Alfentanil HCl	ASZ	55 mcg/mL[e]	DB	0.8 mg/mL[e]	No loss of either drug in 182 days at room temperature or refrigerated	2527	C
Atropine sulfate		0.6 mg/1.5 mL	WY	15 mg/1 mL	Physically compatible for at least 15 min	14	C
	ST	0.4 mg/1 mL	ST	15 mg/1 mL	Physically compatible for at least 15 min	326	C
Bupivacaine HCl	AST	3 mg/mL		1 mg/mL	Little loss of either drug in 30 days at 18 °C	1932	C
	g	2.5 mg/mL[e]	g	5 mg/mL[e]	Physically compatible. Little morphine or bupivacaine loss in 60 days at 23 °C in fluorescent light and at 4 °C	2378	C
	g	25 mg/mL[c]	g	50 mg/mL[a]	Physically compatible. Little morphine or bupivacaine loss in 60 days at 23 °C in fluorescent light and at 4 °C in dark. Slight yellow discoloration at 23 °C not indicative of decomposition	2378	C
Bupivacaine HCl with clonidine HCl	SW BI	1.5 mg/mL 0.03 mg/mL	ES	0.2 mg/mL	Diluted to 5 mL with NS. Visually compatible with no new GC/MS peaks in 1 hr at room temperature	1956	C
Butorphanol tartrate	BR	4 mg/2 mL	AH	15 mg/1 mL	Physically compatible for 30 min at room temperature	566	C
Caffeine citrate		20 mg/1 mL	SW	4 mg/1 mL	Visually compatible for 4 hr at 25 °C	2440	C
Chlorpromazine HCl	SKF	50 mg/2 mL	WY	15 mg/1 mL	Physically compatible for at least 15 min	14	C
	PO	50 mg/2 mL	ST	15 mg/1 mL	Physically compatible for at least 15 min	326	C
Clonidine HCl	FUJ	100 mcg/1 mL	SAN	10 mg/1 mL	Physically and chemically stable for 14 days at room temperature	2069	C
	g	0.25 mg/mL[e]	g	5 mg/mL[e]	Physically compatible. Little morphine or clonidine loss in 60 days at 23 °C in light and at 4 °C in dark	2380	C
	g	4 mg/mL[c]	g	50 mg/mL[a]	Physically compatible. Little morphine or clonidine loss in 60 days at 23 °C in light and at 4 °C in dark. Slight yellow discoloration at 23 °C not indicative of decomposition	2380	C
Clonidine HCl with bupivacaine HCl	BI SW	0.03 mg/mL 1.5 mg/mL	ES	0.2 mg/mL	Diluted to 5 mL with NS. Visually compatible with no new GC/MS peaks in 1 hr at room temperature	1956	C
Dimenhydrinate	HR	50 mg/1 mL	ST	15 mg/1 mL	Physically compatible for at least 15 min	326	C
Diphenhydramine HCl	PD	50 mg/1 mL	WY	15 mg/1 mL	Physically compatible for at least 15 min	14	C
	PD	50 mg/1 mL	ST	15 mg/1 mL	Physically compatible for at least 15 min	326	C
Droperidol	MN	2.5 mg/1 mL	ST	15 mg/1 mL	Physically compatible for at least 15 min	326	C
Fentanyl citrate	MN	0.05 mg/1 mL	ST	15 mg/1 mL	Physically compatible for at least 15 min	326	C

Drugs in Syringe Compatibility (Cont.)

Morphine sulfate

Drug (in syringe)	Mfr	Amt	Mfr	Amt	Remarks	Ref	C/I
Glycopyrrolate	RB	0.2 mg/ 1 mL	LI	15 mg/ 1 mL	Physically compatible. pH in glycopyrrolate stability range for 48 hr at 25 °C	331	C
	RB	0.2 mg/ 1 mL	LI	30 mg/ 2 mL	Physically compatible. pH in glycopyrrolate stability range for 48 hr at 25 °C	331	C
	RB	0.4 mg/ 2 mL	LI	15 mg/ 1 mL	Physically compatible. pH in glycopyrrolate stability range for 48 hr at 25 °C	331	C
Haloperidol lactate	MN	5 mg/ 1 mL		5 and 10 mg/ 1 mL^c	Cloudiness forms immediately, becoming a crystalline precipitate of haloperidol and parabens	1901	I
	MN	2 mg/mL	ME	20 mg/ mL^a	White precipitate of haloperidol forms on mixing	668	I
Heparin sodium	WY	100 and 200 units		1, 2, 5, 10 mg	Brought to 5 mL with NS. Physically compatible with no morphine loss in 24 hr at 23 °C	985	C
	WY	100 and 200 units		1, 2, 5 mg	Brought to 5 mL with W. Physically compatible with no morphine loss in 24 hr at 23 °C	985	C
	WY	100 and 200 units		10 mg	Brought to 5 mL with W. Immediate haze with precipitate and 5 to 7% morphine loss	985	I
Hydroxyzine HCl	PF	100 mg/ 4 mL	WY	15 mg/ 1 mL	Physically compatible for at least 15 min	14	C
	PF	50 mg/ 1 mL	ST	15 mg/ 1 mL	Physically compatible for at least 15 min	326	C
	PF	50 mg/ 1 mL		10 mg/ 0.7 mL	Physically compatible	771	C
	PF	100 mg/ 2 mL		5 mg/ 0.3 mL	Physically compatible	771	C
Ketamine HCl	PD	1 mg/mL^e	SX	1 mg/ mL^e, 10 mg/ mL^e	At least 90% of both drugs retained for 6 days at room temperature	2260	C
	PD	1 mg/mL^e	SX	25 mg/ mL^e	5% morphine loss in 6 days at room temperature. Up to 15% ketamine loss in 2 to 6 days	2260	C
	PD	10, 25 mg/ mL^e	SX	1, 10, 25 mg/ mL^e	At least 90% of both drugs retained for 6 days at room temperature	2260	C
		5, 10, 20 mg/ 1 mL		1 mg/ 1 mL	No substantial change in the concentration of either drug over 4 days	669	C
	SZ	2 mg/mL^e	SZ	2, 5, 10 mg/ mL^e	Physically compatible. Little loss of either drug at 23 and 5 °C in 91 days	2797	C
Ketamine HCl with lidocaine HCl	PD AST	2 mg/mL 2 mg/mL	ES	0.2 mg/ mL	Diluted to 5 mL with NS. Visually compatible with no new GC/MS peaks in 1 hr at room temperature	1956	C
Lidocaine HCl with ketamine HCl	AST PD	2 mg/mL 2 mg/mL	ES	0.2 mg/ mL	Diluted to 5 mL with NS. Visually compatible with no new GC/MS peaks in 1 hr at room temperature	1956	C
Meperidine HCl	WI	50 mg/ 1 mL	ST	15 mg/ 1 mL	Physically incompatible within 15 min	326	I
Metoclopramide HCl	NO	10 mg/ 2 mL	AH	10 mg/ 1 mL	Physically compatible for 15 min at room temperature	565	C

Drugs in Syringe Compatibility (Cont.)

Morphine sulfate

Drug (in syringe)	Mfr	Amt	Mfr	Amt	Remarks	Ref	C/I
	SKB	0.5 mg/mL	EV	1 mg/mL	Diluted with NS. 5% or less loss of both drugs in 35 days at 22 °C and 182 days at 4 °C followed by 7 days at 32 °C	1939	**C**
	RB	5 mg/mL	ME	25 mg/mL[a]	Visually compatible with less than 10% drug loss in 7 days at 8 °C	668	**C**
Midazolam HCl	RC	5 mg/1 mL	WB	10 mg/1 mL	Physically compatible for 4 hr at 25 °C	1145	**C**
	RC	5 mg/1 mL		5 and 10 mg/1 mL[c]	Visually compatible. 9% or less morphine and 8% or less midazolam loss in 14 days at 22 °C in dark. Microprecipitate may form, requiring filtration	1901	**C**
	RC	5 mg/1 mL		5 and 10 mg/1 mL[d]	Visually compatible. 8% or less morphine and 3% or less midazolam loss in 14 days at 22 °C protected from light. Microprecipitate may form, requiring filtration	1901	**C**
Milrinone lactate	STR	5.25 mg/5.25 mL	WI	40 mg/5 mL	Physically compatible. No loss of either drug in 20 min at 23 °C	1410	**C**
Ondansetron HCl	GW	1.33 mg/mL[e]	ES	2.67 mg/mL[e]	Physically compatible. Under 5% ondansetron and under 4% morphine losses in 24 hr at 4 or 23 °C	2199	**C**
Pantoprazole sodium	[b]	4 mg/1 mL		50 mg/1 mL	Yellowish precipitate	2574	**I**
Pentazocine lactate	WI	30 mg/1 mL	ST	15 mg/1 mL	Physically compatible for at least 15 min	326	**C**
Pentobarbital sodium	AB	500 mg/10 mL		16.2 mg/1 mL	Physically compatible	55	**C**
	WY	100 mg/2 mL	WY	15 mg/1 mL	Precipitate forms within 15 min	14	**I**
	AB	50 mg/1 mL	ST	15 mg/1 mL	Physically incompatible within 15 min	326	**I**
Prochlorperazine edisylate	SKF		WY	15 mg/1 mL	Physically compatible for at least 15 min	14	**C**
	PO	5 mg/1 mL	ST	15 mg/1 mL	Physically compatible for at least 15 min	326	**C**
	ES, SKF	10 mg/2 mL	WB	10 mg/1 mL	Precipitates immediately, probably due to phenol in morphine formulation	1006	**I**
	SKF	5 mg/1 mL	WY	8, 10, 15 mg/1 mL	Physically compatible for 24 hr at 25 °C	1086	**C**
Promethazine HCl	WY	50 mg/2 mL	WY	15 mg/1 mL	Physically compatible for at least 15 min	14	**C**
	PO	50 mg/2 mL	ST	15 mg/1 mL	Physically compatible for at least 15 min	326	**C**
	WY	12.5 mg	WY	8 mg	Cloudiness develops	98	**I**
Ranitidine HCl	GL	50 mg/2 mL	AH	10 mg/1 mL	Physically compatible for 1 hr at 25 °C	978	**C**
Salbutamol	GL	2.5 mg/2.5 mL[f]	AB	5 mg/0.5 mL	Physically compatible for 1 hr	1904	**C**
Scopolamine HBr		0.6 mg/1.5 mL	WY	15 mg/1 mL	Physically compatible for at least 15 min	14	**C**

Drugs in Syringe Compatibility (Cont.)

Morphine sulfate

Drug (in syringe)	Mfr	Amt	Mfr	Amt	Remarks	Ref	C/I
	ST	0.4 mg/ 1 mL	ST	15 mg/ 1 mL	Physically compatible for at least 15 min	326	C
	BP	5 mg/ 5 mL	BP	500 mg/ 5 mL	Little scopolamine loss in 14 days at room temperature or 37 °C. Morphine not tested	1609	C
Ziconotide acetate	ELN	25 mcg/ mL	BB	35 mg/ mL[h]	No loss of either drug in 17 days at 5 °C	2702	C

[a]Tested in sterile water for injection.
[b]Test performed using the formulation WITHOUT edetate disodium.
[c]Morphine sulfate powder dissolved in dextrose 5%.
[d]Morphine sulfate powder dissolved in water and sodium chloride 0.9%.
[e]Diluted in sodium chloride 0.9%.
[f]Both preserved (benzyl alcohol 0.9%; benzalkonium chloride 0.01%) and unpreserved sodium chloride 0.9% were used as a diluent.
[g]Extemporaneously compounded from bulk drug powders.
[h]Morphine sulfate powder dissolved in ziconotide acetate injection.

Y-Site Injection Compatibility (1:1 Mixture)

Morphine sulfate

Drug	Mfr	Conc	Mfr	Conc	Remarks	Ref	C/I
Acyclovir sodium	BW	5 mg/mL[a]	WB	0.08 mg/mL[a]	Physically compatible for 4 hr at 25 °C	1157	C
	BW	5 mg/mL[a]	AB	1 mg/mL	Precipitate forms in 2 hr at 25 °C	1397	I
Allopurinol sodium	BW	3 mg/mL[b]	WI	1 mg/mL[b]	Physically compatible for 4 hr at 22 °C	1686	C
Amifostine	USB	10 mg/mL[a]	AST	1 mg/mL[a]	Physically compatible for 4 hr at 23 °C	1845	C
Amikacin sulfate	BR	5 mg/mL[a]	WI	1 mg/mL[a]	Physically compatible for 4 hr at 25 °C	987	C
Aminophylline	ES	4 mg/mL[c]	WY	0.2 mg/mL[c]	Physically compatible for 3 hr	1316	C
Amiodarone HCl	WY	4.8 mg/mL[a]	SX	1 mg/mL[a]	Visually compatible for 24 hr at 23 °C	1877	C
	WY	6 mg/mL[a]	WY	1 mg/mL[a]	Visually compatible for 24 hr at 22 °C	2352	C
	WY	6 mg/mL[a]	WY	10 mg/mL	Visually compatible for 24 hr at 22 °C	2352	C
Amphotericin B cholesteryl sulfate complex	SEQ	0.83 mg/mL[a]	ES	1 mg/mL[a]	Increased turbidity forms immediately	2117	I
Ampicillin sodium	BR	20 mg/mL[b]	WI	1 mg/mL[a]	Physically compatible for 4 hr at 25 °C	987	C
Ampicillin sodium–sulbactam sodium	RR	20 + 10 mg/ mL[b]	ES	1 mg/mL[b]	Physically compatible for 1 hr at 25 °C	1338	C
Amsacrine	NCI	1 mg/mL[a]	ES	1 mg/mL[a]	Visually compatible for 4 hr at 22 °C	1381	C
Anidulafungin	VIC	0.5 mg/mL[a]	ES	15 mg/mL	Physically compatible for 4 hr at 23 °C	2617	C
Argatroban	GSK	1 mg/mL[b]	ES	10 mg/mL	Visually compatible for 24 hr at 23 °C	2391	C
Atracurium besylate	BW	0.5 mg/mL[a]	WY	1 mg/mL[a]	Physically compatible for 24 hr at 28 °C	1337	C
Atropine sulfate	LY	0.4 mg/mL	AST	1 mg/mL[a]	Physically compatible for 48 hr at 22 °C	1706	C
Azithromycin	PF	2 mg/mL[b]	WY	1 mg/mL[q]	White microcrystals found	2368	I
Aztreonam	SQ	20 mg/mL[a]	AB	1 mg/mL	Physically compatible for 4 hr at 25 °C	1397	C
	SQ	40 mg/mL[a]	AST	1 mg/mL[a]	Physically compatible for 4 hr at 23 °C	1758	C
Bivalirudin	TMC	5 mg/mL[a]	AST	1 mg/mL[a]	Physically compatible for 4 hr at 23 °C	2373	C
	TMC	5 mg/mL[a,b]	ES	10 mg/mL	Visually compatible for 6 hr at 23 °C	2680	C
Bumetanide	RC	0.25 mg/mL	AB	1 mg/mL	Physically compatible for 4 hr at 25 °C	1397	C
Calcium chloride	AB	4 mg/mL[c]	WY	0.2 mg/mL[c]	Physically compatible for 3 hr	1316	C

Y-Site Injection Compatibility (1:1 Mixture) (Cont.)

Morphine sulfate

Drug	Mfr	Conc	Mfr	Conc	Remarks	Ref	C/I
Caspofungin acetate	ME	0.7 mg/mL[b]	BA	15 mg/mL	Physically compatible for 4 hr at room temperature	2758	C
	ME	0.5 mg/mL[b]	HOS	2 mg/mL	Physically compatible with morphine sulfate i.v. push over 2 to 5 min	2766	C
Cefazolin sodium	SKF	20 mg/mL[a]	WI	1 mg/mL[a]	Physically compatible for 4 hr at 25 °C	987	C
Cefepime HCl	BMS	120 mg/mL[d]		1 mg/mL	Physically compatible with less than 10% cefepime loss. Morphine not tested	2513	C
Cefotaxime sodium	HO	20 mg/mL[a]	WI	1 mg/mL[a]	Physically compatible for 4 hr at 25 °C	987	C
Cefotetan disodium	STU	20 and 40 mg/mL[a]	ES	1 mg/mL[b]	Physically compatible for 1 hr at 25 °C	1338	C
Cefoxitin sodium	MSD	20 mg/mL[a]	WI	1 mg/mL[a]	Physically compatible for 4 hr at 25 °C	987	C
	MSD	40 mg/mL[a]	ES	1 mg/mL[b]	Physically compatible for 1 hr at 25 °C	1338	C
Ceftaroline fosamil	FOR	2.22 mg/mL[a,b,i]	BA	15 mg/mL	Physically compatible for 4 hr at 23 °C	2826	C
Ceftazidime	LI	20 and 40 mg/mL[a]	AB	1 mg/mL	Physically compatible for 4 hr at 25 °C	1397	C
	GSK	120 mg/mL[d]		1 mg/mL	Physically compatible with less than 10% ceftazidime loss. Morphine not tested	2513	C
Ceftriaxone sodium	RC	20 and 40 mg/mL[a]	AB	1 mg/mL	Physically compatible for 4 hr at 25 °C	1397	C
Cefuroxime sodium	GL	30 mg/mL[a]	WI	1 mg/mL[a]	Physically compatible for 4 hr at 25 °C	987	C
Chloramphenicol sodium succinate	LY	20 mg/mL[a]	WI	1 mg/mL[a]	Physically compatible for 4 hr at 25 °C	987	C
Cisatracurium besylate	GW	0.1, 2, 5 mg/mL[a]	AST	1 mg/mL[a]	Physically compatible for 4 hr at 23 °C	2074	C
Cladribine	ORT	0.015[b] and 0.5[e] mg/mL	AST	1 mg/mL[b]	Physically compatible for 4 hr at 23 °C	1969	C
Clindamycin phosphate	UP	12 mg/mL[a]	WI	1 mg/mL[a]	Physically compatible for 4 hr at 25 °C	987	C
Dexamethasone sodium phosphate	LY	0.2 mg/mL[a]	AB	1 mg/mL	Physically compatible for 4 hr at 25 °C	1397	C
	AMR	1 mg/mL[a]	AST	1 mg/mL[a]	Physically compatible for 48 hr at 22 °C	1706	C
Dexmedetomidine HCl	HOS				Stated to be compatible	1	C
Diazepam	ES	0.5 mg/mL[a]	AST	1 mg/mL[a]	Physically compatible for 48 hr at 22 °C	1706	C
Digoxin	BW	0.25 mg/mL	AB	1 mg/mL	Physically compatible for 4 hr at 25 °C	1397	C
Diltiazem HCl	MMD	1[b] and 5 mg/mL	SCN	15 mg/mL	Visually compatible	1807	C
	MMD	5 mg/mL	SCN	0.4 mg/mL[b]	Visually compatible	1807	C
	MMD	1 mg/mL[a]	SCN	2 mg/mL[a]	Visually compatible for 4 hr at 27 °C	2062	C
Diphenhydramine HCl	SCN	2 mg/mL[a]	AST	1 mg/mL[a]	Physically compatible for 48 hr at 22 °C	1706	C
Dobutamine HCl	LI	4 mg/mL[a]	SCN	2 mg/mL[a]	Visually compatible for 4 hr at 27 °C	2062	C
Docetaxel	RPR	0.9 mg/mL[a]	ES	1 mg/mL[a]	Physically compatible for 4 hr at 23 °C	2224	C
Dopamine HCl	AB	1.6 mg/mL[a]	AB	1 mg/mL	Physically compatible for 4 hr at 25 °C	1397	C
	AB	3.2 mg/mL[a]	SCN	2 mg/mL[a]	Visually compatible for 4 hr at 27 °C	2062	C
Doripenem	JJ	5 mg/mL[a,b]	BA	15 mg/mL	Physically compatible for 4 hr at 23 °C	2743	C
Doxorubicin HCl liposomal	SEQ	0.4 mg/mL[a]	ES	1 mg/mL[a]	Partial loss of measured natural turbidity	2087	I

Y-Site Injection Compatibility (1:1 Mixture) (Cont.)

Morphine sulfate

Drug	Mfr	Conc	Mfr	Conc	Remarks	Ref	C/I
Doxycycline hyclate	ES	1 mg/mL[a]	WI	1 mg/mL[a]	Physically compatible for 4 hr at 25 °C	987	C
Enalaprilat	MSD	0.05 mg/mL[b]	WY	0.2 mg/mL[a]	Physically compatible for 24 hr at room temperature under fluorescent light	1355	C
Epinephrine HCl	AB	0.02 mg/mL[a]	SCN	2 mg/mL[a]	Visually compatible for 4 hr at 27 °C	2062	C
Erythromycin lactobionate	AB	5 mg/mL[a]	WI	1 mg/mL[a]	Physically compatible for 4 hr at 25 °C	987	C
Esmolol HCl	DCC	1 g/100 mL[f]	ES	15 mg/1 mL	Physically compatible when morphine is injected in Y-site[d]	1168	C
	DCC	10 mg/mL[f]	ES	15 mg/mL	Physically compatible. No drug loss in 8 hr at room temperature in light	1168	C
Etomidate	AB	2 mg/mL	ES	10 mg/mL	Visually compatible for 7 days at 25 °C	1801	C
Etoposide phosphate	BR	5 mg/mL[a]	ES	1 mg/mL[a]	Physically compatible for 4 hr at 23 °C	2218	C
Famotidine	MSD	0.2 mg/mL[a]	ES	0.2 mg/mL[a]	Physically compatible for 4 hr at 25 °C	1188	C
	MSD	0.2 mg/mL[a]	AB	1 mg/mL	Physically compatible for 4 hr at 25 °C	1397	C
	ME	2 mg/mL[b]		1 mg/mL[a]	Visually compatible for 4 hr at 22 °C	1936	C
Fenoldopam mesylate	AB	80 mcg/mL[b]	ES	1 mg/mL[b]	Physically compatible for 4 hr at 23 °C	2467	C
Fentanyl citrate	ES	0.05 mg/mL	SCN	2 mg/mL[a]	Visually compatible for 4 hr at 27 °C	2062	C
Filgrastim	AMG	30 mcg/mL[a]	WY	1 mg/mL[a]	Physically compatible for 4 hr at 22 °C	1687	C
Fluconazole	RR	2 mg/mL	IMS	25 mg/mL	Physically compatible for 24 hr at 25 °C	1407	C
	RR	2 mg/mL	AB	1 mg/mL	Physically compatible for 4 hr at 25 °C	1397	C
Fludarabine phosphate	BX	1 mg/mL[a]	WI	1 mg/mL[a]	Visually compatible for 4 hr at 22 °C	1439	C
Foscarnet sodium	AST	24 mg/mL	IMS	1 mg/mL	Physically compatible for 24 hr at room temperature under fluorescent light	1335	C
	AST	24 mg/mL	ES	1 mg/mL[c]	Physically compatible for 24 hr at 25 °C under fluorescent light	1393	C
	AST	24 mg/mL	ES	5[b] and 15 mg/mL	Visually compatible for 24 hr at 23 °C under fluorescent light	1529	C
Furosemide	ES	0.8[a], 2.4[a], 10 mg/mL	AB	1 mg/mL	White precipitate in 1 hr at 25 °C	1397	I
	AMR	10 mg/mL	SCN	2 mg/mL[a]	Visually compatible for 4 hr at 27 °C	2062	C
Gallium nitrate	FUJ	1 mg/mL[b]	SCN	1 mg/mL[b]	Precipitate forms in 24 hr at 25 °C	1673	I
Gemcitabine HCl	LI	10 mg/mL[b]	ES	1 mg/mL[b]	Physically compatible for 4 hr at 23 °C	2226	C
Gentamicin sulfate	TR	0.8 mg/mL[a]	WI	1 mg/mL[a]	Physically compatible for 4 hr at 25 °C	987	C
	ES	1.2 and 2 mg/mL[b]	ES	1 mg/mL[b]	Physically compatible for 1 hr at 25 °C	1338	C
Granisetron HCl	SKB	1 mg/mL	AST	1 mg/mL[b]	Physically compatible with little or no loss of either drug in 4 hr at 22 °C	1883	C
	SKB	0.05 mg/mL[a]	AST	1 mg/mL[a]	Physically compatible for 4 hr at 23 °C	2000	C
Haloperidol lactate	MN	0.2 mg/mL[a]	AST	1 mg/mL[a]	Physically compatible for 48 hr at 22 °C	1706	C
Heparin sodium	UP	1000 units/L[h]	WY	15 mg/mL	Physically compatible for 4 hr at room temperature	534	C
	ES	50 units/mL[c]	WY	0.2 mg/mL[c]	Physically compatible for 3 hr	1316	C
	ES	60 units/mL[a]	ES	1 mg/mL[b]	Physically compatible for 1 hr at 25 °C	1338	C
	ES	100 units/mL[a]	SCN	2 mg/mL[a]	Visually compatible for 4 hr at 27 °C	2062	C
Hetastarch in lactated electrolyte	AB	6%	AST	1 mg/mL[a]	Physically compatible for 4 hr at 23 °C	2339	C

Y-Site Injection Compatibility (1:1 Mixture) (Cont.)

Morphine sulfate

Drug	Mfr	Conc	Mfr	Conc	Remarks	Ref	C/I
Hydrocortisone sodium succinate	UP	10 mg/L[f]	WY	15 mg/mL	Physically compatible for 4 hr at room temperature	534	C
Hydromorphone HCl	KN	1 mg/mL	SCN	2 mg/mL[a]	Visually compatible for 4 hr at 27 °C	2062	C
Hydroxyethyl starch 130/0.4 in sodium chloride 0.9%	FRK	6%	SZ	1, 5, 10 mg/mL[a]	Visually compatible for 24 hr at room temperature	2770	C
Hydroxyzine HCl	WI	4 mg/mL[a]	AST	1 mg/mL[a]	Physically compatible for 48 hr at 22 °C	1706	C
Insulin, regular	LI	0.2 unit/mL[b]	ES	1 mg/mL[b]	Physically compatible for 1 hr at 25 °C	1338	C
	LI	0.2 unit/mL[b]	ES	5 mg/mL[b]	Physically compatible for 2 hr at 25 °C	1395	C
	LI	1 unit/mL[a]	SX	1 mg/mL[a]	Visually compatible for 24 hr at 23 °C	1877	C
Ketorolac tromethamine	WY	1 mg/mL[a]	AST	1 mg/mL[a]	Physically compatible for 48 hr at 22 °C	1706	C
Labetalol HCl	SC	1 mg/mL[a]	WY	1 mg/mL[a]	Physically compatible for 24 hr at 18 °C	1171	C
	GL	5 mg/mL	AB	1 mg/mL	Physically compatible for 4 hr at 25 °C	1397	C
	GL	1 mg/mL[a]	ES	0.5 mg/mL[a]	Visually compatible. Little loss of either drug in 4 hr at room temperature	1762	C
	AH	2 mg/mL[a]	SCN	2 mg/mL[a]	Visually compatible for 4 hr at 27 °C	2062	C
Levofloxacin	OMN	5 mg/mL[a]	SW	4 mg/mL	Visually compatible for 4 hr at 24 °C	2233	C
Lidocaine HCl	AB	1 mg/mL[a]	AB	1 mg/mL	Physically compatible for 4 hr at 25 °C	1397	C
Linezolid	PHU	2 mg/mL	AST	1 mg/mL[a]	Physically compatible for 4 hr at 23 °C	2264	C
Lorazepam	WY	0.5 mg/mL[a]	SCN	2 mg/mL[a]	Visually compatible for 4 hr at 27 °C	2062	C
	WY	0.1 mg/mL[a]	AST	1 mg/mL[a]	Physically compatible for 48 hr at 22 °C	1706	C
Magnesium sulfate	LY	16.7, 33.3, 50, 100 mg/mL[a]	ES	1 mg/mL[a]	Visually compatible for 4 hr at 25 °C	1549	C
	AB	2, 4, 8 mg/mL[b]	j	2 mg/mL[b]	Visually compatible for 8 hr at room temperature	1719	C
Melphalan HCl	BW	0.1 mg/mL[b]	WI	1 mg/mL[b]	Physically compatible for 3 hr at 22 °C	1557	C
Meropenem	ZEN	1 and 50 mg/mL[b]	ES	1 mg/mL[d]	Visually compatible for 4 hr at room temperature	1994	C
Methotrimeprazine HCl	LE	0.2 mg/mL[a]	AST	1 mg/mL[a]	Physically compatible for 48 hr at 22 °C	1706	C
Methyldopate HCl	AMR	2.5 mg/mL[a]	AB	1 mg/mL	Physically compatible for 4 hr at 25 °C	1397	C
Methylprednisolone sodium succinate	UP	2.5 mg/mL[a]	AB	1 mg/mL	Physically compatible for 4 hr at 25 °C	1397	C
Metoclopramide HCl	SN	0.2 mg/mL[a]	AB	1 mg/mL	Physically compatible for 4 hr at 25 °C	1397	C
	DU	5 mg/mL	AST	1 mg/mL[a]	Physically compatible for 48 hr at 22 °C	1706	C
Metoprolol tartrate	CI	1 mg/mL	AB	1 mg/mL	Physically compatible for 4 hr at 25 °C	1397	C
Metronidazole	SE	5 mg/mL	WI	1 mg/mL[a]	Physically compatible for 4 hr at 25 °C	987	C
Micafungin sodium	ASP	1.5 mg/mL[b]	APP	15 mg/mL	White precipitate forms immediately	2683	I
Midazolam HCl	RC	0.2 mg/mL[a]	AST	1 mg/mL[a]	Physically compatible for 48 hr at 22 °C	1706	C
	RC	0.1 and 0.5 mg/mL[a]	ES	0.25 mg/mL[a]	Visually compatible with no loss of either drug in 3 hr at 24 °C	1789	C
	RC	0.1 and 0.5 mg/mL[a]	ES	1 mg/mL[a]	Visually compatible with no loss of either drug in 3 hr at 24 °C	1789	C
	RC	1 mg/mL[a]	SX	1 mg/mL[a]	Visually compatible for 24 hr at 23 °C	1877	C
	RC	2 mg/mL[a]	SCN	2 mg/mL[a]	Visually compatible for 4 hr at 27 °C	2062	C
Milrinone lactate	SW	0.2 mg/mL[a]	SCN	2 mg/mL[a]	Visually compatible for 4 hr at 27 °C	2062	C
	SW	0.4 mg/mL[a]	AST	1 mg/mL[a]	Visually compatible. Little loss of either drug in 4 hr at 23 °C	2214	C

Y-Site Injection Compatibility (1:1 Mixture) (Cont.)

Morphine sulfate

Drug	Mfr	Conc	Mfr	Conc	Remarks	Ref	C/I
	SS	0.2 mg/mL[a]	FAU	25 mg/mL[a]	Visually compatible for 4 hr at 25 °C	2381	C
Nafcillin sodium	WY	20 mg/mL[a]	WI	1 mg/mL[a]	Physically compatible for 4 hr at 25 °C	987	C
	WY	30 mg/mL[a]	ES	1 mg/mL[b]	Physically compatible for 1 hr at 25 °C	1338	C
Nesiritide	SCI	50 mcg/mL[a,b]		15 mg/mL	Physically compatible for 4 hr. May be chemically incompatible with nesiritide[k]	2625	?
Nicardipine HCl	WY	1 mg/mL[a]	SCN	2 mg/mL[a]	Visually compatible for 4 hr at 27 °C	2062	C
	DCC	0.1 mg/mL[a]	WY	0.2 mg/mL[a]	Visually compatible for 24 hr at room temperature	235	C
Nitroglycerin	AB	0.4 mg/mL[a]	SCN	2 mg/mL[a]	Visually compatible for 4 hr at 27 °C	2062	C
Norepinephrine bitartrate	STR	0.064 mg/mL[a]	SX	1 mg/mL[a]	Visually compatible for 24 hr at 23 °C	1877	C
	AB	0.128 mg/mL[a]	SCN	2 mg/mL[a]	Visually compatible for 4 hr at 27 °C	2062	C
Ondansetron HCl	GL	1 mg/mL[b]	WI	1 mg/mL[a]	Visually compatible for 4 hr at 22 °C	1365	C
Oxacillin sodium	BE	20 mg/mL[a]	WI	1 mg/mL[a]	Physically compatible for 4 hr at 25 °C	987	C
Oxaliplatin	SS	0.5 mg/mL[a]	ES	15 mg/mL	Physically compatible for 4 hr at 23 °C	2566	C
Oxytocin	PD	0.02 unit/mL[m]	ES	1 mg/mL[b]	Physically compatible for 1 hr at 25 °C	1338	C
Paclitaxel	NCI	1.2 mg/mL[a]	WY	1 mg/mL[a]	Physically compatible for 4 hr at 22 °C	1556	C
Palonosetron HCl	MGI	50 mcg/mL	BA	15 mg/mL	Physically compatible. No loss of either drug in 4 hr	2720	C
Pancuronium bromide	ES	0.05 mg/mL[a]	WY	1 mg/mL[a]	Physically compatible for 24 hr at 28 °C	1337	C
Pantoprazole sodium	ALT[l]	0.16 to 0.8 mg/mL[b]	AB	1 to 10 mg/mL[a]	Visually compatible for 12 hr at 23 °C	2603	C
Pemetrexed disodium	LI	20 mg/mL[b]	ES	15 mg/mL	Physically compatible for 4 hr at 23 °C	2564	C
Penicillin G potassium	PF	100,000 units/mL[a]	WI	1 mg/mL[a]	Physically compatible for 4 hr at 25 °C	987	C
Phenobarbital sodium	WY	2 mg/mL[a]	AST	1 mg/mL[a]	Physically compatible for 48 hr at 22 °C	1706	C
Phenytoin sodium	ES	2 mg/mL[a,b]	AST	1 mg/mL[a]	Precipitate forms after 1 hr	1706	I
Piperacillin sodium–tazobactam sodium	LE[l]	40 + 5 mg/mL[a]	WY	1 mg/mL[a]	Physically compatible for 4 hr at 22 °C	1688	C
Potassium chloride	AB	40 mEq/L[f]	WY	15 mg/mL	Physically compatible for 4 hr at room temperature	534	C
Propofol	ZEN	10 mg/mL	AST	1 mg/mL[a]	Physically compatible for 1 hr at 23 °C	2066	C
Propranolol HCl	WY	1 mg/mL	AB	1 mg/mL	Physically compatible for 4 hr at 25 °C	1397	C
Ranitidine HCl	GL	0.5 mg/mL[n]	ES	1 mg/mL[b]	Physically compatible for 1 hr at 25 °C	1338	C
	GL	1 mg/mL[a]	SCN	2 mg/mL[a]	Visually compatible for 4 hr at 27 °C	2062	C
Remifentanil HCl	GW	0.025 and 0.25 mg/mL[b]	AST	1 mg/mL[a]	Physically compatible for 4 hr at 23 °C	2075	C
Sargramostim	IMM	10 mcg/mL[b]	WI	1 mg/mL[b]	Slight haze and particles in 1 hr	1436	I
Scopolamine HBr	LY	0.05 mg/mL[a]	AST	1 mg/mL[a]	Physically compatible for 48 hr at 22 °C	1706	C
Sodium bicarbonate	AB	1 mEq/mL	WY	0.2 mg/mL[c]	Physically compatible for 3 hr	1316	C
Sodium nitroprusside	RC	0.2 mg/mL[a]	SX	1 mg/mL[a]	Visually compatible for 24 hr at 23 °C	1877	C
	RC	0.3, 1.2, 3 mg/mL[a]	AB	0.5 mg/mL[g]	Visually compatible for 48 hr at 24 °C protected from light	2357	C

Y-Site Injection Compatibility (1:1 Mixture) (Cont.)

Morphine sulfate

Drug	Mfr	Conc	Mfr	Conc	Remarks	Ref	C/I
	RC	1.2 and 3 mg/mL[a]	AB	1 mg/mL[g]	Visually compatible for 48 hr at 24 °C protected from light	2357	C
Tacrolimus	FUJ	10 and 40 mcg/mL[b]	SCN	1 and 3 mg/mL[b]	Visually compatible. No loss of either drug in 4 hr at 24 °C	2216	C
Teniposide	BR	0.1 mg/mL[a]	AST	1 mg/mL[a]	Physically compatible for 4 hr at 23 °C	1725	C
Thiotepa	IMM[o]	1 mg/mL[a]	AST	1 mg/mL[a]	Physically compatible for 4 hr at 23 °C	1861	C
Ticarcillin disodium–clavulanate potassium	BE	31 mg/mL[b]	ES	1 mg/mL[b]	Physically compatible for 1 hr at 25 °C	1338	C
Tirofiban HCl	ME	50 mcg/mL[a,b]	ES	0.1 and 1 mg/mL[a]	Physically compatible. No loss of either drug in 4 hr at 23 °C	2356	C
TNA #218 to #226[p]			ES	1 mg/mL[a]	Visually compatible for 4 hr at 23 °C	2215	C
			ES	15 mg/mL	Damage to emulsion occurs immediately with free oil formation possible	2215	I
Tobramycin sulfate	DI	0.8 mg/mL[a]	WI	1 mg/mL[a]	Physically compatible for 4 hr at 25 °C	987	C
	LI	1.6, 2, 2.4 mg/mL[a]	ES	1 mg/mL[b]	Physically compatible for 1 hr at 25 °C	1338	C
TPN #131, #132[p]			AB	1 mg/mL	Physically compatible for 4 hr at 25 °C	1397	C
TPN #189[p]			DB	30 mg/mL	Visually compatible for 24 hr at 22 °C	1767	C
TPN #203, #204[p]			ES	1 mg/mL	Visually compatible for 2 hr at 23 °C	1974	C
TPN #212 to #215[p]			AST	1 mg/mL[a]	Physically compatible for 4 hr at 23 °C	2109	C
Trimethoprim–sulfamethoxazole	BW	0.8 + 4 mg/mL[a]	WI	1 mg/mL[a]	Physically compatible for 4 hr at 25 °C	987	C
Vancomycin HCl	LI	5 mg/mL[a]	WI	1 mg/mL[a]	Physically compatible for 4 hr at 25 °C	987	C
Vecuronium bromide	OR	0.1 mg/mL[a]	WY	1 mg/mL[a]	Physically compatible for 24 hr at 28 °C	1337	C
	OR	1 mg/mL	SCN	2 mg/mL[a]	Visually compatible for 4 hr at 27 °C	2062	C
Vinorelbine tartrate	BW	1 mg/mL[b]	WI	1 mg/mL[b]	Physically compatible for 4 hr at 22 °C	1558	C
Warfarin sodium	DU	2 mg/mL[d]	ES	2 mg/mL[a]	Visually compatible with no warfarin loss in 30 min	2010	C
	DME	2 mg/mL[d]	ES	2 mg/mL[a]	Visually compatible for 24 hr at 24 °C	2078	C
Zidovudine	BW	4 mg/mL[a]	ES	1 mg/mL[a]	Physically compatible for 4 hr at 25 °C	1193	C

[a]*Tested in dextrose 5%.*
[b]*Tested in sodium chloride 0.9%.*
[c]*Tested in both dextrose 5% and sodium chloride 0.9%.*
[d]*Tested in sterile water for injection.*
[e]*Tested in bacteriostatic sodium chloride 0.9% preserved with benzyl alcohol 0.9%.*
[f]*Tested in dextrose 5% in sodium chloride 0.9%.*
[g]*Tested in dextrose 5% in sodium chloride 0.2%.*
[h]*Tested in dextrose 5% in Ringer's injection, dextrose 5% in Ringer's injection, lactated, dextrose 5%, Ringer's injection, lactated, and sodium chloride 0.9%.*
[i]*Tested in Ringer's injection, lactated.*
[j]*Extemporaneously prepared product.*
[k]*Nesiritide is incompatible with bisulfite antioxidants used in some drug formulations. The specific formulation of the product to be used should be checked to ensure that no sulfite antioxidants are present.*
[l]*Test performed using the formulation WITHOUT edetate disodium.*
[m]*Tested in dextrose 5% in Ringer's injection, lactated.*
[n]*Tested in sodium chloride 0.45%.*
[o]*Lyophilized formulation tested.*
[p]*Refer to Appendix I for the composition of parenteral nutrition solutions. TNA indicates a 3-in-1 admixture, and TPN indicates a 2-in-1 admixture.*
[q]*Injected via Y-site into an administration set running azithromycin.*

Additional Compatibility Information

Bupivacaine — Bupivacaine hydrochloride 25 mg/mL admixed with morphine sulfate 50 mg/mL in sterile water for injection appeared to prevent the formation of precipitation that occurs with morphine sulfate 50 mg/mL alone when refrigerated. (2378)

Bupivacaine hydrochloride 2.5 mg/mL admixed with morphine sulfate 5 mg/mL in sodium chloride 0.9% and bupivacaine hydrochloride 25 mg/mL admixed with morphine sulfate 50 mg/mL in sterile water for injection exhibited little or no loss of either drug in 60 days at 4 and 23 °C. The slight yellow discoloration that appeared in the high concentration samples was not indicative of drug decomposition. Samples stored for two days at 37 °C and frozen for two days at −20 °C resulted in little or no loss of either drug. However, the frozen samples upon thawing exhibited the formation of large amounts of microparticulates numbering in the thousands per milliliter, possibly shed by the syringe components. (2378)

Clonidine Hydrochloride — Clonidine hydrochloride (Fujisawa) 100 mcg/mL and morphine sulfate (Elkins-Sinn) 10 mg/mL were mixed in equal quantities, transferred to flint glass vials with rubber stoppers, and stored for 14 days at controlled room temperature protected from light. The solutions remained clear and colorless with no increase in particulate content. Little or no change in concentration for either drug occurred. (2069)

Clonidine hydrochloride 0.25 mg/mL admixed with morphine sulfate 5 mg/mL in sodium chloride 0.9% and clonidine hydrochloride 4 mg/mL admixed with morphine sulfate 50 mg/mL in sterile water for injection exhibited little or no loss of either drug at 4 and 23 °C. The slight yellow discoloration that appeared in the high concentration samples was not indicative of drug decomposition. Samples stored for two days at 37 °C and frozen for two days at −20 °C resulted in little or no loss of either drug. However, a precipitate formed in the frozen samples as freezing occurred and in the refrigerated high concentration samples after two to four days. Upon warming to room temperature the precipitate redissolved, but the samples exhibited large amounts of undissolved microparticulates numbering in the thousands per milliliter remaining in the solutions, possibly shed by the syringe components. (2380)

MOXIFLOXACIN HYDROCHLORIDE
AHFS 8:12.18

Products — Moxifloxacin hydrochloride is available as a ready-to-use 1.6 mg/mL clear yellow injection in 250-mL (400-mg) plastic bags with sodium chloride 0.8% in water for injection. Hydrochloric acid and/or sodium hydroxide may have been added during manufacturing to adjust pH. (1)

pH — From 4.1 to 4.6. (1)

Trade Name(s) — Avelox.

Administration — Moxifloxacin hydrochloride is administered by intravenous infusion only over 60 minutes once every 24 hours. No dilution of the injection is necessary. (1)

Stability — Moxifloxacin hydrochloride is stored at controlled room temperature. The manufacturer notes that high humidity should be avoided. The product should not be refrigerated because precipitation may result. Any unused portions should be discarded. (1)

Moxifloxacin hydrochloride 25 mg/mL in two peritoneal dialysis solutions was evaluated for stability. No color change or precipitation occurred. In Dianeal PD1 1.36% and 3.86% moxifloxacin hydrochloride lost 2% and 9%, respectively, in 14 days at 4 °C, and 3% and 11%, respectively, in 7 days at 25 °C. Losses at 37 °C were higher. In Dianeal PD1 1.36%, 10% loss occurred in 3 days; in Dianeal PD1 3.86%, 7% loss occurred in 12 hours and 13% loss occurred in 24 hours. (2712)

Compatibility Information

Solution Compatibility

Moxifloxacin HCl

Solution	Mfr	Mfr	Conc/L	Remarks	Ref	C/I
Dextrose 5%		BAY	[a]	Compatible	1	**C**
Dextrose 10%		BAY	[a]	Compatible	1	**C**
Ringer's injection, lactated		BAY	[a]	Compatible	1	**C**
Sodium chloride 0.9%		BAY	[a]	Compatible	1	**C**

[a]*Combined in ratios of 1:10 and 10:1.*

Y-Site Injection Compatibility (1:1 Mixture)

Moxifloxacin HCl

Drug	Mfr	Conc	Mfr	Conc	Remarks	Ref	C/I
Ceftaroline fosamil	FOR	2.22 mg/mL[a,b,c]	BAY	1.6 mg/mL	Physically compatible for 4 hr at 23 °C	2826	**C**
Doripenem	JJ	5 mg/mL[a,b]	BAY	1.6 mg/mL	Physically compatible for 4 hr at 23 °C	2743	**C**
Hydroxyethyl starch 130/0.4 in sodium chloride 0.9%	FRK	6%	BAY	0.4[a], 0.8[a], 1.6 mg/mL	Visually compatible for 24 hr at room temperature	2770	**C**
Vasopressin	APP	0.2 unit/mL[b]	BAY	1.6 mg/mL	Physically compatible	2641	**C**

[a]*Tested in dextrose 5% in water.*
[b]*Tested in sodium chloride 0.9%.*
[c]*Tested in Ringer's injection, lactated.*

MULTIVITAMINS
AHFS 88:28

Products — Multivitamin products for parenteral administration are available in a variety of compositions and sizes. The following products are representative formulations.

M.V.I. Adult is available as a package of two vials (labeled Vial 1 and Vial 2) that are prepared for use by transferring the contents of Vial 1 into Vial 2 and mixing gently. After mixing, the product contains (1):

Ascorbic acid	200 mg
Vitamin A	1 mg
Vitamin D_3 (ergocalciferol)	5 mcg
Thiamine (as hydrochloride)	6 mg
Riboflavin (as 5′-phosphate sodium)	3.6 mg
Pyridoxine hydrochloride	6 mg
Niacinamide	40 mg
Dexpanthenol	15 mg
Vitamin E (*dl-α* tocopheryl acetate)	10 mg
Vitamin K	150 mcg
Folic acid	600 mcg
Biotin	60 mcg
Vitamin B_{12} (cyanocobalamin)	5 mcg

The product also contains propylene glycol 30%, polysorbate 80 1.4%, citric acid, and sodium hydroxide and/or hydrochloric acid in water for injection. The concentrated vitamins must be diluted for use; do not give undiluted. (1)

M.V.I.-12 has the same vitamin content as M.V.I. Adult except for the absence of vitamin K. (1)

M.V.I. Pediatric is available as a lyophilized powder in vials containing a single dose. Each single dose contains (1):

Ascorbic acid	80 mg
Vitamin A (retinol)	0.7 mg
Vitamin D (ergocalciferol)	10 mcg
Thiamine (as hydrochloride)	1.2 mg
Riboflavin (as 5′-phosphate sodium)	1.4 mg
Pyridoxine (as hydrochloride)	1 mg
Niacinamide	17 mg
Dexpanthenol	5 mg
Vitamin E (*dl*-alpha tocopheryl acetate)	7 mg
Biotin	20 mcg
Folic acid	140 mcg
Cyanocobalamin	1 mcg
Phytonadione	200 mcg

M.V.I. Pediatric also contains, in each vial, mannitol 375 mg, polysorbate 80 50 mg, polysorbate 20 0.8 mg, butylated hydroxytoluene 58 mcg, butylated hydroxyanisole 14 mcg, and sodium hydroxide for pH adjustment. (1)

Reconstitute the single-dose vial with 5 mL of sterile water for injection, dextrose 5%, or sodium chloride 0.9% and swirl gently. The solution is ready within three minutes. This solution must be further diluted for use; do not give it undiluted. (1)

Administration — Multivitamin infusion preparations are administered by intravenous infusion only. They should not be given by direct intravenous injection. M.V.I. Adult is diluted in not less than 500 mL but preferably 1000 mL of intravenous infusion solution for administration. M.V.I. Pediatric should be added to at least 100 mL of a compatible intravenous infusion solution for administration. (1)

Stability — Multivitamin products for infusion should be stored under refrigeration and protected from light. Since some of the vitamins, especially A, D, and riboflavin, are light sensitive, light protection is necessary. After reconstitution of M.V.I. Pediatric, use of the product without delay is recommended. However, if this is not possible, the manufacturer permits use within a maximum of four hours from the initial penetration of the closure. (1)

Light Effects — The effects of photoirradiation on a FreAmine II–dextrose 10% parenteral nutrition solution containing 1 mL/500 mL of multivitamins (USV) were evaluated. During simulated continuous administration to an infant at 0.156 mL/min, the amino acids were stable when the bottle, infusion tubing, and collection bottle were shielded with foil. Only 20 cm of tubing in the incubator was exposed to light. However, if the flow was stopped, marked reductions in methionine (40%), tryptophan (44%), and histidine (22%) occurred in the solution exposed to light for 24 hours. In a similar solution without vitamins, only the tryptophan concentration decreased. The difference was attributed to the presence of riboflavin, a photosensitizer. The authors recommended administering the multivitamins separately and shielding from light. (833)

The stability of five B vitamins was studied over eight hours in representative parenteral nutrition solutions exposed to fluorescent light, indirect sunlight, or direct sunlight. One 5-mL vial of multivitamin concentrate (Lyphomed) and 1 mg of folic acid (Lederle) were added to a liter of parenteral nutrition solution composed of amino acids 4.25% and dextrose 25% (Travenol) with standard electrolytes and trace elements. The five B vitamins were stable for eight hours at room temperature when exposed to fluorescent light. In addition, folic acid and niacinamide were stable over eight hours in direct or indirect sunlight. Exposure to indirect sunlight appeared to have little or no effect on thiamine hydrochloride and pyridoxine hydrochloride in eight hours, but riboflavin-5′-phosphate lost 47%. Direct sunlight caused a 26% loss of thiamine hydrochloride and an 86% loss of pyridoxine hydrochloride in eight hours. A four-hour exposure of riboflavin-5′-phosphate to direct sunlight resulted in a 98% loss. (842)

A parenteral nutrition solution in glass bottles exposed to sunlight was studied. Vitamin A decomposed rapidly, losing more than 50% in three hours. The decomposition could be slowed by covering the bottle with a light-resistant vinyl bag, resulting in about a 25% loss in three hours. Vitamin E was stable in the parenteral nutrition solution in glass bottles exposed to sunlight, with no loss occurring during six hours of exposure. (1040)

Vitamin A rapidly and significantly decomposes when exposed to daylight. The extent and rate of loss were dependent on the degree of exposure to daylight which, in turn, depended on various factors such as the direction of the radiation, time of day, and climatic conditions. Delivery of less than 10% of the expected amount was reported. (1047) In controlled light experiments, the decomposition initially progressed exponentially. Subsequently, the rate of decomposition slowed. This result was attributed to a protective effect of the degradation products on the remaining vitamin A. The presence of amino acids provided greater protection. Compared to degradation rates in dextrose 5%, decomposition was reduced by up to 50% in some amino acid mixtures. (1048)

The stability of several water-soluble vitamins in dextrose 5% and sodium chloride 0.9% in PVC and ClearFlex containers was evaluated. Thiamine, riboflavin, ascorbic acid, and folic acid were stable at 23 °C when protected from light, exhibiting 10% or less loss in 24 hours. When exposed to light, thiamine and folic acid were stable but ascorbic acid was reduced by approximately 50 to 65% and riboflavin was completely lost. (1509)

The stability of phytonadione in a TPN solution containing amino acids 2%, dextrose 12.5%, "standard" electrolytes, and M.V.I. Pediatric over 24 hours while exposed to light was evaluated. Vitamin loss was about 7% in four hours and 27% in 24 hours. Some loss was attributed to the light sensitivity of the phytonadione. (1815)

Substantial loss of retinol all-*trans* palmitate and phytonadione was reported from both TPN and TNA admixtures due to exposure to sunlight. In three hours of exposure to sunlight, essentially total loss of retinol and 50% loss of phytonadione had occurred. The presence or absence of lipids did not affect stability. In contrast, tocopherol concentrations remained essentially unchanged by exposure to sunlight through 12 hours. The container material used to store the nutrition admixtures affected the concentration of the vitamins as well. Losses were greatest (10 to 25%) in PVC containers and were slightly better in EVA and glass containers. (2049)

Sorption — The following vitamins did not reveal significant sorption to a PVC plastic test strip in 24 hours (12):

Ascorbic acid
Niacinamide
Pyridoxine hydrochloride
Riboflavin
Thiamine hydrochloride
Vitamin D
Vitamin E acetate

Riboflavin was shown not to exhibit sorption to PVC bags and tubing, polyethylene tubing, Silastic tubing, and polypropylene syringes. (536; 606)

Vitamin A (as the acetate) (Sigma) 7.5 mg/L displayed 66.7% sorption to a PVC plastic test strip in 24 hours. The presence of dextrose 5% and sodium chloride 0.9% increased the extent of the sorption. (12)

In another report, vitamin A acetate 3 mg/L displayed 78% sorption to 200-mL PVC containers after 24 hours at 25 °C with gentle shaking. The sorption was increased by 10% in sodium chloride 0.9% and by 20% in dextrose 5%. (133)

However, vitamin A delivery is also reduced in glass intravenous containers. At a concentration of 10,000 units/L in glass and PVC plastic containers protected from light with aluminum foil, 77 and 71%, respectively, of the vitamin A were delivered over a 10-hour period. Without light protection, 61% was delivered from glass and 49% from PVC plastic containers over a 10-hour period. (290)

In another test using multivitamin infusion (USV), one ampul per liter of sodium chloride 0.9% in glass and PVC plastic containers not protected from light, 69.4 and 67.9% of the vitamin A were delivered from glass and PVC containers, respectively, over a 10-hour period. The amount of vitamin A was constant over the test period. (282)

The delivery of vitamins A, D, and E from a parenteral nutrition solution composed of 3% amino acid solution (Pharmacia) in dextrose 10% with electrolytes, trace elements, vitamin K, folate, and vitamin B_{12} was evaluated. To this solution was added 6 mL of multivitamin infusion (USV). The solution was prepared in PVC bags (Travenol), and administration was simulated through a fluid chamber (Buretrol) and infusion tubing with a 0.5-μm filter at 10 mL/hr. During the first 60 to 90 minutes, minimal delivery of the vitamins occurred. This was followed by a rise and plateau in the delivered vitamins, which were attributed to an increasing saturation of adsorptive binding sites in the tubing. The total amounts delivered over 24 hours were 31% for vitamin A, 68% for vitamin D, and 64% for vitamin E. Sorption of the vitamins was found in the PVC bag, fluid chamber, and tubing. Decomposition was not a factor. (836)

A patient receiving 3000 I.U. of retinol daily in a parenteral nutrition solution experienced two episodes of night blindness. The pharmacy prepared the parenteral nutrition solution in 1-L PVC bags in weekly batches and stored them at 4 °C in the dark until use. A subsequent in vitro study showed losses of vitamin A of 23 and 77% in three- and 14-day periods, respectively, under these conditions. About 30% of the lost vitamin A could be extracted from the PVC bag. (1038)

Vitamin A was lost from multivitamin infusion (USV) in a neonatal parenteral nutrition solution. The solution was prepared in colorless glass bottles and run through an administration set with a burette (Travenol). The total loss of vitamin A was 75% in 24 hours, with about 16% as decomposition in the glass bottle. The decomposition was not noticeable during the first 12 hours, but then vitamin A levels fell rather precipitously to about one-third of the initial amount. The balance of the loss, averaging about 59%, occurred during transit through the administration set. Removal of the inline filter and treatment of the set with albumin human had no effect on vitamin A delivery. Increasing three- to fourfold the amount of vitamin A was suggested to compensate for the losses. (1039)

A 50% loss of vitamin A from a bottle of parenteral nutrition solution prepared with multivitamin infusion (USV) after 5.5 hours of infusion was noted. The amount delivered through an Ivex-2 filter set was only 6.3% of the added amount. Similar quantities were found after 20 hours of infusion. Vitamin A binding to the infusion bottles and tubing was confirmed. (704)

Solutions containing multivitamin infusion (USV) spiked with ^{3}H-labeled retinol in intravenous tubing protected from light and agitated to simulate flow for five hours were evaluated. About half of the vitamin A was lost in 30 minutes, and 88 to 96% was lost in five hours. (1049)

The stability of vitamin E (alpha-tocopherol acetate from M.V.I.-1000 or Soluzyme) and selenium (from Selepen) in amino acids (Abbott) and dextrose in PVC bags was studied. Exposure to fluorescent light and room temperature (23 °C) for 24 hours and simulated infusion at 50 mL/hr for eight hours through a Medlon TPN administration set with a 0.22-μm filter did not affect the concentrations of vitamin E and selenium. (1224)

The stability of numerous vitamins in parenteral nutrition solutions composed of amino acids (Kabi-Vitrum), dextrose 30%, and fat emulsion 20% (Kabi-Vitrum) in a 2:1:1 ratio with electrolytes, trace elements, and both fat- and water-soluble vitamins was reported. The admixtures were stored in darkness at 2 to 8 °C for 96 hours with no significant loss of retinyl palmitate, alpha-tocopherol, thiamine mononitrate, sodium riboflavin-5'-phosphate, pyridoxine hydrochloride, nicotinamide, folic acid, biotin, sodium pantothenate, and cyanocobalamin. Sodium ascorbate and its biologically active degradation product, dehydroascorbic acid, totaled 59 and 42% of the nominal starting concentration at 24 and 96 hours, respectively. (1225)

When the admixture was subjected to simulated infusion over 24 hours at 20 °C, either exposed to room light or light protected, or stored for six days in the dark under refrigeration and then subjected to the same simulated infusion, once again the retinyl palmitate, alpha-tocopherol, and sodium riboflavin-5'-phosphate did not undergo significant loss. However, sodium ascorbate and its degradation product, dehydroascorbic acid, had initial combined concentrations of 51 to 65% of the nominal initial concentration, with further declines during infusion. Light protection did not significantly alter the loss of total ascorbic acid. (1225)

Neonatal parenteral nutrition solutions containing multivitamin infusion prepared in bags were delivered at 10 mL/hr through Buretrol sets (Travenol). The bags and sets were protected from light. About 26% of the vitamin A was lost before the flow was started. At 10 mL/hr, about 67% was lost from the effluent. More rapid flow reduced the extent of loss. Analysis of clinical samples of parenteral nutrition solutions showed losses of 21 to 57% after 20 hours. Because losses after five hours were of the same magnitude, it was concluded that the loss occurs rapidly and is not due to decomposition. (1049)

Retinol losses of 40% occurred in two hours and 60% in five hours from parenteral nutrition solutions pumped at 10 mL/hr through standard infusion sets at room temperature. The retinol concentration in the bottle remained constant while the retinol in the effluent decreased. Antioxidants had no effect. Much of the vitamin A was recoverable from the tubing. (1050)

To minimize the importance of this sorption, Allwood suggested using vitamin A palmitate instead of acetate; he stated that vitamin A palmitate does not sorb to PVC. However, this does not alter the problem of degradation from exposure to light. (1033)

Plasticizer Leaching — Multivitamins (Lyphomed) 1 mL in 50 mL of dextrose 5% leached insignificant amounts of diethylhexyl phthalate (DEHP) plasticizer due to the surfactant polysorbate 80 in the formulation. This finding is consistent with the low surfactant concentration (0.032%) in the admixture solution. (1683)

Compatibility Information

Solution Compatibility

Multivitamins

Solution	Mfr	Mfr	Conc/L	Remarks	Ref	C/I
Amino acids 2%, dextrose 12.5%, electrolytes		ROR	5 mL[b]	7% phytonadione loss in 4 hr and 27% loss in 24 hr under ambient temperature and light	1815	**I**
Amino acids 4.25%, dextrose 25%	TR	USV	1 vial	No thiamine loss in 22 hr at 30 °C	843	**C**
	MG[c,d]	LY	10 mL	All vitamins stable for 24 hr at 4 °C	926	**C**
Amino acids 2.5%, dextrose 25%	AB[c,d]	LY	10 mL	All vitamins stable for 24 hr at 4 °C	926	**C**
Dextrose 5% in Ringer's injection, lactated	BA	USV	20 mL	Physically compatible for 24 hr	315	**C**
Dextrose 5% in sodium chloride 0.9%	BA	USV	20 mL	Physically compatible for 24 hr	315	**C**
	[b]	LY	10 mL	All vitamins stable for 24 hr at 4 °C	926	**C**
Dextrose 5%	BA	USV	20 mL	Physically compatible for 24 hr	315	**C**
	TR[c]	RC	4 mL[a]	8% or less thiamine loss in 24 hr at 23 °C	774	**C**
	[d]	LY	10 mL	All vitamins stable for 24 hr at 4 °C	926	**C**
Dextrose 10%	BA	USV	20 mL	Physically compatible for 24 hr	315	**C**
	TR[c]	RC	4 mL[a]	5% or less thiamine loss in 24 hr at 23 °C	774	**C**
	MG[d]	RC	4 mL[a]	11% or less thiamine loss in 24 hr at 23 °C	774	**C**
Dextrose 20%	BA	USV	20 mL	Physically compatible for 24 hr	315	**C**

Solution Compatibility (Cont.)

Multivitamins

Solution	Mfr	Mfr	Conc/L	Remarks	Ref	C/I
Ringer's injection, lactated	BA	USV	20 mL	Physically compatible for 24 hr	315	C
	TR[c]	RC	4 mL[a]	5% or less thiamine loss in 24 hr at 23 °C	774	C
Sodium chloride 0.9%	BA	USV	20 mL	Physically compatible for 24 hr	315	C
	TR[c]	RC	4 mL[a]	Thiamine losses of 6 to 11% in 24 hr at 23 °C	774	C
Sodium lactate ⅙ M	BA	USV	20 mL	Physically compatible for 24 hr	315	C

[a] *Berocca Parenteral Nutrition.*
[b] *M.V.I. Pediatric.*
[c] *Tested in both glass and PVC containers.*
[d] *Tested in polyolefin containers.*

Additive Compatibility

Multivitamins

Drug	Mfr	Conc/L	Mfr	Conc/L	Test Soln	Remarks	Ref	C/I
Cefoxitin sodium	MSD	10 g	USV	50 mL[a]	W	5% cefoxitin loss in 24 hr and 10% in 48 hr at 25 °C; 3% in 48 hr at 5 °C	308	C
Fat emulsion, intravenous	VT	10%	USV	4 mL		Physically compatible for 48 hr at 4 °C and room temperature	32	C
	KA	10%	KA			Physically compatible for 24 hr at 26 °C. Little loss of most vitamins; up to 52% ascorbate loss	2050	C
Isoproterenol HCl	WI	4 mg	USV	10 mL		Physically compatible	59	C
Meropenem	ZEN	1 and 20 g	AST	50 mL	NS	Color darkened in 4 hr at room temperature	1994	I
Methyldopate HCl	MSD	1 g	USV	10 mL	D, D–S, S	Physically compatible	23	C
Metoclopramide HCl	RB	20 and 320 mg	USV	20 mL[b]	NS	Physically compatible for 48 hr at room temperature	924	C
	RB	20 and 320 mg	USV	20 mL[c]	NS	Physically compatible for 48 hr at room temperature	924	C
Norepinephrine bitartrate	WI	8 mg	USV	10 mL	D, D–S, S	Physically compatible	77	C
Sodium bicarbonate	AB	4.8 mEq[d]	USV	10 mL	D5W	Physically compatible for 24 hr	772	C
Verapamil HCl	KN	80 mg	USV	10 mL	D5W, NS	Physically compatible for 24 hr	764	C

[a] *Concentrate.*
[b] *M.V.I.*
[c] *M.V.I.-12.*
[d] *Two vials of Neut added to a liter of admixture.*

Y-Site Injection Compatibility (1:1 Mixture)

Multivitamins

Drug	Mfr	Conc	Mfr	Conc	Remarks	Ref	C/I
Acyclovir sodium	BW	5 mg/mL[a]	LY	0.01 mL/mL[a]	Physically compatible for 4 hr at 25 °C	1157	C
Ampicillin sodium	AY	1 g/50 mL[a,b]	USV	5 mL/L[a]	Physically compatible for 24 hr at room temperature	323	C

Y-Site Injection Compatibility (1:1 Mixture) (Cont.)

Multivitamins

Drug	Mfr	Conc	Mfr	Conc	Remarks	Ref	C/I
Cefazolin sodium	SKF	1 g/50 mL[a]	USV	5 mL/L[a]	Physically compatible for 24 hr at room temperature	323	**C**
Ceftaroline fosamil	FOR	2.22 mg/mL[a,b,g]	BA	5 mL/L[a,b,g]	Physically compatible for 4 hr at 23 °C	2826	**C**
Clindamycin phosphate	UP	600 mg/100 mL[a]	USV	5 mL/L[a]	Physically compatible for 24 hr at room temperature	323	**C**
Diltiazem HCl	MMD	5 mg/mL		[c]	Visually compatible	1807	**C**
Erythromycin lactobionate	AB	500 mg/250 mL[b]	USV	5 mL/L[a]	Physically compatible for 24 hr at room temperature	323	**C**
Fludarabine phosphate	BX	1 mg/mL[a]	ROR	0.01 mL/mL[a]	Visually compatible for 4 hr at 22 °C	1439	**C**
Gentamicin sulfate	SC	80 mg/100 mL[a]	USV	5 mL/L[a]	Physically compatible for 24 hr at room temperature	323	**C**
Hydroxyethyl starch 130/0.4 in sodium chloride 0.9%	FRK	6%	SX	2.5, 5, 10 mL/L[a]	Visually compatible for 24 hr at room temperature	2770	**C**
Pantoprazole sodium	[f]	4 mg/mL	SX		Precipitates within 1 hr	2574	**I**
Tacrolimus	FUJ	1 mg/mL[b]	LY	0.001 mL/mL[a]	Visually compatible for 24 hr at 25 °C	1630	**C**
TPN #189[d]			ROR	[e]	Visually compatible for 24 hr at 22 °C	1767	**C**

[a]*Tested in dextrose 5%.*
[b]*Tested in sodium chloride 0.9%.*
[c]*Concentration unspecified.*
[d]*Refer to Appendix I for the composition of parenteral nutrition solutions. TPN indicates a 2-in-1 admixture.*
[e]*M.V.I.-12.*
[f]*Test performed using the formulation WITHOUT edetate disodium.*
[g]*Tested in Ringer's injection, lactated.*

Additional Compatibility Information

Parenteral Nutrition Solutions — In a parenteral nutrition solution composed of amino acids, dextrose, electrolytes, trace elements, and multivitamins in PVC bags stored at 4 and 25 °C, vitamin A rapidly deteriorated to 10% of the initial concentration in eight hours at 25 °C when exposed to light. The decomposition was slowed by light protection and refrigeration, with a loss of about 25% in four days. Folic acid concentration dropped 40% initially on admixture and then remained relatively constant for 28 days of storage. About 35% of the ascorbic acid was lost in 39 hours at 25 °C when exposed to light. The loss was reduced to a negligible amount in four days by refrigeration and light protection. Thiamine content dropped by 50% initially but then remained unchanged over 120 hours of storage. (1063)

The stability of ascorbic acid in parenteral nutrition solutions, with and without fat emulsion, was studied. Both with and without fat emulsion, the total vitamin C content (ascorbic acid plus dehydroascorbic acid) remained above 90% for 12 hours when the solutions were exposed to fluorescent light and for 24 hours when they were protected from light. When stored in a cool dark place, the solutions were stable for seven days. (1227)

Samples from 24 1-L and four 2-L parenteral nutrition solutions, containing one vial each of multivitamin concentrate (USV), were evaluated for thiamine hydrochloride content 48 and 72 hours after mixing. The parenteral nutrition solutions contained amino acids 2.75 to 5%, dextrose 15 to 25%, and electrolytes. Thiamine hydrochloride was stable in all of the solutions tested in spite of approximately 0.05% sulfite content. (843)

The vitamins in Cernevit (Baxter) diluted in three 2-in-1 parenteral nutrition admixtures were tested for stability over 48 hours. Nearly all of the vitamins retained their initial concentrations. However, ascorbic acid exhibited losses of about 5%, 13%, and 17% in TPNs with dextrose concentrations of 10, 15, and 25%, respectively. (2796)

Erythromycin — Erythromycin 5 mg/mL as the lactobionate in pH 8 buffer was combined with riboflavin in concentrations varying from 1 mg/mL to 20 mcg/mL. On exposure to light for four hours, almost total decomposition of the erythromycin occurred, with only 4 to 12% remaining. Protection from light resulted in 12 to 25% decomposition. When no riboflavin was present, 10% or less decomposition of the erythromycin occurred. It was concluded that a photodynamic decomposition reaction was taking place. (564)

Penicillin G — The times to 10% decomposition of combinations of penicillin G potassium buffered with multivitamin infusion concentrate in dextrose 5% and sodium chloride 0.9% have been calculated on the pH of the admixture (304):

Penicillin G Potassium	Multivitamin Infusion Concentrate	pH	Time to 10% Decomposition
1 million units/L	1 mL/L	5.1	6.51 hr
1 million units/L	5 mL/L	4.9	4.56 hr
3 million units/L	1 mL/L	5.4	13.54 hr
3 million units/L	5 mL/L	5.0	6.38 hr
5 million units/L	1 mL/L	5.7	22.01 hr
5 million units/L	5 mL/L	5.1	6.51 hr
10 million units/L	1 mL/L	5.9	over 24 hr
10 million units/L	5 mL/L	5.4	13.54 hr

MYCOPHENOLATE MOFETIL HYDROCHLORIDE
AHFS 92:44

Products — Mycophenolate mofetil hydrochloride is available as a lyophilized powder in vials containing 500 mg of drug along with polysorbate 80 25 mg and citric acid 5 mg. Sodium hydroxide may have been added during manufacturing to adjust pH. (1)

Dextrose 5% is used for reconstitution and dilution for use to a concentration of 6 mg/mL. Using care and precautions to avoid contact with the drug solution, reconstitute each vial with 14 mL of dextrose 5% and gently shake to dissolve the drug. Dilute the reconstituted solution further with dextrose 5% to yield a 6-mg/mL concentration. The volumes of dextrose 5% to be used for 1- and 1.5-g doses are 140 and 210 mL, respectively. The solution should be inspected for particulate matter and discoloration. (1)

pH — From 2.4 to 4.1. (1)

Trade Name(s) — CellCept.

Administration — Mycophenolate mofetil hydrochloride is administered by slow intravenous infusion over a minimum of two hours into either a central line or peripheral vein. The drug should not be administered by rapid or bolus administration. (1)

Stability — The intact vials containing mycophenolate mofetil hydrochloride as white to off-white lyophilized powder should be stored at controlled room temperature. Dextrose 5% is recommended for reconstitution and dilution of mycophenolate mofetil hydrochloride. All other solutions are stated to be incompatible. The reconstituted solution and dilution for use are slightly yellow and may also be kept at room temperature. The manufacturer indicates administration should begin within four hours after reconstitution. (1)

Compatibility Information

Solution Compatibility

Mycophenolate mofetil HCl

Solution	Mfr	Mfr	Conc/L	Remarks	Ref	C/I
Dextrose 5%	MAC[a]	RC	1, 5, 10 g	Physically compatible. No loss in 7 days at 4 and 25 °C	2394	C

[a]Tested in PVC containers.

Y-Site Injection Compatibility (1:1 Mixture)

Mycophenolate mofetil HCl

Drug	Mfr	Conc	Mfr	Conc	Remarks	Ref	C/I
Anidulafungin	VIC	0.5 mg/mL[a]	RC	6 mg/mL[a]	Physically compatible for 4 hr at 23 °C	2617	C
Caspofungin acetate	ME	0.7 mg/mL[b]	RC	6 mg/mL[b]	Physically compatible for 4 hr at room temperature	2758	C

Y-Site Injection Compatibility (1:1 Mixture) (Cont.)

Mycophenolate mofetil HCl

Drug	Mfr	Conc	Mfr	Conc	Remarks	Ref	C/I
Cefepime HCl		20 mg/mL[a]	RC	5.9 mg/mL[a]	Physically compatible with no mycopheno-late mofetil loss in 4 hr	2738	**C**
Cyclosporine	BED	1 mg/mL[a]	RC	5.9 mg/mL[a]	Effervescence reported. No mycophenolate mofetil loss in 4 hr	2738	**?**
Dopamine HCl	AMR	4 mg/mL[a]	RC	5.9 mg/mL[a]	Physically compatible and 4% mycopheno-late mofetil loss in 4 hr	2738	**C**
Micafungin sodium	ASP	1.5 mg/mL[b]	RC	6 mg/mL[a]	White precipitate forms immediately	2683	**I**
Norepinephrine bitartrate		1 mg/mL[a]	RC	5.9 mg/mL[a]	Physically compatible and 2% mycopheno-late mofetil loss in 4 hr	2738	**C**
Tacrolimus	FUJ	0.02 mg/mL[a]	RC	5.9 mg/mL[a]	Physically compatible and 2% mycopheno-late mofetil loss in 4 hr	2738	**C**
Vancomycin HCl		10 mg/mL[a]	RC	5.9 mg/mL[a]	Physically compatible and 3% mycopheno-late mofetil loss in 4 hr	2738	**C**

[a] *Tested in dextrose 5%.*
[b] *Tested in sodium chloride 0.9%.*

NAFCILLIN SODIUM
AHFS 8:12.16.12

Products — Nafcillin sodium is available in vials containing the equivalent of 1 and 2 g of nafcillin. (4) Reconstitute the 1-g vial with 3.4 mL and the 2-g vial with 6.6 mL of sterile water for injection, sodium chloride 0.9%, or bacteriostatic water for injection containing parabens or benzyl alcohol. The solution then contains nafcillin sodium equivalent to nafcillin 250 mg/mL with sodium citrate buffer. The final volumes of the 1- and 2-g vials are 4 and 8 mL, respectively. (4)

A 10-g pharmacy bulk vial is also available and is reconstituted with 93 mL of sterile water for injection or sodium chloride 0.9% to yield a 100-mg/mL solution with sodium citrate buffer 4 mg/mL. (4)

Nafcillin sodium is also available as frozen premixed solutions containing 1 and 2 g of nafcillin per minibag in dextrose 3.6% or 2%, respectively. (1)

pH — The pH of the reconstituted solution and frozen premixed solution is 6 to 8.5. (4)

Osmolality — The osmolality of nafcillin sodium 250 mg/mL in sterile water for injection was 709 mOsm/kg by freezing-point depression and 665 mOsm/kg by vapor pressure. (1071)

The frozen premixed solutions have an osmolality of 300 mOsm/kg. (4)

The osmolality of nafcillin sodium (Wyeth) 40 mg/mL was determined to be 403 mOsm/kg in dextrose 5% and 402 mOsm/kg in sodium chloride 0.9%. (1375)

The osmolality of nafcillin sodium was calculated for the following dilutions (1054):

Diluent	Osmolality (mOsm/kg)	
	50 mL	100 mL
2 g		
Dextrose 5%	399	334
Sodium chloride 0.9%	425	361
3 g		
Dextrose 5%	458	371
Sodium chloride 0.9%	485	398

The following maximum nafcillin sodium concentrations were recommended to achieve osmolalities suitable for peripheral infusion in fluid-restricted patients (1180):

Diluent	Maximum Concentration (mg/mL)	Osmolality (mOsm/kg)
Dextrose 5%	71	491
Sodium chloride 0.9%	64	470
Sterile water for injection	128	319

Sodium Content — Each gram of nafcillin sodium with sodium citrate buffer contains 2.9 mEq (66 mg) of sodium. (4; 27)

Administration — Nafcillin sodium may be administered intramuscularly by deep intragluteal injection, by direct intravenous injection, or by intermittent intravenous infusion. For direct intravenous injection, the dose should be diluted with 15 to 30 mL of sterile water for injection or sodium chloride 0.45 or 0.9% and given over five to 10 minutes into the tubing of a running intravenous infusion. Intermittent intravenous infusion in a concentration between 2 and 40 mg/mL should be administered slowly, over 30 to 60 minutes. (4)

Stability — Intact containers should be stored at controlled room temperature or lower. (4) When reconstituted to a concentration of 250 mg/mL, nafcillin sodium is stable for three days at room temperature or seven days when refrigerated at 2 to 8 °C. (4; 27) At concentrations of 2 to 40 mg/mL, nafcillin sodium is stable for 24 hours at room temperature or 96 hours under refrigeration. (4)

Commercially available frozen premixed nafcillin sodium solutions, thawed at room temperature or under refrigeration, are stable for 72 hours at 25 °C and 21 days at 5 °C. (4)

The activity of nafcillin 100 mg/L was evaluated in peritoneal dialysis fluids containing dextrose 1.5 or 4.25% (Dianeal 137, Travenol). Storage at 25 °C resulted in no loss of antimicrobial activity in 24 hours. (515)

The stability of nafcillin sodium (Wyeth) 100 mg/L in peritoneal dialysis solutions (Dianeal 137 and PD2) with heparin sodium 500 units/L was evaluated. About 98% activity remained after 24 hours at 25 °C. (1228)

pH Effects — The stability of nafcillin sodium is pH dependent, with a maximum stability at pH 6 and a preferred range of pH 5 to 8. Drug decomposition is increased as pH values vary from this range. Additives that may result in a final pH of above 8 or below 5 should not be mixed with nafcillin sodium. (27)

Freezing Solutions — At a concentration of 250 mg/mL in sterile water for injection and frozen at −20 °C, the drug is stable for up to three months. (27; 123)

In one study, however, when nafcillin sodium (Wyeth) 1 g/4 mL was frozen at −20 °C in glass syringes (Hy-Pod), the drug was stable for nine months. (532)

In another study, nafcillin sodium (Wyeth) 1 g/50 mL of dextrose 5% in PVC bags frozen at −20 °C for 30 days and then thawed by exposure to ambient temperature or microwave radiation showed no evidence of precipitation or color change but had a 2 to 3% loss. Subsequent storage of the admixture at room temperature for 24 hours also yielded physically compatible solutions with no additional loss of activity. (555)

Syringes — Nafcillin sodium (Apothecon) 10 mg/mL in sodium chloride 0.9% was packaged in 10-mL polypropylene syringes (Becton Dickinson) and stored at 5 and 25 °C. The solutions remained clear under refrigeration for 44 days and at room temperature for seven days. A yellow color developed after 14 days at room temperature. About 2% loss of nafcillin sodium occurred after seven days and 18% loss in 14 days at 25 °C. Under refrigeration, 1% loss occurred after 44 days. Stability in glass containers was comparable. (2325)

Ambulatory Pumps — Nafcillin sodium (Marsam) 20 mg/mL in sterile water for injection in PVC portable pump reservoirs (Pharmacia Deltec) exhibited no loss in three days stored at 25 °C and in 14 days at 5 °C. However, at a concentration of 120 mg/mL, 6% loss was found in three days at 25 °C, and 2% loss occurred in 14 days at 5 °C. (2080)

Nafcillin sodium 40 and 50 mg/mL in sodium chloride 0.9% precipitated in as little as one day at the simulated ambulatory use temperature of 35 °C. At 20 mg/mL, precipitation appeared in three days. When stored at room temperature, no precipitation appeared at any concentration in three days. (2664)

Compatibility Information

Solution Compatibility

Nafcillin sodium

Solution	Mfr	Mfr	Conc/L	Remarks	Ref	C/I
Dextrose 5% in Ringer's injection	AB	WY	2 and 30 g	Physically compatible and stable for 24 hr at 25 °C	27	C
Dextrose 5% in half-strength Ringer's injection, lactated	AB	WY	2 and 30 g	Physically compatible	27	C
Dextrose 5% in Ringer's injection, lactated	AB	WY	2 and 30 g	Physically compatible	27	C
Dextrose 5% in sodium chloride 0.225%	AB	WY	2 and 30 g	Physically compatible	27	C
Dextrose 5% in sodium chloride 0.45%			2 to 40 g	Under 10% loss in 24 hr at room temperature and 96 hr refrigerated	4	C
	AB	WY	2 and 30 g	Physically compatible and stable for 24 hr at 25 °C	27	C
Dextrose 5% in sodium chloride 0.9%	AB	WY	2 and 30 g	Physically compatible and stable for 24 hr at 25 °C	27	C
Dextrose 5%			2 to 40 g	Under 10% loss in 24 hr at room temperature and 96 hr refrigerated	4	C
		WY	1 g	Stable for 24 hr	109	C
	AB	WY	2 and 30 g	Physically compatible and stable for 24 hr at 25 °C	27	C

Solution Compatibility (Cont.)

Nafcillin sodium

Solution	Mfr	Mfr	Conc/L	Remarks	Ref	C/I
	TRª	WY	20 g	Physically compatible and stable for 24 hr at room temperature	555	C
	TRª	WY	20 g	About 10% loss in 7 days at 24 °C and 8% loss in 15 days at 4 °C	336	C
Dextrose 10% in sodium chloride 0.9%	AB	WY	2 and 30 g	Physically compatible	27	C
Dextrose 10%	AB	WY	2 and 30 g	Physically compatible	27	C
Ionosol T in dextrose 5%	AB	WY	2 and 30 g	Physically compatible	27	C
Normosol M in dextrose 5%	AB	WY	2 and 30 g	Physically compatible and stable for 24 hr at 25 °C	27	C
Normosol R	AB	WY	2 and 30 g	Physically compatible	27	C
Normosol R in dextrose 5%	AB	WY	2 and 30 g	Physically compatible	27	C
Ringer's injection			2 to 40 g	Under 10% loss in 24 hr at room temperature and 96 hr refrigerated	4	C
	AB	WY	2 and 30 g	Physically compatible and stable for 24 hr at 25 °C	27	C
Ringer's injection, lactated	AB	WY	2 and 30 g	Physically compatible and stable for 24 hr at 25 °C	27	C
Sodium chloride 0.9%			2 to 40 g	Under 10% loss in 24 hr at room temperature and 96 hr refrigerated	4	C
		WY	1 g	Stable for 24 hr	109	C
	AB	WY	2 and 30 g	Physically compatible and stable for 24 hr at 25 °C	27	C
	ABᶜ	WY	80 g	5% or less loss with 24-hr storage at 5 °C then 48 hr at 30 °C	1779	C
	TRª	WY	20 g	About 6% loss in 3 days at 24 °C and 6% loss in 24 days at 4 °C	336	C
Sodium lactate ⅙ M			2 to 40 g	Under 10% loss in 24 hr at room temperature and 96 hr refrigerated	4	C
	AB	WY	2 and 30 g	Physically compatible and stable for 24 hr at 25 °C	27	C
TPN #107ᵇ			1 and 2 g	Nafcillin activity retained for 24 hr at 21 °C	1326	C

ªTested in PVC containers.
ᵇRefer to Appendix I for the composition of parenteral nutrition solutions. TPN indicates a 2-in-1 admixture.
ᶜTested in portable pump reservoirs (Pharmacia Deltec).

Additive Compatibility

Nafcillin sodium

Drug	Mfr	Conc/L	Mfr	Conc/L	Test Soln	Remarks	Ref	C/I
Aminophylline	SE	500 mg	WY	30 g	D5W	Nafcillin retained for 24 hr at 25 °C	27	C
	SE	500 mg	WY	2 g	D5W	14% nafcillin loss in 24 hr at 25 °C	27	I

Additive Compatibility (Cont.)

Nafcillin sodium

Drug	Mfr	Conc/L	Mfr	Conc/L	Test Soln	Remarks	Ref	C/I
Ascorbic acid	UP	500 mg	WY	5 g	D5W	Physically incompatible	15	I
Aztreonam	SQ	20 g	BR	20 g	D5W, NS[a]	Cloudiness and precipitate form. 7% aztreonam and 11% nafcillin loss in 24 hr at room temperature	1028	I
Bleomycin sulfate	BR	20 and 30 units	BR	2.5 g	NS	Substantial loss of bleomycin activity in 1 week at 4 °C	763	I
Chloramphenicol sodium succinate	PD	1 g	WY	500 mg		Physically compatible	27	C
Chlorothiazide sodium	MSD	500 mg	WY	500 mg		Physically compatible	27	C
Cytarabine	UP	100 mg		4 g	D5W	Heavy crystalline precipitation	174	I
Dexamethasone sodium phosphate	MSD	4 mg	WY	500 mg		Physically compatible	27	C
Dextran 40	PH	10%	WY	2 and 30 g	D5W	Physically compatible and stable for 24 hr at 25 °C	27	C
Diphenhydramine HCl	PD	50 mg	WY	500 mg		Physically compatible	27	C
Ephedrine sulfate		50 mg	WY	500 mg		Physically compatible	27	C
Gentamicin sulfate		75 mg		1 g	TPN #107[b]	10% gentamicin loss in 24 hr at 21 °C	1326	I
Heparin sodium	AB, WY	20,000 units	WY	500 mg		Physically compatible	27	C
	AB	20,000 units	WY	500 mg		Physically compatible	21	C
Hydrocortisone sodium succinate	UP	250 mg	WY	500 mg		Precipitate forms within 1 hr	27	I
Hydroxyzine HCl	PF	100 mg	WY	500 mg		Physically compatible	27	C
Lidocaine HCl	AST	0.6 g	AP	20 g	D5W[a], NS[c]	Visually compatible. Little nafcillin loss in 48 hr at 23 °C. Lidocaine not tested	1806	C
Methylprednisolone sodium succinate	UP	125 mg	WY	500 mg	D5W	Precipitate forms	329	I
Potassium chloride	TR	40 mEq	WY	30 g	NS	Nafcillin stable for 24 hr at 25 °C	27	C
	AB	40 mEq	WY	500 mg		Physically compatible	27	C
Prochlorperazine edisylate	SKF	10 mg	WY	500 mg		Physically compatible	27	C
Sodium bicarbonate	AB	40 mEq	WY	500 mg		Physically compatible	27	C
Sodium lactate	AB	50 mEq	WY	500 mg		Physically compatible	27	C
Verapamil HCl	KN	80 mg	WY	4 g	D5W, NS	Physically compatible for 24 hr	764	C
	SE	[d]	WY	40 g	D5W, NS	Cloudy solution clears with agitation	1166	?

[a]Tested in PVC containers.
[b]Refer to Appendix I for the composition of parenteral nutrition solutions. TPN indicates a 2-in-1 admixture.
[c]Tested in polyolefin containers.
[d]Final concentration unspecified.

Drugs in Syringe Compatibility

Nafcillin sodium

Drug (in syringe)	Mfr	Amt	Mfr	Amt	Remarks	Ref	C/I
Heparin sodium	AB	20,000 units/ 1 mL	WY	500 mg	Physically compatible for at least 30 min	21	C

Y-Site Injection Compatibility (1:1 Mixture)

Nafcillin sodium

Drug	Mfr	Conc	Mfr	Conc	Remarks	Ref	C/I
Acyclovir sodium	BW	5 mg/mL[a]	WY	20 mg/mL[a]	Physically compatible for 4 hr at 25 °C	1157	C
Atropine sulfate		0.4 mg/mL	WY	33 mg/mL[b]	No precipitation	547	C
Caspofungin acetate	ME	0.7 mg/mL[b]	SZ	20 mg/mL[b]	Transient turbidity becomes white precipitate	2758	I
Cyclophosphamide	MJ	20 mg/mL[a]	WY	20 mg/mL[a]	Physically compatible for 4 hr at 25 °C	1194	C
Diazepam		5 mg/mL	WY	33 mg/mL[b]	No precipitation	547	C
Diltiazem HCl	MMD	5 mg/mL	WY	10 mg/mL[b]	Cloudiness forms and persists	1807	I
	MMD	5 mg/mL	WY	200 mg/mL[b]	Cloudiness forms but clears with swirling	1807	?
	MMD	1 mg/mL[b]	WY	10 and 200 mg/mL[b]	Visually compatible	1807	C
Droperidol		2.5 mg/mL	WY	33 mg/mL[b]	Precipitate forms, probably free nafcillin	547	I
Enalaprilat	MSD	0.05 mg/mL[b]	BR	10 mg/mL[a]	Physically compatible for 24 hr at room temperature under fluorescent light	1355	C
Esmolol HCl	DCC	10 mg/mL[a]	BR	10 mg/mL[a]	Physically compatible for 24 hr at 22 °C	1169	C
Famotidine	MSD	0.2 mg/mL[a]	WY	15 mg/mL[b]	Physically compatible for 14 hr	1196	C
Fentanyl citrate		0.05 mg/mL	WY	33 mg/mL[b]	No precipitation	547	C
Fluconazole	RR	2 mg/mL	BR	20 mg/mL	Physically compatible for 24 hr at 25 °C	1407	C
Foscarnet sodium	AST	24 mg/mL	BR	20 mg/mL[c]	Physically compatible for 24 hr at 25 °C under fluorescent light	1393	C
Heparin sodium	TR	50 units/mL	WY	20 mg/mL[a]	Visually compatible for 4 hr at 25 °C	1793	C
Hydromorphone HCl	WY	0.2 mg/mL[a]	WY	20 mg/mL[a]	Physically compatible for 4 hr at 25 °C	987	C
Insulin, regular	LI	0.2 unit/mL[b]	BA	20 and 40 mg/mL[a]	Precipitates immediately	1395	I
Labetalol HCl	SC	1 mg/mL[a]	BR	10 mg/mL[a]	Cloudy precipitate forms immediately	1171	I
Magnesium sulfate	IX	16.7, 33.3, 66.7, 100 mg/ mL[a]	WY	20 mg/mL[a]	Physically compatible for at least 4 hr at 32 °C	813	C
Meperidine HCl	WY	10 mg/mL[a]	WY	20 mg/mL[a]	Cloudy haze cleared on mixing and remained clear for 4 hr at 25 °C	987	?
	WY	10 mg/mL[b]	WY	20 and 30 mg/mL[a]	Cloudy solution formed immediately and persisted for at least 1 hr at 25 °C	1338	I
Midazolam HCl	RC	1 mg/mL[a]	WY	20 mg/mL[a]	Immediate haze. Particles in 4 hr	1847	I
Morphine sulfate	WI	1 mg/mL[a]	WY	20 mg/mL[a]	Physically compatible for 4 hr at 25 °C	987	C
	ES	1 mg/mL[b]	WY	30 mg/mL[a]	Physically compatible for 1 hr at 25 °C	1338	C
Nalbuphine HCl		10 mg/mL	WY	33 mg/mL[b]	Precipitate forms, probably free nafcillin	547	I

Y-Site Injection Compatibility (1:1 Mixture) (Cont.)

Nafcillin sodium

Drug	Mfr	Conc	Mfr	Conc	Remarks	Ref	C/I
Nicardipine HCl	DCC	0.1 mg/mL[a]	BR	10 mg/mL[a]	Visually compatible for 24 hr at room temperature	235	C
Pentazocine lactate		30 mg/mL	WY	33 mg/mL[b]	Precipitate forms, probably free nafcillin	547	I
Propofol	ZEN	10 mg/mL	MAR	20 mg/mL[a]	Physically compatible for 1 hr at 23 °C	2066	C
Theophylline	TR	4 mg/mL	WY	20 mg/mL[a]	Visually compatible for 6 hr at 25 °C	1793	C
TNA #218 to #226[d]			BE, APC	20 mg/mL[a]	Visually compatible for 4 hr at 23 °C	2215	C
TPN #54[d]				250 mg/mL	Physically compatible and nafcillin activity retained over 6 hr at 22 °C	1045	C
TPN #61[d]		[e]	WY	250 mg/1 mL[f]	Physically compatible	1012	C
		[g]	WY	1.5 g/6 mL[f]	Physically compatible	1012	C
TPN #212 to #215[d]			BE	20 mg/mL[a]	Physically compatible for 4 hr at 23 °C	2109[d]	C
Vancomycin HCl	AB	20 mg/mL[a]	BE	250 mg/mL[i]	Transient precipitate forms followed by a visibly hazy solution	2189	I
	AB	20 mg/mL[a]	BE	10 and 50 mg/mL[b]	Gross white precipitate forms immediately	2189	I
	AB	20 mg/mL[a]	BE	1 mg/mL[b]	Physically compatible for 4 hr at 23 °C	2189	C
	AB	2 mg/mL[a]	BE	10[b], 50[b], 250[i] mg/mL	Subvisible measured haze forms immediately	2189	I
	AB	2 mg/mL[a]	BE	1 mg/mL[b]	Physically compatible for 4 hr at 23 °C	2189	C
Verapamil HCl		[h]			White milky precipitate forms immediately	840; 1303	I
	SE	2.5 mg/mL	WY	40 mg/mL[c]	White precipitate forms immediately. 20% of verapamil precipitated	1166	I
Zidovudine	BW	4 mg/mL[a]	BR	20 mg/mL[a]	Physically compatible for 4 hr at 25 °C	1193	C

[a]Tested in dextrose 5%.
[b]Tested in sodium chloride 0.9%.
[c]Tested in both dextrose 5% and sodium chloride 0.9%.
[d]Refer to Appendix I for the composition of parenteral nutrition solutions. TNA indicates a 3-in-1 admixture, and TPN indicates a 2-in-1 admixture.
[e]Run at 21 mL/hr.
[f]Given over five minutes by syringe pump.
[g]Run at 94 mL/hr.
[h]Injected into a line being used to infuse nafcillin sodium.
[i]Tested in sterile water for injection.

NALBUPHINE HYDROCHLORIDE
AHFS 28:08.12

Products — Nalbuphine hydrochloride is available as a 10-mg/mL concentration in 1-mL ampuls and 10-mL vials and as a 20-mg/mL concentration in 1-mL ampuls and 10-mL vials. Each milliliter of solution in vials also contains sodium citrate hydrous 0.94%, citric acid anhydrous 1.26%, methyl- and propylparabens 0.2%, and hydrochloric acid to adjust pH. The 10-mg/mL solution contains sodium chloride 0.2%. The ampul formulation contains no parabens. (1)

pH — The pH is adjusted to about pH 3.5 to 3.7. (1)

Administration — Nalbuphine hydrochloride is administered by subcutaneous, intramuscular, or intravenous injection. (1; 4)

Stability — Intact vials and ampuls should be protected from excessive light and stored at 15 to 30 °C. (1; 4)

Central Venous Catheter — Nalbuphine hydrochloride (Astra) 1 mg/mL in dextrose 5% was found to be compatible with the ARROWg+ard Blue Plus (Arrow International) chlorhexidine-bearing triple-lumen central catheter. Essentially complete delivery of the drug was found with little or no drug loss occurring. Furthermore, chlorhexidine delivered from the catheter remained at trace amounts with no substantial increase due to the delivery of the drug through the catheter. (2335)

Compatibility Information

Solution Compatibility

Nalbuphine HCl

Solution	Mfr	Mfr	Conc/L	Remarks	Ref	C/I
Dextrose 5% in sodium chloride 0.9%		DU	3.3 to 10 g	Physically compatible for 48 hr	128	**C**
Dextrose 10%		DU	3.3 to 10 g	Physically compatible for 48 hr	128	**C**
Ringer's injection, lactated		DU	3.3 to 10 g	Physically compatible for 48 hr	128	**C**
Sodium chloride 0.9%		DU	3.3 to 10 g	Physically compatible for 48 hr	128	**C**

Drugs in Syringe Compatibility

Nalbuphine HCl

Drug (in syringe)	Mfr	Amt	Mfr	Amt	Remarks	Ref	C/I
Atropine sulfate	WY	0.2 mg	EN	10 mg/ 1 mL	Physically compatible for 36 hr at 27 °C	762	**C**
	WY	0.2 mg	EN	5 mg/ 0.5 mL	Physically compatible for 36 hr at 27 °C	762	**C**
	WY	0.5 mg	EN	10 mg/ 1 mL	Physically compatible for 36 hr at 27 °C	762	**C**
	WY	0.5 mg	EN	5 mg/ 0.5 mL	Physically compatible for 36 hr at 27 °C	762	**C**
		0.4 and 1 mg	DU	10 mg/ 1 mL	Physically compatible for 48 hr	128	**C**
		0.4 and 1 mg	DU	20 mg/ 1 mL	Physically compatible for 48 hr	128	**C**
Diazepam	RC	5 mg/ 1 mL	EN	10 mg/ 1 mL	Immediate milky precipitate that persists for 36 hr at 27 °C	762	**I**
	RC	5 mg/ 1 mL	EN	5 mg/ 0.5 mL	Immediate milky precipitate that clears upon shaking. Clear for 36 hr at 27 °C	762	**?**
	RC	5 mg/ 1 mL	EN	2.5 mg/ 0.25 mL	Immediate milky precipitate that clears upon shaking. Clear for 36 hr at 27 °C	762	**?**
	RC	10 mg/ 2 mL	DU	10 mg/ 1 mL	Physically incompatible	128	**I**
	RC	10 mg/ 2 mL	DU	20 mg/ 1 mL	Physically incompatible	128	**I**
Diphenhydramine HCl	PD	50 mg/ 1 mL	DU	10 mg/ 1 mL	Physically compatible for 48 hr	128	**C**
	PD	50 mg/ 1 mL	DU	20 mg/ 1 mL	Physically compatible for 48 hr	128	**C**
Droperidol	JN	5 mg/ 2 mL	EN	5 mg/ 0.5 mL	Physically compatible for 36 hr at 27 °C	762	**C**
	JN	2.5 mg/ 1 mL	EN	10 mg/ 1 mL	Physically compatible for 36 hr at 27 °C	762	**C**
	JN	2.5 mg/ 1 mL	EN	5 mg/ 0.5 mL	Physically compatible for 36 hr at 27 °C	762	**C**
	JN	5 mg/ 2 mL	DU	10 mg/ 1 mL	Physically compatible for 48 hr	128	**C**
	JN	5 mg/ 2 mL	DU	20 mg/ 1 mL	Physically compatible for 48 hr	128	**C**

Drugs in Syringe Compatibility (Cont.)

Nalbuphine HCl

Drug (in syringe)	Mfr	Amt	Mfr	Amt	Remarks	Ref	C/I
Glycopyrrolate	RB	0.2 mg/ 1 mL	DU	10 mg/ 1 mL	Physically compatible for 48 hr	128	C
	RB	0.2 mg/ 1 mL	DU	20 mg/ 1 mL	Physically compatible for 48 hr	128	C
Hydroxyzine HCl	PF	50 mg	EN	10 mg/ 1 mL	Physically compatible for 36 hr at 27 °C	762	C
	PF	50 mg	EN	5 mg/ 0.5 mL	Physically compatible for 36 hr at 27 °C	762	C
	PF	50 mg	EN	2.5 mg/ 0.25 mL	Physically compatible for 36 hr at 27 °C	762	C
	PF	25 mg/ 1 mL	DU	10 mg/ 1 mL	Physically compatible for 48 hr	128	C
	PF	25 mg/ 1 mL	DU	20 mg/ 1 mL	Physically compatible for 48 hr	128	C
Ketorolac tromethamine	SY	180 mg/ 6 mL	DU	30 mg/ 3 mL	Solid white precipitate forms immediately and settles to bottom	1703	I
Lidocaine HCl		40 mg	DU	10 mg/ 1 mL	Physically compatible for 48 hr	128	C
		40 mg	DU	20 mg/ 1 mL	Physically compatible for 48 hr	128	C
Midazolam HCl	RC	5 mg/ 1 mL	DU	10 mg/ 1 mL	Physically compatible for 4 hr at 25 °C	1145	C
Pentobarbital sodium	WY	50 mg/ 1 mL	EN	10 mg/ 1 mL	Immediate white milky precipitate that persists for 36 hr at 27 °C	762	I
	WY	50 mg/ 1 mL	EN	2.5 mg/ 0.25 mL	Immediate white milky precipitate that clears upon vigorous shaking	762	I
	WY	50 mg/ 1 mL	EN	5 mg/ 0.5 mL	Immediate white milky precipitate that persists for 36 hr at 27 °C	762	I
Prochlorperazine edisylate	WY	5 mg/ 1 mL	EN	10 mg/ 1 mL	Physically compatible for 36 hr at 27 °C	762	C
	WY	5 mg/ 1 mL	EN	5 mg/ 0.5 mL	Physically compatible for 36 hr at 27 °C	762	C
	WY	5 mg/ 1 mL	EN	2.5 mg/ 0.25 mL	Physically compatible for 36 hr at 27 °C	762	C
	SKF	10 mg/ 2 mL	DU	10 mg/ 1 mL	Physically compatible for 48 hr	128	C
	SKF	10 mg/ 2 mL	DU	20 mg/ 1 mL	Physically compatible for 48 hr	128	C
Promethazine HCl	ES	25 mg	EN	10 mg/ 1 mL	Physically compatible for 36 hr at 27 °C	762	C
	ES	25 mg	EN	5 mg/ 0.5 mL	Physically compatible for 36 hr at 27 °C	762	C
	ES	12.5 mg	EN	10 mg/ 1 mL	Physically compatible for 36 hr at 27 °C	762	C
	WY	25 and 50 mg	DU	10 mg/ 1 mL	Physically incompatible	128	I
	WY	25 and 50 mg	DU	20 mg/ 1 mL	Physically incompatible	128	I
	WY	25 mg/ 1 mL	DU	10 mg/ 1 mL	White flocculent precipitate forms immediately	1184	I
	ES	25 mg/ 1 mL	DU	10 mg/ 1 mL	Physically compatible for 24 hr at room temperature	1184	C

Drugs in Syringe Compatibility (Cont.)

Nalbuphine HCl

Drug (in syringe)	Mfr	Amt	Mfr	Amt	Remarks	Ref	C/I
Ranitidine HCl	GL	50 mg/ 2 mL	EN	10 mg/ 1 mL	Physically compatible for 1 hr at 25 °C	978	**C**
Scopolamine HBr	BW	0.86 mg/ 1 mL	EN	10 mg/ 1 mL	Physically compatible for 36 hr at 27 °C	762	**C**
	BW	0.86 mg/ 1 mL	EN	5 mg/ 0.5 mL	Physically compatible for 36 hr at 27 °C	762	**C**
	BW	0.43 mg/ 0.5 mL	EN	10 mg/ 1 mL	Physically compatible for 36 hr at 27 °C	762	**C**
		0.4 mg	DU	10 mg/ 1 mL	Physically compatible for 48 hr	128	**C**
		0.4 mg	DU	20 mg/ 1 mL	Physically compatible for 48 hr	128	**C**
Trimethobenzamide HCl	BE	100 mg/ 1 mL	EN	10 mg/ 1 mL	Physically compatible for 36 hr at 27 °C	762	**C**
	BE	100 mg/ 1 mL	EN	5 mg/ 0.5 mL	Physically compatible for 36 hr at 27 °C	762	**C**
	BE	100 mg/ 1 mL	EN	2.5 mg/ 0.25 mL	Physically compatible for 36 hr at 27 °C	762	**C**
		200 mg/ 2 mL	DU	10 mg/ 1 mL	Physically compatible for 48 hr	128	**C**
		200 mg/ 2 mL	DU	20 mg/ 1 mL	Physically compatible for 48 hr	128	**C**

Y-Site Injection Compatibility (1:1 Mixture)

Nalbuphine HCl

Drug	Mfr	Conc	Mfr	Conc	Remarks	Ref	C/I
Acyclovir sodium	BV	5 mg/mL[b]	HOS	10 mg/mL	Physically compatible	2794	**C**
Allopurinol sodium	BW	3 mg/mL[b]	DU	10 mg/mL	Particles in 1 hr. Crystals in 4 hr	1686	**I**
Amifostine	USB	10 mg/mL[a]	AST	10 mg/mL	Physically compatible for 4 hr at 23 °C	1845	**C**
Amphotericin B cholesteryl sulfate complex	SEQ	0.83 mg/mL[a]	AST	10 mg/mL	Gross precipitate forms	2117	**I**
Aztreonam	SQ	40 mg/mL[a]	AST	10 mg/mL	Physically compatible for 4 hr at 23 °C	1758	**C**
Bivalirudin	TMC	5 mg/mL[a]	AST	10 mg/mL	Physically compatible for 4 hr at 23 °C	2373	**C**
Cisatracurium besylate	GW	0.1, 2, 5 mg/ mL[a]	AST	10 mg/mL	Physically compatible for 4 hr at 23 °C	2074	**C**
Cladribine	ORT	0.015[b] and 0.5[c] mg/mL	AST	10 mg/mL	Physically compatible for 4 hr at 23 °C	1969	**C**
Dexmedetomidine HCl	AB	4 mcg/mL[b]	AST	10 mg/mL	Physically compatible for 4 hr at 23 °C	2383	**C**
Docetaxel	RPR	0.9 mg/mL[a]	AST	10 mg/mL	Increase in measured subvisible turbidity occurs immediately	2224	**I**
Etoposide phosphate	BR	5 mg/mL[a]	AST	10 mg/mL	Physically compatible for 4 hr at 23 °C	2218	**C**
Fenoldopam mesylate	AB	80 mcg/mL[b]	EN	10 mg/mL	Physically compatible for 4 hr at 23 °C	2467	**C**
Filgrastim	AMG	30 mcg/mL[a]	DU	10 mg/mL	Physically compatible for 4 hr at 22 °C	1687	**C**
Fludarabine phosphate	BX	1 mg/mL[a]	DU	10 mg/mL	Visually compatible for 4 hr at 22 °C	1439	**C**
Gemcitabine HCl	LI	10 mg/mL[b]	AST	10 mg/mL	Physically compatible for 4 hr at 23 °C	2226	**C**
Granisetron HCl	SKB	0.05 mg/mL[a]	AB	10 mg/mL	Physically compatible for 4 hr at 23 °C	2000	**C**

Y-Site Injection Compatibility (1:1 Mixture) (Cont.)

Nalbuphine HCl

Drug	Mfr	Conc	Mfr	Conc	Remarks	Ref	C/I
Hetastarch in lactated electrolyte	AB	6%	AST	10 mg/mL	Physically compatible for 4 hr at 23 °C	2339	C
Linezolid	PHU	2 mg/mL	AST	10 mg/mL	Physically compatible for 4 hr at 23 °C	2264	C
Melphalan HCl	BW	0.1 mg/mL[b]	AST	10 mg/mL	Physically compatible for 3 hr at 22 °C	1557	C
Methotrexate sodium		30 mg/mL	DU	10 mg/mL	Yellow precipitate forms immediately	1788	I
Nafcillin sodium	WY	33 mg/mL[b]		10 mg/mL	Precipitate forms, probably free nafcillin	547	I
Oxaliplatin	SS	0.5 mg/mL[a]	EN	10 mg/mL	Physically compatible for 4 hr at 23 °C	2566	C
Paclitaxel	NCI	1.2 mg/mL[a]	AST	10 mg/mL	Physically compatible for 4 hr at 22 °C	1556	C
Pemetrexed disodium	LI	20 mg/mL[b]	EN	10 mg/mL	White precipitate forms immediately	2564	I
Piperacillin sodium–tazobactam sodium	LE[f]	40 + 5 mg/mL[a]	DU	10 mg/mL	Heavy white turbidity forms immediately. Particles form in 4 hr	1688	I
Propofol	ZEN	10 mg/mL	AB	10 mg/mL	Physically compatible for 1 hr at 23 °C	2066	C
Remifentanil HCl	GW	0.025 and 0.25 mg/mL[b]	AST	10 mg/mL	Physically compatible for 4 hr at 23 °C	2075	C
Sargramostim	IMM	10 mcg/mL[b]	DU	10 mg/mL	Haze and filament form	1436	I
Sodium bicarbonate		1.4%	DU	10 mg/mL	Gas evolves	1788	I
Teniposide	BR	0.1 mg/mL[a]	DU	10 mg/mL	Physically compatible for 4 hr at 23 °C	1725	C
Thiotepa	IMM[d]	1 mg/mL[a]	AST	10 mg/mL	Physically compatible for 4 hr at 23 °C	1861	C
TNA #218 to #226[e]			AB, AST	10 mg/mL	Damage to emulsion occurs immediately with free oil formation possible	2215	I
TPN #212 to #215[e]			AB	10 mg/mL	Physically compatible for 4 hr at 23 °C	2109	C
Vinorelbine tartrate	BW	1 mg/mL[b]	AST	10 mg/mL	Physically compatible for 4 hr at 22 °C	1558	C

[a]*Tested in dextrose 5%.*
[b]*Tested in sodium chloride 0.9%.*
[c]*Tested in bacteriostatic sodium chloride 0.9% preserved with benzyl alcohol 0.9%.*
[d]*Lyophilized formulation tested.*
[e]*Refer to Appendix I for the composition of parenteral nutrition solutions. TNA indicates a 3-in-1 admixture, and TPN indicates a 2-in-1 admixture.*
[f]*Test performed using the formulation WITHOUT edetate disodium.*

NALOXONE HYDROCHLORIDE
AHFS 28:10

Products — Naloxone hydrochloride is available in the following formulations (1):

Component	Preserved (mg/mL)		Paraben-Free (mg/mL)		
Naloxone HCl	1	0.4	1	0.4	0.02
Sodium chloride	8.35	8.6	9	9	9
Methyl- and propylparabens (9:1)	2	2			
Sizes (mL)	10	10	2	1	2

pH — The pH is adjusted during manufacturing with hydrochloric acid to a target pH of 3 to 4 (1-6/06) with a range of 3 to 6.5. (17)

Osmolality — The osmolality of the 0.02-mg/mL concentration was determined to be 293 mOsm/kg by freezing-point depression and 289 mOsm/kg by vapor pressure. (1071)

The osmolality of naloxone hydrochloride 0.4 mg/mL was determined to be 301 mOsm/kg. (1233)

Trade Name(s) — Narcan.

Administration — Naloxone hydrochloride may be administered by subcutaneous, intramuscular, or intravenous injection or by continuous intravenous infusion. Solutions for continuous intravenous infusion may be prepared as 2 mg/500 mL (4 mcg/mL) of sodium chloride 0.9% or dextrose 5%. (1; 4)

Stability — Naloxone hydrochloride should be stored at room temperature and protected from excessive light. Naloxone hydrochloride should not be mixed with bisulfite, sulfite, or long-chain or high molecular weight anions or any solution with an alkaline pH. (1; 4)

Naloxone hydrochloride under simulated summer conditions in paramedic vehicles was exposed to 26 to 38 °C over four weeks. Analysis found no loss of the drug under these conditions. (2562)

Syringes — Naloxone hydrochloride (Astra) 0.133 mg/mL in sodium chloride 0.9% packaged in polypropylene syringes (Sherwood) was physically stable and exhibited little or no loss in 24 hours stored at 4 and 23 °C. (2199)

Compatibility Information

Solution Compatibility

Naloxone HCl

Solution	Mfr	Mfr	Conc/L	Remarks	Ref	C/I
Dextrose 5%			4 mg	Discard after 24 hr	1	**C**
Sodium chloride 0.9%			4 mg	Discard after 24 hr	1	**C**

Additive Compatibility

Naloxone HCl

Drug	Mfr	Conc/L	Mfr	Conc/L	Test Soln	Remarks	Ref	C/I
Verapamil HCl	KN	80 mg	EN	0.8 mg	D5W, NS	Physically compatible for 24 hr	764	**C**

Drugs in Syringe Compatibility

Naloxone HCl

Drug (in syringe)	Mfr	Amt	Mfr	Amt	Remarks	Ref	C/I
Dimenhydrinate		10 mg/ 1 mL		0.4 mg/ 1 mL	Clear solution	2569	**C**
Heparin sodium		2500 units/ 1 mL	DU	0.4 mg/ 1 mL	Physically compatible for at least 5 min	1053	**C**
Ondansetron HCl	GW	1.33 mg/ mL[a]	AST	0.133 mg/mL[a]	Physically compatible. Under 6% ondansetron and under 5% naloxone losses in 24 hr at 4 or 23 °C	2199	**C**
Pantoprazole sodium	[b]	4 mg/ 1 mL		0.4 mg/ 1 mL	Precipitates within 4 hr	2574	**I**

[a]*Tested in sodium chloride 0.9%.*
[b]*Test performed using the formulation WITHOUT edetate disodium.*

Y-Site Injection Compatibility (1:1 Mixture)

Naloxone HCl

Drug	Mfr	Conc	Mfr	Conc	Remarks	Ref	C/I
Amphotericin B cholesteryl sulfate complex	SEQ	0.83 mg/mL[a]	AST	0.4 mg/mL	Gross precipitate forms	2117	**I**
Fenoldopam mesylate	AB	80 mcg/mL[b]	AB	0.4 mg/mL[b]	Physically compatible for 4 hr at 23 °C	2467	**C**
Linezolid	PHU	2 mg/mL	DU	0.4 mg/mL	Physically compatible for 4 hr at 23 °C	2264	**C**
Propofol	ZEN	10 mg/mL	AST	0.4 mg/mL	Physically compatible for 1 hr at 23 °C	2066	**C**

[a]*Tested in dextrose 5%.*
[b]*Tested in sodium chloride 0.9%.*

NEOSTIGMINE METHYLSULFATE
AHFS 12:04

Products — Neostigmine methylsulfate is available in concentrations of 0.5 and 1 mg/mL in 10-mL vials with methyl- and propylparabens 0.2%. (1)

pH — The pH is adjusted to near 5.9 with a range of 5 to 6.5. (1; 17)

Administration — Neostigmine methylsulfate may be administered intramuscularly, subcutaneously, or slowly intravenously. (1; 4)

Stability — Neostigmine methylsulfate in intact containers should be stored at controlled room temperature and protected from light, freezing, and temperatures of 40 °C or more. (1; 4)

Syringes — The stability of neostigmine 0.5 mg/mL repackaged in polypropylene syringes was evaluated. Little concentration change was found after four weeks of storage at room temperature not exposed to direct light. (2164)

Neostigmine methylsulfate (Elkins-Sinn) 0.167 mg/mL in sodium chloride 0.9% packaged in polypropylene syringes (Sherwood) was physically stable and exhibited no loss in 24 hours stored at 4 and 23 °C. (2199)

Undiluted neostigmine methylsulfate (American Pharmaceutical Partners) 1 mg/mL was packaged in 6-mL polypropylene syringes (Becton Dickinson) and stored at 23 °C in fluorescent light and at 4 °C for 90 days. The drug remained physically stable and under 2% loss occurred. (2425)

Compatibility Information

Drugs in Syringe Compatibility

Neostigmine methylsulfate

Drug (in syringe)	Mfr	Amt	Mfr	Amt	Remarks	Ref	C/I
Glycopyrrolate	RB	0.2 mg/ 1 mL	RC	0.5 mg/ 1 mL	Physically compatible. pH in glycopyrrolate stability range for 48 hr at 25 °C	331	C
	RB	0.2 mg/ 1 mL	RC	1 mg/ 2 mL	Physically compatible. pH in glycopyrrolate stability range for 48 hr at 25 °C	331	C
	RB	0.4 mg/ 2 mL	RC	0.5 mg/ 1 mL	Physically compatible. pH in glycopyrrolate stability range for 48 hr at 25 °C	331	C
Heparin sodium		2500 units/ 1 mL	RC	0.5 mg/ 1 mL	Physically compatible for at least 5 min	1053	C
Ondansetron HCl	GW	1.33 mg/ mL[a]	ES	0.167 mg/mL[a]	Physically compatible. Under 3% ondansetron and under 5% neostigmine losses in 24 hr at 4 or 23 °C	2199	C
Pentobarbital sodium	AB	500 mg/ 10 mL	RC	0.5 mg/ 1 mL	Physically compatible	55	C

[a]*Tested in sodium chloride 0.9%.*

Y-Site Injection Compatibility (1:1 Mixture)

Neostigmine methylsulfate

Drug	Mfr	Conc	Mfr	Conc	Remarks	Ref	C/I
Heparin sodium	UP	1000 units/L[a]	RC	0.5 mg/mL	Physically compatible for 4 hr at room temperature	534	C
Hydrocortisone sodium succinate	UP	10 mg/L[a]	RC	0.5 mg/mL	Physically compatible for 4 hr at room temperature	534	C
Palonosetron HCl	MGI	50 mcg/mL	BA	0.5 mg/mL	Physically compatible. No loss of either drug in 4 hr	2772	C
Potassium chloride	AB	40 mEq/L[a]	RC	0.5 mg/mL	Physically compatible for 4 hr at room temperature	534	C

[a]*Tested in dextrose 5% in Ringer's injection, dextrose 5% in Ringer's injection, lactated, dextrose 5%, Ringer's injection, lactated, and sodium chloride 0.9%.*

NESIRITIDE
AHFS 24:12.92

Products — Nesiritide is available in 1.5-mg single-use vials containing 1.58 mg of nesiritide with mannitol 20 mg, citric acid monohydrate 2.1 mg, and sodium citrate dihydrate 2.94 mg. (1)

Reconstitute nesiritide using 5 mL of solution from a 250-mL plastic intravenous infusion container of dextrose 5%, sodium chloride 0.9%, dextrose 5% in sodium chloride 0.45%, or dextrose 5% in sodium chloride 0.2%, yielding a nesiritide concentration of 0.32 mg/mL. Gently rock the vial to aid dissolution making sure all surfaces, including the stopper, are in contact with the diluent; do not shake the vial. The reconstituted solution should be clear and colorless. Add the entire contents of the vial into the 250-mL plastic infusion solution container and invert several times to yield a nesiritide infusion concentration of 6 mcg/mL. (1)

Trade Name(s) — Natrecor.

Administration — Nesiritide is administered by an initial intravenous injection drawn from the intravenous infusion solution and given over about one minute followed by continuous intravenous infusion. The intravenous tubing should be primed with 5 mL of the solution before connecting to the patient's access port and before administering the initial bolus dose or beginning the infusion. (1)

Stability — Intact vials should be stored below 25 °C in the original carton to protect from light. Protect the vials from freezing. (1)

The manufacturer states that the reconstituted nesiritide should be used within 24 hours stored between 2 and 25 °C because no antimicrobial preservative is present. (1)

Nesiritide is incompatible with sodium metabisulfite and other bisulfite antioxidants used in some drug formulations. The specific formulation of the product to be used should be checked to ensure that no sulfite antioxidants are present. Drugs that contain sulfite antioxidants should not be administered into the same intravenous infusion line as nesiritide. The line should be flushed between administration of the incompatible drugs and nesiritide. (1; 2625)

Sorption — The official product labeling states that nesiritide may bind to heparin-coated administration catheters decreasing the delivery of nesiritide to the patient and that heparin-coated administration lines must not be used to administer nesiritide. (1)

However, a study of nesiritide delivery through unprimed PVC and polyethylene tubing, a polyurethane central catheter, and a heparin-coated PVC catheter found little alteration of the delivered concentration. About 94 to 98% of the drug was delivered through these devices compared to 98% through primed PVC tubing alone. (2646)

Compatibility Information

Y-Site Injection Compatibility (1:1 Mixture)

Nesiritide

Drug	Mfr	Conc	Mfr	Conc	Remarks	Ref	C/I
Amiodarone HCl		50 mg/mL	SCI	50 mcg/mL[a,b]	Physically compatible for 4 hr	2625	C
Argatroban	SKB	1 mg/mL[a]	SCI	6 mcg/mL[a]	Physically compatible for 24 hr at 23 °C	2572	C
Bumetanide		0.25 mg/mL	SCI	50 mcg/mL[a,b]	Physically incompatible	2625	I
Digoxin		0.25 mg/mL	SCI	50 mcg/mL[a,b]	Physically compatible for 4 hr	2625	C
Diltiazem HCl		5 mg/mL	SCI	50 mcg/mL[a,b]	Physically compatible for 4 hr	2625	C
Dobutamine HCl		12.5 mg/mL	SCI	50 mcg/mL[a,b]	Physically compatible for 4 hr. May be chemically incompatible with nesiritide[c]	2625	?
Dopamine HCl		80 mg/mL	SCI	50 mcg/mL[a,b]	Physically compatible for 4 hr. May be chemically incompatible with nesiritide[c]	2625	?
Enalaprilat		1.25 mg/mL	SCI	50 mcg/mL[a,b]	Physically incompatible	2625	I
Epinephrine HCl		1 mg/mL	SCI	50 mcg/mL[a,b]	Physically compatible for 4 hr. May be chemically incompatible with nesiritide[c]	2625	?
Ethacrynate sodium		1 mg/mL	SCI	50 mcg/mL[a,b]	Physically incompatible	2625	I
Fentanyl citrate		0.05 mg/mL	SCI	50 mcg/mL[a,b]	Physically compatible for 4 hr	2625	C
Furosemide		10 mg/mL	SCI	50 mcg/mL[a,b]	Physically incompatible	2625	I
Heparin sodium		0.1, 1, 10 units/mL	SCI	50 mcg/mL[a,b]	Physically incompatible	2625	I
Hydralazine HCl		20 mg/mL	SCI	50 mcg/mL[a,b]	Physically incompatible	2625	I
Insulin, regular		Up to 100 units/mL	SCI	50 mcg/mL[a,b]	Physically incompatible	2625	I

Y-Site Injection Compatibility (1:1 Mixture) (Cont.)

Nesiritide

Drug	Mfr	Conc	Mfr	Conc	Remarks	Ref	C/I
Lidocaine HCl		20 mg/mL	SCI	50 mcg/mL[a,b]	Physically compatible for 4 hr. May be chemically incompatible with nesiritide[c]	2625	?
Meperidine HCl		100 mg/mL	SCI	50 mcg/mL[a,b]	Physically compatible for 4 hr. May be chemically incompatible with nesiritide[c]	2625	?
Metoprolol tartrate		1 mg/mL	SCI	50 mcg/mL[a,b]	Physically compatible for 4 hr	2625	C
	BED	1 mg/mL	SCI	6 mcg/mL[a]	Trace precipitate in 24 hr at 19 °C	2795	I
Micafungin sodium	ASP	1.5 mg/mL[b]	SCI	6 mcg/mL[a]	Microparticulates form immediately	2683	I
Milrinone lactate		1 mg/mL	SCI	50 mcg/mL[a,b]	Physically compatible for 4 hr	2625	C
Morphine sulfate		15 mg/mL	SCI	50 mcg/mL[a,b]	Physically compatible for 4 hr. May be chemically incompatible with nesiritide[c]	2625	?
Nicardipine HCl		2.5 mg/mL	SCI	50 mcg/mL[a,b]	Physically compatible for 4 hr	2625	C
Nitroglycerin		0.2 mg/mL	SCI	50 mcg/mL[a,b]	Physically compatible for 4 hr	2625	C
Norepinephrine bitartrate		1 mg/mL	SCI	50 mcg/mL[a,b]	Physically compatible for 4 hr. May be chemically incompatible with nesiritide[c]	2625	?
Phenylephrine HCl		10 mg/mL	SCI	50 mcg/mL[a,b]	Physically compatible for 4 hr. May be chemically incompatible with nesiritide[c]	2625	?
Procainamide HCl		500 mg/mL	SCI	50 mcg/mL[a,b]	Physically compatible for 4 hr. May be chemically incompatible with nesiritide[c]	2625	?
Propranolol HCl		1 mg/mL	SCI	50 mcg/mL[a,b]	Physically compatible for 4 hr	2625	C
Quinidine gluconate		80 mg/mL	SCI	50 mcg/mL[a,b]	Physically compatible for 4 hr	2625	C
Sodium nitroprusside		5 mg/mL	SCI	50 mcg/mL[a,b]	Physically compatible for 4 hr	2625	C
Torsemide		10 mg/mL	SCI	50 mcg/mL[a,b]	Physically compatible for 4 hr	2625	C
Verapamil HCl		2.5 mg/mL	SCI	50 mcg/mL[a,b]	Physically compatible for 4 hr	2625	C

[a]*Tested in dextrose 5%.*
[b]*Tested in sodium chloride 0.9%.*
[c]*Nesiritide is incompatible with bisulfite antioxidants used in some drug formulations. The specific formulation of the product to be used should be checked to ensure that no sulfite antioxidants are present.*

NICARDIPINE HYDROCHLORIDE
AHFS 24:28.08

Products — Nicardipine hydrochloride is available as a 2.5-mg/mL concentrate in 10-mL ampuls. Each milliliter also contains sorbitol 48 mg, citric acid monohydrate 0.525 mg, and sodium hydroxide 0.09 mg in water for injection. Additional citric acid and/or sodium hydroxide may have been added to adjust solution pH. (1)

pH — Buffered to pH 3.5. (1)

Trade Name(s) — Cardene I.V.

Administration — Nicardipine hydrochloride must be diluted for use. It is administered as a slow continuous intravenous infusion at a concentration of 0.1 mg/mL. The infusion is prepared by adding 10 mL of nicardipine hydrochloride (25 mg) to 240 mL of compatible infusion solution, making 250 mL of a 0.1-mg/mL solution. If nicardipine hydrochloride is administered via a peripheral vein, the infusion site should be changed every 12 hours to avoid venous irritation. (1; 4)

Stability — Intact ampuls of the clear, yellow solution should be stored at controlled room temperature and protected from light. Freezing does not adversely affect the product, but exposure to elevated temperatures should be avoided. (1)

Light Effects — Deliberate exposure of a 0.1-mg/mL nicardipine hydrochloride solution to daylight resulted in about 8% loss in seven hours and 21% loss in 14 hours. Protection from light may be considered. (2193)

Sorption — Nicardipine hydrochloride (Dupont Merck) 50 and 500 mg/L in a variety of infusion solutions in PVC containers showed a decline in concentration due to sorption to the plastic. Losses were rapid in Ringer's injection, lactated with up to 42% lost in 24 hours. The concentrations were stable in glass containers. (1380)

Compatibility Information

Solution Compatibility

Nicardipine HCl

Solution	Mfr	Mfr	Conc/L	Remarks	Ref	C/I
Dextrose 5% in Ringer's injection, lactated	MG[a]	DME	50 and 500 mg	Physically compatible. 7% loss in 7 days at room temperature in light	1380	C
	TR[b]	DME	500 mg	Physically compatible. 7% loss in 24 hr at room temperature in light	1380	C
	TR[b]	DME	50 mg	Physically compatible. 11% loss in 24 hr at room temperature in light	1380	I
Dextrose 5% in sodium chloride 0.45%	a,b		100 mg	Stable for 24 hr at room temperature	1	C
	MG[a]	DME	50 and 500 mg	Physically compatible. Little loss in 7 days at room temperature in light	1380	C
	TR[b]	DME	50 and 500 mg	Physically compatible. 9% loss in 72 hr at room temperature in light	1380	C
Dextrose 5% in sodium chloride 0.9%	a,b		100 mg	Stable for 24 hr at room temperature	1	C
	MG[a]	DME	50 and 500 mg	Physically compatible. Little loss in 7 days at room temperature in light	1380	C
	TR[b]	DME	50 and 500 mg	Physically compatible. 7% loss in 7 days at room temperature in light	1380	C
Dextrose 5%	a,b		100 mg	Stable for 24 hr at room temperature	1	C
	MG[a]	DME	50 and 500 mg	Physically compatible. Little loss in 7 days at room temperature in light	1380	C
	TR[b]	DME	500 mg	Physically compatible. 6% loss in 7 days at room temperature in light	1380	C
	TR[b]	DME	50 mg	Physically compatible. 13% loss in 24 hr at room temperature in light	1380	I
Ringer's injection, lactated				Incompatible	1	I
	MG[a]	DME	50 and 500 mg	Physically compatible. Little loss in 7 days at room temperature in light	1380	C
	TR[b]	DME	500 mg	Physically compatible. 15% loss in 24 hr at room temperature in light	1380	I
	TR[b]	DME	50 mg	Physically compatible. 42% loss in 24 hr at room temperature in light	1380	I
Sodium chloride 0.45%	a,b		100 mg	Stable for 24 hr at room temperature	1	C
	MG[a]	DME	50 and 500 mg	Physically compatible. Little loss in 7 days at room temperature in light	1380	C
	TR[b]	DME	500 mg	Physically compatible. 3% loss in 7 days at room temperature in light	1380	C
	TR[b]	DME	50 mg	Physically compatible. 11% loss in 24 hr at room temperature in light	1380	I
Sodium chloride 0.9%	a,b		100 mg	Stable for 24 hr at room temperature	1	C
	MG[a]	DME	50 and 500 mg	Physically compatible. Little loss in 7 days at room temperature in light	1380	C
	TR[b]	DME	50 and 500 mg	Physically compatible. 8% loss in 72 hr at room temperature in light	1380	C

[a]Tested in glass containers.
[b]Tested in PVC containers.

Additive Compatibility

Nicardipine HCl

Drug	Mfr	Conc/L	Mfr	Conc/L	Test Soln	Remarks	Ref	C/I
Potassium chloride	ES	40 mEq	DME	50 and 500 mg	D5W[a]	Physically compatible. Little loss in 7 days at room temperature in light	1380	**C**
	ES	40 mEq	DME	50 and 500 mg	D5W[b]	Physically compatible. 12% loss in 7 days at room temperature in light	1380	**C**
Sodium bicarbonate	TR[a]	5%	DME	50 and 500 mg		Precipitate forms immediately	1380	**I**

[a]Tested in glass containers.
[b]Tested in PVC containers.

Y-Site Injection Compatibility (1:1 Mixture)

Nicardipine HCl

Drug	Mfr	Conc	Mfr	Conc	Remarks	Ref	C/I
Amikacin sulfate	BR	2 mg/mL[a]	DCC	0.1 mg/mL[a]	Visually compatible for 24 hr at room temperature	235	**C**
Aminophylline	ES	1 mg/mL[a]	DCC	0.1 mg/mL[a]	Visually compatible for 24 hr at room temperature	235	**C**
Ampicillin sodium	BR	10 mg/mL[a,b]	DCC	0.1 mg/mL[a,b]	Turbidity forms immediately	235	**I**
Ampicillin sodium–sulbactam sodium	PF	10 + 5 mg/mL[a,b]	DCC	0.1 mg/mL[a,b]	Turbidity forms immediately	235	**I**
Aztreonam	SQ	10 mg/mL[a]	DCC	0.1 mg/mL[a]	Visually compatible for 24 hr at room temperature	235	**C**
Butorphanol tartrate	BR	0.4 mg/mL[a]	DCC	0.1 mg/mL[a]	Visually compatible for 24 hr at room temperature	235	**C**
Calcium gluconate	ES	0.092 mEq/mL[a]	DCC	0.1 mg/mL[a]	Visually compatible for 24 hr at room temperature	235	**C**
Cefazolin sodium	SKF	20 mg/mL[a]	DCC	0.1 mg/mL[a]	Visually compatible for 24 hr at room temperature	235	**C**
Cefepime HCl	BMS	120 mg/mL[c]		1 mg/mL	Precipitates	2513	**I**
Ceftazidime	GL	10 mg/mL[a]	DCC	0.1 mg/mL[a]	Visually compatible for 24 hr at room temperature	235	**C**
	SKB	125 mg/mL		1 mg/mL	Precipitates immediately	2434	**I**
	GSK	120 mg/mL[c]		1 mg/mL	Precipitates	2513	**I**
Chloramphenicol sodium succinate	PD	10 mg/mL[a]	DCC	0.1 mg/mL[a]	Visually compatible for 24 hr at room temperature	235	**C**
Clindamycin phosphate	UP	9 mg/mL[a]	DCC	0.1 mg/mL[a]	Visually compatible for 24 hr at room temperature	235	**C**
Dextran 40 in dextrose 5%	TR	10%	DCC	0.1 mg/mL[a]	Visually compatible for 24 hr at room temperature	235	**C**
Diltiazem HCl	MMD	1 mg/mL[a]	WY	1 mg/mL[a]	Visually compatible for 4 hr at 27 °C	2062	**C**
Dobutamine HCl	LI	4 mg/mL[a]	WY	1 mg/mL[a]	Visually compatible for 4 hr at 27 °C	2062	**C**
	LI	1 mg/mL[a]	DCC	0.1 mg/mL[a]	Visually compatible for 24 hr at room temperature	235	**C**
Dopamine HCl	AB	3.2 mg/mL[a]	WY	1 mg/mL[a]	Visually compatible for 4 hr at 27 °C	2062	**C**
	IMS	1.6 mg/mL[a]	DCC	0.1 mg/mL[a]	Visually compatible for 24 hr at room temperature	235	**C**

Y-Site Injection Compatibility (1:1 Mixture) (Cont.)

Nicardipine HCl

Drug	Mfr	Conc	Mfr	Conc	Remarks	Ref	C/I
Enalaprilat	MSD	0.05 mg/mL[b]	DU	0.1 mg/mL[a]	Physically compatible for 24 hr at room temperature under fluorescent light	1355	C
	MSD	0.5 mg/mL[a]	DCC	0.1 mg/mL[a]	Visually compatible for 24 hr at room temperature	235	C
Epinephrine HCl	AB	0.02 mg/mL[a]	WY	1 mg/mL[a]	Visually compatible for 4 hr at 27 °C	2062	C
Erythromycin lactobionate	AB	5 mg/mL[a]	DCC	0.1 mg/mL[a]	Visually compatible for 24 hr at room temperature	235	C
Esmolol HCl	DU	10 mg/mL[a]	DCC	0.1 mg/mL[a]	Visually compatible for 24 hr at room temperature	235	C
Famotidine	MSD	0.2 mg/mL[a]	DCC	0.1 mg/mL[a]	Visually compatible for 24 hr at room temperature	235	C
Fenoldopam mesylate	AB	80 mcg/mL[b]	WAY	1 mg/mL[b]	Physically compatible for 4 hr at 23 °C	2467	C
Fentanyl citrate	ES	0.05 mg/mL	WY	1 mg/mL[a]	Visually compatible for 4 hr at 27 °C	2062	C
	ES	2 mcg/mL[a]	DCC	0.1 mg/mL[a]	Visually compatible for 24 hr at room temperature	235	C
Furosemide	AMR	10 mg/mL	WY	1 mg/mL[a]	Precipitate forms immediately	2062	I
Gentamicin sulfate	ES	0.8 mg/mL[a]	DCC	0.1 mg/mL[a]	Visually compatible for 24 hr at room temperature	235	C
Heparin sodium	ES	100 units/mL[a]	WY	1 mg/mL[a]	Precipitate forms immediately	2062	I
	IX	40 units/mL[a]	DCC	0.1 mg/mL[a]	Visually compatible for 24 hr at room temperature	235	C
Hetastarch in sodium chloride 0.9%	DU	6%	DCC	0.1 mg/mL[a]	Visually compatible for 24 hr at room temperature	235	C
Hydrocortisone sodium succinate	UP	2 mg/mL[a]	DCC	0.1 mg/mL[a]	Visually compatible for 24 hr at room temperature	235	C
Hydromorphone HCl	KN	1 mg/mL	WY	1 mg/mL[a]	Visually compatible for 4 hr at 27 °C	2062	C
Labetalol HCl	AH	2 mg/mL[a]	WY	1 mg/mL[a]	Visually compatible for 4 hr at 27 °C	2062	C
	GL	1 mg/mL[a]	DCC	0.1 mg/mL[a]	Visually compatible for 24 hr at room temperature	235	C
Lidocaine HCl	AST	4 mg/mL[a]	DCC	0.1 mg/mL[a]	Visually compatible for 24 hr at room temperature	235	C
Linezolid	PHU	2 mg/mL	WAY	1 mg/mL[a]	Physically compatible for 4 hr at 23 °C	2264	C
Lorazepam	WY	0.5 mg/mL[a]	WY	1 mg/mL[a]	Visually compatible for 4 hr at 27 °C	2062	C
Magnesium sulfate	LY	10 mg/mL[a]	DCC	0.1 mg/mL[a]	Visually compatible for 24 hr at room temperature	235	C
Methylprednisolone sodium succinate	UP	0.8 mg/mL[a]	DCC	0.1 mg/mL[a]	Visually compatible for 24 hr at room temperature	235	C
Metronidazole	SE	5 mg/mL	DCC	0.1 mg/mL[a]	Visually compatible for 24 hr at room temperature	235	C
Micafungin sodium	ASP	1.5 mg/mL[b]	ESP	1 mg/mL[b]	Precipitate forms immediately	2683	I
Midazolam HCl	RC	2 mg/mL[a]	WY	1 mg/mL[a]	Visually compatible for 4 hr at 27 °C	2062	C
Milrinone lactate	SW	0.2 mg/mL[a]	WY	1 mg/mL[a]	Visually compatible for 4 hr at 27 °C	2062	C
Morphine sulfate	SCN	2 mg/mL[a]	WY	1 mg/mL[a]	Visually compatible for 4 hr at 27 °C	2062	C
	WY	0.2 mg/mL[a]	DCC	0.1 mg/mL[a]	Visually compatible for 24 hr at room temperature	235	C

Y-Site Injection Compatibility (1:1 Mixture) (Cont.)

Nicardipine HCl

Drug	Mfr	Conc	Mfr	Conc	Remarks	Ref	C/I
Nafcillin sodium	BR	10 mg/mL[a]	DCC	0.1 mg/mL[a]	Visually compatible for 24 hr at room temperature	235	C
Nesiritide	SCI	50 mcg/mL[a,b]		2.5 mg/mL	Physically compatible for 4 hr	2625	C
Nitroglycerin	AB	0.4 mg/mL[a]	WY	1 mg/mL[a]	Visually compatible for 4 hr at 27 °C	2062	C
Norepinephrine bitartrate	AB	0.128 mg/mL[a]	WY	1 mg/mL[a]	Visually compatible for 4 hr at 27 °C	2062	C
Penicillin G potassium	PF	50,000 units/mL[a]	DCC	0.1 mg/mL[a]	Visually compatible for 24 hr at room temperature	235	C
Potassium chloride	LY	0.4 mEq/mL[a]	DCC	0.1 mg/mL[a]	Visually compatible for 24 hr at room temperature	235	C
Potassium phosphates	LY	0.44 mEq/mL[a]	DCC	0.1 mg/mL[a]	Visually compatible for 24 hr at room temperature	235	C
Ranitidine HCl	GL	1 mg/mL[a]	WY	1 mg/mL[a]	Visually compatible for 4 hr at 27 °C	2062	C
	GL	0.5 mg/mL[a]	DCC	0.1 mg/mL[a]	Visually compatible for 24 hr at room temperature	235	C
Sodium acetate	LY	0.4 mEq/mL[a]	DCC	0.1 mg/mL[a]	Visually compatible for 24 hr at room temperature	235	C
Sodium nitroprusside	LY	0.2 mg/mL[a]	DCC	0.1 mg/mL[a]	Visually compatible for 24 hr at room temperature	235	C
Tobramycin sulfate	LI	0.8 mg/mL[a]	DCC	0.1 mg/mL[a]	Visually compatible for 24 hr at room temperature	235	C
Trimethoprim–sulfamethoxazole	QU	0.16 + 0.8 mg/mL[a]	DCC	0.1 mg/mL[a]	Visually compatible for 24 hr at room temperature	235	C
Vancomycin HCl	LE	5 mg/mL[a]	DCC	0.1 mg/mL[a]	Visually compatible for 24 hr at room temperature	235	C
Vecuronium bromide	OR	1 mg/mL	WY	1 mg/mL[a]	Visually compatible for 4 hr at 27 °C	2062	C

[a]Tested in dextrose 5%.
[b]Tested in sodium chloride 0.9%.
[c]Tested in sterile water for injection.

NIMODIPINE
AHFS 24:28.08

Products — Nimodipine 0.02% (0.2 mg/mL) is available in 50-mL brown glass vials and 250-mL brown glass bottles. The product also contains ethanol 20% (w/v), polyethylene glycol 400, sodium citrate, citric acid, and water for injection. (38; 115)

Administration — Nimodipine is given by intravenous infusion via a central catheter (38; 115); use of an infusion pump has been recommended. (115) Intracisternal instillation has also been described. (115) The drug must not be added to an infusion bag or bottle. For administration, nimodipine injection is drawn into a 50-mL syringe and connected to a three-way stopcock and polyethylene tube that permits simultaneous administration of the nimodipine and a co-infusion running at a rate of 40 mL/hr. Dextrose 5%, sodium chloride 0.9%, lactated Ringer's injection, lactated Ringer's injection with magnesium, dextran 40, mannitol 10%, albumin human 5%, and hetastarch 6% in sodium chloride 0.9% have been recommended for use as the co-infusion solution. (38; 115)

Stability — Nimodipine injection is a clear yellow solution. Intact containers of the drug should be stored at or below 25 °C. The drug is light sensitive and should be stored in the light-protective container within the carton that is supplied with the product. Nimodipine should not be added to infusion solution bags or bottles or mixed with other drugs. The 250-mL bottles are intended for single use only and should be pierced only once. Once pierced, the bottle should be used for no longer than 25 hours regardless of whether all of the solution has been administered. (38; 115)

Light Effects — Nimodipine is light sensitive. The drug drawn into a syringe for administration must be protected from direct sunlight during administration but is stable for up to 10 hours exposed to diffuse daylight and artificial light. The 250-mL infusion bottle should also be protected from direct sunlight at all times. Opaque coverings for infusion pumps and tubing or black, brown, yellow, or red infusion lines can be used when needed. (38; 115)

Sorption — Nimodipine reacts with PVC equipment but is compatible with polyethylene and polypropylene containers, syringes, and administration sets as well as glass containers. (38; 115)

Nimodipine (Bayer) 0.01 mg/mL in dextrose 5% and sodium chloride 0.9% packaged in PVC, polyethylene, and glass containers exhibited only 3 to 5% loss in glass and polyethylene containers but 94% loss due to sorption in PVC containers when stored at 4 and 22 °C for 24 hours protected from light. (2289)

Compatibility Information

Solution Compatibility

Nimodipine

Solution	Mfr	Mfr	Conc/L	Remarks	Ref	C/I
Dextrose 5%	BA[a]	BAY	10 mg	Visually compatible. 94% loss to PVC at 22 °C and 81% loss at 4 °C in 24 hr	2289	I
	BRN[b,c]	BAY	10 mg	Visually compatible. 3 to 5% loss in 24 hr at 4 and 22 °C	2289	C
Sodium chloride 0.9%	BA[a]	BAY	10 mg	Visually compatible. 94% loss to PVC at 22 °C and 81% loss at 4 °C in 24 hr	2289	I
	BRN[b,c]	BAY	10 mg	Visually compatible. 3 to 5% loss in 24 hr at 4 and 22 °C	2289	C

[a]Tested in PVC containers.
[b]Tested in glass containers.
[c]Tested in polyethylene containers.

NITROGLYCERIN
AHFS 24:12.08

Products — Nitroglycerin injection is available in a 5-mg/mL concentration in 5- and 10-mL vials. The product also contains ethanol 30% and propylene glycol 30% in water for injection. The pH may have been adjusted during manufacture with sodium hydroxide and/or hydrochloric acid. Nitroglycerin injection must be diluted before use. (1; 4)

Nitroglycerin is available premixed in dextrose 5% at concentrations of 100, 200, and 400 mcg/mL in 250- and 500-mL containers. The Baxter premixed infusions contain propylene glycol and ethanol with citric acid as a buffer and sodium hydroxide and/or hydrochloric acid, if necessary, to adjust the pH during manufacturing. The Hospira premixed infusions also contain propylene glycol (but no ethanol) and nitric acid to adjust pH during manufacturing. (1)

pH — The concentrate for injection has a pH of 3 to 6.5. (1; 4) The Baxter premixed infusion solution has a pH of 4 (range 3 to 5). The Hospira premixed infusion solution also has a pH of about 4 but with a range of 3 to 6.5. (1)

Osmolarity — The osmolarities of the nitroglycerin premixed infusions solutions in dextrose 5% vary by manufacturer but are all within the normal range for infusions (1):

Nitroglycerin Concentration	Osmolarity (mOsm/L)	
	Hospira	Baxter
100 mcg/mL	265	428
200 mcg/mL	277	440
400 mcg/mL	301	465

Administration — Nitroglycerin injection is administered by intravenous infusion after dilution in dextrose 5% or sodium chloride 0.9% contained in glass bottles, using an infusion control device. The use of filters should be avoided. Various concentrations and administration rates are utilized, depending on the fluid requirements of the patient and the duration of therapy. An initial concentration of 50 to 100 mcg/mL, with adjustment to the concentration if necessary, has been recommended. The concentration should not exceed 400 mcg/mL. (1; 4)

Because of nitroglycerin sorption into PVC plastic, dosing is higher with standard PVC administration sets and should be reduced when nonabsorbing administration sets are used. (4)

Inaccurate nitroglycerin dosing may occur with nonabsorbing high-density polyethylene plastic administration sets. Such tubing is less pliable than PVC and may not work well with some infusion control devices designed for PVC tubing, resulting in overinfusion. (729; 730; 731; 1120)

Stability — Nitroglycerin injections are practically colorless and stable in the intact containers. The solutions are not explosive. Storage should be at controlled room temperature; the containers should be protected from freezing. (1; 4) Exposure to light, even high intensity light, does not adversely affect nitroglycerin stability. (506; 510; 928; 930; 1941)

pH Effects — The rate of nitroglycerin hydrolysis becomes significant at low pH values and is also quite rapid in alkaline solutions. (933) In neutral to weakly acidic solutions, the drug is stable. No loss was observed over 136 days at room temperature at pH 3 to 5. (1072)

Syringes — Plastic syringes having polypropylene barrels and polyethylene plungers (Pharma-Plast) and all-glass containers were compared in an investigation of the possible sorption of nitroglycerin. After 24 hours of storage of aqueous nitroglycerin solutions (concentrations unspecified), no drug loss was found in either the plastic syringes or glass containers. The authors indicated that these plastic syringes could be substituted for glass syringes for use with syringe pumps. (782)

Nitroglycerin (DuPont) (concentration unspecified) was filled into 3-mL plastic syringes (Becton Dickinson, Sherwood Monoject, and Terumo) and stored at −20, 4, and 25 °C in the dark. Nitroglycerin losses in one day ranged from 10 to 15% at 25 °C, to 2 to 3% at 4 °C, to 2% or less at −20 °C. Long-term storage for seven days at 4 °C and 30 days at −20 °C resulted in losses of 5 to 7% and 2% or less, respectively. The losses were presumably due to sorption to surfaces and/or the elastomeric plunger. (1562)

Nitroglycerin (DuPont) 50 mg/50 mL in dextrose 5% exhibited no change in appearance and about a 3.6% loss when stored in 60-mL plastic syringes (Becton Dickinson) for 24 hours at 25 °C. (1579)

Nitroglycerin concentrate 5 mg/mL from four manufacturers (Abbott, DuPont, Goldline, Marion) was filled as 10 mL in 10-mL glass syringes (Becton Dickinson) and in 10-mL (Becton Dickinson) and 12-mL (Monoject) polypropylene plastic syringes. No loss of nitroglycerin content occurred in 23 hours when stored at 25 °C protected from light. Mean nitroglycerin concentrations were greater than 99% and were the same for both the glass and plastic syringes. (2055)

Sorption — Nitroglycerin readily undergoes sorption to many soft plastics, especially PVC which is commonly used to make infusion solution bags and intravenous tubing.

Plastics such as polyethylene and polypropylene generally do not absorb nitroglycerin. Consequently, it is recommended that only infusion solution containers made from glass or a plastic known to be compatible with nitroglycerin (i.e., polyolefin) be used for mixing infusions.

To circumvent the significant loss to PVC tubing, use of the special high-density polyethylene administration sets provided by the various nitroglycerin injection manufacturers is recommended. Nitroglycerin is not significantly sorbed to these special sets, but the rate of loss to conventional PVC sets is significant (40 to 80%), although not constant nor self-limiting. Many factors including flow rate, concentration, and length of the set affect the extent of sorption. The greatest amount of sorption occurs early in the infusion. A slow rate of flow and long tubing length increase the loss. Simple calculations or corrections cannot be applied to this complex phenomenon to determine or control the actual amount of nitroglycerin delivered through PVC tubing. (1; 4; 503; 506; 508; 509; 510; 511; 721; 723; 724; 725; 726; 727; 728; 769; 770; 797; 930; 931; 932; 934; 943; 1027; 1121; 1122; 1392; 1510; 1511; 1512; 1796; 2143; 2289; 2660; 2792)

In addition to PVC bags and infusion tubing, nitroglycerin has been demonstrated to undergo similar sorption to cellulose propionate drip chambers (725; 931; 1027; 1512), polystyrolbutadiene burettes (1512), PVC pulmonary artery catheters (937) and central venous pressure catheters (Intracath, Deseret) (938), a polyurethane sponge used to defoam blood in a bubble oxygenator (939), a silicone rubber membrane in a membrane oxygenator (940), an infusion pump cassette (Accuset C-924, IMED) (941), and silicone rubber microbore intravenous infusion tubing. (942)

However, the clinical importance of the sorption to PVC has been questioned because nitroglycerin administration is titrated to clinical response, not in a fixed dosage. (1120; 1123; 2015; 2016; 2054) A 25 to 35% loss to PVC tubing was reported at rates of nitroglycerin administration of 80 and 60 mcg/min, respectively. Polyethylene tubing delivered essentially 100% of the nitroglycerin. Nevertheless, there was no statistically significant difference in physiologic response in patients when a variety of parameters were evaluated. The type of tubing used does not influence the ultimate hemodynamic responses significantly, because even the PVC delivered a significant amount of the drug. It was advised that physiologic endpoints be monitored in patients on intravenous nitroglycerin. (1120)

A number of similar results were also reported. (2015; 2016; 2054) Adequate clinical response was achieved using PVC containers and tubing. However, changes in patient hemodynamic status could occur if containers for nitroglycerin infusions were changed during the treatment course; switching from PVC to glass or vice versa could require substantial adjustment in the rate of administration to achieve a similar clinical response. (2016)

Filtration — Some filters absorb nitroglycerin and should be avoided. (4) Filtration of 250 mL of a 485-mcg/mL aqueous solution through three different 142-mm, 0.2-μm filters was performed. A loss of 55% resulted with the Gelman GA filter composed of cellulose triacetate. Losses of only 5% occurred with a Millipore GS filter (a mixture of cellulose acetate and cellulose nitrate), and 2% losses occurred with a Gelman Tuffryn filter (a high-temperature aromatic polymer). (724)

In one study, a filter material specially treated with a proprietary agent was evaluated for a possible reduction in nitroglycerin binding. Nitroglycerin (Abbott) 62.5 mg/250 mL in dextrose 5% and in sodium chloride 0.9% was run through an administration set with a treated 0.22-μm cellulose ester inline filter at a rate of 3 mL/min. Cumulative nitroglycerin losses of less than 6% occurred from 200 mL of either solution. However, equilibrium binding studies showed no significant differences in drug affinity between treated and untreated filter material in either solution. (904) Ivex integral filter and extension sets use the treated filter material. (1074)

Compatibility Information

Solution Compatibility

Nitroglycerin

Solution	Mfr	Mfr	Conc/L	Remarks	Ref	C/I
Dextrose 5% in Ringer's injection, lactated	MG[c,d]	ACC	200 and 400 mg	Physically compatible. Little or no loss after 28 days at 4 °C and room temperature	928	C
Dextrose 5% in sodium chloride 0.45%	MG[c,d]	ACC	200 and 400 mg	Physically compatible. Little or no loss after 28 days at 4 °C and room temperature	928	C
Dextrose 5% in sodium chloride 0.9%	MG[c,d]	ACC	200 and 400 mg	Physically compatible. Little or no loss after 28 days at 4 °C and room temperature	928	C
Dextrose 5%	[c]	LI[c]	32 mg	Negligible loss over 24 hr at room temperature	510	C
	[c]	[a]	100 mg	1% loss in 24 hr at room temperature	509	C
	TR[c]		50 mg	Little change in 2 hr	508	C
	TR[c]	[a]	465 mg	8% loss in 24 hr and 13% in 50 hr at room temperature	506	C
	[c]	[a]	35 mg	Little loss after 70 days at room temperature or under refrigeration	503	C
	MG[c]	ACC	50 mg	0 to 3% loss in 48 hr at 4 and 25 °C	721	C
	MG[d]	ACC	50 mg	1 to 6% loss in 48 hr at 4 and 25 °C	721	C
	MG[c]	[a]	50 mg	Stable for 48 hr at 4 and 25 °C	724	C
	[c]		100 mg	Little or no loss in 8 hr	726	C
	ON[c,d]	[a]	90 mg	No precipitate and negligible loss in 24 hr at 25 °C	797	C
	MG[c,d]	ACC	200 and 400 mg	Physically compatible. Little loss after 28 days at 4 °C and room temperature	928	C
	TR[c]	[a]	200 mg	No loss after 52 hr at 29 °C	930	C
	[c]		200 to 800 mg	Physically compatible. 4% loss in 24 hr in light	1412	C
	[c]		250 mg	3% loss in 24 hr at 6, 20, and 40 °C in light or dark	1512	C
	TR[b]	LI	32 mg	50% loss in 24 hr at room temperature	510	I
	TR[b]		50 mg	Almost 50% loss in 2 hr	508	I
	TR[b]	[a]	465 mg	Over 50% loss in 8 hr and 83% in 50 hr at room temperature	506	I
	[b]	[a]	35 mg	10% loss in 1 hr. In 7 days, 55% loss at room temperature and 30% under refrigeration	503	I
	TR[b]	ACC	50 mg	44% loss in 48 hr at 4 °C and 70% loss at 25 °C	721	I
	TR[b]	[a]	50 mg	43% loss at 4 °C and 64% at 25 °C in 24 hr	724	I
	TR[b]	[a]	100 and 500 mg	50% loss in 24 hr at 20 to 24 °C	725	I
	TR[b]		100 mg	20% loss in 1 hr and 35% in 8 hr	726	I
	[b]	[a]	90 mg	No precipitate but 10% loss in 3 hr and 27% loss in 24 hr at 25 °C	797	I
	BA[c]	AMR	800 mg	No loss in 24 hr at 23 °C	2085	C
	BA[b]	PB	10 mg	Visually compatible. 66% loss at 22 °C and 33% at 4 °C in 24 hr	2289	I
	BRN[c,d]	PB	10 mg	Visually compatible. No loss in 24 hr at 4 and 22 °C	2289	C
	HOS[e]	AMR	400 mg	Less than 2% loss in 24 hr	2660; 2792	C
Ringer's injection, lactated	MG[c,d]	ACC	200 and 400 mg	Physically compatible. Little loss after 28 days at 4 °C and room temperature	928	C
Sodium chloride 0.45%	MG[c,d]	ACC	200 and 400 mg	Physically compatible. Little loss after 28 days at 4 °C and room temperature	928	C
Sodium chloride 0.9%	TR[c]	[a]	465 mg	8% loss in 24 hr and 13% in 50 hr at room temperature	506	C

Solution Compatibility (Cont.)

Nitroglycerin

Solution	Mfr	Mfr	Conc/L	Remarks	Ref	C/I
	c	a	35 to 87 mg	Little loss after 70 days at room temperature or under refrigeration	503	**C**
	MG[c]	ACC	50 mg	5% loss in 48 hr at 4 and 25 °C	721	**C**
	MG[d]	ACC	50 mg	No loss in 48 hr at 4 and 25 °C	721	**C**
	c	a	200 mg	No loss in 24 hr and 5% loss in 3 months at room temperature or under refrigeration	722	**C**
	c	a	3.6 to 95 mg	Little loss in 48 hr at 35 °C	723	**C**
	c	a	0.2 mg	10% loss in 24 hr and 13% in 48 hr at 35 °C	723	**C**
	MG[c]	a	50 mg	Stable for 48 hr at 4 and 25 °C	724	**C**
	ON[c,d]	a	90 mg	No precipitate. 2 to 3% loss in 24 hr at 25 °C	797	**C**
	MG[c,d]	ACC	200 and 400 mg	Physically compatible. Little loss after 28 days at 4 °C and room temperature	928	**C**
	TR[c]	a	200 mg	No loss after 52 hr at 29 °C	930	**C**
	c		200 to 800 mg	Physically compatible. 8% or less loss in 24 hr exposed to light	1412	**C**
	c,d		100 mg	Physically compatible. 2 to 5% loss in 24 hr at 21 °C in the dark	1392	**C**
	c		250 mg	4% loss at 6 °C and 7% loss at 40 °C in 6 hr; no further loss in 24 hr	1512	**C**
	TR[b]	a	465 mg	Over 50% loss in 8 hr and 83% in 50 hr at room temperature	506	**I**
	TR[b]	ACC	50 mg	38% loss in 48 hr at 4 °C and 68% at 25 °C	721	**I**
	TR[b]	a	50 mg	45% loss at 4 °C and 54% at 25 °C in 24 hr	724	**I**
	TR[b]	a	100 and 500 mg	50% loss in 24 hr at 20 to 24 °C	725	**I**
	b	a	90 mg	No precipitate but 10% loss in 3 hr and 28% loss in 24 hr at 25 °C	797	**I**
	TR[b]	a	200 mg	38 to 44% loss in 8 hr at 29 °C. At 6 °C, 14% loss in 8 hr	930	**I**
	b		100 mg	10% loss in 1 hr and 51% loss in 24 hr at 21 °C in the dark	1392	**I**
	c	PD	50, 125, 200 mg	About 14% loss in 8 hr at 24 °C	1510	**I**
	ON[c,d]	ON	100 mg	Visually compatible. No loss in 24 hr at 21 °C	1796	**C**
	ON[b]	ON	100 mg	Visually compatible. 50% loss in 24 hr and 75% loss in 120 hr at 21 °C	1796	**I**
	BA[b]	PB	10 mg	Visually compatible. 66% loss in 24 hr at 4 and 22 °C	2289	**I**
	BRN[c,d]	PB	10 mg	Visually compatible. 4 to 5% loss in 24 hr at 4 and 22 °C	2289	**C**
Sodium lactate ⅙ M	MG[c,d]	ACC	200 and 400 mg	Physically compatible. Little loss after 28 days at 4 °C and room temperature in glass and polyolefin containers	928	**C**

[a] *An extemporaneous preparation was tested.*
[b] *Tested in PVC containers.*
[c] *Tested in glass containers.*
[d] *Tested in polyolefin containers.*
[e] *Tested in VISIV polyolefin containers.*

Additive Compatibility

Nitroglycerin

Drug	Mfr	Conc/L	Mfr	Conc/L	Test Soln	Remarks	Ref	C/I
Alteplase	GEN	0.5 g	ACC	400 mg	D5W, NS	Visually compatible with 2% or less clot-lysis activity loss in 24 hr at 25 °C	1856	C
Aminophylline	IX	1 g	ACC	400 mg	D5W[a]	Physically compatible with 4% nitroglycerin loss in 24 hr and 6% loss in 48 hr at 23 °C. Aminophylline not tested	929	C
	IX	1 g	ACC	400 mg	NS[a]	Physically compatible with no nitroglycerin loss in 24 hr and 5% loss in 48 hr at 23 °C. Aminophylline not tested	929	C
Dobutamine HCl	LI	1 g	AB	120 mg	D5W, NS	Physically compatible for 24 hr at 21 °C	812	C
	LI	500 mg	ACC	100 mg	D5S	Stable with no loss of either drug after 24 hr at 25 °C. Pink color after 4 hr	990	C
Dobutamine HCl with sodium nitroprusside		2 to 8 g 200 to 800 mg		200 to 800 mg	D5W[a]	Pink color with small amount of dark brown precipitate and 11 to 19% nitroglycerin loss in 24 hr exposed to light	1412	I
Dobutamine HCl with sodium nitroprusside		2 to 8 g 200 to 800 mg		200 to 800 mg	NS[a]	Pink color with 8% or less loss for any drug for 24 hr exposed to light	1412	C
Dopamine HCl	ACC	800 mg	ACC	400 mg	D5W, NS[a]	Physically compatible with little or no nitroglycerin loss in 48 hr at 23 °C. Dopamine not tested	929	C
Enalaprilat	MSD	12 mg	DU	200 mg	D5W[a]	Visually compatible. 4% enalaprilat loss in 24 hr at room temperature in light. Nitroglycerin not tested	1572	C
Furosemide	HO	1 g	ACC	400 mg	D5W[a]	Physically compatible with no nitroglycerin loss in 48 hr at 23 °C. Furosemide not tested	929	C
	HO	1 g	ACC	400 mg	NS[a]	Physically compatible with 3% nitroglycerin loss in 48 hr at 23 °C. Furosemide not tested	929	C
Hydralazine HCl	CI	1 g	ACC	400 mg	D5W[a]	Yellow color. 4% nitroglycerin loss in 48 hr at 23 °C. Hydralazine not tested	929	I
	CI	1 g	ACC	400 mg	NS[a]	Yellow color. No nitroglycerin loss in 48 hr at 23 °C. Hydralazine not tested	929	I
Lidocaine HCl	IMS	4 g	ACC	400 mg	D5W, NS[a]	Physically compatible. No nitroglycerin loss in 48 hr at 23 °C. Lidocaine not tested	929	C
Phenytoin sodium	PD	1 g	ACC	400 mg	D5W, NS[a]	Phenytoin crystals in 24 hr. 3 to 4% nitroglycerin loss in 24 hr and 9% in 48 hr at 23 °C. Phenytoin not tested	929	I
Sodium nitroprusside with dobutamine HCl		200 to 800 mg 2 to 8 g		200 to 800 mg	D5W[a]	Pink color with small amount of dark brown precipitate and 11 to 19% nitroglycerin loss in 24 hr exposed to light	1412	I
Sodium nitroprusside with dobutamine HCl		200 to 800 mg 2 to 8 g		200 to 800 mg	NS[a]	Pink color with 8% or less loss for any drug for 24 hr exposed to light	1412	C
Verapamil HCl	KN	80 mg	ACC	100 mg	D5W, NS	Physically compatible for 24 hr	764	C

[a]*Tested in glass containers.*

Drugs in Syringe Compatibility

Nitroglycerin

Drug (in syringe)	Mfr	Amt	Mfr	Amt	Remarks	Ref	C/I
Caffeine citrate		20 mg/ 1 mL	SO	5 mg/ 1 mL	White precipitate forms immediately becoming two layers over time	2440	I
Heparin sodium		2500 units/ 1 mL		25 mg/ 25 mL	Physically compatible for at least 5 min	1053	C
Pantoprazole sodium	[a]	4 mg/ 1 mL		5 mg/ 1 mL	Precipitates	2574	I

[a]*Test performed using the formulation WITHOUT edetate disodium.*

Y-Site Injection Compatibility (1:1 Mixture)

Nitroglycerin

Drug	Mfr	Conc	Mfr	Conc	Remarks	Ref	C/I
Alteplase	GEN	1 mg/mL	DU	0.2 mg/mL[a]	Haze noted in 24 hr	1340	I
Amiodarone HCl	LZ	4 mg/mL[c]	AB	0.24 mg/mL[c]	Physically compatible for 24 hr at 21 °C	1032	C
Amphotericin B cholesteryl sulfate complex	SEQ	0.83 mg/mL[a]	AMR	0.4 mg/mL[a]	Physically compatible for 4 hr at 23 °C	2117	C
Argatroban	SKB	1 mg/mL[a]	BA	0.2 mg/mL[a]	Physically compatible for 24 hr at 23 °C	2572	C
Atracurium besylate	BW	0.5 mg/mL[a]	SO	0.4 mg/mL[a]	Physically compatible for 24 hr at 28 °C	1337	C
Bivalirudin	TMC	5 mg/mL[a]	AMR	0.4 mg/mL[a]	Physically compatible for 4 hr at 23 °C	2373	C
Cisatracurium besylate	GW	0.1, 2, 5 mg/ mL[a]	DU	0.4 mg/mL[a]	Physically compatible for 4 hr at 23 °C	2074	C
Clonidine HCl	BI	18 mcg/mL[b]	NYC	0.4 mg/mL[a]	Visually compatible	2642	C
Dexmedetomidine HCl	AB	4 mcg/mL[b]	AMR	0.4 mg/mL[b]	Physically compatible for 4 hr at 23 °C	2383	C
Diltiazem HCl	MMD	1 mg/mL[a]	DU	0.032 mg/ mL[a]	Visually compatible for 24 hr at 25 °C	1530	C
	MMD	1[b] and 5 mg/ mL	DU	400 mcg/mL[b]	Visually compatible	1807	C
	MMD	5 mg/mL	DU	400 mcg/mL[a]	Visually compatible	1807	C
	MMD	1 mg/mL[a]	AB	0.4 mg/mL[a]	Visually compatible for 4 hr at 27 °C	2062	C
Dobutamine HCl	LI	4 mg/mL[c]	LY	0.4 mg/mL[c]	Physically compatible for 3 hr	1316	C
	LI	4 mg/mL[a]	AB	0.4 mg/mL[a]	Visually compatible for 4 hr at 27 °C	2062	C
Dobutamine HCl with dopamine HCl	LI DCC	4 mg/mL[c] 3.2 mg/mL[c]	LY	0.4 mg/mL[c]	Physically compatible for 3 hr	1316	C
Dobutamine HCl with lidocaine HCl	LI AB	4 mg/mL[c] 8 mg/mL[c]	LY	0.4 mg/mL[c]	Physically compatible for 3 hr	1316	C
Dobutamine HCl with sodium nitroprusside	LI ES	4 mg/mL[c] 0.4 mg/mL[c]	LY	0.4 mg/mL[c]	Physically compatible for 3 hr	1316	C
Dopamine HCl	DCC	3.2 mg/mL[c]	LY	0.4 mg/mL[c]	Physically compatible for 3 hr	1316	C
	AB	3.2 mg/mL[a]	AB	0.4 mg/mL[a]	Visually compatible for 4 hr at 27 °C	2062	C
Dopamine HCl with dobutamine HCl	DCC LI	3.2 mg/mL[c] 4 mg/mL[c]	LY	0.4 mg/mL[c]	Physically compatible for 3 hr	1316	C
Dopamine HCl with lidocaine HCl	DCC AB	3.2 mg/mL[c] 8 mg/mL[c]	LY	0.4 mg/mL[c]	Physically compatible for 3 hr	1316	C
Dopamine HCl with sodium nitroprusside	DCC ES	3.2 mg/mL[c] 0.4 mg/mL[c]	LY	0.4 mg/mL[c]	Physically compatible for 3 hr	1316	C

Y-Site Injection Compatibility (1:1 Mixture) (Cont.)

Nitroglycerin

Drug	Mfr	Conc	Mfr	Conc	Remarks	Ref	C/I
Epinephrine HCl	AB	0.02 mg/mL[a]	AB	0.4 mg/mL[a]	Visually compatible for 4 hr at 27 °C	2062	**C**
Esmolol HCl	DU	40 mg/mL[a]	OM	0.2 mg/mL[a]	Visually compatible for 24 hr at 23 °C	1877	**C**
Famotidine	MSD	0.2 mg/mL[a]	IMS	0.8 mg/mL[a]	Physically compatible for 4 hr at 25 °C	1188	**C**
	MSD	0.2 mg/mL[a]	PD	85 mcg/mL[b]	Physically compatible for 14 hr	1196	**C**
Fenoldopam mesylate	AB	80 mcg/mL[b]	AMR	0.4 mg/mL[b]	Physically compatible for 4 hr at 23 °C	2467	**C**
Fentanyl citrate	ES	0.05 mg/mL	AB	0.4 mg/mL[a]	Visually compatible for 4 hr at 27 °C	2062	**C**
Fluconazole	RR	2 mg/mL	AMR	0.2 mg/mL[a]	Visually compatible for 24 hr at 28 °C under fluorescent light	1760	**C**
Furosemide	AMR	10 mg/mL	AB	0.4 mg/mL[a]	Visually compatible for 4 hr at 27 °C	2062	**C**
	AMR	10 mg/mL	BA	0.1 mg/mL[e]	Precipitation occurs immediately	2725	**I**
	AMR	10 mg/mL	AMR	0.1 mg/mL[a]	Physically compatible for 48 hr at room temperature	2725	**C**
Haloperidol lactate	MN	0.5[a] and 5 mg/mL	DU	0.4 mg/mL[a]	Visually compatible for 24 hr at 21 °C	1523	**C**
Heparin sodium	ES	50 units/mL	BA	0.2 mg/mL	Visually compatible for 24 hr at 23 °C	1794	**C**
	OR	100 units/mL[a]	OM	0.2 mg/mL[a]	Visually compatible for 24 hr at 23 °C	1877	**C**
	ES	100 units/mL[a]	AB	0.4 mg/mL[a]	Visually compatible for 4 hr at 27 °C	2062	**C**
Hetastarch in lactated electrolyte	AB	6%	AMR	0.4 mg/mL[a]	Physically compatible for 4 hr at 23 °C	2339	**C**
Hydralazine HCl	SO	1 mg/mL[a]	LY	0.4 mg/mL[a]	Physically compatible for 3 hr	1316	**C**
	SO	1 mg/mL[b]	LY	0.4 mg/mL[b]	Slight precipitate in 3 hr	1316	**I**
Hydromorphone HCl	KN	1 mg/mL	AB	0.4 mg/mL[a]	Visually compatible for 4 hr at 27 °C	2062	**C**
Hydroxyethyl starch 130/0.4 in sodium chloride 0.9%	FRK	6%	SZ	0.1, 0.25, 0.4 mg/mL[a]	Visually compatible for 24 hr at room temperature	2770	**C**
Insulin, regular	LI	1 unit/mL[a]	OM	0.2 mg/mL[a]	Visually compatible for 24 hr at 23 °C	1877	**C**
Labetalol HCl	GL	1 mg/mL[a]	DU	0.2 mg/mL[a]	Visually compatible. No labetalol loss and 6% nitroglycerin loss in 4 hr at room temperature	1762	**C**
	GL	5 mg/mL	OM	0.2 mg/mL[a]	Visually compatible for 24 hr at 23 °C	1877	**C**
	AH	2 mg/mL[a]	AB	0.4 mg/mL[a]	Visually compatible for 4 hr at 27 °C	2062	**C**
Levofloxacin	OMN	5 mg/mL[a]	AMR	5 mg/mL	Cloudy precipitate forms	2233	**I**
Lidocaine HCl	AB	8 mg/mL[c]	LY	0.4 mg/mL[c]	Physically compatible for 3 hr	1316	**C**
Lidocaine HCl with dobutamine HCl	AB LI	8 mg/mL[c] 4 mg/mL[c]	LY	0.4 mg/mL[c]	Physically compatible for 3 hr	1316	**C**
Lidocaine HCl with dopamine HCl	AB DCC	8 mg/mL[c] 3.2 mg/mL[c]	LY	0.4 mg/mL[c]	Physically compatible for 3 hr	1316	**C**
Lidocaine HCl with sodium nitroprusside	AB ES	8 mg/mL[c] 0.4 mg/mL[c]	LY	0.4 mg/mL[c]	Physically compatible for 3 hr	1316	**C**
Linezolid	PHU	2 mg/mL	FAU	0.4 mg/mL[a]	Physically compatible for 4 hr at 23 °C	2264	**C**
Lorazepam	WY	0.5 mg/mL[a]	AB	0.4 mg/mL[a]	Visually compatible for 4 hr at 27 °C	2062	**C**
Metoprolol tartrate	BED	1 mg/mL	BA	0.2 mg/mL[a]	Trace precipitate in 8 hr at 19 °C	2795	**I**
Micafungin sodium	ASP	1.5 mg/mL[b]	AMR	0.4 mg/mL[b]	Physically compatible for 4 hr at 23 °C	2683	**C**
Midazolam HCl	RC	1 mg/mL[a]	SO	0.2 mg/mL[a]	Visually compatible for 24 hr at 23 °C	1847	**C**
	RC	1 mg/mL[a]	OM	0.2 mg/mL[a]	Visually compatible for 24 hr at 23 °C	1877	**C**
	RC	2 mg/mL[a]	AB	0.4 mg/mL[a]	Visually compatible for 4 hr at 27 °C	2062	**C**

Y-Site Injection Compatibility (1:1 Mixture) (Cont.)

Nitroglycerin

Drug	Mfr	Conc	Mfr	Conc	Remarks	Ref	C/I
Milrinone lactate	SW	0.2 mg/mL[a]	AB	0.4 mg/mL[a]	Visually compatible for 4 hr at 27 °C	2062	C
	SW	0.4 mg/mL[a]	SO	0.8 mg/mL[a]	Visually compatible. Little loss of either drug in 4 hr at 23 °C	2214	C
Morphine sulfate	SCN	2 mg/mL[a]	AB	0.4 mg/mL[a]	Visually compatible for 4 hr at 27 °C	2062	C
Nesiritide	SCI	50 mcg/mL[a,b]		0.2 mg/mL	Physically compatible for 4 hr	2625	C
Nicardipine HCl	WY	1 mg/mL[a]	AB	0.4 mg/mL[a]	Visually compatible for 4 hr at 27 °C	2062	C
Norepinephrine bitartrate	AB	0.128 mg/mL[a]	AB	0.4 mg/mL[a]	Visually compatible for 4 hr at 27 °C	2062	C
Pancuronium bromide	ES	0.05 mg/mL[a]	SO	0.4 mg/mL[a]	Physically compatible for 24 hr at 28 °C	1337	C
Pantoprazole sodium	ALT[h]	0.16 to 0.8 mg/mL[b]	SX	0.1 to 0.4 mg/mL[a]	Visually compatible for 12 hr at 23 °C	2603	C
Propofol	ZEN	10 mg/mL	DU	0.4 mg/mL[a]	Physically compatible for 1 hr at 23 °C	2066	C
Ranitidine HCl	GL	0.5 mg/mL	SO	0.2 mg/mL[a]	Physically compatible for 24 hr	1323	C
	GL	1 mg/mL[a]	AB	0.4 mg/mL[a]	Visually compatible for 4 hr at 27 °C	2062	C
Remifentanil HCl	GW	0.025 and 0.25 mg/mL[b]	DU	0.4 mg/mL[a]	Physically compatible for 4 hr at 23 °C	2075	C
Sodium nitroprusside	ES	0.4 mg/mL[c]	LY	0.4 mg/mL[c]	Physically compatible for 3 hr	1316	C
	RC	1.2 and 3 mg/mL[a]	SX	0.4 and 1.5 mg/mL[g]	Visually compatible for 48 hr at 24 °C protected from light	2357	C
Sodium nitroprusside with dobutamine HCl	ES LI	0.4 mg/mL[c] 4 mg/mL[c]	LY	0.4 mg/mL[c]	Physically compatible for 3 hr	1316	C
Sodium nitroprusside with dopamine HCl	ES DCC	0.4 mg/mL[c] 3.2 mg/mL[c]	LY	0.4 mg/mL[c]	Physically compatible for 3 hr	1316	C
Sodium nitroprusside with lidocaine HCl	ES AB	0.4 mg/mL[c] 8 mg/mL[c]	LY	0.4 mg/mL[c]	Physically compatible for 3 hr	1316	C
Tacrolimus	FUJ	1 mg/mL[b]	DU	0.1 mg/mL[a]	Visually compatible for 24 hr at 25 °C	1630	C
Theophylline	TR	4 mg/mL	LY	0.2 mg/mL[a]	Visually compatible for 6 hr at 25 °C	1793	C
Tirofiban HCl	ME	50 mcg/mL[a,b]	AB	0.1 and 0.4 mg/mL	Physically compatible. No loss of either drug in 4 hr at 23 °C	2356	C
TNA #218 to #226[f]			DU	0.4 mg/mL[a]	Visually compatible for 4 hr at 23 °C	2215	C
TPN #212 to #215[f]			DU	0.4 mg/mL[a]	Physically compatible for 4 hr at 23 °C	2109	C
Vasopressin	AMR	2 and 4 units/mL[b]	BA	0.2 mg/mL[a]	Physically compatible with vasopressin pushed through a Y-site over 5 sec	2478	C
Vecuronium bromide	OR	0.1 mg/mL[a]	SO	0.4 mg/mL[a]	Physically compatible for 24 hr at 28 °C	1337	C
	OR	1 mg/mL	AB	0.4 mg/mL[a]	Visually compatible for 4 hr at 27 °C	2062	C
Warfarin sodium	DU	2 mg/mL[d]	FAU	0.4 mg/mL[a]	Visually compatible with no warfarin loss in 30 min	2010	C
	DME	2 mg/mL[d]	DU	0.4 mg/mL[a]	Visually compatible for 24 hr at 24 °C	2078	C

[a]*Tested in dextrose 5%.*
[b]*Tested in sodium chloride 0.9%.*
[c]*Tested in both dextrose 5% and sodium chloride 0.9%.*
[d]*Tested in sterile water for injection.*
[e]*Tested using Baxter Healthcare premixed nitroglycerin infusion in dextrose 5% with citrate buffer.*
[f]*Refer to Appendix I for the composition of parenteral nutrition solutions. TNA indicates a 3-in-1 admixture, and TPN indicates a 2-in-1 admixture.*
[g]*Tested in dextrose 5% in sodium chloride 0.2%.*
[h]*Test performed using the formulation WITHOUT edetate disodium.*

NOREPINEPHRINE BITARTRATE
(NORADRENALINE ACID TARTRATE)
AHFS 12:12

Products — Norepinephrine bitartrate is available as 1 mg/mL of norepinephrine base in 4-mL vials. Each milliliter of solution also contains sodium metabisulfite 0.2 mg and sodium chloride for isotonicity in water for injection. (1)

pH — From 3 to 4.5. (1; 77)

Osmolality — Norepinephrine bitartrate injection is adjusted to isotonicity with sodium chloride. (1)

Trade Name(s) — Levophed.

Administration — Norepinephrine bitartrate is administered by intravenous infusion into a large vein, using a pump or other flow rate control device. Extravasation may cause tissue damage and should be avoided. A 4-mcg/mL dilution of norepinephrine base for infusion is usually prepared by adding 4 mg of base (4 mL) to 1000 mL of dextrose 5% with or without sodium chloride. The concentration and infusion rate depend on the patient's requirements. (1; 4)

Stability — Norepinephrine bitartrate in intact containers should be stored at controlled room temperature and protected from light. (1; 4) Dextrose 5% and dextrose 5% in sodium chloride 0.9% are the recommended diluents for infusion because their dextrose content provides protection against significant drug loss due to oxidation. The drug gradually darkens upon exposure to light or air and must not be used if it is discolored or has a precipitate. (4)

pH Effects — Norepinephrine bitartrate is stable at pH 3.6 to 6 in dextrose 5%. (48; 77) The pH of a solution is the primary determinant of catecholamine stability in intravenous admixtures. (527) At a concentration of 5 mg/L in dextrose 5% at pH 6.5, norepinephrine bitartrate loses 5% in six hours; at pH 7.5, it loses 5% in four hours. (77) The rate of loss also increases with exposure to increasing temperatures. (1929)

Caution should be employed in mixing additives that may result in a final pH above 6 since norepinephrine bitartrate is alkali labile. (6; 24; 77)

Visual inspection for color change may be inadequate to assess compatibility of admixtures. In one evaluation with aminophylline stored at 25 °C, a color change was not noted until 48 hours had elapsed. However, no intact norepinephrine bitartrate was present in the admixture at 48 hours. (527)

Filtration — Norepinephrine bitartrate 4 mg/L in dextrose 5% and sodium chloride 0.9% was filtered at a rate of 120 mL/hr for six hours through a 0.22-μm cellulose ester membrane filter (Ivex-2). No significant drug loss due to binding to the filter was noted. (533)

Central Venous Catheter — Norepinephrine bitartrate 0.1 mg/mL in dextrose 5% was found to be compatible with the ARROWg+ard Blue Plus (Arrow International) chlorhexidine-bearing triple-lumen central catheter. Essentially complete delivery of the drug was found with little or no drug loss occurring. Furthermore, chlorhexidine delivered from the catheter remained at trace amounts with no substantial increase due to the delivery of the drug through the catheter. (2335)

Compatibility Information

Solution Compatibility

Norepinephrine bitartrate

Solution	Mfr	Mfr	Conc/L	Remarks	Ref	C/I
Amino acids 4.25%, dextrose 25%	MG	WI	4 mg	No increase in particulate matter in 24 hr at 5 °C	349	C
Dextrose 5% in sodium chloride 0.9%		WI	8 mg	Physically compatible	74	C
Dextrose 5%		WI	8 mg	Physically compatible	74	C
	AB	WI	8 mg	Physically compatible. 10% calculated loss in 2500 hr at 25 °C	527	C
	TR[a]	WI	4 and 8 mg	2 to 4% loss in 24 hr at room temperature exposed to light	1163	C
	BA[a]	WI	16 mg	5% loss in 47.2 days at 5 °C in the dark	1610	C
	BA[a]	WI	40 mg	5% loss in 87.7 days at 5 °C in the dark	1610	C
	TR[a]	RC	4 and 8 mg	Visually compatible. No loss in 48 hr at room temperature	1802	C
	BA[a]	SW	42 mg	No loss in 24 hr at 23 °C in the dark	2085	C
	[a]	SX	4 and 16 mg	Less than 4% loss in 7 days at 20 °C	2776	C
	BA[a]	SZ	64 mg	Little loss in 61 days at 4 and 23 °C in the dark	2815	C
Ringer's injection, lactated		WI	8 mg	Physically compatible	74	C
Sodium chloride 0.9%		WI	8 mg	Physically compatible	74	C
	TR[a]	WI	4 and 8 mg	2% loss in 24 hr at room temperature in light	1163	C

Solution Compatibility (Cont.)

Norepinephrine bitartrate

Solution	Mfr	Mfr	Conc/L	Remarks	Ref	C/I
[a]		SX	4 and 16 mg	Less than 3% loss in 7 days at 20 °C	2776	C
	BA[a]	SZ	64 mg	Little loss in 61 days at 4 and 23 °C in the dark	2815	C

[a]Tested in PVC containers.

Additive Compatibility

Norepinephrine bitartrate

Drug	Mfr	Conc/L	Mfr	Conc/L	Test Soln	Remarks	Ref	C/I
Amikacin sulfate	BR	5 g	WI	8 mg	D5LR, D5R, D5S, D5W, D10W, LR, NS, R, SL	Physically compatible and both stable for 24 hr at 25 °C	294	C
Aminophylline	SE	500 mg	WI	8 mg	D5W	10% norepinephrine loss in 3.6 hr at 25 °C	527	I
Calcium chloride	UP	1 g	WI	8 mg	D, D–S, S	Physically compatible	77	C
Calcium gluconate		1 g	WI	8 mg	D5W	Physically compatible	74	C
Ciprofloxacin	BAY	2 g	SW	64 mg	D5W	Visually compatible. No ciprofloxacin loss in 24 hr at 22 °C in light. Norepinephrine not tested	2413	C
Dimenhydrinate	SE	50 mg	WI	8 mg	D5W	Physically compatible	74	C
Dobutamine HCl	LI	1 g	BN	32 mg	D5W, NS	Physically compatible for 24 hr at 21 °C	812	C
Heparin sodium		12,000 units	WI	8 mg	D5W	Physically compatible	74	C
	AB	20,000 units	WI	8 mg	D, D–S, S	Physically compatible	77	C
Hydrocortisone sodium succinate	UP	100 mg	WI	8 mg	D5W	Physically compatible	74	C
Magnesium sulfate		1 g	WI	8 mg	D, D–S, S	Physically compatible	77	C
Meropenem	ZEN	1 and 20 g	WI	8 g	NS	Visually compatible for 4 hr at room temperature	1994	C
Methylprednisolone sodium succinate	UP	40 mg	WI	8 mg	D5S	Physically compatible	329	C
Multivitamins	USV	10 mL	WI	8 mg	D, D–S, S	Physically compatible	77	C
Potassium chloride		3 g	WI	8 mg	D5W	Physically compatible	74	C
	AB	40 mEq	WI	8 mg	D, D–S, S	Physically compatible	77	C
Ranitidine HCl	GL	50 mg	WI	4 and 8 mg	D5W, NS[a]	Physically compatible. 2 to 6% ranitidine loss in 48 hr at room temperature in light. Norepinephrine not tested	1361	C
	GL	50 mg		4 mg	D5W	Physically compatible. Ranitidine stable for 24 hr at 25 °C. Norepinephrine not tested	1515	C
	GL	50 mg	RC	4 and 8 mg	D5W[a]	Visually compatible. 5 to 7% ranitidine loss and little norepinephrine loss in 48 hr at room temperature	1802	C
	GL	2 g	RC	4 mg	D5W[a]	Visually compatible. 7% norepinephrine loss in 4 hr and 13% in 12 hr at room temperature. No ranitidine loss in 48 hr	1802	I

Additive Compatibility (Cont.)

Norepinephrine bitartrate

Drug	Mfr	Conc/L	Mfr	Conc/L	Test Soln	Remarks	Ref	C/I
	GL	2 g	RC	8 mg	D5W[a]	Visually compatible. 6% norepinephrine loss in 12 hr and 11% in 24 hr at room temperature. No ranitidine loss in 48 hr	1802	I
Sodium bicarbonate	AB	80 mEq	WI	2 mg	D5W	Physically incompatible	15	I
	AB	2.4 mEq[b]	BN	8 mg	D5W	Norepinephrine decomposition	772	I
Succinylcholine chloride	AB	2 g	WI	8 mg	D, D–S, S	Physically compatible	77	C
Verapamil HCl	KN	80 mg	BN	8 mg	D5W, NS	Physically compatible for 24 hr	764	C

[a]Tested in PVC containers.
[b]One vial of Neut added to a liter of admixture.

Drugs in Syringe Compatibility

Norepinephrine bitartrate

Drug (in syringe)	Mfr	Amt	Mfr	Amt	Remarks	Ref	C/I
Pantoprazole sodium	[a]	4 mg/ 1 mL		1 mg/ 1 mL	Precipitates within 15 min	2574	I

[a]Test performed using the formulation WITHOUT edetate disodium.

Y-Site Injection Compatibility (1:1 Mixture)

Norepinephrine bitartrate

Drug	Mfr	Conc	Mfr	Conc	Remarks	Ref	C/I
Amiodarone HCl	LZ	4 mg/mL[c]	BN	64 mcg/mL[c]	Physically compatible for 24 hr at 21 °C	1032	C
Anidulafungin	VIC	0.5 mg/mL[a]	BED	0.12 mg/mL[a]	Physically compatible for 4 hr at 23 °C	2617	C
Argatroban	GSK	1 mg/mL[b]	AB	1 mg/mL	Visually compatible for 24 hr at 23 °C	2391	C
Bivalirudin	TMC	5 mg/mL[a]	AB	0.12 mg/mL[a]	Physically compatible for 4 hr at 23 °C	2373	C
Caspofungin acetate	ME	0.7 mg/mL[b]	BED	0.128 mg/mL[b]	Physically compatible for 4 hr at room temperature	2758	C
Ceftaroline fosamil	FOR	2.22 mg/mL[a,b,i]	BED	0.128 mg/mL[a,b,i]	Physically compatible for 4 hr at 23 °C	2826	C
Cisatracurium besylate	GW	0.1, 2, 5 mg/mL[a]	SW	0.12 mg/mL[a]	Physically compatible for 4 hr at 23 °C	2074	C
Clonidine HCl	BI	18 mcg/mL[b]	APO	20 mcg/mL[a]	Visually compatible	2642	C
Dexmedetomidine HCl	AB	4 mcg/mL[b]	AB	0.12 mg/mL[b]	Physically compatible for 4 hr at 23 °C	2383	C
Diltiazem HCl	MMD	1 mg/mL[a]	WI	0.12 mg/mL[a]	Visually compatible for 24 hr at 25 °C	1530	C
	MMD	1 mg/mL[a]	AB	0.128 mg/mL[a]	Visually compatible for 4 hr at 27 °C	2062	C
Dobutamine HCl	LI	4 mg/mL[a]	AB	0.128 mg/mL[a]	Visually compatible for 4 hr at 27 °C	2062	C
Dopamine HCl	DU	3.2 mg/mL[a]	STR	0.064 mg/mL[a]	Visually compatible for 24 hr at 23 °C	1877	C
	AB	3.2 mg/mL[a]	AB	0.128 mg/mL[a]	Visually compatible for 4 hr at 27 °C	2062	C

Y-Site Injection Compatibility (1:1 Mixture) (Cont.)

Norepinephrine bitartrate

Drug	Mfr	Conc	Mfr	Conc	Remarks	Ref	C/I
Doripenem	JJ	5 mg/mL[a,b]	BED	0.128 mg/mL[a,b]	Physically compatible for 4 hr at 23 °C	2743	C
Epinephrine HCl	AB	0.02 mg/mL[a]	AB	0.128 mg/mL[a]	Visually compatible for 4 hr at 27 °C	2062	C
Esmolol HCl	DU	40 mg/mL[a]	STR	0.064 mg/mL[a]	Visually compatible for 24 hr at 23 °C	1877	C
Famotidine	MSD	0.2 mg/mL[a]	WI	0.004 mg/mL[a]	Physically compatible for 4 hr at 25 °C	1188	C
Fenoldopam mesylate	AB	80 mcg/mL[b]	AB	0.12 mg/mL[b]	Physically compatible for 4 hr at 23 °C	2467	C
Fentanyl citrate	ES	0.05 mg/mL	AB	0.128 mg/mL[a]	Visually compatible for 4 hr at 27 °C	2062	C
Furosemide	AMR	10 mg/mL	AB	0.128 mg/mL[a]	Visually compatible for 4 hr at 27 °C	2062	C
Haloperidol lactate	MN	0.5[a] and 5 mg/mL	WI	0.032 mg/mL[a]	Visually compatible for 24 hr at 21 °C	1523	C
Heparin sodium	UP	1000 units/L[d]	WI	1 mg/mL	Physically compatible for 4 hr at room temperature	534	C
	ES	100 units/mL[a]	AB	0.128 mg/mL[a]	Visually compatible for 4 hr at 27 °C	2062	C
Hetastarch in lactated electrolyte	AB	6%	AB	0.12 mg/mL[a]	Physically compatible for 4 hr at 23 °C	2339	C
Hydrocortisone sodium succinate	UP	10 mg/L[d]	WI	1 mg/mL	Physically compatible for 4 hr at room temperature	534	C
Hydromorphone HCl	KN	1 mg/mL	AB	0.128 mg/mL[a]	Visually compatible for 4 hr at 27 °C	2062	C
Hydroxyethyl starch 130/0.4 in sodium chloride 0.9%	FRK	6%	SZ	6, 8, 64 mcg/mL[a]	Visually compatible for 24 hr at room temperature	2770	C
Insulin, regular	LI	1 unit/mL[a]	STR	0.064 mg/mL[a]	White precipitate forms immediately	1877	I
Labetalol HCl	GL	5 mg/mL	STR	64 mcg/mL[a]	Visually compatible for 24 hr at 23 °C	1877	C
	AH	2 mg/mL[a]	AB	0.128 mg/mL[a]	Visually compatible for 4 hr at 27 °C	2062	C
Lorazepam	WY	0.5 mg/mL[a]	AB	0.128 mg/mL[a]	Visually compatible for 4 hr at 27 °C	2062	C
Meropenem	ZEN	1 and 50 mg/mL[b]	WI	1 mg/mL	Visually compatible for 4 hr at room temperature	1994	C
Micafungin sodium	ASP	1.5 mg/mL[b]	BED	0.128 mg/mL[b]	Physically compatible for 4 hr at 23 °C	2683	C
Midazolam HCl	RC	1 mg/mL[a]	STR	0.064 mg/mL[a]	Visually compatible for 24 hr at 23 °C	1877	C
	RC	2 mg/mL[a]	AB	0.128 mg/mL[a]	Visually compatible for 4 hr at 27 °C	2062	C
Milrinone lactate	SW	0.2 mg/mL[a]	AB	0.128 mg/mL[a]	Visually compatible for 4 hr at 27 °C	2062	C
	SW	0.4 mg/mL[a]	SW	0.064 mg/mL[a]	Visually compatible. Little loss of either drug in 4 hr at 23 °C	2214	C
Morphine sulfate	SX	1 mg/mL[a]	STR	0.064 mg/mL[a]	Visually compatible for 24 hr at 23 °C	1877	C

Y-Site Injection Compatibility (1:1 Mixture) (Cont.)

Norepinephrine bitartrate

Drug	Mfr	Conc	Mfr	Conc	Remarks	Ref	C/I
	SCN	2 mg/mL[a]	AB	0.128 mg/mL[a]	Visually compatible for 4 hr at 27 °C	2062	**C**
Mycophenolate mofetil HCl	RC	5.9 mg/mL[a]		1 mg/mL[a]	Physically compatible and 2% mycophenolate mofetil loss in 4 hr	2738	**C**
Nesiritide	SCI	50 mcg/mL[a,b]		1 mg/mL	Physically compatible for 4 hr. May be chemically incompatible with nesiritide[g]	2625	**?**
Nicardipine HCl	WY	1 mg/mL[a]	AB	0.128 mg/mL[a]	Visually compatible for 4 hr at 27 °C	2062	**C**
Nitroglycerin	AB	0.4 mg/mL[a]	AB	0.128 mg/mL[a]	Visually compatible for 4 hr at 27 °C	2062	**C**
Pantoprazole sodium	ALT[h]	0.16 to 0.8 mg/mL[b]	SX	6 to 8 mcg/mL[a]	Visually compatible for 12 hr at 23 °C	2603	**C**
	ALT[h]	0.16 mg/mL[b]	SX	64 mcg/mL[a]	Visually compatible for 12 hr at 23 °C	2603	**C**
	ALT[h]	0.4 to 0.8 mg/mL[b]	SX	64 mcg/mL[a]	Turns cloudy upon mixing	2603	**I**
Potassium chloride	AB	40 mEq/L[d]	WI	1 mg/mL	Physically compatible for 4 hr at room temperature	534	**C**
Propofol	ZEN	10 mg/mL	AB	0.016 mg/mL[a]	Physically compatible for 1 hr at 23 °C	2066	**C**
Ranitidine HCl	GL	1 mg/mL[a]	AB	0.128 mg/mL[a]	Visually compatible for 4 hr at 27 °C	2062	**C**
Remifentanil HCl	GW	0.025 and 0.25 mg/mL[b]	SW	0.12 mg/mL[a]	Physically compatible for 4 hr at 23 °C	2075	**C**
Sodium nitroprusside	RC	0.3, 1.2, 3 mg/mL[a]	SX	0.03, 0.12, 3 mg/mL[f]	Visually compatible for 48 hr at 24 °C protected from light	2357	**C**
Telavancin HCl	ASP	7.5 mg/mL[a,b,i]	BED	0.128 mg/mL[a,b,i]	Physically compatible for 2 hr	2830	**C**
TNA #73[e]			BN	8 mcg/mL[c]	Visually compatible for 4 hr	1009	**C**
TPN #212 to #215[e]			AB	16 mcg/mL[a]	Physically compatible for 4 hr at 23 °C	2109	**C**
Vasopressin	AMR	2 and 4 units/mL[b]	AB	4 mcg/mL[b]	Physically compatible with vasopressin pushed through a Y-site over 5 sec	2478	**C**
	APP	0.2 unit/mL[b]	GNS	16 mcg/mL[b]	Physically compatible	2641	**C**
	APP	0.2 unit/mL[b]	AB	4 mcg/mL[b]	Physically compatible	2641	**C**
Vecuronium bromide	OR	1 mg/mL	AB	0.128 mg/mL[a]	Visually compatible for 4 hr at 27 °C	2062	**C**

[a]*Tested in dextrose 5%.*

[b]*Tested in sodium chloride 0.9%.*

[c]*Tested in both dextrose 5% and sodium chloride 0.9%.*

[d]*Tested in dextrose 5% in Ringer's injection, dextrose 5% in Ringer's injection, lactated, dextrose 5%, Ringer's injection, lactated, and sodium chloride 0.9%.*

[e]*Refer to Appendix I for the composition of parenteral nutrition solutions. TNA indicates a 3-in-1 admixture, and TPN indicates a 2-in-1 admixture.*

[f]*Tested in dextrose 5% in sodium chloride 0.2%.*

[g]*Nesiritide is incompatible with bisulfite antioxidants used in some drug formulations. The specific formulation of the product to be used should be checked to ensure that no sulfite antioxidants are present.*

[h]*Test performed using the formulation WITHOUT edetate disodium.*

[i]*Tested in Ringer's injection, lactated.*

OCTREOTIDE ACETATE
AHFS 92:92

Products — Octreotide acetate injection is available in 1-mL ampuls containing 0.05 mg (50 mcg), 0.1 mg (100 mcg), and 0.5 (500 mcg) mg of octreotide and in 5-mL multiple-dose vials containing 0.2 mg (200 mcg) and 1 (1000 mcg) mg/mL of octreotide. (1)

The Sandostatin (Sandoz) products also contain in each milliliter lactic acid 3.4 mg, mannitol 45 mg, phenol 5 mg (vial only), and sodium bicarbonate to adjust pH in water for injection. (1)

Octreotide acetate (Bedford) has a differing formulation. In addition to the octreotide acetate, the Bedford formulation in ampuls and multidose vials contains in each milliliter l-lactic acid 3 mg and sodium chloride 7 mg with sodium hydroxide for pH adjustment in water for injection. The multidose vials also contain phenol 5 mg/mL as a preservative. (1)

pH — From 3.9 to 4.5. (1)

Trade Name(s) — Sandostatin.

Administration — Octreotide acetate injection is usually administered by subcutaneous injection in the smallest volume that will deliver the dose. Subcutaneous injection sites should be rotated. Multiple subcutaneous injections at the same site within a short time should be avoided. Administration by intravenous injection over three minutes or by infusion over 15 to 30 minutes after further dilution with 50 to 200 mL of dextrose 5% or sodium chloride 0.9% also has been recommended. (1; 4) NOTE: Do not confuse octreotide acetate injection with the injectable depot suspension product, which cannot be given by these routes of administration. (1)

Stability — Octreotide acetate injection is a clear solution. Ampuls and vials should be stored under refrigeration and protected from light. However, octreotide acetate injection can be stored at room temperature for up to 14 days when protected from light. (1; 4)

The manufacturers state that octreotide acetate injection should not be added to total parenteral nutrition solutions because of the formation of a glycosyl octreotide conjugate that may decrease the product's efficacy (1), although the clinical value of this administration approach continues to be debated. (2136)

Syringes — In Travenol, Minimed, and Becton Dickinson plastic syringes of polypropylene and natural rubber, octreotide 100 and 500 mcg/mL as the acetate was stable for 30 days. (1370)

The stability of octreotide acetate injection (Sandoz) 0.2 mg/mL packaged 1 mL in 3-mL polypropylene syringes sealed with tip caps (Becton Dickinson) was evaluated at 3 and 23 °C both exposed to and protected from normal room light. No octreotide acetate loss was found in 29 days stored at 3 °C protected from light but about 7 to 9% loss occurred in 15 to 22 days exposed to light. At 23 °C, the drug was less stable. Although results were variable, more than 10% loss occurred in about two weeks. Maximum storage of one week at 23 °C, whether protected from light or not was recommended. (2020)

In a similar study, the stability of octreotide acetate injection (Sandoz) 0.2 mg/mL was evaluated for 60 days stored at 5 and −20 °C (light conditions were not stated). The undiluted octreotide acetate injection was packaged 1 mL in 3-mL polypropylene syringes (Terumo) and sealed with a cap. A loss of about 6% at both storage conditions after 60 days was found. (2021)

Sorption — The manufacturer indicates that octreotide, a peptide, has the potential for adsorption to plastic and, possibly, glass. (1540) However, in both static and dynamic tests, octreotide did not adsorb to Travenol, Minimed, and Becton Dickinson (Plastipak) syringes of polypropylene and natural rubber, Travenol 3-mL insulin pump containers of polypropylene and polycarbonate, and Microflex PVC and Minimed polyolefin-lined PVC administration tubing. (1370) Neither was it adsorbed to glass infusion bottles or a PVC administration set at a concentration of 5 mcg/mL in sodium chloride 0.9%. (1371)

Compatibility Information

Solution Compatibility

Octreotide acetate

Solution	Mfr	Mfr	Conc/L	Remarks	Ref	C/I
Sodium chloride 0.9%	TR[a]	SZ	1.5 mg	Little octreotide loss over 48 hr at room temperature in ambient room light	1373	C
		SZ	5, 50, 250 mg	Physically compatible with no octreotide loss in 96 hr at room temperature exposed to light	1372	C
TNA #139[b]	[c]	SZ	450 mcg	Physically compatible with no change in lipid particle size in 48 hr at 22 °C under fluorescent light and 7 days at 4 °C. Octreotide activity highly variable	1540	?
TPN #119, #120[b]	[a]	SZ	1.5 mg	Little octreotide loss over 48 hr at room temperature in ambient room light	1373	C

[a]*Tested in PVC containers.*
[b]*Refer to Appendix I for the composition of parenteral nutrition solutions. TNA indicates a 3-in-1 admixture, and TPN indicates a 2-in-1 admixture.*
[c]*Tested in both glass and ethylene vinyl acetate (EVA) containers.*

Additive Compatibility

Octreotide acetate

Drug	Mfr	Conc/L	Mfr	Conc/L	Test Soln	Remarks	Ref	C/I
Fat emulsion, intravenous	KV	10%	SZ	1.5 mg		Octreotide content unstable	1373	I
Heparin sodium	ES	1000 units	SZ	1.5 mg	TPN #120[a]	Little octreotide loss over 48 hr at room temperature in ambient light	1373	C
Insulin, regular		5 units		50 mcg	TPN	Substantial insulin loss	1377	I

[a]*Refer to Appendix I for the composition of parenteral nutrition solutions. TPN indicates a 2-in-1 admixture.*

Drugs in Syringe Compatibility

Octreotide acetate

Drug (in syringe)	Mfr	Amt	Mfr	Amt	Remarks	Ref	C/I
Diamorphine HCl	EV	50 mg/ 8 mL[a]	NVA	300 mcg/ 8 mL[a]	Visually compatible with no octreotide loss in 48 hr. Diamorphine not tested	2709	C
	EV	50 mg/ 8 mL[a]	NVA	600 mcg/ 8 mL[a]	Visually compatible with no octreotide loss in 48 hr. Diamorphine not tested	2709	C
	EV	50 mg/ 8 mL[a]	NVA	900 mcg/ 8 mL[a]	Visually compatible with 1% octreotide loss in 48 hr. Diamorphine not tested	2709	C
	EV	100 mg/ 8 mL[a]	NVA	300 mcg/ 8 mL[a]	Visually compatible with 4% octreotide loss in 48 hr. Diamorphine not tested	2709	C
	EV	100 mg/ 8 mL[a]	NVA	600 mcg/ 8 mL[a]	Visually compatible with 6% octreotide loss in 48 hr. Diamorphine not tested	2709	C
	EV	100 mg/ 8 mL[a]	NVA	900 mcg/ 8 mL[a]	Visually compatible with 5% octreotide loss in 48 hr. Diamorphine not tested	2709	C
	EV	200 mg/ 8 mL[a]	NVA	600 mcg/ 8 mL[a]	Visually compatible with 6% octreotide loss in 48 hr. Diamorphine not tested	2709	C
Dimenhydrinate		10 mg/ 1 mL		0.5 mg/ 1 mL	Precipitate forms in about 1 hr	2569	I
Pantoprazole sodium	[b]	4 mg/ 1 mL		0.5 mcg/ 1 mL	Precipitates	2574	I

[a]*Tested in sterile water for injection.*
[b]*Test performed using the formulation WITHOUT edetate disodium.*

Y-Site Injection Compatibility (1:1 Mixture)

Octreotide acetate

Drug	Mfr	Conc	Mfr	Conc	Remarks	Ref	C/I
Hydroxyethyl starch 130/0.4 in sodium chloride 0.9%	FRK	6%	NVA	5, 7.5, 10 mcg/mL[a]	Visually compatible for 24 hr at room temperature	2770	C
Micafungin sodium	ASP	1.5 mg/mL[b]	NVA	5 mcg/mL[b]	Microparticulates form in 4 hr	2683	I
Pantoprazole sodium	ALT[c]	0.16 to 0.4 mg/mL[b]	NVA	5 to 10 mcg/mL[a]	Yellow discoloration forms	2603	I
	ALT[c]	0.8 mg/mL[b]	NVA	7.5 to 10 mcg/mL[a]	Yellow discoloration forms	2603	I
	ALT[c]	0.8 mg/mL[b]	NVA	5 mcg/mL[a]	Visually compatible for 12 hr at 23 °C	2603	C
TNA #218 to #226[d]			SZ	0.01 mg/mL[a]	Visually compatible for 4 hr at 23 °C	2215	C
TPN #212 to #215[d]			SZ	0.01 mg/mL[a]	Physically compatible for 4 hr at 23 °C	2109	C

[a]*Tested in dextrose 5%.*
[b]*Tested in sodium chloride 0.9%.*
[c]*Test performed using the formulation WITHOUT edetate disodium.*
[d]*Refer to Appendix I for the composition of parenteral nutrition solutions. TNA indicates a 3-in-1 admixture, and TPN indicates a 2-in-1 admixture.*

OMEPRAZOLE
AHFS 56:28.36

Products — Omeprazole infusion is available in vials containing 40 mg of drug as the sodium salt. Also present in the formulation are sodium hydroxide and disodium edetate. Reconstitute the vials with 5 mL from a 100-mL bag or bottle of sodium chloride 0.9% or dextrose 5%. Mix thoroughly, ensuring that all of the omeprazole has dissolved; do not use if any particles remain in the reconstituted solution. The reconstituted solution should be transferred into the infusion bag or bottle making 100 mL of the admixture solution. (38; 115)

Omeprazole injection is also available in vials containing 40 mg of drug as the sodium salt with an accompanying 10-mL ampul of special solvent. Each milliliter of the solvent contains citric acid monohydrate 0.5 mg and polyethylene glycol 400 0.4 g in water for injection. The vial of omeprazole should be reconstituted with 10 mL of the solvent provided in the accompanying ampul in two 5-mL increments withdrawing air pressure back into the syringe between the increments. No other diluent should be used for reconstitution. Rotate and shake the vial to ensure all of the omeprazole has dissolved; do not use if any particles remain in the reconstituted solution. (38; 115)

Sodium Content — Omeprazole 40 mg provides sodium 2.6 mg. (115)

Trade Name(s) — Losec, Mopral, Omeprazen.

Administration — Omeprazole is administered by intravenous infusion and intravenous injection. The drug must not be given by any other route. (38; 115)

After dilution of the omeprazole infusion to 100 mL with sodium chloride 0.9% or dextrose 5%, omeprazole is administered only as a 20- to 30-minute intravenous infusion. (38; 115)

After dilution with the accompanying special diluent, omeprazole injection is administered intravenously over 2.5 to 5 minutes at a maximum rate of 4 mL/min. (38; 115)

Stability — Intact vials of omeprazole infusion and injection should be stored at room temperature not exceeding 25 °C and protected from light. Discoloration of the reconstituted solution may occur if reconstituted incorrectly. Dilution of omeprazole infusion with sodium chloride 0.9% results in a solution that is stable for 12 hours (38; 115); diluted in dextrose 5% omeprazole is stable for three (38) to six (115) hours. Other solutions must not be used for dilution of omeprazole infusion. Omeprazole injection reconstituted with the accompanying special diluent is stable for four hours. Do not use the reconstituted solution if particles are present. (38; 115)

Reconstituted omeprazole has been reported to develop an unacceptable discoloration indicating decomposition within six hours at room temperature exposed to light. (2507)

Compatibility Information

Solution Compatibility

Omeprazole

Solution	Mfr	Mfr	Conc/L	Remarks	Ref	C/I
Dextrose 5%	BA	PH	400 mg	Physically compatible. 10% loss occurs in 2.5 days at 22 °C in light	2696	C
Sodium chloride 0.9%	BA	PH	400 mg	Physically compatible. 10% loss occurs in 10 days at 22 °C in light	2696	C

Y-Site Injection Compatibility (1:1 Mixture)

Omeprazole

Drug	Mfr	Conc	Mfr	Conc	Remarks	Ref	C/I
Lorazepam	WY	0.33 mg/mL[b]	AST	4 mg/mL	Yellow discoloration forms	1855	I
Midazolam HCl	RC	5 mg/mL	AST	4 mg/mL	Brown color then precipitate	1855	I
Vancomycin HCl		10 mg/mL[a]		4 mg/mL	White precipitate forms within 5 min	2173	I

[a]Tested in dextrose 5%.
[b]Tested in sodium chloride 0.9%.

ONDANSETRON HYDROCHLORIDE
AHFS 56:22.20

Products — Ondansetron hydrochloride is available in 20-mL multiple-dose vials and 2-mL single-dose vials. Each milliliter of solution in multiple-dose vials contains ondansetron (as the hydrochloride dihydrate) 2 mg with sodium chloride 8.3 mg, citric acid monohydrate 0.5 mg, sodium citrate dihydrate 0.25 mg, methylparaben 1.2 mg, and propylparaben 0.15 mg. Each milliliter of solution in single-dose vials contains ondansetron (as the hydrochloride dihydrate) 2 mg with sodium chloride 9 mg, citric acid monohydrate 0.5 mg, and sodium citrate dihydrate 0.25 mg. (1)

Ondansetron hydrochloride is also available as a premixed infusion solution in a dextrose or sodium chloride solution containing ondansetron 32 mg/50 mL (as the hydrochloride dihydrate) with citric acid and sodium citrate in water for injection. (1)

pH — Injection from 3.3 to 4. Premixed infusion from 3 to 4. (1)

Osmolality — The osmolarity of the premixed ondansetron hydrochloride 32 mg/50 mL solution is 270 mOsm/L. (1)

Trade Name(s) — Zofran.

Administration — Ondansetron hydrochloride is administered intravenously over 15 minutes after further dilution with 50 mL of sodium chloride 0.9% or dextrose 5%. By intravenous injection, it is administered undiluted over at least 30 seconds and preferably over two to five minutes. It has also been administered intramuscularly. (1)

Stability — Ondansetron hydrochloride is a clear, colorless solution. It should be stored at room temperature and protected from light, excessive heat, and from freezing. (1) Although ondansetron hydrochloride is unstable under intense light, it is stable for about a month in daylight with added fluorescent light. (1366)

Ondansetron hydrochloride (Glaxo) 0.03 and 0.3 mg/mL in dextrose 5% or sodium chloride 0.9% was stable when frozen at −20 °C, exhibiting a 10% or less loss in three months. (1642)

pH Effects — The natural pH of ondansetron hydrochloride solutions is about 4.5 to 4.6. (1366; 1367) If the pH is increased, a precipitate of ondansetron free base has been reported to develop at pH 5.7 (1366) and pH 7. (1513) Redissolution of the ondansetron precipitate occurs at pH 6.2 when titrated with hydrochloric acid. (1513) Precipitation by combination with alkaline drugs has been observed. (1365; 1513)

Syringes — The stability of ondansetron hydrochloride undiluted at 2 mg/mL and diluted in dextrose 5% and sodium chloride 0.9% at 1, 0.5, and 0.25 mg/mL packaged in polypropylene syringes was reported. Representative syringes were stored at 24 °C for 48 hours, 4 °C for 14 days, and frozen at −20 °C for 90 days. Visually, the solutions exhibited no precipitate or color or clarity changes. Ondansetron hydrochloride concentrations in all samples remained above 90%; most samples were above 95%. Sequentially storing sample syringes for 90 days at −20 °C followed by 14 days at 4 °C followed by 48 hours at 24 °C did not alter the stability. (2056)

When diluted with compatible infusion solutions, ondansetron hydrochloride is stable for up to seven days at room temperature or under refrigeration in Plastipak syringes with syringe caps. (1366)

Filtration — Ondansetron hydrochloride (Glaxo) 0.03 and 0.2 mg/mL (30 and 200 mcg/mL) in sodium chloride 0.9% was delivered over 15 minutes through five 0.2-μm inline filters: Continu-Flo Solution Set (Baxter, 2C5561S), Filtered Extension Sets (Burron, PFE-2007 and FE-2024), Universal Primary infusion set (IVAC, 52023), and Ivex-HP Filterset-SL (Abbott, 4524). Little or no ondansetron loss was found. (1678)

Central Venous Catheter — Ondansetron hydrochloride (Glaxo Wellcome) 0.2 mg/mL in dextrose 5% was found to be compatible with the ARROWg+ard Blue Plus (Arrow International) chlorhexidine-bearing triple-lumen central catheter. Essentially complete delivery of the drug was found with little or no drug loss occurring. Furthermore, chlorhexidine delivered from the catheter remained at trace amounts with no substantial increase due to the delivery of the drug through the catheter. (2335)

Compatibility Information

Solution Compatibility

Ondansetron HCl

Solution	Mfr	Mfr	Conc/L	Remarks	Ref	C/I
Dextrose 5% in sodium chloride 0.45%				Stable for 48 hr at room temperature in light	1	C
Dextrose 5% in sodium chloride 0.9%				Stable for 48 hr at room temperature in light	1	C
Dextrose 5%				Stable for 48 hr at room temperature in light	1	C
	BP[a]	GL	16 and 80 mg	Physically compatible and stable for 7 days at room temperature in light and at 4 °C	1366	C
		GL	24 and 96 mg	Visually compatible. No loss in 14 days at 24 °C or 14 days at 5 °C then 2 days at 24 °C	1560	C
	BA[a]	GL	30 and 300 mg	Visually compatible with 5% or less loss in 48 hr at 25 °C or 14 days at 5 °C	1642	C
	MG[b]	GL	0.03 and 0.3 g	Visually compatible with no loss in 14 days at 4 °C in light	1722	C
Dextrose 5% with potassium chloride 0.3%	BP[a]	GL	16 mg	Physically compatible and stable for 7 days at room temperature in light and at 4 °C	1366	C
Ringer's injection	BP[a]	GL	16 mg	Physically compatible and stable for 7 days at room temperature in light and at 4 °C	1366	C
Ringer's injection, lactated		GL	24 and 96 mg	Visually compatible. No loss in 14 days at 24 °C or 14 days at 5 °C then 2 days at 24 °C	1560	C
Sodium chloride 0.9%				Stable for 48 hr at room temperature in light	1	C
	BP[a]	GL	16 and 80 mg	Physically compatible and stable for 7 days at room temperature in light and at 4 °C	1366	C
		GL	24 and 96 mg	Visually compatible. No loss in 14 days at 24 °C or 14 days at 5 °C then 2 days at 24 °C	1560	C
	BA[c]	GL	240 mg	No loss in 24 hr at 30 °C or 30 days at 3 °C then 24 hr at 30 °C	1553	C
	BA[a]	GL	30 and 300 mg	Visually compatible with 4% or less loss in 48 hr at 25 °C or 14 days at 5 °C	1642	C
	MG[b]	GL	0.03 and 0.3 g	Visually compatible with no loss in 14 days at 4 °C in light	1722	C
	BA[a]	CER	100 mg	Visually compatible. 6 to 7% loss after 30 days at 4 °C then 2 days at 23 °C	1882	C
	BA[a]	CER	200, 400, 640 mg	Visually compatible. Up to 4% loss after 30 days at 4 °C then 2 days at 23 °C	1882	C
	AGT[a]	GL	80 mg	Visually compatible with 4% loss in 120 days at 4 and −20 °C	2405	C
Sodium chloride 0.9% with potassium chloride 0.3%	BP[a]	GL	16 mg	Physically compatible and stable for 7 days at room temperature in light and at 4 °C	1366	C
TNA #190[d]		GL	0.03 and 0.3 g	Physically compatible with no loss in 48 hr at 24 °C in light	1766	C

[a]Tested in PVC containers.
[b]Tested in a Kraton polymer elastomeric infusion device (Homepump, Block).
[c]Tested in a medication cassette reservoir (Pharmacia Deltec CADD-1).
[d]Refer to Appendix I for the composition of parenteral nutrition solutions. TNA indicates a 3-in-1 admixture.

Additive Compatibility

Ondansetron HCl

Drug	Mfr	Conc/L	Mfr	Conc/L	Test Soln	Remarks	Ref	C/I
Cisplatin	BR	485 mg	GL	1.031 g	NS[a]	Physically compatible. Little loss of drugs in 24 hr at 4 °C then 7 days at 30 °C	1846	**C**
	BR	219 mg	GL	479 mg	NS[b]	Physically compatible. Little loss of drugs in 7 days at 4 °C then 24 hr at 30 °C	1846	**C**
Cyclophosphamide	MJ	300 mg	GL	50 mg	D5W[a], NS[a]	Visually compatible with 9 to 10% cyclophosphamide loss and no ondansetron loss in 5 days at 24 °C. No loss of either drug in 8 days at 4 °C	1812	**C**
	MJ	2 g	GL	400 mg	D5W[a], NS[a]	Visually compatible with 10% cyclophosphamide loss and no ondansetron loss in 5 days at 24 °C. No loss of either drug in 8 days at 4 °C	1812	**C**
Cytarabine	UP	200 mg	GL	30 and 300 mg	D5W[a]	Physically compatible with little loss of either drug in 48 hr at 23 °C	1876	**C**
	UP	40 g	GL	30 and 300 mg	D5W[a]	Physically compatible with little loss of either drug in 48 hr at 23 °C	1876	**C**
Dacarbazine	MI	1 g	GL	30 and 300 mg	D5W[a]	Physically compatible with little loss of ondansetron in 48 hr at 23 °C. 8 to 12% dacarbazine loss in 24 hr and 20% loss in 48 hr at 23 °C	1876	**C**
	MI	3 g	GL	30 and 300 mg	D5W[a]	Physically compatible with little loss of ondansetron in 48 hr at 23 °C. 8% dacarbazine loss in 24 hr and 15% loss in 48 hr at 23 °C	1876	**C**
Dacarbazine with doxorubicin HCl	LY AD	8 g 800 mg	GL	640 mg	D5W[a]	Visually compatible. Under 10% ondansetron and doxorubicin loss in 24 hr at 30 °C and 7 days at 4 °C then 24 hr at 30 °C. Dacarbazine stable for 8 hr but 13% loss in 24 hr	2092	**I**
Dacarbazine with doxorubicin HCl	LY AD	8 g 800 mg	GL	640 mg	D5W[b]	Visually compatible. Under 10% loss of all drugs in 24 hr at 30 °C and 7 days at 4 °C then 24 hr at 30 °C	2092	**C**
Dacarbazine with doxorubicin HCl	LY AD	20 g 1.5 g	GL	640 mg	D5W[a,b]	Visually compatible. Under 10% loss of all drugs in 24 hr at 30 °C and 7 days at 4 °C then 24 hr at 30 °C	2092	**C**
Dexamethasone sodium phosphate		20 and 40 mg	GL	48 mg	D5W, NS	Visually compatible for 24 hr at 22 °C	1608	**C**
		200 and 400 mg	GL	160 mg	NS	Visually compatible for 24 hr at 22 °C	1608	**C**
	ES	200 mg	CER	100 mg	NS[a]	Visually compatible. No dexamethasone and 8% ondansetron loss in 30 days at 4 °C then 2 days at 23 °C	1882	**C**
	ES	400 mg	CER	100 and 200 mg	NS[a]	Visually compatible. No dexamethasone and 7 to 10% ondansetron loss in 30 days at 4 °C then 2 days at 23 °C	1882	**C**
	ES	200 mg	CER	200, 400, 640 mg	NS[a]	Visually compatible. No dexamethasone and 5% ondansetron loss in 30 days at 4 °C then 2 days at 23 °C	1882	**C**
	ES	400 mg	CER	400 and 640 mg	NS[a]	Visually compatible. No dexamethasone and 3% ondansetron loss in 30 days at 4 °C then 2 days at 23 °C	1882	**C**

Additive Compatibility (Cont.)

Ondansetron HCl

Drug	Mfr	Conc/L	Mfr	Conc/L	Test Soln	Remarks	Ref	C/I
	ES	200 and 400 mg	CER	640 mg	D5W[c]	Visually compatible. 7% dexamethasone and no ondansetron loss in 30 days at 4 °C then 2 days at 23 °C	1882	C
	MSD	400 mg	GL	150 mg	NS[a]	Visually compatible. 4% or less loss of either drug in 28 days at 4 and 22 °C	2084	C
	MSD	400 mg	GL	150 mg	D5W[a]	Visually compatible. 4% or less loss of either drug in 28 days at 4 °C. 10% ondansetron loss in 3 days at 22 °C	2084	C
	MSD	230 mg	GL	750 mg	NS[a]	Visually compatible. 4% or less loss of either drug in 28 days at 4 °C. 10% ondansetron loss in 7 days at 22 °C	2084	C
	MSD	230 mg	GL	750 mg	D5W[a]	Visually compatible. Up to 13% ondansetron loss in 3 days at 4 and 22 °C	2084	?
	OR	100 mg	GSK	80 mg	D5W[d]	Visually compatible. Under 3% ondansetron and 8% dexamethasone loss when frozen for 3 months then stored refrigerated for 30 days	2822	C
Doxorubicin HCl	MJ	100 mg and 2 g	GL	30 and 300 mg	D5W[a]	Physically compatible with little loss of either drug in 48 hr at 23 °C	1876	C
Doxorubicin HCl with dacarbazine	AD LY	800 mg 8 g	GL	640 mg	D5W[a]	Visually compatible. Under 10% ondansetron and doxorubicin loss in 24 hr at 30 °C and 7 days at 4 °C then 24 hr at 30 °C. Dacarbazine stable for 8 hr but 13% loss in 24 hr	2092	I
Doxorubicin HCl with dacarbazine	AD LY	800 mg 8 g	GL	640 mg	D5W[b]	Visually compatible. Under 10% loss of all drugs in 24 hr at 30 °C and 7 days at 4 °C then 24 hr at 30 °C	2092	C
Doxorubicin HCl with dacarbazine	AD LY	1.5 g 20 g	GL	640 mg	D5W[a,b]	Visually compatible. Under 10% loss of all drugs in 24 hr at 30 °C and 7 days at 4 °C then 24 hr at 30 °C	2092	C
Doxorubicin HCl with vincristine sulfate	AD LI	400 mg 14 mg	GL	480 mg	D5W[b]	Visually compatible. Under 10% loss of all drugs in 5 days at 4 °C then 24 hr at 30 °C	2092	C
Doxorubicin HCl with vincristine sulfate	AD LI	800 mg 28 mg	GL	960 mg	D5W[a]	Visually compatible. Under 10% loss of all drugs after 120 hr at 30 °C	2092	C
Etoposide	BR	100 mg	GL	30 and 300 mg	D5W[a]	Physically compatible. Little or no loss of ondansetron in 48 hr at 23 °C. 4% etoposide loss in 24 hr and 6% loss in 48 hr at 23 °C	1876	C
	BR	400 mg	GL	30 and 300 mg	D5W[a]	Physically compatible with little or no loss of either drug in 48 hr at 23 °C	1876	C
Fluconazole with ranitidine HCl	RR GL	2 g 500 mg	GL	100 mg	[a]	Visually compatible with no loss of any drug in 4 hr	1730	C
Hydromorphone HCl	ES	500 mg	GL	100 mg and 1 g	NS	Physically compatible. No loss of either drug in 7 days at 32 °C or 31 days at 4 and 22 °C protected from light	1690	C
Mannitol	BP[a]	10%	GL	16 mg		Physically compatible. Stable for 7 days at room temperature in light and at 4 °C	1366	C
Meperidine HCl	WY	4 g	GL	100 mg and 1 g	NS[a]	Physically compatible. No loss of either drug in 31 days at 4 and 22 °C and in 7 days at 32 °C	1862	C

Additive Compatibility (Cont.)

Ondansetron HCl

Drug	Mfr	Conc/L	Mfr	Conc/L	Test Soln	Remarks	Ref	C/I
Meropenem	ZEN	1 g	GL	1 g	NS	Visually compatible for 4 hr at room temperature	1994	**C**
	ZEN	20 g	GL	1 g	NS	White precipitate forms immediately	1994	**I**
Methotrexate sodium	LE	0.5 and 6 g	GL	30 and 300 mg	D5W[a]	Physically compatible with little or no loss of either drug in 48 hr at 23 °C	1876	**C**
Methylprednisolone sodium succinate	PH	2.4 g	GSK	160 mg	D5W, NS	Transient turbidity forms then clears. 5% or less loss of either drug in 24 hr at 23 °C and 48 hr at 6 °C	2643	**?**
Morphine sulfate	AST	1 g	GL	100 mg and 1 g	NS	Physically compatible. No ondansetron loss and 5% or less morphine loss in 7 days at 32 °C or 31 days at 4 and 22 °C protected from light	1690	**C**
Ranitidine HCl with fluconazole	RR GL	2 g 500 mg	GL	100 mg	[a]	Visually compatible with no loss of any drug in 4 hr	1730	**C**
Tramadol HCl	GRU	400 mg	GL	1.6 mg	NS	Visually compatible with about 7% tramadol loss in 24 hr at room temperature	2652	**C**
Vincristine sulfate with doxorubicin HCl	LI AD	14 mg 400 mg	GL	480 mg	D5W[b]	Visually compatible. Under 10% loss of all drugs in 5 days at 4 °C then 24 hr at 30 °C	2092	**C**
Vincristine sulfate with doxorubicin HCl	AD LI	28 mg 800 mg	GL	960 mg	D5W[a]	Visually compatible. Under 10% loss of all drugs after 120 hr at 30 °C	2092	**C**

[a]Tested in PVC containers.
[b]Tested in polyisoprene reservoirs (Travenol Infusors).
[c]Tested in ondansetron hydrochloride ready-to-use CR3 polyester bags.
[d]Tested in polyolefin containers.

Drugs in Syringe Compatibility

Ondansetron HCl

Drug (in syringe)	Mfr	Amt	Mfr	Amt	Remarks	Ref	C/I
Alfentanil HCl	JN	0.167 mg/mL[b]	GW	1.33 mg/mL[b]	Physically compatible. Little loss of either drug in 24 hr at 4 or 23 °C	2199	**C**
Atropine sulfate	GNS	0.133 mg/mL[b]	GW	1.33 mg/mL[b]	Physically compatible. Under 6% ondansetron and under 7% atropine losses in 24 hr at 4 or 23 °C	2199	**C**
Dexamethasone sodium phosphate	ES	0.33 and 0.67 mg/mL[a]	CER	0.17 mg/mL[a]	Visually compatible. No loss of either drug in 30 days at 4 °C then 2 days at 23 °C	1882	**C**
	ES	0.5 mg/mL[a]	CER	0.25 mg/mL[a]	Visually compatible. No loss of either drug in 30 days at 4 °C then 2 days at 23 °C	1882	**C**
	ES	1 mg/mL[a]	CER	0.25 mg/mL[a]	Visually compatible for 3 days at 4 °C. Precipitation of ondansetron observed at 7 days as opaque white ring	1882	**C**
	ES	0.33 and 0.67 mg/mL[a]	CER	0.33 mg/mL[a]	Visually compatible. No loss of either drug in 30 days at 4 °C then 2 days at 23 °C	1882	**C**
	ES	0.5 mg/mL[a]	CER	0.5 mg/mL[a]	Visually compatible. No loss of either drug in 30 days at 4 °C then 2 days at 23 °C	1882	**C**

Drugs in Syringe Compatibility (Cont.)

Drug (in syringe)	Mfr	Amt	Mfr	Amt	Remarks	Ref	C/I
	ES	1 mg/mL[a]	CER	0.5 mg/mL[a]	Visually compatible for 3 days at 4 °C. Precipitation of ondansetron observed at 5 days as opaque white ring	1882	C
	ES	0.33 and 0.67 mg/mL[a]	CER	0.67 mg/mL[a]	Visually compatible. No loss of either drug in 30 days at 4 °C then 2 days at 23 °C	1882	C
	ES	0.33 mg/mL[a]	CER	1.07 mg/mL[a]	Visually compatible. No loss of either drug in 30 days at 4 °C then 2 days at 23 °C	1882	C
	ES	0.67 mg/mL[a]	CER	1.07 mg/mL[a]	Heavy white precipitate in 72 hr at 4 °C. 25 to 30% loss of both drugs	1882	I
	OM[c]	4 mg/1 mL		4 mg/2 mL	Physically incompatible within 3 min	2767	I
	[d]	4 mg/1 mL		4 mg/2 mL	Physically compatible	2767	C
Droperidol	AMR	1.25 mg/mL[b]	GW	1 mg/mL[b]	Droperidol precipitates at 4 °C. At 23 °C, little or no loss of either drug in 8 hr, but droperidol precipitates after that time	2199	I
Fentanyl citrate	ES	16.7 mcg/mL[b]	GW	1.33 mg/mL[b]	Physically compatible. Little loss of either drug in 24 hr at 4 or 23 °C	2199	C
Glycopyrrolate	AMR	0.1 mg/mL[b]	GW	1 mg/mL[b]	Physically compatible. Little loss of either drug in 24 hr at 4 or 23 °C	2199	C
Meperidine HCl	ES	8.33 mg/mL[b]	GW	1.33 mg/mL[b]	Physically compatible. Little loss of either drug in 24 hr at 4 or 23 °C	2199	C
Metoclopramide HCl	SO	2.5 mg/mL[b]	GW	1 mg/mL[b]	Physically compatible. Under 6% ondansetron and under 5% metoclopramide losses in 24 hr at 4 or 23 °C	2199	C
Midazolam HCl	RC	1.66 mg/mL[b]	GW	1.33 mg/mL[b]	Physically compatible. Under 4% ondansetron and under 7% midazolam losses in 24 hr at 4 or 23 °C	2199	C
Morphine sulfate	ES	2.67 mg/mL[b]	GW	1.33 mg/mL[b]	Physically compatible. Under 5% ondansetron and under 4% morphine losses in 24 hr at 4 or 23 °C	2199	C
Naloxone HCl	AST	0.133 mg/mL[b]	GW	1.33 mg/mL[b]	Physically compatible. Under 6% ondansetron and under 5% naloxone losses in 24 hr at 4 or 23 °C	2199	C
Neostigmine methylsulfate	ES	0.167 mg/mL[b]	GW	1.33 mg/mL[b]	Physically compatible. Under 3% ondansetron and under 5% neostigmine losses in 24 hr at 4 or 23 °C	2199	C
Propofol	STU	1 and 5 mg/mL[b]	GW	1 mg/mL[b]	Physically compatible. Little loss of either drug in 4 hr at 23 °C	2199	C

[a]Diluted with sodium chloride 0.9% drawn into a syringe prior to drugs to yield the concentrations cited.
[b]Tested in sodium chloride 0.9%.
[c]Contained benzyl alcohol as a preservative.
[d]Contained parabens as preservatives.

Y-Site Injection Compatibility (1:1 Mixture)

Ondansetron HCl

Drug	Mfr	Conc	Mfr	Conc	Remarks	Ref	C/I
Acyclovir sodium	BW	7 mg/mL[a]	GL	1 mg/mL[b]	Precipitates immediately	1365	I
Aldesleukin	CHI	33,800 I.U./mL[a]	GL	0.7 mg/mL[a]	Visually compatible with little or no loss of aldesleukin activity	1857	C
	CHI	5 to 40 mcg/mL[k]	GL		Visually compatible. Aldesleukin activity retained if each drug infused at a similar rate. Ondansetron not tested	1890	C
Allopurinol sodium	BW	3 mg/mL[b]	GL	1 mg/mL[b]	Immediate turbidity becoming precipitate	1686	I
Amifostine	USB	10 mg/mL[a]	GL	1 mg/mL[a]	Physically compatible for 4 hr at 23 °C	1845	C
Amikacin sulfate	BR	5 mg/mL[a]	GL	1 mg/mL[b]	Visually compatible for 4 hr at 22 °C	1365	C
Aminophylline	AMR	2.5 mg/mL[a]	GL	1 mg/mL[b]	Immediate turbidity and precipitation	1365	I
Amphotericin B	SQ	0.6 mg/mL[a]	GL	1 mg/mL[a]	Immediate yellow turbid precipitation	1365	I
Amphotericin B cholesteryl sulfate complex	SEQ	0.83 mg/mL[a]	CER	1 mg/mL[a]	Gross precipitate forms	2117	I
Ampicillin sodium	BR	20 mg/mL[b]	GL	1 mg/mL[b]	Immediate turbidity and precipitation	1365	I
Ampicillin sodium–sulbactam sodium	RR	20 + 10 mg/mL[b]	GL	1 mg/mL[b]	Immediate turbidity and precipitation	1365	I
Amsacrine	NCI	1 mg/mL[a]	GL	1 mg/mL[a]	Orange precipitate forms within 30 min	1365	I
Azithromycin	PF	2 mg/mL[b]	GW	2 mg/mL[j]	Visually compatible	2368	C
Aztreonam	SQ	40 mg/mL[a]	GL	1 mg/mL[b]	Visually compatible for 4 hr at 22 °C	1365	C
	SQ	40 mg/mL[a]	GL	0.03 and 0.3 mg/mL[a]	Visually compatible with little loss of either drug in 4 hr at 25 °C	1732	C
	SQ	40 mg/mL[a]	GL	1 mg/mL[a]	Physically compatible for 4 hr at 23 °C	1758	C
Bleomycin sulfate	BR	1 unit/mL[b]	GL	1 mg/mL[b]	Visually compatible for 4 hr at 22 °C	1365	C
Carboplatin	BR	5 mg/mL[a]	GL	1 mg/mL[b]	Visually compatible for 4 hr at 22 °C	1365	C
		0.18 to 9.9 mg/mL	GL	16 to 160 mcg/mL	Physically compatible when carboplatin given over 10 to 60 min via Y-site	1366	C
Carmustine	BR	1.5 mg/mL[a]	GL	1 mg/mL[b]	Visually compatible for 4 hr at 22 °C	1365	C
Caspofungin acetate	ME	0.5 mg/mL[b]	BED	2 mg/mL	Physically compatible with ondansetron HCl i.v. push over 2 to 5 min	2766	C
Cefazolin sodium	LEM	20 mg/mL[a]	GL	1 mg/mL[b]	Visually compatible for 4 hr at 22 °C	1365	C
	LI	20 mg/mL[a]	GL	0.03 and 0.3 mg/mL[a]	Visually compatible with little loss of either drug in 4 hr at 25 °C	1732	C
Cefotaxime sodium	HO	20 mg/mL[a]	GL	1 mg/mL[b]	Visually compatible for 4 hr at 22 °C	1365	C
Cefoxitin sodium	MSD	20 mg/mL[a]	GL	1 mg/mL[b]	Visually compatible for 4 hr at 22 °C	1365	C
Ceftaroline fosamil	FOR	2.22 mg/mL[a,b,i]	WOC	1 mg/mL[a,b,i]	Physically compatible for 4 hr at 23 °C	2826	C
Ceftazidime	GL	40 mg/mL[a]	GL	1 mg/mL[b]	Visually compatible for 4 hr at 22 °C	1365	C
		100 to 200 mg/mL	GL	16 to 160 mcg/mL	Physically compatible when ceftazidime given as 5-min bolus via Y-site	1366	C
	LI	40 mg/mL[a]	GL	0.03 and 0.3 mg/mL[a]	Visually compatible with less than 10% loss of either drug in 4 hr at 25 °C	1732	C
Cefuroxime sodium	LI	30 mg/mL[a]	GL	1 mg/mL[b]	Visually compatible for 4 hr at 22 °C	1365	C
Chlorpromazine HCl	ES	2 mg/mL[a]	GL	1 mg/mL[b]	Visually compatible for 4 hr at 22 °C	1365	C
Cisatracurium besylate	GW	0.1, 2, 5 mg/mL[a]	CER	1 mg/mL[a]	Physically compatible for 4 hr at 23 °C	2074	C

Y-Site Injection Compatibility (1:1 Mixture) (Cont.)

Ondansetron HCl

Drug	Mfr	Conc	Mfr	Conc	Remarks	Ref	C/I
Cisplatin	BR	1 mg/mL	GL	1 mg/mL[b]	Visually compatible for 4 hr at 22 °C	1365	C
		0.48 mg/mL	GL	16 to 160 mcg/mL	Physically compatible when cisplatin given over 1 to 8 hr via Y-site	1366	C
Cladribine	ORT	0.015[b] and 0.5[d] mg/mL	CER	1 mg/mL[b]	Physically compatible for 4 hr at 23 °C	1969	C
Clindamycin phosphate	LY	10 mg/mL[a]	GL	1 mg/mL[b]	Visually compatible for 4 hr at 22 °C	1365	C
Cyclophosphamide	MJ	10 mg/mL[a]	GL	1 mg/mL[b]	Visually compatible for 4 hr at 22 °C	1365	C
		20 mg/mL	GL	16 to 160 mcg/mL	Physically compatible when cyclophosphamide given as 5-min bolus via Y-site	1366	C
Cytarabine	UP	50 mg/mL	GL	1 mg/mL[b]	Visually compatible for 4 hr at 22 °C	1365	C
Dacarbazine	MI	4 mg/mL[a]	GL	1 mg/mL[b]	Visually compatible for 4 hr at 22 °C	1365	C
Dactinomycin	MSD	0.01 mg/mL[a]	GL	1 mg/mL[b]	Visually compatible for 4 hr at 22 °C	1365	C
Daunorubicin HCl	WY	2 mg/mL[a]	GL	1 mg/mL[b]	Visually compatible for 4 hr at 22 °C	1365	C
Dexamethasone sodium phosphate	MSD	1 mg/mL[a]	GL	1 mg/mL[b]	Visually compatible for 4 hr at 22 °C	1365	C
Dexmedetomidine HCl	AB	4 mcg/mL[b]	GW	1 mg/mL[b]	Physically compatible for 4 hr at 23 °C	2383	C
Diphenhydramine HCl	PD	2 mg/mL[a]	GL	1 mg/mL[b]	Visually compatible for 4 hr at 22 °C	1365	C
Docetaxel	RPR	0.9 mg/mL[a]	GW	1 mg/mL[a]	Physically compatible for 4 hr at 23 °C	2224	C
Dopamine HCl	AB	0.8 mg/mL[a]	GL	0.32 mg/mL[c]	Visually compatible for 24 hr at room temperature in test tubes. No precipitate found on filter from Y-site delivery	2063	C
Doripenem	JJ	5 mg/mL[a,b]	WOC	1 mg/mL[a,b]	Physically compatible for 4 hr at 23 °C	2743	C
Doxorubicin HCl	CET	2 mg/mL	GL	1 mg/mL[b]	Visually compatible for 4 hr at 22 °C	1365	C
		2 mg/mL	GL	16 to 160 mcg/mL	Physically compatible when doxorubicin given as 5-min bolus via Y-site	1366	C
Doxorubicin HCl liposomal	SEQ	0.4 mg/mL[a]	CER	1 mg/mL[a]	Physically compatible for 4 hr at 23 °C	2087	C
Doxycycline hyclate	ES	1 mg/mL[a]	GL	1 mg/mL[b]	Visually compatible for 4 hr at 22 °C	1365	C
Droperidol	JN	0.4 mg/mL[a]	GL	1 mg/mL[b]	Visually compatible for 4 hr at 22 °C	1365	C
Etoposide	BR	0.4 mg/mL[a]	GL	1 mg/mL[b]	Visually compatible for 4 hr at 22 °C	1365	C
		0.144 to 0.25 mg/mL	GL	16 to 160 mcg/mL	Physically compatible when etoposide given over 30 to 60 min via Y-site	1366	C
Etoposide phosphate	BR	5 mg/mL[a]	GW	1 mg/mL[a]	Physically compatible for 4 hr at 23 °C	2218	C
Famotidine	MSD	2 mg/mL[a]	GL	1 mg/mL[b]	Visually compatible for 4 hr at 22 °C	1365	C
Fenoldopam mesylate	AB	80 mcg/mL[b]	GW	1 mg/mL[b]	Physically compatible for 4 hr at 23 °C	2467	C
Filgrastim	AMG	30 mcg/mL[a]	GL	1 mg/mL[a]	Physically compatible for 4 hr at 22 °C	1687	C
Floxuridine	RC	3 mg/mL[a]	GL	1 mg/mL[b]	Visually compatible for 4 hr at 22 °C	1365	C
Fluconazole	PF	2 mg/mL	GL	1 mg/mL[b]	Visually compatible for 4 hr at 22 °C	1365	C
	RR	2 mg/mL[b]	GL	0.03 and 0.3 mg/mL[a]	Visually compatible. Little loss of either drug in 4 hr at 25 °C in light	1732	C
	RR	2 mg/mL	GL	0.03, 0.1, 0.3 mg/mL[a,b]	Visually compatible. Little loss of both drugs in 4 hr. 5% or less loss of both in 12 hr at room temperature	2168	C
Fludarabine phosphate	BX	1 mg/mL[a]	GL	0.5 mg/mL[a]	Visually compatible for 4 hr at 22 °C	1439	C
Fluorouracil	SO	16 mg/mL[a]	GL	1 mg/mL[b]	Precipitates immediately	1365	I

Y-Site Injection Compatibility (1:1 Mixture) (Cont.)

Ondansetron HCl

Drug	Mfr	Conc	Mfr	Conc	Remarks	Ref	C/I
		≤0.8 mg/mL	GL	16 to 160 mcg/mL	Physically compatible when fluorouracil given at 20 mL/hr via Y-site	1366	**C**
Furosemide	AB	3 mg/mL[a]	GL	1 mg/mL[b]	Immediate turbidity and precipitation	1365	**I**
Gallium nitrate	FUJ	1 mg/mL[b]	GL	0.3 mg/mL[b]	Visually compatible for 24 hr at 25 °C	1673	**C**
Ganciclovir sodium	SY	20 mg/mL[a]	GL	1 mg/mL[b]	Immediate turbidity and precipitation	1365	**I**
Gemcitabine HCl	LI	10 mg/mL[b]	GW	1 mg/mL[b]	Physically compatible for 4 hr at 23 °C	2226	**C**
Gentamicin sulfate	ES	5 mg/mL[a]	GL	1 mg/mL[b]	Visually compatible for 4 hr at 22 °C	1365	**C**
Haloperidol lactate	LY	0.2 mg/mL[a]	GL	1 mg/mL[b]	Visually compatible for 4 hr at 22 °C	1365	**C**
Heparin sodium	SO	40 units/mL[a]	GL	1 mg/mL[b]	Visually compatible for 4 hr at 22 °C	1365	**C**
Hetastarch in lactated electrolyte	AB	6%	GW	1 mg/mL[a]	Physically compatible for 4 hr at 23 °C	2339	**C**
Hydrocortisone sodium succinate	UP	1 mg/mL[a]	GL	1 mg/mL[b]	Visually compatible for 4 hr at 22 °C	1365	**C**
Hydromorphone HCl	KN	0.5 mg/mL[a]	GL	1 mg/mL[b]	Visually compatible for 4 hr at 22 °C	1365	**C**
Hydroxyzine HCl	WI	4 mg/mL[a]	GL	1 mg/mL[b]	Visually compatible for 4 hr at 22 °C	1365	**C**
Ifosfamide	MJ	25 mg/mL[a]	GL	1 mg/mL[b]	Visually compatible for 4 hr at 22 °C	1365	**C**
Imipenem–cilastatin sodium	MSD	5 mg/mL[b]	GL	1 mg/mL[b]	Visually compatible for 4 hr at 22 °C	1365	**C**
Linezolid	PHU	2 mg/mL	GW	1 mg/mL[a]	Physically compatible for 4 hr at 23 °C	2264	**C**
Lorazepam	WY	0.1 mg/mL[a]	GL	1 mg/mL[b]	Light haze develops immediately	1365	**I**
Magnesium sulfate	SO	100 mg/mL[a]	GL	1 mg/mL[b]	Visually compatible for 4 hr at 22 °C	1365	**C**
Mannitol	BA	15%	GL	1 mg/mL[b]	Visually compatible for 4 hr at 22 °C	1365	**C**
Mechlorethamine HCl	MSD	1 mg/mL	GL	1 mg/mL[b]	Visually compatible for 4 hr at 22 °C	1365	**C**
Melphalan HCl	BW	0.1 mg/mL[b]	GL	1 mg/mL[b]	Physically compatible for 3 hr at 22 °C	1557	**C**
Meperidine HCl	WI	4 mg/mL[a]	GL	1 mg/mL[b]	Visually compatible for 4 hr at 22 °C	1365	**C**
Meropenem	ZEN	1 mg/mL[b]	GL	1 mg/mL[c]	Visually compatible for 4 hr at room temperature	1994	**C**
	ZEN	50 mg/mL[b]	GL	1 mg/mL[c]	White precipitate forms immediately	1994	**I**
Mesna	BR	10 mg/mL[a]	GL	1 mg/mL[b]	Visually compatible for 4 hr at 22 °C	1365	**C**
Methotrexate sodium	CET	15 mg/mL[a]	GL	1 mg/mL[b]	Visually compatible for 4 hr at 22 °C	1365	**C**
		30 mg/mL	GL	2 mg/mL	Visually compatible for 4 hr at room temperature	1788	**C**
Methylprednisolone sodium succinate	UP	5 mg/mL[a]	GL	1 mg/mL[b]	Light haze develops in 30 min	1365	**I**
Metoclopramide HCl	DU	5 mg/mL	GL	1 mg/mL[b]	Visually compatible for 4 hr at 22 °C	1365	**C**
Micafungin sodium	ASP	1.5 mg/mL[b]	GSK	1 mg/mL[b]	White precipitate forms immediately	2683	**I**
Mitomycin	BR	0.5 mg/mL	GL	1 mg/mL[b]	Visually compatible for 4 hr at 22 °C	1365	**C**
Mitoxantrone HCl	LE	0.5 mg/mL[a]	GL	1 mg/mL[b]	Visually compatible for 4 hr at 22 °C	1365	**C**
Morphine sulfate	WI	1 mg/mL[a]	GL	1 mg/mL[b]	Visually compatible for 4 hr at 22 °C	1365	**C**
Oxaliplatin	SS	0.5 mg/mL[a]	GW	1 mg/mL[a]	Physically compatible for 4 hr at 23 °C	2566	**C**
Paclitaxel	NCI	1.2 mg/mL[a]	GL	0.5 mg/mL[a]	Physically compatible for 4 hr at 22 °C	1556	**C**
	BR	0.3 mg/mL[a]	GL	0.03 and 0.3 mg/mL[a]	Visually compatible with no loss of either drug in 4 hr at 23 °C	1741	**C**
	BR	1.2 mg/mL[a]	GL	0.03 and 0.3 mg/mL[a]	Visually compatible with no loss of either drug in 4 hr at 23 °C	1741	**C**

Y-Site Injection Compatibility (1:1 Mixture) (Cont.)

Ondansetron HCl

Drug	Mfr	Conc	Mfr	Conc	Remarks	Ref	C/I
Paclitaxel with ranitidine HCl	BR GL	1.2 mg/mL[a] 2 mg/mL[a]	GL	0.3 mg/mL[a]	Visually compatible with no loss of any drug in 4 hr at 23 °C	1741	C
Pemetrexed disodium	LI	20 mg/mL[b]	GSK	1 mg/mL[a]	Trace haze and microparticulates form immediately. White cloudy precipitate forms in 4 hr	2564	I
Pentostatin	NCI	0.4 mg/mL[b]	GL	1 mg/mL[b]	Visually compatible for 4 hr at 22 °C	1365	C
Piperacillin sodium–tazobactam sodium	LE[h]	40 + 5 mg/mL[a]	GL	1 mg/mL[a]	Physically compatible for 4 hr at 22 °C	1688	C
	LE[h]	40 + 5 mg/mL[b]	GL	0.03, 0.1, 0.3 mg/mL[b]	Visually compatible with no loss of any component in 4 hr	1752	C
	LE[h]	80 + 10 mg/mL[b]	GL	0.03, 0.1, 0.3 mg/mL[b]	Visually compatible with no loss of any component in 4 hr	1752	C
Potassium chloride	AB	0.1 mEq/mL[a]	GL	1 mg/mL[b]	Visually compatible for 4 hr at 22 °C	1365	C
Prochlorperazine edisylate	SKF	0.5 mg/mL[a]	GL	1 mg/mL[b]	Visually compatible for 4 hr at 22 °C	1365	C
Promethazine HCl	ES	2 mg/mL[a]	GL	1 mg/mL[b]	Visually compatible for 4 hr at 22 °C	1365	C
Ranitidine HCl	GL	2 mg/mL[a]	GL	1 mg/mL[b]	Visually compatible for 4 hr at 22 °C	1365	C
	GL	0.5 mg/mL[a]	GL	0.03, 0.1, 0.3 mg/mL[a]	Visually compatible with no loss of either drug in 4 hr	1730	C
	GL	2 mg/mL[a]	GL	0.03, 0.1, 0.3 mg/mL[a]	Visually compatible with no loss of either drug in 4 hr	1730	C
Ranitidine HCl with paclitaxel	GL BR	2 mg/mL[a] 1.2 mg/mL[a]	GL	0.3 mg/mL[a]	Visually compatible with no loss of any drug in 4 hr at 23 °C	1741	C
Remifentanil HCl	GW	0.025 and 0.25 mg/mL[b]	CER	1 mg/mL[a]	Physically compatible for 4 hr at 23 °C	2075	C
Sargramostim	IMM	10 mcg/mL[b]	GL	0.5 mg/mL[b]	Filaments form in 30 to 60 min	1436	I
Sodium acetate		0.1 and 1 mEq/mL[a]	GL	0.1 mg/mL[a]	Physically compatible for 4 hr at room temperature	1661	C
Sodium bicarbonate		0.05 mmol/mL[e]	GL	0.32 mg/mL[a]	White precipitate forms immediately	1513	I
		0.1 mEq/mL[a]	GL	0.1 mg/mL[a]	Visible particles in 30 to 60 min at room temperature	1661	I
		1.4%	GL	2 mg/mL	Heavy white precipitate forms immediately	1788	I
Streptozocin	UP	30 mg/mL[a]	GL	1 mg/mL[b]	Visually compatible for 4 hr at 22 °C	1365	C
Telavancin HCl	ASP	7.5 mg/mL[a,b,i]	BA	1 mg/mL[a,b,i]	Physically compatible for 2 hr	2830	C
Teniposide	BR BR	0.1 mg/mL[a] 0.1 mg/mL[a]	GL GL	1 mg/mL[b] 1 mg/mL[a]	Visually compatible for 4 hr at 22 °C Physically compatible for 4 hr at 23 °C	1365 1725	C C
Thiotepa	IMM[f]	1 mg/mL[a]	GL	1 mg/mL[a]	Physically compatible for 4 hr at 23 °C	1861	C
Ticarcillin disodium–clavulanate potassium	BE	31 mg/mL[a]	GL	1 mg/mL[b]	Visually compatible for 4 hr at 22 °C	1365	C
TNA #218 to #226[g]			CER	1 mg/mL[a]	Damage to emulsion occurs immediately with free oil formation possible	2215	I
Topotecan HCl	SKB	56 mcg/mL[a,b]	CER	0.48 mg/mL[a,b]	Visually compatible. Little loss of either drug in 4 hr at 22 °C	2245	C
TPN #212 to #215[g]			GL	1 mg/mL[a]	Physically compatible for 4 hr at 23 °C	2109	C
Vancomycin HCl	LI	10 mg/mL[a]	GL	1 mg/mL[b]	Visually compatible for 4 hr at 22 °C	1365	C
Vinblastine sulfate	LY	0.12 mg/mL[a]	GL	1 mg/mL[b]	Visually compatible for 4 hr at 22 °C	1365	C

Y-Site Injection Compatibility (1:1 Mixture) (Cont.)

Ondansetron HCl

Drug	Mfr	Conc	Mfr	Conc	Remarks	Ref	C/I
Vincristine sulfate	LY	0.05 mg/mL[a]	GL	1 mg/mL[b]	Visually compatible for 4 hr at 22 °C	1365	C
Vinorelbine tartrate	BW	1 mg/mL[b]	GL	1 mg/mL[b]	Physically compatible for 4 hr at 22 °C	1558	C
Zidovudine	BW	4 mg/mL[a]	GL	1 mg/mL[b]	Visually compatible for 4 hr at 22 °C	1365	C

[a]*Tested in dextrose 5%.*
[b]*Tested in sodium chloride 0.9%.*
[c]*Tested in sterile water for injection.*
[d]*Tested in bacteriostatic sodium chloride 0.9% preserved with benzyl alcohol 0.9%.*
[e]*Tested in dextrose 5% with potassium chloride 0.02 mM/mL.*
[f]*Lyophilized formulation tested.*
[g]*Refer to Appendix I for the composition of parenteral nutrition solutions. TNA indicates a 3-in-1 admixture, and TPN indicates a 2-in-1 admixture.*
[h]*Test performed using the formulation WITHOUT edetate disodium.*
[i]*Tested in Ringer's injection, lactated.*
[j]*Injected via Y-site into an administration set running azithromycin.*
[k]*Tested with albumin human 0.1%.*

OXACILLIN SODIUM
AHFS 8:12.16.12

Products — Oxacillin sodium is available in vials containing the equivalent of oxacillin 1 and 2 g. A 10-g hospital bulk package also is available. The products contain dibasic sodium phosphate 20 mg/g of drug. (4)

For intramuscular use, reconstitute the 1-g vials with 5.7 mL and the 2-g vials with 11.5 mL of sterile water for injection or sodium chloride 0.45 or 0.9% and shake until a clear solution is obtained. A 250-mg/1.5 mL (167 mg/mL) solution results. (4)

For direct intravenous injection, reconstitute the 1- or 2-g vials with 10 or 20 mL, respectively, of sterile water for injection, sodium chloride 0.45%, or sodium chloride 0.9% and shake until a clear solution is obtained to yield a 100-mg/mL concentration. (4)

The 10-g hospital bulk package is reconstituted with 93 mL of sterile water for injection to yield a 100-mg/mL solution. (4)

Frozen premixed solutions of oxacillin 1 g/50 mL in dextrose 3% and 2 g/50 mL in dextrose 0.6% are also available. The solutions also contain sodium citrate buffer and hydrochloric acid and/or sodium hydroxide to adjust the pH. (1; 4)

pH — From 6 to 8.5. (17) At 10 g/L in dextrose 5%, the pH has been variously reported as 7.4 (149) and 7.94. (153) At this concentration in sodium chloride 0.9%, the pH has been reported as 7.73. (153)

Osmolality — The osmolality of oxacillin sodium 250 mg/1.5 mL in sterile water for injection was 596 mOsm/kg by freezing-point depression and 657 mOsm/kg by vapor pressure. (1071)

The osmolality of oxacillin sodium 50 mg/mL was 381 mOsm/kg in dextrose 5% and 396 mOsm/kg in sodium chloride 0.9%. (1375)

The osmolality of oxacillin sodium was calculated for the following dilutions (1054):

Diluent	Osmolality (mOsm/kg)	
	50 mL	100 mL
1 g		
Dextrose 5%	326	295
Sodium chloride 0.9%	353	321
2 g		
Dextrose 5%	379	329
Sodium chloride 0.9%	406	356

The following maximum oxacillin sodium concentrations have been recommended to achieve osmolalities suitable for peripheral infusion in fluid-restricted patients (1180):

Diluent	Maximum Concentration (mg/mL)	Osmolality (mOsm/kg)
Dextrose 5%	59	530
Sodium chloride 0.9%	53	519
Sterile water for injection	106	422

The frozen premixed solutions are iso-osmotic, having an osmolality of about 300 mOsm/kg. (4)

Sodium Content — Each gram of oxacillin sodium powder contains approximately 2.5 to 3.1 mEq of sodium. (4)

Administration — Oxacillin sodium may be administered by deep intramuscular injection, direct intravenous injection, or by continuous or intermittent intravenous infusion. By direct intravenous injection, the dose should be given over a 10-minute period. To minimize vein irritation, intravenous injections should be made as slowly as possible.

For intermittent infusion, the drug should be further diluted with a compatible solution to a concentration of 0.5 to 40 mg/mL. (4)

Stability — Oxacillin sodium in intact vials should be stored at controlled room temperature. After reconstitution, oxacillin sodium is stable for three days at room temperature and for one week under refrigeration at concentrations used for intramuscular or direct intravenous injection. The reconstituted hospital bulk package is stable for 24 hours at room temperature. (4)

The frozen premixed injection is stable at −20 °C for at least 90 days after shipping. The frozen premixed infusions should be thawed at room temperature or under refrigeration and should not be refrozen after being thawed. The thawed solutions are stated to be stable for 48 hours at room temperature and 21 days under refrigeration. (4)

Freezing Solutions — Oxacillin sodium, 500 mg/2.5 mL and 1 g/5 mL in sterile water for injection in glass and plastic syringes and 200 mg/mL in the original vial, was frozen at −20 °C. Adequate stability was maintained over three months. (303)

In another study, oxacillin sodium 1 g/100 mL of dextrose 5% in PVC bags was frozen at −20 °C for 30 days. The bags were then thawed by exposure to ambient temperature or microwave radiation. The solutions had no precipitation or color change and no drug loss. Subsequent storage at room temperature for 24 hours yielded a physically compatible solution, which exhibited a 3 to 4% loss. (554)

Syringes — Oxacillin sodium (Bristol) 8.33, 16.7, and 33.3 mg/mL in dextrose 5% and in sodium chloride 0.9% packaged in plastic syringes was reported to be stable for 24 hours at room temperature, 8 days refrigerated, and 30 days frozen at −20 °C. (31)

Ambulatory Pumps — The stability of oxacillin sodium 120 mg/mL in sterile water for injection was evaluated in PVC portable infusion pump reservoirs (Pharmacia Deltec). No oxacillin loss in three days at 25 °C and 5% loss in 14 days at 5 °C was found. (2080)

Sorption — Little loss due to sorption of oxacillin sodium (Bristol) 1 g/100 mL in dextrose 5% and sodium chloride 0.9% in trilayer solution bags (Bieffe Medital) composed of polyethylene, polyamide, and polypropylene occurred in two hours. Similarly, no loss was found during a one-hour simulated infusion. (1918)

Compatibility Information

Solution Compatibility

Oxacillin sodium

Solution	Mfr	Mfr	Conc/L	Remarks	Ref	C/I
Amino acids 4.25%, dextrose 25%	MG	BR	500 mg	No increase in particulate matter in 24 hr at 5 °C	349	C
Dextrose 5% in Ringer's injection, lactated	TR[a]	BR	1 g	Stable for 24 hr at 5 °C	282	C
Dextrose 5% in sodium chloride 0.45%			10 to 30 g	Stable for 24 hr at 25 °C, 4 days at 4 °C, and 30 days at −20 °C	1	C
Dextrose 5% in sodium chloride 0.9%			0.5 to 2 g	Under 10% loss in 6 hr at room temperature	1	C
	TR[a]	BR	1 g	Stable for 24 hr at 5 °C	282	C
		BR	2 g	12% decomposition in 12 hr and 14% in 24 hr	109	I
Dextrose 5%			10 to 30 g	Stable for 4 days at 4 °C and 30 days at −20 °C	1	C
			0.5 to 2 g	Stable for 6 hr at room temperature	1	C
		BR	2 g	Stable for 24 hr	109	C
		BR	1, 10, 50 g	4 to 9% decomposition in 24 hr at 23 °C	153	C
	TR[a]	BR	1 g	Stable for 24 hr at 5 °C	282	C
	TR[b]	BR	10 g	Physically compatible with 8% loss in 24 hr at room temperature	554	C
			4 g	8% loss in 6 hr and 14% loss in 24 hr at room temperature	768	I
	[b]	BR	20 g	No drug loss during 2-hr storage and 1-hr simulated infusion	1774	C
Dextrose 10%		BR	2 g	Stable for 24 hr	109	C
Ringer's injection, lactated			0.5 to 2 g	Stable for 6 hr at room temperature	1	C
			10 to 30 g	Stable for 4 days at 4 °C and 30 days at −20 °C	1	C
	TR[a]	BR	1 g	Stable for 24 hr at 5 °C	282	C

Solution Compatibility (Cont.)

Oxacillin sodium

Solution	Mfr	Mfr	Conc/L	Remarks	Ref	C/I
Sodium chloride 0.9%			10 to 100 g	Stable for 4 days at 25 °C, 7 days at 4 °C, and 30 days at −20 °C	1	**C**
		BR	2 g	Stable for 24 hr	109	**C**
		BR	1, 10, 50 g	2 to 4% decomposition in 24 hr at 23 °C	153	**C**
	TR[a]	BR	1 g	Stable for 24 hr at 5 °C	282	**C**
			4 g	10% loss in 8 hr and 12% loss in 24 hr at room temperature	768	**I**
	[b]	BR	20 g	No drug loss during 2-hr storage and 1-hr simulated infusion	1774	**C**
Sodium lactate ⅙ M			10 to 30 g	Stable for 24 hr at 25 °C, 4 days at 4 °C, and 30 days at −20 °C	1	**C**

[a]Tests performed in both glass and PVC containers.
[b]Tested in PVC containers.

Additive Compatibility

Oxacillin sodium

Drug	Mfr	Conc/L	Mfr	Conc/L	Test Soln	Remarks	Ref	C/I
Amikacin sulfate	BR	5 g	BR	2 g	D5LR, D5R, D5S, D5W, D10W, LR, NS, R	Physically compatible and both stable for 24 hr at 25 °C	293	**C**
	BR	5 g	BR	2 g	NR, SL	Oxacillin stable for 8 hr at 25 °C. Over 10% loss in 24 hr	293	**I**
Chloramphenicol sodium succinate	PD	500 mg	BR	500 mg	D5S, D5W	Therapeutic availability maintained	110	**C**
	PD	1 g	BR	2 g	D5S, D5W	Therapeutic availability maintained	110	**C**
	PD	1 g	BR	2 g		Physically compatible	6	**C**
Cytarabine	UP	100 mg		2 g	D5W	pH outside stability range for oxacillin	174	**I**
Dextran 40		10%		4 g	D5W	3% loss in 24 hr at 20 °C	834	**C**
Dopamine HCl	AS	800 mg	BR	2 g	D5W	No dopamine and 2% oxacillin loss in 24 hr at 25 °C	312	**C**
Hetastarch in sodium chloride 0.9%		6%		4 g		1% oxacillin loss in 24 hr at 20 °C	834	**C**
Potassium chloride		20, 40, 80 mEq	BR	1, 2.5, 4 g	D5S, D5W	Therapeutic availability maintained	110	**C**
Verapamil HCl	KN	80 mg	BR	4 g	D5W, NS	Physically compatible for 24 hr	764	**C**
	SE	[a]	BR	40 g	D5W, NS	Cloudy solution clears with agitation	1166	**?**

[a]Final concentration unspecified.

Drugs in Syringe Compatibility

Oxacillin sodium

Drug (in syringe)	Mfr	Amt	Mfr	Amt	Remarks	Ref	C/I
Caffeine citrate		20 mg/1 mL	APC	50 mg/1 mL	White precipitate forms immediately becoming two layers over time	2440	**I**

Y-Site Injection Compatibility (1:1 Mixture)

Oxacillin sodium

Drug	Mfr	Conc	Mfr	Conc	Remarks	Ref	C/I
Acyclovir sodium	BW	5 mg/mL[a]	BE	20 mg/mL[a]	Physically compatible for 4 hr at 25 °C	1157	**C**
Cyclophosphamide	MJ	20 mg/mL[a]	BE	20 mg/mL[a]	Physically compatible for 4 hr at 25 °C	1194	**C**
Diltiazem HCl	MMD	1[b] and 5 mg/mL		100 mg/mL[b]	Visually compatible	1807	**C**
	MMD	5 mg/mL		10 mg/mL[b]	Visually compatible	1807	**C**
Doxapram HCl	RB	2 mg/mL[a]	APO	20 mg/mL[a]	Visually compatible for 4 hr at 23 °C	2470	**C**
Famotidine	MSD	0.2 mg/mL[a]	BE	20 mg/mL[b]	Physically compatible for 14 hr	1196	**C**
Fluconazole	RR	2 mg/mL	BE	40 mg/mL	Physically compatible for 24 hr at 25 °C	1407	**C**
Foscarnet sodium	AST	24 mg/mL	BR	40 mg/mL	Physically compatible for 24 hr at room temperature under fluorescent light	1335	**C**
	AST	24 mg/mL	BE	20 mg/mL[c]	Physically compatible for 24 hr at 25 °C under fluorescent light	1393	**C**
Heparin sodium	UP	1000 units/L[d]	BR	100 mg/mL	Physically compatible for 4 hr at room temperature	534	**C**
Hydrocortisone sodium succinate	UP	10 mg/L[d]	BR	100 mg/mL	Physically compatible for 4 hr at room temperature	534	**C**
Hydromorphone HCl	WY	0.2 mg/mL[a]	BE	20 mg/mL[a]	Physically compatible for 4 hr at 25 °C	987	**C**
Labetalol HCl	SC	1 mg/mL[a]	BR	10 mg/mL[a]	Physically compatible for 24 hr at 18 °C	1171	**C**
Levofloxacin	OMN	5 mg/mL[a]	APC	167 mg/mL	Visually compatible for 4 hr at 24 °C	2233	**C**
Magnesium sulfate	IX	16.7, 33.3, 66.7, 100 mg/mL[a]	BE	20 mg/mL[a]	Physically compatible for at least 4 hr at 32 °C	813	**C**
Meperidine HCl	WY	10 mg/mL[a]	BE	20 mg/mL[a]	Physically compatible for 4 hr at 25 °C	987	**C**
Methotrexate sodium		30 mg/mL	BR	250 mg/mL	Visually compatible for 4 hr at room temperature	1788	**C**
Milrinone lactate	SS	0.2 mg/mL[a]	APO	100 mg/mL[a]	Visually compatible for 4 hr at 25 °C	2381	**C**
Morphine sulfate	WI	1 mg/mL[a]	BE	20 mg/mL[a]	Physically compatible for 4 hr at 25 °C	987	**C**
Potassium chloride	AB	40 mEq/L[d]	BR	100 mg/mL	Physically compatible for 4 hr at room temperature	534	**C**
Sodium bicarbonate		1.4%	BR	250 mg/mL	Gas evolves	1788	**I**
Tacrolimus	FUJ	1 mg/mL[b]	BR	40 mg/mL[a]	Visually compatible for 24 hr at 25 °C	1630	**C**
TNA #73[e]		32.5 mL[f]	BE	20 mg/mL[a]	Visually compatible for 4 hr at 25 °C	1008	**C**
TPN #54[e]				100 and 150 mg/mL	Physically compatible with 88 to 94% oxacillin activity retained over 6 hr at 22 °C	1045	**C**
TPN #61[e]		[g]	BE	250 mg/1.5 mL[h]	Physically compatible	1012	**C**
		[i]	BE	1.5 g/9 mL[h]	Physically compatible	1012	**C**

Y-Site Injection Compatibility (1:1 Mixture) (Cont.)

Oxacillin sodium

Drug	Mfr	Conc	Mfr	Conc	Remarks	Ref	C/I
Verapamil HCl	SE	2.5 mg/mL	BR	40 mg/mL[c]	White precipitate forms immediately. 39% of verapamil precipitated	1166	**I**
Zidovudine	BW	4 mg/mL[a]	BR	20 mg/mL[a]	Physically compatible for 4 hr at 25 °C	1193	**C**

[a]*Tested in dextrose 5%.*
[b]*Tested in sodium chloride 0.9%.*
[c]*Tested in both dextrose 5% and sodium chloride 0.9%.*
[d]*Tested in dextrose 5% in Ringer's injection, dextrose 5% in Ringer's injection, lactated, dextrose 5%, Ringer's injection, lactated, and sodium chloride 0.9%.*
[e]*Refer to Appendix I for the composition of parenteral nutrition solutions. TNA indicates a 3-in-1 admixture, and TPN indicates a 2-in-1 admixture.*
[f]*A 32.5-mL sample of parenteral nutrition solution mixed with 50 mL of antibiotic solution.*
[g]*Run at 21 mL/hr.*
[h]*Given over five minutes by syringe pump.*
[i]*Run at 94 mL/hr.*

OXALIPLATIN
AHFS 10:00

Products — Oxaliplatin is available as a 5-mg/mL concentrated solution in 10- and 20-mL sizes. (1)

Trade Name(s) — Eloxatin.

Administration — For intravenous infusion, the liquid concentrated injection must be diluted in 250 to 500 mL of dextrose 5%. Chloride-containing solutions must not be used for dilution. (1)

Contact of oxaliplatin solutions with aluminum in needles or metal parts of administration equipment should be avoided. Aluminum has caused degradation of some platinum compounds. (1)

Stability — Intact vials are stored at controlled room temperature and protected from freezing and light kept in the outer carton. (1)

After dilution for administration in dextrose 5%, the manufacturer indicates that the drug is stable for six hours at room temperature and for 24 hours under refrigeration. (1) However, Sanofi stated that oxaliplatin diluted in dextrose 5% for infusion was stable for 24 hours at room temperature. At a concentration of 3 g/L, the drug was stated to be stable for at least five days at room temperature. (2623)

pH Effects — Oxaliplatin is incompatible with alkaline drugs and solutions and should not be mixed with or administered simultaneously with them. Administration lines should be flushed with dextrose 5% prior to administering other medications. (1)

Compatibility Information

Solution Compatibility

Oxaliplatin

Solution	Mfr	Mfr	Conc/L	Remarks	Ref	C/I
Dextrose 5%	KA[a]	SAA	700 mg	Visually compatible and 5% or less drug loss in 30 days refrigerated or at room temperature	2744	**C**
	KA[b]	AVE	250 mg	Visually compatible and less than 4% drug loss in 90 days refrigerated or at room temperature	2782	**C**

[a]*Tested in MacoFlex N polyolefin containers.*
[b]*Tested in FreeFlex polyolefin containers.*

Y-Site Injection Compatibility (1:1 Mixture)

Oxaliplatin

Drug	Mfr	Conc	Mfr	Conc	Remarks	Ref	C/I
Bumetanide	BA	0.04 mg/mL[a]	SS	0.5 mg/mL[a]	Physically compatible for 4 hr at 23 °C	2566	C
Buprenorphine HCl	RKC	0.04 mg/mL[a]	SS	0.5 mg/mL[a]	Physically compatible for 4 hr at 23 °C	2566	C
Butorphanol tartrate	APO	0.04 mg/mL[a]	SS	0.5 mg/mL[a]	Physically compatible for 4 hr at 23 °C	2566	C
Calcium gluconate	APP	40 mg/mL[a]	SS	0.5 mg/mL[a]	Physically compatible for 4 hr at 23 °C	2566	C
Carboplatin	BR	5 mg/mL[a]	SS	0.5 mg/mL[a]	Physically compatible for 4 hr at 23 °C	2566	C
Chlorpromazine HCl	ES	2 mg/mL[a]	SS	0.5 mg/mL[a]	Physically compatible for 4 hr at 23 °C	2566	C
Cyclophosphamide	MJ	10 mg/mL[a]	SS	0.5 mg/mL[a]	Physically compatible for 4 hr at 23 °C	2566	C
Dexamethasone sodium phosphate	AMR	1 mg/mL[a]	SS	0.5 mg/mL[a]	Physically compatible for 4 hr at 23 °C	2566	C
Diazepam	AB	5 mg/mL	SS	0.5 mg/mL[a]	Gross white turbidity forms immediately	2566	I
Diphenhydramine HCl	ES	2 mg/mL[a]	SS	0.5 mg/mL[a]	Physically compatible for 4 hr at 23 °C	2566	C
Dobutamine HCl	BED	4 mg/mL[a]	SS	0.5 mg/mL[a]	Physically compatible for 4 hr at 23 °C	2566	C
Docetaxel	AVE	2 mg/mL[a]	SS	0.5 mg/mL[a]	Physically compatible for 4 hr at 23 °C	2566	C
Dolasetron mesylate	AVE	2 mg/mL[a]	SS	0.5 mg/mL[a]	Physically compatible for 4 hr at 23 °C	2566	C
Dopamine HCl	AB	3.2 mg/mL[a]	SS	0.5 mg/mL[a]	Physically compatible for 4 hr at 23 °C	2566	C
Doxorubicin HCl	APP	1 mg/mL[a]	SS	0.5 mg/mL[a]	Physically compatible for 4 hr at 23 °C	2566	C
Droperidol	AB	2.5 mg/mL	SS	0.5 mg/mL[a]	Physically compatible for 4 hr at 23 °C	2566	C
Enalaprilat	BA	0.1 mg/mL[a]	SS	0.5 mg/mL[a]	Physically compatible for 4 hr at 23 °C	2566	C
Epirubicin HCl	PHU	0.5 mg/mL[a]	SS	0.5 mg/mL[a]	Physically compatible for 4 hr at 23 °C	2566	C
Etoposide phosphate	BR	5 mg/mL[a]	SS	0.5 mg/mL[a]	Physically compatible for 4 hr at 23 °C	2566	C
Famotidine	ESL	2 mg/mL[a]	SS	0.5 mg/mL[a]	Physically compatible for 4 hr at 23 °C	2566	C
Fentanyl citrate	AB	0.05 mg/mL[a]	SS	0.5 mg/mL[a]	Physically compatible for 4 hr at 23 °C	2566	C
Furosemide	AMR	3 mg/mL[a]	SS	0.5 mg/mL[a]	Physically compatible for 4 hr at 23 °C	2566	C
Gemcitabine HCl	LI	10 mg/mL[a]	SS	0.5 mg/mL[a]	Physically compatible for 4 hr at 23 °C	2566	C
Granisetron HCl	SKB	0.05 mg/mL[a]	SS	0.5 mg/mL[a]	Physically compatible for 4 hr at 23 °C	2566	C
Haloperidol lactate	APP	0.2 mg/mL[a]	SS	0.5 mg/mL[a]	Physically compatible for 4 hr at 23 °C	2566	C
Heparin sodium	AB	100 units/mL	SS	0.5 mg/mL[a]	Physically compatible for 4 hr at 23 °C	2566	C
Hydrocortisone sodium succinate	PHU	1 mg/mL[a]	SS	0.5 mg/mL[a]	Physically compatible for 4 hr at 23 °C	2566	C
Hydromorphone HCl	ES	0.5 mg/mL[a]	SS	0.5 mg/mL[a]	Physically compatible for 4 hr at 23 °C	2566	C
Hydroxyzine HCl	ES	2 mg/mL[a]	SS	0.5 mg/mL[a]	Physically compatible for 4 hr at 23 °C	2566	C
Ifosfamide	MJ	20 mg/mL[a]	SS	0.5 mg/mL[a]	Physically compatible for 4 hr at 23 °C	2566	C
Irinotecan HCl	PHU	1 mg/mL[a]	SS	0.5 mg/mL[a]	Physically compatible for 4 hr at 23 °C	2566	C
Leucovorin calcium	BED	2 mg/mL[a]	SS	0.5 mg/mL[a]	Physically compatible for 4 hr at 23 °C	2566	C
Lorazepam	ESL	0.5 mg/mL[a]	SS	0.5 mg/mL[a]	Physically compatible for 4 hr at 23 °C	2566	C
Magnesium sulfate	APP	100 mg/mL[a]	SS	0.5 mg/mL[a]	Physically compatible for 4 hr at 23 °C	2566	C
Mannitol	BA	15%	SS	0.5 mg/mL[a]	Physically compatible for 4 hr at 23 °C	2566	C
Meperidine HCl	AB	10 mg/mL[a]	SS	0.5 mg/mL[a]	Physically compatible for 4 hr at 23 °C	2566	C
Mesna	MJ	10 mg/mL[a]	SS	0.5 mg/mL[a]	Physically compatible for 4 hr at 23 °C	2566	C
Methotrexate sodium	BED	12.5 mg/mL[a]	SS	0.5 mg/mL[a]	Physically compatible for 4 hr at 23 °C	2566	C

Y-Site Injection Compatibility (1:1 Mixture) (Cont.)

Oxaliplatin

Drug	Mfr	Conc	Mfr	Conc	Remarks	Ref	C/I
Methylprednisolone sodium succinate	PHU	5 mg/mL[a]	SS	0.5 mg/mL[a]	Physically compatible for 4 hr at 23 °C	2566	C
Metoclopramide HCl	RB	5 mg/mL	SS	0.5 mg/mL[a]	Physically compatible for 4 hr at 23 °C	2566	C
Mitoxantrone HCl	IMM	0.5 mg/mL[a]	SS	0.5 mg/mL[a]	Physically compatible for 4 hr at 23 °C	2566	C
Morphine sulfate	ES	15 mg/mL	SS	0.5 mg/mL[a]	Physically compatible for 4 hr at 23 °C	2566	C
Nalbuphine HCl	EN	10 mg/mL	SS	0.5 mg/mL[a]	Physically compatible for 4 hr at 23 °C	2566	C
Ondansetron HCl	GW	1 mg/mL[a]	SS	0.5 mg/mL[a]	Physically compatible for 4 hr at 23 °C	2566	C
Paclitaxel	MJ	0.6 mg/mL[a]	SS	0.5 mg/mL[a]	Physically compatible for 4 hr at 23 °C	2566	C
Palonosetron HCl	MGI	50 mcg/mL	SS	0.5 mg/mL[a]	Physically compatible. No loss of either drug in 4 hr	2579	C
Potassium chloride	APP	0.1 mEq/mL[a]	SS	0.5 mg/mL[a]	Physically compatible for 4 hr at 23 °C	2566	C
Prochlorperazine edisylate	SKB	0.5 mg/mL[a]	SS	0.5 mg/mL[a]	Physically compatible for 4 hr at 23 °C	2566	C
Promethazine HCl	ES	2 mg/mL[a]	SS	0.5 mg/mL[a]	Physically compatible for 4 hr at 23 °C	2566	C
Ranitidine HCl	GW	2 mg/mL[a]	SS	0.5 mg/mL[a]	Physically compatible for 4 hr at 23 °C	2566	C
Theophylline	AB	4 mg/mL	SS	0.5 mg/mL[a]	Physically compatible for 4 hr at 23 °C	2566	C
Topotecan HCl	SKB	0.1 mg/mL[a]	SS	0.5 mg/mL[a]	Physically compatible for 4 hr at 23 °C	2566	C
Verapamil HCl	AB	1.25 mg/mL[a]	SS	0.5 mg/mL[a]	Physically compatible for 4 hr at 23 °C	2566	C
Vincristine sulfate	FAU	0.05 mg/mL[a]	SS	0.5 mg/mL[a]	Physically compatible for 4 hr at 23 °C	2566	C
Vinorelbine tartrate	GW	1 mg/mL[a]	SS	0.5 mg/mL[a]	Physically compatible for 4 hr at 23 °C	2566	C

[a]Tested in dextrose 5%.

OXYCODONE HYDROCHLORIDE
AHFS 28:08.08

Products — Oxycodone hydrochloride is available as a 10-mg/mL injection (equivalent to 9 mg of oxycodone base per milliliter) in 1- and 2-mL ampuls. Also present in the formulation are citric acid monohydrate, sodium citrate, sodium chloride, and hydrochloric acid and/or sodium hydroxide to adjust pH in water for injection. (38)

Administration — Oxycodone hydrochloride is administered by subcutaneous or intravenous injection or infusion. For infusion, the drug may be diluted to a concentration of 1 mg/mL in dextrose 5% or sodium chloride 0.9%. (38)

Stability — Intact vials should be stored at controlled room temperature. The ampuls should be used immediately upon opening; unused portions should be discarded immediately. The manufacturer states that oxycodone hydrochloride diluted for infusion is stable for 24 hours under refrigeration. (38)

Compatibility Information

Solution Compatibility

Oxycodone HCl

Solution	Mfr	Mfr	Conc/L	Remarks	Ref	C/I
Dextrose 5%	BA[b]		5 and 50 g	Visually compatible with little or no loss in 35 days at 4 and 24 °C	2590	C
	BA[a]	NAP	1 g	Visually compatible with less than 4% change in concentration in 14 days at 4 and 25 °C	2600	C
	BA[b,c]	NAP	1 g	Visually compatible with less than 4% change in concentration in 7 days at 4 and 25 °C	2600	C
	[b]	MUN	1 g	Visually compatible. No drug loss in 28 days at 25 °C	2827	C
Sodium chloride 0.9%	BA[b]		5 and 50 g	Visually compatible with little or no loss in 35 days at 4 and 24 °C	2590	C
	BA[a]	NAP	1 g	Visually compatible with less than 4% change in concentration in 14 days at 4 and 25 °C	2600	C
	BA[b,c]	NAP	1 g	Visually compatible with less than 4% change in concentration in 7 days at 4 and 25 °C	2600	C
	[b]	MUN	1 g	Visually compatible. No drug loss in 28 days at 25 °C	2827	C

[a]Tested in glass containers.
[b]Tested in PVC containers.
[c]Tested in EVA containers.

Additive Compatibility

Oxycodone HCl

Drug	Mfr	Conc/L	Mfr	Conc/L	Test Soln	Remarks	Ref	C/I
Cyclizine lactate	GW	1 g	NAP	1 g	NS	Crystals form in a few hours	2600	I
	GW	1 g	NAP	1 g	W	Visually compatible. Under 4% concentration change in 24 hr at 25 °C	2600	C
	GW	500 mg	NAP	1 g	NS	Crystals form in a few hours	2600	I
	GW	500 mg	NAP	1 g	W	Visually compatible. Under 4% concentration change in 24 hr at 25 °C	2600	C
Dexamethasone sodium phosphate	FAU	0.8 g	NAP	0.8 g	NS, W	Visually compatible. Under 4% concentration change in 24 hr at 25 °C	2600	C
Haloperidol lactate	JC	125 mg	NAP	1 g	NS, W	Visually compatible. Under 4% concentration change in 24 hr at 25 °C	2600	C
Methotrimeprazine HCl		250 mg	NAP	1 g	NS, W	Visually compatible. Under 4% concentration change in 24 hr at 25 °C	2600	C
Metoclopramide HCl		1.2 g	NAP	770 mg	NS, W	Visually compatible. Under 4% concentration change in 24 hr at 25 °C	2600	C
Midazolam HCl	RC	830 mg	NAP	830 mg	NS, W	Visually compatible. Under 4% concentration change in 24 hr at 25 °C	2600	C
Prochlorperazine mesylate		600 mg	NAP	1 g	NS, W	Substantial change in prochlorperazine concentration in 24 hr at 25 °C	2600	I
Scopolamine butylbromide	BI	1 g	NAP	1 g	NS, W	Visually compatible. Under 4% concentration change in 24 hr at 25 °C	2600	C
Scopolamine HBr		30 mg	NAP	1 g	NS, W	Visually compatible. Under 4% concentration change in 24 hr at 25 °C	2600	C

Drugs in Syringe Compatibility

Oxycodone HCl

Drug (in syringe)	Mfr	Amt	Mfr	Amt	Remarks	Ref	C/I
Cyclizine lactate	GW	150 mg/ 3 mL	NAP	200 mg/ 20 mL	Crystals form in 5 hr	2600	I
	GW	50 mg/ 1 mL	NAP	70 mg/ 7 mL	Crystals form in 5 hr	2600	I
	GW	50 mg/ 1 mL	NAP	100 mg/ 10 mL	Visually compatible. Under 4% concentration change in 24 hr at 25 °C	2600	C
	GW	50 mg/ 1 mL	NAP	150 mg/ 15 mL	Visually compatible. Under 4% concentration change in 24 hr at 25 °C	2600	C
	GW	50 mg/ 1 mL	NAP	200 mg/ 20 mL	Visually compatible. Under 4% concentration change in 24 hr at 25 °C	2600	C
	GW	100 mg/ 2 mL	NAP	200 mg/ 20 mL	Visually compatible. Under 4% concentration change in 24 hr at 25 °C	2600	C
Dexamethasone sodium phosphate	FAU	40 mg/ 10 mL	NAP	200 mg/ 20 mL	Visually compatible. Under 4% concentration change in 24 hr at 25 °C	2600	C
Haloperidol lactate	JC	15 mg/ 3 mL	NAP	200 mg/ 20 mL	Visually compatible. Under 4% concentration change in 24 hr at 25 °C	2600	C
Methotrimeprazine HCl		200 mg/ 8 mL	NAP	200 mg/ 20 mL	Visually compatible. Under 4% concentration change in 24 hr at 25 °C	2600	C
Metoclopramide HCl		100 mg/ 20 mL	NAP	200 mg/ 20 mL	Visually compatible. Under 4% concentration change in 24 hr at 25 °C	2600	C
Midazolam HCl	RC	100 mg/ 20 mL	NAP	200 mg/ 20 mL	Visually compatible. Under 4% concentration change in 24 hr at 25 °C	2600	C
Prochlorperazine mesylate		12.5 mg/ 1 mL	NAP	200 mg/ 20 mL	Substantial change in prochlorperazine concentration in 24 hr at 25 °C	2600	I
Scopolamine butylbromide	BI	60 mg/ 3 mL	NAP	200 mg/ 20 mL	Visually compatible. Under 4% concentration change in 24 hr at 25 °C	2600	C
Scopolamine HBr		2.4 mg/ 6 mL	NAP	200 mg/ 20 mL	Visually compatible. Under 4% concentration change in 24 hr at 25 °C	2600	C

OXYTOCIN
AHFS 76:00

Products — Oxytocin is available in 1-mL ampuls and 1- and 10-mL vials. Each milliliter contains oxytocin 10 units with chlorobutanol 0.5%. Acetic acid may have been added to adjust the pH during manufacture. (1; 4)

Units — One unit of oxytocin is equivalent to 2 to 2.2 mcg of pure oxytocin. (4)

pH — The pH range is 3 to 5. (1; 17)

Trade Name(s) — Pitocin.

Administration — Oxytocin is administered by intravenous infusion using an infusion control device (1; 4) or intramuscular injection (1), although intramuscular injection is usually not recommended for induction or augmentation of labor because the drug's effects are unpredictable and difficult to control. (4) For intravenous administration the injection should be diluted to a usual concentration of 10 milliunits/mL by adding 10 units (1 mL) to 1000 mL of dextrose 5%, Ringer's injection, lactated, or sodium chloride 0.9%. (1; 4) A higher concentration range of 10 to 40 milliunits/mL has been cited to control postpartum uterine bleeding. (1)

Stability — Oxytocin injection should be stored at controlled room temperature and protected from freezing. Do not use the solution if it is discolored or contains a precipitate. (1; 4)

Oxytocin appears to be rapidly decomposed in the presence of sodium bisulfite. (333)

Filtration — Oxytocin (Parke-Davis) 25 units/100 mL in dextrose 5% and sodium chloride 0.9% was filtered at about 3 mL/min through a 0.22-μm cellulose ester membrane filter (Ivex-2). At this concentration, 25 times higher than normally used, oxytocin appeared to bind initially to the filter from the sodium chloride 0.9% solution. Results in dextrose 5% were equivocal. From these data, it is not possible to draw a definite conclusion regarding substantial binding of oxytocin during normal usage. (533)

Compatibility Information

Solution Compatibility

Oxytocin

Solution	Mfr	Mfr	Conc/L	Remarks	Ref	C/I
Dextrose–Ringer's injection combinations	AB	PD	5 units	Physically compatible	3	C
Dextrose–Ringer's injection, lactated, combinations	AB	PD	5 units	Physically compatible	3	C
Dextrose–saline combinations	AB	PD	5 units	Physically compatible	3	C
Dextrose 2.5%	AB	PD	5 units	Physically compatible	3	C
Dextrose 5%	AB	PD	5 units	Physically compatible	3	C
		CN	10.4 units	Stable for at least 6 hr at room temperature	333	C
	BA[a]	APP	80 units	Physically compatible with little or no loss of oxytocin in 90 days at 23 °C protected from light	2671	C
Dextrose 10%	AB	PD	5 units	Physically compatible	3	C
Ionosol products	AB	PD	5 units	Physically compatible	3	C
Ringer's injection	AB	PD	5 units	Physically compatible	3	C
Ringer's injection, lactated	AB	PD	5 units	Physically compatible	3	C
	BA[a]	APP	80 units	Physically compatible with little or no loss of oxytocin in 28 days at 23 °C protected from light. Microprecipitate forms and loss of oxytocin occurs after that time	2671	C
	BA[a]	APP	20 units	Highly variable results. Oxytocin concentrations after 31 days of 99% at 4 °C and 106% at 25 °C. Physical stability not evaluated	2688	?
	BA[a]	APP	50 units	Highly variable results. Oxytocin concentrations after 31 days of 91% at 4 °C and 108% at 25 °C. Physical stability not evaluated	2688	?
Sodium chloride 0.45%	AB	PD	5 units	Physically compatible	3	C
Sodium chloride 0.9%	AB	PD	5 units	Physically compatible	3	C
	BA[a]	APP	80 units	Physically compatible with little or no loss of oxytocin in 90 days at 23 °C protected from light	2671	C
Sodium lactate ⅙ M	AB	PD	5 units	Physically compatible	3	C

[a]Tested in PVC containers.

Additive Compatibility

Oxytocin

Drug	Mfr	Conc/L	Mfr	Conc/L	Test Soln	Remarks	Ref	C/I
Chloramphenicol sodium succinate	PD	1 g	PD	5 units		Physically compatible	6	C
Sodium bicarbonate	AB	2.4 mEq[a]	PD	5 units	D5W	Physically compatible for 24 hr	772	C
Verapamil HCl	KN	80 mg	SZ	40 units	D5W, NS	Physically compatible for 24 hr	764	C

[a] One vial of Neut added to a liter of admixture.

Drugs in Syringe Compatibility

Oxytocin

Drug (in syringe)	Mfr	Amt	Mfr	Amt	Remarks	Ref	C/I
Dimenhydrinate		10 mg/ 1 mL		10 units/ 1 mL	Precipitate forms	2569	I
Pantoprazole sodium	[a]	4 mg/ 1 mL		10 units/ 1 mL	Orange precipitate	2574	I

[a] Test performed using the formulation WITHOUT edetate disodium.

Y-Site Injection Compatibility (1:1 Mixture)

Oxytocin

Drug	Mfr	Conc	Mfr	Conc	Remarks	Ref	C/I
Heparin sodium	UP	1000 units/L[d]	SZ	1 unit/mL	Physically compatible for 4 hr at room temperature	534	C
Hydrocortisone sodium succinate	UP	10 mg/L[d]	SZ	1 unit/mL	Physically compatible for 4 hr at room temperature	534	C
Insulin, regular	LI	0.2 unit/mL[b]	PD	0.02 unit/mL[c]	Physically compatible for 2 hr at 25 °C	1395	C
Meperidine HCl	WY	10 mg/mL[b]	PD	0.02 unit/mL[c]	Physically compatible for 1 hr at 25 °C	1338	C
Morphine sulfate	ES	1 mg/mL[b]	PD	0.02 unit/mL[c]	Physically compatible for 1 hr at 25 °C	1338	C
Potassium chloride	AB	40 mEq/L[d]	SZ	1 unit/mL	Physically compatible for 4 hr at room temperature	534	C
Warfarin sodium	DU	0.1[a,b] and 2[e] mg/mL	FUJ	1 unit/mL[a,b]	Physically compatible for 24 hr at 23 °C	2011	C
Zidovudine	GSK	2 mg/mL[a]	NVA	10 milliunits/ mL[a]	Visually compatible with no zidovudine loss in 6 hr at 20 °C	2491	C
	GSK	4 mg/mL[a]	NVA	10 milliunits/ mL[a]	Visually compatible with no zidovudine loss in 6 hr at 20 °C	2491	C

[a] Tested in dextrose 5%.
[b] Tested in sodium chloride 0.9%.
[c] Tested in dextrose 5% in Ringer's injection, lactated.
[d] Tested in dextrose 5% in Ringer's injection, dextrose 5% in Ringer's injection, lactated, dextrose 5%, Ringer's injection, lactated, and sodium chloride 0.9%.
[e] Tested in sterile water for injection.

PACLITAXEL
AHFS 10:00

Products — Paclitaxel is available as 6-mg/mL non-aqueous concentrated solution that must be diluted for use and is available in 5-, 16.7-, 25-, and 50-mL multiple-dose vials. One milliliter provides paclitaxel 6 mg with polyoxyl 35 castor oil (Cremophor EL; polyoxyethylated castor oil) surfactant 527 mg and dehydrated alcohol 49.7% (v/v). Some formulations also incorporate citric acid anhydrous 2 mg/mL. (1; 4)

CAUTION: Care should be taken to ensure that the correct drug product, dose, and administration procedure are used and that no confusion with other products occurs.

Although Abraxane, a protein-bound paclitaxel suspension (1), exists it is sufficiently different from conventional solvent-formulated paclitaxel that extrapolating information to or from it would be inappropriate.

pH — Paclitaxel admixtures at concentrations of 0.6 and 1.2 mg/mL in dextrose 5%, sodium chloride 0.9%, and dextrose 5% in lactated Ringer's injection have a pH of 4.4 to 5.6. (4)

Administration — Paclitaxel is administered by intravenous infusion. The concentrate must be diluted to a final paclitaxel concentration of 0.3 to 1.2 mg/mL in dextrose 5%, sodium chloride 0.9%, dextrose 5% in sodium chloride 0.9%, or dextrose 5% in lactated Ringer's injection. Administration over three hours is often recommended (1; 4), although other duration periods have been used. (4) An inline 0.22-μm filter should be used for administration. The intravenous solution containers and administration sets should be free of the plasticizer diethylhexyl phthalate (DEHP). (1)

Use of self-venting sets spiked into glass bottles of paclitaxel admixtures has occasionally resulted in solution dripping from the air vent. Presumably, the surfactant content wetted the hydrophobic filter, allowing the solution to drip. (1843) In another observation, the spikes of administration sets were made sufficiently slippery by surfactant in the paclitaxel formulation that the spike slipped out after it had been seated through the rubber bung of the glass bottle. The admixture also leaked due to a poor seal. The authors recommend use of non-PVC plastic solution containers to avoid the problem. (2052)

Stability — Intact vials should be stored between 20 and 25 °C and protected from light. Stability is not adversely affected by refrigeration or freezing. Refrigeration may result in the precipitation of formulation components. However, warming to room temperature redissolves the material and does not adversely affect the product. If a precipitate is insoluble, the product should be discarded. (1)

Paclitaxel 0.7 mg/mL diluted in sodium chloride 0.9% did not exhibit an antimicrobial effect on the growth of three of four organisms (*Enterococcus faecium, Staphylococcus aureus, Pseudomonas aeruginosa,* and *Candida albicans*) inoculated into the solution. *S. aureus* remained viable for 4 hours. *E. faecium* and *P. aeruginosa* remained viable for 48 hours, and *C. albicans* remained viable to the end of the study at 120 hours. Diluted solutions of paclitaxel should be stored under refrigeration whenever possible, and the potential for microbiological growth should be considered when assigning expiration periods. (2160)

Turbidity — Paclitaxel is a clear, colorless to slightly yellow viscous liquid. After dilution in an infusion solution, the drug may exhibit haziness because of the surfactant content of the formulation. (1528)

Precipitation — Although paclitaxel in aqueous solutions is chemically stable for 27 hours (1) or longer (1746; 1842; 2708), precipitation has occurred irregularly and unpredictably. Such precipitation occurs within the recommended range of 0.3 to 1.2 mg/mL and at lower paclitaxel concentrations. These precipitates have been observed in the infusion tubing distal to the pump chamber. (1716) Although precipitation of insoluble drugs in an aqueous medium is a foregone conclusion, the time to precipitation is irregular. It may be accelerated by the presence or formation of crystallization nuclei, agitation, and contact with incompatible drugs or materials. (1374; 1521) Since the mechanism of this irregular precipitation has not been identified (1739), vigilance throughout its infusion is required.

Sorption — No paclitaxel loss due to sorption to containers or sets has been observed. (1520; 2230; 2231; 2232)

Plasticizer Leaching — Contact of undiluted paclitaxel concentrate with plasticized PVC equipment and devices is not recommended. (1; 4) With use of infusion bags and tubing that are free of DEHP plasticizer and the elimination of PVC precision flow regulators, a reduction in leached DEHP of up to 96% has been reported. (2679)

Paclitaxel vehicle equivalent to paclitaxel 1.2 mg/mL in dextrose 5% in VISIV polyolefin bags was tested at room temperature near 23 °C for 24 hours. No plastic components leached within the 24-hour study period. (2660; 2792)

Paclitaxel itself does not contribute to the extraction of the plasticizer DEHP. (1520) However, the surfactant, Cremophor EL, in the paclitaxel formulation extracts DEHP from PVC containers and sets. The amount of DEHP extracted increases with time and drug concentration. (1520; 1683; 2146) Consequently, the use of DEHP-plasticized PVC containers and sets is not recommended for infusion of paclitaxel solutions. Instead, the manufacturer recommends the use of glass, polypropylene, or polyolefin containers and non-PVC administration sets such as those that are polyethylene lined. (1-2/06)

The use of inline filters, such as the Ivex-2 filter set that incorporates about 10 inches of PVC inlet and outlet tubing, has resulted in a small amount of DEHP extraction. Since the extracted DEHP is at a sufficiently low level, however, the manufacturer considers the Ivex-2 filter set to be acceptable. (1-2/06)

A study was performed on the compatibility of paclitaxel 0.3- and 1.2-mg/mL infusions with various non-PVC infusion sets. The paclitaxel infusions were run through the study sets, and the effluent was then analyzed for leached DEHP plasticizer. The following sets had significant and unacceptable amounts of leached DEHP: Baxter vented nitroglycerin (2C7552S), Baxter vented basic solution (1C8355S), McGaw Horizon pump vented nitroglycerin (V7450), and McGaw Intelligent pump vented nitroglycerin (V7150). Although these sets were largely non-PVC, their highly plasticized pumping segments contributed the DEHP. The administration and extension sets cited in Tables 1 and 2 exhibited no more leached DEHP than the Ivex-2 filter set specified in the product labeling. (1843)

Paclitaxel 0.3 and 1.2 mg/mL was prepared in PVC bags dextrose 5% and in sodium chloride 0.9%. Leaching of the plasticizer was found to be time and concentration dependent; however, there was little difference between the two infusion solutions. After storage for eight hours at 21 °C, leached DEHP in the range from 73 to 108 mcg/mL was found for the 1.2 mg/mL concentration and from 21 to 30 mcg/mL for the 0.3 mg/mL concentration. During a simulated one-hour infusion using DEHP plasticized administration sets, the amount of leached DEHP did not exceed 18 mcg/mL at the 0.3 mg/mL pac-

Table 1. Administration Sets Compatible with Paclitaxel Infusions by Manufacturer (1843)

Abbott	LifeCare 5000 Plum PVC specialty set (11594)
	Life Shield anesthesia pump set OL with cartridge (13503)
	LifeCare model 4P specialty set, non-PVC (11434)
	Omni-Flow universal primary intravenous pump short minibore patient line (40527)
Baxter	Vented volumetric pump nitroglycerin set (2C1042)
Block Medical	Verifuse nonvented administration set with 0.22-μm filter, check valve, injection site, and non-DEHP PVC tubing (V021015)
I-Flow	Vivus-4000 polyethylene-lined infusion set (5000-784)
IMED	Standard PVC set (9215)
	Closed-system non-PVC fluid path nonvented quick-spike administration set (9635)
	Non-PVC set with inline filter (9986)
	Gemini 20 nonvented primary administration set for nitroglycerin and emulsions (2262)
IVAC	Universal set with low-sorbing tubing (52053, 59953, and S75053)
Ivion/Medex	WalkMed spike set (SP-06) with pump set (PS-401, PS-360, FPS-560, or FPX-560)
Siemens	Reduced-PVC full set MiniMed Uni-Set macrobore (28-60-190)

Table 2. Extension Sets Compatible with Paclitaxel Infusions by Manufacturer (1843)

Abbott	Ivex-HP filter set (4524)
	Ivex-2 filter set (2679)
Becton Dickinson	Intima intravenous catheter placement set (38-6918-1)
	J-loop connector (38-1252-2)
	E-Z infusion set shorty (38-53741)
	E-Z infusion set (38-53121)
Baxter	Polyethylene-lined extension set with 0.22-μm air-eliminating filter (1C8363)
Braun	0.2-μm filter extension set (FE-2012L)
	Small-bore 0.2-μm filter extension set (PFE-2007)
	Whin-winged extension set with 90° Huber needle (HW-2267)
	Whin extension set with Y-site and Huber needle (HW-2276 YHR)
	Y-extension set with valve (ET-08-YL)
	Small-bore extension set with T-fitting (ET-04T)
	Small-bore extension set with reflux valve (ET-116L)
Gish Biomedical	VasTack noncoring portal-access needle system (VT-2022)
IMED	0.2-μm add-on filter set (9400 XL)
IVAC	Spec-Sets extension set with 0.22-μm inline filter (C20028 and C20350)
Ivion/Medex	Extension set with 0.22-μm filter (IV4A07-IV3)
PALL	SetSaver extended-life disposable set with 0.2-μm filter (ELD-96P and ELD-96LL)
	SetSaver extended-life disposable microbore extension tubing with 0.2-μm Posidyne filter (ELD-96LYL and ELD-96LYLN)
Pfizer/Strato Medical	Lifeport vascular-access system infusion set with Y-site (LPS 3009)

litaxel concentration but resulted in a maximum of 114 mcg/mL with the 1.2 mg/mL concentration. (1825)

DEHP plasticizer leaching from PVC containers and administration sets, and the amount of DEHP leached was reported to depend on surfactant concentration and length of contact period. They also reported leaching of up to 30 mg of DEHP per dose from Flo-Gard Low Adsorption Sets (Baxter), a set with a reduced amount of PVC present in its construction. (2146)

An acceptability limit of no more than 5 parts per million (5 mcg/mL) for DEHP plasticizer released from PVC containers, administration sets, and other equipment has been proposed. The limit was based on a review of metabolic and toxicologic considerations. (2185)

Two reduced-phthalate administration sets for the Acclaim (Abbott) pump were evaluated. Administration set model 11993-48 (Abbott) is composed of polyethylene tubing but has a DEHP-plasticized pumping segment. Administration set model L-12060 (Abbott) is composed of tris(2-ethylhexyl)trimellitate (TOTM)–plasticized PVC tubing and a DEHP-plasticized pumping segment. Paclitaxel diluent at concentrations equivalent to 0.3 and 1.2 mg/mL in dextrose 5% delivered rapidly over three hours at 23 °C did not leach detectable levels of TOTM from model L-12060 or DEHP from either set. Similarly, slow delivery over four days of the 0.3-mg/mL concentration yielded detectable but not quantifiable amounts of plasticizer. However, slow delivery of the equivalent of 1.2 mg/mL over four days yielded large but variable amounts of DEHP from both sets; DEHP concentrations ranged from 30 to 150 mcg/mL. Consequently, these two reduced-phthalate sets are suitable for short-term delivery up to three hours of paclitaxel at concentrations up to 1.2 mg/mL. However, these sets should not be used for slow delivery of paclitaxel. (2198)

Paclitaxel vehicle equivalent to paclitaxel 0.3 and 1.2 mg/mL in dextrose 5% did not leach TOTM plasticizer from a TOTM-plasticized PVC set (SoloPak) during simulated three-hour administration. During extremely slow delivery at 5.2 mL/hr for four days, no detectable TOTM was found in the 0.3-mg/mL equivalent concentration, and only a barely detectable, unquantifiable amount of TOTM was found with the 1.2-mg/mL equivalent solution. (2232)

Paclitaxel 0.3 and 1.2 mg/mL in dextrose 5% or in sodium chloride 0.9% in ethylene vinyl acetate (EVA) containers was found to leach an unknown material stored at 25 and 32 °C for 24 hours. (2182)

Filtration — The manufacturer recommends the use of a 0.22-μm inline filter for paclitaxel administration. (1) No loss of paclitaxel due to filtration through 0.22-μm filters occurs. (1; 1520)

The acceptability of the 0.22-μm IV Express Filter Unit (Millipore) for the administration of paclitaxel was evaluated. Paclitaxel vehicle equivalent to paclitaxel 1.2 mg/mL (for plasticizer leaching) and paclitaxel 0.3 mg/mL (for sorption potential) in 500 mL of dextrose 5% in polyolefin containers was delivered through the filter units over a three-hour period at a rate of 167 mL/hr at about 23 °C to simulate paclitaxel administration. No leached plasticizer and no loss of paclitaxel due to sorption was found. (2231)

Central Venous Catheter — The acceptability of the Arrow-Howes triple-lumen, 7 French, 30-cm polyurethane central catheter (Arrow International) for the administration of paclitaxel was evaluated. Pac-

litaxel vehicle equivalent to paclitaxel 0.3 and 1.2 mg/mL (for catheter component leaching) and paclitaxel 0.3 mg/mL (for sorption potential) were prepared in polyolefin bags of dextrose 5%. The solutions were delivered through the polyurethane central venous catheters for periods of three hours and of 24 hours at 23 °C to simulate rapid and slow administration. No leached catheter components were found in the effluent solution and no loss of paclitaxel occurred. (2230)

Compatibility Information

Solution Compatibility

Paclitaxel

Solution	Mfr	Mfr	Conc/L	Remarks	Ref	C/I
Dextrose 5%	MG, TR[a]	NCI	0.3, 0.6, 0.9 g	Visually compatible. No loss in 12 hr at 22 °C	1520	C
	MG[b]	NCI	0.6 g	Visually compatible. No loss in 25 hr at 22 °C	1520	C
	MG, TR[c]	NCI	1.2 g	Visually compatible. No loss in 12 hr at 22 °C	1520	C
		BR	0.2 to 0.58 g	Fluffy, white precipitate forms occasionally in administration set just distal to pump chamber	1716	I
	MG[b]	BR	0.1 and 1 g	Physically compatible. Stable for 3 days at 4, 22, and 32 °C. Crystals after 3 days	1746	C
	MG[b]	BR	0.3 and 1.2 g	Physically compatible and chemically stable for 48 hr at 22 °C	1842	C
	BA[d]	FAU	0.3 and 1.2 g	Physically compatible. Stable for 3 days at 25 and 32 °C. Unknown material leached from EVA container by 24 hr	2182	?
	BA[b], BRN[b], FRE[b], MAC[b]	BMS	0.3 and 1.2 g	Physically compatible with less than 5% loss in 72 hr at 37 °C in the dark	2669	C
	BRN[e]	BMS	0.4 and 1.2 g	Physically compatible. Little loss in 5 days at 23 and 4 °C. Precipitation occurred after this	2673	C
	BA[f]	TE	0.3 mg/mL	Chemically stable until precipitation. Precipitate after 3 days at 25 °C and 13 days at 5 °C	2708	C
	BRN[e]	TE	0.3 mg/mL	Chemically stable until precipitation. Precipitate found after 3 days at 25 °C and 18 days at 5 °C	2708	C
	BRN[g]	TE	0.3 mg/mL	Chemically stable until precipitation. Precipitate found after 7 days at 25 °C and 20 days at 5 °C	2708	C
	BA[f]	TE	1.2 mg/mL	Chemically stable until precipitation. Precipitate found after 3 days at 25 °C and 10 days at 5 °C	2708	C
	BRN[e]	TE	1.2 mg/mL	Chemically stable until precipitation. Precipitate found after 3 days at 25 °C and 12 days at 5 °C	2708	C
	BRN[g]	TE	1.2 mg/mL	Chemically stable until precipitation. Precipitate found after 7 days at 25 °C and 10 days at 5 °C	2708	C
	FRE	MAY	0.3 g	Chemically stable for 8 days at 25 °C and 28 days at 5 °C; then precipitation	2729	C
	FRE	MAY	0.75 g	Chemically stable for 4 days at 25 °C and 20 days at 5 °C; then precipitation	2729	C
	FRE	MAY	1.2 g	Chemically stable for 4 days at 25 °C and 12 days at 5 °C; then precipitation	2729	C
Sodium chloride 0.9%	MG, TR[a]	NCI	0.3, 0.6, 0.9, 1.2 g	Visually compatible. No loss over 12 hr at 22 °C	1520	C
	MG[b]	NCI	0.6 and 1.2 g	Visually compatible. No loss over 26 hr at 22 °C	1520	C

Solution Compatibility (Cont.)

Paclitaxel

Solution	Mfr	Mfr	Conc/L	Remarks	Ref	C/I
	MG[b]	BR	0.1 and 1 g	Physically compatible. Stable for 3 days at 4, 22, and 32 °C. Crystals after 3 days	1746	C
	MG[b]	BR	0.3 and 1.2 g	Physically compatible and chemically stable for 48 hr at 22 °C	1842	C
	BA[d]	FAU	0.3 and 1.2 g	Physically compatible. Stable for 3 days at 25 and 32 °C. Unknown material leached from EVA container by 24 hr	2182	?
	BA[b], BRN[b], FRE[b], MAC[b]	BMS	0.3 and 1.2 g	Physically compatible with less than 5% loss in 72 hr at 37 °C in the dark	2669	C
	BA[f]	TE	0.3 mg/mL	Chemically stable until precipitation. Precipitate found after 3 days at 25 °C and 13 days at 5 °C	2708	C
	BRN[e]	TE	0.3 mg/mL	Chemically stable until precipitation. Precipitate found after 3 days at 25 °C and 16 days at 5 °C	2708	C
	BRN[g]	TE	0.3 mg/mL	Chemically stable until precipitation. Precipitate found after 3 days at 25 °C and 13 days at 5 °C	2708	C
	BA[f]	TE	1.2 mg/mL	Chemically stable until precipitation. Precipitate found after 3 days at 25 °C and 9 days at 5 °C	2708	C
	BRN[e]	TE	1.2 mg/mL	Chemically stable until precipitation. Precipitate found after 3 days at 25 °C and 12 days at 5 °C	2708	C
	BRN[g]	TE	1.2 mg/mL	Chemically stable until precipitation. Precipitate found after 5 days at 25 °C and 8 days at 5 °C	2708	C
	FRE	MAY	0.3 g	Chemically stable for 6 days at 25 °C and 28 days at 5 °C; then precipitation	2729	C
	FRE	MAY	0.75 g	Chemically stable for 6 days at 25 °C and 20 days at 5 °C; then precipitation	2729	C
	FRE	MAY	1.2 g	Chemically stable for 4 days at 25 °C and 12 days at 5 °C; then precipitation	2729	C

[a]Tested in both glass and PVC containers.
[b]Tested in polyolefin containers.
[c]Tested in glass, PVC, and polyolefin containers.
[d]Tested in Baxter ethylene vinyl acetate (EVA) containers.
[e]Tested in ECOFLAC low-density polyethylene plastic containers.
[f]Tested in polyolefin containers.
[g]Tested in glass containers.

Additive Compatibility

Paclitaxel

Drug	Mfr	Conc/L	Mfr	Conc/L	Test Soln	Remarks	Ref	C/I
Carboplatin	BMS	2 g	BMS	300 mg and 1.2 g	NS	No paclitaxel loss but carboplatin losses of less than 2, 5, and 6 to 7% at 4, 24, and 32 °C, respectively, in 24 hr. Physically compatible for 24 hr but microparticles of paclitaxel form after 3 to 5 days	2094	C
	BMS	2 g	BMS	300 mg and 1.2 g	D5W	No paclitaxel and carboplatin loss at 4, 24, and 32 °C in 24 hr. Physically compatible for 24 hr but microparticles of paclitaxel form after 3 to 5 days	2094	C

Additive Compatibility (Cont.)

Paclitaxel

Drug	Mfr	Conc/L	Mfr	Conc/L	Test Soln	Remarks	Ref	C/I
Cisplatin	BMS	200 mg	BMS	300 mg	NS	No paclitaxel loss and cisplatin losses of 1, 4, and 5% at 4, 24, and 32 °C, respectively, in 24 hr. Physically compatible for 24 hr but microparticles of paclitaxel form after 3 to 5 days	2094	**C**
	BMS	200 mg	BMS	1.2 g	NS	No paclitaxel loss but cisplatin losses of 10, 19, and 22% at 4, 24, and 32 °C, respectively, in 24 hr. Physically compatible for 24 hr but microparticles of paclitaxel form after 3 to 5 days	2094	**I**
Doxorubicin HCl	PH	200 mg	BMS	300 mg	D5W, NS	Visually compatible for 1 day with microprecipitation in 3 to 5 days and gross precipitation in 7 days at 4, 23, and 32 °C in the dark. No paclitaxel and under 8% doxorubicin loss in 7 days	2247	**C**
	PH	200 mg	BMS	1.2 g	D5W, NS	Visually compatible for 1 day with microprecipitation in 3 to 5 days and gross precipitation in 7 days at 4, 23, and 32 °C in the dark. No paclitaxel and less than 7% doxorubicin loss in 7 days	2247	**C**

Y-Site Injection Compatibility (1:1 Mixture)

Paclitaxel

Drug	Mfr	Conc	Mfr	Conc	Remarks	Ref	C/I
Acyclovir sodium	BW	7 mg/mL[a]	NCI	1.2 mg/mL[a]	Physically compatible for 4 hr at 22 °C	1556	**C**
Amikacin sulfate	BR	5 mg/mL[a]	NCI	1.2 mg/mL[a]	Physically compatible for 4 hr at 22 °C	1556	**C**
Aminophylline	AB	2.5 mg/mL[a]	NCI	1.2 mg/mL[a]	Physically compatible for 4 hr at 22 °C	1556	**C**
Amphotericin B	SQ	0.6 mg/mL[a]	NCI	1.2 mg/mL[a]	Immediate increase in measured turbidity followed by separation into two layers in 24 hr at 22 °C	1556	**I**
Amphotericin B cholesteryl sulfate complex	SEQ	0.83 mg/mL[a]	MJ	0.6 mg/mL[a]	Decreased natural turbidity occurs	2117	**I**
Ampicillin sodium–sulbactam sodium	RR	20 + 10 mg/mL[b]	NCI	1.2 mg/mL[a]	Physically compatible for 4 hr at 22 °C	1556	**C**
Anidulafungin	VIC	0.5 mg/mL[a]	MJ	0.6 mg/mL[a]	Physically compatible for 4 hr at 23 °C	2617	**C**
Bleomycin sulfate	MJ	1 unit/mL[a]	NCI	1.2 mg/mL[a]	Physically compatible for 4 hr at 22 °C	1556	**C**
Butorphanol tartrate	BR	0.04 mg/mL[a]	NCI	1.2 mg/mL[a]	Physically compatible for 4 hr at 22 °C	1556	**C**
Calcium chloride	AST	20 mg/mL[a]	NCI	1.2 mg/mL[a]	Physically compatible for 4 hr at 22 °C	1556	**C**
Carboplatin		5 mg/mL[a]	NCI	1.2 mg/mL[a]	Physically compatible for 4 hr at 22 °C	1528	**C**
Cefotetan disodium	STU	20 mg/mL[a]	NCI	1.2 mg/mL[a]	Physically compatible for 4 hr at 22 °C	1556	**C**
Ceftazidime	LI	40 mg/mL[a]	NCI	1.2 mg/mL[a]	Physically compatible for 4 hr at 22 °C	1556	**C**
Ceftriaxone sodium	RC	20 mg/mL[a]	NCI	1.2 mg/mL[a]	Physically compatible for 4 hr at 22 °C	1556	**C**
Chlorpromazine HCl	ES	2 mg/mL[a]	NCI	1.2 mg/mL[a]	Normal inherent haze from paclitaxel decreases immediately	1556	**I**
Cisplatin		1 mg/mL	NCI	1.2 mg/mL[a]	Physically compatible for 4 hr at 22 °C	1528	**C**

Y-Site Injection Compatibility (1:1 Mixture) (Cont.)

Paclitaxel

Drug	Mfr	Conc	Mfr	Conc	Remarks	Ref	C/I
Cladribine	ORT	0.015[b] and 0.5[c] mg/mL	BR	0.6 mg/mL[b]	Physically compatible for 4 hr at 23 °C	1969	C
Cyclophosphamide		10 mg/mL[a]	NCI	1.2 mg/mL[a]	Physically compatible for 4 hr at 22 °C	1528	C
Cytarabine		50 mg/mL	NCI	1.2 mg/mL[a]	Physically compatible for 4 hr at 22 °C	1528	C
Dacarbazine	MI	4 mg/mL[a]	NCI	1.2 mg/mL[a]	Physically compatible for 4 hr at 22 °C	1556	C
Dexamethasone sodium phosphate		1 mg/mL[a]	NCI	1.2 mg/mL[a]	Physically compatible for 4 hr at 22 °C	1528	C
Diphenhydramine HCl		2 mg/mL[a]	NCI	1.2 mg/mL[a]	Physically compatible for 4 hr at 22 °C	1528	C
Doripenem	JJ	5 mg/mL[a,b]	MAY	0.6 mg/mL[a,b]	Physically compatible for 4 hr at 23 °C	2743	C
Doxorubicin HCl		2 mg/mL	NCI	1.2 mg/mL[a]	Physically compatible for 4 hr at 22 °C	1528	C
Doxorubicin HCl liposomal	SEQ	0.4 mg/mL[a]	MJ	0.6 mg/mL[a]	Partial loss of measured natural turbidity	2087	I
Droperidol	JN	0.4 mg/mL[a]	NCI	1.2 mg/mL[a]	Physically compatible for 4 hr at 22 °C	1556	C
Etoposide		0.4 mg/mL[a]	NCI	1.2 mg/mL[a]	Physically compatible for 4 hr at 22 °C	1528	C
Etoposide phosphate	BR	5 mg/mL[a]	MJ	1.2 mg/mL[a]	Physically compatible for 4 hr at 23 °C	2218	C
Famotidine	MSD	2 mg/mL[a]	NCI	1.2 mg/mL[a]	Physically compatible for 4 hr at 22 °C	1556	C
Floxuridine	RC	3 mg/mL[a]	NCI	1.2 mg/mL[a]	Physically compatible for 4 hr at 22 °C	1556	C
Fluconazole	RR	2 mg/mL	NCI	1.2 mg/mL[a]	Physically compatible for 4 hr at 22 °C	1556	C
	PF	2 mg/mL	BR	0.3 and 1.2 mg/mL[a]	Visually compatible. No loss of either drug in 4 hr at 23 °C	1790	C
Fluorouracil		16 mg/mL[a]	NCI	1.2 mg/mL[a]	Physically compatible for 4 hr at 22 °C	1528	C
Furosemide	AST	3 mg/mL[a]	NCI	1.2 mg/mL[a]	Physically compatible for 4 hr at 22 °C	1556	C
Ganciclovir sodium	SY	20 mg/mL[a]	NCI	1.2 mg/mL[a]	Physically compatible for 4 hr at 22 °C	1556	C
Gemcitabine HCl	LI	10 mg/mL[b]	MJ	1.2 mg/mL[a]	Physically compatible for 4 hr at 23 °C	2226	C
Gentamicin sulfate	ES	5 mg/mL[a]	NCI	1.2 mg/mL[a]	Physically compatible for 4 hr at 22 °C	1556	C
Granisetron HCl	SKB	1 mg/mL	MJ	0.3 mg/mL[b]	Physically compatible with little or no loss of either drug in 4 hr at 22 °C	1883	C
	SKB	0.05 mg/mL[a]	MJ	1.2 mg/mL[a]	Physically compatible for 4 hr at 23 °C	2000	C
Haloperidol lactate		0.2 mg/mL[a]	NCI	1.2 mg/mL[a]	Physically compatible for 4 hr at 22 °C	1528	C
Heparin sodium	WY	100 units/mL[a]	NCI	1.2 mg/mL[a]	Physically compatible for 4 hr at 22 °C	1556	C
Hydrocortisone sodium succinate	AB	1 mg/mL[a]	NCI	1.2 mg/mL[a]	Physically compatible for 4 hr at 22 °C	1556	C
Hydromorphone HCl	KN	0.5 mg/mL[a]	NCI	1.2 mg/mL[a]	Physically compatible for 4 hr at 22 °C	1556	C
Hydroxyzine HCl	ES	4 mg/mL[a]	NCI	1.2 mg/mL[a]	Normal inherent haze from paclitaxel decreases immediately	1556	I
Ifosfamide	BR	25 mg/mL[a]	NCI	1.2 mg/mL[a]	Physically compatible for 4 hr at 22 °C	1556	C
Linezolid	PHU	2 mg/mL	MJ	0.6 mg/mL[a]	Physically compatible for 4 hr at 23 °C	2264	C
Lorazepam		0.1 mg/mL[a]	NCI	1.2 mg/mL[a]	Physically compatible for 4 hr at 22 °C	1528	C
Magnesium sulfate	AST	100 mg/mL[a]	NCI	1.2 mg/mL[a]	Physically compatible for 4 hr at 22 °C	1556	C
Mannitol	BA	15%	NCI	1.2 mg/mL[a]	Physically compatible for 4 hr at 22 °C	1556	C
Meperidine HCl	WY	4 mg/mL[a]	NCI	1.2 mg/mL[a]	Physically compatible for 4 hr at 22 °C	1556	C
Mesna	MJ	10 mg/mL[a]	NCI	1.2 mg/mL[a]	Physically compatible for 4 hr at 22 °C	1556	C
Methotrexate sodium		15 mg/mL[a]	NCI	1.2 mg/mL[a]	Physically compatible for 4 hr at 22 °C	1528	C

Y-Site Injection Compatibility (1:1 Mixture) (Cont.)

Paclitaxel

Drug	Mfr	Conc	Mfr	Conc	Remarks	Ref	C/I
Methylprednisolone sodium succinate	UP	5 mg/mL[a]	NCI	1.2 mg/mL[a]	Normal inherent haze from paclitaxel decreases immediately	1556	I
Metoclopramide HCl		5 mg/mL	NCI	1.2 mg/mL[a]	Physically compatible for 4 hr at 22 °C	1528	C
Mitoxantrone HCl	LE	0.5 mg/mL[a]	NCI	1.2 mg/mL[a]	Normal inherent haze from paclitaxel decreases immediately	1556	I
Morphine sulfate	WY	1 mg/mL[a]	NCI	1.2 mg/mL[a]	Physically compatible for 4 hr at 22 °C	1556	C
Nalbuphine HCl	AST	10 mg/mL	NCI	1.2 mg/mL[a]	Physically compatible for 4 hr at 22 °C	1556	C
Ondansetron HCl	GL	0.5 mg/mL[a]	NCI	1.2 mg/mL[a]	Physically compatible for 4 hr at 22 °C	1556	C
	GL	0.03 and 0.3 mg/mL[a]	BR	0.3 mg/mL[a]	Visually compatible with no loss of either drug in 4 hr at 23 °C	1741	C
	GL	0.03 and 0.3 mg/mL[a]	BR	1.2 mg/mL[a]	Visually compatible with no loss of either drug in 4 hr at 23 °C	1741	C
Ondansetron HCl with ranitidine HCl	GL GL	0.3 mg/mL[a] 2 mg/mL[a]	BR	1.2 mg/mL[a]	Visually compatible with no loss of any drug in 4 hr at 23 °C	1741	C
Oxaliplatin	SS	0.5 mg/mL[a]	MJ	0.6 mg/mL[a]	Physically compatible for 4 hr at 23 °C	2566	C
Palonosetron HCl	MGI	50 mcg/mL	MJ	1.2 mg/mL[a]	Physically compatible. Little loss of either drug in 4 hr	2533	C
Pemetrexed disodium	LI	20 mg/mL[b]	MJ	0.6 mg/mL[a]	Physically compatible for 4 hr at 23 °C	2564	C
Pentostatin	NCI	0.4 mg/mL[b]	NCI	1.2 mg/mL[a]	Physically compatible for 4 hr at 22 °C	1556	C
Potassium chloride	AB	0.1 mEq/mL[a]	NCI	1.2 mg/mL[a]	Physically compatible for 4 hr at 22 °C	1556	C
Prochlorperazine edisylate		0.5 mg/mL[a]	NCI	1.2 mg/mL[a]	Physically compatible for 4 hr at 22 °C	1528	C
Propofol	ZEN	10 mg/mL	MJ	1.2 mg/mL[a]	Physically compatible for 1 hr at 23 °C	2066	C
Ranitidine HCl		2 mg/mL[a]	NCI	1.2 mg/mL[a]	Physically compatible for 4 hr at 22 °C	1528	C
	GL	0.5 and 2 mg/mL[a]	BR	0.3 and 1.2 mg/mL[a]	Visually compatible. No loss of either drug in 4 hr at 23 °C	1741	C
Ranitidine HCl with ondansetron HCl	GL GL	2 mg/mL[a] 0.3 mg/mL[a]	BR	1.2 mg/mL[a]	Visually compatible with no loss of any drug in 4 hr at 23 °C	1741	C
Sodium bicarbonate	LY	1 mEq/mL	NCI	1.2 mg/mL[a]	Physically compatible for 4 hr at 22 °C	1556	C
Thiotepa	IMM[d]	1 mg/mL[a]	MJ	0.6 mg/mL[a]	Physically compatible for 4 hr at 23 °C	1861	C
TNA #218 to #226[e]			MJ	1.2 mg/mL[a]	Visually compatible for 4 hr at 23 °C	2215	C
Topotecan HCl	SKB	56 mcg/mL[a,b]	MJ	0.54 mg/mL[a,b]	Visually compatible. Little loss of either drug in 4 hr at 22 °C	2245	C
TPN #212 to #215[e]			MJ	1.2 mg/mL[a]	Physically compatible for 4 hr at 23 °C	2109	C
Vancomycin HCl		10 mg/mL[a]	NCI	1.2 mg/mL[a]	Physically compatible for 4 hr at 22 °C	1528	C
Vinblastine sulfate	LI	0.12 mg/mL[b]	NCI	1.2 mg/mL[a]	Physically compatible for 4 hr at 22 °C	1556	C
Vincristine sulfate	LI	0.05 mg/mL[a]	NCI	1.2 mg/mL[a]	Physically compatible for 4 hr at 22 °C	1556	C
Zidovudine	BW	4 mg/mL[a]	NCI	1.2 mg/mL[a]	Physically compatible for 4 hr at 22 °C	1556	C

[a]Tested in dextrose 5%.
[b]Tested in sodium chloride 0.9%.
[c]Tested in bacteriostatic sodium chloride 0.9% preserved with benzyl alcohol 0.9%.
[d]Lyophilized formulation tested.
[e]Refer to Appendix I for the composition of parenteral nutrition solutions. TNA indicates a 3-in-1 admixture, and TPN indicates a 2-in-1 admixture.

PALONOSETRON HYDROCHLORIDE
AHFS 56:22.20

Products — Palonosetron hydrochloride is available in vials containing palonosetron base 0.25 mg in 5 mL as the hydrochloride. The product also contains mannitol 207.5 mg per 5 mL, disodium edetate, and citrate buffer. (1)

pH — From 4.5 to 5.5. (1)

Tonicity — Palonosetron hydrochloride injection is isotonic. (1)

Trade Name(s) — Aloxi.

Administration — Palonosetron hydrochloride is administered intravenously over 30 seconds. The manufacturer recommends that the infusion line be flushed with sodium chloride 0.9% before and after palonosetron hydrochloride is administered. (1)

Stability — Intact vials of palonosetron hydrochloride injection should be stored at controlled room temperature and should be protected from light and freezing. (1)

Compatibility Information

Solution Compatibility

Palonosetron HCl

Solution	Mfr	Mfr	Conc/L	Remarks	Ref	C/I
Dextrose 5% in Ringer's injection, lactated	BA[a]	MGI	5 and 30 mg	Physically compatible. Stable for 48 hr at 23 °C in light and 14 days at 4 °C	2535	C
Dextrose 5% in sodium chloride 0.45%	BA[a]	MGI	5 and 30 mg	Physically compatible. Stable for 48 hr at 23 °C in light and 14 days at 4 °C	2535	C
Dextrose 5%	BA[a]	MGI	5 and 30 mg	Physically compatible. Stable for 48 hr at 23 °C in light and 14 days at 4 °C	2535	C
Sodium chloride 0.9%	BA[a]	MGI	5 and 30 mg	Physically compatible. Stable for 48 hr at 23 °C in light and 14 days at 4 °C	2535	C

[a]Tested in PVC containers.

Additive Compatibility

Palonosetron HCl

Drug	Mfr	Conc/L	Mfr	Conc/L	Test Soln	Remarks	Ref	C/I
Dexamethasone sodium phosphate	AMR	200 and 400 mg	MGI	5 mg	D5W, NS[a]	Physically compatible. Little loss of either drug in 48 hr at 23 °C in light and 14 days at 4 °C	2552	C

[a]Tested in PVC containers.

Drugs in Syringe Compatibility

Palonosetron HCl

Drug (in syringe)	Mfr	Amt	Mfr	Amt	Remarks	Ref	C/I
Dexamethasone sodium phosphate	AMR	3.3 mg/ 5 mL[a,b]	MGI	0.25 mg/ 5 mL	Physically compatible. Little loss of either drug in 48 hr at 23 °C in light and 14 days at 4 °C	2552	C

[a]Tested in dextrose 5%.
[b]Tested in sodium chloride 0.9%.

Y-Site Injection Compatibility (1:1 Mixture)

Palonosetron HCl

Drug	Mfr	Conc	Mfr	Conc	Remarks	Ref	C/I
Ampicillin sodium–sulbactam sodium	RR	20 + 10 mg/mL[b]	MGI	50 mcg/mL	Physically compatible and no loss of either drug in 4 hr at room temperature	2749	**C**
Atropine sulfate	AMR	0.4 mg/mL	MGI	50 mcg/mL	Physically compatible and no loss of either drug in 4 hr at room temperature	2771	**C**
Carboplatin	BMS	5 mg/mL[a]	MGI	50 mcg/mL	Physically compatible. No palonosetron and 2% carboplatin loss in 4 hr	2579	**C**
Cefazolin sodium	WAT	20 mg/mL[a]	MGI	50 mcg/mL	Physically compatible and no loss of either drug in 4 hr at room temperature	2749	**C**
Cefotetan disodium	ASZ	20 mg/mL[b]	MGI	50 mcg/mL	Physically compatible and no loss of either drug in 4 hr at room temperature	2749	**C**
Cisatracurium besylate	AB	0.5 mg/mL[a]	MGI	50 mcg/mL	Physically compatible with no loss of either drug in 4 hr at room temperature	2764	**C**
Cisplatin	BMS	0.5 mg/mL[b]	MGI	50 mcg/mL	Physically compatible. No palonosetron and 5% cisplatin loss in 4 hr	2579	**C**
Cyclophosphamide	MJ	10 mg/mL[a]	MGI	50 mcg/mL	Physically compatible and no loss of either drug in 4 hr	2640	**C**
Dacarbazine	BV	4 mg/mL[a]	MGI	50 mcg/mL	Physically compatible and no loss of either drug in 4 hr	2681	**C**
Docetaxel	AVE	0.8 mg/mL[a]	MGI	50 mcg/mL	Physically compatible and no loss of either drug in 4 hr	2533	**C**
Famotidine	BED	2 mg/mL[a]	MGI	50 mcg/mL	Physically compatible and no loss of either drug in 4 hr at room temperature	2771	**C**
Fentanyl citrate	AB	50 mcg/mL	MGI	50 mcg/mL	Physically compatible and no loss of either drug in 4 hr	2720	**C**
Fluorouracil	APP	16 mg/mL[a]	MGI	50 mcg/mL	Physically compatible and no loss of either drug in 4 hr	2627	**C**
Gemcitabine HCl	LI	10 mg/mL[a]	MGI	50 mcg/mL	Physically compatible and no loss of either drug in 4 hr	2627	**C**
Gentamicin sulfate	APP	5 mg/mL[a]	MGI	50 mcg/mL	Physically compatible. No loss of either drug in 4 hr at room temperature	2765	**C**
Glycopyrrolate	BA	0.2 mg/mL	MGI	50 mcg/mL	Physically compatible. No loss of either drug in 4 hr at room temperature	2773	**C**
Heparin sodium	HOS	100 units/mL	MGI	50 mcg/mL	Physically compatible. No loss of either drug in 4 hr at room temperature	2771	**C**
Hetastarch in lactated electrolyte	HOS	6%	MGI	50 mcg/mL	Physically compatible. No palonosetron loss in 4 hr at room temperature	2775	**C**
Hydromorphone HCl	BA	0.5 mg/mL[a]	MGI	50 mcg/mL	Physically compatible and no loss of either drug in 4 hr	2720	**C**
Ifosfamide	MJ	10 mg/mL[a]	MGI	50 mcg/mL	Physically compatible and no loss of either drug in 4 hr	2640	**C**
Irinotecan HCl	PHU	1 mg/mL[a]	MGI	50 mcg/mL	Physically compatible. No palonosetron and 5% irinotecan loss in 4 hr	2609	**C**
Lidocaine HCl	AB	10 mg/mL[a]	MGI	50 mcg/mL	Physically compatible. No loss of either drug in 4 hr at room temperature	2771	**C**
Lorazepam	BA	0.5 mg/mL[a]	MGI	50 mcg/mL	Physically compatible. No loss of either drug in 4 hr	2608	**C**

Y-Site Injection Compatibility (1:1 Mixture) (Cont.)

Palonosetron HCl

Drug	Mfr	Conc	Mfr	Conc	Remarks	Ref	C/I
Mannitol	HOS	15%	MGI	50 mcg/mL	Physically compatible. No palonosetron loss in 4 hr at room temperature	2775	C
Meperidine HCl	AB	10 mg/mL[a]	MGI	50 mcg/mL	Physically compatible. No loss of either drug in 4 hr	2720	C
Methylprednisolone sodium succinate	PHU	5 mg/mL[a]	MGI	50 mcg/mL	Microprecipitate begins to form immediately and becomes visible within 4 hr	2681	I
Metoclopramide HCl	BA	5 mg/mL	MGI	50 mcg/mL	Physically compatible. No loss of either drug in 4 hr	2716	C
Metronidazole	BA	5 mg/mL	MGI	50 mcg/mL	Physically compatible. No loss of either drug in 4 hr at room temperature	2765	C
Midazolam HCl	BA	2 mg/mL[a]	MGI	50 mcg/mL	Physically compatible. No loss of either drug in 4 hr	2608	C
Morphine sulfate	BA	15 mg/mL	MGI	50 mcg/mL	Physically compatible. No loss of either drug in 4 hr	2720	C
Neostigmine methylsulfate	BA	0.5 mg/mL	MGI	50 mcg/mL	Physically compatible. No loss of either drug in 4 hr	2772	C
Oxaliplatin	SS	0.5 mg/mL[a]	MGI	50 mcg/mL	Physically compatible. No loss of either drug in 4 hr	2579	C
Paclitaxel	MJ	1.2 mg/mL[a]	MGI	50 mcg/mL	Physically compatible. Little loss of either drug in 4 hr	2533	C
Potassium chloride	AB	0.1 mEq/mL[a]	MGI	50 mcg/mL	Physically compatible. No loss of either drug in 4 hr at room temperature	2771	C
Promethazine HCl	PAD	2 mg/mL[a]	MGI	50 mcg/mL	Physically compatible. No loss of either drug in 4 hr	2716	C
Rocuronium bromide	BA	1 mg/mL[a]	MGI	50 mcg/mL	Physically compatible and no loss of either drug in 4 hr at room temperature	2764	C
Succinylcholine chloride	SZ	2 mg/mL[a]	MGI	50 mcg/mL	Physically compatible and no loss of either drug in 4 hr at room temperature	2764	C
Sufentanil citrate	HOS	12.5 mcg/mL[a]	MGI	50 mcg/mL	Physically compatible. No loss of either drug in 4 hr	2720	C
Topotecan HCl	GSK	0.1 mg/mL[a]	MGI	50 mcg/mL	Physically compatible. Little loss of either drug in 4 hr	2609	C
Vancomycin HCl	HOS	5 mg/mL[a]	MGI	50 mcg/mL	Physically compatible and no loss of either drug in 4 hr at room temperature	2765	C
Vecuronium bromide	BED	1 mg/mL	MGI	50 mcg/mL	Physically compatible and no loss of either drug in 4 hr at room temperature	2764	C

[a]Tested in dextrose 5%.
[b]Tested in sodium chloride 0.9%.

PANCURONIUM BROMIDE
AHFS 12:20.20

Products — Pancuronium bromide is available in 2- and 5-mL ampuls and vials containing 2 mg/mL of drug. It is also available in 10-mL vials at a concentration of 1 mg/mL. Each milliliter also contains sodium acetate anhydrous 1.2 mg, benzyl alcohol 1%, and sodium chloride 4 mg for isotonicity. Acetic acid and/or sodium hydroxide is added to adjust the pH. (1; 4)

pH — The solution has been adjusted to pH 3.8 to 4.2 by the manufacturer. (1; 4)

Osmolality — The osmolality of pancuronium bromide (Organon) 1 mg/mL was determined to be 277 mOsm/kg by freezing-point depression and 273 mOsm/kg by vapor pressure. (1071)

The osmolality of pancuronium bromide 2 mg/mL was determined to be 338 mOsm/kg. (1233)

Administration — Pancuronium bromide is administered intravenously. (1; 4)

Stability — Pancuronium bromide should be stored under refrigeration at 2 to 8 °C. (4) However, the manufacturer indicates that the drug is stable for six months at room temperature. (1; 853; 1181; 1433)

Sorption — The manufacturer indicates that pancuronium bromide in compatible infusion solutions does not undergo sorption to glass or plastic containers during short-term storage over 48 hours at room temperature. (1; 4) However, the drug may exhibit sorption to plastic containers with prolonged contact. (4)

Compatibility Information

Solution Compatibility

Pancuronium bromide

Solution	Mfr	Mfr	Conc/L	Remarks	Ref	C/I
Dextrose 5% in sodium chloride 0.45%				No loss in 48 hr	1	C
Dextrose 5% in sodium chloride 0.9%				No loss in 48 hr	1	C
Dextrose 5%				No loss in 48 hr	1	C
Ringer's injection, lactated				No loss in 48 hr	1	C
Sodium chloride 0.9%				No loss in 48 hr	1	C

Additive Compatibility

Pancuronium bromide

Drug	Mfr	Conc/L	Mfr	Conc/L	Test Soln	Remarks	Ref	C/I
Ciprofloxacin	BAY	1.6 g	OR	200 mg	D5W	Visually compatible with no loss of ciprofloxacin in 24 hr at 22 °C under fluorescent light. Pancuronium not tested	2413	C
Verapamil HCl	KN	80 mg	OR	8 mg	D5W, NS	Physically compatible for 24 hr	764	C

Drugs in Syringe Compatibility

Pancuronium bromide

Drug (in syringe)	Mfr	Amt	Mfr	Amt	Remarks	Ref	C/I
Caffeine citrate		20 mg/1 mL	GNS	1 mg/1 mL	Visually compatible for 4 hr at 25 °C	2440	C
Heparin sodium		2500 units/1 mL		4 mg/2 mL	Physically compatible for at least 5 min	1053	C
Pantoprazole sodium	a	4 mg/1 mL		2 mg/1 mL	Orange precipitate	2574	I

aTest performed using the formulation WITHOUT edetate disodium.

Y-Site Injection Compatibility (1:1 Mixture)

Pancuronium bromide

Drug	Mfr	Conc	Mfr	Conc	Remarks	Ref	C/I
Aminophylline	AB	1 mg/mL[a]	ES	0.05 mg/mL[a]	Physically compatible for 24 hr at 28 °C	1337	C
Cefazolin sodium	LY	10 mg/mL[a]	ES	0.05 mg/mL[a]	Physically compatible for 24 hr at 28 °C	1337	C
Cefuroxime sodium	GL	7.5 mg/mL[a]	ES	0.05 mg/mL[a]	Physically compatible for 24 hr at 28 °C	1337	C
Dexmedetomidine HCl	HOS				Stated to be compatible	1	C
Diazepam	ES	5 mg/mL	ES	0.05 mg/mL[a]	Cloudy solution forms immediately	1337	I
Dobutamine HCl	LI	1 mg/mL[a]	ES	0.05 mg/mL[a]	Physically compatible for 24 hr at 28 °C	1337	C
Dopamine HCl	SO	1.6 mg/mL[a]	ES	0.05 mg/mL[a]	Physically compatible for 24 hr at 28 °C	1337	C
Epinephrine HCl	AB	4 mcg/mL[a]	ES	0.05 mg/mL[a]	Physically compatible for 24 hr at 28 °C	1337	C
Esmolol HCl	DCC	10 mg/mL[a]	ES	0.05 mg/mL[a]	Physically compatible for 24 hr at 28 °C	1337	C
Etomidate	AB	2 mg/mL	GNS	2 mg/mL	Visually compatible for 7 days at 25 °C	1801	C
Fenoldopam mesylate	AB	80 mcg/mL[b]	BA	0.1 mg/mL[b]	Physically compatible for 4 hr at 23 °C	2467	C
Fentanyl citrate	ES	10 mcg/mL[a]	ES	0.05 mg/mL[a]	Physically compatible for 24 hr at 28 °C	1337	C
Fluconazole	RR	2 mg/mL	GNS	0.5 mg/mL[b]	Visually compatible for 24 hr at 28 °C under fluorescent light	1760	C
Gentamicin sulfate	ES	2 mg/mL[a]	ES	0.05 mg/mL[a]	Physically compatible for 24 hr at 28 °C	1337	C
Heparin sodium	SO	40 units/mL[a]	ES	0.05 mg/mL[a]	Physically compatible for 24 hr at 28 °C	1337	C
Hetastarch in lactated electrolyte	AB	6%	ES	0.1 mg/mL[a]	Physically compatible for 4 hr at 23 °C	2339	C
Hydrocortisone sodium succinate	AB	1 mg/mL[a]	ES	0.05 mg/mL[a]	Physically compatible for 24 hr at 28 °C	1337	C
Isoproterenol HCl	ES	4 mcg/mL	ES	0.05 mg/mL[a]	Physically compatible for 24 hr at 28 °C	1337	C
Levofloxacin	OMN	5 mg/mL[a]	ES	1 mg/mL	Visually compatible for 4 hr at 24 °C	2233	C
Lorazepam	WY	0.5 mg/mL[a]	ES	0.05 mg/mL[a]	Physically compatible for 24 hr at 28 °C	1337	C
Midazolam HCl	RC	0.05 mg/mL[a]	ES	0.05 mg/mL[a]	Physically compatible for 24 hr at 28 °C	1337	C
Milrinone lactate	SW	0.4 mg/mL[a]	GNS	1 mg/mL	Visually compatible. Little loss of either drug in 4 hr at 23 °C	2214	C
Morphine sulfate	WY	1 mg/mL[a]	ES	0.05 mg/mL[a]	Physically compatible for 24 hr at 28 °C	1337	C
Nitroglycerin	SO	0.4 mg/mL[a]	ES	0.05 mg/mL[a]	Physically compatible for 24 hr at 28 °C	1337	C
Propofol	STU	2 mg/mL	GNS	2 mg/mL	Oil droplets form within 7 days at 25 °C. No visible change in 24 hr	1801	?
	ZEN	10 mg/mL	AST	1 mg/mL	Physically compatible for 1 hr at 23 °C	2066	C
Ranitidine HCl	GL	0.5 mg/mL[a]	ES	0.05 mg/mL[a]	Physically compatible for 24 hr at 28 °C	1337	C
Sodium nitroprusside	ES	0.2 mg/mL[a]	ES	0.05 mg/mL[a]	Physically compatible for 24 hr at 28 °C	1337	C
Trimethoprim–sulfamethoxazole	ES	0.64 + 3.2 mg/mL[a]	ES	0.05 mg/mL[a]	Physically compatible for 24 hr at 28 °C	1337	C
Vancomycin HCl	ES	5 mg/mL[a]	ES	0.05 mg/mL[a]	Physically compatible for 24 hr at 28 °C	1337	C

[a]*Tested in dextrose 5%.*
[b]*Tested in sodium chloride 0.9%.*

PANTOPRAZOLE SODIUM
AHFS 56:28.36

Products — Pantoprazole sodium is available as a lyophilized powder in vials containing pantoprazole 40 mg as the sodium salt with edetate disodium 1 mg and sodium hydroxide to adjust pH during manufacturing. (1)

Reconstitute the vials with 10 mL of sodium chloride 0.9% to a concentration of 4 mg/mL. For intravenous infusion, one vial of the reconstituted drug solution may be diluted further with 100 mL or two vials may be diluted with 80 mL of sodium chloride 0.9%, dextrose 5%, or Ringer's injection, lactated to yield concentrations of about 0.4 or 0.8 mg/mL, respectively. (1)

pH — From 9.0 to 10.5. (1)

Trade Name(s) — Protonix I.V.

Administration — Pantoprazole sodium injection reconstituted as directed to a concentration of 4 mg/mL may be administered by intra-venous injection over a period of at least two minutes. The reconstituted solution may also be diluted further in a compatible infusion solution to a concentration of about 0.4 mg/mL and administered by intravenous infusion over about 15 minutes. (1)

Stability — Intact vials of pantoprazole sodium should be stored at controlled room temperature and should be protected from light during storage. (1)

After reconstitution as directed, pantoprazole sodium injection may be stored for up to six hours at room temperature before use. The manufacturer notes that the reconstituted solution should not be frozen. After dilution in a compatible infusion solution, the drug may be stored for up to 24 hours prior to use at room temperature. Protection from light exposure is not required. (1) Pantoprazole sodium admixtures prepared for infusion did not undergo discoloration over 24 hours at room temperature exposed to light. (2507)

Reconstituted pantoprazole sodium (Wyeth) 4 mg/mL in sodium chloride 0.9% in polypropylene syringes (Terumo) has been found to be physically and chemically stable for at least 96 hours at room temperature of 24 °C exposed to light and refrigerated at 4 °C. (2656)

Compatibility Information

Solution Compatibility

Pantoprazole sodium

Solution	Mfr	Mfr	Conc/L	Remarks	Ref	C/I
Dextrose 5%	BA	PH[a]	400 mg	Physically compatible. 10% loss occurs in 4 days at 22 °C in light	2696	**C**
	BA	ALT[b]	160 mg	10% loss in 24 hr at 23 °C. 5% loss in 14 days and 11% in 21 days at 4 °C	2798	**C**
	BA	ALT[b]	800 mg	9% loss in 4 days at 23 °C. Little loss in 21 days at 4 °C	2798	**C**
Sodium chloride 0.9%	AB	WY[b]	4 g	Physically and chemically stable for 96 hr at 24 °C in light and 4 °C	2656	**C**
	BA	PH[a]	400 mg	Physically compatible. 10% loss occurs in 8 days at 22 °C in light	2696	**C**
	HOS	ALT[b]	160 mg	6% loss in 48 hr and 11% in 4 days at 23 °C. 5% loss in 21 days at 4 °C	2797	**C**
	HOS	ALT[b]	800 mg	4% loss in 7 days and 11% in 9 days at 23 °C. Little loss in 21 days at 4 °C	2797	**C**
TPN #275[c]		ALT[b]	13.3 mg	Yellow color and losses of 12% in 3 hr at room temperature in dark	2789	**I**

[a] *Test performed using the formulation WITHOUT edetate disodium.*
[b] *Test performed using the formulation WITH edetate disodium.*
[c] *Refer to Appendix I for the composition of parenteral nutrition solutions. TPN indicates a 2-in-1 admixture.*

Drugs in Syringe Compatibility

Pantoprazole sodium

Drug (in syringe)	Mfr	Amt	Mfr	Amt	Remarks	Ref	C/I
Acetazolamide sodium		100 mg/ 1 mL	[a]	4 mg/ 1 mL	Clear solution	2574	**C**
Acyclovir sodium		50 mg/ 1 mL	[a]	4 mg/ 1 mL	Precipitates within 4 hr	2574	**I**

Drugs in Syringe Compatibility (Cont.)

Pantoprazole sodium

Drug (in syringe)	Mfr	Amt	Mfr	Amt	Remarks	Ref	C/I
Alprostadil		0.5 mg/ 1 mL	a	4 mg/ 1 mL	Clear solution	2574	C
Amikacin sulfate		250 mg/ 1 mL	a	4 mg/ 1 mL	Precipitates	2574	I
Aminophylline		50 mg/ 1 mL	a	4 mg/ 1 mL	Clear solution	2574	C
Amiodarone HCl		50 mg/ 1 mL	a	4 mg/ 1 mL	Precipitates	2574	I
Amphotericin B		5 mg/ 1 mL	a	4 mg/ 1 mL	Opacity within 1 hr	2574	I
Ampicillin sodium		250 mg/ 1 mL	a	4 mg/ 1 mL	Clear solution	2574	C
Atropine sulfate		0.4 mg/ 1 mL	a	4 mg/ 1 mL	Incompatible after 4 hr	2574	I
Caffeine citrate		10 mg/ 1 mL	a	4 mg/ 1 mL	Precipitates	2574	I
Calcium chloride		100 mg/ 1 mL	a	4 mg/ 1 mL	Precipitates	2574	I
Calcium gluconate		100 mg/ 1 mL	a	4 mg/ 1 mL	Precipitates	2574	I
Cefazolin sodium		100 mg/ 1 mL	a	4 mg/ 1 mL	Precipitates immediately	2574	I
Cefotaxime sodium		100 mg/ 1 mL	a	4 mg/ 1 mL	Precipitates immediately	2574	I
Cefoxitin sodium		100 mg/ 1 mL	a	4 mg/ 1 mL	Precipitates immediately	2574	I
Ceftazidime		100 mg/ 1 mL	a	4 mg/ 1 mL	Precipitates immediately	2574	I
Cefuroxime sodium		100 mg/ 1 mL	a	4 mg/ 1 mL	Precipitates immediately	2574	I
Chlorpromazine HCl		25 mg/ 1 mL	a	4 mg/ 1 mL	Precipitates immediately	2574	I
Ciprofloxacin		2 mg/ 1 mL	a	4 mg/ 1 mL	Precipitates immediately	2574	I
Clindamycin phosphate		150 mg/ 1 mL	a	4 mg/ 1 mL	Precipitates within 1 hr	2574	I
Cloxacillin sodium		100 mg/ 1 mL	a	4 mg/ 1 mL	Precipitates immediately	2574	I
Cyclosporine		50 mg/ 1 mL	a	4 mg/ 1 mL	Precipitates	2574	I
Dexamethasone sodium phosphate		10 mg/ 1 mL	a	4 mg/ 1 mL	Precipitates immediately	2574	I
Diazepam		5 mg/ 1 mL	a	4 mg/ 1 mL	Red precipitate forms immediately	2574	I
Digoxin		0.05 mg/ 1 mL	a	4 mg/ 1 mL	Precipitates within 4 hr	2574	I

Drugs in Syringe Compatibility (Cont.)

Pantoprazole sodium

Drug (in syringe)	Mfr	Amt	Mfr	Amt	Remarks	Ref	C/I
Dimenhydrinate		50 mg/ 1 mL	a	4 mg/ 1 mL	White precipitate	2574	**I**
Diphenhydramine HCl		50 mg/ 1 mL	a	4 mg/ 1 mL	Precipitates immediately	2574	**I**
Dobutamine HCl		12.5 mg/ 1 mL	a	4 mg/ 1 mL	White precipitate forms within 1 hr	2574	**I**
Dopamine HCl		40 mg/ 1 mL	a	4 mg/ 1 mL	Whitish precipitate forms within 1 hr	2574	**I**
Enalaprilat		1.25 mg/ 1 mL	a	4 mg/ 1 mL	Precipitate forms within 1 hr	2574	**I**
Epinephrine HCl		1 mg/ 1 mL	a	4 mg/ 1 mL	Precipitates	2574	**I**
Estrogens, conjugated		5 mg/ 1 mL	a	4 mg/ 1 mL	Possible precipitate within 1 hr	2574	**I**
Fentanyl citrate		50 mcg/ 1 mL	a	4 mg/ 1 mL	Possible precipitate within 15 min	2574	**I**
Fluconazole		2 mg/ 1 mL	a	4 mg/ 1 mL	Possible precipitate within 4 hr	2574	**I**
Furosemide		10 mg/ 1 mL	a	4 mg/ 1 mL	Possible precipitate within 15 min	2574	**I**
Gentamicin sulfate		40 mg/ 1 mL	a	4 mg/ 1 mL	Whitish precipitate	2574	**I**
Heparin sodium		25,000 units/ 1 mL	a	4 mg/ 1 mL	Precipitates within 1 hr	2574	**I**
Hydralazine HCl		20 mg/ 1 mL	a	4 mg/ 1 mL	Precipitates within 4 hr	2574	**I**
Hydrocortisone sodium succinate		125 mg/ 1 mL	a	4 mg/ 1 mL	Possible precipitate within 15 min	2574	**I**
Hydromorphone HCl		10 mg/ 1 mL	a	4 mg/ 1 mL	Whitish precipitate forms within 4 hr	2574	**I**
Indomethacin sodium trihydrate		0.5 mg/ 1 mL	a	4 mg/ 1 mL	Precipitates within 1 hr	2574	**I**
Insulin, regular		100 units/ 1 mL	a	4 mg/ 1 mL	Precipitates within 1 hr	2574	**I**
Isoproterenol HCl		0.2 mg/ 1 mL	a	4 mg/ 1 mL	Whitish precipitate	2574	**I**
Labetalol HCl		5 mg/ 1 mL	a	4 mg/ 1 mL	Whitish precipitate	2574	**I**
Lidocaine HCl		200 mg/ 1 mL	a	4 mg/ 1 mL	Precipitates within 4 hr	2574	**I**
Lorazepam		4 mg/ 1 mL	a	4 mg/ 1 mL	Precipitates	2574	**I**
Magnesium sulfate		500 mg/ 1 mL	a	4 mg/ 1 mL	Whitish precipitate	2574	**I**

Drugs in Syringe Compatibility (Cont.)

Pantoprazole sodium

Drug (in syringe)	Mfr	Amt	Mfr	Amt	Remarks	Ref	C/I
Meperidine HCl		100 mg/ 1 mL	a	4 mg/ 1 mL	Yellowish precipitate within 15 min	2574	I
Meropenem		50 mg/ 1 mL	a	4 mg/ 1 mL	Precipitates within 15 min	2574	I
Methylprednisolone sodium succinate		62.5 mg/ 1 mL	a	4 mg/ 1 mL	Precipitates within 15 min	2574	I
Metoclopramide HCl		5 mg/ 1 mL	a	4 mg/ 1 mL	Precipitates within 15 min	2574	I
Midazolam HCl		5 mg/ 1 mL	a	4 mg/ 1 mL	Precipitates immediately	2574	I
Morphine sulfate		50 mg/ 1 mL	a	4 mg/ 1 mL	Yellowish precipitate	2574	I
Naloxone HCl		0.4 mg/ 1 mL	a	4 mg/ 1 mL	Precipitates within 4 hr	2574	I
Nitroglycerin		5 mg/ 1 mL	a	4 mg/ 1 mL	Precipitates	2574	I
Norepinephrine bitartrate		1 mg/ 1 mL	a	4 mg/ 1 mL	Precipitates within 15 min	2574	I
Octreotide acetate		0.5 mcg/ 1 mL	a	4 mg/ 1 mL	Precipitates	2574	I
Oxytocin		10 units/ 1 mL	a	4 mg/ 1 mL	Orange precipitate	2574	I
Pancuronium bromide		2 mg/ 1 mL	a	4 mg/ 1 mL	Orange precipitate	2574	I
Penicillin G sodium		500,000 units/ 1 mL	a	4 mg/ 1 mL	Clear solution	2574	C
Phenobarbital sodium		120 mg/ 1 mL	a	4 mg/ 1 mL	Precipitates within 4 hr	2574	I
Phenytoin sodium		50 mg/ 1 mL	a	4 mg/ 1 mL	Precipitates within 1 hr	2574	I
Piperacillin sodium–tazobactam sodium	a	200 + 25 mg/ 1 mL	a	4 mg/ 1 mL	Precipitates within 1 hr	2574	I
Potassium chloride		2 mEq/ 1 mL	a	4 mg/ 1 mL	Clear solution	2574	C
Potassium phosphates		4 mmol/ 1 mL	a	4 mg/ 1 mL	Precipitates	2574	I
Procainamide HCl		100 mg/ 1 mL	a	4 mg/ 1 mL	Clear solution	2574	C
Prochlorperazine edisylate		5 mg/ 1 mL	a	4 mg/ 1 mL	Yellowish precipitate forms	2574	I
Propofol		10 mg/ 1 mL	a	4 mg/ 1 mL	No change seen	2574	?
Propranolol HCl		1 mg/ 1 mL	a	4 mg/ 1 mL	Precipitates	2574	I

Drugs in Syringe Compatibility (Cont.)

Pantoprazole sodium

Drug (in syringe)	Mfr	Amt	Mfr	Amt	Remarks	Ref	C/I
Ranitidine HCl		25 mg/ 1 mL	a	4 mg/ 1 mL	Possible precipitate within 4 hr	2574	I
Salbutamol		1 mg/ 1 mL	a	4 mg/ 1 mL	Precipitates immediately	2574	I
Sodium bicarbonate		1 mEq/ 1 mL	a	4 mg/ 1 mL	Precipitates after 1 hr	2574	I
Sodium nitroprusside		10 mg/ 1 mL	a	4 mg/ 1 mL	Precipitates within 15 min	2574	I
Ticarcillin disodium–clavulanate potassium		200 mg/ 1 mL	a	4 mg/ 1 mL	Clear solution	2574	C
Tobramycin sulfate		40 mg/ 1 mL	a	4 mg/ 1 mL	Precipitates immediately	2574	I
Trimethoprim–sulfamethoxazole		16 + 80 mg/ 1 mL	a	4 mg/ 1 mL	Possible precipitate within 1 hr	2574	I
Vancomycin HCl		50 mg/ 1 mL	a	4 mg/ 1 mL	Clear solution	2574	C
Vecuronium bromide		1 mg/ 1 mL	a	4 mg/ 1 mL	Precipitates	2574	I
Verapamil HCl		2.5 mg/ 1 mL	a	4 mg/ 1 mL	Whitish precipitate	2574	I
Zidovudine		10 mg/ 1 mL	a	4 mg/ 1 mL	Clear solution	2574	C

[a]*Test performed using the formulation WITHOUT edetate disodium.*

Y-Site Injection Compatibility (1:1 Mixture)

Pantoprazole sodium

Drug	Mfr	Conc	Mfr	Conc	Remarks	Ref	C/I
Ampicillin sodium	NVP	10 to 40 mg/ mL[a]	ALT[c]	0.16 to 0.8 mg/mL[b]	Visually compatible for 12 hr at 23 °C	2603	C
Anidulafungin	VIC	0.5 mg/mL[a]	WAY[c]	0.4 mg/mL[a]	Physically compatible for 4 hr at 23 °C	2617	C
Caspofungin acetate	ME	0.7 mg/mL[b]	WY[d]	0.4 mg/mL[b]	Physically compatible for 4 hr at room temperature	2758	C
	ME	0.5 mg/mL[b]	WY[d]	0.4 mg/mL[b]	White particles reported	2766	I
Cefazolin sodium	NOP	20 to 40 mg/ mL[a]	ALT[c]	0.16 to 0.8 mg/mL[b]	Visually compatible for 12 hr at 23 °C	2603	C
Ceftaroline fosamil	FOR	2.22 mg/ mL[a,b,e]	WY[d]	0.4 mg/mL[a,b,e]	Physically compatible for 4 hr at 23 °C	2826	C
Ceftriaxone sodium	RC	20 to 40 mg/ mL[a]	ALT[c]	0.16 to 0.8 mg/mL[b]	Visually compatible for 12 hr at 23 °C	2603	C
Dimenhydrinate	AST	0.5 to 1 mg/ mL[a]	ALT[c]	0.16 to 0.8 mg/mL[b]	Visually compatible for 12 hr at 23 °C	2603	C
Dobutamine HCl	LI	1 to 4 mg/ mL[a]	ALT[c]	0.16 to 0.8 mg/mL[b]	Cloudiness forms over time	2603	I

Y-Site Injection Compatibility (1:1 Mixture) (Cont.)

Pantoprazole sodium

Drug	*Mfr*	*Conc*	*Mfr*	*Conc*	*Remarks*	*Ref*	*C/I*
Dopamine HCl	DU	0.8 to 3.2 mg/mL[a]	ALT[c]	0.16 to 0.8 mg/mL[b]	Visually compatible for 12 hr at 23 °C	2603	**C**
Doripenem	JJ	5 mg/mL[a,b]	WY[d]	0.4 mg/mL[a,b]	Physically compatible for 4 hr at 23 °C	2743	**C**
Epinephrine HCl	AB	16 to 32 mcg/mL[a]	ALT[c]	0.16 to 0.8 mg/mL[b]	Visually compatible for 12 hr at 23 °C	2603	**C**
Esmolol HCl	BA	10 to 20 mg/mL[a]	ALT[c]	0.16 to 0.8 mg/mL[b]	Discoloration and reddish-brown precipitate form	2603	**I**
Furosemide	SX	1 to 2 mg/mL[a]	ALT[c]	0.16 to 0.8 mg/mL[b]	Visually compatible for 12 hr at 23 °C	2603	**C**
Insulin, regular	LI	5 to 50 units/mL[a]	ALT[c]	0.16 to 0.8 mg/mL[b]	Visually compatible for 12 hr at 23 °C	2603	**C**
Mannitol		25%	[c]	4 mg/mL	Precipitates	2574	**I**
Midazolam HCl	SX	1 to 2 mg/mL[a]	ALT[c]	0.16 to 0.8 mg/mL[b]	Discoloration and reddish-brown precipitate form	2603	**I**
	RC	0.1 mg/mL	ALT[c]	8 mg/mL	Yellow color forms immediately	2727	**I**
Morphine sulfate	AB	1 to 10 mg/mL[a]	ALT[c]	0.16 to 0.8 mg/mL[b]	Visually compatible for 12 hr at 23 °C	2603	**C**
Multivitamins	SX		[c]	4 mg/mL	Precipitates within 1 hr	2574	**I**
Nitroglycerin	SX	0.1 to 0.4 mg/mL[a]	ALT[c]	0.16 to 0.8 mg/mL[b]	Visually compatible for 12 hr at 23 °C	2603	**C**
Norepinephrine bitartrate	SX	6 to 8 mcg/mL[a]	ALT[c]	0.16 to 0.8 mg/mL[b]	Visually compatible for 12 hr at 23 °C	2603	**C**
	SX	64 mcg/mL[a]	ALT[c]	0.16 mg/mL[b]	Visually compatible for 12 hr at 23 °C	2603	**C**
	SX	64 mcg/mL[a]	ALT[c]	0.4 to 0.8 mg/mL[b]	Turns cloudy upon mixing	2603	**I**
Octreotide acetate	NVA	5 to 10 mcg/mL[a]	ALT[c]	0.16 to 0.4 mg/mL[b]	Yellow discoloration forms	2603	**I**
	NVA	7.5 to 10 mcg/mL[a]	ALT[c]	0.8 mg/mL[b]	Yellow discoloration forms	2603	**I**
	NVA	5 mcg/mL[a]	ALT[c]	0.8 mg/mL[b]	Visually compatible for 12 hr at 23 °C	2603	**C**
Potassium chloride	AST	20 to 210 mEq/L[a]	ALT[c]	0.16 to 0.8 mg/mL[b]	Visually compatible for 12 hr at 23 °C	2603	**C**
Telavancin HCl	ASP	7.5 mg/mL[a,b,e]	WY[d]	0.4 mg/mL[a,b,e]	Physically compatible for 2 hr	2830	**C**
Vancomycin HCl	ME	40 mg/mL	ALT[c]	8 mg/mL	Color change after 10 hr	2727	**I**
Vasopressin	FER	0.4 to 1 unit/mL[a]	ALT[c]	0.16 to 0.8 mg/mL[b]	Visually compatible for 12 hr at 23 °C	2603	**C**

[a]Tested in dextrose 5%

[b]Tested in sodium chloride 0.9%.

[c]Test performed using the formulation WITHOUT edetate disodium.

[d]Test performed using the formulation WITH edetate disodium.

[e]Tested in Ringer's injection, lactated.

PAPAVERINE HYDROCHLORIDE
AHFS 24:12.92

Products — Papaverine hydrochloride is available in 2-mL single-dose ampuls and vials and 10-mL multiple-dose vials. Each milliliter of solution contains 30 mg of papaverine as the hydrochloride. (1; 4) The multiple-dose vials also contain edetate disodium 0.005%, chlorobutanol 0.5%, and sodium hydroxide to adjust the pH. (1) The single-dose containers are preservative free. (4)

pH — Not below 3. (17)

Administration — Papaverine hydrochloride may be administered by intramuscular or slow intravenous injection over one to two minutes. (1; 4)

Stability — Papaverine hydrochloride injection should be stored at controlled room temperature and protected from light, temperatures of 40 °C or higher, and from freezing. (1; 4) It should not be refrigerated because of a reduction in solubility with possible precipitation. (593) The solutions should be clear and colorless to pale yellow. (1) The yellow discoloration of papaverine hydrochloride injection does not appear to be related to drug decomposition. Analysis of a yellow injection found nearly 100% of the drug. Furthermore, yellow discoloration is not produced by intentional degradation from boiling with acid or base. (1996)

Compatibility Information

Solution Compatibility

Papaverine HCl

Solution	Mfr	Mfr	Conc/L	Remarks	Ref	C/I
Dextrose–Ringer's injection combinations	AB		96 mg	Physically compatible	3	C
Dextrose–saline combinations	AB		96 mg	Physically compatible	3	C
Dextrose 2.5%	AB		96 mg	Physically compatible	3	C
Dextrose 5%	AB		96 mg	Physically compatible	3	C
Dextrose 10%	AB		96 mg	Physically compatible	3	C
Ionosol products	AB		96 mg	Physically compatible	3	C
Ringer's injection	AB		96 mg	Physically compatible	3	C
Ringer's injection, lactated				Precipitation occurs	4	I
Sodium chloride 0.45%	AB		96 mg	Physically compatible	3	C
Sodium chloride 0.9%	AB		96 mg	Physically compatible	3	C
Sodium lactate ⅙ M	AB		96 mg	Physically compatible	3	C

Additive Compatibility

Papaverine HCl

Drug	Mfr	Conc/L	Mfr	Conc/L	Test Soln	Remarks	Ref	C/I
Theophylline		2 g		160 mg	D5W	Visually compatible with little or no loss of either drug in 48 hr	1909	C

Drugs in Syringe Compatibility

Papaverine HCl

Drug (in syringe)	Mfr	Amt	Mfr	Amt	Remarks	Ref	C/I
Iohexol	WI	64.7%, 5 mL	LI	30 mg/ 1 mL	Physically compatible for at least 2 hr	1438	C
Iopamidol	SQ	61%, 5 mL	LI	30 mg/ 1 mL	Physically compatible for at least 2 hr	1438	C

Drugs in Syringe Compatibility (Cont.)

Papaverine HCl

Drug (in syringe)	Mfr	Amt	Mfr	Amt	Remarks	Ref	C/I
Iothalamate meglumine	MA	60%, 5 mL	LI	30 mg/ 1 mL	Physically compatible for at least 2 hr	1438	**C**
Ioxaglate meglumine–ioxaglate sodium	MA	5 mL	ME	32 mg/ 1 mL	Precipitate forms immediately and persists for at least 2 hr	1438	**I**
	MA	3 and 5 mL	LI	30 mg/ 1 mL	White amorphous precipitate forms immediately and persists for 24 hr. If shaken, it dissolves in 20 to 30 min	1437	**I**
	MA	5 mL	LI	30 mg/2 to 6 mL[a]	Precipitate forms	1437	**I**
	MA	5 mL	LI	30 mg/11 and 16 mL[a]	Precipitate forms and then redissolves	1437	**?**
	MA	5 mL	LI	30 mg/ 21 mL[a]	Physically compatible	1437	**C**
	MA	15 and 30 mL	LI	30 mg/ 11 mL[a]	Physically compatible	1437	**C**
	MA	5 mL	LI	60 mg/12 and 17 mL[a]	Precipitate forms	1437	**I**
	MA	5 mL	LI	60 mg/ 22 mL[a]	Precipitate forms	1437	**I**
Phentolamine mesylate	BV, CI	0.5 mg/ mL[b]	LI	30 mg/ mL	Physically compatible. Little papaverine loss at 5 and 25 °C. 1 to 3% phentolamine loss at 5 °C and 4 to 5% at 25 °C in 30 days	1161	**C**

[a]*Diluted in sodium chloride 0.9%.*
[b]*Reconstituted with the papaverine hydrochloride injection.*

PEMETREXED DISODIUM
AHFS 10:00

Products — Pemetrexed disodium is available in vials containing pemetrexed 500 mg as the disodium salt. The vials also contain mannitol 500 mg with hydrochloric acid and/or sodium hydroxide to adjust pH during manufacturing. The vials should be reconstituted with 20 mL of sodium chloride 0.9% (without preservatives) and swirled gently to yield a 25-mg/mL solution. (1)

pH — From 6.6 to 7.8. (1)

Trade Name(s) — Alimta.

Administration — Pemetrexed disodium reconstituted as directed must be diluted to 100 mL with additional sodium chloride 0.9% for administration by intravenous infusion over 10 minutes. (1)

Stability — Intact vials of pemetrexed disodium may be stored at controlled room temperature. The reconstituted solution is chemically and physically stable for up to 24 hours at ambient room temperature and lighting and also under refrigeration. Pemetrexed disodium diluted in sodium chloride 0.9% for intravenous infusion is also stable for 24 hours at ambient room temperature and lighting and under refrigeration. The drug is not sensitive to light. (1)

Pemetrexed disodium (Lilly) 9 mg/mL in sodium chloride 0.9% did not result in the loss of viability of *Pseudomonas aeruginosa* within 120 hours at room temperature of 22 °C. A slight antimicrobial effect against *Staphylococcus aureus* was reported after 120 hours at room temperature; this slight effect cannot be regarded as sufficient for patient protection from growth of this microorganism. Diluted solutions should be stored under refrigeration whenever possible, and the potential for microbiological growth should be considered when assigning expiration periods. (2740)

Pemetrexed disodium (Lilly) 25 mg/mL reconstituted with sodium chloride 0.9% was reported to be stable for 48 hours at 23 °C exposed to or protected from light and for 31 days at 4 °C exhibiting little or no drug loss when packaged in polypropylene syringes (Becton Dickinson) with Red Cap tip seals (Burron). (2676)

Freezing Solutions — Pemetrexed disodium (Lilly) 2 to 20 mg/mL in dextrose 5% and also in sodium chloride 0.9% frozen at –20 °C in PVC bags developed substantial amounts of microparticulates, up to 30,000/mL, at all time points in the study up to 90 days. Especially concerning was the presence of hundreds of particles of 10 μm and larger, which may adversely impact patient safety. Although little loss of the drug occurred, the formation of such large quantities of microparticulates made the solutions unacceptable for use. The microparticulates that formed appeared to be related to the PVC containers because upon repeating the study in glass laboratory vessels few microparticulates appeared. (2693)

Compatibility Information

Solution Compatibility

Pemetrexed disodium

Solution	Mfr	Mfr	Conc/L	Remarks	Ref	C/I
Dextrose 5%	BA[a]	LI	2, 10, 20 g	Physically compatible for 48 hr at 23 °C. At 4 °C, microprecipitation occurs after 24 hr. No loss in 48 hr at 23 °C and in 31 days at 4 °C	2689	**C**
Ringer's injection				Physically incompatible	1	**I**
Ringer's injection, lactated				Physically incompatible	1	**I**
Sodium chloride 0.9%		LI		Physically compatible and stable for 24 hr at room temperature and refrigerated	1	**C**
	BA[a]	LI	2, 10, 20 g	Physically compatible for 48 hr at 23 °C. At 4 °C, microprecipitation occurs after 24 hr. No loss in 48 hr at 23 °C and in 31 days at 4 °C	2689	**C**
	MAC[a]	LI	5 g	About 5% loss in 28 days at 2 to 8 °C. No visible precipitation, but possible microprecipitation not evaluated	2733	**?**

[a]Tested in PVC containers.

Y-Site Injection Compatibility (1:1 Mixture)

Pemetrexed disodium

Drug	Mfr	Conc	Mfr	Conc	Remarks	Ref	C/I
Acyclovir sodium	APP	7 mg/mL[a]	LI	20 mg/mL[b]	Physically compatible for 4 hr at 23 °C	2564	**C**
Amifostine	MDI	10 mg/mL[b]	LI	20 mg/mL[b]	Physically compatible for 4 hr at 23 °C	2564	**C**
Amikacin sulfate	APC	5 mg/mL[a]	LI	20 mg/mL[b]	Physically compatible for 4 hr at 23 °C	2564	**C**
Aminophylline	AB	2.5 mg/mL[a]	LI	20 mg/mL[b]	Physically compatible for 4 hr at 23 °C	2564	**C**
Amphotericin B	PHT	0.6 mg/mL[a]	LI	20 mg/mL[b]	Yellow precipitate forms immediately	2564	**I**
Ampicillin sodium	APC	20 mg/mL[b]	LI	20 mg/mL[b]	Physically compatible for 4 hr at 23 °C	2564	**C**
Ampicillin sodium–sulbactam sodium	LE	20 + 10 mg/mL[b]	LI	20 mg/mL[b]	Physically compatible for 4 hr at 23 °C	2564	**C**
Aztreonam	BMS	40 mg/mL[a]	LI	20 mg/mL[b]	Physically compatible for 4 hr at 23 °C	2564	**C**
Bumetanide	BA	0.04 mg/mL[a]	LI	20 mg/mL[b]	Physically compatible for 4 hr at 23 °C	2564	**C**
Buprenorphine HCl	RKB	0.04 mg/mL[a]	LI	20 mg/mL[b]	Physically compatible for 4 hr at 23 °C	2564	**C**
Butorphanol tartrate	BMS	0.04 mg/mL[a]	LI	20 mg/mL[b]	Physically compatible for 4 hr at 23 °C	2564	**C**
Calcium gluconate	APP	40 mg/mL[a]	LI	20 mg/mL[b]	White microparticulates form within 4 hr	2564	**I**
Carboplatin	BMS	5 mg/mL[a]	LI	20 mg/mL[b]	Physically compatible for 4 hr at 23 °C	2564	**C**
Cefazolin sodium	GVA	20 mg/mL[a]	LI	20 mg/mL[b]	Slight color darkening occurs over 4 hr	2564	**I**
Cefotaxime sodium	APP	20 mg/mL[a]	LI	20 mg/mL[b]	Slight color darkening occurs over 4 hr	2564	**I**

Y-Site Injection Compatibility (1:1 Mixture) (Cont.)

Pemetrexed disodium

Drug	Mfr	Conc	Mfr	Conc	Remarks	Ref	C/I
Cefotetan disodium	ASZ	20 mg/mL[a]	LI	20 mg/mL[b]	Color darkening and brownish discoloration occur immediately	2564	I
Cefoxitin sodium	APP	20 mg/mL[a]	LI	20 mg/mL[b]	Immediate brown discoloration	2564	I
Ceftazidime	GW	40 mg/mL[a]	LI	20 mg/mL[b]	Color darkening and brownish discoloration occur over 4 hr	2564	I
Ceftriaxone sodium	RC	20 mg/mL[a]	LI	20 mg/mL[b]	Physically compatible for 4 hr at 23 °C	2564	C
Cefuroxime sodium	GSK	30 mg/mL[a]	LI	20 mg/mL[b]	Physically compatible for 4 hr at 23 °C	2564	C
Chlorpromazine HCl	ES	2 mg/mL[a]	LI	20 mg/mL[b]	Cloudy precipitate forms immediately	2564	I
Ciprofloxacin	BAY	2 mg/mL[a]	LI	20 mg/mL[b]	Slight color darkening occurs over 4 hr	2564	I
Cisplatin	BMS	0.5 mg/mL[b]	LI	20 mg/mL[b]	Physically compatible for 4 hr at 23 °C	2564	C
Clindamycin phosphate	PHU	10 mg/mL[a]	LI	20 mg/mL[b]	Physically compatible for 4 hr at 23 °C	2564	C
Cyclophosphamide	MJ	10 mg/mL[a]	LI	20 mg/mL[b]	Physically compatible for 4 hr at 23 °C	2564	C
Cytarabine	PHU	50 mg/mL	LI	20 mg/mL[b]	Physically compatible for 4 hr at 23 °C	2564	C
Dexamethasone sodium phosphate	AMR	1 mg/mL[a]	LI	20 mg/mL[b]	Physically compatible for 4 hr at 23 °C	2564	C
Dexrazoxane	PHU	5 mg/mL[a]	LI	20 mg/mL[b]	Physically compatible for 4 hr at 23 °C	2564	C
Diphenhydramine HCl	ES	2 mg/mL[a]	LI	20 mg/mL[b]	Physically compatible for 4 hr at 23 °C	2564	C
Dobutamine HCl	AB	4 mg/mL[a]	LI	20 mg/mL[b]	White cloudy precipitate with microparticulates forms immediately	2564	I
Docetaxel	AVE	0.8 mg/mL[a]	LI	20 mg/mL[b]	Physically compatible for 4 hr at 23 °C	2564	C
Dopamine HCl	AB	3.2 mg/mL[a]	LI	20 mg/mL[b]	Physically compatible for 4 hr at 23 °C	2564	C
Doxorubicin HCl	BED	1 mg/mL[a]	LI	20 mg/mL[b]	Dark-red discoloration forms immediately	2564	I
Doxycycline hyclate	APP	1 mg/mL[a]	LI	20 mg/mL[b]	Cloudy precipitate forms immediately	2564	I
Droperidol	AB	2.5 mg/mL	LI	20 mg/mL[b]	Gross white precipitate forms immediately	2564	I
Enalaprilat	BED	0.1 mg/mL[a]	LI	20 mg/mL[b]	Physically compatible for 4 hr at 23 °C	2564	C
Famotidine	ESL	2 mg/mL[a]	LI	20 mg/mL[b]	Physically compatible for 4 hr at 23 °C	2564	C
Fluconazole	PF	2 mg/mL	LI	20 mg/mL[b]	Physically compatible for 4 hr at 23 °C	2564	C
Fluorouracil	APP	16 mg/mL[a]	LI	20 mg/mL[b]	Physically compatible for 4 hr at 23 °C	2564	C
Ganciclovir sodium	RC	20 mg/mL[a]	LI	20 mg/mL[b]	Physically compatible for 4 hr at 23 °C	2564	C
Gemcitabine HCl	LI	10 mg/mL[a]	LI	20 mg/mL[b]	Cloudy precipitate forms immediately	2564	I
Gentamicin sulfate	AB	5 mg/mL[a]	LI	20 mg/mL[b]	Gross white precipitate forms immediately	2564	I
Granisetron HCl	RC	0.05 mg/mL[a]	LI	20 mg/mL[b]	Physically compatible for 4 hr at 23 °C	2564	C
Haloperidol lactate	APP	0.2 mg/mL[a]	LI	20 mg/mL[b]	Physically compatible for 4 hr at 23 °C	2564	C
Heparin sodium	AB	100 units/mL	LI	20 mg/mL[b]	Physically compatible for 4 hr at 23 °C	2564	C
Hydromorphone HCl	ES	0.5 mg/mL[a]	LI	20 mg/mL[b]	Physically compatible for 4 hr at 23 °C	2564	C
Hydroxyzine HCl	APP	2 mg/mL[a]	LI	20 mg/mL[b]	Physically compatible for 4 hr at 23 °C	2564	C
Ifosfamide	MJ	20 mg/mL[a]	LI	20 mg/mL[b]	Physically compatible for 4 hr at 23 °C	2564	C
Irinotecan HCl	PHU	1 mg/mL[a]	LI	20 mg/mL[b]	Color darkening occurs over 4 hr	2564	I
Leucovorin calcium	SIC	2 mg/mL[a]	LI	20 mg/mL[b]	Physically compatible for 4 hr at 23 °C	2564	C
Lorazepam	ES	0.5 mg/mL[a]	LI	20 mg/mL[b]	Physically compatible for 4 hr at 23 °C	2564	C

Y-Site Injection Compatibility (1:1 Mixture) (Cont.)

Pemetrexed disodium

Drug	Mfr	Conc	Mfr	Conc	Remarks	Ref	C/I
Mannitol	BA	15%	LI	20 mg/mL[b]	Physically compatible for 4 hr at 23 °C	2564	C
Meperidine HCl	AB	10 mg/mL[a]	LI	20 mg/mL[b]	Physically compatible for 4 hr at 23 °C	2564	C
Mesna	APP	10 mg/mL[a]	LI	20 mg/mL[b]	Physically compatible for 4 hr at 23 °C	2564	C
Methylprednisolone sodium succinate	PHU	5 mg/mL[a]	LI	20 mg/mL[b]	Physically compatible for 4 hr at 23 °C	2564	C
Metoclopramide HCl	RB	5 mg/mL	LI	20 mg/mL[b]	Physically compatible for 4 hr at 23 °C	2564	C
Metronidazole	BA	5 mg/mL	LI	20 mg/mL[b]	Color darkening and brownish discoloration occur immediately	2564	I
Mitoxantrone HCl	IMM	0.5 mg/mL[a]	LI	20 mg/mL[b]	Dark-blue precipitate forms immediately	2564	I
Morphine sulfate	ES	15 mg/mL	LI	20 mg/mL[b]	Physically compatible for 4 hr at 23 °C	2564	C
Nalbuphine HCl	EN	10 mg/mL	LI	20 mg/mL[b]	White precipitate forms immediately	2564	I
Ondansetron HCl	GSK	1 mg/mL[a]	LI	20 mg/mL[b]	Trace haze and microparticulates form immediately. White cloudy precipitate forms in 4 hr	2564	I
Paclitaxel	MJ	0.6 mg/mL[a]	LI	20 mg/mL[b]	Physically compatible for 4 hr at 23 °C	2564	C
Potassium chloride	APP	0.1 mEq/mL[a]	LI	20 mg/mL[b]	Physically compatible for 4 hr at 23 °C	2564	C
Prochlorperazine edisylate	SKB	0.5 mg/mL[a]	LI	20 mg/mL[b]	Cloudy precipitate forms immediately	2564	I
Promethazine HCl	SIC	0.5 mg/mL[a]	LI	20 mg/mL[b]	Physically compatible for 4 hr at 23 °C	2564	C
Ranitidine HCl	GSK	2 mg/mL[a]	LI	20 mg/mL[b]	Physically compatible for 4 hr at 23 °C	2564	C
Sodium bicarbonate	AB	1 mEq/mL	LI	20 mg/mL[b]	Physically compatible for 4 hr at 23 °C	2564	C
Ticarcillin disodium–clavulanate potassium	GSK	31 mg/mL[a]	LI	20 mg/mL[b]	Physically compatible for 4 hr at 23 °C	2564	C
Tobramycin sulfate	AB	5 mg/mL[a]	LI	20 mg/mL[b]	White precipitate forms immediately	2564	I
Topotecan HCl	GSK	0.1 mg/mL[a]	LI	20 mg/mL[b]	Color darkening occurs immediately	2564	I
Trimethoprim–sulfamethoxazole	ES	0.8 + 4 mg/mL[a]	LI	20 mg/mL[b]	Physically compatible for 4 hr at 23 °C	2564	C
Vancomycin HCl	AB	10 mg/mL[a]	LI	20 mg/mL[b]	Physically compatible for 4 hr at 23 °C	2564	C
Vinblastine sulfate	APP	0.12 mg/mL[a]	LI	20 mg/mL[b]	Physically compatible for 4 hr at 23 °C	2564	C
Vincristine sulfate	SIC	0.05 mg/mL[a]	LI	20 mg/mL[b]	Physically compatible for 4 hr at 23 °C	2564	C
Zidovudine	GSK	4 mg/mL[a]	LI	20 mg/mL[b]	Physically compatible for 4 hr at 23 °C	2564	C

[a]Tested in dextrose 5%.
[b]Tested in sodium chloride 0.9%.

PENICILLIN G POTASSIUM (BENZYLPENICILLIN POTASSIUM)
AHFS 8:12.16.04

Products — Penicillin G potassium is available in vial sizes of 5 million and 20 million units. (1) The commercial products contain sodium citrate and citric acid as buffers. Depending on the route of administration, reconstitute the vials with sterile water for injection, dextrose 5%, or sodium chloride 0.9%. The recommended reconstitution volumes may vary slightly among manufacturers; the amount of diluent recommended by the manufacturer should be used for reconstitution. To reconstitute the product, loosen the powder in the vials. While holding the vial horizontally, rotate it and add the diluent slowly, directing the stream against the wall of the vial. Shake the vial vigorously. When the required volume of solvent is greater than the capacity of the vial, a portion of the total volume of diluent may be added to the vial first to dissolve the drug. The resulting solution should then be withdrawn and mixed with the remainder of the needed diluent in a larger container. (1; 4)

Penicillin G potassium is also available as frozen premixed infusion solutions of 1, 2, and 3 million units in 50 mL of dextrose 4, 2.3, and 0.7%, respectively. The products also contain sodium citrate buffer; hydrochloric acid and/or sodium hydroxide may have been used to adjust the pH during manufacture. (1)

Units — Each milligram of penicillin G potassium has 1440 to 1680 USP units. Each milligram of the powder for injection (which contains sodium citrate buffer) has 1355 to 1595 USP units. (4)

pH — The reconstituted powder for injection has a pH of 6 to 8.5. (1) The frozen premixed infusion solutions have a pH of 5.5 to 8. (1; 4)

Osmolality — The frozen premixed penicillin G potassium infusion solutions are iso-osmotic with an osmolality of 300 mOsm/kg. (1)

The osmolality of penicillin G potassium (Pfizer) 250,000 units/mL in sterile water for injection was determined to be 776 mOsm/kg by freezing-point depression and 767 mOsm/kg by vapor pressure. (1071) Another report cited the osmolality of this concentration as 749 mOsm/kg. (50)

The osmolality of penicillin G potassium 50,000 units/mL was 402 mOsm/kg in dextrose 5% and 414 mOsm/kg in sodium chloride 0.9%. At 100,000 units/mL, the osmolality was 535 mOsm/kg in dextrose 5% and 554 mOsm/kg in sodium chloride 0.9%. (1375)

The osmolality of penicillin G potassium was calculated for the following dilutions (1054):

Diluent	Osmolality (mOsm/kg)	
	50 mL	100 mL
3 million units		
Dextrose 5%	411	340
Sodium chloride 0.9%	437	367
5 million units		
Dextrose 5%	501	394
Sodium chloride 0.9%	527	420

The following maximum penicillin G potassium concentrations were recommended to achieve osmolalities suitable for peripheral infusion in fluid-restricted patients (1180):

Diluent	Maximum Concentration (units/mL)	Osmolality (mOsm/kg)
Dextrose 5%	81,568	566
Sodium chloride 0.9%	73,455	545
Sterile water for injection	147,205	513

Sodium and Potassium Content — Penicillin G potassium contains, in each million units, 1.7 mEq of potassium and 0.3 mEq of sodium. (1)

Administration — NOTE: Do not confuse other forms of penicillin G with penicillin G potassium.

Penicillin G potassium is administered by intramuscular injection or continuous or intermittent intravenous infusion. It may also be administered by intrathecal, intra-articular, and intrapleural injections and other local instillations. Vials containing 20 million units are intended for intravenous administration. For intramuscular injections, concentrations of up to 100,000 units/mL will cause a minimum of discomfort. Higher concentrations may be used when needed. (1; 4)

In high doses, intravenous administration should be performed slowly to avoid electrolyte imbalance from the potassium content. For daily doses of 10 million units or more, the drug may be diluted in 1 or 2 L of infusion solution and administered in a 24-hour period. By intermittent intravenous infusion, one-fourth or one-sixth of the daily dose may be given over one to two hours and repeated every six to four hours, respectively. Divided doses are generally infused over 15 to 30 minutes in children and neonates. (4)

Stability — The drug powder is stable at room temperature. After reconstitution, the drug is stable for seven days under refrigeration. (1; 4)

However, penicillin G potassium 500,000 units/mL was stored at room temperature and 4 °C. After 24 hours at room temperature, a new compound formed, which increased by 72 hours. Storage at 4 °C substantially reduced the rate of formation. Although the activity of penicillin G potassium was retained over the time period, its potential as an antigen may change due to formation of polymers or conjugation products that may cause allergic reactions. It was recommended that the drug be freshly prepared before use or refrigerated during storage. (785)

Another study found increased formation of specific antipenicillin antibodies in patients administered aged penicillin solutions, not only at room temperature but also 4 °C. The causative antigens were degradation or transformation products of penicillin G. Freshly prepared solutions did not seem to be immunogenic. (946)

The activity of penicillin G 6 mg/L was evaluated in peritoneal dialysis fluids containing dextrose 1.5 and 4.25% (Dianeal 137, Travenol). Storage at 25 °C resulted in about a 25% loss of antimicrobial activity in 24 hours. The loss of activity was attributed to the pH (5.2) of the dialysis fluids. (515)

However, penicillin G potassium (Parke-Davis) 500,000 units/L in peritoneal dialysis concentrate (Travenol) containing dextrose 30% with and without heparin sodium 2500 units/L underwent substantial reduction in activity within as little as 10 minutes. (273)

pH Effects — The stability of penicillin G potassium 500,000 units/mL is greatest at pH 7. (160) Penicillin G activity rapidly declines at pH 5.5 and below and at pH values above 8. (47)

Penicillin G potassium is both an acid- and alkali-labile drug. It should not be mixed with drugs that may result in a final pH outside of its stability range of pH 5.5 to 8. (47) Unfortunately, the citrate buffer is of little value in the presence of strongly acidic or alkaline drugs. (48)

The times to 10% decomposition of combinations of penicillin G potassium buffered with multivitamin infusion concentrate in dextrose 5% and sodium chloride 0.9% have been calculated on the basis of the final pH of the admixture (304):

Penicillin G Potassium	Multivitamin Infusion Concentrate	pH	Time to 10% Decomposition
1 million units/L	1 mL/L	5.1	6.51 hr
1 million units/L	5 mL/L	4.9	4.56 hr
3 million units/L	1 mL/L	5.4	13.54 hr
3 million units/L	5 mL/L	5.0	6.38 hr
5 million units/L	1 mL/L	5.7	22.01 hr
5 million units/L	5 mL/L	5.1	6.51 hr
10 million units/L	1 mL/L	5.9	over 24 hr
10 million units/L	5 mL/L	5.4	13.54 hr

Freezing Solutions — Frozen premixed infusion solutions of penicillin G potassium are stable for at least 90 days from shipping stored at −20 °C. The frozen solutions should be thawed at room temperature or under refrigeration and, once thawed, should not be refrozen. Thawing should not be performed using a warm water bath or microwave radiation. Thawed solutions are stated to be stable for 24 hours at room temperature and for 14 days under refrigeration. (4)

Penicillin G potassium 1 million units/100 mL of dextrose 5% in PVC bags was frozen at −20 °C for 30 days and then thawed by exposure to ambient temperature or microwave radiation. No evidence of precipitation or color change was observed, and a 3 to 4% loss was reported. The thawed solution at room temperature was physically compatible and exhibited no further loss over 24 hours. (554)

A fivefold increase in particles of 2 to 60 μm was produced by freezing and thawing penicillin G potassium (Squibb) 2 million units/ 100 mL of dextrose 5% (Travenol). The constituted drug was filtered through a 0.45-μm filter into PVC bags of solution and frozen for seven days at −20 °C. Thawing was performed at 29 °C for 12 hours. Although the total number of particles increased significantly, no particles greater than 60 μm were observed; the solutions complied with USP standards for particle sizes and numbers in large volume parenteral solutions. (822)

Penicillin G potassium 1 million units/50 mL of sodium chloride 0.9% lost 5% in 16 days and 7% in 25 days when frozen at −7 °C. However, samples of the same solution stored at 4 °C showed similar results, indicating a lack of advantage for frozen storage. (1035)

Ambulatory Pumps — The stability of penicillin G potassium 100,000 and 200,000 units/mL in sterile water for injection was evaluated in PVC portable pump reservoirs (Pharmacia Deltec). A 6% loss occurred in three days at 25 °C. The 200,000-unit/mL concentration was also tested stored at 5 °C. A 3% loss occurred in 14 days. (2080)

Elastomeric Reservoir Pumps — Penicillin G potassium (Pfizer) 40,000 units/mL in both dextrose 5% and sodium chloride 0.9% was evaluated for binding potential to natural rubber elastomeric reservoirs (Baxter). No binding was found after storage for two weeks at 35 °C with gentle agitation. (2014)

Filtration — Filtering penicillin G potassium (Pfizer) through 5-μm stainless steel and 0.22-μm cellulose ester inline filters resulted in no significant reduction in activity under conditions of varying doses, temperatures, flow rates, and administration methods. (167)

Compatibility Information

Solution Compatibility

Penicillin G potassium

Solution	Mfr	Mfr	Conc/L	Remarks	Ref	C/I
Amino acids 4.25%, dextrose 25%	MG	LI	1 MU[b]	No increase in particulate matter in 24 hr at 5 °C	349	C
Dextrose–Ringer's injection combinations	AB		1 MU[b]	Physically compatible	3	C
Dextrose–Ringer's injection, lactated, combinations	AB		1 MU[b]	Physically compatible	3	C
Dextrose 5% in Ringer's injection, lactated	TR[c]	SQ	10 MU[b]	Stable for 24 hr at 5 °C	282	C
Dextrose–saline combinations	AB		1 MU[b]	Physically compatible	3	C
Dextrose 5% in sodium chloride 0.9%	MG	SQ	5 MU[b]	Stable for 24 hr at 4 and 25 °C	105	C
		SQ	2 MU[b]	Stable for 24 hr	109	C
	AB, BA, CU	[a]	5 MU[b]	Stable for 48 hr at 25 °C	164	C
			1 MU[b]	Physically compatible	74	C
	TR[c]	SQ	10 MU[b]	Stable for 24 hr at 5 °C	282	C
Dextrose 2.5%	AB		1 MU[b]	Physically compatible	3	C
Dextrose 5%	AB		1 MU[b]	Physically compatible	3	C
			10 MU[b]	No decomposition in 12 hr	165	C
			100 MU[b]	7.5% decomposition in 48 hr at 25 °C and none at 5 °C	141	C
	MG	SQ	5 MU[b]	Stable for 24 hr at 4 and 25 °C	105	C
		SQ	2 MU[b]	Stable for 24 hr	109	C
		[a]	900,000 units	Stable for 24 hr at 25 °C	48	C
			1 MU[b]	Physically compatible	74	C
	TR[c]	SQ	10 MU[b]	Stable for 24 hr at 5 °C	282	C
	BA[c], TR	AY	40 MU[b]	Stable for 24 hr at 5 and 22 °C	298	C
	TR[d]	SQ	10 MU[b]	Physically compatible. 5% loss in 24 hr at room temperature	554	C

Solution Compatibility (Cont.)

Penicillin G potassium

Solution	Mfr	Mfr	Conc/L	Remarks	Ref	C/I
Dextrose 10%	AB		1 MU[b]	Physically compatible	3	C
	MG	SQ	5 MU[b]	Stable for 24 hr at 4 and 25 °C	105	C
		SQ	2 MU[b]	Stable for 24 hr	109	C
Isolyte M in dextrose 5%	MG	SQ	5 MU[b]	Stable for 24 hr at 4 and 25 °C	105	C
Isolyte P in dextrose 5%	MG	SQ	5 MU[b]	Stable for 24 hr at 4 and 25 °C	105	C
Ionosol products	AB		1 MU[b]	Physically compatible	3	C
Ringer's injection	AB		1 MU[b]	Physically compatible	3	C
Ringer's injection, lactated	AB		1 MU[b]	Physically compatible	3	C
	MG	SQ	5 MU[b]	Stable for 24 hr at 4 and 25 °C	105	C
			1 MU[b]	Physically compatible	74	C
	TR[c]	SQ	10 MU[b]	Stable for 24 hr at 5 °C	282	C
Sodium chloride 0.45%	AB		1 MU[b]	Physically compatible	3	C
Sodium chloride 0.9%	AB		1 MU[b]	Physically compatible	3	C
			100 MU[b]	Stable for 48 hr at 5 °C	141	C
	MG	SQ	5 MU[b]	Stable for 24 hr at 4 and 25 °C	105	C
		SQ	2 MU[b]	Stable for 24 hr	109	C
	AB, BA, CU	[a]	5 MU[b]	Stable for 48 hr at 25 °C	164	C
			1 MU[b]	Physically compatible	74	C
	TR[c]	SQ	10 MU[b]	Stable for 24 hr at 5 °C	282	C
	BA[c], TR	AY	40 MU[b]	Stable for 24 hr at 5 and 22 °C	298	C
	TR[d]	PD	20 MU[b]	5% loss at 24 °C and no loss at 4 °C in 4 days	1035	C
TPN #21[e]		SQ	5 MU[b]	Activity retained for 24 hr at 4 and 25 °C	87	C
TPN #22[e]		AY	25 MU[b]	Physically compatible with no loss of activity in 24 hr at 22 °C in dark	837	C
TPN #107[e]			2 g	Activity retained for 24 hr at 21 °C	1326	C

[a] Indicate a buffered preparation.
[b] Million units.
[c] Tested in both glass and PVC containers.
[d] Tested in PVC containers.
[e] Refer to Appendix I for the composition of parenteral nutrition solutions. TPN indicates a 2-in-1 admixture.

Additive Compatibility

Penicillin G potassium

Drug	Mfr	Conc/L	Mfr	Conc/L	Test Soln	Remarks	Ref	C/I
Amikacin sulfate	BR	5 g	LI	20 million units	D5LR, D5R, D5S, D5W, D10W, LR, NS, R, SL	Physically compatible and both stable for 24 hr at 25 °C	293	C
Aminophylline	SE	500 mg	[a]	900,000 units	D5W	22% penicillin loss in 6 hr at 25 °C	48	I
	SE	500 mg	SQ	1 million units	D5W	44% penicillin loss in 24 hr at 25 °C	47	I

Additive Compatibility (Cont.)

Penicillin G potassium

Drug	Mfr	Conc/L	Mfr	Conc/L	Test Soln	Remarks	Ref	C/I
Amphotericin B		200 mg	BP	10 million units	D5W	Haze develops over 3 hr	26	I
	SQ	50 mg	SQ	5 million units		Precipitate forms within 1 hr	47	I
	SQ	100 mg	SQ	20 million units	D5W	Physically incompatible	15	I
Ascorbic acid	AB	1 g		1 million units		Physically compatible	3	C
	PD	500 mg	SQ	10 million units	D5W	1% penicillin loss in 8 hr	166	C
Calcium chloride	UP	1 g	SQ	20 million units	D5W	Physically compatible	15	C
Calcium gluconate	UP	1 g	SQ	20 million units	D5W	Physically compatible	15	C
		1 g		1 million units	D5W	Physically compatible	74	C
Chloramphenicol sodium succinate	PD	10 g	SQ	20 million units	D5W	Physically compatible	15	C
	PD	1 g	SQ	5 million units		Physically compatible	47	C
	PD	500 mg	SQ	1 million units	D5S, D5W	Therapeutic availability maintained	110	C
	PD	1 g	SQ	5 and 10 million units	D5S, D5W	Therapeutic availability maintained	110	C
	PD	1 g		1 million units		Physically compatible	3	C
	PD	1 g	SQ	10 million units		Physically compatible	6	C
Chlorpromazine HCl	BP	200 mg	BP	10 million units	NS	Haze develops over 3 hr	26	I
Colistimethate sodium	WC	500 mg	SQ	20 million units	D5W	Physically compatible	15	C
	WC	500 mg	SQ	5 million units	D	Physically compatible	47	C
Dextran 40		10%		6 million units	D5W	34% loss in 24 hr at 20 °C	834	I
Dimenhydrinate	SE	50 mg		1 million units	D5W	Physically compatible	74	C
Diphenhydramine HCl	PD	80 mg	SQ	20 million units	D5W	Physically compatible	15	C

Additive Compatibility (Cont.)

Penicillin G potassium

Drug	Mfr	Conc/L	Mfr	Conc/L	Test Soln	Remarks	Ref	C/I
	PD	50 mg	SQ	1 million units	D5W	Physically compatible. Penicillin stable for 24 hr at 25 °C	47	C
Dopamine HCl	AS	800 mg	LI	20 million units	D5W	14% penicillin loss in 24 hr at 25 °C. Dopamine stable for 24 hr	78	I
Ephedrine sulfate		50 mg		1 million units		Physically compatible	3	C
	AB	50 mg	SQ	5 million units		Physically compatible	47	C
Erythromycin lactobionate	AB	5 g	SQ	20 million units	D5W	Physically compatible	15	C
	AB	1 g	SQ	5 million units		Physically compatible	20; 47	C
	AB	1 g		1 million units		Physically compatible	3	C
Heparin sodium		12,000 units		1 million units	D5W	Physically compatible	74	C
	AB	20,000 units	SQ	1 million units	D5W	Penicillin stable for 24 hr at 25 °C	47	C
	UP	4000 units	SQ	20 million units	D5W	Physically incompatible	15	I
Hydrocortisone sodium succinate	UP	500 mg	SQ	20 million units	D5W	Physically compatible	15	C
	UP	250 mg	SQ	5 million units	D	Physically compatible	47	C
	UP	100 mg		1 million units	D5W	Physically compatible	74	C
Hydroxyzine HCl	RR	250 mg	SQ	20 million units	D5W	Physically incompatible	15	I
Lidocaine HCl	AST	2 g	SQ	1 million units		Physically compatible	24	C
Lincomycin HCl	UP	6 g	SQ	20 million units	D5W	Physically compatible	15	C
	UP	600 mg	SQ	5 million units	D	Physically compatible	47	C
Magnesium sulfate		1 g	PF	500 mg	W	5% penicillin loss in 1 day and 13% in 2 days at 24 °C	999	C
		2 to 8 g	PF	500 mg	W	7 to 8% penicillin loss in 1 day and 20 to 25% in 2 days at 24 °C	999	C
Methylprednisolone sodium succinate	UP	80 mg		2 to 10 million units	D5S, D5W, LR	Clear solution for 24 hr	329	C
Metronidazole	SE	5 g	PF	200 million units		5% penicillin loss in 22 hr and 8% in 72 hr at 25 °C. 2% penicillin loss in 12 days at 5 °C. No metronidazole loss	993	C

Additive Compatibility (Cont.)

Penicillin G potassium

Drug	Mfr	Conc/L	Mfr	Conc/L	Test Soln	Remarks	Ref	C/I
Pentobarbital sodium	AB	500 mg	a	900,000 units	D5W	17% penicillin loss in 6 hr at 25 °C	48	I
	AB	500 mg	SQ	1 million units	D5W	42% penicillin loss in 24 hr at 25 °C	47	I
Polymyxin B sulfate	BW	200 mg	SQ	20 million units	D5W	Physically compatible	15	C
	BW	200 mg	SQ	5 million units	D	Physically compatible	47	C
Potassium chloride		20 mEq	SQ	1 million units	D5S, D5W	Therapeutic availability maintained	110	C
		40 mEq	SQ	5 million units	D5S, D5W	Therapeutic availability maintained	110	C
	AB	40 mEq	SQ	5 million units		Physically compatible	47	C
Prochlorperazine edisylate	SKF	10 mg	SQ	5 million units	D5W	Physically compatible. Penicillin stable for 24 hr at 25 °C	47	C
	SKF	10 mg	a	900,000 units	D5W	Penicillin stable for 24 hr at 25 °C	48	C
Prochlorperazine mesylate	BP	100 mg	BP	10 million units	NS	Haze develops over 3 hr	26	I
Promethazine HCl	WY	100 mg	SQ	5 million units		Physically compatible	47	C
	WY	100 mg		1 million units		Physically compatible	3	C
	WY	250 mg	SQ	20 million units	D5W	Physically incompatible	15	I
Ranitidine HCl	GL	50 mg and 2 g		24 million units	D5W, NS	Physically compatible. Ranitidine stable for 24 hr at 25 °C. Penicillin not tested	1515	C
Sodium bicarbonate		0.5 and 0.75 g	SQ	1 million units	D5W	Penicillin loss at 20 °C due to pH	135	I
		3.75 g	a	900,000 units	D5W	26% penicillin loss in 24 hr at 25 °C	48	I
	AB	3.75 g	SQ	1 million units	D5W	26% penicillin loss in 24 hr at 25 °C	47	I
	AB	2.4 mEq[b]	SQ	100 million units	D5W	Physically compatible for 24 hr	772	C
Verapamil HCl	KN	80 mg	SQ	10 million units	D5W, NS	Physically compatible for 24 hr	764	C
	SE	c	PD	62.5 g	D5W, NS	Physically compatible for 24 hr at 21 °C under fluorescent light	1166	C

[a]*Indicate a buffered preparation.*
[b]*One vial of Neut added to a liter of admixture.*
[c]*Final concentration unspecified.*

Drugs in Syringe Compatibility

Penicillin G potassium

Drug (in syringe)	Mfr	Amt	Mfr	Amt	Remarks	Ref	C/I
Metoclopramide HCl	RB	10 mg/ 2 mL	SQ	250,000 units/ 1 mL	Incompatible. If mixed, use immediately	924; 1167	**I**
	RB	10 mg/ 2 mL	SQ	1 million units/ 4 mL	Incompatible. If mixed, use immediately	924; 1167	**I**

Y-Site Injection Compatibility (1:1 Mixture)

Penicillin G potassium

Drug	Mfr	Conc	Mfr	Conc	Remarks	Ref	C/I
Acyclovir sodium	BW	5 mg/mL[a]	PF	40,000 units/ mL[a]	Physically compatible for 4 hr at 25 °C	1157	C
Amiodarone HCl	LZ	4 mg/mL[c]	PF	100,000 units/mL[c]	Physically compatible for 4 hr at room temperature	1444	C
Cyclophosphamide	MJ	20 mg/mL[a]	PF	100,000 units/mL[a]	Physically compatible for 4 hr at 25 °C	1194	C
Diltiazem HCl	MMD	1[b] and 5 mg/ mL	RR	1 million units/mL	Visually compatible	1807	C
	MMD	5 mg/mL	RR	100,000 units/mL[b]	Visually compatible	1807	C
Enalaprilat	MSD	0.05 mg/mL[b]	PF	50,000 units/ mL[a]	Physically compatible for 24 hr at room temperature under fluorescent light	1355	C
Esmolol HCl	DCC	10 mg/mL[a]	PF	50,000 units/ mL[a]	Physically compatible for 24 hr at 22 °C	1169	C
Fluconazole	RR	2 mg/mL	RR	100,000 units/mL	Physically compatible for 24 hr at 25 °C	1407	C
Foscarnet sodium	AST	24 mg/mL	SQ	100,000 units/mL	Physically compatible for 24 hr at room temperature under fluorescent light	1335	C
Heparin sodium	TR	50 units/mL	RR	40,000 units/ mL[b]	Visually compatible for 4 hr at 25 °C	1793	C
Heparin sodium[j]	RI	1000 units/L[d]	LI	200,000 units/mL	Physically compatible for 4 hr at room temperature	322	C
Hydrocortisone sodium succinate[k]	UP	100 mg/L[d]	LI	200,000 units/mL	Physically compatible for 4 hr at room temperature	322	C
Hydromorphone HCl	WY	0.2 mg/mL[a]	PF	100,000 units/mL[a]	Physically compatible for 4 hr at 25 °C	987	C
Labetalol HCl	SC	1 mg/mL[a]	PF	50,000 units/ mL[a]	Physically compatible for 24 hr at 18 °C	1171	C
Magnesium sulfate	IX	16.7, 33.3, 66.7, 100 mg/ mL[a]	SQ	100,000 units/mL[a]	Physically compatible for at least 4 hr at 32 °C	813	C
Meperidine HCl	WY	10 mg/mL[a]	PF	100,000 units/mL[a]	Physically compatible for 4 hr at 25 °C	987	C
Morphine sulfate	WI	1 mg/mL[a]	PF	100,000 units/mL[a]	Physically compatible for 4 hr at 25 °C	987	C

Y-Site Injection Compatibility (1:1 Mixture) (Cont.)

Penicillin G potassium

Drug	Mfr	Conc	Mfr	Conc	Remarks	Ref	C/I
Nicardipine HCl	DCC	0.1 mg/mL[a]	PF	50,000 units/mL[a]	Visually compatible for 24 hr at room temperature	235	C
Potassium chloride		40 mEq/L[d]	LI	200,000 units/mL	Physically compatible for 4 hr at room temperature	322	C
Tacrolimus	FUJ	1 mg/mL[b]	BR	100,000 units/mL[a]	Visually compatible for 24 hr at 25 °C	1630	C
Theophylline	TR	4 mg/mL	RR	40,000 units/mL[b]	Visually compatible for 6 hr at 25 °C	1793	C
TNA #73[e]		32.5 mL[f]	SQ	40,000 units/mL[a]	Visually compatible for 4 hr at 25 °C	1008	C
TPN #54[e]				320,000 and 500,000 units/mL	Physically compatible and 88% penicillin activity retained over 6 hr at 22 °C	1045	C
TPN #61[e]		[g]	PF	200,000 units/2 mL[h]	Physically compatible	1012	C
		[i]	PF	1.2 million units/1.2 mL[h]	Physically compatible	1012	C
TPN #189[e]				300 mg/mL[b]	Visually compatible for 24 hr at 22 °C	1767	C
TPN #203, #204[e]			MAR	500,000 units/mL	Visually compatible for 2 hr at 23 °C	1974	C
Verapamil HCl	SE	2.5 mg/mL	PD	62.5 mg/mL[c]	Physically compatible for 15 min at 21 °C	1166	C

[a]*Tested in dextrose 5%.*
[b]*Tested in sodium chloride 0.9%.*
[c]*Tested in both dextrose 5% and sodium chloride 0.9%.*
[d]*Tested in dextrose 5%, Ringer's injection, lactated, and sodium chloride 0.9%.*
[e]*Refer to Appendix I for the composition of parenteral nutrition solutions. TNA indicates a 3-in-1 admixture, and TPN indicates a 2-in-1 admixture.*
[f]*A 32.5-mL sample of parenteral nutrition solution mixed with 50 mL of antibiotic solution.*
[g]*Run at 21 mL/hr.*
[h]*Given over five minutes by syringe pump.*
[i]*Run at 94 mL/hr.*
[j]*Tested in combination with hydrocortisone sodium succinate (Upjohn) 100 mg/L.*
[k]*Tested in combination with heparin sodium (Riker) 1000 units/L.*

PENICILLIN G SODIUM
(BENZYLPENICILLIN SODIUM)
AHFS 8:12.16.04

Products — Penicillin G sodium is available in vials containing 5 million units of drug with sodium citrate and citric acid as buffers. Depending on the route of administration, reconstitute the vials with sterile water for injection, dextrose 5%, or sodium chloride 0.9%; reconstitution of the 5 million-unit vial with 3 or 8 mL of diluent results in a final concentration of 1 million or 500,000 units/mL, respectively. Loosen the powder in the vial while holding the vial horizontally, rotate it and add the diluent slowly, directing the stream against the wall of the vial. Shake the vial vigorously. (1; 4)

Units — Each milligram of penicillin G sodium has 1500 to 1750 USP units. Each milligram of the powder for injection (which contains sodium citrate buffer) has 1420 to 1667 USP units. (4)

pH — From 5 to 7.5. (1)

Osmolality — Penicillin G sodium 250,000 units/mL in sterile water for injection has an osmolality of 795 mOsm/kg. (50)

The osmolality of penicillin G sodium was calculated for the following dilutions (1054):

Diluent	Osmolality (mOsm/kg)	
	50 mL	100 mL
3 million units		
Dextrose 5%	413	341
Sodium chloride 0.9%	439	368
5 million units		
Dextrose 5%	502	394
Sodium chloride 0.9%	529	421

The following maximum penicillin G sodium concentrations were recommended to achieve osmolalities suitable for peripheral infusion in fluid-restricted patients (1180):

Diluent	Maximum Concentration (units/mL)	Osmolality (mOsm/kg)
Dextrose 5%	85,383	573
Sodium chloride 0.9%	76,891	563
Sterile water for injection	154,091	545

Sodium Content — Penicillin G sodium contains 1.68 mEq of sodium per million units. (1)

Administration — NOTE: Do not confuse other forms of penicillin G with penicillin G sodium.

Penicillin G sodium is administered by intramuscular injection or by continuous or intermittent intravenous infusion. For intramuscular injections, concentrations of up to 100,000 units/mL will cause a minimum of discomfort. Higher concentrations may be used when needed. In high doses, intravenous administration should be performed slowly to avoid electrolyte imbalance from the sodium content. For daily doses of 10 million units or more, the drug may be diluted in 1 or 2 L of infusion solution and administered in a 24-hour period. By intermittent intravenous infusion, one-fourth or one-sixth of the daily dose may be given over one to two hours and repeated every six to four hours, respectively. Divided doses are generally infused over 15 to 30 minutes in children and neonates. (4)

Stability — The dry powder may be stored at controlled room temperature. After reconstitution, solutions may be stored for three days (1) to seven days (4) under refrigeration. Intravenous infusions containing this drug are stable at room temperature for at least 24 hours. (4)

The activity of penicillin G 6 mg/L was evaluated in peritoneal dialysis fluids containing dextrose 1.5 and 4.25% (Dianeal 137, Travenol). Storage at 25 °C resulted in about a 25% loss of antimicrobial activity in 24 hours. The loss of activity was attributed to the pH (5.2) of the dialysis fluids. (515)

pH Effects — At 25 °C, the maximum stability of penicillin G sodium is attained at pH 6.8 (131), but little difference in the rate of decomposition occurs in the pH range of 6.5 to 7.5. (1947) Not more than 10% loss occurs in 24 hours in a pH range of 5.4 to 8.5. (131) Unbuffered penicillin G sodium injection 12 and 48 mg/mL in sodium chloride 0.9% had an initial pH between 5.4 and 5.8. A 7% loss occurred in two days in samples stored at 5 °C. However, reconstituting with citrate buffers having pH values of 6.5, 7.0, and 7.5 resulted in great stability improvement. At these same concentrations in sodium chloride 0.9% in minibags stored at 5 °C, losses of 5 to 7% occurred in 28 days and 10% in 56 days. (1671)

Freezing Solutions — It has been shown that penicillin G sodium in concentrations of 1 to 10%, buffered to pH 6.85, loses not more than 1% in one month when frozen at −20 °C. (99) Another report stated that solutions of penicillin G sodium at a concentration of 50,000 units/mL in water, sodium chloride 0.9%, and 0.05 M citrate buffer and also at a concentration of 500,000 units/mL with sodium citrate 15 mg are stable for at least 12 weeks when frozen at −25 °C. At −5 °C in the citrate buffer, the rate of decomposition is considerably higher than at either −25 or 5 °C. (156)

Penicillin G sodium 2.5 million units/50 mL of dextrose 5% in PVC containers was physically compatible and stable for 39 days frozen at −20 °C. Subsequent thawing and storage at 4 °C resulted in a 3 to 4% loss in 10 to 15 days and up to a 10% loss in 31 days. (1125)

Little penicillin G sodium loss occurred in a solution containing 180,000 units/mL in sterile water for injection in PVC and glass containers after 30 days at −20 °C. Subsequent thawing and storage for four days at 5 °C, followed by 24 hours at 37 °C to simulate the use of a portable infusion pump, resulted in about a 12 to 16% penicillin loss. (1391)

Ambulatory Pumps — The stability of penicillin G sodium 100,000 and 200,000 units/mL in sterile water for injection was evaluated in PVC portable pump reservoirs (Pharmacia Deltec). A 4 to 6% loss occurred in three days at 25 °C. (2080)

Compatibility Information

Solution Compatibility

Penicillin G sodium

Solution	Mfr	Mfr	Conc/L	Remarks	Ref	C/I
Dextrose 5%		KA	6 MU[a]	Stable for 24 hr at 25 °C	131	**C**
		BE	20 MU[a]	25% loss in 24 hr at 25 °C	113	**I**
			4 MU[a,b]	7% loss in 6 hr and 29% in 24 hr at room temperature	768	**I**
	TR[c]	AY	50 MU[a]	No loss in 39 days at −20 °C. Then up to 10% loss in 31 days at 5 °C	1125	**C**

Solution Compatibility (Cont.)

Penicillin G sodium

Solution	Mfr	Mfr	Conc/L	Remarks	Ref	C/I
Sodium chloride 0.9%		KA	20 MU[a]	Stable for 24 hr at 25 °C	131	C
			4 MU[a,b]	10% loss in 8 hr and 16% in 24 hr at room temperature	768	I
	TR[c]	GL	20 and 80 MU[a]	In unbuffered solution. 7 to 8% loss in 48 hr and 18% in 96 hr at 5 °C	1671	C
	TR[c]	GL	20 MU[a]	Reconstituted with citrate buffer (pH 6.5 to 7.5). 5% loss in 28 days and 10% in 56 days at 5 °C	1671	C
	BA[e]	CSL	133 MU[a]	Losses of 10% in 13 hr at 22 °C and 5 hr at 36 °C. More than 10% loss in 7 days at 4 °C	2547	I
TPN #107[d]			2 g	Activity retained for 24 hr at 21 °C	1326	C

[a]Million units.
[b]An unbuffered preparation was specified.
[c]Tested in PVC containers.
[d]Refer to Appendix I for the composition of parenteral nutrition solutions. TPN indicates a 2-in-1 admixture.
[e]Tested in IntraVia polypropylene containers.

Additive Compatibility

Penicillin G sodium

Drug	Mfr	Conc/L	Mfr	Conc/L	Test Soln	Remarks	Ref	C/I
Amphotericin B	SQ	100 mg	UP	20 million units	D5W	Physically incompatible	15	I
		200 mg	BP	10 million units	D5W	Haze develops over 3 hr	26	I
Bleomycin sulfate	BR	20 and 30 units	SQ	2 million units	NS	77% loss of bleomycin activity in 1 week at 4 °C	763	I
	BR	20 and 30 units	SQ	5 million units	NS	41% loss of bleomycin activity in 1 week at 4 °C	763	I
Calcium chloride	UP	1 g	UP	20 million units	D5W	Physically compatible	15	C
Calcium gluconate	UP	1 g	UP	20 million units	D5W	Physically compatible	15	C
Chloramphenicol sodium succinate	PD	10 g	UP	20 million units	D5W	Physically compatible	15	C
Chlorpromazine HCl	BP	200 mg	BP	10 million units	NS	Haze develops over 3 hr	26	I
Colistimethate sodium	WC	500 mg	UP	20 million units	D5W	Physically compatible	15	C
Cytarabine	UP	200 mg		2 million units	D5W	pH outside stability range for penicillin G	174	I
Dextran 40	PH	10%	KA	6 million units		Stable for 24 hr at 25 °C	131	C

Additive Compatibility (Cont.)

Penicillin G sodium

Drug	Mfr	Conc/L	Mfr	Conc/L	Test Soln	Remarks	Ref	C/I
Diphenhydramine HCl	PD	80 mg	UP	20 million units	D5W	Physically compatible	15	C
Erythromycin lactobionate	AB	5 g	UP	20 million units	D5W	Physically compatible	15	C
Gentamicin sulfate	RS	160 mg	GL	13 and 40 million units	D5¼S, D5W, NS	Gentamicin stable for 24 hr at room temperature	157	C
Heparin sodium	OR	20,000 units	BE	20 million units	NS	Both stable for 24 hr at 25 °C	113	C
	UP	4000 units	UP	20 million units	D5W	Physically incompatible	15	I
Hydrocortisone sodium succinate	UP	500 mg	UP	20 million units	D5W	Physically compatible	15	C
Hydroxyzine HCl	RR	250 mg	UP	20 million units	D5W	Physically incompatible	15	I
Lincomycin HCl	UP	6 g	UP	20 million units	D5W	Physically compatible	15	C
Methylprednisolone sodium succinate	UP	125 mg		5 million units	D5W, LR	Precipitate forms	329	I
Polymyxin B sulfate	BW	200 mg	UP	20 million units	D5W	Physically compatible	15	C
Potassium chloride		40 mEq	KA	6 million units	D5W	Penicillin stable for 24 hr at 25 °C	131	C
		40 mEq	KA	5 million units	IS10	pH outside stability range for penicillin	131	I
Prochlorperazine mesylate	BP	100 mg	BP	10 million units	NS	Haze develops over 3 hr	26	I
Promethazine HCl	WY	250 mg	UP	20 million units	D5W	Physically incompatible	15	I
Ranitidine HCl	GL	100 mg		2.4 million units	D5W	Physically compatible for 24 hr at ambient temperature in light	1151	C
Verapamil HCl	KN	80 mg	SQ	10 million units	D5W, NS	Physically compatible for 24 hr	764	C

Drugs in Syringe Compatibility

Penicillin G sodium

Drug (in syringe)	Mfr	Amt	Mfr	Amt	Remarks	Ref	C/I
Chloramphenicol sodium succinate	PD	250 and 400 mg in 1.5 to 2 mL		1 million units	No precipitate or color change within 1 hr at room temperature	99	C
Colistimethate sodium	PX	40 mg/ 2 mL		1 million units	No precipitate or color change within 1 hr at room temperature	99	C
Dimenhydrinate		10 mg/ 1 mL		500,000 units/ 1 mL	Clear solution	2569	C
Gentamicin sulfate		80 mg/ 2 mL		1 million units	No precipitate or color change within 1 hr at room temperature	99	C
Lincomycin HCl	UP	600 mg/ 2 mL		1 million units	No precipitate or color change within 1 hr at room temperature	99	C
Pantoprazole sodium	[a]	4 mg/ 1 mL		500,000 units/ 1 mL	Clear solution	2574	C
Polymyxin B sulfate	BW	25 mg/ 1.5 to 2 mL		1 million units	No precipitate or color change within 1 hr at room temperature	99	C
Streptomycin sulfate		1 g/2 mL		1 million units	No precipitate or color change within 1 hr at room temperature	99	C

[a]Test performed using the formulation WITHOUT edetate disodium.

Y-Site Injection Compatibility (1:1 Mixture)

Penicillin G sodium

Drug	Mfr	Conc	Mfr	Conc	Remarks	Ref	C/I
Clarithromycin	AB	4 mg/mL[a]	BRT	24 mg/mL[a]	Visually compatible for 72 hr at both 30 and 17 °C	2174	C
Levofloxacin	OMN	5 mg/mL[a]	MAR	500,000 units/mL	Visually compatible for 4 hr at 24 °C	2233	C
TPN #54[e]				320,000 and 500,000 units/mL	Physically compatible and 88% penicillin activity retained over 6 hr at 22 °C	1045	C
TPN #61[e]		[b]	PF	200,000 units/2 mL[c]	Physically compatible	1012	C
		[d]	PF	1.2 million units/12 mL[c]	Physically compatible	1012	C
TPN #189[e]				300 mg/mL[f]	Visually compatible for 24 hr at 22 °C	1767	C

[a]Tested in dextrose 5%.
[b]Run at 21 mL/hr.
[c]Given over five minutes by syringe pump.
[d]Run at 94 mL/hr.
[e]Refer to Appendix I for the composition of parenteral nutrition solutions. TPN indicates a 2-in-1 admixture.
[f]Tested in sodium chloride 0.9%.

PENTAMIDINE ISETHIONATE
AHFS 8:30.92

Products — Pentamidine isethionate is available in vials containing 300 mg in lyophilized form; sodium hydroxide and/or hydrochloric acid may have been added during manufacture to adjust the pH. (1) For intramuscular injection, the contents of a vial should be reconstituted with 3 mL of sterile water for injection to yield a 100-mg/mL concentration. For intravenous administration, the contents of a vial should be reconstituted with 3, 4, or 5 mL of sterile water for injection or dextrose 5% to yield solutions containing 100, 75, or 60 mg/mL, respectively. The dose should be withdrawn and further diluted in 50 to 250 mL of dextrose 5% for administration. (1; 4)

Do not use sodium chloride 0.9% to reconstitute pentamidine isethionate because precipitation will occur. (1)

pH — Reconstituted solutions of 60 to 100 mg/mL have a pH of approximately 5.4 in sterile water for injection and of 4.09 to 4.38 in dextrose 5%. (4)

Osmolality — At 100 mg/mL in sterile water for injection and dextrose 5%, the osmolalities are 160 and 455 mOsm/kg, respectively. (4)

Equivalency — Pentamidine isethionate 1.74 mg is equivalent to pentamidine 1 mg. (4)

Trade Name(s) — Pentam 300.

Administration — Pentamidine isethionate injection may be administered by slow intravenous infusion or deep intramuscular injection using the Z-track technique. Intravenously, the calculated dose should be diluted in 50 to 250 mL of dextrose 5% and infused over 60 to 120 minutes. The drug should not be administered by rapid intravenous injection or infusion. (4)

Stability — The sterile dry powder should be stored at controlled room temperature and protected from light. (1; 4)

Reconstituted solutions containing 60 to 100 mg/mL are stable for 48 hours at room temperature protected from light. The reconstituted solution should be kept between 22 and 30 °C to avoid crystallization. (1; 4) Because no preservative is present, the manufacturer recommends discarding remaining solution. (4)

Pentamidine isethionate in concentrations ranging from about 0.8 to 97 mg/mL in dextrose 5% and about 0.9 to 93 mg/mL in sterile water for injection is reported to be stable for 30 days stored under refrigeration. (31)

Freezing Solutions — The manufacturer states that crystals may form in pentamidine isethionate solutions if stored below room temperature. (1)

Elastomeric Reservoir Pumps — Pentamidine isethionate (Fujisawa) 3 mg/mL in dextrose 5% and 2 mg/mL in sodium chloride 0.9% was evaluated for binding potential to natural rubber elastomeric reservoirs (Baxter). No binding was found after storage for two weeks at 35 °C with gentle agitation. (2014)

Compatibility Information

Solution Compatibility

Pentamidine isethionate

Solution	Mfr	Mfr	Conc/L	Remarks	Ref	C/I
Dextrose 5%	TR[a]	LY	1 g	Physically compatible with 3% loss in 48 hr at 24 °C under fluorescent light	1142	C
	TR[a]	LY	2 g	Physically compatible with 1% loss in 48 hr at 24 °C under fluorescent light	1142	C
	TR[a]	MB	2 g	Physically compatible with little or no loss in 24 hr at 20 °C	1311	C
Sodium chloride 0.9%	TR[a]	LY	1 g	Physically compatible with 2% loss in 48 hr at 24 °C under fluorescent light	1142	C
	TR[a]	LY	2 g	Physically compatible with no loss in 48 hr at 24 °C under fluorescent light	1142	C
	TR[a]	MB	2 g	Physically compatible with little or no loss in 24 hr at 20 °C	1311	C

[a]Tested in PVC containers.

Y-Site Injection Compatibility (1:1 Mixture)

Pentamidine isethionate

Drug	Mfr	Conc	Mfr	Conc	Remarks	Ref	C/I
Aldesleukin	CHI	33,800 I.U./mL[a]	FUJ	6 mg/mL[a]	Aldesleukin bioactivity inhibited	1857	I
Cefazolin sodium	SKB	20 mg/mL[a]	FUJ	3 mg/mL[a]	Cloudy precipitation forms immediately	1880	I
Cefotaxime sodium	HO	20 mg/mL[a]	FUJ	3 mg/mL[a]	Fine precipitate forms immediately	1880	I
Cefoxitin sodium	ME	20 mg/mL[c]	FUJ	3 mg/mL[a]	Immediate cloudy precipitation	1880	I
Ceftazidime	LI	20 mg/mL[a]	FUJ	3 mg/mL[a]	Fine precipitate forms immediately	1880	I
Ceftriaxone sodium	RC	20 mg/mL[a]	FUJ	3 mg/mL[a]	Heavy white precipitate forms immediately	1880	I
Diltiazem HCl	MMD	5 mg/mL	LY	6 and 30 mg/mL[a]	Visually compatible	1807	C
Fluconazole	RR	2 mg/mL	LY	6 mg/mL	Cloudiness develops	1407	I
Foscarnet sodium	AST	24 mg/mL	LY	6 mg/mL	Precipitates immediately	1335	I
	AST	24 mg/mL	LY	6 mg/mL[a,b]	Pentamidine crystals form immediately	1393	I
Linezolid	PHU	2 mg/mL	FUJ	6 mg/mL[a]	Crystalline precipitate forms in 1 to 4 hr	2264	I
Zidovudine	BW	4 mg/mL[a]	LY	6 mg/mL[a]	Physically compatible for 4 hr at 25 °C	1193	C

[a] *Tested in dextrose 5%.*
[b] *Tested in sodium chloride 0.9%.*
[c] *Tested in dextrose 4%.*

PENTAZOCINE LACTATE
AHFS 28:08.12

Products — Pentazocine lactate is supplied in 1-mL ampuls, 1- and 2-mL syringe cartridges, and 10-mL multiple-dose vials. Each milliliter of solution contains (1):

Component	Ampul	Cartridge Unit	Vial
Pentazocine (as lactate)	30 mg	30 mg	30 mg
Sodium chloride	2.8 mg	2.2 mg	1.5 mg
Acetone sodium bisulfite		1 mg	2 mg
Methylparaben			1 mg
Water for injection	qs 1 mL	qs 1 mL	qs 1 mL

pH — The pH is adjusted to 4 to 5 with lactic acid or sodium hydroxide. (1)

Osmolality — The osmolality of pentazocine lactate 30 mg/mL was determined to be 307 mOsm/kg. (1233)

Trade Name(s) — Talwin.

Administration — Pentazocine lactate may be administered by intramuscular, subcutaneous, or intravenous injection. For repeated administration, intramuscular injection with constant rotation of the injection sites should be used. Subcutaneous injection should be used only when necessary because of possible tissue damage. (1; 4)

Stability — Pentazocine lactate injection should be stored at controlled room temperature (1) and protected from temperatures of 40 °C or above and from freezing. Pentazocine lactate is incompatible with alkaline substances. (4)

Syringes — Pentazocine lactate (Winthrop) 30 mg/1 mL, repackaged in 3-mL clear glass syringes (Hy-Pod) and stored at 25 °C, exhibited no significant changes in pH, physical appearance, or drug concentration during 360 days of storage. (535)

Compatibility Information

Additive Compatibility

Pentazocine lactate

Drug	Mfr	Conc/L	Mfr	Conc/L	Test Soln	Remarks	Ref	C/I
Aminophylline	SE	1 g	WI	300 mg	D5W	Physically incompatible	15	I
Pentobarbital sodium	AB	1 g	WI	300 mg	D5W	Physically incompatible	15	I
Phenobarbital sodium	WI	200 mg	WI	300 mg	D5W	Physically incompatible	15	I
Sodium bicarbonate	AB	80 mEq	WI	300 mg	D5W	Physically incompatible	15	I

Drugs in Syringe Compatibility

Pentazocine lactate

Drug (in syringe)	Mfr	Amt	Mfr	Amt	Remarks	Ref	C/I
Atropine sulfate		0.6 mg/ 1.5 mL	WI	30 mg/ 1 mL	Physically compatible for at least 15 min	14	C
	ST	0.4 mg/ 1 mL	WI	30 mg/ 1 mL	Physically compatible for at least 15 min	326	C
Butorphanol tartrate	BR	4 mg/ 2 mL	WI	30 mg/ 1 mL	Physically compatible for 30 min at room temperature	566	C
Chlorpromazine HCl	SKF	50 mg/ 2 mL	WI	30 mg/ 1 mL	Physically compatible for at least 15 min	14	C
	PO	50 mg/ 2 mL	WI	30 mg/ 1 mL	Physically compatible for at least 15 min	326	C
Dimenhydrinate	HR	50 mg/ 1 mL	WI	30 mg/ 1 mL	Physically compatible for at least 15 min	326	C
Diphenhydramine HCl	PD	50 mg/ 1 mL	WI	30 mg/ 1 mL	Physically compatible for at least 15 min	326	C
Droperidol	MN	2.5 mg/ 1 mL	WI	30 mg/ 1 mL	Physically compatible for at least 15 min	326	C
Fentanyl citrate	MN	0.05 mg/ 1 mL	WI	30 mg/ 1 mL	Physically compatible for at least 15 min	326	C
Glycopyrrolate	RB	0.2 mg/ 1 mL	WI	30 mg/ 1 mL	Precipitates immediately	331	I
	RB	0.2 mg/ 1 mL	WI	60 mg/ 2 mL	Precipitates immediately	331	I
	RB	0.4 mg/ 2 mL	WI	30 mg/ 1 mL	Precipitates immediately	331	I
Heparin sodium		2500 units/ 1 mL	WI	30 mg/ 1 mL	Turbidity or precipitate forms within 5 min	1053	I
Hydromorphone HCl	KN	4 mg/ 2 mL	WI	30 mg/ 1 mL	Physically compatible for 30 min	517	C
Hydroxyzine HCl	PF	100 mg/ 4 mL	WI	30 mg/ 1 mL	Physically compatible for at least 15 min	14	C
	PF	50 mg/ 1 mL	WI	30 mg/ 1 mL	Physically compatible for at least 15 min	326	C
	PF	50 mg/ 1 mL	WI	60 mg/ 2 mL	Physically compatible	771	C
	PF	100 mg/ 2 mL	WI	30 mg/ 1 mL	Physically compatible	771	C

Drugs in Syringe Compatibility (Cont.)

Pentazocine lactate

Drug (in syringe)	Mfr	Amt	Mfr	Amt	Remarks	Ref	C/I
Meperidine HCl	WI	50 mg/ 1 mL	WI	30 mg/ 1 mL	Physically compatible for at least 15 min	326	C
Metoclopramide HCl	NO	10 mg/ 2 mL	WI	30 mg/ 1 mL	Physically compatible for 15 min at room temperature	565	C
Morphine sulfate	ST	15 mg/ 1 mL	WI	30 mg/ 1 mL	Physically compatible for at least 15 min	326	C
Pentobarbital sodium	WY	100 mg/ 2 mL	WI	30 mg/ 1 mL	Precipitate forms within 15 min	14	I
	AB	50 mg/ 1 mL	WI	30 mg/ 1 mL	Physically incompatible within 15 min	326	I
Prochlorperazine edisylate	PO	5 mg/ 1 mL	WI	30 mg/ 1 mL	Physically compatible for at least 15 min	326	C
Promethazine HCl	WY	50 mg/ 2 mL	WI	30 mg/ 1 mL	Physically compatible for at least 15 min	14	C
	PO	50 mg/ 2 mL	WI	30 mg/ 1 mL	Physically compatible for at least 15 min	326	C
Ranitidine HCl	GL	50 mg/ 2 mL	WI	60 mg/ 2 mL	Physically compatible for 1 hr at 25 °C	978	C
Scopolamine HBr		0.6 mg/ 1.5 mL	WI	30 mg/ 1 mL	Physically compatible for at least 15 min	14	C
	ST	0.4 mg/ 1 mL	WI	30 mg/ 1 mL	Physically compatible for at least 15 min	326	C

Y-Site Injection Compatibility (1:1 Mixture)

Pentazocine lactate

Drug	Mfr	Conc	Mfr	Conc	Remarks	Ref	C/I
Heparin sodium	UP	1000 units/L[a]	WI	30 mg/mL	Physically compatible for 4 hr at room temperature	534	C
Hydrocortisone sodium succinate	UP	10 mg/L[a]	WI	30 mg/mL	Physically compatible for 4 hr at room temperature	534	C
Nafcillin sodium	WY	33 mg/mL[b]		30 mg/mL	Precipitate forms, probably free nafcillin	547	I
Potassium chloride	AB	40 mEq/L[a]	WI	30 mg/mL	Physically compatible for 4 hr at room temperature	534	C

[a]Tested in dextrose 5% in Ringer's injection, dextrose 5% in Ringer's injection, lactated, dextrose 5%, Ringer's injection, lactated, and sodium chloride 0.9%.
[b]Tested in sodium chloride 0.9%.

PENTOBARBITAL SODIUM
AHFS 28:24.04

Products — Pentobarbital sodium 50 mg/mL is available in 20- and 50-mL multiple-dose vials. Each milliliter of solution also contains propylene glycol 40% (v/v), alcohol 10%, and hydrochloric acid and/ or sodium hydroxide to adjust pH in water for injection. (1)

pH — Adjusted to approximately 9.5. (1); range 9 to 10.5. (17)

Trade Name(s) — Nembutal.

Administration — Pentobarbital sodium may be administered by deep intramuscular injection into a large muscle or by slow intravenous injection. The rate of intravenous administration should not exceed

50 mg/min. No more than 5 mL of solution (250 mg) should be injected intramuscularly at any one site. (1; 4) .

Stability — Intact vials of pentobarbital sodium should be stored at controlled room temperature and protected from excessive heat and freezing. Brief exposures to temperatures up to 40 °C does not adversely affect the product. (1)

Aqueous solutions of pentobarbital sodium are not stable. The commercially available pentobarbital sodium in a propylene glycol vehicle is more stable. In an acidic medium, pentobarbital sodium may precipitate. (4) No solution containing a precipitate or that is cloudy should be used. (1; 4)

Pentobarbital sodium may raise the pH of admixture solutions to the alkaline range and, therefore, should not be mixed with alkali-labile drugs. (47)

Syringes — Pentobarbital sodium 50 mg/mL was packaged in 1-mL glass and polypropylene syringes and 3-mL polypropylene syringes (Becton Dickinson) and stored at 25 °C. No loss occurred in 31 days. (2429)

Sorption — Pentobarbital sodium did not undergo sorption to a PVC plastic test strip or PVC infusion solution bag. (12; 770)

Plasticizer Leaching — Pentobarbital sodium 2 mg/mL in dextrose 5% did not leach diethylhexyl phthalate (DEHP) plasticizer from 50-mL PVC bags in 24 hours at 24 °C. (1683)

Filtration — Pentobarbital sodium 600 mg/L and 1.25 g/L in dextrose 5% and also sodium chloride 0.9% was filtered through a 0.45-μm filter. The delivered concentration did not decrease. (754)

Compatibility Information

Solution Compatibility

Pentobarbital sodium

Solution	Mfr	Mfr	Conc/L	Remarks	Ref	C/I
Dextrose–Ringer's injection combinations	AB	AB	500 mg	Physically compatible	3	C
Dextrose–Ringer's injection, lactated, combinations	AB	AB	500 mg	Physically compatible	3	C
Dextrose–saline combinations	AB	AB	500 mg	Physically compatible	3	C
Dextrose 2.5%	AB	AB	500 mg	Physically compatible	3	C
Dextrose 5%	AB	AB	500 mg	Physically compatible	3	C
	MG[a]	AB	600 mg and 1.25 g	Physically compatible and chemically stable for 12-hr study period	754	C
	BA[b]	AB	4 and 8 g	Visually compatible with no loss in 24 hr	1590	C
	BA[b]	AB	>8 g	Occasional visible precipitation	1590	I
Dextrose 10%	AB	AB	500 mg	Physically compatible	3	C
Ionosol products	AB	AB	500 mg	Physically compatible	3	C
Ringer's injection	AB	AB	500 mg	Physically compatible	3	C
Ringer's injection, lactated	AB	AB	500 mg	Physically compatible	3	C
Sodium chloride 0.45%	AB	AB	500 mg	Physically compatible	3	C
Sodium chloride 0.9%	AB	AB	500 mg	Physically compatible	3	C
	MG[a]	AB	600 mg and 1.25 g	Physically compatible and chemically stable for 12-hr study period	754	C
	BA[b]	AB	4 and 8 g	Visually compatible with no loss in 24 hr	1590	C
	BA[b]	AB	>8 g	Occasional visible precipitation	1590	I
	BA	AB	10 g	Crystals form in less than 24 hr at 25 °C	2429	I
Sodium lactate ⅙ M	AB	AB	500 mg	Physically compatible	3	C

[a] *Tested in polyolefin containers.*
[b] *Tested in PVC containers.*

Additive Compatibility

Pentobarbital sodium

Drug	Mfr	Conc/L	Mfr	Conc/L	Test Soln	Remarks	Ref	C/I
Amikacin sulfate	BR	5 g	AB	100 mg	D5LR, D5R, D5S, D5W, D10W, LR, NS, R, SL	Physically compatible and both stable for 24 hr at 25 °C	294	C
Aminophylline		500 mg	AB	500 mg		Physically compatible	3	C
	SE	500 mg	AB	500 mg		Physically compatible	6	C
	SE	1 g	AB	1 g	D5W	Physically compatible	15	C
Calcium chloride	UP	1 g	AB	1 g	D5W	Physically compatible	15	C
Chloramphenicol sodium succinate	PD	1 g	AB	200 mg		Physically compatible	6	C
Dimenhydrinate	SE	500 mg	AB	1 g	D5W	Physically compatible	15	C
Ephedrine sulfate	LI	250 mg	AB	1 g	D5W	Physically incompatible	15	I
Erythromycin lactobionate	AB	1 g	AB	500 mg		Physically compatible. Erythromycin stable for 24 hr at 25 °C	20	C
Hydrocortisone sodium succinate	UP	500 mg	AB	1 g	D5W	Physically incompatible	15	I
Hydroxyzine HCl	RR	250 mg	AB	1 g	D5W	Physically incompatible	15	I
Lidocaine HCl	AST	2 g	AB	500 mg		Physically compatible	24	C
Penicillin G potassium	[a]	900,000 units	AB	500 mg	D5W	17% penicillin loss in 6 hr at 25 °C	48	I
	SQ	1 million units	AB	500 mg	D5W	42% penicillin loss in 24 hr at 25 °C	47	I
Pentazocine lactate	WI	300 mg	AB	1 g	D5W	Physically incompatible	15	I
Promethazine HCl	WY	250 mg	AB	1 g	D5W	Physically incompatible	15	I
Sodium bicarbonate	AB	80 mEq	AB	1 g	D5W	Physically incompatible	15	I
Succinylcholine chloride						Pentobarbital precipitates or succinylcholine hydrolyzes	4	I
Verapamil HCl	KN	80 mg	AB	200 mg	D5W, NS	Physically compatible for 24 hr	764	C

[a] *A buffered preparation was specified.*

Drugs in Syringe Compatibility

Pentobarbital sodium

Drug (in syringe)	Mfr	Amt	Mfr	Amt	Remarks	Ref	C/I
Aminophylline		500 mg/ 2 mL	AB	500 mg/ 10 mL	Physically compatible	55	C
Atropine sulfate		0.6 mg/ 1.5 mL	WY	100 mg/ 2 mL	Physically compatible for at least 15 min	14	C
	ST	0.4 mg/ 1 mL	AB	50 mg/ 1 mL	Physically compatible for at least 15 min	326	C
	LI	0.6 mg/ 1.5 mL	AB	100 mg/ 2 mL	Precipitate forms in 24 hr at room temperature	542	I

Drugs in Syringe Compatibility (Cont.)

Pentobarbital sodium

Drug (in syringe)	Mfr	Amt	Mfr	Amt	Remarks	Ref	C/I
Butorphanol tartrate	BR	4 mg/ 2 mL	AB	50 mg/ 1 mL	Precipitates immediately	761	I
Chlorpromazine HCl	SKF	50 mg/ 2 mL	AB	500 mg/ 10 mL	Physically incompatible	55	I
	SKF	50 mg/ 2 mL	WY	100 mg/ 2 mL	Precipitate forms within 15 min	14	I
	PO	50 mg/ 2 mL	AB	50 mg/ 1 mL	Physically incompatible within 15 min	326	I
Dimenhydrinate	SE	50 mg/ 1 mL	AB	500 mg/ 10 mL	Physically incompatible	55	I
	HR	50 mg/ 1 mL	AB	50 mg/ 1 mL	Physically incompatible within 15 min	326	I
Diphenhydramine HCl	PD	50 mg/ 1 mL	WY	100 mg/ 2 mL	Precipitate observed within 15 min	14	I
	PD	50 mg/ 1 mL	AB	500 mg/ 10 mL	Physically incompatible	55	I
	PD	50 mg/ 1 mL	AB	50 mg/ 1 mL	Physically incompatible within 15 min	326	I
Droperidol	MN	2.5 mg/ 1 mL	AB	50 mg/ 1 mL	Physically incompatible within 15 min	326	I
Ephedrine sulfate		50 mg/ 1 mL	AB	500 mg/ 10 mL	Physically compatible	55	C
Fentanyl citrate	MN	0.05 mg/ 1 mL	AB	50 mg/ 1 mL	Physically incompatible within 15 min	326	I
Glycopyrrolate	RB	0.2 mg/ 1 mL	AB	50 mg/ 1 mL	Precipitates immediately	331	I
	RB	0.4 mg/ 2 mL	AB	50 mg/ 1 mL	Precipitates immediately	331	I
	RB	0.2 mg/ 1 mL	AB	100 mg/ 2 mL	Precipitates immediately	331	I
Hyaluronidase	AB	150 units	AB	500 mg/ 10 mL	Physically compatible	55	C
Hydromorphone HCl	KN	4 mg/ 2 mL[a]	AB	50 mg/ 1 mL	Physically compatible for 30 min	517	C
	KN	4 mg/ 2 mL[b]	AB	50 mg/ 1 mL	Transient precipitate that dissipates after mixing and stays clear for 30 min	517	?
Hydroxyzine HCl	PF	100 mg/ 4 mL	WY	100 mg/ 2 mL	Precipitate forms within 15 min	14	I
	PF	50 mg/ 1 mL	AB	50 mg/ 1 mL	Physically incompatible within 15 min	326	I
Meperidine HCl	WI	100 mg/ 2 mL	AB	500 mg/ 10 mL	Physically incompatible	55	I
	WY	100 mg/ 1 mL	WY	100 mg/ 2 mL	Precipitate forms within 15 min	14	I
	WI	50 mg/ 1 mL	AB	50 mg/ 1 mL	Physically incompatible within 15 min	326	I
Midazolam HCl	RC	5 mg/ 1 mL	WY	100 mg/ 2 mL	White precipitate forms immediately	1145	I
Morphine sulfate		16.2 mg/ 1 mL	AB	500 mg/ 10 mL	Physically compatible	55	C

Drugs in Syringe Compatibility (Cont.)

Pentobarbital sodium

Drug (in syringe)	Mfr	Amt	Mfr	Amt	Remarks	Ref	C/I
	WY	15 mg/ 1 mL	WY	100 mg/ 2 mL	Precipitate forms within 15 min	14	I
	ST	15 mg/ 1 mL	AB	50 mg/ 1 mL	Physically incompatible within 15 min	326	I
Nalbuphine HCl	EN	10 mg/ 1 mL	WY	50 mg/ 1 mL	Immediate white milky precipitate that persists for 36 hr at 27 °C	762	I
	EN	2.5 mg/ 0.25 mL	WY	50 mg/ 1 mL	Immediate white milky precipitate that clears upon vigorous shaking	762	I
	EN	5 mg/ 0.5 mL	WY	50 mg/ 1 mL	Immediate white milky precipitate that persists for 36 hr at 27 °C	762	I
Neostigmine methylsulfate	RC	0.5 mg/ 1 mL	AB	500 mg/ 10 mL	Physically compatible	55	C
Pentazocine lactate	WI	30 mg/ 1 mL	WY	100 mg/ 2 mL	Precipitate forms within 15 min	14	I
	WI	30 mg/ 1 mL	AB	50 mg/ 1 mL	Physically incompatible within 15 min	326	I
Prochlorperazine edisylate	SKF	10 mg/ 2 mL	AB	500 mg/ 10 mL	Physically incompatible	55	I
	SKF		WY	100 mg/ 2 mL	Precipitate forms within 15 min	14	I
	PO	5 mg/ 1 mL	AB	50 mg/ 1 mL	Physically incompatible within 15 min	326	I
Promethazine HCl	WY	100 mg/ 4 mL	AB	500 mg/ 10 mL	Physically incompatible	55	I
	WY	50 mg/ 2 mL	WY	100 mg/ 2 mL	Precipitate forms within 15 min	14	I
	PO	50 mg/ 2 mL	AB	50 mg/ 1 mL	Physically incompatible within 15 min	326	I
Ranitidine HCl	GL	50 mg/ 5 mL	AB	100 mg	Precipitates immediately	1151	I
Scopolamine HBr		0.6 mg/ 1.5 mL	WY	100 mg/ 2 mL	Physically compatible for at least 15 min	14	C
		0.13 mg/ 0.26 mL	AB	500 mg/ 10 mL	Physically compatible	55	C
	ST	0.4 mg/ 1 mL	AB	50 mg/ 1 mL	Physically compatible for at least 15 min	326	C
Sodium bicarbonate		3.75 g/ 50 mL	AB	500 mg/ 10 mL	Physically compatible	55	C

[a]Vial formulation was tested.
[b]Ampul formulation was tested.

Y-Site Injection Compatibility (1:1 Mixture)

Pentobarbital sodium

Drug	Mfr	Conc	Mfr	Conc	Remarks	Ref	C/I
Acyclovir sodium	BW	5 mg/mL[a]	WY	2 mg/mL[a]	Physically compatible for 4 hr at 25 °C	1157	C
Amphotericin B cholesteryl sulfate complex	SEQ	0.83 mg/mL[a]	AB	5 mg/mL[a]	Decreased natural turbidity occurs	2117	I
Fenoldopam mesylate	AB	80 mcg/mL[b]	AB	5 mg/mL[b]	Trace haze and microparticulates form immediately	2467	I
Insulin, regular	LI	1 unit/mL[b]	WY	2 mg/mL[b]	Physically compatible for 3 hr	1316	C
Linezolid	PHU	2 mg/mL	AB	5 mg/mL[a]	Physically compatible for 4 hr at 23 °C	2264	C
Propofol	ZEN	10 mg/mL	WY	5 mg/mL[a]	Physically compatible for 1 hr at 23 °C	2066	C
TNA #218 to #226[c]			AB	5 mg/mL[a]	Damage to emulsion occurs immediately with free oil formation possible	2215	I
TPN #212 to #215[c]			AB	5 mg/mL[a]	Physically compatible for 4 hr at 23 °C	2109	C

[a]Tested in dextrose 5%.
[b]Tested in sodium chloride 0.9%.
[c]Refer to Appendix I for the composition of parenteral nutrition solutions. TNA indicates a 3-in-1 admixture, and TPN indicates a 2-in-1 admixture.

PENTOSTATIN
AHFS 10:00

Products — Pentostatin is available as a lyophilized powder in vials containing 10 mg of drug. Also present are 50 mg of mannitol and sodium hydroxide or hydrochloric acid to adjust the pH. Reconstitute the vial contents with 5 mL of sterile water for injection and shake well to yield a 2-mg/mL solution. (1)

pH — From 7 to 8.5. (1)

Trade Name(s) — Nipent.

Administration — Pentostatin is administered intravenously by injection over five minutes or by infusion over 20 to 30 minutes when diluted in 25 to 50 mL of dextrose 5% or sodium chloride 0.9%. Adequate hydration is necessary prior to administering pentostatin. Administration of 500 to 1000 mL of dextrose 5% in sodium chloride 0.45% or similar solution prior to drug administration with an additional 500 mL of dextrose 5% or similar solution after drug administration is recommended. (1; 4)

Stability — The manufacturer recommends that pentostatin be stored under refrigeration (1), but other information indicates that the drug in intact vials is stable for at least three years at room temperature. (234)

The white to off-white powder yields a colorless solution when reconstituted. The manufacturer states that reconstituted pentostatin solutions are stable at room temperature for up to eight hours only because of the absence of antibacterial preservatives. (1) Other information indicates that the reconstituted solution is stable for 72 hours at room temperature, exhibiting a 2 to 4% loss. (234; 1453)

Pentostatin (Parke-Davis) 0.03 mg/mL diluted in sodium chloride 0.9% and stored at 22 °C did not exhibit a substantial antimicrobial effect on the growth of four organisms (*Enterococcus faecium, Staphylococcus aureus, Pseudomonas aeruginosa,* and *Candida albicans*) inoculated into the solution. *C. albicans* maintained viability for 24 hours, and the others were viable for 48 to 120 hours. The author recommended that diluted solutions of pentostatin be stored under refrigeration whenever possible and that the potential for microbiological growth be considered when assigning expiration periods. (2160)

pH Effects — Pentostatin displays greater decomposition under acidic conditions compared to alkaline conditions. The pH range of maximum stability is about 6.5 to 11.5. At pH 6 to 8, hydrolysis is not sensitive to the ionic strength of the solution. (1453)

Sorption — Pentostatin does not undergo sorption to PVC containers or administration sets at concentrations between 0.18 and 0.33 mg/mL in dextrose 5% water or sodium chloride 0.9%. (1)

Compatibility Information

Solution Compatibility

Pentostatin

Solution	Mfr	Mfr	Conc/L	Remarks	Ref	C/I
Dextrose 5%		NCI	20 mg	2% loss in 24 hr and 8 to 10% in 48 hr at room temperature. No loss in 96 hr refrigerated	234	C
	TRᵃ, BAᵇ	NCI	20 mg	10% loss in 54 hr at 23 °C	1453	C
	TRᵃ, BAᵇ	NCI	2 mg	10% loss in 11 hr at 23 °C	1453	I
Ringer's injection, lactated		NCI	20 mg	Up to 4% loss in 48 hr at room temperature	234	C
Sodium chloride 0.9%		NCI	20 mg	Up to 4% loss in 48 hr at room temperature. No loss in 96 hr under refrigeration	234	C
	ABᵃ, BAᵇ	NCI	20 mg	1 to 4% loss in about 49 hr at 23 °C	1453	C
	ABᵃ, BAᵇ	NCI	2 mg	3 to 6% loss in 48 hr at 23 °C	1453	C

ᵃTested in glass containers.
ᵇTested in PVC containers.

Y-Site Injection Compatibility (1:1 Mixture)

Pentostatin

Drug	Mfr	Conc	Mfr	Conc	Remarks	Ref	C/I
Fludarabine phosphate	BX	1 mg/mLᵃ	NCI	0.4 mg/mLᵇ	Visually compatible for 4 hr at 22 °C	1439	C
Melphalan HCl	BW	0.1 mg/mLᵇ	PD	0.4 mg/mLᵇ	Physically compatible for 3 hr at 22 °C	1557	C
Ondansetron HCl	GL	1 mg/mLᵇ	NCI	0.4 mg/mLᵇ	Visually compatible for 4 hr at 22 °C	1365	C
Paclitaxel	NCI	1.2 mg/mLᵃ	NCI	0.4 mg/mLᵇ	Physically compatible for 4 hr at 22 °C	1556	C
Sargramostim	IMM	10 mcg/mLᵇ	NCI	0.4 mg/mLᵇ	Visually compatible for 4 hr at 22 °C	1436	C

ᵃTested in dextrose 5%.
ᵇTested in sodium chloride 0.9%.

PHENOBARBITAL SODIUM
AHFS 28:12.04

Products — Phenobarbital sodium injection is available in various dosage forms and sizes, including 30, 60, 65, and 130 mg/mL, from several manufacturers. The product formulations also contain ethanol 10%, propylene glycol 67.8 to 75%, and water for injection. Some products also contain benzyl alcohol 1.5% as a preservative. (1; 4)

pH — The USP cites the official pH range as 9.2 to 10.2. (17)

Osmolality — The osmolality of phenobarbital sodium 65 mg/mL was 15,570 mOsm/kg by freezing-point depression and 9285 mOsm/kg by vapor pressure. (1071) The osmolality of phenobarbital sodium 200 mg/mL was 10,800 mOsm/kg.

The osmolality of phenobarbital sodium 100 mg was calculated for the following dilutions (1054):

Diluent	Osmolality (mOsm/kg)	
	50 mL	100 mL
Dextrose 5%	296	289
Sodium chloride 0.9%	325	317

Trade Name(s) — Luminal Sodium.

Administration — Phenobarbital sodium is administered by intramuscular injection into a large muscle and slow intravenous injection. The commercial injection is highly alkaline and may cause local tissue damage. Do not administer subcutaneously. When given intravenously, the rate of injection should not exceed 60 mg/min. (1; 4)

Stability — Phenobarbital sodium injection in intact containers should be stored at controlled room temperature and protected from light. (1)

Phenobarbital sodium under simulated summer conditions in paramedic vehicles was exposed to temperatures ranging from 26 to 38 °C over four weeks. Analysis found no loss of the drug under these conditions. (2562)

Phenobarbital sodium is not generally considered stable in aqueous solutions. (4) However, a test of phenobarbital sodium 10% (w/v) in aqueous solution showed 7% decomposition in four weeks when stored at 20 °C. There was no measurable decomposition in eight weeks with storage at −25 °C. (233)

In addition, the stability of phenobarbital sodium diluted to a 10-mg/mL concentration in sodium chloride 0.9% for use in infants was studied. When stored at 4 °C, the dilution was physically compatible with no loss of drug over 28 days. (1294)

Phenobarbital may precipitate from solutions of phenobarbital sodium, depending on the concentration and acidic pH. (4) No solution containing a precipitate or that is more than slightly discolored should be used. (1; 4)

Phenobarbital sodium may raise the pH of admixture solutions to the alkaline range and, therefore, should not be mixed with alkali-labile drugs. (47)

Plasticizer Leaching — Phenobarbital sodium 6 mg/mL in dextrose 5% did not leach diethylhexyl phthalate (DEHP) plasticizer from 50-mL PVC bags in 24 hours at 24 °C. (1683)

Filtration — Phenobarbital sodium 130 mg/L in dextrose 5%, sodium chloride 0.9%, and Ringer's injection, lactated, filtered over 12 hours through a 5-μm stainless steel depth filter (Argyle Filter Connector), a 0.22-μm cellulose ester membrane filter (Ivex-2 Filter Set), and a 0.22-μm polycarbonate membrane filter (In-Sure Filter Set), showed no loss due to binding to the filters. (320)

Compatibility Information

Solution Compatibility

Phenobarbital sodium

Solution	Mfr	Mfr	Conc/L	Remarks	Ref	C/I
Dextrose–Ringer's injection combinations	AB		320 mg	Physically compatible	3	C
Dextrose–Ringer's injection, lactated, combinations	AB		320 mg	Physically compatible	3	C
Dextrose–saline combinations	AB		320 mg	Physically compatible	3	C
Dextrose 2.5%	AB		320 mg	Physically compatible	3	C
Dextrose 5%	AB		320 mg	Physically compatible	3	C
Dextrose 10%	AB		320 mg	Physically compatible	3	C
Ionosol products	AB		320 mg	Physically compatible	3	C
Ringer's injection	AB		320 mg	Physically compatible	3	C
Ringer's injection, lactated	AB		320 mg	Physically compatible	3	C
Sodium chloride 0.45%	AB		320 mg	Physically compatible	3	C
Sodium chloride 0.9%	AB		320 mg	Physically compatible	3	C
Sodium lactate ⅙ M	AB		320 mg	Physically compatible	3	C

Additive Compatibility

Phenobarbital sodium

Drug	Mfr	Conc/L	Mfr	Conc/L	Test Soln	Remarks	Ref	C/I
Amikacin sulfate	BR	5 g	LI	300 mg	D5LR, D5R, D5S, D5W, D10W, LR, NS, R, SL	Physically compatible and both stable for 24 hr at 25 °C	294	C
Aminophylline	SE	500 mg	AB	100 mg		Physically compatible	6	C
	SE	1 g	WI	200 mg	D5W	Physically compatible	15	C

Additive Compatibility (Cont.)

Phenobarbital sodium

Drug	Mfr	Conc/L	Mfr	Conc/L	Test Soln	Remarks	Ref	C/I
Calcium chloride	UP	1 g	WI	200 mg	D5W	Physically compatible	15	C
Calcium gluconate	UP	1 g	WI	200 mg	D5W	Physically compatible	15	C
Chlorpromazine HCl	BP	200 mg	BP	800 mg	D5W, NS	Precipitates immediately	26	I
Colistimethate sodium	WC	500 mg	WI	200 mg	D5W	Physically compatible	15	C
Dimenhydrinate	SE	500 mg	WI	200 mg	D5W	Physically compatible	15	C
Ephedrine sulfate	LI	250 mg	WI	200 mg	D5W	Physically incompatible	15	I
Hydralazine HCl	BP	80 mg	BP	800 mg	D5W	Yellow color and precipitate in 3 hr	26	I
Hydrocortisone sodium succinate	UP	500 mg	WI	200 mg	D5W	Physically incompatible	15	I
Hydroxyzine HCl	RR	250 mg	WI	200 mg	D5W	Physically incompatible	15	I
Meropenem	ZEN	1 and 20 g	ES	200 mg	NS	Visually compatible for 4 hr at room temperature	1994	C
Pentazocine lactate	WI	300 mg	WI	200 mg	D5W	Physically incompatible	15	I
Polymyxin B sulfate	BW	200 mg	WI	200 mg	D5W	Physically compatible	15	C
Prochlorperazine mesylate	BP	100 mg	BP	800 mg	D5W	Haze develops over 3 hr	26	I
	BP	100 mg	BP	800 mg	NS	Precipitates immediately	26	I
Promethazine HCl	WY	250 mg	WI	200 mg	D5W	Physically incompatible	15	I
	BP	100 mg	BP	800 mg	D5W	Haze develops over 3 hr	26	I
	BP	100 mg	BP	800 mg	NS	Precipitates immediately	26	I
Succinylcholine chloride						Phenobarbital precipitates or succinylcholine hydrolyzes	4	I
Verapamil HCl	KN	80 mg	ES	260 mg	D5W, NS	Physically compatible for 24 hr	764	C

Drugs in Syringe Compatibility

Phenobarbital sodium

Drug (in syringe)	Mfr	Amt	Mfr	Amt	Remarks	Ref	C/I
Caffeine citrate		20 mg/ 1 mL	ES	130 mg/ 1 mL	Visually compatible for 4 hr at 25 °C	2440	C
Heparin sodium		2500 units/ 1 mL		200 mg/ 1 mL	Physically compatible for at least 5 min	1053	C
Hydromorphone HCl	KN	2, 10, 40 mg/ 1 mL	AB	120 mg/ 1 mL	Precipitate forms immediately but dissipates with shaking. Phenobarbital precipitates after 6 hr at room temperature	2082	I
Pantoprazole sodium	a	4 mg/ 1 mL		120 mg/ 1 mL	Precipitates within 4 hr	2574	I
Ranitidine HCl	GL	50 mg/ 2 mL	AB	120 mg/ 1 mL	Immediate white haze	978	I

[a] *Test performed using the formulation WITHOUT edetate disodium.*

Y-Site Injection Compatibility (1:1 Mixture)

Phenobarbital sodium

Drug	Mfr	Conc	Mfr	Conc	Remarks	Ref	C/I
Amphotericin B cholesteryl sulfate complex	SEQ	0.83 mg/mL[a]	WY	5 mg/mL[a]	Increased turbidity forms immediately	2117	I
Doripenem	JJ	5 mg/mL[a,b]	BA	5 mg/mL[a,b]	Physically compatible for 4 hr at 23 °C	2743	C
Doxapram HCl	RB	2 mg/mL[a]	ES	10 mg/mL[b]	Visually compatible for 4 hr at 23 °C	2470	C
Enalaprilat	MSD	1.25 mg/mL	WY	0.32 mg/mL[a,b]	Physically compatible for 4 hr at 21 °C	1409	C
Fentanyl citrate	JN	0.025 mg/mL[a]	WY	2 mg/mL[a]	Physically compatible for 48 hr at 22 °C	1706	C
Fosphenytoin sodium	PD	10 mg PE/mL[b,e]		130 mg/mL	Visually compatible with no loss of either drug in 8 hr at room temperature	2212	C
Hydromorphone HCl	KN	2, 10, 40 mg/mL	AB	120 mg/mL	Turbidity forms but dissipates; phenobarbital precipitates in 6 hr	1532	I
	AST	0.5 mg/mL[a]	WY	2 mg/mL[a]	Physically compatible for 48 hr at 22 °C	1706	C
Levofloxacin	OMN	5 mg/mL[a]	ES	130 mg/mL	Visually compatible for 4 hr at 24 °C	2233	C
Linezolid	PHU	2 mg/mL	WY	5 mg/mL[a]	Physically compatible for 4 hr at 23 °C	2264	C
Meropenem	ZEN	1 and 50 mg/mL[b]	ES	0.32 mg/mL[c]	Visually compatible for 4 hr at room temperature	1994	C
Methadone HCl	LI	1 mg/mL[a]	WY	2 mg/mL[a]	Physically compatible for 48 hr at 22 °C	1706	C
Morphine sulfate	AST	1 mg/mL[a]	WY	2 mg/mL[a]	Physically compatible for 48 hr at 22 °C	1706	C
Propofol	ZEN	10 mg/mL	WY	5 mg/mL[a]	Physically compatible for 1 hr at 23 °C	2066	C
TNA #218 to #226[d]			WY	5 mg/mL[a]	Damage to emulsion occurs immediately with free oil formation possible	2215	I
TPN #212 to #215[d]			WY	5 mg/mL[a]	Physically compatible for 4 hr at 23 °C	2109	C

[a]*Tested in dextrose 5%.*
[b]*Tested in sodium chloride 0.9%.*
[c]*Tested in sterile water for injection.*
[d]*Refer to Appendix I for the composition of parenteral nutrition solutions. TNA indicates a 3-in-1 admixture, and TPN indicates a 2-in-1 admixture.*
[e]*Concentration expressed in milligrams of phenytoin sodium equivalents (PE) per milliliter.*

PHENTOLAMINE MESYLATE
AHFS 12:16.04.04

Products — Phentolamine mesylate is available in vials containing 5 mg of drug with 25 mg of mannitol as a lyophilized powder. Reconstitution with 1 mL of sterile water for injection results in a 5-mg/mL solution. (1; 4)

pH — From 4.5 to 6.5. (4)

Administration — Phentolamine mesylate may be administered by intramuscular or intravenous injection. (1; 4)

Stability — The intact vials should be stored at controlled room temperature. (1; 4) Although the manufacturer recommends that reconstituted solutions be used immediately and not stored (1), other information indicates that such solutions are stable for 48 hours at room temperature and one week at 2 to 8 °C. (4)

Sorption — Phentolamine mesylate was shown not to exhibit sorption to PVC bags and tubing, polyethylene tubing, Silastic tubing, and polypropylene syringes. (536; 606)

Compatibility Information

Additive Compatibility

Phentolamine mesylate

Drug	Mfr	Conc/L	Mfr	Conc/L	Test Soln	Remarks	Ref	C/I
Dobutamine HCl	LI	1 g	CI	20 mg	D5W, NS	Physically compatible for 24 hr at 21 °C	812	C
Verapamil HCl	KN	80 mg	RC	10 mg	D5W, NS	Physically compatible for 24 hr	764	C

Drugs in Syringe Compatibility

Phentolamine mesylate

Drug (in syringe)	Mfr	Amt	Mfr	Amt	Remarks	Ref	C/I
Papaverine HCl	LI	30 mg/mL	BV, CI	0.5 mg/mL[a]	Physically compatible. Little papaverine loss at 5 and 25 °C. 1 to 3% phentolamine loss at 5 °C and 4 to 5% at 25 °C in 30 days	1161	C

[a]Constituted with the papaverine hydrochloride injection.

Y-Site Injection Compatibility (1:1 Mixture)

Phentolamine mesylate

Drug	Mfr	Conc	Mfr	Conc	Remarks	Ref	C/I
Amiodarone HCl	LZ	4 mg/mL[a,b]	CI	0.04 mg/mL[a,b]	Physically compatible for 24 hr at 21 °C under fluorescent light	1032	C

[a]Tested in dextrose 5%.
[b]Tested in sodium chloride 0.9%.

PHENYLEPHRINE HYDROCHLORIDE
AHFS 12:12.04

Products — Phenylephrine hydrochloride is available as a 1% solution in 1-mL ampuls and 1- and 5-mL vials. Each milliliter of solution contains phenylephrine hydrochloride 10 mg with sodium citrate and citric acid buffer, sodium chloride, and sodium metabisulfite antioxidant. The pH may have been adjusted during manufacture. (1; 4)

pH — From 3 to 6.5. (17)

Administration — Phenylephrine hydrochloride is administered by subcutaneous, intramuscular, or direct slow intravenous injection or by intravenous infusion. For direct intravenous injection, a 0.1% solution (1 mg/mL) may be prepared by diluting 1 mL of phenylephrine hydrochloride with 9 mL of sterile water for injection. Solutions for intravenous infusion are usually prepared by adding 10 mg of drug to 500 mL of dextrose 5% or sodium chloride 0.9%. (1; 4)

Stability — Intact containers of phenylephrine hydrochloride should be stored at controlled room temperature and protected from light. (1; 4) Solutions of the drug must not be used if they are brown or contain a precipitate. However, oxidation may occur, resulting in loss of activity even though no color change is evident. (4)

Phenylephrine hydrochloride was stable for 84 days at 60 °C in a 250-mg/100 mL concentration in sterile water for injection. (132)

Phenylephrine hydrochloride in dextrose 5% is stated to be stable for at least 48 hours at pH 3.5 to 7.5. (4)

Syringes — Phenylephrine hydrochloride (Gensia Sicor) 0.1 mg/mL packaged in polypropylene plastic syringes fitted with tip seals and stored at 23 to 25 °C in fluorescent light and at 3 to 5 °C and at –20 °C in the dark for 30 days exhibited no precipitation, cloudiness, or color change and virtually no loss of drug. (2737)

Central Venous Catheter — Phenylephrine hydrochloride (Ohmeda) 1 mg/mL in dextrose 5% was found to be compatible with the ARROWg+ard Blue Plus (Arrow International) chlorhexidine-bearing triple-lumen central catheter. Essentially complete delivery of the drug was found with little or no drug loss occurring. Furthermore, chlorhexidine delivered from the catheter remained at trace amounts with no substantial increase due to the delivery of the drug through the catheter. (2335)

Compatibility Information

Solution Compatibility

Phenylephrine HCl

Solution	Mfr	Mfr	Conc/L	Remarks	Ref	C/I
Dextrose–Ringer's injection combinations	AB	WI	1 mg	Physically compatible	3	C
Dextrose–Ringer's injection, lactated, combinations	AB	WI	1 mg	Physically compatible	3	C
Dextrose–saline combinations	AB	WI	1 mg	Physically compatible	3	C
Dextrose 2.5%	AB	WI	1 mg	Physically compatible	3	C
Dextrose 5%	AB	WI	1 mg	Physically compatible	3	C
Dextrose 10%	AB	WI	1 mg	Physically compatible	3	C
Ionosol products	AB	WI	1 mg	Physically compatible	3	C
Ringer's injection	AB	WI	1 mg	Physically compatible	3	C
Ringer's injection, lactated	AB	WI	1 mg	Physically compatible	3	C
Sodium chloride 0.45%	AB	WI	1 mg	Physically compatible	3	C
Sodium chloride 0.9%		WI	2.5 g	Stable for 24 hr at 22 °C	132	C
	AB	WI	1 mg	Physically compatible	3	C
	BA[a]	BA	100 and 200 mg	Physically compatible with no loss in 14 days at 25 °C	2524	C
Sodium lactate ⅙ M	AB	WI	1 mg	Physically compatible	3	C

[a]Tested in PVC containers.

Additive Compatibility

Phenylephrine HCl

Drug	Mfr	Conc/L	Mfr	Conc/L	Test Soln	Remarks	Ref	C/I
Chloramphenicol sodium succinate[b]	PD	500 mg	WI	2.5 g	D5W, NS	Phenylephrine stable for 24 hr at 22 °C	132	C
Dobutamine HCl	LI	1 g	WI	20 mg	D5W, NS	Physically compatible for 24 hr at 21 °C	812	C
Lidocaine HCl	AST	2 g	WI	20 mg		Physically compatible	24	C
Potassium chloride	AB	40 mEq	WI	2.5 g	D5W	Phenylephrine stable for 24 hr at 22 °C	132	C
Sodium bicarbonate	AB	2.4 mEq[a]	WI	10 mg	D5W	Physically compatible for 24 hr	772	C
		5%	WI	20 mg		Stable for 24 hr at 25 °C	48	C

[a]One vial of Neut added to a liter of admixture.
[b]Tested both with and without sodium bicarbonate 7.5 g/L.

Drugs in Syringe Compatibility

Phenylephrine HCl

Drug (in syringe)	Mfr	Amt	Mfr	Amt	Remarks	Ref	C/I
Caffeine citrate		20 mg/1 mL	ES	10 mg/1 mL	Visually compatible for 4 hr at 25 °C	2440	C
Lidocaine HCl		2%		0.25%	No loss of either drug in 66 days at 25 °C	1278	C

Y-Site Injection Compatibility (1:1 Mixture)

Phenylephrine HCl

Drug	Mfr	Conc	Mfr	Conc	Remarks	Ref	C/I
Amiodarone HCl	LZ	4 mg/mL[a,b]	WI	0.04 mg/mL[a,b]	Physically compatible for 24 hr at 21 °C	1032	C
Anidulafungin	VIC	0.5 mg/mL[a]	BA	1 mg/mL[a]	Physically compatible for 4 hr at 23 °C	2617	C
Argatroban	GSK	1 mg/mL[b]	AMR	10 mg/mL	Visually compatible for 24 hr at 23 °C	2391	C
Bivalirudin	TMC	5 mg/mL[a]	AMR	1 mg/mL[a]	Physically compatible for 4 hr at 23 °C	2373	C
	TMC	5 mg/mL[a,b]	AMR	10 mg/mL	Visually compatible for 6 hr at 23 °C	2680	C
Caspofungin acetate	ME	0.7 mg/mL[b]	BA	1 mg/mL[b]	Physically compatible for 4 hr at room temperature	2758	C
Cisatracurium besylate	GW	0.1, 2, 5 mg/mL[a]	GNS	1 mg/mL[a]	Physically compatible for 4 hr at 23 °C	2074	C
Dexmedetomidine HCl	HOS				Stated to be compatible	1	C
Doripenem	JJ	5 mg/mL[a,b]	GNS	1 mg/mL[a,b]	Physically compatible for 4 hr at 23 °C	2743	C
Etomidate	AB	2 mg/mL	ES	10 mg/mL	Visually compatible for 7 days at 25 °C	1801	C
Famotidine	MSD	0.2 mg/mL[a]	WI	0.02 mg/mL[a]	Physically compatible for 4 hr at 25 °C	1188	C
Fenoldopam mesylate	AB	80 mcg/mL[b]	AMR	1 mg/mL[b]	Physically compatible for 4 hr at 23 °C	2467	C
Furosemide	AB	4 mg/mL[a,b]	BA	0.64 mg/mL[a,b]	Precipitates in 5 to 15 min	2687	I
Haloperidol lactate	MN	0.5[a] and 5 mg/mL	WB	0.02 mg/mL[a]	Visually compatible for 24 hr at 21 °C	1523	C
Hetastarch in lactated electrolyte	AB	6%	OHM	1 mg/mL[a]	Physically compatible for 4 hr at 23 °C	2339	C
Levofloxacin	OMN	5 mg/mL[a]	AMR	10 mg/mL	Visually compatible for 4 hr at 24 °C	2233	C
Micafungin sodium	ASP	1.5 mg/mL[b]	BA	1 mg/mL[b]	Physically compatible for 4 hr at 23 °C	2683	C
Nesiritide	SCI	50 mcg/mL[a,b]		10 mg/mL	Physically compatible for 4 hr. May be chemically incompatible with nesiritide[c]	2625	?
Propofol	STU	2 mg/mL	ES	10 mg/mL	Yellow discoloration forms within 7 days at 25 °C. No visible change in 24 hr	1801	?
	ZEN	10 mg/mL	ES	0.1 mg/mL[a]	Physically compatible for 1 hr at 23 °C	2066	C
Remifentanil HCl	GW	0.025 and 0.25 mg/mL[b]	AMR	1 mg/mL[a]	Physically compatible for 4 hr at 23 °C	2075	C
Telavancin HCl	ASP	7.5 mg/mL[a,b,d]	SZ	1 mg/mL[a,b,d]	Physically compatible for 2 hr	2830	C
Vasopressin	AMR	2 and 4 units/mL[b]	AMR	40 mcg/mL[b]	Physically compatible with vasopressin pushed through a Y-site over 5 sec	2478	C
Zidovudine	BW	4 mg/mL[a]	WI	1 mg/mL[a]	Physically compatible for 4 hr at 25 °C	1193	C

[a]*Tested in dextrose 5%.*
[b]*Tested in sodium chloride 0.9%.*
[c]*Nesiritide is incompatible with bisulfite antioxidants used in some drug formulations. The specific formulation of the product to be used should be checked to ensure that no sulfite antioxidants are present.*
[d]*Tested in Ringer's injection, lactated.*

PHENYTOIN SODIUM
AHFS 28:12.12

Products — Phenytoin sodium 50 mg/mL is available as a ready-mixed solution in 2 mL vials, ampuls, and syringe cartridges and 5 mL vials. Each milliliter of solution also contains propylene glycol 40%, alcohol 10%, and sodium hydroxide to adjust pH in water for injection. (1)

CAUTION: Care should be taken to avoid confusion between phenytoin sodium and fosphenytoin sodium to prevent dosing errors.

pH — From 10 to 12.3. (1; 17) The pH is adjusted to about 12 during manufacture. (4)

Osmolality — The osmolality of phenytoin sodium 50 mg/mL was 9740 mOsm/kg by freezing-point depression and 6175 mOsm/kg by vapor pressure. (1071) Another report indicated that the osmolality was 3035 mOsm/kg by freezing-point depression. (1233)

The osmolality of phenytoin sodium 500 mg in 50 and 100 mL of sodium chloride 0.9% was calculated to be 336 and 312 mOsm/kg, respectively. (1054)

Sodium Content — Each milliliter of phenytoin sodium injection contains 0.2 mEq of sodium. (4)

Administration — Phenytoin sodium is preferably administered by direct intravenous injection into a large vein through a large-gauge needle or intravenous catheter. Although intramuscular injection can be used, erratic or delayed absorption may occur. Subcutaneous injection should be avoided because of the possibility of local tissue damage. The rate of intravenous injection should not exceed 50 mg/min in adults or 1 to 3 mg/kg/min in neonates. Following intravenous injection, sodium chloride 0.9% should be injected through the same needle or catheter to reduce irritation. (1; 4)

Because of the drug's low solubility and possible precipitation, intravenous infusion is usually not recommended. However, some clinicians have suggested that intravenous infusion is reasonable in an appropriately diluted, compatible infusion solution for short periods using inline filtration; they have advocated infusion to circumvent the adverse effects associated with direct intravenous injection. (1; 4)

Stability — Intact containers should be stored at controlled room temperature and protected from freezing. Phenytoin sodium is stable as long as it remains free of haziness and precipitation. If refrigerated or frozen, a precipitate may form, but it dissolves on standing at room temperature. On dissolution of the precipitate, the product is still suitable for use. Also, a faint yellow color, which has no effect on concentration, may sometimes develop in the injection. (1; 4)

Precipitation — Precipitation of free phenytoin occurs at pH 11.5 or less. (4)

The mixing of phenytoin sodium with other drugs or with intravenous infusion solutions is not recommended (1; 4) because the solubility of phenytoin sodium is such that crystallization or precipitation may result if the special vehicle is altered or the pH is lowered. (62; 63; 613) Unfortunately, direct intravenous injection of phenytoin sodium is inconvenient and is occasionally associated with significant cardiovascular side effects. (1; 4) In spite of the caveat against dilution, some clinicians have advocated the infusion of phenytoin sodium (443; 448; 611; 947; 948; 949; 950; 1295) or administration into the tubing of a running infusion solution. (63; 65; 338; 445)

There are a number of reports of phenytoin crystallization in infusion solutions within varying periods after dilution. While the time to crystal formation may be variable and difficult to predict, crystal formation is nonetheless inevitable. (65; 66; 305; 306; 447; 449; 450; 451; 708; 709; 710; 1421)

The relationship of phenytoin sodium solubility to various solution characteristics was explored. It was noted that the effect of the special solvent system could be disregarded in dilutions of 1:5 or more. The pH of the admixture was stated to be the primary determinant of the occurrence or absence of crystallization. With a given solution, the pH is dependent on the volume of dilution, with a lower pH resulting from greater dilution. Phenytoin becomes less soluble in aqueous solution as the pH drops. Equations for predicting the compatibility of phenytoin sodium in admixture solutions were presented, but it was noted that it is not possible to predict the time required to develop precipitation. (713)

Although some may feel that infusion of phenytoin sodium is, perhaps, too dangerous to perform clinically (452), others indicate that such administration may be feasible provided proper precautions are taken such as using a suitable vehicle (i.e., sodium chloride 0.9% or Ringer's injection, lactated), using a sufficiently concentrated solution, starting the infusion immediately after preparation and completing administration within a relatively short time, using a 0.22-μm inline filter, and watching the admixture very carefully. (305; 306; 453; 611; 612; 613; 708; 709; 710; 947; 948; 949; 950; 1295)

Phenytoin precipitate may form if the injection contacts more acidic drugs or infusion solutions such as dextrose 5% during administration. Such precipitation has been found to occlude catheters. Instilling 5 mL of 8.4% sodium bicarbonate injection at 15- to 30-minute intervals has cleared catheters occluded with phenytoin precipitate. The sodium bicarbonate apparently raised the pH enough to result in dissolution of a sufficient amount of the phenytoin precipitate to reopen the catheter. (2299; 2300) However, the safety is uncertain because it is not known if some of the precipitated phenytoin is delivered into the bloodstream upon opening the occlusion.

Sorption — Phenytoin sodium was shown not to exhibit sorption to PVC bags and tubing, polyethylene tubing, Silastic tubing, and polypropylene syringes. (536; 606)

Plasticizer Leaching — Phenytoin sodium 10 mg/mL in sodium chloride 0.9% did not leach diethylhexyl phthalate (DEHP) plasticizer from 50-mL PVC bags in 24 hours at 24 °C. (1683)

Filtration — Phenytoin sodium 250 mg/5 mL was filtered at a rate of 1 mL/min through a 5-μm stainless steel depth filter (Argyle Filter Connector). No reduction due to binding to the filter was observed. (320)

Compatibility Information

Solution Compatibility

Phenytoin sodium

Solution	Mfr	Mfr	Conc/L	Remarks	Ref	C/I
Dextrose 5% in sodium chloride 0.9%	TR	PD	1 g	Visible crystals in minutes. 21% crystallized in 8 hr and 38% in 24 hr	306	I
Dextrose 5%	TR	PD	1 g	Visible crystals in minutes. 15% crystallized in 8 hr and 36% in 24 hr	306	I
	TR	PD	4.6, 9.2, 18.4 g	Crystal formation. Erratic concentrations through 0.2-μm filter over 24 hr at 29 °C	305	I
	MG	PD	1 g	No precipitate or drug loss in 8 hr at room temperature. Precipitate forms within 24 hr with 15% drug	446	I
	TR	PD	1 g	Crystal formation in 1 hr	450; 451	I
	AB	PD	1 g	Visible crystals in less than 12 min. 18% loss of phenytoin in 14 hr and 22% in 24 hr	452	I
			1 g	10% of phenytoin removed by filtration in 2 hr and 15 to 18% in 4 hr	453	I
		PD	670 mg to 4 g	Phenytoin crystals within 5 to 25 min. Reduced phenytoin concentration	708	I
	AB, CU, MG, TR	ES, PD	0.4 to 4.55 g	Visible precipitate in 10 to 60 min with drug loss in 20 to 45 min	710	I
	TR	PD	1, 1.5, 2, 4, 10 g	Visible crystals in 30 min. 12 to 20% crystallized in 4 hr	951	I
Ringer's injection, lactated	TR	PD	4.6, 9.2, 18.4 g	Crystal formation. Erratic concentration through 0.2-μm filter over 24 hr at 29 °C	305	I
	TR	PD	1 g	Visible crystals in 6 to 9 hr. Approximately 0.8% crystallized in 8 hr and 7% in 24 hr	306	I
	TR	ES, PD	0.4 to 4.55 g	No drug loss for 12 to 24 hr at 23 °C. Inconsistent precipitate	710	I
Sodium chloride 0.45%	TR	PD	4.6, 9.2, 18.4 g	Crystal formation. Under 10% drug loss through 0.2-μm filter over 24 hr at 29 °C	305	I
Sodium chloride 0.9%		PD	1 to 10 g	Phenytoin crystal formation in 20 to 30 min	63	I
		PD	200 mg to 10 g	Phenytoin crystal formation in 30 min	65; 447	I
		PD	2 and 4 g	Phenytoin crystal formation in 10 to 15 min	66	I
	TR	PD	1 g	Visible crystals in 6 to 9 hr. Approximately 0.8% crystallized in 8 hr and 7% in 24 hr	306	I
	TR	PD	4.6, 9.2, 18.4 g	Crystal formation. Under 10% drug loss through 0.2-μm filter over 24 hr at 29 °C	305	I
			1 g	10% of phenytoin removed by filtration in 4 hr	453	I
		PD	670 mg to 4 g	No crystals observed during 1-hr study period	708	C
	TR	PD	1 to 10 g	Crystals formed in unfiltered solutions in 18 hr. Filtered solutions stored at 6 °C had no crystals and no reduction in phenytoin in 24 hr	709	I
	TR	ES, PD	0.4 to 4.55 g	No reduction in phenytoin for 8 to 24 hr at 23 °C. Inconsistent precipitate	710	I
	TR	PD	1, 1.5, 2, 4, 10 g	Visible precipitation appeared in some samples in 3 hr	951	I

Solution Compatibility (Cont.)

Phenytoin sodium

Solution	Mfr	Mfr	Conc/L	Remarks	Ref	C/I
	TR	PD	9.2 and 18.4 g	Physically compatible for 2 hr. Filtration did not reduce drug concentration	1514	C
	TR	ES, LY, SO	9.2 and 18.4 g	Microcrystals formed repeatedly, but inconsistently, over 2 hr. Filtration did not reduce drug concentration	1514	?

Additive Compatibility

Phenytoin sodium

Drug	Mfr	Conc/L	Mfr	Conc/L	Test Soln	Remarks	Ref	C/I
Amikacin sulfate	BR	5 g	PD	250 mg	D5LR, D5R, D5S, D5W, D10W, LR, NS, R, SL	Precipitates immediately	294	I
Dobutamine HCl	LI	1 g	ES	1 g	D5W, NS	White precipitate forms within 5 to 10 min	789	I
	LI	1 g	AHP	25 g	D5W, NS	White precipitate forms rapidly, with brown solution in 6 hr at 21 °C	812	I
Fat emulsion, intravenous	VT	10%	PD	1 g		Phenytoin crystal precipitation	32	I
Lidocaine HCl	AST	2 g	ES	1 g	D5W, LR, NS	Immediate formation of a white cloudy precipitate	775	I
Nitroglycerin	ACC	400 mg	PD	1 g	D5W, NS[a]	Phenytoin crystals in 24 hr. 3 to 4% nitroglycerin loss in 24 hr and 9% in 48 hr at 23 °C. Phenytoin not tested	929	I
Verapamil HCl	KN	80 mg	PD	500 mg	D5W, NS	Physically compatible for 48 hr	739	C

[a]Tested in glass containers.

Drugs in Syringe Compatibility

Phenytoin sodium

Drug (in syringe)	Mfr	Amt	Mfr	Amt	Remarks	Ref	C/I
Hydromorphone HCl	KN	2, 10, 40 mg/ 1 mL	AB	50 mg/ 1 mL	White precipitate of phenytoin forms immediately	2082	I
Pantoprazole sodium	[a]	4 mg/ 1 mL		50 mg/ 1 mL	Precipitates within 1 hr	2574	I

[a]Test performed using the formulation WITHOUT edetate disodium.

Y-Site Injection Compatibility (1:1 Mixture)

Phenytoin sodium

Drug	Mfr	Conc	Mfr	Conc	Remarks	Ref	C/I
Amphotericin B cholesteryl sulfate complex	SEQ	0.83 mg/mL[a]	ES	50 mg/mL[a]	Gross precipitate forms	2117	I
Cefepime HCl	BMS	120 mg/mL[h]		50 mg/mL	Precipitates	2513	I
Ceftazidime	GSK	120 mg/mL[h]		50 mg/mL	Precipitates	2513	I
Ciprofloxacin	MI	2 mg/mL[c]	PD	50 mg/mL	Immediate crystal formation	1655	I
Clarithromycin	AB	4 mg/mL[a]	ANT	20 mg/mL[a]	White cloudy precipitate in 1 hr at both 30 and 17 °C	2174	I
Diltiazem HCl	MMD	1 mg/mL[b]	PD	50 mg/mL	Precipitate forms	1807	I
Enalaprilat	MSD	1.25 mg/mL	PD	1 mg/mL[b]	Crystalline precipitate forms immediately	1409	I
Esmolol HCl	DCC	10 mg/mL[a]	IX	1 mg/mL[a]	Physically compatible for 24 hr at 22 °C	1169	C
Famotidine	MSD	0.2 mg/mL[a]	PD	50 mg/mL	Physically compatible for 14 hr	1196	C
Fenoldopam mesylate	AB	80 mcg/mL[b]	ES	50 mg/mL	Microcrystals and yellowish darkening form immediately	2467	I
Fentanyl citrate	JN	0.025 mg/mL[a]	ES	2 mg/mL[a,b]	Precipitate forms within 1 hr	1706	I
Fluconazole	RR	2 mg/mL	PD	50 mg/mL	Physically compatible for 24 hr at 25 °C	1407	C
Heparin sodium	TR	50 units/mL	ES	2 mg/mL[b]	Cloudy immediately and becomes white precipitate in 4 hr at 25 °C	1793	I
Heparin sodium[i]	RI	1000 units/L[d]	PD	50 mg/mL	Immediate crystal formation	322	I
Hydrocortisone sodium succinate[g]	UP	100 mg/L[d]	PD	50 mg/mL	Immediate crystal formation	322	I
Hydromorphone HCl	KN	2, 10, 40 mg/mL	AB	50 mg/mL	Turbidity forms immediately and phenytoin precipitate develops	1532	I
	AST	0.5 mg/mL[a]	ES	2 mg/mL[a,b]	Precipitate forms within 1 hr	1706	I
Hydroxyethyl starch 130/0.4 in sodium chloride 0.9%	FRK	6%	SZ	6, 7.5, 9 mg/mL[a]	White precipitate forms immediately	2770	I
Linezolid	PHU	2 mg/mL	ES	50 mg/mL	Crystalline precipitate forms immediately	2264	I
Methadone HCl	LI	1 mg/mL[a]	ES	2 mg/mL[a,b]	Precipitate forms immediately	1706	I
Micafungin sodium	ASP	1.5 mg/mL[b]	HOS	50 mg/mL	Measured haze increases within 1 hr	2683	I
Morphine sulfate	AST	1 mg/mL[a]	ES	2 mg/mL[a,b]	Precipitate forms after 1 hr	1706	I
Potassium chloride		40 mEq/L[a]	PD	50 mg/mL	Immediate formation of phenytoin crystals	322	I
		40 mEq/L[e]	PD	50 mg/mL	Crystals in 4 hr at room temperature	322	I
Propofol	ZEN	10 mg/mL	ES	50 mg/mL	Needle-like crystals form immediately	2066	I
Tacrolimus	FUJ	1 mg/mL[b]	ES	5 mg/mL[a]	Visually compatible for 4 hr at 25 °C. White haze forms by 24 hr	1630	C
Theophylline	TR	4 mg/mL	ES	2 mg/mL[b]	Immediately cloudy. Dense precipitate in 6 hr at 25 °C	1793	I

Y-Site Injection Compatibility (1:1 Mixture) (Cont.)

Phenytoin sodium

Drug	Mfr	Conc	Mfr	Conc	Remarks	Ref	C/I
TPN #189ᶠ			PD	50 mg/mL	Heavy white precipitate forms immediately	1767	I
Vasopressin	APP	0.2 unit/mLᵇ	ES	50 mg/mL	Crystals form immediately	2641	I

ᵃ*Tested in dextrose 5%.*
ᵇ*Tested in sodium chloride 0.9%.*
ᶜ*Tested in both dextrose 5% and sodium chloride 0.9%.*
ᵈ*Tested in dextrose 5%, Ringer's injection, lactated, and sodium chloride 0.9%.*
ᵉ*Tested in both Ringer's injection, lactated and sodium chloride 0.9%.*
ᶠ*Refer to Appendix I for the composition of parenteral nutrition solutions. TPN indicates a 2-in-1 admixture.*
ᵍ*Tested in combination with heparin sodium (Riker) 1000 units/L.*
ʰ*Tested in sterile water for injection.*
ⁱ*Tested in combination with hydrocortisone sodium succinate (Upjohn) 100 mg/L.*

PHYTONADIONE
(PHYTOMENADIONE)
AHFS 88:24

Products — Phytonadione is available as a 2-mg/mL aqueous dispersion in 0.5-mL ampuls and as a 10-mg/mL aqueous dispersion in 1-mL ampuls and 5-mL vials. Each milliliter also contains polyoxyethylated fatty acid 70 mg, dextrose 37.5 mg, and benzyl alcohol 0.9% in water for injection. (1)

pH — The USP cites the official pH range as 3.5 to 7. (17) Phytonadione (Hospira) has a pH of 5 to 7. (1)

Osmolality — The osmolality of phytonadione 10 mg/mL was 325 mOsm/kg by freezing-point depression and 303 mOsm/kg by vapor pressure. (1071)

Administration — The intramuscular or subcutaneous routes are preferred for phytonadione. If intravenous injection is unavoidable, phytonadione may be given by direct intravenous injection at a rate not exceeding 1 mg/min or by intravenous infusion. (1; 4)

Stability — Phytonadione injection is available as an essentially clear yellow liquid. Phytonadione is photosensitive and should be protected from light at all times. (1; 4) When dilutions are indicated, administration should start immediately after mixing with the diluent; unused portions of the dilution, as well as unused contents of the ampul, should be discarded. (4)

Light Effects — A study of phytonadione in intravenous solutions showed 50% decomposition in 15 days under fluorescent light and 43 to 63% in three hours on exposure to sunlight. (463) A 10 to 15% loss occurs over 24 hours on exposure to fluorescent light or sunlight. (854) It has been recommended that infusion solutions containing phytonadione require wrapping the container with aluminum foil or other opaque material for light protection. (4)

The loss of phytonadione (Roche) 0.05 to 0.1 mg/mL from solutions in glass and polypropylene containers unprotected or packaged in light-protective overwraps when exposed to neon light and daylight was evaluated. Losses approached 80% in one day unprotected from light exposure. A brown polyethylene light protection bag provided the best protection, yielding no phytonadione loss during a seven-day exposure period. A white "light-tight" light-protective overwrap and a black plastic waste disposal bag failed to protect the phytonadione completely. In the black bag, phytonadione losses of over 30% occurred in seven days; the white light-protective overwrap was worse, allowing loss of nearly half of the phytonadione in one day. Substantial differences in light protection are afforded by the different materials and the efficacy of purported light-protection barriers for light-sensitive drugs should be validated prior to use. (1923)

Substantial loss of phytonadione from both TPN and TNA admixtures due to exposure to sunlight was reported. In three hours of exposure to sunlight, 50% loss of phytonadione had occurred. The presence or absence of lipids did not affect stability. (2049)

Filtration — The manufacturer states that phytonadione passes through an inline filter with negligible loss occurring. (854)

Compatibility Information

Solution Compatibility

Phytonadione

Solution	Mfr	Mfr	Conc/L	Remarks	Ref	C/I
Amino acids 2%, dextrose 12.5%		ROR	5 mL	7% phytonadione loss in 4 hr and 27% loss in 24 hr under ambient temperature and light	1815	**I**
Amino acids 4.25%, dextrose 25%	MG	MSD	10 mg	No increase in particulate matter in 24 hr at 4 °C	349	**C**
Dextrose 2.5%	AB	AB	50 mg	Physically compatible	3	**C**
Dextrose 5%	AB	AB	50 mg	Physically compatible	3	**C**
Dextrose 10%	AB	AB	50 mg	Physically compatible	3	**C**
Dextrose–Ringer's injection combinations	AB	AB	50 mg	Physically compatible	3	**C**
Dextrose–Ringer's injection, lactated, combinations	AB	AB	50 mg	Physically compatible	3	**C**
Dextrose–saline combinations	AB	AB	50 mg	Physically compatible	3	**C**
Ionosol products	AB	AB	50 mg	Physically compatible	3	**C**
Ringer's injection	AB	AB	50 mg	Physically compatible	3	**C**
Ringer's injection, lactated	AB	AB	50 mg	Physically compatible	3	**C**
Sodium chloride 0.45%	AB	AB	50 mg	Physically compatible	3	**C**
Sodium chloride 0.9%	AB	AB	50 mg	Physically compatible	3	**C**
Sodium lactate ⅙ M	AB	AB	50 mg	Physically compatible	3	**C**

Additive Compatibility

Phytonadione

Drug	Mfr	Conc/L	Mfr	Conc/L	Test Soln	Remarks	Ref	C/I
Amikacin sulfate	BR	5 g	MSD	200 mg	D5LR, D5R, D5S, D5W, D10W, LR, NS, R, SL	Physically compatible and amikacin stable for 24 hr at 25 °C. Phytonadione not analyzed	294	**C**
Chloramphenicol sodium succinate	PD	1 g	MSD	50 mg		Physically compatible	6	**C**
Ranitidine HCl	GL	50 mg and 2 g		100 mg	D5W	Ranitidine stable for only 6 hr at 25 °C. Phytonadione not tested	1515	**I**
Sodium bicarbonate	AB	2.4 mEq[a]	MSD	10 mg	D5W	Physically compatible for 24 hr	772	**C**

[a] One vial of Neut added to a liter of admixture.

Drugs in Syringe Compatibility

Phytonadione

Drug (in syringe)	Mfr	Amt	Mfr	Amt	Remarks	Ref	C/I
Doxapram HCl	RB	400 mg/ 20 mL		10 mg/ 1 mL	Physically compatible with no doxapram loss in 24 hr	1177	**C**

Y-Site Injection Compatibility (1:1 Mixture)

Phytonadione

Drug	Mfr	Conc	Mfr	Conc	Remarks	Ref	C/I
Ampicillin sodium	WY	40 mg/mL[b]	MSD	0.4 mg/mL[c]	Physically compatible for 3 hr	1316	**C**
Dobutamine HCl	LI	4 mg/mL[c]	MSD	0.4 mg/mL[c]	Slight haze in 3 hr	1316	**I**
Epinephrine HCl	ES	0.032 mg/mL[c]	MSD	0.4 mg/mL[c]	Physically compatible for 3 hr	1316	**C**
Famotidine	MSD	0.2 mg/mL[a]	MSD	2 mg/mL	Physically compatible for 14 hr	1196	**C**
Heparin sodium	UP	1000 units/L[d]	RC	10 mg/mL	Physically compatible for 4 hr at room temperature	534	**C**
Hydrocortisone sodium succinate	UP	10 mg/L[d]	RC	10 mg/mL	Physically compatible for 4 hr at room temperature	534	**C**
Potassium chloride	AB	40 mEq/L[d]	RC	10 mg/mL	Physically compatible for 4 hr at room temperature	534	**C**

[a] *Tested in dextrose 5%.*
[b] *Tested in sodium chloride 0.9%.*
[c] *Tested in both dextrose 5% and sodium chloride 0.9%.*
[d] *Tested in dextrose 5% in Ringer's injection, dextrose 5% in Ringer's injection, lactated, dextrose 5%, Ringer's injection, lactated, and sodium chloride 0.9%.*

PIPERACILLIN SODIUM–TAZOBACTAM SODIUM
AHFS 8:12.16.16

Products — Piperacillin sodium–tazobactam sodium is available in vials containing 2.25 g (piperacillin 2 g plus tazobactam 250 mg), 3.375 g (piperacillin 3 g plus tazobactam 375 mg), and 4.5 g (piperacillin 4 g plus tazobactam 500 mg) as sodium salts. The drug is also available in a pharmacy bulk package containing 40.5 g (piperacillin 36 plus tazobactam 4.5) as sodium salts. The Zosyn products contain EDTA 0.25 mg per gram of piperacillin. Other products do not have EDTA in their formulations. The pH may have been adjusted during manufacture with sodium bicarbonate and hydrochloric acid. (1; 4)

Each gram of piperacillin should be reconstituted with at least 5 mL of sterile water for injection, sodium chloride 0.9%, bacteriostatic water for injection or bacteriostatic sodium chloride 0.9% (preserved with benzyl alcohol or parabens), or dextrose 5% and shaken well until dissolved. Dilute in at least 50 mL of compatible infusion solution for intermittent infusion. (1)

The pharmacy bulk package is reconstituted with 152 mL of compatible diluent to yield a solution containing 200 mg/mL of piperacillin and 25 mg/mL of tazobactam. The reconstituted pharmacy bulk package solution must be diluted further for use. (4)

Piperacillin sodium–tazobactam sodium (Zosyn) is also available as frozen iso-osmotic injections containing piperacillin sodium 40 mg/mL with tazobactam 5 mg/mL and piperacillin sodium 60 mg/mL with tazobactam sodium 7.5 mg/mL and EDTA. (1; 4)

pH — Vials: From 4.5 to 6.8. (4) Frozen premixed solution: From 5.5 to 6.8. (1)

Trade Name(s) — Zosyn.

Administration — Piperacillin sodium–tazobactam sodium should be administered by intravenous infusion over at least 30 minutes after dilution to at least 50 mL in a compatible diluent. It can also be infused using ambulatory infusion pumps. (1; 4)

Stability — The white to off-white lyophilized powder in intact vials should be stored at controlled room temperature. (1)

Single-dose vials of the solution should be used immediately after reconstitution. Any remaining portion should be discarded after 24 hours at room temperature or 48 hours under refrigeration at 2 to 8 °C. (1; 4)

In compatible infusion solutions, the drug is stable for up to 24 hours at room temperature or one week under refrigeration. Glass and plastic (including syringes, intravenous solution bags, and tubing) do not affect stability. (1)

The physical and chemical stability of piperacillin sodium–tazobactam sodium at concentrations of 200 and 25 mcg/mL, respectively, were evaluated in Dianeal PD-2 with dextrose 1.5% and Dianeal PD-2 with dextrose 4.25%. Samples were stored at 4 °C for 14 days, 23 °C for seven days, and 37 °C for one day. The samples were physically and chemically stable. Little or no loss of either component occurred in the 4 °C samples throughout the 14-day period. At 23 °C, losses of each component were in the range of 3 to 6% in seven days. The one-day losses at 37 °C were similarly small, (2018)

Freezing Solutions — The commercially available frozen injections should be stored at or below −20 °C. Thaw at room temperature or under refrigeration but not in a warm water bath or by microwave radiation. Thawed solutions should not be refrozen. After thawing, the solutions are stable for 24 hours at room temperature or 14 days refrigerated. (1; 4)

Piperacillin sodium–tazobactam sodium 80 + 10 mg/mL in PVC bags of dextrose 5% and sodium chloride 0.9% was frozen at −15 °C for 30 days and thawed by microwave radiation for 45 seconds with no loss of either component. (1768)

Piperacillin sodium–tazobactam sodium 150 + 18.75 mg/mL and 200 + 25 mg/mL in dextrose 5% and sodium chloride 0.9% was drawn as 20-mL aliquots into polypropylene syringes (Becton Dickinson). The syringes were frozen at −15 °C for 30 days and then stored at 4 °C for seven days with no loss of either component. (1768)

Piperacillin sodium–tazobactam sodium 40 + 5 mg/mL in dextrose 5% lost less than 3% after three months stored at −20 °C. After microwave thawing, refrigerated storage resulted in 10% loss in 35 days. (2614)

Syringes — Piperacillin sodium–tazobactam sodium 150 + 18.75 mg/mL and 200 + 25 mg/mL in dextrose 5% and sodium chloride 0.9% was drawn as 20-mL aliquots into polypropylene syringes (Becton Dickinson). The syringes were stored at 25 °C for one day and at 4 °C

for seven days with no loss of either drug in the dextrose 5% samples. Similarly, no tazobactam loss occurred in the sodium chloride 0.9% solutions. However, piperacillin losses of 7% in one day at 25 °C and 4% in seven days at 4 °C were found in the sodium chloride 0.9% solutions. (1768)

Ambulatory Pumps — The product was shown to be stable for up to 12 hours in an ambulatory infusion pump. Each dose was diluted to 25 or 37.5 mL, and stability was not affected. (1)

Central Venous Catheter — Piperacillin sodium–tazobactam sodium (Lederle) 10 + 1.25 mg/mL in dextrose 5% was found to be compatible with the ARROWg+ard Blue Plus (Arrow International) chlorhexidine-bearing triple-lumen central catheter. Essentially complete delivery of the drug was found with little or no drug loss occurring. Furthermore, chlorhexidine delivered from the catheter remained at trace amounts with no substantial increase due to the delivery of the drug through the catheter. (2335)

Compatibility Information

Solution Compatibility

Piperacillin sodium–tazobactam sodium

Solution	Mfr	Mfr	Conc/L	Remarks	Ref	C/I
Dextrose 5%				Compatible	1	C
	BA[a]	WY[d]	20 + 2.5, 80 + 10 g	Visually compatible. Little loss of either drug in 28 days at 5 °C then 72 hr at 23 °C in light	2806	C
Ringer's injection, lactated	[c]			Incompatible	1	I
	WY[d]			Compatible	1	C
Sodium chloride 0.9%				Compatible	1	C
	BA[a]	WY[c]	40 + 5 g	Calculated 10% loss in 5.8 days at 7 °C and 3.8 days at room temperature in light	2667	C
	BA[b]	WY[c]	40 + 5 g	Calculated 10% loss in 17.7 days at 7 °C and 2.8 days at room temperature in light	2667	C
	BA[a]	WY[d]	20 + 2.5, 80 + 10 g	Visually compatible. 5% tazobactam and 2% piperacillin loss in 28 days at 5 °C then 72 hr at 23 °C in light	2806	C

[a]*Tested in PVC containers.*
[b]*Tested in polyolefin containers.*
[c]*Test performed using the formulation WITHOUT edetate disodium.*
[d]*Test performed using the formulation WITH edetate disodium.*

Drugs in Syringe Compatibility

Piperacillin sodium–tazobactam sodium

Drug (in syringe)	Mfr	Amt	Mfr	Amt	Remarks	Ref	C/I
Dimenhydrinate		10 mg/ 1 mL	[a]	200 + 25 mg/ 1 mL	Clear solution	2569	C
Pantoprazole sodium	[a]	4 mg/ 1 mL	[a]	200 + 25 mg/ 1 mL	Precipitates within 1 hr	2574	I

[a]*Test performed using the formulation WITHOUT edetate disodium.*

Y-Site Injection Compatibility (1:1 Mixture)

Piperacillin sodium–tazobactam sodium

Drug	Mfr	Conc	Mfr	Conc	Remarks	Ref	C/I
Acyclovir sodium	BW	7 mg/mL[a]	LE[g]	40 + 5 mg/mL[a]	Particles form in 1 hr	1688	I
Aminophylline	AB	2.5 mg/mL[a]	LE[g]	40 + 5 mg/mL[a]	Physically compatible for 4 hr at 22 °C	1688	C
Amiodarone HCl	WY	6 mg/mL[a]	LE[g]	60 + 7.5 mg/mL[a]	White haze in 24 hr at 22 °C	2352	I
Amphotericin B	SQ	0.6 mg/mL[a]	LE[g]	40 + 5 mg/mL[a]	Yellow precipitate forms immediately	1688	I
Amphotericin B cholesteryl sulfate complex	SEQ	0.83 mg/mL[a]	CY[g]	40 + 5 mg/mL[a]	Microprecipitate forms immediately	2117	I
Anidulafungin	VIC	0.5 mg/mL[a]	LE[g]	40 + 5 mg/mL[a]	Physically compatible for 4 hr at 23 °C	2617	C
Azithromycin	PF	2 mg/mL[b]	LE[g]	100 + 12.5 mg/mL[b,f]	White microcrystals found	2368	I
Aztreonam	SQ	40 mg/mL[a]	LE[g]	40 + 5 mg/mL[a]	Physically compatible for 4 hr at 22 °C	1688	C
Bivalirudin	TMC	5 mg/mL[a]	LE[g]	40 + 5 mg/mL[a]	Physically compatible for 4 hr at 23 °C	2373	C
Bleomycin sulfate	BR	1 unit/mL[b]	LE[g]	40 + 5 mg/mL[a]	Physically compatible for 4 hr at 22 °C	1688	C
Bumetanide	RC	0.04 mg/mL[a]	LE[g]	40 + 5 mg/mL[a]	Physically compatible for 4 hr at 22 °C	1688	C
Buprenorphine HCl	RKC	0.04 mg/mL[a]	LE[g]	40 + 5 mg/mL[a]	Physically compatible for 4 hr at 22 °C	1688	C
Butorphanol tartrate	BR	0.04 mg/mL[a]	LE[g]	40 + 5 mg/mL[a]	Physically compatible for 4 hr at 23 °C	1688	C
Calcium gluconate	AMR	40 mg/mL[a]	LE[g]	40 + 5 mg/mL[a]	Physically compatible for 4 hr at 22 °C	1688	C
Carboplatin	BR	5 mg/mL[a]	LE[g]	40 + 5 mg/mL[a]	Physically compatible for 4 hr at 22 °C	1688	C
Carmustine	BR	1.5 mg/mL[a]	LE[g]	40 + 5 mg/mL[a]	Physically compatible for 4 hr at 22 °C	1688	C
Caspofungin acetate	ME	0.7 mg/mL[b]	WY[h]	40 + 5 mg/mL[b]	Immediate white turbid precipitate forms	2758	I
	ME	0.5 mg/mL[b]	WY[g]	80 + 10 mg/mL[b]	Black particles reported	2766	I
Chlorpromazine HCl	RU	2 mg/mL[a]	LE[g]	40 + 5 mg/mL[a]	Heavy white turbidity forms immediately. White precipitate forms in 4 hr	1688	I
Cisatracurium besylate	GW	0.1 and 2 mg/mL[a]	CY[g]	40 + 5 mg/mL[a]	Physically compatible for 4 hr at 23 °C	2074	C
	GW	5 mg/mL[a]	CY[g]	40 + 5 mg/mL[a]	Particles and subvisible haze within 4 hr	2074	I
Cisplatin	BR	1 mg/mL	LE[g]	40 + 5 mg/mL[a]	Haze and particles form in 1 hr	1688	I
Clindamycin phosphate	AB	10 mg/mL[a]	LE[g]	40 + 5 mg/mL[a]	Physically compatible for 4 hr at 22 °C	1688	C

Y-Site Injection Compatibility (1:1 Mixture) (Cont.)

Piperacillin sodium–tazobactam sodium

Drug	Mfr	Conc	Mfr	Conc	Remarks	Ref	C/I
Cyclophosphamide	MJ	10 mg/mL[a]	LE[g]	40 + 5 mg/mL[a]	Physically compatible for 4 hr at 22 °C	1688	C
Cytarabine	SCN	50 mg/mL	LE[g]	40 + 5 mg/mL[a]	Physically compatible for 4 hr at 22 °C	1688	C
Dacarbazine	MI	4 mg/mL[a]	LE[g]	40 + 5 mg/mL[a]	Turbidity and particles form immediately and increase over 4 hr	1688	I
Daunorubicin HCl	WY	1 mg/mL[a]	LE[g]	40 + 5 mg/mL[a]	Turbidity increases immediately	1688	I
Dexamethasone sodium phosphate	LY	1 mg/mL[a]	LE[g]	40 + 5 mg/mL[a]	Physically compatible for 4 hr at 22 °C	1688	C
Dexmedetomidine HCl	AB	4 mcg/mL[b]	LE[g]	40 + 5 mg/mL[b]	Physically compatible for 4 hr at 23 °C	2383	C
Diphenhydramine HCl	WY	2 mg/mL[a]	LE[g]	40 + 5 mg/mL[a]	Physically compatible for 4 hr at 22 °C	1688	C
Dobutamine HCl	LI	4 mg/mL[a]	LE[g]	40 + 5 mg/mL[a]	Heavy white turbidity forms immediately	1688	I
Docetaxel	RPR	0.9 mg/mL[a]	CY[g]	40 + 5 mg/mL[a]	Physically compatible for 4 hr at 23 °C	2224	C
Dopamine HCl	AST	3.2 mg/mL[a]	LE[g]	40 + 5 mg/mL[a]	Physically compatible for 4 hr at 22 °C	1688	C
Doxorubicin HCl	CET	2 mg/mL	LE[g]	40 + 5 mg/mL[a]	Turbidity forms immediately	1688	I
Doxorubicin HCl liposomal	SEQ	0.4 mg/mL[a]	CY[g]	40 + 5 mg/mL[a]	Partial loss of measured natural turbidity	2087	I
Doxycycline hyclate	ES	1 mg/mL[a]	LE[g]	40 + 5 mg/mL[a]	Heavy white turbidity forms immediately	1688	I
Droperidol	JN	0.4 mg/mL[a]	LE[g]	40 + 5 mg/mL[a]	Heavy white turbidity with white precipitate forms immediately	1688	I
Enalaprilat	MSD	0.1 mg/mL[a]	LE[g]	40 + 5 mg/mL[a]	Physically compatible for 4 hr at 22 °C	1688	C
Etoposide	BR	0.4 mg/mL[a]	LE[g]	40 + 5 mg/mL[a]	Physically compatible for 4 hr at 22 °C	1688	C
Etoposide phosphate	BR	5 mg/mL[a]	LE[g]	40 + 5 mg/mL[b]	Physically compatible for 4 hr at 23 °C	2218	C
Famotidine	MSD	2 mg/mL[a]	LE[g]	40 + 5 mg/mL[a]	Particles form immediately	1688	I
Fenoldopam mesylate	AB	80 mcg/mL[b]	LE[g]	40 + 5 mg/mL[b]	Physically compatible for 4 hr at 23 °C	2467	C
Floxuridine	RC	3 mg/mL[a]	LE[g]	40 + 5 mg/mL[a]	Physically compatible for 4 hr at 22 °C	1688	C
Fluconazole	RR	2 mg/mL	LE[g]	40 + 5 mg/mL[a]	Physically compatible for 4 hr at 22 °C	1688	C
Fludarabine phosphate	BX	1 mg/mL[a]	LE[g]	40 + 5 mg/mL[a]	Physically compatible for 4 hr at 22 °C	1688	C
Fluorouracil	LY	16 mg/mL[a]	LE[g]	40 + 5 mg/mL[a]	Physically compatible for 4 hr at 22 °C	1688	C

Y-Site Injection Compatibility (1:1 Mixture) (Cont.)

Piperacillin sodium–tazobactam sodium

Drug	Mfr	Conc	Mfr	Conc	Remarks	Ref	C/I
Furosemide	AB	3 mg/mL[a]	LE[g]	40 + 5 mg/mL[a]	Physically compatible for 4 hr at 22 °C	1688	C
Gallium nitrate	FUJ	0.4 mg/mL[a]	LE[g]	40 + 5 mg/mL[a]	Physically compatible for 4 hr at 22 °C	1688	C
Ganciclovir sodium	SY	20 mg/mL[a]	LE[g]	40 + 5 mg/mL[a]	Large crystals form in 1 hr and become heavy white precipitate in 4 hr	1688	I
Gemcitabine HCl	LI	10 mg/mL[b]	LE[g]	40 + 5 mg/mL[b]	Cloudiness forms immediately, becoming flocculent precipitate in 1 hr	2226	I
Granisetron HCl	SKB	0.05 mg/mL[a]	CY[g]	40 + 5 mg/mL[a]	Physically compatible for 4 hr at 23 °C	2000	C
Haloperidol lactate	MN	0.2 mg/mL[a]	LE[g]	40 + 5 mg/mL[a]	White turbidity and particles form immediately	1688	I
Heparin sodium	ES	100 units/mL[a]	LE[g]	40 + 5 mg/mL[a]	Physically compatible for 4 hr at 22 °C	1688	C
Hetastarch in lactated electrolyte	AB	6%	LE[g]	40 + 5 mg/mL[a]	Physically compatible for 4 hr at 23 °C	2339	C
Hydrocortisone sodium succinate	UP	1 mg/mL[a]	LE[g]	40 + 5 mg/mL[a]	Physically compatible for 4 hr at 22 °C	1688	C
Hydromorphone HCl	ES	0.5 mg/mL[a]	LE[g]	40 + 5 mg/mL[a]	Physically compatible for 4 hr at 22 °C	1688	C
Hydroxyzine HCl	WI	4 mg/mL[a]	LE[g]	40 + 5 mg/mL[a]	Haze and particles form immediately	1688	I
Idarubicin HCl	AD	0.5 mg/mL[a]	LE[g]	40 + 5 mg/mL[a]	Immediate increase in haze	1688	I
Ifosfamide	MJ	25 mg/mL[a]	LE[g]	40 + 5 mg/mL[a]	Physically compatible for 4 hr at 22 °C	1688	C
Leucovorin calcium	LE	2 mg/mL[a]	LE[g]	40 + 5 mg/mL[a]	Physically compatible for 4 hr at 22 °C	1688	C
Linezolid	PHU	2 mg/mL	LE[g]	40 + 5 mg/mL[a]	Physically compatible for 4 hr at 23 °C	2264	C
Lorazepam	WY	0.1 mg/mL[a]	LE[g]	40 + 5 mg/mL[a]	Physically compatible for 4 hr at 22 °C	1688	C
Magnesium sulfate	AST	100 mg/mL	LE[g]	40 + 5 mg/mL[a]	Physically compatible for 4 hr at 22 °C	1688	C
Mannitol	BA	15%	LE[g]	40 + 5 mg/mL[a]	Physically compatible for 4 hr at 22 °C	1688	C
Meperidine HCl	WY	4 mg/mL[a]	LE[g]	40 + 5 mg/mL[a]	Physically compatible for 4 hr at 22 °C	1688	C
Mesna	MJ	10 mg/mL[a]	LE[g]	40 + 5 mg/mL[a]	Physically compatible for 4 hr at 22 °C	1688	C
Methotrexate sodium	LE	15 mg/mL[a]	LE[g]	40 + 5 mg/mL[a]	Physically compatible for 4 hr at 22 °C	1688	C
Methylprednisolone sodium succinate	AB	5 mg/mL[a]	LE[g]	40 + 5 mg/mL[a]	Physically compatible for 4 hr at 22 °C	1688	C
Metoclopramide HCl	RB	5 mg/mL	LE[g]	40 + 5 mg/mL[a]	Physically compatible for 4 hr at 22 °C	1688	C

Y-Site Injection Compatibility (1:1 Mixture) (Cont.)

Piperacillin sodium–tazobactam sodium

Drug	Mfr	Conc	Mfr	Conc	Remarks	Ref	C/I
Metronidazole	BA	5 mg/mL	LE[g]	40 + 5 mg/mL[a]	Physically compatible for 4 hr at 22 °C	1688	C
Milrinone lactate	SS	0.2 mg/mL[a]	LE[g]	200 + 25 mg/mL	Visually compatible for 4 hr at 25 °C	2381	C
Mitomycin	BR	0.5 mg/mL	LE[g]	40 + 5 mg/mL[a]	Blue color darkens in 4 hr, becoming reddish purple in 24 hr	1688	I
Mitoxantrone HCl	LE	0.5 mg/mL[a]	LE[g]	40 + 5 mg/mL[a]	Haze and particles form immediately. Large particles form in 4 hr	1688	I
Morphine sulfate	WY	1 mg/mL[a]	LE[g]	40 + 5 mg/mL[a]	Physically compatible for 4 hr at 22 °C	1688	C
Nalbuphine HCl	DU	10 mg/mL	LE[g]	40 + 5 mg/mL[a]	Heavy white turbidity forms immediately. Particles form in 4 hr	1688	I
Ondansetron HCl	GL	1 mg/mL[a]	LE[g]	40 + 5 mg/mL[a]	Physically compatible for 4 hr at 22 °C	1688	C
	GL	0.03, 0.1, 0.3 mg/mL[b]	LE[g]	40 + 5 mg/mL[b]	Visually compatible with no loss of any component in 4 hr	1752	C
	GL	0.03, 0.1, 0.3 mg/mL[b]	LE[g]	80 + 10 mg/mL[b]	Visually compatible with no loss of any component in 4 hr	1752	C
Potassium chloride	AB	0.1 mEq/mL[a]	LE[g]	40 + 5 mg/mL[a]	Physically compatible for 4 hr at 22 °C	1688	C
Prochlorperazine edisylate	SCN	0.5 mg/mL[a]	LE[g]	40 + 5 mg/mL[a]	White turbidity forms immediately	1688	I
Promethazine HCl	SCN	2 mg/mL[a]	LE[g]	40 + 5 mg/mL[a]	Heavy white turbidity forms immediately. Particles form in 4 hr	1688	I
Ranitidine HCl	GL	2 mg/mL[a]	LE[g]	40 + 5 mg/mL[a]	Physically compatible for 4 hr at 22 °C	1688	C
	GL	0.5 and 2 mg/mL[b]	LE[g]	80 + 10 mg/mL[b]	Visually compatible. Little loss of any component in 4 hr at 23 °C	1759	C
	GL	0.5 and 2 mg/mL[b]	LE[g]	40 + 5 mg/mL[b]	Visually compatible. Little loss of ranitidine and tazobactam in 4 hr at 23 °C. Piperacillin not tested	1759	C
Remifentanil HCl	GW	0.025 and 0.25 mg/mL[b]	CY[g]	40 + 5 mg/mL[a]	Physically compatible for 4 hr at 23 °C	2075	C
Sargramostim	HO	10 mcg/mL[a]	LE[g]	40 + 5 mg/mL[a]	Physically compatible for 4 hr at 22 °C	1688	C
Sodium bicarbonate	AB	1 mEq/mL	LE[g]	40 + 5 mg/mL[a]	Physically compatible for 4 hr at 22 °C	1688	C
Streptozocin	UP	40 mg/mL[a]	LE[g]	40 + 5 mg/mL[a]	Particles form in 1 hr	1688	I
Telavancin HCl	ASP	7.5 mg/mL[a,b,e]	WY[h]	40 + 5 mg/mL[a,b,e]	Physically compatible for 2 hr	2830	C
Thiotepa	LE	1 mg/mL[a]	LE[g]	40 + 5 mg/mL[a]	Physically compatible for 4 hr at 22 °C	1688	C
Tigecycline	WY	1 mg/mL[b]		3 + 0.375 mg/mL[b]	Physically compatible for 4 hr	2714	C
TNA #218 to #226[c]			LE[g]	40 + 5 mg/mL[a]	Visually compatible for 4 hr at 23 °C	2215	C

Y-Site Injection Compatibility (1:1 Mixture) (Cont.)

Piperacillin sodium–tazobactam sodium

Drug	Mfr	Conc	Mfr	Conc	Remarks	Ref	C/I
Tobramycin sulfate					Incompatible	1	**I**
TPN #212 to #215[c]			CY[g]	40 + 5 mg/mL[a]	Physically compatible for 4 hr at 23 °C	2109	**C**
Trimethoprim–sulfamethoxazole	ES	0.8 + 4 mg/mL[a]	LE[g]	40 + 5 mg/mL[a]	Physically compatible for 4 hr at 22 °C	1688	**C**
Vancomycin HCl	AB	10 mg/mL[a]	LE[g]	40 + 5 mg/mL[a]	White turbidity forms immediately and white precipitate forms in 4 hr	1688	**I**
	AB	20 mg/mL[a]	LE[g]	200 + 25 mg/mL[d]	Transient precipitate forms	2189	**?**
	AB	20 mg/mL[a]	LE[g]	10 + 1.25 and 50 + 6.25 mg/mL[a]	Gross white precipitate forms immediately	2189	**I**
	AB	20 mg/mL[a]	LE[g]	1 + 0.125 mg/mL[a]	Physically compatible for 4 hr at 23 °C	2189	**C**
	AB	2 mg/mL[a]	LE[g]	1 + 0.125[a], 10 + 1.25[a], 50 + 6.25[a], 200 + 25[d] mg/mL	Physically compatible for 4 hr at 23 °C	2189	**C**
Vasopressin	APP	0.2 unit/mL[b]	WY[g]	100 + 12.5 mg/mL	Physically compatible	2641	**C**
Vinblastine sulfate	LI	0.12 mg/mL[a]	LE[g]	40 + 5 mg/mL[a]	Physically compatible for 4 hr at 22 °C	1688	**C**
Vincristine sulfate	LI	0.05 mg/mL[a]	LE[g]	40 + 5 mg/mL[a]	Physically compatible for 4 hr at 22 °C	1688	**C**
Zidovudine	BW	4 mg/mL[a]	LE[g]	40 + 5 mg/mL[a]	Physically compatible for 4 hr at 22 °C	1688	**C**

[a]*Tested in dextrose 5%.*
[b]*Tested in sodium chloride 0.9%.*
[c]*Refer to Appendix I for the composition of parenteral nutrition solutions. TNA indicates a 3-in-1 admixture, and TPN indicates a 2-in-1 admixture.*
[d]*Tested in sterile water for injection.*
[e]*Tested in Ringer's injection, lactated.*
[f]*Injected via Y-site into an administration set running azithromycin.*
[g]*Test performed using the formulation WITHOUT edetate disodium.*
[h]*Test performed using the formulation WITH edetate disodium.*

POLYMYXIN B SULFATE
AHFS 8:12.28.28

Products — Polymyxin B sulfate is available in 10-mL vials containing 500,000 units of polymyxin B. For intramuscular injection, reconstitute the vial with 2 mL of sterile water for injection or sodium chloride 0.9%. For intravenous infusion, dilute 500,000 units in 300 to 500 mL of dextrose 5%. For intrathecal administration, reconstitute the vial with 10 mL of sodium chloride 0.9%. (1; 4)

Units — Each milligram of polymyxin base is equivalent to 10,000 units. Each microgram is equivalent to 10 units. (4)

pH — From 5 to 7.5. (4)

Administration — Polymyxin B sulfate is usually administered by intravenous infusion; 500,000 units is added to 300 to 500 mL of dextrose 5% (providing 1667 to 1000 units/mL) and is administered over 60 to 90 minutes. The drug may also be administered intrathecally as a 50,000-units/mL solution in sodium chloride 0.9%. Although it may be administered by deep intramuscular injection in the upper outer quadrant of the gluteal muscles, this route is generally not recommended, because severe pain at the injection site results. (4)

Stability — Intact vials should be stored at controlled room temperature and protected from light. Aqueous solutions in the pH range of 5 to 7.5 are stable for six to 12 months under refrigeration. However, it is recommended that unused portions of the reconstituted solution be discarded after 72 hours. Polymyxin B sulfate is inactivated in strongly acidic or alkaline solutions. (4) The pH of maximum stability is pH 3.4. (2422) In the pH range of 2 to 7, pH has little effect on the rate of decomposition. However, as pH values become more alkaline, the rate of decomposition increases markedly. (1946)

Compatibility Information

Solution Compatibility

Polymyxin B sulfate

Solution	Mfr	Mfr	Conc/L	Remarks	Ref	C/I
Sodium chloride 0.9%	HOS	APP, BED, XGN	56 to 78 mg	Under 10% loss in 24 hr at 4 and 23 °C	2816	C
TPN #52, #53[a]		NOV	40 mg	Physically compatible with no polymyxin loss in 24 hr at 29 °C	440	C

[a]*Refer to Appendix I for the composition of parenteral nutrition solutions. TPN indicates a 2-in-1 admixture.*

Additive Compatibility

Polymyxin B sulfate

Drug	Mfr	Conc/L	Mfr	Conc/L	Test Soln	Remarks	Ref	C/I
Amikacin sulfate	BR	5 g	BW	200 mg	D5LR, D5R, D5S, D5W, D10W, LR, NS, R, SL	Physically compatible and amikacin stable for 24 hr at 25 °C. Polymyxin not analyzed	293	C
Amphotericin B		200 mg	BP	20 mg	D5W	Haze develops over 3 hr	26	I
Ascorbic acid	UP	500 mg	BW	200 mg	D5W	Physically compatible	15	C
Chloramphenicol sodium succinate	PD PD	10 g 10 g	BW BW	200 mg 200 mg	D5W	Physically incompatible Precipitate forms within 1 hr	15 6	I I
Chlorothiazide sodium	BP	2 g	BP	20 mg	D5W	Yellow color produced	26	I
Colistimethate sodium	WC	500 mg	BW	200 mg	D5W	Physically compatible	15	C
Diphenhydramine HCl	PD	80 mg	BW	200 mg	D5W	Physically compatible	15	C
Erythromycin lactobionate	AB	5 g	BW	200 mg	D5W	Physically compatible	15	C
Heparin sodium	BP	20,000 units	BP	20 mg	D5W	Precipitates immediately	26	I
	BP	20,000 units	BP	20 mg	NS	Haze develops over 3 hr	26	I
Hydrocortisone sodium succinate	UP	500 mg	BW	200 mg	D5W	Physically compatible	15	C
Lincomycin HCl						Physically compatible for 24 hr at room temperature	1	C
Magnesium sulfate	LI	16 mEq	BW	200 mg	D5W	Physically incompatible	15	I
Penicillin G potassium	SQ	20 million units	BW	200 mg	D5W	Physically compatible	15	C

Additive Compatibility (Cont.)

Polymyxin B sulfate

Drug	Mfr	Conc/L	Mfr	Conc/L	Test Soln	Remarks	Ref	C/I
	SQ	5 million units	BW	200 mg	D	Physically compatible	47	**C**
Penicillin G sodium	UP	20 million units	BW	200 mg	D5W	Physically compatible	15	**C**
Phenobarbital sodium	WI	200 mg	BW	200 mg	D5W	Physically compatible	15	**C**
Ranitidine HCl	GL	50 mg and 2 g		1 million units	D5W	Physically compatible. Ranitidine stable for 24 hr at 25 °C. Polymyxin B not tested	1515	**C**

Drugs in Syringe Compatibility

Polymyxin B sulfate

Drug (in syringe)	Mfr	Amt	Mfr	Amt	Remarks	Ref	C/I
Ampicillin sodium	AY	500 mg	BW	25 mg/ 1.5 mL	Physically compatible for 1 hr at room temperature	300	**C**
	AY	250 mg	BW	25 mg/ 1.5 mL	Precipitate forms within 1 hr at room temperature	300	**I**
Cloxacillin sodium	BE	250 mg	BE	250,000 units/1.5 to 2 mL	Physically incompatible within 1 hr at room temperature	99	**I**
Penicillin G sodium		1 million units	BW	25 mg/ 1.5 to 2 mL	No precipitate or color change within 1 hr at room temperature	99	**C**

Y-Site Injection Compatibility (1:1 Mixture)

Polymyxin B sulfate

Drug	Mfr	Conc	Mfr	Conc	Remarks	Ref	C/I
Esmolol HCl	DCC	10 mg/mL[a]	PF	0.005 unit/ mL[a]	Physically compatible for 24 hr at 22 °C	1169	**C**

[a]Tested in dextrose 5%.

POTASSIUM ACETATE
AHFS 40:12

Products — Potassium acetate additive solution is available in 20-, 50-, and 100-mL single-dose vials at a concentration of 2 mEq/mL in water for injection. Each milliliter provides potassium acetate 196 mg. It is also available in 50-mL vials at a concentration of 4 mEq/mL in water for injection. Each milliliter provides 392 mg of potassium acetate. The pH of the solutions may have been adjusted with acetic acid when necessary. These concentrated solutions must be diluted for administration. (1)

pH — The pH of potassium acetate additive solution has been stated to be approximately 7.1 to 7.7 (4) with a range of 5.5 to 8. (1)

Osmolarity — The osmolarity of the 2-mEq/mL solution is 4000 mOsm/ L and the 4-mEq/mL solution is 8000 mOsm/L. (1)

Administration — Potassium acetate is administered as a dilute solution by slow intravenous infusion. It must not be administered undiluted. (1; 4) In most cases, the maximum recommended concentration is 40 mEq/L. Solutions generally may be infused at a rate up to 20 mEq/hr. (4)

Stability — Potassium acetate additive solution should be stored at room temperature and protected from freezing. It should not be administered unless the solution is clear. (1)

Compatibility Information

Additive Compatibility

Potassium acetate

Drug	Mfr	Conc/L	Mfr	Conc/L	Test Soln	Remarks	Ref	C/I
Magnesium sulfate		10 mmol		25 mmol	TPN	Transient precipitate forms	2266	?
Metoclopramide HCl	RB	10 and 160 mg	IX	20 mEq	NS	Physically compatible for 48 hr at room temperature	924	C

Y-Site Injection Compatibility (1:1 Mixture)

Potassium acetate

Drug	Mfr	Conc	Mfr	Conc	Remarks	Ref	C/I
Ciprofloxacin	MI	2 mg/mL[a]	LY	2 mEq/mL	Visually compatible for 2 hr at 25 °C	1628	C

[a]Tested in dextrose 5%.

POTASSIUM CHLORIDE
AHFS 40:12

Products — Potassium chloride is available as concentrated solutions of 1.5 and 2 mEq/mL in 10-, 20-, 30-, and 40-mEq sizes in water for injection in ampuls, vials, and syringes. It is also available in a 30-mL (60-mEq) multiple-dose vial containing methylparaben 0.05% and propylparaben 0.005% as preservatives and 250-mL pharmacy bulk packages. The pH may have been adjusted with hydrochloric acid and if necessary potassium hydroxide during manufacture. The concentrated solutions must be diluted for use. (1)

Potassium chloride is also available premixed in infusion solutions in concentrations of 10, 20, 30, and 40 mEq/L. (4)

pH — The pH is usually near 4.6 with a range of 4 to 8. (1; 17)

Osmolarity — The injections are very hypertonic; the 2-mEq/mL concentration has an osmolarity of 4000 mOsm/L. The injection must be diluted for use. (1)

The osmolality of potassium chloride (Abbott) 2 mEq/mL was determined to be 4355 mOsm/kg by freezing-point depression and 3440 mOsm/kg by vapor pressure. (1071)

The osmolality of a potassium chloride 7.5% solution was determined to be 1895 mOsm/kg. (1233)

Administration — Potassium chloride in the concentrated injections must be diluted before slow intravenous administration. Mix potassium chloride injection thoroughly with the infusion solution before administration. The usual maximum concentration is 40 mEq/L. Extravasation should be avoided. (1; 4)

Great care is required when adding potassium chloride to infusion solutions, whether in flexible plastic containers or in rigid bottles. Adding potassium chloride to running infusion solutions hanging in the use position, especially in flexible containers, has resulted in the pooling of potassium chloride and a resultant high-concentration bolus of the drug being administered to patients, with serious and even fatal consequences. Attempts to mix adequately the potassium chloride in flexible containers by squeezing the container in the hanging position were unsuccessful. It is recommended that drugs be admixed with solutions in flexible containers when positioned with the injection arm of the container uppermost. With both rigid bottles and flexible containers, subsequent repeated inversion and agitation to effect thorough mixture are necessary. (85; 130; 454; 455; 456; 714; 715; 1127; 1778; 2151)

Stability — The solution should be stored at controlled room temperature and used only if it is clear. (1)

Potassium chloride injection 80 mEq/L added to dextrose 5% contained in glass bottles results in a leaching of precipitates consisting of silica and alumina. (129)

Compatibility Information

Solution Compatibility

Potassium chloride

Solution	Mfr	Mfr	Conc/L	Remarks	Ref	C/I
Dextrose–Ringer's injection combinations	AB	AB	160 mEq	Physically compatible	3	**C**
Dextrose–Ringer's injection, lactated, combinations	AB	AB	160 mEq	Physically compatible	3	**C**
Dextrose 5% in Ringer's injection, lactated	BA	LI	80 mEq	Physically compatible for 24 hr	315	**C**
Dextrose–saline combinations	AB	AB	160 mEq	Physically compatible	3	**C**
Dextrose 5% in sodium chloride 0.9%			3 g	Physically compatible	74	**C**
	BA	LI	80 mEq	Physically compatible for 24 hr	315	**C**
Dextrose 2.5%	AB	AB	160 mEq	Physically compatible	3	**C**
Dextrose 5%			3 g	Physically compatible	74	**C**
	AB	AB	160 mEq	Physically compatible	3	**C**
	BA	LI	80 mEq	Physically compatible for 24 hr	315	**C**
Dextrose 10%	AB	AB	160 mEq	Physically compatible	3	**C**
	BA	LI	80 mEq	Physically compatible for 24 hr	315	**C**
Dextrose 20%	BA	LI	80 mEq	Physically compatible for 24 hr	315	**C**
Ionosol products	AB	AB	160 mEq	Physically compatible	3	**C**
Ringer's injection	AB	AB	160 mEq	Physically compatible	3	**C**
			3 g	Physically compatible	74	**C**
Ringer's injection, lactated	AB	AB	160 mEq	Physically compatible	3	**C**
	BA	LI	80 mEq	Physically compatible for 24 hr	315	**C**
Sodium chloride 0.45%	AB	AB	160 mEq	Physically compatible	3	**C**
Sodium chloride 0.9%			3 g	Physically compatible	74	**C**
	AB	AB	160 mEq	Physically compatible	3	**C**
	BA	LI	80 mEq	Physically compatible for 24 hr	315	**C**
Sodium lactate ⅙ M	AB	AB	160 mEq	Physically compatible	3	**C**
	BA	LI	80 mEq	Physically compatible for 24 hr	315	**C**

Additive Compatibility

Potassium chloride

Drug	Mfr	Conc/L	Mfr	Conc/L	Test Soln	Remarks	Ref	C/I
Amikacin sulfate	BR	5 g	LI	3 g	D5LR, D5R, D5S, D5W, D10W, LR, NS, R, SL	Physically compatible and both stable for 24 hr at 25 °C	294	C
Aminophylline		250 mg	AB	3 g	D5W	Physically compatible	74	C
	SE	500 mg	AB	40 mEq		Physically compatible	6	C
Amiodarone HCl	LZ	1.8 g	AB	40 mEq	D5W, NS[a]	Physically compatible. No amiodarone loss in 24 hr at 24 °C in light	1031	C
Amphotericin B		200 mg	BP	4 g	D5W	Haze develops over 3 hr	26	I
	SQ	100 mg	AB	100 mEq	D5W	Physically incompatible	15	I
Atracurium besylate	BW	500 mg		80 mEq	D5W	Physically compatible and atracurium stable for 24 hr at 5 and 30 °C	1694	C
Calcium gluconate		1 g		3 g	D5W	Physically compatible	74	C
Cefepime HCl	BR	4 g	AB	10 and 40 mEq	D5W, NS	Visually compatible with 2% cefepime loss in 24 hr at room temperature or 7 days at 5 °C	1681	C
Ceftazidime		4 g		10 and 40 mEq	D5W, NS	Ceftazidime stable for 24 hr at room temperature and 7 days refrigerated	4	C
Chloramphenicol sodium succinate	PD	500 mg		3 g	D5W	Physically compatible	74	C
	PD	1 g	AB	40 mEq		Physically compatible	6	C
	PD	500 mg and 1 g		20 and 40 mEq	D2.5½S, D5W	Therapeutic availability maintained	110	C
Ciprofloxacin	MI	2 g		40 mEq	NS	Compatible for 24 hr at 25 °C	888	C
	BAY	2 g	AB	40 mEq	NS	Visually compatible with little or no ciprofloxacin loss in 24 hr at 25 °C	1934	C
	BAY	2 g	LY	2.9 g	D5W	Visually compatible with no loss of ciprofloxacin in 24 hr at 22 °C under fluorescent light. Potassium chloride not tested	2413	C
Clindamycin phosphate	UP	600 mg		40 mEq	D5½S	Physically compatible and clindamycin stable for 24 hr at room temperature	104	C
	UP	600 mg		100 mEq	D5W, NS	Physically compatible	101	C
	UP	6 g		400 mEq	D5½S	Clindamycin stable for 24 hr	101	C
Cloxacillin sodium	AST	2.25 g		60 mEq	D5W	10% cloxacillin loss in 48 hr at 25 °C	1476	C
Cytarabine	UP	2 g		100 mEq	D5S	Physically compatible. Stable for 8 days	174	C
	UP	170 mg		80 mEq	D5S	Physically compatible for 24 hr	174	C
Dimenhydrinate	SE	50 mg		3 g	D5W	Physically compatible	74	C
Dobutamine HCl	LI	1 g	ES	160 mEq	D5W, NS	Slightly pink in 24 hr at 25 °C	789	I
	LI	1 g	AB	20 mEq	D5W, NS	Physically compatible for 24 hr at 21 °C	812	C
Dopamine HCl	AS	800 mg	MG		D5W	No dopamine loss in 24 hr at 25 °C	312	C
Enalaprilat	MSD	12 mg	AB	3 g	D5W[a]	Visually compatible. Little enalaprilat loss in 24 hr at room temperature in light	1572	C
Erythromycin lactobionate	AB	1 g	AB	40 mEq		Physically compatible	20	C
Fat emulsion, intravenous	VT	10%		100 mEq		Physically compatible for 48 hr at 4 °C and room temperature	32	C

Additive Compatibility (Cont.)

Potassium chloride

Drug	Mfr	Conc/L	Mfr	Conc/L	Test Soln	Remarks	Ref	C/I
	CU	10%		100 mEq		No change in 24 hr at room temperature, but lipid coalescence in 48 hr	656	C
	CU	10%		200 mEq		Coalescence with surface creaming in 4 hr at room temperature. Oil globules on surface at 48 hr	656	I
	VT	10%	DB	4 g		Lipid coalescence in 24 hr at 8 and 25 °C	825	I
Floxacillin sodium	BE	20 g	ANT	40 mM	W	Physically compatible for 72 hr at 15 and 30 °C	1479	C
Fluconazole	PF	1 g	AB	10 mEq	D5W[a]	Fluconazole stable for 24 hr at 25 °C in fluorescent light	1676	C
Foscarnet sodium	AST	12 g		20 to 120 mmol	NS	Foscarnet concentrations of 93 to 99% were maintained for at least 65 hr	2156	C
Fosphenytoin sodium	PD	1, 8, 20 mg PE/mL[c]	BA	20 and 40 mEq	D5½S[a]	Visually compatible with little or no loss in 7 days at 25 °C under fluorescent light	2083	C
Furosemide	HO	1 g	ANT	40 mmol	W	Physically compatible for 72 hr at 15 and 30 °C	1479	C
Heparin sodium		12,000 units		3 g	D5W	Physically compatible	74	C
	AB	20,000 units	AB	40 mEq		Physically compatible	21	C
		32,000 units		80 mEq	NS	Physically compatible and heparin activity retained for 24 hr	57	C
Hydrocortisone sodium succinate	UP	100 mg		3 g	D5W	Physically compatible	74	C
Hydromorphone HCl	KN	2 and 20 mg/mL	AST	0.5 and 1 mEq/mL	D5W[a]	Visually compatible with no loss of hydromorphone in 18 days at 4 and 23 °C. Potassium chloride not tested	2410	C
Isoproterenol HCl	WI	4 mg	AB	40 mEq		Physically compatible	59	C
Lidocaine HCl	AST	2 g	AB	40 mEq		Physically compatible	24	C
Magnesium sulfate	DB	3.9 g	BRN	80 mEq	D5W, NS	Visually compatible. Under 5% loss of ions in 24 hr at 22 °C	2360	C
Methyldopa HCl	MSD	1 g		40 mEq	D, D–S, S	Physically compatible	23	C
Metoclopramide HCl	RB	10 and 160 mg	ES	30 mEq	NS	Physically compatible for 48 hr at room temperature	924	C
Mitoxantrone HCl	LE	500 mg		50 mEq	D5W	Visually compatible. Mitoxantrone stable for 24 hr at room temperature	1531	C
Nafcillin sodium	WY	500 mg	AB	40 mEq		Physically compatible	27	C
	WY	30 g	TR	40 mEq	NS	Nafcillin stable for 24 hr at 25 °C	27	C
Nicardipine HCl	DME	50 and 500 mg	ES	40 mEq	D5W[b]	Physically compatible. Little loss in 7 days at room temperature in light	1380	C
	DME	50 and 500 mg	ES	40 mEq	D5W[a]	Physically compatible. 12% loss in 7 days at room temperature in light	1380	C
Norepinephrine bitartrate	WI	8 mg		3 g	D5W	Physically compatible	74	C
	WI	8 mg	AB	40 mEq	D, D–S, S	Physically compatible	77	C
Oxacillin sodium	BR	1, 2.5, 4 g		20, 40, 80 mEq	D5S, D5W	Therapeutic availability maintained	110	C

Additive Compatibility (Cont.)

Potassium chloride

Drug	Mfr	Conc/L	Mfr	Conc/L	Test Soln	Remarks	Ref	C/I
Penicillin G potassium	SQ	5 million units	AB	40 mEq		Physically compatible	47	C
	SQ	5 million units		40 mEq	D5S, D5W	Therapeutic availability maintained	110	C
	SQ	1 million units		20 mEq	D5S, D5W	Therapeutic availability maintained	110	C
Penicillin G sodium	KA	6 million units		40 mEq	D5W	Penicillin stable for 24 hr at 25 °C	131	C
	KA	5 million units		40 mEq	IS10	pH outside stability range for penicillin	131	I
Phenylephrine HCl	WI	2.5 g	AB	40 mEq	D5W	Phenylephrine stable for 24 hr at 22 °C	132	C
Ranitidine HCl	GL	2 g	LY	10 and 60 mEq	D5W, NS[a]	Physically compatible. 2% ranitidine loss in 48 hr at room temperature in light	1361	C
	GL	50 mg	LY	10 and 60 mEq	NS[a]	Physically compatible. No ranitidine loss in 48 hr at room temperature in light	1361	C
	GL	50 mg	LY	10 and 60 mEq	D5W[a]	Physically compatible. 7% ranitidine loss in 48 hr at room temperature in light	1361	C
	GL	50 mg and 2 g		80 mEq	D5S, D5W, NS	Physically compatible. Ranitidine stable for 24 hr at 25 °C	1515	C
Sodium bicarbonate	AB	2.4 mEq[d]		120 mEq	D5W	Physically compatible for 24 hr	772	C
Vancomycin HCl	LI	1 g		3 g	D5W	Physically compatible	74	C
Verapamil HCl	KN	80 mg	TR	80 mEq	D5W, NS	Physically compatible for 24 hr	764	C

[a]Tested in PVC containers.
[b]Tested in glass containers.
[c]Concentration expressed in milligrams of phenytoin sodium equivalents (PE) per milliliter.
[d]One vial of Neut added to a liter of admixture.

Drugs in Syringe Compatibility

Potassium chloride

Drug (in syringe)	Mfr	Amt	Mfr	Amt	Remarks	Ref	C/I
Dimenhydrinate		10 mg/ 1 mL		2 mEq/ 1 mL	Precipitate forms in about 1 hr	2569	I
Hydromorphone HCl	KN	50 mg/ 1 mL	AST	2 mEq/ 1 mL	Visually compatible for 24 hr at room temperature	2410	C
Pantoprazole sodium	[a]	4 mg/ 1 mL		2 mEq/ 1 mL	Clear solution	2574	C

[a]Test performed using the formulation WITHOUT edetate disodium.

Y-Site Injection Compatibility (1:1 Mixture)

Potassium chloride

Drug	Mfr	Conc	Mfr	Conc	Remarks	Ref	C/I
Acyclovir sodium	BW	5 mg/mL[a]	IX	0.04 mEq/mL[a]	Physically compatible for 4 hr at 25 °C	1157	C
Aldesleukin	CHI	33,800 I.U./mL[a]	AB	0.2 mEq/mL	Visually compatible with little or no loss of aldesleukin activity	1857	C
	CHI	[a,p]			Loss of aldesleukin activity	1890	I
Allopurinol sodium	BW	3 mg/mL[b]	AB	0.1 mEq/mL[b]	Physically compatible for 4 hr at 22 °C	1686	C
Amifostine	USB	10 mg/mL[a]	AB	0.1 mEq/mL[a]	Physically compatible for 4 hr at 23 °C	1845	C
Aminophylline	SE	25 mg/mL		40 mEq/L[c]	Physically compatible for 4 hr at room temperature	322	C
Amiodarone HCl	LZ	4 mg/mL[d]	AB	0.04 mEq/mL[d]	Physically compatible for 24 hr at 21 °C	1032	C
Amphotericin B cholesteryl sulfate complex	SEQ	0.83 mg/mL[a]	AB	0.1 mEq/mL[a]	Gross precipitate forms	2117	I
Ampicillin sodium	BR	25, 50, 100, 125 mg/mL		40 mEq/L[c]	Physically compatible for 4 hr at room temperature	322	C
Anidulafungin	VIC	0.5 mg/mL[a]	APP	0.1 mEq/mL[a]	Physically compatible for 4 hr at 23 °C	2617	C
Atropine sulfate	BW	0.5 mg/mL	AB	40 mEq/L[f]	Physically compatible for 4 hr at room temperature	534	C
Azithromycin	PF	2 mg/mL[b]	BA	20 mEq/L[n]	White microcrystals found	2368	I
Aztreonam	SQ	40 mg/mL[a]	AB	0.1 mEq/mL[a]	Physically compatible for 4 hr at 23 °C	1758	C
Bivalirudin	TMC	5 mg/mL[a]	APP	0.1 mEq/mL[a]	Physically compatible for 4 hr at 23 °C	2373	C
Calcium gluconate	ES	100 mg/mL		40 mEq/L[c]	Physically compatible for 4 hr at room temperature	322	C
Caspofungin acetate	ME	0.7 mg/mL[b]	APP	0.1 mEq/mL[b]	Physically compatible for 4 hr at room temperature	2758	C
	ME	0.5 mg/mL[b]	BA	0.04 mEq/mL[b]	Physically compatible over 60 min	2766	C
Ceftaroline fosamil	FOR	2.22 mg/mL[c]	HOS	0.1 mEq/mL[c]	Physically compatible for 4 hr at 23 °C	2826	C
Chlorpromazine HCl	SKF	25 mg/mL	AB	40 mEq/L[f]	Physically compatible for 4 hr at room temperature	534	C
	RPR	0.13 mg/mL[a]	BRN	0.625 mEq/mL[a]	Visually compatible for 150 min	2244	C
Ciprofloxacin	MI	2 mg/mL[d]	LY	0.04 mEq/mL	Visually compatible for 24 hr at 24 °C	1655	C
	MI	2 mg/mL[a]	AMR	2 mEq/mL	Visually compatible for 2 hr at 25 °C	1628	C
Cisatracurium besylate	GW	0.1, 2, 5 mg/mL[a]	AB	0.1 mEq/mL[a]	Physically compatible for 4 hr at 23 °C	2074	C
Cladribine	ORT	0.015[b] and 0.5[h] mg/mL	AB	0.1 mEq/mL[b]	Physically compatible for 4 hr at 23 °C	1969	C
Clarithromycin	AB	4 mg/mL[a]	ANT	0.08 mmol/mL[a]	Visually compatible for 72 hr at both 30 and 17 °C	2174	C
Clonidine HCl	BI	18 mcg/mL[b]	BRN	1 mEq/mL	Visually compatible	2642	C
Cyanocobalamin	PD	0.1 mg/mL	AB	40 mEq/L[f]	Physically compatible for 4 hr at room temperature	534	C
Dexamethasone sodium phosphate	MSD	4 mg/mL		40 mEq/L[c]	Physically compatible for 4 hr at room temperature	322	C

Y-Site Injection Compatibility (1:1 Mixture) (Cont.)

Potassium chloride

Drug	Mfr	Conc	Mfr	Conc	Remarks	Ref	C/I
Dexmedetomidine HCl	AB	4 mcg/mL[b]	AB	0.1 mEq/mL[b]	Physically compatible for 4 hr at 23 °C	2383	C
Diazepam	RC	5 mg/mL		40 mEq/L[c]	Immediate haziness and globule formation	322	I
Digoxin	BW	0.25 mg/mL		40 mEq/L[c]	Physically compatible for 4 hr at room temperature	322	C
Diltiazem HCl	MMD	5 mg/mL	LY	0.08[a] and 2 mEq/mL	Visually compatible	1807	C
Diphenhydramine HCl	PD	50 mg/mL	AB	40 mEq/L[f]	Physically compatible for 4 hr at room temperature	534	C
Dobutamine HCl	LI	4 mg/mL[d]	AB	0.06 mEq/mL[d]	Physically compatible for 3 hr	1316	C
Docetaxel	RPR	0.9 mg/mL[a]	AB	0.1 mEq/mL[a]	Physically compatible for 4 hr at 23 °C	2224	C
Dopamine HCl	ACC	40 mg/mL	AB	40 mEq/L[f]	Physically compatible for 4 hr at room temperature	534	C
Doripenem	JJ	5 mg/mL[a,b]	APP	0.1 mEq/mL[a,b]	Physically compatible for 4 hr at 23 °C	2743	C
Doxorubicin HCl liposomal	SEQ	0.4 mg/mL[a]	AB	0.1 mEq/mL[a]	Physically compatible for 4 hr at 23 °C	2087	C
Droperidol	CR	1.25 mg/mL	AB	40 mEq/L[f]	Physically compatible for 4 hr at room temperature	534	C
Edrophonium chloride	RC	10 mg/mL	AB	40 mEq/L[f]	Physically compatible for 4 hr at room temperature	534	C
Enalaprilat	MSD	0.05 mg/mL[b]	LY	0.4 mEq/mL[a]	Physically compatible for 24 hr at room temperature under fluorescent light	1355	C
Epinephrine HCl	AB	0.1 mg/mL	AB	40 mEq/L[f]	Physically compatible for 4 hr at room temperature	534	C
Ergotamine tartrate	SZ	0.5 mg/mL	AB	40 mEq/L[f]	Crystal formation and brown discoloration in 4 hr at room temperature	534	I
Ertapenem sodium	ME	10 mg/mL[b]	AB	0.01 and 0.04 mEq/mL[g]	Visually compatible with about 2% ertapenem loss in 4 hr	2487	C
Esmolol HCl	DCC	10 mg/mL[a]	IX	0.4 mEq/mL[a]	Physically compatible for 24 hr at 22 °C	1169	C
Estrogens, conjugated	AY	5 mg/mL		40 mEq/L[c]	Physically compatible for 4 hr at room temperature	322	C
Ethacrynate sodium	MSD	1 mg/mL		40 mEq/L[c]	Physically compatible for 4 hr at room temperature	322	C
Etoposide phosphate	BR	5 mg/mL[a]	AB	0.1 mEq/mL[a]	Physically compatible for 4 hr at 23 °C	2218	C
Famotidine	MSD	0.2 mg/mL[a]	AB	0.04 mEq/mL[a]	Physically compatible for 4 hr at 25 °C	1188	C
	ME	2 mg/mL[b]		0.1 mEq/mL[a]	Visually compatible for 4 hr at 22 °C	1936	C
Fenoldopam mesylate	AB	80 mcg/mL[b]	APP	0.1 mEq/mL[b]	Physically compatible for 4 hr at 23 °C	2467	C
Fentanyl citrate	MN	0.05 mg/mL	AB	40 mEq/L[f]	Physically compatible for 4 hr at room temperature	534	C
Filgrastim	AMG	30 mcg/mL[a]	AB	0.1 mEq/mL[a]	Physically compatible for 4 hr at 22 °C	1687	C
Fludarabine phosphate	BX	1 mg/mL[a]	AB	0.1 mEq/mL[a]	Visually compatible for 4 hr at 22 °C	1439	C
Fluorouracil	RC	50 mg/mL	AB	40 mEq/L[f]	Physically compatible for 4 hr at room temperature	534	C

Y-Site Injection Compatibility (1:1 Mixture) (Cont.)

Potassium chloride

Drug	Mfr	Conc	Mfr	Conc	Remarks	Ref	C/I
Furosemide	HO	10 mg/mL	AB	40 mEq/L[f]	Physically compatible for 4 hr at room temperature	534	C
	HMR	2.6 mg/mL[a]	BRN	0.625 mEq/mL[a]	Visually compatible for 150 min	2244	C
Gallium nitrate	FUJ	1 mg/mL[b]	AB	0.3 mEq/mL[b]	Visually compatible for 24 hr at 25 °C	1673	C
Gemcitabine HCl	LI	10 mg/mL[b]	AB	0.1 mEq/mL[b]	Physically compatible for 4 hr at 23 °C	2226	C
Gentamicin sulfate	AMS	30 mg/mL[e]	BA	0.02 mEq/mL[o]	Physically compatible	2794	C
Granisetron HCl	SKB	1 mg/mL	LY	0.04 mEq/mL[b]	Physically compatible with little or no loss of granisetron in 4 hr at 22 °C	1883	C
Heparin sodium	TR	50 units/mL	AB	0.2 mEq/mL[a]	Visually compatible for 4 hr at 25 °C	1793	C
	NOV	29.2 units/mL[a]	BRN	0.625 mEq/mL[a]	Visually compatible for 150 min	2244	C
Hetastarch in lactated electrolyte	AB	6%	AB	0.1 mEq/mL[a]	Physically compatible for 4 hr at 23 °C	2339	C
Hydralazine HCl	CI	20 mg/mL	AB	40 mEq/L[f]	Physically compatible for 4 hr at room temperature	534	C
Hydroxyethyl starch 130/0.4 in sodium chloride 0.9%	FRK	6%	HOS	0.02, 0.4, 0.8 mEq/mL[a]	Visually compatible for 24 hr at room temperature	2770	C
Idarubicin HCl	AD	1 mg/mL[b]	AB	0.03 mEq/mL[b]	Visually compatible for 24 hr at 25 °C	1525	C
Indomethacin sodium trihydrate	MSD	1 mg/mL[b]	AB	0.2 mEq/mL[a]	Visually compatible for 24 hr at 28 °C	1527	C
Isoproterenol HCl	WI	0.2 mg/mL	AB	40 mEq/L[f]	Physically compatible for 4 hr at room temperature	534	C
Labetalol HCl	SC	1 mg/mL[a]	IX	0.4 mEq/mL[a]	Physically compatible for 24 hr at 18 °C	1171	C
Levofloxacin	OMN	5 mg/mL[a]	HOS	0.04 mEq/mL[a]	Physically compatible	2794	C
Lidocaine HCl	AST	20 mg/mL		40 mEq/L[c]	Physically compatible for 4 hr at room temperature	322	C
Linezolid	PHU	2 mg/mL	FUJ	0.1 mEq/mL[a]	Physically compatible for 4 hr at 23 °C	2264	C
Lorazepam	WY	0.33 mg/mL[b]	BRN	1 mEq/mL	Visually compatible for 24 hr at 22 °C	1855	C
Magnesium sulfate	AB	500 mg/mL	AB	40 mEq/L[f]	Physically compatible for 4 hr at room temperature	534	C
Melphalan HCl	BW	0.1 mg/mL[b]	AB	0.1 mEq/mL[b]	Physically compatible for 3 hr at 22 °C	1557	C
Meperidine HCl	AB	10 mg/mL	AB	0.4 mEq/mL[a]	Physically compatible for 4 hr at 25 °C	1397	C
Meropenem	ZEN	1 mg/mL[a]		10 and 40 mEq/L[a]	Visually compatible. Calculated 10% meropenem loss in 3.3 hr at 23 °C	2492	C
	ZEN	1 mg/mL[a]		10 and 40 mEq/L[b]	Visually compatible. Calculated 10% meropenem loss in 5 hr at 23 °C	2492	C
	ZEN	1 mg/mL[b]		10 and 40 mEq/L[a]	Visually compatible. Calculated 10% meropenem loss in 5.8 hr at 23 °C	2492	C
	ZEN	1 mg/mL[b]		10 and 40 mEq/L[b]	Visually compatible. Calculated 10% meropenem loss in 22 hr at 23 °C	2492	C
	ZEN	22 mg/mL[a]		10 and 40 mEq/L[a]	Visually compatible. Calculated 10% meropenem loss in 7.7 hr at 23 °C	2492	C

Y-Site Injection Compatibility (1:1 Mixture) (Cont.)

Potassium chloride

Drug	Mfr	Conc	Mfr	Conc	Remarks	Ref	C/I
	ZEN	22 mg/mL[a]		10 and 40 mEq/L[b]	Visually compatible. Calculated 10% meropenem loss in 13 hr at 23 °C	2492	C
	ZEN	22 mg/mL[b]		10 and 40 mEq/L[a]	Visually compatible. Calculated 10% meropenem loss in 8 hr at 23 °C	2492	C
	ZEN	22 mg/mL[b]		10 and 40 mEq/L[b]	Visually compatible. Calculated 10% meropenem loss in 20 hr at 23 °C	2492	C
Methylprednisolone sodium succinate	UP	40 mg/mL		40 mEq/L[a]	Physically compatible for 4 hr at room temperature	322	C
	UP	40 mg/mL		40 mEq/L[b]	Physically compatible initially but haze forms in 4 hr at room temperature	322	I
	UP	40 mg/mL		40 mEq/L[i]	Immediate haze formation	322	I
Micafungin sodium	ASP	1.5 mg/mL[b]	AB	0.1 mEq/mL[b]	Physically compatible for 4 hr at 23 °C	2683	C
Midazolam HCl	RC	5 mg/mL	BRN	1 mEq/mL	Visually compatible for 24 hr at 22 °C	1855	C
Milrinone lactate	SW	0.4 mg/mL[a]	AB	1 mEq/mL[a]	Visually compatible. No milrinone loss in 4 hr at 23 °C	2214	C
Morphine sulfate	WY	15 mg/mL	AB	40 mEq/L[f]	Physically compatible for 4 hr at room temperature	534	C
Neostigmine methylsulfate	RC	0.5 mg/mL	AB	40 mEq/L[f]	Physically compatible for 4 hr at room temperature	534	C
Nicardipine HCl	DCC	0.1 mg/mL[a]	LY	0.4 mEq/mL[a]	Visually compatible for 24 hr at room temperature	235	C
Norepinephrine bitartrate	WI	1 mg/mL	AB	40 mEq/L[f]	Physically compatible for 4 hr at room temperature	534	C
Ondansetron HCl	GL	1 mg/mL[b]	AB	0.1 mEq/mL[a]	Visually compatible for 4 hr at 22 °C	1365	C
Oxacillin sodium	BR	100 mg/mL	AB	40 mEq/L[f]	Physically compatible for 4 hr at room temperature	534	C
Oxaliplatin	SS	0.5 mg/mL[a]	APP	0.1 mEq/mL[a]	Physically compatible for 4 hr at 23 °C	2566	C
Oxytocin	SZ	1 unit/mL	AB	40 mEq/L[f]	Physically compatible for 4 hr at room temperature	534	C
Paclitaxel	NCI	1.2 mg/mL[a]	AB	0.1 mEq/mL[a]	Physically compatible for 4 hr at 22 °C	1556	C
Palonosetron HCl	MGI	50 mcg/mL	AB	0.1 mEq/mL[a]	Physically compatible. No loss of either drug in 4 hr at room temperature	2771	C
Pantoprazole sodium	ALT[q]	0.16 to 0.8 mg/mL[b]	AST	20 to 210 mEq/L[a]	Visually compatible for 12 hr at 23 °C	2603	C
Pemetrexed disodium	LI	20 mg/mL[b]	APP	0.1 mEq/mL[a]	Physically compatible for 4 hr at 23 °C	2564	C
Penicillin G potassium	LI	200,000 units/mL		40 mEq/L[c]	Physically compatible for 4 hr at room temperature	322	C
Pentazocine lactate	WI	30 mg/mL	AB	40 mEq/L[f]	Physically compatible for 4 hr at room temperature	534	C
Phenytoin sodium	PD	50 mg/mL		40 mEq/L[a]	Immediate formation of phenytoin crystals	322	I
	PD	50 mg/mL		40 mEq/L[b,i]	Crystals in 4 hr at room temperature	322	I

Y-Site Injection Compatibility (1:1 Mixture) (Cont.)

Potassium chloride

Drug	Mfr	Conc	Mfr	Conc	Remarks	Ref	C/I
Phytonadione	RC	10 mg/mL	AB	40 mEq/L[f]	Physically compatible for 4 hr at room temperature	534	C
Piperacillin sodium–tazobactam sodium	LE[q]	40 + 5 mg/mL[a]	AB	0.1 mEq/mL[a]	Physically compatible for 4 hr at 22 °C	1688	C
Procainamide HCl	SQ	100 mg/mL	AB	40 mEq/L[f]	Physically compatible for 4 hr at room temperature	534	C
Prochlorperazine edisylate	SKF	5 mg/mL	AB	40 mEq/L[f]	Physically compatible for 4 hr at room temperature	534	C
Promethazine HCl	SV	50 mg/mL	AB	40 mEq/L[j]	Clear initially, but cloudiness develops in 4 hr at room temperature	534	I
	SV	50 mg/mL	AB	40 mEq/L[k]	Physically compatible for 4 hr at room temperature	534	C
Propofol	ZEN	10 mg/mL	AB	0.1 mEq/mL[a]	Physically compatible for 1 hr at 23 °C	2066	C
Propranolol HCl	AY	1 mg/mL	AB	40 mEq/L[f]	Physically compatible for 4 hr at room temperature	534	C
Quinupristin–dalfopristin	AVE	2 mg/mL[a]		0.04 mEq/mL[a]	Physically compatible	1	C
Remifentanil HCl	GW	0.025 and 0.25 mg/mL[b]	AB	0.1 mEq/mL[a]	Physically compatible for 4 hr at 23 °C	2075	C
Sargramostim	IMM	10 mcg/mL[b]	AB	0.1 mEq/mL[b]	Visually compatible for 4 hr at 22 °C	1436	C
Scopolamine HBr	BW	0.86 mg/mL	AB	40 mEq/L[f]	Physically compatible for 4 hr at room temperature	534	C
Sodium bicarbonate	BR	75 mg/mL		40 mEq/L[c]	Physically compatible for 4 hr at room temperature	322	C
Sodium nitroprusside	RC	0.3, 1.2, 3 mg/mL[a]	AST	0.04 and 0.5 mEq/mL[o]	Visually compatible for 48 hr at 24 °C protected from light	2357	C
Succinylcholine chloride	BW	20 mg/mL		40 mEq/L[c]	Physically compatible for 4 hr at room temperature	322	C
Tacrolimus	FUJ	1 mg/mL[b]	AB	2 mEq/mL	Visually compatible for 24 hr at 25 °C	1630	C
Telavancin HCl	ASP	7.5 mg/mL[c]	HOS	0.1 mEq/mL[c]	Physically compatible for 2 hr	2830	C
Teniposide	BR	0.1 mg/mL[a]	AB	0.1 mEq/mL[a]	Physically compatible for 4 hr at 23 °C	1725	C
Theophylline	TR	4 mg/mL	AB	0.2 mEq/mL[a]	Visually compatible for 6 hr at 25 °C	1793	C
Thiotepa	IMM[l]	1 mg/mL[a]	AMR	0.1 mEq/mL[a]	Physically compatible for 4 hr at 23 °C	1861	C
Tigecycline	WY	1 mg/mL[b]		0.3 mEq/mL[b]	Physically compatible for 4 hr	2714	C
Tirofiban HCl	ME	0.05 mg/mL[a,b]	AB	0.01 and 0.04 mEq/mL[a,b]	Physically compatible. No tirofiban loss in 4 hr at room temperature	2250	C
TNA #218 to #226[m]			AB	0.1 mEq/mL[a]	Visually compatible for 4 hr at 23 °C	2215	C
TPN #189[m]			AST	30 mg/mL[b]	Visually compatible for 24 hr at 22 °C	1767	C
TPN #212 to #215[m]			AB	0.1 mEq/mL[a]	Physically compatible for 4 hr at 23 °C	2109	C
Trimethobenzamide HCl	RC	100 mg/mL	AB	40 mEq/L[f]	Physically compatible for 4 hr at room temperature	534	C
Vinorelbine tartrate	BW	1 mg/mL[b]	AB	0.1 mEq/mL[b]	Physically compatible for 4 hr at 22 °C	1558	C
Warfarin sodium	DME	2 mg/mL[g]	BA	0.04 mEq/mL[n]	Visually compatible for 24 hr at 24 °C	2078	C

Y-Site Injection Compatibility (1:1 Mixture) (Cont.)

Potassium chloride

Drug	Mfr	Conc	Mfr	Conc	Remarks	Ref	C/I
Zidovudine	BW	4 mg/mL[a]	IMS	0.67 mEq/ mL[a]	Physically compatible for 4 hr at 25 °C	1193	C

[a]*Tested in dextrose 5%.*
[b]*Tested in sodium chloride 0.9%.*
[c]*Tested in dextrose 5%, sodium chloride 0.9%, and Ringer's injection, lactated.*
[d]*Tested in both dextrose 5% and sodium chloride 0.9%.*
[e]*Tested in sodium chloride 0.45%.*
[f]*Tested in dextrose 5% in Ringer's injection, dextrose 5% in Ringer's injection, lactated, dextrose 5%, Ringer's injection, lactated, and sodium chloride 0.9%.*
[g]*Tested in sterile water for injection.*
[h]*Tested in bacteriostatic sodium chloride 0.9% preserved with benzyl alcohol 0.9%.*
[i]*Tested in Ringer's injection, lactated.*
[j]*Tested in dextrose 5% in Ringer's injection.*
[k]*Tested in dextrose 5% in Ringer's injection, lactated, dextrose 5%, Ringer's injection, lactated, and sodium chloride 0.9%.*
[l]*Lyophilized formulation tested.*
[m]*Refer to Appendix I for the composition of parenteral nutrition solutions. TNA indicates a 3-in-1 admixture, and TPN indicates a 2-in-1 admixture.*
[n]*Tested in dextrose 5% in sodium chloride 0.45%.*
[o]*Tested in dextrose 5% in sodium chloride 0.2%.*
[p]*Tested with albumin human 0.1%.*
[q]*Test performed using the formulation WITHOUT edetate disodium.*

Additional Compatibility Information

Methylprednisolone — The compatibility of methylprednisolone sodium succinate (Upjohn) with potassium chloride added to an auxiliary medication infusion unit has been studied. Primary admixtures were prepared by adding potassium chloride 40 mEq/L to dextrose 5%, dextrose 5% in sodium chloride 0.9%, and Ringer's injection, lactated. The primary admixture was added along with methylprednisolone sodium succinate (Upjohn) to the auxiliary medication infusion unit with the following results (329):

Methylprednisolone Sodium Succinate	Potassium Chloride 40 mEq/L Primary Solution	Results
500 mg	D5S, D5W, LR qs 100 mL	Clear solution for 24 hr
1000 mg	D5W qs 100 mL	Clear solution for 24 hr
1000 mg	D5S, LR qs 100 mL	Clear solution for 6 hr
2000 mg	D5S, D5W, LR qs 100 mL	Clear solution for 24 hr

POTASSIUM PHOSPHATES
AHFS 40:12

Products — Potassium phosphates injection is available in single-dose vials containing 5 or 15 mL of solution and 50-mL bulk additive solution containers. Each milliliter of solution contains monobasic potassium phosphate 224 mg and dibasic potassium phosphate 236 mg in water for injection. The phosphate concentration of the solution is 3 mmol/mL, and the potassium content is 4.4 mEq/mL. This concentrated solution must be diluted for use. (1; 4)

pH — Potassium phosphates injection is stated to have a pH of approximately 7 to 7.8. (4) However, some products cite a pH range of 6.2 to 6.8. (1)

Osmolarity — The osmolarity is 7.4 mOsm/mL. (1)

Administration — Potassium phosphates injection is administered slowly intravenously diluted in infusion solutions. (4)

The relationship between milliequivalents and millimoles of phosphate is expressed in the following equation:

$$mEq\ phosphate = mmol\ phosphate \times valence$$

However, the average valence of phosphate changes with changes in pH. Consequently, it is necessary to specify a pH before the valence, and therefore the milliequivalents, can be determined. To avoid this problem, it has been suggested that doses of phosphate be expressed in terms of millimoles, which is independent of valence. (178; 716; 717; 718) Alternatively, the dose may be expressed in terms of milligrams of phosphorus. One millimole of phosphorus equals 31 mg. (205; 717)

Stability — Potassium phosphates injection should be stored at controlled room temperature. The solutions should be clear and free of particulate matter. Unused portions should be discarded. (1)

Compatibility Information

Solution Compatibility

Potassium phosphates

Solution	Mfr	Mfr	Conc/L	Remarks	Ref	C/I
Dextrose 5% in Ringer's injection	AB	AB	160 mEq	Haze or precipitate forms within 1 hr	3	**I**
Dextrose 2.5% in half-strength Ringer's injection, lactated	AB	AB	160 mEq	Haze or precipitate forms within 24 hr	3	**I**
Dextrose 5% in Ringer's injection, lactated	AB	AB	160 mEq	Haze or precipitate forms within 24 hr	3	**I**
Dextrose–saline combinations (except as noted below)	AB	AB	160 mEq	Physically compatible	3	**C**
Dextrose 10% in sodium chloride 0.9%	AB	AB	160 mEq	Haze or precipitate forms within 24 hr	3	**I**
Dextrose 2.5%	AB	AB	160 mEq	Physically compatible	3	**C**
Dextrose 5%	AB	AB	160 mEq	Physically compatible	3	**C**
Dextrose 10%	AB	AB	160 mEq	Physically compatible	3	**C**
Ionosol products	AB	AB	160 mEq	Physically compatible	3	**C**
Ringer's injection	AB	AB	160 mEq	Haze or precipitate forms within 1 hr	3	**I**
Ringer's injection, lactated	AB	AB	160 mEq	Haze or precipitate forms within 24 hr	3	**I**
Sodium chloride 0.45%	AB	AB	160 mEq	Physically compatible	3	**C**
Sodium chloride 0.9%	AB	AB	160 mEq	Physically compatible	3	**C**
Sodium lactate ⅙ M	AB	AB	160 mEq	Physically compatible	3	**C**

Additive Compatibility

Potassium phosphates

Drug	Mfr	Conc/L	Mfr	Conc/L	Test Soln	Remarks	Ref	C/I
Ciprofloxacin		2 g		60 mg	D5W	Precipitation occurs	671	**I**
Dobutamine HCl	LI	200 mg	AB	100 mmol	NS	Small particles form after 1 hr. White precipitate noted after 15 hr	552	**I**
Metoclopramide HCl	RB	10 and 160 mg	IX	15 mmol	NS	Physically compatible for 48 hr at room temperature	924	**C**
Verapamil HCl	KN	80 mg	AB	88 mEq	D5W, NS	Physically compatible for 24 hr	764	**C**

Drugs in Syringe Compatibility

Potassium phosphates

Drug (in syringe)	Mfr	Amt	Mfr	Amt	Remarks	Ref	C/I
Pantoprazole sodium	a	4 mg/ 1 mL		4 mmol/ 1 mL	Precipitates	2574	I

[a]Test performed using the formulation WITHOUT edetate disodium.

Y-Site Injection Compatibility (1:1 Mixture)

Potassium phosphates

Drug	Mfr	Conc	Mfr	Conc	Remarks	Ref	C/I
Amiodarone HCl	WY	6 mg/mL[a]	APP[a]	0.12 mmol/ mL	Immediate white cloudiness	2352	I
Caspofungin acetate	ME	0.7 mg/mL[b]	APP	0.5 mmol/ mL[b]	Immediate white turbid precipitate forms	2758	I
Ceftaroline fosamil	FOR	2.22 mg/mL[a]	HOS	0.5 mmol/ mL[a]	Increase in measured haze and microparti-culates	2826	I
	FOR	2.22 mg/ mL[b,e]	HOS	0.5 mmol/ mL[b,e]	Increase in measured haze	2826	I
Diltiazem HCl	MMD	5 mg/mL	AMR	0.015 mmol/ mL	Visually compatible	1807	C
Doripenem	JJ	5 mg/mL[a,b]	APP	0.5 mmol/ mL[a,b]	Measured haze increases after 1 hr	2743	I
Enalaprilat	MSD	0.05 mg/mL[b]	LY	0.44 mEq/ mL[a]	Physically compatible for 24 hr at room temperature under fluorescent light	1355	C
Esmolol HCl	DCC	10 mg/mL[a]	LY	0.44 mEq/ mL[a]	Physically compatible for 24 hr at 22 °C	1169	C
Famotidine	MSD	0.2 mg/mL[a]	LY	0.03 mmol/ mL[b]	Physically compatible for 14 hr	1196	C
Hydroxyethyl starch 130/0.4 in sodium chloride 0.9%	FRK	6%	SX	0.003, 0.0765, 0.15 mmol/mL[a]	Visually compatible for 24 hr at room temperature	2770	C
Labetalol HCl	SC	1 mg/mL[a]	LY	0.44 mEq/ mL[a]	Physically compatible for 24 hr at 18 °C	1171	C
Micafungin sodium	ASP	1.5 mg/mL[b]	APP	0.5 mmol/ mL[b]	Physically compatible for 4 hr at 23 °C	2683	C
Nicardipine HCl	DCC	0.1 mg/mL[a]	LY	0.44 mEq/ mL[a]	Visually compatible for 24 hr at room temperature	235	C
Sodium nitroprusside	RC	0.3, 1.2, 3 mg/mL[a]	AB	0.3 mmol/ mL[d]	Visually compatible for 48 hr at 24 °C protected from light	2357	C
Telavancin HCl	ASP	7.5 mg/mL[a,b,e]	AMR	0.5 mmol/ mL[a,b,e]	Physically compatible for 2 hr	2830	C

Y-Site Injection Compatibility (1:1 Mixture) (Cont.)

Potassium phosphates

Drug	Mfr	Conc	Mfr	Conc	Remarks	Ref	C/I
TNA #218 to #226[c]			AB	3 mmol/mL	Damage to emulsion occurs immediately with free oil formation possible	2215	I
TPN #212 to #215[c]			AB	3 mmol/mL	Increased turbidity forms immediately	2109	I

[a]Tested in dextrose 5%.
[b]Tested in sodium chloride 0.9%.
[c]Refer to Appendix I for the composition of parenteral nutrition solutions. TNA indicates a 3-in-1 admixture, and TPN indicates a 2-in-1 admixture.
[d]Tested in dextrose 5% in sodium chloride 0.2%.
[e]Tested in Ringer's injection, lactated.

Additional Compatibility Information

Calcium and Phosphate — UNRECOGNIZED CALCIUM PHOSPHATE PRECIPITATION IN A 3-IN-1 PARENTERAL NUTRITION MIXTURE RESULTED IN PATIENT DEATH.

The potential for the formation of a calcium phosphate precipitate in parenteral nutrition solutions is well studied and documented (1771; 1777), but the information is complex and difficult to apply to the clinical situation. (1770; 1772; 1777) The incorporation of fat emulsion in 3-in-1 parenteral nutrition solutions obscures any precipitate that is present which has led to substantial debate on the dangers associated with 3-in-1 parenteral nutrition mixtures and when or if the danger to the patient is warranted therapeutically. (1770; 1771; 1772; 2031; 2032; 2033; 2034; 2035; 2036) Because such precipitation may be life-threatening to patients (2037; 2291), the Food and Drug Administration issued a Safety Alert containing the following recommendations (1769):

1. The amounts of phosphorus and of calcium added to the admixture are critical. The solubility of the added calcium should be calculated from the volume at the time the calcium is added. It should not be based upon the final volume.

   Some amino acid injections for TPN admixtures contain phosphate ions (as a phosphoric acid buffer). These phosphate ions and the volume at the time the phosphate is added should be considered when calculating the concentration of phosphate additives. Also, when adding calcium and phosphate to an admixture, the phosphate should be added first.

   The line should be flushed between the addition of any potentially incompatible components.

2. A lipid emulsion in a three-in-one admixture obscures the presence of a precipitate. Therefore, if a lipid emulsion is needed, either (1) use a two-in-one admixture with the lipid infused separately, or (2) if a three-in-one admixture is medically necessary, then add the calcium before the lipid emulsion and according to the recommendations in number 1 above.

   If the amount of calcium or phosphate which must be added is likely to cause a precipitate, some or all of the calcium should be administered separately. Such separate infusions must be properly diluted and slowly infused to avoid serious adverse events related to the calcium.

3. When using an automated compounding device, the above steps should be considered when programming the device. In addition, automated compounders should be maintained and operated according to the manufacturer's recommendations.

   Any printout should be checked against the programmed admixture and weight of components.

4. During the mixing process, pharmacists who mix parenteral nutrition admixtures should periodically agitate the admixture and check for precipitates. Medical or home care personnel who start and monitor these infusions should carefully inspect for the presence of precipitates both before and during infusion. Patients and care givers should be trained to visually inspect for signs of precipitation. They also should be advised to stop the infusion and seek medical assistance if precipitates are noted.

5. A filter should be used when infusing either central or peripheral parenteral nutrition admixtures. At this time, data have not been submitted to document which size filter is most effective in trapping precipitates.

   Standards of practice vary, but the following is suggested: a 1.2-μm air-eliminating filter for lipid-containing admixtures and a 0.22-μm air-eliminating filter for non-lipid-containing admixtures.

6. Parenteral nutrition admixtures should be administered within the following time frames: if stored at room temperature, the infusion should be started within 24 hours after mixing; if stored at refrigerated temperatures, the infusion should be started within 24 hours of rewarming. Because warming parenteral nutrition admixtures may contribute to the formation of precipitates, once administration begins, care should be taken to avoid excessive warming of the admixture.

   Persons administering home care parenteral nutrition admixtures may need to deviate from these time frames. Pharmacists who initially prepare these admixtures should check a reserve sample for precipitates over the duration and under the conditions of storage.

7. If symptoms of acute respiratory distress, pulmonary emboli, or interstitial pneumonitis develop, the infusion should be stopped immediately and thoroughly checked for precipitates. Appropriate medical interventions should be instituted. Home care personnel and patients should immediately seek medical assistance."

Calcium Phosphate Precipitation Fatalities — Fatal cases of paroxysmal respiratory failure in two previously healthy women receiving peripheral vein parenteral nutrition were reported. The patients experienced sudden cardiopulmonary arrest consistent with pulmonary emboli. The authors used in vitro simulations and an animal model to conclude that unrecognized calcium phosphate precipitation in a 3-in-1 total nutrition admixture caused the fatalities. The precipitation resulted during compounding by introducing calcium and phosphate near to one another in the compounding sequence and prior to complete fluid addition. This resulted in a temporarily high concentration of the drugs and precipitation of calcium phosphate. Observation of the precipitate was obscured by the incorporation of 20% fat emulsion, intravenous, into the nutrition mixture. No filter was used during infusion of the fatal nutrition admixtures. (2037)

In a follow-up retrospective review, five patients were identified who had respiratory distress associated with the infusion of the 3-in-1 admixtures at around the same time. Four of these five patients died, although the cause of death could be definitively determined for only two. (2291)

Calcium and Phosphate Conditional Compatibility — Calcium salts are conditionally compatible with phosphate in parenteral nutrition solutions. The incompatibility is dependent on a solubility and concentration phenomenon and is not entirely predictable. Precipitation may occur during compounding or at some time after compounding is completed.

NOTE: Some amino acids solutions inherently contain calcium and phosphate, which must be considered in any projection of compatibility.

The compatibility of calcium and phosphate in several parenteral nutrition formulas for newborn infants was evaluated. Calcium gluconate 10% (Cutter) and potassium phosphate (Abbott) were used to achieve concentrations of 2.5 to 100 mEq/L of calcium and 2.5 to 100 mmol/L of phosphorus added. The parenteral nutrition solutions evaluated were as shown in Table 1. The results were reported as graphic depictions.

The pH dependence of the phosphate–calcium precipitation has been noted. Dibasic calcium phosphate is very insoluble, while monobasic calcium phosphate is relatively soluble. At low pH, the soluble monobasic form predominates; but as the pH increases, more dibasic phosphate becomes available to bind with calcium and precipitate. Therefore, the lower the pH of the parenteral nutrition solution, the more calcium and phosphate can be solubilized. Once again, the effects of temperature were observed. As the temperature is increased, more calcium ion becomes available and more dibasic calcium phosphate is formed. Therefore, temperature increases will increase the amount of precipitate. (609)

Similar calcium and phosphate solubility curves were reported for neonatal parenteral nutrition solutions using TrophAmine (McGaw) 2, 1.5, and 0.8% as the sources of amino acids. The solutions also contained dextrose 10%, with cysteine and pH adjustment being used in some admixtures. Calcium and phosphate solubility followed the patterns reported previously. (609) A slightly greater concentration of phosphate could be used in some mixtures, but this finding was not consistent. (1024)

Using a similar study design, six neonatal parenteral nutrition solutions based on Aminosyn-PF (Abbott) 2, 1.5, and 0.8%, with and without added cysteine hydrochloride and dextrose 10% were studied. Calcium concentrations ranged from 2.5 to 50 mEq/L, and phosphate concentrations ranged from 2.5 to 50 mmol/L. Solutions sat for 18 hours at 25 °C and then were warmed to 37 °C in a water bath to simulate the clinical situation of warming prior to infusion into a child. Solubility curves were markedly different than those for TrophAmine in the previous study. (1024) Solubilities were reported to decrease by 15 mEq/L for calcium and 15 mmol/L for phosphate. The solutions remained clear during room temperature storage, but crystals often formed on warming to 37 °C. (1211)

However, these data were questioned. The similarities between the Aminosyn-PF and TrophAmine products were noted, and little difference was found in calcium and phosphate solubilities in a preliminary report. (1212) In the full report (1213), parenteral nutrition solutions containing Aminosyn-PF or TrophAmine 1 or 2.5% with dextrose 10 or 25%, respectively, plus electrolytes and trace metals, with or without cysteine hydrochloride, were evaluated under the same conditions. Calcium concentrations ranged from 2.5 to 50 mEq/L, and phosphate concentrations ranged from 5 to 50 mmol/L. In contrast to the previous results (1024), the solubility curves were very similar for the Aminosyn-PF and TrophAmine parenteral nutrition solutions but very different from those of the previous Aminosyn-PF study. (1211) The authors again showed that the solubility of calcium and phosphate is greater in solutions containing higher concentrations of amino acids and dextrose. (1213)

Calcium and phosphate solubility curves for TrophAmine 1 and 2% with dextrose 10% and electrolytes, vitamins, heparin, and trace elements were reported. Calcium concentrations ranged from 10 to 60 mEq/L, and phosphorus concentrations ranged from 10 to 40 mmol/L. Calcium and phosphate solubilities were assessed by analysis of the calcium concentrations and followed patterns similar to those reported previously. (608; 609) The higher percentage of amino acids (TrophAmine 2%) permitted a slightly greater solubility of calcium and phosphate, especially in the 10 to 50-mEq/L and 10 to 35-mmol/L ranges, respectively. (1614)

The maximal product of the amount of calcium (as gluconate) times phosphate (as potassium) that can be added to a parenteral nutrition solution, composed of amino acids 1% (Travenol) and dextrose 10%, for preterm infants was reported. Turbidity was observed on initial mixing when the solubility product was around 115 to 130 mmol² or greater. After storage at 7 °C for 20 hours, visible precipitates formed at solubility products of 130 mmol² or greater. If the solution was administered through a barium-impregnated silicone rubber catheter, crystalline precipitates obstructed the catheters in 12 hours at a solubility product of 100 mmol² and in 10 days at 79 mmol², much lower than the in vitro results. (1041)

The solubility of calcium and phosphorus in neonatal parenteral nutrition solutions composed of amino acids (Abbott) 1.25 and 2.5% with dextrose 5 and 10%, respectively, was evaluated. Also present were multivitamins and trace elements. The solutions contained calcium (as gluconate) in amounts ranging from 25 to 200 mg/100 mL. The phosphorus (as potassium phosphate) concentrations evaluated ranged from 25 to 150 mg/100 mL. If calcium gluconate was added first, cloudiness occurred immediately. If potassium phosphate was added first, substantial quantities could be added with no precipitate formation in 48 hours at 4 °C (Table 2). However, if stored at 22 °C, the solutions were stable for only 24 hours, and all contained precipitates after 48 hours. (1210)

The physical compatibility of calcium gluconate 10 to 40 mEq/L and potassium phosphates 10 to 40 mmol/L in three neonatal parenteral nutrition solutions (TPN #123 to #125 in Appendix I), alone and with retrograde administration of aminophylline 7.5 mg diluted with 1.5 mL of sterile water for injection was reported. Contact of the alkaline aminophylline solution with the parenteral nutrition solutions resulted in the precipitation of calcium phosphate at much lower con-

Table 1. Parenteral Nutrition Solutions Evaluated (609)

| Component | Solution Number | | | |
	#1	#2	#3	#4
FreAmine III	4%	2%	1%	1%
Dextrose	25%	20%	10%	10%
pH	6.3	6.4	6.6	7.0[a]

[a] *Adjusted with sodium hydroxide.*

Table 2. Maximum Calcium and Phosphorus Concentrations Physically Compatible for 48 Hours at 4 °C (1210)

Calcium (mg/100 mL)	Phosphorus (mg/100 mL)	
	Amino Acids 1.25% + Dextrose 5%[a]	Amino Acids 2.5% + Dextrose 10%[a]
200[b]	50	75
150	50	100
100	75	100
50	100	125
25	150[b]	150[b]

[a] Plus multivitamins and trace elements.
[b] Maximum concentration tested.

Table 3. Maximum Amount of Phosphate (as Sodium) (mmol/L) Not Resulting in Precipitation. (2039) See CAUTION below.[a]

Calcium (as Gluconate)	Amino Acid (as TrophAmine) with Cysteine HCl 40 mg/g of Amino Acid				
	0%	0.4%	1%	2%	3%
9.8 mEq/L	0	27	42	60	66
14.7 mEq/L	0	15	18	30	36
19.6 mEq/L	0	6	15	27	30
29.4 mEq/L	0	3	6	21	24

[a] CAUTION: The results cannot be safely extrapolated to other solutions. See text.

centrations than were compatible in the parenteral nutrition solutions alone. (1404)

Koorenhof and Timmer reported the maximum allowable concentrations of calcium and phosphate in a 3-in-1 parenteral nutrition mixture for children (TNA #192 in Appendix I). Added calcium was varied from 1.5 to 150 mmol/L, while added phosphate was varied from 21 to 300 mmol/L. The mixtures were stable for 48 hours at 22 and 37 °C as long as the pH was not greater than 5.7, the calcium concentration was below 16 mmol/L, the phosphate concentration was below 52 mmol/L, and the product of the calcium and phosphate concentrations was below 250 $mmol^2/L^2$. (1773)

Additional calcium and phosphate solubility curves were reported for specialty parenteral nutrition solutions based on NephrAmine and also HepatAmine at concentrations of 0.8, 1.5, and 2% as the sources of amino acids. The solutions also contained dextrose 10%, with cysteine and pH adjustment to simulate addition of fat emulsion used in some admixtures. Calcium and phosphate solubility followed the hyperbolic patterns previously reported. (609) Temperature, time, and pH affected calcium and phosphate solubility, with pH having the greatest effect. (2038)

The maximum sodium phosphate concentrations were reported for given amounts of calcium gluconate that could be admixed in parenteral nutrition solutions containing TrophAmine in varying quantities (with cysteine hydrochloride 40 mg/g of amino acid) and dextrose 10%. The solutions also contained magnesium sulfate 4 mEq/L, potassium acetate 24 mEq/L, sodium chloride 32 mEq/L, pediatric multivitamins, and trace elements. The presence of cysteine hydrochloride reduces the solution pH and increases the amount of calcium and phosphate that can be incorporated before precipitation occurs. The results of this study cannot be safely extrapolated to TPN solutions with compositions other than the ones tested. The admixtures were compounded with the sodium phosphate added last after thorough mixing of all other components. The authors noted that this is not the preferred order of mixing (usually phosphate is added first and thoroughly mixed before adding calcium last); however, they believed this reversed order of mixing would provide a margin of error in cases in which the proper order is not followed. After compounding, the solutions were stored for 24 hours at 40 °C. The maximum calcium and phosphate amounts that could be mixed in the various solutions were reported tabularly and are shown in Table 3. (2039) However, these results are not entirely consistent with another study. See Table 4.

The temperature dependence of the calcium–phosphate precipitation has resulted in the occlusion of a subclavian catheter by a solution apparently free of precipitation. The parenteral nutrition solution consisted of FreAmine III 500 mL, dextrose 70% 500 mL, sodium chlo-

ride 50 mEq, sodium phosphate 40 mmol, potassium acetate 10 mEq, potassium phosphate 40 mmol, calcium gluconate 10 mEq, magnesium sulfate 10 mEq, and Shil's trace metals solution 1 mL. Although there was no evidence of precipitation in the bottle, tubing and pump cassette, and filter (all at approximately 26 °C) during administration, the occluded catheter and Vicra Loop Lock (next to the patient's body at 37 °C) had numerous crystals identified as calcium phosphate. In vitro, this parenteral nutrition solution had a precipitate in 12 hours at 37 °C but was clear for 24 hours at 26 °C. (610)

Similarly, a parenteral nutrition solution that was clear and free of particulates after two weeks under refrigeration developed a precipitate in four to six hours when stored at room temperature. When the solution was warmed in a 37 °C water bath, precipitation occurred in one hour. Administration of the solution before the precipitate was noticed led to interstitial pneumonitis due to deposition of calcium phosphate crystals. (1427)

Calcium phosphate precipitation phenomena was evaluated in a series of parenteral nutrition admixtures composed of dextrose 22%, amino acids (FreAmine III) 2.7%, and fat emulsion (Abbott) 0, 1, and 3.2%. Incorporation of calcium gluconate 19 to 24 mEq/L and phosphate (as sodium) 22 to 28 mmol/L resulted in visible precipitation in the fat-free admixtures. New precipitate continued to form over 14 days, even after repeated filtrations of the solutions through 0.2-μm filters. The presence of the amino acids increased calcium and phosphate solubility, compared with simple aqueous solutions. However, the incorporation of the fat emulsion did not result in a statistically significant increase in calcium and phosphate solubility. The authors noted that the kinetics of calcium phosphate precipitate formation do not appear to be entirely predictable; both transient and permanent precipitation can occur either during the compounding process or at some time afterward. Because calcium phosphate precipitation can be very dangerous clinically, the use of inline filters was recommended. The authors suggested that the filters should have a porosity appropriate to the parenteral nutrition admixture—1.2 μm for fat-containing and 0.2 or 0.45 μm for fat-free nutrition mixtures. (2061)

Laser particle analysis was used to evaluate the formation of calcium phosphate precipitation in pediatric TPN solutions containing TrophAmine in concentrations ranging from 0.5 to 3% with dextrose 10% and also containing L-cysteine hydrochloride 1 g/L. The solutions also contained in each liter sodium chloride 20 mEq, sodium acetate 20 mEq, magnesium sulfate 3 mEq, trace elements 3 mL, and heparin sodium 500 units. The presence of L-cysteine hydrochloride reduces the solution pH and increases the amount of calcium and phosphate that can be incorporated before precipitation occurs. The results of this study cannot be safely extrapolated to TPN solutions with compositions other than the ones tested. The maximum amount of phosphate that was incorporated without the appearance of a measurable increase in particulates in 24 hours at 37 °C for each of the amino acids concentrations is shown in Table 4. (2196) These results are not entirely consistent with previous results. (2039) See above. The use of more sensitive electronic particle measurement for the formation of subvisible particulates in this study may contribute to the differences in the results.

Calcium and phosphate compatibility was evaluated in a series of adult formula parenteral nutrition admixtures composed of FreAmine III, in concentrations ranging from 1 to 5% (TPN #258 through #262). The solutions also contained dextrose ranging from 15% up to 25%. Also present were sodium chloride, potassium chloride, and magnesium sulfate in common amounts. Cysteine hydrochloride was added in an amount of 25 mg/g of amino acids from FreAmine III to reduce the pH by about 0.5 pH unit and thereby increase the amount of calcium and phosphates that can be added to the TPN admixtures as has been done with pediatric parenteral nutrition admixtures. Phosphates as the potassium salts and calcium as the gluconate salt were added in variable quantities to determine the maximum amounts of calcium and phosphates that could be added to the test admixtures. The samples were evaluated at 23 and 37 °C over 48 hours by visual inspection in ambient light and using a Tyndall beam and electronic measurement of turbidity and microparticulates. The addition of the cysteine hydrochloride resulted in an increase of calcium and phosphates solubility of about 30% by lowering the solution pH 0.5 pH unit. The boundaries between the compatible and incompatible concentrations were presented graphically as hyperbolic curves. (2469)

The presence of magnesium in solutions may also influence the reaction between calcium and phosphate, including the nature and extent of precipitation. (158; 159)

The interaction of calcium and phosphate in parenteral nutrition solutions is a complex phenomenon. Various factors have been identified as playing a role in the solubility or precipitation of a given combination, including (608; 609; 1042; 1063; 1404; 1427; 2778):

1. Concentration of calcium
2. Salt form of calcium
3. Concentration of phosphate
4. Concentration of amino acids
5. Amino acids composition
6. Concentration of dextrose
7. Temperature of solution

8. pH of solution
9. Presence of other additives
10. Order of mixing

Enhanced precipitate formation would be expected from such factors as high concentrations of calcium and phosphate, increases in solution pH, decreased amino acid concentrations, increases in temperature, addition of calcium prior to the phosphate, lengthy standing times or slow infusion rates, and use of calcium as the chloride salt. (854)

Even if precipitation does not occur in the container, it has been reported that crystallization of calcium phosphate may occur in a Silastic infusion pump chamber or tubing if the rate of administration is slow, as for premature infants. Water vapor may be transmitted outward and be replaced by air rapidly enough to produce supersaturation. (202) Several other cases of catheter occlusion have been reported. (610; 1427; 1428; 1429)

Table 4. Maximum Amount of Phosphate (as Potassium) (mmol/L) Not Resulting in Precipitation. (2196) See CAUTION below.[a]

Calcium (as Gluconate) (mEq/L)	Amino Acid (as TrophAmine) plus Cysteine HCl 1 g/L					
	0.5%	1%	1.5%	2%	2.5%	3%
10	22	28	38	38	38	43
14	18	18	18	38	38	43
19	18	18	18	33	33	38
24	12	18	18	22	28	28
28	12	18	18	18	18	18
33	12	12	12	12	12	12
37	12	12	12	12	12	12
41	9	9	9	12	12	12
45	0	9	9	12	12	12
49	0	9	9	9	12	12
53	0	9	9	9	9	9

[a]CAUTION: The results cannot be safely extrapolated to solutions with formulas other than the ones tested. See text.

PRALIDOXIME CHLORIDE
AHFS 92:12

Products — Pralidoxime chloride is available as a dry powder in 1-g vials with sodium hydroxide to adjust pH during manufacturing. Reconstitute with 20 mL of sterile water for injection to yield 50 mg/mL. For intravenous infusion, a concentration of 10 to 20 mg/mL in sodium chloride 0.9% is recommended. For intramuscular injection when intravenous administration is not feasible, reconstitute each vial with 3.3 mL of sterile water for injection to yield 300 mg/mL. (1)

Pralidoxime chloride is also available as 600 mg/2 mL in autoinjectors. Also present in the formulation are benzyl alcohol 20 mg/mL and glycine 11.26 mg/mL in water for injection. (1)

pH — Vials- From 3.5 to 4.5. Autoinjectors- From 2.0 to 3.0. (1)

Administration — Pralidoxime chloride in vials is given by intravenous infusion at a concentration of 10 to 20 mg/mL in sodium chloride 0.9%. If necessary, the 50-mg/mL reconstituted drug may be given by slow intravenous injection over not less than five minutes. For intramuscular injection when intravenous administration is not feasible, a 300-mg/mL concentration may be used. Pralidoxime chloride in the autoinjectors is intended for intramuscular administration only. (1)

Stability — Pralidoxime chloride vials should be stored at controlled room temperature. Autoinjectors should be stored at room temperature and protected from freezing. (1)

Compatibility Information

Solution Compatibility

Pralidoxime chloride

Solution	Mfr	Mfr	Conc/L	Remarks	Ref	C/I
Sodium chloride 0.9%		MMT	8 and 10 g	Physically compatible with less than 10% loss in 28 days at –20, 4, 25, and 50 °C	2685	C

PROCAINAMIDE HYDROCHLORIDE
AHFS 24:04.04.04

Products — Procainamide hydrochloride is available in 10-mL vials providing 100 mg/mL or 2-mL vials providing 500 mg/mL. The 100-mg/mL form also contains in each milliliter methylparaben 1 mg and sodium metabisulfite 0.8 mg. The 500-mg/mL form also contains in each milliliter methylparaben 1 mg and sodium metabisulfite 1.8 mg. In both forms, the pH is adjusted with hydrochloric acid and/or sodium hydroxide. (1; 4)

pH — From 4 to 6. (1)

Administration — Procainamide hydrochloride may be administered by intramuscular or direct intravenous injection or intravenous infusion. Both forms may be diluted prior to intravenous use to facilitate control of the administration rate. The intravenous rate of administration should not exceed 50 mg/min. (1; 4)

Stability — Procainamide hydrochloride may be stored at controlled room temperature. (1; 4) However, refrigeration retards oxidation, which causes color formation. The solution is initially colorless but may turn slightly yellow on standing. Injection of air into the vial causes the solution to darken. Solutions darker than a light amber should be discarded. (4)

Procainamide hydrochloride forms α- and β-glucosylamine compounds with dextrose. The reaction proceeds rapidly, with about 10% procainamide loss in dextrose 5% occurring in about five hours and 30% loss in 24 hours at 25 °C. Equilibrium is achieved with about 62% of the procainamide present as glucosylamines. (1896) The bioavailability, activity, and metabolic fate of these compounds is not known. (546; 1896) The α- and β-glucosylamine compounds that form are reversible (1422; 1896), although the extent of reversibility in plasma has been questioned. (2051) The rate and extent of complex formation are dependent on the dextrose concentration and the solution pH but are independent of the procainamide hydrochloride concentration. (1422) In dextrose concentrations ranging from 1 to 5%, the extent of procainamide complex formation ranged from 6% in two days in dextrose 1% up to 35% (1422) to 60% (1896) in dextrose 5%. Lowering the pH from the normal 4.5 to 1.4 with 0.01 N hydrochloric acid completely prevented complex formation. (1422) Similarly, increasing the solution pH to 8 is reported to block complexation. (1423) Maximum complex formation occurred at pH 3 to 5 (1423) or 4 to 5.2 (1358), the natural pH of procainamide hydrochloride admixtures in dextrose 5%. The clinical importance of this complexation, if any, is uncertain.

Sorption — Procainamide hydrochloride was shown not to exhibit sorption to PVC bags and tubing, polyethylene tubing, Silastic tubing, and polypropylene syringes. (536; 606)

Compatibility Information

Solution Compatibility

Procainamide HCl

Solution	Mfr	Mfr	Conc/L	Remarks	Ref	C/I
Dextrose 5% in sodium chloride 0.9%	MG[a,b]	SQ	4 g	17% loss at room temperature and 5% loss at 4 °C in 24 hr	522	I
Dextrose 5%			2 to 4 g	Stable for 24 hr at room temperature and 7 days refrigerated	4	C
Dextrose 5%[c]	BA[b]	ASC	4 and 8 g	10% or less loss in 24 hr at room temperature and under refrigeration	1327	C
Dextrose 5%	TR[a]	SQ	1 g	No loss in 8 hr but 12% loss in 24 hr at room temperature	545	I
	BA[b]	ASC	4 and 8 g	12 to 14% loss in 12 hr at room temperature. 6 to 10% loss in 24 hr under refrigeration	1327	I

Solution Compatibility (Cont.)

Procainamide HCl

Solution	Mfr	Mfr	Conc/L	Remarks	Ref	C/I
	TR	ES	4 g	24% loss in 24 hr at room temperature in light	1358	I
		LY	4 and 10 g	Physically compatible with 14 to 15% loss in 4 hr at 22 °C	1419	I
	AB	SQ	2 g	10% loss in 5 hr and 30% loss in 24 hr at 25 °C due to reaction with dextrose	1896	I
Sodium chloride 0.45%		LY	4 and 10 g	Physically compatible with no loss in 4 hr at 22 °C	1419	C
Sodium chloride 0.9%	TR[a]	SQ	1 g	No decomposition in 24 hr at room temperature	545	C
			2 to 4 g	Stable for 24 hr at room temperature and 7 days refrigerated	4	C

[a]Tested in glass containers.
[b]Tested in PVC containers.
[c]Adjusted to approximately pH 7.5 with sodium bicarbonate 8.4%.

Additive Compatibility

Procainamide HCl

Drug	Mfr	Conc/L	Mfr	Conc/L	Test Soln	Remarks	Ref	C/I
Amiodarone HCl	LZ	1.8 g	SQ	4 g	D5W, NS[a]	Physically compatible. 5% or less amiodarone loss in 24 hr at 24 °C in light	1031	C
Atracurium besylate	BW	500 mg		4 g	D5W	Physically compatible and atracurium stable for 24 hr at 5 and 30 °C	1694	C
Dobutamine HCl	LI	1 g	SQ	1 g	D5W, NS	Physically compatible with no color change in 24 hr at 25 °C	789	C
	LI	1 g	AHP	4 and 50 g	D5W, NS	Physically compatible for 24 hr at 21 °C	812	C
Esmolol HCl	DU	6 g	ES	4 g	D5W	43% procainamide loss in 24 hr at room temperature under fluorescent light	1358	I
Ethacrynate sodium	MSD	50 mg	SQ	1 g	NS	Altered UV spectra at room temperature	16	I
Flumazenil	RC	20 mg	ES	4 g	D5W[b]	Visually compatible. No flumazenil loss in 24 hr at 23 °C in fluorescent light. Procainamide not tested	1710	C
Lidocaine HCl	AST	2 g	SQ	1 g	D5W, LR, NS	Physically compatible for 24 hr at 25 °C	775	C
Milrinone lactate	WI	200 mg	SQ	2 and 4 g	D5W	3% procainamide loss in 1 hr and 11% in 4 hr at 23 °C. No milrinone loss	1191	I
Verapamil HCl	KN	80 mg	SQ	2 g	D5W, NS	Physically compatible for 48 hr	739	C

[a]Tested in both polyolefin and PVC containers.
[b]Tested in PVC containers.

Drugs in Syringe Compatibility

Procainamide HCl

Drug (in syringe)	Mfr	Amt	Mfr	Amt	Remarks	Ref	C/I
Pantoprazole sodium	a	4 mg/ 1 mL		100 mg/ 1 mL	Clear solution	2574	**C**

[a]Test performed using the formulation WITHOUT edetate disodium.

Y-Site Injection Compatibility (1:1 Mixture)

Procainamide HCl

Drug	Mfr	Conc	Mfr	Conc	Remarks	Ref	C/I
Amiodarone HCl	LZ	4 mg/mL[c]	AHP	8 mg/mL[c]	Physically compatible for 24 hr at 21 °C	1032	**C**
Bivalirudin	TMC	5 mg/mL[a]	ES	10 mg/mL[a]	Physically compatible for 4 hr at 23 °C	2373	**C**
Cisatracurium besylate	GW	0.1, 2, 5 mg/ mL[a]	ES	10 mg/mL[a]	Physically compatible for 4 hr at 23 °C	2074	**C**
Dexmedetomidine HCl	AB	4 mcg/mL[b]	ES	10 mg/mL[b]	Physically compatible for 4 hr at 23 °C	2383	**C**
Diltiazem HCl	MMD	5 mg/mL	ES	500 mg/mL	Cloudiness forms but clears within 2 min	1807	**?**
	MMD	1 mg/mL[b]	ES	50 mg/mL[a]	Visually compatible	1807	**C**
	MMD	5 mg/mL	ES	2 mg/mL[a]	Visually compatible	1807	**C**
Famotidine	MSD	0.2 mg/mL[a]	ASC	5 mg/mL[a]	Physically compatible for 4 hr at 25 °C	1188	**C**
Fenoldopam mesylate	AB	80 mcg/mL[b]	ES	10 mg/mL[b]	Physically compatible for 4 hr at 23 °C	2467	**C**
Heparin sodium	UP	1000 units/L[e]	SQ	100 mg/mL	Physically compatible for 4 hr at room temperature	534	**C**
Hetastarch in lactated electrolyte	AB	6%	ES	10 mg/mL[a]	Physically compatible for 4 hr at 23 °C	2339	**C**
Hydrocortisone sodium succinate	UP	10 mg/L[e]	SQ	100 mg/mL	Physically compatible for 4 hr at room temperature	534	**C**
Metoprolol tartrate	BED	1 mg/mL	HOS	8 mg/mL[b]	Visually compatible for 24 hr at 19 °C	2795	**C**
Milrinone lactate	WI	350 mcg/mL[a]	SQ	2 and 4 mg/ mL[a]	3 to 6% procainamide loss in 1 hr and 10 to 13% in 4 hr at 23 °C. No milrinone loss	1191	**I**
Nesiritide	SCI	50 mcg/mL[a,b]		500 mg/mL	Physically compatible for 4 hr. May be chemically incompatible with nesiritide[d]	2625	**?**
Potassium chloride	AB	40 mEq/L[e]	SQ	100 mg/mL	Physically compatible for 4 hr at room temperature	534	**C**
Ranitidine HCl	GL	0.5 mg/mL	BA	4 mg/mL[a]	Physically compatible for 24 hr	1323	**C**
Remifentanil HCl	GW	0.025 and 0.25 mg/mL[b]	ES	10 mg/mL[a]	Physically compatible for 4 hr at 23 °C	2075	**C**
Sodium nitroprusside	RC	0.3, 1.2, 3 mg/mL[a]	SX	6, 20, 40 mg/ mL[b]	Visually compatible for 48 hr at 24 °C protected from light	2357	**C**
Vasopressin	AMR	2 and 4 units/ mL[b]	AB	4 mg/mL[b]	Physically compatible with vasopressin pushed through a Y-site over 5 sec	2478	**C**

[a]Tested in dextrose 5%.
[b]Tested in sodium chloride 0.9%.
[c]Tested in dextrose 5% and sodium chloride 0.9%.
[d]Nesiritide is incompatible with bisulfite antioxidants used in some drug formulations. The specific formulation of the product to be used should be checked to ensure that no sulfite antioxidants are present.
[e]Tested in dextrose 5% in Ringer's injection, dextrose 5% in Ringer's injection, lactated, dextrose 5%, Ringer's injection, lactated, and sodium chloride 0.9%.

PROCHLORPERAZINE EDISYLATE
AHFS 28:16.08.24

Products — Prochlorperazine 5 mg/mL (as edisylate) is available in 2-mL vials and 10-mL multiple-dose vials. Each milliliter of solution also contains sodium biphosphate 5 mg, sodium tartrate 12 mg, sodium saccharin 0.9 mg, and benzyl alcohol 0.75% in water for injection. (1)

pH — From 4.2 to 6.2. (1)

Administration — Prochlorperazine edisylate may be given intramuscularly deep into the upper outer quadrant of the buttock. It may also be given by direct intravenous injection at a rate not exceeding 5 mg/min. It can be given undiluted or diluted in a compatible diluent. It should not be given as a bolus intravenous injection. (1; 4) For intravenous infusion, dilution of 20 mg in a liter of compatible infusion solution is recommended. (4) Because the drug causes local irritation, subcutaneous injection is not recommended. (1; 4)

Stability — Intact containers should be stored at controlled room temperature and protected from temperatures of 40 °C or more and from freezing. Solutions of prochlorperazine edisylate are light sensitive and, therefore, should be protected from light. A slightly yellow solution has not had its concentration altered. However, a markedly discolored solution should be discarded. (1; 4)

Dilution of prochlorperazine edisylate to a 1-mg/mL concentration with bacteriostatic sodium chloride 0.9% containing methyl- and propylparabens resulted in a distinctly cloudy solution. This cloudiness did not occur when sodium chloride 0.9% preserved with benzyl alcohol was used for the dilution. (752)

Light Effects — Prochlorperazine edisylate (Wyeth) 20 mg/L in dextrose 5% exhibited about 20% loss in two hours at room temperature when exposed to light. More rapid and extensive decomposition occurred when sodium chloride 0.9% was used as the diluent. (2412)

Filtration — Prochlorperazine edisylate (SKF) 5 mg/L in dextrose 5% and sodium chloride 0.9% did not display significant sorption to a 0.45-μm cellulose membrane filter. (567)

Central Venous Catheter — Prochlorperazine edisylate (SoloPak) 0.5 mg/mL in dextrose 5% was found to be compatible with the ARROWg+ard Blue Plus (Arrow International) chlorhexidine-bearing triple-lumen central catheter. Essentially complete delivery of the drug was found with little or no drug loss occurring. Furthermore, chlorhexidine delivered from the catheter remained at trace amounts with no substantial increase due to the delivery of the drug through the catheter. (2335)

Compatibility Information

Solution Compatibility

Prochlorperazine edisylate

Solution	Mfr	Mfr	Conc/L	Remarks	Ref	C/I
Dextrose–Ringer's injection combinations	AB	SKF	10 mg	Physically compatible	3	C
Dextrose–Ringer's injection, lactated, combinations	AB	SKF	10 mg	Physically compatible	3	C
Dextrose–saline combinations	AB	SKF	10 mg	Physically compatible	3	C
Dextrose 2.5%	AB	SKF	10 mg	Physically compatible	3	C
Dextrose 5%	AB	SKF	10 mg	Physically compatible	3	C
Dextrose 10%	AB	SKF	10 mg	Physically compatible	3	C
Ionosol products	AB	SKF	10 mg	Physically compatible	3	C
Ringer's injection	AB	SKF	10 mg	Physically compatible	3	C
Ringer's injection, lactated	AB	SKF	10 mg	Physically compatible	3	C
Sodium chloride 0.45%	AB	SKF	10 mg	Physically compatible	3	C
Sodium chloride 0.9%	AB	SKF	10 mg	Physically compatible	3	C
Sodium lactate ⅙ M	AB	SKF	10 mg	Physically compatible	3	C

Additive Compatibility

Prochlorperazine edisylate

Drug	Mfr	Conc/L	Mfr	Conc/L	Test Soln	Remarks	Ref	C/I
Amikacin sulfate	BR	5 g	SKF	20 mg	D5LR, D5R, D5S, D5W, D10W, LR, NS, R, SL	Physically compatible and both stable for 24 hr at 25 °C	294	C
Aminophylline	SE	1 g	SKF	100 mg	D5W	Physically incompatible	15	I
Ascorbic acid	UP	500 mg	SKF	100 mg	D5W	Physically compatible	15	C
Calcium gluconate	UP	1 g	SKF	100 mg	D5W	Physically compatible	15	C
Chloramphenicol sodium succinate	PD	10 g	SKF	100 mg	D5W	Physically incompatible	15	I
Dexamethasone sodium phosphate	MSD	20 mg	SKF	100 mg	D5W	Physically compatible	15	C
Dimenhydrinate	SE	500 mg	SKF	100 mg	D5W	Physically compatible	15	C
Erythromycin lactobionate	AB	1 g	SKF	10 mg		Physically compatible. Erythromycin stable for 24 hr at 25 °C	20	C
Ethacrynate sodium	MSD	80 mg	SKF	20 mg	NS	Little alteration of UV spectra within 8 hr at room temperature	16	C
Floxacillin sodium	BE	20 g	MB	1.25 g	W	Precipitates immediately	1479	I
Furosemide	HO	1 g	MB	1.25 g	W	Yellow precipitate forms immediately	1479	I
Lidocaine HCl	AST	2 g	SKF	10 mg		Physically compatible	24	C
Nafcillin sodium	WY	500 mg	SKF	10 mg		Physically compatible	27	C
Penicillin G potassium	SQ	5 million units	SKF	10 mg	D5W	Physically compatible. Penicillin stable for 24 hr at 25 °C	47	C
	[a]	900,000 units	SKF	10 mg	D5W	Penicillin stable for 24 hr at 25 °C	48	C
Sodium bicarbonate	AB	2.4 mEq[b]	SKF	10 mg	D5W	Physically compatible for 24 hr	772	C

[a] A buffered preparation was specified.
[b] One vial of Neut added to a liter of admixture.

Drugs in Syringe Compatibility

Prochlorperazine edisylate

Drug (in syringe)	Mfr	Amt	Mfr	Amt	Remarks	Ref	C/I
Atropine sulfate		0.6 mg/ 1.5 mL	SKF		Physically compatible for at least 15 min	14	C
	ST	0.4 mg/ 1 mL	PO	5 mg/ 1 mL	Physically compatible for at least 15 min	326	C
Butorphanol tartrate	BR	4 mg/ 2 mL	MB	5 mg/ 1 mL	Physically compatible for 30 min at room temperature	566	C
Chlorpromazine HCl	SKF	50 mg/ 2 mL	SKF		Physically compatible for at least 15 min	14	C
	PO	50 mg/ 2 mL	PO	5 mg/ 1 mL	Physically compatible for at least 15 min	326	C

Drugs in Syringe Compatibility (Cont.)

Prochlorperazine edisylate

Drug (in syringe)	Mfr	Amt	Mfr	Amt	Remarks	Ref	C/I
Diamorphine HCl	MB	10, 25, 50 mg/ 1 mL	MB	1.25 mg/ 1 mL[a]	Physically compatible and diamorphine content retained for 24 hr at room temperature	1454	C
Dimenhydrinate	HR	50 mg/ 1 mL	PO	5 mg/ 1 mL	Physically incompatible within 15 min	326	I
Diphenhydramine HCl	PD	50 mg/ 1 mL	PO	5 mg/ 1 mL	Physically compatible for at least 15 min	326	C
Droperidol	MN	2.5 mg/ 1 mL	PO	5 mg/ 1 mL	Physically compatible for at least 15 min	326	C
Fentanyl citrate	MN	0.05 mg/ 1 mL	PO	5 mg/ 1 mL	Physically compatible for at least 15 min	326	C
Glycopyrrolate	RB	0.2 mg/ 1 mL	SKF	5 mg/ 1 mL	Physically compatible. pH in glycopyrrolate stability range for 48 hr at 25 °C	331	C
	RB	0.2 mg/ 1 mL	SKF	10 mg/ 2 mL	Physically compatible. pH in glycopyrrolate stability range for 48 hr at 25 °C	331	C
	RB	0.4 mg/ 2 mL	SKF	5 mg/ 1 mL	Physically compatible. pH in glycopyrrolate stability range for 48 hr at 25 °C	331	C
Hydromorphone HCl	KN	4 mg/ 2 mL[b]	SKF	5 mg/ 1 mL	Precipitates immediately	517	I
	KN	4 mg/ 2 mL[c]	SKF	5 mg/ 1 mL	Physically compatible for 30 min	517	C
Hydroxyzine HCl	PF	50 mg/ 1 mL	PO	5 mg/ 1 mL	Physically compatible for at least 15 min	326	C
Ketorolac tromethamine	SY	180 mg/ 6 mL	STS	15 mg/ 3 mL	Heavy white precipitate forms immediately, separating into two layers over time	1703	I
Meperidine HCl	WY	100 mg/ 1 mL	SKF		Physically compatible for at least 15 min	14	C
	WI	50 mg/ 1 mL	PO	5 mg/ 1 mL	Physically compatible for at least 15 min	326	C
Metoclopramide HCl	NO	10 mg/ 2 mL	MB	10 mg/ 2 mL	Physically compatible for 15 min at room temperature	565	C
Midazolam HCl	RC	5 mg/ 1 mL	SKF	10 mg/ 2 mL	White precipitate forms immediately	1145	I
Morphine sulfate	WY	15 mg/ 1 mL	SKF		Physically compatible for at least 15 min	14	C
	ST	15 mg/ 1 mL	PO	5 mg/ 1 mL	Physically compatible for at least 15 min	326	C
	WB	10 mg/ 1 mL	ES, SKF	10 mg/ 2 mL	Precipitates immediately, probably due to phenol in morphine formulation	1006	I
	WY	8, 10, 15 mg/ 1 mL	SKF	5 mg/ 1 mL	Physically compatible for 24 hr at 25 °C	1086	C
Nalbuphine HCl	EN	10 mg/ 1 mL	WY	5 mg/ 1 mL	Physically compatible for 36 hr at 27 °C	762	C
	EN	5 mg/ 0.5 mL	WY	5 mg/ 1 mL	Physically compatible for 36 hr at 27 °C	762	C
	EN	2.5 mg/ 0.25 mL	WY	5 mg/ 1 mL	Physically compatible for 36 hr at 27 °C	762	C
	DU	10 mg/ 1 mL	SKF	10 mg/ 2 mL	Physically compatible for 48 hr	128	C

Drugs in Syringe Compatibility (Cont.)

Prochlorperazine edisylate

Drug (in syringe)	Mfr	Amt	Mfr	Amt	Remarks	Ref	C/I
	DU	20 mg/ 1 mL	SKF	10 mg/ 2 mL	Physically compatible for 48 hr	128	**C**
Pantoprazole sodium	d	4 mg/ 1 mL		5 mg/ 1 mL	Yellowish precipitate forms	2574	**I**
Pentazocine lactate	WI	30 mg/ 1 mL	PO	5 mg/ 1 mL	Physically compatible for at least 15 min	326	**C**
Pentobarbital sodium	WY	100 mg/ 2 mL	SKF		Precipitate forms within 15 min	14	**I**
	AB	500 mg/ 10 mL	SKF	10 mg/ 2 mL	Physically incompatible	55	**I**
	AB	50 mg/ 1 mL	PO	5 mg/ 1 mL	Physically incompatible within 15 min	326	**I**
Promethazine HCl	PO	50 mg/ 2 mL	PO	5 mg/ 1 mL	Physically compatible for at least 15 min	326	**C**
Ranitidine HCl	GL	50 mg/ 2 mL	RP	10 mg/ 2 mL	Physically compatible for 1 hr at 25 °C	978	**C**
Scopolamine HBr		0.6 mg/ 1.5 mL	SKF		Physically compatible for at least 15 min	14	**C**
	ST	0.4 mg/ 1 mL	PO	5 mg/ 1 mL	Physically compatible for at least 15 min	326	**C**

[a]Diluted with sterile water for injection.
[b]The vial formulation was tested.
[c]The ampul formulation was tested.
[d]Test performed using the formulation WITHOUT edetate disodium.

Y-Site Injection Compatibility (1:1 Mixture)

Prochlorperazine edisylate

Drug	Mfr	Conc	Mfr	Conc	Remarks	Ref	C/I
Aldesleukin	CHI	33,800 I.U./ mL[a]	SKB	5 mg/mL	Aldesleukin bioactivity inhibited	1857	**I**
Allopurinol sodium	BW	3 mg/mL[b]	SKB	0.5 mg/mL[b]	Heavy turbidity forms immediately	1686	**I**
Amifostine	USB	10 mg/mL[a]	SN	0.5 mg/mL[a]	Immediate increase in measured haze	1845	**I**
Amphotericin B cholesteryl sulfate complex	SEQ	0.83 mg/mL[a]	SKB	0.5 mg/mL[a]	Gross precipitate forms	2117	**I**
Amsacrine	NCI	1 mg/mL[a]	SKF	0.5 mg/mL[a]	Visually compatible for 4 hr at 22 °C	1381	**C**
Aztreonam	SQ	40 mg/mL[a]	ES	0.5 mg/mL[a]	Haze and tiny particles form within 4 hr	1758	**I**
Bivalirudin	TMC	5 mg/mL[a]	SKB	0.5 mg/mL[a]	Gross white precipitate forms immediately	2373	**I**
Calcium gluconate	AMR	10 mg/mL[b]	SCN	5 mg/mL	Visually compatible for 24 hr at room temperature	2063	**C**
Cisatracurium besylate	GW	0.1, 2, 5 mg/ mL[a]	SO	0.5 mg/mL[a]	Physically compatible for 4 hr at 23 °C	2074	**C**
Cladribine	ORT	0.015[b] and 0.5[d] mg/mL	SCN	0.5 mg/mL[b]	Physically compatible for 4 hr at 23 °C	1969	**C**
Dexmedetomidine HCl	AB	4 mcg/mL[b]	SKB	0.5 mg/mL[b]	Physically compatible for 4 hr at 23 °C	2383	**C**
Docetaxel	RPR	0.9 mg/mL[a]	SO	0.5 mg/mL[a]	Physically compatible for 4 hr at 23 °C	2224	**C**
Doxorubicin HCl liposomal	SEQ	0.4 mg/mL[a]	SO	0.5 mg/mL[a]	Physically compatible for 4 hr at 23 °C	2087	**C**

Y-Site Injection Compatibility (1:1 Mixture) (Cont.)

Prochlorperazine edisylate

Drug	Mfr	Conc	Mfr	Conc	Remarks	Ref	C/I
Etoposide phosphate	BR	5 mg/mL[a]	ES	0.5 mg/mL[a]	White cloudy solution forms immediately with precipitate in 4 hr	2218	I
Fenoldopam mesylate	AB	80 mcg/mL[b]	SKB	0.5 mg/mL[b]	Trace haze forms in 4 hr	2467	I
Filgrastim	AMG	30 mcg/mL[a]	SCN	0.5 mg/mL[a]	Particles form immediately. Filaments form in 1 hr	1687	I
Fluconazole	RR	2 mg/mL	SKF	5 mg/mL	Physically compatible for 24 hr at 25 °C	1407	C
Fludarabine phosphate	BX	1 mg/mL[a]	WY	0.5 mg/mL[a]	Slight haze forms within 30 min	1439	I
Foscarnet sodium	AST	24 mg/mL	SKF	5 mg/mL	Cloudy brown solution	1335	I
Gallium nitrate	FUJ	1 mg/mL[b]	SCN	5 mg/mL	Precipitates immediately	1673	I
Gemcitabine HCl	LI	10 mg/mL[b]	SCN	0.5 mg/mL[b]	Subvisible haze forms immediately	2226	I
Granisetron HCl	SKB	0.05 mg/mL[a]	SCN	0.5 mg/mL[a]	Physically compatible for 4 hr at 23 °C	2000	C
Heparin sodium	UP	1000 units/L[e]	SKF	5 mg/mL	Physically compatible for 4 hr at room temperature	534	C
Hetastarch in lactated electrolyte	AB	6%	SO	0.5 mg/mL[a]	Physically compatible for 4 hr at 23 °C	2339	C
Hydrocortisone sodium succinate	UP	10 mg/L[e]	SKF	5 mg/mL	Physically compatible for 4 hr at room temperature	534	C
Linezolid	PHU	2 mg/mL	SO	0.5 mg/mL[a]	Physically compatible for 4 hr at 23 °C	2264	C
Melphalan HCl	BW	0.1 mg/mL[b]	SKB	0.5 mg/mL[b]	Physically compatible for 3 hr at 22 °C	1557	C
Ondansetron HCl	GL	1 mg/mL[b]	SKF	0.5 mg/mL[a]	Visually compatible for 4 hr at 22 °C	1365	C
Oxaliplatin	SS	0.5 mg/mL[a]	SKB	0.5 mg/mL[a]	Physically compatible for 4 hr at 23 °C	2566	C
Paclitaxel	NCI	1.2 mg/mL[a]		0.5 mg/mL[a]	Physically compatible for 4 hr at 22 °C	1528	C
Pemetrexed disodium	LI	20 mg/mL[b]	SKB	0.5 mg/mL[a]	Cloudy precipitate forms immediately	2564	I
Piperacillin sodium–tazobactam sodium	LE[f]	40 + 5 mg/mL[a]	SCN	0.5 mg/mL[a]	White turbidity forms immediately	1688	I
Potassium chloride	AB	40 mEq/L[e]	SKF	5 mg/mL	Physically compatible for 4 hr at room temperature	534	C
Propofol	ZEN	10 mg/mL	SCN	0.5 mg/mL[a]	Physically compatible for 1 hr at 23 °C	2066	C
Remifentanil HCl	GW	0.025 and 0.25 mg/mL[b]	SO	0.5 mg/mL[a]	Physically compatible for 4 hr at 23 °C	2075	C
Sargramostim	IMM	10 mcg/mL[b]	ES	0.5 mg/mL[b]	Visually compatible for 4 hr at 22 °C	1436	C
Teniposide	BR	0.1 mg/mL[a]	SCN	0.5 mg/mL[a]	Physically compatible for 4 hr at 23 °C	1725	C
Thiotepa	IMM[g]	1 mg/mL[a]	SCN	0.5 mg/mL[a]	Physically compatible for 4 hr at 23 °C	1861	C
TNA #218 to #226[c]			SCN, SO	0.5 mg/mL[a]	Visually compatible for 4 hr at 23 °C	2215	C
Topotecan HCl	SKB	56 mcg/mL[a,b]	SKB	0.192 mg/mL[a,b]	Visually compatible. Little loss of either drug in 4 hr at 22 °C	2245	C
TPN #212 to #215[c]			SCN	0.5 mg/mL[a]	Physically compatible for 4 hr at 23 °C	2109	C
Vinorelbine tartrate	BW	1 mg/mL[b]	SKB	0.5 mg/mL[b]	Physically compatible for 4 hr at 22 °C	1558	C

[a]Tested in dextrose 5%.
[b]Tested in sodium chloride 0.9%.
[c]Refer to Appendix I for the composition of parenteral nutrition solutions. TNA indicates a 3-in-1 admixture, and TPN indicates a 2-in-1 admixture.
[d]Tested in bacteriostatic sodium chloride 0.9% preserved with benzyl alcohol 0.9%.
[e]Tested in dextrose 5% in Ringer's injection, dextrose 5% in Ringer's injection, lactated, dextrose 5%, Ringer's injection, lactated, and sodium chloride 0.9%.
[f]Test performed using the formulation WITHOUT edetate disodium.
[g]Lyophilized formulation tested.

PROCHLORPERAZINE MESYLATE
AHFS 28:16.08.24

Products — Prochlorperazine mesylate injection is available in 1- and 2-mL glass ampuls. Each milliliter of solution contains prochlorperazine mesylate 12.5 mg with sodium sulfite, sodium metabisulfite, sodium chloride, ethanolamine, and water for injection. (38; 115)

Trade Name(s) — Stemetil.

Administration — Prochlorperazine mesylate injection is given by deep intramuscular injection. (38; 115)

Stability — Intact ampuls should be stored at controlled room temperature and protected from light. Exposure to light results in discoloration. Discolored injection should be discarded. (38; 115)

Compatibility Information

Additive Compatibility

Prochlorperazine mesylate

Drug	Mfr	Conc/L	Mfr	Conc/L	Test Soln	Remarks	Ref	C/I
Aminophylline	BP	1 g	BP	100 mg	D5W, NS	Precipitates immediately	26	I
Amphotericin B		200 mg	BP	100 mg	D5W	Haze develops over 3 hr	26	I
Ampicillin sodium	BP	2 g	BP	100 mg	D5W, NS	Precipitates immediately	26	I
Chloramphenicol sodium succinate	BP	4 g	BP	100 mg	NS	Haze develops over 3 hr	26	I
Chlorothiazide sodium	BP	2 g	BP	100 mg	D5W	Precipitates immediately	26	I
	BP	2 g	BP	100 mg	NS	Haze develops over 3 hr	26	I
Methohexital sodium	BP	2 g	BP	100 mg	D5W	Haze develops over 3 hr	26	I
Oxycodone HCl	NAP	1 g		600 mg	NS, W	Substantial change in prochlorperazine concentration in 24 hr at 25 °C	2600	I
Penicillin G potassium	BP	10 million units	BP	100 mg	NS	Haze develops over 3 hr	26	I
Penicillin G sodium	BP	10 million units	BP	100 mg	NS	Haze develops over 3 hr	26	I
Phenobarbital sodium	BP	800 mg	BP	100 mg	D5W	Haze develops over 3 hr	26	I
	BP	800 mg	BP	100 mg	NS	Precipitates immediately	26	I

Drugs in Syringe Compatibility

Prochlorperazine mesylate

Drug (in syringe)	Mfr	Amt	Mfr	Amt	Remarks	Ref	C/I
Hydromorphone HCl	KN	2, 10, 40 mg/1 mL	RP	5 mg/1 mL	Visually compatible. Little or no loss of either drug in 7 days at 4, 23, and 37 °C	1776	C
	SX	0.5 mg/mL[a]	RP	1.5 mg/mL[a]	Physically compatible for 96 hr at room temperature exposed to light	2171	C
Ketoprofen		50 mg/mL		12.5 mg/mL	White precipitate forms but then disappears	2495	?
Oxycodone HCl	NAP	200 mg/20 mL		12.5 mg/1 mL	Substantial change in prochlorperazine concentration in 24 hr at 25 °C	2600	I

[a] Diluted in sodium chloride 0.9%.

Y-Site Injection Compatibility (1:1 Mixture)

Prochlorperazine mesylate

Drug	Mfr	Conc	Mfr	Conc	Remarks	Ref	C/I
Clarithromycin	AB	4 mg/mL[a]	ANT	12.5 mg/mL	Visually compatible for 72 hr at both 30 and 17 °C	2174	C

[a]*Tested in dextrose 5%.*

PROMETHAZINE HYDROCHLORIDE
AHFS 28:24.92

Products — Promethazine hydrochloride is available in vials, ampuls, and syringe cartridges in concentrations of 25 and 50 mg/mL. Each milliliter also contains disodium edetate 0.1 mg, calcium chloride 0.04 mg, sodium metabisulfite 0.25 mg, phenol 5 mg, and acetic acid–sodium acetate buffer in water for injection. (1)

pH — From 4 to 5.5. (1)

Osmolality — The osmolality of promethazine hydrochloride 25 mg/mL was determined to be 291 mOsm/kg. (1233)

Administration — Promethazine hydrochloride is administered preferably by deep intramuscular injection. It should not be given subcutaneously or intra-arterially. If given by intravenous injection, a concentration not exceeding 25 mg/mL should be given into the tubing of a running infusion solution at a rate not exceeding 25 mg/min. (1; 4) Extravasation should be avoided. (4; 2312)

Stability — Store at controlled room temperature and protect from freezing and light. Inspect prior to administration for particulate matter formation and discoloration; discard if particulate matter or discoloration is observed. (1; 4) Promethazine hydrochloride exhibits increasing stability with decreasing pH. (1072)

Syringes — Promethazine hydrochloride 25 mg/mL repackaged in 3-mL amber glass syringes (Hy-Pod) and stored at 25 °C exhibited no changes in pH or appearance over 360 days. A possible reduction in concentration to 95% of initial was noted. (535)

Sorption — Promethazine hydrochloride (May & Baker) 8 mg/L in sodium chloride 0.9% (Travenol) in PVC bags exhibited only about 5% sorption to the plastic during one week of storage at room temperature (15 to 20 °C). However, when the solution was buffered from its initial pH of 5 to 7.4, approximately 59% of the drug was lost in one week due to sorption. (536)

In another study, promethazine hydrochloride (May & Baker) 8 mg/L in sodium chloride 0.9% exhibited a cumulative 22% loss during a seven-hour simulated infusion through an infusion set (Travenol) consisting of a cellulose propionate burette chamber and 170 cm of PVC tubing due to sorption. Both the burette and the tubing contributed to the loss. The extent of sorption was found to be independent of concentration. (606)

The drug was also tested as a simulated infusion over at least one hour by a syringe pump system. A glass syringe on a syringe pump was fitted with 20 cm of polyethylene tubing or 50 cm of Silastic tubing. Only 5% of the drug was lost with the polyethylene tubing, but a cumulative loss of 72% occurred during the one-hour infusion through the Silastic tubing. (606)

A 25-mL aliquot of promethazine hydrochloride (May & Baker) 8 mg/L in sodium chloride 0.9% was stored in all-plastic syringes composed of polypropylene barrels and polyethylene plungers for 24 hours at room temperature in the dark. No loss due to sorption occurred. (606)

Central Venous Catheter — Promethazine hydrochloride (Schein) 2 mg/mL in dextrose 5% was found to be compatible with the ARROWg+ard Blue Plus (Arrow International) chlorhexidine-bearing triple-lumen central catheter. Essentially complete delivery of the drug was found with little or no drug loss occurring. Furthermore, chlorhexidine delivered from the catheter remained at trace amounts with no substantial increase due to the delivery of the drug through the catheter. (2335)

Compatibility Information

Solution Compatibility

Promethazine HCl

Solution	Mfr	Mfr	Conc/L	Remarks	Ref	C/I
Dextrose–Ringer's injection combinations	AB	WY	100 mg	Physically compatible	3	C
Dextrose–Ringer's injection, lactated, combinations	AB	WY	100 mg	Physically compatible	3	C

Solution Compatibility (Cont.)

Promethazine HCl

Solution	Mfr	Mfr	Conc/L	Remarks	Ref	C/I
Dextrose–saline combinations	AB	WY	100 mg	Physically compatible	3	C
Dextrose 2.5%	AB	WY	100 mg	Physically compatible	3	C
Dextrose 5%	AB	WY	100 mg	Physically compatible	3	C
Dextrose 10%	AB	WY	100 mg	Physically compatible	3	C
Ionosol products	AB	WY	100 mg	Physically compatible	3	C
Ringer's injection	AB	WY	100 mg	Physically compatible	3	C
Ringer's injection, lactated	AB	WY	100 mg	Physically compatible	3	C
Sodium chloride 0.45%	AB	WY	100 mg	Physically compatible	3	C
Sodium chloride 0.9%	AB	WY	100 mg	Physically compatible	3	C
	[a]		100 mg	Physically compatible with little or no drug loss in 24 hr at 21 °C in the dark	1392	C
Sodium lactate ⅙ M	AB	WY	100 mg	Physically compatible	3	C

[a]Tested in PVC, glass, and polyethylene-lined laminated containers.

Additive Compatibility

Promethazine HCl

Drug	Mfr	Conc/L	Mfr	Conc/L	Test Soln	Remarks	Ref	C/I
Amikacin sulfate	BR	5 g	WY	100 mg	D5LR, D5R, D5S, D5W, D10W, LR, NS, R, SL	Physically compatible and both stable for 24 hr at 25 °C	294	C
Aminophylline	SE	1 g	WY	250 mg	D5W	Physically incompatible	15	I
	BP	1 g	BP	100 mg	D5W, NS	Precipitates immediately	26	I
Ascorbic acid	UP	500 mg	WY	250 mg	D5W	Physically compatible	15	C
Chloramphenicol sodium succinate	PD	10 g	WY	250 mg	D5W	Physically incompatible	15	I
Chlorothiazide sodium	BP	2 g	BP	100 mg	D5W, NS	Precipitates immediately	26	I
Floxacillin sodium	BE	20 g	MB	5 g	W	White precipitate forms immediately	1479	I
Furosemide	HO	1 g	MB	5 g	W	White precipitate forms immediately	1479	I
Heparin sodium	UP	4000 units	WY	250 mg	D5W	Physically incompatible	15	I
Hydrocortisone sodium succinate	UP	500 mg	WY	250 mg	D5W	Physically incompatible	15	I
Hydromorphone HCl	KN	1 g	ES	300 mg	NS[a]	Visually compatible for 21 days at 4 and 25 °C	1992	C
Methohexital sodium	BP	2 g	BP	100 mg	D5W, NS	Precipitates immediately	26	I
Penicillin G potassium	SQ	20 million units	WY	250 mg	D5W	Physically incompatible	15	I
		1 million units	WY	100 mg		Physically compatible	3	C

Additive Compatibility (Cont.)

Promethazine HCl

Drug	Mfr	Conc/L	Mfr	Conc/L	Test Soln	Remarks	Ref	C/I
	SQ	5 million units	WY	100 mg		Physically compatible	47	C
Penicillin G sodium	UP	20 million units	WY	250 mg	D5W	Physically incompatible	15	I
Pentobarbital sodium	AB	1 g	WY	250 mg	D5W	Physically incompatible	15	I
Phenobarbital sodium	WI	200 mg	WY	250 mg	D5W	Physically incompatible	15	I
	BP	800 mg	BP	100 mg	D5W	Haze develops over 3 hr	26	I
	BP	800 mg	BP	100 mg	NS	Precipitates immediately	26	I

ªTested in PVC containers.

Drugs in Syringe Compatibility

Promethazine HCl

Drug (in syringe)	Mfr	Amt	Mfr	Amt	Remarks	Ref	C/I
Atropine sulfate		0.6 mg/ 1.5 mL	WY	50 mg/ 2 mL	Physically compatible for at least 15 min	14	C
	ST	0.4 mg/ 1 mL	PO	50 mg/ 2 mL	Physically compatible for at least 15 min	326	C
Buprenorphine HCl					Physically and chemically compatible	4	C
Butorphanol tartrate	BR	4 mg/ 2 mL	WY	25 mg/ 1 mL	Physically compatible for 30 min at room temperature	566	C
Cefotetan disodium	ZEN	10 mg/ mLª	ES	25 mg/ 1 mL	White precipitate, resembling cottage cheese, forms immediately	1753	I
Chlorpromazine HCl	PO	50 mg/ 2 mL	PO	50 mg/ 2 mL	Physically compatible for at least 15 min	326	C
Dimenhydrinate	HR	50 mg/ 1 mL	PO	50 mg/ 2 mL	Physically incompatible within 15 min	326	I
		10 mg/ 1 mL		25 mg/ 1 mL	Solution discolors	2569	I
Diphenhydramine HCl	PD	50 mg/ 1 mL	WY	50 mg/ 2 mL	Physically compatible for at least 15 min	14	C
	PD	50 mg/ 1 mL	PO	50 mg/ 2 mL	Physically compatible for at least 15 min	326	C
Droperidol	MN	2.5 mg/ 1 mL	PO	50 mg/ 2 mL	Physically compatible for at least 15 min	326	C
Fentanyl citrate	MN	0.05 mg/ 1 mL	PO	50 mg/ 2 mL	Physically compatible for at least 15 min	326	C
Glycopyrrolate	RB	0.2 mg/ 1 mL	WY	25 mg/ 1 mL	Physically compatible. pH in glycopyrrolate stability range for 48 hr at 25 °C	331	C
	RB	0.2 mg/ 1 mL	WY	50 mg/ 2 mL	Physically compatible. pH in glycopyrrolate stability range for 48 hr at 25 °C	331	C
	RB	0.4 mg/ 2 mL	WY	25 mg/ 1 mL	Physically compatible. pH in glycopyrrolate stability range for 48 hr at 25 °C	331	C

Drugs in Syringe Compatibility (Cont.)

Promethazine HCl

Drug (in syringe)	Mfr	Amt	Mfr	Amt	Remarks	Ref	C/I
Heparin sodium		2500 units/ 1 mL		50 mg/ 2 mL	Turbidity or precipitate forms within 5 min	1053	I
Hydromorphone HCl	KN	4 mg/ 2 mL	WY	50 mg/ 1 mL	Physically compatible for 30 min	517	C
	KN	4 mg/ 2 mL	WY	25 mg/ 1 mL	Physically compatible for 30 min	517	C
Hydroxyzine HCl	PF	100 mg/ 4 mL	WY	50 mg/ 2 mL	Physically compatible for at least 15 min	14	C
	PF	50 mg/ 1 mL	PO	50 mg/ 2 mL	Physically compatible for at least 15 min	326	C
Iodipamide meglumine	SQ	52%, 40 and 20 mL	WY	1 mL	Forms a precipitate initially but clears within 1 hr and remains clear for 48 hr	530	?
	SQ	52%, 10 to 1 mL	WY	1 mL	Precipitates immediately	530	I
Iothalamate meglumine	MA	60%, 40 to 1 mL	WY	1 mL	Precipitates immediately	530	I
Ketorolac tromethamine	SY	180 mg/ 6 mL	ES	75 mg/ 3 mL	Heavy white precipitate forms immediately, separating into two layers over time	1703	I
Meperidine HCl	WY	100 mg/ 1 mL	WY	50 mg/ 2 mL	Physically compatible for at least 15 min	14	C
	WI	50 mg/ 1 mL	PO	50 mg/ 2 mL	Physically compatible for at least 15 min	326	C
Metoclopramide HCl	NO	10 mg/ 2 mL	WY	25 mg/ 1 mL	Physically compatible for 15 min at room temperature	565	C
Midazolam HCl	RC	5 mg/ 1 mL	WY	25 mg/ 1 mL	Physically compatible for 4 hr at 25 °C	1145	C
Morphine sulfate	WY	15 mg/ 1 mL	WY	50 mg/ 2 mL	Physically compatible for at least 15 min	14	C
	ST	15 mg/ 1 mL	PO	50 mg/ 2 mL	Physically compatible for at least 15 min	326	C
	WY	8 mg	WY	12.5 mg	Cloudiness develops	98	I
Nalbuphine HCl	EN	10 mg/ 1 mL	ES	25 mg	Physically compatible for 36 hr at 27 °C	762	C
	EN	5 mg/ 0.5 mL	ES	25 mg	Physically compatible for 36 hr at 27 °C	762	C
	EN	10 mg/ 1 mL	ES	12.5 mg	Physically compatible for 36 hr at 27 °C	762	C
	DU	10 mg/ 1 mL	WY	25 and 50 mg	Physically incompatible	128	I
	DU	20 mg/ 1 mL	WY	25 and 50 mg	Physically incompatible	128	I
	DU	10 mg/ 1 mL	WY	25 mg/ 1 mL	White flocculent precipitate forms immediately	1184	I
	DU	10 mg/ 1 mL	ES	25 mg/ 1 mL	Physically compatible for 24 hr at room temperature	1184	C
Pentazocine lactate	WI	30 mg/ 1 mL	WY	50 mg/ 2 mL	Physically compatible for at least 15 min	14	C
	WI	30 mg/ 1 mL	PO	50 mg/ 2 mL	Physically compatible for at least 15 min	326	C

Drugs in Syringe Compatibility (Cont.)

Promethazine HCl

Drug (in syringe)	Mfr	Amt	Mfr	Amt	Remarks	Ref	C/I
Pentobarbital sodium	AB	500 mg/ 10 mL	WY	100 mg/ 4 mL	Physically incompatible	55	I
	WY	100 mg/ 2 mL	WY	50 mg/ 2 mL	Precipitate forms within 15 min	14	I
	AB	50 mg/ 1 mL	PO	50 mg/ 2 mL	Physically incompatible within 15 min	326	I
Prochlorperazine edisylate	PO	5 mg/ 1 mL	PO	50 mg/ 2 mL	Physically compatible for at least 15 min	326	C
Ranitidine HCl	GL	50 mg/ 2 mL	RP	25 mg/ 1 mL	Physically compatible for 1 hr at 25 °C	978	C
	GL	50 mg/ 5 mL	RP	25 mg	Physically compatible for 4 hr	1151	C
Scopolamine HBr		0.6 mg/ 1.5 mL	WY	50 mg/ 2 mL	Physically compatible for at least 15 min	14	C
	ST	0.4 mg/ 1 mL	PO	50 mg/ 2 mL	Physically compatible for at least 15 min	326	C

[a]Tested in dextrose 5%.

Y-Site Injection Compatibility (1:1 Mixture)

Promethazine HCl

Drug	Mfr	Conc	Mfr	Conc	Remarks	Ref	C/I
Aldesleukin	CHI	33,800 I.U./ mL[a]	ES	25 mg/mL	Aldesleukin bioactivity inhibited	1857	I
Allopurinol sodium	BW	3 mg/mL[b]	WY	2 mg/mL[b]	Immediate turbidity. Particles in 4 hr	1686	I
Amifostine	USB	10 mg/mL[a]	ES	2 mg/mL[a]	Physically compatible for 4 hr at 23 °C	1845	C
Amphotericin B cholesteryl sulfate complex	SEQ	0.83 mg/mL[a]	ES	2 mg/mL[a]	Gross precipitate forms	2117	I
Amsacrine	NCI	1 mg/mL[a]	ES	2 mg/mL[a]	Visually compatible for 4 hr at 22 °C	1381	C
Aztreonam	SQ	40 mg/mL[a]	SCN	2 mg/mL[a]	Physically compatible for 4 hr at 23 °C	1758	C
Bivalirudin	TMC	5 mg/mL[a]	ES	2 mg/mL[a]	Physically compatible for 4 hr at 23 °C	2373	C
Cefazolin sodium	LI	10 mg/mL[a]	ES	25 mg	Cloudiness forms then dissipates	1753	?
Cefotetan disodium	ZEN	10 mg/mL[a]	ES	25 mg	White precipitate forms immediately	1753	I
Ceftaroline fosamil	FOR	2.22 mg/ mL[a,b,h]	SIC	2 mg/mL[a,b,h]	Physically compatible for 4 hr at 23 °C	2826	C
Ciprofloxacin	MI	2 mg/mL[a,b]	ES	25 mg/mL	Visually compatible for 24 hr at 24 °C	1655	C
Cisatracurium besylate	GW	0.1, 2, 5 mg/ mL[a]	ES	2 mg/mL[a]	Physically compatible for 4 hr at 23 °C	2074	C
Cladribine	ORT	0.015[b] and 0.5[d] mg/mL	SCN	2 mg/mL[b]	Physically compatible for 4 hr at 23 °C	1969	C
Dexmedetomidine HCl	AB	4 mcg/mL[b]	ES	2 mg/mL[b]	Physically compatible for 4 hr at 23 °C	2383	C
Docetaxel	RPR	0.9 mg/mL[a]	SCN	2 mg/mL[a]	Physically compatible for 4 hr at 23 °C	2224	C
Doxorubicin HCl liposomal	SEQ	0.4 mg/mL[a]	ES	2 mg/mL[a]	Increase in measured turbidity	2087	I
Etoposide phosphate	BR	5 mg/mL[a]	SCN	2 mg/mL[a]	Physically compatible for 4 hr at 23 °C	2218	C
Fenoldopam mesylate	AB	80 mcg/mL[b]	ES	2 mg/mL[b]	Physically compatible for 4 hr at 23 °C	2467	C

Y-Site Injection Compatibility (1:1 Mixture) (Cont.)

Promethazine HCl

Drug	Mfr	Conc	Mfr	Conc	Remarks	Ref	C/I
Filgrastim	AMG	30 mcg/mL[a]	SCN	2 mg/mL[a]	Physically compatible for 4 hr at 22 °C	1687	**C**
Fluconazole	RR	2 mg/mL	ES	50 mg/mL	Physically compatible for 24 hr at 25 °C	1407	**C**
Fludarabine phosphate	BX	1 mg/mL[a]	WY	2 mg/mL[a]	Visually compatible for 4 hr at 22 °C	1439	**C**
Foscarnet sodium	AST	24 mg/mL	ES	50 mg/mL	Gas production	1335	**I**
Gemcitabine HCl	LI	10 mg/mL[b]	SCN	2 mg/mL[b]	Physically compatible for 4 hr at 23 °C	2226	**C**
Granisetron HCl	SKB	0.05 mg/mL[a]	WY	2 mg/mL[a]	Physically compatible for 4 hr at 23 °C	2000	**C**
Heparin sodium	UP	1000 units/L[f]	SV	50 mg/mL	Physically compatible for 4 hr at room temperature	534	**C**
	UP	1000 units/L[g]	SV	50 mg/mL	Clear initially, but cloudiness develops in 4 hr at room temperature	534	**I**
Hetastarch in lactated electrolyte	AB	6%	SCN	2 mg/mL[a]	Physically compatible for 4 hr at 23 °C	2339	**C**
Hydrocortisone sodium succinate	UP	10 mg/L[f]	SV	50 mg/mL	Physically compatible for 4 hr at room temperature	534	**C**
	UP	10 mg/L[g]	SV	50 mg/mL	Clear initially, but cloudiness develops in 4 hr at room temperature	534	**I**
Linezolid	PHU	2 mg/mL	SCN	2 mg/mL[a]	Physically compatible for 4 hr at 23 °C	2264	**C**
Melphalan HCl	BW	0.1 mg/mL[b]	WY	2 mg/mL[b]	Physically compatible for 3 hr at 22 °C	1557	**C**
Ondansetron HCl	GL	1 mg/mL[b]	ES	2 mg/mL[a]	Visually compatible for 4 hr at 22 °C	1365	**C**
Oxaliplatin	SS	0.5 mg/mL[a]	ES	2 mg/mL[a]	Physically compatible for 4 hr at 23 °C	2566	**C**
Palonosetron HCl	MGI	50 mcg/mL	PAD	2 mg/mL[a]	Physically compatible. No loss of either drug in 4 hr	2716	**C**
Pemetrexed disodium	LI	20 mg/mL[b]	SIC	0.5 mg/mL[a]	Physically compatible for 4 hr at 23 °C	2564	**C**
Piperacillin sodium–tazobactam sodium	LE[c]	40 + 5 mg/mL[a]	SCN	2 mg/mL[a]	Heavy white turbidity forms immediately. Particles form in 4 hr	1688	**I**
Potassium chloride	AB	40 mEq/L[f]	SV	50 mg/mL	Physically compatible for 4 hr at room temperature	534	**C**
	AB	40 mEq/L[g]	SV	50 mg/mL	Clear initially, but cloudiness develops in 4 hr at room temperature	534	**I**
Remifentanil HCl	GW	0.025 and 0.25 mg/mL[b]	SCN	2 mg/mL[a]	Physically compatible for 4 hr at 23 °C	2075	**C**
Sargramostim	IMM	10 mcg/mL[b]	ES	2 mg/mL[b]	Visually compatible for 4 hr at 22 °C	1436	**C**
Teniposide	BR	0.1 mg/mL[a]	WY	2 mg/mL[a]	Physically compatible for 4 hr at 23 °C	1725	**C**
Thiotepa	IMM[i]	1 mg/mL[a]	WY	2 mg/mL[a]	Physically compatible for 4 hr at 23 °C	1861	**C**
TNA #218 to #226[e]			SCN	2 mg/mL[a]	Visually compatible for 4 hr at 23 °C	2215	**C**
TPN #212, #214[e]			SCN	2 mg/mL[a]	Physically compatible for 4 hr at 23 °C	2109	**C**
TPN #213, #215[e]			SCN	2 mg/mL[a]	Amber discoloration forms in 4 hr	2109	**I**
Vinorelbine tartrate	BW	1 mg/mL[b]	ES	2 mg/mL[b]	Physically compatible for 4 hr at 22 °C	1558	**C**

[a]Tested in dextrose 5%.
[b]Tested in sodium chloride 0.9%.
[c]Test performed using the formulation WITHOUT edetate disodium.
[d]Tested in bacteriostatic sodium chloride 0.9% preserved with benzyl alcohol 0.9%.
[e]Refer to Appendix I for the composition of parenteral nutrition solutions. TNA indicates a 3-in-1 admixture, and TPN indicates a 2-in-1 admixture.
[f]Tested in dextrose 5% in Ringer's injection, lactated, dextrose 5%, Ringer's injection, lactated, and sodium chloride 0.9%.
[g]Tested in dextrose 5% in Ringer's injection.
[h]Tested in Ringer's injection, lactated.
[i]Lyophilized formulation tested.

Additional Compatibility Information

Chlorpromazine and Meperidine — Chlorpromazine hydrochloride, meperidine hydrochloride, and promethazine hydrochloride combined as an extemporaneous mixture for preoperative sedation, developed a brownish-yellow color after two weeks of storage with protection from light. The discoloration was attributed to the meta-cresol preservative content of the meperidine hydrochloride product used. Use of meperidine hydrochloride which contains a different preservative resulted in a solution that remained clear and colorless for at least three months when protected from light. (1148)

PROPOFOL
AHFS 28:04.92

Products — Propofol (Diprivan) 1% is available as a ready-to-use oil-in-water emulsion in 20-mL ampuls, and 50- and 100-mL infusion vials. Each milliliter contains propofol 10 mg along with soybean oil 100 mg, glycerol 22.5 mg, egg lecithin 12 mg, and disodium edetate 0.005% with sodium hydroxide to adjust the pH. (1)

Generic propofol 1% formulations are also available as ready-to-use oil-in-water emulsion in 20-mL vials and 50- and 100-mL infusion vials. However, the products differ from the Diprivan formulation. Each milliliter contains propofol 10 mg along with soybean oil 100 mg, glycerol 22.5 mg, and egg yolk phospholipid 12 mg, but incorporates sodium metabisulfite 0.25 mg or benzyl alcohol 1 mg/mL. Sodium hydroxide is used to adjust the pH during manufacture. (1)

The propofol products are not identical. Diprivan utilizes disodium edetate as an antimicrobial agent; the generic products utilize sodium metabisulfite or benzyl alcohol for this purpose. Diprivan and the generic propofol with benzyl alcohol have pH values in the range of 7 to 8.5. For the sodium metabisulfite in the propofol formulations to be comparable to the other two formulations as an antimicrobial agent, the pH of the products has been adjusted to 4.5 to 6.4 during manufacture. (2348; 2349)

NOTE: Most of the compatibility information for propofol with other drugs has been developed using Diprivan and cannot be automatically extrapolated to the other products because of the formulation differences. The formulation differences have been demonstrated to result in some differing compatibilities with other drugs. (2336)

pH — Diprivan and the benzyl alcohol-containing formulation have a pH in the range of 7 to 8.5. The metabisulfite-containing formulation has a pH of 4.5 to 6.6. (1)

Tonicity — Propofol 1% injectable emulsion is isotonic. (1)

Trade Name(s) — Diprivan.

Administration — Before use, propofol should be shaken well. It may be administered undiluted by intravenous injection or infusion or diluted with dextrose 5% to no less than 2 mg/mL. (1)

Numerous outbreaks of serious postoperative infections have resulted from inadvertent contamination of propofol. The contamination resulted from risky preparation practices and lapses in aseptic technique. The lipid base supports microbiological growth. (1; 1930) The disodium edetate, sodium metabisulfite, or benzyl alcohol in the formulations retard the growth of microorganisms, but the products can still support growth and are not antimicrobially preserved. Strict aseptic procedures are required during preparation. (1)

Stability — Propofol 1% injection is a white, oil-in-water emulsion. Intact containers should be stored between 4 and 22 °C and protected from freezing. The emulsion should not be used if phase separation is evident. (1)

Propofol undergoes oxidative degradation when exposed to oxygen. Intact containers are packaged using nitrogen to avoid oxygen exposure. If propofol is administered directly from the vial, administration should be completed within 12 hours after the vial is spiked. The tubing and any unused propofol should be discarded after 12 hours. (1)

Propofol formulated with sodium metabisulfite antioxidant is subject to a differing decomposition reaction compared to the edetate-containing Diprivan. Exposure to air results in the formation of a yellow discoloration in about six to seven hours, which does not occur with Diprivan. The yellow discoloration is a result of the formation of oxidized propofol dimer quinone from sulfite radicals that form in the generic product and may be associated with increased adverse effects. This oxidation product does not form in Diprivan with EDTA. (2344; 2575; 2576) Stability information developed for the Diprivan formulation should not be extrapolated to the sodium metabisulfite-containing generic formulation. (2344)

The physical stability of Diprivan and propofol with sodium metabisulfite was evaluated. The formulation differences, principally pH, resulted in a much higher zeta potential for Diprivan, making it a more rugged emulsion and less subject to damage from physical agitation and thermal insult. Physical agitation resulted in no increase in fat droplet size in Diprivan after 16 hours, but a substantial increase in fat droplets larger than 5 μm occurred in as little as four hours in the generic formulation. (2445)

The benzyl alcohol-containing form of propofol has the same pH as Diprivan (pH 7 to 8.5) and exhibits the same degree of ruggedness and resistance to emulsion disruption. (2659)

In another study, Diprivan was again reported to be a more rugged emulsion than the generic form with sodium metabisulfite. Diprivan had a very low quantity of fat globules exceeding 5 μm throughout its shelf life. The generic formulation formed much greater amounts of globules of 5 μm and larger within a few months after manufacture and well before the expiration date. This 5-μm globule size and larger is an important threshold because this size globule may occlude capillaries and lead to embolic syndrome. The safety of using the generic formulation of propofol was questioned, especially as the product nears its expiration date. (2589)

If propofol emulsion is transferred to a syringe or other container prior to use, administration should be begun promptly and completed within six hours after the container is opened. After six hours, the product should be discarded and the lines should be flushed or discarded. (1)

Propofol emulsion is a single-use product and can support the growth of microorganisms. (1; 1930) Propofol strongly supports the growth of *Escherichia coli* and *Candida albicans*. (2411) Strict adherence to proper aseptic procedures, including wiping of the ampul neck or vial stopper with isopropanol 70%, is required (1) and discarding after six hours has been recommended. (2411)

Plastic and Glass Containers — Diluted in dextrose 5%, propofol has been shown to be more stable in glass than in plastic containers. The manufacturers indicate that only 95% remains after only two hours in plastic. However, the type of plastic container subject to this increased rate of loss is not specified. (1)

Syringes — Propofol (Diprivan) 10 mg/mL was repackaged into 60-mL polypropylene syringes (Monoject, Sherwood Medical) and stored at 23 °C under fluorescent light and at 4 °C protected from light. No visually apparent changes occurred to the emulsion under either storage condition. Propofol losses were 7% in five days and 12% in seven days in the room-temperature samples. No propofol losses occurred in 13 days in the refrigerated samples. (1984)

Propofol (Diprivan) 1% was repackaged into 2- and 10-mL Plastipak (Becton Dickinson) and 2-mL Inject (B. Braun) plastic syringes and was stored at 5 °C. Propofol losses were about 7 to 8% in the Plastipak syringes and about 2% in the Inject syringes after 28 days of refrigerated storage. (2118)

Sorption — Diprivan injection was diluted to 2 mg/mL with dextrose 5% and stored in PVC tubing (Kendall-McGaw). A propofol loss exceeding 31% occurred after static storage for two hours. In simulated infusions using the same initial concentration, administration through 72-inch PVC administration sets at a rate of 1.75 mL/min

resulted in an average propofol loss of 7.7% over the two-hour period. (2057)

When tested undiluted at 10 mg/mL, propofol (Diprivan) sorption to administration tubing composed principally of PVC did not represent a substantial portion of the total amount of drug delivered. Any losses that did occur were within the error of the method and were not clinically relevant. (2297)

Propofol (Diprivan) was delivered at rates of 1 and 10 mL/hr through PVC tubing. Little loss occurred at the higher rate of delivery. However, at the slower rate, up to 6% propofol loss due to sorption occurred. (2468)

Plasticizer Leaching — As happens with other surfactant-containing drug formulations, propofol emulsion also has been shown to leach diethylhexyl phthalate (DEHP) plasticizer from PVC equipment such as administration sets. Non-PVC administration sets should be used to deliver this drug. (2424)

Filtration — The manufacturers recommend that filters with a pore size less than 5 μm should not be used with propofol emulsion. These filters may restrict its administration and/or cause the breakdown of the emulsion. (1) Propofol (Diprivan) 1% 10 mL filtered through a 5-μm filter needle (Burron Medical) underwent no loss. (2057)

Opening propofol packaged in glass ampuls has been shown to yield a substantially higher amount of larger particulates compared to the vials. The larger particulates are probably glass shards associated with opening the ampuls. Drawing the propofol into a syringe using a 5-μm filter significantly reduced the amount of these particles in the product. (2311)

Compatibility Information

Solution Compatibility

Propofol

Solution	Mfr	Mfr	Conc/L	Remarks	Ref	C/I
Dextrose 5% in Ringer's injection, lactated				Compatible	1	**C**
Dextrose 5% in sodium chloride 0.2%				Compatible	1	**C**
Dextrose 5% in sodium chloride 0.45%				Compatible	1	**C**
Dextrose 5%				Compatible	1	**C**
Ringer's injection, lactated				Compatible	1	**C**

Drugs in Syringe Compatibility

Propofol

Drug (in syringe)	Mfr	Amt	Mfr	Amt	Remarks	Ref	C/I
Ketamine HCl	SZ	50 mg/ 5 mL	NOP	50 mg/ 5 mL	Physically compatible. Little loss of either drug in 3 hr at room temperature	2790	**C**
	SZ	30 mg/ 3 mL	NOP	70 mg/ 7 mL	Physically compatible. Little loss of either drug in 3 hr at room temperature	2790	**C**
Lidocaine HCl		5 and 10 mg		1%	Physically compatible for 24 hr	2490	**C**
		20 and 40 mg		1%	Physically incompatible. Increased fat droplet size and layering in 3 hr	2490	**I**

Drugs in Syringe Compatibility (Cont.)

Drug (in syringe)	Mfr	Amt	Propofol Mfr	Amt	Remarks	Ref	C/I
		10 mg	ZEN	1%, 20 mL	Physically compatible for 6 hr	2543	**C**
		30 to 50 mg	ZEN	1%, 20 mL	Increased fat droplet size	2543	**I**
Ondansetron HCl	GW	1 mg/mL[b]	STU	1 and 5 mg/mL[b]	Physically compatible. Little loss of either drug in 4 hr at 23 °C	2199	**C**
Pantoprazole sodium	[a]	4 mg/1 mL		10 mg/1 mL	No change seen	2574	**?**

[a]Test performed using the formulation WITHOUT edetate disodium.
[b]Tested in sodium chloride 0.9%.

Y-Site Injection Compatibility (1:1 Mixture)

Drug	Mfr	Conc	Propofol Mfr	Conc	Remarks	Ref	C/I
Acyclovir sodium	BW	7 mg/mL[a]	ZEN	10 mg/mL	Physically compatible for 1 hr at 23 °C	2066	**C**
Alfentanil HCl	JN	0.5 mg/mL	ZEN	10 mg/mL	Physically compatible for 1 hr at 23 °C	2066	**C**
Amikacin sulfate	DU	5 mg/mL[a]	ZEN	10 mg/mL	Immediate precipitate and yellow color	2066	**I**
Aminophylline	AMR	2.5 mg/mL[a]	ZEN	10 mg/mL	Physically compatible for 1 hr at 23 °C	2066	**C**
Amphotericin B	APC	0.6 mg/mL[a]	ZEN	10 mg/mL	Gel-like precipitate forms immediately	2066	**I**
Ampicillin sodium	WY	20 mg/mL[b]	ZEN	10 mg/mL	Physically compatible for 1 hr at 23 °C	2066	**C**
Ascorbic acid	AB	500 mg/mL	STU	2 mg/mL	No visible change in 24 hr at 25 °C. Yellow color forms within 7 days	1801	**?**
Atracurium besylate	BW	10 mg/mL	STU	2 mg/mL	Oil droplets form within 24 hr, followed by phase separation at 25 °C	1801	**I**
	BW	10 mg/mL	ZEN	10 mg/mL	Emulsion broke and oiled out	2066	**I**
		10 mg/mL	ASZ, BA	10 mg/mL	Emulsion disruption upon mixing	2336	**I**
		5 mg/mL[a]	ASZ, BA	10 mg/mL	Emulsion disruption upon mixing	2336	**I**
		0.5 mg/mL[a]	BA	10 mg/mL	Emulsion disruption upon mixing	2336	**I**
		0.5 mg/mL[a]	ASZ	10 mg/mL	Physically compatible for at least 1 hr at room temperature	2336	**C**
Atropine sulfate	GNS	0.4 mg/mL	STU	2 mg/mL	Oil droplets form within 7 days at 25 °C. No visible change in 24 hr	1801	**?**
	AST	0.1 mg/mL[a]	ZEN	10 mg/mL	Physically compatible for 1 hr at 23 °C	2066	**C**
Aztreonam	SQ	40 mg/mL[a]	ZEN	10 mg/mL	Physically compatible for 1 hr at 23 °C	2066	**C**
Bumetanide	RC	0.04 mg/mL[a]	ZEN	10 mg/mL	Physically compatible for 1 hr at 23 °C	2066	**C**
Buprenorphine HCl	RKC	0.04 mg/mL[a]	ZEN	10 mg/mL	Physically compatible for 1 hr at 23 °C	2066	**C**
Butorphanol tartrate	APC	0.04 mg/mL[a]	ZEN	10 mg/mL	Physically compatible for 1 hr at 23 °C	2066	**C**
Calcium chloride	AST	40 mg/mL[a]	ZEN	10 mg/mL	White precipitate forms in 1 hr	2066	**I**
Calcium gluconate	AMR	40 mg/mL[a]	ZEN	10 mg/mL	Physically compatible for 1 hr at 23 °C	2066	**C**
Carboplatin	BR	5 mg/mL[a]	ZEN	10 mg/mL	Physically compatible for 1 hr at 23 °C	2066	**C**
Cefazolin sodium	MAR	20 mg/mL[a]	ZEN	10 mg/mL	Physically compatible for 1 hr at 23 °C	2066	**C**

Y-Site Injection Compatibility (1:1 Mixture) (Cont.)

Propofol

Drug	Mfr	Conc	Mfr	Conc	Remarks	Ref	C/I
Cefepime HCl	BMS	120 mg/mL[c]		1 mg/mL	Precipitates	2513	I
Cefotaxime sodium	HO	20 mg/mL[a]	ZEN	10 mg/mL	Physically compatible for 1 hr at 23 °C	2066	C
Cefotetan disodium	STU	20 mg/mL[a]	ZEN	10 mg/mL	Physically compatible for 1 hr at 23 °C	2066	C
Cefoxitin sodium	ME	20 mg/mL[a]	ZEN	10 mg/mL	Physically compatible for 1 hr at 23 °C	2066	C
Ceftaroline fosamil	FOR	2.22 mg/mL[a,b,c]	HOS	10 mg/mL	Physically compatible for 4 hr at 23 °C	2826	C
Ceftazidime	SKB	40 mg/mL[a]	ZEN	10 mg/mL	Physically compatible for 1 hr at 23 °C	2066	C
	SKB	125 mg/mL		1 mg/mL	Physically incompatible	2434	I
	GSK	120 mg/mL		1 mg/mL	Precipitates	2513	I
Ceftriaxone sodium	RC	20 mg/mL[a]	ZEN	10 mg/mL	Physically compatible for 1 hr at 23 °C	2066	C
Cefuroxime sodium	LI	30 mg/mL[a]	ZEN	10 mg/mL	Physically compatible for 1 hr at 23 °C	2066	C
Chlorpromazine HCl	SCN	2 mg/mL[a]	ZEN	10 mg/mL	Physically compatible for 1 hr at 23 °C	2066	C
Cisatracurium besylate	GW	5 mg/mL[a]	ASZ, BA	10 mg/mL	Emulsion disruption upon mixing	2336	I
	GW	0.5 mg/mL[a]	BA	10 mg/mL	Emulsion disruption upon mixing	2336	I
	GW	0.5 mg/mL[a]	ASZ	10 mg/mL	Physically compatible for at least 1 hr at room temperature	2336	C
Cisplatin	BR	1 mg/mL	ZEN	10 mg/mL	Physically compatible for 1 hr at 23 °C	2066	C
Clindamycin phosphate	AST	10 mg/mL[a]	ZEN	10 mg/mL	Physically compatible for 1 hr at 23 °C	2066	C
Cyclophosphamide	MJ	10 mg/mL[a]	ZEN	10 mg/mL	Physically compatible for 1 hr at 23 °C	2066	C
Cyclosporine	SZ	5 mg/mL[a]	ZEN	10 mg/mL	Physically compatible for 1 hr at 23 °C	2066	C
Cytarabine	CHI	50 mg/mL	ZEN	10 mg/mL	Physically compatible for 1 hr at 23 °C	2066	C
Dexamethasone sodium phosphate	AMR	1 mg/mL[a]	ZEN	10 mg/mL	Physically compatible for 1 hr at 23 °C	2066	C
Dexmedetomidine HCl	AB	4 mcg/mL[b]	ASZ	10 mg/mL	Physically compatible for 4 hr at 23 °C	2383	C
Diazepam	ES	5 mg/mL	ZEN	10 mg/mL	Emulsion broke and oiled out	2066	I
Diphenhydramine HCl	SCN	2 mg/mL[a]	ZEN	10 mg/mL	Physically compatible for 1 hr at 23 °C	2066	C
Dobutamine HCl	LI	4 mg/mL[a]	ZEN	10 mg/mL	Physically compatible for 1 hr at 23 °C	2066	C
Dopamine HCl	AST	3.2 mg/mL[a]	ZEN	10 mg/mL	Physically compatible for 1 hr at 23 °C	2066	C
Doripenem	JJ	5 mg/mL[a,b]	BED	10 mg/mL	Precipitation forms immediately	2743	I
Doxycycline hyclate	LY	1 mg/mL[a]	ZEN	10 mg/mL	Physically compatible for 1 hr at 23 °C	2066	C
Droperidol	JN	0.4 mg/mL[c]	ZEN	10 mg/mL	Physically compatible for 1 hr at 23 °C	2066	C
Enalaprilat	MSD	0.1 mg/mL[a]	ZEN	10 mg/mL	Physically compatible for 1 hr at 23 °C	2066	C
Ephedrine sulfate	AB	5 mg/mL[a]	ZEN	10 mg/mL	Physically compatible for 1 hr at 23 °C	2066	C
Epinephrine HCl	AMR	0.1 mg/mL	ZEN	10 mg/mL	Physically compatible for 1 hr at 23 °C	2066	C
Esmolol HCl	OHM	10 mg/mL	ZEN	10 mg/mL	Physically compatible for 1 hr at 23 °C	2066	C
Famotidine	ME	2 mg/mL[a]	ZEN	10 mg/mL	Physically compatible for 1 hr at 23 °C	2066	C
Fenoldopam mesylate	AB	80 mcg/mL[b]	ASZ	10 mg/mL	Physically compatible for 4 hr at 23 °C	2467	C
Fentanyl citrate	AB	0.05 mg/mL	ZEN	10 mg/mL	Physically compatible for 1 hr at 23 °C	2066	C
Fluconazole	PF	2 mg/mL[a]	ZEN	10 mg/mL	Physically compatible for 1 hr at 23 °C	2066	C
Fluorouracil	AD	16 mg/mL[a]	ZEN	10 mg/mL	Physically compatible for 1 hr at 23 °C	2066	C

Y-Site Injection Compatibility (1:1 Mixture) (Cont.)

					Propofol		
Drug	Mfr	Conc	Mfr	Conc	Remarks	Ref	C/I
Furosemide	AB	3 mg/mL[a]	ZEN	10 mg/mL	Physically compatible for 1 hr at 23 °C	2066	**C**
Ganciclovir sodium	SY	20 mg/mL[a]	ZEN	10 mg/mL	Physically compatible for 1 hr at 23 °C	2066	**C**
Gentamicin sulfate	ES	5 mg/mL[a]	ZEN	10 mg/mL	White precipitate forms immediately	2066	**I**
Glycopyrrolate	RB	0.2 mg/mL	ZEN	10 mg/mL	Physically compatible for 1 hr at 23 °C	2066	**C**
Granisetron HCl	SKB	0.05 mg/mL[a]	ZEN	10 mg/mL	Physically compatible for 1 hr at 23 °C	2066	**C**
Haloperidol lactate	MN	0.2 mg/mL[a]	ZEN	10 mg/mL	Physically compatible for 1 hr at 23 °C	2066	**C**
Heparin sodium	ES	100 units/mL[a]	ZEN	10 mg/mL	Physically compatible for 1 hr at 23 °C	2066	**C**
Hydrocortisone sodium succinate	UP	1 mg/mL[a]	ZEN	10 mg/mL	Physically compatible for 1 hr at 23 °C	2066	**C**
Hydromorphone HCl	AST	0.5 mg/mL[a]	ZEN	10 mg/mL	Physically compatible for 1 hr at 23 °C	2066	**C**
Hydroxyethyl starch 130/0.4 in sodium chloride 0.9%	FRK	6%	NOP	2.5[a], 5[a], 10 mg/mL	Visually compatible for 24 hr at room temperature	2770	**C**
Hydroxyzine HCl	ES	2 mg/mL[a]	ZEN	10 mg/mL	Physically compatible for 1 hr at 23 °C	2066	**C**
Ifosfamide	MJ	25 mg/mL[a]	ZEN	10 mg/mL	Physically compatible for 1 hr at 23 °C	2066	**C**
Imipenem–cilastatin sodium	ME	10 mg/mL[b]	ZEN	10 mg/mL	Physically compatible for 1 hr at 23 °C	2066	**C**
Insulin	NOV	1 unit/mL[a]	ZEN	10 mg/mL	Physically compatible for 1 hr at 23 °C	2066	**C**
Isoproterenol HCl	AB	0.004 mg/mL[a]	ZEN	10 mg/mL	Physically compatible for 1 hr at 23 °C	2066	**C**
Ketamine HCl	PD	10 mg/mL	ZEN	10 mg/mL	Physically compatible for 1 hr at 23 °C	2066	**C**
Labetalol HCl	AH	5 mg/mL	ZEN	10 mg/mL	Physically compatible for 1 hr at 23 °C	2066	**C**
Lidocaine HCl	AST	10 mg/mL	ZEN	10 mg/mL	Physically compatible for 1 hr at 23 °C	2066	**C**
Lorazepam	WY	0.1 mg/mL[a]	ZEN	10 mg/mL	Physically compatible for 1 hr at 23 °C	2066	**C**
Magnesium sulfate	AST	100 mg/mL[a]	ZEN	10 mg/mL	Physically compatible for 1 hr at 23 °C	2066	**C**
Mannitol	BA	15%	ZEN	10 mg/mL	Physically compatible for 1 hr at 23 °C	2066	**C**
Meperidine HCl	WY	4 mg/mL[a]	ZEN	10 mg/mL	Physically compatible for 1 hr at 23 °C	2066	**C**
Methotrexate sodium	LE	15 mg/mL[a]	ZEN	10 mg/mL	White precipitate forms in 1 hr	2066	**I**
Methylprednisolone sodium succinate	AB	5 mg/mL[a]	ZEN	10 mg/mL	White precipitate forms immediately	2066	**I**
Midazolam HCl	RC	5 mg/mL	STU	2 mg/mL	Oil droplets form within 7 days at 25 °C. No visible change in 24 hr	1801	**?**
	RC	2 mg/mL[a]	ZEN	10 mg/mL	Physically compatible for 1 hr at 23 °C	2066	**C**
Milrinone lactate	SW	0.4 mg/mL[a]	ZEN	10 mg/mL	Little loss of either drug in 4 hr at 23 °C	2214	**C**
Mitoxantrone HCl	IMM	0.5 mg/mL[a]	ZEN	10 mg/mL	Particles form immediately	2066	**I**
Morphine sulfate	AST	1 mg/mL[a]	ZEN	10 mg/mL	Physically compatible for 1 hr at 23 °C	2066	**C**
Nafcillin sodium	MAR	20 mg/mL[a]	ZEN	10 mg/mL	Physically compatible for 1 hr at 23 °C	2066	**C**
Nalbuphine HCl	AB	10 mg/mL	ZEN	10 mg/mL	Physically compatible for 1 hr at 23 °C	2066	**C**
Naloxone HCl	AST	0.4 mg/mL	ZEN	10 mg/mL	Physically compatible for 1 hr at 23 °C	2066	**C**
Nitroglycerin	DU	0.4 mg/mL[a]	ZEN	10 mg/mL	Physically compatible for 1 hr at 23 °C	2066	**C**
Norepinephrine bitartrate	AB	0.016 mg/mL[a]	ZEN	10 mg/mL	Physically compatible for 1 hr at 23 °C	2066	**C**
Paclitaxel	MJ	1.2 mg/mL[a]	ZEN	10 mg/mL	Physically compatible for 1 hr at 23 °C	2066	**C**

Y-Site Injection Compatibility (1:1 Mixture) (Cont.)

Propofol

Drug	Mfr	Conc	Mfr	Conc	Remarks	Ref	C/I
Pancuronium bromide	GNS	2 mg/mL	STU	2 mg/mL	Oil droplets form within 7 days at 25 °C. No visible change in 24 hr	1801	?
	AST	1 mg/mL	ZEN	10 mg/mL	Physically compatible for 1 hr at 23 °C	2066	C
Pentobarbital sodium	WY	5 mg/mL[a]	ZEN	10 mg/mL	Physically compatible for 1 hr at 23 °C	2066	C
Phenobarbital sodium	WY	5 mg/mL[a]	ZEN	10 mg/mL	Physically compatible for 1 hr at 23 °C	2066	C
Phenylephrine HCl	ES	10 mg/mL	STU	2 mg/mL	Yellow discoloration forms within 7 days at 25 °C. No visible change in 24 hr	1801	?
	ES	0.1 mg/mL[a]	ZEN	10 mg/mL	Physically compatible for 1 hr at 23 °C	2066	C
Phenytoin sodium	ES	50 mg/mL	ZEN	10 mg/mL	Needle-like crystals form immediately	2066	I
Potassium chloride	AB	0.1 mEq/mL[a]	ZEN	10 mg/mL	Physically compatible for 1 hr at 23 °C	2066	C
Prochlorperazine edisylate	SCN	0.5 mg/mL[a]	ZEN	10 mg/mL	Physically compatible for 1 hr at 23 °C	2066	C
Propranolol HCl	SO	1 mg/mL	ZEN	10 mg/mL	Physically compatible for 1 hr at 23 °C	2066	C
Ranitidine HCl	GL	2 mg/mL[a]	ZEN	10 mg/mL	Physically compatible for 1 hr at 23 °C	2066	C
Scopolamine HBr	LY	0.4 mg/mL	ZEN	10 mg/mL	Physically compatible for 1 hr at 23 °C	2066	C
Sodium bicarbonate	AB	1 mEq/mL	ZEN	10 mg/mL	Physically compatible for 1 hr at 23 °C	2066	C
Sodium nitroprusside	ES	0.4 mg/mL[a]	ZEN	10 mg/mL	Physically compatible for 1 hr at 23 °C	2066	C
Succinylcholine chloride	AB	20 mg/mL	ZEN	10 mg/mL	Physically compatible for 1 hr at 23 °C	2066	C
Sufentanil citrate	JN	0.05 mg/mL	ZEN	10 mg/mL	Physically compatible for 1 hr at 23 °C	2066	C
Telavancin HCl	ASP	7.5 mg/mL[a]	APP	10 mg/mL	Physically compatible for 2 hr	2830	C
	ASP	7.5 mg/mL[b,c]	APP	10 mg/mL	Emulsion broke and oiled out	2830	I
Ticarcillin disodium–clavulanate potassium	SKB	31 mg/mL[a]	ZEN	10 mg/mL	Physically compatible for 1 hr at 23 °C	2066	C
Tobramycin sulfate	AB	5 mg/mL[a]	ZEN	10 mg/mL	Precipitate forms immediately	2066	I
TPN #186[d]			STU	500 mg	Physically compatible but 28% propofol loss in 5 hr at 22 °C	1805	I
TPN #187, #188[d]			STU	500 mg	Physically compatible and 6% or less propofol loss in 5 hr at 22 °C	1805	C
TPN #186 to #188[d]			STU	2 and 3 g	Physically compatible and 6% or less propofol loss in 5 hr at 22 °C	1805	C
Vancomycin HCl		10 mg/mL[a]	BA	10 mg/mL	Emulsion disruption within 1 to 4 hr at room temperature	2336	I
	AB	10 mg/mL[a]	ZEN	10 mg/mL	Physically compatible for 1 hr at 23 °C	2066	C
		10 mg/mL[a]	ASZ	10 mg/mL	Physically compatible for up to 30 days at room temperature	2336	C
Vecuronium bromide	OR	1 mg/mL	ZEN	10 mg/mL	Physically compatible for 1 hr at 23 °C	2066	C
Verapamil HCl	AMR	2.5 mg/mL	ZEN	10 mg/mL	Emulsion broke and oiled out	1916	I

[a]Tested in dextrose 5%.
[b]Tested in sodium chloride 0.9%.
[c]Tested in Ringer's injection, lactated.
[d]Refer to Appendix I for the composition of parenteral nutrition solutions. TPN indicates a 2-in-1 admixture.

PROPRANOLOL HYDROCHLORIDE
AHFS 24:24

Products — Propranolol hydrochloride is available in 1-mL ampuls containing 1 mg of the drug with citric acid to adjust the pH in water for injection. (1)

pH — From 2.8 to 4. (1)

Osmolality — The osmolality of propranolol hydrochloride 1 mg/mL was determined to be 12 mOsm/kg. (1233)

Trade Name(s) — Inderal.

Administration — Propranolol hydrochloride is administered by intravenous injection at a rate not exceeding 1 mg/min for life-threatening arrhythmias or those occurring during anesthesia. (1; 4)

Stability — Propranolol hydrochloride should be stored at controlled room temperature around 25 °C and protected from light, freezing, or excessive heat. (1; 4) Solutions of the drug have maximum stability at pH 3 and decompose rapidly at alkaline pH. Decomposition in aqueous solutions is accompanied by a lowered pH and discoloration. Solutions fluoresce at pH 4 to 5. (4)

Sorption — Propranolol hydrochloride was shown not to exhibit sorption to PVC bags and tubing, polyolefin containers, polyethylene tubing, Silastic tubing, and polypropylene syringes. (536; 606; 746)

Compatibility Information

Solution Compatibility

Propranolol HCl

Solution	Mfr	Mfr	Conc/L	Remarks	Ref	C/I
Dextrose 5% in sodium chloride 0.45%	ABᵃ, TRᵃ	AY	0.5 and 20 mg	Physically compatible and chemically stable for 24 hr at room temperature	746	C
	MGᵇ	AY	0.5 and 20 mg	Physically compatible and chemically stable for 24 hr at room temperature	746	C
Dextrose 5% in sodium chloride 0.9%	ABᵃ, TRᵃ	AY	0.5 and 20 mg	Physically compatible and chemically stable for 24 hr at room temperature	746	C
	MGᵇ	AY	0.5 and 20 mg	Physically compatible and chemically stable for 24 hr at room temperature	746	C
Dextrose 5%	ABᵃ, TRᵃ	AY	0.5 and 20 mg	Physically compatible and chemically stable for 24 hr at room temperature	746	C
	MGᵇ	AY	0.5 and 20 mg	Physically compatible and chemically stable for 24 hr at room temperature	746	C
Ringer's injection, lactated	ABᵃ, TRᵃ	AY	0.5 and 20 mg	Physically compatible and chemically stable for 24 hr at room temperature	746	C
	MGᵇ	AY	0.5 and 20 mg	Physically compatible and chemically stable for 24 hr at room temperature	746	C
Sodium chloride 0.45%		LY	500 mg	Physically compatible with no loss in 4 hr at 22 °C	1419	C
Sodium chloride 0.9%	ABᵃ, TRᵃ	AY	0.5 and 20 mg	Physically compatible and chemically stable for 24 hr at room temperature	746	C
	MGᵇ	AY	0.5 and 20 mg	Physically compatible and chemically stable for 24 hr at room temperature	746	C

ᵃTested in PVC containers.
ᵇTested in polyolefin containers.

Additive Compatibility

Propranolol HCl

Drug	Mfr	Conc/L	Mfr	Conc/L	Test Soln	Remarks	Ref	C/I
Dobutamine HCl	LI	1 g	AY	50 mg	D5W, NS	Physically compatible for 24 hr at 21 °C	812	C
Verapamil HCl	KN	80 mg	AY	4 mg	D5W, NS	Physically compatible for 24 hr	764	C

Drugs in Syringe Compatibility

Propranolol HCl

Drug (in syringe)	Mfr	Amt	Mfr	Amt	Remarks	Ref	C/I
Milrinone lactate	WI	3.5 mg/ 3.5 mL	AY	3 mg/ 3 mL	Brought to 10-mL total volume with D5W. Physically compatible with no loss of either drug in 4 hr at 23 °C	1191	**C**
Pantoprazole sodium	a	4 mg/ 1 mL		1 mg/ 1 mL	Precipitates	2574	**I**

[a]*Test performed using the formulation WITHOUT edetate disodium.*

Y-Site Injection Compatibility (1:1 Mixture)

Propranolol HCl

Drug	Mfr	Conc	Mfr	Conc	Remarks	Ref	C/I
Alteplase	GEN	1 mg/mL	AY	1 mg/mL	Visually compatible. 2% clot-lysis activity loss in 24 hr at 25 °C	1856	**C**
Amphotericin B cholesteryl sulfate complex	SEQ	0.83 mg/mL[a]	WY	1 mg/mL	Gross precipitate forms	2117	**I**
Fenoldopam mesylate	AB	80 mcg/mL[b]	WAY	1 mg/mL	Physically compatible for 4 hr at 23 °C	2467	**C**
Heparin sodium	UP	1000 units/L[c]	AY	1 mg/mL	Physically compatible for 4 hr at room temperature	534	**C**
Hydrocortisone sodium succinate	UP	10 mg/L[c]	AY	1 mg/mL	Physically compatible for 4 hr at room temperature	534	**C**
Linezolid	PHU	2 mg/mL	WAY	1 mg/mL	Physically compatible for 4 hr at 23 °C	2264	**C**
Meperidine HCl	AB	10 mg/mL	WY	1 mg/mL	Physically compatible for 4 hr at 25 °C	1397	**C**
Milrinone lactate	WI	200 mcg/mL[a]	AY	1 mg/mL	Physically compatible with no loss of either drug in 4 hr at 23 °C	1191	**C**
Morphine sulfate	AB	1 mg/mL	WY	1 mg/mL	Physically compatible for 4 hr at 25 °C	1397	**C**
Nesiritide	SCI	50 mcg/mL[a,b]		1 mg/mL	Physically compatible for 4 hr	2625	**C**
Potassium chloride	AB	40 mEq/L[c]	AY	1 mg/mL	Physically compatible for 4 hr at room temperature	534	**C**
Propofol	ZEN	10 mg/mL	SO	1 mg/mL	Physically compatible for 1 hr at 23 °C	2066	**C**
Tacrolimus	FUJ	1 mg/mL[b]	AY	1 mg/mL	Visually compatible for 24 hr at 25 °C	1630	**C**
Tirofiban HCl	ME	50 mcg/mL[a,b]	WAY	1 mg/mL	Physically compatible. No loss of either drug in 4 hr at 23 °C	2356	**C**

[a]*Tested in dextrose 5%.*
[b]*Tested in sodium chloride 0.9%.*
[c]*Tested in dextrose 5% in Ringer's injection, dextrose 5% in Ringer's injection, lactated, dextrose 5%, Ringer's injection, lactated, and sodium chloride 0.9%.*

PROTAMINE SULFATE
AHFS 20:28.08

Products — Protamine sulfate is available in 5- and 25-mL vials. Each milliliter contains protamine sulfate 10 mg with sodium chloride 0.9% and sodium phosphate and/or sulfuric acid to adjust the pH. (1)

pH — From 6 to 7. (1)

Osmolality — The osmolality of protamine sulfate 10 mg/mL was determined to be 290 mOsm/kg by freezing-point depression and 292 mOsm/kg by vapor pressure. (1071)

Administration — Protamine sulfate 10 mg/mL is administered by slow intravenous injection undiluted. No more than 50 mg should be administered in any 10-minute period. It has also been given by intravenous infusion after dilution in sodium chloride 0.9% or dextrose 5%. (1; 4)

Stability — Protamine sulfate should be stored under refrigeration; freezing should be avoided. (1) However, protamine sulfate has been stated to be stable for 10 days (1433) to two weeks (853) at room temperature.

Protamine sulfate is incompatible with some antibiotics including cephalosporins and penicillins. (1)

Filtration — Protamine sulfate (Fournier Freres) 0.2 mg/mL in dextrose 5% and sodium chloride 0.9% was filtered through a 0.22-μm cellulose ester membrane filter (Ivex-HP, Millipore) over six hours. No significant drug loss due to binding to the filter was noted. (1034)

Compatibility Information

Additive Compatibility

Protamine sulfate

Drug	Mfr	Conc/L	Mfr	Conc/L	Test Soln	Remarks	Ref	C/I
Ranitidine HCl	GL	50 mg and 2 g		500 mg	D5W	Physically compatible. Ranitidine stable for 24 hr at 25 °C. Protamine not tested	1515	C
Verapamil HCl	KN	80 mg	LI	100 mg	D5W, NS	Physically compatible for 24 hr	764	C

Drugs in Syringe Compatibility

Protamine sulfate

Drug (in syringe)	Mfr	Amt	Mfr	Amt	Remarks	Ref	C/I
Iohexol	WI	64.7%, 5 mL	LI	10 mg/ 1 mL	Physically compatible for at least 2 hr	1438	C
Iopamidol	SQ	61%, 5 mL	LI	10 mg/ 1 mL	Physically compatible for at least 2 hr	1438	C
Iothalamate meglumine	MA	60%, 5 mL	LI	10 mg/ 1 mL	Physically compatible for at least 2 hr	1438	C
Ioxaglate meglumine–ioxaglate sodium	MA	5 mL	LI	10 mg/ 1 mL	Precipitate forms immediately and persists for at least 2 hr	1438	I

PYRIDOXINE HYDROCHLORIDE
AHFS 88:08

Products — Pyridoxine hydrochloride 100 mg/mL is available in 1-, 10-, and 30-mL multiple-dose vials. Antimicrobial preservatives, such as benzyl alcohol 1.5% or chlorobutanol 0.5%, may also be present. Sodium hydroxide and/or hydrochloric acid may have been used to adjust pH. (1; 4)

pH — From 2 to 3.8. (1; 4)

Osmolality — The osmolality of pyridoxine hydrochloride 100 mg/mL was determined to be 870 mOsm/kg by freezing-point depression and 852 mOsm/kg by vapor pressure. (1071)

Administration — Pyridoxine hydrochloride may be administered by intramuscular, subcutaneous, or intravenous injection. (4)

Stability — The product should be stored at controlled room temperature and protected from freezing and from light. (1; 4)

Because pyridoxine hydrochloride is photosensitive and degrades slowly when exposed to light, protection from light has been recommended. (4)

Syringes — Pyridoxine hydrochloride 100 mg/mL was stable for six months at room temperature packaged in 5-, 10-, and 20-mL polypropylene syringes (Becton Dickinson). (2692)

Sorption — Pyridoxine hydrochloride (Sigma) 40 mg/L did not display significant sorption to a PVC plastic test strip in 24 hours. (12)

Compatibility Information

Drugs in Syringe Compatibility

Pyridoxine HCl

Drug (in syringe)	Mfr	Amt	Mfr	Amt	Remarks	Ref	C/I
Doxapram HCl	RB	400 mg/ 20 mL		10 mg/ 1 mL	Physically compatible with 6% doxapram loss in 24 hr	1177	C

Additional Compatibility Information

Parenteral Nutrition Solutions — The stability of pyridoxine hydrochloride 15 mg/L was studied in representative parenteral nutrition solutions exposed to fluorescent light, indirect sunlight, and direct sunlight for eight hours. One 5-mL vial of multivitamin concentrate (Lyphomed) containing 15 mg of pyridoxine hydrochloride and also 1 mg of folic acid (Lederle) was added to a liter of parenteral nutrition solution composed of amino acids 4.25%–dextrose 25% (Travenol) with standard electrolytes and trace elements. Pyridoxine hydrochloride was stable over the eight-hour study at room temperature under fluorescent light and indirect sunlight. However, eight hours of exposure to direct sunlight caused an 86% loss of pyridoxine hydrochloride. (842)

The stability of numerous vitamins in parenteral nutrition solutions composed of amino acids (Kabi-Vitrum), dextrose 30%, and fat emulsion 20% (Kabi-Vitrum) in a 2:1:1 ratio with electrolytes, trace elements, and both fat- and water-soluble vitamins was reported. The admixtures were stored in darkness at 2 to 8 °C for 96 hours with no significant loss of pyridoxine hydrochloride. (1225)

The vitamins in Cernevit (Baxter) diluted in three 2-in-1 parenteral nutrition admixtures were tested for stability over 48 hours. Most of the other vitamins, including pyridoxine hydrochloride, retained their initial concentrations. (2796)

QUINIDINE GLUCONATE
AHFS 24:04.04.04

Products — Quinidine gluconate is available in 10-mL vials. Each milliliter contains 80 mg of drug with edetate disodium 0.005% and phenol 0.25% in water for injection. D-gluconic acid delta-lactone may have been added to adjust the pH. (1)

Equivalency — Quinidine gluconate 800 mg is equivalent to 500 mg of anhydrous quinidine. (1)

pH — Quinidine gluconate injection has a pH of 5.5 to 7. (4)

Administration — Quinidine gluconate injection may be given by intermittent or continuous intravenous administration. (4) For intravenous administration in treating arrhythmias, 800 mg (10 mL) is diluted with 40 mL of dextrose 5% for a total of 50 mL to yield a 16-mg/mL solution. The drug has also been given by intramuscular injection, but this route is not recommended because of variable absorption. (1; 4)

For the treatment of malaria, continuous and intermittent infusion regimens have been used. A loading dose is prepared as a dilution in 250 mL of sodium chloride 0.9% and given as a one- or two-hour (continuous regimen) or four-hour (intermittent regimen) infusion. (4)

Infusions of quinidine gluconate must be delivered slowly at a rate no faster than 0.25 mg/kg/min, preferably using a volumetric pump to control the rate of administration. (1)

Stability — Quinidine gluconate should be stored at controlled room temperature. (1) Quinidine salts slowly discolor on exposure to light, acquiring a brownish tint. Only clear, colorless solutions are suitable for injection. (4)

Sorption — A substantial loss of quinidine (as the gluconate) was noted due to sorption to PVC containers and administration sets. Quinidine gluconate 6 mg/mL in dextrose 5% in 100-mL PVC bags (Baxter) exhibited about 5 to 7% loss. Administration of the solution over 30 minutes through 112-inch PVC administration sets (Gemini, IMED) resulted in an additional loss of over 30% of the quinidine gluconate from the delivered solution. Losses totaled over 40% for both bag and catheter. Use of a glass syringe on a syringe pump and a winged administration catheter having only 12 inches of PVC tubing reduced the loss to about 3%. (2005)

In two studies, quinidine (as the sulfate) was shown not to exhibit sorption to PVC bags and tubing, polyethylene tubing, Silastic tubing, and polypropylene syringes. (536; 606)

Compatibility Information

Solution Compatibility

Quinidine gluconate

Solution	Mfr	Mfr	Conc/L	Remarks	Ref	C/I
Dextrose 5%			16 g	Stable for 24 hr at room temperature and 48 hr refrigerated	4	C

Additive Compatibility

Quinidine gluconate

Drug	Mfr	Conc/L	Mfr	Conc/L	Test Soln	Remarks	Ref	C/I
Amiodarone HCl	LZ	1.8 g	LI	1 g	D5W[a]	Milky precipitation. 13% amiodarone loss in 6 hr and 23% in 24 hr at 24 °C in light	1031	I
	LZ	1.8 g	LI	1 g	D5W[b]	Milky precipitation. No amiodarone loss in 24 hr at 24 °C in light	1031	I
	LZ	1.8 g	LI	1 g	NS[a]	Physically compatible. 13% amiodarone loss in 24 hr at 24 °C in light	1031	I
	LZ	1.8 g	LI	1 g	NS[b]	Physically compatible. No amiodarone loss in 24 hr at 24 °C in light	1031	C
Atracurium besylate	BW	500 mg		8.3 g	D5W	Particles form and atracurium unstable at 5 and 30 °C	1694	I
Milrinone lactate	WI	200 mg	LI	16 g	D5W	Physically compatible with no loss of either drug in 4 hr at 23 °C	1191	C
Ranitidine HCl	GL	50 mg and 2 g		3.2 g	D5W	Physically compatible. Ranitidine stable for 24 hr at 25 °C. Quinidine not tested	1515	C
Verapamil HCl	KN	80 mg	LI	800 mg	D5W, NS	Physically compatible for 48 hr	739	C

[a]Tested in PVC containers.
[b]Tested in polyolefin containers.

Y-Site Injection Compatibility (1:1 Mixture)

Quinidine gluconate

Drug	Mfr	Conc	Mfr	Conc	Remarks	Ref	C/I
Diazepam	ES	0.2 mg/mL[a,b]	LI	6 mg/mL[a,b]	Physically compatible for 3 hr	1316	C
Furosemide	ES	4 mg/mL[a,b]	LI	6 mg/mL[a,b]	Immediate gross precipitation	1316	I
Heparin sodium	ES	50 units/mL[b]	LI	6 mg/mL[b]	Physically compatible for 3 hr	1316	C
	ES	50 units/mL[a]	LI	6 mg/mL[a]	Immediate gross haze	1316	I
Milrinone lactate	WI	350 mcg/mL[a]	LI	16 mg/mL[a]	Physically compatible with no loss of either drug in 4 hr at 23 °C	1191	C
Nesiritide	SCI	50 mcg/mL[a,b]		80 mg/mL	Physically compatible for 4 hr	2625	C

[a]Tested in dextrose 5%.
[b]Tested in sodium chloride 0.9%.

QUINUPRISTIN–DALFOPRISTIN
AHFS 8:12.28.32

Products — Quinupristin–dalfopristin is available as a lyophilized powder in vials containing a total of 500 mg of the two pristinamycin derivatives (quinupristin 150 mg and dalfopristin 350 mg) and vials containing 600 mg of the two drugs (quinupristin 180 mg and dalfopristin 420 mg). Reconstitute the 500- and 600-mg vials with 5 and 6 mL, respectively, of sterile water for injection or dextrose 5% and gently swirl (without shaking) to effect dissolution. The reconstituted solution should be allowed to sit for a few minutes until the foam has dissipated and a clear 100-mg/mL solution has formed; this solution must be diluted for administration. (1)

Trade Name(s) — Synercid.

Administration — Quinupristin–dalfopristin is administered by intravenous infusion after suitable dilution in dextrose 5%. For peripheral line administration, the dose should be diluted to about 2 mg/mL in 250 mL of dextrose 5%; for central line administration, 100 mL of diluent may be used. If moderate-to-severe venous irritation occurs during peripheral administration, dilution in 500 or 750 mL should be considered along with changing the infusion site, use of a central catheter, or use of a peripherally inserted central catheter (PICC). The dose is usually administered over 60 minutes. For intermittent infusion of quinupristin–dalfopristin and other drugs through a common line, the manufacturer recommends flushing the line before and after administration with dextrose 5%. (1)

Stability — Intact vials of quinupristin–dalfopristin should be stored under refrigeration. (1) Although refrigerated storage is required, the manufacturer has stated the drug may be stored at room temperature for 7 days. (2745) Because no antimicrobial preservative is present, the manufacturer recommends dilution of the reconstituted solution within 30 minutes. The drug diluted for infusion in dextrose 5% is stated to be stable for up to five hours at room temperature and 54 hours under refrigeration. It should not be frozen. The use of sodium chloride-containing solutions is not recommended because of incompatibility. (1)

Compatibility Information

Y-Site Injection Compatibility (1:1 Mixture)

Quinupristin–dalfopristin

Drug	Mfr	Conc	Mfr	Conc	Remarks	Ref	C/I
Anidulafungin	VIC	0.5 mg/mL[a]	AVE	5 mg/mL[a]	Physically compatible for 4 hr at 23 °C	2617	C
Aztreonam		20 mg/mL[a]	AVE	2 mg/mL[a]	Physically compatible	1	C
Caspofungin acetate	ME	0.7 mg/mL[b]	MON	5 mg/mL[b]	Physically compatible for 4 hr at room temperature	2758	C
Ciprofloxacin		1 mg/mL[a]	AVE	2 mg/mL[a]	Physically compatible	1	C
Fenoldopam mesylate	AB	80 mcg/mL[b]	AVE	5 mg/mL[b]	Physically compatible for 4 hr at 23 °C	2467	C
Fluconazole		2 mg/mL	AVE	2 mg/mL[a]	Physically compatible	1	C
Haloperidol lactate		0.2 mg/mL[a]	AVE	2 mg/mL[a]	Physically compatible	1	C
Metoclopramide HCl		5 mg/mL	AVE	2 mg/mL[a]	Physically compatible	1	C
Potassium chloride		0.04 mEq/mL[a]	AVE	2 mg/mL[a]	Physically compatible	1	C

[a]*Tested in dextrose 5%.*
[b]*Tested in sodium chloride 0.9%.*

RANITIDINE HYDROCHLORIDE
AHFS 56:28.12

Products — Ranitidine hydrochloride 25 mg/mL is available in 2-mL single-dose vials, 6-mL multiple-dose vials, and 40-mL pharmacy bulk packages. Each milliliter of solution also contains phenol 5 mg, dibasic sodium phosphate 2.4 mg, and monobasic sodium phosphate 0.96 mg in water for injection. (1)

Ranitidine hydrochloride is also available at a 1-mg/mL concentration in 50-mL (50 mg) plastic containers premixed in sodium chloride 0.45%. The solution also contains citric acid 15 mg and dibasic sodium phosphate 90 mg as buffers. (1)

Equivalency — Ranitidine hydrochloride 168 mg is approximately equivalent to 150 mg of ranitidine. (4)

pH — From 6.7 to 7.3. (1; 4)

Osmolality — The osmolality of ranitidine hydrochloride 10 mg/mL was determined to be 59 mOsm/kg. (1233)

The osmolality of ranitidine hydrochloride 1 mg/mL was 260 mOsm/kg in dextrose 5% and 302 mOsm/kg in sodium chloride 0.9%. At 2 mg/mL, the osmolality was 257 mOsm/kg in dextrose 5% and 294 mOsm/kg in sodium chloride 0.9%. (1375)

The premixed ranitidine 1-mg/mL solution in sodium chloride 0.45% has an osmolarity of 180 mOsm/L. (1)

Trade Name(s) — Zantac.

Administration — Ranitidine hydrochloride is administered intramuscularly undiluted or slowly intravenously after dilution. For direct intravenous injection, 50 mg is usually diluted to a total of at least 20 mL with a compatible intravenous infusion fluid and given over at least five minutes. For intermittent intravenous infusion, 50 mg may be added to at least 100 mL of intravenous solution and infused over 15 to 20 minutes. For continuous intravenous infusion, 150 mg of ranitidine hydrochloride may be diluted in 250 mL of intravenous fluid and infused at 6.25 mg/hr for 24 hours. (1; 4)

Stability — Ranitidine hydrochloride injection should be stored between 4 and 25 °C and protected from light and excessive heat. Brief exposure to temperatures up to 30 °C will not adversely affect the stability of the injection. (1; 4) However, ranitidine hydrochloride injection is reported to form an unacceptable brown discoloration if stored at 40 °C or higher for several months. (2505) The product is a clear, colorless to yellow solution. Slight darkening does not indicate concentration change. (1; 4)

Ranitidine hydrochloride was diluted to a concentration of 2.5 mg/mL with bacteriostatic water for injection and repackaged in 30-mL glass vials and 10-mL polypropylene syringes (Becton Dickinson). The vials and syringes were stored at 4 °C for 91 days. Approximately 5 to 6% loss occurred after 91 days of storage under refrigeration. Freshly prepared syringes and syringes stored at 4 °C for 91 days were also stored at 22 °C for 72 hours. No loss was found in the freshly prepared syringes, and about 2% additional loss was found in syringes stored under refrigeration for 91 days. (1965)

Freezing Solutions — Ranitidine hydrochloride (Glaxo) 0.5, 1, and 2 mg/mL in dextrose 5% and sodium chloride 0.9% in PVC bags showed no change in appearance or concentration when frozen for 30 days at −30 °C. An additional 14 days of refrigerated storage at 4 °C for these previously frozen solutions also resulted in no loss. (1143)

At a concentration of 2 mg/mL in dextrose 5% and sodium chloride 0.9% in PVC containers, no change in appearance or drug loss occurred after 100 days of storage at −30 °C. (1143)

The stability of ranitidine hydrochloride (Glaxo) 0.5, 1, and 2 mg/mL in several infusion fluids frozen at −20 °C for 60 days followed by seven days at 23 °C or 14 days at 4 °C was studied. In dextrose 5% in sodium chloride 0.45%, dextrose 5%, dextrose 10%, and sodium chloride 0.9%, ranitidine was physically compatible and chemically stable, retaining more than 90% of the initial concentration under these storage conditions. However, in dextrose 5% in Ringer's injection, lactated, the thawed solutions were slightly yellow with ranitidine hydrochloride losses of 25, 16, and 9% at 0.5, 1, and 2 mg/mL, respectively. (1516)

Ranitidine hydrochloride (Glaxo) 1.5 mg/mL in dextrose 5% or in sodium chloride 0.9% was packaged in PVC infusion pump reservoirs. The reservoirs were stored at −20 °C for 30 days. The frozen solutions were then thawed by storing at 3 °C for 24 hours followed by 24 hours at 30 °C to simulate use conditions. No loss was found. (1865)

Filtration — Filtration of ranitidine hydrochloride (Glaxo) 0.25, 0.5, and 2.5 mg/mL in sodium chloride 0.9% through 0.2-μm polysulfone filters (IVS Set-P Supor Filter, Codan) at a rate of 4 mL/hr for five hours did not result in any loss of drug due to sorption to the filter. (2229)

Central Venous Catheter — Ranitidine hydrochloride (Glaxo Wellcome) 0.2 mg/mL in dextrose 5% was found to be compatible with the ARROWg+ard Blue Plus (Arrow International) chlorhexidine-bearing triple-lumen central catheter. Essentially complete delivery of the drug was found with little or no drug loss occurring. Furthermore, chlorhexidine delivered from the catheter remained at trace amounts with no substantial increase due to the delivery of the drug through the catheter. (2335)

Compatibility Information

Solution Compatibility

Ranitidine HCl

Solution	Mfr	Mfr	Conc/L	Remarks	Ref	C/I
Dextrose 5% in Ringer's injection, lactated	TR[a]	GL	50 mg	15% loss in 2 days at room temperature in light	1362	**I**
	TR[a]	GL	500 mg, 1 g, 2 g	Physically compatible. Up to 5% loss in 7 days at 23 °C and 8% loss in 30 days at 4 °C	1516	**C**
Dextrose 5% in sodium chloride 0.45%	TR[a]	GL	50 mg	10% loss in 7 days at room temperature in light	1362	**C**
	TR[a]	GL	500 mg, 1 g, 2 g	Physically compatible. Up to 5% loss in 7 days at 23 °C and 8% loss in 30 days at 4 °C	1516	**C**
Dextrose 5%				Stable for 48 hr at room temperature	1	**C**
	TR[a]	GL	1 g	Little or no loss in 10 days at 4 °C	1143	**C**
	TR[a]		1 g	Physically compatible. 8% loss in 18 days at 25 °C and 3% loss in 66 days at 5 °C	1342	**C**
	TR[a]	GL	1 g	Physically compatible. No loss in 92 days at 4 °C	1350	**C**
	TR[a]	GL	50 mg and 2 g	Physically compatible. 6% or less loss in 48 hr at room temperature in light	1361	**C**

Solution Compatibility (Cont.)

Ranitidine HCl

Solution	Mfr	Mfr	Conc/L	Remarks	Ref	C/I
	TR[a]	GL	500 mg, 1 g, 2 g	5% or less loss in 28 days at room temperature in light	1362	C
	TR[a]	GL	50 mg	10% loss in 7 days at room temperature in light	1362	C
	TR[a]	GL	500 mg, 1 g, 2 g	Physically compatible. Up to 5% loss in 7 days at 23 °C and 6% loss in 30 days at 4 °C	1516	C
	MG	GL	441 mg	Visually compatible. No loss after 30 days at −20 °C then 10 days at 4 °C	1539	C
	TR[a]	GL	50 mg and 2 g	Visually compatible. 6% or less loss in 48 hr at room temperature	1802	C
	AB[a]	GL	1.5 g	Little loss in 24 hr at 30 °C and for 7 days at 3 °C then 24 hr at 30 °C	1865	C
	BA[a], BRN[b]	GW	250 mg	Visually compatible. 5% or less loss in 24 hr at 4 and 22 °C	2289	C
Dextrose 10%				Stable for 48 hr at room temperature	1	C
	TR[a]	GL	50 mg	7% loss in 2 days at room temperature in light	1362	C
	TR[a]	GL	500 mg, 1 g, 2 g	Physically compatible. Up to 4% loss in 7 days at 23 °C and 8% loss in 30 days at 4 °C	1516	C
Ringer's injection, lactated				Stable for 48 hr at room temperature	1	C
Sodium chloride 0.9%				Stable for 48 hr at room temperature	1	C
	TR	GL	50 and 100 mg	No loss in 48 hr at 24 °C in light	1010	C
	TR[a]	GL	1 g	Little loss in 10 days at 4 °C	1143	C
	TR[a]		1 g	Physically compatible with no loss in 18 days at 25 °C and in 66 days at 5 °C	1342	C
	TR[a]	GL	1 g	Physically compatible. No loss in 92 days at 4 °C	1350	C
	TR	GL	50 mg	Physically compatible. No loss in 48 hr at 25 °C	1360	C
	TR	GL	100 mg	Physically compatible. No loss in 48 hr at 25 °C and refrigerated for 24 hr then 24 hr at 25 °C	1360	C
	TR[a]	GL	50 mg and 2 g	Physically compatible. No loss in 48 hr at room temperature in light	1361	C
	TR[a]	GL	50 mg to 2 g	3% or less loss in 28 days at room temperature in light	1362	C
	TR[a]	GL	500 mg, 1 g, 2 g	Physically compatible. No loss in 7 days at 23 °C and 3% loss in 30 days at 4 °C	1516	C
	TR[a]	GL	50 mg and 2 g	Visually compatible. Little loss in 48 hr at room temperature	1802	C
	AB[a]	GL	1.5 g	Little loss in 24 hr at 30 °C and for 7 days at 3 °C then 24 hr at 30 °C	1865	C
	BA[a]	GL	0.6 and 1 g	Visually compatible. Little loss in 24 hr at ambient temperature	2079	C
	BA[a], BRN[b]	GW	250 mg	Visually compatible. 5% or less loss in 24 hr at 4 and 22 °C	2289	C
TNA #92[d]	[c]	GL	50 and 100 mg	7 to 10% ranitidine loss in 12 hr and 20 to 28% loss in 24 hr at 23 °C in light	1183	I
TNA #118[d]		GL	50 and 100 mg	Physically compatible. 6 to 10% ranitidine loss in 36 hr under refrigeration and at 25 °C	1360	C
TNA #197 to #200[d]		GL	75 mg	Physically compatible with 7% or less ranitidine loss in 24 hr at 22 °C in light. About 15% loss in 48 hr	1921	C
TNA #245[d]			200 mg	No ranitidine loss and no lipid change in 24 hr at room temperature	486	C

Solution Compatibility (Cont.)

Ranitidine HCl

Solution	Mfr	Mfr	Conc/L	Remarks	Ref	C/I
TNA #246[d]		GL	72 mg	Less than 7% ranitidine loss and no change in emulsion integrity in 14 days at 4 °C	501	C
TPN #58[d]		GL	83, 167, 250 mg	10% ranitidine loss in 48 hr at 23 °C	997	C
TPN #59, #60[d]	[a]	GL	50 and 100 mg	No color change and 7 to 9% ranitidine loss in 24 hr at 24 °C in light. Amino acids unaffected. Darkened color and 10 to 12% ranitidine loss in 48 hr	1010	C
TPN #117[d]		GL	50 and 100 mg	Physically compatible and 5% ranitidine loss in 48 hr refrigerated and at 25 °C	1360	C
TPN #196[d]		GL	75 mg	Physically compatible with 7% or less ranitidine loss in 24 hr at 22 °C in light. About 12% loss in 48 hr	1921	C
TPN #247[d]		GL	72 mg	2% ranitidine loss in 14 days at 4 °C	501	C

[a]Tested in PVC containers.
[b]Tested in polyethylene and glass containers.
[c]Tested in ethylene vinyl acetate containers.
[d]Refer to Appendix I for the composition of parenteral nutrition solutions. TNA indicates a 3-in-1 admixture, and TPN indicates a 2-in-1 admixture.

Additive Compatibility

Ranitidine HCl

Drug	Mfr	Conc/L	Mfr	Conc/L	Test Soln	Remarks	Ref	C/I
Acetazolamide sodium		5 g	GL	50 mg and 2 g	D5W	Physically compatible. Ranitidine stable for 24 hr at 25 °C. Acetazolamide not tested	1515	C
Amikacin sulfate	BR	1 g	GL	100 mg	D5W	Physically compatible for 24 hr at ambient temperature in light	1151	C
		2.5 g	GL	50 mg and 2 g	D5W	Physically compatible. Ranitidine stable for 24 hr at 25 °C. Amikacin not tested	1515	C
Aminophylline	ES	500 mg and 2 g	GL	50 mg and 2 g	D5W, NS[a]	Physically compatible. 4% or less ranitidine loss in 24 hr at room temperature in light. Aminophylline not tested	1361	C
	ES	0.5 and 2 g	GL	50 mg and 2 g	D5W, NS[a]	Visually compatible. Little loss of either drug in 48 hr at room temperature	1802	C
Amphotericin B	SQ	200 mg	GL	100 mg	D5W	Color change and particle formation	1151	I
Ampicillin sodium		2 g	GL	100 mg	D5W	Physically compatible for 24 hr at ambient temperature under fluorescent light. Ampicillin instability is determining factor	1151	?
		1 g	GL	50 mg and 2 g	NS	Physically compatible. Ranitidine stable for 24 hr at 25 °C. Ampicillin not tested	1515	C
Atracurium besylate	BW	500 mg		500 mg	D5W	Atracurium unstable due to high pH	1694	I
Cefazolin sodium		2 g	GL	100 mg	D5W	Color change within 24 hr	1151	?
		1 g	GL	50 mg and 2 g	D5W	Ranitidine stable for only 6 hr at 25 °C. Cefazolin not tested	1515	I
Cefoxitin sodium		10 g	GL	50 mg and 2 g	D5W	Ranitidine stable for only 4 hr at 25 °C. Cefoxitin not tested	1515	I
Ceftazidime	GL	10 g	GL	500 mg	D2.5½S	8% ranitidine loss in 4 hr and 37% loss in 24 hr at 22 °C	1632	I

Additive Compatibility (Cont.)

Ranitidine HCl

Drug	Mfr	Conc/L	Mfr	Conc/L	Test Soln	Remarks	Ref	C/I
Cefuroxime sodium	GL	1.5 g	GL	100 mg	D5W	Color change in 24 hr at ambient temperature in light	1151	?
		6 g	GL	50 mg and 2 g	D5W	Ranitidine stable for only 6 hr at 25 °C. Cefuroxime not tested	1515	I
Chloramphenicol sodium succinate		2 g	GL	100 mg	D5W	Physically compatible for 24 hr at ambient temperature	1151	C
Chlorothiazide sodium		5 g	GL	50 mg and 2 g	D5W	Physically compatible. Ranitidine stable for 24 hr at 25 °C. Chlorothiazide not tested	1515	C
Ciprofloxacin	BAY	2 g	GL	500 mg and 1 g	NS	Visually compatible. Little ciprofloxacin loss in 24 hr at 25 °C. Ranitidine not tested	1934	C
Clindamycin phosphate	UP	1.2 g	GL	100 mg	D5W	Color change and gas formation	1151	I
		1.2 g	GL	50 mg and 2 g	D5W, NS	Physically compatible. Ranitidine stable for 24 hr at 25 °C. Clindamycin not tested	1515	C
Colistimethate sodium		1.5 g	GL	50 mg and 2 g	D5W	Physically compatible. Ranitidine stable for 24 hr at 25 °C. Colistimethate not tested	1515	C
Dexamethasone sodium phosphate		40 mg	GL	50 mg and 2 g	D5W	Physically compatible. Ranitidine stable for 24 hr at 25 °C. Dexamethasone not tested	1515	C
Digoxin		2.5 mg	GL	50 mg and 2 g	D5W	Physically compatible. Ranitidine stable for 24 hr at 25 °C. Digoxin not tested	1515	C
Dobutamine HCl	LI	250 mg and 1 g	GL	2 g	D5W, NS[a]	Physically compatible. No ranitidine loss in 48 hr at room temperature in light. Dobutamine not tested	1361	C
	LI	250 mg and 1 g	GL	50 mg	D5W[a]	Physically compatible. 7% ranitidine loss in 48 hr at room temperature in light. Dobutamine not tested	1361	C
	LI	250 mg and 1 g	GL	50 mg	NS[a]	Physically compatible. No ranitidine loss in 48 hr at room temperature in light. Dobutamine not tested	1361	C
	LI	0.25 and 1 g	GL	50 mg and 2 g	D5W, NS[a]	Visually compatible. Little loss of either drug in 48 hr at room temperature	1802	C
Dopamine HCl	ES	400 mg and 3.2 g	GL	50 mg and 2 g	D5W, NS[a]	Physically compatible. 6% ranitidine loss in 48 hr at room temperature in light. Dopamine not tested	1361	C
	ES	0.4 and 3.2 g	GL	50 mg and 2 g	D5W, NS[a]	Visually compatible. No dopamine and 7% ranitidine loss in 48 hr at room temperature	1802	C
Doxycycline hyclate	PF	200 mg	GL	100 mg	D5W	Physically compatible for 24 hr at ambient temperature in light	1151	C
Epinephrine HCl		50 mg	GL	50 mg and 2 g	D5W	Physically compatible. Ranitidine stable for 24 hr at 25 °C. Epinephrine not tested	1515	C
Erythromycin lactobionate		5 g	GL	50 mg and 2 g	NS	Physically compatible. Ranitidine stable for 24 hr at 25 °C. Erythromycin not tested	1515	C
Ethacrynate sodium		500 mg	GL	50 mg and 2 g	D5W	Ranitidine stable for only 6 hr at 25 °C. Ethacrynate not tested	1515	I
Fat emulsion, intravenous	KV	10%	GL	50 and 100 mg		Physically compatible. 4% or less ranitidine loss in 48 hr at 25 °C in light or dark	1360	C

Additive Compatibility (Cont.)

Ranitidine HCl

Drug	Mfr	Conc/L	Mfr	Conc/L	Test Soln	Remarks	Ref	C/I
Floxacillin sodium	BE	20 g	GL	500 mg	NS	Physically compatible for 72 hr at 15 and 30 °C	1479	C
Fluconazole with ondansetron HCl	RR GL	2 g 100 mg	GL	500 mg	[a]	Visually compatible with no loss of any drug in 4 hr	1730	C
Flumazenil	RC	20 mg	GL	300 mg	D5W[a]	Visually compatible. 3% flumazenil loss in 24 hr at 23 °C in light. Ranitidine not tested	1710	C
Furosemide	HO	1 g	GL	500 mg	NS	Physically compatible for 72 hr at 15 and 30 °C	1479	C
		400 mg	GL	50 mg and 2 g	D5W	Physically compatible. Ranitidine stable for 24 hr at 25 °C. Furosemide not tested	1515	C
Gentamicin sulfate		160 mg	GL	100 mg	D5W	Physically compatible for 24 hr at ambient temperature in light	1151	C
		80 mg	GL	50 mg and 2 g	D5W, NS	Physically compatible. Ranitidine stable for 24 hr at 25 °C. Gentamicin not tested	1515	C
Heparin sodium	ES	10,000 and 40,000 units	GL	2 g	D5W, NS[a]	Physically compatible. 2% ranitidine loss in 48 hr at room temperature in light. Heparin not tested	1361	C
	ES	10,000 and 40,000 units	GL	50 mg	NS[a]	Physically compatible. No ranitidine loss in 48 hr at room temperature in light. Heparin not tested	1361	C
	ES	10,000 and 40,000 units	GL	50 mg	D5W[a]	Physically compatible. 7% ranitidine loss in 24 hr and 12% loss in 48 hr at room temperature in light. Heparin not tested	1361	C
Insulin, regular	LI	1000 units	GL	600 mg	NS[a]	Visually compatible. Little ranitidine loss in 24 hr at ambient temperature but insulin losses of 9% in 4 hr and 14% in 24 hr, presumably due to sorption	2079	I
Isoproterenol HCl		20 mg	GL	50 mg and 2 g	D5W	Physically compatible. Ranitidine stable for 24 hr at 25 °C. Isoproterenol not tested	1515	C
Lidocaine HCl	AST	1 and 8 g	GL	50 mg and 2 g	D5W, NS[a]	Physically compatible. 3% ranitidine loss in 24 hr at room temperature in light. Lidocaine not tested	1361	C
		2.5 g	GL	50 mg and 2 g	D5W	Physically compatible. Ranitidine stable for 24 hr at 25 °C. Lidocaine not tested	1515	C
	AST	1 and 8 g	GL	50 mg and 2 g	D5W, NS[a]	Visually compatible. Little loss of either drug in 48 hr at room temperature	1802	C
Lincomycin HCl		2.4 g	GL	50 mg and 2 g	D5W	Physically compatible. Ranitidine stable for 24 hr at 25 °C. Lincomycin not tested	1515	C
Meropenem	ZEN	1 and 20 g	GL	100 mg	NS	Visually compatible for 4 hr at room temperature	1994	C
Methylprednisolone sodium succinate	UP	40 mg	GL	50 mg	D5W[a]	Visually compatible with 7% ranitidine loss and no methylprednisolone loss in 48 hr at room temperature	1802	C
	UP	2 g	GL	50 mg	D5W[a]	Visually compatible with 6% ranitidine loss and 10% methylprednisolone loss in 48 hr at room temperature	1802	C

Additive Compatibility (Cont.)

Ranitidine HCl

Drug	Mfr	Conc/L	Mfr	Conc/L	Test Soln	Remarks	Ref	C/I
	UP	40 mg and 2 g	GL	2 g	D5W[a]	Visually compatible with no loss of either drug in 48 hr at room temperature	1802	C
	UP	40 mg and 2 g	GL	50 mg and 2 g	NS[a]	Visually compatible with no ranitidine loss and about 10% methylprednisolone loss in 48 hr at room temperature	1802	C
Midazolam HCl	RC	50 and 250 mg	GL	400 mg	NS	Visually compatible for 4 hr	355	C
Norepinephrine bitartrate	WI	4 and 8 mg	GL	50 mg	D5W, NS[a]	Physically compatible. 2 to 6% ranitidine loss in 48 hr at room temperature in light. Norepinephrine not tested	1361	C
		4 mg	GL	50 mg	D5W	Physically compatible. Ranitidine stable for 24 hr at 25 °C. Norepinephrine not tested	1515	C
	RC	4 and 8 mg	GL	50 mg	D5W[a]	Visually compatible. 5 to 7% ranitidine loss and little norepinephrine loss in 48 hr at room temperature	1802	C
	RC	4 mg	GL	2 g	D5W[a]	Visually compatible. 7% norepinephrine loss in 4 hr and 13% in 12 hr at room temperature. No ranitidine loss in 48 hr	1802	I
	RC	8 mg	GL	2 g	D5W[a]	Visually compatible. 6% norepinephrine loss in 12 hr and 11% in 24 hr at room temperature. No ranitidine loss in 48 hr	1802	I
Ondansetron HCl with fluconazole	GL RR	100 mg 2 g	GL	500 mg	[a]	Visually compatible with no loss of any drug in 4 hr	1730	C
Penicillin G potassium		24 million units	GL	50 mg and 2 g	D5W, NS	Physically compatible. Ranitidine stable for 24 hr at 25 °C. Penicillin not tested	1515	C
Penicillin G sodium		2.4 million units	GL	100 mg	D5W	Physically compatible for 24 hr at ambient temperature in light	1151	C
Phytonadione		100 mg	GL	50 mg and 2 g	D5W	Ranitidine stable for only 6 hr at 25 °C. Phytonadione not tested	1515	I
Polymyxin B sulfate		1 million units	GL	50 mg and 2 g	D5W	Physically compatible. Ranitidine stable for 24 hr at 25 °C. Polymyxin B not tested	1515	C
Potassium chloride	LY	10 and 60 mEq	GL	2 g	D5W, NS[a]	Physically compatible. 2% ranitidine loss in 48 hr at room temperature in light	1361	C
	LY	10 and 60 mEq	GL	50 mg	NS[a]	Physically compatible. No ranitidine loss in 48 hr at room temperature in light	1361	C
	LY	10 and 60 mEq	GL	50 mg	D5W[a]	Physically compatible. 7% ranitidine loss in 48 hr at room temperature in light	1361	C
		80 mEq	GL	50 mg and 2 g	D5S, D5W, NS	Physically compatible. Ranitidine stable for 24 hr at 25 °C	1515	C
Protamine sulfate		500 mg	GL	50 mg and 2 g	D5W	Physically compatible. Ranitidine stable for 24 hr at 25 °C. Protamine not tested	1515	C
Quinidine gluconate		3.2 g	GL	50 mg and 2 g	D5W	Physically compatible. Ranitidine stable for 24 hr at 25 °C. Quinidine not tested	1515	C
Sodium nitroprusside	RC	50 and 400 mg	GL	2 g	D5W, NS[a]	Physically compatible. No ranitidine loss in 48 hr at room temperature light protected. Nitroprusside not tested	1361	C

Additive Compatibility (Cont.)

Ranitidine HCl

Drug	Mfr	Conc/L	Mfr	Conc/L	Test Soln	Remarks	Ref	C/I
	RC	50 and 400 mg	GL	50 mg	NS[a]	Physically compatible. No ranitidine loss in 48 hr at room temperature light protected. Nitroprusside not tested	1361	C
	RC	50 and 400 mg	GL	50 mg	D5W[a]	Physically compatible with 7% or less ranitidine loss in 48 hr protected from light. Nitroprusside not tested	1361	C
		50 mg and 1 g	GL	50 mg and 2 g	D5W, NS	Physically compatible. Both drugs stable for 48 hr at room temperature protected from light	1515	C
		100 mg	GL	50 mg and 2 g	D5W	Physically compatible. Ranitidine stable for 24 hr at 25 °C. Sodium nitroprusside not tested	1515	C
	RC	50 and 400 mg	GL	50 mg and 2 g	D5W[a]	Visually compatible. 7% ranitidine and 8% nitroprusside loss in 48 hr at room temperature protected from light	1802	C
	RC	50 and 400 mg	GL	50 mg and 2 g	NS[a]	Visually compatible. No loss of either drug in 48 hr at room temperature protected from light	1802	C
Tobramycin sulfate	DI	200 mg	GL	100 mg	D5W	Physically compatible for 24 hr at ambient temperature in light	1151	C
Tramadol HCl	GRU	400 mg	AB	0.5 g	NS	Visually compatible with little or no tramadol loss in 24 hr at room temperature	2652	C
Vancomycin HCl	DI	1 g	GL	100 mg	D5W	Physically compatible for 24 hr at ambient temperature in light	1151	C
		5 g	GL	50 mg and 2 g	D5W	Physically compatible. Ranitidine stable for 24 hr at 25 °C. Vancomycin not tested	1515	C
Zidovudine	GSK	2 g	GSK	500 mg	NS	Physically compatible with no loss of either drug in 24 hr at 4 and 23 °C	2523	C
	GSK	2 g	GSK	500 mg	D5W	Physically compatible. Up to 8% ranitidine loss at 23 °C and 2% at 4 °C in 24 hr. Zidovudine losses of 5 to 6% in 24 hr at 4 and 23 °C	2523	C

[a]*Tested in PVC containers.*

Drugs in Syringe Compatibility

Ranitidine HCl

Drug (in syringe)	Mfr	Amt	Mfr	Amt	Remarks	Ref	C/I
Atropine sulfate	GL	0.4 mg/ 1 mL	GL	50 mg/ 2 mL	Physically compatible for 1 hr at 25 °C	978	C
Chlorpromazine HCl	RP	25 mg/ 1 mL	GL	50 mg/ 2 mL	Physically compatible for 1 hr at 25 °C	978	C
	RP	25 mg	GL	50 mg/ 5 mL	Gas formation	1151	I
Cyclizine lactate	CA	50 mg/ 1 mL	GL	50 mg/ 2 mL	Physically compatible for 1 hr at 25 °C	978	C
Dexamethasone sodium phosphate	ME	4 mg	GL	50 mg/ 5 mL	Physically compatible for 4 hr at ambient temperature under fluorescent light	1151	C
Diazepam	RC	10 mg/ 2 mL	GL	50 mg/ 2 mL	Immediate white haze that disappears following vortex mixing	978	?

Drugs in Syringe Compatibility (Cont.)

Ranitidine HCl

Drug (in syringe)	Mfr	Amt	Mfr	Amt	Remarks	Ref	C/I
		10 mg	GL	50 mg/ 5 mL	Physically compatible for 4 hr at ambient temperature under fluorescent light	1151	C
Dimenhydrinate	HR	50 mg/ 1 mL	GL	50 mg/ 2 mL	Physically compatible for 1 hr at 25 °C	978	C
Diphenhydramine HCl	PD	50 mg/ 1 mL	GL	50 mg/ 2 mL	Physically compatible for 1 hr at 25 °C	978	C
Dobutamine HCl	LI	25 mg	GL	50 mg/ 5 mL	Physically compatible for 4 hr at ambient temperature under fluorescent light	1151	C
Dopamine HCl		40 mg	GL	50 mg/ 5 mL	Physically compatible for 4 hr at ambient temperature under fluorescent light	1151	C
Fentanyl citrate	JN	0.1 mg/ 2 mL	GL	50 mg/ 2 mL	Physically compatible for 1 hr at 25 °C	978	C
Glycopyrrolate	RB	0.2 mg/ 1 mL	GL	50 mg/ 2 mL	Physically compatible for 1 hr at 25 °C	978	C
Heparin sodium		2500 units/ 1 mL	GL	50 mg/ 5 mL	Visually compatible for at least 5 min	1053	C
Hydromorphone HCl	PE	2 mg/ 1 mL	GL	50 mg/ 2 mL	Physically compatible for 1 hr at 25 °C	978	C
Hydroxyzine HCl	PF	50 mg/ 1 mL	GL	50 mg/ 2 mL	Immediate white haze that disappears following vortex mixing	978	I
Lorazepam	WY	4 mg/ 1 mL	GL	50 mg/ 2 mL	Poor mixing and layering, which disappears following vortex mixing	978	?
Meperidine HCl	WI	100 mg/ 1 mL	GL	50 mg/ 2 mL	Physically compatible for 1 hr at 25 °C	978	C
Methotrimeprazine HCl	RP	25 mg/ 1 mL	GL	50 mg/ 2 mL	Immediate white turbidity	978	I
Metoclopramide HCl	RB	10 mg/ 1 mL	GL	50 mg/ 2 mL	Physically compatible for 1 hr at 25 °C	978	C
Midazolam HCl	RC	5 mg/ 1 mL	GL	50 mg/ 2 mL	White precipitate forms immediately	1145	I
Morphine sulfate	AH	10 mg/ 1 mL	GL	50 mg/ 2 mL	Physically compatible for 1 hr at 25 °C	978	C
Nalbuphine HCl	EN	10 mg/ 1 mL	GL	50 mg/ 2 mL	Physically compatible for 1 hr at 25 °C	978	C
Pantoprazole sodium	a	4 mg/ 1 mL		25 mg/ 1 mL	Possible precipitate within 4 hr	2574	I
Pentazocine lactate	WI	60 mg/ 2 mL	GL	50 mg/ 2 mL	Physically compatible for 1 hr at 25 °C	978	C
Pentobarbital sodium	AB	100 mg	GL	50 mg/ 5 mL	Precipitates immediately	1151	I
Phenobarbital sodium	AB	120 mg/ 1 mL	GL	50 mg/ 2 mL	Immediate white haze	978	I
Prochlorperazine edisylate	RP	10 mg/ 2 mL	GL	50 mg/ 2 mL	Physically compatible for 1 hr at 25 °C	978	C

Drugs in Syringe Compatibility (Cont.)

Ranitidine HCl

Drug (in syringe)	Mfr	Amt	Mfr	Amt	Remarks	Ref	C/I
Promethazine HCl	RP	25 mg/ 1 mL	GL	50 mg/ 2 mL	Physically compatible for 1 hr at 25 °C	978	C
	RP	25 mg	GL	50 mg/ 5 mL	Physically compatible for 4 hr	1151	C
Scopolamine HBr	AB	0.4 mg/ 1 mL	GL	50 mg/ 2 mL	Physically compatible for 1 hr at 25 °C	978	C
		0.5 mg	GL	50 mg/ 5 mL	Physically compatible for 4 hr at ambient temperature under fluorescent light	1151	C

[a]Test performed using the formulation WITHOUT edetate disodium.

Y-Site Injection Compatibility (1:1 Mixture)

Ranitidine HCl

Drug	Mfr	Conc	Mfr	Conc	Remarks	Ref	C/I
Acyclovir sodium	BW	5 mg/mL[a]	GL	1 mg/mL[a]	Physically compatible for 4 hr at 25 °C	1157	C
Aldesleukin	CHI	33,800 I.U./ mL[a]	AB	1 mg/mL[c]	Visually compatible with little or no loss of aldesleukin activity	1857	C
Allopurinol sodium	BW	3 mg/mL[b]	GL	2 mg/mL[b]	Physically compatible for 4 hr at 22 °C	1686	C
Amifostine	USB	10 mg/mL[a]	GL	2 mg/mL[a]	Physically compatible for 4 hr at 23 °C	1845	C
Aminophylline	LY	4 mg/mL[a]	GL	0.5 mg/mL	Physically compatible for 24 hr	1323	C
Amphotericin B cholesteryl sulfate complex	SEQ	0.83 mg/mL[a]	GL	2 mg/mL[a]	Microprecipitate and increased turbidity form immediately	2117	I
Amsacrine	NCI	1 mg/mL[a]	GL	2 mg/mL[a]	Visually compatible for 4 hr at 22 °C	1381	C
Anidulafungin	VIC	0.5 mg/mL[a]	GSK	2 mg/mL[a]	Physically compatible for 4 hr at 23 °C	2617	C
Atracurium besylate	BW	0.5 mg/mL[a]	GL	0.5 mg/mL[a]	Physically compatible for 24 hr at 28 °C	1337	C
Aztreonam	SQ	16.7 mg/mL[b]	GL	1 mg/mL[b]	No loss of either drug in 4 hr at 22 °C	1632	C
	SQ	40 mg/mL[a]	GL	2 mg/mL[a]	Physically compatible for 4 hr at 23 °C	1758	C
Bivalirudin	TMC	5 mg/mL[a]	GW	2 mg/mL[a]	Physically compatible for 4 hr at 23 °C	2373	C
Cefazolin sodium	FUJ	20 mg/mL[b]	GL	1 mg/mL[b]	Visually compatible with little loss of either drug in 4 hr at 25 °C	2259	C
	FUJ	20 mg/mL[b]	GL	1 mg/mL[b]	Visually compatible with no cefazolin loss and 3% ranitidine loss in 4 hr	2362	C
Cefoxitin sodium	BAN	20 mg/mL[b]	GL	1 mg/mL[b]	Visually compatible. No cefoxitin loss. Under 8% ranitidine loss in 4 hr at 25 °C	2259	C
	BAN	20 mg/mL[b]	GL	1 mg/mL[b]	Visually compatible with no cefoxitin loss and 7% ranitidine loss in 4 hr	2362	C
Ceftaroline fosamil	FOR	2.22 mg/ mL[a,b,d]	BED	2 mg/mL[a,b,d]	Physically compatible for 4 hr at 23 °C	2826	C
Ceftazidime	GL	20 mg/mL[a]	GL	1 mg/mL[b]	8% ranitidine loss and no ceftazidime loss in 4 hr at 22 °C	1632	C
Ciprofloxacin	MI	2 mg/mL[e]	GL	0.5 mg/mL[e]	Visually compatible for 24 hr at 24 °C	1655	C
Cisatracurium besylate	GW	0.1, 2, 5 mg/ mL[a]	GL	2 mg/mL[a]	Physically compatible for 4 hr at 23 °C	2074	C
Cladribine	ORT	0.015[b] and 0.5[f] mg/mL	GL	2 mg/mL[b]	Physically compatible for 4 hr at 23 °C	1969	C

Y-Site Injection Compatibility (1:1 Mixture) (Cont.)

Ranitidine HCl

Drug	Mfr	Conc	Mfr	Conc	Remarks	Ref	C/I
Clarithromycin	AB	4 mg/mL[a]	GW	5 mg/mL[a]	Visually compatible for 72 hr at both 30 and 17 °C	2174	C
Dexmedetomidine HCl	AB	4 mcg/mL[b]	GW	2 mg/mL[b]	Physically compatible for 4 hr at 23 °C	2383	C
Diltiazem HCl	MMD	1[b] and 5 mg/mL	GL	25 mg/mL	Visually compatible	1807	C
	MMD	5 mg/mL	GL	0.5[c] and 1[b] mg/mL	Visually compatible	1807	C
	MMD	1 mg/mL[a]	GL	1 mg/mL[a]	Visually compatible for 4 hr at 27 °C	2062	C
Dobutamine HCl	LI	1 mg/mL[a]	GL	0.5 mg/mL	Physically compatible for 24 hr	1323	C
	LI	4 mg/mL[a]	GL	1 mg/mL[a]	Visually compatible for 4 hr at 27 °C	2062	C
Docetaxel	RPR	0.9 mg/mL[a]	GL	2 mg/mL[a]	Physically compatible for 4 hr at 23 °C	2224	C
Dopamine HCl	ES	1.6 mg/mL[a]	GL	0.5 mg/mL	Physically compatible for 24 hr	1323	C
	AB	3.2 mg/mL[a]	GL	1 mg/mL[a]	Visually compatible for 4 hr at 27 °C	2062	C
Doripenem	JJ	5 mg/mL[a,b]	BED	2 mg/mL[a,b]	Physically compatible for 4 hr at 23 °C	2743	C
Doxapram HCl	RB	2 mg/mL[a]	GSK	5 mg/mL[a]	Visually compatible for 4 hr at 23 °C	2470	C
Doxorubicin HCl liposomal	SEQ	0.4 mg/mL[a]	GL	2 mg/mL[a]	Physically compatible for 4 hr at 23 °C	2087	C
Enalaprilat	MSD	0.05 mg/mL[b]	GL	0.5 mg/mL[a]	Physically compatible for 24 hr at room temperature under fluorescent light	1355	C
Epinephrine HCl	AB	0.02 mg/mL[a]	GL	1 mg/mL[a]	Visually compatible for 4 hr at 27 °C	2062	C
Esmolol HCl	DCC	10 mg/mL[a]	GL	0.5 mg/mL[a]	Physically compatible for 24 hr at 22 °C	1169	C
Etoposide phosphate	BR	5 mg/mL[a]	GL	2 mg/mL[a]	Physically compatible for 4 hr at 23 °C	2218	C
Fenoldopam mesylate	AB	80 mcg/mL[b]	GW	2 mg/mL[b]	Physically compatible for 4 hr at 23 °C	2467	C
Fentanyl citrate	ES	0.05 mg/mL	GL	1 mg/mL[a]	Visually compatible for 4 hr at 27 °C	2062	C
Filgrastim	AMG	30 mcg/mL[a]	GL	2 mg/mL[a]	Physically compatible for 4 hr at 22 °C	1687	C
Fluconazole	RR	2 mg/mL[b]	GL	0.5 and 2 mg/mL[a]	Visually compatible. No loss of either drug in 4 hr	1730	C
Fludarabine phosphate	BX	1 mg/mL[a]	GL	2 mg/mL[a]	Visually compatible for 4 hr at 22 °C	1439	C
Foscarnet sodium	AST	24 mg/mL	GL	2 mg/mL[e]	Physically compatible for 24 hr at 25 °C under fluorescent light	1393	C
Furosemide	AMR	10 mg/mL	GL	1 mg/mL[a]	Visually compatible for 4 hr at 27 °C	2062	C
Gallium nitrate	FUJ	1 mg/mL[b]	GL	2.5 mg/mL[b]	Visually compatible for 24 hr at 25 °C	1673	C
Gemcitabine HCl	LI	10 mg/mL[b]	GL	2 mg/mL[b]	Physically compatible for 4 hr at 23 °C	2226	C
Granisetron HCl	SKB	0.05 mg/mL[a]	GL	2 mg/mL[a]	Physically compatible for 4 hr at 23 °C	2000	C
Heparin sodium	LY	50 units/mL[a]	GL	0.5 mg/mL	Physically compatible for 24 hr	1323	C
	TR	50 units/mL	GL	1 mg/mL	Visually compatible for 4 hr at 25 °C	1793	C
	ES	100 units/mL[a]	GL	1 mg/mL[a]	Visually compatible for 4 hr at 27 °C	2062	C
Hetastarch in lactated electrolyte	AB	6%	GW	2 mg/mL[a]	Physically compatible for 4 hr at 23 °C	2339	C
Hetastarch in sodium chloride 0.9%	DCC	6%	GL	0.5 mg/mL	Barely visible single particle appeared after 1 hr but disappeared	1313	?
	DCC	6%	GL	0.5 mg/mL	Barely visible particles appeared and disappeared	1314	I
	DCC	6%	GL	0.5 mg/mL	Small white particles and white fiber	1315	I
Hydromorphone HCl	KN	1 mg/mL	GL	1 mg/mL[a]	Visually compatible for 4 hr at 27 °C	2062	C

Y-Site Injection Compatibility (1:1 Mixture) (Cont.)

Ranitidine HCl

Drug	Mfr	Conc	Mfr	Conc	Remarks	Ref	C/I
Idarubicin HCl	AD	1 mg/mL[b]	GL	1 mg/mL[a]	Visually compatible for 24 hr at 25 °C	1525	C
Insulin, regular	LI	1 unit/mL[b]	GL	1 mg/mL[b]	Visually compatible. Little loss of ranitidine in 4 hr but insulin losses of 9% in 1 hr and 20% in 4 hr, presumably due to sorption	2079	I
Labetalol HCl	SC	1 mg/mL[a]	GL	0.5 mg/mL[a]	Physically compatible for 24 hr at 18 °C	1171	C
	GL	1 mg/mL[a]	GL	0.6 mg/mL[a]	Visually compatible. Little rantidine and 5% labetalol loss in 4 hr at room temperature	1762	C
	AH	2 mg/mL[a]	GL	1 mg/mL[a]	Visually compatible for 4 hr at 27 °C	2062	C
Linezolid	PHU	2 mg/mL	GW	2 mg/mL[a]	Physically compatible for 4 hr at 23 °C	2264	C
Lorazepam	WY	0.33 mg/mL[b]	GL	0.5 mg/mL	Visually compatible for 24 hr at 22 °C	1855	C
	WY	0.5 mg/mL[a]	GL	1 mg/mL[a]	Visually compatible for 4 hr at 27 °C	2062	C
Melphalan HCl	BW	0.1 mg/mL[b]	GL	2 mg/mL[b]	Physically compatible for 3 hr at 22 °C	1557	C
Meperidine HCl	WY	10 mg/mL[b]	GL	0.5 mg/mL[c]	Physically compatible for 1 hr at 25 °C	1338	C
Midazolam HCl	RC	5 mg/mL	GL	0.5 mg/mL	Visually compatible for 24 hr at 22 °C	1855	C
	RC	2 mg/mL[a]	GL	1 mg/mL[a]	Visually compatible for 4 hr at 27 °C	2062	C
Milrinone lactate	SW	0.2 mg/mL[a]	GL	1 mg/mL[a]	Visually compatible for 4 hr at 27 °C	2062	C
	SW	0.4 mg/mL[a]	GL	2 mg/mL[a]	Visually compatible. Little loss of either drug in 4 hr at 23 °C	2214	C
Morphine sulfate	ES	1 mg/mL[b]	GL	0.5 mg/mL[c]	Physically compatible for 1 hr at 25 °C	1338	C
	SCN	2 mg/mL[a]	GL	1 mg/mL[a]	Visually compatible for 4 hr at 27 °C	2062	C
Nicardipine HCl	DCC	0.1 mg/mL[a]	GL	0.5 mg/mL[a]	Visually compatible for 24 hr at room temperature	235	C
	WY	1 mg/mL[a]	GL	1 mg/mL[a]	Visually compatible for 4 hr at 27 °C	2062	C
Nitroglycerin	SO	0.2 mg/mL[a]	GL	0.5 mg/mL	Physically compatible for 24 hr	1323	C
	AB	0.4 mg/mL[a]	GL	1 mg/mL[a]	Visually compatible for 4 hr at 27 °C	2062	C
Norepinephrine bitartrate	AB	0.128 mg/mL[a]	GL	1 mg/mL[a]	Visually compatible for 4 hr at 27 °C	2062	C
Ondansetron HCl	GL	1 mg/mL[b]	GL	2 mg/mL[a]	Visually compatible for 4 hr at 22 °C	1365	C
	GL	0.03, 0.1, 0.3 mg/mL[a]	GL	0.5 mg/mL[a]	Visually compatible with no loss of either drug in 4 hr	1730	C
	GL	0.03, 0.1, 0.3 mg/mL[a]	GL	2 mg/mL[a]	Visually compatible with no loss of either drug in 4 hr	1730	C
Ondansetron HCl with paclitaxel	GL BR	0.3 mg/mL[a] 1.2 mg/mL[a]	GL	2 mg/mL[a]	Visually compatible with no loss of any drug in 4 hr at 23 °C	1741	C
Oxaliplatin	SS	0.5 mg/mL[a]	GW	2 mg/mL[a]	Physically compatible for 4 hr at 23 °C	2566	C
Paclitaxel	NCI	1.2 mg/mL[a]		2 mg/mL[a]	Physically compatible for 4 hr at 22 °C	1528	C
	BR	0.3 and 1.2 mg/mL[a]	GL	0.5 and 2 mg/mL[a]	Visually compatible. No loss of either drug in 4 hr at 23 °C	1741	C
Paclitaxel with ondansetron HCl	BR GL	1.2 mg/mL[a] 0.3 mg/mL[a]	GL	2 mg/mL[a]	Visually compatible with no loss of any drug in 4 hr at 23 °C	1741	C
Pancuronium bromide	ES	0.05 mg/mL[a]	GL	0.5 mg/mL[a]	Physically compatible for 24 hr at 28 °C	1337	C
Pemetrexed disodium	LI	20 mg/mL[b]	GSK	2 mg/mL[a]	Physically compatible for 4 hr at 23 °C	2564	C
Piperacillin sodium–tazobactam sodium	LE[g]	40 + 5 mg/mL[a]	GL	2 mg/mL[a]	Physically compatible for 4 hr at 22 °C	1688	C

Y-Site Injection Compatibility (1:1 Mixture) (Cont.)

Ranitidine HCl

Drug	Mfr	Conc	Mfr	Conc	Remarks	Ref	C/I
	LE[g]	80 + 10 mg/mL[b]	GL	0.5 and 2 mg/mL[b]	Visually compatible. Little loss of any component in 4 hr at 23 °C	1759	C
	LE[g]	40 + 5 mg/mL[b]	GL	0.5 and 2 mg/mL[b]	Visually compatible. Little loss of ranitidine and tazobactam in 4 hr at 23 °C. Piperacillin not tested	1759	C
Procainamide HCl	BA	4 mg/mL[a]	GL	0.5 mg/mL	Physically compatible for 24 hr	1323	C
Propofol	ZEN	10 mg/mL	GL	2 mg/mL[a]	Physically compatible for 1 hr at 23 °C	2066	C
Remifentanil HCl	GW	0.025 and 0.25 mg/mL[b]	GL	2 mg/mL[a]	Physically compatible for 4 hr at 23 °C	2075	C
Sargramostim	IMM	10 mcg/mL[b]	GL	2 mg/mL[b]	Visually compatible for 4 hr at 22 °C	1436	C
Tacrolimus	FUJ	1 mg/mL[b]	GL	25 mg/mL	Visually compatible for 24 hr at 25 °C	1630	C
Telavancin HCl	ASP	7.5 mg/mL[a,b,d]	BED	2 mg/mL[a,b,d]	Physically compatible for 2 hr	2830	C
Teniposide	BR	0.1 mg/mL[a]	GL	2 mg/mL[a]	Physically compatible for 4 hr at 23 °C	1725	C
Theophylline	TR	4 mg/mL	GL	1 mg/mL	Visually compatible for 6 hr at 25 °C	1793	C
Thiotepa	IMM[i]	1 mg/mL[a]	GL	2 mg/mL[a]	Physically compatible for 4 hr at 23 °C	1861	C
Tigecycline	WY	1 mg/mL[b]		0.6 mg/mL[b]	Physically compatible for 4 hr	2714	C
TNA #218 to #226[j]			GL	2 mg/mL[a]	Visually compatible for 4 hr at 23 °C	2215	C
TPN #189[j]			GL	2.5 mg/mL[b]	Visually compatible for 24 hr at 22 °C	1767	C
TPN #203, #204[j]			GL	25 mg/mL	Visually compatible for 2 hr at 23 °C	1974	C
TPN #212 to #215[j]			GL	2 mg/mL[a]	Physically compatible for 4 hr at 23 °C	2109	C
Vecuronium bromide	OR	0.1 mg/mL[a]	GL	0.5 mg/mL[a]	Physically compatible for 24 hr at 28 °C	1337	C
	OR	1 mg/mL	GL	1 mg/mL[a]	Visually compatible for 4 hr at 27 °C	2062	C
Vinorelbine tartrate	BW	1 mg/mL[b]	GL	2 mg/mL[b]	Physically compatible for 4 hr at 22 °C	1558	C
Warfarin sodium	DU	2 mg/mL[h]	GL	1 mg/mL[a]	Visually compatible with no warfarin loss in 30 min	2010	C
	DME	2 mg/mL[h]	GL	1 mg/mL[a]	Visually compatible for 24 hr at 24 °C	2078	C
Zidovudine	BW	4 mg/mL[a]	GL	1 mg/mL[a]	Physically compatible for 4 hr at 25 °C	1193	C

[a]Tested in dextrose 5%.
[b]Tested in sodium chloride 0.9%.
[c]Tested in sodium chloride 0.45%.
[d]Tested in Ringer's injection, lactated.
[e]Tested in both dextrose 5% and sodium chloride 0.9%.
[f]Tested in bacteriostatic sodium chloride 0.9% preserved with benzyl alcohol 0.9%.
[g]Test performed using the formulation WITHOUT edetate disodium.
[h]Tested in sterile water for injection.
[i]Lyophilized formulation tested.
[j]Refer to Appendix I for the composition of parenteral nutrition solutions. TNA indicates a 3-in-1 admixture, and TPN indicates a 2-in-1 admixture.

REMIFENTANIL HYDROCHLORIDE
AHFS 28:08.08

Products — Remifentanil hydrochloride is available in vials containing 1, 2, or 5 mg of remifentanil base present as the hydrochloride. Each vial also contains glycine 15 mg and hydrochloric acid for pH adjustment. The contents of the vials should be reconstituted with 1 mL of compatible diluent per milligram of remifentanil to yield a 1-mg/mL solution. (1)

pH — From 2.5 to 3.5. (1)

Trade Name(s) — Ultiva.

Administration — Remifentanil hydrochloride is administered intravenously only. Single doses may be given over 30 to 60 seconds.

Remifentanil hydrochloride may also be given by continuous intravenous infusion using an infusion device. The manufacturer recommends that the injection site be near the venous cannula and that all tubing be cleared at the time the infusion is discontinued. Bolus doses and continuous infusion should not be administered simultaneously to spontaneously breathing patients. (1)

For intravenous administration, remifentanil hydrochloride should be diluted to a final concentration of 20, 25, 50, or 250 mcg/mL. It should not be administered without dilution. (1)

Stability — Remifentanil hydrochloride is a white to off-white lyophilized powder that forms a clear, colorless solution upon reconstitution. Intact vials should be stored between 2 and 25 °C. (1)

Compatibility Information

Solution Compatibility

Remifentanil HCl

Solution	Mfr	Mfr	Conc/L	Remarks	Ref	C/I
Dextrose 5% in Ringer's injection, lactated			20 to 250 mg	Compatible and stable for 24 hr	1	C
Dextrose 5% in sodium chloride 0.9%			20 to 250 mg	Compatible and stable for 24 hr	1	C
Dextrose 5%			20 to 250 mg	Compatible and stable for 24 hr	1	C
Ringer's injection, lactated			20 to 250 mg	Stable for 4 hr	1	C
Sodium chloride 0.45%			20 to 250 mg	Compatible and stable for 24 hr	1	C
Sodium chloride 0.9%			20 to 250 mg	Compatible and stable for 24 hr	1	C

Y-Site Injection Compatibility (1:1 Mixture)

Remifentanil HCl

Drug	Mfr	Conc	Mfr	Conc	Remarks	Ref	C/I
Acyclovir sodium	BW	7 mg/mL[a]	GW	0.025 and 0.25 mg/mL[b]	Physically compatible for 4 hr at 23 °C	2075	C
Alfentanil HCl	JN	0.125 mg/mL[a]	GW	0.025 and 0.25 mg/mL[b]	Physically compatible for 4 hr at 23 °C	2075	C
Amikacin sulfate	AB	5 mg/mL[a]	GW	0.025 and 0.25 mg/mL[b]	Physically compatible for 4 hr at 23 °C	2075	C
Aminophylline	AB	2.5 mg/mL[a]	GW	0.025 and 0.25 mg/mL[b]	Physically compatible for 4 hr at 23 °C	2075	C
Amphotericin B	PHT	0.6 mg/mL[a]	GW	0.025 mg/mL[a]	Physically compatible for 4 hr at 23 °C	2075	C
	PHT	0.6 mg/mL[a]	GW	0.25 mg/mL[a]	Yellow precipitate forms immediately	2075	I
Amphotericin B cholesteryl sulfate complex	SEQ	0.83 mg/mL[a]	GW	0.5 mg/mL[a]	Gross precipitate forms	2117	I

Y-Site Injection Compatibility (1:1 Mixture) (Cont.)

Remifentanil HCl

Drug	Mfr	Conc	Mfr	Conc	Remarks	Ref	C/I
Ampicillin sodium	SKB	20 mg/mL[b]	GW	0.025 and 0.25 mg/mL[b]	Physically compatible for 4 hr at 23 °C	2075	C
Ampicillin sodium–sulbactam sodium	RR	20 + 10 mg/mL[b]	GW	0.025 and 0.25 mg/mL[b]	Physically compatible for 4 hr at 23 °C	2075	C
Aztreonam	SQ	40 mg/mL[a]	GW	0.025 and 0.25 mg/mL[b]	Physically compatible for 4 hr at 23 °C	2075	C
Bumetanide	RC	0.04 mg/mL[a]	GW	0.025 and 0.25 mg/mL[b]	Physically compatible for 4 hr at 23 °C	2075	C
Buprenorphine HCl	RKC	0.04 mg/mL[a]	GW	0.025 and 0.25 mg/mL[b]	Physically compatible for 4 hr at 23 °C	2075	C
Butorphanol tartrate	APC	0.04 mg/mL[a]	GW	0.025 and 0.25 mg/mL[b]	Physically compatible for 4 hr at 23 °C	2075	C
Calcium gluconate	AB	40 mg/mL[a]	GW	0.025 and 0.25 mg/mL[b]	Physically compatible for 4 hr at 23 °C	2075	C
Cefazolin sodium	SKB	20 mg/mL[a]	GW	0.025 and 0.25 mg/mL[b]	Physically compatible for 4 hr at 23 °C	2075	C
Cefepime HCl	BMS	120 mg/mL[c]		0.2 mg/mL	Physically compatible with less than 10% cefepime loss. Remifentanil not tested	2513	C
Cefotaxime sodium	HO	20 mg/mL[a]	GW	0.025 and 0.25 mg/mL[b]	Physically compatible for 4 hr at 23 °C	2075	C
Cefotetan disodium	ZEN	20 mg/mL[a]	GW	0.025 and 0.25 mg/mL[b]	Physically compatible for 4 hr at 23 °C	2075	C
Cefoxitin sodium	ME	20 mg/mL[a]	GW	0.025 and 0.25 mg/mL[b]	Physically compatible for 4 hr at 23 °C	2075	C
Ceftaroline fosamil	FOR	2.22 mg/mL[a,b,e]	HOS	0.25 mg/mL[a,b,e]	Physically compatible for 4 hr at 23 °C	2826	C
Ceftazidime	GSK	120 mg/mL[c]		0.2 mg/mL	Physically compatible with less than 10% ceftazidime loss. Remifentanil not tested	2513	C
Ceftriaxone sodium	RC	20 mg/mL[a]	GW	0.025 and 0.25 mg/mL[b]	Physically compatible for 4 hr at 23 °C	2075	C
Cefuroxime sodium	LI	30 mg/mL[a]	GW	0.025 and 0.25 mg/mL[b]	Physically compatible for 4 hr at 23 °C	2075	C
Chlorpromazine HCl	SCN	2 mg/mL[a]	GW	0.025 mg/mL[b]	Slight haze forms in 1 hr	2075	I
	SCN	2 mg/mL[a]	GW	0.25 mg/mL[b]	Physically compatible for 4 hr at 23 °C	2075	C
Ciprofloxacin	BAY	1 mg/mL[a]	GW	0.025 and 0.25 mg/mL[b]	Physically compatible for 4 hr at 23 °C	2075	C
Cisatracurium besylate	GW	2 mg/mL[a]	GW	0.025 and 0.25 mg/mL[b]	Physically compatible for 4 hr at 23 °C	2075	C
Clindamycin phosphate	AST	10 mg/mL[a]	GW	0.025 and 0.25 mg/mL[b]	Physically compatible for 4 hr at 23 °C	2075	C
Dexamethasone sodium phosphate	FUJ	2 mg/mL[a]	GW	0.025 and 0.25 mg/mL[b]	Physically compatible for 4 hr at 23 °C	2075	C
Dexmedetomidine HCl	AB	4 mcg/mL[b]	AB	0.25 mg/mL[b]	Physically compatible for 4 hr at 23 °C	2383	C
Diazepam	ES	5 mg/mL	GW	0.025 and 0.25 mg/mL[b]	White turbidity forms immediately	2075	I

Y-Site Injection Compatibility (1:1 Mixture) (Cont.)

Remifentanil HCl

Drug	Mfr	Conc	Mfr	Conc	Remarks	Ref	C/I
	ES	0.25 mg/mL[a]	GW	0.025 and 0.25 mg/mL[b]	Physically compatible for 4 hr at 23 °C	2075	C
Digoxin	ES	0.25 mg/mL	GW	0.025 and 0.25 mg/mL[b]	Physically compatible for 4 hr at 23 °C	2075	C
Diphenhydramine HCl	SCN	2 mg/mL[a]	GW	0.025 and 0.25 mg/mL[b]	Physically compatible for 4 hr at 23 °C	2075	C
Dobutamine HCl	LI	4 mg/mL[a]	GW	0.025 and 0.25 mg/mL[b]	Physically compatible for 4 hr at 23 °C	2075	C
Dopamine HCl	AB	3.2 mg/mL[a]	GW	0.025 and 0.25 mg/mL[b]	Physically compatible for 4 hr at 23 °C	2075	C
Doxycycline hyclate	FUJ	1 mg/mL[a]	GW	0.025 and 0.25 mg/mL[b]	Physically compatible for 4 hr at 23 °C	2075	C
Droperidol	AST	2.5 mg/mL	GW	0.025 and 0.25 mg/mL[b]	Physically compatible for 4 hr at 23 °C	2075	C
Enalaprilat	ME	0.1 mg/mL[a]	GW	0.025 and 0.25 mg/mL[b]	Physically compatible for 4 hr at 23 °C	2075	C
Epinephrine HCl	AMR	0.05 mg/mL[a]	GW	0.025 and 0.25 mg/mL[b]	Physically compatible for 4 hr at 23 °C	2075	C
Esmolol HCl	OHM	10 mg/mL[a]	GW	0.025 and 0.25 mg/mL[b]	Physically compatible for 4 hr at 23 °C	2075	C
Famotidine	MSD	2 mg/mL[a]	GW	0.025 and 0.25 mg/mL[b]	Physically compatible for 4 hr at 23 °C	2075	C
Fenoldopam mesylate	AB	80 mcg/mL[b]	AB	0.2 mg/mL[b]	Physically compatible for 4 hr at 23 °C	2467	C
Fentanyl citrate	ES	12.5 mcg/mL[a]	GW	0.025 and 0.25 mg/mL[b]	Physically compatible for 4 hr at 23 °C	2075	C
Fluconazole	RR	2 mg/mL	GW	0.025 and 0.25 mg/mL[b]	Physically compatible for 4 hr at 23 °C	2075	C
Furosemide	AMR	3 mg/mL[a]	GW	0.025 and 0.25 mg/mL[b]	Physically compatible for 4 hr at 23 °C	2075	C
Ganciclovir sodium	SY	20 mg/mL[a]	GW	0.025 and 0.25 mg/mL[b]	Physically compatible for 4 hr at 23 °C	2075	C
Gentamicin sulfate	ES	5 mg/mL[a]	GW	0.025 and 0.25 mg/mL[b]	Physically compatible for 4 hr at 23 °C	2075	C
Haloperidol lactate	MN	0.2 mg/mL[a]	GW	0.025 and 0.25 mg/mL[b]	Physically compatible for 4 hr at 23 °C	2075	C
Heparin sodium	AB	100 units/mL	GW	0.025 and 0.25 mg/mL[b]	Physically compatible for 4 hr at 23 °C	2075	C
Hydrocortisone sodium succinate	AB	1 mg/mL[a]	GW	0.025 and 0.25 mg/mL[b]	Physically compatible for 4 hr at 23 °C	2075	C
Hydromorphone HCl	ES	0.5 mg/mL[a]	GW	0.025 and 0.25 mg/mL[b]	Physically compatible for 4 hr at 23 °C	2075	C
Hydroxyzine HCl	ES	2 mg/mL[a]	GW	0.025 and 0.25 mg/mL[b]	Physically compatible for 4 hr at 23 °C	2075	C
Imipenem–cilastatin sodium	ME	10 mg/mL[a]	GW	0.025 and 0.25 mg/mL[b]	Physically compatible for 4 hr at 23 °C	2075	C

Y-Site Injection Compatibility (1:1 Mixture) (Cont.)

Remifentanil HCl

Drug	Mfr	Conc	Mfr	Conc	Remarks	Ref	C/I
Isoproterenol HCl	SW	0.02 mg/mL[a]	GW	0.025 and 0.25 mg/mL[b]	Physically compatible for 4 hr at 23 °C	2075	**C**
Ketorolac tromethamine	RC	15 mg/mL[a]	GW	0.025 and 0.25 mg/mL[b]	Physically compatible for 4 hr at 23 °C	2075	**C**
Lidocaine HCl	AST	8 mg/mL[a]	GW	0.025 and 0.25 mg/mL[b]	Physically compatible for 4 hr at 23 °C	2075	**C**
Linezolid	PHU	2 mg/mL	GW	0.5 mg/mL[a]	Physically compatible for 4 hr at 23 °C	2264	**C**
Lorazepam	WY	0.5 mg/mL[a]	GW	0.025 and 0.25 mg/mL[b]	Physically compatible for 4 hr at 23 °C	2075	**C**
Magnesium sulfate	AB	100 mg/mL[a]	GW	0.025 and 0.25 mg/mL[b]	Physically compatible for 4 hr at 23 °C	2075	**C**
Mannitol	BA	15%	GW	0.025 and 0.25 mg/mL[b]	Physically compatible for 4 hr at 23 °C	2075	**C**
Meperidine HCl	AST	4 mg/mL[a]	GW	0.025 and 0.25 mg/mL[b]	Physically compatible for 4 hr at 23 °C	2075	**C**
Methylprednisolone sodium succinate	AB	5 mg/mL[a]	GW	0.025 and 0.25 mg/mL[b]	Physically compatible for 4 hr at 23 °C	2075	**C**
Metoclopramide HCl	AB	5 mg/mL	GW	0.025 and 0.25 mg/mL[b]	Physically compatible for 4 hr at 23 °C	2075	**C**
Metronidazole	AB	5 mg/mL	GW	0.025 and 0.25 mg/mL[b]	Physically compatible for 4 hr at 23 °C	2075	**C**
Midazolam HCl	RC	1 mg/mL[a]	GW	0.025 and 0.25 mg/mL[b]	Physically compatible for 4 hr at 23 °C	2075	**C**
Morphine sulfate	AST	1 mg/mL[a]	GW	0.025 and 0.25 mg/mL[b]	Physically compatible for 4 hr at 23 °C	2075	**C**
Nalbuphine HCl	AST	10 mg/mL	GW	0.025 and 0.25 mg/mL[b]	Physically compatible for 4 hr at 23 °C	2075	**C**
Nitroglycerin	DU	0.4 mg/mL[a]	GW	0.025 and 0.25 mg/mL[b]	Physically compatible for 4 hr at 23 °C	2075	**C**
Norepinephrine bitartrate	SW	0.12 mg/mL[a]	GW	0.025 and 0.25 mg/mL[b]	Physically compatible for 4 hr at 23 °C	2075	**C**
Ondansetron HCl	CER	1 mg/mL[a]	GW	0.025 and 0.25 mg/mL[b]	Physically compatible for 4 hr at 23 °C	2075	**C**
Phenylephrine HCl	AMR	1 mg/mL[a]	GW	0.025 and 0.25 mg/mL[b]	Physically compatible for 4 hr at 23 °C	2075	**C**
Piperacillin sodium–tazobactam sodium	CY[d]	40 + 5 mg/mL[a]	GW	0.025 and 0.25 mg/mL[b]	Physically compatible for 4 hr at 23 °C	2075	**C**
Potassium chloride	AB	0.1 mEq/mL[a]	GW	0.025 and 0.25 mg/mL[b]	Physically compatible for 4 hr at 23 °C	2075	**C**
Procainamide HCl	ES	10 mg/mL[a]	GW	0.025 and 0.25 mg/mL[b]	Physically compatible for 4 hr at 23 °C	2075	**C**
Prochlorperazine edisylate	SO	0.5 mg/mL[a]	GW	0.025 and 0.25 mg/mL[b]	Physically compatible for 4 hr at 23 °C	2075	**C**
Promethazine HCl	SCN	2 mg/mL[a]	GW	0.025 and 0.25 mg/mL[b]	Physically compatible for 4 hr at 23 °C	2075	**C**

Y-Site Injection Compatibility (1:1 Mixture) (Cont.)

Remifentanil HCl

Drug	Mfr	Conc	Mfr	Conc	Remarks	Ref	C/I
Ranitidine HCl	GL	2 mg/mL[a]	GW	0.025 and 0.25 mg/mL[b]	Physically compatible for 4 hr at 23 °C	2075	C
Sodium bicarbonate	AB	1 mEq/mL	GW	0.025 and 0.25 mg/mL[b]	Physically compatible for 4 hr at 23 °C	2075	C
Sufentanil citrate	ES	0.0125 mg/ mL[a]	GW	0.025 and 0.25 mg/mL[b]	Physically compatible for 4 hr at 23 °C	2075	C
Theophylline	AB	3.2 mg/mL[a]	GW	0.025 and 0.25 mg/mL[b]	Physically compatible for 4 hr at 23 °C	2075	C
Ticarcillin disodium–clavulanate potassium	SKB	31 mg/mL[a]	GW	0.025 and 0.25 mg/mL[b]	Physically compatible for 4 hr at 23 °C	2075	C
Tobramycin sulfate	AB	5 mg/mL[a]	GW	0.025 and 0.25 mg/mL[b]	Physically compatible for 4 hr at 23 °C	2075	C
Trimethoprim–sulfamethoxazole	ES	0.8 + 4 mg/ mL[a]	GW	0.025 and 0.25 mg/mL[b]	Physically compatible for 4 hr at 23 °C	2075	C
Vancomycin HCl	AB	10 mg/mL[a]	GW	0.025 and 0.25 mg/mL[b]	Physically compatible for 4 hr at 23 °C	2075	C
Zidovudine	BW	4 mg/mL[a]	GW	0.025 and 0.25 mg/mL[b]	Physically compatible for 4 hr at 23 °C	2075	C

[a]*Tested in dextrose 5%.*
[b]*Tested in sodium chloride 0.9%.*
[c]*Tested in sterile water for injection.*
[d]*Test performed using the formulation WITHOUT edetate disodium.*
[e]*Tested in Ringer's injection, lactated.*

RETEPLASE
AHFS 20:12.20

Products — Reteplase is available as a lyophilized powder in 10.4-unit (18.1-mg) vials; the slight overfill is to ensure that 10 units of drug can be delivered. The vials are packaged with sterile water for injection diluent in kits containing two vials of drug and diluent along with syringes, needles, alcohol swabs, and dispensing pins and in half-kits with a single vial of drug and diluent with a dispensing pin. Each vial also contains tranexamic acid 8.32 mg, dipotassium hydrogen phosphate 136.24 mg, phosphoric acid 51.27 mg, sucrose 364 mg, and polysorbate 80 5.2 mg. (1)

Reconstitute the reteplase vials using the diluent and dispensing pin provided. Other solutions should not be used to reconstitute the drug. Swirl gently to dissolve the drug yielding a 1-unit/mL solution. Do not shake. If slight foaming occurs, the vials should be allowed to stand for several minutes to dissipate large bubbles. (1; 4)

pH — The reconstituted solution has a pH from 5.7 to 6.3. (1)

Trade Name(s) — Retavase.

Administration — Reteplase is administered intravenously as a double bolus injection, each injection delivered over two minutes. The second injection is given 30 minutes after completion of the first injection. The manufacturer recommends no other drugs be administered in the line used to deliver reteplase. (1)

Stability — Intact packages should be stored between 2 and 25 °C. The boxes should stay sealed until use to protect from light. Because no antimicrobial preservatives are present, the manufacturer recommends reconstitution immediately before use. The colorless reconstituted solution may be used for up to four hours after reconstitution when stored between 2 and 30 °C. (1)

Reteplase is incompatible with heparin sodium. If mixed in the same container or run into the same line as heparin sodium, a solid or semisolid mass may form. However, heparin sodium may be administered sequentially with reteplase into the same line used to deliver reteplase if the line is adequately flushed with sodium chloride 0.9% or dextrose 5% both before and after reteplase administration. (1)

Compatibility Information

Y-Site Injection Compatibility (1:1 Mixture)

Reteplase

Drug	Mfr	Conc	Mfr	Conc	Remarks	Ref	C/I
Bivalirudin	TMC	5 mg/mL[a]	CEN	1 unit/mL[a]	Small aggregates form immediately	2373	I

[a]Tested in dextrose 5%.

RIFAMPIN
AHFS 8:16.04

Products — Rifampin is available as a lyophilized powder in vials containing rifampin 600 mg, sodium formaldehyde sulfoxylate 10 mg, and sodium hydroxide to adjust the pH. Reconstitute with 10 mL of sterile water for injection; swirl gently to dissolve the vial contents for a 60-mg/mL solution. (1)

Trade Name(s) — Rifadin I.V.

Administration — Rifampin is administered by intravenous infusion. It must not be given intramuscularly or subcutaneously, and extravasation should be avoided. The reconstituted solution may be diluted in 500 mL of dextrose 5% or sodium chloride 0.9% and infused over three hours. Alternatively, the desired dose may be diluted in 100 mL and administered over 30 minutes. (1; 4)

Stability — Rifampin powder is reddish brown. Intact vials should be stored at room temperature and protected from excessive heat and light. The reconstituted solution is stable for 24 hours at room temperature. (1)

Compatibility Information

Solution Compatibility

Rifampin

Solution	Mfr	Mfr	Conc/L	Remarks	Ref	C/I
Dextrose 5%				Use within 4 hr	1	C
	AB	MMD	6 g	Gelatinous precipitate after overnight room temperature storage	1543	I
	AB	MMD	1.2 g	Clear with no visible precipitation over 3 hr	1543	C
	BA[a]	MMD	0.1 g	Brownish color in 4 hr. 5% rifampin loss in 8 hr and 17% loss in 24 hr at 24 °C. 8% loss in 3 days at 4 °C	1559	I[b]
Sodium chloride 0.9%				Use within 24 hr	1	C
	BA[a]	MMD	0.1 g	Brownish color in 4 hr. 7% rifampin loss in 8 hr and 13% loss in 24 hr at 24 °C. 7% loss in 3 days at 4 °C	1559	I[b]

[a]Tested in PVC containers.
[b]Incompatible by conventional standards. May be used in shorter time periods.

Y-Site Injection Compatibility (1:1 Mixture)

Rifampin

Drug	Mfr	Conc	Mfr	Conc	Remarks	Ref	C/I
Diltiazem HCl	MMD	1[a] and 5 mg/mL	MMD	6 mg/mL[a]	Precipitate forms	1807	I
Tramadol HCl	GRU	8.33 mg/mL	AVE	6 mg/mL	Immediate red-orange turbid precipitate	2727	I

[a]Tested in sodium chloride 0.9%.

ROCURONIUM BROMIDE
AHFS 12:20.20

Products — Rocuronium bromide is available in 5- and 10-mL vials. Each milliliter contains rocuronium bromide 10 mg with sodium acetate 2 mg, sodium chloride for isotonicity, and acetic acid and/or sodium hydroxide to adjust the pH. (1)

pH — Adjusted during manufacture to pH 4. (1)

Osmolality — The injection is isotonic. (1)

Trade Name(s) — Zemuron.

Administration — Rocuronium bromide is administered intravenously only by rapid intravenous injection or by intravenous infusion when admixed in an appropriate intravenous infusion solution. Infusion rates should be individualized for each patient according to the requirements and response. (1; 4)

Stability — Intact vials of rocuronium bromide should be stored under refrigeration at 2 to 8 °C and protected from freezing. Intact vials stored at room temperature should be used within 60 days. Opened vials should be used within 30 days. (1)

Compatibility Information

Solution Compatibility

Rocuronium bromide

Solution	Mfr	Mfr	Conc/L	Remarks	Ref	C/I
Dextrose 5% in sodium chloride 0.9%				Compatible and stable for 24 hr	1	**C**
Dextrose 5%				Compatible and stable for 24 hr	1	**C**
Ringer's injection, lactated				Compatible and stable for 24 hr	1	**C**
Sodium chloride 0.9%				Compatible and stable for 24 hr	1	**C**

Y-Site Injection Compatibility (1:1 Mixture)

Rocuronium bromide

Drug	Mfr	Conc	Mfr	Conc	Remarks	Ref	C/I
Dexmedetomidine HCl	AB	4 mcg/mL[b]	OR	1 mg/mL[b]	Physically compatible for 4 hr at 23 °C	2383	**C**
Fenoldopam mesylate	AB	80 mcg/mL[b]	OR	1 mg/mL[b]	Physically compatible for 4 hr at 23 °C	2467	**C**
Hetastarch in lactated electrolyte	AB	6%	OR	1 mg/mL[a]	Physically compatible for 4 hr at 23 °C	2339	**C**
Micafungin sodium	ASP	1.5 mg/mL[b]	OR	1 mg/mL[b]	White precipitate forms immediately	2683	**I**
Milrinone lactate	SW	0.4 mg/mL[a]	OR	2 mg/mL[a]	Visually compatible. Little loss of either drug in 4 hr at 23 °C	2214	**C**
Palonosetron HCl	MGI	50 mcg/mL	BA	1 mg/mL[a]	Physically compatible and no loss of either drug in 4 hr at room temperature	2764	**C**

[a]Tested in dextrose 5%.
[b]Tested in sodium chloride 0.9%.

ROPIVACAINE HYDROCHLORIDE
AHFS 72:00

Products — Ropivacaine hydrochloride is available in concentrations of 2 mg/mL (0.2%), 5 mg/mL (0.5%), 7.5 mg/mL (0.75%), and 10 mg/mL (1%) along with sodium chloride for isotonicity and sodium hydroxide and/or hydrochloric acid for pH adjustment in water for injection. The products are packaged in single-dose glass vials and in polypropylene plastic ampuls designed to fit Luer-lock and Luer-slip syringes. The 2-mg/mL concentration is also available in 100 and 200-mL infusion bottles. Sterile-Pak products should be selected when a container having a sterile outside is required. (1)

pH — From 4 to 6.5. (404)

Tonicity — Ropivacaine hydrochloride injections are isotonic. (1)

Specific Gravity — The specific gravities of ropivacaine hydrochloride injections range from 1.002 to 1.005 at 25 °C. (1)

Trade Name(s) — Naropin.

Administration — Ropivacaine hydrochloride is administered parenterally by lumbar epidural injection or infusion, by thoracic epidural infusion, by injection for nerve block, and by infiltration. (1)

Stability — Intact containers of ropivacaine hydrochloride should be stored at controlled room temperature. The single-dose containers have no antimicrobial preservatives. The manufacturer recommends that any remaining solution in an opened container be discarded promptly. The continuous infusion bottles should not be left in place for more than 24 hours. (1)

Autoclaving — Ropivacaine hydrochloride in glass containers is stable during one autoclaving to sterilize the container. (1)

pH Effects — The solubility of ropivacaine hydrochloride is reduced above pH 6. Consequently, contact with alkaline solutions may result in precipitation. (1)

Compatibility Information

Additive Compatibility

Ropivacaine HCl

Drug	Mfr	Conc/L	Mfr	Conc/L	Test Soln	Remarks	Ref	C/I
Clonidine HCl	BI	5 and 50 mg	ASZ	1 g	NS[a]	Physically compatible. No loss of either drug in 30 days at 30 °C in the dark	2433	C
	BI	5 mg	ASZ	2 g	[a]	Physically compatible. No loss of either drug in 30 days at 30 °C in the dark	2433	C
Diamorphine HCl		25 mg	ASZ	2 g	[d]	No ropivacaine and 10% diamorphine loss in 70 days at 4 °C and 28 days at 21 °C	2517	C
Fentanyl citrate	JN	1 mg	ASZ	1 g	NS[a]	Physically compatible. No loss of either drug in 30 days at 30 °C in the dark	2433	C
	JN	1 and 10 mg	ASZ	2 g	[a]	Physically compatible. No loss of either drug in 30 days at 30 °C in the dark	2433	C
	CUR	3 mg	ASZ	1.5 g	NS[b,c]	Physically compatible. No loss of either drug in 51 days at 20 and 4 °C	2498	C
	CUR	3 mg	ASZ	1.5 g	NS[d]	Physically compatible. No loss of either drug in 7 days at 20 and 4 °C	2498	C
Morphine sulfate	AST	20 mg	ASZ	1 g	NS[a]	Physically compatible. Little loss of either drug in 30 days at 30 °C in the dark	2433	C
	AST	20 and 100 mg	ASZ	2 g	[a]	Physically compatible. Little loss of either drug in 30 days at 30 °C in the dark	2433	C
Sufentanil citrate	JN	0.4 mg	ASZ	1 g	NS[a]	Physically compatible. No loss of either drug in 30 days at 30 °C in the dark	2433	C
	JN	0.4 and 4 mg	ASZ	2 g	[a]	Physically compatible. No loss of either drug in 30 days at 30 °C in the dark	2433	C
	JC	0.5, 0.75, 1 mg	ASZ	2 mg	NS[b,d]	Physically compatible with no major sufentanil loss in 96 hr at 25 °C. Ropivacaine not tested	2506	C

[a]Tested in polypropylene bags (Mark II Polybags).
[b]Tested in glass containers.
[c]Tested in ethylene vinyl acetate (EVA) containers.
[d]Tested in PVC containers.

Drugs in Syringe Compatibility

Ropivacaine HCl

Drug (in syringe)	Mfr	Amt	Mfr	Amt	Remarks	Ref	C/I
Diamorphine HCl		45 mg	ASZ	10 g	No ropivacaine loss and 10% diamorphine loss in 30 days at 4 °C and 16 days at 21 °C	2517	C
Methylprednisolone acetate	PHU	80 mg/ 2 mL	AST	6 mg/ 3 mL	Little loss of either drug in 30 days at 4 and 24 °C in light or dark	2367	C

SALBUTAMOL
AHFS 12:12.08.12

Products — Salbutamol injection is available as a 500-mcg/mL solution in 1-mL ampuls as the sulfate. In addition, the product contains sodium chloride, sodium hydroxide, and sulfuric acid in water for injection. (38; 115)

Salbutamol infusion is available as a 1-mg/mL solution as the sulfate in 5-mL containers for use in infusions. In addition, the product for infusion also contains sodium chloride, sodium hydroxide, and sulfuric acid in water for injection. This concentrate must be diluted in a suitable intravenous infusion solution for use. (38; 115)

pH — About 3.5. (115)

Tonicity — Both salbutamol injection and infusion are isotonic. (38; 115)

Trade Name(s) — Salbumol, Ventolin, others.

Administration — Salbutamol injection is administered by subcutaneous, intramuscular, or slow intravenous injection. A 50-mcg/mL concentration is suitable for slow intravenous injection; dilution of the 500-mcg/mL concentration with water for injection has been recommended for intravenous injection, (38; 115) although it is likely to be hypotonic.

Salbutamol 1-mg/mL for intravenous infusion is used to prepare intravenous infusion solutions of the drug. It should not be given undiluted. It should be diluted to a concentration of 10 or 20 mcg/mL with a compatible infusion solution. Dextrose 5% is recommended but sodium chloride 0.9% may also be used. (38; 115)

Stability — Salbutamol injection and infusion are clear, colorless, or pale straw-colored solutions. The intact containers should be stored below 30 °C and protected from light. (38; 115)

Compatibility Information

Solution Compatibility

Salbutamol

Solution	Mfr	Mfr	Conc/L	Remarks	Ref	C/I
Dextrose 5%				Stable for 24 hr	38	C
Sodium chloride 0.9%				Stable for 24 hr	38	C

Drugs in Syringe Compatibility

Salbutamol

Drug (in syringe)	Mfr	Amt	Mfr	Amt	Remarks	Ref	C/I
Dimenhydrinate		10 mg/ 1 mL		1 mg/ 1 mL	Precipitate forms	2569	I
Hydromorphone HCl	KN	1 mg/ 0.5 mL	GL	2.5 mg/ 2.5 mL[a]	Physically compatible for 1 hr	1904	C
Morphine sulfate	AB	5 mg/ 0.5 mL	GL	2.5 mg/ 2.5 mL[a]	Physically compatible for 1 hr	1904	C
Pantoprazole sodium	[b]	4 mg/ 1 mL		1 mg/ 1 mL	Precipitates immediately	2574	I

[a]*Both preserved (benzyl alcohol 0.9%; benzalkonium chloride 0.01%) and unpreserved sodium chloride 0.9% were used as a diluent.*
[b]*Test performed using the formulation WITHOUT edetate disodium.*

SARGRAMOSTIM
(GM-CSF)
AHFS 20:16

Products — Sargramostim is available in single-dose vials labeled as 250 mcg. Reconstitute the vial with 1 mL of sterile water for injection or bacteriostatic water for injection containing benzyl alcohol 0.9% directed at the sides of the vial. Gently swirl to avoid foaming during dissolution, and do not shake. Each milliliter of the reconstituted solution contains sargramostim 250 mcg, mannitol 40 mg, sucrose 10 mg, and tromethamine 1.2 mg. (1; 4) The contents of vials reconstituted with different diluents should not be mixed. (1)

Sargramostim is also available as a preserved liquid formulation in 1-mL vials containing in each milliliter sargramostim 500 mcg along with mannitol 40 mg, sucrose 10 mg, tromethamine 1.2 mg, and benzyl alcohol 1.1% as an antimicrobial preservative. (1; 4)

Specific Activity — The specific activity is approximately 5.6×10^6 units per milligram. (1)

pH — From 7.1 to 7.7. (1; 17)

Trade Name(s) — Leukine.

Administration — Sargramostim may be administered by subcutaneous injection undiluted or by intravenous infusion usually over two to four hours after dilution in sodium chloride 0.9%. (1; 4) Intravenous infusion also has been performed. (4) For infusion concentrations below 10 mcg/mL, albumin human at a final concentration of 0.1% should be added to the intravenous solution prior to the addition of sargramostim to prevent adsorption. (1; 4)

The preparations containing benzyl alcohol (Leukine liquid, and lyophilized Leukine reconstituted with bacteriostatic water for injection containing benzyl alcohol) should not be used in neonates. (1)

Stability — Intact vials, reconstituted solutions, and sargramostim diluted in sodium chloride 0.9% should be stored under refrigeration. Solutions should be protected from freezing and not shaken. The liquid formulation is a clear, colorless solution. The white lyophilized powder forms a clear, colorless solution on reconstitution. The manufacturer recommends administration within six hours following reconstitution with sterile water for injection and/or dilution in an infusion solution and discarding any unused solution. When reconstituted with bacteriostatic water for injection preserved with benzyl alcohol 0.9%, the manufacturer states that the solution may be stored for up to 20 days under refrigeration. (1)

Other information indicates that sargramostim reconstituted with sterile water for injection or bacteriostatic water for injection is stable for 30 days at 25 °C or under refrigeration. (226)

Syringes — Sargramostim 250 mcg and 500 mcg reconstituted with 1 mL of bacteriostatic water for injection with benzyl alcohol 0.9% and repackaged in 1-mL tuberculin syringes (Becton Dickinson) is stated to be stable for 14 days when stored under refrigeration. (226)

Sorption — Sargramostim will adsorb to containers and tubing if the concentration is below 10 mcg/mL. Albumin human 0.1% should be added to the intravenous solution to prevent this. (1)

Filtration — Sargramostim should not be infused through an inline filter because of possible absorption. (1; 4)

Compatibility Information

Solution Compatibility

Sargramostim

Solution	Mfr	Mfr	Conc/L	Remarks	Ref	C/I
Sodium chloride 0.9%			10 mg or more	Use within 6 hr	1	C

Y-Site Injection Compatibility (1:1 Mixture)

Sargramostim

Drug	Mfr	Conc	Mfr	Conc	Remarks	Ref	C/I
Acyclovir sodium	BW	7 mg/mL[b]	IMM	10 mcg/mL[b]	Few small white particles form in 4 hr	1436	I
Amikacin sulfate	BR	5 mg/mL[b]	IMM	10 mcg/mL[b]	Visually compatible for 4 hr at 22 °C	1436	C
Aminophylline	ES	2.5 mg/mL[b]	IMM	10 mcg/mL[b]	Visually compatible for 4 hr at 22 °C	1436	C
Amphotericin B	SQ	0.6 mg/mL[a]	IMM	10 mcg/mL[b]	Yellow precipitate forms immediately	1436	I
	SQ	0.6 mg/mL[a]	IMM	10 mcg/mL[a]	Visually compatible for 4 hr at 22 °C	1436	C
Ampicillin sodium	BR	20 mg/mL[b]	IMM	10 mcg/mL[b]	Few small particles form in 4 hr	1436	I
Ampicillin sodium–sulbactam sodium	RR	20 + 10 mg/mL[b]	IMM	10 mcg/mL[b]	Few small particles form in 4 hr	1436	I
Amsacrine	NCI	1 mg/mL[a]	IMM	10 mcg/mL[a]	Visually compatible for 4 hr at 22 °C	1436	C
	NCI	1 mg/mL[a]	IMM	10 mcg/mL[b]	Haze and yellow precipitate form	1436	I
Aztreonam	SQ	40 mg/mL[b]	IMM	10 mcg/mL[b]	Visually compatible for 4 hr at 22 °C	1436	C
	SQ	40 mg/mL[a]	IMM	10 mcg/mL[b]	Physically compatible for 4 hr at 23 °C	1758	C
Bleomycin sulfate	MJ	1 unit/mL[b]	IMM	10 mcg/mL[b]	Visually compatible for 4 hr at 22 °C	1436	C
Butorphanol tartrate	BR	0.04 mg/mL[b]	IMM	10 mcg/mL[b]	Visually compatible for 4 hr at 22 °C	1436	C
Calcium gluconate	AMR	40 mg/mL[b]	IMM	10 mcg/mL[b]	Visually compatible for 4 hr at 22 °C	1436	C
Carboplatin	BR	5 mg/mL[b]	IMM	10 mcg/mL[b]	Visually compatible for 4 hr at 22 °C	1436	C

Y-Site Injection Compatibility (1:1 Mixture) (Cont.)

Sargramostim

Drug	Mfr	Conc	Mfr	Conc	Remarks	Ref	C/I
Carmustine	BR	1.5 mg/mL[b]	IMM	10 mcg/mL[b]	Visually compatible for 4 hr at 22 °C	1436	C
Cefazolin sodium	LEM	20 mg/mL[b]	IMM	10 mcg/mL[b]	Visually compatible for 4 hr at 22 °C	1436	C
Cefotaxime sodium	HO	20 mg/mL[b]	IMM	10 mcg/mL[b]	Visually compatible for 4 hr at 22 °C	1436	C
Cefotetan disodium	STU	20 mg/mL[b]	IMM	10 mcg/mL[b]	Visually compatible for 4 hr at 22 °C	1436	C
Ceftazidime	GL	40 mg/mL[b]	IMM	10 mcg/mL[b]	Particles and filaments form in 4 hr	1436	I
	LI	40 mg/mL[d]	IMM	6[b,e] and 15[b] mcg/mL	Visually compatible for 2 hr	1618	C
Ceftriaxone sodium	RC	20 mg/mL[b]	IMM	10 mcg/mL[b]	Visually compatible for 4 hr at 22 °C	1436	C
Cefuroxime sodium	GL	30 mg/mL[b]	IMM	10 mcg/mL[b]	Visually compatible for 4 hr at 22 °C	1436	C
Chlorpromazine HCl	ES	2 mg/mL[b]	IMM	10 mcg/mL[b]	Slight haze forms immediately	1436	I
Cisplatin	BR	1 mg/mL	IMM	10 mcg/mL[b]	Visually compatible for 4 hr at 22 °C	1436	C
Clindamycin phosphate	LY	10 mg/mL[b]	IMM	10 mcg/mL[b]	Visually compatible for 4 hr at 22 °C	1436	C
Cyclophosphamide	MJ	10 mg/mL[b]	IMM	10 mcg/mL[b]	Visually compatible for 4 hr at 22 °C	1436	C
Cyclosporine	SZ	5 mg/mL[b]	IMM	6[b,e] and 15[b] mcg/mL	Visually compatible for 2 hr	1618	C
Cytarabine	SCN	50 mg/mL	IMM	10 mcg/mL[b]	Visually compatible for 4 hr at 22 °C	1436	C
Dacarbazine	MI	4 mg/mL[b]	IMM	10 mcg/mL[b]	Visually compatible for 4 hr at 22 °C	1436	C
Dactinomycin	MSD	0.01 mg/mL[b]	IMM	10 mcg/mL[b]	Visually compatible for 4 hr at 22 °C	1436	C
Dexamethasone sodium phosphate	ES	1 mg/mL[b]	IMM	10 mcg/mL[b]	Visually compatible for 4 hr at 22 °C	1436	C
Diphenhydramine HCl	RU	1 mg/mL[b]	IMM	10 mcg/mL[b]	Visually compatible for 4 hr at 22 °C	1436	C
Dopamine HCl	DU	1.6 mg/mL[d]	IMM	6[b,e] and 15[b] mcg/mL	Visually compatible for 2 hr	1618	C
Doxorubicin HCl	CET	2 mg/mL	IMM	10 mcg/mL[b]	Visually compatible for 4 hr at 22 °C	1436	C
Doxycycline hyclate	LY	1 mg/mL[b]	IMM	10 mcg/mL[b]	Visually compatible for 4 hr at 22 °C	1436	C
Droperidol	DU	0.4 mg/mL[b]	IMM	10 mcg/mL[b]	Visually compatible for 4 hr at 22 °C	1436	C
Etoposide	BR	0.4 mg/mL[b]	IMM	10 mcg/mL[b]	Visually compatible for 4 hr at 22 °C	1436	C
Famotidine	MSD	2 mg/mL	IMM	10 mcg/mL[b]	Visually compatible for 4 hr at 22 °C	1436	C
Fentanyl citrate	ES	50 mcg/mL	IMM	6[b,e] and 15[b] mcg/mL	Visually compatible for 2 hr	1618	C
Floxuridine	RC	3 mg/mL[b]	IMM	10 mcg/mL[b]	Visually compatible for 4 hr at 22 °C	1436	C
Fluconazole	RR	2 mg/mL	IMM	10 mcg/mL[b]	Visually compatible for 4 hr at 22 °C	1436	C
Fluorouracil	SO	16 mg/mL	IMM	10 mcg/mL[b]	Visually compatible for 4 hr at 22 °C	1436	C
Furosemide	AB	3 mg/mL[b]	IMM	10 mcg/mL[b]	Visually compatible for 4 hr at 22 °C	1436	C
Ganciclovir sodium	SY	20 mg/mL[b]	IMM	10 mcg/mL[b]	Small particles form in 4 hr	1436	I
Gentamicin sulfate	SO	5 mg/mL[a]	IMM	10 mcg/mL[b]	Visually compatible for 4 hr at 22 °C	1436	C
Granisetron HCl	SKB	0.05 mg/mL[a]	IMM	10 mcg/mL[b]	Physically compatible for 4 hr at 23 °C	2000	C
Haloperidol lactate	LY	0.2 mg/mL[b]	IMM	10 mcg/mL[b]	Small particles form in 4 hr	1436	I
Heparin sodium	WY	100 units/mL[b]	IMM	10 mcg/mL[b]	Visually compatible for 4 hr at 22 °C	1436	C
	ES	100 units/mL[d]	IMM	6[b,e] and 15[b] mcg/mL	Visually compatible for 2 hr	1618	C

Y-Site Injection Compatibility (1:1 Mixture) (Cont.)

Sargramostim

Drug	Mfr	Conc	Mfr	Conc	Remarks	Ref	C/I
Hydrocortisone sodium succinate	UP	1 mg/mL[b]	IMM	10 mcg/mL[b]	Few small particles in 1 hr	1436	**I**
Hydromorphone HCl	WI	0.5 mg/mL[b]	IMM	10 mcg/mL[b]	Few small particles in 30 min	1436	**I**
Hydroxyzine HCl	ES	4 mg/mL[b]	IMM	10 mcg/mL[b]	Slight haze and particles form in 4 hr	1436	**I**
Idarubicin HCl	AD	0.5 mg/mL[b]	IMM	10 mcg/mL[b]	Physically compatible	1675	**C**
Ifosfamide	MJ	25 mg/mL[b]	IMM	10 mcg/mL[b]	Visually compatible for 4 hr at 22 °C	1436	**C**
Imipenem–cilastatin sodium	MSD	5 mg/mL[b]	IMM	10 mcg/mL[b]	Large particle and clump form in 4 hr	1436	**I**
Immune globulin intravenous	CU	50 mg/mL	IMM	6[b,e] and 15[b] mcg/mL	Visually compatible for 2 hr	1618	**C**
Lorazepam	WY	0.1 mg/mL[b]	IMM	10 mcg/mL[b]	Slightly bluish haze forms in 1 hr	1436	**I**
Magnesium sulfate	LY	100 mg/mL[b]	IMM	10 mcg/mL[b]	Visually compatible for 4 hr at 22 °C	1436	**C**
Mannitol	BA	15%	IMM	10 mcg/mL[b]	Visually compatible for 4 hr at 22 °C	1436	**C**
Mechlorethamine HCl	MSD	1 mg/mL	IMM	10 mcg/mL[b]	Visually compatible for 4 hr at 22 °C	1436	**C**
Meperidine HCl	WI	4 mg/mL[b]	IMM	10 mcg/mL[b]	Visually compatible for 4 hr at 22 °C	1436	**C**
Mesna	MJ	10 mg/mL[b]	IMM	10 mcg/mL[b]	Visually compatible for 4 hr at 22 °C	1436	**C**
Methotrexate sodium	CET	15 mg/mL[b]	IMM	10 mcg/mL[b]	Visually compatible for 4 hr at 22 °C	1436	**C**
Methylprednisolone sodium succinate	UP	5 mg/mL[b]	IMM	10 mcg/mL[b]	Small amounts of particles and filaments form in 4 hr	1436	**I**
Metoclopramide HCl	DU	5 mg/mL[b]	IMM	10 mcg/mL[b]	Visually compatible for 4 hr at 22 °C	1436	**C**
Metronidazole	MG	5 mg/mL	IMM	10 mcg/mL[b]	Visually compatible for 4 hr at 22 °C	1436	**C**
Mitomycin	BR	0.5 mg/mL	IMM	10 mcg/mL[b]	Slight haze in 30 min	1436	**I**
Mitoxantrone HCl	LE	0.5 mg/mL[b]	IMM	10 mcg/mL[b]	Visually compatible for 4 hr at 22 °C	1436	**C**
Morphine sulfate	WI	1 mg/mL[b]	IMM	10 mcg/mL[b]	Slight haze and particles in 1 hr	1436	**I**
Nalbuphine HCl	DU	10 mg/mL	IMM	10 mcg/mL[b]	Haze and filament form	1436	**I**
Ondansetron HCl	GL	0.5 mg/mL[b]	IMM	10 mcg/mL[b]	Filaments form in 30 to 60 min	1436	**I**
Pentostatin	NCI	0.4 mg/mL[b]	IMM	10 mcg/mL[b]	Visually compatible for 4 hr at 22 °C	1436	**C**
Piperacillin sodium–tazobactam sodium	LE[c]	40 + 5 mg/mL[a]	HO	10 mcg/mL[a]	Physically compatible for 4 hr at 22 °C	1688	**C**
Potassium chloride	AB	0.1 mEq/mL[b]	IMM	10 mcg/mL[b]	Visually compatible for 4 hr at 22 °C	1436	**C**
Prochlorperazine edisylate	ES	0.5 mg/mL[b]	IMM	10 mcg/mL[b]	Visually compatible for 4 hr at 22 °C	1436	**C**
Promethazine HCl	ES	2 mg/mL[b]	IMM	10 mcg/mL[b]	Visually compatible for 4 hr at 22 °C	1436	**C**
Ranitidine HCl	GL	2 mg/mL[b]	IMM	10 mcg/mL[b]	Visually compatible for 4 hr at 22 °C	1436	**C**
Sodium bicarbonate	LY	1 mEq/mL	IMM	10 mcg/mL[b]	Small amount of particles forms in 4 hr	1436	**I**
Teniposide	BR	0.1 mg/mL[b]	IMM	10 mcg/mL[b]	Visually compatible for 4 hr at 22 °C	1436	**C**
Ticarcillin disodium–clavulanate potassium	BE	31 mg/mL[b]	IMM	10 mcg/mL[b]	Visually compatible for 4 hr at 22 °C	1436	**C**
Tobramycin sulfate	LI	5 mg/mL[b]	IMM	10 mcg/mL[b]	Particles and filaments form in 4 hr	1436	**I**
TPN #133[f]			IMM	10 mcg/mL[b]	Visually compatible for 4 hr at 22 °C	1436	**C**
TPN #181[f]			IMM	6[b,e] and 15[b] mcg/mL	Visually compatible for 2 hr	1618	**C**
Trimethoprim–sulfamethoxazole	ES	0.8 + 4 mg/mL[b]	IMM	10 mcg/mL[b]	Visually compatible for 4 hr at 22 °C	1436	**C**

Y-Site Injection Compatibility (1:1 Mixture) (Cont.)

Sargramostim

Drug	Mfr	Conc	Mfr	Conc	Remarks	Ref	C/I
Vancomycin HCl	LI	10 mg/mL[b]	IMM	10 mcg/mL[b]	Visually compatible for 4 hr at 22 °C	1436	C
	LI	20 mg/mL[d]	IMM	15 mcg/mL[b]	Visually compatible for 2 hr	1618	C
	LI	20 mg/mL[d]	IMM	6 mcg/mL[b,e]	Haze forms within 15 min and increases due to vancomycin incompatibility with albumin human	1618; 1701	I
Vinblastine sulfate	LY	0.12 mg/mL[b]	IMM	10 mcg/mL[b]	Visually compatible for 4 hr at 22 °C	1436	C
Vincristine sulfate	LY	0.05 mg/mL[b]	IMM	10 mcg/mL[b]	Visually compatible for 4 hr at 22 °C	1436	C
Zidovudine	BW	4 mg/mL[b]	IMM	10 mcg/mL[b]	Visually compatible for 4 hr at 22 °C	1436	C

[a]Tested in dextrose 5%.
[b]Tested in sodium chloride 0.9%.
[c]Test performed using the formulation WITHOUT edetate disodium.
[d]Tested in both dextrose 5% and sodium chloride 0.9%.
[e]Tested with 0.1% albumin human added.
[f]Refer to Appendix I for the composition of parenteral nutrition solutions. TPN indicates a 2-in-1 admixture.

SCOPOLAMINE BUTYLBROMIDE (HYOSCINE BUTYLBROMIDE) AHFS 12:08.08

Products — Scopolamine butylbromide 20 mg/mL with sodium chloride in water for injection is available in 1-mL ampuls. (115)

Trade Name(s) — Buscopan, Scoburen.

Administration — Scopolamine butylbromide is administered by intramuscular or subcutaneous injection or slowly intravenously. Dextrose 5% and sodium chloride 0.9% are recommended for dilution if needed. (115)

Stability — Scopolamine butylbromide injection is a clear, colorless or nearly colorless solution. Intact containers should be stored below 30 °C and protected from light. (115)

Compatibility Information

Additive Compatibility

Scopolamine butylbromide

Drug	Mfr	Conc/L	Mfr	Conc/L	Test Soln	Remarks	Ref	C/I
Floxacillin sodium	BE	20 g	BI	2 g	W	Physically compatible for 24 hr at 15 and 30 °C. Precipitate forms in 48 hr at 30 °C. No change in 48 hr at 15 °C	1479	C
Furosemide	HO	1 g	BI	2 g	W	Physically compatible for 72 hr at 15 and 30 °C	1479	C
Oxycodone HCl	NAP	1 g	BI	1 g	NS, W	Visually compatible. Under 4% concentration change in 24 hr at 25 °C	2600	C
Tramadol HCl	AND	11.18 g	BI	1.68 g	NS[a]	Visually compatible for 7 days at 25 °C protected from light	2701	C
	AND	5 g	BI	5 g	NS[a]	Visually compatible for 7 days at 25 °C protected from light	2701	C

[a]Tested in elastomeric pump reservoirs (Baxter).

Drugs in Syringe Compatibility

Scopolamine butylbromide

Drug (in syringe)	Mfr	Amt	Mfr	Amt	Remarks	Ref	C/I
Diamorphine HCl	EV	50 and 150 mg/ 1 mL	BI	20 mg/ 1 mL	Physically compatible with no scopolamine loss and 4% diamorphine loss in 7 days at room temperature	1455	C
Haloperidol lactate		0.3125 mg/mL	BI	2.5, 5, 10 mg/ mL	Physically compatible. Less than 10% loss of both drugs in 15 days at 4 and 25 °C	2521	C
		0.625 mg/mL	BI	2.5, 5, 10 mg/ mL	Physically compatible. Less than 10% loss of both drugs in 7 days at 4 and 25 °C. Over 10% loss of scopolamine in 15 days at both temperatures	2521	C
		1.25 mg/ mL	BI	2.5, 5, 10 mg/ mL	Physically incompatible. Haloperidol precipitates in 15 days at 25 °C and 7 days at 4 °C	2521	I
Oxycodone HCl	NAP	200 mg/ 20 mL	BI	60 mg/ 3 mL	Visually compatible. Under 4% concentration change in 24 hr at 25 °C	2600	C
Tramadol HCl	GRU	8.33, 16.67, 33.33 mg/mL[a]	BI	3.33, 4.99, 6.67 mg/ mL[a]	Physically compatible with no loss of tramadol HCl and about 5 to 6% loss of scopolamine butylbromide in 15 days at 4 and 25 °C protected from light	2632	C

[a]Diluted with sodium chloride 0.9%.

SCOPOLAMINE HYDROBROMIDE (HYOSCINE HYDROBROMIDE)
AHFS 12:08.08

Products — Scopolamine hydrobromide is available in 1-mL multiple-dose vials containing 0.4- and 1-mg/mL concentrations. Also present in the products are methylparaben 0.18% and propylparaben 0.02%. Hydrobromic acid may have been used to adjust the pH. (1; 4)

pH — From 3.5 to 6.5. (1; 4)

Osmolality — The osmolality of scopolamine hydrobromide 0.5 mg/mL was determined to be 303 mOsm/kg. (1233)

Administration — Scopolamine hydrobromide may be administered subcutaneously, intramuscularly, or intravenously by direct intravenous injection after dilution with sterile water for injection. (1; 4)

Stability — The product should be stored at controlled room temperature and protected from light. (1) Scopolamine hydrobromide is stated to be incompatible with alkalies. (4) Scopolamine hydrobromide decomposition is primarily due to hydrolysis below pH 3 and to both hydrolysis and inversion about the chiral carbon above pH 3. The minimum rate of decomposition occurs at pH 3.5. (1072)

Compatibility Information

Additive Compatibility

Scopolamine HBr

Drug	Mfr	Conc/L	Mfr	Conc/L	Test Soln	Remarks	Ref	C/I
Meperidine HCl	WI	100 mg		0.43 mg		Physically compatible	3	C
Oxycodone HCl	NAP	1 g		30 mg	NS, W	Visually compatible. Under 4% concentration change in 24 hr at 25 °C	2600	C
Succinylcholine chloride	AB	2 g		0.43 mg		Physically compatible	3	C

Drugs in Syringe Compatibility

Scopolamine HBr

Drug (in syringe)	Mfr	Amt	Mfr	Amt	Remarks	Ref	C/I
Atropine sulfate	ST	0.4 mg/ 1 mL	ST	0.4 mg/ 1 mL	Physically compatible for at least 15 min	326	C
Buprenorphine HCl					Physically and chemically compatible	4	C
Butorphanol tartrate	BR	4 mg/ 2 mL	ST	0.4 mg/ 1 mL	Physically compatible for 30 min at room temperature	566	C
Chlorpromazine HCl	SKF	50 mg/ 2 mL		0.6 mg/ 1.5 mL	Physically compatible for at least 15 min	14	C
	PO	50 mg/ 2 mL	ST	0.4 mg/ 1 mL	Physically compatible for at least 15 min	326	C
Diamorphine HCl	MB	10, 25, 50 mg/ 1 mL	EV	60 mcg/ 1 mL[a]	Physically compatible and diamorphine stable for 24 hr at room temperature	1454	C
	EV	50 and 150 mg/ 1 mL	EV	0.4 mg/ 1 mL	Physically compatible with 7% diamorphine loss in 7 days at room temperature	1455	C
Dimenhydrinate	HR	50 mg/ 1 mL	ST	0.4 mg/ 1 mL	Physically compatible for at least 15 min	326	C
Diphenhydramine HCl	PD	50 mg/ 1 mL	ST	0.4 mg/ 1 mL	Physically compatible for at least 15 min	326	C
Droperidol	MN	2.5 mg/ 1 mL	ST	0.4 mg/ 1 mL	Physically compatible for at least 15 min	326	C
Fentanyl citrate	MN	100 mcg/ 1 mL		0.6 mg/ 1.5 mL	Physically compatible for at least 15 min	14	C
	MN	0.05 mg/ 1 mL	ST	0.4 mg/ 1 mL	Physically compatible for at least 15 min	326	C
Glycopyrrolate	RB	0.2 mg/ 1 mL	ES	0.4 mg/ 1 mL	Physically compatible. pH in glycopyrrolate stability range for 48 hr at 25 °C	331	C
	RB	0.2 mg/ 1 mL	ES	0.8 mg/ 2 mL	Physically compatible. pH in glycopyrrolate stability range for 48 hr at 25 °C	331	C
	RB	0.4 mg/ 2 mL	ES	0.4 mg/ 1 mL	Physically compatible. pH in glycopyrrolate stability range for 48 hr at 25 °C	331	C
Hydromorphone HCl	KN	4 mg/ 2 mL	BW	0.43 mg/ 0.5 mL	Physically compatible for 30 min	517	C
Hydroxyzine HCl	PF	100 mg/ 4 mL		0.6 mg/ 1.5 mL	Physically compatible for at least 15 min	14	C
	PF	50 mg/ 1 mL	ST	0.4 mg/ 1 mL	Physically compatible for at least 15 min	326	C

Drugs in Syringe Compatibility (Cont.)

Scopolamine HBr

Drug (in syringe)	Mfr	Amt	Mfr	Amt	Remarks	Ref	C/I
	PF	100 mg/ 2 mL		0.65 mg/ 1 mL	Physically compatible	771	C
	PF	50 mg/ 1 mL		0.65 mg/ 1 mL	Physically compatible	771	C
Meperidine HCl	WY	100 mg/ 1 mL		0.6 mg/ 1.5 mL	Physically compatible for at least 15 min	14	C
	WI	50 mg/ 1 mL	ST	0.4 mg/ 1 mL	Physically compatible for at least 15 min	326	C
Methohexital sodium					Haze forms in 1 hr	4	I
Metoclopramide HCl	NO	10 mg/ 2 mL	ST	0.4 mg/ 1 mL	Physically compatible for 15 min at room temperature	565	C
Midazolam HCl	RC	5 mg/ 1 mL	BW	0.43 mg/ 0.5 mL	Physically compatible for 4 hr at 25 °C	1145	C
Morphine sulfate	WY	15 mg/ 1 mL		0.6 mg/ 1.5 mL	Physically compatible for at least 15 min	14	C
	ST	15 mg/ 1 mL	ST	0.4 mg/ 1 mL	Physically compatible for at least 15 min	326	C
	BP	500 mg/ 5 mL	BP	5 mg/ 5 mL	Little scopolamine loss in 14 days at room temperature or 37 °C. Morphine not tested	1609	C
Nalbuphine HCl	EN	10 mg/ 1 mL	BW	0.86 mg/ 1 mL	Physically compatible for 36 hr at 27 °C	762	C
	EN	5 mg/ 0.5 mL	BW	0.86 mg/ 1 mL	Physically compatible for 36 hr at 27 °C	762	C
	EN	10 mg/ 1 mL	BW	0.43 mg/ 0.5 mL	Physically compatible for 36 hr at 27 °C	762	C
	DU	10 mg/ 1 mL		0.4 mg	Physically compatible for 48 hr	128	C
	DU	20 mg/ 1 mL		0.4 mg	Physically compatible for 48 hr	128	C
Oxycodone HCl	NAP	200 mg/ 20 mL		2.4 mg/ 6 mL	Visually compatible. Under 4% concentration change in 24 hr at 25 °C	2600	C
Pentazocine lactate	WI	30 mg/ 1 mL		0.6 mg/ 1.5 mL	Physically compatible for at least 15 min	14	C
	WI	30 mg/ 1 mL	ST	0.4 mg/ 1 mL	Physically compatible for at least 15 min	326	C
Pentobarbital sodium	AB	500 mg/ 10 mL		0.13 mg/ 0.26 mL	Physically compatible	55	C
	WY	100 mg/ 2 mL		0.6 mg/ 1.5 mL	Physically compatible for at least 15 min	14	C
	AB	50 mg/ 1 mL	ST	0.4 mg/ 1 mL	Physically compatible for at least 15 min	326	C
Prochlorperazine edisylate	SKF			0.6 mg/ 1.5 mL	Physically compatible for at least 15 min	14	C
	PO	5 mg/ 1 mL	ST	0.4 mg/ 1 mL	Physically compatible for at least 15 min	326	C
Promethazine HCl	WY	50 mg/ 2 mL		0.6 mg/ 1.5 mL	Physically compatible for at least 15 min	14	C
	PO	50 mg/ 2 mL	ST	0.4 mg/ 1 mL	Physically compatible for at least 15 min	326	C
Ranitidine HCl	GL	50 mg/ 2 mL	AB	0.4 mg/ 1 mL	Physically compatible for 1 hr at 25 °C	978	C

Drugs in Syringe Compatibility (Cont.)

Scopolamine HBr

Drug (in syringe)	Mfr	Amt	Mfr	Amt	Remarks	Ref	C/I
	GL	50 mg/ 5 mL		0.5 mg	Physically compatible for 4 hr at ambient temperature under fluorescent light	1151	C

[a]Diluted with sterile water for injection.

Y-Site Injection Compatibility (1:1 Mixture)

Scopolamine HBr

Drug	Mfr	Conc	Mfr	Conc	Remarks	Ref	C/I
Fentanyl citrate	JN	0.025 mg/ mL[a]	LY	0.05 mg/mL[a]	Physically compatible for 48 hr at 22 °C	1706	C
Heparin sodium	UP	1000 units/L[b]	BW	0.86 mg/mL	Physically compatible for 4 hr at room temperature	534	C
Hydrocortisone sodium succinate	UP	10 mg/L[b]	BW	0.86 mg/mL	Physically compatible for 4 hr at room temperature	534	C
Hydromorphone HCl	AST	0.5 mg/mL[a]	LY	0.05 mg/mL[a]	Physically compatible for 48 hr at 22 °C	1706	C
Methadone HCl	LI	1 mg/mL[a]	LY	0.05 mg/mL[a]	Physically compatible for 48 hr at 22 °C	1706	C
Morphine sulfate	AST	1 mg/mL[a]	LY	0.05 mg/mL[a]	Physically compatible for 48 hr at 22 °C	1706	C
Potassium chloride	AB	40 mEq/L[b]	BW	0.86 mg/mL	Physically compatible for 4 hr at room temperature	534	C
Propofol	ZEN	10 mg/mL	LY	0.4 mg/mL	Physically compatible for 1 hr at 23 °C	2066	C

[a]Tested in dextrose 5%.
[b]Tested in dextrose 5% in Ringer's injection, lactated, dextrose 5% in Ringer's injection, dextrose 5%, Ringer's injection, lactated, and sodium chloride 0.9%.

SODIUM ACETATE
AHFS 40:08

Products — Sodium acetate is available as a 16.4% solution in 20-, 50-, 100-, and 250-mL vials. Each milliliter of solution contains 2 mEq of sodium acetate in water for injection. Sodium acetate is also available as a 32.8% solution in 50- and 100-mL vials. Each milliliter of solution contains 4 mEq of sodium acetate in water for injection. The pH may have been adjusted with acetic acid. (1)

pH — From 6 to 7. (1; 17)

Osmolarity — Sodium acetate injection is very hypertonic and must be diluted for use. The 2-mEq/mL concentration has a calculated os-molarity of 4 mOsm/mL, and the 4-mEq/mL concentration has a calculated osmolarity of 8 mOsm/mL. (1)

Administration — Sodium acetate is administered by slow intravenous infusion after addition to a larger volume of fluid. It must not be given undiluted. (1)

Stability — The product should be stored at controlled room temperature and protected from freezing and excessive heat. Discarding the vials four hours after initial entry has been recommended. (1)

Compatibility Information

Y-Site Injection Compatibility (1:1 Mixture)

Sodium acetate

Drug	Mfr	Conc	Mfr	Conc	Remarks	Ref	C/I
Enalaprilat	MSD	0.05 mg/mL[b]	LY	0.4 mEq/mL[a]	Physically compatible for 24 hr at room temperature under fluorescent light	1355	**C**
Esmolol HCl	DCC	10 mg/mL[a]	LY	0.4 mEq/mL[a]	Physically compatible for 24 hr at 22 °C	1169	**C**
Labetalol HCl	SC	1 mg/mL[a]	LY	0.4 mEq/mL[a]	Physically compatible for 24 hr at 18 °C	1171	**C**
Nicardipine HCl	DCC	0.1 mg/mL[a]	LY	0.4 mEq/mL[a]	Visually compatible for 24 hr at room temperature	235	**C**
Ondansetron HCl	GL	0.1 mg/mL[a]		0.1 and 1 mEq/mL[a]	Physically compatible for 4 hr at room temperature	1661	**C**

[a]Tested in dextrose 5%.
[b]Tested in sodium chloride 0.9%.

SODIUM BICARBONATE
AHFS 40:08

Products — Sodium bicarbonate injections are available from various manufacturers in vials, ampuls, bottles, and disposable syringes as aqueous solutions in concentrations ranging from 4.2% to 8.4%. (1; 4)

Concentration	Bicarbonate (and Sodium) Concentration	Total Container Content	Osmolarity
8.4%	1 mEq/mL	10 mEq/10 mL 50 mEq/50 mL	2000 mOsm/L
7.5%	0.892 mEq/mL	44.6 mEq/50 mL	1790 mOsm/L
5.0%	0.595 mEq/mL	297.5 mEq/500 mL	1200 mOsm/L
4.2%	0.5 mEq/mL	5 mEq/10 mL	1000 mOsm/L

Sodium bicarbonate 4 and 4.2% neutralizing additive solutions are available in 5-mL vials. Each milliliter of solution provides 0.48 or 0.5 mEq of bicarbonate and sodium, respectively. (1; 4) The sodium bicarbonate-neutralizing additive solutions are used to raise the pH of acidic solutions.

Equivalency — Each 84 mg of sodium bicarbonate provides 1 mEq of sodium and bicarbonate ions. Each gram of sodium bicarbonate provides about 12 mEq of sodium and bicarbonate ions. (4)

pH — From 7 to 8.5. (17)

Administration — Sodium bicarbonate is administered intravenously, either undiluted or diluted in other fluids. It may also be given subcutaneously if diluted to isotonicity (1.5%). (4)

Stability — Sodium bicarbonate injection should be stored at controlled room temperature and protected from freezing and excessive temperatures of 40 °C or above. Do not use a solution that is unclear or that contains a precipitate. (4)

Sodium bicarbonate injection under simulated summer conditions in paramedic vehicles was exposed to temperatures ranging from 26 to 38 °C over four weeks. Analysis found no loss of the drug under these conditions. (2562)

Combining sodium bicarbonate with acids in aqueous solutions results in the liberation of carbon dioxide gas. The bubbles can be evolved in sufficient quantity to cause effervescence. (4)

The stability of sodium bicarbonate 7.5% in polypropylene syringes is inversely related to the storage temperature. (136) Estimates of room temperature stability range from one week (137) to one month. (136) Refrigeration may increase the stability to 60 (137) to 90 days. (136) Stability may also be increased by refrigerating the sodium bicarbonate injection and the syringes before preparation, rinsing the syringes twice with refrigerated sterile water for injection, minimizing the contact of the solution with the air by expelling the air from the syringes, and taping the plunger in place to minimize its movement from escaping carbon dioxide. (137)

pH Effects — Drugs such as sodium bicarbonate that may raise the pH of an admixture above 6 may cause significant decomposition of alkali-labile drugs. (59; 77; 79)

The change in pH that occurs when 5 mL of Neut is added to a liter of 10 common infusion solutions was reported:

Solution	Initial pH	pH after Neut Added	pH Increase
Dextrose 5% in Electrolyte #48	5.0	6.1	1.1
Dextrose 5% in Electrolyte #75	4.7	5.5	0.8
Dextrose 5% in Ringer's injection	4.3	7.3	3.0
Dextrose 5% in Ringer's injection, lactated	5.0	6.2	1.2
Dextrose 5%	4.4	7.5	3.1
Dextrose 10%	3.9	7.1	3.2
Ringer's injection	5.6	7.5	1.9
Ringer's injection, lactated	6.3	7.4	1.1
Sodium chloride 0.45%	5.6	7.8	2.2
Sodium chloride 0.9%	5.4	7.6	2.2

Compatibility Information

Solution Compatibility

Sodium bicarbonate

Solution	Mfr	Mfr	Conc/L	Remarks	Ref	C/I
Dextrose–Ringer's injection combinations	AB		3.75 g	Physically compatible	3	C
Dextrose–Ringer's injection, lactated, combinations	AB		3.75 g	Physically compatible	3	C
Dextrose 5% in Ringer's injection, lactated	AB	AB	80 mEq	Physically incompatible	15	I
Dextrose–saline combinations	AB		3.75 g	Physically compatible	3	C
Dextrose 5% in sodium chloride 0.9%	TR[a]	AB	4 g	Stable for 24 hr at 5 °C	282	C
Dextrose 2.5%	AB		3.75 g	Physically compatible	3	C
Dextrose 5%	AB		3.75 g	Physically compatible	3	C
	TR[a]	AB	4 g	Stable for 24 hr at 5 °C	282	C
	BRN[c]	HOS	50, 100, 150 mEq	Physically compatible. Bicarbonate and pH remained stable over 7 days at 4 and 24 °C	2817	C
Dextrose 10%	AB		3.75 g	Physically compatible	3	C
Ionosol products	AB		3.75 g	Physically compatible	3	C
Ringer's injection	AB		3.75 g	Physically compatible	3	C
Ringer's injection, lactated	AB		3.75 g	Physically compatible	3	C
	AB	AB	80 mEq	Physically incompatible	15	I
Sodium chloride 0.45%	AB		3.75 g	Physically compatible	3	C
Sodium chloride 0.9%	AB		3.75 g	Physically compatible	3	C
	TR[a]	AB	4 g	Stable for 24 hr at 5 °C	282	C
Sodium lactate ⅙ M	AB		3.75 g	Physically compatible	3	C
TNA #66 to #68[b]			100 mEq	Physically compatible with 10% or less carbon dioxide loss and unchanged pH in 7 days at 25 °C protected from light	1011	C
TPN #62 to #65[b]			50 and 150 mEq	Physically compatible with 10% or less carbon dioxide loss and unchanged pH in 7 days at 25 °C protected from light	1011	C

[a]Tested in both glass and PVC containers.
[b]Refer to Appendix I for the composition of parenteral nutrition solutions. TNA indicates a 3-in-1 admixture, and TPN indicates a 2-in-1 admixture.
[c]Tested in polyolefin containers.

Additive Compatibility

Sodium bicarbonate

Drug	Mfr	Conc/L	Mfr	Conc/L	Test Soln	Remarks	Ref	C/I
Amikacin sulfate	BR	5 g	BR	15 g	D5LR, D5R, D5S, D5W, D10W, LR, NS, R, SL	Physically compatible and both stable for 24 hr at 25 °C	294	C
Aminophylline	SE	1 g	AB	80 mEq	D5W	Physically compatible	15	C
	SE	500 mg	AB	40 mEq		Physically compatible	6	C

Additive Compatibility (Cont.)

Sodium bicarbonate

Drug	Mfr	Conc/L	Mfr	Conc/L	Test Soln	Remarks	Ref	C/I
Amoxicillin sodium		10, 20, 50 g		2.74%		9% amoxicillin loss in 6 and 4 hr at 10 and 20 g/L, respectively, and 15% loss in 4 hr at 50 g/L at 25 °C	1469	I
		10, 20, 50 g		8.4%		10 and 13% amoxicillin loss in 4 hr at 10 and 20 g/L, respectively, and 17% loss in 3 hr at 50 g/L at 25 °C	1469	I
Amphotericin B	SQ	50 mg	AB	2.4 mEq[a]	D5W	Physically compatible for 24 hr	772	C
Ampicillin sodium	AY	2 and 4 g		1.4%		10% ampicillin loss in 6 hr at room temperature	99	I
	BAY	15 g		1.4%		10% ampicillin loss in 10 hr at 25 °C	604	I
	BAY	2 g		1.4%		10% ampicillin loss in 17 hr at 25 °C	604	I
	BAY	5 g		1.4%		10% ampicillin loss in 14 hr at 25 °C	604	I
Amsacrine	NCI			2 mEq	D5W	Amsacrine chemically stable for 96 hr at room temperature	234	C
Ascorbic acid	UP	500 mg	AB	80 mEq	D5W	Physically incompatible	15	I
Atropine sulfate		0.4 mg	AB	2.4 mEq[a]	D5W	Physically compatible for 24 hr	772	C
Calcium chloride	UP		AB		D5W	Conditionally compatible depending on concentrations	15	?
		1 g	AB	2.4 mEq[a]	D5W	Physically compatible for 24 hr	772	C
Calcium gluconate	UP		AB		D5W	Conditionally compatible depending on concentrations	15	?
Carboplatin		1 g		200 mmol		13% carboplatin loss in 24 hr at 27 °C	1379	I
Carmustine	BR	100 mg	AB	100 mEq	D5W, NS	10% carmustine loss in 15 min and 27% in 90 min	523	I
Cefoxitin sodium	MSD	1 g	AB	200 mg	W	5 to 6% cefoxitin loss in 24 hr and 11 to 12% in 48 hr at 25 °C. 2 to 3% loss in 7 days at 5 °C	308	C
Ceftazidime	GL	20 g		4.2%		11% ceftazidime loss in 24 hr at 25 °C. 3% loss in 48 hr at 4 °C	1136	C
Ceftriaxone sodium	RC	10 to 40 g		5%		Less than 10% loss in 24 hr at 25 °C	1	C
Chloramphenicol sodium succinate	PD	10 g	AB	80 mEq	D5W	Physically compatible	15	C
	PD	1 g	AB	80 mEq		Physically compatible	6	C
Ciprofloxacin	MI	2 g		[i]	D5W	Physically incompatible	888	I
	BAY	2 g	AST	4 g	D5W	Precipitates immediately	2413	I
Cisplatin		50 and 500 mg		5%		Bright gold precipitate forms in 8 to 24 hr at 25 °C	635	I
Clindamycin phosphate	UP	1.2 g		44 mEq	D5S, D5W	Clindamycin stable for 24 hr	101	C
Cytarabine	UP	200 mg and 1 g	AB	50 mEq	D5W[b]	Physically compatible with no cytarabine loss in 7 days at 8 and 22 °C	748	C
	UP	200 mg	AB	50 mEq	D5¼S[b,c]	Physically compatible with no cytarabine loss in 7 days at 8 and 22 °C	748	C
Dobutamine HCl	LI	1 g	MG	5%		Cloudy brown with precipitate in 3 hr at 25 °C. 18% dobutamine loss in 24 hr	789	I
	LI	1 g	IX	500 mEq	D5W, NS	White precipitate in 6 hr at 21 °C	812	I
Dopamine HCl	AS	800 mg	MG	5%		Color change 5 min after mixing	79	I

Additive Compatibility (Cont.)

Sodium bicarbonate

Drug	Mfr	Conc/L	Mfr	Conc/L	Test Soln	Remarks	Ref	C/I
Epinephrine HCl		4 mg	AB	2.4 mEq[a]	D5W	Epinephrine inactivated	772	I
		4 mg		5%		Epinephrine rapidly decomposes. 58% loss immediately after mixing	48	I
Ertapenem sodium	ME	10 and 20 g	AB	5%		Visually compatible. 11% loss in 3 hr at 25 °C. 16 to 19% loss in 1 day at 4 °C	2487	I
Erythromycin lactobionate	AB	1 g	AB	3.75 g		Physically compatible. Erythromycin stable for 24 hr at 25 °C	20	C
	AB	1 g	AB	2.4 mEq[a]	D5W	Physically compatible for 24 hr	772	C
Esmolol HCl	ACC	10 g	MG[c]	5%		Visually compatible. 5 and 8% esmolol losses in 7 days at 4 and 27 °C, respectively	1831	C
Fat emulsion, intravenous	VT	10%	BR	7.5 g		Physically compatible for 48 hr at 4 °C and room temperature	32	C
	VT	10%		3.4 g		Lipid coalescence in 24 hr at 8 and 25 °C	825	I
Furosemide	HO	1 g	IMS	8.4%		Physically compatible for 72 hr at 15 and 30 °C	1479	C
Heparin sodium	AB	20,000 units	AB	2.4 mEq[a]	D5W	Physically compatible for 24 hr	772	C
Hyaluronidase	WY	150 units	AB	2.4 mEq[a]	D5W	Physically compatible for 24 hr	772	C
Imipenem–cilastatin sodium	MSD	2.5 g	AB	5%		43% imipenem loss in 3 hr at 25 °C and 52% in 24 hr at 4 °C	1141	I
	MSD	5 g	AB	5%		45% imipenem loss in 3 hr at 25 °C and 50% in 24 hr at 4 °C	1141	I
Isoproterenol HCl	WI	5 mg		5%		Isoproterenol decomposition	48	I
	BN	1 mg	AB	2.4 mEq[a]	D5W	Isoproterenol decomposition	772	I
Labetalol HCl	SC	1.25, 2.5, 3.75 g	TR	5%		White precipitate forms within 6 hr after mixing at 4 and 25 °C	757	I
Levofloxacin	OMJ	0.5 g	BA	5%[b]		Physically compatible. No loss in 3 days at 25 °C, 14 days at 5 °C, in dark	1986	C
	OMJ	0.5 g	BA	5%[b]		Precipitate forms within 13 weeks at −20 °C	1986	I
	OMJ	5 g	BA	5%[b]		Physically compatible. No loss in 3 days at 25 °C, 14 days at 5 °C, 26 weeks at −20 °C, in dark	1986	C
Lidocaine HCl	AST	2 g	AB	40 mEq		Physically compatible	24	C
		1 g	AB	2.4 mEq[a]	D5W	Physically compatible for 24 hr	772	C
Magnesium sulfate	LI	16 mEq	AB	80 mEq	D5W	Physically incompatible	15	I
	HOS	1.5 and 15 mEq	BA	50 mEq	[h]	Physically compatible. No loss of ions for 48 hr at 23 °C	2814	C
Mannitol	AMR	25 g	AB	44.6 mEq	D5LR, D5¼S, D5½S, D5S, D5W, D10W, NS, ½S[d]	Visually compatible for 24 hr at 24 °C	1853; 1973	C

Additive Compatibility (Cont.)

Sodium bicarbonate

Drug	Mfr	Conc/L	Mfr	Conc/L	Test Soln	Remarks	Ref	C/I
Meperidine HCl	WI	100 mg	AB	2.4 mEq[a]	D5W	Physically compatible for 24 hr	772	C
Meropenem	ZEN	1 g	BA	5%		10% meropenem loss in 4 hr at 24 °C and 18 hr at 4 °C	2089	I[g]
	ZEN	20 g	BA	5%		9 to 10% meropenem loss in 3 hr at 24 °C and 18 hr at 4 °C	2089	I[g]
Methotrexate sodium		2 g		50 mEq		No photodegradation products in 12 hr in room light	433	C
	LE	750 mg		50 mEq	D5W	6% methotrexate loss in 1 week at 5 °C in dark. At 23 °C in light, 6% loss in 72 hr and 15% in 1 week	465	C
Methyldopate HCl	MSD	1 g		50 mEq	D, D–S, S	Physically compatible	23	C
	MSD	1 g	AB	5%		Stable for 24 hr	23	C
Midazolam HCl	RC	100 mg	c	5%		Transient precipitation upon mixing	355	?
	RC	500 mg	c	5%		Precipitation upon mixing	355	I
Multivitamins	USV	10 mL	AB	4.8 mEq[e]	D5W	Physically compatible for 24 hr	772	C
Nafcillin sodium	WY	500 mg	AB	40 mEq		Physically compatible	27	C
Nicardipine HCl	DME	50 and 500 mg	TR[c]	5%		Precipitate forms immediately	1380	I
Norepinephrine bitartrate	WI	2 mg	AB	80 mEq	D5W	Physically incompatible	15	I
	BN	8 mg	AB	2.4 mEq[a]	D5W	Norepinephrine decomposition	772	I
Oxytocin	PD	5 units	AB	2.4 mEq[a]	D5W	Physically compatible for 24 hr	772	C
Penicillin G potassium		100 million units	AB	2.4 mEq[a]	D5W	Physically compatible for 24 hr	772	C
	SQ	1 million units	AB	3.75 g	D5W	26% penicillin loss in 24 hr at 25 °C	47	I
	SQ	1 million units		0.5 and 0.75 g	D5W	Penicillin loss at 20 °C due to pH	135	I
	f	900,000 units		3.75 g	D5W	26% penicillin loss in 24 hr at 25 °C	48	I
Pentazocine lactate	WI	300 mg	AB	80 mEq	D5W	Physically incompatible	15	I
Pentobarbital sodium	AB	1 g	AB	80 mEq	D5W	Physically incompatible	15	I
Phenylephrine HCl	WI	10 mg	AB	2.4 mEq[a]	D5W	Physically compatible for 24 hr	772	C
	WI	20 mg		5%		Stable for 24 hr at 25 °C	48	C
Phytonadione	MSD	10 mg	AB	2.4 mEq[a]	D5W	Physically compatible for 24 hr	772	C
Potassium chloride		120 mEq	AB	2.4 mEq[a]	D5W	Physically compatible for 24 hr	772	C
Prochlorperazine edisylate	SKF	10 mg	AB	2.4 mEq[a]	D5W	Physically compatible for 24 hr	772	C
Succinylcholine chloride	AB	1 g	AB	2.4 mEq[a]	D5W	Succinylcholine decomposition	772	I
Verapamil HCl	KN	80 mg	BR	89.2 mEq	D5W, NS	Physically compatible for 24 hr	764	C

Additive Compatibility (Cont.)

Sodium bicarbonate

Drug	Mfr	Conc/L	Mfr	Conc/L	Test Soln	Remarks	Ref	C/I
Voriconazole	PF			4.2%		Voriconazole slightly decomposes at room temperature	1	**I**

[a] One vial of Neut added to a liter of admixture.
[b] Tested in PVC containers.
[c] Tested in glass containers.
[d] Tested in polyolefin containers.
[e] Two vials of Neut added to a liter of admixture.
[f] A buffered preparation was specified.
[g] Incompatible by conventional standards but may be used in shorter periods of time.
[h] Tested in an extemporaneously-compounded hemofiltration solution.
[i] Final sodium bicarbonate concentration not specified.

Drugs in Syringe Compatibility

Sodium bicarbonate

Drug (in syringe)	Mfr	Amt	Mfr	Amt	Remarks	Ref	C/I
Bupivacaine HCl	AST, WI	0.25, 0.5[a], 0.75%[a], 20 mL	AB	4%, 0.05 to 0.6 mL	Precipitate forms in 1 to 2 min up to 2 hr at lowest amount of bicarbonate	1724	**I**
	BEL	0.5%[b], 20 mL		1.4%, 1.5 mL	No epinephrine loss in 7 days at room temperature. Bupivacaine not tested	1743	**C**
	BEL	0.5%[b], 20 mL		4.2 and 8.4%, 1.5 mL	5 to 7% epinephrine loss in 7 days at room temperature. Bupivacaine not tested	1743	**C**
Caffeine citrate		20 mg/ 1 mL	AST	4.2%, 1 mL	Visually compatible for 4 hr at 25 °C	2440	**C**
Dimenhydrinate		10 mg/ 1 mL		1 mEq/ 1 mL	Precipitates immediately	2569	**I**
Glycopyrrolate	RB	0.2 mg/ 1 mL	AB	75 mg/ 1 mL	Gas evolves	331	**I**
	RB	0.2 mg/ 1 mL	AB	150 mg/ 2 mL	Gas evolves	331	**I**
	RB	0.4 mg/ 2 mL	AB	75 mg/ 1 mL	Gas evolves	331	**I**
Lidocaine HCl	ES	2%[c], 30 mL	AB	3 mEq/ 3 mL	11% lidocaine and 28% epinephrine loss in 1 week at 25 °C	1712	**I**
	ES	2%[c], 30 mL	AB	3 mEq/ 3 mL	6% lidocaine loss in 4 weeks at 4 °C. 12% epinephrine loss in 3 weeks at 4 °C	1712	**C**
	AST	1%[c]	LY	0.1 mEq/ mL	25% epinephrine loss in 1 week at room temperature. Lidocaine not tested	1713	**I**
		0.9%		0.088 mEq/mL	11% lidocaine loss in 7 days at room temperature	1723	**C**
	AST	1 and 1.5%[a], 20 mL	AST	8.4%/ 2 mL	Visually compatible for up to 5 hr at room temperature	1724	**C**
	AST	2%[a], 20 mL	AST	8.4%/ 2 mL	Haze forms but dissipates with gentle agitation	1724	**?**

Drugs in Syringe Compatibility (Cont.)

Sodium bicarbonate

Drug (in syringe)	Mfr	Amt	Mfr	Amt	Remarks	Ref	C/I
	AST	1 and 1.5%[a], 20 mL	AB	4%/4 mL	Visually compatible for up to 5 hr at room temperature	1724	C
	AST	2%[a], 20 mL	AB	4%/4 mL	Haze forms but dissipates with gentle agitation	1724	?
	BEL	2%[d], 20 mL		1.4 and 8.4%/ 1.5 mL	8% epinephrine loss in 7 days at room temperature. Lidocaine not tested	1743	C
		2%/ 10 mL		8.4%/ 1 mL	Physically compatible. No loss of lidocaine in 6 hr	1401	C
		2%[c], 10 mL		8.4%/ 1.5 mL	Physically compatible. No loss of lidocaine or epinephrine in 6 hr	1401	C
		2%[c], 10 mL		1.4%/ 1.5 mL	Physically compatible. No loss of lidocaine or epinephrine in 6 hr	1401	C
		1%[c], 10 mL		8.4%/ 1 mL	Cloudiness in some samples with no epinephrine loss for 72 hr in the dark. Exposed to light and air, precipitation and 20% epinephrine loss in 24 hr. Lidocaine not tested	2408	?
	ASZ	1 and 2%[c], 2.7 mL	HOS	8.4%/ 0.3 mL	Physically compatible. 10% epinephrine loss in 7 days and 5% lidocaine loss in 28 days at 5 °C in dark	2815	C
Mepivacaine HCl	AST, WI	1 and 1.5%/ 20 mL	AST	8.4%; 0.5, 1, 2 mL	Precipitate forms within approximately 1 hr	1724	I
	AST, WI	1 and 1.5%/ 20 mL	AB	4%; 1, 2, 4 mL	Precipitate forms within approximately 1 hr	1724	I
Metoclopramide HCl	RB	10 mg/ 2 mL	AB	100 mEq/ 100 mL	Gas evolves	1167	I
	RB	160 mg/ 32 mL	AB	100 mEq/ 100 mL	Gas evolves	1167	I
Milrinone lactate	STR	5.25 mg/ 5.25 mL	AB	3.75 g/ 50 mL	Physically compatible. No milrinone loss in 20 min at 23 °C	1410	C
Pantoprazole sodium	[e]	4 mg/ 1 mL		1 mEq/ 1 mL	Precipitates after 1 hr	2574	I
Pentobarbital sodium	AB	500 mg/ 10 mL		3.75 g/ 50 mL	Physically compatible	55	C

[a]Tested with and without epinephrine hydrochloride 1:200,000 added.
[b]Tested with epinephrine hydrochloride 1:200,000 added.
[c]Tested with epinephrine hydrochloride 1:100,000 added.
[d]Tested with epinephrine hydrochloride 1:80,000 added.
[e]Test performed using the formulation WITHOUT edetate disodium.

Y-Site Injection Compatibility (1:1 Mixture)

Sodium bicarbonate

Drug	Mfr	Conc	Mfr	Conc	Remarks	Ref	C/I
Acyclovir sodium	BW	5 mg/mL[a]	IX	0.5 mEq/mL[a]	Physically compatible for 4 hr at 25 °C	1157	C
Allopurinol sodium	BW	3 mg/mL[b]	AB	1 mEq/mL	Small and large crystals form in 1 hr	1686	I
Amifostine	USB	10 mg/mL[a]	AST	1 mEq/mL	Physically compatible for 4 hr at 23 °C	1845	C

Y-Site Injection Compatibility (1:1 Mixture) (Cont.)

Sodium bicarbonate

Drug	Mfr	Conc	Mfr	Conc	Remarks	Ref	C/I
Amiodarone HCl	WY	3 mg/mL[a]	AB	1 mEq/mL	Precipitate forms immediately	1851	**I**
	WY	6 mg/mL[a]	AB	1 mEq/mL	Translucent haze in 1 hr	2352	**I**
Amphotericin B cholesteryl sulfate complex	SEQ	0.83 mg/mL[a]	AB	1 mEq/mL	Gross precipitate forms	2117	**I**
Anidulafungin	VIC	0.5 mg/mL[a]	APP	1 mEq/mL	Haze increases immediately and microparticulates occur in 4 hr	2617	**I**
Asparaginase	BEL	120 I.U./mL[a]		1.4%	Visually compatible for 4 hr at room temperature	1788	**C**
Aztreonam	SQ	40 mg/mL[a]	AB	1 mEq/mL	Physically compatible for 4 hr at 23 °C	1758	**C**
Bivalirudin	TMC	5 mg/mL[a]	AMR	1 mEq/mL	Physically compatible for 4 hr at 23 °C	2373	**C**
Calcium chloride	AB	4 mg/mL[d]	AB	1 mEq/mL	Slight haze or precipitate in 1 hr	1316	**I**
Ceftaroline fosamil	FOR	2.22 mg/mL[h]	HOS	1 mEq/mL	Physically compatible for 4 hr at 23 °C	2826	**C**
Ceftriaxone sodium	RC	100 mg/mL		1.4%	Visually compatible for 4 hr at room temperature	1788	**C**
Ciprofloxacin	MI	2 mg/mL[a]	AB	1 mEq/mL	Visually compatible for 24 hr at 24 °C	1655	**C**
	MI	2 mg/mL[b]	AB	1 mEq/mL	Very fine crystals form in 20 min in NS	1655	**I**
	MI	2 mg/mL[a]	AB	1 mEq/mL	Physically compatible for 4 hr at 23 °C	1869	**C**
	MI	2 mg/mL[a]	AB	0.1 mEq/mL[a]	Subvisible haze forms immediately. Crystalline precipitate in 4 hr at 23 °C	1869	**I**
	BAY	1 and 2 mg/mL[a]	AB	1 and 0.75[a] mEq/mL	Physically compatible for 4 hr at 23 °C	2065	**C**
	BAY	1 mg/mL[b]	AB	1 and 0.75[b] mEq/mL	Physically compatible for 4 hr at 23 °C	2065	**C**
	BAY	2 mg/mL[b]	AB	1 and 0.75[b] mEq/mL	Particles form immediately, becoming more numerous over 4 hr at 23 °C	2065	**I**
	BAY	1 and 2 mg/mL[a]	AB	0.5, 0.25, 0.1 mEq/mL[a]	Particles form immediately, becoming more numerous over 4 hr at 23 °C	2065	**I**
	BAY	1 mg/mL[b]	AB	0.5, 0.25, 0.1 mEq/mL[b]	Particles form immediately, becoming more numerous over 4 hr at 23 °C	2065	**I**
	BAY	2 mg/mL[b]	AB	0.5, 0.25, 0.1 mEq/mL[b]	Precipitate forms immediately	2065	**I**
Cisatracurium besylate	GW	0.1 mg/mL[a]	AB	1 mEq/mL	Physically compatible for 4 hr at 23 °C	2074	**C**
	GW	2 mg/mL[a]	AB	1 mEq/mL	Subvisible brown color and haze in 1 hr	2074	**I**
	GW	5 mg/mL[a]	AB	1 mEq/mL	Subvisible haze forms immediately with brown color and turbidity in 4 hr	2074	**I**
Cladribine	ORT	0.015[b] and 0.5[f] mg/mL	AB	1 mEq/mL	Physically compatible for 4 hr at 23 °C	1969	**C**
Cyclophosphamide		20 mg/mL[a]		1.4%	Visually compatible for 4 hr at room temperature	1788	**C**
Cytarabine	UP	0.6 mg/mL[a]		1.4%	Visually compatible for 4 hr at room temperature	1788	**C**
Daunorubicin HCl	BEL	0.52 mg/mL[a]		1.4%	Visually compatible for 4 hr at room temperature	1788	**C**
Dexamethasone sodium phosphate	MSD	4 mg/mL		1.4%	Visually compatible for 4 hr at room temperature	1788	**C**
Dexmedetomidine HCl	AB	4 mcg/mL[b]	AMR	1 mEq/mL	Physically compatible for 4 hr at 23 °C	2383	**C**
Diltiazem HCl	MMD	5 mg/mL	LY	1 mEq/mL	Precipitate forms	1807	**I**
	MMD	1 mg/mL[b]	LY	1 mEq/mL	Visually compatible	1807	**C**

Y-Site Injection Compatibility (1:1 Mixture) (Cont.)

Sodium bicarbonate

Drug	Mfr	Conc	Mfr	Conc	Remarks	Ref	C/I
	MMD	5 mg/mL	AMR	0.05 mEq/mL[a]	Visually compatible	1807	**C**
Docetaxel	RPR	0.9 mg/mL[a]	AB	1 mEq/mL	Physically compatible for 4 hr at 23 °C	2224	**C**
Doripenem	JJ	5 mg/mL[a,b]	HOS	1 mEq/mL	Physically compatible for 4 hr at 23 °C	2743	**C**
Doxorubicin HCl	FA	0.4 mg/mL[a]		1.4%	Visually compatible for 2 hr at room temperature	1788	**C**
Doxorubicin HCl liposomal	SEQ	0.4 mg/mL[a]	AB	1 mEq/mL	Partial loss of measured natural turbidity	2087	**I**
Etoposide	BR	0.6 mg/mL[b]		1.4%	Visually compatible for 4 hr at room temperature	1788	**C**
Etoposide phosphate	BR	5 mg/mL[a]	AB	1 mEq/mL	Physically compatible for 4 hr at 23 °C	2218	**C**
Famotidine	MSD	0.2 mg/mL[a]	AB	1 mEq/mL	Physically compatible for 4 hr at 25 °C	1188	**C**
Fenoldopam mesylate	AB	80 mcg/mL[b]	APP	1 mEq/mL	Trace haze and microparticulates form immediately with turbidity in 4 hr	2467	**I**
Filgrastim	AMG	30 mcg/mL[a]	AB	1 mEq/mL	Physically compatible for 4 hr at 22 °C	1687	**C**
Fludarabine phosphate	BX	1 mg/mL[a]	AB	1 mEq/mL	Visually compatible for 4 hr at 22 °C	1439	**C**
Gallium nitrate	FUJ	1 mg/mL[b]	AB	1 mEq/mL	Visually compatible for 24 hr at 25 °C	1673	**C**
Gemcitabine HCl	LI	10 mg/mL[b]	AB	1 mEq/mL	Physically compatible for 4 hr at 23 °C	2226	**C**
Granisetron HCl	SKB	0.05 mg/mL[a]	AB	1 mEq/mL	Physically compatible for 4 hr at 23 °C	1804	**C**
	SKB	1 mg/mL	AB	0.33 mEq/mL[b]	Physically compatible with 8% loss of granisetron in 4 hr at 22 °C	1883	**C**
	SKB	0.05 mg/mL[a]	AB	1 mEq/mL	Physically compatible for 4 hr at 23 °C	2000	**C**
Heparin sodium	CH	500 units/mL[b]		1.4%	Visually compatible for 4 hr at room temperature	1788	**C**
Heparin sodium[g]	RI	1000 units/L[h]	BR	75 mg/mL	Physically compatible for 4 hr at room temperature	322	**C**
Hetastarch in lactated electrolyte	AB	6%	AB	1 mEq/mL	Microprecipitate develops rapidly	2339	**I**
Hydrocortisone sodium succinate[e]	UP	100 mg/L[h]	BR	75 mg/mL	Physically compatible for 4 hr at room temperature	322	**C**
Hydroxyethyl starch 130/0.4 in sodium chloride 0.9%	FRK	6%	HOS	0.25[a], 0.5[a], 1 mmol/mL	Visually compatible for 24 hr at room temperature	2770	**C**
Idarubicin HCl	AD	1 mg/mL[b]	AB	0.09 mEq/mL[a]	Haze forms and color changes immediately. Precipitate forms in 20 min	1525	**I**
Ifosfamide		36 mg/mL[a]		1.4%	Visually compatible for 4 hr at room temperature	1788	**C**
Imipenem–cilastatin sodium	MSD	5 mg/mL[a]		1.4%	Pale yellow precipitate forms in 1 hr at room temperature	1788	**I**
Indomethacin sodium trihydrate	MSD	1 mg/mL[b]	AB	0.5 mEq/mL[a]	Visually compatible for 24 hr at 28 °C	1527	**C**
Insulin, regular	LI	1 unit/mL[d]	AB	1 mEq/mL	Physically compatible for 3 hr	1316	**C**
Leucovorin calcium	LE	10 mg/mL		1.4%	Yellow precipitate forms in 0.5 hr at room temperature	1788	**I**
Levofloxacin	OMN	5 mg/mL[a]	AB	0.5 mEq/mL	Visually compatible for 4 hr at 24 °C	2233	**C**
Linezolid	PHU	2 mg/mL	AB	1 mEq/mL	Physically compatible for 4 hr at 23 °C	2264	**C**
Melphalan HCl	BW	0.1 mg/mL[b]	AB	1 mEq/mL	Physically compatible for 3 hr at 22 °C	1557	**C**

Y-Site Injection Compatibility (1:1 Mixture) (Cont.)

Sodium bicarbonate

Drug	Mfr	Conc	Mfr	Conc	Remarks	Ref	C/I
Mesna		1.8 mg/mL[a]		1.4%	Visually compatible for 4 hr at room temperature	1788	C
Methylprednisolone sodium succinate	UP	20 mg/mL		1.4%	Visually compatible for 4 hr at room temperature	1788	C
Midazolam HCl	RC	5 mg/mL		1.4%	White precipitate forms immediately	1788	I
	RC	1 mg/mL[a]	IMS	1 mEq/mL	Immediate haze. Precipitate in 2 hr	1847	I
Milrinone lactate	SW	0.4 mg/mL[a]	AB	1 mEq/mL	Visually compatible with 4% loss of milrinone in 4 hr at 23 °C	2214	C
Morphine sulfate	WY	0.2 mg/mL[d]	AB	1 mEq/mL	Physically compatible for 3 hr	1316	C
Nalbuphine HCl	DU	10 mg/mL		1.4%	Gas evolves	1788	I
Ondansetron HCl	GL	0.32 mg/mL[a]		0.05 mmol/mL[i]	White precipitate forms immediately	1513	I
	GL	0.1 mg/mL[a]		0.1 mEq/mL[a]	Visible particles in 30 to 60 min at room temperature	1661	I
	GL	2 mg/mL		1.4%	Heavy white precipitate forms immediately	1788	I
Oxacillin sodium	BR	250 mg/mL		1.4%	Gas evolves	1788	I
Paclitaxel	NCI	1.2 mg/mL[a]	LY	1 mEq/mL	Physically compatible for 4 hr at 22 °C	1556	C
Pemetrexed disodium	LI	20 mg/mL[b]	AB	1 mEq/mL	Physically compatible for 4 hr at 23 °C	2564	C
Piperacillin sodium–tazobactam sodium	LE[l]	40 + 5 mg/mL[a]	AB	1 mEq/mL	Physically compatible for 4 hr at 22 °C	1688	C
Potassium chloride		40 mEq/L[h]	BR	75 mg/mL	Physically compatible for 4 hr at room temperature	322	C
Propofol	ZEN	10 mg/mL	AB	1 mEq/mL	Physically compatible for 1 hr at 23 °C	2066	C
Remifentanil HCl	GW	0.025 and 0.25 mg/mL[b]	AB	1 mEq/mL	Physically compatible for 4 hr at 23 °C	2075	C
Sargramostim	IMM	10 mcg/mL[b]	LY	1 mEq/mL	Small amount of particles forms in 4 hr	1436	I
Tacrolimus	FUJ	1 mg/mL[b]	AB	1 mEq/mL	Visually compatible for 24 hr at 25 °C	1630	C
Telavancin HCl	ASP	7.5 mg/mL[h]	HOS	1 mEq/mL	Physically compatible for 2 hr	2830	C
Teniposide	BR	0.1 mg/mL[a]	AB	1 mEq/mL	Physically compatible for 4 hr at 23 °C	1725	C
Thiotepa	IMM[j]	1 mg/mL[a]	AB	1 mEq/mL	Physically compatible for 4 hr at 23 °C	1861	C
TNA #218 to #226[k]			AB	1 mEq/mL	Visually compatible for 4 hr at 23 °C	2215	C
TPN #212, #214[k]			AB	1 mEq/mL	Microprecipitate in 1 hr	2109	I
TPN #213, #215[k]			AB	1 mEq/mL	Physically compatible for 4 hr at 23 °C	2109	C
Vancomycin HCl		5 mg/mL[a]		1.4%	Visually compatible for 4 hr at room temperature	1788	C
Vasopressin	APP	0.2 unit/mL[b]	AB	0.15 mEq/mL[b]	Physically compatible	2641	C
Verapamil HCl	SE	5 mg/2 mL		88 mEq/L[c]	Crystalline precipitate forms when verapamil injected into infusion line	839	I
Vincristine sulfate	LI	0.1 mg/mL		1.4%	White precipitate forms in 30 min at room temperature	1788	I

Y-Site Injection Compatibility (1:1 Mixture) (Cont.)

Sodium bicarbonate

Drug	Mfr	Conc	Mfr	Conc	Remarks	Ref	C/I
Vinorelbine tartrate	BW	1 mg/mL[b]	AB	1 mEq/mL	Tiny particles and haze form immediately. Large particles in 4 hr at 22 °C	1558	I

[a]*Tested in dextrose 5%.*
[b]*Tested in sodium chloride 0.9%.*
[c]*Tested in sodium chloride 0.45%.*
[d]*Tested in both dextrose 5% and sodium chloride 0.9%.*
[e]*Tested in combination with heparin sodium (Riker) 1000 units/L.*
[f]*Tested in bacteriostatic sodium chloride 0.9% preserved with benzyl alcohol 0.9%.*
[g]*Tested in combination with hydrocortisone sodium succinate (Upjohn) 100 mg/L.*
[h]*Tested in dextrose 5%, sodium chloride 0.9%, and Ringer's injection, lactated.*
[i]*Tested in dextrose 5% with potassium chloride 0.02 mM/mL.*
[j]*Lyophilized formulation tested.*
[k]*Refer to Appendix I for the composition of parenteral nutrition solutions. TNA indicates a 3-in-1 admixture, and TPN indicates a 2-in-1 admixture.*
[l]*Test performed using the formulation WITHOUT edetate disodium.*

Additional Compatibility Information

Methylprednisolone — The compatibility of methylprednisolone sodium succinate (Upjohn) with sodium bicarbonate added to an auxiliary medication infusion unit has been studied. Primary admixtures were prepared by adding sodium bicarbonate 44.6 mEq/L to dextrose 5%, dextrose 5% in sodium chloride 0.9%, and Ringer's injection, lactated. Up to 100 mL of the primary admixture was added along with methylprednisolone sodium succinate (Upjohn) to the auxiliary medication infusion unit with the following results (329):

Methylprednisolone Sodium Succinate	Sodium Bicarbonate 44.6 mEq/L Primary Solution	Results
500 mg	D5S, D5W qs 100 mL	Clear solution for 24 hr
500 mg	LR qs 100 mL or added to 100 mL LR	Clear solution for 1 hr
1000 mg	D5W qs 100 mL	Clear solution for 24 hr
1000 mg	D5S qs 100 mL or added to 100 mL D5S	Clear solution for 24 hr
1000 mg	LR qs 100 mL	Clear solution for 1 hr
1000 mg	Added to 100 mL LR	Clear solution for 4 hr
2000 mg	D5S, D5W qs 100 mL	Clear solution for 24 hr
2000 mg	LR qs 100 mL	Clear solution for 30 min
2000 mg	Added to 100 mL LR	Clear solution for 4 hr

SODIUM CHLORIDE
AHFS 40:12

Products — Sodium chloride additive solution is available in various size containers in concentrations of 14.6 and 23.4%. The 14.6% concentration contains sodium chloride 146 mg/mL and provides 2.5 mEq/mL of sodium and chloride ions. The 23.4% concentration contains sodium chloride 234 mg/mL and provides 4 mEq/mL of sodium and chloride ions. (1)

NOTE: Do not confuse these high concentration additive solutions with other sodium chloride products with lower concentrations.

Sodium chloride 0.45 and 0.9% infusion solutions are available in a variety of sizes from 25 to 1000 mL. The 0.45 and 0.9% concentrations provide 77 and 154 mEq of sodium and chloride per liter, respectively. (1; 4)

pH — From 4.5 to 7. (17)

Osmolarity — Sodium chloride additive solutions are very hypertonic and must be diluted for use. The osmolarities of the 14.6 and 23.4% concentrations have been calculated to be about 5000 and 8000 mOsm/L, respectively. (4) The osmolality of the 14.6% concentration was determined to be 5370 mOsm/kg by freezing-point depression and 4783 mOsm/kg by vapor pressure. (1071) A 0.9% sodium chloride solution is isotonic, having an osmolarity of 308 mOsm/L. A 0.45% sodium chloride solution is hypotonic, having a calculated osmolarity of 154 mOsm/L. (4)

Administration — Sodium chloride additive solutions of 14.6 and 23.4% are administered by intravenous infusion only after dilution in a larger volume of fluid. (4) Dextrose 5% has been recommended for this dilution. (1) When concentrations of 3 or 5% are indicated, these hypertonic solutions should be administered into a large vein, at a rate not exceeding 100 mL/hr. Infiltration should be avoided. (4)

Stability — Sodium chloride additive solution should be stored at controlled room temperature and protected from excessive heat and freezing. (1)

Elastomeric Reservoir Pumps — Sodium chloride 0.9% (Baxter) 250 mL was filled into Intermate LV 250 (Baxter) elastomeric infusion devices and stored at 5 and 23 °C for 90 days. The solution remained visually compatible with no change in pH and sodium or chloride concentration and less than 0.1% water loss. (1993)

Compatibility Information

Solution Compatibility

Sodium chloride

Solution	Mfr	Mfr	Conc/L	Remarks	Ref	C/I
Dextrose–Ringer's injection combinations	AB	AB	200 mEq	Physically compatible	3	C
Dextrose–Ringer's injection, lactated, combinations	AB	AB	200 mEq	Physically compatible	3	C
Dextrose–saline combinations	AB	AB	200 mEq	Physically compatible	3	C
Dextrose 2.5%	AB	AB	200 mEq	Physically compatible	3	C
Dextrose 5%	AB	AB	200 mEq	Physically compatible	3	C
Dextrose 10%	AB	AB	200 mEq	Physically compatible	3	C
Ionosol products	AB	AB	200 mEq	Physically compatible	3	C
Ringer's injection	AB	AB	200 mEq	Physically compatible	3	C
Ringer's injection, lactated	AB	AB	200 mEq	Physically compatible	3	C
Sodium chloride 0.45%	AB	AB	200 mEq	Physically compatible	3	C
Sodium chloride 0.9%	AB	AB	200 mEq	Physically compatible	3	C
Sodium lactate ⅙ M	AB	AB	200 mEq	Physically compatible	3	C

Additive Compatibility

Sodium chloride

Drug	Mfr	Conc/L	Mfr	Conc/L	Test Soln	Remarks	Ref	C/I
Fat emulsion, intravenous	CU	10%		100 mEq		No change for 24 hr at room temperature, but lipid coalescence in 48 hr	656	C

Additive Compatibility (Cont.)

Sodium chloride

Drug	Mfr	Conc/L	Mfr	Conc/L	Test Soln	Remarks	Ref	C/I
	CU	10%		200 mEq		Lipid coalescence with surface creaming in 4 hr at room temperature. Oil globules on surface at 48 hr	656	I

Y-Site Injection Compatibility (1:1 Mixture)

Sodium chloride

Drug	Mfr	Conc	Mfr	Conc	Remarks	Ref	C/I
Ciprofloxacin	MI	2 mg/mL[a]	AMR	4 mEq/mL	Visually compatible for 2 hr at 25 °C	1628	C

[a]*Tested in dextrose 5%.*

SODIUM LACTATE
AHFS 40:08

Products — Sodium lactate additive solution is available in 10-mL vials. Each milliliter of solution contains 5 mEq of sodium lactate. The 10-mL vial contains a total of 50 mEq each of Na$^+$ and lactate ion (5.6 g of sodium lactate). The pH is adjusted with hydrochloric acid, lactic acid, or sodium hydroxide if necessary. (1; 4)

Sodium lactate ⅙ M (1.9%) infusion solution is available in 500- and 1000-mL containers. It provides 167 mEq of sodium and lactate per liter. (4)

pH — From 6 to 7.3. (1; 17)

Osmolality — Sodium lactate additive solution is very hypertonic and must be diluted for use. The osmolarity was calculated to be about 10,000 mOsm/L. (1) The osmolality was determined to be 11,490 mOsm/kg by freezing-point depression and 10,665 mOsm/kg by vapor pressure. (1071)

Sodium lactate ⅙ M (1.9%) is approximately isotonic with a calculated osmolarity of 330 mOsm/L. (4)

Administration — Sodium lactate additive solution is administered by intravenous infusion only after dilution in a larger volume of fluid. A ⅙ M (1.9%) solution may be prepared by diluting 50 mEq of the additive solution to 300 mL with a nonelectrolyte solution or sterile water for injection. Sodium lactate ⅙ M infusion solution does not require dilution prior to use. The rate of infusion should not exceed 300 mL/hr in adults. (1; 4)

Stability — Sodium lactate additive solution should be stored at controlled room temperature and protected from freezing and excessive temperatures of 40 °C or more. (1; 4)

Compatibility Information

Solution Compatibility

Sodium lactate

Solution	Mfr	Mfr	Conc/L	Remarks	Ref	C/I
Dextrose–Ringer's injection combinations	AB	AB	200 mEq	Physically compatible	3	C
Dextrose–Ringer's injection, lactated, combinations	AB	AB	200 mEq	Physically compatible	3	C
Dextrose–saline combinations	AB	AB	200 mEq	Physically compatible	3	C
Dextrose 2.5%	AB	AB	200 mEq	Physically compatible	3	C

Solution Compatibility (Cont.)

Sodium lactate

Solution	Mfr	Mfr	Conc/L	Remarks	Ref	C/I
Dextrose 5%	AB	AB	200 mEq	Physically compatible	3	C
Dextrose 10%	AB	AB	200 mEq	Physically compatible	3	C
Ionosol products	AB	AB	200 mEq	Physically compatible	3	C
Ringer's injection	AB	AB	200 mEq	Physically compatible	3	C
Ringer's injection, lactated	AB	AB	200 mEq	Physically compatible	3	C
Sodium chloride 0.45%	AB	AB	200 mEq	Physically compatible	3	C
Sodium chloride 0.9%	AB	AB	200 mEq	Physically compatible	3	C

Additive Compatibility

Sodium lactate

Drug	Mfr	Conc/L	Mfr	Conc/L	Test Soln	Remarks	Ref	C/I
Lidocaine HCl	AST	2 g	AB	50 mEq		Physically compatible	24	C
Nafcillin sodium	WY	500 mg	AB	50 mEq		Physically compatible	27	C

SODIUM NITROPRUSSIDE
AHFS 24:08.20

Products — Sodium nitroprusside (Nitropress) is available in vials containing 50 mg of sodium nitroprusside dihydrate. Reconstitute with 2 to 3 mL of dextrose 5% or sterile water for injection (without preservative). Bacteriostatic water for injection should not be used, because preservatives increase the rate of decomposition. (4; 457)

Sodium nitroprusside is also available in 2-mL vials as a 25-mg/mL solution of sodium nitroprusside dihydrate in water for injection. (1)

For administration, dilute the reconstituted solution or the liquid form in dextrose 5%. The infusion containers should be wrapped in aluminum foil or other opaque material for light protection. The manufacturer states that it is not necessary to cover the infusion drip chamber or tubing. However, AHFS recommends covering the tubing. (1; 4)

pH — The pH in dextrose 5% is 3.5 to 6. (4)

Sodium Content — Contains sodium 0.335 mEq/50 mg of drug. (846)

Trade Name(s) — Nitropress.

Administration — Sodium nitroprusside is administered only as an intravenous infusion by freshly reconstituting the drug and diluting 50 mg in 250 to 1000 mL of dextrose 5%. An infusion pump, microdrip regulator, or similar device should be used to control the flow rate precisely. Extravasation should be avoided. (1; 4)

Stability — Sodium nitroprusside is a reddish-brown color. Sodium nitroprusside in intact containers should be stored at controlled room temperature and protected from light and heat and from freezing for the liquid product. (1; 4)

Sodium nitroprusside protected from light has been reported to be stable for 12 to 24 hours (93; 460; 1296; 1579), to 48 hours (958), to 13 days (95), or even longer. (94; 458; 459; 732) It is recommended that reconstituted sodium nitroprusside solutions be used within 24 hours when stored adequately protected from light. (4)

Sodium nitroprusside reacts with even minute quantities of a wide variety of inorganic and organic substances, forming highly colored reaction products (usually blue, green, or dark red). Such solutions should not be used. It is, therefore, recommended that no drug or preservative be added to sodium nitroprusside solutions. (4)

Dextrose 5% is the recommended infusion solution for admixture (1; 4; 90; 91) although it turns blue more rapidly than the drug in saline solution. (732)

Sodium nitroprusside 1 mg/mL in six solutions in PVC bags was evaluated for production of cyanide, produced by sodium nitroprusside degradation from exposure to 300 foot-candles of light for 72 hours. The solutions tested included three nonelectrolyte solutions (dextrose 5%, dextrose 10%, distilled water) and three electrolyte solutions (sodium chloride 0.9%, Ringer's injection, lactated, Ringer's injection, lactated, with dextrose 5%). There was no difference in the amount of cyanide produced among the solutions throughout the first 24 hours. However, the electrolyte solutions exhibited statistically significant lower mean cyanide ion concentrations, about 2 to 5 ppm, than the nonelectrolyte solutions (about 7 to 9 ppm). These levels of cyanide are an order of magnitude greater than in light-protected solutions. It was concluded that electrolyte solutions may be preferable to dextrose 5% for sodium nitroprusside administration and that all doses should be prepared as fresh as possible and protected from light. (2023)

Temperature Effects — Sodium nitroprusside solutions are heat sensitive. Autoclaving a solution of 100 mg/250 mL in dextrose 5% at 115 °C for 30 minutes results in decomposition to a pale blue-green precipitate. (458) It has been stated that autoclaving is less deleterious than even moderate exposure to light. (94)

Light Effects — Solutions of sodium nitroprusside exhibit a color variously described as brownish (4), brown (90), brownish-pink (91), light orange (95), and straw. (92) These solutions are highly sensitive to light. Exposure to light causes decomposition, resulting in a highly colored solution of orange (92), dark brown (91), or blue. (4; 90; 91; 92) A blue color indicates almost complete degradation. (92)

The rate of decomposition of sodium nitroprusside when exposed to light is dependent on such factors as the wavelength and intensity of light, temperature, infusion fluid, pH, and container material. The amount of loss occurring in the administration tubing can be affected additionally by the nature and thickness of the tubing wall, duration of light exposure, volume of fluid, and flow rate. (1297)

In one study, sodium nitroprusside 0.01% in both water and dextrose 5% in glass bottles exhibited 9 to 10% decomposition in two hours and 18 to 20% decomposition in four hours on exposure to fluorescent light. No decomposition was detected in either solution in 24 hours when protected from light. In PVC bags, even greater decomposition occurred on exposure to light. (460)

In another study, 10-mg/mL aqueous solutions of sodium nitroprusside lost 3% in 24 hours on exposure to fluorescent light and 10% in 24 hours when exposed to both fluorescent light and indirect daylight. At a concentration of 200 mg/L in infusion solutions, exposure to bright daylight increased the loss to approximately 15 to 30% in five hours. The rate of breakdown was related to the amount of illumination. When the containers were protected from light by wrapping with foil, no decomposition was observed in infusion solutions for seven days at room temperature and for two years at 10 mg/mL in glass tubes at room temperature or 4 °C. (732)

The rate of decomposition of sodium nitroprusside (David Bull Laboratories) 1 mg/mL in dextrose 5% was studied when exposed to

fluorescent light and natural daylight. The solutions were stored at 23 °C in the burette chambers of an amber light-protective set, a clear colorless set, and a clear set covered with a foil overwrap. With exposure to fluorescent light, losses in the clear burette chamber totaled 11% in 150 minutes and 100% in 24 hours. Both the amber and foil-wrapped clear sets sustained virtually no loss in four hours and about a 3 to 4% loss in 24 hours. Natural daylight caused a more rapid drug loss in the unprotected burette; essentially all drug was lost in 30 to 150 minutes, depending on the daylight intensity. The amber set slowed the degradation rate, but 32% was still lost in two hours with exposure to intense direct sunlight. (1296)

Solutions of sodium nitroprusside should be protected from light by wrapping the container with aluminum foil or some other opaque material. (4; 90; 91; 1297) The container should be wrapped as soon as practical without delaying therapy. (959) Amber plastic bags, which are often used for light protection, have been stated not to provide sufficient protection for sodium nitroprusside against photodegradation. Only opaque materials should be used. (733)

The effect of the light exposure that sodium nitroprusside infusions receive while flowing through a 3-m long PVC infusion set tubing was evaluated. Sodium nitroprusside infusions in dextrose 5%, sodium chloride 0.9%, and Ringer's injection, lactated, were studied for 24 and eight hours at flow rates of 10 and 50 mL/hr, respectively. The delivered amount of sodium nitroprusside was not reduced. (958)

The stability of sodium nitroprusside (Roche) 100 mcg/mL in dextrose 5% was studied when delivered through tubing exposed to normal room light. No degradation occurred in the infusion container wrapped in foil, but concentration differences in the delivered solution of about 2% were noted at each time point sampled over the five-hour study. When the effects of different light sources on a 50-mcg/mL solution in dextrose 5% were compared, about a 7% loss occurred on exposure to fluorescent light for six hours but a 32% loss occurred in one hour on exposure to direct sunlight. (1131)

The stability of sodium nitroprusside (Roche) 0.5 and 1.67 mg/mL in dextrose 5% administered by a syringe pump system was evaluated. In polypropylene syringes (Sherwood Medical) exposed to both artificial light and daylight, sodium nitroprusside losses after 24 hours were 26.0 and 18.7% at 0.5 and 1.67 mg/mL, respectively. The level of free cyanide exceeded 2 mcg/mL. The time to 10% decomposition was about four hours. Syringes wrapped in foil exhibited less than a 5% loss in 24 hours. A comparison of the decomposition occurring in the delivery tubing showed that about 10.3 and 3.7% were lost from the 0.5- and 1.67-mg/mL concentrations, respectively, when delivered by pumps at 3 mL/hr through tubing exposed to the light. Wrapping the line with foil prevented any decomposition over the 24-hour study. (1130)

Sodium nitroprusside (Roche) 50 mg/50 mL in dextrose 5% exhibited no change in appearance and no loss when stored for 24 hours at 25 °C in 60-mL plastic syringes (Becton Dickinson) wrapped in foil. However, if the syringes were not wrapped in foil for light protection, the solution turned yellow in 12 hours and had 11 and 17% losses in six and 12 hours, respectively. (1579)

Sorption — Sodium nitroprusside was shown not to exhibit sorption to PVC bags and tubing, polyethylene tubing, Silastic tubing, and polypropylene syringes. (536; 606; 1131)

Compatibility Information

Solution Compatibility

Sodium nitroprusside

Solution	Mfr	Mfr	Conc/L	Remarks	Ref	C/I
Dextrose 5%			100 mg	No decomposition in 24 hr protected from light	460	C
			100 mg	9 to 10% decomposition in 2 hr exposed to light	460	I
	TR		200 mg	No decomposition in 7 days at room temperature in foil-wrapped bottles	732	C
	TR		200 mg	14 to 16% decomposition in 5 hr exposed to bright daylight	732	I
	TRᵃ		88 mg	18% loss in 24 hr when bag was exposed to both daylight and fluorescent light	732	I
	TR	RC	165 mg	4% loss in 65 min in bright daylight	732	I
	ABᵇ	RC	50 and 100 mg	No decomposition in 48 hr in foil-wrapped bottles and bags at room temperature	958	C
	MG	RC	50 mg	Little or no loss over 6 days at room temperature protected from light	1131	C
	MG	RC	50 mg	10% loss in 7 hr at room temperature exposed to fluorescent light. 32% loss in 1 hr exposed to direct sunlight	1131	I
	BTᶜ	DB	100 mg	11% loss in 2.5 hr and 100% in 24 hr at 23 °C under fluorescent light. 100% loss in 0.5 to 2.5 hr in daylight	1296	I
	BTᶜ	DB	100 mg	3 to 4% loss in 24 hr at 23 °C protected from light with foil wrapping or amber light-protective set	1296	C
	BTᶜ	DB	100 mg	32% loss in 2 hr at 23 °C in intense daylight in amber light-protective set	1296	I
	ᵈ		200 to 800 mg	Physically compatible with 7% or less loss in 24 hr exposed to light	1412	C
	TRᵃ	RC	50 and 400 mg	Visually compatible with little or no drug loss in 48 hr at room temperature	1802	C
Ringer's injection, lactated	ABᵇ	RC	50 and 100 mg	No decomposition in 48 hr in foil-wrapped bottles and bags at room temperature	958	C
Sodium chloride 0.9%	TR		200 mg	No decomposition in 7 days at room temperature in foil-wrapped bottles	732	C
	TR		200 mg	24 to 28% decomposition in 5 hr exposed to bright daylight	732	I
	TR		289 mg	4% loss in 3 hr exposed to both daylight and fluorescent light	732	I
	TR		206 mg	2% loss in 60 min exposed to both daylight and fluorescent light	732	I
	TR		183 mg	1% loss in 2 hr in fluorescent light only	732	I
	ABᵇ	RC	50 and 100 mg	No decomposition in 48 hr in foil-wrapped bottles and bags at room temperature	958	C
	ᵈ		200 to 800 mg	Physically compatible with 8% or less loss in 24 hr exposed to light	1412	C
	TRᵃ	RC	50 and 400 mg	Visually compatible with little or no drug loss in 48 hr at room temperature	1802	C

ᵃTested in PVC containers.
ᵇTested in both glass and PVC containers.
ᶜTested in burette chambers of administration sets.
ᵈTested in glass containers.

Additive Compatibility

Sodium nitroprusside

Drug	Mfr	Conc/L	Mfr	Conc/L	Test Soln	Remarks	Ref	C/I
Atracurium besylate	BW	500 mg		2 g	D5W	Physically incompatible. Haze, particles, and yellow color form	1694	**I**
Dobutamine HCl with nitroglycerin		2 to 8 g 200 to 800 mg		200 to 800 mg	D5W[a]	Pink color with small amount of dark brown precipitate and 11 to 19% nitroglycerin loss in 24 hr exposed to light	1412	**I**
Dobutamine HCl with nitroglycerin		2 to 8 g 200 to 800 mg		200 to 800 mg	NS[a]	Pink color with 8% or less loss for any drug for 24 hr exposed to light	1412	**C**
Enalaprilat	MSD	12 mg	ES	1 g	D5W[b]	Visually compatible. Little enalaprilat loss in 24 hr at room temperature under fluorescent light. Sodium nitroprusside not tested	1572	**C**
Nitroglycerin with dobutamine HCl		200 to 800 mg 2 to 8 g		200 to 800 mg	D5W[a]	Pink color with small amount of dark brown precipitate and 11 to 19% nitroglycerin loss in 24 hr exposed to light	1412	**I**
Nitroglycerin with dobutamine HCl		200 to 800 mg 2 to 8 g		200 to 800 mg	NS[a]	Pink color with 8% or less loss for any drug for 24 hr exposed to light	1412	**C**
Ranitidine HCl	GL	2 g	RC	50 and 400 mg	D5W, NS[b]	Physically compatible. No ranitidine loss in 48 hr at room temperature light protected. Nitroprusside not tested	1361	**C**
	GL	50 mg	RC	50 and 400 mg	NS[b]	Physically compatible. No ranitidine loss in 48 hr at room temperature light protected. Nitroprusside not tested	1361	**C**
	GL	50 mg	RC	50 and 400 mg	D5W[b]	Physically compatible with 7% or less ranitidine loss in 48 hr protected from light. Nitroprusside not tested	1361	**C**
	GL	50 mg and 2 g		50 mg and 1 g	D5W, NS	Physically compatible. Both drugs stable for 48 hr at room temperature protected from light	1515	**C**
	GL	50 mg and 2 g		100 mg	D5W	Physically compatible. Ranitidine stable for 24 hr at 25 °C. Sodium nitroprusside not tested	1515	**C**
	GL	50 mg and 2 g	RC	50 and 400 mg	D5W[a]	Visually compatible. 7% ranitidine and 8% nitroprusside loss in 48 hr at room temperature protected from light	1802	**C**
	GL	50 mg and 2 g	RC	50 and 400 mg	NS[a]	Visually compatible. No loss of either drug in 48 hr at room temperature protected from light	1802	**C**
Verapamil HCl	KN	80 mg	RC	100 mg	D5W, NS	Physically compatible for 24 hr	764	**C**

[a]*Tested in glass containers.*
[b]*Tested in PVC containers.*

Drugs in Syringe Compatibility

					Sodium nitroprusside		
Drug (in syringe)	*Mfr*	*Amt*	*Mfr*	*Amt*	*Remarks*	*Ref*	*C/I*
Caffeine citrate		20 mg/ 1 mL	ES	25 mg/ 1 mL	Visually compatible for 4 hr at 25 °C	2440	**C**
Heparin sodium		2500 units/ 1 mL		60 mg/ 5 mL	Physically compatible for at least 5 min	1053	**C**
Pantoprazole sodium	[a]	4 mg/ 1 mL		10 mg/ 1 mL	Precipitates within 15 min	2574	**I**

[a]*Test performed using the formulation WITHOUT edetate disodium.*

Y-Site Injection Compatibility (1:1 Mixture)

					Sodium nitroprusside		
Drug	*Mfr*	*Conc*	*Mfr*	*Conc*	*Remarks*	*Ref*	*C/I*
Alprostadil	UP	2 mcg/mL[a]	RC	0.3, 1.2, 3 mg/mL[a]	Visually compatible for 48 hr at 24 °C protected from light	2357	**C**
	UP	10 mcg/mL[a]	RC	0.3, 1.2, 3 mg/mL[a]	Visually compatible for 48 hr at 24 °C protected from light	2357	**C**
Amiodarone HCl	WY	6 mg/mL[a]	BA	0.4 mg/mL[a]	Visually compatible for 24 hr at 22 °C	2352	**C**
	WAY	1.5 mg/mL[a]	RC	0.3 mg/mL[a]	Cloudy precipitate forms within 4 hr at 24 °C protected from light	2357	**I**
	WAY	1.5 mg/mL[a]	RC	1.2 and 3 mg/ mL[a]	Cloudy precipitate forms immediately	2357	**I**
	WAY	6 and 15 mg/ mL[a]	RC	0.3 mg/mL[a]	Visually compatible for 48 hr at 24 °C protected from light	2357	**C**
	WAY	6 and 15 mg/ mL[a]	RC	1.2 and 3 mg/ mL[a]	Cloudy precipitate forms immediately	2357	**I**
Argatroban	SKB	1 mg/mL[a]	AB	0.2 mg/mL[a]	Physically compatible for 24 hr at 23 °C	2572	**C**
Atracurium besylate	BW	0.5 mg/mL[a]	ES	0.2 mg/mL[a]	Physically compatible for 24 hr at 28 °C	1337	**C**
Bivalirudin	TMC	5 mg/mL[a]	BA	2 mg/mL[a]	Physically compatible for 4 hr at 23 °C protected from light	2373	**C**
Calcium chloride	AST	0.4 and 1.36 mEq/ mL[d]	RC	0.3, 1.2, 3 mg/mL[a]	Visually compatible for 48 hr at 24 °C protected from light	2357	**C**
	AST	0.8 mEq/mL[d]	RC	1.2 and 3 mg/ mL[a]	Visually compatible for 48 hr at 24 °C protected from light	2357	**C**
Cisatracurium besylate	GW	0.1 mg/mL[a]	AB	2 mg/mL[a]	Physically compatible for 4 hr at 23 °C protected from light	2074	**C**
	GW	2 and 5 mg/ mL[a]	AB	2 mg/mL[a]	White cloudiness forms immediately	2074	**I**
Dexmedetomidine HCl	AB	4 mcg/mL[b]	BA	2 mg/mL[b]	Physically compatible for 4 hr at 23 °C protected from light	2383	**C**
Diltiazem HCl	MMD	5 mg/mL	AB	0.2 mg/mL[a]	Visually compatible	1807	**C**
Dobutamine HCl	LI	4 mg/mL[c]	ES	0.4 mg/mL[c]	Physically compatible for 3 hr	1316	**C**
	LI	1.5 mg/mL[d]	RC	0.3, 1.2, 3 mg/mL[a]	Visually compatible for 48 hr at 24 °C protected from light	2357	**C**
	LI	6 mg/mL[d]	RC	1.2 and 3 mg/ mL[a]	Color darkening occurs over 48 hr at 24 °C protected from light	2357	**?**
	LI	12.5 mg/mL[d]	RC	0.3 and 1.2 mg/mL[a]	Visually compatible for 48 hr at 24 °C protected from light	2357	**C**

Y-Site Injection Compatibility (1:1 Mixture) (Cont.)

Sodium nitroprusside

Drug	Mfr	Conc	Mfr	Conc	Remarks	Ref	C/I
	LI	12.5 mg/mL[d]	RC	3 mg/mL[a]	Color darkening occurs over 48 hr at 24 °C protected from light	2357	?
Dobutamine HCl with dopamine HCl	LI DCC	4 mg/mL[c] 3.2 mg/mL[c]	ES	0.4 mg/mL[c]	Physically compatible for 3 hr	1316	C
Dobutamine HCl with lidocaine HCl	LI AB	4 mg/mL[c] 8 mg/mL[c]	ES	0.4 mg/mL[c]	Physically compatible for 3 hr	1316	C
Dobutamine HCl with nitroglycerin	LI LY	4 mg/mL[c] 0.4 mg/mL[c]	ES	0.4 mg/mL[c]	Physically compatible for 3 hr	1316	C
Dopamine HCl	DCC DU	3.2 mg/mL[c] 1.5, 6, 15 mg/ mL[d]	ES RC	0.4 mg/mL[c] 0.3, 1.2, 3 mg/mL[a]	Physically compatible for 3 hr Visually compatible for 48 hr at 24 °C protected from light	1316 2357	C C
Dopamine HCl with dobutamine HCl	DCC LI	3.2 mg/mL[c] 4 mg/mL[c]	ES	0.4 mg/mL[c]	Physically compatible for 3 hr	1316	C
Dopamine HCl with lidocaine HCl	DCC AB	3.2 mg/mL[c] 8 mg/mL[c]	ES	0.4 mg/mL[c]	Physically compatible for 3 hr	1316	C
Dopamine HCl with nitroglycerin	DCC LY	3.2 mg/mL[c] 0.4 mg/mL[c]	ES	0.4 mg/mL[c]	Physically compatible for 3 hr	1316	C
Enalaprilat	MSD	0.05 mg/mL[b]	LY	0.2 mg/mL[a]	Physically compatible for 24 hr at room temperature protected from light	1355	C
Epinephrine HCl	AB	0.03, 0.12, 0.3 mg/mL[d]	RC	1.2 and 3 mg/ mL[a]	Visually compatible for 48 hr at 24 °C protected from light	2357	C
Esmolol HCl	DU	40 mg/mL[a]	RC	0.2 mg/mL[a]	Visually compatible for 24 hr at 23 °C	1877	C
Famotidine	MSD	0.2 mg/mL[a]	ES	0.2 mg/mL[a]	Physically compatible for 4 hr at 25 °C protected from light	1188	C
Furosemide	SX SX	1.2[d] and 10 mg/mL 5 mg/mL[a]	RC RC	0.3, 1.2, 3 mg/mL[a] 1.2 and 3 mg/ mL[a]	Visually compatible for 48 hr at 24 °C protected from light Visually compatible for 48 hr at 24 °C protected from light	2357 2357	C C
Haloperidol lactate	MN MN	5 mg/mL 0.5 mg/mL[a]	AB AB	0.2 mg/mL[a] 0.2 mg/mL[a]	Immediate turbidity. Precipitate in 24 hr at 21 °C in fluorescent light Visually compatible for 24 hr at 21 °C	1523 1523	I C
Heparin sodium	TR OR OR OR	50 units/mL 100 units/ mL[a] 48, 200, 480 units/mL[d] 480 units/ mL[d]	ES RC RC RC	0.2 mg/mL[a] 0.2 mg/mL[a] 1.2 and 3 mg/ mL[a] 0.3 mg/mL[a]	Visually compatible for 4 hr at 25 °C protected from light Visually compatible for 24 hr at 23 °C Visually compatible for 48 hr at 24 °C protected from light Visually compatible for 48 hr at 24 °C protected from light	1793 1877 2357 2357	C C C C
Hetastarch in lactated electrolyte	AB	6%	OHM	2 mg/mL[a]	Physically compatible for 4 hr at 23 °C protected from light	2339	C
Indomethacin sodium trihydrate	MSD	1 mg/mL[b]	AB	0.2 mg/mL[a]	Visually compatible for 24 hr at 28 °C	1527	C
Insulin, regular	LI LI	1 unit/mL[a] 1 and 2 units/ mL[b]	RC RC	0.2 mg/mL[a] 1.2 and 3 mg/ mL[a]	Visually compatible for 24 hr at 23 °C Visually compatible for 48 hr at 24 °C protected from light	1877 2357	C C
Isoproterenol HCl	SX	20 mcg/mL[d]	RC	0.3, 1.2, 3 mg/mL[a]	Visually compatible for 48 hr at 24 °C protected from light	2357	C

Y-Site Injection Compatibility (1:1 Mixture) (Cont.)

Drug	Mfr	Conc	Mfr	Conc	Remarks	Ref	C/I
	SX	80 mcg/mL[d]	RC	1.2 and 3 mg/mL[a]	Visually compatible for 48 hr at 24 °C protected from light	2357	C
Labetalol HCl	GL	5 mg/mL	RC	0.2 mg/mL[a]	Visually compatible for 24 hr at 23 °C	1877	C
Levofloxacin	OMN	5 mg/mL[a]	ES	10 mg/mL[b]	Fluffy precipitate forms	2233	I
Lidocaine HCl	AB	8 mg/mL[c]	ES	0.4 mg/mL[c]	Physically compatible for 3 hr	1316	C
	AST	6 mg/mL[d]	RC	1.2 and 3 mg/mL[a]	Visually compatible for 48 hr at 24 °C protected from light	2357	C
	AST	20 and 40 mg/mL[d]	RC	0.3, 1.2, 3 mg/mL[a]	Visually compatible for 48 hr at 24 °C protected from light	2357	C
Lidocaine HCl with dobutamine HCl	AB LI	8 mg/mL[c] 4 mg/mL[c]	ES	0.4 mg/mL[c]	Physically compatible for 3 hr	1316	C
Lidocaine HCl with dopamine HCl	AB DCC	8 mg/mL[c] 3.2 mg/mL[c]	ES	0.4 mg/mL[c]	Physically compatible for 3 hr	1316	C
Lidocaine HCl with nitroglycerin	AB LY	8 mg/mL[c] 0.4 mg/mL[a]	ES	0.4 mg/mL[c]	Physically compatible for 3 hr	1316	C
Magnesium sulfate	SX	0.4 and 0.8 mEq/mL[d]	RC	0.3, 1.2, 3 mg/mL[a]	Visually compatible for 48 hr at 24 °C protected from light	2357	C
Metoprolol tartrate	BED	1 mg/mL	HOS	0.4 mg/mL[a]	Visually compatible for 24 hr at 19 °C	2795	C
Micafungin sodium	ASP	1.5 mg/mL[b]	AB	2 mg/mL[b]	Physically compatible for 4 hr at 23 °C protected from light	2683	C
Midazolam HCl	RC	1 mg/mL[a]	ES	0.2 mg/mL[a]	Visually compatible for 24 hr at 23 °C	1847	C
	RC	1 mg/mL[a]	RC	0.2 mg/mL[a]	Visually compatible for 24 hr at 23 °C	1877	C
	RC	1.2 and 2.4 mg/mL[d]	RC	1.2 and 3 mg/mL[a]	Visually compatible for 48 hr at 24 °C protected from light	2357	C
	RC	5 mg/mL[d]	RC	0.3, 1.2, 3 mg/mL[a]	Visually compatible for 48 hr at 24 °C protected from light	2357	C
Milrinone lactate	SW	0.4 mg/mL[a]	AB	0.8 mg/mL[a]	Visually compatible. Little loss of either drug in 4 hr at 23 °C protected from light	2214	C
	SW	0.1[d], 0.4[d], 1 mg/mL	RC	0.3, 1.2, 3 mg/mL[a]	Visually compatible for 48 hr at 24 °C protected from light	2357	C
Morphine sulfate	SX	1 mg/mL[a]	RC	0.2 mg/mL[a]	Visually compatible for 24 hr at 23 °C	1877	C
	AB	0.5 mg/mL[d]	RC	0.3, 1.2, 3 mg/mL[a]	Visually compatible for 48 hr at 24 °C protected from light	2357	C
	AB	1 mg/mL[d]	RC	1.2 and 3 mg/mL[a]	Visually compatible for 48 hr at 24 °C protected from light	2357	C
Nesiritide	SCI	50 mcg/mL[a,b]		5 mg/mL	Physically compatible for 4 hr	2625	C
Nicardipine HCl	DCC	0.1 mg/mL[a]	LY	0.2 mg/mL[a]	Visually compatible for 24 hr at room temperature	235	C
Nitroglycerin	LY	0.4 mg/mL[c]	ES	0.4 mg/mL[c]	Physically compatible for 3 hr	1316	C
	SX	0.4 and 1.5 mg/mL[d]	RC	1.2 and 3 mg/mL[a]	Visually compatible for 48 hr at 24 °C protected from light	2357	C
Nitroglycerin with dobutamine HCl	LY LI	0.4 mg/mL[c] 4 mg/mL[c]	ES	0.4 mg/mL[c]	Physically compatible for 3 hr	1316	C
Nitroglycerin with dopamine HCl	LY DCC	0.4 mg/mL[c] 3.2 mg/mL[c]	ES	0.4 mg/mL[c]	Physically compatible for 3 hr	1316	C
Nitroglycerin with lidocaine HCl	LY AB	0.4 mg/mL[c] 8 mg/mL[c]	ES	0.4 mg/mL[c]	Physically compatible for 3 hr	1316	C

Y-Site Injection Compatibility (1:1 Mixture) (Cont.)

Sodium nitroprusside

Drug	Mfr	Conc	Mfr	Conc	Remarks	Ref	C/I
Norepinephrine bitartrate	SX	0.03, 0.12, 3 mg/mL[d]	RC	0.3, 1.2, 3 mg/mL[a]	Visually compatible for 48 hr at 24 °C protected from light	2357	C
Pancuronium bromide	ES	0.05 mg/mL[a]	ES	0.2 mg/mL[a]	Physically compatible for 24 hr at 28 °C	1337	C
Potassium chloride	AST	0.04 and 0.5 mEq/mL[d]	RC	0.3, 1.2, 3 mg/mL[a]	Visually compatible for 48 hr at 24 °C protected from light	2357	C
Potassium phosphates	AB	0.3 mmol/mL[d]	RC	0.3, 1.2, 3 mg/mL[a]	Visually compatible for 48 hr at 24 °C protected from light	2357	C
Procainamide HCl	SX	6, 20, 40 mg/mL[b]	RC	0.3, 1.2, 3 mg/mL[a]	Visually compatible for 48 hr at 24 °C protected from light	2357	C
Propofol	ZEN	10 mg/mL	ES	0.4 mg/mL[a]	Physically compatible for 1 hr at 23 °C	2066	C
Tacrolimus	FUJ	1 mg/mL[b]	ES	0.004 mg/mL[a]	Visually compatible for 24 hr at 25 °C	1630	C
Theophylline	TR	4 mg/mL	ES	0.2 mg/mL[a]	Visually compatible for 6 hr at 25 °C protected from light	1793	C
TNA #218 to #226[e]			AB	0.4 mg/mL[a]	Visually compatible for 4 hr at 23 °C protected from light	2215	C
TPN #212 to #215[e]			AB	0.4 mg/mL[a]	Physically compatible for 4 hr at 23 °C protected from light	2109	C
Vecuronium bromide	OR	0.1 mg/mL[a]	ES	0.2 mg/mL[a]	Physically compatible for 24 hr at 28 °C	1337	C

[a]*Tested in dextrose 5%.*
[b]*Tested in sodium chloride 0.9%.*
[c]*Tested in both dextrose 5% and sodium chloride 0.9%.*
[d]*Tested in dextrose 5% in sodium chloride 0.2%.*
[e]*Refer to Appendix I for the composition of parenteral nutrition solutions. TNA indicates a 3-in-1 admixture, and TPN indicates a 2-in-1 admixture.*

SODIUM PHOSPHATES
AHFS 40:12

Products — Sodium phosphates additive solution is available in 5-, 15-, and 50-mL vials. Each milliliter contains monobasic sodium phosphate monohydrate 276 mg and dibasic sodium phosphate anhydrous 142 mg. The phosphorus concentration is 3 mmol/mL (93 mg/mL), and the sodium content is 4 mEq/mL (92 mg/mL). The additive solution is a concentrate and must be diluted for use. (1)

pH — From 5.0 to 6.0. (1)

Osmolarity — Sodium phosphates additive solution is very hypertonic. The osmolarity of sodium phosphates additive solution is calculated to be 12 mOsm/mL. (1)

Administration — Sodium phosphates additive solution must be diluted and thoroughly mixed in a larger volume of fluid before use. (1)

Stability — Sodium phosphates additive solution should be stored at room temperature. The solution should be inspected for discoloration or particulate matter prior to use and should be used only if it is clear. The injection contains no antibacterial preservative. After the vials have been entered, discard any unused portions. (1)

Compatibility Information

Y-Site Injection Compatibility (1:1 Mixture)

Sodium phosphates

Drug	Mfr	Conc	Mfr	Conc	Remarks	Ref	C/I
Amiodarone HCl	WY	6 mg/mL[a]	APP	0.12 mmol/mL[a]	Immediate white cloudiness	2352	I
Ceftaroline fosamil	FOR	2.22 mg/mL[a,b,e]	HOS	0.5 mmol/mL[a,b,e]	Increase in measured haze	2826	I
Ciprofloxacin	BAY	2 mg/mL[a]	AB	3 mmol/mL	Microcrystals form in 1 hr at 23 °C	1972	I
	BAY	2 mg/mL[c]	AB	3 mmol/mL	White crystalline precipitate forms immediately	1971; 1972	I
Doripenem	JJ	5 mg/mL[a,b]	AMR	0.5 mmol/mL[a,b]	Physically compatible for 4 hr at 23 °C	2743	C
Micafungin sodium	ASP	1.5 mg/mL[b]	AMR	0.5 mmol/mL[b]	Physically compatible for 4 hr at 23 °C	2683	C
Telavancin HCl	ASP	7.5 mg/mL[a,b,e]	HOS	0.5 mmol/mL[a,b,e]	Physically compatible for 2 hr	2830	C
TNA #218 to #226[d]			AB	3 mmol/mL	Damage to emulsion occurs immediately with free oil formation possible	2215	I
TPN #212 to #215[d]			AB	3 mmol/mL	Increased turbidity forms immediately	2109	I

[a]*Tested in dextrose 5%.*
[b]*Tested in sodium chloride 0.9%.*
[c]*Tested in both sodium chloride 0.9% and 0.45%.*
[d]*Refer to Appendix I for the composition of parenteral nutrition solutions. TNA indicates a 3-in-1 admixture, and TPN indicates a 2-in-1 admixture.*
[e]*Tested in Ringer's injection, lactated.*

Additional Compatibility Information

Calcium and Phosphate — Phosphates may be incompatible with metal ions such as magnesium and calcium. A number of studies using potassium phosphate have been performed. For additional information, refer to the potassium phosphate monograph.

UNRECOGNIZED CALCIUM PHOSPHATE PRECIPITATION IN A 3-IN-1 PARENTERAL NUTRITION MIXTURE RESULTED IN PATIENT DEATH.

The potential for the formation of a calcium phosphate precipitate in parenteral nutrition solutions is well studied and documented (1771; 1777), but the information is complex and difficult to apply to the clinical situation. (1770; 1772; 1777) The incorporation of fat emulsion in 3-in-1 parenteral nutrition solutions obscures any precipitate that is present, which has led to substantial debate on the dangers associated with 3-in-1 parenteral nutrition mixtures and when or if the danger to the patient is warranted therapeutically. (1770; 1771; 1772; 2031; 2032; 2033; 2034; 2035; 2036) Because such precipitation may be life-threatening to patients (2037; 2291), the Food and Drug Administration issued a Safety Alert containing the following recommendations (1769):

"1. The amounts of phosphorus and of calcium added to the admixture are critical. The solubility of the added calcium should be calculated from the volume at the time the calcium is added. It should not be based upon the final volume.

Some amino acid injections for TPN admixtures contain phosphate ions (as a phosphoric acid buffer). These phosphate ions and the volume at the time the phosphate is added should be considered when calculating the concentration of phosphate additives. Also, when adding calcium and phosphate to an admixture, the phosphate should be added first.

The line should be flushed between the addition of any potentially incompatible components.

2. A lipid emulsion in a three-in-one admixture obscures the presence of a precipitate. Therefore, if a lipid emulsion is needed, either (1) use a two-in-one admixture with the lipid infused separately, or (2) if a three-in-one admixture is medically necessary, then add the calcium before the lipid emulsion and according to the recommendations in number 1 above.

If the amount of calcium or phosphate which must be added is likely to cause a precipitate, some or all of the calcium should be administered separately. Such separate infusions must be properly diluted and slowly infused to avoid serious adverse events related to the calcium.

3. When using an automated compounding device, the above steps should be considered when programming the device. In addition, automated compounders should be maintained and operated according to the manufacturer's recommendations.

Any printout should be checked against the programmed admixture and weight of components.

4. During the mixing process, pharmacists who mix parenteral nutrition admixtures should periodically agitate the admixture and check for precipitates. Medical or home care personnel who start and monitor these infusions should carefully inspect for the presence of precipitates both before and during infusion. Patients and care givers should be trained to visually

inspect for signs of precipitation. They also should be advised to stop the infusion and seek medical assistance if precipitates are noted.

5. A filter should be used when infusing either central or peripheral parenteral nutrition admixtures. At this time, data have not been submitted to document which size filter is most effective in trapping precipitates.

Standards of practice vary, but the following is suggested: a 1.2-μm air-eliminating filter for lipid-containing admixtures and a 0.22-μm air-eliminating filter for non-lipid-containing admixtures.

6. Parenteral nutrition admixtures should be administered within the following time frames: if stored at room temperature, the infusion should be started within 24 hours after mixing; if stored at refrigerated temperatures, the infusion should be started within 24 hours of rewarming. Because warming parenteral nutrition admixtures may contribute to the formation of precipitates, once administration begins, care should be taken to avoid excessive warming of the admixture.

Persons administering home care parenteral nutrition admixtures may need to deviate from these time frames. Pharmacists who initially prepare these admixtures should check a reserve sample for precipitates over the duration and under the conditions of storage.

7. If symptoms of acute respiratory distress, pulmonary emboli, or interstitial pneumonitis develop, the infusion should be stopped immediately and thoroughly checked for precipitates. Appropriate medical interventions should be instituted. Home care personnel and patients should immediately seek medical assistance."

Calcium Phosphate Precipitation Fatalities — Fatal cases of paroxysmal respiratory failure in two previously healthy women receiving peripheral vein parenteral nutrition were reported. The patients experienced sudden cardiopulmonary arrest consistent with pulmonary emboli. The authors used in vitro simulations and an animal model to conclude that unrecognized calcium phosphate precipitation in a 3-in-1 total nutrition admixture caused the fatalities. The precipitation resulted during compounding by introducing calcium and phosphate near to one another in the compounding sequence and prior to complete fluid addition. This resulted in a temporarily high concentration of the drugs and precipitation of calcium phosphate. Observation of the precipitate was obscured by the incorporation of 20% fat emulsion, intravenous, into the nutrition mixture. No filter was used during infusion of the fatal nutrition admixtures. (2037)

In a follow-up retrospective review, five patients were identified who had respiratory distress associated with the infusion of the 3-in-1 admixtures at around the same time. Four of these five patients died, although the cause of death could be definitively determined for only two. (2291)

Calcium and Phosphate Conditional Compatibility — Calcium salts are conditionally compatible with phosphates in parenteral nutrition solutions. The incompatibility is dependent on a solubility and concentration phenomenon and is not entirely predictable. Precipitation may occur during compounding or at some time after compounding is completed.

NOTE: Some amino acid solutions inherently contain calcium and phosphate, which must be considered in any projection of compatibility.

A study determined the maximum concentrations of calcium (as chloride and gluconate) and phosphate that can be maintained without precipitation in a parenteral nutrition solution consisting of FreAmine II 4.25% and dextrose 25% for 24 hours at 30 °C. It was noted that the amino acids in parenteral nutrition solutions form soluble complexes with calcium and phosphate, reducing the available free calcium and phosphate that can form insoluble precipitates. The concentration of calcium available for precipitation is greater with the chloride salt compared to the gluconate salt, at least in part because of differences in dissociation characteristics. Consequently, a greater concentration of calcium gluconate than calcium chloride can be mixed with sodium phosphate. (608)

In addition to the concentrations of phosphate and calcium and the salt form of the calcium, the concentration of amino acids and the time and temperature of storage altered the formation of calcium phosphate in parenteral nutrition solutions. As the temperature was increased, the incidence of precipitate formation also increased. This finding was attributed, at least in part, to a greater degree of dissociation of the calcium and phosphate complexes and the decreased solubility of calcium phosphate. Therefore, a solution possibly may be stored at 4 °C with no precipitation, but on warming to room temperature a precipitate will form over time. (608)

The solubility characteristics of calcium and phosphate in pediatric parenteral nutrition solutions composed of Aminosyn 0.5, 2, and 4% with dextrose 10 to 25% were reported. Also present were electrolytes and vitamins. Sodium phosphate was added sequentially in phosphorus concentrations from 10 to 30 mmol/L. Calcium gluconate was added last in amounts ranging from 1 to 10 g/L. The solutions were stored at 25 °C for 30 hours and examined visually and microscopically for precipitation. The authors found that higher concentrations of Aminosyn increased the solubility of calcium and phosphate. Precipitation occurred at lower calcium and phosphate concentrations in the 0.5% solution compared to the 2 and 4% solutions. For example, at a phosphorus concentration of 30 mmol/L, precipitation occurred at calcium gluconate concentrations of about 1, 2, and 4 g/L in the 0.5, 2, and 4% Aminosyn mixtures, respectively. Similarly, at a calcium gluconate concentration of 8 g/L and above, precipitation occurred at phosphorus concentrations of about 13, 17, and 22 mmol/L in the 0.5, 2, and 4% solutions, respectively. The dextrose concentration did not appear to affect the calcium and phosphate solubility significantly. (1042)

The maximum allowable concentrations of calcium and phosphate in a 3-in-1 parenteral nutrition mixture for children (TNA #192 in Appendix I) were reported. Added calcium was varied from 1.5 to 150 mmol/L, and added phosphate was varied from 21 to 300 mmol/L. These mixtures were stable for 48 hours at 22 and 37 °C as long as the pH was not greater than 5.7, the calcium concentration was below 16 mmol/L, the phosphate concentration was below 52 mmol/L, and the product of the calcium and phosphate concentrations was below 250 $mmol^2/L^2$. (1773)

Additional calcium and phosphate solubility curves were reported for specialty parenteral nutrition solutions based on NephrAmine and also HepatAmine at concentrations of 0.8, 1.5, and 2% as the sources of amino acids. The solutions also contained dextrose 10%, with cysteine and pH adjustment to simulate addition of fat emulsion used in some admixtures. Calcium and phosphate solubility followed the hyperbolic patterns previously reported. (609) Temperature, time, and pH affected calcium and phosphate solubility, with pH having the greatest effect. (2038)

The maximum sodium phosphate concentrations were reported for given amounts of calcium gluconate that could be admixed in parenteral nutrition solutions containing TrophAmine in varying quantities (with cysteine hydrochloride 40 mg/g of amino acid) and dextrose

Table 1. Maximum Amount of Phosphate (as Sodium) (mmol/L) Not Resulting in Precipitation. (2039) See CAUTION below.[a]

Calcium (as Gluconate)	Amino Acid (as TrophAmine) plus Cysteine HCl 40 mg/g of Amino Acid				
	0%	0.4%	1%	2%	3%
9.8 mEq/L	0	27	42	60	66
14.7 mEq/L	0	15	18	30	36
19.6 mEq/L	0	6	15	27	30
29.4 mEq/L	0	3	6	21	24

[a]*CAUTION: The results cannot be safely extrapolated to solutions with formulas other than the ones tested. See text.*

10%. The solutions also contained magnesium sulfate 4 mEq/L, potassium acetate 24 mEq/L, sodium chloride 32 mEq/L, pediatric multivitamins, and trace elements. The presence of cysteine hydrochloride reduces the solution pH and increases the amount of calcium and phosphate that can be incorporated before precipitation occurs. The results of this study cannot be safely extrapolated to TPN solutions with compositions other than the ones tested. The admixtures were compounded with the sodium phosphate added last after thorough mixing of all other components. The authors noted that this is not the preferred order of mixing (usually phosphate is added first and thoroughly mixed before adding calcium last); however, they believed this reversed order of mixing would provide a margin of error in cases in which the proper order is not followed. After compounding, the solutions were stored for 24 hours at 40 °C. The maximum calcium and phosphate amounts that could be mixed in the various solutions were reported tabularly and are shown in Table 1. (2039) However, these results are not entirely consistent with another study. (2196)

Calcium phosphate precipitation phenomena was evaluated in a series of parenteral nutrition admixtures composed of dextrose 22%, amino acids (FreAmine III) 2.7%, and fat emulsion (Abbott) 0, 1, and 3.2%. Incorporation of calcium gluconate 19 to 24 mEq/L and phosphate (as sodium) 22 to 28 mmol/L resulted in visible precipitation in the fat-free admixtures. New precipitate continued to form over 14 days, even after repeated filtrations of the solutions through 0.2-μm filters. The presence of the amino acids increased calcium and phosphate solubility, compared with simple aqueous solutions. However, the incorporation of the fat emulsion did not result in a statistically significant increase in calcium and phosphate solubility. The authors noted that the kinetics of calcium phosphate precipitate formation do not appear to be entirely predictable; both transient and permanent precipitation can occur either during the compounding process or at some time afterward. Because calcium phosphate precipitation can be very dangerous clinically, the use of inline filters was recommended. The authors suggested that the filters should have a porosity appropriate to the parenteral nutrition admixture—1.2 μm for fat-containing and 0.2 or 0.45 μm for fat-free nutrition mixtures. (2061)

A 2-mL fluid barrier of dextrose 5% in a microbore retrograde infusion set failed to prevent precipitation when used between calcium gluconate 200 mg/2 mL and sodium phosphate 0.3 mmol/0.1 mL. (1385)

A 2-in-1 parenteral nutrition admixture with final concentrations of TrophAmine 0.5%, dextrose 5%, L-cysteine hydrochloride 40 mg/g of amino acids, calcium gluconate 60 mg/100 mL, and sodium phosphates 46.5 mg/mL was found to result in visible precipitation of calcium phosphate within 30 hours stored at 23 to 27 °C. Despite the presence of the acidifying l-cysteine hydrochloride, precipitation occurred at clinically utilized amounts of calcium and phosphates. (2622)

The presence of magnesium in solutions may also influence the reaction between calcium and phosphate, including the nature and extent of precipitation. (158; 159)

The interaction of calcium and phosphate in parenteral nutrition solutions is a complex phenomenon. Various factors have been identified as playing a role in the solubility or precipitation of a given combination, including (608; 609; 1042; 1063; 1427; 2778):

1. Concentration of calcium
2. Salt form of calcium
3. Concentration of phosphate
4. Concentration of amino acids
5. Amino acids composition
6. Concentration of dextrose
7. Temperature of solution
8. pH of solution
9. Presence of other additives
10. Order of mixing

Enhanced precipitate formation would be expected from such factors as high concentrations of calcium and phosphate, increases in solution pH, decreased amino acid concentrations, increases in temperature, addition of calcium prior to phosphate, lengthy standing times or slow infusion rates, and use of calcium as the chloride salt. (854)

SOMATROPIN
AHFS 68:28

Products — Somatropin derived from *Escherichia coli* is available in vials and cartridges in sizes ranging from 1.5 to 24 mg, depending on the specific product. Each milligram represents about three units of activity. The commercially available dosage forms are variable in components and concentrations; care should be taken to follow the directions for the specific product being used. Most products are supplied in dry form requiring reconstitution using a diluent that is supplied with the product. Manufacturers' specific reconstitution instructions for each product should be followed. For products in vials, the specified amount of the diluent is injected into the somatropin container, aiming the stream at the container wall. The drug is reconstituted by gentle swirling using a rotary motion for most products but vigorous swirling for two minutes for Nutropin Depot. Vial inversion is recommended for reconstitution of Norditropin. Shaking is not recommended for any product and may damage the product. (1)

Norditropin Cartridges and Nutropin AQ are available as liquid injections not requiring dilution for use. (1)

Somatropin derived from mammalian cells (Saizen; Serostim) is available in vials in varying sizes from 4 to 8.8 mg, depending on the specific product. The manufacturer's specific reconstitution instructions for each product using the diluents provided should be followed. The specified amount of the diluent is injected into the somatropin container, aiming the stream at the container wall. The drug is dissolved by gentle swirling using a rotary motion, *not* shaking. Shaking is not recommended for any product and may damage the protein. (1)

pH — The pH values cited by the manufacturers are as follows (1):

Products	pH
Genotropin	about 6.7
Humatrope	about 7.5
Norditropin	about 7.3
Nutropin	about 7.4
Nutropin AQ	about 6.0
Saizen	6.5 to 8.5
Serostim	7.4 to 8.5

Administration — Somatropin products are usually administered by subcutaneous injection. Humatrope and Saizen may also be administered intramuscularly. (1)

Stability — Intact containers of somatropin products derived from *E. coli* should be stored under refrigeration and protected from freezing. Genotropin and Norditropin should also be protected from light during storage. Most somatropin products result in clear solutions when reconstituted correctly. Shaking may result in cloudiness, rendering the products unacceptable for use. Reconstituted Nutropin Depot is a thick, milky suspension. (1)

Stability after reconstitution is variable among the products and depends on whether a preservative-containing diluent is used. See Table 1. Unpreserved reconstituted products of Genotropin and Humatrope should be stored under refrigeration and used within 24 hours. Nutropin Depot suspension should be used immediately upon reconstitution, discarding any unused remainder. Products reconstituted with the specified preserved diluents are stable for longer periods. After reconstitution with the appropriate preserved diluent, Norditropin and Nutropin are stable for 14 days, Genotropin for 21 days, and Humatrope for 28 days stored under refrigeration. Nutropin AQ is stable for 28 days after initial stopper penetration when stored under refrigeration. (1)

Table 1. Recommended Stability Periods for Somatropin Products Using Diluents with and without Preservatives and Stored under Refrigeration (1)

Product	Stability Period
Diluent with Preservative	
Genotropin 5.8 and 13.8 mg	21 days
Humatrope	28 days
Norditropin	14 days
Nutropin	14 days
Nutropin AQ	28 days[a]
Saizen	14 days
Diluent without Preservative	
Genotropin 1.5 mg	24 hr
Humatrope	24 hr
Serostim	24 hr

[a] *Period after initial penetration of the vial stopper of this liquid product.*

Intact containers of somatropin products derived from mammalian cells should be stored at controlled room temperature. Saizen reconstituted with the preserved diluent provided is stable for 14 days after reconstitution when stored under refrigeration. Serostim reconstituted with the unpreserved diluent provided is stable for 24 hours stored under refrigeration. Freezing of reconstituted solutions should be avoided. (1)

Syringes — Somatropin (Humatrope) was reconstituted to concentrations of 1 and 3.33 mg/mL with the accompanying diluent; the diluent contains glycerin 1.7% and *m*-cresol 0.3% as a preservative. The reconstituted product at each concentration was packaged in 1-mL plastic syringes with barrels composed of polypropylene (Becton Dickinson) or propylene–ethylene copolymer (Terumo) and capped and stored under refrigeration at about 5 °C for 28 days. Little or no loss of somatropin occurred stored in either syringe. The solutions remained visually acceptable for 28 days in the polypropylene syringes, but an unacceptable turbidity formed within 21 days in the propylene–ethylene copolymer syringes, which became a precipitate by 28 days. The preservative, *m*-cresol, concentrations fell up to 4% but remained above the minimum acceptable concentration. Somatropin should be stored no more than 14 days at 5 °C in propylene–ethylene copolymer syringes. Storage up to 28 days was acceptable in the polypropylene syringes. (2210)

STERILE WATER FOR INJECTION
AHFS 96:00

Products — Sterile water for injection is available in ampuls, vials, and plastic bags in sizes ranging from 5 mL to 5 L. This diluent is a pharmaceutical aid that contains no antimicrobial preservative or any other solute but must have drugs or other solutes added prior to administration. (1)

pH — From 5 to 7. (1; 17)

Osmolality — Sterile water for injection has an osmolality of 0 mOsm/kg. It is incompatible with blood and will cause hemolysis if administered intravenously in sufficient quantity. (1)

Administration — Sterile water for injection is intended for use as a pharmaceutical aid in dissolving or diluting drugs for subcutaneous, intramuscular, and intravenous injection. It must not be administered intravenously without the addition of a sufficient amount of drugs or other solutes to provide adequate osmolality to make the solution approximately isotonic. (1) Death and injury have resulted from hemolysis caused by intravenous administration of a sufficient volume of sterile water for injection and other low-osmolality solutions. (4; 1942; 2072; 2073; 2481; 2482)

For patient safety, medical orders for large volumes of sterile water for injection, especially plastic bags of any size, without the addition of sufficient drug or solute to render the solutions approximately iso-

tonic (about 308 mOsm/kg) should not be permitted. Immediate consultation with the prescriber or referral to the institutional medical peer review process may be necessary to avoid possible patient harm. Large-volume containers of sterile water for injection should be stored only in pharmacies and not in patient care areas. Suitable warnings near the stored product and computer system alerts should remind staff that sterile water for injection is for diluent use only. (2481)

Stability — The intact single-use containers of sterile water for injection should be stored at controlled room temperature. (1)

STREPTOMYCIN SULFATE
AHFS 8:12.02

Products — Streptomycin sulfate is available as a lyophilized powder for injection in vials containing 1 g of drug with no preservatives. Reconstitute with 4.2, 3.2, or 1.8 mL of sterile water for injection to yield solutions containing 200, 250, or 400 mg/mL, respectively. (4)

pH — The reconstituted injection at a concentration of 200 mg/mL has a pH of 4.5 to 7. (1; 4)

Administration — Streptomycin sulfate is administered by deep intramuscular injection well within the body of a relatively large muscle,

such as the upper outer quadrant of the buttock in adults or the mid-lateral thigh in adults or children. Injection sites should be alternated. (1; 4) Intravenous injection is not recommended (4), although it has been performed. (1603)

Stability — Intact vials of streptomycin sulfate lyophilized powder should be stored at controlled room temperature and protected from light. (1; 4)

Reconstituted solutions of streptomycin sulfate are stated to be stable for one week at room temperature and protected from light. However, no preservatives are present and the possibility of microbiological contamination must be considered. (1; 4)

Compatibility Information

Additive Compatibility

Streptomycin sulfate

Drug	Mfr	Conc/L	Mfr	Conc/L	Test Soln	Remarks	Ref	C/I
Amphotericin B		200 mg	BP	4 g	D5W	Haze develops over 3 hr	26	I
Bleomycin sulfate	BR	20 and 30 units	PF	4 g	NS	Physically compatible and bleomycin activity retained for 1 week at 4 °C. Streptomycin not tested	763	C
Heparin sodium	AB	20,000 units		1 g		Precipitate forms within 1 hr	21	I
	BP	20,000 units	BP	4 g	D5W, NS	Precipitates immediately	26	I
Methohexital sodium	BP	2 g	BP	4 g	NS	Crystals produced	26	I

Drugs in Syringe Compatibility

Streptomycin sulfate

Drug (in syringe)	Mfr	Amt	Mfr	Amt	Remarks	Ref	C/I
Ampicillin sodium	AY	500 mg		1 g/2 mL	No precipitate or color change within 1 hr at room temperature	99	C
	AY	500 mg	BP	1 g/2 mL	Physically compatible for 1 hr at room temperature	300	C

Drugs in Syringe Compatibility (Cont.)

Streptomycin sulfate

Drug (in syringe)	Mfr	Amt	Mfr	Amt	Remarks	Ref	C/I
	AY	500 mg	BP	1 g/1.5 mL	Syrupy solution forms	300	I
Cloxacillin sodium	BE	250 mg		1 g/2 mL	No precipitate or color change within 1 hr at room temperature	99	C
	AY	250 mg	BP	1 g/1.5 mL	Syrupy solution forms	300	I
	AY	250 mg	BP	1 g/2 mL	Physically compatible for 1 hr at room temperature	300	C
	AY	250 mg	BP	750 mg/1.5 mL	Precipitate forms within 1 hr at room temperature	300	I
Heparin sodium	AB	20,000 units/1 mL		1 g	Physically incompatible	21	I
Penicillin G sodium		1 million units		1 g/2 mL	No precipitate or color change within 1 hr at room temperature	99	C

Y-Site Injection Compatibility (1:1 Mixture)

Streptomycin sulfate

Drug	Mfr	Conc	Mfr	Conc	Remarks	Ref	C/I
Esmolol HCl	DCC	10 mg/mL[a]	PF	10 mg/mL[a]	Physically compatible for 24 hr at 22 °C	1169	C

[a]*Tested in dextrose 5%.*

STREPTOZOCIN
AHFS 10:00

Products — Streptozocin is available in single-dose vials containing 1 g of drug and 220 mg of citric acid anhydrous. Sodium hydroxide may have been used to adjust the pH. (1)

Reconstitute with 9.5 mL of sodium chloride 0.9% or dextrose 5% to provide a 100-mg/mL solution. (1; 4)

pH — From 3.5 to 4.5. (1)

Trade Name(s) — Zanosar.

Administration — Streptozocin may be administered by rapid intravenous injection or intravenous infusion over 15 minutes to six hours. (1; 4)

Stability — Intact vials containing a pale yellow powder should be refrigerated and protected from light. (1; 4)

The pale gold reconstituted solution is stable for 48 hours at room temperature or 96 hours under refrigeration. (4) However, the manufacturer recommends use within 12 hours because the product does not contain an antibacterial preservative. (1; 4)

Streptozocin (Upjohn) 3 mg/mL in sodium chloride 0.9% did not support the growth of *Staphylococcus aureus*, *Enterococcus faecium*, *Pseudomonas aeruginosa*, and *Candida albicans* with loss of viability over 24 hours at room temperature. Even so, admixtures should be stored under refrigeration whenever possible, and the potential for microbiological growth should be considered when assigning expiration periods. (2740)

Filtration — Streptozocin 10 to 200 mcg/mL exhibited no loss due to sorption to either cellulose nitrate/cellulose acetate ester (Millex OR) or Teflon (Millex FG) filters. (1415; 1416)

Compatibility Information

Solution Compatibility

Streptozocin

Solution	Mfr	Mfr	Conc/L	Remarks	Ref	C/I
Dextrose 5%			2 g	Stable for 48 hr at room temperature and 96 hr refrigerated	4	C
Sodium chloride 0.9%			2 g	Stable for 48 hr at room temperature and 96 hr refrigerated	4	C

Y-Site Injection Compatibility (1:1 Mixture)

Streptozocin

Drug	Mfr	Conc	Mfr	Conc	Remarks	Ref	C/I
Allopurinol sodium	BW	3 mg/mL[b]	UP	40 mg/mL[b]	Haze and small particles in 1 hr	1686	I
Amifostine	USB	10 mg/mL[a]	UP	40 mg/mL[a]	Physically compatible for 4 hr at 23 °C	1845	C
Aztreonam	SQ	40 mg/mL[a]	UP	40 mg/mL[a]	Red color forms in 1 hr	1758	I
Etoposide phosphate	BR	5 mg/mL[a]	UP	40 mg/mL[a]	Physically compatible for 4 hr at 23 °C	2218	C
Filgrastim	AMG	30 mcg/mL[a]	UP	40 mg/mL[a]	Physically compatible for 4 hr at 22 °C	1687	C
Gemcitabine HCl	LI	10 mg/mL[b]	UP	40 mg/mL[b]	Physically compatible for 4 hr at 23 °C	2226	C
Granisetron HCl	SKB	1 mg/mL	UP	9.1 mg/mL[b]	Physically compatible with little or no loss of either drug in 4 hr at 22 °C	1883	C
Melphalan HCl	BW	0.1 mg/mL[b]	UP	40 mg/mL[b]	Physically compatible for 3 hr at 22 °C	1557	C
Ondansetron HCl	GL	1 mg/mL[b]	UP	30 mg/mL[a]	Visually compatible for 4 hr at 22 °C	1365	C
Piperacillin sodium–tazobactam sodium	LE[d]	40 + 5 mg/mL[a]	UP	40 mg/mL[a]	Particles form in 1 hr	1688	I
Teniposide	BR	0.1 mg/mL[a]	UP	40 mg/mL[a]	Physically compatible for 4 hr at 23 °C	1725	C
Thiotepa	IMM[c]	1 mg/mL[a]	UP	40 mg/mL[a]	Physically compatible for 4 hr at 23 °C	1861	C
Vinorelbine tartrate	BW	1 mg/mL[b]	UP	40 mg/mL[b]	Physically compatible for 4 hr at 22 °C	1558	C

[a]Tested in dextrose 5%.
[b]Tested in sodium chloride 0.9%.
[c]Lyophilized formulation tested.
[d]Test performed using the formulation WITHOUT edetate disodium.

SUCCINYLCHOLINE CHLORIDE
AHFS 12:20.20

Products — Succinylcholine chloride is available in a concentration of 20 mg/mL in 5- and 10-mL multiple-dose vials and 5-mL syringes. The vials are preserved with parabens or benzyl alcohol and may contain sodium chloride for isotonicity and hydrochloric acid for pH adjustment. Succinylcholine chloride is also available in higher concentrations of 50 mg/mL in 10-mL ampuls and 100 mg/mL in 10-mL single-dose vials. (1; 4)

pH — From 3 to 4.5. (1; 4)

Osmolality — The osmolality of succinylcholine chloride 50 mg/mL was determined to be 409 mOsm/kg. (1233)

Trade Name(s) — Anectine, Quelicin.

Administration — Succinylcholine chloride is usually administered by direct intermittent intravenous injection or intravenous infusion. For continuous intravenous infusion, a 1- to 2-mg/mL (0.1 to 0.2%) solution is prepared, usually in 250 to 1000 mL of compatible fluid. If necessary, when a suitable vein is inaccessible, a maximum of 150 mg of the drug may be administered by deep intramuscular injection, preferably high into the deltoid muscle. (1; 4)

Stability — Commercially available injections of succinylcholine chloride should be stored at 2 to 8 °C to retard loss. (1; 4) Succinylcholine chloride injection in the original unopened containers is stated in the labeling to be stable for 14 days at room temperature. (1; 1433)

Studies indicate that succinylcholine chloride injection in original unopened containers may be stable at room temperature for longer periods. The manufacturer of Quelicin has stated that the drug was stable for three months at temperatures up to 25 °C. (1239; 2745) More recently, Hospira has stated that Quelicin is stable only for 30 days at room temperature. (2783)

Research studies have also looked at the stability of succinylcholine chloride above refrigeration temperature. In one study, storage for seven days at 40 °C followed by storage at 25 °C for four weeks was used to simulate the worst case of shipping followed by storage on an emergency cart. Calculated loss at room temperature was 1%/week; at 40 °C, it was 3.2%/week. Therefore, the loss was estimated to be about 7% under such conditions. (960)

In another study, similar results were found. The decomposition rate of succinylcholine chloride was dependent on both concentration and temperature. The calculated degradation rates at room temperature were all higher for the 50-mg/mL concentration (2.1%/month) compared to the 20-mg/mL injection (1.2%/month). The time to 10% decomposition on an emergency cart was about 4.8 months for the 50-mg/mL concentration and was about 8.3 months for the 20-mg/mL concentration. Refrigeration cut the decomposition rates to 0.3 and 0.18% per month, respectively. (2742)

However, a somewhat shorter time to 10% decomposition at room temperature has also been reported. Commercial vials of succinylcholine chloride 20 mg/mL (Quelicin) stored at room temperature were found to decompose about 10 to 11% drug in 6 months. The authors recommended limiting room temperature storage to not more than 6 months. (2763)

After dilution of succinylcholine chloride to a concentration of 1 or 2 mg/mL in sodium chloride 0.9%, the drug is stated to be chemically stable for four weeks at 5 °C and one week at 25 °C. However, use within 24 hours of preparation is recommended along with discarding any unused solution. (1; 4)

pH Effects — Succinylcholine chloride is unstable in alkaline solutions (1; 4) and decomposes in solutions with a pH greater than 4.5. (4) The pH of maximum stability was found to be 3.75 to 4.50. (960)

In combination with barbiturates, either free barbituric acid will precipitate or the succinylcholine chloride will be hydrolyzed, depending on the final pH of the admixture. (1; 4; 21) Succinylcholine chloride should not be mixed with barbiturates in the same syringe or given simultaneously through the same needle. (1)

Syringes — Succinylcholine chloride (Abbott) 20 mg/mL was packaged in both glass and polypropylene syringes (Becton Dickinson) sealed with rubber luer-tip caps (Becton Dickinson). The syringes were stored for 45 days at 4 °C, 22 °C and 50% relative humidity, and 37 °C and 85% relative humidity. At 4 °C, there was little or no succinylcholine chloride loss after 45 days in either glass or plastic syringes. At 22 °C and 50% relative humidity, about a 5% loss occurred in 45 days. However, at 37 °C and 85% relative humidity, the drug concentration fell below the acceptable USP limit after about 30 days. (1209)

Succinylcholine chloride (Burroughs Wellcome) 20 mg/mL in dextrose 5% and in sodium chloride 0.9% (Baxter) was packaged as 10 mL in 12-mL plastic syringes (Monoject) and wrapped in aluminum foil. Little or no loss of succinylcholine chloride occurred during 107 days of storage at 5 °C. At 25 °C, about 5 to 6% loss occurred in 100 days. Samples at an elevated temperature of 40 °C were stable through 22 days with only 3 to 4% loss but exhibited 12 to 14% loss at 63 days. (1892)

Succinylcholine chloride (Abbott) 20 mg/mL was packaged as 8 mL of undiluted injection in 12-mL polypropylene syringes (Becton Dickinson) and was stored at 4 °C and 25 °C exposed to fluorescent light. The injection remained visually clear at both temperatures. Little or no loss of succinylcholine chloride occurred in 90 days when stored at 4 °C. However, at 25 °C losses of about 6, 10, and 12% occurred in 45, 60, and 90 days, respectively. (2438)

Syringes prefilled with succinylcholine chloride injection for emergency use have been reported to freeze upon storage under refrigeration. Care should be taken to make sure that refrigerators are operating within compendial temperature ranges to ensure the availability of stored drugs in emergencies. (2698; 2699)

Compatibility Information

Solution Compatibility

Succinylcholine chloride

Solution	Mfr	Mfr	Conc/L	Remarks	Ref	C/I
Dextrose–Ringer's injection combinations	AB	AB	2 g	Physically compatible	3	**C**
Dextrose–Ringer's injection, lactated, combinations	AB	AB	2 g	Physically compatible	3	**C**
Dextrose 5% in Ringer's injection, lactated	TRª	TR	1 g	Stable for 24 hr at 5 °C	282	**C**
Dextrose–saline combinations	AB	AB	2 g	Physically compatible	3	**C**
Dextrose 5% in sodium chloride 0.9%	TRª	TR	1 g	Stable for 24 hr at 5 °C	282	**C**
Dextrose 2.5%	AB	AB	2 g	Physically compatible	3	**C**

Solution Compatibility (Cont.)

Succinylcholine chloride

Solution	Mfr	Mfr	Conc/L	Remarks	Ref	C/I
Dextrose 5%	AB	AB	2 g	Physically compatible	3	C
	TR[a]	TR	1 g	Stable for 24 hr at 5 °C	282	C
Dextrose 10%	AB	AB	2 g	Physically compatible	3	C
Ionosol products	AB	AB	2 g	Physically compatible	3	C
Ringer's injection	AB	AB	2 g	Physically compatible	3	C
Ringer's injection, lactated	AB	AB	2 g	Physically compatible	3	C
	TR[a]	TR	1 g	Stable for 24 hr at 5 °C	282	C
Sodium chloride 0.45%	AB	AB	2 g	Physically compatible	3	C
Sodium chloride 0.9%	AB	AB	2 g	Physically compatible	3	C
	TR[a]	TR	1 g	Stable for 24 hr at 5 °C	282	C
Sodium lactate ⅙ M	AB	AB	2 g	Physically compatible	3	C

[a]Tested in both glass and PVC containers.

Additive Compatibility

Succinylcholine chloride

Drug	Mfr	Conc/L	Mfr	Conc/L	Test Soln	Remarks	Ref	C/I
Amikacin sulfate	BR	5 g	SQ	2 g	D5LR, D5R, D5S, D5W, D10W, LR, NS, R, SL	Physically compatible and both stable for 24 hr at 25 °C	294	C
Isoproterenol HCl	WI	4 mg	AB	2 g		Physically compatible	59	C
Meperidine HCl	WI	100 mg	AB	2 g		Physically compatible	3	C
Methyldopate HCl	MSD	1 g	AB	2 g	D, D–S, S	Physically compatible	23	C
Morphine sulfate		16.2 mg	AB	2 g		Physically compatible	3	C
Norepinephrine bitartrate	WI	8 mg	AB	2 g	D, D–S, S	Physically compatible	77	C
Pentobarbital sodium						Pentobarbital precipitates or succinylcholine hydrolyzes	4	I
Phenobarbital sodium						Phenobarbital precipitates or succinylcholine hydrolyzes	4	I
Scopolamine HBr		0.43 mg	AB	2 g		Physically compatible	3	C
Sodium bicarbonate	AB	2.4 mEq[a]	AB	1 g	D5W	Succinylcholine decomposition	772	I

[a]One vial of Neut added to a liter of admixture.

Drugs in Syringe Compatibility

Succinylcholine chloride

Drug (in syringe)	Mfr	Amt	Mfr	Amt	Remarks	Ref	C/I
Heparin sodium		2500 units/ 1 mL		100 mg/ 5 mL	Physically compatible for at least 5 min	1053	C

Y-Site Injection Compatibility (1:1 Mixture)

Succinylcholine chloride

Drug	Mfr	Conc	Mfr	Conc	Remarks	Ref	C/I
Dexmedetomidine HCl	HOS				Stated to be compatible	1	**C**
Etomidate	AB	2 mg/mL	AB	20 mg/mL	Visually compatible for 7 days at 25 °C	1801	**C**
Heparin sodium[d]	RI	1000 units/L[a,b,c]	BW	20 mg/mL	Physically compatible for 4 hr at room temperature	322	**C**
Hetastarch in lactated electrolyte	AB	6%	AB	2 mg/mL[a]	Physically compatible for 4 hr at 23 °C	2339	**C**
Hydrocortisone sodium succinate[e]	UP	100 mg/L[a,b,c]	BW	20 mg/mL	Physically compatible for 4 hr at room temperature	322	**C**
Palonosetron HCl	MGI	50 mcg/mL	SZ	2 mg/mL[a]	Physically compatible and no loss of either drug in 4 hr at room temperature	2764	**C**
Potassium chloride		40 mEq/L[a,b,c]	BW	20 mg/mL	Physically compatible for 4 hr at room temperature	322	**C**
Propofol	ZEN	10 mg/mL	AB	20 mg/mL	Physically compatible for 1 hr at 23 °C	2066	**C**

[a]*Tested in dextrose 5%.*
[b]*Tested in sodium chloride 0.9%.*
[c]*Tested in Ringer's injection, lactated.*
[d]*Tested in combination with hydrocortisone sodium succinate (Upjohn) 100 mg/L.*
[e]*Tested in combination with heparin sodium (Riker) 1000 units/L.*

SUFENTANIL CITRATE
AHFS 28:08.08

Products — Sufentanil citrate is available as a preservative-free aqueous injection in 1-, 2-, and 5-mL ampuls and vials. Each milliliter of solution contains sufentanil citrate equivalent to 50 mcg of sufentanil base. (1)

pH — From 3.5 to 6. (1)

Trade Name(s) — Sufenta.

Administration — Sufentanil citrate is administered intravenously by slow injection or infusion. For labor and delivery, it may be administered epidurally. The drug has also been given intramuscularly. (1; 4)

Stability — Sufentanil citrate is a stable, clear, aqueous, preservative-free injection. The product should be stored at controlled room temperature and protected from light. (1; 4)

pH Effects — Sufentanil citrate is hydrolyzed in acidic solutions. A 5 mcg/mL solution with a pH greater than 3 lost less than 1% in 48 weeks at 90 °C. However, at a pH of less than 2, the drug loss was 14% at 60 °C and 32% at 90 °C in 48 weeks. (1755)

Freezing Solutions — Sufentanil citrate (Janssen) 5 mcg/mL in sodium chloride 0.9% became nonhomogeneous and difficult to restore to homogeneity when frozen at −20 °C. (1755)

Syringes — Sufentanil citrate (Janssen) 2 mcg/mL in sodium chloride 0.9% was packaged in 50-mL polypropylene syringes (Omnifix, B. Braun) and stored at 21 °C. Less than 10% sufentanil loss occurred in 24 hours. (2201)

Ambulatory Pumps — Sufentanil citrate 50 mcg/mL was evaluated in CADD-1 and CADD-PRIZM medication cassettes. About 4% drug loss occurred in 14 days at room and refrigeration temperatures. (2717)

Sorption — Sufentanil citrate (Janssen) demonstrated loss from solutions in concentrations from 1 to 20 mcg/mL due to sorption to PVC/Kalex 3000 reservoirs for use with CADD pumps (Pharmacia Deltec) and administration tubing. (790)

Sufentanil citrate (Janssen) 2 mcg/mL in sodium chloride 0.9% was delivered from 50-mL polypropylene syringes (Omnifix, B. Braun) by a syringe pump (JMS-Syringe-Pump Model SP-100, Japan Medical Supply Company) through polyethylene extension sets (Original-Perfusor-Leitung, Type PE, B. Braun) or polyvinyl chloride extension sets (Original-Perfusor-Leitung, Type N, B. Braun), 0.2-μm epidural filters (Sterifix, B. Braun), and epidural catheters (Perifix, B. Braun) over 24 hours. The pump, syringes, and extension sets were kept at 21 °C while the filters and epidural catheters were kept at 36 °C. Running at 1 mL/hr, the delivered sufentanil concentration using PVC tubing was about 7 to 10% below the theoretical concentration throughout 24 hours. Using polyethylene tubing, losses were about 16% initially but the concentration returned to expected levels within one to two hours and remained stable throughout the 24-hour delivery. (2201)

Filtration — Sufentanil citrate (Janssen) 50 mcg/10 mL in sodium chloride 0.9% was evaluated for drug loss when administered through filters or epidural catheters; 2.5-g cellulose acetate/cellulose nitrate 0.2-μm filters (Millex, Millipore) were utilized. Approximately 20% of the sufentanil was lost to the void volume and/or adsorption. This loss should be considered when a new filter is used. (1667)

Sufentanil citrate (Janssen) 2 mcg/mL in sodium chloride 0.9% delivered at 1 mL/hr through 0.2-μm epidural filters (Sterifix, B. Braun) during the first hour was 83% of the theoretical concentration and remained at reduced concentrations of 85 to 89% of theoretical through at least six hours. By 24 hours the concentration was near 96% of theoretical. The authors attributed the lower concentrations to sorption of sufentanil onto the filter. (2201)

In addition, sufentanil citrate (Janssen) demonstrated varying amounts of loss from solutions in concentrations from 1 to 20 mcg/mL due to sorption to several filters including Millex-OR, Minisart NML, Schleicher & Schuell FP 30/3, and Sterifix EF. (790)

Sufentanil citrate was found to undergo sorption to 0.22-μm polyamide epidural filters (Perifix, Braun Melsungen). Delivery of a 5-mcg/mL solution through the filter resulted in nearly total loss of the drug from the first milliliter. Three milliliters had to be passed through the filter before the delivered drug concentration was near the original concentration. (2545)

Compatibility Information

Solution Compatibility

Sufentanil citrate

Solution	Mfr	Mfr	Conc/L	Remarks	Ref	C/I
Dextrose 5%	a	JN	5 mg	10% loss in 30 days at 32 °C and little loss in 30 days at 4 °C	1756	C
	HOS[d]	AKN, BA	5 mg	No loss in 24 hr	2660; 2792	C
Sodium chloride 0.9%	a	JN	20 mg	10 and 18% losses in 24 hr at 26 and 37 °C, respectively, due to sorption. 5% loss in 10 days at 5 °C	1751	I
	a	JN	5 mg	13% loss in 2 days at 32 °C due to sorption. Little loss in 25 days at 4 °C. Precipitate in 6 days	1755	I
	FRE[b]	JN	5 mg	No loss in 21 days at 4 and 32 °C	1755	C
	c	JN	5 mg	No loss in 21 days at 4 and 32 °C	1755	C
	a	JN	5 mg	Visually compatible. 11% loss in 48 hr at 32 °C. 5% loss in 48 hr when buffered to pH 4.6	2042	C
	AB	AB	1 mg	Visually compatible with little drug loss in 23 days at 4 °C and in 3 days at 21 °C	2550	C

[a]Tested in PVC/Kalex 3000 (phthalate ester) CADD pump reservoirs.
[b]Tested in glass containers.
[c]Tested in high-density polyethylene containers.
[d]Tested in VISIV polyolefin containers.

Additive Compatibility

Sufentanil citrate

Drug	Mfr	Conc/L	Mfr	Conc/L	Test Soln	Remarks	Ref	C/I
Bupivacaine HCl		3 g	JN	20 mg	NS[a]	5% sufentanil loss and no bupivacaine loss in 10 days at 5, 26, and 37 °C	1751	C
	AST	2 g	JN	5 mg	NS[a]	9% sufentanil loss and 5% bupivacaine loss in 30 days at 32 °C. No loss of either drug in 30 days at 4 °C	1756	C
	AST	2 g	JN	5 mg	NS[a]	Buffered with pH 4.6 citrate buffer. Visually compatible with no loss of either drug in 48 hr at 32 °C	2042	C
	AST	40 mg	JN	12 mg	NS[b]	Visually compatible with no loss of either drug in 43 days at 4 and 25 °C	2455	C
Ropivacaine HCl	ASZ	1 g	JN	0.4 mg	NS[c]	Physically compatible. No loss of either drug in 30 days at 30 °C in the dark	2433	C

Additive Compatibility (Cont.)

Sufentanil citrate

Drug	Mfr	Conc/L	Mfr	Conc/L	Test Soln	Remarks	Ref	C/I
	ASZ	2 g	JN	0.4 and 4 mg	c	Physically compatible. No loss of either drug in 30 days at 30 °C in the dark	2433	C
	ASZ	2 mg	JC	0.5, 0.75, 1 mg	NS[d,e]	Physically compatible with no major sufentanil loss in 96 hr at 25 °C. Ropivacaine not tested	2506	C
Ziconotide acetate	ELN	25 mg[f]	BB	1 g[g]		10% ziconotide loss in 33 days. No sufentanil loss in 40 days at 37 °C	2772	C

[a]Tested in PVC/Kalex 3000 (phthalate ester) CADD pump reservoirs.
[b]Tested in PVC containers.
[c]Tested in polypropylene bags (Mark II Polybags).
[d]Tested in glass containers.
[e]Tested in PVC containers.
[f]Tested in SynchroMed II implantable pumps.
[g]Sufentanil citrate powder dissolved in ziconotide acetate injection.

Drugs in Syringe Compatibility

Sufentanil citrate

Drug (in syringe)	Mfr	Amt	Mfr	Amt	Remarks	Ref	C/I
Atracurium besylate	BW	10 mg/mL		50 mcg/mL	Physically compatible and atracurium stable for 24 hr at 5 and 30 °C	1694	C

Y-Site Injection Compatibility (1:1 Mixture)

Sufentanil citrate

Drug	Mfr	Conc	Mfr	Conc	Remarks	Ref	C/I
Amphotericin B cholesteryl sulfate complex	SEQ	0.83 mg/mL[a]	JN	0.05 mg/mL	Physically compatible for 4 hr at 23 °C	2117	C
Bivalirudin	TMC	5 mg/mL[a]	ES	50 mcg/mL	Physically compatible for 4 hr at 23 °C	2373	C
Cefepime HCl	BMS	120 mg/mL[c]		5 mcg/mL	Physically compatible with less than 10% cefepime loss. Sufentanil not tested	2513	C
Ceftazidime	SKB	125 mg/mL		50 mcg/mL	Visually compatible with less than 10% loss of ceftazidime in 24 hr. Sufentanil not tested	2434	C
	GSK	120 mg/mL[c]		5 mcg/mL	Physically compatible with less than 10% ceftazidime loss. Sufentanil not tested	2513	C
Cisatracurium besylate	GW	0.1, 2, 5 mg/mL[a]	ES	0.0125 mg/mL[a]	Physically compatible for 4 hr at 23 °C	2074	C
Dexmedetomidine HCl	AB	4 mcg/mL[b]	AB	50 mcg/mL	Physically compatible for 4 hr at 23 °C	2383	C
Etomidate	AB	2 mg/mL	JN	0.05 mg/mL	Visually compatible for 7 days at 25 °C	1801	C
Fenoldopam mesylate	AB	80 mcg/mL[b]	BA	12.5 mcg/mL[b]	Physically compatible for 4 hr at 23 °C	2467	C
Hetastarch in lactated electrolyte	AB	6%	BA	12.5 mcg/mL[a]	Physically compatible for 4 hr at 23 °C	2339	C
Linezolid	PHU	2 mg/mL	ES	0.05 mg/mL	Physically compatible for 4 hr at 23 °C	2264	C
Palonosetron HCl	MGI	50 mcg/mL	HOS	12.5 mcg/mL[a]	Physically compatible. No loss of either drug in 4 hr	2720	C

Y-Site Injection Compatibility (1:1 Mixture) (Cont.)

Sufentanil citrate

Drug	Mfr	Conc	Mfr	Conc	Remarks	Ref	C/I
Propofol	ZEN	10 mg/mL	JN	0.05 mg/mL	Physically compatible for 1 hr at 23 °C	2066	C
Remifentanil HCl	GW	0.025 and 0.25 mg/mL[b]	ES	0.0125 mg/mL[a]	Physically compatible for 4 hr at 23 °C	2075	C

[a]*Tested in dextrose 5%.*
[b]*Tested in sodium chloride 0.9%.*
[c]*Tested in sterile water for injection.*

SUMATRIPTAN SUCCINATE
AHFS 28:32.28

Products — Sumatriptan succinate is available at a concentration of 6 mg/0.5 mL with sodium chloride 3.5 mg/0.5 mL in water for injection in single-dose vials and prefilled syringes. The drug is also available at a concentration of 4 mg/0.5 mL with sodium chloride 3.8 mg/0.5 mL in water for injection in prefilled syringes. (1)

pH — Approximately 4.2 to 5.3. (1)

Osmolality — The solution is nearly isotonic with an osmolality of 291 mOsm/kg. (1)

Trade Name(s) — Imitrex.

Administration — Sumatriptan succinate is administered subcutaneously. It should not be given by other routes of administration. (1)

Stability — Intact containers of sumatriptan succinate should be stored between 2 and 30 °C and protected from light. The injection is a clear, colorless to light yellow solution. (1)

Syringes — The stability of sumatriptan succinate (Glaxo Wellcome) 12 mg/mL packaged as 1 mL of solution drawn into 1-mL polypropylene tuberculin syringes was evaluated stored under refrigeration and at room temperature of 25 °C both exposed to and protected from fluorescent light. The room temperature samples were evaluated over 24 hours while the refrigerated samples were evaluated over 72 hours. No visible indications of physical instability were observed, and no loss of sumatriptan was found. (2276)

TACROLIMUS
AHFS 92:44

Products — Tacrolimus injection is available in 1-mL ampuls containing the equivalent of 5 mg of anhydrous tacrolimus per milliliter. In addition to tacrolimus, each milliliter contains polyoxyl 60 hydrogenated castor oil (surfactant) 200 mg and dehydrated alcohol, USP, 80% (v/v). The product is a concentrate that must be diluted for use in dextrose 5% or sodium chloride 0.9%. (1)

Trade Name(s) — Prograf.

Administration — Tacrolimus is administered by intravenous infusion diluted to a final concentration of 0.004 to 0.02 mg/mL (4 to 20 mcg/mL) in dextrose 5% or sodium chloride 0.9%. Intravenous solution containers should be made of glass or polyethylene; PVC containers plasticized with diethylhexyl phthalate (DEHP) should be avoided due to leaching of plasticizer and decreased stability. For dilute solutions of tacrolimus, non-PVC tubing should also be used to minimize the potential for significant drug sorption. (1)

Stability — Intact ampuls should be stored at temperatures between 5 and 25 °C. (1) Tacrolimus exhibits a minimum rate of decomposition at pH values between 2 and 6; the rate of decomposition increases substantially at higher pH values (1926) and is unstable above pH 9. (2216) The manufacturer recommends that tacrolimus not be mixed with or even co-infused with solutions having a pH of 9 or greater. (1)

Syringes — Tacrolimus (Fujisawa) 100 mcg/mL in sodium chloride 0.9% was packaged 20 mL in 30-mL plastic syringes (Becton Dickinson) and stored at 24 °C exposed to normal room light and protected from light. No decrease in tacrolimus concentration was found after storage for 24 hours. (1864)

Sorption — Tacrolimus (Fujisawa) 100 mcg/mL in dextrose 5% was delivered through PVC anesthesia extension tubing (Abbott), PVC intravenous administration set tubing (Venoset, Abbott), and fat emulsion tubing (Abbott). The delivered solutions had no loss of tacrolimus using the PVC administration set tubing and the fat emulsion tubing and only 2.5% drug loss from the PVC anesthesia extension tubing. (1864)

Tacrolimus 50 mcg/mL delivered through 100 cm of PVC tubing at a rate of 5 mL/hr resulted in the delivery of 76% of the tacrolimus concentration. No loss due to sorption occurred when the tacrolimus solution was delivered through polyolefin tubing. (2452)

Plasticizer Leaching — Parenteral products containing a large amount of surfactant in the formulation such as tacrolimus injection will extract the plasticizer DEHP from PVC containers and administration sets. Consequently, their use should be avoided for tacrolimus. Instead, glass or polyethylene containers and non-DEHP plasticized administration sets are recommended. (1; 4; 1683)

Tacrolimus 50 mcg/mL delivered through 100 cm of PVC tubing at a rate of 5 mL/hr leached 12 mcg/mL of DEHP into the drug solution. No plasticizer leached when the tacrolimus solution was delivered through similar polyolefin tubing. (2452)

Tacrolimus 0.02 mg/mL in dextrose 5% in VISIV polyolefin bags was tested at room temperature near 23 °C for 24 hours. No leached plastic components were found within the 24-hour study period. (2660; 2792)

Compatibility Information

Solution Compatibility

Tacrolimus

Solution	Mfr	Mfr	Conc/L	Remarks	Ref	C/I
Dextrose 5%			4 to 20 mg	Stable for 24 hr	1	**C**
	AB[a]	FUJ	100 mg	5 to 8% loss in 48 hr at 24 °C	1864	**C**
	AB[b]	FUJ	100 mg	15% loss in 6 hr and 19% loss in 24 hr at 24 °C	1864	**I**
Sodium chloride 0.9%			4 to 20 mg	Stable for 24 hr	1	**C**
	BA[c]	FUJ	10 mg	Visually compatible with 4% loss in 48 hr	1854	**C**
	AB[c]	FUJ	100 mg	10 to 12% loss in 24 hr at 24 °C	1864	**C**
	AB[b]	FUJ	100 mg	12% loss in 6 hr and 16% loss in 24 hr at 24 °C	1864	**I**
TPN #201[d]	c	FUJ	100 mg	Visually compatible with no loss in 24 hr at 24 °C	1922	**C**

[a]*Tested in glass and polyolefin containers.*
[b]*Tested in PVC containers.*
[c]*Tested in glass containers.*
[d]*Refer to Appendix I for the composition of parenteral nutrition solutions. TPN indicates a 2-in-1 admixture.*

Y-Site Injection Compatibility (1:1 Mixture)

Tacrolimus

Drug	Mfr	Conc	Mfr	Conc	Remarks	Ref	C/I
Acyclovir sodium			FUJ		Significant tacrolimus loss within 15 min	191	**I**
Aminophylline	ES	2 mg/mL[a]	FUJ	1 mg/mL[b]	Visually compatible for 24 hr at 25 °C	1630	**C**
Amphotericin B	LY	5 mg/mL[a]	FUJ	1 mg/mL[c]	Visually compatible for 24 hr at 25 °C	1630	**C**
Ampicillin sodium	WY	20 mg/mL[a]	FUJ	1 mg/mL[b]	Visually compatible for 24 hr at 25 °C	1630	**C**
Ampicillin sodium–sulbactam sodium	RR	33.3 + 16.7 mg/mL[a]	FUJ	1 mg/mL[b]	Visually compatible for 24 hr at 25 °C	1630	**C**
Anidulafungin	VIC	0.5 mg/mL[a]	FUJ	20 mcg/mL[a]	Physically compatible for 4 hr at 23 °C	2617	**C**
Benztropine mesylate	MSD	1 mg/mL[a]	FUJ	1 mg/mL[b]	Visually compatible for 24 hr at 25 °C	1630	**C**
Calcium gluconate	ES	100 mg/mL	FUJ	1 mg/mL[b]	Visually compatible for 24 hr at 25 °C	1630	**C**
Caspofungin acetate	ME	0.7 mg/mL[b]	AST	0.02 mg/mL[b]	Physically compatible for 4 hr at room temperature	2758	**C**
Cefazolin sodium	BR	40 mg/mL[a]	FUJ	1 mg/mL[b]	Visually compatible for 24 hr at 25 °C	1630	**C**
Cefotetan disodium	STU	40 mg/mL[a]	FUJ	1 mg/mL[b]	Visually compatible for 24 hr at 25 °C	1630	**C**
Ceftazidime	GL	20 mg/mL[a]	FUJ	1 mg/mL[b]	Visually compatible for 24 hr at 25 °C	1630	**C**

Y-Site Injection Compatibility (1:1 Mixture) (Cont.)

Tacrolimus

Drug	Mfr	Conc	Mfr	Conc	Remarks	Ref	C/I
	GW	40 and 200 mg/mL[a]	FUJ	10 and 40 mcg/mL[a]	Visually compatible with no loss of either drug in 4 hr at 24 °C	2216	C
Ceftriaxone sodium	RC	40 mg/mL[a]	FUJ	1 mg/mL[b]	Visually compatible for 24 hr at 25 °C	1630	C
Cefuroxime sodium	LI	30 mg/mL[a]	FUJ	1 mg/mL[b]	Visually compatible for 24 hr at 25 °C	1630	C
Chloramphenicol sodium succinate	PD	20 mg/mL[a]	FUJ	1 mg/mL[b]	Visually compatible for 24 hr at 25 °C	1630	C
Ciprofloxacin	MI	1 mg/mL[a]	FUJ	1 mg/mL[b]	Visually compatible for 24 hr at 25 °C	1630	C
Clindamycin phosphate	ES	12 mg/mL[a]	FUJ	1 mg/mL[b]	Visually compatible for 24 hr at 25 °C	1630	C
Dexamethasone sodium phosphate	ES	4 mg/mL[a]	FUJ	1 mg/mL[b]	Visually compatible for 24 hr at 25 °C	1630	C
Digoxin	WY	0.25 mg/mL	FUJ	1 mg/mL[b]	Visually compatible for 24 hr at 25 °C	1630	C
Diphenhydramine HCl	ES	1 mg/mL[a]	FUJ	1 mg/mL[b]	Visually compatible for 24 hr at 25 °C	1630	C
Dobutamine HCl	LI	1 mg/mL[a]	FUJ	1 mg/mL[b]	Visually compatible for 24 hr at 25 °C	1630	C
Dopamine HCl	ES	1.6 mg/mL[a]	FUJ	1 mg/mL[b]	Visually compatible for 24 hr at 25 °C	1630	C
Doripenem	JJ	5 mg/mL[a,b]	ASP	0.02 mg/mL[a,b]	Physically compatible for 4 hr at 23 °C	2743	C
Doxycycline hyclate	RR	5 mg/mL[a]	FUJ	1 mg/mL[b]	Visually compatible for 24 hr at 25 °C	1630	C
Erythromycin lactobionate	AB	20 mg/mL[a]	FUJ	1 mg/mL[b]	Visually compatible for 24 hr at 25 °C	1630	C
Esmolol HCl	DU	10 mg/mL[a]	FUJ	1 mg/mL[b]	Visually compatible for 24 hr at 25 °C	1630	C
Fluconazole	RR	2 mg/mL[a]	FUJ	1 mg/mL[b]	Visually compatible for 24 hr at 25 °C	1630	C
	PF	0.5 and 1.5 mg/mL[b]	FUJ	5 and 20 mcg/mL[b]	Visually compatible. No loss of either drug in 3 hr at 24 °C	2236	C
Furosemide	ES	10 mg/mL	FUJ	1 mg/mL[b]	Visually compatible for 24 hr at 25 °C	1630	C
Ganciclovir sodium			FUJ		Significant tacrolimus loss within 15 min	191	I
Gentamicin sulfate	SCN	4 mg/mL[a]	FUJ	1 mg/mL[b]	Visually compatible for 24 hr at 25 °C	1630	C
Haloperidol lactate	SO	2.5 mg/mL[a]	FUJ	1 mg/mL[b]	Visually compatible for 24 hr at 25 °C	1630	C
Heparin sodium	ES	10 units/mL[a]	FUJ	1 mg/mL[b]	Visually compatible for 24 hr at 25 °C	1630	C
Hydrocortisone sodium succinate	AB	50 mg/mL[a]	FUJ	1 mg/mL[b]	Visually compatible for 24 hr at 25 °C	1630	C
Hydromorphone HCl	KN	2 and 0.2 mg/mL[a]	FUJ	10 and 40 mcg/mL[a]	Visually compatible. No loss of either drug in 4 hr at 24 °C	2216	C
Imipenem–cilastatin sodium	MSD	10 mg/mL[b]	FUJ	1 mg/mL[b]	Visually compatible for 24 hr at 25 °C	1630	C
Insulin, regular	LI	0.1 unit/mL[a]	FUJ	1 mg/mL[b]	Visually compatible for 24 hr at 25 °C	1630	C
Isoproterenol HCl	ES	0.04 mg/mL[a]	FUJ	1 mg/mL[b]	Visually compatible for 24 hr at 25 °C	1630	C
Leucovorin calcium	ES	10 mg/mL[a]	FUJ	1 mg/mL[b]	Visually compatible for 24 hr at 25 °C	1630	C
Lorazepam	WY	1 mg/mL[a]	FUJ	1 mg/mL[b]	Visually compatible for 24 hr at 25 °C	1630	C
Methylprednisolone sodium succinate	UP	0.8 mg/mL[a]	FUJ	1 mg/mL[b]	Visually compatible for 24 hr at 25 °C	1630	C
Metoclopramide HCl	DU	0.2 mg/mL[a]	FUJ	1 mg/mL[b]	Visually compatible for 24 hr at 25 °C	1630	C
Metronidazole	AB	5 mg/mL	FUJ	1 mg/mL[b]	Visually compatible for 24 hr at 25 °C	1630	C
Micafungin sodium	ASP	1.5 mg/mL[b]	FUJ	20 mcg/mL[b]	Physically compatible for 4 hr at 23 °C	2683	C
Morphine sulfate	SCN	1 and 3 mg/mL[b]	FUJ	10 and 40 mcg/mL[b]	Visually compatible. No loss of either drug in 4 hr at 24 °C	2216	C

Y-Site Injection Compatibility (1:1 Mixture) (Cont.)

Tacrolimus

Drug	Mfr	Conc	Mfr	Conc	Remarks	Ref	C/I
Multivitamins	LY	0.001 mL/mL[a]	FUJ	1 mg/mL[b]	Visually compatible for 24 hr at 25 °C	1630	C
Mycophenolate mofetil HCl	RC	5.9 mg/mL[a]	FUJ	0.02 mg/mL[a]	Physically compatible and 2% mycophenolate mofetil loss in 4 hr	2738	C
Nitroglycerin	DU	0.1 mg/mL[a]	FUJ	1 mg/mL[b]	Visually compatible for 24 hr at 25 °C	1630	C
Oxacillin sodium	BR	40 mg/mL[a]	FUJ	1 mg/mL[b]	Visually compatible for 24 hr at 25 °C	1630	C
Penicillin G potassium	BR	100,000 units/mL[a]	FUJ	1 mg/mL[b]	Visually compatible for 24 hr at 25 °C	1630	C
Phenytoin sodium	ES	5 mg/mL[a]	FUJ	1 mg/mL[b]	Visually compatible for 4 hr at 25 °C. White haze forms by 24 hr	1630	C
Potassium chloride	AB	2 mEq/mL	FUJ	1 mg/mL[b]	Visually compatible for 24 hr at 25 °C	1630	C
Propranolol HCl	AY	1 mg/mL	FUJ	1 mg/mL[b]	Visually compatible for 24 hr at 25 °C	1630	C
Ranitidine HCl	GL	25 mg/mL	FUJ	1 mg/mL[b]	Visually compatible for 24 hr at 25 °C	1630	C
Sodium bicarbonate	AB	1 mEq/mL	FUJ	1 mg/mL[b]	Visually compatible for 24 hr at 25 °C	1630	C
Sodium nitroprusside	ES	0.004 mg/mL[a]	FUJ	1 mg/mL[b]	Visually compatible for 24 hr at 25 °C	1630	C
TNA #218 to #226[d]			FUJ	1 mg/mL[a]	Visually compatible for 4 hr at 23 °C	2215	C
Tobramycin sulfate	BR	40 mg/mL	FUJ	1 mg/mL[b]	Visually compatible for 24 hr at 25 °C	1630	C
TPN #212 to #215[d]			FUJ	1 mg/mL[a]	Physically compatible for 4 hr at 23 °C	2109	C
Trimethoprim–sulfamethoxazole	RC	1.6 + 8 mg/mL[a]	FUJ	1 mg/mL[b]	Visually compatible for 24 hr at 25 °C	1630	C
Vancomycin HCl	LI	5 mg/mL[a]	FUJ	1 mg/mL[b]	Visually compatible for 24 hr at 25 °C	1630	C

[a]Tested in dextrose 5%.
[b]Tested in sodium chloride 0.9%.
[c]Diluted with sterile water for injection.
[d]Refer to Appendix I for the composition of parenteral nutrition solutions. TNA indicates a 3-in-1 admixture, and TPN indicates a 2-in-1 admixture.

TEICOPLANIN
AHFS 8:12.28.16

Products — Teicoplanin is available as a lyophilized powder in vials containing teicoplanin 200 and 400 mg. The vials are accompanied by an ampul of water for injection for use as a diluent. Reconstitute by adding the diluent slowly down the side of the vial of teicoplanin and then rolling the vial gently until the powder is completely dissolved. Do not shake the vial. Care should be taken to avoid the formation of foam; if foam does form, the solution should stand for about 15 minutes for the foam to subside. The teicoplanin vials contain a calculated excess so that when reconstituted as directed the full amount of drug can be withdrawn from the vial using a syringe and needle. The concentration is 100 mg in 1.5 mL (from the 200-mg vials) and 400 mg in 3 mL (from the 400-mg vial). (38; 115)

Trade Name(s) — Targocid.

Administration — Teicoplanin may be administered after reconstitution either intramuscularly with a maximum of 3 mL in a single site or by direct intravenous injection as a bolus over 3 to 5 minutes. It may also be administered as an intravenous infusion over 30 minutes after dilution in a compatible infusion solution. The manufacturer recommends dextrose 5%, dextrose 4% and sodium chloride 0.18%, Ringer's injection, lactated, and sodium chloride 0.9% for dilution for intravenous infusion. (38; 115)

Stability — Intact vials of teicoplanin should be stored below 25 °C. The manufacturer recommends that reconstituted teicoplanin be used immediately after preparation and any unused portion be discarded. However, the manufacturer also states that the reconstituted solution may be stored under refrigeration at 4 °C for up to 24 hours if the situation makes discarding the reconstituted drug impractical. Do not store in syringes. (38; 115)

Teicoplanin forms dextrose aldehyde adducts when diluted in dextrose-containing solutions. Equilibrium is reached faster at room temperature (seven days) than with refrigerated storage (30 days). The equilibrium concentration of the adduct is directly related to the dextrose concentration. The reaction is reversible with dilution. (2046)

The stability of catheter flush solutions composed of teicoplanin 133 mg/mL in water for injection, or heparin sodium 10 units/mL or 100 units/mL, was evaluated in Hickman catheters at 25 °C over 24 hours. No decomposition products formed, and no loss was found. Indeed, a small (11%) increase in teicoplanin concentration was observed which was attributed to loss of water. (2165)

The manufacturer recommends use of peritoneal dialysis solutions containing 1.36 or 3.86% dextrose. (38)

Teicoplanin (Marion Merrell Dow) 0.025 mg/mL in Dianeal PD-2 with dextrose 1.5% in PVC containers was physically and chemically stable for 24 hours at 25 °C exposed to light, exhibiting no loss; additional storage for eight hours at 37 °C resulted in losses of 6% or less. Under refrigeration at 4 °C protected from light, no loss occurred in seven days. Additional storage for 16 hours at 25 °C followed by eight hours at 37 °C resulted in about 7% loss. (1989)

Ceftazidime (Glaxo) 0.1 mg/mL admixed with teicoplanin (Marion Merrell Dow) 0.025 mg/mL in Dianeal PD-2 with dextrose 1.5% in PVC containers did not result in a stable mixture. Large (but variable) teicoplanin losses generally in the 20% range were noted in as little as two hours at 25 °C exposed to light. Ceftazidime losses of about 9% occurred in 16 hours. Refrigeration and protection from light of the peritoneal dialysis admixture reduced losses of both drugs to negligible levels. Even so, admixing these two drugs was not recommended because of the high levels of teicoplanin loss at room temperature. (1989)

Teicoplanin (Merrell Dow) 25 mg/L in Dianeal 137 with dextrose 1.36% (Baxter) was evaluated for stability over 42 days. Stored at 4 °C, teicoplanin retained stability with a loss of less than 5% in 42 days. At 20 °C, 10% loss occurred in about 25 days with 17% loss in 42 days. At an elevated temperature of 37 °C, a much greater rate of decomposition occurs with over 40% loss occurring in 42 days. (2145)

Compatibility Information

Solution Compatibility

Teicoplanin

Solution	Mfr	Mfr	Conc/L	Remarks	Ref	C/I
Dextrose 5%	BA[a]	HO	2 g	Visually compatible. No loss in 24 hr at 25 °C	2165	C
	BA[b]	HO	4 g	Visually compatible. 10% loss in 6 days at 4 °C	2364	C
Sodium chloride 0.9%	BA[a]	HO	2 g	Visually compatible. No loss in 24 hr at 25 °C	2165	C

[a]Tested in glass containers.
[b]Tested in PVC containers.

Additive Compatibility

Teicoplanin

Drug	Mfr	Conc/L	Mfr	Conc/L	Test Soln	Remarks	Ref	C/I
Heparin sodium	CPP	20,000 and 40,000 units	HO	2 g	D5W, NS	Visually compatible. No loss of teicoplanin and heparin in 24 hr at 25 °C	2165	C

Y-Site Injection Compatibility (1:1 Mixture)

Teicoplanin

Drug	Mfr	Conc	Mfr	Conc	Remarks	Ref	C/I
Ciprofloxacin	BAY	2 mg/mL[a]	GRP	60 mg/mL	White precipitate forms immediately but disappears with shaking	1934	?

[a]Tested in sodium chloride 0.9%.

TELAVANCIN HYDROCHLORIDE
AHFS 8:12.28.16

Products — Telavancin hydrochloride is available as a lyophilized powder in single-use vials containing telavancin 250 and 750 mg as the hydrochloride. Also present are hydroxypropyl-beta-cyclodextrin, mannitol, and sodium hydroxide and hydrochloric acid to adjust pH. (1)

   Reconstitute the 250-mg vial with 15 mL and the 750-mg vial with 45 mL of dextrose 5%, sterile water for injection, or sodium chloride 0.9% and mix thoroughly to yield a telavancin concentration of 15 mg/mL. Dissolution may occasionally require up to 20 minutes. Discard any vial that does not have a vacuum. (1)

pH — From 4.0 to 5.0. (1)

Trade Name(s) — Vibativ.

Administration — Telavancin hydrochloride is administered by intravenous infusion over 60 minutes after dilution in a compatible infusion solution. For telavancin doses of 150 to 800 mg, dilution in 100 to 250 mL is recommended. For doses outside this range, dilution to a concentration of 0.6 to 8 mg/mL is recommended. The manufacturer recommends dilution in dextrose 5%, sodium chloride 0.9%, or Ringer's injection, lactated. (1)

Stability — Intact vials of telavancin hydrochloride should be stored under refrigeration. The manufacturer recommends that the reconstituted drug should be used within four hours at room temperature or 72 hours under refrigeration. After dilution in a compatible infusion solution, the total time for the reconstituted drug and the diluted solution together should not exceed four hours at room temperature or 72 hours under refrigeration. (1)

Compatibility Information

Solution Compatibility

Telavancin HCl

Solution	Mfr	Mfr	Conc/L	Remarks	Ref	C/I
Dextrose 5%		ASP		Use within 4 hr at room temperature or 72 hr refrigerated	1	C
Ringer's injection, lactated		ASP		Use within 4 hr at room temperature or 72 hr refrigerated	1	C
Sodium chloride 0.9%		FOR		Use within 4 hr at room temperature or 72 hr refrigerated	1	C

Y-Site Injection Compatibility (1:1 Mixture)

Telavancin HCl

Drug	Mfr	Conc	Mfr	Conc	Remarks	Ref	C/I
Amphotericin B	XGN	0.1 mg/mL[a]	ASP	7.5 mg/mL[a]	Increase in measured turbidity	2830	I
Amphotericin B lipid complex	ENZ	1 mg/mL[a]	ASP	7.5 mg/mL[a]	Physically compatible for 2 hr	2830	C
Amphotericin B liposomal	ASP	1 mg/mL[a]	ASP	7.5 mg/mL[a]	Increase in measured turbidity	2830	I
Ampicillin sodium–sulbactam sodium	BA	20 + 10 mg/mL[a,b,c]	ASP	7.5 mg/mL[a,b,c]	Physically compatible for 2 hr	2830	C
Azithromycin	APP	2 mg/mL[a,b,c]	ASP	7.5 mg/mL[a,b,c]	Physically compatible for 2 hr	2830	C
Calcium gluconate	APP	40 mg/mL[a,b,c]	ASP	7.5 mg/mL[a,b,c]	Physically compatible for 2 hr	2830	C
Caspofungin acetate	ME	0.5 mg/mL[b]	ASP	7.5 mg/mL[b]	Physically compatible for 2 hr	2830	C
Cefepime HCl	SAG	40 mg/mL[a,b,c]	ASP	7.5 mg/mL[a,b,c]	Physically compatible for 2 hr	2830	C
Ceftazidime	HOS	40 mg/mL[a,b,c]	ASP	7.5 mg/mL[a,b,c]	Physically compatible for 2 hr	2830	C
Ceftriaxone sodium	HOS	20 mg/mL[a,b]	ASP	7.5 mg/mL[a,b]	Physically compatible for 2 hr	2830	C
Ciprofloxacin	BED	2 mg/mL[a]	ASP	7.5 mg/mL[a]	Physically compatible for 2 hr	2830	C
Colistimethate sodium	PAD	4.5 mg/mL[a]	ASP	7.5 mg/mL[a]	Visible turbidity formed	2830	I
	PAD	4.5 mg/mL[b,c]	ASP	7.5 mg/mL[b,c]	Physically compatible for 2 hr	2830	C
Cyclosporine	BED	5 mg/mL[b,c]	ASP	7.5 mg/mL[b,c]	Increase in measured turbidity	2830	I
	BED	5 mg/mL[a]	ASP	7.5 mg/mL[a]	Physically compatible for 2 hr	2830	C

Y-Site Injection Compatibility (1:1 Mixture) (Cont.)

Telavancin HCl

Drug	Mfr	Conc	Mfr	Conc	Remarks	Ref	C/I
Dexamethasone sodium phosphate	AMR	1 mg/mL[a,b,c]	ASP	7.5 mg/mL[a,b,c]	Physically compatible for 2 hr	2830	**C**
Digoxin	BA	0.25 mg/mL	ASP	7.5 mg/mL[a,b,c]	Visible turbidity formed	2830	**I**
Diltiazem HCl	BED	5 mg/mL	ASP	7.5 mg/mL[a,b,c]	Physically compatible for 2 hr	2830	**C**
Dobutamine HCl	HOS	4 mg/mL[a,b,c]	ASP	7.5 mg/mL[a,b,c]	Physically compatible for 2 hr	2830	**C**
Dopamine HCl	HOS	3.2 mg/mL[a,b,c]	ASP	7.5 mg/mL[a,b,c]	Physically compatible for 2 hr	2830	**C**
Doripenem	OMN	10 mg/mL[a,b]	ASP	7.5 mg/mL[a,b]	Physically compatible for 2 hr	2830	**C**
Doxycycline hyclate	APP	1 mg/mL[a,b,c]	ASP	7.5 mg/mL[a,b,c]	Physically compatible for 2 hr	2830	**C**
Ertapenem sodium	ME	20 mg/mL[b]	ASP	7.5 mg/mL[b]	Physically compatible for 2 hr	2830	**C**
Esomeprazole sodium	ASZ	0.4 mg/mL[a,b,c]	ASP	7.5 mg/mL[a,b,c]	Discoloration and increase in measured turbidity	2830	**I**
Famotidine	BED	2 mg/mL[a,b,c]	ASP	7.5 mg/mL[a,b,c]	Physically compatible for 2 hr	2830	**C**
Fluconazole	SAG	2 mg/mL[b]	ASP	7.5 mg/mL[b]	Physically compatible for 2 hr	2830	**C**
Furosemide	HOS	3 mg/mL[a,b,c]	ASP	7.5 mg/mL[a,b,c]	Immediate precipitation	2830	**I**
Gentamicin sulfate	HOS	5 mg/mL[a,b,c]	ASP	7.5 mg/mL[a,b,c]	Physically compatible for 2 hr	2830	**C**
Heparin sodium	APP	1000 units/mL[a,b]	ASP	7.5 mg/mL[a,b]	Measured turbidity increased	2830	**I**
	APP	1000 units/mL[c]	ASP	7.5 mg/mL[c]	Physically compatible for 2 hr	2830	**C**
Hydrocortisone sodium succinate	PF	1 mg/mL[a,b,c]	ASP	7.5 mg/mL[a,b,c]	Physically compatible for 2 hr	2830	**C**
Imipenem–cilastatin sodium	ME	5 mg/mL[a]	ASP	7.5 mg/mL[a]	Slight measured turbidity increase	2830	**I**
	ME	5 mg/mL[b]	ASP	7.5 mg/mL[b]	Physically compatible for 2 hr	2830	**C**
Labetalol HCl	BED	5 mg/mL	ASP	7.5 mg/mL[a,b,c]	Physically compatible for 2 hr	2830	**C**
Levofloxacin	OMN	5 mg/mL[a,b,c]	ASP	7.5 mg/mL[a,b,c]	Discoloration and measured haze increase	2830	**I**
Magnesium sulfate	AMR	100 mg/mL[a,b,c]	ASP	7.5 mg/mL[a,b,c]	Physically compatible for 2 hr	2830	**C**
Mannitol	HOS	20%	ASP	7.5 mg/mL[a,b,c]	Physically compatible for 2 hr	2830	**C**
Meropenem	ASZ	10 mg/mL[a,b,c]	ASP	7.5 mg/mL[a,b,c]	Physically compatible for 2 hr	2830	**C**
Methylprednisolone sodium succinate	PF	5 mg/mL[a]	ASP	7.5 mg/mL[a]	Slight measured turbidity increase	2830	**I**
	PF	5 mg/mL[b,c]	ASP	7.5 mg/mL[b,c]	Physically compatible for 2 hr	2830	**C**
Metoclopramide HCl	HOS	1 mg/mL[a,b,c]	ASP	7.5 mg/mL[a,b,c]	Physically compatible for 2 hr	2830	**C**
Micafungin sodium	ASP	5 mg/mL[a,b]	ASP	7.5 mg/mL[a,b]	Visible haze forms	2830	**I**
Milrinone lactate	BED	0.2 mg/mL[a,b,c]	ASP	7.5 mg/mL[a,b,c]	Physically compatible for 2 hr	2830	**C**
Norepinephrine bitartrate	BED	0.128 mg/mL[a,b,c]	ASP	7.5 mg/mL[a,b,c]	Physically compatible for 2 hr	2830	**C**
Ondansetron HCl	BA	1 mg/mL[a,b,c]	ASP	7.5 mg/mL[a,b,c]	Physically compatible for 2 hr	2830	**C**
Pantoprazole sodium	WY[d]	0.4 mg/mL[a,b,c]	ASP	7.5 mg/mL[a,b,c]	Physically compatible for 2 hr	2830	**C**
Phenylephrine HCl	SZ	1 mg/mL[a,b,c]	ASP	7.5 mg/mL[a,b,c]	Physically compatible for 2 hr	2830	**C**
Piperacillin sodium–tazobactam sodium	WY[d]	40 + 5 mg/mL[a,b,c]	ASP	7.5 mg/mL[a,b,c]	Physically compatible for 2 hr	2830	**C**
Potassium chloride	HOS	0.1 mEq/mL[a,b,c]	ASP	7.5 mg/mL[a,b,c]	Physically compatible for 2 hr	2830	**C**

Y-Site Injection Compatibility (1:1 Mixture) (Cont.)

Telavancin HCl

Drug	Mfr	Conc	Mfr	Conc	Remarks	Ref	C/I
Potassium phosphates	AMR	0.5 mmol/mL[a,b,c]	ASP	7.5 mg/mL[a,b,c]	Physically compatible for 2 hr	2830	**C**
Propofol	APP	10 mg/mL	ASP	7.5 mg/mL[a]	Physically compatible for 2 hr	2830	**C**
	APP	10 mg/mL	ASP	7.5 mg/mL[b,c]	Emulsion broke and oiled out	2830	**I**
Ranitidine HCl	BED	2 mg/mL[a,b,c]	ASP	7.5 mg/mL[a,b,c]	Physically compatible for 2 hr	2830	**C**
Sodium bicarbonate	HOS	1 mEq/mL	ASP	7.5 mg/mL[a,b,c]	Physically compatible for 2 hr	2830	**C**
Sodium phosphates	HOS	0.5 mmol/mL[a,b,c]	ASP	7.5 mg/mL[a,b,c]	Physically compatible for 2 hr	2830	**C**
Tigecycline	WY	1 mg/mL[a,b,c]	ASP	7.5 mg/mL[a,b,c]	Physically compatible for 2 hr	2830	**C**
Tobramycin sulfate	HOS	5 mg/mL[a,b]	ASP	7.5 mg/mL[a,b]	Physically compatible for 2 hr	2830	**C**
Vasopressin	AMR	1 unit/mL[a,b,c]	ASP	7.5 mg/mL[a,b,c]	Physically compatible for 2 hr	2830	**C**

[a]*Tested in dextrose 5%.*
[b]*Tested in sodium chloride 0.9%.*
[c]*Tested in Ringer's injection, lactated.*
[d]*Test performed using the formulation WITH edetate disodium.*

TENIPOSIDE
(VM-26)
AHFS 10:00

Products — Teniposide is available in 5-mL ampuls containing 50 mg of drug. Each milliliter of solution contains teniposide 10 mg, benzyl alcohol 30 mg, *N,N*-dimethylacetamide 60 mg, polyoxyethylated castor oil (Cremophor EL) 500 mg, and dehydrated alcohol 42.7% (v/v). The pH is adjusted with maleic acid. The product is a concentrate that must be diluted for use. (1)

pH — Approximately 5. (1)

Trade Name(s) — Vumon.

Administration — Teniposide is administered by slow intravenous infusion over at least 30 to 60 minutes after dilution in dextrose 5% or sodium chloride 0.9% to a final concentration of 0.1, 0.2, 0.4, or 1 mg/mL. (1) Extended infusions of 0.1- and 0.2-mg/mL solutions over 24 hours have resulted in precipitation. (1; 1502; 1521) The intravenous solution containers and sets used to administer teniposide should not contain the plasticizer diethylhexyl phthalate (DEHP). Extravasation should be avoided because of local tissue irritation and phlebitis. (1; 4)

Heparin sodium can cause precipitation of teniposide. Administration apparatus should be thoroughly flushed before and after teniposide administration with dextrose 5% or sodium chloride 0.9%. (1; 1502)

Contact of the undiluted teniposide concentrate with plastic equipment and devices during preparation has resulted in softening of the plastic, cracking, and leakage. Damage to plastic equipment has not been reported with diluted solutions. (1)

Stability — The teniposide concentrate is clear (1) but may exhibit a slight opalescence when diluted in infusion solutions due to the surfactant content. (234)

Intact ampuls should be stored under refrigeration in the original package to protect from light. Teniposide stability is not adversely affected by freezing (1) or exposure to normal room fluorescent light during administration. (1374)

The manufacturer does not recommend refrigeration of teniposide diluted in infusion solutions. (1)

Precipitation — Although teniposide is chemically stable for at least 24 hours, precipitation from aqueous solutions has occurred irregularly and unpredictably even at 0.1 and 0.2 mg/mL, the lowest recommended concentrations. (1; 1502; 1521) The precipitation rate depends on the formation of crystallization nuclei. Precipitation then proceeds rapidly. The formation of crystallization nuclei may be accelerated by agitation, contact with incompatible drugs or material surfaces, and, possibly, other factors. (1374; 1502; 1521) The manufacturer recommends avoiding an inordinate amount of agitation during preparation, minimizing storage time prior to administration, and avoiding contact with other drugs and solutions. Even the compatibility of teniposide infusions with some infusion set materials and pumps cannot be assured. (1; 1502; 1521)

Sorption — No teniposide loss due to sorption to PVC containers has been observed. (1374; 2053)

Plasticizer Leaching — The surfactant, Cremophor EL, in the teniposide formulation leaches the plasticizer DEHP from PVC containers and sets. The amount leached increases with time and drug concentration and is similar for sodium chloride 0.9% and dextrose 5%. The use of non-PVC containers, such as glass bottles and polyolefin bags, and non-PVC administration sets, such as lipid administration sets and nitroglycerin sets, is recommended. (1)

Teniposide (Bristol) 0.1 mg/mL in dextrose 5% leached relatively large amounts of DEHP from PVC bags due to the Cremophor EL surfactant in the formulation. After eight hours at 24 °C, the DEHP concentration in 50-mL bags of infusion solution was as much as 7.5 mcg/mL; it continued to increase through 24 hours to 22.2 mcg/mL. This finding is consistent with the surfactant concentration (1%) of the final admixture solution. The actual amount of DEHP leached from PVC containers and administration sets may vary in clinical situations, depending on surfactant concentration, bag size, and contact time. (1683)

Substantial leaching of DEHP plasticizer was reported from PVC bags of dextrose 5% and sodium chloride 0.9% and PVC administration sets by teniposide admixtures containing 0.4 mg/mL of the drug due to the Cremophor EL surfactant used in the formulation. DEHP levels increased throughout the one-hour infusion time to over 20 mcg/mL from both the bags and sets. There was no difference in plasticizer leaching between the two infusion solutions. Storage of the teniposide 0.4-mg/mL admixtures for 48 hours at both 4 and 24 °C resulted in substantially greater DEHP leaching. DEHP concentrations ranged from about 60 mcg/mL in the refrigerated samples to over 200 mcg/mL (a total of 52 mg) in the room temperature samples. The actual amount of DEHP a patient will receive is dependent on a number of factors, including Cremophor EL concentration, storage temperature, and contact time. No plasticizer was leached from glass bottles or polyolefin infusion containers. To minimize plasticizer leaching if PVC containers and sets must be used, it is recommended that teniposide admixtures be used immediately after preparation and administered over no more than one hour. (2053)

An acceptability limit of no more than 5 parts per million (5 mcg/mL) for DEHP plasticizer released from PVC containers, administration sets, and other equipment has been proposed. The limit was based on a review of metabolic and toxicologic considerations. (2185)

Teniposide 0.1 mg/mL in dextrose 5% in VISIV polyolefin bags was tested at room temperature near 23 °C for 24 hours. No leached plastic components were found within the 24-hour study period. (2660; 2792)

Compatibility Information

Solution Compatibility

Teniposide

Solution	Mfr	Mfr	Conc/L	Remarks	Ref	C/I
Dextrose 5%			100, 200, 400 mg	Stable for 24 hr at room temperature	1	C
			1 g	May precipitate in 4 hr	1	?
	a	BR	400 mg	Physically compatible. 6% loss in 4 days at 21 °C in light or dark	1374	C
Ringer's injection, lactated	a	BR	400 mg	Physically compatible. 3% loss in 4 days at 21 °C in light or dark	1374	C
Sodium chloride 0.9%			100, 200, 400 mg	Stable for 24 hr at room temperature	1	C
			1 g	May precipitate in 4 hr	1	?
	b	BR	400 mg	Physically compatible. 4% loss in 4 days at 21 °C in light or dark	1374	C
	a	BR	500, 600, 700 mg	Physically compatible for 4 days at 21 °C	1374	C

[a]Tested in glass containers.
[b]Tested in both glass and PVC containers.

Y-Site Injection Compatibility (1:1 Mixture)

Teniposide

Drug	Mfr	Conc	Mfr	Conc	Remarks	Ref	C/I
Acyclovir sodium	BW	7 mg/mL[a]	BR	0.1 mg/mL[a]	Physically compatible for 4 hr at 23 °C	1725	C
Allopurinol sodium	BW	3 mg/mL[a]	BR	0.1 mg/mL[a]	Physically compatible for 4 hr at 23 °C	1725	C

Y-Site Injection Compatibility (1:1 Mixture) (Cont.)

Teniposide

Drug	Mfr	Conc	Mfr	Conc	Remarks	Ref	C/I
Amifostine	USB	10 mg/mL[a]	BR	0.1 mg/mL[a]	Physically compatible for 4 hr at 23 °C	1845	C
Amikacin sulfate	BR	5 mg/mL[a]	BR	0.1 mg/mL[a]	Physically compatible for 4 hr at 23 °C	1725	C
Aminophylline	AB	2.5 mg/mL[a]	BR	0.1 mg/mL[a]	Physically compatible for 4 hr at 23 °C	1725	C
Amphotericin B	SQ	0.6 mg/mL[a]	BR	0.1 mg/mL[a]	Physically compatible for 4 hr at 23 °C	1725	C
Ampicillin sodium	WY	20 mg/mL[b]	BR	0.1 mg/mL[a]	Physically compatible for 4 hr at 23 °C	1725	C
Ampicillin sodium–sulbactam sodium	RR	20 + 10 mg/mL[b]	BR	0.1 mg/mL[a]	Physically compatible for 4 hr at 23 °C	1725	C
Aztreonam	SQ	40 mg/mL[a]	BR	0.1 mg/mL[a]	Physically compatible for 4 hr at 23 °C	1725; 1758	C
Bleomycin sulfate	BR	1 unit/mL[b]	BR	0.1 mg/mL[a]	Physically compatible for 4 hr at 23 °C	1725	C
Bumetanide	RC	0.04 mg/mL[a]	BR	0.1 mg/mL[a]	Physically compatible for 4 hr at 23 °C	1725	C
Buprenorphine HCl	RKC	0.04 mg/mL[a]	BR	0.1 mg/mL[a]	Physically compatible for 4 hr at 23 °C	1725	C
Butorphanol tartrate	BR	0.04 mg/mL[a]	BR	0.1 mg/mL[a]	Physically compatible for 4 hr at 23 °C	1725	C
Calcium gluconate	AMR	40 mg/mL[a]	BR	0.1 mg/mL[a]	Physically compatible for 4 hr at 23 °C	1725	C
Carboplatin	BR	5 mg/mL[a]	BR	0.1 mg/mL[a]	Physically compatible for 4 hr at 23 °C	1725	C
Carmustine	BR	1.5 mg/mL[a]	BR	0.1 mg/mL[a]	Physically compatible for 4 hr at 23 °C	1725	C
Cefazolin sodium	MAR	20 mg/mL[a]	BR	0.1 mg/mL[a]	Physically compatible for 4 hr at 23 °C	1725	C
Cefotaxime sodium	HO	20 mg/mL[a]	BR	0.1 mg/mL[a]	Physically compatible for 1 hr at 23 °C	1725	C
Cefotetan disodium	STU	20 mg/mL[a]	BR	0.1 mg/mL[a]	Physically compatible for 4 hr at 23 °C	1725	C
Cefoxitin sodium	MSD	20 mg/mL[a]	BR	0.1 mg/mL[a]	Physically compatible for 4 hr at 23 °C	1725	C
Ceftazidime	LI	40 mg/mL[a]	BR	0.1 mg/mL[a]	Physically compatible for 4 hr at 23 °C	1725	C
Ceftriaxone sodium	RC	20 mg/mL[a]	BR	0.1 mg/mL[a]	Physically compatible for 4 hr at 23 °C	1725	C
Cefuroxime sodium	GL	20 mg/mL[a]	BR	0.1 mg/mL[a]	Physically compatible for 4 hr at 23 °C	1725	C
Chlorpromazine HCl	SCN	2 mg/mL[a]	BR	0.1 mg/mL[a]	Physically compatible for 4 hr at 23 °C	1725	C
Ciprofloxacin	MI	2 mg/mL[a]	BR	0.1 mg/mL[a]	Physically compatible for 4 hr at 23 °C	1725	C
Cisplatin	BR	1 mg/mL	BR	0.1 mg/mL[a]	Physically compatible for 4 hr at 23 °C	1725	C
Cladribine	ORT	0.015[b] and 0.5[c] mg/mL	BR	0.1 mg/mL[b]	Physically compatible for 4 hr at 23 °C	1969	C
Clindamycin phosphate	AST	10 mg/mL[a]	BR	0.1 mg/mL[a]	Physically compatible for 4 hr at 23 °C	1725	C
Cyclophosphamide	MJ	10 mg/mL[a]	BR	0.1 mg/mL[a]	Physically compatible for 4 hr at 23 °C	1725	C
Cytarabine	CET	50 mg/mL	BR	0.1 mg/mL[a]	Physically compatible for 4 hr at 23 °C	1725	C
Dacarbazine	MI	4 mg/mL[a]	BR	0.1 mg/mL[a]	Physically compatible for 4 hr at 23 °C	1725	C
Dactinomycin	MSD	0.01 mg/mL[a]	BR	0.1 mg/mL[a]	Physically compatible for 4 hr at 23 °C	1725	C
Daunorubicin HCl	WY	1 mg/mL[a]	BR	0.1 mg/mL[a]	Physically compatible for 4 hr at 23 °C	1725	C
Dexamethasone sodium phosphate	LY	1 mg/mL[a]	BR	0.1 mg/mL[a]	Physically compatible for 4 hr at 23 °C	1725	C
Diphenhydramine HCl	ES	2 mg/mL[a]	BR	0.1 mg/mL[a]	Physically compatible for 4 hr at 23 °C	1725	C
Doxorubicin HCl	CET	2 mg/mL	BR	0.1 mg/mL[a]	Physically compatible for 4 hr at 23 °C	1725	C
Doxycycline hyclate	LY	1 mg/mL[a]	BR	0.1 mg/mL[a]	Physically compatible for 4 hr at 23 °C	1725	C
Droperidol	JN	0.4 mg/mL[a]	BR	0.1 mg/mL[a]	Physically compatible for 4 hr at 23 °C	1725	C
Enalaprilat	MSD	0.1 mg/mL[a]	BR	0.1 mg/mL[a]	Physically compatible for 4 hr at 23 °C	1725	C

Y-Site Injection Compatibility (1:1 Mixture) (Cont.)

Teniposide

Drug	Mfr	Conc	Mfr	Conc	Remarks	Ref	C/I
Etoposide	BR	0.4 mg/mL[a]	BR	0.1 mg/mL[a]	Physically compatible for 4 hr at 23 °C	1725	C
Etoposide phosphate	BR	5 mg/mL[a]	BR	0.1 mg/mL[a]	Physically compatible for 4 hr at 23 °C	2218	C
Famotidine	MSD	2 mg/mL[a]	BR	0.1 mg/mL[a]	Physically compatible for 4 hr at 23 °C	1725	C
Floxuridine	RC	3 mg/mL[a]	BR	0.1 mg/mL[a]	Physically compatible for 4 hr at 23 °C	1725	C
Fluconazole	RR	2 mg/mL	BR	0.1 mg/mL[a]	Physically compatible for 4 hr at 23 °C	1725	C
Fludarabine phosphate	BX	1 mg/mL[a]	BR	0.1 mg/mL[a]	Physically compatible for 4 hr at 23 °C	1725	C
Fluorouracil	AD	16 mg/mL[a]	BR	0.1 mg/mL[a]	Physically compatible for 4 hr at 23 °C	1725	C
Furosemide	AB	3 mg/mL[a]	BR	0.1 mg/mL[a]	Physically compatible for 4 hr at 23 °C	1725	C
Gallium nitrate	FUJ	0.4 mg/mL[a]	BR	0.1 mg/mL[a]	Physically compatible for 4 hr at 23 °C	1725	C
Ganciclovir sodium	SY	20 mg/mL[a]	BR	0.1 mg/mL[a]	Physically compatible for 4 hr at 23 °C	1725	C
Gemcitabine HCl	LI	10 mg/mL[b]	BR	0.1 mg/mL[a]	Physically compatible for 4 hr at 23 °C	2226	C
Gentamicin sulfate	LY	5 mg/mL[a]	BR	0.1 mg/mL[a]	Physically compatible for 4 hr at 23 °C	1725	C
Granisetron HCl	SKB	0.05 mg/mL[a]	BMS	0.1 mg/mL[a]	Physically compatible for 4 hr at 23 °C	2000	C
Haloperidol lactate	MN	0.2 mg/mL[a]	BR	0.1 mg/mL[a]	Physically compatible for 4 hr at 23 °C	1725	C
Hydrocortisone sodium succinate	UP	1 mg/mL[a]	BR	0.1 mg/mL[a]	Physically compatible for 4 hr at 23 °C	1725	C
Hydromorphone HCl	KN	0.5 mg/mL[a]	BR	0.1 mg/mL[a]	Physically compatible for 4 hr at 23 °C	1725	C
Hydroxyzine HCl	WI	4 mg/mL[a]	BR	0.1 mg/mL[a]	Physically compatible for 4 hr at 23 °C	1725	C
Idarubicin HCl	AD	0.5 mg/mL[a]	BR	0.1 mg/mL[a]	Unacceptable increase in turbidity	1725	I
Ifosfamide	MJ	25 mg/mL[a]	BR	0.1 mg/mL[a]	Physically compatible for 4 hr at 23 °C	1725	C
Imipenem–cilastatin sodium	MSD	10 mg/mL[b]	BR	0.1 mg/mL[a]	Physically compatible for 4 hr at 23 °C	1725	C
Leucovorin calcium	LE	2 mg/mL[a]	BR	0.1 mg/mL[a]	Physically compatible for 4 hr at 23 °C	1725	C
Lorazepam	WY	0.1 mg/mL[a]	BR	0.1 mg/mL[a]	Physically compatible for 4 hr at 23 °C	1725	C
Mannitol	BA	15%	BR	0.1 mg/mL[a]	Physically compatible for 4 hr at 23 °C	1725	C
Mechlorethamine HCl	MSD	1 mg/mL	BR	0.1 mg/mL[a]	Physically compatible for 4 hr at 23 °C	1725	C
Melphalan HCl	BW	0.1 mg/mL[a]	BR	0.1 mg/mL[a]	Physically compatible for 4 hr at 23 °C	1725	C
Meperidine HCl	WY	4 mg/mL[a]	BR	0.1 mg/mL[a]	Physically compatible for 4 hr at 23 °C	1725	C
Mesna	MJ	10 mg/mL[a]	BR	0.1 mg/mL[a]	Physically compatible for 4 hr at 23 °C	1725	C
Methotrexate sodium	LE	15 mg/mL[a]	BR	0.1 mg/mL[a]	Physically compatible for 4 hr at 23 °C	1725	C
Methylprednisolone sodium succinate	AB	5 mg/mL[a]	BR	0.1 mg/mL[a]	Physically compatible for 4 hr at 23 °C	1725	C
Metoclopramide HCl	ES	5 mg/mL	BR	0.1 mg/mL[a]	Physically compatible for 4 hr at 23 °C	1725	C
Metronidazole	BA	5 mg/mL	BR	0.1 mg/mL[a]	Physically compatible for 4 hr at 23 °C	1725	C
Mitomycin	BR	0.5 mg/mL	BR	0.1 mg/mL[a]	Physically compatible for 4 hr at 23 °C	1725	C
Mitoxantrone HCl	LE	0.5 mg/mL[a]	BR	0.1 mg/mL[a]	Physically compatible for 4 hr at 23 °C	1725	C
Morphine sulfate	AST	1 mg/mL[a]	BR	0.1 mg/mL[a]	Physically compatible for 4 hr at 23 °C	1725	C
Nalbuphine HCl	DU	10 mg/mL	BR	0.1 mg/mL[a]	Physically compatible for 4 hr at 23 °C	1725	C
Ondansetron HCl	GL	1 mg/mL[b]	BR	0.1 mg/mL[a]	Visually compatible for 4 hr at 22 °C	1365	C
	GL	1 mg/mL[a]	BR	0.1 mg/mL[a]	Physically compatible for 4 hr at 23 °C	1725	C
Potassium chloride	AB	0.1 mEq/mL[a]	BR	0.1 mg/mL[a]	Physically compatible for 4 hr at 23 °C	1725	C
Prochlorperazine edisylate	SCN	0.5 mg/mL[a]	BR	0.1 mg/mL[a]	Physically compatible for 4 hr at 23 °C	1725	C

Y-Site Injection Compatibility (1:1 Mixture) (Cont.)

Teniposide

Drug	Mfr	Conc	Mfr	Conc	Remarks	Ref	C/I
Promethazine HCl	WY	2 mg/mL[a]	BR	0.1 mg/mL[a]	Physically compatible for 4 hr at 23 °C	1725	C
Ranitidine HCl	GL	2 mg/mL[a]	BR	0.1 mg/mL[a]	Physically compatible for 4 hr at 23 °C	1725	C
Sargramostim	IMM	10 mcg/mL[b]	BR	0.1 mg/mL[b]	Visually compatible for 4 hr at 22 °C	1436	C
Sodium bicarbonate	AB	1 mEq/mL	BR	0.1 mg/mL[a]	Physically compatible for 4 hr at 23 °C	1725	C
Streptozocin	UP	40 mg/mL[a]	BR	0.1 mg/mL[a]	Physically compatible for 4 hr at 23 °C	1725	C
Thiotepa	LE	1 mg/mL[a]	BR	0.1 mg/mL[a]	Physically compatible for 4 hr at 23 °C	1725	C
Ticarcillin disodium–clavulanate potassium	SKB	31 mg/mL[a]	BR	0.1 mg/mL[a]	Physically compatible for 4 hr at 23 °C	1725	C
Tobramycin sulfate	LI	5 mg/mL[a]	BR	0.1 mg/mL[a]	Physically compatible for 4 hr at 23 °C	1725	C
Trimethoprim–sulfamethoxazole	ES	0.8 + 4 mg/mL[a]	BR	0.1 mg/mL[a]	Physically compatible for 4 hr at 23 °C	1725	C
Vancomycin HCl	AB	10 mg/mL[a]	BR	0.1 mg/mL[a]	Physically compatible for 4 hr at 23 °C	1725	C
Vinblastine sulfate	LI	0.12 mg/mL[a]	BR	0.1 mg/mL[a]	Physically compatible for 4 hr at 23 °C	1725	C
Vincristine sulfate	LI	0.05 mg/mL[a]	BR	0.1 mg/mL[a]	Physically compatible for 4 hr at 23 °C	1725	C
Vinorelbine tartrate	BW	1 mg/mL[a]	BR	0.1 mg/mL[a]	Physically compatible for 4 hr at 23 °C	1725	C
Zidovudine	BW	4 mg/mL[a]	BR	0.1 mg/mL[a]	Physically compatible for 4 hr at 23 °C	1725	C

[a]*Tested in dextrose 5%.*
[b]*Tested in sodium chloride 0.9%.*
[c]*Tested in bacteriostatic sodium chloride 0.9% preserved with benzyl alcohol 0.9%.*

TENOXICAM
AHFS 28:08.04

Products — Tenoxicam is available as a lyophilized powder for injection in vials containing 20 and 40 mg of drug. Also present in the vials are mannitol, ascorbic acid, disodium edetate, tromethamine, and sodium hydroxide or hydrochloric acid. The lyophilized powder should be reconstituted using the 2-mL ampuls of sterile water for injection provided for that purpose. (38; 115)

Trade Name(s) — Mobiflex, Tilcotil.

Administration — Tenoxicam is administered by intramuscular (38; 115) or intravenous bolus injection. (38; 115) Addition to infusion solutions is not recommended. (38; 115)

Stability — The greenish-yellow lyophilized powder in intact vials should be stored at controlled room temperature at or below 25 °C (38) to 30 °C (115) and protected from freezing. The drug is stable for 24 hours after reconstitution, but administration immediately after preparation is recommended. It should not be added to infusion solutions because of the possibility of precipitation. (38; 115)

Compatibility Information

Additive Compatibility

Tenoxicam

Drug	Mfr	Conc/L	Mfr	Conc/L	Test Soln	Remarks	Ref	C/I
Cefazolin sodium	FUJ	5 g	RC	200 mg	D5W	Visually compatible with less than 10% loss of both drugs in 48 hr at 25 °C and in 72 hr at 4 °C in the dark	2441	C

Additive Compatibility (Cont.)

Tenoxicam

Drug	Mfr	Conc/L	Mfr	Conc/L	Test Soln	Remarks	Ref	C/I
Ceftazidime	LI	5 g	RC	200 mg	D5W[a]	Visually compatible for up to 72 hr with yellow discoloration. 10% loss of ceftazidime in 96 hr and of tenoxicam in 168 hr at 4 and 25 °C	2557	C
	LI	5 g	RC	200 mg	D5W[b]	Visually compatible with about 10% loss of both drugs in 168 hr at 4 and 25 °C	2557	C

[a]Tested in PVC containers.
[b]Tested in glass containers.

TERBUTALINE SULFATE
AHFS 12:12.08.12

Products — Terbutaline sulfate is available in 1-mL ampuls. Each milliliter contains terbutaline sulfate 1 mg, sodium chloride for isotonicity, and hydrochloric acid to adjust the pH. (1)

pH — The pH is adjusted to 3 to 5. (1; 4)

Osmolality — The injection is isotonic. (1)

Administration — Terbutaline sulfate injection is administered subcutaneously only, usually into the lateral deltoid area. (1; 4) Intravenous administration is not recommended by the manufacturer (1) but has been used in selected patients with careful monitoring. (4)

Stability — Although relatively stable compared to corresponding catecholamines (738), terbutaline sulfate is nonetheless sensitive to light and excessive heat. The injection should be stored at controlled room temperature and protected from light and freezing. Discolored solutions should not be used. (1; 4) Terbutaline sulfate is stated to be stable over the pH range of 1 to 7. (4)

Syringes — The stability of terbutaline sulfate (Geigy) 1 mg/mL was studied packaged in polypropylene syringes (Becton Dickinson) fitted with luer-tip caps (Becton Dickinson). The samples were stored at 4 °C in the dark, 25 °C in the dark, and 25 °C with exposure to fluorescent light. Samples stored in the dark at both temperatures were stable, exhibiting a 5 to 6% drug loss in 60 days. The 25 °C samples exposed to light showed a 5% loss in 28 days and an 11% loss in 60 days with a yellow discoloration. (1298)

The stability of terbutaline sulfate (Geigy) 1 mg/mL repackaged in syringes was evaluated. A 0.25-mL sample was drawn into each plastic tuberculin syringe (Becton Dickinson) and sealed with a luer-tip cap (Becton Dickinson). Samples were stored at 4 and 24 °C with exposure to light and light protection. Little difference was reported in the terbutaline sulfate content among the four storage conditions. Drug losses of 5% or less were observed after seven weeks of storage. Although no discoloration was reported, it may not have been observed in the small sample present in the tuberculin syringe. (1299)

Compatibility Information

Solution Compatibility

Terbutaline sulfate

Solution	Mfr	Mfr	Conc/L	Remarks	Ref	C/I
Dextrose 5%	AB	CI	4 mg	Physically compatible. Calculated 10% loss in 328 hr at 25 °C in light	527	C
	TR[a]	MRD	30 mg	Under 10% loss in 7 days at 25 °C in light	1133	C
Sodium chloride 0.45%	TR[a]	MRD	30 mg	Under 5% loss in 7 days at 25 °C in light or at 4 °C	1133	C
Sodium chloride 0.9%	TR[a]	MRD	30 mg	Under 6% loss in 7 days at 25 °C in light	1133	C
	BA[a]	NVA	100 mg	Solution remained clear with no loss in 23 days at 25 °C	2551	C

[a]Tested in PVC containers.

Additive Compatibility

Terbutaline sulfate

Drug	Mfr	Conc/L	Mfr	Conc/L	Test Soln	Remarks	Ref	C/I
Aminophylline	SE	500 mg	CI	4 mg	D5W	Physically compatible. At 25 °C, 10% terbutaline loss in 44 hr in light	527	C
Bleomycin sulfate	BR	20 and 30 units	GG	7.5 mg	NS	36% loss of bleomycin activity in 1 week at 4 °C	763	I

Drugs in Syringe Compatibility

Terbutaline sulfate

Drug (in syringe)	Mfr	Amt	Mfr	Amt	Remarks	Ref	C/I
Doxapram HCl	RB	400 mg/ 20 mL		0.2 mg/ 1 mL	Physically compatible with 6% doxapram loss in 24 hr	1177	C

Y-Site Injection Compatibility (1:1 Mixture)

Terbutaline sulfate

Drug	Mfr	Conc	Mfr	Conc	Remarks	Ref	C/I
Insulin, regular	LI	0.2 unit/mL[b]	CI	0.02 mg/mL[a]	Physically compatible for 2 hr at 25 °C	1395	C

[a]*Tested in dextrose 5%.*
[b]*Tested in sodium chloride 0.9%.*

TETRACAINE HYDROCHLORIDE
AHFS 72:00

Products — Tetracaine hydrochloride is available as a preservative-free solution in a concentration of 10 mg/mL (1%) in 2-mL ampules. The product also contains sodium chloride and hydrochloric acid and/or sodium hydroxide to adjust pH in water for injection. (1)

Pontocaine brand of tetracaine hydrochloride 10 mg/mL also contains acetone sodium bisulfite. (4)

Tetracaine hydrochloride hyperbaric solutions are available in concentrations of 0.2 and 0.3% in dextrose 6%. (4)

pH — Tetracaine hydrochloride injection has a pH ranging from 3.2 to 6.0. (1) Reconstituted tetracaine hydrochloride powder has a pH ranging from 5 to 6 after reconstitution. (4)

Osmolality — Tetracaine hydrochloride 10-mg/mL injection is isotonic. (1)

Trade Name(s) — Pontocaine Hydrochloride.

Administration — Tetracaine hydrochloride injection is used for prolonged spinal anesthesia. The injection is isobaric having a specific gravity of 1.0060 to 1.0074 at 25 °C, which is very similar to spinal fluid. A hyperbaric solution of tetracaine hydrochloride may be prepared by diluting the 10-mg/mL injection in dextrose 10%. (1; 4)

Tetracaine hydrochloride powder for injection dissolved in spinal fluid is slightly hyperbaric. A hypobaric solution with a specific gravity of 1.000 at 25 °C may be prepared by dissolving the tetracaine hydrochloride powder in sterile water for injection at a concentration of 0.1%. A hyperbaric solution of tetracaine hydrochloride may be prepared by dissolving the powder in dextrose 10% to yield a 10-mg/mL solution. The resulting solution is further diluted with an equal volume of cerebrospinal fluid to yield 5 mg/mL of tetracaine hydrochloride and dextrose. (4)

Stability — Tetracaine hydrochloride injection in intact vials should be stored under refrigeration and protected from light. Freezing should be avoided. The injection should not be used if crystals, cloudiness, or discoloration is present. (1; 4)

Tetracaine hydrochloride 10-mg/mL injection and tetracaine hydrochloride powder in intact containers can be autoclaved at 121 °C for 15 minutes to sterilize the exterior of the ampuls. However, autoclaving may increase the occurrence of crystal formation. Ampuls that have been autoclaved but are not used must be discarded and may not be returned to stock. (1; 4)

Tetracaine hydrochloride in aqueous solutions undergoes hydrolysis slowly that results in the formation of *p*-butylaminobenzoic acid crystals. Solutions containing crystals should not be used. (4)

Tetracaine hydrochloride stability in aqueous solution was evaluated. Accelerated degradation at elevated temperatures led to a determination that tetracaine hydrochloride in aqueous solution was stable for at least 12 months at 25 °C with about 96% remaining. After two years, the concentration had declined to about 89%. (2453) When stored under refrigeration at 4 to 6 °C, no loss of tetracaine hydrochloride was detected after 365 days of storage. (2705)

pH Effects — Tetracaine hydrochloride is unstable in both acidic and alkaline media. The pH of maximum stability was found to be 3.8. (2666; 2705) Tetracaine hydrochloride mixed with alkali hydroxides or carbonates results in the precipitation of tetracaine base as an oily liquid. (4)

Compatibility Information

Drugs in Syringe Compatibility

Tetracaine HCl

Drug (in syringe)	Mfr	Amt	Mfr	Amt	Remarks	Ref	C/I
Clonidine HCl with ketamine HCl	BI PD	0.03 mg/mL 2 mg/mL	SW	2 mg/mL	Diluted to 5 mL with NS. Visually compatible with no new GC/MS peaks in 1 hr at room temperature	1956	C
Ketamine HCl with clonidine HCl	PD BI	2 mg/mL 0.03 mg/mL	SW	2 mg/mL	Diluted to 5 mL with NS. Visually compatible with no new GC/MS peaks in 1 hr at room temperature	1956	C

THEOPHYLLINE
AHFS 86:16

Products — Theophylline is available, premixed in dextrose 5%, in concentrations from 0.8 to 4 mg/mL (expressed as anhydrous theophylline). (1)

pH — From 3.5 to 6.5. (1)

Osmolality — Theophylline premixed in dextrose 5% products have osmolalities in the range of 255 to 275 mOsm/kg. (1)

Administration — Theophylline may be administered by continuous or intermittent intravenous infusion. Slow administration, not exceeding 20 mg/min, has been recommended. Loading doses are usually given over 20 to 30 minutes. (1)

Stability — Theophylline injection should be stored at controlled room temperature and protected from freezing. Avoid excessive heat. (1)

At a concentration of 1 g/L in dextrose 5%, theophylline was stable during autoclaving for 20 minutes at 120 °C. No decrease in the theophylline content was detected. (1173)

Compatibility Information

Additive Compatibility

Theophylline

Drug	Mfr	Conc/L	Mfr	Conc/L	Test Soln	Remarks	Ref	C/I
Ascorbic acid		1.9 g		2 g	D5W	Yellow discoloration. 8% ascorbic acid loss in 6 hr and 15% in 24 hr. No theophylline loss	1909	I
Cefepime HCl	BR	4 g	BA	800 mg	D5W	Visually compatible. 3% cefepime loss in 24 hr at room temperature and 7 days at 5 °C. No theophylline loss	1681	C
Ceftriaxone sodium	RC	40 g	BAa	4 g		Yellow color forms immediately. 14% ceftriaxone loss and no theophylline loss in 24 hr	1727	I

Additive Compatibility (Cont.)

Theophylline

Drug	Mfr	Conc/L	Mfr	Conc/L	Test Soln	Remarks	Ref	C/I
Chlorpromazine HCl		200 mg		2 g	D5W	Visually compatible. 7% chlorpromazine and no theophylline loss in 48 hr	1909	C
Fluconazole	PF	1 g	BA	0.4 g	D5W	Fluconazole stable for 72 hr at 25 °C in fluorescent light. Theophylline not tested	1676	C
Furosemide		330 mg		2 g	D5W	Visually compatible. Little theophylline and 10% furosemide loss in 48 hr	1909	C
Lidocaine HCl		380 mg		2 g	D5W	Visually compatible with little or no loss of either drug in 48 hr	1909	C
Methylprednisolone sodium succinate	UP	500 mg and 2 g	AB	4 g	D5W	Physically compatible. Little theophylline or methylprednisolone alcohol loss in 24 hr at room temperature, but 8% ester hydrolysis	1150	C
	UP	500 mg and 2 g	AB	400 mg	D5W	Physically compatible. Little theophylline or methylprednisolone alcohol loss in 24 hr at room temperature, but 11% ester hydrolysis	1150	C
Papaverine HCl		160 mg		2 g	D5W	Visually compatible with little or no loss of either drug in 48 hr	1909	C
Verapamil HCl	KN	100 and 400 mg	AB	400 mg and 4 g	D5W	Physically compatible. Little loss of either drug in 24 hr at 24 °C in light	1172	C

[a]Tested in PVC containers.

Y-Site Injection Compatibility (1:1 Mixture)

Theophylline

Drug	Mfr	Conc	Mfr	Conc	Remarks	Ref	C/I
Acyclovir sodium	BW	5 mg/mL[a]	TR	1.6 mg/mL[a]	Physically compatible for 4 hr at 25 °C	1157	C
Ampicillin sodium	WY	20 mg/mL[b]	TR	4 mg/mL	Visually compatible for 6 hr at 25 °C	1793	C
Ampicillin sodium–sulbactam sodium	PF	20 + 10 mg/mL[b]	TR	4 mg/mL	Visually compatible for 6 hr at 25 °C	1793	C
Aztreonam	BV	20 mg/mL[a]	TR	4 mg/mL	Visually compatible for 6 hr at 25 °C	1793	C
Bivalirudin	TMC	5 mg/mL[a]	BA	4 mg/mL[a]	Physically compatible for 4 hr at 23 °C	2373	C
Cefazolin sodium	SKB	20 mg/mL	TR	4 mg/mL	Visually compatible for 6 hr at 25 °C	1793	C
Cefepime HCl	BMS	120 mg/mL[d]		20 mg/mL	Over 25% cefepime loss in 1 hr	2513	I
Cefotetan disodium	STU	40 mg/mL[a]	TR	4 mg/mL	Visually compatible for 6 hr at 25 °C	1793	C
Ceftazidime	LI	20 mg/mL	TR	4 mg/mL	Visually compatible for 6 hr at 25 °C	1793	C
	GSK	120 mg/mL[d]		20 mg/mL	Over 25% ceftazidime loss in 1 hr	2513	I
Ceftriaxone sodium	RC	20 mg/mL	TR	4 mg/mL	Visually compatible for 6 hr at 25 °C	1793	C
Cisatracurium besylate	GW	0.1, 2, 5 mg/mL[a]	AB	3.2 mg/mL	Physically compatible for 4 hr at 23 °C	2074	C
Clindamycin phosphate	UP	12 mg/mL[a]	TR	4 mg/mL	Visually compatible for 6 hr at 25 °C	1793	C
Clonidine HCl	BI	18 mcg/mL[b]	ASZ	1 mg/mL	Visually compatible	2642	C
Dexamethasone sodium phosphate	ES	0.08 mg/mL[a]	TR	4 mg/mL	Visually compatible for 6 hr at 25 °C	1793	C

Y-Site Injection Compatibility (1:1 Mixture) (Cont.)

Theophylline

Drug	Mfr	Conc	Mfr	Conc	Remarks	Ref	C/I
Dexmedetomidine HCl	AB	4 mcg/mL[b]	AB	4 mg/mL[a]	Physically compatible for 4 hr at 23 °C	2383	C
Diltiazem HCl	MMD	5 mg/mL	AB	0.8 mg/mL[a]	Visually compatible	1807	C
Dobutamine HCl	LI	1 mg/mL[a]	TR	4 mg/mL	Visually compatible for 6 hr at 25 °C	1793	C
Dopamine HCl	BA	1.6 mg/mL	TR	4 mg/mL	Visually compatible for 6 hr at 25 °C	1793	C
Doxycycline hyclate	ES	1 mg/mL[a]	TR	4 mg/mL	Visually compatible for 6 hr at 25 °C	1793	C
Erythromycin lactobionate	AB	3.3 mg/mL[b]	TR	4 mg/mL	Visually compatible for 6 hr at 25 °C	1793	C
Famotidine	MSD	0.2 mg/mL[a]	TR	1.6 mg/mL[a]	Physically compatible for 4 hr at 25 °C	1188	C
Fenoldopam mesylate	AB	80 mcg/mL[b]	BA	4 mg/mL[a]	Physically compatible for 4 hr at 23 °C	2467	C
Fluconazole	RR	2 mg/mL	AMR	1.6 mg/mL[a]	Visually compatible for 24 hr at 28 °C under fluorescent light	1760	C
	PF	2 mg/mL	TR	4 mg/mL	Visually compatible for 6 hr at 25 °C	1793	C
Gentamicin sulfate	TR	2 mg/mL	TR	4 mg/mL	Visually compatible for 6 hr at 25 °C	1793	C
Haloperidol lactate	MN	0.5[a] and 5 mg/mL	TR	1.6 mg/mL[a]	Visually compatible for 24 hr at 21 °C	1523	C
Heparin sodium	TR	50 units/mL	TR	4 mg/mL	Visually compatible for 4 hr at 25 °C	1793	C
Hetastarch in lactated electrolyte	AB	6%	BA	4 mg/mL[a]	Physically compatible for 4 hr at 23 °C	2339	C
Hetastarch in sodium chloride 0.9%	DCC	6%	TR[c]	4 mg/mL	Precipitates after 2 hr at room temperature	1313	I
Hydrocortisone sodium succinate	UP	2 mg/mL[a]	TR	4 mg/mL	Visually compatible for 6 hr at 25 °C	1793	C
Lidocaine HCl	TR	4 mg/mL	TR	4 mg/mL	Visually compatible for 6 hr at 25 °C	1793	C
Linezolid	PHU	2 mg/mL	BA	4 mg/mL[a]	Physically compatible for 4 hr at 23 °C	2264	C
Methyldopate HCl	ES	5 mg/mL[a]	TR	4 mg/mL	Visually compatible for 6 hr at 25 °C	1793	C
Methylprednisolone sodium succinate	UP	2.5 mg/mL[a]	TR	4 mg/mL	Visually compatible for 6 hr at 25 °C	1793	C
Metronidazole	MG	5 mg/mL	TR	4 mg/mL	Visually compatible for 6 hr at 25 °C	1793	C
Micafungin sodium	ASP	1.5 mg/mL[b]	AB	4 mg/mL	Physically compatible for 4 hr at 23 °C	2683	C
Midazolam HCl	RC	1 mg/mL[a]	BA	1.6 mg/mL[a]	Visually compatible for 24 hr at 23 °C	1847	C
Milrinone lactate	SW	0.4 mg/mL[a]	AB	1.6 mg/mL[a]	Visually compatible. Little loss of either drug in 4 hr at 23 °C	2214	C
Nafcillin sodium	WY	20 mg/mL[a]	TR	4 mg/mL	Visually compatible for 6 hr at 25 °C	1793	C
Nitroglycerin	LY	0.2 mg/mL[a]	TR	4 mg/mL	Visually compatible for 6 hr at 25 °C	1793	C
Oxaliplatin	SS	0.5 mg/mL[a]	AB	4 mg/mL	Physically compatible for 4 hr at 23 °C	2566	C
Penicillin G potassium	RR	40,000 units/mL[a]	TR	4 mg/mL	Visually compatible for 6 hr at 25 °C	1793	C
Phenytoin sodium	ES	2 mg/mL[b]	TR	4 mg/mL	Immediately cloudy. Dense precipitate in 6 hr at 25 °C	1793	I
Potassium chloride	AB	0.2 mEq/mL[a]	TR	4 mg/mL	Visually compatible for 6 hr at 25 °C	1793	C
Ranitidine HCl	GL	1 mg/mL	TR	4 mg/mL	Visually compatible for 6 hr at 25 °C	1793	C
Remifentanil HCl	GW	0.025 and 0.25 mg/mL[b]	AB	3.2 mg/mL[a]	Physically compatible for 4 hr at 23 °C	2075	C
Sodium nitroprusside	ES	0.2 mg/mL[a]	TR	4 mg/mL	Visually compatible for 6 hr at 25 °C protected from light	1793	C

Y-Site Injection Compatibility (1:1 Mixture) (Cont.)

Theophylline

Drug	Mfr	Conc	Mfr	Conc	Remarks	Ref	C/I
Ticarcillin disodium–clavulanate potassium	BE	31 mg/mL[a]	TR	4 mg/mL	Visually compatible for 6 hr at 25 °C	1793	**C**
Tigecycline	WY	1 mg/mL[b]		1.6 mg/mL[a]	Physically compatible for 4 hr	2714	**C**
Tobramycin sulfate	LI	0.8 mg/mL[a]	TR	4 mg/mL	Visually compatible for 6 hr at 25 °C	1793	**C**
Vancomycin HCl	LI	6.6 mg/mL[a]	TR	4 mg/mL	Visually compatible for 6 hr at 25 °C	1793	**C**

[a]Tested in dextrose 5%.
[b]Tested in sodium chloride 0.9%.
[c]Tested in premixed infusion solution.
[d]Tested in sterile water for injection.

THIAMINE HYDROCHLORIDE
AHFS 88:08

Products — Thiamine hydrochloride is available in a concentration of 100 mg/mL in 1- and 2-mL vials. Each milliliter of solution may also contain chlorobutanol 0.5% as an antibacterial preservative and monothioglycerol 0.5%. Sodium hydroxide and/or hydrochloric acid may be added to adjust the pH. (1; 4)

pH — From 2.5 to 4.5. (1; 17)

Administration — Thiamine hydrochloride injection may be administered by intramuscular or slow intravenous injection. An intradermal test dose has been recommended for patients with suspected thiamine sensitivity. (1; 4)

Stability — Thiamine hydrochloride in intact containers should be stored at controlled room temperature and protected from light and freezing. (1; 4)

Thiamine hydrochloride under simulated summer conditions in paramedic vehicles was exposed to temperatures ranging from 26 to 38 °C over four weeks. Analysis found no loss of the drug under these conditions. (2562)

Thiamine hydrochloride is stated to be incompatible with oxidizing and reducing agents. (4) In solutions with sulfites or bisulfites, it is rapidly inactivated. (52; 1072; 1925) Oxidation of thiamine hydrochloride results in the formation of the highly blue-colored and biologically inactive compound thiochrome. (734; 1072)

pH Effects — Thiamine hydrochloride is stable in acid solutions, losing activity very slowly at pH 4 or less. It is maximally stable at pH 2. (1072) Thiamine hydrochloride is unstable in neutral or alkaline solutions. (1; 4; 1072)

Syringes — Thiamine hydrochloride (Lilly) 100 mg/mL was repackaged in glass syringes (Glaspak), back-fill glass syringes (Hy-Pod), and plastic syringes (Stylex). Half of the syringes were filled with thiamine hydrochloride injection filtered through 5-μm stainless steel depth filters (Extemp filter pin), and the rest were filled with unfiltered drug. The syringes containing 1 mL of thiamine hydrochloride injection were stored protected from light (amber UV-light-inhibiting plastic bags) at 22 to 24 °C for 84 days. No color changes were observed, and changes in pH were minimal. Furthermore, no differences between filtered or unfiltered samples occurred, with all solutions retaining approximately 100% over the 84 days. (734)

Sorption — Thiamine hydrochloride (Merck) 30 mg/L did not display significant sorption to a PVC plastic test strip in 24 hours. (12)

Compatibility Information

Solution Compatibility

Thiamine HCl

Solution	Mfr	Mfr	Conc/L	Remarks	Ref	C/I
Dextrose–Ringer's injection combinations	AB		100 mg	Physically compatible	3	**C**
Dextrose–Ringer's injection, lactated, combinations	AB		100 mg	Physically compatible	3	**C**
Dextrose–saline combinations	AB		100 mg	Physically compatible	3	**C**

Solution Compatibility (Cont.)

Thiamine HCl

Solution	Mfr	Mfr	Conc/L	Remarks	Ref	C/I
Dextrose 2.5%	AB		100 mg	Physically compatible	3	C
Dextrose 5%	AB		100 mg	Physically compatible	3	C
Dextrose 10%	AB		100 mg	Physically compatible	3	C
Ionosol products	AB		100 mg	Physically compatible	3	C
Ringer's injection	AB		100 mg	Physically compatible	3	C
Ringer's injection, lactated	AB		100 mg	Physically compatible	3	C
Sodium chloride 0.45%	AB		100 mg	Physically compatible	3	C
Sodium chloride 0.9%	AB		100 mg	Physically compatible	3	C
Sodium lactate ⅙ M	AB		100 mg	Physically compatible	3	C

Drugs in Syringe Compatibility

Thiamine HCl

Drug (in syringe)	Mfr	Amt	Mfr	Amt	Remarks	Ref	C/I
Doxapram HCl	RB	400 mg/ 20 mL		10 mg/ 2 mL	Physically compatible with 6% doxapram loss in 24 hr	1177	C

Y-Site Injection Compatibility (1:1 Mixture)

Thiamine HCl

Drug	Mfr	Conc	Mfr	Conc	Remarks	Ref	C/I
Famotidine	MSD	0.2 mg/mL[a]	ES	100 mg/mL	Physically compatible for 14 hr	1196	C

[a] *Tested in dextrose 5%.*

Additional Compatibility Information

Parenteral Nutrition Solutions — The stability of thiamine hydrochloride 50 mg/L was studied in representative parenteral nutrition solutions exposed to fluorescent light, indirect sunlight, and direct sunlight for eight hours. One 5-mL vial of multivitamin concentrate (Lyphomed) containing 50 mg of thiamine hydrochloride and also 1 mg of folic acid (Lederle) were added to a liter of parenteral nutrition solution composed of amino acids 4.25%–dextrose 25% (Travenol) with standard electrolytes and trace elements. Thiamine hydrochloride was stable over the eight-hour study period at room temperature under fluorescent light and indirect sunlight, but direct sunlight caused a 26% loss. (842)

A 50% initial drop in thiamine concentration immediately after admixture of multivitamins in a parenteral nutrition solution composed of amino acids, dextrose, electrolytes, and trace elements in PVC bags was reported. The thiamine concentration then remained relatively constant for 120 hours when stored at both 4 and 25 °C. (1063)

The stability of numerous vitamins in parenteral nutrition solutions composed of amino acids (Kabi-Vitrum), dextrose 30%, and fat emulsion 20% (Kabi-Vitrum) in a 2:1:1 ratio with electrolytes, trace elements, and both fat- and water-soluble vitamins was reported. The admixtures were stored in darkness at 2 to 8 °C for 96 hours with no significant loss of thiamine mononitrate. (1225)

The stability of several vitamins from M.V.I.-12 (Armour) admixed in parenteral nutrition solutions composed of different amino acid products, with or without Intralipid 10%, when stored in glass bottles and PVC bags at 25 and 5 °C for 48 hours was reported. Thiamine hydrochloride was stable in the parenteral nutrition solutions prepared with amino acid products without bisulfite. (1431)

The stability of several vitamins following admixture (as M.V.I-12) with four different amino acid products (Novamine, Neopham, FreAmine III, Travasol) with or without Intralipid when stored in glass bottles or PVC bags at 25 °C for 48 hours was reported. Exposure to high intensity phototherapy light did not affect thiamine. (487)

The stability of thiamine hydrochloride from a multiple vitamin product in dextrose 5% and sodium chloride 0.9% in PVC and ClearFlex containers was evaluated. Thiamine hydrochloride was stable at 23 °C when exposed to or protected from light, exhibiting losses of 11% or less in 24 hours. (1509)

The degradation of vitamins A, B_1, C, and E from Cernevit (Roche) multivitamins in NuTRIflex Lipid Plus (B. Braun) admixtures prepared in ethylene vinyl acetate (EVA) bags and in multilayer bags was evaluated. After storage for up to 72 hours at 4, 21, and 40 °C, greater vitamin losses occurred in the EVA bags. Thiamine hydrochloride losses were 25%. In the multilayer bags (presumably a better barrier to oxygen transfer), losses were less. Thiamine hydrochloride losses were 10%. (2618)

The vitamins in Cernevit (Baxter) diluted in three 2-in-1 parenteral nutrition admixtures were tested for stability over 48 hours. Most of the other vitamins, including thiamine hydrochloride, retained their initial concentrations. (2796)

THIOTEPA
AHFS 10:00

Products — Thiotepa is available in vials containing 15 mg of drug and sodium carbonate 0.03 mg as a lyophilized powder. Reconstitute the vials with 1.5 mL of sterile water for injection. The withdrawable volume is about 1.4 mL. Because of a small excess of drug, the reconstituted solution contains thiotepa 10.4 mg/mL, yielding a withdrawable amount of approximately 14.7 mg from each vial. (1)

pH — Approximately 5.5 to 7.5. (1)

Tonicity — Reconstitution with sterile water for injection results in a hypotonic solution; it should be diluted in sodium chloride 0.9% prior to use. (1) Reconstitution with other diluents may result in a hypertonic solution which can cause mild to moderate discomfort upon administration. (4)

Thiotepa concentrations, 0.5 and 1 mg/mL diluted in sodium chloride 0.9%, are nearly isotonic, having osmolalities of 277 and 269 mOsm/kg, respectively. However, thiotepa concentrations of 3 and 5 mg/mL in sodium chloride 0.9% are hypotonic. (2006)

Trade Name(s) — Thioplex.

Administration — Thiotepa is usually given by rapid intravenous administration but may also be given by the intracavitary or intravesical route. (1; 4) The drug has also been given by intramuscular, intrathecal, and intratumoral administration. (4)

Stability — Intact vials should be stored under refrigeration and protected from light at all times. Reconstituted solutions should be stored under refrigeration and protected from light until used. (1; 4) The reconstituted solution in sterile water for injection is stated to be stable for up to 28 days stored under refrigeration or frozen and seven days at room temperature. (1369) However, the manufacturer recommends storage under refrigeration and use within eight hours because of the absence of an antimicrobial preservative. (1; 4) Thiotepa may undergo polymerization forming inactive and insoluble derivatives (1369), especially at high temperatures. (4) Solutions that are grossly opaque or contain a precipitate should not be used. (1; 4)

Thiotepa is stable in alkaline media but unstable in acidic media (1; 4), undergoing increased rates of hydrolysis. (1389)

Syringes — Thiotepa reconstituted to a concentration of 10 mg/mL with sterile water for injection was found to be stable for 24 hours under refrigeration at 8 °C and at room temperature of 23 °C in both the original vials and transferred to plastic syringes. (2006)

Filtration — Thiotepa 10 to 300 mcg/mL exhibited no loss due to sorption to either cellulose nitrate/cellulose acetate ester (Millex OR) or Teflon (Millex FG) filters. (1415; 1416)

Compatibility Information

Solution Compatibility

Thiotepa

Solution	Mfr	Mfr	Conc/L	Remarks	Ref	C/I
Dextrose 5%	BA[a], MG[b]	IMM	0.5 g	Physically stable. Losses of 10% or less in 8 hr at 4 and 23 °C and 17% in 24 hr	2007	I
	BA[a], MG[b]	IMM	5 g	Physically stable with losses of less than 10% in 14 days at 4 °C and in 3 days at 23 °C	2007	C
Sodium chloride 0.9%	BA[a]	IMM	1 and 3 g	Physically stable with 7 to 10% loss in 24 hr at 25 °C and 4% or less in 48 hr at 4 °C	2077	C
	BA[a]	IMM	0.5 g	Physically stable but up to 7% loss in 8 hr with substantial chloro-adduct formation. Up to 13% loss in 24 hr at 25 °C	2077	I
	BA[a]	IMM	0.5 g	Physically stable with 4% or less loss in 48 hr at 8 °C	2077	C

[a]*Tested in PVC containers.*
[b]*Tested in polyolefin containers.*

Additive Compatibility

Thiotepa

Drug	Mfr	Conc/L	Mfr	Conc/L	Test Soln	Remarks	Ref	C/I
Cisplatin		200 mg		1 g	NS	Yellow precipitation	1379	**I**

Y-Site Injection Compatibility (1:1 Mixture)

Thiotepa

Drug	Mfr	Conc	Mfr	Conc	Remarks	Ref	C/I
Acyclovir sodium	BW	7 mg/mL[a]	IMM[c]	1 mg/mL[a]	Physically compatible for 4 hr at 23 °C	1861	**C**
Allopurinol sodium	BW	3 mg/mL[b]	LE[d]	1 mg/mL[c]	Physically compatible for 4 hr at 22 °C	1686	**C**
Amifostine	USB	10 mg/mL[a]	LE[d]	1 mg/mL[a]	Physically compatible for 4 hr at 23 °C	1845	**C**
Amikacin sulfate	DU	5 mg/mL[a]	IMM[c]	1 mg/mL[a]	Physically compatible for 4 hr at 23 °C	1861	**C**
Aminophylline	AMR	2.5 mg/mL[a]	IMM[c]	1 mg/mL[a]	Physically compatible for 4 hr at 23 °C	1861	**C**
Amphotericin B	APC	0.6 mg/mL[a]	IMM[c]	1 mg/mL[a]	Physically compatible for 4 hr at 23 °C	1861	**C**
Ampicillin sodium	WY	20 mg/mL[b]	IMM[c]	1 mg/mL[a]	Physically compatible for 4 hr at 23 °C	1861	**C**
Ampicillin sodium–sulbactam sodium	RR	20 + 10 mg/mL[b]	IMM[c]	1 mg/mL[a]	Physically compatible for 4 hr at 23 °C	1861	**C**
Aztreonam	SQ	40 mg/mL[a]	LE[d]	1 mg/mL[a]	Physically compatible for 4 hr at 23 °C	1758	**C**
	SQ	40 mg/mL[a]	IMM[c]	1 mg/mL[a]	Physically compatible for 4 hr at 23 °C	1861	**C**
Bleomycin sulfate	MJ	1 unit/mL[b]	IMM[c]	1 mg/mL[a]	Physically compatible for 4 hr at 23 °C	1861	**C**
Bumetanide	RC	0.04 mg/mL[a]	IMM[c]	1 mg/mL[a]	Physically compatible for 4 hr at 23 °C	1861	**C**
Buprenorphine HCl	RKC	0.04 mg/mL[a]	IMM[c]	1 mg/mL[a]	Physically compatible for 4 hr at 23 °C	1861	**C**
Butorphanol tartrate	APC	0.04 mg/mL[a]	IMM[c]	1 mg/mL[a]	Physically compatible for 4 hr at 23 °C	1861	**C**
Calcium gluconate	AMR	40 mg/mL[a]	IMM[c]	1 mg/mL[a]	Physically compatible for 4 hr at 23 °C	1861	**C**
Carboplatin	BMS	5 mg/mL[a]	IMM[c]	1 mg/mL[a]	Physically compatible for 4 hr at 23 °C	1861	**C**
Carmustine	BMS	1.5 mg/mL[a]	IMM[c]	1 mg/mL[a]	Physically compatible for 4 hr at 23 °C	1861	**C**
Cefazolin sodium	MAR	20 mg/mL[a]	IMM[c]	1 mg/mL[a]	Physically compatible for 4 hr at 23 °C	1861	**C**
Cefotaxime sodium	HO	20 mg/mL[a]	IMM[c]	1 mg/mL[a]	Physically compatible for 1 hr at 23 °C	1861	**C**
Cefotetan disodium	STU	20 mg/mL[a]	IMM[c]	1 mg/mL[a]	Physically compatible for 4 hr at 23 °C	1861	**C**
Cefoxitin sodium	ME	20 mg/mL[a]	IMM[c]	1 mg/mL[a]	Physically compatible for 4 hr at 23 °C	1861	**C**
Ceftazidime	LI	40 mg/mL[a]	IMM[c]	1 mg/mL[a]	Physically compatible for 4 hr at 23 °C	1861	**C**
Ceftriaxone sodium	RC	20 mg/mL[a]	IMM[c]	1 mg/mL[a]	Physically compatible for 4 hr at 23 °C	1861	**C**
Cefuroxime sodium	LI	30 mg/mL[a]	IMM[c]	1 mg/mL[a]	Physically compatible for 4 hr at 23 °C	1861	**C**
Chlorpromazine HCl	SCN	2 mg/mL[a]	IMM[c]	1 mg/mL[a]	Physically compatible for 4 hr at 23 °C	1861	**C**
Ciprofloxacin	MI	1 mg/mL[a]	IMM[c]	1 mg/mL[a]	Physically compatible for 4 hr at 23 °C	1861	**C**
Cisplatin	BMS	1 mg/mL	IMM[c]	1 mg/mL[a]	White cloudiness appears in 4 hr at 23 °C	1861	**I**
Clindamycin phosphate	AST	10 mg/mL[a]	IMM[c]	1 mg/mL[a]	Physically compatible for 4 hr at 23 °C	1861	**C**
Cyclophosphamide	MJ	10 mg/mL[a]	IMM[c]	1 mg/mL[a]	Physically compatible for 4 hr at 23 °C	1861	**C**
Cytarabine	CET	50 mg/mL	IMM[c]	1 mg/mL[a]	Physically compatible for 4 hr at 23 °C	1861	**C**
Dacarbazine	MI	4 mg/mL[a]	IMM[c]	1 mg/mL[a]	Physically compatible for 4 hr at 23 °C	1861	**C**
Dactinomycin	ME	0.01 mg/mL[a]	IMM[c]	1 mg/mL[a]	Physically compatible for 4 hr at 23 °C	1861	**C**

Y-Site Injection Compatibility (1:1 Mixture) (Cont.)

Thiotepa

Drug	Mfr	Conc	Mfr	Conc	Remarks	Ref	C/I
Daunorubicin HCl	WY	1 mg/mL[a]	IMM[c]	1 mg/mL[a]	Physically compatible for 4 hr at 23 °C	1861	C
Dexamethasone sodium phosphate	AMR	1 mg/mL[a]	IMM[c]	1 mg/mL[a]	Physically compatible for 4 hr at 23 °C	1861	C
Diphenhydramine HCl	WY	2 mg/mL[a]	IMM[c]	1 mg/mL[a]	Physically compatible for 4 hr at 23 °C	1861	C
Dobutamine HCl	LI	4 mg/mL[a]	IMM[c]	1 mg/mL[a]	Physically compatible for 4 hr at 23 °C	1861	C
Dopamine HCl	AST	3.2 mg/mL[a]	IMM[c]	1 mg/mL[a]	Physically compatible for 4 hr at 23 °C	1861	C
Doxorubicin HCl	CHI	2 mg/mL	IMM[c]	1 mg/mL[a]	Physically compatible for 4 hr at 23 °C	1861	C
Doxycycline hyclate	LY	1 mg/mL[a]	IMM[c]	1 mg/mL[a]	Physically compatible for 4 hr at 23 °C	1861	C
Droperidol	JN	0.4 mg/mL[a]	IMM[c]	1 mg/mL[a]	Physically compatible for 4 hr at 23 °C	1861	C
Enalaprilat	ME	0.1 mg/mL[a]	IMM[c]	1 mg/mL[a]	Physically compatible for 4 hr at 23 °C	1861	C
Etoposide	BR	0.4 mg/mL[a]	IMM[c]	1 mg/mL[a]	Physically compatible for 4 hr at 23 °C	1861	C
Etoposide phosphate	BR	5 mg/mL[a]	IMM[c]	1 mg/mL[a]	Physically compatible for 4 hr at 23 °C	2218	C
Famotidine	ME	2 mg/mL[a]	IMM[c]	1 mg/mL[a]	Physically compatible for 4 hr at 23 °C	1861	C
Filgrastim	AMG	30 mcg/mL[a]	LE[d]	1 mg/mL[a]	Particles and filaments form immediately	1687	I
Floxuridine	RC	3 mg/mL[a]	IMM[c]	1 mg/mL[a]	Physically compatible for 4 hr at 23 °C	1861	C
Fluconazole	RR	2 mg/mL	IMM[c]	1 mg/mL[a]	Physically compatible for 4 hr at 23 °C	1861	C
Fludarabine phosphate	BX	1 mg/mL[a]	IMM[c]	1 mg/mL[a]	Physically compatible for 4 hr at 23 °C	1861	C
Fluorouracil	AD	16 mg/mL[a]	IMM[c]	1 mg/mL[a]	Physically compatible for 4 hr at 23 °C	1861	C
Furosemide	AMR	3 mg/mL[a]	IMM[c]	1 mg/mL[a]	Physically compatible for 4 hr at 23 °C	1861	C
Gallium nitrate	FUJ	0.4 mg/mL[a]	IMM[c]	1 mg/mL[a]	Physically compatible for 4 hr at 23 °C	1861	C
Ganciclovir sodium	SY	20 mg/mL[a]	IMM[c]	1 mg/mL[a]	Physically compatible for 4 hr at 23 °C	1861	C
Gemcitabine HCl	LI	10 mg/mL[b]	IMM[c]	1 mg/mL[b]	Physically compatible for 4 hr at 23 °C	2226	C
Gentamicin sulfate	ES	5 mg/mL[a]	IMM[c]	1 mg/mL[a]	Physically compatible for 4 hr at 23 °C	1861	C
Granisetron HCl	SKB	0.05 mg/mL[a]	IMM[c]	1 mg/mL[a]	Physically compatible for 4 hr at 23 °C	1861	C
Haloperidol lactate	MN	0.2 mg/mL[a]	IMM[c]	1 mg/mL[a]	Physically compatible for 4 hr at 23 °C	1861	C
Heparin sodium	ES	100 units/mL[a]	IMM[c]	1 mg/mL[a]	Physically compatible for 4 hr at 23 °C	1861	C
Hydrocortisone sodium succinate	UP	1 mg/mL[a]	IMM[c]	1 mg/mL[a]	Physically compatible for 4 hr at 23 °C	1861	C
Hydromorphone HCl	AST	0.5 mg/mL[a]	IMM[c]	1 mg/mL[a]	Physically compatible for 4 hr at 23 °C	1861	C
Hydroxyzine HCl	ES	4 mg/mL[a]	IMM[c]	1 mg/mL[a]	Physically compatible for 4 hr at 23 °C	1861	C
Idarubicin HCl	AD	0.5 mg/mL[a]	IMM[c]	1 mg/mL[a]	Physically compatible for 4 hr at 23 °C	1861	C
Ifosfamide	MJ	25 mg/mL[a]	IMM[c]	1 mg/mL[a]	Physically compatible for 4 hr at 23 °C	1861	C
Imipenem–cilastatin sodium	ME	10 mg/mL[a]	IMM[c]	1 mg/mL[a]	Physically compatible for 4 hr at 23 °C	1861	C
Leucovorin calcium	LE	2 mg/mL[a]	IMM[c]	1 mg/mL[a]	Physically compatible for 4 hr at 23 °C	1861	C
Lorazepam	WY	0.1 mg/mL[a]	IMM[c]	1 mg/mL[a]	Physically compatible for 4 hr at 23 °C	1861	C
Magnesium sulfate	AST	100 mg/mL[a]	IMM[c]	1 mg/mL[a]	Physically compatible for 4 hr at 23 °C	1861	C
Mannitol	BA	15%	IMM[c]	1 mg/mL[a]	Physically compatible for 4 hr at 23 °C	1861	C
Melphalan HCl	BW	0.1 mg/mL[b]	LE[d]	10 mg/mL[b]	Physically compatible for 3 hr at 22 °C	1557	C
Meperidine HCl	WY	4 mg/mL[a]	IMM[c]	1 mg/mL[a]	Physically compatible for 4 hr at 23 °C	1861	C

Y-Site Injection Compatibility (1:1 Mixture) (Cont.)

Thiotepa

Drug	Mfr	Conc	Mfr	Conc	Remarks	Ref	C/I
Mesna	MJ	10 mg/mL[a]	IMM[c]	1 mg/mL[a]	Physically compatible for 4 hr at 23 °C	1861	C
Methotrexate sodium	LE	15 mg/mL[a]	IMM[c]	1 mg/mL[a]	Physically compatible for 4 hr at 23 °C	1861	C
Methylprednisolone sodium succinate	AB	5 mg/mL[a]	IMM[c]	1 mg/mL[a]	Physically compatible for 4 hr at 23 °C	1861	C
Metoclopramide HCl	RB	5 mg/mL	IMM[c]	1 mg/mL[a]	Physically compatible for 4 hr at 23 °C	1861	C
Metronidazole	BA	5 mg/mL	IMM[c]	1 mg/mL[a]	Physically compatible for 4 hr at 23 °C	1861	C
Mitomycin	BMS	0.5 mg/mL	IMM[c]	1 mg/mL[a]	Physically compatible for 4 hr at 23 °C	1861	C
Mitoxantrone HCl	IMM	0.5 mg/mL[a]	IMM[c]	1 mg/mL[a]	Physically compatible for 4 hr at 23 °C	1861	C
Morphine sulfate	AST	1 mg/mL[a]	IMM[c]	1 mg/mL[a]	Physically compatible for 4 hr at 23 °C	1861	C
Nalbuphine HCl	AST	10 mg/mL	IMM[c]	1 mg/mL[a]	Physically compatible for 4 hr at 23 °C	1861	C
Ondansetron HCl	GL	1 mg/mL[a]	IMM[c]	1 mg/mL[a]	Physically compatible for 4 hr at 23 °C	1861	C
Paclitaxel	MJ	0.6 mg/mL[a]	IMM[c]	1 mg/mL[b]	Physically compatible for 4 hr at 23 °C	1861	C
Piperacillin sodium–tazobactam sodium	LE[e]	40 + 5 mg/mL[a]	LE[d]	1 mg/mL[a]	Physically compatible for 4 hr at 22 °C	1688	C
Potassium chloride	AMR	0.1 mEq/mL[a]	IMM[c]	1 mg/mL[a]	Physically compatible for 4 hr at 23 °C	1861	C
Prochlorperazine edisylate	SCN	0.5 mg/mL[a]	IMM[c]	1 mg/mL[a]	Physically compatible for 4 hr at 23 °C	1861	C
Promethazine HCl	WY	2 mg/mL[a]	IMM[c]	1 mg/mL[a]	Physically compatible for 4 hr at 23 °C	1861	C
Ranitidine HCl	GL	2 mg/mL[a]	IMM[c]	1 mg/mL[a]	Physically compatible for 4 hr at 23 °C	1861	C
Sodium bicarbonate	AB	1 mEq/mL	IMM[c]	1 mg/mL[a]	Physically compatible for 4 hr at 23 °C	1861	C
Streptozocin	UP	40 mg/mL[a]	IMM[c]	1 mg/mL[a]	Physically compatible for 4 hr at 23 °C	1861	C
Teniposide	BR	0.1 mg/mL[a]	LE[d]	1 mg/mL[a]	Physically compatible for 4 hr at 23 °C	1725	C
Ticarcillin disodium–clavulanate potassium	SKB	31 mg/mL[a]	IMM[c]	1 mg/mL[a]	Physically compatible for 4 hr at 23 °C	1861	C
Tobramycin sulfate	LI	5 mg/mL[a]	IMM[c]	1 mg/mL[a]	Physically compatible for 4 hr at 23 °C	1861	C
TPN #193[f]			IMM[c]	1 mg/mL[a]	Physically compatible for 4 hr at 23 °C	1861	C
Trimethoprim–sulfamethoxazole	ES	0.8 + 4 mg/mL[a]	IMM[c]	1 mg/mL[a]	Physically compatible for 4 hr at 23 °C	1861	C
Vancomycin HCl	AB	10 mg/mL[a]	IMM[c]	1 mg/mL[a]	Physically compatible for 4 hr at 23 °C	1861	C
Vinblastine sulfate	LI	0.12 mg/mL[a]	IMM[c]	1 mg/mL[a]	Physically compatible for 4 hr at 23 °C	1861	C
Vincristine sulfate	LI	0.05 mg/mL[a]	IMM[c]	1 mg/mL[a]	Physically compatible for 4 hr at 23 °C	1861	C
Vinorelbine tartrate	BW	1 mg/mL[b]	LE[d]	10 mg/mL[b]	Immediate cloudiness with particles	1558	I
Zidovudine	BW	4 mg/mL[a]	IMM[c]	1 mg/mL[a]	Physically compatible for 4 hr at 23 °C	1861	C

[a]Tested in dextrose 5%.
[b]Tested in sodium chloride 0.9%.
[c]Lyophilized formulation tested.
[d]Powder fill formulation tested.
[e]Test performed using the formulation WITHOUT edetate disodium.
[f]Refer to Appendix I for the composition of parenteral nutrition solutions. TPN indicates a 2-in-1 admixture.

TICARCILLIN DISODIUM–CLAVULANATE POTASSIUM
AHFS 8:12.16.16

Products — Ticarcillin disodium–clavulanate potassium is available in vials containing 3.1 g (ticarcillin 3 g as the disodium salt plus clavulanic acid 100 mg as the potassium salt). Reconstitute the vials with 13 mL of sterile water for injection or sodium chloride 0.9% and shake well. When dissolution is completed, the solution will contain ticarcillin 200 mg/mL with clavulanic acid 6.7 mg/mL. (1)

The product is also available in a pharmacy bulk package containing 31 g (ticarcillin 30 g as the disodium salt plus clavulanic acid 1 g as the potassium salt). It should be reconstituted with 76 mL of sterile water for injection or sodium chloride 0.9%, added in two portions, and shaken well. Each milliliter of this concentrate contains ticarcillin 300 mg plus clavulanic acid 10 mg. (4)

Ticarcillin disodium–clavulanate potassium is available as a frozen premixed infusion containing 3.1 g in 100 mL of water (30 mg/mL of ticarcillin plus 1 mg/mL of clavulanic acid) with sodium citrate buffer and hydrochloric acid or sodium hydroxide to adjust pH. Thawing for use should be performed at room temperature or under refrigeration and not by warming in a water bath or by exposure to microwave radiation. Any precipitate that has formed during freezing should redissolve upon reaching room temperature. The container and ports should be checked for leaking by squeezing the bag. (4)

pH — From 5.5 to 7.5. (1)

Osmolality — The following maximum ticarcillin disodium–clavulanate potassium concentrations were recommended to achieve osmolalities suitable for peripheral infusion in fluid-restricted patients (1180):

Diluent	Maximum Concentration[a] (mg/mL)	Osmolality (mOsm/kg)
Dextrose 5%	48	562
Sodium chloride 0.9%	43	546
Sterile water for injection	86	573

[a]*Ticarcillin concentration.*

Sodium and Potassium Content — Each gram of this combination product contains 4.51 mEq of sodium and 0.15 mEq of potassium. (1)
The 3.1 g/100 mL frozen injection contains 0.187 mEq/mL of sodium and 0.005 mEq/mL of potassium. (4)

Trade Name(s) — Timentin.

Administration — Reconstituted ticarcillin disodium–clavulanate potassium solutions should be further diluted to concentrations of 10 to 100 mg/mL of ticarcillin and given over 30 minutes by intermittent intravenous infusion directly into a vein or through a Y-type administration set. Other solutions should be temporarily discontinued during the infusion of ticarcillin disodium–clavulanate potassium. (1; 4)

Stability — The commercially available combination product as a powder is white to pale yellow. It should be stored at 24 °C or less. Higher temperatures may cause darkening, an indication of clavulanate potassium degradation. (4)

The concentrated reconstituted solutions, which are colorless to pale yellow, are stable for up to six hours after reconstitution when stored at room temperatures of 21 to 24 °C or for up to 72 hours when refrigerated at 4 °C. (1; 4)

The frozen premixed infusion solutions should be stored at −20 °C. After thawing at room temperature or under refrigeration, the solutions are stable for 24 hours at room temperature or seven days under refrigeration. Thawed solutions should not be refrozen. (4)

pH Effects — Clavulanic acid exhibits maximum stability at pH 6.4. (1797)

Freezing Solutions — Ticarcillin disodium–clavulanate potassium solutions of 10 to 100 mg/mL (ticarcillin content) in sodium chloride 0.9% or Ringer's injection, lactated, are stable for up to 30 days when frozen at −18 °C. Diluted to this concentration range in dextrose 5%, the drug is stable for up to seven days when frozen. Frozen solutions should be thawed at room temperature, and thawed solutions should be used within eight hours and not be refrozen. (1; 4)

Elastomeric Reservoir Pumps — Ticarcillin disodium–clavulanate potassium (Beecham) 15 mg/mL in both dextrose 5% and sodium chloride 0.9% was evaluated for binding potential to natural rubber elastomeric reservoirs (Baxter). No binding was found after storage for two weeks at 35 °C with gentle agitation. (2014)

Central Venous Catheter — Ticarcillin disodium–clavulanate potassium (SmithKline Beecham) 10.33 mg/mL in dextrose 5% was found to be compatible with the ARROWg+ard Blue Plus (Arrow International) chlorhexidine-bearing triple-lumen central catheter. Essentially complete delivery of the drug was found with little or no drug loss occurring. Furthermore, chlorhexidine delivered from the catheter remained at trace amounts with no substantial increase due to the delivery of the drug through the catheter. (2335)

Compatibility Information

Solution Compatibility

Ticarcillin disodium–clavulanate potassium

Solution	Mfr	Mfr	Conc/L	Remarks	Ref	C/I
Dextrose 5%			10 to 100 g	Stable for 24 hr at room temperature and 3 days refrigerated	1	**C**
Ringer's injection, lactated			10 to 100 g	Stable for 24 hr at room temperature and 7[a] or 4[b] days refrigerated	1	**C**

Solution Compatibility (Cont.)

Ticarcillin disodium–clavulanate potassium

Solution	Mfr	Mfr	Conc/L	Remarks	Ref	C/I
Sodium chloride 0.9%			10 to 100 g	Stable for 24 hr at room temperature and 7[a] or 4[b] days refrigerated	1	**C**

[a] Prepared from the 200-mg/mL reconstituted solution.
[b] Prepared from the 300-mg/mL reconstituted bulk solution.

Additive Compatibility

Ticarcillin disodium–clavulanate potassium

Drug	Mfr	Conc/L	Mfr	Conc/L	Test Soln	Remarks	Ref	C/I
Ciprofloxacin	BAY	2 g	SKB	30 g	D5W	Visually compatible but pH changed by more than 1 unit	2413	**?**

Drugs in Syringe Compatibility

Ticarcillin disodium–clavulanate potassium

Drug (in syringe)	Mfr	Amt	Mfr	Amt	Remarks	Ref	C/I
Pantoprazole sodium	[a]	4 mg/ 1 mL		200 mg/ 1 mL	Clear solution	2574	**C**

[a] Test performed using the formulation WITHOUT edetate disodium.

Y-Site Injection Compatibility (1:1 Mixture)

Ticarcillin disodium–clavulanate potassium

Drug	Mfr	Conc	Mfr	Conc	Remarks	Ref	C/I
Allopurinol sodium	BW	3 mg/mL[b]	SKB	31 mg/mL[b]	Physically compatible for 4 hr at 22 °C	1686	**C**
Amifostine	USB	10 mg/mL[a]	SKB	31 mg/mL[a]	Physically compatible for 4 hr at 23 °C	1845	**C**
Amphotericin B cholesteryl sulfate complex	SEQ	0.83 mg/mL[a]	SKB	31 mg/mL[a]	Gross precipitate forms	2117	**I**
Anidulafungin	VIC	0.5 mg/mL[a]	GSK	31 mg/mL[a]	Physically compatible for 4 hr at 23 °C	2617	**C**
Azithromycin	PF	2 mg/mL[b]	SKB	103.3 mg/ mL[b,g]	Amber microcrystals found	2368	**I**
Aztreonam	SQ	40 mg/mL[a]	SKB	31 mg/mL[a]	Physically compatible for 4 hr at 23 °C	1758	**C**
Bivalirudin	TMC	5 mg/mL[a]	SKB	31 mg/mL[a]	Physically compatible for 4 hr at 23 °C	2373	**C**
Cisatracurium besylate	GW	0.1 and 2 mg/ mL[a]	SKB	31 mg/mL[a]	Physically compatible for 4 hr at 23 °C	2074	**C**
	GW	5 mg/mL[a]	SKB	31 mg/mL[a]	Subvisible haze forms immediately	2074	**I**
Clarithromycin	AB	4 mg/mL[a]	BE	32 mg/mL[a]	Visually compatible for 72 hr at both 30 and 17 °C	2174	**C**
Cyclophosphamide	MJ	20 mg/mL[a]	BE	31 mg/mL[a]	Physically compatible for 4 hr at 25 °C	1194	**C**
Dexmedetomidine HCl	AB	4 mcg/mL[b]	SKB	31 mg/mL[b]	Physically compatible for 4 hr at 23 °C	2383	**C**
Diltiazem HCl	MMD	1[b] and 5 mg/ mL	BE	200 mg/mL[b]	Visually compatible	1807	**C**
	MMD	5 mg/mL	BE	10 mg/mL[b]	Visually compatible	1807	**C**

Y-Site Injection Compatibility (1:1 Mixture) (Cont.)

Ticarcillin disodium–clavulanate potassium

Drug	Mfr	Conc	Mfr	Conc	Remarks	Ref	C/I
Docetaxel	RPR	0.9 mg/mL[a]	SKB	31 mg/mL[a]	Physically compatible for 4 hr at 23 °C	2224	C
Doxorubicin HCl liposomal	SEQ	0.4 mg/mL[a]	SKB	31 mg/mL[a]	Physically compatible for 4 hr at 23 °C	2087	C
Etoposide phosphate	BR	5 mg/mL[a]	SKB	31 mg/mL[a]	Physically compatible for 4 hr at 23 °C	2218	C
Famotidine	MSD	0.2 mg/mL[a]	BE	31 mg/mL[b]	Physically compatible for 14 hr	1196	C
Fenoldopam mesylate	AB	80 mcg/mL[b]	SKB	31 mg/mL[b]	Physically compatible for 4 hr at 23 °C	2467	C
Filgrastim	AMG	30 mcg/mL[a]	SKB	31 mg/mL[a]	Physically compatible for 4 hr at 22 °C	1687	C
Fluconazole	RR	2 mg/mL	BE	60 mg/mL	Physically compatible for 24 hr at 25 °C	1407	C
Fludarabine phosphate	BX	1 mg/mL[a]	BE	31 mg/mL[a]	Visually compatible for 4 hr at 22 °C	1439	C
Foscarnet sodium	AST	24 mg/mL	BE	100 mg/mL[c]	Physically compatible for 24 hr at 25 °C under fluorescent light	1393	C
Gallium nitrate	FUJ	1 mg/mL[b]	SKB	103.3 mg/mL[b]	Visually compatible for 24 hr at 25 °C	1673	C
Gemcitabine HCl	LI	10 mg/mL[b]	SKB	31 mg/mL[b]	Physically compatible for 4 hr at 23 °C	2226	C
Granisetron HCl	SKB	1 mg/mL	SKB	27 mg/mL[b]	Physically compatible with little or no loss of either drug in 4 hr at 22 °C	1883	C
	SKB	0.05 mg/mL[a]	SKB	31 mg/mL[a]	Physically compatible for 4 hr at 23 °C	2000	C
Heparin sodium	TR	50 units/mL	BE	31 mg/mL[b]	Visually compatible for 4 hr at 25 °C	1793	C
Hetastarch in lactated electrolyte	AB	6%	SKB	31 mg/mL[a]	Physically compatible for 4 hr at 23 °C	2339	C
Insulin, regular	LI	0.2 unit/mL[b]	BE	31 mg/mL[b]	Physically compatible for 2 hr at 25 °C	1395	C
Melphalan HCl	BW	0.1 mg/mL[b]	SKB	31 mg/mL[b]	Physically compatible for 3 hr at 22 °C	1557	C
Meperidine HCl	WY	10 mg/mL[b]	BE	31 mg/mL[b]	Physically compatible for 1 hr at 25 °C	1338	C
Milrinone lactate	SS	0.2 mg/mL[a]	SKB	100 mg/mL[a]	Visually compatible for 4 hr at 25 °C	2381	C
Morphine sulfate	ES	1 mg/mL[b]	BE	31 mg/mL[b]	Physically compatible for 1 hr at 25 °C	1338	C
Ondansetron HCl	GL	1 mg/mL[b]	BE	31 mg/mL[a]	Visually compatible for 4 hr at 22 °C	1365	C
Pemetrexed disodium	LI	20 mg/mL[b]	GSK	31 mg/mL[a]	Physically compatible for 4 hr at 23 °C	2564	C
Propofol	ZEN	10 mg/mL	SKB	31 mg/mL[a]	Physically compatible for 1 hr at 23 °C	2066	C
Remifentanil HCl	GW	0.025 and 0.25 mg/mL[b]	SKB	31 mg/mL[a]	Physically compatible for 4 hr at 23 °C	2075	C
Sargramostim	IMM	10 mcg/mL[b]	BE	31 mg/mL[b]	Visually compatible for 4 hr at 22 °C	1436	C
Teniposide	BR	0.1 mg/mL[a]	SKB	31 mg/mL[a]	Physically compatible for 4 hr at 23 °C	1725	C
Theophylline	TR	4 mg/mL	BE	31 mg/mL[b]	Visually compatible for 6 hr at 25 °C	1793	C
Thiotepa	IMM[d]	1 mg/mL[a]	SKB	31 mg/mL[a]	Physically compatible for 4 hr at 23 °C	1861	C
TNA #218 to #226[e]			SKB	31 mg/mL[a]	Visually compatible for 4 hr at 23 °C	2215	C
Topotecan HCl	SKB	56 mcg/mL[a]	SKB	24.6 mg/mL[a]	Immediate yellow color. 11% topotecan loss in 4 hr at 22 °C	2245	I
	SKB	56 mcg/mL[b]	SKB	24.6 mg/mL[b]	Immediate yellow color. Under 5% loss of all components in 4 hr at 22 °C	2245	C
TPN #189[e]			BE	30 mg/mL[b]	Visually compatible for 24 hr at 22 °C	1767	C
TPN #212 to #215[e]			SKB	31 mg/mL[a]	Physically compatible for 4 hr at 23 °C	2109	C
Vancomycin HCl	AB	20 mg/mL[a]	SKB	206.7 mg/mL[f]	Transient precipitate forms	2189	?

Y-Site Injection Compatibility (1:1 Mixture) (Cont.)

Ticarcillin disodium–clavulanate potassium

Drug	Mfr	Conc	Mfr	Conc	Remarks	Ref	C/I
	AB	20 mg/mL[a]	SKB	1.034, 10.335, 51.675 mg/mL[a]	Gross white precipitate forms	2189	**I**
	AB	5 mg/mL[b]	SKB	31 mg/mL[b]	White precipitate formed sporadically	2167	**I**
	AB	2 mg/mL[a]	SKB	1.034[a], 10.335[a], 51.675[a], 206.7[f] mg/mL	Physically compatible for 4 hr at 23 °C	2189	**C**
Vinorelbine tartrate	BW	1 mg/mL[b]	SKB	31 mg/mL[b]	Physically compatible for 4 hr at 22 °C	1558	**C**

[a]*Tested in dextrose 5%.*
[b]*Tested in sodium chloride 0.9%.*
[c]*Tested in both dextrose 5% and sodium chloride 0.9%.*
[d]*Lyophilized formulation tested.*
[e]*Refer to Appendix I for the composition of parenteral nutrition solutions. TNA indicates a 3-in-1 admixture, and TPN indicates a 2-in-1 admixture.*
[f]*Tested in sterile water for injection.*
[g]*Injected via Y-site into an administration set running azithromycin.*

TIGECYCLINE
AHFS 8:12.24.12

Products — Tigecycline is available as a 50-mg lyophilized powder in vials with lactose monohydrate 100 mg as an excipient. The pH is adjusted with hydrochloric acid and, if necessary, sodium hydroxide. (1)

Reconstitute the vials with 5.3 mL of sodium chloride 0.9% or dextrose 5% and gently swirl to aid dissolution. The vials contain an excess of drug, and this reconstitution volume yields a 10-mg/mL solution. The reconstituted solution must be diluted for administration. (1)

Trade Name(s) — Tygacil.

Administration — Tigecycline is administered by intravenous infusion over 30 to 60 minutes after dilution of the reconstituted solution in 100 mL of dextrose 5% or sodium chloride 0.9%. The concentration should not exceed 1 mg/mL. The solution should be yellow to orange. Discard if the solution does not have the correct color. (1)

Stability — Intact vials of tigecycline should be stored at controlled room temperature. Tigecycline reconstituted as directed may be stored at room temperature for up to six hours with an additional 18 hours after dilution in the infusion solution. Alternatively, the dilution for infusion may be stored for up to 48 hours under refrigeration if mixed immediately after reconstitution. The solution should be yellow to orange and should be inspected for the formation of a green or black discoloration. Discolored solutions should be discarded. (1)

Compatibility Information

Solution Compatibility

Tigecycline

Solution	Mfr	Mfr	Conc/L	Remarks	Ref	C/I
Dextrose 5%		WY	1 g	Physically compatible for 4 hr	2714	**C**
Dextrose 5% in Ringer's injection, lactated		WY	1 g	Physically compatible for 4 hr	2714	**C**
Dextrose 5% in sodium chloride 0.9%		WY	1 g	Physically compatible for 4 hr	2714	**C**

Solution Compatibility (Cont.)

Tigecycline

Solution	Mfr	Mfr	Conc/L	Remarks	Ref	C/I
Plasma-Lyte 56 in dextrose 5%	BA	WY	1 g	Physically compatible for 4 hr	2714	**C**
Ringer's injection, lactated		WY	1 g	Physically compatible for 4 hr	2714	**C**

Y-Site Injection Compatibility (1:1 Mixture)

Tigecycline

Drug	Mfr	Conc	Mfr	Conc	Remarks	Ref	C/I
Amikacin sulfate		5 mg/mL[b]	WY	1 mg/mL[b]	Physically compatible for 4 hr	2714	**C**
Amphotericin B		2 mg/mL[a]	WY	1 mg/mL[b]	Immediate cloudiness with particulates in 1 hr	2714	**I**
Amphotericin B lipid complex	ENZ	2 mg/mL[a]	WY	1 mg/mL[b]	Incompatible with sodium chloride diluent	2714	**I**
Azithromycin		2 mg/mL[b]	WY	1 mg/mL[b]	Physically compatible for 4 hr	2714	**C**
Aztreonam		20 mg/mL[b]	WY	1 mg/mL[b]	Physically compatible for 4 hr	2714	**C**
Cefepime HCl	ELN	40 mg/mL[b]	WY	1 mg/mL[b]	Physically compatible for 4 hr	2714	**C**
Cefotaxime sodium		40 mg/mL[b]	WY	1 mg/mL[b]	Physically compatible for 4 hr	2714	**C**
Ceftazidime		40 mg/mL[b]	WY	1 mg/mL[b]	Physically compatible for 4 hr	2714	**C**
Ceftriaxone sodium		40 mg/mL[b]	WY	1 mg/mL[b]	Physically compatible for 4 hr	2714	**C**
Chlorpromazine HCl		1 mg/mL[b]	WY	1 mg/mL[b]	Precipitates immediately	2714	**I**
Ciprofloxacin		1 mg/mL[b]	WY	1 mg/mL[b]	Physically compatible for 4 hr	2714	**C**
Dobutamine HCl		0.2 and 1 mg/mL[b]	WY	1 mg/mL[b]	Physically compatible for 4 hr	2714	**C**
Dopamine HCl		1.6 mg/mL[b]	WY	1 mg/mL[b]	Physically compatible for 4 hr	2714	**C**
Doripenem	JJ	5 mg/mL[a,b]	WY	1 mg/mL[a,b]	Physically compatible for 4 hr at 23 °C	2743	**C**
Epinephrine HCl		4 mcg/mL[b]	WY	1 mg/mL[b]	Physically compatible for 4 hr	2714	**C**
Ertapenem sodium		20 mg/mL[b]	WY	1 mg/mL[b]	Physically compatible for 4 hr	2714	**C**
Fluconazole		2 mg/mL	WY	1 mg/mL[b]	Physically compatible for 4 hr	2714	**C**
Gentamicin sulfate		1.4 mg/mL[b]	WY	1 mg/mL[b]	Physically compatible for 4 hr	2714	**C**
Haloperidol lactate		0.2 mg/mL[b]	WY	1 mg/mL[b]	Physically compatible for 4 hr	2714	**C**
Heparin sodium		10 units/mL	WY	1 mg/mL[b]	Physically compatible for 4 hr	2714	**C**
		100 units/mL[b]	WY	1 mg/mL[b]	Physically compatible for 4 hr	2714	**C**
Imipenem–cilastatin sodium		5 mg/mL[b]	WY	1 mg/mL[b]	Physically compatible for 4 hr	2714	**C**
Lidocaine HCl		200 mg/mL	WY	1 mg/mL[b]	Physically compatible for 4 hr	2714	**C**
Linezolid	PF	2 mg/mL	WY	1 mg/mL[b]	Physically compatible for 4 hr	2714	**C**
Methylprednisolone sodium succinate		20 mg/mL[b]	WY	1 mg/mL[b]	Microparticulates form	2714	**I**
Metoclopramide HCl		5 mg/mL	WY	1 mg/mL[b]	Physically compatible for 4 hr	2714	**C**
Piperacillin sodium–tazobactam sodium	c	3 + 0.375 mg/mL[b]	WY	1 mg/mL[b]	Physically compatible for 4 hr	2714	**C**
Potassium chloride		0.3 mEq/mL[b]	WY	1 mg/mL[b]	Physically compatible for 4 hr	2714	**C**

Y-Site Injection Compatibility (1:1 Mixture) (Cont.)

Tigecycline

Drug	Mfr	Conc	Mfr	Conc	Remarks	Ref	C/I
Ranitidine HCl		0.6 mg/mL[b]	WY	1 mg/mL[b]	Physically compatible for 4 hr	2714	C
Telavancin HCl	ASP	7.5 mg/mL[a,b,d]	WY	1 mg/mL[a,b,d]	Physically compatible for 2 hr	2830	C
Theophylline		1.6 mg/mL[a]	WY	1 mg/mL[b]	Physically compatible for 4 hr	2714	C
Tobramycin sulfate		2.5 mg/mL[b]	WY	1 mg/mL[b]	Physically compatible for 4 hr	2714	C
Vancomycin HCl		5 mg/mL[b]	WY	1 mg/mL[b]	Physically compatible for 4 hr	2714	C
Voriconazole	PF	2 mg/mL[b]	WY	1 mg/mL[b]	Microparticulates form	2714	I

[a]Tested in dextrose 5%.
[b]Tested in sodium chloride 0.9%.
[c]Test performed using the formulation WITHOUT edetate disodium.
[d]Tested in Ringer's injection, lactated.

TIROFIBAN HYDROCHLORIDE
AHFS 20:12.18

Products — Tirofiban hydrochloride is available premixed as a ready-to-use solution for infusion in 100- and 250-mL (IntraVia) plastic containers. Each milliliter of the ready-to-use infusion provides tirofiban 0.05 mg (50 mcg) as the hydrochloride monohydrate along with sodium chloride 9 mg, sodium citrate dihydrate 0.54 mg, citric acid anhydrous 0.032 mg, and sodium hydroxide and/or hydrochloric acid to adjust pH in water for injection. (1)

pH — From 5.5 to 6.5. (1)

Osmolality — The osmolality of tirofiban hydrochloride premixed infusion solution is approximately 300 mOsm/kg. (4)

Trade Name(s) — Aggrastat.

Administration — Tirofiban hydrochloride is administered only by intravenous infusion. The premixed infusion solution is ready to use and does not require dilution. (1)

Stability — Tirofiban hydrochloride ready-to-use infusion is clear and colorless. Intact plastic containers should be stored at controlled room temperature of 25 °C, with temperature excursions in the range of 15 to 30 °C permitted, and protected from light and freezing. (1)

Compatibility Information

Solution Compatibility

Tirofiban HCl

Solution	Mfr	Mfr	Conc/L	Remarks	Ref	C/I
Dextrose 5% in sodium chloride 0.45%	AB[a]	ME	50 mg	Visually compatible. No loss in 24 hr at 23 °C in light	2249	C
Dextrose 5%	BA[a]	ME	50 mg	Visually compatible. No loss in 24 hr at 23 °C in light	2249	C
Sodium chloride 0.9%	AB[a]	ME	50 mg	Visually compatible. No loss in 24 hr at 23 °C in light	2249	C
	[b]	MSD	50 mg	Visually compatible. No loss in 30 days at room temperature	2355	C

[a]Tested in PVC containers.
[b]Tested in glass and polyethylene containers.

Y-Site Injection Compatibility (1:1 Mixture)

Tirofiban HCl

Drug	Mfr	Conc	Mfr	Conc	Remarks	Ref	C/I
Amiodarone HCl	WY	6 mg/mL[a]	ME	0.25 mg/mL[a]	Visually compatible for 24 hr at 22 °C	2352	**C**
Argatroban	GSK	1 mg/mL[a,b,c]	ME	0.05 mg/mL[c]	Physically compatible with no loss of either drug in 4 hr at 23 °C	2630	**C**
Atropine sulfate	APP	0.4 mg/mL	ME	50 mcg/mL[a,b]	Physically compatible with no loss of either drug in 4 hr at 23 °C	2356	**C**
	AMR	1 mg/mL	ME	50 mcg/mL[a,b]	Physically compatible with no loss of either drug in 4 hr at 23 °C	2356	**C**
Bivalirudin	TMC	5 mg/mL[a]	ME	50 mcg/mL[a]	Physically compatible for 4 hr at 23 °C	2373	**C**
Diazepam	ES	5 mg/mL	ME	50 mcg/mL[a,b]	Precipitate forms immediately	2356	**I**
Dobutamine HCl	AB	0.25 and 5 mg/mL[a,b]	ME	50 mcg/mL[a,b]	Physically compatible with no loss of either drug in 4 hr at 23 °C	2356	**C**
Dopamine HCl	AMR	0.2 and 3.2 mg/mL[a,b]	ME	0.05 mg/mL[a,b]	Physically compatible. Little loss of either drug in 4 hr at room temperature	2250	**C**
Epinephrine HCl	AMR	2 and 100 mcg/mL[a,b]	ME	50 mcg/mL[a,b]	Physically compatible. No loss of either drug in 4 hr at 23 °C	2356	**C**
Famotidine	ME	2 and 4 mg/mL[a]	ME	0.05 mg/mL[b]	Physically compatible. Little loss of either drug in 4 hr at room temperature	2250	**C**
	ME	2 and 4 mg/mL[b]	ME	0.05 mg/mL[a]	Physically compatible. Little loss of either drug in 4 hr at room temperature	2250	**C**
Furosemide	AB	0.5[a,b] and 10 mg/mL	ME	50 mcg/mL[a,b]	Physically compatible with no loss of either drug in 4 hr at 23 °C	2356	**C**
Heparin sodium	AB	40 units/mL[a]	ME	0.05 mg/mL[a,b]	Physically compatible. No tirofiban or heparin loss in 4 hr at room temperature	2250	**C**
	AB	50 units/mL[b]	ME	0.05 mg/mL[b]	Physically compatible. No tirofiban or heparin loss in 4 hr at room temperature	2250	**C**
	AB	100 units/mL[a,b]	ME	0.05 mg/mL[a,b]	Physically compatible. No tirofiban or heparin loss in 4 hr at room temperature	2250	**C**
Lidocaine HCl	AB	1 and 20 mg/mL[a,b]	ME	0.05 mg/mL[a,b]	Physically compatible. Little loss of either drug in 4 hr at room temperature	2250	**C**
Midazolam HCl	RC	5 and 0.05[a,b] mg/mL	ME	50 mcg/mL[a,b]	Physically compatible. No loss of either drug in 4 hr at 23 °C	2356	**C**
Morphine sulfate	ES	0.1 and 1 mg/mL[a]	ME	50 mcg/mL[a,b]	Physically compatible. No loss of either drug in 4 hr at 23 °C	2356	**C**
Nitroglycerin	AB	0.1 and 0.4 mg/mL	ME	50 mcg/mL[a,b]	Physically compatible. No loss of either drug in 4 hr at 23 °C	2356	**C**
Potassium chloride	AB	0.01 and 0.04 mEq/mL[a,b]	ME	0.05 mg/mL[a,b]	Physically compatible. No tirofiban loss in 4 hr at room temperature	2250	**C**
Propranolol HCl	WAY	1 mg/mL	ME	50 mcg/mL[a,b]	Physically compatible. No loss of either drug in 4 hr at 23 °C	2356	**C**

[a] Tested in dextrose 5%.
[b] Tested in sodium chloride 0.9%.
[c] Mixed argatroban:tirofiban hydrochloride 1:1 and 8:1.

TOBRAMYCIN SULFATE
AHFS 8:12.02

Products — Tobramycin sulfate is available in a concentration equivalent to tobramycin base 40 mg/mL in 2-mL vials as well as 50-mL bulk vials. It is also available as a pediatric injection containing tobramycin sulfate equivalent to tobramycin base 10 mg/mL in 2-, 6-, and 8-mL vials. In addition to tobramycin sulfate, other components may be present in the formulations including varying amounts of sodium metabisulfite, and disodium edetate 0.1 mg in water for injection. Phenol 5 mg is present in some formulations. Sodium hydroxide and/or sulfuric acid may have been added during manufacture for pH adjustment. (1)

Tobramycin sulfate is also available premixed in sodium chloride 0.9% in 0.8-mg/mL (80 mg) and 1.2-mg/mL (60 mg) concentrations. (4)

Tobramycin sulfate is also available in a pharmacy bulk package as a dry powder in vials containing the equivalent of tobramycin 1.2 g. (1) The vial contents should be diluted with 30 mL of sterile water for injection to yield a 40-mg/mL solution. The reconstituted solution is intended to be diluted in a suitable intravenous infusion solution for administration. (4)

pH — The pH of the injection is adjusted to 3 to 6.5. (1)

Osmolality — The osmolality of tobramycin sulfate 10 mg/mL was 133 mOsm/kg by freezing-point depression and 213 mOsm/kg by vapor pressure. (1071)

The osmolality of tobramycin sulfate 1 mg/mL was 254 mOsm/kg in dextrose 5% and 288 mOsm/kg in sodium chloride 0.9%. At 2.5 mg/mL, the osmolality was 261 mOsm/kg in dextrose 5% and 283 mOsm/kg in sodium chloride 0.9%. (1375)

The osmolality of tobramycin sulfate 80 mg was calculated for the following dilutions (1054):

Diluent	Osmolality (mOsm/kg) 50 mL	100 mL
Dextrose 5%	289	285
Sodium chloride 0.9%	319	315

The premixed products in sodium chloride 0.9% have an osmolarity of approximately 316 mOsm/kg. (4)

Sodium Content — The premixed products contain about 15.4 mEq of sodium per 100 mL of solution. (4)

Administration — Tobramycin sulfate may be administered by intramuscular injection or intermittent intravenous infusion. Intramuscular doses should be withdrawn only from multiple-dose vials; alternatively, the commercial prefilled syringes may be used. When given by intravenous infusion, the dose should be added to 50 to 100 mL of infusion solution and administered over 20 to 60 minutes. In children, the volume should be proportionately less but should allow an infusion period of 20 to 60 minutes. Infusion periods should not be less than 20 minutes; such shorter periods could result in excessive peak serum concentrations. (1; 4)

Stability — Tobramycin sulfate is stable at room temperature. Intact containers should be stored at controlled room temperature between 15 and 30 °C; premixed infusion solutions may be stored at temperatures up to 25 °C. Freezing and excessive temperatures above 40 °C should be avoided. The injections should not be used if they are discolored. The manufacturer recommends use of the 40-mg/mL reconstituted solution within 24 hours when stored at room temperature or 96 hours if refrigerated. (1; 4) Tobramycin sulfate is stable for several weeks at pH 1 to 11 at temperatures from 5 to 27 °C. It can be autoclaved without loss. (145)

Freezing Solutions — Tobramycin sulfate reconstituted to a concentration of 40 mg/mL and immediately frozen in the original container is stable for up to 12 weeks when stored at −10 to −20 °C. (4)

Tobramycin sulfate (Lilly) 160 mg/50 mL of dextrose 5% in PVC bags frozen at −20 °C for 30 days and then thawed by exposure to ambient temperature or microwave radiation was evaluated. The solutions showed no evidence of precipitation or color change and showed 6% or less loss. Subsequent storage of the admixture at room temperature for 24 hours also yielded a physically compatible solution which exhibited little or no additional loss. (555)

Tobramycin sulfate (Dista) 120 mg/50 mL in dextrose 5% and sodium chloride 0.9% in PVC bags lost 9% activity in 28 days when frozen at −20 °C. (981)

Minibags of tobramycin sulfate in dextrose 5% or sodium chloride 0.9%, frozen at −20 °C for up to 35 days, were thawed at room temperature and in a microwave oven, with care taken that the thawed solution temperature never exceeded 25 °C. No significant differences in tobramycin sulfate concentrations occurred between the two thawing methods. (1192)

Syringes — Samples of a 40-mg/mL solution of tobramycin sulfate (Lilly) from a reconstituted 1.2-g vial were stored in Monoject plastic syringes at both 25 and 4 °C. After two months, no significant change in concentration was detected in samples at either storage temperature. The authors did note that the manufacturer does not recommend storage in plastic syringes because of possible incompatibility with the plunger heads. (736)

Tobramycin sulfate (Dista) 120 mg diluted with 1 mL of sodium chloride 0.9% to a final volume of 4 mL was stable (less than a 10% loss) when stored in polypropylene syringes (Becton-Dickinson) for 48 hours at 25 °C under fluorescent light. (1159)

Elastomeric Reservoir Pumps — Tobramycin sulfate (Lilly) 0.8 mg/mL in both dextrose 5% and sodium chloride 0.9% was evaluated for binding potential to natural rubber elastomeric reservoirs (Baxter). No binding was found after storage for two weeks at 35 °C with gentle agitation. (2014)

Sorption — Tobramycin sulfate was shown not to exhibit sorption to PVC bags and tubing, polyethylene tubing, Silastic tubing, and polypropylene syringes. (536; 606)

Tobramycin sulfate (Qualimed) 1.5 mg/mL in dextrose 5% and in sodium chloride 0.9% was packaged in PVC bags (Macropharma) and in multilayer bags composed of polyethylene, polyamide, and polypropylene (Bieffe Medital). The solutions were delivered through PVC administration sets (Abbott) over one hour and evaluated for drug loss. No loss due to sorption to any of the plastic materials was found. (2269)

Filtration — Tobramycin sulfate (Lilly) 0.3 mg/mL in dextrose 5% and sodium chloride 0.9% was filtered through a 0.22-μm cellulose ester membrane filter (Ivex-HP, Millipore) over six hours. No significant drug loss due to binding to the filter was noted. (1034)

Tobramycin sulfate 5 and 10 mg/55 mL in dextrose 5% and sodium chloride 0.9% filtered over 20 minutes through a 0.22-μm cellulose ester filter set (Ivex-2, Millipore) was evaluated. Little or no binding of the drug to the filter occurred. (1003)

No significant loss due to sorption to a 0.22-μm cellulose ester filter (Continu-Flo 2C0252s, Travenol) occurred from a solution containing tobramycin sulfate (Dista) 80 mg/100 mL of dextrose 5% administered over 30 minutes. No difference in drug recovery was found between filtered and unfiltered solutions. However, 10% or more of the solution may remain in the tubing unless the sets are flushed. (1132)

Central Venous Catheter — Tobramycin sulfate (Lilly) 1 mg/mL in dextrose 5% was found to be compatible with the ARROWg+ard Blue Plus (Arrow International) chlorhexidine-bearing triple-lumen central catheter. Essentially complete delivery of the drug was found with little or no drug loss occurring. Furthermore, chlorhexidine delivered from the catheter remained at trace amounts with no substantial increase due to the delivery of the drug through the catheter. (2335)

Compatibility Information

Solution Compatibility

Tobramycin sulfate

Solution	Mfr	Mfr	Conc/L	Remarks	Ref	C/I
Amino acids 4.25%, dextrose 25%	MG	LI	80 mg	No increase in particulate matter in 24 hr at 25 °C	349	C
Dextrose 5% in sodium chloride 0.9%	TR[a]	LI	200 mg and 1 g	Physically compatible and chemically stable for 48 hr at 25 °C. Not more than 7% loss occurs	147	C
Dextrose 5%	TR[a]	LI	200 mg and 1 g	Physically compatible and chemically stable for 48 hr at 25 °C. Not more than 4% loss occurs	147	C
	TR[a]	LI	3.2 g	Physically compatible and no loss in 24 hr at room temperature	555	C
		LI	1 and 5 g	Physically compatible with no loss of activity in 60 min at room temperature	984	C
	AB[a]	DI	1.2 g	Visually compatible and stable for 48 hr at 25 °C under fluorescent light and 4 °C in the dark	1541	C
Dextrose 10%	TR[a]	LI	200 mg and 1 g	Physically compatible and chemically stable for 48 hr at 25 °C. Not more than 4% loss occurs	147	C
	SO	LI	60 mg/ 2- 1.5 mL[b]	Visually compatible with little or no tobramycin loss in 30 days at 5 °C in the dark	1731	C
	SO	LI	60 mg/ 1- 8.5 mL[b]	Visually compatible with little or no tobramycin loss in 30 days at 5 °C in the dark	1731	C
	SO	LI	120 mg/ 23 mL[b]	Visually compatible with little or no tobramycin loss in 30 days at 5 °C in the dark	1731	C
	SO	LI	120 mg/ 20 mL[b]	Visually compatible with little or no tobramycin loss in 30 days at 5 °C in the dark	1731	C
Isolyte E in dextrose 5%	MG	LI	1 g	12% loss in 24 hr at 25 °C. Stable for 4 hr	147	I
Isolyte M in dextrose 5%	MG	LI	200 mg and 1 g	12% loss in 24 hr at 25 °C. Stable for 4 hr	147	I
Isolyte P in dextrose 5%	MG	LI	200 mg and 1 g	12% loss in 24 hr at 25 °C. Stable for 4 hr	147	I
Normosol M in dextrose 5%	AB	LI	200 mg and 1 g	Physically compatible and chemically stable for 24 hr at 25 °C. Not more than 10% loss occurs	147	C
Normosol R	AB	LI	200 mg and 1 g	Physically compatible and chemically stable for 24 hr at 25 °C	147	C
Normosol R in dextrose 5%	AB	LI	200 mg and 1 g	Physically compatible and chemically stable for 24 hr at 25 °C. Not more than 8% loss occurs	147	C
Normosol R, pH 7.4	AB	LI	200 mg and 1 g	Physically compatible and chemically stable for 24 hr at 25 °C	147	C

Solution Compatibility (Cont.)

Tobramycin sulfate

Solution	Mfr	Mfr	Conc/L	Remarks	Ref	C/I
Ringer's injection	TR[a]	LI	200 mg and 1 g	Physically compatible and chemically stable for 24 hr at 25 °C	147	**C**
Ringer's injection, lactated		LI	200 mg and 1 g	Physically compatible and chemically stable for 24 hr at 25 °C	147	**C**
Sodium chloride 0.9%	TR[a]	LI	200 mg and 1 g	Physically compatible and chemically stable for 48 hr at 25 °C	147	**C**
	AB[a]	DI	1.2 g	Visually compatible and stable for 48 hr at 25 °C under fluorescent light and 4 °C in the dark	1541	**C**
	AB[c]	MAR	1 and 10 g	Little loss in 3 days at 25 °C and 14 days at 5 °C in PVC	2080	**C**
Sodium lactate ⅙ M		LI	200 mg and 1 g	Physically compatible and chemically stable for 48 hr at 25 °C	147	**C**

[a]Tested in PVC containers.
[b]Tested in glass vials as a concentrate.
[c]Tested in PVC portable pump reservoirs (Pharmacia Deltec).

Additive Compatibility

Tobramycin sulfate

Drug	Mfr	Conc/L	Mfr	Conc/L	Test Soln	Remarks	Ref	C/I
Aztreonam	SQ	10 and 20 g	LI	200 and 800 mg	D5W, NS	Little or no loss of either drug in 48 hr at 25 °C and 7 days at 4 °C	1023	**C**
Bleomycin sulfate	BR	20 and 30 units	LI	500 mg	NS	Physically compatible and bleomycin activity retained for 1 week at 4 °C. Tobramycin not tested	763	**C**
Calcium gluconate		16 g	LI	5 g	D5W	Physically compatible. No tobramycin loss in 60 min at room temperature	984	**C**
		33 g	LI	1 g	D5W	Physically compatible. No tobramycin loss in 60 min at room temperature	984	**C**
Cefepime HCl	BR	40 g	AB	0.4 g	D5W, NS	Cloudiness forms immediately	1682	**I**
	BR	2.5 g	AB	2 g	D5W, NS	Cloudiness forms immediately	1682	**I**
Cefoxitin sodium	MSD	5 g	LI	400 mg	D5S	5% cefoxitin loss in 24 hr and 11% in 48 hr at 25 °C. 3% in 48 hr at 5 °C. 8% tobramycin loss in 24 hr and 37% in 48 hr at 25 °C. 3% in 48 hr at 5 °C	308	**C**
Ciprofloxacin	MI	1.6 g	LI	1 g	D5W, NS	Visually compatible and both drugs stable for 48 hr at 25 °C under fluorescent light and 4 °C in the dark	1541	**C**
	BAY	2 g	LI	1.6 g	D5W	Visually compatible with no loss of ciprofloxacin in 24 hr at 22 °C under fluorescent light. Tobramycin not tested	2413	**C**
Clindamycin phosphate	UP	18 g	DI	2.4 g	D5W[a]	8% tobramycin lost in 14 days and 17% in 28 days at −20 °C. Clindamycin stable	981	**C**
	UP	18 g	DI	2.4 g	NS[a]	Both drugs stable for 28 days frozen at −20 °C	981	**C**
	UP	9 g	DI	1 g	D5W, NS[b]	Physically compatible and both drugs stable for 48 hr at room temperature exposed to light and for 1 week frozen	174	**C**

Additive Compatibility (Cont.)

Tobramycin sulfate

Drug	Mfr	Conc/L	Mfr	Conc/L	Test Soln	Remarks	Ref	C/I
	UP	9 g	DI	1.2 g	D5W[c]	Physically compatible and clindamycin stable for 28 days frozen. 8% tobramycin loss in 14 days and 17% in 28 days	174	C
	UP	9 g	DI	1.2 g	NS[c]	Physically compatible and both drugs stable for 28 days frozen	174	C
Dextran 40	TR	10%	LI	200 mg and 1 g	D5W	Physically compatible and stable for 24 hr at 25 °C. Not more than 9% loss	147	C
Floxacillin sodium	BE	20 g	LI	8 g	NS	White precipitate forms in 7 hr	1479	I
Furosemide	HO	1 g	LI	8 g	NS	Physically compatible for 72 hr at 15 and 30 °C	1479	C
	HO	800 mg	DI	1.6 g	D5W, NS	Transient cloudiness then physically compatible for 24 hr at 21 °C	876	?
Imipenem–cilastatin sodium		100 mg		10 mg	W	Little or no loss of antibiotic activity in 24 hr at 37 °C	498	C
Linezolid	PHU	2 g	GNS	800 mg	[d]	Physically compatible. Little linezolid loss in 7 days at 4 and 23 °C in dark. No tobramycin loss in 7 days at 4 °C but losses of 4% in 1 day and 12% in 3 days at 23 °C	2332	C
Mannitol		20%	LI	200 mg and 1 g		Physically compatible and chemically stable for 48 hr at 25 °C	147	C
Metronidazole	RP	5 g	LI	1 g		Visually compatible with no loss of metronidazole in 15 days at 5 and 25 °C. 10% tobramycin loss in 73 hr at 25 °C and 12.1 days at 5 °C	1931	C
Ranitidine HCl	GL	100 mg	DI	200 mg	D5W	Physically compatible for 24 hr at ambient temperature in light	1151	C
Verapamil HCl	KN	80 mg	LI	160 mg	D5W, NS	Physically compatible for 24 hr	764	C

[a]*Tested in PVC containers.*
[b]*Tested in both glass and PVC containers.*
[c]*Tested in glass containers.*
[d]*Admixed in the linezolid infusion container.*

Drugs in Syringe Compatibility

Tobramycin sulfate

Drug (in syringe)	Mfr	Amt	Mfr	Amt	Remarks	Ref	C/I
Clindamycin phosphate	UP	900 mg/ 6 mL	DI	120 mg/ 4 mL[a]	Cloudy white precipitate forms immediately and changes to gel-like precipitate	1159	I
Dimenhydrinate		10 mg/ 1 mL		40 mg/ 1 mL	Clear solution	2569	C
Doxapram HCl	RB	400 mg/ 20 mL		60 mg/ 1.5 mL	Physically compatible with no doxapram loss in 24 hr	1177	C
Heparin sodium		10 units/ 1 mL		80 mg/ 2 mL	Turbidity or fine white precipitate due to formation of an insoluble salt	845	I
		2500 units/ 1 mL	LI	40 mg	Turbidity or precipitate forms within 5 min	1053	I

Drugs in Syringe Compatibility (Cont.)

Tobramycin sulfate

Drug (in syringe)	Mfr	Amt	Mfr	Amt	Remarks	Ref	C/I
Pantoprazole sodium	b	4 mg/ 1 mL		40 mg/ 1 mL	Precipitates immediately	2574	I

[a] Diluted to 4 mL with 1 mL of sodium chloride 0.9%.
[b] Test performed using the formulation WITHOUT edetate disodium.

Y-Site Injection Compatibility (1:1 Mixture)

Tobramycin sulfate

Drug	Mfr	Conc	Mfr	Conc	Remarks	Ref	C/I
Acyclovir sodium	BW	5 mg/mL[a]	DI	1.6 mg/mL[a]	Physically compatible for 4 hr at 25 °C	1157	C
Allopurinol sodium	BW	3 mg/mL[b]	LI	5 mg/mL[b]	Haze and crystals form in 1 hr	1686	I
Alprostadil	BED	7.5 mcg/mL[s,n]	LI	1 mg/mL[r]	Visually compatible for 1 hr	2746	C
Amifostine	USB	10 mg/mL[a]	LI	5 mg/mL[a]	Physically compatible for 4 hr at 23 °C	1845	C
Amiodarone HCl	LZ	4 mg/mL[c]	LI	0.8 mg/mL[c]	Physically compatible for 4 hr at room temperature	1444	C
	WY	6 mg/mL[a]	LI	5 mg/mL[a]	Visually compatible for 24 hr at 22 °C	2352	C
Amphotericin B cholesteryl sulfate complex	SEQ	0.83 mg/mL[a]	AB	5 mg/mL[a]	Gross precipitate forms	2117	I
Amsacrine	NCI	1 mg/mL[a]	LI	5 mg/mL[a]	Visually compatible for 4 hr at 22 °C	1381	C
Anidulafungin	VIC	0.5 mg/mL[a]	AB	5 mg/mL[a]	Physically compatible for 4 hr at 23 °C	2617	C
Azithromycin	PF	2 mg/mL[b]		21 mg/mL[p]	White microcrystals found	2368	I
Aztreonam	SQ	40 mg/mL[a]	LI	5 mg/mL[a]	Physically compatible for 4 hr at 23 °C	1758	C
Bivalirudin	TMC	5 mg/mL[a]	GNS	5 mg/mL[a]	Physically compatible for 4 hr at 23 °C	2373	C
Caspofungin acetate	ME	0.7 mg/mL[b]	SIC	5 mg/mL[b]	Physically compatible for 4 hr at room temperature	2758	C
Cefepime HCl	BMS	120 mg/mL[q]		6 mg/mL	Physically compatible with less than 10% cefepime loss. Tobramycin not tested	2513	C
Ceftaroline fosamil	FOR	2.22 mg/ml[a,b,o]	SIC	5 mg/mL[a,b,o]	Physically compatible for 4 hr at 23 °C	2826	C
Ceftazidime	SKB	125 mg/mL		0.6 mg/mL	Visually compatible with less than 10% loss of both drugs in 1 hr	2434	C
	GSK	120 mg/mL[q]		6 mg/mL	Physically compatible with less than 10% ceftazidime loss. Tobramycin not tested	2513	C
Ciprofloxacin	MI	1 mg/mL[a]	LI	1.6 mg/mL[c]	Physically compatible for 24 hr at 22 °C	1189	C
Cisatracurium besylate	GW	0.1, 2, 5 mg/mL[a]	AB	5 mg/mL[a]	Physically compatible for 4 hr at 23 °C	2074	C
Cyclophosphamide	MJ	20 mg/mL[a]	DI	0.8 mg/mL[a]	Physically compatible for 4 hr at 25 °C	1194	C
Dexmedetomidine HCl	AB	4 mcg/mL[b]	GNS	5 mg/mL[b]	Physically compatible for 4 hr at 23 °C	2383	C
Diltiazem HCl	MMD	5 mg/mL	LI	2.4[b] and 40 mg/mL	Visually compatible	1807	C
Docetaxel	RPR	0.9 mg/mL[a]	LI	5 mg/mL[a]	Physically compatible for 4 hr at 23 °C	2224	C
Doripenem	JJ	5 mg/mL[a,b]	SIC	5 mg/mL[a,b]	Physically compatible for 4 hr at 23 °C	2743	C
Doxorubicin HCl liposomal	SEQ	0.4 mg/mL[a]	AB	5 mg/mL[a]	Physically compatible for 4 hr at 23 °C	2087	C

Y-Site Injection Compatibility (1:1 Mixture) (Cont.)

Tobramycin sulfate

Drug	Mfr	Conc	Mfr	Conc	Remarks	Ref	C/I
Enalaprilat	MSD	0.05 mg/mL[b]	LI	0.8 mg/mL[a]	Physically compatible for 24 hr at room temperature under fluorescent light	1355	C
Esmolol HCl	DCC	10 mg/mL[a]	LI	0.8 mg/mL[a]	Physically compatible for 24 hr at 22 °C	1169	C
Etoposide phosphate	BR	5 mg/mL[a]	LI	5 mg/mL[a]	Physically compatible for 4 hr at 23 °C	2218	C
Fenoldopam mesylate	AB	80 mcg/mL[b]	LI	5 mg/mL[b]	Physically compatible for 4 hr at 23 °C	2467	C
Filgrastim	AMG	30 mcg/mL[a]	LI	5 mg/mL[a]	Physically compatible for 4 hr at 22 °C	1687	C
	AMG	10[d] and 40[a] mcg/mL	LI	1.6 mg/mL[a]	Visually compatible. Little loss of filgrastim and tobramycin in 4 hr at 25 °C	2060	C
Fluconazole	RR	2 mg/mL	LI	40 mg/mL	Physically compatible for 24 hr at 25 °C	1407	C
Fludarabine phosphate	BX	1 mg/mL[a]	LI	5 mg/mL[a]	Visually compatible for 4 hr at 22 °C	1439	C
Foscarnet sodium	AST	24 mg/mL	LI	40 mg/mL	Physically compatible for 24 hr at room temperature under fluorescent light	1335	C
Furosemide	HO	10 mg/mL	DI	1.6 mg/mL[c]	Physically compatible for 24 hr at 21 °C	876	C
Gemcitabine HCl	LI	10 mg/mL[b]	LI	5 mg/mL[b]	Physically compatible for 4 hr at 23 °C	2226	C
Granisetron HCl	SKB	0.05 mg/mL[a]	AB	5 mg/mL[a]	Physically compatible for 4 hr at 23 °C	2000	C
Heparin sodium	ES	50 units/mL[c]	LI	3.2 mg/mL[c]	Immediate gross haze	1316	I
	TR	50 units/mL	LI	0.8 mg/mL[a]	Visually incompatible within 4 hr at 25 °C	1793	I
Hetastarch in lactated electrolyte	AB	6%	GNS	5 mg/mL[a]	Physically compatible for 4 hr at 23 °C	2339	C
Hetastarch in sodium chloride 0.9%	DCC	6%	LI[e]	0.8 mg/mL	Small crystals form immediately after mixing and persist for 4 hr	1313	I
Hydromorphone HCl	WY	0.2 mg/mL[a]	DI	0.8 mg/mL[a]	Physically compatible for 4 hr at 25 °C	987	C
Indomethacin sodium trihydrate	MSD	0.5 and 1 mg/mL[a]		1 mg/mL[a]	White turbidity forms immediately and becomes white flakes in 1 hr	1550	I
Insulin, regular	LI	0.2 unit/mL[b]	LI	1.6 and 2 mg/mL[a]	Physically compatible for 2 hr at 25 °C	1395	C
Labetalol HCl	SC	1 mg/mL[a]	LI	0.8 mg/mL[a]	Physically compatible for 24 hr at 18 °C	1171	C
Linezolid	PHU	2 mg/mL	AB	5 mg/mL[a]	Physically compatible for 4 hr at 23 °C	2264	C
Magnesium sulfate	IX	16.7, 33.3, 66.7, 100 mg/mL[a]	DI	0.8 mg/mL[a]	Physically compatible for at least 4 hr at 32 °C	813	C
Melphalan HCl	BW	0.1 mg/mL[b]	LI	5 mg/mL[b]	Physically compatible for 3 hr at 22 °C	1557	C
Meperidine HCl	WY	10 mg/mL[a]	DI	0.8 mg/mL[a]	Physically compatible for 4 hr at 25 °C	987	C
	WY	10 mg/mL[b]	LI	1.6, 2, 2.4 mg/mL[a]	Physically compatible for 1 hr at 25 °C	1338	C
Midazolam HCl	RC	1 mg/mL[a]	LI	10 mg/mL	Visually compatible for 24 hr at 23 °C	1847	C
Milrinone lactate	SS	0.2 mg/mL[a]	LI	10 mg/mL	Visually compatible for 4 hr at 25 °C	2381	C
Morphine sulfate	WI	1 mg/mL[a]	DI	0.8 mg/mL[a]	Physically compatible for 4 hr at 25 °C	987	C
	ES	1 mg/mL[b]	LI	1.6, 2, 2.4 mg/mL[a]	Physically compatible for 1 hr at 25 °C	1338	C
Nicardipine HCl	DCC	0.1 mg/mL[a]	LI	0.8 mg/mL[a]	Visually compatible for 24 hr at room temperature	235	C
Pemetrexed disodium	LI	20 mg/mL[b]	AB	5 mg/mL[a]	White precipitate forms immediately	2564	I
Piperacillin sodium–tazobactam sodium					Incompatible	1	I

Y-Site Injection Compatibility (1:1 Mixture) (Cont.)

Tobramycin sulfate

Drug	Mfr	Conc	Mfr	Conc	Remarks	Ref	C/I
Propofol	ZEN	10 mg/mL	AB	5 mg/mL[a]	Precipitate forms immediately	2066	**I**
Remifentanil HCl	GW	0.025 and 0.25 mg/mL[b]	AB	5 mg/mL[a]	Physically compatible for 4 hr at 23 °C	2075	**C**
Sargramostim	IMM	10 mcg/mL[b]	LI	5 mg/mL[b]	Particles and filaments form in 4 hr	1436	**I**
Tacrolimus	FUJ	1 mg/mL[b]	BR	40 mg/mL	Visually compatible for 24 hr at 25 °C	1630	**C**
Telavancin HCl	ASP	7.5 mg/mL[a,b]	HOS	5 mg/mL[a,b]	Physically compatible for 2 hr	2830	**C**
Teniposide	BR	0.1 mg/mL[a]	LI	5 mg/mL[a]	Physically compatible for 4 hr at 23 °C	1725	**C**
Theophylline	TR	4 mg/mL	LI	0.8 mg/mL[a]	Visually compatible for 6 hr at 25 °C	1793	**C**
Thiotepa	IMM[c]	1 mg/mL[a]	LI	5 mg/mL[a]	Physically compatible for 4 hr at 23 °C	1861	**C**
Tigecycline	WY	1 mg/mL[b]		2.5 mg/mL[b]	Physically compatible for 4 hr	2714	**C**
TNA #73[g]		32.5 mL[h]	LI	1.6 mg/mL[a]	Visually compatible for 4 hr at 25 °C	1008	**C**
TNA #97 to #104[g]			LI	40 mg/mL	Physically compatible and tobramycin content retained for 6 hr at 21 °C	1324	**C**
TNA #218 to #226[g]			AB	5 mg/mL[a]	Visually compatible for 4 hr at 23 °C	2215	**C**
TPN #54[g]				20 mg/mL	Physically compatible and tobramycin activity retained over 6 hr at 22 °C	1045	**C**
TPN #61[g]		[i]	DI	12.5 mg/ 1.25 mL[j]	Physically compatible	1012	**C**
		[k]	DI	75 mg/ 1.9 mL[j]	Physically compatible	1012	**C**
TPN #91[g]		[l]	LI	5 mg[m]	Physically compatible	1170	**C**
TPN #212 to #215[g]			AB	5 mg/mL[a]	Physically compatible for 4 hr at 23 °C	2109	**C**
Vinorelbine tartrate	BW	1 mg/mL[b]	LI	5 mg/mL[b]	Physically compatible for 4 hr at 22 °C	1558	**C**
Zidovudine	BW	4 mg/mL[a]	LI	2 mg/mL[a]	Physically compatible for 4 hr at 25 °C	1193	**C**

[a]*Tested in dextrose 5%.*
[b]*Tested in sodium chloride 0.9%.*
[c]*Tested in both dextrose 5% and sodium chloride 0.9%.*
[d]*Tested in dextrose 5% with albumin human 2 mg/mL.*
[e]*Tested in premixed infusion solution.*
[f]*Lyophilized formulation tested.*
[g]*Refer to Appendix I for the composition of parenteral nutrition solutions. TNA indicates a 3-in-1 admixture, and TPN indicates a 2-in-1 admixture.*
[h]*A 32.5-mL sample of parenteral nutrition solution mixed with 50 mL of antibiotic solution.*
[i]*Run at 21 mL/hr.*
[j]*Given over 30 minutes by syringe pump.*
[k]*Run at 94 mL/hr.*
[l]*Run at 10 mL/hr.*
[m]*Given over one hour by syringe pump.*
[n]*Tested in a 1:1 mixture of dextrose 5% and TPN #274 (see Appendix I).*
[o]*Tested in Ringer's injection, lactated.*
[p]*Injected via Y-site into an administration set running azithromycin.*
[q]*Tested in sterile water for injection.*
[r]*Tested in either dextrose 5% or in sodium chloride 0.9%, but the report did not specify which solution.*
[s]*Tested in a 1:1 mixture of (1) dextrose 5% and dextrose 5% in sodium chloride 0.45% with and without potassium chloride 20 mEq/L and also in (2) dextrose 10% in sodium chloride 0.45% with and without potassium chloride 20 mEq/L.*

Additional Compatibility Information

Peritoneal Dialysis Solutions — Tobramycin base (Lilly) 3 and 10 mg/L in peritoneal dialysis concentrate with dextrose 50% (McGaw) retained about 50 to 60% of initial activity in seven hours and about 15 to 30% in 24 hours at room temperature. (1044)

The stability of tobramycin sulfate (Lilly) 10 mg/L in peritoneal dialysis solutions (Dianeal 137 and PD2) with heparin sodium 500 units/L was evaluated. Approximately $102 \pm 20\%$ activity remained after 24 hours at 25 °C. (1228)

In another study, the stability of tobramycin sulfate (Lilly) was evaluated in peritoneal dialysis concentrates containing dextrose 30 and 50% (Dianeal) as well as in a diluted solution containing dextrose 2.5%. The tobramycin sulfate concentrations were 100 and 160 mg/L in the peritoneal dialysate concentrates and 5 and 8 mg/L in the diluted solution. Tobramycin sulfate was found to be stable in the diluted peritoneal dialysis solution for at least 24 hours at 23 °C. However, greater decomposition occurred in the concentrates, with a 10% loss in as little as 9 to 15 hours. (1229)

The retention of antimicrobial activity of tobramycin sulfate (Lilly) 120 mg/L alone and with vancomycin hydrochloride (Lilly) 1 g/L was evaluated in Dianeal PD-2 (Travenol) with dextrose 1.5%. Little or no loss of either antibiotic occurred in eight hours at 37 °C. Tobramycin sulfate alone retained activity for at least 48 hours at 4 and 25 °C. With vancomycin hydrochloride, the activity of both antibiotics was retained for up to 48 hours; however, the authors recommended refrigeration at 4 °C for storage longer than 24 hours. (1414)

Ceftazidime (Fortaz) 125 mg/L and tobramycin sulfate (Lilly) 8 mg/L in Dianeal PD-2 with dextrose 2.5% (Baxter) were visually compatible and chemically stable. After 16 hours of storage at 25 °C under fluorescent light, the loss of both drugs was less than 3%. Additional storage for eight hours at 37 °C, to simulate the maximum peritoneal dwell time, showed tobramycin sulfate concentrations of 96% and ceftazidime concentrations of 92 to 96%. (1652)

Tobramycin sulfate (Lilly) 25 mcg/mL combined separately with the cephalosporins cefazolin sodium (Lilly) and cefoxitin (MSD) at a concentration of 125 mcg/mL in peritoneal dialysis solution (Dianeal 1.5%) exhibited enhanced rates of lethality to *Staphylococcus aureus*, *Escherichia coli*, and *Pseudomonas aeruginosa* compared to any of the drugs alone. (1623)

β-Lactam Antibiotics — In common with other aminoglycoside antibiotics, tobramycin sulfate activity may be impaired by the β-lactam antibiotics. The inactivation is dependent on concentration, temperature, and time of exposure. (68; 497; 498; 574; 575; 654; 740; 814; 816; 817; 832; 824; 973; 1005; 1052; 1420)

The clinical significance of these interactions appears to be primarily confined to patients with renal failure. (218; 334; 361; 364; 616; 737; 816; 847; 952) Literature reports of greatly reduced aminoglycoside levels in such patients have appeared frequently. (363; 365; 366; 367; 614; 666; 962) In addition, the interaction may be clinically important if assays for aminoglycoside levels in serum are sufficiently delayed. (576; 618; 735; 824; 832; 847; 1052)

Most authors believe that in vitro mixing of penicillins with aminoglycoside antibiotics should be avoided but that clinical use of the drugs in combination can be of great value. It is generally recommended that the drugs be given separately in such combined therapy. (157; 218; 222; 224; 361; 364; 368; 369; 370)

TOPOTECAN HYDROCHLORIDE
AHFS 10:00

Products — Topotecan hydrochloride is available in vials containing 4 mg of topotecan base (present as the hydrochloride) as a lyophilized powder. Reconstitute with 4 mL of sterile water for injection to yield a 1-mg/mL topotecan solution. In addition to topotecan hydrochloride, each milliliter of the reconstituted solution contains mannitol 12 mg and tartaric acid 5 mg. Hydrochloric acid and sodium hydroxide may have been used during manufacture to adjust the pH. The reconstituted solution must be diluted for use. (1)

pH — From 2.5 to 3.5. (1)

Trade Name(s) — Hycamtin.

Administration — Topotecan hydrochloride is administered by intravenous infusion over 30 minutes after dilution in 50 to 250 mL of either sodium chloride 0.9% or dextrose 5%. Extravasation should be avoided; local reactions including erythema and bruising may result. (1; 4)

As for other toxic drugs, topotecan hydrochloride should be prepared and administered using protective measures to avoid inadvertent contact with the drug. The use of gloves, protective clothing, and vertical laminar flow hoods or biological safety cabinets is recommended. If skin contact with the drug does occur, wash the area thoroughly with soap and water. For mucous membrane contact, flush thoroughly with water. Disposal should also be performed safely to avoid inadvertent exposure. (1; 4)

Stability — Topotecan hydrochloride in intact vials should be stored in the original cartons at controlled room temperature and protected from light. The lyophilized drug is a light yellow to greenish powder. The reconstituted solution is yellow to yellow-green in color. (1) The reconstituted solution should be inspected for particulate matter in the vial and again in the transferring syringe prior to preparing admixtures. As for all parenteral products, the admixtures should also be inspected for particulate matter and discoloration prior to administration. (4)

Reconstituted topotecan hydrochloride is stated to be stable for 24 hours at 20 to 25 °C exposed to ambient light. (4) However, the manufacturer recommends use immediately after reconstitution because the product contains no antibacterial preservative. (1)

Other information indicates the reconstituted drug may be stable for longer periods. Vials of reconstituted topotecan hydrochloride at a concentration of 1 mg/mL were stored at 5, 25, and 30 °C both upright and inverted for 28 days. The solutions remained visually clear with no change in color, and little or no loss of topotecan hydrochloride occurred at any condition. (2211)

Topotecan hydrochloride 1 mg/mL reconstituted with sterile water for injection was physically and chemically stable for 28 days at 4 and 25 °C protected from light. No loss of topotecan was found, and no visible precipitation or color change occurred. (2243)

Whether any antimicrobial effect of topotecan hydrochloride exists is uncertain but could be concentration dependent. Two studies that have been performed seem to have different results, perhaps due to the very different topotecan hydrochloride concentrations being tested.

Topotecan hydrochloride 0.01 mg/mL diluted in sodium chloride 0.9% and stored at 22 °C did not exhibit an antimicrobial effect on the growth of four organisms (*Enterococcus faecium, Staphylococcus aureus, Pseudomonas aeruginosa,* and *Candida albicans*) inoculated into the solution. The author recommended that diluted solutions of

topotecan hydrochloride be stored under refrigeration whenever possible and that the potential for microbiological growth be considered when assigning expiration periods. (2160)

Topotecan hydrochloride 1 mg/mL reconstituted with sterile water did not support the growth of five organisms inoculated into the solution. The USP Preservative Effectiveness Test found that *Pseudomonas aeruginosa, Staphylococcus aureus,* and *Escherichia coli* were not viable after 16 hours, 24 hours, and 28 days, respectively. *Candida albicans* and *Aspergillus niger* did not lose viability but did not exhibit growth during the test. (2211)

pH Effects — Topotecan hydrochloride has a pH near 3 maintained with tartaric acid to ensure adequate solubility of greater than 2.5 mg/mL. The solubility decreases as the pH increases, becoming virtually insoluble at pH 4.5. (1747) Hydrolysis of the topotecan hydrochloride lactone ring is known to occur at pH values above 4. (2140)

Compatibility Information

Solution Compatibility

Topotecan HCl

Solution	Mfr	Mfr	Conc/L	Remarks	Ref	C/I
Dextrose 5%	BA[a], MG[b], MG[c]	SKB	50 mg	Visually compatible. No loss in 24 hr at 24 °C in light and 7 days at 5 °C in dark	2140	**C**
	BA[a]	SKB	25 mg	Visually compatible. No loss in 24 hr at 24 °C in light and 7 days at 5 °C in dark	2140	**C**
	BA[a]	SKB	10, 25, 50 mg	Visually compatible. Little loss in 28 days at 4 and 25 °C in dark	2243	**C**
	BA[d]	SKB	10, 25, 50 mg	Visually compatible. Little loss in 28 days at 4 and 25 °C in dark followed by 5 days at 37 °C	2243	**C**
Sodium chloride 0.9%	BA[a], MG[b], MG[c]	SKB	50 mg	Visually compatible. No loss in 24 hr at 24 °C in light and 7 days at 5 °C in dark	2140	**C**
	BA[a]	SKB	25 mg	Visually compatible. No loss in 24 hr at 24 °C in light and 7 days at 5 °C in dark	2140	**C**
	BA[a]	SKB	10, 25, 50 mg	Visually compatible. Little loss in 28 days at 4 and 25 °C in dark	2243	**C**
	BA[d]	SKB	10, 25, 50 mg	Visually compatible. Little loss in 28 days at 4 and 25 °C in dark followed by 5 days at 37 °C	2243	**C**
	BA[a]	SKB	10 mg	Visually compatible. 10% loss due to photodegradation in 17 days at room temperature in mixed daylight and fluorescent light	2243	**C**

[a]*Tested in PVC containers.*
[b]*Tested in polyolefin containers.*
[c]*Tested in glass containers.*
[d]*Tested in elastomeric infusion devices (Infusors LV 2, Baxter)*

Y-Site Injection Compatibility (1:1 Mixture)

Topotecan HCl

Drug	Mfr	Conc	Mfr	Conc	Remarks	Ref	C/I
Carboplatin	BR	0.9 mg/mL[a,b]	SKB	56 mcg/mL[a,b]	Visually compatible. Little loss of either drug in 4 hr at 22 °C	2245	**C**

Y-Site Injection Compatibility (1:1 Mixture) (Cont.)

Topotecan HCl

Drug	Mfr	Conc	Mfr	Conc	Remarks	Ref	C/I
Cisplatin	BR	0.168 mg/mL[b]	SKB	56 mcg/mL[b]	Visually compatible. Little loss of either drug in 4 hr at 22 °C	2245	**C**
Cyclophosphamide	MJ	20 mg/mL	SKB	56 mcg/mL[a,b]	Visually compatible. Little loss of either drug in 4 hr at 22 °C	2245	**C**
Dexamethasone sodium phosphate	RU	4 mg/mL	SKB	56 mcg/mL[b]	Haze and color change to intense yellow occur immediately	2245	**I**
Doxorubicin HCl	PH	2 mg/mL	SKB	56 mcg/mL[a,b]	Visually compatible. Little loss of either drug in 4 hr at 22 °C	2245	**C**
Etoposide	BR	0.4 mg/mL[a,b]	SKB	56 mcg/mL[a,b]	Visually compatible. Little loss of either drug in 4 hr at 22 °C	2245	**C**
Fluorouracil	RC	50 mg/mL	SKB	56 mcg/mL[b]	Immediate haze and yellow color	2245	**I**
Gemcitabine HCl	LI	10 mg/mL[b]	SKB	0.1 mg/mL[b]	Physically compatible for 4 hr at 23 °C	2226	**C**
Granisetron HCl	SKB	20 mcg/mL[a,b]	SKB	56 mcg/mL[a,b]	Visually compatible. Little loss of either drug in 4 hr at 22 °C	2245	**C**
Ifosfamide	MJ	14.28 mg/mL[a,b]	SKB	56 mcg/mL[a,b]	Visually compatible. Little loss of either drug in 4 hr at 22 °C	2245	**C**
Methylprednisolone sodium succinate	UP	2.4 mg/mL[a,b]	SKB	56 mcg/mL[a,b]	Yellow color forms. Little loss of either drug in 4 hr at 22 °C	2245	**C**
Metoclopramide HCl	RB	1.72 mg/mL[a,b]	SKB	56 mcg/mL[a,b]	Visually compatible. Little loss of either drug in 4 hr at 22 °C	2245	**C**
Mitomycin	BR	84 mcg/mL[a,b]	SKB	56 mcg/mL[a,b]	Pale purple color forms immediately becoming a dark pinkish-lavender in 4 hr. 15 to 20% mitomycin loss in 4 hr at 22 °C	2245	**I**
Ondansetron HCl	CER	0.48 mg/mL[a,b]	SKB	56 mcg/mL[a,b]	Visually compatible. Little loss of either drug in 4 hr at 22 °C	2245	**C**
Oxaliplatin	SS	0.5 mg/mL[a]	SKB	0.1 mg/mL[a]	Physically compatible for 4 hr at 23 °C	2566	**C**
Paclitaxel	MJ	0.54 mg/mL[a,b]	SKB	56 mcg/mL[a,b]	Visually compatible. Little loss of either drug in 4 hr at 22 °C	2245	**C**
Palonosetron HCl	MGI	50 mcg/mL	GSK	0.1 mg/mL[a]	Physically compatible. Little loss of either drug in 4 hr	2609	**C**
Pemetrexed disodium	LI	20 mg/mL[b]	GSK	0.1 mg/mL[a]	Color darkening occurs immediately	2564	**I**
Prochlorperazine edisylate	SKB	0.192 mg/mL[a,b]	SKB	56 mcg/mL[a,b]	Visually compatible. Little loss of either drug in 4 hr at 22 °C	2245	**C**
Ticarcillin disodium–clavulanate potassium	SKB	24.6 mg/mL[a]	SKB	56 mcg/mL[a]	Immediate yellow color. 11% topotecan loss in 4 hr at 22 °C	2245	**I**
	SKB	24.6 mg/mL[b]	SKB	56 mcg/mL[b]	Immediate yellow color. Under 5% loss of all components in 4 hr at 22 °C	2245	**C**
Vincristine sulfate	LI	1 mg/mL	SKB	56 mcg/mL[a,b]	Visually compatible. Little loss of either drug in 4 hr at 22 °C	2245	**C**

[a]*Tested in dextrose 5%.*
[b]*Tested in sodium chloride 0.9%.*

TORSEMIDE
AHFS 40:28

Products — Torsemide is available in 2- and 5-mL ampuls. Each milliliter of solution contains torsemide 10 mg along with polyethylene glycol 400, tromethamine, water for injection, and sodium hydroxide if needed to adjust pH during manufacture. (1)

pH — Approximately 8.3. (1)

Administration — Torsemide is administered intravenously either slowly as a bolus over two minutes or as a continuous infusion. If given through an intravenous line, flushing with sodium chloride 0.9% before and after torsemide administration is recommended. (1)

Stability — Intact containers of torsemide should be stored at controlled room temperature and protected from freezing. (1)

Compatibility Information

Solution Compatibility

Torsemide

Solution	Mfr	Mfr	Conc/L	Remarks	Ref	C/I
Dextrose 5%			0.1 to 0.8 g	Stable for 24 hr at room temperature	1	**C**
	AB[a]	BM	200 mg	6% loss in 72 hr at 24 °C	2108	**C**
	AB[a]	BM	5 g	3% loss in 72 hr at 24 °C	2108	**C**
Sodium chloride 0.45%			0.1 to 0.4 g	Stable for 24 hr at room temperature	1	**C**
Sodium chloride 0.9%			0.1 to 0.8 g	Stable for 24 hr at room temperature	1	**C**

[a]*Tested in PVC containers.*

Y-Site Injection Compatibility (1:1 Mixture)

Torsemide

Drug	Mfr	Conc	Mfr	Conc	Remarks	Ref	C/I
Milrinone lactate	SW	0.4 mg/mL[a]	BM	10 mg/mL	Visually compatible. Little loss of either drug in 4 hr at 23 °C	2214	**C**
Nesiritide	SCI	50 mcg/mL[a,b]		10 mg/mL	Physically compatible for 4 hr	2625	**C**

[a]*Tested in dextrose 5%.*
[b]*Tested in sodium chloride 0.9%.*

TRAMADOL HYDROCHLORIDE
AHFS 28:08.08

Products — Tramadol hydrochloride is available as a 50-mg/mL aqueous solution in 1- and 2-mL (50- and 100-mg) ampuls. Sodium acetate and water for injection are also present in the formulation. (38; 115)

Trade Name(s) — Contramal, Topalgic, Tramal, Zamadol, Zydol.

Administration — Tramadol hydrochloride is administered intramuscularly, by direct intravenous injection slowly over two to three minutes, or by intravenous infusion after dilution. (38; 115)

Stability — Tramadol hydrochloride is a clear, colorless solution. The intact ampuls should be stored below 30 °C. (38; 115)

Exposure to or protection from light did not affect the stability of tramadol hydrochloride 0.5- and 4-mg/mL infusion solutions in dextrose 5% or sodium chloride 0.9%. (434)

Freezing Solutions — Tramadol hydrochloride (Searle) 1 mg/mL in dextrose 5% in PVC bags was stored frozen at −20 °C for 120 days, microwave thawed, and stored refrigerated at 4 °C for 60 days. No visual changes and 5% loss of tramadol hydrochloride was found. (2450; 2526)

Compatibility Information

Solution Compatibility

Tramadol HCl

Solution	Mfr	Mfr	Conc/L	Remarks	Ref	C/I
Dextrose 5%		MUN		Physically compatible and chemically stable for 5 days	38	**C**
	[a]	MUN	0.5 and 4 g	Visually compatible. No loss in 14 days at 4 °C and 7 days at room temperature or 40 °C	434	**C**
	BA[a]	GRU	0.4 g	Visually compatible with no loss in 24 hr at room temperature and 4 °C	2652	**C**
Ringer's injection, lactated		MUN		Physically compatible and chemically stable for 5 days	38	**C**
		GRU	0.4 g	Visually compatible with no loss in 24 hr at room temperature and 4 °C	2652	**C**
Sodium chloride 0.9%		MUN		Physically compatible and chemically stable for 5 days	38	**C**
	[a]	MUN	0.5 and 4 g	Visually compatible with little or no loss in 14 days at 4 °C and 7 days at room temperature. 3 to 5% loss in 7 days at 40 °C	434	**C**
	BA[a]	GRU	0.4 g	Visually compatible with no loss in 24 hr at room temperature and 4 °C	2652	**C**

[a]Tested in PVC containers.

Additive Compatibility

Tramadol HCl

Drug	Mfr	Conc/L	Mfr	Conc/L	Test Soln	Remarks	Ref	C/I
Acyclovir sodium	WEL	5 g	GRU	400 mg	NS	Precipitation and 20% tramadol loss in 1 hr	2652	**I**
Ampicillin sodium–sulbactam sodium	PF	20 + 10 g	GRU	400 mg	NS	Visually compatible with up to 9% tramadol loss in 24 hr at room temperature	2652	**C**
Clindamycin phosphate	AB	6 g	GRU	400 mg	NS	Tramadol losses of 20% in 4 hr at room temperature with precipitate	2652	**I**
Dexamethasone sodium phosphate	ME	440 mg	AND	11.18 g	NS[a]	Visually compatible for 7 days at 25 °C protected from light	2701	**C**
	ME	1.33 g	AND	33.3 g	NS[a]	Visually compatible for 7 days at 25 °C protected from light	2701	**C**
Haloperidol lactate	EST	210 mg	AND	11.18 g	NS[a]	Visually compatible for 7 days at 25 °C protected from light	2701	**C**
	EST	620 mg	AND	33.3 g	NS[a]	Visually compatible for 7 days at 25 °C protected from light	2701	**C**
Mannitol		20%	GRU	0.4 g		Visually compatible with no tramadol loss in 24 hr at room temperature and 4 °C	2652	**C**
Metoclopramide HCl	SYO	1.11 g	AND	1.118 g	NS[a]	Visually compatible for 7 days at 25 °C protected from light	2701	**C**
	SYO	3.33 g	AND	3.33 g	NS[a]	Visually compatible for 7 days at 25 °C protected from light	2701	**C**
Midazolam HCl	RC	500 mg	AND	11.18 g	NS[a]	Visually compatible for 7 days at 25 °C protected from light	2701	**C**
	RC	1.5 g	AND	33.3 g	NS[a]	Visually compatible for 7 days at 25 °C protected from light	2701	**C**

Additive Compatibility (Cont.)

Tramadol HCl

Drug	Mfr	Conc/L	Mfr	Conc/L	Test Soln	Remarks	Ref	C/I
Ondansetron HCl	GL	1.6 mg	GRU	400 mg	NS	Visually compatible with about 7% tramadol loss in 24 hr at room temperature	2652	C
Ranitidine HCl	AB	0.5 g	GRU	400 mg	NS	Visually compatible with little or no tramadol loss in 24 hr at room temperature	2652	C
Scopolamine butylbromide	BI	1.68 g	AND	11.18 g	NS[a]	Visually compatible for 7 days at 25 °C protected from light	2701	C
	BI	5 g	AND	5 g	NS[a]	Visually compatible for 7 days at 25 °C protected from light	2701	C

[a]*Tested in elastomeric pump reservoirs (Baxter).*

Drugs in Syringe Compatibility

Tramadol HCl

Drug (in syringe)	Mfr	Amt	Mfr	Amt	Remarks	Ref	C/I
Dexamethasone sodium phosphate	ME	3.33, 1.67, 1.33, 0.33 mg/mL[a]	GRU	33.33, 16.66, 8.33 mg/mL[a]	Physically compatible and both drugs chemically stable for 5 days at 25 °C protected from light	2747	C
Haloperidol lactate	EST	0.208 mg/mL[a]	GRU	8.33, 16.67, 33.33 mg/mL[a]	Physically compatible with no loss of either drug in 15 days at 4 and 25 °C protected from light	2672	C
Heparin sodium		2500 units/ 1 mL	GRU	100 mg/ 2 mL	Visually compatible for at least 5 min	1053	C
Scopolamine butylbromide	BI	3.33, 4.99, 6.67 mg/mL[a]	GRU	8.33, 16.67, 33.33 mg/mL[a]	Physically compatible with no loss of tramadol HCl and about 5 to 6% loss of scopolamine butylbromide in 15 days at 4 and 25 °C protected from light	2632	C

[a]*Tested in sodium chloride 0.9%.*

Y-Site Injection Compatibility (1:1 Mixture)

Tramadol HCl

Drug	Mfr	Conc	Mfr	Conc	Remarks	Ref	C/I
Rifampin	AVE	6 mg/mL	GRU	8.33 mg/mL	Immediate red-orange turbid precipitate	2727	I

TREPROSTINIL SODIUM
AHFS 24:12.92

Products — Treprostinil is available as 1-, 2.5-, 5-, and 10-mg/mL (as sodium) in 20-mL multiple-dose vials. Each milliliter also contains sodium chloride 5.3 mg (except the 10-mg/mL concentration which contains 4 mg), metacresol 3 mg, and sodium citrate 6.3 mg in water for injection. Sodium hydroxide and/or hydrochloridic acid may have been added during manufacturing to adjust the pH. (1)

pH — From 6.0 to 7.2. (1)

Trade Name(s) — Remodulin.

Administration — Treprostinil sodium is preferably administered by continuous subcutaneous infusion using a syringe pump designed for subcutaneous administration. The drug may also be administered via a central venous catheter only after dilution in sterile water for injection, sodium chloride 0.9%, or Flolan special diluent using an intravenous infusion pump. The subcutaneous or intravenous infusion pump must have a reservoir made of polypropylene, polyvinyl chloride, or glass. (1)

Stability — Intact vials should be stored at controlled room temperature. The drug is stable at room temperature and neutral pH. The manufacturer recommends using the vials for no more than 14 days after initial stopper penetration. The undiluted drug is stable for up to 72 hours at 37 °C during administration in syringe reservoirs. The manufacturer states that after dilution in sterile water for injection, sodium chloride 0.9%, or Flolan special diluent, the drug is stable for 48 hours at 37 °C at concentrations as low as 4 mcg/mL. (1)

Using proper technique to penetrate the vial stopper with a needle, limiting the number of punctures of a vial stopper to 10, and using a Clave Connector Multidose Vial Adapter were shown to reduce the amount of particulate matter from the stopper that was found upon multiple-day use of treprostinil sodium 1- and 10-mg/mL vials and to be within the USP limit for such particulate matter over the 30-day test period. No loss of treprostinil sodium occurred during this period as well. Improper needle technique and numerous stopper penetrations were found to result in unacceptable particulate matter from the vial stopper. (2611)

Syringes — The chemical and physical stability of undiluted treprostinil sodium (United Therapeutics) 1, 2.5, 5, and 10 mg/mL was evaluated packaged in 3-mL MiniMed plastic syringe pump reservoirs sealed with plastic tip caps. The samples were stored at 37, 23, 4, and −20 °C for 60 days. The samples were clear and colorless, and treprostinil was stable at all four storage temperatures, exhibiting concentrations of 95% or more over 60 days. (2528)

Compatibility Information

Solution Compatibility

Treprostinil sodium

Solution	Mfr	Mfr	Conc/L	Remarks	Ref	C/I
Dextrose 5%	BAª	UT	4 mcg/mL	Treprostinil loss of 15 to 20% in 24 to 48 hr at 40 °C. Up to 70% loss of metacresol preservative	2476	I
	BAª	UT	20 and 130 mcg/mL	Treprostinil loss of 5% or less in 48 hr at 40 °C. Up to 70% loss of metacresol preservative	2476	C
Sodium chloride 0.9%	BAª	UT	4 and 130 mcg/mL	Little or no treprostinil loss in 48 hr at 40 °C. Up to 70% loss of metacresol preservative	2476	C

ªTested in medication cassette reservoirs (SIMS-Deltec).

TRIMETHOBENZAMIDE HYDROCHLORIDE
AHFS 56:22.08

Products — Trimethobenzamide hydrochloride 100 mg/mL is available in 2-mL single-dose and 20-mL multiple-dose vials. Each milliliter of solution also contains sodium citrate, citric acid, and sodium hydroxide to adjust pH. Some products may contain edetate disodium. The multiple-dose vials also contain phenol 0.45%. (1)

pH — The official pH range is 4.5 to 5.5. (17) The manufacturer indicates the actual pH is approximately 5. (1)

Trade Name(s) — Tigan.

Administration — Trimethobenzamide hydrochloride is administered by intramuscular injection deep into the upper outer quadrant of the gluteal region. Intravenous injection is not recommended. (1; 4)

Stability — Trimethobenzamide hydrochloride should be stored at controlled room temperature and protected from freezing. (1; 4)

Compatibility Information

Drugs in Syringe Compatibility

Trimethobenzamide HCl

Drug (in syringe)	Mfr	Amt	Mfr	Amt	Remarks	Ref	C/I
Glycopyrrolate	RB	0.2 mg/ 1 mL	BE	100 mg/ 1 mL	Physically compatible. pH in glycopyrrolate stability range for 48 hr at 25 °C	331	C
	RB	0.2 mg/ 1 mL	BE	200 mg/ 2 mL	Physically compatible. pH in glycopyrrolate stability range for 48 hr at 25 °C	331	C
	RB	0.4 mg/ 2 mL	BE	100 mg/ 1 mL	Physically compatible. pH in glycopyrrolate stability range for 48 hr at 25 °C	331	C
Hydromorphone HCl	KN	4 mg/ 2 mL	BE	100 mg/ 1 mL	Physically compatible for 30 min	517	C
Midazolam HCl	RC	5 mg/ 1 mL	BE	200 mg/ 2 mL	Physically compatible for 4 hr at 25 °C	1145	C
Nalbuphine HCl	EN	10 mg/ 1 mL	BE	100 mg/ 1 mL	Physically compatible for 36 hr at 27 °C	762	C
	EN	5 mg/ 0.5 mL	BE	100 mg/ 1 mL	Physically compatible for 36 hr at 27 °C	762	C
	EN	2.5 mg/ 0.25 mL	BE	100 mg/ 1 mL	Physically compatible for 36 hr at 27 °C	762	C
	DU	10 mg/ 1 mL		200 mg/ 2 mL	Physically compatible for 48 hr	128	C
	DU	20 mg/ 1 mL		200 mg/ 2 mL	Physically compatible for 48 hr	128	C

Y-Site Injection Compatibility (1:1 Mixture)

Trimethobenzamide HCl

Drug	Mfr	Conc	Mfr	Conc	Remarks	Ref	C/I
Heparin sodium	UP	1000 units/L[a]	RC	100 mg/mL	Physically compatible for 4 hr at room temperature	534	C
Hydrocortisone sodium succinate	UP	10 mg/L[a]	RC	100 mg/mL	Physically compatible for 4 hr at room temperature	534	C
Potassium chloride	AB	40 mEq/L[a]	RC	100 mg/mL	Physically compatible for 4 hr at room temperature	534	C

[a]Tested in dextrose 5% in Ringer's injection, dextrose 5% in Ringer's injection, lactated, dextrose 5%, Ringer's injection, lactated, and sodium chloride 0.9%.

TRIMETHOPRIM–SULFAMETHOXAZOLE (CO-TRIMOXAZOLE)
AHFS 8:12.20

Products — Trimethoprim–sulfamethoxazole 16 + 80 mg/mL is available as a concentrate in 5-, 10-, and 30-mL vials. Each milliliter also contains propylene glycol, ethyl alcohol, diethanolamine, benzyl alcohol, sodium metabisulfite, and sodium hydroxide to adjust pH in water for injection. (1)

pH — From 9.5 to 10.5 (1)

Osmolality — The osmolalities of trimethoprim–sulfamethoxazole (Burroughs Wellcome) in concentrations of 0.8 + 4, 1.1 + 5.5, and 1.6 + 8 mg/mL in dextrose 5% were determined to be 541, 669, and 798 mOsm/kg, respectively. At 1.6 + 8 mg/mL in sodium chloride 0.9%, the osmolality was determined to be 833 mOsm/kg. (1375)

Administration — Trimethoprim–sulfamethoxazole is administered by intravenous infusion only after dilution in dextrose 5%. The drug should not be injected intramuscularly. Infusion over 60 to 90 minutes is recommended; rapid or direct intravenous injection must not be used. It is recommended that each 5 mL be diluted in 125 mL or, if fluid restriction is required, in 75 mL of dextrose 5%. Infusion admixtures should be inspected for cloudiness or crystallization before and during administration. (1; 4)

Stability — Trimethoprim–sulfamethoxazole in intact vials should be stored at controlled room temperature and not refrigerated. The multiple-dose vials should be used within 48 hours of initial entry. (1)

The solubility of trimethoprim in aqueous solutions is partially dependent on the pH of the solution. Trimethoprim is a weak base, and its solubility is lower in solutions with a more alkaline pH. (553)

Precipitation occurs in the diluted infusion solution in varying time periods, depending on the final concentration. For dilutions of 5 mL per 125 mL of dextrose 5% (trimethoprim 640 mg/L, sulfamethoxazole 3.2 g/L), use within six hours is recommended. (1) However, precipitation within four hours has been observed at this concentration. (553) For dilutions of 5 mL per 100 mL of dextrose 5% (trimethoprim 800 mg/L, sulfamethoxazole 4 g/L), use within four hours is recommended. For dilutions of 5 mL per 75 mL of dextrose 5% (trimethoprim 1.067 g/L, sulfamethoxazole 5.33 g/L), use within two hours is recommended. All infusions should be inspected carefully and watched closely for turbidity and precipitation. Infusion admixtures in dextrose 5% should not be refrigerated. (1; 4)

The nature of the precipitate that forms from seven infusion solutions containing trimethoprim–sulfamethoxazole (Roche) was evaluated. In all cases, the sulfamethoxazole concentrations were within 5% of expected values, but the trimethoprim concentrations dropped to about 30% of the initial values. Further evaluation of the solid phases showed them to be trimethoprim alone or with trimethoprim monohydrate. (1895)

Syringes — Undiluted trimethoprim–sulfamethoxazole (Elkins-Sinn) (16 + 80 mg/mL) was stored in polypropylene syringes (Becton Dickinson) for 2.5 days at room temperature. The syringes were exposed to fluorescent light during the day but kept in the dark at night. No loss was observed. (1582)

Sorption — Trimethoprim was shown not to exhibit sorption to PVC bags and tubing, polyethylene tubing, Silastic tubing, and polypropylene syringes. (536; 606)

Plasticizer Leaching — Trimethoprim–sulfamethoxazole (Elkins-Sinn) 0.8 + 4 mg/mL in dextrose 5% did not leach diethylhexyl phthalate (DEHP) plasticizer from 50-mL PVC bags in 24 hours at 24 °C. (1683)

Filtration — Filtration of dilutions of trimethoprim–sulfamethoxazole (Roche), ranging from 1:25 (v/v) to 1:10 (v/v) in several common intravenous infusion solutions, did not appear to result in loss of either drug because of sorption to the filter. Filtration of a visibly precipitated solution resulted in a substantial loss of trimethoprim. (747)

Trimethoprim–sulfamethoxazole (Roche) 1.88 mg/mL in dextrose 5% and sodium chloride 0.9% was filtered through a 0.22-μm cellulose ester membrane filter (Ivex-HP, Millipore) over six hours. No significant drug loss due to binding to the filter was noted. (1034)

Compatibility Information

Solution Compatibility

Trimethoprim + Sulfamethoxazole

Solution	Mfr	Mfr	Conc/L	Remarks	Ref	C/I
Dextrose 5% in sodium chloride 0.45%	AB	RC	640 mg + 3.2 g	Physically compatible. 6% trimethoprim loss and little sulfamethoxazole loss in 24 hr at 25 °C	747	**C**
	AB	RC	800 mg + 4 g	Physically compatible. 4% trimethoprim loss and little sulfamethoxazole loss in 24 hr at 25 °C	747	**C**
Dextrose 5%	AB	RC	640 mg + 3.2 g	Physically compatible. Little trimethoprim and sulfamethoxazole loss in 24 hr at 25 °C	747	**C**
	AB	RC	800 mg + 4 g	Physically compatible. Little trimethoprim and sulfamethoxazole loss in 24 hr at 25 °C	747	**C**
	TR	RC	640 mg + 3.2 g	Admixture clear and colorless for 4 hr at 22 °C. Turbidity and precipitation appear after this time. 5% trimethoprim loss in 4 hr and 28% in 24 hr. About 1% sulfamethoxazole loss in 24 hr	553	**I**[a]
	TR	RC	1.6 + 8 g	Admixture clear and colorless for 2 hr at 22 °C. Turbidity and precipitation appear after this time. 5% trimethoprim loss in 2 hr and 64% in 24 hr. About 3% sulfamethoxazole loss in 24 hr	553	**I**[a]
	TR	RC	3.2 + 16 g	Rapid precipitation and 32% trimethoprim loss in 1 hr. 9% sulfamethoxazole loss in 24 hr	553	**I**
	AB[b]	BW, RC	640 mg + 3.2 g	Physically compatible. Little trimethoprim and sulfamethoxazole loss in 48 hr at 24 °C	1201	**C**
	AB[b]	BW, RC	800 mg + 4 g	Physically compatible. Little or no trimethoprim and sulfamethoxazole loss in 24 hr at 24 °C. Precipitate in 48 hr	1201	**C**

Solution Compatibility (Cont.)

Trimethoprim + Sulfamethoxazole

Solution	Mfr	Mfr	Conc/L	Remarks	Ref	C/I
	AB[b]	BW, RC	1.07 + 5.33 g	Physically compatible. Little or no trimethoprim and sulfamethoxazole loss in 4 hr at 24 °C. Precipitate in 8 hr	1201	I[a]
	AB[b]	BW, RC	1.6 + 8 g	Precipitate forms as early as 2 hr at 24 °C. Up to 75% trimethoprim loss in 4 hr	1201	I
	BA[b]	ES	1.08 + 5.4 mg/mL	4 of 20 samples precipitated. No loss of trimethoprim in 24 hr at 23 °C. Sulfamethoxazole not tested	2536	I
	BA[c]	ES	1.08 + 5.4 mg/mL	Physically compatible. No loss of trimethoprim in 24 hr at 23 °C. Sulfamethoxazole not tested	2536	C
	BA[b]	ES	1.6 + 8 mg/mL	4 of 20 samples precipitated. No loss of trimethoprim in 24 hr at 23 °C. Sulfamethoxazole not tested	2536	I
	BA[c]	ES	1.6 + 8 mg/mL	Physically compatible. No loss of trimethoprim in 24 hr at 23 °C. Sulfamethoxazole not tested	2536	C
Ringer's injection, lactated	AB	RC	640 mg + 3.2 g	Physically compatible. 4% trimethoprim loss and little sulfamethoxazole loss in 24 hr at 25 °C	747	C
	AB	RC	800 mg + 4 g	Physically compatible. Little trimethoprim loss and 4% sulfamethoxazole loss in 24 hr at 25 °C	747	C
Sodium chloride 0.45%	AB	RC	640 mg + 3.2 g	Physically compatible. Little trimethoprim and sulfamethoxazole loss in 24 hr at 25 °C	747	C
	AB	RC	800 mg + 4 g	Physically compatible. 4% trimethoprim loss and little sulfamethoxazole loss in 24 hr at 25 °C	747	C
Sodium chloride 0.9%	AB	RC	640 mg + 3.2 g	Physically compatible. 5% trimethoprim loss and 4% sulfamethoxazole loss in 24 hr at 25 °C	747	C
	AB	RC	800 mg + 4 g	Physically compatible. Little trimethoprim and sulfamethoxazole loss in 24 hr at 25 °C	747	C
	TR	RC	640 mg + 3.2 g	Admixture clear and colorless for 4 hr at 22 °C. Turbidity and precipitation appear after this time. 1% trimethoprim loss in 4 hr and 36% in 24 hr. No sulfamethoxazole loss in 24 hr	553	I[a]
	TR	RC	1.6 + 8 g	Admixture clear and colorless for 1 to 2 hr at 22 °C. Turbidity appears after this time. 15% trimethoprim loss in 2 hr and 76% in 24 hr. 5% sulfamethoxazole loss in 24 hr	553	I
	TR	RC	3.2 + 16 g	Rapid precipitation and 74% trimethoprim loss in 1 hr. 6% sulfamethoxazole loss in 24 hr	553	I
	AB[b]	BW, RC	640 mg + 3.2 g	Physically compatible. Little trimethoprim and sulfamethoxazole loss in 48 hr at 24 °C	1201	C
	AB[b]	BW, RC	800 mg + 4 g	Physically compatible. Little trimethoprim and sulfamethoxazole loss in 14 hr at 24 °C. Precipitate forms within 24 hr	1201	I[a]
	AB[b]	BW, RC	1.07 + 5.33 g	Physically compatible. Little trimethoprim and sulfamethoxazole loss in 2 hr at 24 °C. Precipitate forms within 4 hr	1201	I[a]
	AB[b]	BW, RC	1.6 + 8 g	Precipitate forms as early as 2 hr at 24 °C. Up to 18% trimethoprim loss in 4 hr	1201	I
	[b]	BW	1.6 + 8 mg	Precipitate forms in 1.5 hr at 20 °C. 10% trimethoprim loss in 1.5 hr, 21% loss in 3 hr, and 60% loss in 24 hr	1555	I

Solution Compatibility (Cont.)

Trimethoprim + Sulfamethoxazole

Solution	Mfr	Mfr	Conc/L	Remarks	Ref	C/I
	BA[b]	ES	1.08 + 5.4 mg/ mL	2 of 20 samples precipitated. 4% loss of trimetho- prim in 24 hr at 23 °C. Sulfamethoxazole not tested	2536	**I**
	BA[c]	ES	1.08 + 5.4 mg/ mL	Physically compatible. No loss of trimethoprim in 24 hr at 23 °C. Sulfamethoxazole not tested	2536	**C**
	BA[b]	ES	1.6 + 8 mg/ mL	14 of 20 samples precipitated. 4% loss of trimeth- oprim in 24 hr at 23 °C. Sulfamethoxazole not tested	2536	**I**
	BA[c]	ES	1.6 + 8 mg/ mL	Physically compatible. No loss of trimethoprim in 24 hr at 23 °C. Sulfamethoxazole not tested	2536	**C**

[a]*Incompatible by conventional standards. May be used in shorter time periods.*
[b]*Tested in glass containers.*
[c]*Tested in PVC containers.*

Additive Compatibility

Trimethoprim + Sulfamethoxazole

Drug	Mfr	Conc/L	Mfr	Conc/L	Test Soln	Remarks	Ref	C/I
Fluconazole	PF	1 g	ES	0.4 + 2 g	D5W	Delayed cloudiness and precipitation. No fluconazole loss in 72 hr at 25 °C under fluorescent light	1677	**I**
Linezolid	PHU	2 g	ES	800 mg + 4 g	[a]	A large amount of white needle-like crys- tals forms immediately	2333	**I**
Verapamil HCl	KN	80 mg	BW	160 + 800 mg	D5W, NS	Transient precipitate	764	**I**

[a]*Admixed in the linezolid infusion container.*

Drugs in Syringe Compatibility

Trimethoprim + Sulfamethoxazole

Drug (in syringe)	Mfr	Amt	Mfr	Amt	Remarks	Ref	C/I
Dimenhydrinate		10 mg/ 1 mL		16 + 80 mg/ 1 mL	Clear solution	2569	**C**
Heparin sodium		2500 units/ 1 mL		80 + 400 mg/ 5 mL	Physically compatible for at least 5 min	1053	**C**
Pantoprazole sodium	[a]	4 mg/ 1 mL		16 + 80 mg/ 1 mL	Possible precipitate within 1 hr	2574	**I**

[a]*Test performed using the formulation WITHOUT edetate disodium.*

Y-Site Injection Compatibility (1:1 Mixture)

Trimethoprim + Sulfamethoxazole

Drug	Mfr	Conc	Mfr	Conc	Remarks	Ref	C/I
Acyclovir sodium	BW	5 mg/mL[a]	RC	0.8 + 4 mg/mL[a]	Physically compatible for 4 hr at 25 °C	1157	C
Aldesleukin	CHI	33,800 I.U./mL[a]	BW	1.6 + 8 mg/mL[a]	Visually compatible with little or no loss of aldesleukin activity	1857	C
Allopurinol sodium	BW	3 mg/mL[b]	ES	0.8 + 4 mg/mL[b]	Physically compatible for 4 hr at 22 °C	1686	C
Amifostine	USB	10 mg/mL[a]	ES	0.8 + 4 mg/mL[a]	Physically compatible for 4 hr at 23 °C	1845	C
Amphotericin B cholesteryl sulfate complex	SEQ	0.83 mg/mL[a]	ES	0.8 + 4 mg/mL[a]	Physically compatible for 4 hr at 23 °C	2117	C
Anidulafungin	VIC	0.5 mg/mL[a]	ES	0.8 + 4 mg/mL[a]	Physically compatible for 4 hr at 23 °C	2617	C
Atracurium besylate	BW	0.5 mg/mL[a]	ES	0.64 + 3.2 mg/mL[a]	Physically compatible for 24 hr at 28 °C	1337	C
Aztreonam	SQ	40 mg/mL[a]	ES	0.8 + 4 mg/mL[a]	Physically compatible for 4 hr at 23 °C	1758	C
Bivalirudin	TMC	5 mg/mL[a]	GNS	0.8 + 4 mg/mL[a]	Physically compatible for 4 hr at 23 °C	2373	C
Caspofungin acetate	ME	0.7 mg/mL[b]	SIC	0.8 + 4 mg/mL[b]	Immediate white turbid precipitate forms	2758	I
Ceftaroline fosamil	FOR	2.22 mg/mL[a,b,f]	SIC	0.8 + 4 mg/mL[a,b,f]	Physically compatible for 4 hr at 23 °C	2826	C
Cisatracurium besylate	GW	0.1 mg/mL[a]	ES	0.8 + 4 mg/mL[a]	Physically compatible for 4 hr at 23 °C	2074	C
	GW	2 mg/mL[a]	ES	0.8 + 4 mg/mL[a]	Subvisible haze forms in 1 hr	2074	I
	GW	5 mg/mL[a]	ES	0.8 + 4 mg/mL[a]	Subvisible haze forms immediately	2074	I
Cyclophosphamide	MJ	20 mg/mL[a]	BW	0.8 + 4 mg/mL[a]	Physically compatible for 4 hr at 25 °C	1194	C
Dexmedetomidine HCl	AB	4 mcg/mL[b]	GNS	0.8 + 4 mg/mL[b]	Physically compatible for 4 hr at 23 °C	2383	C
Diltiazem HCl	MMD	5 mg/mL	BW, RC	0.21 + 1[a] and 0.63 + 3.2 mg/mL[a]	Visually compatible	1807	C
Docetaxel	RPR	0.9 mg/mL[a]	ES	0.8 + 4 mg/mL[a]	Physically compatible for 4 hr at 23 °C	2224	C
Doxorubicin HCl liposomal	SEQ	0.4 mg/mL[a]	ES	0.8 + 4 mg/mL[a]	Physically compatible for 4 hr at 23 °C	2087	C
Enalaprilat	MSD	0.05 mg/mL[b]	QU	0.16 + 0.8 mg/mL[a]	Physically compatible for 24 hr at room temperature under fluorescent light	1355	C
Esmolol HCl	DCC	10 mg/mL[a]	BW	0.64 + 3.2 mg/mL[a]	Physically compatible for 24 hr at 22 °C	1169	C
Etoposide phosphate	BR	5 mg/mL[a]	ES	0.8 + 4 mg/mL[a]	Physically compatible for 4 hr at 23 °C	2218	C
Fenoldopam mesylate	AB	80 mcg/mL[b]	ES	0.8 + 4 mg/mL[b]	Physically compatible for 4 hr at 23 °C	2467	C

Y-Site Injection Compatibility (1:1 Mixture) (Cont.)

Trimethoprim + Sulfamethoxazole

Drug	Mfr	Conc	Mfr	Conc	Remarks	Ref	C/I
Filgrastim	AMG	30 mcg/mL[a]	ES	0.8 + 4 mg/mL[a]	Physically compatible for 4 hr at 22 °C	1687	C
Fluconazole	RR	2 mg/mL	BW	16 + 80 mg/mL	Viscous gel-like substance forms	1407	I
Fludarabine phosphate	BX	1 mg/mL[a]	ES	0.8 + 4 mg/mL[a]	Visually compatible for 4 hr at 22 °C	1439	C
Foscarnet sodium	AST	24 mg/mL	RC	16 + 80 mg/mL	Precipitates immediately and gas production	1335	I
	AST	24 mg/mL	BW	0.53 + 2.6 mg/mL[a]	Physically compatible for 24 hr at 25 °C under fluorescent light	1393	C
Gallium nitrate	FUJ	1 mg/mL[b]	ES	0.8 + 4 mg/mL[b]	Visually compatible for 24 hr at 25 °C	1673	C
Gemcitabine HCl	LI	10 mg/mL[b]	ES	0.8 + 4 mg/mL[b]	Physically compatible for 4 hr at 23 °C	2226	C
Granisetron HCl	SKB	0.05 mg/mL[a]	ES	0.8 + 4 mg/mL[a]	Physically compatible for 4 hr at 23 °C	2000	C
Hetastarch in lactated electrolyte	AB	6%	ES	0.8 + 4 mg/mL[a]	Physically compatible for 4 hr at 23 °C	2339	C
Hydromorphone HCl	WY	0.2 mg/mL[a]	BW	0.8 + 4 mg/mL[a]	Physically compatible for 4 hr at 25 °C	987	C
Labetalol HCl	SC	1 mg/mL[a]	BW	0.8 + 4 mg/mL[a]	Physically compatible for 24 hr at 18 °C	1171	C
Lorazepam	WY	0.33 mg/mL[b]	RC	0.8 + 4 mg/mL	Visually compatible for 24 hr at 22 °C	1855	C
Magnesium sulfate	IX	16.7, 33.3, 66.7, 100 mg/mL[a]	RC	0.8 + 4 mg/mL[a]	Physically compatible for at least 4 hr at 32 °C	813	C
Melphalan HCl	BW	0.1 mg/mL[b]	ES	0.8 + 4 mg/mL[b]	Physically compatible for 3 hr at 22 °C	1557	C
Meperidine HCl	WY	10 mg/mL[a]	BW	0.8 + 4 mg/mL[a]	Physically compatible for 4 hr at 25 °C	987	C
Midazolam HCl	RC	5 mg/mL	RC	0.8 + 4 mg/mL	White precipitate forms immediately	1855	I
Morphine sulfate	WI	1 mg/mL[a]	BW	0.8 + 4 mg/mL[a]	Physically compatible for 4 hr at 25 °C	987	C
Nicardipine HCl	DCC	0.1 mg/mL[a]	QU	0.16 + 0.8 mg/mL[a]	Visually compatible for 24 hr at room temperature	235	C
Pancuronium bromide	ES	0.05 mg/mL[a]	ES	0.64 + 3.2 mg/mL[a]	Physically compatible for 24 hr at 28 °C	1337	C
Pemetrexed disodium	LI	20 mg/mL[b]	ES	0.8 + 4 mg/mL[a]	Physically compatible for 4 hr at 23 °C	2564	C
Piperacillin sodium–tazobactam sodium	LE[e]	40 + 5 mg/mL[a]	ES	0.8 + 4 mg/mL[a]	Physically compatible for 4 hr at 22 °C	1688	C

V-Site Injection Compatibility (1:1 Mixture) (Cont.)

Trimethoprim + Sulfamethoxazole

Drug	Mfr	Conc	Mfr	Conc	Remarks	Ref	C/I
Remifentanil HCl	GW	0.025 and 0.25 mg/mL[b]	ES	0.8 + 4 mg/mL[a]	Physically compatible for 4 hr at 23 °C	2075	C
Sargramostim	IMM	10 mcg/mL[b]	ES	0.8 + 4 mg/mL[b]	Visually compatible for 4 hr at 22 °C	1436	C
Tacrolimus	FUJ	1 mg/mL[b]	RC	1.6 + 8 mg/mL[a]	Visually compatible for 24 hr at 25 °C	1630	C
Teniposide	BR	0.1 mg/mL[a]	ES	0.8 + 4 mg/mL[a]	Physically compatible for 4 hr at 23 °C	1725	C
Thiotepa	IMM[c]	1 mg/mL[a]	ES	0.8 + 4 mg/mL[a]	Physically compatible for 4 hr at 23 °C	1861	C
TNA #218 to #226[d]			ES	0.8 + 4 mg/mL[a]	Visually compatible for 4 hr at 23 °C	2215	C
TPN #212 to #215[d]			ES	0.8 + 4 mg/mL[a]	Physically compatible for 4 hr at 23 °C	2109	C
Vecuronium bromide	OR	0.1 mg/mL[a]	ES	0.64 + 3.2 mg/mL[a]	Physically compatible for 24 hr at 28 °C	1337	C
Vinorelbine tartrate	BW	1 mg/mL[b]	ES	0.8 + 4 mg/mL[b]	Heavy white turbidity forms immediately, developing particles in 1 hr	1558	I
Zidovudine	BW	4 mg/mL[a]	BW	0.53 + 2.6 mg/mL[a]	Physically compatible for 4 hr at 25 °C	1193	C

[a]*Tested in dextrose 5%.*
[b]*Tested in sodium chloride 0.9%.*
[c]*Lyophilized formulation tested.*
[d]*Refer to Appendix I for the composition of parenteral nutrition solutions. TNA indicates a 3-in-1 admixture, and TPN indicates a 2-in-1 admixture.*
[e]*Test performed using the formulation WITHOUT edetate disodium.*
[f]*Tested in Ringer's injection, lactated.*

TROPISETRON HYDROCHLORIDE
AHFS 56:22.20

Products — Tropisetron hydrochloride is available as an aqueous solution in 2- and 5-mL ampuls. Each milliliter of solution provides 1 mg of tropisetron (present as 1.13 mg of the hydrochloride). Also present in the formulation are acetic acid, sodium acetate, sodium chloride, and water for injection. (38; 115)

Trade Name(s) — Navoban.

Administration — Tropisetron hydrochloride is administered either as a slow intravenous injection over not less than 30 seconds for a 2-mg dose (38; 115) or one minute for a 5-mg dose (115) or as an intravenous infusion over 15 minutes. (38)

Stability — Tropisetron hydrochloride injection is a colorless or faintly brown-yellow solution. Intact ampuls should be stored at room temperature. (38)

Syringes — Tropisetron hydrochloride (Sandoz) 1 mg/mL was packaged in polypropylene syringes (Becton Dickinson) and stored under refrigeration at 4 °C and at room temperature about 23 °C exposed to daylight and protected from light for 15 days. About 4% loss of tropisetron hydrochloride occurred in 15 days under any of the storage conditions. (2298)

Sorption — The manufacturer indicates that tropisetron hydrochloride solutions are compatible with both glass and PVC containers and infusion sets. (38)

Compatibility Information

Solution Compatibility

Tropisetron HCl

Solution	Mfr	Mfr	Conc/L	Remarks	Ref	C/I
Dextrose 5%		SZ	50 mg	Compatible and stable for 24 hr refrigerated	38	C
	AGT[a], BFM[b]	SZ	50 mg	Visually compatible with no loss in 90 days at 4 and −20 °C	470	C
	BA[a], BRN[c]	SZ	50 mg	10% or less change in concentration in 15 days at 4 and 23 °C in light or dark	2298	C
Ringer's injection		SZ	50 mg	Compatible and stable for 24 hr refrigerated	38	C
Sodium chloride 0.9%		SZ	50 mg	Compatible and stable for 24 hr refrigerated	38	C
	AGT[a], BFM[b]	SZ	50 mg	Visually compatible with no loss in 90 days at 4 and −20 °C	470	C
	BA[a], BRN[c]	SZ	50 mg	10% or less change in concentration in 15 days at 4 and 23 °C in light or dark	2298	C

[a]Tested in PVC containers.
[b]Tested in three-layer (Clear-Flex) laminate containers having a polyethylene inner surface.
[c]Tested in glass and polyethylene containers.

VALPROATE SODIUM
AHFS 28:12.92

Products — Valproate sodium is available in 5-mL single-dose vials. Each milliliter of solution contains valproate sodium equivalent to valproic acid 100 mg and edetate disodium 0.4 mg in water for injection. Sodium hydroxide and/or hydrochloric acid may have been used to adjust pH during manufacture. The product should be diluted for use. (1)

pH — 7.6. (1; 4)

Trade Name(s) — Depacon.

Administration — Valproate sodium is usually administered as an intravenous infusion over 60 minutes at a rate that does not exceed 20 mg/min diluted in at least 50 mL of a compatible infusion solution. More rapid infusion at a rate of 1.5 to 3 mg/kg/min over 5 to 10 minutes has been used in one study. (1)

Stability — Intact vials should be stored at controlled room temperature. The injection is a clear, colorless solution. Because no antibacterial preservatives are present in the formulation, any unused solution remaining in a vial after entry should be discarded. (1)

Compatibility Information

Solution Compatibility

Valproate sodium

Solution	Mfr	Mfr	Conc/L	Remarks	Ref	C/I
Dextrose 5%	a			Compatible and stable for at least 24 hr	1	C
	GRI[b]	SW	1.6 g	Under 10% loss in 6 days at room temperature	2287	C
Ringer's injection, lactated	a			Compatible and stable for at least 24 hr	1	C
	GRI[b]	SW	1.6 g	Under 10% loss in 6 days at room temperature	2287	C
Sodium chloride 0.9%	a			Compatible and stable for at least 24 hr	1	C
	GRI[b]	SW	1.6 g	Under 10% loss in 6 days at room temperature	2287	C

[a]Tested in PVC and glass containers.
[b]Tested in glass, polyethylene (polyolefin), and PVC containers.

Y-Site Injection Compatibility (1:1 Mixture)

			Valproate sodium				
Drug	*Mfr*	*Conc*	*Mfr*	*Conc*	*Remarks*	*Ref*	*C/I*
Cefepime HCl	BMS	120 mg/mL[a]		100 mg/mL	Physically compatible. Under 10% cefepime loss. Valproate not tested	2513	C
Ceftazidime	SKB	125 mg/mL		100 mg/mL	Physically compatible. Under 10% ceftazidime loss. Valproate not tested	2434	C
	GSK	120 mg/mL[a]		100 mg/mL	Physically compatible. Under 10% ceftazidime loss. Valproate not tested	2513	C

[a]*Tested in sterile water for injection.*

VANCOMYCIN HYDROCHLORIDE
AHFS 8:12.28.16

Products — Vancomycin hydrochloride is available in vials containing drug equivalent to 500 mg or 1 g of vancomycin base. Reconstitute the vials with 10 or 20 mL, respectively, of sterile water for injection to yield a solution containing 50 mg of base (as the hydrochloride) per milliliter. Vancomycin hydrochloride is also available in 5- and 10-g pharmacy bulk packages. (1; 4)

pH — A 5% solution in water has a pH of 2.5 to 4.5. (1)

Osmolality — Vancomycin hydrochloride (Lilly) 50 mg/mL in sterile water for injection has an osmolality of 57 mOsm/kg. (50)

The osmolality of vancomycin hydrochloride (Lederle) 5 mg/mL was determined to be 249 mOsm/kg in dextrose 5% and 291 mOsm/kg in sodium chloride 0.9%. (1375)

Administration — Vancomycin hydrochloride is administered by intermittent (1; 4) or continuous (4) intravenous infusion. The drug is extremely irritating to tissue and may cause necrosis. Therefore, it should not be given by intramuscular injection, and extravasation should be avoided during intravenous administration. For intermittent intravenous infusion, 500 mg to 1 g should be added to 100 to 200 mL, respectively, of dextrose 5% or sodium chloride 0.9% and administered over at least one hour. (1; 4) For continuous infusion, 1 to 2 g may be added to a fluid volume sufficient to permit administration of the daily dose over 24 hours. (4) Thrombophlebitis can be minimized by using dilute solutions of 2.5 to 5 mg/mL and rotating injection sites. (1; 4)

Stability — Intact vials should be stored at controlled room temperature. The manufacturer indicates that reconstituted solutions of vancomycin hydrochloride are stable for 14 days under refrigeration (1); other information indicates that the drug is also stable in solution for 14 days at room temperature. (4; 141)

pH Effects — In the pH range of 2 to 10, vancomycin hydrochloride degradation is principally deamidation. (1927) Vancomycin hydrochloride has been reported to be most stable at pH 3 to 5 (141) and at pH 5.5 (1927), with relatively pH-independent decomposition in the range of 3 to 8. (1927) The stability of a 1-mg/mL concentration was evaluated in buffer solutions having pH values of 1.4, 5.6, and 7.1 at 24 °C. Little or no loss occurred in 24 hours in any solution. However, the pH 1.4 buffer had a 19% loss in five days, the pH 5.6 buffer had a 10% loss in 17 days, and the pH 7.1 buffer had an 11% loss in five days. (1134)

In an accelerated study at 66 °C, the half-life of vancomycin B (the largest component of the commercial product) was 400 minutes in a phosphate buffer with a pH of 2.2 and 650 minutes in a phosphate buffer with a pH of 7. (1354)

Vancomycin hydrochloride has a low pH and may cause a physical incompatibility with other drugs, especially drugs with an alkaline pH. (1; 4; 873)

The concentration dependency of compatibility or incompatibility of vancomycin hydrochloride mixed with or administered simultaneously with a number of penicillins and cephalosporins has been demonstrated. (2189) Vancomycin hydrochloride has a low pH and is variably compatible with drugs having neutral to mildly alkaline pH, including cephalosporins and penicillins. The compatibility may depend on a number of factors including concentration of each drug, dilution vehicle, actual pH of solutions, and completeness of mixing during administration. Combinations that are compatible when well mixed may result in precipitation if only partially mixed, presumably due to regionally different concentrations and pH values. If attempting to administer vancomycin hydrochloride with another drug product, care should be taken to ensure that the specific combination and concentrations are compatible under the exact administration conditions to be used. An inline filter should be used as a final safety measure. (2189)

Freezing Solutions — Vancomycin hydrochloride (Lilly) at a concentration of 5 mg/mL in dextrose 5% or sodium chloride 0.9% exhibited no loss after 63 days of storage when frozen at −10 °C. However, neither did a loss occur in the same time period when the solution was stored at 5 °C. (1134)

In one study, vancomycin hydrochloride (Lilly) 5 mg/mL in dextrose 5% was stored frozen at −20 °C for 105 days. After thawing in a microwave, the samples were stored for 56 more days under refrigeration. The samples remained clear and had no color change. In addition, no loss of vancomycin occurred throughout the entire test period. (2682)

Syringes — The stability of vancomycin hydrochloride (Lilly) 5 mg/mL in dextrose concentrations ranging from 5 to 30% and packaged in plastic syringes was studied. The syringes were stored at 4 °C for 24 hours followed by two hours at room temperature. Little change in the concentration occurred. (1301)

The stability of vancomycin hydrochloride (Lilly) reconstituted to a concentration of 10 mg/mL with sterile water for injection, dextrose 5%, and 0.9% sodium chloride repackaged into plastic syringes was studied. Five milliliters of the solutions were filled into three-piece Plastipak (Becton Dickinson) and two-piece Injekt (Braun) syringes that were then sealed with Luer-Lok hubs (Vigon) and stored at 4 and 25 °C for 84 days. Under refrigeration, vancomycin hydrochloride prepared with all three solutions and packaged in both kinds of syringes was physically and chemically stable for the 84-day period; losses were 4% or less. (1893)

However, stored at 25 °C in the Plastipak syringes, 10% loss occurred in about 47 days in water, 55 days in dextrose 5%, and 62 days in sodium chloride 0.9%. In the Injekt syringes, stability was less; 10% loss occurred in 29 days in water, 33 days in dextrose 5%, and 34 days in sodium chloride 0.9%. In addition, a degradation product appeared as a white flocculent precipitate in all room temperature samples after about eight weeks of storage. (1893)

Vancomycin hydrochloride 5 mg/mL in dextrose 5% and in sodium chloride 0.9% packaged in polypropylene syringes (Becton Dickinson) exhibited less than 10% loss in 14 days at room temperature and in 6 months under refrigeration. Refrigerated solutions warmed to room temperature were stable for 48 hours. (2730)

Elastomeric Reservoir Pumps — Vancomycin hydrochloride (Lilly) 10 mg/mL in both dextrose 5% and sodium chloride 0.9% was evaluated for binding potential to natural rubber elastomeric reservoirs (Baxter). No binding was found after storage for two weeks at 35 °C with gentle agitation. (2014)

Implantable Pumps — Vancomycin hydrochloride (Lilly) 1 mg/mL in water in an implantable pump (Infusaid model 100) was incubated in a water bath at 37 °C for 28 days. Vancomycin losses were substantial—about 25% in seven days and 40% in 28 days. At the end of the test period, a colloidal precipitate also was found in the pumps. (1302)

Sorption — Vancomycin hydrochloride (Lilly) 15 mg/mL in dextrose 5% is reported to undergo substantial sorption to Teflon tubing used in an automatic dilutor (Syva). The vancomycin hydrochloride was apparently released from the tubing into subsequent solutions resulting in vancomycin toxicity. (2153)

Vancomycin hydrochloride 10 mg/mL with heparin sodium 5000 units/mL as an antibiotic lock in polyurethane central hemodialysis catheters lost about 50% of the antibiotic over 72 hours at 37 °C. The loss was attributed to sorption to the catheters, although precipitation is also possible. Nevertheless, the reduced antibiotic concentration (about 5 mg/mL) remained effective against common microorganisms in catheter-related bacteremia in hemodialysis patients. (2515; 2516)

Plasticizer Leaching — Vancomycin hydrochloride (Qualimed Laboratories) 8 mg/mL in dextrose 5% and sodium chloride 0.9% in PVC containers (Macropharma) did not leach detectable amounts of DEHP plasticizer during simulated administration over 24 hours. If any DEHP was present, the concentration was less than 1 mcg/mL, the limit of detection in this study. (2148)

Filtration — Vancomycin hydrochloride (Lilly) 2 mg/mL in dextrose 5% or sodium chloride 0.9% was filtered through a 0.22-μm cellulose ester filter (Ivex-HP, Millipore) over six hours. No significant drug loss due to binding to the filter was noted. (1034)

Central Venous Catheter — Vancomycin hydrochloride (Fujisawa) 2 mg/mL in dextrose 5% was found to be compatible with the ARROWg+ard Blue Plus (Arrow International) chlorhexidine-bearing triple-lumen central catheter. Essentially complete delivery of the drug was found with little or no drug loss occurring. Furthermore, chlorhexidine delivered from the catheter remained at trace amounts with no substantial increase due to the delivery of the drug through the catheter. (2335)

Compatibility Information

Solution Compatibility

Vancomycin HCl

Solution	Mfr	Mfr	Conc/L	Remarks	Ref	C/I
Dextrose 5% in Ringer's injection, lactated			5 g	Stable for 96 hr refrigerated	1	C
Dextrose 5% in sodium chloride 0.9%			5 g	Stable for 96 hr refrigerated	1	C
		LI	1 g	Physically compatible	74	C
Dextrose 5%			5 g	Stable for 14 days refrigerated	1	C
		LI	1 g	Physically compatible	74	C
		LI	5 g	Stable for 7 days at 5 and 25 °C	141	C
	TR[a]	LI	5 g	Physically compatible and stability for 24 hr at room temperature	518	C
	TR[b]	LI	5 g	Physically compatible with no loss in 7 days and 5% loss in 17 days at 24 °C. In glass containers, no loss in 63 days at 5 °C	1134	C
	TR	LI	4 and 5 g	Physically compatible with 8% loss in 17 days at 23 °C and 11% loss in 30 days at 4 °C	1354	C

Solution Compatibility (Cont.)

Vancomycin HCl

Solution	Mfr	Mfr	Conc/L	Remarks	Ref	C/I
	AB[e]	AB	20 and 40 g	Little loss in 96 hr at 25 °C and in 30 days at 5 °C	2097	C
	[a]	QLM	8 g	Visually compatible and no loss during a 24 hr simulated infusion at 22 °C	2148	C
	[a]	QLM	5 g	Visually compatible and no loss during a 1 hr simulated infusion at 22 °C	2148	C
	[a]	QLM	5 g	Visually compatible and no loss during storage for 48 hr at 22 °C in light and 7 days at 4 °C in dark	2148	C
	BA[a]	LI	5 and 10 g	Visually compatible with less than 3% loss in 58 days at 4 °C	2252	C
	BA[f]	QLM	2 g	Visually compatible with no loss at 4 °C and 4 to 6% loss at room temperature in 48 hr	2278	C
	BG[g]	HOS	1 and 5 g	Under 10% loss in 7 days at 23 °C and 31 days at 4 °C	2819	C
Dextrose 10%		LI	5 g	Physically compatible	143	C
Normosol M in dextrose 5%			5 g	Stable for 96 hr refrigerated	1	C
Ringer's injection, lactated			5 g	Stable for 96 hr refrigerated	1	C
		LI	5 g	Physically compatible	143	C
		LI	1 g	Physically compatible	74	C
Sodium chloride 0.9%			5 g	Stable for 14 days refrigerated	1	C
		LI	5 g	Stable for at least 7 days at 5 and 25 °C	141	C
		LI	1 g	Physically compatible	74	C
	TR[a]	LI	5 g	Physically compatible and stable for 24 hr at room temperature	518	C
	TR[b]	LI	5 g	Physically compatible with no loss in 7 days and 5% loss in 17 days at 24 °C. In glass containers, no loss in 63 days at 5 °C	1134	C
	TR	LI	4 and 5 g	Physically compatible with 9% loss in 24 days at 23 °C and 5 to 6% loss in 30 days at 4 °C	1354	C
	AB[c]	ES	10 g	Little loss with 24-hr storage at 5 °C followed by 24-hr simulated administration at 30 °C via portable pump	1779	C
	[a]	QLM	8 g	Visually compatible and no loss during a 24 hr simulated infusion at 22 °C	2148	C
	[a]	QLM	5 g	Visually compatible and no loss during a 1 hr simulated infusion at 22 °C	2148	C
	[a]	QLM	5 g	Visually compatible and no loss during storage for 48 hr at 22 °C in light and 7 days at 4 °C in dark	2148	C
	BA[f]	QLM	2 g	Visually compatible with no loss at 4 °C and at room temperature in 48 hr	2278	C
	HOS[g]	HOS	1 and 5 g	Under 10% loss in 7 days at 23 °C and 31 days at 4 °C	2819	C
Sodium lactate 1/6 M		LI	5 g	Physically compatible	143	C
TPN #95, #96[d]		LE	400 mg	Physically compatible and no vancomycin loss for 8 days at room temperature and refrigerated	1321	C
TPN #105, #106[d]		LI	1 and 6 g	Physically compatible with little or no vancomycin loss in 4 hr at 22 °C	1325	C

Solution Compatibility (Cont.)

Vancomycin HCl

Solution	Mfr	Mfr	Conc/L	Remarks	Ref	C/I
TPN #107[d]			200 mg	Activity retained for 24 hr at 21 °C	1326	**C**
TPN #202[a,d]		LI	500 mg and 1 g	Visually compatible and activity retained for 35 days at 4 °C plus 24 hr at 22 °C	1933	**C**

[a]Tested in PVC containers.
[b]Tested in both glass and PVC containers.
[c]Tested in portable pump reservoirs (Pharmacia Deltec).
[d]Refer to Appendix I for the composition of parenteral nutrition solutions. TPN indicates a 2-in-1 admixture.
[e]Tested in SIMS Deltec Medication Cassette reservoirs.
[f]Tested in PVC, polyolefin, and glass containers.
[g]Tested in Accufusor reservoirs.

Additive Compatibility

Vancomycin HCl

Drug	Mfr	Conc/L	Mfr	Conc/L	Test Soln	Remarks	Ref	C/I
Amikacin sulfate	BR	5 g	LI	2 g	D5LR, D5R, D5S, D5W, D10W, LR, NS, R, SL	Physically compatible and amikacin stable for 24 hr at 25 °C. Vancomycin not tested	293	**C**
Aminophylline		250 mg	LI	1 g	D5W	Physically compatible	74	**C**
	SE	1 g	LI	5 g	D5W	Physically incompatible	15	**I**
Atracurium besylate	BW	500 mg		5 g	D5W	Physically compatible and atracurium stable for 24 hr at 5 and 30 °C	1694	**C**
Aztreonam	SQ	40 g	AB	10 g	D5W, NS	Immediate microcrystalline precipitate. Turbidity and precipitate over 24 hr	1848	**I**
	SQ	4 g	AB	1 g	D5W	Physically compatible. Little loss of either drug in 31 days at 4 °C. 10% aztreonam loss in 14 days at 23 °C and 7 days at 32 °C	1848	**C**
	SQ	4 g	AB	1 g	NS	Physically compatible. Little loss of either drug in 31 days at 4 °C. 8% aztreonam loss in 31 days at 23 °C and 7 days at 32 °C	1848	**C**
Calcium gluconate		1 g	LI	1 g	D5W	Physically compatible	74	**C**
Cefepime HCl	BR	4 g	LI	5 g	D5W, NS	4% cefepime loss in 24 hr at room temperature in light and 2% loss in 7 days at 5 °C. No vancomycin loss. Cloudiness in 5 days at 5 °C	1682	**C**
	BR	40 g	LI	1 g	D5W, NS	4% cefepime loss in 24 hr at room temperature in light and 2% loss in 7 days at 5 °C. No vancomycin loss and no cloudiness	1682	**C**
Chloramphenicol sodium succinate	PD	10 g	LI	5 g	D5W	Physically incompatible	15	**I**
Dimenhydrinate	SE	50 mg	LI	1 g	D5W	Physically compatible	74	**C**

Additive Compatibility (Cont.)

Vancomycin HCl

Drug	Mfr	Conc/L	Mfr	Conc/L	Test Soln	Remarks	Ref	C/I
Famotidine	YAM	200 mg	AB	5 g	D5W[b]	Visually compatible. 9% vancomycin and 6% famotidine loss in 14 days at 25 °C. At 4 °C, 4% loss of both drugs in 14 days	2111	C
Fusidate sodium	LEO	500 mg		25 g	D–S	Physically incompatible	1800	I
Heparin sodium		12,000 units	LI	1 g	D5W	Precipitates immediately	74	I
	IX	1000 units	LE	400 mg	TPN #95[a]	Physically compatible and vancomycin stable for 8 days at room temperature and under refrigeration	1321	C
	ES	100,000 units	LI	25 mg	NS	Physically compatible. Under 10% vancomycin loss and no heparin loss in 30 days at 28 °C and 63 days at 4 °C	2542	C
Hydrocortisone sodium succinate	UP	100 mg	LI	1 g	D5W	Physically compatible	74	C
Meropenem	ZEN	1 and 20 g	LI	1 g	NS	Visually compatible for 4 hr at room temperature	1994	C
Potassium chloride		3 g	LI	1 g	D5W	Physically compatible	74	C
Ranitidine HCl	GL	100 mg	DI	1 g	D5W	Physically compatible for 24 hr at ambient temperature in light	1151	C
	GL	50 mg and 2 g		5 g	D5W	Physically compatible. Ranitidine stable for 24 hr at 25 °C. Vancomycin not tested	1515	C
Verapamil HCl	KN	80 mg	LI	1 g	D5W, NS	Physically compatible for 24 hr	764	C

[a]*Refer to Appendix I for the composition of parenteral nutrition solutions. TPN indicates a 2-in-1 admixture.*
[b]*Tested in methyl-methacrylate-butadiene-styrene plastic containers.*

Drugs in Syringe Compatibility

Vancomycin HCl

Drug (in syringe)	Mfr	Amt	Mfr	Amt	Remarks	Ref	C/I
Caffeine citrate		20 mg/ 1 mL	LI	50 mg/ 1 mL	Visually compatible for 4 hr at 25 °C	2440	C
Dimenhydrinate		10 mg/ 1 mL		50 mg/ 1 mL	Precipitate forms	2569	I
Heparin sodium		2500 units/ 1 mL	LI	500 mg	Turbidity or precipitate forms within 5 min	1053	I
Pantoprazole sodium	[a]	4 mg/ 1 mL		50 mg/ 1 mL	Clear solution	2574	C

[a]*Test performed using the formulation WITHOUT edetate disodium.*

Y-Site Injection Compatibility (1:1 Mixture)

Vancomycin HCl

Drug	Mfr	Conc	Mfr	Conc	Remarks	Ref	C/I
Acyclovir sodium	BW	5 mg/mL[a]	LI	5 mg/mL[a]	Physically compatible for 4 hr at 25 °C	1157	C
Albumin human		0.1 and 1%[b]		20 mg/mL[a]	Heavy turbidity forms immediately and precipitate develops subsequently	1701	I
Aldesleukin	CHI[q]	[a]			Visually compatible. Aldesleukin activity retained. Vancomycin not tested	1890	C
Allopurinol sodium	BW	3 mg/mL[b]	LY	10 mg/mL[b]	Physically compatible for 4 hr at 22 °C	1686	C
Alprostadil	BED	7.5 mcg/mL[p,e]	LI	5 mg/mL[s]	Visually compatible for 1 hr	2746	C
Amifostine	USB	10 mg/mL[a]	AB	10 mg/mL[a]	Physically compatible for 4 hr at 23 °C	1845	C
Amiodarone HCl	LZ	4 mg/mL[c]	LI	5 mg/mL[c]	Physically compatible for 4 hr at room temperature	1444	C
	WY	6 mg/mL[a]	APP	4 mg/mL[a]	Visually compatible for 24 hr at 22 °C	2352	C
	WY	6 mg/mL[a]	APP	10 mg/mL[a]	Visually compatible for 24 hr at 22 °C	2352	C
Amphotericin B cholesteryl sulfate complex	SEQ	0.83 mg/mL[a]	AB	10 mg/mL[a]	Gross precipitate forms	2117	I
Ampicillin sodium	SKB	250 mg/mL[d]	AB	20 mg/mL[a]	Transient precipitate forms	2189	?
	SKB	1, 10, 50 mg/mL[b]	AB	20 mg/mL[a]	Physically compatible for 4 hr at 23 °C	2189	C
	SKB	1[b], 10[b], 50[b], 250[d] mg/mL	AB	2 mg/mL[a]	Physically compatible for 4 hr at 23 °C	2189	C
Ampicillin sodium–sulbactam sodium	PF	250 + 125 mg/mL[d]	AB	20 mg/mL[a]	Transient precipitate forms	2189	?
	PF	1 + 0.5, 10 + 5, 50 + 25 mg/mL[b]	AB	20 mg/mL[a]	Physically compatible for 4 hr at 23 °C	2189	C
	PF	1 + 0.5[b], 10 + 5[b], 50 + 25[b], 250 + 125[d] mg/mL	AB	2 mg/mL[a]	Physically compatible for 4 hr at 23 °C	2189	C
Amsacrine	NCI	1 mg/mL[a]	LI	10 mg/mL[a]	Visually compatible for 4 hr at 22 °C	1381	C
Anidulafungin	VIC	0.5 mg/mL[a]	APP	10 mg/mL[a]	Physically compatible for 4 hr at 23 °C	2617	C
Atracurium besylate	BW	0.5 mg/mL[a]	ES	5 mg/mL[a]	Physically compatible for 24 hr at 28 °C	1337	C
Aztreonam	SQ	200 mg/mL[b]	LI	67 mg/mL[b]	White granular precipitate forms immediately in tubing when given sequentially	1364	I
	SQ	40 mg/mL[a]	AB	10 mg/mL[a]	Physically compatible for 4 hr at 23 °C	1758	C
Bivalirudin	TMC	5 mg/mL[a]	AB	10 mg/mL[a]	Gross white precipitate forms immediately	2373	I
Caspofungin acetate	ME	0.7 mg/mL[b]	HOS	10 mg/mL[b]	Physically compatible for 4 hr at room temperature	2758	C
	ME	0.5 mg/mL[b]	HOS	4 mg/mL[b]	Physically compatible over 60 min	2766	C
Cefazolin sodium	SKB	200 mg/mL[d]	AB	20 mg/mL[a]	Transient precipitate forms	2189	?
	SKB	10 and 50 mg/mL[a]	AB	20 mg/mL[a]	Gross white precipitate forms immediately	2189	I
	SKB	1 mg/mL[a]	AB	20 mg/mL[a]	Physically compatible for 4 hr at 23 °C	2189	C
	SKB	200 mg/mL[d]	AB	2 mg/mL[a]	Physically compatible for 4 hr at 23 °C	2189	C
	SKB	50 mg/mL[a]	AB	2 mg/mL[a]	Subvisible haze forms immediately	2189	I
	SKB	1 and 10 mg/mL[a]	AB	2 mg/mL[a]	Physically compatible for 4 hr at 23 °C	2189	C

Y-Site Injection Compatibility (1:1 Mixture) (Cont.)

		Vancomycin HCl					
Drug	*Mfr*	*Conc*	*Mfr*	*Conc*	*Remarks*	*Ref*	*C/I*
Cefepime HCl	BMS	120 mg/mL[d]		30 mg/mL	Physically compatible with less than 10% cefepime loss. Vancomycin not tested	2513	C
Cefotaxime sodium		100 mg/mL[d]		12.5, 25, 30, 50 mg/mL[d]	White precipitate forms immediately	1721	I
		100 mg/mL[d]		5 mg/mL[d]	No precipitate visually observed over 7 days at room temperature, but nonvisible incompatibility cannot be ruled out	1721	?
	HO	200 mg/mL[d]	AB	20 mg/mL[a]	Transient precipitate forms	2189	?
	HO	50 mg/mL[a]	AB	20 mg/mL[a]	White cloudiness forms immediately	2189	I
	HO	1 and 10 mg/mL[a]	AB	20 mg/mL[a]	Physically compatible for 4 hr at 23 °C	2189	C
	HO	1[a], 10[a], 50[a], 200[d] mg/mL	AB	2 mg/mL[a]	Physically compatible for 4 hr at 23 °C	2189	C
Cefotetan disodium	ZEN	200 mg/mL[d]	AB	20 mg/mL[a]	Transient precipitate forms followed by white precipitate in 4 hr	2189	I
	ZEN	10 and 50 mg/mL[a]	AB	20 mg/mL[a]	Gross white precipitate forms immediately	2189	I
	ZEN	1 mg/mL[a]	AB	20 mg/mL[a]	Subvisible haze forms immediately. White precipitate in 4 hr	2189	I
	ZEN	1[a], 10[a], 50[a], 200[d] mg/mL	AB	2 mg/mL[a]	Physically compatible for 4 hr at 23 °C	2189	C
Cefoxitin sodium	ME	180 mg/mL[d]	AB	20 mg/mL[a]	Transient precipitate forms	2189	?
	ME	50 mg/mL[a]	AB	20 mg/mL[a]	Immediate gross white precipitate	2189	I
	ME	10 mg/mL[a]	AB	20 mg/mL[a]	Visible haze forms in 4 hr at 23 °C	2189	I
	ME	1 mg/mL[a]	AB	20 mg/mL[a]	Physically compatible for 4 hr at 23 °C	2189	C
	ME	1[a], 10[a], 50[a], 180[d] mg/mL	AB	2 mg/mL[a]	Physically compatible for 4 hr at 23 °C	2189	C
Ceftazidime		50 mg/mL[d]		10 mg/mL[a]	Precipitates immediately	873	I
	SKB	10[a], 50[a], 200[d] mg/mL	AB	20 mg/mL[a]	Gross white precipitate forms immediately	2189	I
	SKB	1 mg/mL[a]	AB	20 mg/mL[a]	Physically compatible for 4 hr at 23 °C	2189	C
	SKB	1[a], 10[a], 50[a], 200[d] mg/mL	AB	2 mg/mL[a]	Physically compatible for 4 hr at 23 °C	2189	C
	SKB	125 mg/mL		30 mg/mL	Precipitates immediately	2434	I
	GSK	120 mg/mL[d]		30 mg/mL	Precipitates	2513	I
Ceftriaxone sodium	RC	100 mg/mL	LI	20 mg/mL	White precipitate forms immediately	1398	I
	RC	250 mg/mL[d]	AB	20 mg/mL[a]	Transient precipitate forms	2189	?
	RC	10 and 50 mg/mL[a]	AB	20 mg/mL[a]	Gross white precipitate forms immediately	2189	I
	RC	1 mg/mL[a]	AB	20 mg/mL[a]	Subvisible haze forms immediately	2189	I
	RC	1[a], 10[a], 50[a], 250[d] mg/mL	AB	2 mg/mL[a]	Physically compatible for 4 hr at 23 °C	2189	C
Cefuroxime sodium	GW	150 mg/mL[d]	AB	20 mg/mL[a]	Transient precipitate forms followed by a subvisible haze	2189	I
	GW	50 mg/mL[a]	AB	20 mg/mL[a]	Gross white precipitate forms immediately	2189	I
	GW	10 mg/mL[a]	AB	20 mg/mL[a]	Subvisible haze forms immediately	2189	I
	GW	1 mg/mL[a]	AB	20 mg/mL[a]	Physically compatible for 4 hr at 23 °C	2189	C
	GW	1[a], 10[a], 50[a], 150[d] mg/mL	AB	2 mg/mL[a]	Physically compatible for 4 hr at 23 °C	2189	C
Cisatracurium besylate	GW	0.1, 2, 5 mg/mL[a]	AB	10 mg/mL[a]	Physically compatible for 4 hr at 23 °C	2074	C

Y-Site Injection Compatibility (1:1 Mixture) (Cont.)

Vancomycin HCl

Drug	Mfr	Conc	Mfr	Conc	Remarks	Ref	C/I
Clarithromycin	AB	4 mg/mL[a]	DB	10 mg/mL[a]	Visually compatible for 72 hr at both 30 and 17 °C	2174	C
Cyclophosphamide	MJ	20 mg/mL[a]	LI	5 mg/mL[a]	Physically compatible for 4 hr at 25 °C	1194	C
Dexmedetomidine HCl	AB	4 mcg/mL[b]	AB	10 mg/mL[b]	Physically compatible for 4 hr at 23 °C	2383	C
Diltiazem HCl	MMD	5 mg/mL	LI	5 and 50 mg/mL[b]	Visually compatible	1807	C
Docetaxel	RPR	0.9 mg/mL[a]	LI	10 mg/mL[a]	Physically compatible for 4 hr at 23 °C	2224	C
Doripenem	JJ	5 mg/mL[a,b]	HOS	10 mg/mL[a,b]	Physically compatible for 4 hr at 23 °C	2743	C
Doxapram HCl	RB	2 mg/mL[a]	APP	5 mg/mL[a]	Visually compatible for 4 hr at 23 °C	2470	C
Doxorubicin HCl liposomal	SEQ	0.4 mg/mL[a]	AB	10 mg/mL[a]	Physically compatible for 4 hr at 23 °C	2087	C
Enalaprilat	MSD	0.05 mg/mL[b]	LE	5 mg/mL[a]	Physically compatible for 24 hr at room temperature under fluorescent light	1355	C
Esmolol HCl	DCC	10 mg/mL[a]	LE	5 mg/mL[a]	Physically compatible for 24 hr at 22 °C	1169	C
Etoposide phosphate	BR	5 mg/mL[a]	LI	10 mg/mL[a]	Physically compatible for 4 hr at 23 °C	2218	C
Fenoldopam mesylate	AB	80 mcg/mL[b]	APP	10 mg/mL[b]	Physically compatible for 4 hr at 23 °C	2467	C
Filgrastim	AMG	30 mcg/mL[a]	AB	10 mg/mL[a]	Physically compatible for 4 hr at 22 °C	1687	C
Fluconazole	RR	2 mg/mL	LY	20 mg/mL	Physically compatible for 24 hr at 25 °C	1407	C
Fludarabine phosphate	BX	1 mg/mL[a]	LI	10 mg/mL[a]	Visually compatible for 4 hr at 22 °C	1439	C
Foscarnet sodium	AST	24 mg/mL	LE	20 mg/mL	Precipitates immediately	1335	I
	AST	24 mg/mL	LE	15 mg/mL[c]	Physically compatible for 24 hr at 25 °C under fluorescent light	1393	C
	AST	24 mg/mL	LE	10 mg/mL[b]	Visually compatible for 24 hr at room temperature. No precipitate found	2063	C
Gallium nitrate	FUJ	1 mg/mL[b]	AB	5 mg/mL[b]	Visually compatible for 24 hr at 25 °C	1673	C
Gemcitabine HCl	LI	10 mg/mL[b]	LI	10 mg/mL[b]	Physically compatible for 4 hr at 23 °C	2226	C
Granisetron HCl	SKB	0.05 mg/mL[a]	AB	10 mg/mL[a]	Physically compatible for 4 hr at 23 °C	2000	C
Heparin sodium	TR	50 units/mL	LI	6.6 mg/mL[a]	Visually incompatible within 4 hr at 25 °C	1793	I
	ES	100 units/mL[c]	LE	10 mg/mL[b]	Precipitate forms	2063	I
	LEO	10 and 5000 units/mL[b]	PHS	2.5 mg/mL[b]	Physically compatible with little change in heparin activity in 14 days at 4 and 37 °C. Antibiotic not tested	2684	C
	LEO	10 units/mL[b]	PHS	2 mg/mL[b]	Physically compatible with little change in heparin activity in 14 days at 4 and 37 °C. Antibiotic not tested	2684	C
Hetastarch in lactated electrolyte	AB	6%	LI	10 mg/mL[a]	Physically compatible for 4 hr at 23 °C	2339	C
Hydromorphone HCl	WY	0.2 mg/mL[a]	LI	5 mg/mL[a]	Physically compatible for 4 hr at 25 °C	987	C
	HOS	2 mg/mL	HOS	4 mg/mL[b]	Physically compatible	2794	C
Idarubicin HCl	AD	1 mg/mL[b]	AD	4 mg/mL[a]	Color changes immediately	1525	I
Insulin, regular	LI	0.2 unit/mL[b]	LI	4 mg/mL[a]	Physically compatible for 2 hr at 25 °C	1395	C
Labetalol HCl	SC	1 mg/mL[a]	LE	5 mg/mL[a]	Physically compatible for 24 hr at 18 °C	1171	C
Levofloxacin	OMN	5 mg/mL[a]	LI	50 mg/mL	Visually compatible for 4 hr at 24 °C	2233	C
Linezolid	PHU	2 mg/mL	FUJ	10 mg/mL[a]	Physically compatible for 4 hr at 23 °C	2264	C
Lorazepam	WY	0.33 mg/mL[b]	LI	5 mg/mL	Visually compatible for 24 hr at 22 °C	1855	C

Y-Site Injection Compatibility (1:1 Mixture) (Cont.)

Vancomycin HCl

Drug	Mfr	Conc	Mfr	Conc	Remarks	Ref	C/I
Magnesium sulfate	IX	16.7, 33.3, 66.7, 100 mg/mL[a]	LI	5 mg/mL[a]	Physically compatible for at least 4 hr at 32 °C	813	C
Melphalan HCl	BW	0.1 mg/mL[b]	LY	10 mg/mL[b]	Physically compatible for 3 hr at 22 °C	1557	C
Meperidine HCl	WY	10 mg/mL[a]	LI	5 mg/mL[a]	Physically compatible for 4 hr at 25 °C	987	C
Meropenem	ZEN	1 and 50 mg/mL[b]	LI	5 mg/mL[d]	Visually compatible for 4 hr at room temperature	1994	C
Methotrexate sodium	LE	[a,f]	AB	510 mg[g]	Physically compatible during 1-hr simultaneous infusion	1405	C
		30 mg/mL		5 mg/mL[a]	Visually compatible for 2 hr at room temperature. Yellow precipitate in 4 hr	1788	I
Midazolam HCl	RC	1 mg/mL[a]	LI	5 mg/mL[a]	Visually compatible for 24 hr at 23 °C	1847	C
	RC	5 mg/mL	LI	5 mg/mL	Visually compatible for 24 hr at 22 °C	1855	C
Milrinone lactate	SS	0.2 mg/mL[a]	OR	5 mg/mL[a]	Visually compatible for 4 hr at 25 °C	2381	C
Morphine sulfate	WI	1 mg/mL[a]	LI	5 mg/mL[a]	Physically compatible for 4 hr at 25 °C	987	C
Mycophenolate mofetil HCl	RC	5.9 mg/mL[a]		10 mg/mL[a]	Physically compatible and 3% mycophenolate mofetil loss in 4 hr	2738	C
Nafcillin sodium	BE	250 mg/mL[d]	AB	20 mg/mL[a]	Transient precipitate forms followed by a visibly hazy solution	2189	I
	BE	10 and 50 mg/mL[b]	AB	20 mg/mL[a]	Gross white precipitate forms immediately	2189	I
	BE	1 mg/mL[b]	AB	20 mg/mL[a]	Physically compatible for 4 hr at 23 °C	2189	C
	BE	10[b], 50[b], 250[d] mg/mL	AB	2 mg/mL[a]	Subvisible measured haze forms immediately	2189	I
	BE	1 mg/mL[b]	AB	2 mg/mL[a]	Physically compatible for 4 hr at 23 °C	2189	C
Nicardipine HCl	DCC	0.1 mg/mL[a]	LE	5 mg/mL[a]	Visually compatible for 24 hr at room temperature	235	C
Omeprazole		4 mg/mL		10 mg/mL[a]	White precipitate forms within 5 min	2173	I
Ondansetron HCl	GL	1 mg/mL[b]	LI	10 mg/mL[a]	Visually compatible for 4 hr at 22 °C	1365	C
Paclitaxel	NCI	1.2 mg/mL[a]		10 mg/mL[a]	Physically compatible for 4 hr at 22 °C	1528	C
Palonosetron HCl	MGI	50 mcg/mL	HOS	5 mg/mL[a]	Physically compatible and no loss of either drug in 4 hr at room temperature	2765	C
Pancuronium bromide	ES	0.05 mg/mL[a]	ES	5 mg/mL[a]	Physically compatible for 24 hr at 28 °C	1337	C
Pantoprazole sodium	ALT[r]	8 mg/mL	ME	40 mg/mL	Color change after 10 hr	2727	I
Pemetrexed disodium	LI	20 mg/mL[b]	AB	10 mg/mL[a]	Physically compatible for 4 hr at 23 °C	2564	C
Piperacillin sodium–tazobactam sodium	LE[r]	40 + 5 mg/mL[a]	AB	10 mg/mL[a]	White turbidity forms immediately and white precipitate forms in 4 hr	1688	I
	LE[r]	200 + 25 mg/mL[d]	AB	20 mg/mL[a]	Transient precipitate forms	2189	?
	LE[r]	10 + 1.25 and 50 + 6.25 mg/mL[a]	AB	20 mg/mL[a]	Gross white precipitate forms immediately	2189	I
	LE[r]	1 + 0.125 mg/mL[a]	AB	20 mg/mL[a]	Physically compatible for 4 hr at 23 °C	2189	C

Y-Site Injection Compatibility (1:1 Mixture) (Cont.)

Vancomycin HCl

Drug	Mfr	Conc	Mfr	Conc	Remarks	Ref	C/I
	LE[r]	1 + 0.125[a], 10 + 1.25[a], 50 + 6.25[a], 200 + 25[d] mg/mL	AB	2 mg/mL[a]	Physically compatible for 4 hr at 23 °C	2189	**C**
Propofol	ZEN	10 mg/mL	AB	10 mg/mL[a]	Physically compatible for 1 hr at 23 °C	2066	**C**
	BA	10 mg/mL		10 mg/mL[a]	Emulsion disruption within 1 to 4 hr at room temperature	2336	**I**
	ASZ	10 mg/mL		10 mg/mL[a]	Physically compatible for up to 30 days at room temperature	2336	**C**
Remifentanil HCl	GW	0.025 and 0.25 mg/mL[b]	AB	10 mg/mL[a]	Physically compatible for 4 hr at 23 °C	2075	**C**
Sargramostim	IMM	10 mcg/mL[b]	LI	10 mg/mL[b]	Visually compatible for 4 hr at 22 °C	1436	**C**
	IMM	15 mcg/mL[b]	LI	20 mg/mL[c]	Visually compatible for 2 hr	1618	**C**
	IMM	6 mcg/mL[b,h]	LI	20 mg/mL[c]	Haze forms within 15 min and increases due to vancomycin incompatibility with albumin human	1618; 1701	**I**
Sodium bicarbonate		1.4%		5 mg/mL[a]	Visually compatible for 4 hr at room temperature	1788	**C**
Tacrolimus	FUJ	1 mg/mL[b]	LI	5 mg/mL[a]	Visually compatible for 24 hr at 25 °C	1630	**C**
Teniposide	BR	0.1 mg/mL[a]	AB	10 mg/mL[a]	Physically compatible for 4 hr at 23 °C	1725	**C**
Theophylline	TR	4 mg/mL	LI	6.6 mg/mL[a]	Visually compatible for 6 hr at 25 °C	1793	**C**
Thiotepa	IMM[i]	1 mg/mL[a]	AB	10 mg/mL[a]	Physically compatible for 4 hr at 23 °C	1861	**C**
Ticarcillin disodium–clavulanate potassium	SKB	206.7 mg/mL[d]	AB	20 mg/mL[a]	Transient precipitate forms	2189	**?**
	SKB	1.034, 10.335, 51.675 mg/mL[a]	AB	20 mg/mL[a]	Gross white precipitate forms	2189	**I**
	SKB	31 mg/mL[b]		5 mg/mL[b]	White precipitate formed sporadically	2167	**I**
	SKB	1.034[a], 10.335[a], 51.675[a], 206.7[d] mg/mL	AB	2 mg/mL[a]	Physically compatible for 4 hr at 23 °C	2189	**C**
Tigecycline	WY	1 mg/mL[b]		5 mg/mL[b]	Physically compatible for 4 hr	2714	**C**
TNA #218 to #226[j]			AB	10 mg/mL[a]	Visually compatible for 4 hr at 23 °C	2215	**C**
TPN #61[j]		[k]	LI	50 mg/1 mL[l]	Physically compatible	1012	**C**
		[m]	LI	300 mg/6 mL[l]	Physically compatible	1012	**C**
TPN #91[j]		[n]	LI	30 mg[o]	Physically compatible	1170	**C**
TPN #189[j]			DB	10 mg/mL[b]	Visually compatible for 24 hr at 22 °C	1767	**C**
TPN #212 to #215[j]			AB	10 mg/mL[a]	Physically compatible for 4 hr at 23 °C	2109	**C**
Vecuronium bromide	OR	0.1 mg/mL[a]	ES	5 mg/mL[a]	Physically compatible for 24 hr at 28 °C	1337	**C**
Vinorelbine tartrate	BW	1 mg/mL[b]	LY	10 mg/mL[b]	Physically compatible for 4 hr at 22 °C	1558	**C**

Y-Site Injection Compatibility (1:1 Mixture) (Cont.)

Vancomycin HCl

Drug	Mfr	Conc	Mfr	Conc	Remarks	Ref	C/I
Warfarin sodium	DU	2 mg/mL[d]	LI	4 mg/mL[a]	Haze forms immediately	2010	I
	DU	0.1 mg/mL[c]	AB	10 mg/mL[c]	Physically compatible for 24 hr at 23 °C	2011	C
	DU	2 mg/mL[d]	AB	10 mg/mL[c]	Heavy white turbidity forms immediately	2011	I
	DME	2 mg/mL[d]	LI	4 mg/mL[a]	Haze forms immediately	2078	I
Zidovudine	BW	4 mg/mL[a]	LI	15 mg/mL[a]	Physically compatible for 4 hr at 25 °C	1193	C

[a]*Tested in dextrose 5%.*
[b]*Tested in sodium chloride 0.9%.*
[c]*Tested in both dextrose 5% and sodium chloride 0.9%.*
[d]*Tested in sterile water for injection.*
[e]*Tested in a 1:1 mixture of dextrose 5% and TPN #274 (see Appendix I).*
[f]*Concentration unspecified.*
[g]*Infused over one hour simultaneously with methotrexate.*
[h]*Tested with 0.1% albumin human added.*
[i]*Lyophilized formulation tested.*
[j]*Refer to Appendix I for the composition of parenteral nutrition solutions. TNA indicates a 3-in-1 admixture, and TPN indicates a 2-in-1 admixture.*
[k]*Run at 21 mL/hr.*
[l]*Given over 30 minutes by syringe pump.*
[m]*Run at 94 mL/hr.*
[n]*Run at 10 mL/hr.*
[o]*Given over one hour by syringe pump.*
[p]*Tested in a 1:1 mixture of (1) dextrose 5% and dextrose 5% in sodium chloride 0.45% with and without potassium chloride 20 mEq/L and also in (2) dextrose 10% in sodium chloride 0.45% with and without potassium chloride 20 mEq/L.*
[q]*Tested with albumin human 0.1%.*
[r]*Test performed using the formulation WITHOUT edetate disodium.*
[s]*Tested in either dextrose 5% or in sodium chloride 0.9%, but the report did not specify which solution.*

Additional Compatibility Information

Peritoneal Dialysis Solutions — The activity of vancomycin 15 mg/L was evaluated in peritoneal dialysis fluids containing dextrose 1.5 or 4.25% (Dianeal 137, Travenol). Storage at 25 °C resulted in virtually no loss of antimicrobial activity in 24 hours. (515)

Vancomycin hydrochloride with aztreonam admixed in Dianeal 137 with dextrose 4.25% is stated to be stable for 24 hours at room temperature. (1)

Vancomycin hydrochloride (Lilly) 10 and 50 mg/L in peritoneal dialysis concentrate with dextrose 50% (McGaw) retained 93 to 100% of its initial activity after 24 hours of storage at room temperature. (1044)

The stability of vancomycin hydrochloride (Lilly) 20 mg/L in peritoneal dialysis solutions (Dianeal 137 and PD2) with heparin sodium 500 units/L was evaluated. Approximately 95 ± 12% activity remained after 24 hours at 25 °C. (1228)

Vancomycin hydrochloride (Lilly) 15 mg/L to 5.3 g/L in Dianeal with dextrose 2.5 or 4.25% was physically compatible with heparin sodium (Organon) 500 to 14,300 units/L for 24 hours at 25 °C under fluorescent light. However, a white precipitate formed immediately in combinations of heparin sodium with vancomycin hydrochloride 6.9 to 14.3 g/L. (1322)

The retention of antimicrobial activity of vancomycin hydrochloride (Lilly) 1 g/L alone and with each of the aminoglycosides gentamicin sulfate (SoloPak) 120 mg/L and tobramycin sulfate (Lilly) 120 mg/L in Dianeal PD-2 (Travenol) with dextrose 1.5% was evaluated. Little or no loss of any antibiotic occurred in eight hours at 37 °C. Vancomycin hydrochloride alone retained activity for at least 48 hours at 4 and 25 °C. In combination with gentamicin sulfate and tobramycin sul-

fate, antimicrobial activity of both vancomycin and the aminoglycosides was retained for up to 48 hours. However, refrigeration at 4 °C was recommended for storage periods greater than 24 hours. (1414)

The stability of vancomycin hydrochloride (Lilly) 25 mg/L in Dianeal 137 (Baxter) with dextrose 1.36 and 3.86%, while protected from direct sunlight, was evaluated. At both dextrose concentrations, less than 4% vancomycin hydrochloride was lost in 42 days at 4 °C. At 20 °C, a 5% or less loss occurred in 28 days. At 37 °C, a 10% loss occurred in six to seven days. (1654)

Vancomycin hydrochloride (Lilly) 1 mg/mL admixed with ceftazidime (Lilly) 0.5 mg/mL in Dianeal PD-2 (Baxter) with 1.5% and also 4.25% dextrose were evaluated for compatibility and stability. Samples were stored under fluorescent light at 4 and 24 °C for 24 hours and at 37 °C for 12 hours. No precipitation or other change was observed by visual inspection in any sample. No loss of either drug was found in the samples stored at 4 °C and no loss of vancomycin hydrochloride and about 4 to 5% ceftazidime loss in the samples stored at 24 °C in 24 hours. Vancomycin hydrochloride losses of 3% or less and ceftazidime loss of about 6% were found in the samples stored at 37 °C for 12 hours. No difference in stability was found between samples at either dextrose concentration. (2217)

Vancomycin hydrochloride (Lederle) 0.05 mg/mL in Dianeal PD-2 with dextrose 1.5% with or without heparin sodium 1 unit/mL in PVC bags was chemically stable for up to six days at 4 °C (about 3 to 5% loss) and 25 °C (up to 7% loss) and five days at body temperature of 37 °C. (866)

The addition of ceftazidime (Glaxo) 0.1 mg/mL to this peritoneal dialysis solution demonstrated a somewhat reduced stability with the ceftazidime being the defining component. The ceftazidime was chemically stable for up to six days at 4 °C (about 3% loss), three days at 25 °C (about 9 to 10% loss), and 12 hours at body temperature of 37 °C with the vancomycin exhibiting less loss throughout. (866)

Vancomycin hydrochloride (Lederle) 25 mcg/mL in Delflex peritoneal dialysis solution bags with 2.5% dextrose (Fresenius) was stable with little loss occurring in 14 days refrigerated and at room temperature. (2573)

Gentamicin sulfate (American Pharmaceutical Partners) 8 mcg/mL with vancomycin hydrochloride (Lederle) 25 mcg/mL in Delflex peritoneal dialysis solution bags with 2.5% dextrose (Fresenius) was stable with little or no loss of either drug occurring in 14 days refrigerated and at room temperature. (2573)

Vancomycin hydrochloride (Abbott) 1 mg/mL in icodextrin 7.5% PD (Baxter) was tested for stability at 5, 24, and 37 °C. The solutions remained clear and colorless. Little or no loss at 5 °C and about 3% loss at 24 °C after seven days of storage was found. At 37 °C, about 6% loss occurred in 24 hours. (2650)

Heparin Locks — Vancomycin hydrochloride (Lilly) 25 mcg/mL and heparin sodium (Elkins-Sinn) 100 units/mL in 0.9% sodium chloride injection as a catheter flush solution was evaluated for stability when stored at 4 °C for 14 days. The flush solution was visually clear, and the vancomycin activity and heparin activity were retained throughout the storage period. However, an additional 24 hours at 37 °C to simulate use conditions resulted in losses of both agents ranging from 20 to 37%. (1933)

Vancomycin hydrochloride (Lilly) 25 mcg/mL and preservative-free heparin sodium (Elkins-Sinn) 100 units/mL in 0.9% sodium chloride in 2-mL glass vials for use as a central catheter flush solution were evaluated for compatibility and stability at 4 and 28 °C. Visual inspection found no evidence of color change or particulate formation throughout the study. Heparin activity remained unchanged for 100 days. Acceptable vancomycin levels were maintained for 30 days at 28 °C and for 63 days at 4 °C. However, unacceptable losses occurred after those times. The activity of both drugs was unaffected by the presence of the other when compared to the activity of single drug controls. (2279)

Vancomycin hydrochloride 25 mcg/mL combined with heparin sodium (Hospira) 10 units/mL in sterile water for injection for use as a lock solution was found to be physically compatible. Little or no vancomycin loss occurred in 3 days at 4 °C. However, losses of 8% occurred in 3 days at 27 °C and 1 day at 40 °C. (2820)

If ciprofloxacin (Sicor) 2 mg/mL was added to this flush solution, a white precipitate appeared within 1 day. Losses of both ciprofloxacin and vancomycin occurred as well. (2820)

VASOPRESSIN
AHFS 68:28

Products — Vasopressin is available in 0.5-, 1-, and 10-mL vials. Each milliliter of solution contains vasopressin 20 pressor units, sodium chloride 0.9%, chlorobutanol 0.5%, in water for injection. Acetic acid and/or sodium hydroxide may have been used to adjust pH during manufacture. (1)

pH — From 2.5 to 4.5. (1; 4)

Administration — Vasopressin may be given subcutaneously or intramuscularly. (1; 4) or by continuous intravenous or intra-arterial infusion using a controlled infusion device. For infusion, the drug is usually diluted to a concentration of 0.1 to 1 unit/mL with sodium chloride 0.9% or dextrose 5%. (4)

Stability — Vasopressin injection is a clear, colorless or practically colorless solution. Intact containers should be stored at controlled room temperature and protected from freezing. (1; 4)

Compatibility Information

Additive Compatibility

Vasopressin

Drug	Mfr	Conc/L	Mfr	Conc/L	Test Soln	Remarks	Ref	C/I
Verapamil HCl	KN	80 mg	PD	40 units	D5W, NS	Physically compatible for 24 hr	764	C

Y-Site Injection Compatibility (1:1 Mixture)

Vasopressin

Drug	Mfr	Conc	Mfr	Conc	Remarks	Ref	C/I
Amiodarone HCl	WY	6 mg/mL[a]	AMR	0.2 unit/mL[b]	Visually compatible for 24 hr at 22 °C	2352	C
	WY	1.5 mg/mL[a]	AMR	2 and 4 units/mL[b]	Physically compatible with vasopressin pushed through a Y-site over 5 sec	2478	C

Y-Site Injection Compatibility (1:1 Mixture) (Cont.)

Vasopressin

Drug	Mfr	Conc	Mfr	Conc	Remarks	Ref	C/I
Argatroban	SKB	1 mg/mL[a]	AMR	0.4 unit/mL[a]	Physically compatible for 24 hr at 23 °C	2572	C
Caspofungin acetate	ME	0.5 mg/mL[b]	APP	0.2 unit/mL[b]	Physically compatible	2641	C
Ceftaroline fosamil	FOR	2.22 mg/mL[a,b,e]	APP	1 unit/mL[a,b,e]	Physically compatible for 4 hr at 23 °C	2826	C
Ciprofloxacin	BAY	2 mg/mL[a]	APP	0.2 unit/mL[b]	Physically compatible	2641	C
Diltiazem HCl	NVP	1 mg/mL[b]	AMR	2 and 4 units/mL[b]	Physically compatible with vasopressin pushed through a Y-site over 5 sec	2478	C
Dobutamine HCl	AB	4.2 mg/mL[a]	AMR	2 and 4 units/mL[b]	Physically compatible with vasopressin pushed through a Y-site over 5 sec	2478	C
Dopamine HCl	AMR	4.2 mg/mL[a]	AMR	2 and 4 units/mL[b]	Physically compatible with vasopressin pushed through a Y-site over 5 sec	2478	C
	BA	3.2 mg/mL[a]	APP	0.2 unit/mL[b]	Physically compatible	2641	C
Epinephrine HCl	AMR	4 mcg/mL[b]	AMR	2 and 4 units/mL[b]	Physically compatible with vasopressin pushed through a Y-site over 5 sec	2478	C
Fluconazole	PF	2 mg/mL	APP	0.2 unit/mL[b]	Physically compatible	2641	C
Furosemide	AB	4 mg/mL[a,b]	APP	0.4 unit/mL[a,b]	Precipitates in 5 to 15 min	2687	I
Gentamicin sulfate	APP	1.2 mg/mL[c]	APP	0.2 unit/mL[b]	Physically compatible	2641	C
Heparin sodium	BA	100 units/mL[a]	AMR	2 and 4 units/mL[b]	Physically compatible with vasopressin pushed through a Y-site over 5 sec	2478	C
Hydroxyethyl starch 130/0.4 in sodium chloride 0.9%	FRK	6%	SZ	0.4, 0.7, 1 unit/mL[a]	Visually compatible for 24 hr at room temperature	2770	C
Imipenem–cilastatin sodium	ME	5 mg/mL[a]	APP	0.2 unit/mL[b]	Physically compatible	2641	C
Insulin, regular	NOV	1 unit/mL[b]	APP	0.2 unit/mL[b]	Physically compatible	2641	C
Lidocaine HCl	BA	4 mg/mL[a]	AMR	2 and 4 units/mL[b]	Physically compatible with vasopressin pushed into a Y-site over 5 sec	2478	C
Linezolid	PHU	2 mg/mL	APP	0.2 unit/mL[b]	Physically compatible	2641	C
Meropenem	ASZ	5 mg/mL[a]	APP	0.2 unit/mL[b]	Physically compatible	2641	C
Metronidazole	AB	5 mg/mL	APP	0.2 unit/mL[b]	Physically compatible	2641	C
Micafungin sodium	ASP	1.5 mg/mL[b]	AMR	1 unit/mL	Physically compatible for 4 hr at 23 °C	2683	C
Milrinone lactate	AB	0.2 mg/mL[a]	AMR	2 and 4 units/mL[b]	Physically compatible with vasopressin pushed through a Y-site over 5 sec	2478	C
Moxifloxacin HCl	BAY	1.6 mg/mL	APP	0.2 unit/mL[b]	Physically compatible	2641	C
Nitroglycerin	BA	0.2 mg/mL[a]	AMR	2 and 4 units/mL[b]	Physically compatible with vasopressin pushed through a Y-site over 5 sec	2478	C
Norepinephrine bitartrate	AB	4 mcg/mL[b]	AMR	2 and 4 units/mL[b]	Physically compatible with vasopressin pushed through a Y-site over 5 sec	2478	C
	GNS	16 mcg/mL[b]	APP	0.2 unit/mL[b]	Physically compatible	2641	C
	AB	4 mcg/mL[b]	APP	0.2 unit/mL[b]	Physically compatible	2641	C
Pantoprazole sodium	ALT[d]	0.16 to 0.8 mg/mL[b]	FER	0.4 to 1 unit/mL[a]	Visually compatible for 12 hr at 23 °C	2603	C
Phenylephrine HCl	AMR	40 mcg/mL[b]	AMR	2 and 4 units/mL[b]	Physically compatible with vasopressin pushed through a Y-site over 5 sec	2478	C
Phenytoin sodium	ES	50 mg/mL	APP	0.2 unit/mL[b]	Crystals form immediately	2641	I

Y-Site Injection Compatibility (1:1 Mixture) (Cont.)

Vasopressin

Drug	Mfr	Conc	Mfr	Conc	Remarks	Ref	C/I
Piperacillin sodium–tazobactam sodium	WY[d]	100 + 12.5 mg/mL	APP	0.2 unit/mL[b]	Physically compatible	2641	**C**
Procainamide HCl	AB	4 mg/mL[b]	AMR	2 and 4 units/mL[b]	Physically compatible with vasopressin pushed through a Y-site over 5 sec	2478	**C**
Sodium bicarbonate	AB	0.15 mEq/mL[c]	APP	0.2 unit/mL[b]	Physically compatible	2641	**C**
Telavancin HCl	ASP	7.5 mg/mL[a,b,e]	AMR	1 unit/mL[a,b,e]	Physically compatible for 2 hr	2830	**C**
Voriconazole	PF	3 mg/mL[c]	APP	0.2 unit/mL[b]	Physically compatible	2641	**C**

[a]*Tested in dextrose 5%.*
[b]*Tested in sodium chloride 0.9%.*
[c]*Tested in sodium chloride 0.45%.*
[d]*Test performed using the formulation WITHOUT edetate disodium.*
[e]*Tested in Ringer's injection, lactated.*

VECURONIUM BROMIDE
AHFS 12:20.20

Products — Vecuronium bromide is available in 10-mg vials as a lyophilized cake, both with and without accompanying bacteriostatic water for injection with benzyl alcohol 0.9% for use as a diluent. It also is available in 20-mg vials without a diluent. The vials also contain citric acid anhydrous, mannitol, and sodium phosphate dibasic anhydrous. Sodium hydroxide and/or phosphoric acid also may be present to adjust the pH. (1)

The 10- and 20-mg vials should be reconstituted with 10 and 20 mL, respectively, of the accompanying bacteriostatic water for injection or sterile water for injection to yield a 1-mg/mL solution. (1; 4) The bacteriostatic water for injection, which contains benzyl alcohol 0.9%, is not for use in newborns. (1)

pH — From 3.5 to 4.5 (1)

Osmolality — The osmolality of vecuronium bromide 4 mg/mL was determined to be 292 mOsm/kg. (1233)

Administration — Vecuronium bromide may be administered by rapid intravenous injection or by intravenous infusion using an infusion control device at a concentration of 0.1 to 0.2 mg/mL in a compatible solution. It should not be administered intramuscularly. (4)

Stability — Vecuronium bromide should be stored at room temperature and protected from light. The reconstituted solution is clear and colorless. When reconstituted with bacteriostatic water for injection, the solution may be used for up to five days when stored at room temperature or under refrigeration. When reconstituted with sterile water for injection, the vial is a single-use container and should be stored under refrigeration and used within 24 hours. (1)

pH Effects — Vecuronium bromide is unstable in the presence of bases and should not be combined with alkaline drugs or simultaneously administered through the same line as an alkaline solution. (4)

Syringes — Vecuronium bromide 1 mg/mL in sterile water for injection and packaged in plastic syringes was found to be stable with no loss of drug for 21 days at room temperature and refrigerated. (2735)

Compatibility Information

Solution Compatibility

Vecuronium bromide

Solution	Mfr	Mfr	Conc/L	Remarks	Ref	C/I
Dextrose 5% in sodium chloride 0.9%				Compatible and stable for 24 hr	1	**C**
Dextrose 5%				Compatible and stable for 24 hr	1	**C**
Ringer's injection, lactated				Compatible and stable for 24 hr	1	**C**
Sodium chloride 0.9%				Compatible and stable for 24 hr	1	**C**

Additive Compatibility

Vecuronium bromide

Drug	Mfr	Conc/L	Mfr	Conc/L	Test Soln	Remarks	Ref	C/I
Ciprofloxacin	BAY	1.6 g	OR	200 mg	D5W	Visually compatible with no loss of ciprofloxacin in 24 hr at 22 °C under fluorescent light. Vecuronium not tested	2413	C

Drugs in Syringe Compatibility

Vecuronium bromide

Drug (in syringe)	Mfr	Amt	Mfr	Amt	Remarks	Ref	C/I
Pantoprazole sodium	a	4 mg/1 mL		1 mg/1 mL	Precipitates	2574	I

[a]*Test performed using the formulation WITHOUT edetate disodium.*

Y-Site Injection Compatibility (1:1 Mixture)

Vecuronium bromide

Drug	Mfr	Conc	Mfr	Conc	Remarks	Ref	C/I
Alprostadil	BED	7.5 mcg/mL[d,f]	OR	1 mg/mL[e]	Visually compatible for 1 hr	2746	C
Aminophylline	AB	1 mg/mL[a]	OR	0.1 mg/mL[a]	Physically compatible for 24 hr at 28 °C	1337	C
Amiodarone HCl	WY	6 mg/mL[a]	OR	1 mg/mL[a]	Visually compatible for 24 hr at 22 °C	2352	C
Amphotericin B cholesteryl sulfate complex	SEQ	0.83 mg/mL[a]	MAR	1 mg/mL[a]	Gross precipitate forms	2117	I
Cefazolin sodium	LY	10 mg/mL[a]	OR	0.1 mg/mL[a]	Physically compatible for 24 hr at 28 °C	1337	C
Cefuroxime sodium	GL	7.5 mg/mL[a]	OR	0.1 mg/mL[a]	Physically compatible for 24 hr at 28 °C	1337	C
Clarithromycin	AB	4 mg/mL[a]	OR	2 mg/mL[a]	Visually compatible for 72 hr at both 30 and 17 °C	2174	C
Dexmedetomidine HCl	HOS				Stated to be compatible	1	C
Diazepam	ES	5 mg/mL[a]	OR	0.1 mg/mL[a]	Cloudy solution forms immediately	1337	I
Diltiazem HCl	MMD	1 mg/mL[a]	OR	1 mg/mL	Visually compatible for 4 hr at 27 °C	2062	C
Dobutamine HCl	LI	1 mg/mL[a]	OR	0.1 mg/mL[a]	Physically compatible for 24 hr at 28 °C	1337	C
	LI	4 mg/mL[a]	OR	1 mg/mL	Visually compatible for 4 hr at 27 °C	2062	C
Dopamine HCl	SO	1.6 mg/mL[a]	OR	0.1 mg/mL[a]	Physically compatible for 24 hr at 28 °C	1337	C
	AB	3.2 mg/mL[a]	OR	1 mg/mL	Visually compatible for 4 hr at 27 °C	2062	C
Epinephrine HCl	AB	4 mcg/mL[a]	OR	0.1 mg/mL[a]	Physically compatible for 24 hr at 28 °C	1337	C
	AB	0.02 mg/mL[a]	OR	1 mg/mL	Visually compatible for 4 hr at 27 °C	2062	C
Esmolol HCl	DCC	10 mg/mL[a]	OR	0.1 mg/mL[a]	Physically compatible for 24 hr at 28 °C	1337	C
Etomidate	AB	2 mg/mL	OR	1 mg/mL	Slight turbidity and white particles form	1801	I
Fenoldopam mesylate	AB	80 mcg/mL[b]	ES	0.2 mg/mL[b]	Physically compatible for 4 hr at 23 °C	2467	C
Fentanyl citrate	ES	10 mcg/mL[a]	OR	0.1 mg/mL[a]	Physically compatible for 24 hr at 28 °C	1337	C
	ES	0.05 mg/mL	OR	1 mg/mL	Visually compatible for 4 hr at 27 °C	2062	C
Fluconazole	RR	2 mg/mL	OR	1 mg/mL[a]	Visually compatible for 24 hr at 28 °C under fluorescent light	1760	C
Furosemide	AMR	10 mg/mL	OR	1 mg/mL	Precipitate forms immediately	2062	I

Y-Site Injection Compatibility (1:1 Mixture) (Cont.)

Vecuronium bromide

Drug	Mfr	Conc	Mfr	Conc	Remarks	Ref	C/I
Gentamicin sulfate	ES	2 mg/mL[a]	OR	0.1 mg/mL[a]	Physically compatible for 24 hr at 28 °C	1337	C
Heparin sodium	SO	40 units/mL[a]	OR	0.1 mg/mL[a]	Physically compatible for 24 hr at 28 °C	1337	C
	ES	100 units/mL[a]	OR	1 mg/mL	Visually compatible for 4 hr at 27 °C	2062	C
Hetastarch in lactated electrolyte	AB	6%	OR	0.2 mg/mL[a]	Physically compatible for 4 hr at 23 °C	2339	C
Hydrocortisone sodium succinate	AB	1 mg/mL[a]	OR	0.1 mg/mL[a]	Physically compatible for 24 hr at 28 °C	1337	C
Hydromorphone HCl	KN	1 mg/mL	OR	1 mg/mL	Visually compatible for 4 hr at 27 °C	2062	C
Isoproterenol HCl	ES	4 mcg/mL[a]	OR	0.1 mg/mL[a]	Physically compatible for 24 hr at 28 °C	1337	C
Labetalol HCl	AH	2 mg/mL[a]	OR	1 mg/mL	Visually compatible for 4 hr at 27 °C	2062	C
Linezolid	PHU	2 mg/mL	OR	1 mg/mL	Physically compatible for 4 hr at 23 °C	2264	C
Lorazepam	WY	0.5 mg/mL[a]	OR	0.1 mg/mL[a]	Physically compatible for 24 hr at 28 °C	1337	C
	WY	0.33 mg/mL[a]	OR	4 mg/mL	Visually compatible for 24 hr at 22 °C	1855	C
	WY	0.5 mg/mL[a]	OR	1 mg/mL	Visually compatible for 4 hr at 27 °C	2062	C
Micafungin sodium	ASP	1.5 mg/mL[b]	BED	1 mg/mL	White precipitate forms immediately	2683	I
Midazolam HCl	RC	0.05 mg/mL[a]	OR	0.1 mg/mL[a]	Physically compatible for 24 hr at 28 °C	1337	C
	RC	5 mg/mL	OR	4 mg/mL	Visually compatible for 24 hr at 22 °C	1855	C
	RC	2 mg/mL[a]	OR	1 mg/mL	Visually compatible for 4 hr at 27 °C	2062	C
Milrinone lactate	SW	0.2 mg/mL[a]	OR	1 mg/mL	Visually compatible for 4 hr at 27 °C	2062	C
	SW	0.4 mg/mL[a]	OR	1 mg/mL	Visually compatible. Little loss of either drug in 4 hr at 23 °C	2214	C
Morphine sulfate	WY	1 mg/mL[a]	OR	0.1 mg/mL[a]	Physically compatible for 24 hr at 28 °C	1337	C
	SCN	2 mg/mL[a]	OR	1 mg/mL	Visually compatible for 4 hr at 27 °C	2062	C
Nicardipine HCl	WY	1 mg/mL[a]	OR	1 mg/mL	Visually compatible for 4 hr at 27 °C	2062	C
Nitroglycerin	SO	0.4 mg/mL[a]	OR	0.1 mg/mL[a]	Physically compatible for 24 hr at 28 °C	1337	C
	AB	0.4 mg/mL[a]	OR	1 mg/mL	Visually compatible for 4 hr at 27 °C	2062	C
Norepinephrine bitartrate	AB	0.128 mg/mL[a]	OR	1 mg/mL	Visually compatible for 4 hr at 27 °C	2062	C
Palonosetron HCl	MGI	50 mcg/mL	BED	1 mg/mL	Physically compatible and no loss of either drug in 4 hr at room temperature	2764	C
Propofol	ZEN	10 mg/mL	OR	1 mg/mL	Physically compatible for 1 hr at 23 °C	2066	C
Ranitidine HCl	GL	0.5 mg/mL[a]	OR	0.1 mg/mL[a]	Physically compatible for 24 hr at 28 °C	1337	C
	GL	1 mg/mL[a]	OR	1 mg/mL	Visually compatible for 4 hr at 27 °C	2062	C
Sodium nitroprusside	ES	0.2 mg/mL[a]	OR	0.1 mg/mL[a]	Physically compatible for 24 hr at 28 °C	1337	C
TPN #189[c]			OR	2 mg/mL[b]	Visually compatible for 24 hr at 22 °C	1767	C
Trimethoprim–sulfamethoxazole	ES	0.64 + 3.2 mg/mL[a]	OR	0.1 mg/mL[a]	Physically compatible for 24 hr at 28 °C	1337	C
Vancomycin HCl	ES	5 mg/mL[a]	OR	0.1 mg/mL[a]	Physically compatible for 24 hr at 28 °C	1337	C

[a]Tested in dextrose 5%.

[b]Tested in sodium chloride 0.9%.

[c]Refer to Appendix I for the composition of parenteral nutrition solutions. TPN indicates a 2-in-1 admixture.

[d]Tested in a 1:1 mixture of dextrose 5% and TPN #274 (see Appendix I).

[e]Tested in either dextrose 5% or in sodium chloride 0.9%, but the report did not specify which solution.

[f]Tested in a 1:1 mixture of (1) dextrose 5% and dextrose 5% in sodium chloride 0.45% with and without potassium chloride 20 mEq/L and also in (2) dextrose 10% in sodium chloride 0.45% with and without potassium chloride 20 mEq/L.

VERAPAMIL HYDROCHLORIDE
AHFS 24:28.92

Products — Verapamil hydrochloride is available in single-dose containers including 2-mL ampuls, vials, and syringes and in 4-mL vials and syringes. Each milliliter contains verapamil hydrochloride 2.5 mg with sodium chloride 8.5 mg in water for injection. Hydrochloric acid may have been used to adjust pH during manufacture. (1)

pH — From 4 to 6.5. (1)

Osmolality — The osmolality of verapamil hydrochloride 2.5 mg/mL was determined to be 290 mOsm/kg. (1233)

Administration — Verapamil hydrochloride is administered slowly intravenously. Direct intravenous injection should be performed over at least two minutes and at least three minutes in older patients. (1; 4) Intravenous infusion has also been performed. (4)

Stability — Verapamil hydrochloride should be stored at controlled room temperature and protected from light. (1) Freezing should be avoided. (4) It is physically compatible in solution over a pH range of 3 to 6 but may precipitate in solutions having a pH greater than 6 (1; 4) or 7. (1384)

Verapamil hydrochloride under simulated summer conditions in paramedic vehicles was exposed to temperatures ranging from 26 to 38 °C over four weeks. Analysis found no loss of the drug under these conditions. (2562)

Compatibility Information

Solution Compatibility

Verapamil HCl

Solution	Mfr	Mfr	Conc/L	Remarks	Ref	C/I
Dextrose 5% in Ringer's injection	MG	KN	40 mg	Physically compatible and chemically stable for 48 hr at 25 °C protected from light	548	C
Dextrose 5% in Ringer's injection, lactated	MG	KN	40 mg	Physically compatible and chemically stable for 24 hr at 25 °C protected from light	548	C
Dextrose 5% in sodium chloride 0.45%	MG	KN	40 mg	Physically compatible and chemically stable for 24 hr at 25 °C protected from light	548	C
Dextrose 5% in sodium chloride 0.9%	MG	KN	40 mg	Physically compatible and chemically stable for 24 hr at 25 °C protected from light	548	C
Dextrose 5%	CU	KN	40 mg	Physically compatible and chemically stable for 48 hr at 25 °C protected from light	548	C
	MG[a]	KN	40 mg	Physically compatible and chemically stable for 24 hr at 25 °C protected from light	548	C
	TR[b]	KN	40 mg	Physically compatible and chemically stable for 24 hr at 25 °C protected from light	548	C
	TR[b]	KN	160 mg	Physically compatible. No loss in 7 days at 24 °C	811	C
	AB	KN	100 and 400 mg	Physically compatible. No loss in 24 hr at 24 °C under fluorescent light	1198	C
Ringer's injection	MG	KN	40 mg	Physically compatible and chemically stable for 24 hr at 25 °C protected from light	548	C
Ringer's injection, lactated	MG	KN	40 mg	Physically compatible and chemically stable for 24 hr at 25 °C protected from light	548	C
Sodium chloride 0.45%	MG	KN	40 mg	Physically compatible and chemically stable for 24 hr at 25 °C protected from light	548	C
		LY	1.25 and 2 g	Physically compatible with no drug loss in 4 hr at 22 °C	1419	C
Sodium chloride 0.9%	CU	KN	40 mg	Physically compatible and chemically stable for 48 hr at 25 °C protected from light	548	C
	MG[a]	KN	40 mg	Physically compatible and chemically stable for 24 hr at 25 °C protected from light	548	C
	TR[b]	KN	40 mg	Physically compatible and chemically stable for 24 hr at 25 °C protected from light	548	C
	TR[b]	KN	160 mg	Physically compatible. Little loss in 7 days at 24 °C	811	C

Solution Compatibility (Cont.)

Verapamil HCl

Solution	Mfr	Mfr	Conc/L	Remarks	Ref	C/I
Sodium lactate ⅙ M	MG	KN	40 mg	Physically compatible and chemically stable for 48 hr at 25 °C protected from light	548	C

[a]Tested in polyolefin containers.
[b]Tested in PVC containers.

Additive Compatibility

Verapamil HCl

Drug	Mfr	Conc/L	Mfr	Conc/L	Test Soln	Remarks	Ref	C/I
Albumin human	ARC	25 g	KN	80 mg	D5W, NS	Cloudiness develops within 8 hr	764	I
Amikacin sulfate	BR	2 g	KN	80 mg	D5W, NS	Physically compatible for 24 hr	764	C
Aminophylline	SE	1 g	KN	80 mg	D5W, NS	Transient precipitate clears rapidly, then clear for 48 hr	739	?
	SE	1 g	KN	400 mg	D5W	Visible turbidity forms immediately. Filtration removes all verapamil	1198	I
	SE	1 g	KN	100 mg	D5W	Visually clear, but precipitate found by microscopic examination. Filtration removes all verapamil	1198	I
Amiodarone HCl	LZ	1.8 g	KN	50 mg	D5W, NS[a]	Physically compatible. 8% or less amiodarone loss in 24 hr at 24 °C in light	1031	C
Amphotericin B	SQ	100 mg	KN	80 mg	D5W	Physically incompatible after 8 hr	764	I
	SQ	100 mg	KN	80 mg	NS	Immediate physical incompatibility	764	I
Ampicillin sodium	BR	4 g	KN	80 mg	D5W, NS	Physically compatible for 24 hr	764	C
	WY	40 g	SE	[b]	D5W, NS	Cloudy solution clears with agitation	1166	?
Ascorbic acid	LI	1 g	KN	80 mg	D5W, NS	Physically compatible for 24 hr	764	C
Atropine sulfate	IX	0.8 mg	KN	80 mg	D5W, NS	Physically compatible for 24 hr	764	C
Calcium chloride	ES	2 g	KN	80 mg	D5W, NS	Physically compatible for 24 hr	764	C
Calcium gluconate	IX	2 g	KN	80 mg	D5W, NS	Physically compatible for 48 hr	739	C
Cefazolin sodium	SKF	2 g	KN	80 mg	D5W, NS	Physically compatible for 24 hr	764	C
Cefotaxime sodium	HO	4 g	KN	80 mg	D5W, NS	Physically compatible for 24 hr	764	C
Cefoxitin sodium	MSD	4 g	KN	80 mg	D5W, NS	Physically compatible for 24 hr	764	C
Chloramphenicol sodium succinate	PD	2 g	KN	80 mg	D5W, NS	Physically compatible for 24 hr	764	C
Clindamycin phosphate	UP	1.2 g	KN	80 mg	D5W, NS	Physically compatible for 24 hr	764	C
Dexamethasone sodium phosphate	MSD	40 mg	KN	80 mg	D5W, NS	Physically compatible for 24 hr	764	C
Dextran 40	TR	10%	KN	80 mg	NS	Physically compatible for 24 hr	764	C
Diazepam	RC	20 mg	KN	80 mg	D5W, NS	Physically compatible for 24 hr	764	C
Digoxin	BW	2 mg	KN	80 mg	D5W, NS	Physically compatible for 48 hr	739	C
Dobutamine HCl	LI	500 mg	KN	80 mg	D5W, NS	Slight pink color develops after 24 hr because of dobutamine oxidation	764	I
	LI	250 mg	KN	160 mg	D5W	No loss of either drug in 48 hr at 24 °C or 7 days at 5 °C. Transient pink color	811	C

Additive Compatibility (Cont.)

Verapamil HCl

Drug	Mfr	Conc/L	Mfr	Conc/L	Test Soln	Remarks	Ref	C/I
	LI	250 mg	KN	160 mg	NS	Pink color and no verapamil and 3% dobutamine loss in 48 hr at 24 °C. At 5 °C, no loss of either drug in 7 days	811	C
	LI	1 g	KN	1.25 g	D5W, NS	Physically compatible for 24 hr at 21 °C	812	C
Dopamine HCl	ES	400 mg	KN	80 mg	D5W, NS	Physically compatible for 24 hr	764	C
Epinephrine HCl	PD	2 mg	KN	80 mg	D5W, NS	Physically compatible for 24 hr	764	C
Erythromycin lactobionate	AB	2 g	KN	80 mg	D5W, NS	Physically compatible for 24 hr	764	C
Floxacillin sodium	BE	20 g	AB	500 mg	NS	Haze and precipitate form in 24 hr at 30 °C. No change at 15 °C	1479	I
Furosemide	HO	200 mg	KN	80 mg	D5W, NS	Physically compatible for 24 hr	764	C
	HO	1 g	AB	500 mg	NS	Slight precipitate forms but dissipates	1479	?
Gentamicin sulfate	SC	160 mg	KN	80 mg	D5W, NS	Physically compatible for 24 hr	764	C
Heparin sodium	ES	20,000 units	KN	80 mg	D5W, NS	Physically compatible for 24 hr	764	C
Hydralazine HCl	CI	40 mg	KN	80 mg	D5W, NS	Yellow discoloration	764	I
Hydrocortisone sodium succinate	UP	200 mg	KN	80 mg	D5W, NS	Physically compatible for 24 hr	764	C
Hydromorphone HCl	KN	16 mg	KN	80 mg	D5W, NS	Physically compatible for 24 hr	764	C
Isoproterenol HCl	BN	10 mg	KN	80 mg	D5W, NS	Physically compatible for 24 hr	764	C
Lidocaine HCl	IMS	2 g	KN	80 mg	D5W, NS	Physically compatible for 48 hr	739	C
Magnesium sulfate	IX	10 g	KN	80 mg	D5W, NS	Physically compatible for 24 hr	764	C
Mannitol	IX	25 g	KN	80 mg	D5W, NS	Physically compatible for 24 hr	764	C
Meperidine HCl	WI	150 mg	KN	80 mg	D5W, NS	Physically compatible for 24 hr	764	C
Methyldopate HCl	MSD	500 mg	KN	80 mg	D5W, NS	Physically compatible for 24 hr	764	C
Methylprednisolone sodium succinate	UP	250 mg	KN	80 mg	D5W, NS	Physically compatible for 24 hr	764	C
Metoclopramide HCl	RB	20 mg	KN	80 mg	D5W, NS	Physically compatible for 24 hr	764	C
Morphine sulfate	KN	30 mg	KN	80 mg	D5W, NS	Physically compatible for 24 hr	764	C
Multivitamins	USV	10 mL	KN	80 mg	D5W, NS	Physically compatible for 24 hr	764	C
Nafcillin sodium	WY	4 g	KN	80 mg	D5W, NS	Physically compatible for 24 hr	764	C
	WY	40 g	SE	b	D5W, NS	Cloudy solution clears with agitation	1166	?
Naloxone HCl	EN	0.8 mg	KN	80 mg	D5W, NS	Physically compatible for 24 hr	764	C
Nitroglycerin	ACC	100 mg	KN	80 mg	D5W, NS	Physically compatible for 24 hr	764	C
Norepinephrine bitartrate	BN	8 mg	KN	80 mg	D5W, NS	Physically compatible for 24 hr	764	C
Oxacillin sodium	BR	4 g	KN	80 mg	D5W, NS	Physically compatible for 24 hr	764	C
	BR	40 g	SE	b	D5W, NS	Cloudy solution clears with agitation	1166	?
Oxytocin	SZ	40 units	KN	80 mg	D5W, NS	Physically compatible for 24 hr	764	C
Pancuronium bromide	OR	8 mg	KN	80 mg	D5W, NS	Physically compatible for 24 hr	764	C
Penicillin G potassium	SQ	10 million units	KN	80 mg	D5W, NS	Physically compatible for 24 hr	764	C
	PD	62.5 g	SE	b	D5W, NS	Physically compatible for 24 hr at 21 °C under fluorescent light	1166	C

Additive Compatibility (Cont.)

Verapamil HCl

Drug	Mfr	Conc/L	Mfr	Conc/L	Test Soln	Remarks	Ref	C/I
Penicillin G sodium	SQ	10 million units	KN	80 mg	D5W, NS	Physically compatible for 24 hr	764	C
Pentobarbital sodium	AB	200 mg	KN	80 mg	D5W, NS	Physically compatible for 24 hr	764	C
Phenobarbital sodium	ES	260 mg	KN	80 mg	D5W, NS	Physically compatible for 24 hr	764	C
Phentolamine mesylate	RC	10 mg	KN	80 mg	D5W, NS	Physically compatible for 24 hr	764	C
Phenytoin sodium	PD	500 mg	KN	80 mg	D5W, NS	Physically compatible for 48 hr	739	C
Potassium chloride	TR	80 mEq	KN	80 mg	D5W, NS	Physically compatible for 24 hr	764	C
Potassium phosphates	AB	88 mEq	KN	80 mg	D5W, NS	Physically compatible for 24 hr	764	C
Procainamide HCl	SQ	2 g	KN	80 mg	D5W, NS	Physically compatible for 48 hr	739	C
Propranolol HCl	AY	4 mg	KN	80 mg	D5W, NS	Physically compatible for 24 hr	764	C
Protamine sulfate	LI	100 mg	KN	80 mg	D5W, NS	Physically compatible for 24 hr	764	C
Quinidine gluconate	LI	800 mg	KN	80 mg	D5W, NS	Physically compatible for 48 hr	739	C
Sodium bicarbonate	BR	89.2 mEq	KN	80 mg	D5W, NS	Physically compatible for 24 hr	764	C
Sodium nitroprusside	RC	100 mg	KN	80 mg	D5W, NS	Physically compatible for 24 hr	764	C
Theophylline	AB	400 mg and 4 g	KN	100 and 400 mg	D5W	Physically compatible. Little loss of either drug in 24 hr at 24 °C in light	1172	C
Tobramycin sulfate	LI	160 mg	KN	80 mg	D5W, NS	Physically compatible for 24 hr	764	C
Trimethoprim–sulfamethoxazole	BW	160 + 800 mg	KN	80 mg	D5W, NS	Transient precipitate	764	I
Vancomycin HCl	LI	1 g	KN	80 mg	D5W, NS	Physically compatible for 24 hr	764	C
Vasopressin	PD	40 units	KN	80 mg	D5W, NS	Physically compatible for 24 hr	764	C

[a]Tested in both polyolefin and PVC containers.
[b]Final concentration unspecified.

Drugs in Syringe Compatibility

Verapamil HCl

Drug (in syringe)	Mfr	Amt	Mfr	Amt	Remarks	Ref	C/I
Dimenhydrinate		10 mg/ 1 mL		2.5 mg/ 1 mL	Clear solution	2569	C
Heparin sodium		2500 units/ 1 mL	KN	5 mg/ 2 mL	Physically compatible for at least 5 min	1053	C
Milrinone lactate	WI	3.5 mg/ 3.5 mL	KN	10 mg/ 4 mL	Brought to 10-mL total volume with D5W. Physically compatible with no loss of either drug in 4 hr at 23 °C	1191	C
Pantoprazole sodium	[a]	4 mg/ 1 mL		2.5 mg/ 1 mL	Whitish precipitate	2574	I

[a]Test performed using the formulation WITHOUT edetate disodium.

Y-Site Injection Compatibility (1:1 Mixture)

Verapamil HCl

Drug	Mfr	Conc	Mfr	Conc	Remarks	Ref	C/I
Albumin human	HY	250 mg/mL[a]	LY	0.2 mg/mL[a]	Slight haze in 1 hr	1316	I
	HY	250 mg/mL[b]	LY	0.2 mg/mL[b]	Slight haze in 3 hr	1316	I
Amphotericin B cholesteryl sulfate complex	SEQ	0.83 mg/mL[a]	AMR	2.5 mg/mL	Gross precipitate forms	2117	I
Ampicillin sodium	WY	40 mg/mL[c]	SE	2.5 mg/mL	White precipitate forms immediately. 91% of verapamil precipitated	1166	I
Argatroban	GSK	1 mg/mL[b]	AMR	2.5 mg/mL	Visually compatible for 24 hr at 23 °C	2391	C
Bivalirudin	TMC	5 mg/mL[a]	AB	1.25 mg/mL[a]	Physically compatible for 4 hr at 23 °C	2373	C
	TMC	5 mg/mL[a,b]	AMR	2.5 mg/mL	Visually compatible for 6 hr at 23 °C	2680	C
Ciprofloxacin	MI	2 mg/mL[c]	KN	2.5 mg/mL	Visually compatible for 24 hr at 24 °C	1655	C
Clarithromycin	AB	4 mg/mL[a]	BKN	2.5 mg/mL	Visually compatible for 72 hr at both 30 and 17 °C	2174	C
Clonidine HCl	BI	18 mcg/mL[b]	AB	2.5 mg/mL	Visually compatible	2642	C
Dexmedetomidine HCl	AB	4 mcg/mL[b]	AB	1.25 mg/mL[b]	Physically compatible for 4 hr at 23 °C	2383	C
Dobutamine HCl	LI	4 mg/mL[c]	LY	0.2 mg/mL[c]	Physically compatible for 3 hr	1316	C
Dopamine HCl				e	Physically compatible	840	C
Famotidine	MSD	0.2 mg/mL[a]	KN	0.1 mg/mL[a]	Physically compatible for 4 hr at 25 °C	1188	C
Fenoldopam mesylate	AB	80 mcg/mL[b]	AB	1.25 mg/mL[b]	Physically compatible for 4 hr at 23 °C	2467	C
Hetastarch in lactated electrolyte	AB	6%	AMR	1.25 mg/mL[a]	Physically compatible for 4 hr at 23 °C	2339	C
Hydralazine HCl	SO	1 mg/mL[c]	LY	0.2 mg/mL[c]	Physically compatible for 3 hr	1316	C
Linezolid	PHU	2 mg/mL	AB	2.5 mg/mL	Physically compatible for 4 hr at 23 °C	2264	C
Meperidine HCl	AB	10 mg/mL	DU	2.5 mg/mL	Physically compatible for 4 hr at 25 °C	1397	C
Milrinone lactate	WI	200 mcg/mL[a]	KN	2.5 mg/mL[a]	Physically compatible with no loss of either drug in 4 hr at 23 °C	1191	C
Nafcillin sodium				f	White milky precipitate forms immediately	840; 1303	I
	WY	40 mg/mL[c]	SE	2.5 mg/mL	White precipitate forms immediately. 20% of verapamil precipitated	1166	I
Nesiritide	SCI	50 mcg/mL[a,b]		2.5 mg/mL	Physically compatible for 4 hr	2625	C
Oxacillin sodium	BR	40 mg/mL[c]	SE	2.5 mg/mL	White precipitate forms immediately. 39% of verapamil precipitated	1166	I
Oxaliplatin	SS	0.5 mg/mL[a]	AB	1.25 mg/mL[a]	Physically compatible for 4 hr at 23 °C	2566	C
Penicillin G potassium	PD	62.5 mg/mL[c]	SE	2.5 mg/mL	Physically compatible for 15 min at 21 °C	1166	C
Propofol	ZEN	10 mg/mL	AMR	2.5 mg/mL	Emulsion broke and oiled out	1916	I
Sodium bicarbonate		88 mEq/L[d]	SE	5 mg/2 mL	Crystalline precipitate forms when verapamil injected into infusion line	839	I

[a]*Tested in dextrose 5%.*
[b]*Tested in sodium chloride 0.9%.*
[c]*Tested in both dextrose 5% and sodium chloride 0.9%.*
[d]*Tested in sodium chloride 0.45%.*
[e]*Injected into a line being used to infuse dopamine hydrochloride in dextrose 5% in sodium chloride 0.3% with potassium chloride 20 mEq.*
[f]*Injected into a line being used to infuse nafcillin sodium.*

VINBLASTINE SULFATE
AHFS 10:00

Products — Vinblastine sulfate is available in 10-mL vials containing 10 mg of lyophilized drug without excipients. It should be reconstituted with 10 mL of sodium chloride 0.9% or bacteriostatic sodium chloride 0.9% (preserved with benzyl alcohol) to yield a 1-mg/mL solution. (1)

Vinblastine sulfate is also available as a 1-mg/mL solution with benzyl alcohol 0.9% in 10-mL vials. (1; 4)

pH — The pH of the reconstituted lyophilized product is 3.5 to 5. (1) The pH of the vinblastine sulfate injection is 3 to 5.5. (4)

Administration — Vinblastine sulfate is administered intravenously only. It should not be given by any other route. A sticker is provided in the vinblastine sulfate package that must be affixed directly to the container of the individual dose that states (1):

Fatal if given intrathecally. For intravenous use only.

In addition, the container holding an individual dose must be enclosed in an overwrap which is labeled (1):

Do not remove covering until moment of injection.
Fatal if given intrathecally. For intravenous use only.

The drug may be administered over one minute directly into a vein or into the tubing of a running infusion solution. Generally, dilution of vinblastine sulfate in larger amounts of intravenous fluid and administration over longer time periods are not recommended. Extravasation should be avoided. (1; 4)

In the event of spills or leaks, sodium hypochlorite 5% (household bleach) has been used to inactivate vinblastine sulfate. (1200)

Stability — The vials should be refrigerated to ensure extended stability. (1) Room temperature stability of intact vials has been variously reported for the Lilly product to be at least one month (853) and only 14 days. (1433) The Lyphomed product has been reported to be stable for up to three months (1181) and for less than two months. (1433) The solution reconstituted with bacteriostatic sodium chloride injection is stable under refrigeration for 28 days. If reconstituted with unpreserved sodium chloride injection, any remaining unused drug should be discarded immediately. (1)

Vinblastine sulfate 0.015 and 0.5 mg/mL in sodium chloride 0.9% did not inhibit the growth of deliberately inoculated *Staphylococcus epidermidis* (10^6 to 10^7 CFU/mL) during 21 days at 35 °C (representing near body temperature). (1659)

Immersion of a needle with an aluminum component in vinblastine sulfate 1 mg/mL resulted in no visually apparent reaction after seven days at 24 °C. (988)

pH Effects — Maximum stability for vinblastine sulfate in aqueous solutions was determined to be pH 2 to 4. Vinblastine sulfate in solution at pH 3 retained 90% after 39 days at 20 °C. (1307)

Vinblastine sulfate in solutions having a pH above 6 may form a precipitate of vinblastine base. (1369)

Freezing Solutions — Vinblastine sulfate (Lilly) 20 mcg/mL in dextrose 5%, Ringer's injection, lactated, and sodium chloride 0.9% underwent no degradation after four weeks when frozen at −20 °C. (1195)

Light Effects — It is recommended that vinblastine sulfate, both in the dry state and in solution, be protected from light. (4)

The effects of light exposure on a 1.197-mg/mL vinblastine sulfate solution in sterile water for injection was studied. Samples at 25 °C were exposed to indirect incandescent (not fluorescent) light intermittently for 12 hours each day; another group was exposed to direct incandescent light intermittently for 12 hours daily with at least two additional hours of exposure to sunlight. A third group of samples at 30 °C were exposed to continuous direct incandescent light. Both groups of samples exposed directly to light showed substantial losses of vinblastine sulfate. Samples exposed to continuous direct light sustained a 10% loss in about one day and a 71% loss in 14 days. Samples intermittently exposed to direct light and sunlight sustained a 10% loss in eight days and a 23% loss in 15 days. However, samples exposed to intermittent indirect light showed no drug loss in 70 days. (1306)

Under 6% vinblastine loss occurred in 48 hours from a 3-mcg/mL solution in sodium chloride 0.9% contained as a static solution in polybutadiene tubing when exposed to normal mixed daylight and fluorescent light. It was concluded that photodegradation is not a problem with vinblastine sulfate. (1378)

Syringes — Vinblastine sulfate (David Bull Laboratories) 1 mg/mL in polypropylene syringes was stable for 31 days at 8 °C and for at least 23 days at 21 °C in the dark; little or no loss occurred. (1566)

Vinblastine sulfate (Lilly) 1 mg/mL in sodium chloride 0.9% was packaged in polypropylene syringes (Plastipak, Becton Dickinson) and stored at 25 °C protected from light. No vinblastine sulfate loss was found after storage for 30 days. (2155)

Elastomeric Reservoir Pumps — Vinblastine sulfate 0.2 mg/mL in both dextrose 5% and sodium chloride 0.9% was evaluated for binding potential to natural rubber elastomeric reservoirs (Baxter). Less than 1% binding was found after storage for two weeks at 35 °C with gentle agitation. (2014)

Implantable Pumps — Vinblastine sulfate (Lilly) 1 mg/mL in bacteriostatic sodium chloride 0.9% was evaluated for stability in an implantable pump (Infusaid model 400). In this in vitro assessment, a 24% vinblastine loss occurred in 24 hours at 37 °C with mild agitation. In 12 days, the loss totaled 48%. In comparison, control solutions in glass vials had no drug loss in 24 hours and a 20% loss in 12 days at 37 °C. The authors believed that this indicated an interaction of vinblastine with some component of the Infusaid model 400, rendering it unsuitable for administration with this infusion device. (767)

Sorption — The stability of vinblastine sulfate (Lilly) 3 mcg/mL in methacrylate butadiene styrene (Avon A2001 Sureset) and cellulose propionate (Avon A200 standard and A2000 Amberset) when exposed to normal mixed daylight and fluorescent light for up to 48 hours was evaluated. A maximum vinblastine loss of about 5% resulted in the Sureset, with as little as a 2.25% loss occurring with foil wrapping. However, significant losses occurred in both cellulose propionate burettes in 24 hours, and losses of 15 to 20% occurred in 48 hours. The vinblastine sulfate solution in the polybutadiene tubing of the Sureset showed no more than a 6% drug loss with or without light protection. However, in the PVC tubing of the standard or Amberset, losses were significant within four hours; at 48 hours, losses were 42 to 44%. (1378)

Vinblastine sulfate (Lilly) 10 mg/250 mL in dextrose 5% or sodium chloride 0.9%, in PVC bags at 22 °C with protection from light, was infused over two hours at 2.08 mL/min through PVC sets. No loss due to sorption was found. (1631)

Vinblastine sulfate (Lederle) 250 mcg/mL in sodium chloride 0.9% exhibited no loss due to sorption to PVC and polyethylene administration lines during simulated infusions at 0.875 mL/hr for 2.5 hours via a syringe pump. (1795)

Filtration — Vinblastine sulfate (Lilly) 10 mg/50 mL in dextrose 5% and sodium chloride 0.9%, filtered at a rate of about 3 mL/min through a 0.22-μm cellulose ester membrane filter (Ivex-2), showed no significant reduction due to binding to the filter. (533)

Vinblastine sulfate 10 to 300 mcg/mL exhibited no loss due to sorption to either cellulose nitrate/cellulose acetate ester (Millex OR) or Teflon (Millex FG) filters. (1415; 1416)

Vinblastine sulfate (Lederle) 250 mcg/mL in sodium chloride 0.9% exhibited no loss due to sorption to cellulose acetate (Minisart 45, Sartorius) and polysulfone (Acrodisc 45, Gelman) filters. However, a

10 to 20% loss due to sorption occurred during the first 30 to 60 minutes of infusion through nylon filters (Nylaflo, Gelman, and Utipore, Pall). About a 30% loss was found during the first hour using a positively-charged nylon filter (Posidyne ELD96, Pall). The delivered concentrations gradually returned to the full concentrations within 2 to 2.5 hours. (1795)

Central Venous Catheter — Vinblastine sulfate (Lilly) 0.12 mg/mL in dextrose 5% was found to be compatible with the ARROWg+ard Blue Plus (Arrow International) chlorhexidine-bearing triple-lumen central catheter. Essentially complete delivery of the drug was found with little or no drug loss occurring. Furthermore, chlorhexidine delivered from the catheter remained at trace amounts with no substantial increase due to the delivery of the drug through the catheter. (2335)

Compatibility Information

Solution Compatibility

Vinblastine sulfate

Solution	Mfr	Mfr	Conc/L	Remarks	Ref	C/I
Dextrose 5%	TR[a]	LI	170 mg	Under 10% loss in 24 hr at room temperature	519	C
		LI	20 mg	Physically compatible with little loss in 21 days at 4 and 25 °C in the dark	1195	C
	[b]	LI	100 mg	8% loss in 7 days at 4 °C protected from light	1631	C
	MG[c]		170 mg	Under 10% loss in 24 hr at room temperature exposed to light	1658	C
Ringer's injection, lactated		LI	20 mg	Physically compatible with 2 to 3% drug loss in 21 days at 4 and 25 °C in the dark	1195	C
Sodium chloride 0.9%		LI	20 mg	Physically compatible with little loss in 21 days at 4 and 25 °C in the dark	1195	C
	[b]	LI	100 mg	No loss in 7 days at 4 °C protected from light	1631	C
	[d]		50 mg	5% loss at 23 °C and 3% loss at 4 °C in 21 days protected from light	2256	C

[a]*Tested in both glass and PVC containers.*
[b]*Tested in PVC containers.*
[c]*Tested in both glass and polyolefin containers.*
[d]*Tested in glass containers.*

Additive Compatibility

Vinblastine sulfate

Drug	Mfr	Conc/L	Mfr	Conc/L	Test Soln	Remarks	Ref	C/I
Bleomycin sulfate	BR	20 and 30 units	LI	10 and 100 mg	NS	Physically compatible and bleomycin activity retained for 1 week at 4 °C. Vinblastine not tested	763	C
Doxorubicin HCl	AD	500 mg	LI	75 mg	NS[a]	Physically compatible for 10 days at 8, 25, and 32 °C. Assays highly erratic	838	?
	AD	1.5 g	LI	150 mg	NS[a]	Physically compatible for 10 days at 8, 25, and 32 °C. Assays highly erratic	838	?

[a]*Tested in PVC containers.*

Drugs in Syringe Compatibility

Vinblastine sulfate

Drug (in syringe)	Mfr	Amt	Mfr	Amt	Remarks	Ref	C/I
Bleomycin sulfate		1.5 units/ 0.5 mL		0.5 mg/ 0.5 mL	Physically compatible for 5 min at room temperature followed by 8 min of centrifugation	980	C
Cisplatin		0.5 mg/ 0.5 mL		0.5 mg/ 0.5 mL	Physically compatible for 5 min at room temperature followed by 8 min of centrifugation	980	C
Cyclophosphamide		10 mg/ 0.5 mL		0.5 mg/ 0.5 mL	Physically compatible for 5 min at room temperature followed by 8 min of centrifugation	980	C
Doxorubicin HCl	AD	45 mg/ 22.5 mL	LI	4.5 mg/ 4.5 mL	Brought to 30-mL total volume with NS. Physically compatible for 10 days at 8, 25, and 32 °C. Assays highly erratic	838	?
	AD	15 mg/ 7.5 mL	LI	2.25 mg/ 2.25 mL	Brought to 30-mL total volume with NS. Physically compatible for 10 days at 8, 25, and 32 °C. Assays highly erratic	838	?
		1 mg/ 0.5 mL		0.5 mg/ 0.5 mL	Physically compatible for 5 min at room temperature followed by 8 min of centrifugation	980	C
Droperidol		1.25 mg/ 0.5 mL		0.5 mg/ 0.5 mL	Physically compatible for 5 min at room temperature followed by 8 min of centrifugation	980	C
Fluorouracil		25 mg/ 0.5 mL		0.5 mg/ 0.5 mL	Physically compatible for 5 min at room temperature followed by 8 min of centrifugation	980	C
Furosemide		5 mg/ 0.5 mL		0.5 mg/ 0.5 mL	Precipitates immediately	980	I
Heparin sodium		200 units/ 1 mL[a]	LI	1 mg/ 1 mL	Turbidity appears in 2 to 3 min	767	I
		500 units/ 0.5 mL		0.5 mg/ 0.5 mL	Physically compatible for 5 min at room temperature followed by 8 min of centrifugation	980	C
Leucovorin calcium		5 mg/ 0.5 mL		0.5 mg/ 0.5 mL	Physically compatible for 5 min at room temperature followed by 8 min of centrifugation	980	C
Methotrexate sodium		12.5 mg/ 0.5 mL		0.5 mg/ 0.5 mL	Physically compatible for 5 min at room temperature followed by 8 min of centrifugation	980	C
Metoclopramide HCl		2.5 mg/ 0.5 mL		0.5 mg/ 0.5 mL	Physically compatible for 5 min at room temperature followed by 8 min of centrifugation	980	C
Mitomycin		0.25 mg/ 0.5 mL		0.5 mg/ 0.5 mL	Physically compatible for 5 min at room temperature followed by 8 min of centrifugation	980	C
Vincristine sulfate		0.5 mg/ 0.5 mL		0.5 mg/ 0.5 mL	Physically compatible for 5 min at room temperature followed by 8 min of centrifugation	980	C

[a]*Tested in bacteriostatic sodium chloride 0.9%.*

Y-Site Injection Compatibility (1:1 Mixture)

Vinblastine sulfate

Drug	Mfr	Conc	Mfr	Conc	Remarks	Ref	C/I
Allopurinol sodium	BW	3 mg/mL[b]	LI	0.12 mg/mL[b]	Physically compatible for 4 hr at 22 °C	1686	C
Amifostine	USB	10 mg/mL[a]	LI	0.12 mg/mL[a]	Physically compatible for 4 hr at 23 °C	1845	C
Amphotericin B cholesteryl sulfate complex	SEQ	0.83 mg/mL[a]	FAU	0.12 mg/mL[a]	Physically compatible for 4 hr at 23 °C	2117	C
Aztreonam	SQ	40 mg/mL[a]	LI	0.12 mg/mL[a]	Physically compatible for 4 hr at 23 °C	1758	C

Y-Site Injection Compatibility (1:1 Mixture) (Cont.)

Vinblastine sulfate

Drug	Mfr	Conc	Mfr	Conc	Remarks	Ref	C/I
Bleomycin sulfate		3 units/mL		1 mg/mL	Drugs injected sequentially in Y-site with no flush. No precipitate seen	980	C
Cisplatin		1 mg/mL		1 mg/mL	Drugs injected sequentially in Y-site with no flush. No precipitate seen	980	C
Cyclophosphamide		20 mg/mL		1 mg/mL	Drugs injected sequentially in Y-site with no flush. No precipitate seen	980	C
Doxorubicin HCl		2 mg/mL		1 mg/mL	Drugs injected sequentially in Y-site with no flush. No precipitate seen	980	C
Doxorubicin HCl liposomal	SEQ	0.4 mg/mL[a]	FAU	0.12 mg/mL[a]	Physically compatible for 4 hr at 23 °C	2087	C
Droperidol		2.5 mg/mL		1 mg/mL	Drugs injected sequentially in Y-site with no flush. No precipitate seen	980	C
Etoposide phosphate	BR	5 mg/mL[a]	FAU	0.12 mg/mL[a]	Physically compatible for 4 hr at 23 °C	2218	C
Filgrastim	AMG	30 mcg/mL[a]	LI	0.12 mg/mL[a]	Physically compatible for 4 hr at 22 °C	1687	C
Fludarabine phosphate	BX	1 mg/mL[a]	LY	0.12 mg/mL[a]	Visually compatible for 4 hr at 22 °C	1439	C
Fluorouracil		50 mg/mL		1 mg/mL	Drugs injected sequentially in Y-site with no flush. No precipitate seen	980	C
Furosemide		10 mg/mL		1 mg/mL	Drugs injected sequentially in Y-site with no flush. Precipitates immediately	980	I
Gemcitabine HCl	LI	10 mg/mL[b]	FAU	0.12 mg/mL[b]	Physically compatible for 4 hr at 23 °C	2226	C
Granisetron HCl	SKB	0.05 mg/mL[a]	LI	0.12 mg/mL[a]	Physically compatible for 4 hr at 23 °C	2000	C
Heparin sodium		1000 units/mL		1 mg/mL	Drugs injected sequentially in Y-site with no flush. No precipitate seen	980	C
Leucovorin calcium		10 mg/mL		1 mg/mL	Drugs injected sequentially in Y-site with no flush. No precipitate seen	980	C
Melphalan HCl	BW	0.1 mg/mL[b]	LI	0.12 mg/mL[b]	Physically compatible for 3 hr at 22 °C	1557	C
Methotrexate sodium		25 mg/mL		1 mg/mL	Drugs injected sequentially in Y-site with no flush. No precipitate seen	980	C
Metoclopramide HCl		5 mg/mL		1 mg/mL	Drugs injected sequentially in Y-site with no flush. No precipitate seen	980	C
Mitomycin		0.5 mg/mL		1 mg/mL	Drugs injected sequentially in Y-site with no flush. No precipitate seen	980	C
Ondansetron HCl	GL	1 mg/mL[b]	LY	0.12 mg/mL[a]	Visually compatible for 4 hr at 22 °C	1365	C
Paclitaxel	NCI	1.2 mg/mL[a]	LI	0.12 mg/mL[b]	Physically compatible for 4 hr at 22 °C	1556	C
Pemetrexed disodium	LI	20 mg/mL[b]	APP	0.12 mg/mL[a]	Physically compatible for 4 hr at 23 °C	2564	C
Piperacillin sodium–tazobactam sodium	LE[d]	40 + 5 mg/mL[a]	LI	0.12 mg/mL[a]	Physically compatible for 4 hr at 22 °C	1688	C
Sargramostim	IMM	10 mcg/mL[b]	LY	0.12 mg/mL[b]	Visually compatible for 4 hr at 22 °C	1436	C
Teniposide	BR	0.1 mg/mL[a]	LI	0.12 mg/mL[a]	Physically compatible for 4 hr at 23 °C	1725	C
Thiotepa	IMM[c]	1 mg/mL[a]	LI	0.12 mg/mL[a]	Physically compatible for 4 hr at 23 °C	1861	C
Vincristine sulfate		1 mg/mL		1 mg/mL	Drugs injected sequentially in Y-site with no flush. No precipitate seen	980	C
Vinorelbine tartrate	BW	1 mg/mL[b]	LI	0.12 mg/mL[b]	Physically compatible for 4 hr at 22 °C	1558	C

[a]*Tested in dextrose 5%.*
[b]*Tested in sodium chloride 0.9%.*
[c]*Lyophilized formulation tested.*
[d]*Test performed using the formulation WITHOUT edetate disodium.*

VINCRISTINE SULFATE
AHFS 10:00

Products — Vincristine sulfate is available as a preservative-free solution in a 1-mg/mL concentration with mannitol 100 mg/mL and sulfuric acid or sodium hydroxide to adjust pH during manufacturing. The ready-to-use solution is available in 1- and 2-mL single-dose vials. (1; 4)

pH — The official pH range is 3.5 to 5.5. (17) A narrower range of pH 4.0 to 5.0 has been cited by a manufacturer. (1)

Administration — Vincristine sulfate is administered intravenously only. It should not be given by any other route. A sticker is provided in the vincristine sulfate package that must be affixed directly to the container of the individual dose that states (1):

> *Fatal if given intrathecally. For intravenous use only.*

In addition, the container holding an individual dose must be enclosed in an overwrap which is labeled (1):

> *Do not remove covering until moment of injection.*
> *Fatal if given intrathecally. For intravenous use only.*

The drug may be administered over one minute directly into a vein or into the tubing of a running infusion solution. (1; 4) It can also be diluted in dextrose 5% or sodium chloride 0.9% and given by intermittent or continuous intravenous infusion. (4) Extravasation should be avoided. (1; 4)

In the event of spills or leaks, sodium hypochlorite 5% (household bleach) has been used to inactivate vincristine sulfate. (1200)

Stability — The ready-to-use solution should be stored under refrigeration, kept upright, and protected from light. Unused drug solution should be discarded. (1) The pH range of maximum stability is 4 to 6. (1195) Precipitation may occur at alkaline pH values. (1369) Vincristine sulfate should not be added to solutions that would raise or lower the pH outside the 3.5 to 5.5 range. Only dextrose 5% and sodium chloride 0.9% are recommended. (1)

Admixtures containing doxorubicin hydrochloride, etoposide phosphate, and vincristine sulfate in a variety of concentration combinations in sodium chloride 0.9% were unable to pass the USP test for antimicrobial growth effectiveness. Mixtures of these drugs are not "self-preserving" and will permit microbial growth. (2343)

Immersion of a needle with an aluminum component in vincristine sulfate 1 mg/mL resulted in no visually apparent reaction after seven days at 24 °C. (988)

Freezing Solutions — Vincristine sulfate (Lilly) 20 mcg/mL in dextrose 5%, Ringer's injection, lactated, and sodium chloride 0.9% underwent no degradation after four weeks when frozen at −20 °C. (1195)

Syringes — Vincristine sulfate (Lilly) 0.5, 1, 2, and 3 mg diluted to 20 mL with sodium chloride 0.9% and packaged in 30-mL polypropylene syringes (Becton Dickinson) was stored for seven days at 4 °C followed by two days at 23 °C. All samples remained physically compatible with no increase in measured turbidity or particle content. No loss occurred after seven days at 4 °C and not more than 5% loss after two additional days at room temperature. (2350)

Sorption — Vincristine sulfate 2 mg/250 mL in dextrose 5% or sodium chloride 0.9%, in PVC bags at 22 °C with protection from light, was infused over two hours at 2.08 mL/min through PVC sets. No loss due to sorption was found. (1631)

Vincristine sulfate 25 mcg/mL in sodium chloride 0.9% exhibited no loss due to sorption to a polyethylene administration line (Vygon) during simulated infusions at 0.875 mL/hr for 2.5 hours via a syringe pump. However, about a 9% loss of delivered concentration due to sorption occurred during the first hour using a PVC administration line (Baxter). The delivered concentration returned to the full concentration within 1.5 hours. (1795)

Filtration — Vincristine sulfate (Lilly) 1 mg/50 mL in dextrose 5% and sodium chloride 0.9% was filtered at about 3 mL/min through a 0.22-μm cellulose ester membrane filter (Ivex-2). Losses of vincristine sulfate due to binding to the filters were noted in both solutions. In dextrose 5%, about 6.5% of the vincristine sulfate was bound; about 12% of the drug was lost from the sodium chloride 0.9% solution. (533)

In static equilibrium experiments, 100 mg of 0.22-μm cellulose ester membrane filter (Ivex-2) was soaked in 25 mL of vincristine sulfate (Lilly) 10 and 20 mcg/mL in both dextrose 5% and sodium chloride 0.9%. The higher concentration exhibited about 20 to 30% binding to the filter in 24 to 48 hours. The lower concentration had about 30 to 45% binding in the same period. (533)

A filter material specially treated with a proprietary agent was evaluated for a reduction in vincristine sulfate binding. Vincristine sulfate (Lilly) 1 mg/50 mL in dextrose 5% and sodium chloride 0.9% was run through an administration set with a treated 0.22-μm cellulose ester inline filter at a rate of 3 mL/min. Cumulative vincristine sulfate losses of about 1% occurred from both solutions compared to the much higher losses previously reported for untreated cellulose ester filter material. Furthermore, equilibrium binding studies showed five- and sevenfold reductions in binding from dextrose 5% and sodium chloride 0.9%, respectively. (904) All Abbott Ivex integral filter and extension sets use this treated filter material. (1074)

Vincristine sulfate 1.5 mg/3 mL was injected through a 0.2-μm nylon, air-eliminating, filter (Ultipor, Pall) to evaluate the effect of filtration on simulated intravenous push delivery. About 90% of the drug was delivered through the filter after flushing with 10 mL of sodium chloride 0.9%. (809)

Vincristine sulfate 10 to 200 mcg/mL exhibited a 10 to 15% loss due to sorption to both cellulose nitrate/cellulose acetate ester (Millex OR) and Teflon (Millex FG) filters. (1415; 1416)

Vincristine sulfate (David Bull Laboratories) 250 mcg/mL in sodium chloride 0.9% exhibited little loss due to sorption to cellulose acetate (Minisart 45, Sartorius) and polysulfone (Acrodisc 45, Gelman) filters. However, a 5 to 20% loss due to sorption occurred during the first 30 to 60 minutes of infusion through nylon filters (Nylaflo, Gelman, and Utipore, Pall). About a 20 to 25% loss was found during the first hour using a nylon filter (Posidyne ELD96, Pall). The delivered concentrations gradually returned to the full concentrations within 2 to 2.5 hours. (1795)

Central Venous Catheter — Vincristine sulfate (Lilly) 0.05 mg/mL in dextrose 5% was found to be compatible with the ARROWg+ard Blue Plus (Arrow International) chlorhexidine-bearing triple-lumen central catheter. Essentially complete delivery of the drug was found with little or no drug loss occurring. Furthermore, chlorhexidine delivered from the catheter remained at trace amounts with no substantial increase due to the delivery of the drug through the catheter. (2335)

Compatibility Information

Solution Compatibility

Vincristine sulfate

Solution	Mfr	Mfr	Conc/L	Remarks	Ref	C/I
Dextrose 5%	TR[a]	LI	16.7 mg	No loss in 24 hr at room temperature	806	C
		LI	20 mg	Physically compatible. 5% loss in 21 days at 4 and 25 °C in dark	1195	C
	[b]	LI	20 mg	Little loss in 7 days at 4 °C in dark	1631	C
	MG, TR[c]		20 mg	Under 10% loss in 24 hr at room temperature in light	1658	C
Ringer's injection, lactated		LI	20 mg	Physically compatible. Little loss in 21 days at 4 and 25 °C in dark	1195	C
Sodium chloride 0.9%		LI	20 mg	Physically compatible. Little loss in 21 days at 4 and 25 °C in dark	1195	C
	[b]	LI	20 mg	8% or less loss in 7 days at 4 °C in dark	1631	C
	BA[b]	LI	10, 20, 40, 60, 80, 120 mg	Physically compatible. No loss after 7 days at 4 °C followed by 2 days at 23 °C	2350	C

[a]*Tested in both glass and PVC containers.*
[b]*Tested in PVC containers.*
[c]*Tested in glass, polyolefin, and PVC containers.*

Additive Compatibility

Vincristine sulfate

Drug	Mfr	Conc/L	Mfr	Conc/L	Test Soln	Remarks	Ref	C/I
Bleomycin sulfate	BR	20 and 30 units	LI	50 and 100 mg	NS	Physically compatible and bleomycin activity retained for 1 week at 4 °C. Vincristine not tested	763	C
Cytarabine	UP	16 mg	LI	4 mg	D5W	Physically compatible. No alteration in UV spectra in 8 hr at room temperature	207	C
Doxorubicin HCl	FA	1.4 g	LI	33 mg	D5½S, NS	Visually compatible. Less than 10% loss of both drugs for 14 days at 25, 30, and 37 °C	1030	C
	FA	1.88 and 2.37 g	LI	50 mg	D5½S, NS	Visually compatible. Less than 10% loss of both drugs for 14 days at 25 and 30 °C. Up to 16% doxorubicin loss at 37 °C in 14 days	1030	C
	NYC	1.67 g	LI	36 mg	NS[a,b]	Visually compatible and both drugs stable for 7 days at 4 °C then 4 days at 37 °C	1874	C
	PHU	2 g	FAU	200 mg	W[c]	Physically compatible. No loss of either drug in 7 days at 37 °C. 4% loss of both drugs in 14 days at 4 °C	2288	C
	PHC	1.4 g	PHC	33 mg	D5½S	Physically compatible. Little loss of either drug in 14 days at 4 and 25 °C. 12% loss of both drugs at 37 °C	2674	C
	PHC	1.4 g	PHC	33 mg	NS	Physically compatible. Little loss of either drug in 14 days at 4 and 25 °C. 4% loss of both drugs at 37 °C	2674	C
	PHC	1.4 g	PHC	53 mg	D5½S	Physically compatible. Little loss of either drug in 14 days at 4 and 25 °C. 8% loss of both drugs at 37 °C	2674	C

Additive Compatibility (Cont.)

Vincristine sulfate

Drug	Mfr	Conc/L	Mfr	Conc/L	Test Soln	Remarks	Ref	C/I
	PHC	1.4 g	PHC	53 mg	NS	Physically compatible. Little loss of either drug in 14 days at 4 and 25 °C. 9% loss of both drugs at 37 °C	2674	C
Doxorubicin HCl with etoposide	PHU BMS	40 mg 200 mg	LI	1.6 mg	NS[d]	Visually compatible. All drugs stable for 72 hr at 30 °C in the dark	2239	C
Doxorubicin HCl with etoposide	PHU BMS	25 mg 125 mg	LI	1 mg	NS[d]	Visually compatible. All drugs stable for 96 hr at 24 °C in light or dark	2239	C
Doxorubicin HCl with etoposide	PHU BMS	35 mg 175 mg	LI	1.4 mg	NS[d]	Visually compatible. All drugs stable for 96 hr at 24 °C in light or dark	2239	C
Doxorubicin HCl with etoposide	PHU BMS	50 mg 250 mg	LI	2 mg	NS[d]	Visually compatible. All drugs stable for 48 hr at 24 °C in light or dark. Etoposide precipitate in 72 hr	2239	C
Doxorubicin HCl with etoposide	PHU BMS	70 mg 350 mg	LI	2.8 mg	NS[d]	Visually compatible. All drugs stable for 24 hr at 24 °C in light or dark. Etoposide precipitate in 36 hr	2239	C
Doxorubicin HCl with etoposide	PHU BMS	100 mg 500 mg	LI	4 mg	NS[d]	Etoposide precipitate formed in 12 hr at 24 °C in light or dark	2239	I
Doxorubicin HCl with etoposide phosphate	PHU BMS	120 mg 600 mg	LI	5 mg	NS[d]	Physically compatible. Little loss of any drug in 124 hr at 4 and 40 °C	2343	C
Doxorubicin HCl with etoposide phosphate	PHU BMS	240 mg 1.2 g	LI	10 mg	NS[d]	Physically compatible. Little loss of any drug in 124 hr at 4 and 40 °C	2343	C
Doxorubicin HCl with etoposide phosphate	PHU BMS	400 mg 2 g	LI	16 mg	NS[d]	Physically compatible. Under 4% loss of any drug in 124 hr at 4 and 40 °C	2343	C
Doxorubicin HCl with ondansetron HCl	AD GL	400 mg 480 mg	LI	14 mg	D5W[b]	Visually compatible. Under 10% loss of all drugs in 5 days at 4 °C then 24 hr at 30 °C	2092	C
Doxorubicin HCl with ondansetron HCl	AD GL	800 mg 960 mg	LI	28 mg	D5W[a]	Visually compatible. Under 10% loss of all drugs after 120 hr at 30 °C	2092	C
Etoposide with doxorubicin HCl	BMS PHU	200 mg 40 mg	LI	1.6 mg	NS[d]	Visually compatible. All drugs stable for 72 hr at 30 °C in the dark	2239	C
Etoposide with doxorubicin HCl	BMS PHU	125 mg 25 mg	LI	1 mg	NS[d]	Visually compatible. All drugs stable for 96 hr at 24 °C in light or dark	2239	C
Etoposide with doxorubicin HCl	BMS PHU	175 mg 35 mg	LI	1.4 mg	NS[d]	Visually compatible. All drugs stable for 96 hr at 24 °C in light or dark	2239	C
Etoposide with doxorubicin HCl	BMS PHU	250 mg 50 mg	LI	2 mg	NS[d]	Visually compatible. All drugs stable for 48 hr at 24 °C in light or dark. Etoposide precipitate in 72 hr	2239	C
Etoposide with doxorubicin HCl	BMS PHU	350 mg 70 mg	LI	2.8 mg	NS[d]	Visually compatible. All drugs stable for 24 hr at 24 °C in light or dark. Etoposide precipitate in 36 hr	2239	C
Etoposide with doxorubicin HCl	BMS PHU	500 mg 100 mg	LI	4 mg	NS[d]	Etoposide precipitate formed in 12 hr at 24 °C in light or dark	2239	I
Etoposide phosphate with doxorubicin HCl	BMS PHU	600 mg 120 mg	LI	5 mg	NS[d]	Physically compatible. Little loss of any drug in 124 hr at 4 and 40 °C	2343	C
Etoposide phosphate with doxorubicin HCl	BMS PHU	1.2 g 240 mg	LI	10 mg	NS[d]	Physically compatible. Little loss of any drug in 124 hr at 4 and 40 °C	2343	C
Etoposide phosphate with doxorubicin HCl	BMS PHU	2 g 400 mg	LI	16 mg	NS[d]	Physically compatible. Under 4% loss of any drug in 124 hr at 4 and 40 °C	2343	C
Fluorouracil	RC	10 mg	LI	4 mg	D5W	Physically compatible. No alteration in UV spectra in 8 hr at room temperature	207	C
Methotrexate sodium	LE	100 mg	LI	10 mg	D5W	Physically compatible	15	C

Additive Compatibility (Cont.)

Vincristine sulfate

Drug	Mfr	Conc/L	Mfr	Conc/L	Test Soln	Remarks	Ref	C/I
	LE	8 mg	LI	4 mg	D5W	Physically compatible. No change in UV spectra in 8 hr at room temperature	207	C
Ondansetron HCl with doxorubicin HCl	GL AD	480 mg 400 mg	LI	14 mg	D5W[b]	Visually compatible. Under 10% loss of all drugs in 5 days at 4 °C then 24 hr at 30 °C	2092	C
Ondansetron HCl with doxorubicin HCl	GL AD	960 mg 800 mg	LI	28 mg	D5W[a]	Visually compatible. Under 10% loss of all drugs after 120 hr at 30 °C	2092	C

[a]Tested in PVC containers.
[b]Tested in polyisoprene infusion pump reservoirs.
[c]Tested in PVC reservoirs for the Graseby 9000 ambulatory pumps.
[d]Tested in polyolefin-lined plastic bags.

Drugs in Syringe Compatibility

Vincristine sulfate

Drug (in syringe)	Mfr	Amt	Mfr	Amt	Remarks	Ref	C/I
Bleomycin sulfate		1.5 units/ 0.5 mL		0.5 mg/ 0.5 mL	Physically compatible for 5 min at room temperature followed by 8 min of centrifugation	980	C
Cisplatin		0.5 mg/ 0.5 mL		0.5 mg/ 0.5 mL	Physically compatible for 5 min at room temperature followed by 8 min of centrifugation	980	C
Cyclophosphamide		10 mg/ 0.5 mL		0.5 mg/ 0.5 mL	Physically compatible for 5 min at room temperature followed by 8 min of centrifugation	980	C
Doxapram HCl	RB	400 mg/ 20 mL		1 mg/ 10 mL	Physically compatible with 7% doxapram loss in 24 hr	1177	C
Doxorubicin HCl		1 mg/ 0.5 mL		0.5 mg/ 0.5 mL	Physically compatible for 5 min at room temperature followed by 8 min of centrifugation	980	C
Droperidol		1.25 mg/ 0.5 mL		0.5 mg/ 0.5 mL	Physically compatible for 5 min at room temperature followed by 8 min of centrifugation	980	C
Fluorouracil		25 mg/ 0.5 mL		0.5 mg/ 0.5 mL	Physically compatible for 5 min at room temperature followed by 8 min of centrifugation	980	C
Furosemide		5 mg/ 0.5 mL		0.5 mg/ 0.5 mL	Precipitates immediately	980	I
Heparin sodium		500 units/ 0.5 mL		0.5 mg/ 0.5 mL	Physically compatible for 5 min at room temperature followed by 8 min of centrifugation	980	C
Leucovorin calcium		5 mg/ 0.5 mL		0.5 mg/ 0.5 mL	Physically compatible for 5 min at room temperature followed by 8 min of centrifugation	980	C
Methotrexate sodium		12.5 mg/ 0.5 mL		0.5 mg/ 0.5 mL	Physically compatible for 5 min at room temperature followed by 8 min of centrifugation	980	C
Metoclopramide HCl		2.5 mg/ 0.5 mL		0.5 mg/ 0.5 mL	Physically compatible for 5 min at room temperature followed by 8 min of centrifugation	980	C
Mitomycin		0.25 mg/ 0.5 mL		0.5 mg/ 0.5 mL	Physically compatible for 5 min at room temperature followed by 8 min of centrifugation	980	C
Vinblastine sulfate		0.5 mg/ 0.5 mL		0.5 mg/ 0.5 mL	Physically compatible for 5 min at room temperature followed by 8 min of centrifugation	980	C

Y-Site Injection Compatibility (1:1 Mixture)

Vincristine sulfate

Drug	Mfr	Conc	Mfr	Conc	Remarks	Ref	C/I
Allopurinol sodium	BW	3 mg/mL[b]	LI	0.05 mg/mL[b]	Physically compatible for 4 hr at 22 °C	1686	C
Amifostine	USB	10 mg/mL[a]	LI	0.05 mg/mL[a]	Physically compatible for 4 hr at 23 °C	1845	C
Amphotericin B cholesteryl sulfate complex	SEQ	0.83 mg/mL[a]	FAU	0.05 mg/mL[a]	Physically compatible for 4 hr at 23 °C	2117	C
Anidulafungin	VIC	0.5 mg/mL[a]	FAU	50 mcg/mL[a]	Physically compatible for 4 hr at 23 °C	2617	C
Aztreonam	SQ	40 mg/mL[a]	LI	0.05 mg/mL[a]	Physically compatible for 4 hr at 23 °C	1758	C
Bleomycin sulfate		3 units/mL		1 mg/mL	Drugs injected sequentially in Y-site with no flush. No precipitate seen	980	C
Caspofungin acetate	ME	0.7 mg/mL[b]	MAY	0.05 mg/mL[b]	Physically compatible for 4 hr at room temperature	2758	C
Cisplatin		1 mg/mL		1 mg/mL	Drugs injected sequentially in Y-site with no flush. No precipitate seen	980	C
Cladribine	ORT	0.015[b] and 0.5[c] mg/mL	LI	0.05 mg/mL[b]	Physically compatible for 4 hr at 23 °C	1969	C
Cyclophosphamide		20 mg/mL		1 mg/mL	Drugs injected sequentially in Y-site with no flush. No precipitate seen	980	C
Doxorubicin HCl		2 mg/mL		1 mg/mL	Drugs injected sequentially in Y-site with no flush. No precipitate seen	980	C
Doxorubicin HCl liposomal	SEQ	0.4 mg/mL[a]	FAU	0.05 mg/mL[a]	Physically compatible for 4 hr at 23 °C	2087	C
Droperidol		2.5 mg/mL		1 mg/mL	Drugs injected sequentially in Y-site with no flush. No precipitate seen	980	C
Etoposide phosphate	BR	5 mg/mL[a]	FAU	0.05 mg/mL[a]	Physically compatible for 4 hr at 23 °C	2218	C
Filgrastim	AMG	30 mcg/mL[a]	LI	0.05 mg/mL[a]	Physically compatible for 4 hr at 22 °C	1687	C
Fludarabine phosphate	BX	1 mg/mL[a]	LY	1 mg/mL[a]	Visually compatible for 4 hr at 22 °C	1439	C
Fluorouracil		50 mg/mL		1 mg/mL	Drugs injected sequentially in Y-site with no flush. No precipitate seen	980	C
Furosemide		10 mg/mL		1 mg/mL	Drugs injected sequentially in Y-site with no flush. Precipitates immediately	980	I
Gemcitabine HCl	LI	10 mg/mL[b]	FAU	0.05 mg/mL[b]	Physically compatible for 4 hr at 23 °C	2226	C
Granisetron HCl	SKB	1 mg/mL	LI	0.01 and 0.34 mg/mL[b]	Physically compatible with little or no loss of either drug in 4 hr at 22 °C	1883	C
Heparin sodium		1000 units/mL		1 mg/mL	Drugs injected sequentially in Y-site with no flush. No precipitate seen	980	C
Idarubicin HCl	AD	1 mg/mL[b]	AD	1 mg/mL	Color changes immediately	1525	I
Leucovorin calcium		10 mg/mL		1 mg/mL	Drugs injected sequentially in Y-site with no flush. No precipitate seen	980	C
Linezolid	PHU	2 mg/mL	LI	0.05 mg/mL[a]	Physically compatible for 4 hr at 23 °C	2264	C
Melphalan HCl	BW	0.1 mg/mL[b]	LI	0.05 mg/mL[b]	Physically compatible for 3 hr at 22 °C	1557	C
Methotrexate sodium		25 mg/mL		1 mg/mL	Drugs injected sequentially in Y-site with no flush. No precipitate seen	980	C
		30 mg/mL	LI	0.1 mg/mL	Visually compatible for 4 hr at room temperature	1788	C
Metoclopramide HCl		5 mg/mL		1 mg/mL	Drugs injected sequentially in Y-site with no flush. No precipitate seen	980	C

Y-Site Injection Compatibility (1:1 Mixture) (Cont.)

Vincristine sulfate

Drug	Mfr	Conc	Mfr	Conc	Remarks	Ref	C/I
Mitomycin		0.5 mg/mL		1 mg/mL	Drugs injected sequentially in Y-site with no flush. No precipitate seen	980	C
Ondansetron HCl	GL	1 mg/mL[b]	LY	0.05 mg/mL[a]	Visually compatible for 4 hr at 22 °C	1365	C
Oxaliplatin	SS	0.5 mg/mL[a]	FAU	0.05 mg/mL[a]	Physically compatible for 4 hr at 23 °C	2566	C
Paclitaxel	NCI	1.2 mg/mL[a]	LI	0.05 mg/mL[a]	Physically compatible for 4 hr at 22 °C	1556	C
Pemetrexed disodium	LI	20 mg/mL[b]	SIC	0.05 mg/mL[a]	Physically compatible for 4 hr at 23 °C	2564	C
Piperacillin sodium–tazobactam sodium	LE[e]	40 + 5 mg/mL[a]	LI	0.05 mg/mL[a]	Physically compatible for 4 hr at 22 °C	1688	C
Sargramostim	IMM	10 mcg/mL[b]	LY	0.05 mg/mL[b]	Visually compatible for 4 hr at 22 °C	1436	C
Sodium bicarbonate		1.4%	LI	0.1 mg/mL	White precipitate forms in 30 min at room temperature	1788	I
Teniposide	BR	0.1 mg/mL[a]	LI	0.05 mg/mL[a]	Physically compatible for 4 hr at 23 °C	1725	C
Thiotepa	IMM[d]	1 mg/mL[a]	LI	0.05 mg/mL[a]	Physically compatible for 4 hr at 23 °C	1861	C
Topotecan HCl	SKB	56 mcg/mL[a,b]	LI	1 mg/mL	Visually compatible. Little loss of either drug in 4 hr at 22 °C	2245	C
Vinblastine sulfate		1 mg/mL		1 mg/mL	Drugs injected sequentially in Y-site with no flush. No precipitate seen	980	C
Vinorelbine tartrate	BW	1 mg/mL[b]	LI	0.05 mg/mL[b]	Physically compatible for 4 hr at 22 °C	1558	C

[a]*Tested in dextrose 5%.*
[b]*Tested in sodium chloride 0.9%.*
[c]*Tested in bacteriostatic sodium chloride 0.9% preserved with benzyl alcohol 0.9%.*
[d]*Lyophilized formulation tested.*
[e]*Test performed using the formulation WITHOUT edetate disodium.*

VINORELBINE TARTRATE
AHFS 10:00

Products — Vinorelbine tartrate is available in a 10-mg/mL concentration in water for injection in 1- and 5-mL single-use vials. No preservatives or other additives are present. (1)

Vinorelbine tartrate should be diluted with a compatible diluent for administration. Because skin reactions may occur, gloves should be worn during preparation. (1)

pH — The injection has a pH of approximately 3.5. (1)

Administration — Vinorelbine tartrate is administered intravenously, after dilution, from a syringe (at a concentration of 1.5 to 3 mg/mL) or infusion solution minibag (at a concentration of 0.5 to 2 mg/mL) over six to 10 minutes into the side port of a free-flowing infusion solution closest to the infusion container. After administration, 75 to 125 mL of solution should be used as a flush. Extravasation should be avoided due to tissue irritation, necrosis, and thrombophlebitis. (1) A literature review for the period 1966 through 2004 did not find a statistically significant difference in the rate of venous irritation from one- to two-minute intravenous pushes and six- to 10-minute intravenous infusions. (2637)

Intrathecal injection of vinca alkaloids has resulted in death. When vinorelbine tartrate is dispensed in a syringe containing an individual dose, the syringe must be labeled with this statement (1):

WARNING – FOR IV USE ONLY. FATAL if given intrathecally

Stability — Vinorelbine tartrate injection is a colorless to pale yellow clear solution. Intact vials should be refrigerated at 2 to 8 °C and protected from light (by storage in the carton) and freezing. Intact vials are stable at room temperature (up to 25 °C) for 72 hours. (1)

When diluted to 1.5 to 3 mg/mL in polypropylene syringes or to 0.5 to 2 mg/mL in PVC infusion containers, vinorelbine tartrate is stable for 24 hours at 5 to 30 °C with exposure to normal room light. (1)

Vinorelbine tartrate 0.1 mg/mL diluted in sodium chloride 0.9% and stored at 22 °C did not exhibit an antimicrobial effect on the growth of four organisms (*Enterococcus faecium, Staphylococcus aureus, Pseudomonas aeruginosa,* and *Candida albicans*) inoculated into the solution. The author recommended that diluted solutions of vinorelbine tartrate be stored under refrigeration whenever possible and that the potential for microbiological growth be considered when assigning expiration periods. (2160)

Sorption — Vinorelbine tartrate was shown not to exhibit sorption to PVC bags and tubing as well as polyethylene and glass containers. (1631; 2420; 2430)

Compatibility Information

Solution Compatibility

Vinorelbine tartrate

Solution	Mfr	Mfr	Conc/L	Remarks	Ref	C/I
Dextrose 5% in sodium chloride 0.45%			0.5 to 2 g	Stable for 24 hr at 5 to 30 °C in light	1	**C**
Dextrose 5%			0.5 to 3 g	Stable for 24 hr at 5 to 30 °C in light	1	**C**
	[a]		500 mg	Little loss in 7 days at 4 °C in dark	1631	**C**
	[a]	GW	0.5 and 2 g	Visually compatible. 6% or less loss in 120 hr at 24 °C in light	2213	**C**
Ringer's injection			0.5 to 2 g	Stable for 24 hr at 5 to 30 °C in light	1	**C**
Ringer's injection, lactated			0.5 to 2 g	Stable for 24 hr at 5 to 30 °C in light	1	**C**
Sodium chloride 0.45%			0.5 to 2 g	Stable for 24 hr at 5 to 30 °C in light	1	**C**
Sodium chloride 0.9%			0.5 to 3 g	Stable for 24 hr at 5 to 30 °C in light	1	**C**
	[a]		500 mg	4% loss in 3 days and 14% loss in 7 days at 4 °C protected from light	1631	**C**
	[a]	GW	0.5 and 2 g	Visually compatible. 3% or less loss in 120 hr at 24 °C in light	2213	**C**

[a]Tested in PVC containers.

Y-Site Injection Compatibility (1:1 Mixture)

Vinorelbine tartrate

Drug	Mfr	Conc	Mfr	Conc	Remarks	Ref	C/I
Acyclovir sodium	BW	7 mg/mL[b]	BW	1 mg/mL[b]	Immediate white precipitate	1558	**I**
Allopurinol sodium	BW	3 mg/mL[b]	BW	1 mg/mL[b]	Immediate white precipitate	1686	**I**
Amikacin sulfate	BR	5 mg/mL[b]	BW	1 mg/mL[b]	Physically compatible for 4 hr at 22 °C	1558	**C**
Aminophylline	AB	2.5 mg/mL[b]	BW	1 mg/mL[b]	Visible haze with large particles in 1 hr	1558	**I**
Amphotericin B	SQ	0.6 mg/mL[a,b]	BW	1 mg/mL[b]	Yellow precipitate forms immediately	1558	**I**
Amphotericin B cholesteryl sulfate complex	SEQ	0.83 mg/mL[a]	BW	1 mg/mL[a]	Gross precipitate forms	2117	**I**
Ampicillin sodium	WY	20 mg/mL[b]	BW	1 mg/mL[b]	Tiny particles form immediately. White particles in turbidity in 1 hr	1558	**I**
Aztreonam	SQ	40 mg/mL[b]	BW	1 mg/mL[b]	Physically compatible for 4 hr at 23 °C	1558	**C**
Bleomycin sulfate	BR	1 unit/mL[b]	BW	1 mg/mL[b]	Physically compatible for 4 hr at 22 °C	1558	**C**
Bumetanide	RC	0.04 mg/mL[b]	BW	1 mg/mL[b]	Physically compatible for 4 hr at 22 °C	1558	**C**
Buprenorphine HCl	RKC	0.04 mg/mL[b]	BW	1 mg/mL[b]	Physically compatible for 4 hr at 22 °C	1558	**C**
Butorphanol tartrate	BR	0.04 mg/mL[b]	BW	1 mg/mL[b]	Physically compatible for 4 hr at 22 °C	1558	**C**
Calcium gluconate	AMR	40 mg/mL[b]	BW	1 mg/mL[b]	Physically compatible for 4 hr at 22 °C	1558	**C**
Carboplatin	BR	5 mg/mL[b]	BW	1 mg/mL[b]	Physically compatible for 4 hr at 22 °C	1558	**C**
Carmustine	BR	1.5 mg/mL[b]	BW	1 mg/mL[b]	Physically compatible for 4 hr at 22 °C	1558	**C**
Cefazolin sodium	GEM	20 mg/mL[b]	BW	1 mg/mL[b]	Measured turbidity increases immediately	1558	**I**

Y-Site Injection Compatibility (1:1 Mixture) (Cont.)

Vinorelbine tartrate

Drug	Mfr	Conc	Mfr	Conc	Remarks	Ref	C/I
Cefotaxime sodium	HO	20 mg/mL[b]	BW	1 mg/mL[b]	Physically compatible for 4 hr at 22 °C	1558	**C**
Cefotetan disodium	STU	20 mg/mL[b]	BW	1 mg/mL[b]	Tiny particles form immediately. Turbidity in 4 hr	1558	**I**
Ceftazidime	LI	40 mg/mL[b]	BW	1 mg/mL[b]	Physically compatible for 4 hr at 22 °C	1558	**C**
Ceftriaxone sodium	RC	20 mg/mL[b]	BW	1 mg/mL[b]	Tiny particles form immediately, becoming more numerous in 4 hr at 22 °C	1558	**I**
Cefuroxime sodium	GL	20 mg/mL[b]	BW	1 mg/mL[b]	Large increase in measured turbidity occurs immediately	1558	**I**
Chlorpromazine HCl	RU	2 mg/mL[b]	BW	1 mg/mL[b]	Physically compatible for 4 hr at 22 °C	1558	**C**
Cisplatin	BR	1 mg/mL	BW	1 mg/mL[b]	Physically compatible for 4 hr at 22 °C	1558	**C**
Clindamycin phosphate	AB	10 mg/mL[b]	BW	1 mg/mL[b]	Physically compatible for 4 hr at 22 °C	1558	**C**
Cyclophosphamide	MJ	10 mg/mL[b]	BW	1 mg/mL[b]	Physically compatible for 4 hr at 22 °C	1558	**C**
Cytarabine	CET	50 mg/mL	BW	1 mg/mL[b]	Physically compatible for 4 hr at 22 °C	1558	**C**
Dacarbazine	MI	4 mg/mL[b]	BW	1 mg/mL[b]	Physically compatible for 4 hr at 22 °C	1558	**C**
Dactinomycin	MSD	0.01 mg/mL[b]	BW	1 mg/mL[b]	Physically compatible for 4 hr at 22 °C	1558	**C**
Daunorubicin HCl	WY	1 mg/mL[b]	BW	1 mg/mL[b]	Physically compatible for 4 hr at 22 °C	1558	**C**
Dexamethasone sodium phosphate	LY	1 mg/mL[b]	BW	1 mg/mL[b]	Physically compatible for 4 hr at 22 °C	1558	**C**
Diphenhydramine HCl	ES	2 mg/mL[b]	BW	1 mg/mL[b]	Physically compatible for 4 hr at 22 °C	1558	**C**
Doxorubicin HCl	CET	2 mg/mL	BW	1 mg/mL[b]	Physically compatible for 4 hr at 22 °C	1558	**C**
Doxorubicin HCl liposomal	SEQ	0.4 mg/mL[a]	BW	1 mg/mL[a]	Physically compatible for 4 hr at 23 °C	2087	**C**
Doxycycline hyclate	ES	1 mg/mL[b]	BW	1 mg/mL[b]	Physically compatible for 4 hr at 22 °C	1558	**C**
Droperidol	JN	0.4 mg/mL[b]	BW	1 mg/mL[b]	Physically compatible for 4 hr at 22 °C	1558	**C**
Enalaprilat	MSD	0.1 mg/mL[b]	BW	1 mg/mL[b]	Physically compatible for 4 hr at 22 °C	1558	**C**
Etoposide	BR	0.4 mg/mL[b]	BW	1 mg/mL[b]	Physically compatible for 4 hr at 22 °C	1558	**C**
Famotidine	MSD	2 mg/mL[b]	BW	1 mg/mL[b]	Physically compatible for 4 hr at 22 °C	1558	**C**
Filgrastim	AMG	30 mcg/mL[a]	BW	1 mg/mL[b]	Physically compatible for 4 hr at 22 °C	1687	**C**
Floxuridine	RC	3 mg/mL[b]	BW	1 mg/mL[b]	Physically compatible for 4 hr at 22 °C	1558	**C**
Fluconazole	RR	2 mg/mL	BW	1 mg/mL[b]	Physically compatible for 4 hr at 22 °C	1558	**C**
Fludarabine phosphate	BX	1 mg/mL[b]	BW	1 mg/mL[b]	Physically compatible for 4 hr at 22 °C	1558	**C**
Fluorouracil	RC	16 mg/mL[b]	BW	1 mg/mL[b]	Heavy white precipitate forms immediately	1558	**I**
Furosemide	ES	3 mg/mL[b]	BW	1 mg/mL[b]	Heavy white precipitate forms immediately	1558	**I**
Gallium nitrate	FUJ	0.4 mg/mL[b]	BW	1 mg/mL[b]	Physically compatible for 4 hr at 22 °C	1558	**C**
Ganciclovir sodium	SY	20 mg/mL[b]	BW	1 mg/mL[b]	Turbid precipitate forms immediately	1558	**I**
Gemcitabine HCl	LI	10 mg/mL[b]	GW	1 mg/mL[b]	Physically compatible for 4 hr at 23 °C	2226	**C**
Gentamicin sulfate	ES	5 mg/mL[b]	BW	1 mg/mL[b]	Physically compatible for 4 hr at 22 °C	1558	**C**
Granisetron HCl	SKB	0.05 mg/mL[a]	BW	1 mg/mL[a]	Physically compatible for 4 hr at 23 °C	2000	**C**
Haloperidol lactate	MN	0.2 mg/mL[b]	BW	1 mg/mL[b]	Physically compatible for 4 hr at 22 °C	1558	**C**
Heparin sodium	ES	100 units/mL[b]	BW	1 mg/mL[b]	Physically compatible for 4 hr at 22 °C	1558	**C**
		100 units/mL[b]	GW	3 mg/mL[b]	A fine haze forms immediately, becoming cloudy in 15 min	2238	**I**

Y-Site Injection Compatibility (1:1 Mixture) (Cont.)

Vinorelbine tartrate

Drug	Mfr	Conc	Mfr	Conc	Remarks	Ref	C/I
		100 units/mL[b]	GW	2 mg/mL[b]	Visually compatible for at least 15 min	2238	C
		100 units/mL[b]	GW	1 mg/mL[b]	Visually compatible for at least 15 min	2238	C
		100 units/1 mL[b]	GW	4 mg/4 mL[b]	Volumes mixed as cited. Visually compatible for at least 15 min	2238	C
		100 units/1 mL[b]	GW	8 mg/4 mL[b]	Volumes mixed as cited. Precipitate forms	2238	I
		100 units/1 mL[b]	GW	12 mg/4 mL[b]	Volumes mixed as cited. Precipitate forms	2238	I
Hydrocortisone sodium succinate	UP	1 mg/mL[b]	BW	1 mg/mL[b]	Physically compatible for 4 hr at 22 °C	1558	C
Hydromorphone HCl	KN	0.5 mg/mL[b]	BW	1 mg/mL[b]	Physically compatible for 4 hr at 22 °C	1558	C
Hydroxyzine HCl	ES	4 mg/mL[b]	BW	1 mg/mL[b]	Physically compatible for 4 hr at 22 °C	1558	C
Idarubicin HCl	AD	0.5 mg/mL[b]	BW	1 mg/mL[b]	Physically compatible for 4 hr at 22 °C	1558; 1675	C
Ifosfamide	MJ	25 mg/mL[b]	BW	1 mg/mL[b]	Physically compatible for 4 hr at 22 °C	1558	C
Imipenem–cilastatin sodium	MSD	10 mg/mL[b]	BW	1 mg/mL[b]	Physically compatible for 4 hr at 22 °C	1558	C
Lorazepam	WY	0.1 mg/mL[b]	BW	1 mg/mL[b]	Physically compatible for 4 hr at 22 °C	1558	C
Mannitol	BA	15%	BW	1 mg/mL[b]	Physically compatible for 4 hr at 22 °C	1558	C
Mechlorethamine HCl	MSD	1 mg/mL	BW	1 mg/mL[b]	Physically compatible for 4 hr at 22 °C	1558	C
Melphalan HCl	BW	0.1 mg/mL[b]	BW	1 mg/mL[b]	Physically compatible for 4 hr at 22 °C	1558	C
Meperidine HCl	WY	4 mg/mL[b]	BW	1 mg/mL[b]	Physically compatible for 4 hr at 22 °C	1558	C
Mesna	MJ	10 mg/mL[b]	BW	1 mg/mL[b]	Physically compatible for 4 hr at 22 °C	1558	C
Methotrexate sodium	LE	15 mg/mL[b]	BW	1 mg/mL[b]	Physically compatible for 4 hr at 22 °C	1558	C
Methylprednisolone sodium succinate	AB	5 mg/mL[b]	BW	1 mg/mL[b]	Heavy white precipitate forms immediately	1558	I
Metoclopramide HCl	RB	5 mg/mL	BW	1 mg/mL[b]	Physically compatible for 4 hr at 22 °C	1558	C
Metronidazole	BA	5 mg/mL	BW	1 mg/mL[b]	Physically compatible for 4 hr at 22 °C	1558	C
Mitomycin	BR	0.5 mg/mL	BW	1 mg/mL[b]	Reddish-purple color in 1 hr	1558	I
Mitoxantrone HCl	LE	0.5 mg/mL[b]	BW	1 mg/mL[b]	Physically compatible for 4 hr at 22 °C	1558	C
Morphine sulfate	WI	1 mg/mL[b]	BW	1 mg/mL[b]	Physically compatible for 4 hr at 22 °C	1558	C
Nalbuphine HCl	AST	10 mg/mL	BW	1 mg/mL[b]	Physically compatible for 4 hr at 22 °C	1558	C
Ondansetron HCl	GL	1 mg/mL[b]	BW	1 mg/mL[b]	Physically compatible for 4 hr at 22 °C	1558	C
Oxaliplatin	SS	0.5 mg/mL[a]	GW	1 mg/mL[a]	Physically compatible for 4 hr at 23 °C	2566	C
Potassium chloride	AB	0.1 mEq/mL[b]	BW	1 mg/mL[b]	Physically compatible for 4 hr at 22 °C	1558	C
Prochlorperazine edisylate	SKB	0.5 mg/mL[b]	BW	1 mg/mL[b]	Physically compatible for 4 hr at 22 °C	1558	C
Promethazine HCl	ES	2 mg/mL[b]	BW	1 mg/mL[b]	Physically compatible for 4 hr at 22 °C	1558	C
Ranitidine HCl	GL	2 mg/mL[b]	BW	1 mg/mL[b]	Physically compatible for 4 hr at 22 °C	1558	C
Sodium bicarbonate	AB	1 mEq/mL	BW	1 mg/mL[b]	Tiny particles and haze form immediately. Large particles in 4 hr at 22 °C	1558	I
Streptozocin	UP	40 mg/mL[b]	BW	1 mg/mL[b]	Physically compatible for 4 hr at 22 °C	1558	C
Teniposide	BR	0.1 mg/mL[a]	BW	1 mg/mL[a]	Physically compatible for 4 hr at 23 °C	1725	C
Thiotepa	LE	10 mg/mL[b]	BW	1 mg/mL[b]	Immediate cloudiness with particles	1558	I

Y-Site Injection Compatibility (1:1 Mixture) (Cont.)

Vinorelbine tartrate

Drug	Mfr	Conc	Mfr	Conc	Remarks	Ref	C/I
Ticarcillin disodium–clavulanate potassium	SKB	31 mg/mL[b]	BW	1 mg/mL[b]	Physically compatible for 4 hr at 22 °C	1558	**C**
Tobramycin sulfate	LI	5 mg/mL[b]	BW	1 mg/mL[b]	Physically compatible for 4 hr at 22 °C	1558	**C**
Trimethoprim–sulfamethoxazole	ES	0.8 + 4 mg/mL[b]	BW	1 mg/mL[b]	Heavy white turbidity forms immediately, developing particles in 1 hr	1558	**I**
Vancomycin HCl	LY	10 mg/mL[b]	BW	1 mg/mL[b]	Physically compatible for 4 hr at 22 °C	1558	**C**
Vinblastine sulfate	LI	0.12 mg/mL[b]	BW	1 mg/mL[b]	Physically compatible for 4 hr at 22 °C	1558	**C**
Vincristine sulfate	LI	0.05 mg/mL[b]	BW	1 mg/mL[b]	Physically compatible for 4 hr at 22 °C	1558	**C**
Zidovudine	BW	4 mg/mL[b]	BW	1 mg/mL[b]	Physically compatible for 4 hr at 22 °C	1558	**C**

[a]*Tested in dextrose 5%.*
[b]*Tested in sodium chloride 0.9%.*

VITAMIN A
AHFS 88:04

Products — Vitamin A 50,000 I.U./mL is available in 2-mL single-dose vials. Each milliliter also contains polysorbate 80, chlorobutanol, citric acid, and sodium hydroxide to adjust pH. (1)

pH — From 6.5 to 7.1. (4)

Trade Name(s) — Aquasol A Parenteral.

Administration — Vitamin A is administered intramuscularly. (1; 4) Intravenous administration is not recommended. (1)

Stability — Vitamin A is a light yellow to amber or red oil. It is sensitive to, and should be protected from, light and air. (4) Intact vials should be stored under refrigeration and protected from light and freezing. (1; 4) Although refrigerated storage is required, the manufacturer has stated the drug may be stored at room temperature for 4 weeks. (2745)

The stability of retinol palmitate and tocopherols (δ, γ, and α) in 3-in-1 admixtures of amino acids 4%, dextrose 10%, fat emulsion 3% (Intralipid, Liposyn, and ClinOleic), various electrolytes, vitamins, and trace elements in ethylene vinyl acetate (EVA) bags over three days at 4, 25, and 37 °C was determined. Retinol palmitate was unstable at room temperature with 33 and 50% degradation at 24 and 72 hours after compounding, respectively. Refrigeration of the admixture reduced the degradation to 29% at 72 hours. (2460)

The degradation of vitamins A, B₁, C, and E from Cernevit (Roche) multivitamins was evaluated in NuTRIflex Lipid Plus (B. Braun) admixtures prepared in ethylene vinyl acetate (EVA) bags and in multilayer bags. After storage for up to 72 hours at 4, 21, and 40 °C, greater vitamin losses occurred in the EVA bags. Vitamin A (retinyl palmitate) losses were 20%. In the multilayer bags (presumably a better barrier to oxygen transfer), vitamin A (retinyl palmitate) losses were 5%. (2618)

The vitamins in Cernevit (Baxter) diluted in three 2-in-1 parenteral nutrition admixtures were tested for stability over 48 hours. Most of the other vitamins, including vitamin A, retained their initial concentrations. (2796)

Light Effects — A parenteral nutrition solution in glass bottles exposed to sunlight was evaluated. Vitamin A decomposed rapidly, losing more than 50% in three hours. The decomposition could be slowed to approximately a 25% loss in three hours by covering the bottle with a light-resistant vinyl bag. (1040)

Vitamin A was rapidly and significantly decomposed when exposed to daylight. The extent and rate of loss were dependent on the degree of exposure to daylight which, in turn, depended on various factors such as the direction of the radiation, time of day, and climatic conditions. Delivery of less than 10% of the expected amount was reported. (1047) In controlled light experiments, the decomposition initially progressed exponentially. Subsequently, the rate of decomposition slowed. This result was attributed to a protective effect of the degradation products on the remaining vitamin A. The presence of amino acids provided greater protection. Compared to degradation rates in dextrose 5%, decomposition was reduced by up to 50% in some amino acid mixtures. (1048)

In a parenteral nutrition solution composed of amino acids, dextrose, electrolytes, trace elements, and multivitamins in PVC bags stored at 4 and 25 °C, vitamin A rapidly deteriorated to 10% of the initial concentration in eight hours at 25 °C while exposed to light. The decomposition was slowed by light protection and refrigeration, with a loss of about 25% in four days. (1063)

Substantial loss of retinol all-*trans* palmitate was reported from both TPN and TNA admixtures due to exposure to sunlight. In three hours' exposure to sunlight, essentially total loss of retinol had occurred. The presence or absence of lipids did not affect stability. The container material used to store the nutrition admixtures affected the concentration of the vitamins as well. Losses were greatest in PVC containers and were slightly better in EVA and glass containers. (2049)

The photodegradation of vitamin A in 2-in-1 (Synthamin 9, Glucose 20%) and 3-in-1 (Synthamin 9, Glucose 20%, Intralipid 20%, electrolytes, vitamins, trace elements) admixtures was reported after exposure to six hours of indirect daylight. The compounded admixtures were prepared in multilayer bags protected from light and stored at 5 °C for a minimum of five days. The same admixtures were prepared in EVA bags 24 hours prior to use with vitamins added prior to study. Vitamin A decreased to 60 to 80% of the initial concentrations in two to six hours. The type of bag had no influence on the photodegradation of vitamin A. Despite fat emulsion, no significant light protection was noted with the 3-in-1 admixture. The authors concluded that light protection can minimize vitamin A losses. (2459)

Sorption — Vitamin A (as the acetate) (Sigma) 7.5 mg/L displayed 66.7% sorption to a PVC plastic test strip in 24 hours. The presence of dextrose 5% and sodium chloride 0.9% increased the extent of sorption. (12)

Vitamin A acetate displayed 78% sorption to 200-mL PVC containers after 24 hours at 25 °C with gentle shaking. The initial concentration was 3 mg/L. The sorption was increased by approximately 10% in sodium chloride 0.9% and by 20% in dextrose 5%. (133)

However, vitamin A delivery is also reduced in glass intravenous containers. At a concentration of 10,000 units/L in glass and PVC plastic containers protected from light with aluminum foil, 77 and 71%, respectively, of the vitamin A were delivered in 10 hours. Without light protection, 61% was delivered from glass and 49% from PVC plastic containers over a 10-hour period. (290)

In another test using multivitamin infusion (USV), one ampul/L of sodium chloride 0.9% in glass and PVC containers not protected from light, 69.4 and 67.9% of the vitamin A were delivered from the glass and PVC containers, respectively, in 10 hours. The amount of vitamin A was constant over this test period, not decreasing with time. (282)

The delivery of vitamins A, D, and E from a parenteral nutrition solution composed of 3% amino acid solution (Pharmacia) in dextrose 10% with electrolytes, trace elements, vitamin K, folate, and vitamin B$_{12}$ was evaluated. To this solution was added 6 mL of multivitamin infusion (USV). The solution was prepared in PVC bags (Travenol), and administration was simulated through a fluid chamber (Buretrol) and infusion tubing with a 0.5-μm filter at 10 mL/hr. During the first 60 to 90 minutes, minimal delivery of the vitamins occurred. Then a rise and a plateau in the delivered vitamins followed and were attributed to an increasing saturation of adsorptive binding sites in the tubing. Total amounts delivered over 24 hours were: vitamin A, 31%; vitamin D, 68%; and vitamin E, 64%. Sorption of the vitamins was found in the PVC bag, fluid chamber, and tubing. Decomposition was not a factor. (836)

A patient receiving 3000 I.U. of retinol daily in a parenteral nutrition solution nevertheless experienced two episodes of night blindness. The pharmacy prepared the parenteral nutrition solution in 1-L PVC bags in weekly batches and stored them at 4 °C in the dark until use. A subsequent in vitro study showed losses of vitamin A of 23 and 77% in three- and 14-day periods, respectively, under these conditions. About 30% of the lost vitamin A could be extracted from the PVC bag. (1038)

Losses of vitamin A from neonatal parenteral nutrition solutions containing multivitamins (USV) was reported. The solution was prepared in colorless glass bottles and run through an administration set with a burette (Travenol). The total loss of vitamin A was 75% in 24 hours, with about 16% as decomposition in the glass bottle. The decomposition was not noticeable during the first 12 hours, but then vitamin A levels fell rather precipitously to about one-third of the initial amount.

The balance of the loss, averaging about 59%, occurred during transit through the administration set. Removal of the inline filter and treatment of the set with albumin had no effect on vitamin A delivery. The authors recommended a three- to fourfold increase in the amount of vitamin A to compensate for the losses. (1039)

A 50% loss of vitamin A was noted from a bottle of parenteral nutrition solution prepared with multivitamin infusion (USV) after 5.5 hours of infusion. The amount delivered through an Ivex-2 filter set was only 6.3% of the added amount. Similar quantities were found after 20 hours of infusion. A reduced light exposure and use of ^{3}H-labeled vitamin A confirmed binding to the infusion bottles and tubing. (704)

Solutions containing multivitamins (USV) spiked with ^{3}H-labeled retinol in intravenous tubing protected from light and agitated to simulate flow for five hours were evaluated. About half of the vitamin A was lost in 30 minutes, and 88 to 96% was lost in five hours. Hexane rinses and radioactivity determinations on the tubing accounted for the decrease in radioactivity. (1049)

Neonatal parenteral nutrition solutions containing multivitamins prepared in bags were delivered at 10 mL/hr through Buretrol sets (Travenol). The bags and sets were protected from light. About 26% of the vitamin A was lost before the flow was started. At 10 mL/hr, about 67% was lost from the effluent. More rapid flow reduced the extent of loss. Analysis of clinical samples of parenteral nutrition solutions showed losses of 21 to 57% after 20 hours. Because losses after five hours were of the same magnitude, the authors concluded that the loss occurs rapidly and is not due to gradual decomposition. (1049)

The stability of numerous vitamins in parenteral nutrition solutions composed of amino acids (Kabi-Vitrum), dextrose 30%, and fat emulsion 20% (Kabi-Vitrum) in a 2:1:1 ratio with electrolytes, trace elements, and both fat- and water-soluble vitamins was reported. The admixtures were stored in darkness at 2 to 8 °C for 96 hours with no significant loss of retinyl palmitate. (1225)

When the admixture was subjected to simulated infusion over 24 hours at 20 °C, either exposed to room light or light protected, or stored for six days in the dark under refrigeration and then subjected to the same simulated infusion, once again the retinyl palmitate did not undergo significant loss. (1225)

Retinol losses of 40% occurred in two hours and 60% in five hours from parenteral nutrition solutions pumped at 10 mL/hr through standard infusion sets at room temperature. The retinol concentration in the bottle remained constant while the retinol in the effluent decreased. Antioxidants had no effect. Much of the vitamin A was recoverable from hexane washings of the tubing. (1050)

The stability of several vitamins from M.V.I.-12 (Armour) admixed in parenteral nutrition solutions composed of different amino acid products, with or without Intralipid 10%, when stored in glass bottles and PVC bags at 25 and 5 °C for 48 hours was reported. No vitamin A was lost from any formula in glass bottles, but samples in PVC containers lost as much as 35 and 60% at 5 and 25 °C, respectively, in 48 hours. (1431)

The stability of vitamin A was studied in two parenteral nutrition solutions. In TPN #172 (see Appendix I), a 10% loss of vitamin A palmitate occurred in about 20 days in PVC bags while no loss occurred in Buretrol chambers in 21 days at 30 °C with exposure to normal ward light. In TPN #173 (see Appendix I), a 10% loss of vitamin A palmitate occurred in about 12 days in both glass and PVC containers at 2 to 8 °C with protection from light. (1606)

The effects of the fat emulsion concentration on vitamin A stability in several parenteral nutrition solutions were evaluated. Vitamin A palmitate was not absorbed into PVC containers from Intralipid 10%. Among TPN solutions with lower Intralipid contents, no correlation existed between the fat emulsion content and the extent of vitamin A loss during refrigerated storage. The fat emulsion content afforded vitamin A some protection from decomposition due to light exposure at 30 °C. (1607)

The quantity of retinol delivered from an M.V.I.-containing 2-in-1 parenteral nutrition solution and when M.V.I. was added to Intralipid 10% was evaluated during simulated administration through a PVC administration set. The parenteral nutrition solution was composed of amino acids 2.8%, dextrose 10%, and standard electrolytes; M.V.I. was added to yield a nominal retinol concentration of 455 mcg/150 mL. Retinol losses were about 80% of the admixed amount after being delivered through the PVC set. When M.V.I. was added to Intralipid 10% in a retinol concentration of 455 mcg/20 mL, retinol losses were reduced to about 10% of the admixed amount. The fat emulsion provided retinol protection from sorption to the PVC administration set. (2027)

Substantially higher amounts of retinol were found to be delivered using polyolefin administration set tubing than with PVC tubing during simulated neonatal intensive care administration. Retinol was added to a 2-in-1 parenteral nutrition solution (TPN #206) in concentrations of 25 and 50 I.U./mL and run at 4 and 10 mL/hr through three meter lengths of polyolefin (MiniMed) and PVC (Baxter) intravenous extension set tubing protected from light and passed through a 37 °C water bath. Delivered quantities of retinol varied from 19 to 74% through the PVC tubing and 47 to 87% through the polyolefin tubing. The loss of retinol to the PVC tubing appeared to be saturable. Even so, the use of polyolefin tubing increases the amount of retinol delivered during simulated neonatal administration. (2028)

To minimize the importance of sorption, use vitamin A palmitate, which does not sorb as extensively to PVC (1033; 1606; 2026), instead of the acetate. However, this change does not alter the problem of degradation from exposure to light. Alternatively, an excess of vitamin A could be used. (1033)

Plasticizer Leaching — Vitamin A leached significant amounts of diethylhexyl phthalate (DEHP) plasticizer from PVC bags and administration set tubing. (1621)

VORICONAZOLE
AHFS 8:14.08

Products — Voriconazole is available as a lyophilized powder in single-use vials containing 200 mg with 3.2 g of sulfobutyl ether β-cyclodextrin sodium and bearing a vacuum. Reconstitute with 19 mL of sterile water for injection and shake well to yield 20 mL of a voriconazole 10-mg/mL solution. Do not use the vial if a vacuum does not draw in the diluent for reconstitution. (1)

The reconstituted solution is a concentrate that must be diluted in a compatible solution to a concentration of 0.5 to 5 mg/mL before intravenous administration. The manufacturer recommends removing a volume equivalent to the volume of drug before addition to the bag. (1)

Trade Name(s) — Vfend.

Administration — Voriconazole is administered by intravenous infusion in a compatible infusion solution at a concentration between 0.5 and 5 mg/mL over one to two hours at a maximum rate of 3 mg/kg/hr. (1)

Stability — Intact vials should be stored at controlled room temperature. Voriconazole reconstituted as directed is chemically and physically stable for 24 hours under refrigeration. However, because no antimicrobial preservative is present, the manufacturer recommends use immediately after reconstitution. Voriconazole is intended for single use, and any remaining drug should be discarded. (1)

Compatibility Information

Solution Compatibility

Voriconazole

Solution	Mfr	Mfr	Conc/L	Remarks	Ref	C/I
Dextrose 5% in Ringer's injection, lactated		PF		Compatible and stable for 24 hr	1	C
Dextrose 5% in sodium chloride 0.45%		PF		Compatible and stable for 24 hr	1	C
Dextrose 5% in sodium chloride 0.9%		PF		Compatible and stable for 24 hr	1	C
Dextrose 5%		PF		Compatible and stable for 24 hr	1	C
	a	PF	4 g	Visually compatible. 3% loss in 15 days at 4 °C	2662	C
	MAC[b]	PF	2 g	Visually compatible. 9% loss in 6 days at 4 °C and in 5 days at 25 °C	2694	C
Sodium chloride 0.45%		PF		Compatible and stable for 24 hr	1	C
Sodium chloride 0.9%		PF		Compatible and stable for 24 hr	1	C
	MAC[b]	PF	2 g	No loss over 32 days at 4 °C	2624	C

Solution Compatibility (Cont.)

Voriconazole

Solution	Mfr	Mfr	Conc/L	Remarks	Ref	C/I
	MAC[b]	PF	2 g	Visually compatible. No loss at 4 °C and 5% loss at 25 °C in 8 days	2694	C

[a]*Tested in PVC containers.*
[b]*Tested in polyolefin containers.*

Additive Compatibility

Voriconazole

Drug	Mfr	Conc/L	Mfr	Conc/L	Test Soln	Remarks	Ref	C/I
Sodium bicarbonate		4.2%	PF			Voriconazole slightly decomposes at room temperature	1	I

Y-Site Injection Compatibility (1:1 Mixture)

Voriconazole

Drug	Mfr	Conc	Mfr	Conc	Remarks	Ref	C/I
Anidulafungin	VIC	0.5 mg/mL[a]	PF	4 mg/mL[a]	Physically compatible for 4 hr at 23 °C	2617	C
Caspofungin acetate	ME	0.7 mg/mL[b]	PF	4 mg/mL[b]	Physically compatible for 4 hr at room temperature	2758	C
	ME	0.5 mg/mL[b]	PF	2 mg/mL[b]	Physically compatible over 60 min	2766	C
Ceftaroline fosamil	FOR	2.22 mg/mL[a,b,d]	PF	4 mg/mL[a,b,d]	Physically compatible for 4 hr at 23 °C	2826	C
Doripenem	JJ	5 mg/mL[a,b]	PF	4 mg/mL[a,b]	Physically compatible for 4 hr at 23 °C	2743	C
Tigecycline	WY	1 mg/mL[b]	PF	2 mg/mL[b]	Microparticulates form	2714	I
Vasopressin	APP	0.2 unit/mL[b]	PF	3 mg/mL[c]	Physically compatible	2641	C

[a]*Tested in dextrose 5%.*
[b]*Tested in sodium chloride 0.9%.*
[c]*Tested in sodium chloride 0.45%.*
[d]*Tested in Ringer's injection, lactated.*

WARFARIN SODIUM
AHFS 20:12.04.08

Products — Warfarin sodium is available as a lyophilized powder in vials containing a total of 5.4 mg of drug. When reconstituted with 2.7 mL of sterile water for injection, each milliliter of solution contains warfarin sodium 2 mg with sodium phosphate salts, sodium chloride, mannitol, and sodium hydroxide to adjust pH. The maximum amount of withdrawable solution is about 2.5 mL. (1)

pH — From 8.1 to 8.3. (1)

Trade Name(s) — Coumadin.

Administration — Warfarin sodium is administered by slow intravenous injection over one to two minutes into a peripheral vein. It should not be given intramuscularly. (1)

Stability — Intact vials should be stored at controlled room temperature and protected from exposure to light. After reconstitution, warfarin sodium is physically and chemically stable for only four hours at room temperature. The reconstituted solution should not be refrigerated. If either particulates or discoloration is noted, the drug should be discarded. Unused solution also should be discarded. (1)

pH Effects — A precipitate may form in solution due to formation of the poorly soluble enol form of warfarin at pH values below 8. At pH

8 or higher, clear stable solutions result because the warfarin is in the soluble enolate form. (964)

Sorption — Warfarin sodium (Abbott) 25 mg/L displayed 11.7% sorption to a PVC plastic test strip in 24 hours. The presence of dextrose 5% increased the extent of the sorption. (12)

Warfarin sodium 22 mg/L in sodium chloride 0.9% (Travenol) in PVC bags exhibited approximately a 15% loss in one week at room temperature (15 to 20 °C) due to sorption. However, when the solution was buffered from its initial pH of 6.7 to 7.4, no significant loss of drug due to sorption was observed over the one-week study period. (536)

In another study, warfarin sodium 22 mg/L in sodium chloride 0.9% did not exhibit any loss due to sorption during a seven-hour simulated infusion through an infusion set (Travenol) consisting of a cellulose propionate burette chamber and 170 cm of PVC tubing. (606)

The drug was also tested as a simulated infusion over at least one hour by a syringe pump system. A glass syringe on a syringe pump was fitted with 20 cm of polyethylene tubing or 50 cm of Silastic tubing. No loss of drug due to sorption was observed with either tubing. (606)

In addition, a 25-mL aliquot of warfarin sodium 22 mg/L in sodium chloride 0.9% was stored in all-plastic syringes composed of polypropylene barrels and polyethylene plungers for 24 hours at room temperature in the dark. No loss due to sorption occurred. (606)

The sorption of warfarin sodium 20 mg/L in sodium chloride 0.9% was evaluated in 100-mL PVC infusion bags (Travenol). After eight

Table 1. Extent of Equilibrium Sorption of Warfarin Sodium in Sodium Chloride 0.9% in PVC Bags (770)

Initial Concentration (mg/mL)	pH	Extent of Sorption (%)
1.31	6.95	4
0.433	6.55	6
0.190	6.27	18
0.093	6.04	24
0.048	5.90	30
0.024	5.78	45
0.009	5.65	66

hours at 20 to 24 °C, 29% of the warfarin was lost. Adjusting the pH of the solution to 2 or 4 increased the sorption in eight hours to 49% because of the increased amount of un-ionized warfarin present in the solution at these low pH values. The un-ionized form is most favorably sorbed by the plastic. The concentration of warfarin sodium in solution also affects the pH and, thereby, the extent of sorption. Table 1 shows that as the warfarin sodium concentration is reduced, small changes in the pH of the solution occur. Even these small pH changes result in a greatly increased extent of sorption at equilibrium (about 100 hours of exposure). (770)

Warfarin sodium showed a negligible (less than 3%) loss if the aqueous solutions at pH 2 to 7 were stored in polypropylene infusion bags. (770)

Compatibility Information

Solution Compatibility

Warfarin sodium

Solution	Mfr	Mfr	Conc/L	Remarks	Ref	C/I
Dextrose 5% in Ringer's injection, lactated	BA	DU	100 mg	Physically compatible for 24 hr at 23 °C	2011	C
Dextrose 5% in sodium chloride 0.45%	BA	DU	100 mg	Physically compatible for 24 hr at 23 °C	2011	C
Dextrose 5% in sodium chloride 0.9%	BA	DU	100 mg	Physically compatible for 24 hr at 23 °C	2011	C
Dextrose 5%	a	DU	20 mg	Visually compatible. 2.4% loss due to sorption in 6 hr	2010	C
	b	DU	20 mg	Visually compatible with no loss in 6 hr	2010	C
	a	DU	600 mg	Visually compatible with no loss in 6 hr	2010	C
	MG	DU	100 mg	Physically compatible for 24 hr at 23 °C	2011	C
Dextrose 10%	BA	DU	100 mg	Physically compatible for 24 hr at 23 °C	2011	C
Ringer's injection		DU	1 g	Haze forms immediately	2010	I
	BA	DME	1 g	Haze forms immediately	2078	I
Ringer's injection, lactated	BA	DU	100 mg	Physically compatible for 24 hr at 23 °C	2011	C
	BA	DME	1 g	Slight haze may form in 1 hr	2078	I
Sodium chloride 0.9%	c	ON	100 mg	Visually compatible. No loss in 24 hr at 21 °C	1796	C
	a	ON	100 mg	Visually compatible. 50% loss in 24 hr and 70% loss in 120 hr at 21 °C due to sorption	1796	I
	a	DU	20 mg	Visually compatible. 1% loss due to sorption in 6 hr	2010	C
	b	DU	20 mg	Visually compatible with no loss in 6 hr	2010	C
	a	DU	600 mg	Visually compatible with no loss in 6 hr	2010	C
	MG	DU	100 mg	Physically compatible for 24 hr at 23 °C	2011	C

Solution Compatibility (Cont.)

Warfarin sodium

Solution	Mfr	Mfr	Conc/L	Remarks	Ref	C/I
	AB	DME	1 g	Haze may form in 24 hr	2078	**I**

[a]Tested in PVC containers.
[b]Tested in glass containers.
[c]Tested in glass containers and polypropylene trilayer containers.

Drugs in Syringe Compatibility

Warfarin sodium

Drug (in syringe)	Mfr	Amt	Mfr	Amt	Remarks	Ref	C/I
Heparin sodium	ES	5000 units/ 1 mL	DU	2 mg/ 1 mL[a]	Low-level haze forms immediately and becomes visible in ambient light in 1 hr	2010	**I**

[a]Tested in sterile water for injection.

Y-Site Injection Compatibility (1:1 Mixture)

Warfarin sodium

Drug	Mfr	Conc	Mfr	Conc	Remarks	Ref	C/I
Amikacin sulfate	AB	5 mg/mL[a,b]	DU	0.1[a,b] and 2[d] mg/mL	Physically compatible for 24 hr at 23 °C	2011	**C**
Aminophylline	ES	4 mg/mL[a]	DME	2 mg/mL[d]	Haze forms in 4 hr	2078	**I**
Ammonium chloride	AB	5 mEq/mL	DU	0.1 mg/mL[a]	Subvisible haze forms immediately	2011	**I**
	AB	5 mEq/mL	DU	0.1 mg/mL[b]	Physically compatible for 24 hr at 23 °C	2011	**C**
	AB	5 mEq/mL	DU	2 mg/mL[d]	Immediate turbidity becoming a precipitate in 24 hr at 23 °C	2011	**I**
Ascorbic acid	SCN	0.5 mg/mL[a,b]	DU	0.1[a,b] and 2[d] mg/mL	Physically compatible for 24 hr at 23 °C	2011	**C**
Bivalirudin	TMC	5 mg/mL[a]	DU	2 mg/mL	Physically compatible for 4 hr at 23 °C	2373	**C**
Cefazolin sodium	SKB	20 mg/mL[a]	DU	2 mg/mL[d]	Visually compatible with no warfarin loss in 30 min	2010	**C**
	SKB	20 mg/mL[a]	DME	2 mg/mL[d]	Visually compatible for 24 hr at 24 °C	2078	**C**
Ceftazidime	SKB	20 mg/mL[a]	DME	2 mg/mL[d]	Haze forms in 24 hr at 24 °C	2078	**I**
Ceftriaxone sodium	RC	20 mg/mL[a]	DME	2 mg/mL[d]	Visually compatible for 24 hr at 24 °C	2078	**C**
Ciprofloxacin	MI	2 mg/mL[a]	DU	2 mg/mL[d]	Immediate haze; crystals form in 1 hr	2010	**I**
	MI	2 mg/mL[a]	DME	2 mg/mL[d]	Immediate haze; crystals form in 1 hr	2078	**I**
Dobutamine HCl	LI	1 mg/mL[a]	DU	2 mg/mL[d]	Haze and precipitate form immediately	2010	**I**
	LI	1 mg/mL[a]	DME	2 mg/mL[d]	Haze and precipitate form immediately	2078	**I**
Dopamine HCl	FAU	1.6 mg/mL[a]	DU	2 mg/mL[d]	Visually compatible with no warfarin loss in 30 min	2010	**C**
	DU	1.6 mg/mL[a]	DME	2 mg/mL[d]	Visually compatible for 24 hr at 24 °C	2078	**C**
Epinephrine HCl	AMR	0.1 mg/mL[a,b]	DU	0.1[a,b] and 2[d] mg/mL	Physically compatible for 24 hr at 23 °C	2011	**C**
Esmolol HCl	OHM	10 mg/mL[a]	DU	2 mg/mL[d]	Haze forms immediately	2010	**I**
	OHM	10 mg/mL[a]	DME	2 mg/mL[d]	Haze forms immediately	2078	**I**
Gentamicin sulfate	SC	1.6 mg/mL[a]	DU	2 mg/mL[d]	Haze forms immediately	2010	**I**
	SC	1.6 mg/mL[a]	DME	2 mg/mL[d]	Haze forms immediately	2078	**I**

Y-Site Injection Compatibility (1:1 Mixture) (Cont.)

Warfarin sodium

Drug	Mfr	Conc	Mfr	Conc	Remarks	Ref	C/I
Heparin sodium	AB	100 units/mL[a]	DU	2 mg/mL[d]	Visually compatible with no warfarin loss in 30 min	2010	C
	AB	100 units/mL[a]	DME	2 mg/mL[d]	Visually compatible for 24 hr at 24 °C	2078	C
Labetalol HCl	SC	0.8 mg/mL[a]	DU	2 mg/mL[d]	Haze forms immediately	2010	I
	SC	0.8 mg/mL[a]	DME	2 mg/mL[d]	Haze forms immediately	2078	I
Lidocaine HCl	AST	2 mg/mL[a]	DU	2 mg/mL[d]	Visually compatible with no warfarin loss in 30 min	2010	C
	AST	2 mg/mL[a]	DME	2 mg/mL[d]	Visually compatible for 24 hr at 24 °C	2078	C
Morphine sulfate	ES	2 mg/mL[a]	DU	2 mg/mL[d]	Visually compatible with no warfarin loss in 30 min	2010	C
	ES	2 mg/mL[a]	DME	2 mg/mL[d]	Visually compatible for 24 hr at 24 °C	2078	C
Nitroglycerin	FAU	0.4 mg/mL[a]	DU	2 mg/mL[d]	Visually compatible with no warfarin loss in 30 min	2010	C
	DU	0.4 mg/mL[a]	DME	2 mg/mL[d]	Visually compatible for 24 hr at 24 °C	2078	C
Oxytocin	FUJ	1 unit/mL[a,b]	DU	0.1[a,b] and 2[d] mg/mL	Physically compatible for 24 hr at 23 °C	2011	C
Potassium chloride	BA	0.04 mEq/mL[c]	DME	2 mg/mL[d]	Visually compatible for 24 hr at 24 °C	2078	C
Ranitidine HCl	GL	1 mg/mL[a]	DU	2 mg/mL[d]	Visually compatible with no warfarin loss in 30 min	2010	C
	GL	1 mg/mL[a]	DME	2 mg/mL[d]	Visually compatible for 24 hr at 24 °C	2078	C
Vancomycin HCl	LI	4 mg/mL[a]	DU	2 mg/mL[d]	Haze forms immediately	2010	I
	AB	10 mg/mL[a,b]	DU	0.1 mg/mL[a,b]	Physically compatible for 24 hr at 23 °C	2011	C
	AB	10 mg/mL[a,b]	DU	2 mg/mL[d]	Heavy white turbidity forms immediately	2011	I
	LI	4 mg/mL[a]	DME	2 mg/mL[d]	Haze forms immediately	2078	I

[a]Tested in dextrose 5%.
[b]Tested in sodium chloride 0.9%.
[c]Tested in dextrose 5% in sodium chloride 0.45%.
[d]Tested in sterile water for injection.

ZICONOTIDE ACETATE
AHFS 28:08.92

Products — Ziconotide acetate is available as a 100-mcg/mL solution in 1-, 2-, and 5-mL single-use vials and as a 25-mcg/mL solution in 20-mL single-use vials. The formulation also contains L-methionine and sodium chloride excipients. (1)

pH — From 4 to 5. (1)

Trade Name(s) — Prialt.

Administration — Ziconotide acetate is administered intrathecally either undiluted or diluted in preservative-free sodium chloride 0.9% using a programmable implanted variable-rate microinfusion device or an external microinfusion device and catheter. The drug is intended for use only with the following infusion devices: Medtronic Synchromed EL, SynchroMed II Infusion System, and the CADD-Micro ambulatory infusion pump. (1)

When using the Medtronic Synchromed pumps, only the undiluted 25-mcg/mL concentration should be used for the initial priming of a new pump. Three 2-mL rinses of the new pump should be performed using the 25-mcg/mL concentration. After performing the initial rinses of a new pump, only the 25-mcg/mL concentration should be used for the first fill. (1)

It should be refilled within 14 days because of initial loss of drug due to sorption to titanium internal surfaces and residual spaces in the pump. These losses do not persist after the initial use. (1)

Subsequently, the pumps may be filled with undiluted ziconotide acetate at least every 84 days or every 40 days if the drug is diluted using a Medtronic refill kit to assist in maintaining asepsis. The pumps should be emptied of any remaining solution prior to refilling. (1)

When using the CADD-Micro ambulatory infusion pump, the pump should be initially filled with ziconotide acetate 5 mcg/mL diluted in preservative-free sodium chloride 0.9%. The pump manufacturer's instructions for pump filling and refilling of the pump reservoir should be followed. (1)

Stability — Intact vials of ziconotide acetate should be stored under refrigeration and protected from light and freezing. Ziconotide acetate diluted in preservative-free sodium chloride 0.9% is stable for 24 hours under refrigeration. (1)

Implantable Pumps — Clonidine hydrochloride and morphine sulfate powders were dissolved in ziconotide acetate (Elan) injection to yield concentrations of 2 and 35 mg/mL and 25 mcg/mL, respectively. Stored at 37 °C, 11% ziconotide loss in 7 days, 4% clonidine loss in 20 days, and no morphine loss in 28 days occurred. (2752)

Compatibility Information

Additive Compatibility

Ziconotide acetate

Drug	Mfr	Conc/L	Mfr	Conc/L	Test Soln	Remarks	Ref	C/I
Bupivacaine HCl	BB	5 g[b]	ELN	25 mg[a]		90% ziconotide retained for 22 days at 37 °C. No bupivacaine loss in 30 days	2751	C
Clonidine HCl	BB	2 g[b]	ELN	25 mg[a]		No loss of either drug in 28 days at 37 °C	2703	C
Fentanyl citrate	BB	1 g[b]	ELN	25 mg[a]		10% ziconotide loss in 26 days. No fentanyl loss in 40 days at 37 °C	2772	C
Hydromorphone HCl	BB	35 g[b]	ELN	25 mg[a]		90% ziconotide retained for 19 days at 37 °C. No hydromorphone loss in 25 days	2702	C
Morphine sulfate	BB	35 g[b]	ELN	25 mg[a]		90% ziconotide retained for 8 days at 37 °C. No morphine loss in 17 days	2702	C
	BB	20 g[b]	ELN	25 mg[a]		90% ziconotide retained for 19 days at 37 °C. No morphine loss in 28 days	2713	C
	BB	20 g[b]	ELN	25 mg[a]		10% ziconotide loss in 19 days. No morphine loss in 28 days at 37 °C	2780	C
	BB	10 g[b]	ELN	25 mg[a]		10% ziconotide loss in 34 days. No morphine loss in 60 days at 37 °C	2780	C
Sufentanil citrate	BB	1 g[b]	ELN	25 mg[a]		10% ziconotide loss in 33 days. No sufentanil loss in 40 days at 37 °C	2772	C

[a]Tested in SynchroMed II implantable pumps.
[b]Drug powder dissolved in ziconotide acetate injection.

Drugs in Syringe Compatibility

Ziconotide acetate

Drug (in syringe)	Mfr	Amt	Mfr	Amt	Remarks	Ref	C/I
Clonidine HCl	BB	2 mg/mL[a]	ELN	25 mcg/mL	No loss of either drug in 28 days at 5 °C	2703	C
Hydromorphone HCl	BB	35 mg/mL[a]	ELN	25 mcg/mL	No loss of either drug in 25 days at 5 °C	2702	C
Morphine sulfate	BB	35 mg/mL[a]	ELN	25 mcg/mL	No loss of either drug in 17 days at 5 °C	2702	C

[a]Test drug powder dissolved in ziconotide acetate injection.

ZIDOVUDINE
AHFS 8:18.08.20

Products — Zidovudine is available in 20-mL single-use vials. Each milliliter of solution contains zidovudine 10 mg in water for injection. Hydrochloric acid and/or sodium hydroxide may be present to adjust the pH. (1)

pH — Approximately 5.5. (1)

Trade Name(s) — Retrovir.

Administration — Zidovudine must be diluted in dextrose 5% to a concentration no greater than 4 mg/mL prior to administration. The drug is administered by intravenous infusion at a constant rate over one hour. (1; 4) Zidovudine has also been administered by continuous intravenous infusion. (4) Intramuscular injection, intravenous bolus, and rapid intravenous infusion should be avoided. (1; 4)

Stability — Intact vials of zidovudine should be stored at 15 to 25 °C and protected from light. (1)

Central Venous Catheter — Zidovudine (Glaxo Wellcome) 1 mg/mL in dextrose 5% was found to be compatible with the ARROWg+ard Blue Plus (Arrow International) chlorhexidine-bearing triple-lumen central catheter. Essentially complete delivery of the drug was found with little or no drug loss occurring. Furthermore, chlorhexidine delivered from the catheter remained at trace amounts with no substantial increase due to the delivery of the drug through the catheter. (2335)

Compatibility Information

Solution Compatibility

Zidovudine

Solution	Mfr	Mfr	Conc/L	Remarks	Ref	C/I
Dextrose 5%				Stable for 24 hr at room temperature and 48 hr refrigerated. Use within 8 hr at room temperature and 24 hr refrigerated recommended	1	C
	a	BW	4 g	Physically compatible. No loss in 8 days at 4 and 25 °C	1411	C
Sodium chloride 0.9%	a	BW	4 g	Physically compatible. No loss in 8 days at 4 and 25 °C	1411	C

ᵃTested in PVC containers.

Additive Compatibility

Zidovudine

Drug	Mfr	Conc/L	Mfr	Conc/L	Test Soln	Remarks	Ref	C/I
Dobutamine HCl	AB	1 g	GW	2 g	D5W	No more than 5% loss for either drug at 23 °C and 2% loss at 4 °C in 24 hr	2489	C
	AB	1 g	GW	2 g	NS	No more than 4% loss for either drug at 23 °C and 2% loss at 4 °C in 24 hr	2489	C
Meropenem	ZEN	1 g	BW	4 g	NS	Visually compatible for 4 hr at room temperature	1994	C
	ZEN	20 g	BW	4 g	NS	Dark yellow discoloration forms in 4 hr at room temperature	1994	I
Ranitidine HCl	GSK	500 mg	GSK	2 g	NS	Physically compatible with no loss of either drug in 24 hr at 4 and 23 °C	2523	C
	GSK	500 mg	GSK	2 g	D5W	Physically compatible. Up to 8% ranitidine loss at 23 °C and 2% at 4 °C in 24 hr. Zidovudine losses of 5 to 6% in 24 hr at 4 and 23 °C	2523	C

Drugs in Syringe Compatibility

Zidovudine

Drug (in syringe)	Mfr	Amt	Mfr	Amt	Remarks	Ref	C/I
Pantoprazole sodium	a	4 mg/ 1 mL		10 mg/ 1 mL	Clear solution	2574	C

[a]Test performed using the formulation WITHOUT edetate disodium.

Y-Site Injection Compatibility (1:1 Mixture)

Zidovudine

Drug	Mfr	Conc	Mfr	Conc	Remarks	Ref	C/I
Acyclovir sodium	BW	7 mg/mL[a]	BW	4 mg/mL[a]	Physically compatible for 4 hr at 25 °C	1193	C
Allopurinol sodium	BW	3 mg/mL[b]	BW	4 mg/mL[b]	Physically compatible for 4 hr at 22 °C	1686	C
Amifostine	USB	10 mg/mL[a]	BW	4 mg/mL[a]	Physically compatible for 4 hr at 23 °C	1845	C
Amikacin sulfate	BR	4 mg/mL[a]	BW	4 mg/mL[a]	Physically compatible for 4 hr at 25 °C	1193	C
Amphotericin B	SQ	600 mcg/mL[a]	BW	4 mg/mL[a]	Physically compatible for 4 hr at 25 °C	1193	C
Amphotericin B cholesteryl sulfate complex	SEQ	0.83 mg/mL[a]	BW	4 mg/mL[a]	Physically compatible for 4 hr at 23 °C	2117	C
Anidulafungin	VIC	0.5 mg/mL[a]	GSK	4 mg/mL[a]	Physically compatible for 4 hr at 23 °C	2617	C
Aztreonam	SQ	40 mg/mL[a]	BW	4 mg/mL[a]	Physically compatible for 4 hr at 25 °C	1193	C
	SQ	40 mg/mL[a]	BW	4 mg/mL[a]	Physically compatible for 4 hr at 23 °C	1758	C
Ceftazidime	GL	20 mg/mL[a]	BW	4 mg/mL[a]	Physically compatible for 4 hr at 25 °C	1193	C
Ceftriaxone sodium	RC	20 mg/mL[a]	BW	4 mg/mL[a]	Physically compatible for 4 hr at 25 °C	1193	C
Cisatracurium besylate	GW	0.1, 2, 5 mg/ mL[a]	BW	4 mg/mL[a]	Physically compatible for 4 hr at 23 °C	2074	C
Clindamycin phosphate	UP	12 mg/mL[a]	BW	4 mg/mL[a]	Physically compatible for 4 hr at 25 °C	1193	C
Dexamethasone sodium phosphate	ES	0.16 mg/mL[a]	BW	4 mg/mL[a]	Physically compatible for 4 hr at 25 °C	1193	C
Dobutamine HCl	LI	5 mg/mL[a]	BW	4 mg/mL[a]	Physically compatible for 4 hr at 25 °C	1193	C
Docetaxel	RPR	0.9 mg/mL[a]	GW	4 mg/mL[a]	Physically compatible for 4 hr at 23 °C	2224	C
Dopamine HCl	AB	1.6 mg/mL[a]	BW	4 mg/mL[a]	Physically compatible for 4 hr at 25 °C	1193	C
Doripenem	JJ	5 mg/mL[a,b]	GSK	4 mg/mL[a,b]	Physically compatible for 4 hr at 23 °C	2743	C
Doxorubicin HCl liposomal	SEQ	0.4 mg/mL[a]	BW	4 mg/mL[a]	Physically compatible for 4 hr at 23 °C	2087	C
Erythromycin lactobionate	AB	20 mg/mL[a,c]	BW	4 mg/mL[a]	Physically compatible for 4 hr at 25 °C	1193	C
Etoposide phosphate	BR	5 mg/mL[a]	BW	4 mg/mL[a]	Physically compatible for 4 hr at 23 °C	2218	C
Filgrastim	AMG	30 mcg/mL[a]	BW	4 mg/mL[a]	Physically compatible for 4 hr at 22 °C	1687	C
Fluconazole	RR	2 mg/mL	BW	10 mg/mL	Physically compatible for 24 hr at 25 °C	1407	C
Fludarabine phosphate	BX	1 mg/mL[a]	BW	4 mg/mL[a]	Visually compatible for 4 hr at 22 °C	1439	C
Gemcitabine HCl	LI	10 mg/mL[b]	GW	4 mg/mL[b]	Physically compatible for 4 hr at 23 °C	2226	C
Gentamicin sulfate	IMS	2 mg/mL[a]	BW	4 mg/mL[a]	Physically compatible for 4 hr at 25 °C	1193	C
Granisetron HCl	SKB	0.05 mg/mL[a]	BW	4 mg/mL[a]	Physically compatible for 4 hr at 23 °C	2000	C
Heparin sodium	LY	100 units/ mL[a]	BW	4 mg/mL[a]	Physically compatible for 4 hr at 25 °C	1193	C
Imipenem–cilastatin sodium	MSD	5 mg/mL[a]	BW	4 mg/mL[a]	Physically compatible for 4 hr at 25 °C	1193	C

Y-Site Injection Compatibility (1:1 Mixture) (Cont.)

Zidovudine

Drug	Mfr	Conc	Mfr	Conc	Remarks	Ref	C/I
Linezolid	PHU	2 mg/mL	GW	4 mg/mL[a]	Physically compatible for 4 hr at 23 °C	2264	C
Lorazepam	WY	80 mcg/mL[a]	BW	4 mg/mL[a]	Physically compatible for 4 hr at 25 °C	1193	C
Melphalan HCl	BW	0.1 mg/mL[b]	BW	4 mg/mL[b]	Physically compatible for 3 hr at 22 °C	1557	C
Meropenem	ZEN	1 mg/mL[b]	BW	4 mg/mL[d]	Visually compatible for 4 hr at room temperature	1994	C
	ZEN	50 mg/mL[b]	BW	4 mg/mL[d]	Yellow color in 4 hr at room temperature	1994	I
Metoclopramide HCl	RB	2 mg/mL[a]	BW	4 mg/mL[a]	Physically compatible for 4 hr at 25 °C	1193	C
Morphine sulfate	ES	1 mg/mL[a]	BW	4 mg/mL[a]	Physically compatible for 4 hr at 25 °C	1193	C
Nafcillin sodium	BR	20 mg/mL[a]	BW	4 mg/mL[a]	Physically compatible for 4 hr at 25 °C	1193	C
Ondansetron HCl	GL	1 mg/mL[b]	BW	4 mg/mL[a]	Visually compatible for 4 hr at 22 °C	1365	C
Oxacillin sodium	BR	20 mg/mL[a]	BW	4 mg/mL[a]	Physically compatible for 4 hr at 25 °C	1193	C
Oxytocin	NVA	10 milliunits/mL[a]	GSK	2 mg/mL[a]	Visually compatible with no zidovudine loss in 6 hr at 20 °C	2491	C
	NVA	10 milliunits/mL[a]	GSK	4 mg/mL[a]	Visually compatible with no zidovudine loss in 6 hr at 20 °C	2491	C
Paclitaxel	NCI	1.2 mg/mL[a]	BW	4 mg/mL[a]	Physically compatible for 4 hr at 22 °C	1556	C
Pemetrexed disodium	LI	20 mg/mL[b]	GSK	4 mg/mL[a]	Physically compatible for 4 hr at 23 °C	2564	C
Pentamidine isethionate	LY	6 mg/mL[a]	BW	4 mg/mL[a]	Physically compatible for 4 hr at 25 °C	1193	C
Phenylephrine HCl	WI	1 mg/mL[a]	BW	4 mg/mL[a]	Physically compatible for 4 hr at 25 °C	1193	C
Piperacillin sodium–tazobactam sodium	LE[g]	40 + 5 mg/mL[a]	BW	4 mg/mL[a]	Physically compatible for 4 hr at 22 °C	1688	C
Potassium chloride	IMS	0.67 mEq/mL[a]	BW	4 mg/mL[a]	Physically compatible for 4 hr at 25 °C	1193	C
Ranitidine HCl	GL	1 mg/mL[a]	BW	4 mg/mL[a]	Physically compatible for 4 hr at 25 °C	1193	C
Remifentanil HCl	GW	0.025 and 0.25 mg/mL[b]	BW	4 mg/mL[a]	Physically compatible for 4 hr at 23 °C	2075	C
Sargramostim	IMM	10 mcg/mL[b]	BW	4 mg/mL[b]	Visually compatible for 4 hr at 22 °C	1436	C
Teniposide	BR	0.1 mg/mL[a]	BW	4 mg/mL[a]	Physically compatible for 4 hr at 23 °C	1725	C
Thiotepa	IMM[e]	1 mg/mL[a]	BW	4 mg/mL[a]	Physically compatible for 4 hr at 23 °C	1861	C
TNA #218 to #226[f]			GW	4 mg/mL[a]	Visually compatible for 4 hr at 23 °C	2215	C
Tobramycin sulfate	LI	2 mg/mL[a]	BW	4 mg/mL[a]	Physically compatible for 4 hr at 25 °C	1193	C
TPN #212 to #215[f]			BW	4 mg/mL[a]	Physically compatible for 4 hr at 23 °C	2109	C
Trimethoprim–sulfamethoxazole	BW	0.53 + 2.6 mg/mL[a]	BW	4 mg/mL[a]	Physically compatible for 4 hr at 25 °C	1193	C
Vancomycin HCl	LI	15 mg/mL[a]	BW	4 mg/mL[a]	Physically compatible for 4 hr at 25 °C	1193	C
Vinorelbine tartrate	BW	1 mg/mL[b]	BW	4 mg/mL[b]	Physically compatible for 4 hr at 22 °C	1558	C

[a]*Tested in dextrose 5%.*
[b]*Tested in sodium chloride 0.9%.*
[c]*Sodium bicarbonate 2.5 mEq added to adjust pH.*
[d]*Tested in sterile water for injection.*
[e]*Lyophilized formulation tested.*
[f]*Refer to Appendix I for the composition of parenteral nutrition solutions. TNA indicates a 3-in-1 admixture, and TPN indicates a 2-in-1 admixture.*
[g]*Test performed using the formulation WITHOUT edetate disodium.*

APPENDIX I: Parenteral Nutrition Formulas

The following tables summarize the composition of the total parenteral nutrition mixtures that are referenced throughout the *Handbook on Injectable Drugs*. Each unique formula that has been tested for stability and/or compatibility characteristics, alone or in combination with other drugs, is described and assigned a code number. These code numbers are used in the drug monographs to denote the TNA (3-in-1) or TPN (2-in-1) formulation being discussed (i.e., TPN #183, TPN #184, etc.). The TNA and TPN formulations are described as completely as possible from the original published sources.

The consolidation of the formulations into a single appendix is designed to avoid unnecessary repetition and to facilitate comparisons among different mixtures.

Component	Mfr	Concentration per Liter			
		#21	#22	#23	#24
Amino acids	MG	200 mL			
Amino acids 8.5% with electrolytes	TR		500 mL	500 mL	500 mL
Dextrose 50%		400 mL		500 mL	500 mL
Dextrose 33.3% in water			500 mL		
Phosphate		15 mEq[a]	30 mEq		30 mEq[a]
Acetate		15 mEq[a]	67.5 mEq		
Calcium gluconate		2 g	9 mEq	1 g	
Calcium chloride			7.2 mEq		
Potassium chloride			70 mEq		20 mEq
Sodium chloride		40 mEq	55 mEq		60 mEq
Magnesium sulfate		8.1 mEq			
Multivitamins		10 mL			
Multivitamin concentrate				5 mL	
Water for injection		qs 1000 mL			
Trace elements			present		

[a] *Potassium salt.*

Component	Mfr	Concentration per Liter					
		#25	#26	#27	#28	#29	#30
Amino acids (Aminosyn)	AB	3.5%			1%		
Amino acids (FreAmine III)	MG		4.25%			1%	
Amino acids (Travasol)	TR			4.25%			1%
Dextrose		25%	25%	25%	25%	25%	25%
Sodium phosphate	AB	10 mmol	10 mmol	10 mmol	10 mmol	10 mmol	10 mmol
Multivitamins (M.V.I.-12)	USV	10 mL	10 mL	10 mL	10 mL	10 mL	10 mL
Multielectrolyte concentrate[a]	SE	25 mL	25 mL	25 mL	25 mL	25 mL	25 mL
Trace mineral injection[b]		3.5 mL	3.5 mL	3.5 mL	3.5 mL	3.5 mL	3.5 mL

[a] *Each 25 mL provides: sodium, 25 mEq; potassium, 40.5 mEq; calcium, 5 mEq; magnesium, 8 mEq; chloride, 33.5 mEq; acetate, 40.6 mEq; and gluconate, 5 mEq.*
[b] *Each 3.5 mL provides: zinc, 2 mg; copper, 1 mg; manganese, 0.5 mg; and chromium, 10 mcg.*

Component	Mfr	Concentration per Liter						
		#31	#32	#33	#34	#35	#36	#37
Amino acids	TR	4.2%	4.2%	4.2%	4.2%	4.2%	4.2%	4.2%
Dextrose		25%	25%	25%	25%	25%	25%	25%
Sodium		29 mEq	29 mEq	29 mEq	29 mEq	69 mEq	69 mEq	69 mEq
Potassium		25 mEq	25 mEq	25 mEq	25 mEq	46 mEq	46 mEq	46 mEq
Calcium		9 mEq	9 mEq	9 mEq	4.5 mEq	9.5 mEq	9.5 mEq	9.5 mEq
Magnesium		4 mEq	4 mEq	4 mEq	4 mEq	12 mEq	12 mEq	12 mEq
Phosphorus		388 mg	388 mg	388 mg	388 mg	388 mg	388 mg	388 mg
Chloride		29 mEq	29 mEq	29 mEq	29 mEq	103 mEq	103 mEq	103 mEq
Acetate		63 mEq	63 mEq	63 mEq	63 mEq	63 mEq	63 mEq	63 mEq
Trace elements		[a,b]	[a]			[a,b]	[a,b]	[a,b]
Multivitamins	USV		10 mL				5 mL	5 mL
Vitamin B complex with C plus folic acid (Soluzyme)	UP		5 mL					5 mL

[a]Trace elements: selenium, 120 mcg; chromium, 2 mcg; zinc, 3 mg; and manganese, 0.7 mg.
[b]Trace elements: iodine, 120 mcg; and copper, 1 mg.

Component	Concentration per Liter			
	#48	#49	#50	#51
Amino acids	5%	5%	5%	5%
Dextrose	5%	5%	25%	25%
Vitamins	present		present	
Trace elements		present		present

Component	Mfr	Concentration per Liter				
		#52	#53	#54	#55	#56
Amino acids	VT	7%	2.3%			
Amino acids	AB			1.5%		
Amino acids (FreAmine III)	MG				3%	3%
Dextrose			6.5%	15%	25%	25%
Fructose		10%	3.2%			
Sodium		50 mmol	16.2 mmol	[a]	35 mEq	35 mEq
Potassium		20 mmol	18.4 mmol	[a]		
Calcium		2.5 mmol	4.9 mmol	300 mg	5 mEq[b]	5 mEq[b]
Magnesium		1.5 mmol	2.1 mmol		8 mEq	8 mEq
Phosphorus				155 mg		
Phosphate			12.1 mmol[c]		40 mEq[d]	40 mEq[d]
Chloride		55 mmol	17.8 mmol	[e]	35 mEq	35 mEq
Laevulate calcium			9.8 mmol			
Folic acid				0.5 mg		
Cyanocobalamin				[f]		
Phytonadione				0.2 mg		
Multivitamins			present	4 mL		10 mL
Vitamin B complex with C (Berocca-C)				0.2 mL		

[a]Adjusted to provide 2.5 mEq/kg/day.
[b]Present as the gluconate.
[c]Anion not specified.
[d]Present as the potassium salt.
[e]Adjusted to provide 5 mEq/kg/day.
[f]Present but concentration not specified.

Component	Mfr	Concentration per Liter				
		#57	#58[a]	#59	#60	#61
Amino acids	MG	2.125%	4.25%			
Amino acids	TR			2.125%		
Amino acids	AB				3%	
Amino acids with electrolytes	TR			4.25%		
Dextrose		10%	25%	25%	25%	20%
Sodium		40 mEq	100 mmol	50 mEq	50 mEq	30 mEq
Potassium		30 mEq	60 to 80 mmol			25 mEq
Calcium		15 mEq	5 mmol	5 mEq	5 mEq	15 mEq
Magnesium		12.5 mEq	5 mmol	5 mEq	5 mEq	10 mEq
Phosphorus		6 mmol	10 mmol	465 mg	465 mg	15 mmol
Chloride		40 mEq	100 mmol	50 mEq	50 mEq	
Heparin sodium			1000 units	500 units	500 units	
Phytonadione				1 mg	1 mg	
Multivitamins			10 mL	10 mL	10 mL	2 mL
Multivitamin concentrate		2 mL				
Iron			1 mg			
Trace elements		present	present	present	present	present

[a]Concentration per 1200 mL.

Component	Mfr	Component Amounts						
		#62	#63	#64	#65	#66	#67	#68
Amino acids 8.5% (FreAmine III)	MG	500 mL	500 mL			500 mL		
Amino acids 5.4% (Nephramine)	MG			500 mL			500 mL	
Amino acids 5.2% (Aminosyn RF)	AB				500 mL			500 mL
Dextrose 50%	MG	500 mL	500 mL	500 mL	500 mL	500 mL	500 mL	500 mL
Hyperlyte (electrolyte) concentrate	MG		25 mL					
Fat emulsion 10%, intravenous	CU					500 mL	500 mL	500 mL
Multivitamins (M.V.I.-12)	USV	a	a	a	a	a	a	a

[a]Tested both with and without multivitamins.

Component	Mfr	Component Amounts		
		#69	#70	#71
Amino acids 8.5% (FreAmine II)	MG	1000 mL		
Amino acids 8.5% with electrolytes	TR			1500 mL[a]
Amino acids 7%	AB		500 mL	
Dextrose 50%		500 mL	500 mL	1500 mL
Dextrose 20% with electrolyte pattern A	TR	500 mL[b]		
Dextrose 20%		500 mL		
Sodium chloride 0.9%		500 mL		
Potassium chloride		20 mmol		
Calcium gluconate 10%				30 mL
Multivitamins		1 ampul		10 mL
Multivitamin concentrate			5 mL	
Folic acid		1 mg	0.25, 0.5, 0.75, 1 mg	
Trace elements				present

[a]Each 1500 mL provides: sodium, 105 mEq; potassium, 90 mEq; magnesium, 15 mEq; chloride, 105 mEq; acetate, 203 mEq; and phosphate, 45 mmol.
[b]Each 500 mL provides: magnesium, 14 mmol; calcium, 13 mmol; chloride, 54 mmol; acetate, 0.08 mmol; zinc, 0.04 mmol; and manganese, 0.02 mmol.

Component	Mfr	Component Amounts			
		#72	#73	#74	#75
Amino acids 10%	TR	750 mL	750 mL		
Amino acids 8.5%	TR			500 mL	
Amino acids 8.5%	MG				500 mL
Dextrose 70%		429 mL	429 mL		300 mL
Dextrose 50%				500 mL	
Fat emulsion 20%, intravenous	TR	225 mL	225 mL		
Sterile water for injection		24.2 mL	15 mL		300 mL
Calcium gluconate 10%		20 mL	20 mL		
Calcium gluceptate					8 mEq
Sodium phosphate			15 mmol		
Potassium phosphate		20 mmol		30 mEq	18 mEq
Potassium chloride		30 mEq	40 mEq	20 mEq	20 mEq
Magnesium sulfate 50%		2 mL	2 mL		8 mEq
Sodium chloride		60 mEq	60 mEq	40 mEq	60 mEq
Sodium acetate					5 mEq
Heparin sodium			6000 units		
Multivitamins		10 mL	10 mL		
Trace elements		present	present		

Component	Mfr	Concentration per Liter		
		#86	#87	#88
Amino acids (Aminosyn)	AB	2.5%	4.25%	5%
Dextrose		10%	25%	35%
Calcium		4.5 mEq	4.5 mEq	4.5 mEq
Magnesium		5 mEq	5 mEq	5 mEq
Potassium		23 mEq	40 mEq	40 mEq
Sodium		47 mEq	35 mEq	35 mEq
Acetate		82 mEq	74.5 mEq	74.5 mEq
Chloride		35 mEq	52.5 mEq	52.5 mEq
Phosphorus		9 mmol	12 mmol	12 mmol
Heparin sodium		1000 units	1000 units	1000 units
Insulin		[a]	[a]	[a]

[a] *Insulin 10 to 40 units/L.*

Component	Concentration per Liter	
	#89	#90
Amino acids (Travasol)	4.25%	
Amino acids with electrolytes (Travasol with electrolytes)		4.25%
Dextrose	25%	25%

Component	Mfr	Concentration per 100 mL #91	Concentration per 2 L #92
Amino acids 10%		1.6 mL	
Nitrogen (from amino acids)	PFM		14 g
Dextrose 5%		15 mL	
Dextrose 50%			500 mL
Fat emulsion 20%, intravenous	KA		500 mL
Sodium		3 mEq	150 mEq
Potassium		2.2 mEq	120 mEq
Calcium		1 mEq	15 mEq
Magnesium		0.3 mEq	30 mEq
Phosphate		0.5 mmol	30 mmol
Chloride		2.5 mEq	150 mEq
Sulfate			30 mEq
Acetate			90 mEq
Pediatric multivitamins		5 mL	
Multivitamins			present
Trace elements		[a]	present
Heparin sodium		100 units	
Water for injection			qs 2000 mL

[a]*Trace elements: zinc, 600 mcg; copper, 40 mcg; manganese, 10 mcg; and chromium, 0.4 mcg.*

Component	Mfr	Concentration per Liter #93	#94	#95	#96
Amino acids	TR	4.25%	4.25%		
Amino acids	AB			3%	3%
Dextrose		25%	25%	20%	20%
Potassium chloride		15 mEq	15 mEq	25 mEq	25 mEq
Sodium chloride		15 mEq	15 mEq	30 mEq	30 mEq
Calcium gluconate		4.7 mEq	4.7 mEq	15 mEq	15 mEq
Magnesium sulfate		4.05 mEq	4.05 mEq	10 mEq	10 mEq
Potassium phosphate		5 mEq	5 mEq	15 mmol	15 mmol
Sodium phosphate		10 mEq	10 mEq		
Zinc		1.5 mg	1.5 mg	3 mg	3 mg
Manganese		150 mcg	150 mcg	50 mcg	50 mcg
Chromium		6 mcg	6 mcg	2 mcg	2 mcg
Selenium		30 mcg	30 mcg		
Copper			600 mcg	200 mcg	200 mcg
Multivitamins	LY			2 mL	2 mL
Heparin sodium	IX			1000 units	

Component	Mfr	Milliliters per Container #97	#98	#99	#100	#101	#102	#103	#104
Amino acids 8.5% (FreAmine III)	MG	10	10	10	10	75	75	75	75
Dextrose 70%		89	36	89	36	89	36	89	36
Fat emulsion 20%, intravenous (Intralipid)	KV	5	5	75	75	5	5	50	50
Sterile water qs ad		250	250	250	250	250	250	250	250
Other components		[a]	[a]	[a]	[a]	[a]	[a]	[a]	[a]

[a]*Each TNA admixture also contained: sodium, 25 mEq; potassium, 25 mEq; calcium, 5 mEq; magnesium, 25 mEq; chloride, 30 mEq; acetate, 7.5 mEq; lactate, 10.5 mEq; phosphate, 1.5 mmol; multivitamins (M.V.I. Pediatric), 2.5 mL; trace elements; and heparin sodium, 250 units.*

Component	Mfr	Concentration per Liter			
		#105	#106	#107	#108
Amino acids	TR	1.65%	4.25%	1.5%	1.5%
Dextrose		10%	10%	15%	15%
Sodium		21 mEq	35 mEq		
Potassium		18 mEq	30 mEq		
Magnesium		3 mEq	5 mEq		
Calcium		15 mEq	10 mEq		
Phosphate		10 mmol	15 mmol		
Chloride		21 mEq	35 mEq		
Acetate		30 mEq	68 mEq		
Pediatric multivitamins		1 mL	1 mL		
Trace elements		0.1 mL	0.1 mL		
Unspecified electrolytes and vitamins				present	present

Component	Mfr	Concentration per Liter				
		#109	#110	#111	#112	#113
Amino acids (FreAmine III)	MG	4.25%	2%	4.25%	2.125%	
Amino acids (Travasol)	TR					4.25%
Fat emulsion 20%, intravenous (Intralipid)	KV			200 mL	125 mL	
Dextrose		25%	25%	20%	25%	25%
Sodium		50 mEq	50 mEq	50 mEq	50 mEq	35 mEq
Potassium		40 mEq	40 mEq	40 mEq	40 mEq	30 mEq
Chloride		40 mEq	40 mEq	a	a	35 mEq
Phosphorus		13 mmol	13 mmol	6 mmol	6 mmol	15 mmol
Acetate		31 mEq	31 mEq	a	a	70.5 mEq
Calcium		16.7 mEq	16.7 mEq	10 mEq	10 mEq	4.7 mEq
Magnesium		10 mEq	10 mEq	5 mEq	5 mEq	5 mEq
Multivitamins		4 mL	4 mL	3.33 mL	3.33 mL	
Trace elements		present	present	present	present	present
Heparin sodium		1000 units	1000 units	1000 units	1000 units	
Sterile water		qs	qs	qs	qs	

[a] Not cited.

Component	Concentration per Liter				
	#114	#115	#116	#117	#118
Nitrogen (from amino acids)	7 g				
Amino acids (Travasol)		4.2%	4.2%	4.5%	3.7%
Dextrose	12.5%	4.2%	21%	22.7%	18.5%
Fat emulsion, intravenous	50 g[a]				3.7%
Sodium	75 mEq	66.7 mmol	66.7 mmol	40.9 mEq	45 mEq
Potassium	60 mEq	50 mmol	50 mmol	36.4 mEq	40 mEq
Magnesium	15 mEq	4.16 mmol	4.16 mmol	7.3 mEq	8 mEq
Calcium	7.5 mEq	4.16 mmol	4.16 mmol	4.5 mEq	5 mEq
Chloride	75 mEq	66.7 mmol	66.7 mmol	48.2 mEq	53 mEq
Phosphorus	15 mmol	8.3 mmol	8.3 mmol	13.6 mmol	15 mmol
Sulfate	15 mEq				
Acetate	45 mEq	90.8 mmol	90.8 mmol	76.4 mEq	84 mEq
Trace elements	present	present	present		
Multivitamins	present	8.3 mL	8.3 mL		
Sterile water for injection	qs				
Iron		833 mcg	833 mcg		
Heparin sodium		1000 units	1000 units		

[a] Both Intralipid (long-chain triglycerides) and MCT/LCT (medium- and long-chain triglycerides) tested.

Component	Mfr	Concentration per Liter						
		#119	#120	#121	#122	#123	#124	#125
Amino acids		4.25%	4.25%	5%	5%	1%	2%	
Amino acids (TrophAmine)	MG							2%
Dextrose		35%	35%	20%	14.3%	10%	10%	10%
Fat emulsion					5.7%			
Sodium chloride		50 mEq	50 mEq	20 mEq	4 mEq	16 mEq	16 mEq	16 mEq
Potassium chloride				20 mEq	30 mEq	5 mEq	5 mEq	5 mEq
Potassium phosphate		30 mEq	30 mEq		3 mmol	10 to 40 mmol	10 to 40 mmol	10 to 40 mmol
Magnesium sulfate		10 mEq	10 mEq	8 mEq	12 mEq	4 mEq	4 mEq	4 mEq
Calcium gluconate		4.7 mEq	4.7 mEq	4.8 mEq	4 mEq	10 to 40 mEq	10 to 40 mEq	10 to 40 mEq
Sodium phosphates				20 mEq				
Sodium acetate					20 mEq	10 mEq	10 mEq	10 mEq
Cysteine HCl								1 g
Mixed electrolytes	LY				27 mL			
Trace Elements		1 mL	1 mL	present	3 mL			
Heparin sodium			1000 units					
Multivitamins				10 mL	10 mL			
Phytonadione					1 mg			
Cimetidine HCl					1 g			

Component	Mfr	Concentration per Liter							
		#126	#127	#128	#129	#130	#131	#132	#133
Amino acids (Aminosyn II)	AB	2%	3.3%	3.6%	3.6%	5%	3.5%	3.5%	
Amino acids (Travasol)	TR								4.25%
Dextrose		14.8%	3.3%	23.3%	20.8%	10%	25%	25%	25%
Fat emulsion, intravenous (Liposyn II)	AB	1.2%	3.3%	3.3%	2%	7.1%			
Sodium		39.5 mEq	51.7 mEq	48.4 mEq	96.3 mEq	49.4 mEq	33.6 mEq	33.6 mEq	75 mEq
Potassium		27 mEq	13.3 mEq	21.4 mEq	60 mEq	78.6 mEq	35.6 mEq	35.6 mEq	20 mEq
Calcium		6.6 mEq	3 mEq	6.7 mEq	10 mEq	13.4 mEq	4.5 mEq	4.5 mEq	9.6 mEq
Magnesium		3.2 mEq	3.3 mEq	10 mEq	12 mEq	14.5 mEq	5 mEq	5 mEq	10 mEq
Phosphate		5.5 mmol	10 mmol	10 mmol	15 mmol	21.4 mmol	12 mmol	12 mmol	10 mEq
Chloride		57.9 mEq	23.3 mEq	40 mEq	80 mEq	73.9 mEq	35 mEq	35 mEq	85 mEq
Acetate		21.9 mEq	43.6 mEq	23.9 mEq	65.8 mEq	35.9 mEq	35.7 mEq	35.7 mEq	
Trace elements		present	present	present	present	present		present	3 mL
Multivitamins (M.V.I.-12)								present	10 mL

Component	Mfr	Concentration per Liter						
		#134	#135	#136	#137	#138	#139	#140
Amino acids (Travasol)		5.8%	5.8%	5.8%	5.8%	5.8%	4.26%	6%
Dextrose	BA	23.7%	23.7%	23.7%	23.7%	23.7%	17.5%	25%
Fat emulsion, intravenous (Intralipid)	KV			3%	5%		3%	
Fat emulsion, intravenous (Liposyn II)	AB					3%	5%	
Potassium chloride		54.2 mEq	54.2 mEq	54.2 mEq	54.2 mEq	54.2 mEq	40.2 mEq	30 mEq
Sodium chloride		108 mEq	108 mEq	108 mEq	108 mEq	108 mEq	80.5 mEq	110 mEq
Calcium gluconate 10%		13.6 mL	13.6 mL	13.6 mL	13.6 mL	13.6 mL	4.65 mEq	10 mL
Magnesium sulfate 50%		1.4 mL	1.4 mL	1.4 mL	1.4 mL	1.4 mL	4 mEq	4 mL
Potassium phosphate		20.3 mmol	20.3 mmol	20.3 mmol	20.3 mmol	20.3 mmol	45 mmol	
Multivitamins		6.8 mL	6.8 mL	6.8 mL	6.8 mL	6.8 mL	5 mL	1 vial
Trace elements		present	present	present	present	present	present	present
Phytonadione								1 mg

Component	Mfr	Concentration per Liter			
		#141	#142	#143	#144
Amino acids	AB		2.5%	5%	
Amino acids (Travasol)	TR				4.25%
Dextrose		25%	25%	25%	25%
Sodium				50 mEq	22.5 mEq
Potassium			40 mEq	40 mEq	20 mEq
Magnesium			5 mEq	5 mEq	2.85 mEq
Calcium			5 mEq	5 mEq	4.25 mEq
Phosphorus			15 mmol	15 mmol	15.75 mmol
Chloride			58 mEq	58 mEq	17 mEq
Acetate					58 mEq
Multivitamins			10 mL	10 mL	
Trace elements			1 mL	1 mL	present
Heparin sodium	UP		500 units	500 units	
Sterile water for injection					qs

Component	Mfr	Concentration per Liter			
		#145	#146	#147	#148
Amino acids (Travasol)	BA	5%			
Amino acids	AB		5%	2.5%	1%
Dextrose		15%	25%	25%	25%
Sodium		45 mEq	35 mEq	35 mEq	35 mEq
Potassium		15 mEq	40 mEq	40 mEq	40 mEq
Chloride		20 mEq	35 mEq	35 mEq	35 mEq
Phosphorus		16 mmol	12 mmol	12 mmol	12 mmol
Acetate		81 mEq	82 mEq	82 mEq	82 mEq
Calcium		20 mEq	9 mEq	9 mEq	9 mEq
Magnesium			5 mEq	5 mEq	5 mEq

Component	Component Amounts									
	#149	#150	#151	#152	#153	#154	#155	#156	#157	#158
Amino acids 10% (TrophAmine)	50 mL	50 mL	50 mL	50 mL	350 mL	350 mL	350 mL	350 mL	50 mL	350 mL
Dextrose	10%	10%	10%	10%	25%	25%	25%	25%	25%	25%
Fat emulsion 20%, intravenous[a]	25 mL	25 mL	70 mL	70 mL	25 mL	25 mL	70 mL	70 mL	100 mL	100 mL
Sodium	25 mEq	100 mEq	25 mEq	100 mEq	25 mEq	100 mEq	25 mEq	100 mEq	100 mEq	100 mEq
Potassium	15 mEq	80 mEq	15 mEq	80 mEq	15 mEq	80 mEq	15 mEq	80 mEq	80 mEq	80 mEq
Chloride	25 mEq	100 mEq	25 mEq	100 mEq	25 mEq	100 mEq	25 mEq	100 mEq	100 mEq	100 mEq
Calcium	7 mEq	18 mEq	7 mEq	18 mEq	7 mEq	18 mEq	7 mEq	18 mEq	18 mEq	18 mEq
Magnesium	2.5 mEq	13 mEq	2.5 mEq	13 mEq	2.5 mEq	13 mEq	2.5 mEq	13 mEq	13 mEq	13 mEq
Phosphate	3.4 mmol	9 mmol	3.4 mmol	9 mmol	3.4 mmol	9 mmol	3.4 mmol	9 mmol	9 mmol	9 mmol
Trace elements	present	present	present	present	present	present	present	present	present	present
Multivitamins (M.V.I. Pediatric)	5 mL	5 mL	5 mL	5 mL	5 mL	5 mL	5 mL	5 mL	5 mL	5 mL
Heparin	1000 units	1000 units	1000 units	1000 units	1000 units	1000 units	1000 units	1000 units	1000 units	1000 units

[a]*Intralipid 20%, Liposyn II 20%, and Nutrilipid 20% were each tested.*

Component	Mfr	Component Amounts							
		#159	#160	#161	#162	#163	#164	#165	#166
Amino acids 5.5% with electrolytes (Travasol)	BA	100 mL	100 mL	400 mL	400 mL	400 mL	400 mL	100 mL	100 mL
Fat emulsion 20%, intravenous (Intralipid)	KV	100 mL		200 mL		100 mL		200 mL	
Fat emulsion 20%, intravenous (Liposyn II)	AB		100 mL		200 mL		100 mL		200 mL
Heparin sodium 1000 units/mL	ES	5 mL	5 mL	5 mL	5 mL	5 mL	5 mL	5 mL	5 mL
Dextrose 10%		795 mL	795 mL					695 mL	695 mL
Dextrose 20%				395 mL	395 mL	495 mL	495 mL		

Component	Component Amounts						
	#167	#168	#169	#170	#171	#172	#173
Aminoplex 12			500 mL		1000 mL		
Aminoplex 24	500 mL	500 mL	500 mL	500 mL			
Vamin glucose							1000 mL
Lipofundin S 20%	500 mL	500 mL	500 mL	500 mL	500 mL		
Fat emulsion 10%, intravenous (Intralipid)						300 mL	
Glucoplex 1000	1000 mL						
Glucoplex 1600		1000 mL	1000 mL		500 mL		
Dextrose 5%					1000 mL		
Dextrose 50%				500 mL			1000 mL
Potassium chloride 15%		37.5 mL		10 mL			
Potassium phosphate 17%	20 mL	20 mL	20 mL	20 mL	10 mL		
Sodium chloride 30%		27 mL		15 mL			
Addamel	10 mL	10 mL	10 mL	10 mL	10 mL		10 mL
Soluvit						7.5 mL	
Vitalipid infant						15 mL	
Pancebrin							10 mL

Component	Mfr	Concentration per Liter					
		#174	#175	#176	#177	#178	#179
Amino acids	AB	25 g	50 g	15 g			
Amino acids	TR				3%		
Nitrogen						7.9 g	7 g
Dextrose		125 g	250 g	100 g	5%	100 g	125 g
Fat emulsion, intravenous (Intralipid)	KV					50 g	5 g
TPN II electrolytes	AB	20 mL	20 mL				
Sodium		26.3 mEq	37.5 mEq	40 mEq	46 mEq	24 mmol	75 mEq
Potassium		35.5 mEq	40 mEq	50 mEq	40 mEq	12.5 mmol	60 mEq
Magnesium		5 mEq	5 mEq	10 mEq	8 mEq	2.5 mmol	15 mEq
Calcium		9 mEq	4.5 mEq	10 mEq	5 mEq		7.5 mEq
Phosphorus		12 mmol	45 mmol	5 mmol	12 mmol	4.5 mmol	15 mmol
Chloride		35 mEq	35 mEq	47.6 mEq	57 mEq	7 mmol	75 mEq
Acetate		25 mEq	43 mEq	31.8 mEq	61 mEq	40.5 mmol	45 mEq
Gluconate				10 mEq			
Sulfate				10 mEq			15 mEq
Trace elements			present	present	present	present	present
Multivitamins (M.V.I. Pediatric)		3 mL			3 mL		
Multivitamins (M.V.I. 9+3)			10 mL				
Multivitamins					10 mL	present	present
Vitamin K			5 mg				
Heparin sodium		1000 units	1000 units	1000 units	1000 units		
Sterile water qs ad		1000 mL	1000 mL	1000 mL		1000 mL	1000 mL

Component		Component Amounts	
		#180	#181
Amino acids 10%		1000 mL	400 mL
Dextrose 50%		500 mL	500 mL
Fat emulsion 20%, intravenous (Intralipid)		500 mL	
Sodium		40 mmol	41 mEq
Potassium		70 mmol	22.7 mEq
Calcium		4.6 mmol	5 mEq
Magnesium		5 mmol	5 mEq
Phosphorus		17.5 mmol	12 mmol
Chloride		120 mmol	30 mEq
Acetate		45 mmol	89 mEq
Trace elements			present
Multivitamins			10 mL

Component	Mfr	Concentration per Liter
		#182
Amino acids	KV	5%
Dextrose		25%
Fat emulsion, intravenous (Intralipid)	KV	2.25%
Potassium phosphate		10 mmol
Potassium chloride		45 mEq
Sodium chloride		75 mEq
Magnesium sulfate		8 mEq
Calcium gluconate		47 mg
Trace elements		present
Multivitamins		5 mL
Sterile water qs ad		1000 mL

Component	Mfr	Component Amounts						
		#183	#184	#185	#186[a]	#187[b]	#188[c]	#189
Amino acids (Aminosyn II)	AB	1%	2.5%	5%				
Amino acids (Aminosyn)	AB				15 g	25 g	50 g	
Amino acids 10% with electrolytes (Synthamin 17 with electrolytes)								500 mL
Dextrose	AB	10%	10%	25%	125 g	125 g	250 g	
Dextrose 50%								500 mL
TPN II electrolytes						1 mL	1 mL	
Calcium		9 mEq	4.4 mEq	5 mEq	1 mEq	9 mEq	4.5 mEq	2.2 mmol
Magnesium		5 mEq	5 mEq	5 mEq	1 mEq	5 mEq	5 mEq	2.5 mmol
Potassium		27 mEq	18 mEq	40 mEq	5 mEq	30 mEq	40 mEq	42.5 mmol
Sodium		24 mEq	38 mEq	42 mEq	4 mEq	35 mEq	37.65 mEq	45 mmol
Phosphorus		6 mmol	9 mmol	15 mmol	2 mmol	6 mmol	12 mmol	15 mmol
Chloride		35 mEq	35 mEq	43 mEq	5.7 mEq	46.9 mEq	39.4 mEq	55.65 mmol
Acetate		22 mEq	25 mEq	38 mEq	11.1 mEq	25.6 mEq	43.5 mEq	81.25 mmol
Gluconate					1.1 mEq	2.5 mEq	0.05 mEq	
Sulfate					1.1 mEq			
Trace elements		1 mL	1 mL	1 mL	0.6 mL	1 mL	1 mL	present
Multivitamins (M.V.I. Pediatric)	AST				3 mL	3 mL		
Multivitamins (M.V.I. 9+3)	AST						10 mL	
Heparin sodium	ES				1000 units	1000 units	1000 units	
Sterile water					qs	qs	qs	

[a]Neonatal formula.
[b]Pediatric formula.
[c]Adult formula.

Component	Mfr	Component Amounts		
		#190	#191	#192
Amino acids (Aminosyn II 15%)	AB	333 mL		
Amino acids (Azonutril 25)			500 mL	
Amino acids				17 g
Dextrose 70%		500 mL		
Dextrose 50%			250 mL	
Dextrose 30%			750 mL	
Dextrose				42.4 g
Fat emulsion 20%, intravenous (Intralipid)			500 mL	24.2 g
Fat emulsion 20%, intravenous (Liposyn II)	AB	400 mL		
Sterile water		133 mL		
Sodium				55.7 mmol
Potassium				19.4 mmol
Magnesium				2.3 mmol
Calcium				1.5 to 150 mmol
Phosphate				21 to 300 mmol
Unspecified electrolytes		present		
Vitamins		present		present
Trace elements			present	present

Component	Mfr	Component Amounts
		#193
Amino acids 10%	CL	1000 mL
Dextrose 50%	CL	750 mL
Sodium chloride	AB	140 mEq
Potassium phosphates	AB	20 mmol
Calcium gluconate		4.8 mEq
Magnesium sulfate		40 mEq
Multivitamins	AST	10 mL
Trace elements	LY	3 mL
Famotidine		40 mg

Component	Concentration per Liter	
	#194	#195
Amino acids	2.2%	2.2%
Dextrose	12.5%	20%
Sodium chloride	26 mEq	26 mEq
Potassium phosphates	15 mmol	15 mmol
Calcium gluconate	25 mEq	25 mEq
Magnesium sulfate	8 mEq	8 mEq
Potassium chloride	2 mEq	2 mEq
Heparin sodium	1000 units	1000 units
Cysteine	660 mg	660 mg
Trace elements	present	present
Multivitamins	20 mL	20 mL

Component	Mfr	Concentration per Liter				
		#196	#197	#198	#199	#200
Amino acids	BA	6%	6%	6%	6%	6%
Dextrose	BA	24%	24%	24%	24%	24%
Intralipid	KV		3%	5%		
Liposyn II	AB				3%	5%
Sodium chloride	LY	108 mEq	108 mEq	108 mEq	108 mEq	108 mEq
Potassium phosphates	AB	20 mmol	20 mmol	20 mmol	20 mmol	20 mmol
Calcium gluconate	LY	6.3 mEq	6.3 mEq	6.3 mEq	6.3 mEq	6.3 mEq
Magnesium sulfate	AST	5.6 mEq	5.6 mEq	5.6 mEq	5.6 mEq	5.6 mEq
Potassium chloride	AB	54 mEq	54 mEq	54 mEq	54 mEq	54 mEq
Trace elements	SO	present	present	present	present	present
Multivitamins	AR	6.8 mL	6.8 mL	6.8 mL	6.8 mL	6.8 mL

Component	Mfr	Concentration per Liter			
		#201	#202	#203[a]	#204[b]
Amino acids	BA	4.25%			
Amino acids	AB		4.25%		
Amino acids (TrophAmine)	MG			2%	3%
Dextrose		25%	25%	10%	20%
Sodium		35 mEq	35 mEq	38 mEq	77 mEq
Potassium		30 mEq	30 mEq	20 mEq	40 mEq
Calcium		5 mEq	9.4 mEq	600 mg	600 mg
Magnesium		3 mEq	10 mEq	2.5 mEq	2.5 mEq
Chloride		47 mEq	[c]	38 mEq	77 mEq
Phosphate		14.3 mEq	15 mmol	400 mg	400 mg
Acetate		67 mEq	50 mEq	29 mEq	58 mEq
L-Cysteine				200 mg	300 mg
Trace elements			present	present	present
Multivitamins			present	present	present
Heparin					500 units

[a]Calculated quantities from a pediatric peripheral line formula.
[b]Calculated quantities from a pediatric central line formula.
[c]Unspecified.

Component	Mfr	Concentration per Liter	
		#205	#206
Amino acids	BA	5%	
Aminosyn	AB		2.125%
Dextrose		25%	20%
Intralipid	KA		
Liposyn II	AB		
Sodium chloride		75 mEq	30 mEq
Potassium chloride		60 mEq	30 mEq
Potassium phosphates		20 mmol	
Sodium phosphates			15 mmol
Calcium gluconate		10 mEq	14 mEq
Magnesium sulfate		10 mEq	50 mg
Trace elements		present	present
Multivitamins			
Heparin sodium		3000 to 20,000 units	

Component	Mfr	Concentration per Liter				
		#207	#208	#209	#210	#211
Amino acids (TrophAmine)	MG	0.5%	1%	1.5%	2%	2.5%
Dextrose		10%	10%	10%	10%	10%
Sodium chloride		20 mEq	20 mEq	20 mEq	20 mEq	20 mEq
Sodium acetate		10 mEq	10 mEq	10 mEq	10 mEq	10 mEq
Potassium acetate		5 mEq	5 mEq	5 mEq	5 mEq	5 mEq
Potassium phosphates		10 mmol	10 mmol	10 mmol	10 mmol	10 mmol
Calcium gluconate		20 mEq	20 mEq	20 mEq	20 mEq	20 mEq
Magnesium sulfate		4 mEq	4 mEq	4 mEq	4 mEq	4 mEq
Trace elements	FUJ	[a]	[a]	[a]	[a]	[a]
Multivitamins	AST	[b]	[b]	[b]	[b]	[b]
Heparin sodium		1000 units	1000 units	1000 units	1000 units	1000 units
L-Cysteine[c]		200 mg	400 mg	600 mg	800 mg	1 g

[a]Tested with and without trace elements (Neotrace, Fujisawa).
[b]Tested with and without multivitamins (M.V.I. Pediatric, Astra) 3.5 mL/L.
[c]40 mg/g of protein.

Component	Mfr	Concentration per Liter				
		#212	#213	#214	#215	#216[a]
Amino acids (Aminosyn II)	AB	3.5%		4.25%		
Amino acids (FreAmine III)	MG		3.5%		4.25%	
Amino acids (Travasol)	BA					0.5 to 5%
Dextrose		5%	5%	25%	25%	10 to 20%
Sterile water for injection		516.8 mL	516.75 mL	161 mL	158.6 mL	q.s.
Potassium phosphates		3.5 mmol	[b]	15 mmol	5.75 mmol[c]	0 to 20 mEq K[d]
Sodium chloride		25 mEq	37.5 mEq	25 mEq	40 mEq	0 to 44 mEq
Sodium acetate						0 to 40 mEq
Potassium chloride		35 mEq	40 mEq	18 mEq	25 mEq	0 to 20 mEq
Magnesium sulfate		8 mEq	8 mEq	8 mEq	8 mEq	4 mEq
Calcium gluconate		9.3 mEq	5 mEq	9.15 mEq	7.5 mEq	19.2 to 28.8 mEq
Multivitamins	AST	10 mL	10 mL	10 mL	10 mL	14 mL
Trace elements		present	present	present	present	present
Heparin sodium	ES					500 units
Ranitidine (as HCl)	GL					0 to 84 mg

[a]Forty parenteral nutrition formulations within the ranges cited were tested. Specific formulations were not reported.
[b]No phosphates added. Phosphates from FreAmine III formulation yielded 3.5 mmol/L.
[c]Added phosphates indicated. All phosphates from addition plus FreAmine III formulation totaled 10 mmol/L.
[d]Reported as potassium concentration.

Component	Mfr	Concentration per Liter			
		#217	#218	#219	#220
Amino acids		5%			
Amino acids	MG		3%	3%	
Amino acids	AB				3%
Dextrose		25%	5%	5%	5%
Intralipid	KA		2%		
Liposyn II	AB			2%	
Liposyn III	AB				2%
Sodium		50 mEq	43 mEq	43 mEq	41.6 mEq
Potassium		40 mEq	40 mEq	40 mEq	40 mEq
Chloride		58 mEq	45 mEq	45 mEq	35 mEq
Phosphorus		15 mmol	7.5 mmol	7.5 mmol	15 mmol
Calcium		5 mEq	5 mEq	5 mEq	9.15 mEq
Magnesium		8 mEq	8 mEq	8 mEq	8 mEq
Acetate			51.7 mEq	51.7 mEq	42 mEq
Heparin sodium		1000 units			
Multivitamins		10 mL	10 mL	10 mL	10 mL
Phytonadione		1 mg			
Trace elements		2 mL	1 mL	1 mL	1 mL
Sterile water for injection			qs	qs	qs

Component	Mfr	Concentration per Liter					
		#221	#222	#223	#224	#225	#226
Amino acids	MG	4.9%	4.9%			6%	6%
Amino acids	AB			4.9%	6%		
Dextrose		20%	20%	20%	11%	10.7%	10.7%
Intralipid	KA		3.5%				4%
Liposyn II	AB	3.5%				4%	
Liposyn III	AB			3.5%	4%		
Sodium		39.8 mEq	39.8 mEq	39.7 mEq	45 mEq	45 mEq	45 mEq
Potassium		40 mEq	40 mEq	40 mEq	40 mEq	40.2 mEq	40.2 mEq
Calcium		7.5 mEq	7.5 mEq	9.15 mEq	9.15 mEq	7.5 mEq	7.5 mEq
Magnesium		8 mEq	8 mEq	8 mEq	8 mEq	8 mEq	8 mEq
Chloride		45 mEq	45 mEq	35 mEq	35 mEq	51 mEq	51 mEq
Acetate		67.7 mEq	67.7 mEq	45 mEq	53.2 mEq	78.4 mEq	78.4 mEq
Phosphate		10 mmol	10 mmol	15 mmol	15 mmol	10 mmol	10 mmol
Multivitamins		10 mL	10 mL	10 mL	10 mL	10 mL	10 mL
Trace elements		1 mL	1 mL	1 mL	1 mL	1 mL	1 mL

Component	Mfr	Concentration per Liter				
		#227	#228	#229	#230	#231
Aminosyn II	AB	2%	3.5%	4.25%	4.25%	5%
Dextrose	AB	10%	10%	15%	25%	25%
Sodium (as chloride)	AB	40 mEq	40 mEq	70 mEq	70 mEq	70 mEq
Potassium (as chloride)	AB	20 mEq	20 mEq	50 mEq	50 mEq	50 mEq
Magnesium (as sulfate)	AB	8 mEq	8 mEq	12 mEq	12 mEq	12 mEq
Phosphates (as potassium)	AB	up to 40 mmol	up to 40 mmol	up to 40 mmol	up to 40 mmol	up to 40 mmol
Calcium (as acetate)	AB	up to 40 mEq	up to 40 mEq	up to 40 mEq	up to 40 mEq	up to 40 mEq

Component	Mfr	Component Amounts					
		#232	#233	#234	#235	#236	#237
Synthamin 17		500 mL	500 mL	500 mL	500 mL		
Vaminolact	FRE					150 mL	150 mL
Dextrose 50%		500 mL	500 mL	500 mL	500 mL	180 mL	154 mL
Sterile water for injection		500 mL	500 mL	500 mL	500 mL		
Intralipid 20%		500 mL	500 mL	500 mL	500 mL		
Medialipide	BRN						50 mL
Albumin, human		100 mL	100 mL	200 mL	200 mL		
Sodium chloride 10%						6.08 mL	6.08 mL
Potassium chloride 10%						18.66 mL	18.66 mL
Calcium chloride			7 mmol		7 mmol		
Calcium gluconate/glucoheptonate						16.1 mL	16.1 mL
Magnesium sulfate			10 mmol		10 mmol		
Magnesium sulfate 15%						1.64 mL	1.64 mL
Phosphorus (Phocytan)						14.56 mL	14.56 mL
Vitamins (Soluvit)						5 mL	5 mL
Trace elements, pediatric (OEP)						10 mL	10 mL

Component	Mfr	Component Amounts		
		#238	#239	#240
Aminoplex 12	GEI	200 mL		
FreAmine III	FRE		200 mL	
Vamin 14	PH			200 mL
Dextrose 20%	BA	300 mL	300 mL	300 mL
Addiphos	PH	4 mL	4 mL	4 mL
Additrace	PH	2 mL	2 mL	2 mL

Component	Mfr	Concentration per Liter	
		#241	#242
Aminosyn	AB	4.25%	5%
Dextrose		25%	25%
Calcium		4.5 mEq	4.5 mEq
Magnesium		5 mEq	5 mEq
Potassium		40 mEq	40 mEq
Sodium		35 mEq	35 mEq
Acetate		74.5 mEq	74.5 mEq
Chloride		52.5 mEq	52.5 mEq
Phosphorus		12 mmol	12 mmol
Heparin sodium		1000 units	1000 units

Component	Concentration per Liter		
	#243	#244	#245
Amino acids (Aminosyn)	4%		
Amino acids (TrophAmine)		3%	
Nitrogen			0.8%
Dextrose	20%	20%	12.5%
Fat emulsion			5%
Sodium chloride	93 mEq	48 mEq	20 mEq
Potassium (from acetate and phosphate)	60 mEq	40 mEq	35 mEq
Calcium (as gluconate)	330 mg	600 mg	4.6 mEq
Chloride			60 mEq
Acetate			22.5 mEq
Magnesium sulfate	8 mEq	4.3 mEq	5 mEq
Trace elements (pediatric)	3 mL	3 mL	
L-Cysteine HCl (40 mg/g amino acids)		1.2 g	
Multivitamin injection (M.V.I. Pediatric)	5 mL	5 mL	present
Heparin sodium	500 units	500 units	

Component	Concentration per Liter	
	#246	#247
Amino acids (Aminoplasmal L10)	1000 mL	1000 mL
Dextrose 37.5% with electrolytes	500 mL	500 mL
Dextrose 10%	500 mL	500 mL
Fat emulsion (Lipofundin-S 20%)	500 mL	
Sterile water for injection		500 mL
Calcium gluconate	2.5 mmol	2.5 mmol
Magnesium sulfate	2 mmol	2 mmol
Addamel	10 mL	10 mL
Potassium phosphate	20 mL[a]	20 mL[a]
Sodium chloride 30%	8 mL	8 mL
Folic acid	15 mg	15 mg
Multivitamins	present	present
Trace elements	present	present

[a] Provided potassium 20 mEq and phosphate 10 mmol.

Component	Concentration per Liter	
	#248	#249
Amino acids (Aminotripa 2)	3.3%	
Amino Acids (Unicaliq N)		3%
Dextrose	19.4%	17.5%
Sodium	38.9 mEq	40 mEq
Potassium	30 mEq	27 mEq
Magnesium	5.6 mEq	6 mEq
Calcium	5.6 mEq	6 mEq
Chloride	38.9 mEq	59 mEq
Sulfate	5.6 mEq	
Acetate	60 mEq	10 mEq
Gluconate	5.6 mEq	6 mEq
Citrate	12.2 mEq	
L-Malate		17 mEq
L-Lactate		35 mEq
Phosphorus	206.7 mg	250 mg
Zinc	11.1 mcmol	20 mcmol

Component	Concentration per Liter							
	#250	#251	#252	#253	#254	#255	#256	#257
Aminosyn II	4%	4%	3.7%	3.7%	2.8%	2.8%	2.5%	2.5%
Dextrose	17.6%	17.6%	16.1%	16.1%	17.6%	17.6%	16.1%	16.1%
Liposyn II	6.0%		5.5%		6.0%		5.5%	
Intralipid		6.0%		5.5%		6.0%		5.5%
Sodium chloride			104 mEq	104 mEq			109 mEq	109 mEq
Potassium chloride			47 mEq	47 mEq			47 mEq	47 mEq
Potassium acetate			43 mEq	43 mEq			43 mEq	43 mEq
Sodium phosphates			11 mmol	11 mmol			11 mmol	11 mmol
Magnesium sulfate			6 mEq	6 mEq			6 mEq	6 mEq
Calcium gluconate			5.1 mEq	5.1 mEq			5 mEq	5 mEq
Sterile water for injection	qs	qs	qs	qs	qs	qs	qs	qs

Component	Concentration per Liter				
	#258	#259	#260	#261	#262
FreAmine III	1%	2%	3%	4%	5%
Dextrose	15%	15%	25%	25%	25%
Cysteine HCl	250 mg	500 mg	750 mg	1 g	1.25 g
Sodium chloride	40 mEq	40 mEq	40 mEq	70 mEq	70 mEq
Potassium chloride	20 mEq	20 mEq	20 mEq	50 mEq	50 mEq
Magnesium sulfate	8 mEq	8 mEq	8 mEq	12 mEq	12 mEq
Sterile water for injection	qs	qs	qs	qs	qs

Component	Concentration per Liter				
	#263	#264	#265	#266	#267
Travasol 10%	267 mL				
Fravasol 10%		250 mL			
Livaframine 10%			250 mL		
Synthamin 10%				500 mL	
Amino acids 17%					1000 mL
Dextrose 70%	347 mL				
Dextrose 50%				500 mL	500 mL
Dextrose 10%		250 mL	250 mL		
Sterile water for injection	367 mL				
Fat emulsion 20%					500 mL
Sodium	36.6 mEq		5 mmoL		
Potassium	26.6 mEq				
Calcium	5 mEq				
Chloride	50 mEq	20 mmoL	4.5 mmoL		
Acetate		41 mmoL	31 mmoL		
Phosphate	9 mmoL		5 mmoL		
Trace elements	present				

| | Concentration per Liter |
Component	#268
Aminosyn 15%	29.75 mL
Dextrose 70%	37.5 mL
Sterile water for injection	33.65 mL
Sodium chloride	4.7 mEq
Potassium chloride	2.1 mEq
Potassium phosphates	1.05 mmol
Magnesium sulfate	80 mg
Calcium gluconate	137 mg

| | Concentration per Liter | | | | |
Component	#269	#270	#271	#272	#273
Amino acids (Aminoplasmal 16%)	7.12%	7.34%	7.49%	7.6%	7.68%
Dextrose 70%	19.69%	20.35%	20.82%	21.0%	21.32%
Fat emulsion 20% (Lipofundin MCT)	2.49%	2.54%	2.58%	2.68%	2.69%
Sodium	118.6 mEq	97.8 mEq	83.3 mEq	72.4 mEq	64 mEq
Potassium	71.2 mEq	58.7 mEq	49.9 mEq	43.5 mEq	38.4 mEq
Calcium	11.9 mEq	9.8 mEq	8.3 mEq	7.2 mEq	6.4 mEq
Magnesium	11.9 mEq	9.8 mEq	8.3 mEq	7.2 mEq	6.4 mEq
Phosphate	28.5 mmol	23.5 mmol	19.9 mmol	17.4 mmol	15.4 mmol
Chloride	118.6 mEq	97.8 mEq	83.3 mmol	72.4 mEq	64.0 mEq
Trace elements	3.6 mL	2.9 mL	2.5 mL	2.2 mL	1.9 mL
Multivitamins	11.9 mL	9.8 mL	8.3 mL	7.2 mL	6.4 mL

| | Concentration per Liter | |
Component	#274	#275
TrophAmine	3.75%	
Amino acids		3.6%
Dextrose	17.5%	10.6%
Sodium	25 mEq	36 mEq
Potassium	19 mEq	25.5 mEq
Calcium	19 mEq	6.4 mEq
Magnesium	3.8 mEq	6.4 mEq
Phosphates	12.5 mEq	5.5 mmol
Acetate	25 mEq	70 mEq
M.V.I.-Pediatric	52 mL	
Trace elements (pediatric)	2.5 mL	
Ranitidine HCl	73 mL	

| | Concentration per Liter |
Component	#276
Aminosyn	4.25%
Dextrose	25%
Sterile water for injection	97.68 mL
Sodium chloride	50 mEq
Potassium chloride	40 mEq
Potassium phosphates	10 mmol
Magnesium sulfate	8 mEq
Calcium chloride and gluconate	10 mEq

HID REFERENCES

1. Package insert (for brands listed after the nonproprietary name heading a monograph; date of package insert given as part of citation).

2. Physicians' desk reference. 63rd ed. Montvale, NJ: Thomson PDR; 2009.

3. Kirkland WD, Jones RW, Ellis JR, et al. Compatibility studies of parenteral admixtures. *Am J Hosp Pharm.* 1961; 18:694–9.

4. McEvoy GK, ed. AHFS drug information 2011. Bethesda, MD: American Society of Health-System Pharmacists; 2011.

5. Sweetman SC, ed. Martindale: the complete drug reference. 37th ed. London, England: The Pharmaceutical Press; 2011.

6. Parker EA. Staphcillin injection. *Am J Hosp Pharm.* 1970; 27: 67–8.

7. Parker EA. Compatibility digest. *Am J Hosp Pharm.* 1970; 27: 672–3.

8. Trissel LA. Trissel's stability of compounded formulations. 4th ed. Washington, DC: American Pharmacists Association; 2009.

9. Patel JA, Phillips GL. Guide to physical compatibility of intravenous drug admixtures. *Am J Hosp Pharm.* 1966; 23:409–11.

10. Bogash RC. Compatibilities and incompatibilities of some parenteral medication. *Bull Am Soc Hosp Pharm.* 1955; 12: 445–8.

11. Dunworth RD, Kenna FR. Preliminary report: incompatibility of combinations of medications in intravenous solutions. *Am J Hosp Pharm.* 1965; 22:190–1.

12. Moorhatch P, Chiou WL. Interactions between drugs and plastic intravenous fluid bags, part i: sorption studies on 17 drugs. *Am J Hosp Pharm.* 1974; 31:72–8.

13. Levin HJ, Fieber RA. Stability data for Tubex filled by hospital pharmacists. *Hosp Pharm.* 1973; 8:310–1.

14. Powers S. Incompatibilities of pre-op medications. *Hosp Formul Manage.* 1970; 5:22.

15. Intravenous additive incompatibilities. Bethesda, MD: Pharmacy Department, National Institutes of Health; 1970 Jan.

16. Cantania PN, King JC. Physico-chemical incompatibilities of selected cardiovascular and psychotherapeutic agents with sodium ethacrynate. *Am J Hosp Pharm.* 1972; 29:141–6.

17. The United States Pharmacopeia, 34th rev. Rockville, MD: United States Pharmacopeial Convention; 2011.

18. Kramer W, Inglott A. Some physical and chemical incompatibilities of drugs for i.v. administration. *Drug Intell Clin Pharm.* 1971; 5:211–28.

19. McEvoy GK, ed. American hospital formulary service drug information. Bethesda, MD: American Society of Health-System Pharmacists; prior editions.

20. Parker EA. Compatibility digest. *Am J Hosp Pharm.* 1969; 26: 412–3.

21. Parker EA. Compatibility digest. *Am J Hosp Pharm.* 1969; 26: 653–5.

22. Parker EA. Compatibility digest. *Am J Hosp Pharm.* 1970; 27: 327–9.

23. Parker EA. Compatibility digest. *Am J Hosp Pharm.* 1974; 31: 1076.

24. Parker EA. Compatibility digest. *Am J Hosp Pharm.* 1971; 28: 805.

25. Souney PF, Solomon MA. Visual compatibility of cimetidine hydrochloride with common preoperative injectable medications. *Am J Hosp Pharm.* 1984; 41:1840–1.

26. Riley BB. Incompatibilities in intravenous solutions. *J Hosp Pharm.* 1970; 28:228–40.

27. Parker EA, Levin HJ. Compatibility digest. *Am J Hosp Pharm.* 1975; 32:943–4.

28. Misgen R. Compatibilities and incompatibilities of some intravenous solution admixtures. *Am J Hosp Pharm.* 1965; 22: 92–4.

29. Reference number not in use.

30. Reference number not in use.

31. Reference number not in use.

32. Frank JT. Intralipid compatibility study. *Drug Intell Clin Pharm.* 1973; 7:351–2.

33. Yeo MT, Gazzaniga AB, Bartlett RH, et al. Total intravenous nutrition experience with fat emulsions and hypertonic glucose. *Arch Surg.* 1973; 106:792–6.

34. Melly MA, Meng HC. Microbial growth in lipid emulsions used in parenteral nutrition. *Arch Surg.* 1975; 110:1479–81.

35. Deitel M, Kaminsky V. Total nutrition by peripheral vein—the lipid system. *Can Med Assoc J.* 1974; 111:152–4.

36. Cashore WJ, Sedaghatian MR. Nutritional supplements with intravenously administered lipid, protein hydrolysate, and glucose in small premature infants. *Pediatrics.* 1975; 56:8–16.

37. Lynn B. Intralipid compatibility study. *Drug Intell Clin Pharm.* 1974; 8:75.

38. Electronic Medicines Compendium. London, England: Datapharm Communications Ltd.

39. Fortner CL, Grove WR, Bowie D, et al. Fat emulsion vehicle for intravenous administration of an aqueous insoluble drug. *Am J Hosp Pharm.* 1975; 32:582–4.

40. Riffkin C. Incompatibilities of manufactured parenteral products. *Am J Hosp Pharm.* 1963; 20:19–22.

41. Edward M. pH—an important factor in the compatibility of additives in intravenous therapy. *Am J Hosp Pharm.* 1967; 24: 440–9.

42. Turner FE, King JC. Spectrophotometric analysis of intravenous admixtures containing metaraminol and corticosteroids. *Am J Hosp Pharm.* 1970; 27:540–7.

43. Anderson RW, Latiolais CJ. Physico-chemical incompatibilities of parenteral admixtures—Aramine and Solu-Cortef. *Am J Hosp Pharm.* 1973; 30:128–33.

44. Smith MC. The dextrans. *Am J Hosp Pharm.* 1965; 22:273–5.

45. Stokes TF, Sumner ED. Particulate contamination and stability of three additives in 0.9% sodium chloride injection in plastic and glass large-volume containers. *Am J Hosp Pharm.* 1975; 32:821–6.

46. Parker EA. Solution additive chemical incompatibility study. *Am J Hosp Pharm.* 1967; 24:434–9.

47. Parker EA. Compatibility digest. *Am J Hosp Pharm.* 1969; 26: 543–4.

48. Parker EA. Parenteral incompatibilities. *Hosp Pharm.* 1969; 4: 14–22.

49. Beatrice MG, Stanaszek WF, Allen LV, et al. Physicochemical stability of a preanesthetic mixture of hydroxyzine hydrochloride and atropine sulfate. *Am J Hosp Pharm.* 1975; 32: 1133–7.

50. Leff RD, Roberts RJ. Effect of intravenous fluid and drug solution coadministration on final-infusate osmolality, specific gravity, and pH. *Am J Hosp Pharm.* 1982; 39:468–71.

51. Crevar GE, Slotnick IJ. A note on the stability of actinomycin D. *J Pharm Pharmacol.* 1964; 16:429.

52. Coles CLJ, Lees KA. Additives to intravenous fluids. *Pharm J.* 1971; 206:153–4.

53. Rudd L. Pethidine stability in intravenous solutions. *Med J Aust.* 1978; 2:34.

54. Webb JW. A pH pattern for i.v. additives. *Am J Hosp Pharm.* 1969; 26:31–5.

55. Jones RW, Stanko GL. Pharmaceutical compatibilities of Pentothal and Nembutal. *Am J Hosp Pharm.* 1961; 18:700–4.

56. Turco SJ, Sherman NE, Zagar L, et al. Stability of aminophylline in 5% dextrose in water. *Hosp Pharm.* 1975; 10:374–5.

57. Hodby ED, Hirsch J. Influence of drugs upon the anticoagulant activity of heparin. *Can Med Assoc J.* 1972; 106:562–4.

58. Pamperl H, Kleinberger G. Morphologic changes of Intralipid 20% liposomes in all-in-one solutions during prolonged storage. *Infusiontherapie.* 1982; 9:86–91.

59. Parker EA. Compatibility digest. *Am J Hosp Pharm.* 1974; 31: 775.

60. Wolfert RR, Cox RM. Room temperature stability of drug products labeled for refrigerated storage. *Am J Hosp Pharm.* 1975; 32:585–7.

61. Anon. Intravenous fat. *Lancet.* 1976; 1:1059–60.

62. Sachtler G. Dilantin for i.v. use. *Drug Intell Clin Pharm.* 1973; 7:418.

63. Burke WA. I.V. drug incompatibilities—Dilantin. *Am J IV Ther.* 1975; 2:16–8.

64. Baldwin J, Amerson AB. Intramuscular use of diphenylhydantoin. *Am J Hosp Pharm.* 1973; 30:837–8.

65. Tobias DC, Kellick KA. Dilantin for i.v. use. *Drug Intell Clin Pharm.* 1973; 7:418.

66. Chan NL. Dilantin for i.v. use. *Drug Intell Clin Pharm.* 1973; 7:419.

67. Ammar HO, Salama HA. Studies on the stability of injectable solutions of some phenothiazines, part i: effect of pH and buffer systems. *Pharmazie.* 1975; 30:368–9.

68. Pickering LK, Rutherford I. Effect of concentration and time upon inactivation of tobramycin, gentamicin, netilmicin, and amikacin by azlocillin, carbenicillin, mecillinam, mezlocillin, and piperacillin. *J Pharmacol Exp Ther.* 1981; 217:345–9.

69. Ho NFH, Goeman JA. Prediction of pharmaceutical stability of parenteral solutions. *Drug Intell Clin Pharm.* 1970; 4:69-71.

70. Reference number not in use.

71. Reference number not in use.

72. Trissel LA, Davignon JP, Kleinman LM, et al. NCI investigational drugs pharmaceutical data. Bethesda, MD: National Cancer Institute; 1988.

73. Muhlhauser I, Broermann C, Tsotsalas M, et al. Miscibility of human and bovine ultralente insulin with soluble insulin. *BMJ.* 1984; 289:1656–7.

74. Grant HR. Compatibilities of intravenous admixtures. *Hosp Pharmacist.* 94 (Mar-Apr) 1962; 15:67–70.

75. Hanson DB, Hendeles L. Guide to total dose intravenous iron dextran therapy. *Am J Hosp Pharm.* 1974; 31:592–5.

76. Duke AB, Kelleher J. Serum iron and iron binding capacity after total dose infusion of iron-dextran for iron deficiency anaemia in pregnancy. *J Obstet Gynaecol Br Commonw.* 1974; 81(11): 895–900.

77. Parker EA. Compatibility digest. *Am J Hosp Pharm.* 1975; 32: 214.

78. Gardella LA, Kesler H, Carter JE, et al. Intropin (dopamine hydrochloride) intravenous admixture compatibility, part ii: stability with some commonly used antibiotics in 5% dextrose injection. *Am J Hosp Pharm.* 1976; 33:537–40.

79. Gardella LA, Zaroslinski JF. Intropin (dopamine hydrochloride) intravenous admixture compatibility, part i: stability with common intravenous fluids. *Am J Hosp Pharm.* 1975; 32:575–8.

80. Garnett W. Diluents for antineoplastic drugs. *Drug Intell Clin Pharm.* 1971; 5:261.

81. Landersjo L, Stjernstrom G. Studies on the stability and compatibility of drugs in infusion fluids V. Effect of lactate and metal ions on the stability of benzylpenicillin. *Acta Pharm Suec.* 1978; 15:161–8.

82. Notari RE, Chin ML. Arabinosylcytosine stability in aqueous solutions: pH profile and shelf life predictions. *J Pharm Sci.* 1972; 61:1189–96.

83. Murty BSR, Kapoor JN. Properties of mannitol injection (25%) after repeated autoclavings. *Am J Hosp Pharm.* 1975; 32: 826–7.

84. Rosch JM, Pazin GJ, Fireman P. Reduction of amphotericin B nephrotoxicity with mannitol. *JAMA.* 1976; 235:1995–6.

85. Bergman N, Vellar ID. Potential life-threatening variations of drug concentrations in intravenous infusion systems—potassium chloride, insulin, and heparin. *Med J Aust.* 1982; 2: 270–2.

86. Parker EA. Compatibility digest. *Am J Hosp Pharm.* 1970; 27: 492–3.

87. Feigen RD, Moss KS. Antibiotic stability in solutions used for intravenous nutrition and fluid therapy. *Pediatrics.* 1973; 51: 1016–26.

88. Zost ED, Yanchick VA. Compatibility and stability of disodium carbenicillin in combination with other drugs and large volume parenteral solutions. *Am J Hosp Pharm.* 1972; 29:135–40.

89. Lynn B. Recent work on parenteral penicillins. *J Hosp Pharm.* 1971; 29:183–194.

90. Tourville J. Sodium nitroprusside. *Drug Intell Clin Pharm.* 1975; 9:361–4.

91. Anon. Editorial: Sodium nitroprusside in anaesthesia. *Br Med J.* 1975; 2:524–5.

92. Hargrave RE. Degradation of solutions of sodium nitroprusside. *J Hosp Pharm.* 1974; 32:188–9.

93. Anon. Sodium nitroprusside for hypertensive crisis. *Med Lett Drugs Ther.* 1975; 17:82–3.

94. Anderson RA, Rae W. Stability of sodium nitroprusside solutions. *Aust J Pharm Sci NS1.* 1972; (July):45–6.

95. Schumacher GE. Sodium nitroprusside injection. *Am J Hosp Pharm.* 1966; 23:532.

96. Cruz JE, Maness DD, Yakatan GJ. Kinetics and mechanism of hydrolysis of furosemide. *Int J Pharm.* 1979; 2:275–81.

97. Thomas R. Meperidine HCl and heparin sodium precipitation. *Hosp Pharm.* 1979; 2:275–81.

98. Fleischer NM. Promethazine hydrochloride-morphine sulfate incompatibility. *Am J Hosp Pharm.* 1973; 30:665.

99. Lynn B. Pharmaceutical aspects of semi-synthetic penicillins. *J Hosp Pharm.* 1970; 28:71–86.

100. Meisler JM, Skolaut MW. Extemporaneous sterile compounding in intravenous additives. *Am J Hosp Pharm.* 1966; 23: 557–63.

101. Guthaus MR (Medical Services, The Upjohn Company, Kalamazoo, MI): Personal communication; 1973 Aug 9.

102. HamLin WE, Riebe KW, Scothorn WW, et al. Pharmacy profile of cleocin phosphate. Presented at 10th annual ASHP midyear clinical meeting. Washington, DC: 1975 Dec 11.

103. Riebe KW, Oesterling TO. Parenteral development of clindamycin-2–phosphate. *Bull Parenter Drug Assoc.* 1972; 26: 139–45.

104. Therapeutic profile: cleocin phosphate. Kalamazoo, MI: The Upjohn Company; 1973.

105. Wyatt RG, Okamato GA. Stability of antibiotics in parenteral solutions. *Pediatrics.* 1972; 49:22–9.

106. Halasi S, Nairn JD. Stability studies of hydralazine hydrochloride in aqueous solutions. *J Parenter Sci Technol.* 1990; 44: 30–4.

107. Whiting DA. Treatment of chromoblastomycosis with local concentrations of amphotericin B. *Br J Dermatol.* 1967; 79: 345–51.

108. Kirschenbaum BE, Latiolais CJ. Injectable medications—a guide to stability and reconstitution. New York, NY: McMahon Group; 1993.

109. Bair JN, Carew DP. Therapeutic availability of antibiotics in parenteral solutions. *Bull Parenter Drug Assoc.* 1965; 19: 153–63.

110. Dancey JW, Carew DP. Availability of antibiotics in combination with other additives in intravenous solutions. *Am J Hosp Pharm.* 1966; 23:543–51.

111. Prasad VK, Granatek AP. Physical compatibility and chemical stability of cephapirin sodium in combination with antibiotics and large-volume parenteral solutions, part i. *Curr Ther Res Clin Exp.* 1974; 16:505–39.

112. Lynn B. Carbenicillin plus gentamicin. *Lancet.* 1971; 1:654.

113. Jacobs J, Kletter D, Superstine E, et al. Intravenous infusions of heparin and penicillins. *J Clin Pathol.* 1973; 26:742–6.

114. Lynn B. Penicillin instability in infusions. *Br Med J.* 1971; 1: 174.

115. Information for health professionals. Wellington, New Zealand: New Zealand Medicines and Medical Devices Safety Authority.

116. Reference number not in use.

117. McEvoy GK, ed. American hospital formulary service drug information 95. Bethesda, MD: American Society of Health-System Pharmacists; 1995.

118. Harrison DC. Practical guidelines for the use of lidocaine. Prevention and treatment of cardiac arrhythmias. *JAMA.* 1975; 233: 1202–4.

119. Collinsworth K. Clinical pharmacology of lidocaine as an antiarrhythmic drug. *West J Med.* 1976; 124:36–43.

120. Anon. Prophylactic use of lidocaine in myocardial infarction. *Med Lett Drugs Ther.* 1976; 18:1–2.

121. Dundee JW, Gamble JA, Assaf RA. Plasma diazepam levels following intramuscular injection by nurses and doctors. *Lancet.* 1974; 2:1461.

122. Reference number not in use.

123. Tortorici MP. Stability data on frozen i.m. and i.v. solutions. *Pharm Times.* 1975; 41:68–72.

124. Barbara AC, Clemente C. Physical incompatibility of sulfonamide compounds and polyionic solutions. *N Engl J Med.* 1966; 274:1316–7.

125. Brooke D, Bequette RJ. Chemical stability of cyclophosphamide in parenteral solutions. *Am J Hosp Pharm.* 1973; 30: 134–7.

126. Brooke D, Scott JA. Effect of briefly heating cyclophosphamide solutions. *Am J Hosp Pharm.* 1975; 32:44–5.

127. Gallelli JF. Stability studies of drugs used in intravenous solutions, part i. *Am J Hosp Pharm.* 1967; 24:425–33.

128. Dupont Pharmaceuticals. Nubain, physical compatibility. Wilmington, DE; undated.

129. Kramer W, Tanja JJ. Precipitates found in admixtures of potassium chloride and dextrose 5% in water. *Am J Hosp Pharm.* 1970; 27:548–53.

130. Lawson DH. Clinical use of potassium supplements. *Am J Hosp Pharm.* 1975; 32:708–11.

131. Lundgren P, Landersjo L. Studies on the stability and compatibility of drugs in infusion fluids, ii: factors affecting the stability of benzylpenicillin. *Acta Pharm Suec.* 1970; 7:509–26.

132. Weber CR, Gupta VD. Stability of phenylephrine hydrochloride in intravenous solutions. *J Hosp Pharm.* 1970; 28:200–8.

133. Chiou WL, Moorhatch P. Interaction between vitamin A and plastic intravenous fluid bags. *J Am Med Assoc.* 1973; 223: 328.

134. Komesaroff D, Field JE. Pancuronium bromide: a new nondepolarizing muscle relaxant. *Med J Aust.* 1969; 1:908–11.

135. Simberkoff MS, Thomas L, McGregor D, et al. Inactivation of penicillins by carbohydrate solutions at alkaline pH. *N Engl J Med.* 1970; 283:116–9.

136. Hicks CI, Gallardo JPB. Stability of sodium bicarbonate injection stored in polypropylene syringes. *Am J Hosp Pharm.* 1972; 29:210–6.

137. DeLuca PP, Kowalski RJ. Problems arising from the transfer of sodium bicarbonate injection from ampuls to plastic disposable syringes. *Am J Hosp Pharm.* 1972; 29:217–22.

138. D'Arcy PF, Thompson KM. Stability of chlorpromazine hydrochloride added to intravenous infusion fluids. *Pharm J.* 1973; 210:28.

139. Nahata MC, Zingarelli JR, Hipple TF. Stability of caffeine injection stored in plastic and glass syringes. *DICP.* 1989; 23: 1035.

140. Murabito AS (Smith Kline & French Laboratories, Philadelphia, PA): Personal communication; 1986 Dec 15.

141. Mann JM, Coleman DL. Stability of parenteral solutions of sodium cephalothin, cephaloridine, potassium penicillin G (buffered), and vancomycin HCl. *Am J Hosp Pharm.* 1971; 28: 760–3.

142. Appleby DH, John JF. Effect of peritoneal dialysis solution on the antimicrobial activity of cephalosporins. *Nephron.* 1982; 30: 341–4.

143. Upshaw MD (Medical Information Services, Eli Lilly and Company, Indianapolis, IN): Personal communication; 1972 Jan 10.

144. Gallelli JF, MacLowry JD. Stability of antibiotics in parenteral solutions. *Am J Hosp Pharm.* 1969; 26:630–5.

145. Dienstag JL, Neu HC. Tobramycin: new aminoglycoside antibiotic. *Clin Med.* 1975; 82:13–9.

146. Struhar M, Heinrich J. K sorpcii pentoxifyllinu na infuznu supravu Luer. *Farm Obz.* 1988; 57:405–10.

147. Bergstrom RF, Fites AL. Stability of parenteral solutions of tobramycin sulfate. *Am J Hosp Pharm.* 1975; 32:887–8.

148. Huber RC, Riffkin C. Inline final filters for removing particles from amphotericin B infusions. *Am J Hosp Pharm.* 1975; 32: 173–6.

149. Rebagay T, Rapp R, Bivins B, et al. Residues in antibiotic preparations, i: scanning electron microscopic studies of surface topography. *Am J Hosp Pharm.* 1976; 33:433–43.

150. Gallelli JF. Assay and stability of amphotericin B in aqueous solutions. *Drug Intell.* 1967; 1:102–5.

151. Piecoro JJ, Goodman NL, Wheeler WE, et al. Particulate matter in reconstituted amphotericin B and assay of filtered solutions of amphotericin B. *Am J Hosp Pharm.* 1975; 32:381–4.

152. Gotz V, Simon W. Inline filtration of amphotericin B infusions. *Am J Hosp Pharm.* 1975; 32:458.

153. Chatterji D, Hiranaka PK. Stability of sodium oxacillin in intravenous solutions. *Am J Hosp Pharm.* 1975; 32:1130–2.

154. Facts and Comparisons, Inc. Drug facts and comparisons. St. Louis, MO; 2003.

155. Parodi JF. Stability of frozen antibiotic solutions in Viaflex infusion containers. *Hosp Pharm.* 1976; 11:178–9.

156. Larsen SS. Studies on stability of drugs in frozen systems. IV. The stability of benzylpenicillin sodium in frozen aqueous solutions. *Dan Tidsskr Farm.* 1971; 45:307–16.

157. Noone P, Pattison JR. Therapeutic implications of interaction of gentamicin and penicillins. *Lancet.* 1971; 2:575–8.

158. Boulet M, Marier JR. Effect of magnesium on formation of calcium phosphate precipitates. *Arch Biochem Biophys.* 1962; 96:629–36.

159. van den Berg L, Soliman FS. Composition and pH changes during freezing of solutions containing calcium and magnesium phosphate. *Cryobiology.* 1969; 6:10–4.

160. Ong JTH, Kostenbauder HB. Effect of self-association on rate of penicillin G degradation in concentrated aqueous solutions. *J Pharm Sci.* 1975; 64:1378–80.

161. Shoup LK, Thur MP. Stability of frozen buffered penicillin G potassium injection. *Hosp Formul Manage.* 1968; 3:38–9.

162. Boylan JC, Simmons JL. Stability of frozen solutions of sodium cephalothin and cephaloridine. *Am J Hosp Pharm.* 1972; 29: 687–9.

163. Grant NH, Clark DE. Imidazole- and base-catalyzed hydrolysis of penicillin in frozen systems. *J Am Chem Soc.* 1961; 83: 4476–7.

164. Lindsay RE, Hem SL. Dosage form for potassium penicillin G intravenous infusion solutions. *Drug Devel Commun.* 1974–5; 1:211–222.

165. Im S, Latiolais CJ. Physico-chemical incompatibilities of parenteral admixtures—penicillin and tetracyclines. *Am J Hosp Pharm.* 1966; 23:333–43.

166. Pfeifer HJ, Webb JW. Compatibility of penicillin and ascorbic acid injection. *Am J Hosp Pharm.* 1976; 33:448–50.

167. Rusmin S, DeLuca PP. Effect of inline filtration on the potency of potassium penicillin G. *Bull Parenter Drug Assoc.* 1976; 30: 64–71.

168. Stolar MH, Carlin HS. Effect of freezing on the stability of sodium methicillin injection. *Am J Hosp Pharm.* 1968; 25: 32–5.

169. Lynn B. Stability of methicillin in dextrose solutions at alkaline pH. *J Hosp Pharm.* 1972; 30:81–3.

170. Lynn B. Pharmaceutics of the semi-synthetic penicillins. *Chem Drug.* 1967; 187:134–6.

171. Lynn B. Inactivation of methicillin in dextrose solutions at alkaline pH. *N Engl J Med.* 1971; 285:690.

172. Mattson CJ, Clark ST, Colangelo A. Stability of clindamycin phosphate in plastic syringes. Presented at 20th annual ASHP midyear clinical meeting. New Orleans, LA: 1985 Dec.

173. Clark ST, Colangelo A. Stability of clindamycin phosphate in plastic syringes. Presented at 20th annual ASHP midyear clinical meeting. New Orleans, LA: 1985 Dec.

174. Cohon MS (Drug Information Services, Upjohn Company, Kalamazoo, MI): Personal communications; 1986 Dec 12, 1988 Jan 27, 1988 Feb 3.

175. Reference number not in use.

176. Owen RT (UK Medical Information Section, The Wellcome Foundation Ltd., Cheshire, England): Personal communication; 1993 Aug 19.

177. Lesson LJ, Weidenheimer JF. Stability of tetracycline and riboflavin. *J Pharm Sci.* 1969; 58:355–7.

178. Turco SJ, Burke WA. Methods of ordering and use of intravenous phosphate (mEq vs mM). *Hosp Pharm.* 322, 326 (Aug) 1975; 10:320.

179. Pinkus TF, Jeffrey LP. Incompatibility of calcium and phosphate in parenteral alimentation solutions. *Am J IV Ther.* 1976; 3:22–4.

180. Kaminski MV, Harris DF, Collin CF, et al. Electrolyte compatibility in synthetic amino acid hyperalimentation solution. *Am J Hosp Pharm.* 1974; 31:244–6.

181. Schlicht JR. Adjustments in etoposide infusion flow rates when using controllers. *Am J Hosp Pharm.* 1990; 47:2656.

182. FASS, Karolinska Institutet, Huddinge, Sweden. Available at http://edu.ofa.ki.effica/.

183. Lee FA, Gwinn JL. Roentgen patterns of extravasation of calcium gluconate in the tissues of the neonate. *J Pediatr.* 1975; 86:598–601.

184. Weiss Y, Ackerman C. Localized necrosis of scalp in neonates due to calcium gluconate infusions: a cautionary note. *Pediatrics.* 1975; 56:1084–6.

185. Ramamurthy RS, Harris V. Subcutaneous calcium deposition in the neonate associated with intravenous administration of calcium gluconate. *Pediatrics.* 1975; 55:802–6.

186. Laegeler WL, Tio JM. Stability of certain amino acids in a parenteral nutrition solution. *Am J Hosp Pharm.* 1974; 31: 776–9.

187. Kleinman LM, Tangrea JA, Gallelli JF, et al. Stability of solutions of essential amino acids. *Am J Hosp Pharm.* 1973; 30: 1054–7.

188. Rowlands DA. Compatibility of calcium and phosphate in amino acids solution. *Am J Hosp Pharm.* 1975; 32:360.

189. Saudek EC (The Upjohn Company): Personal communication; 1973 Jan 3.

190. Rowlands DA, Wilkinson WR. Storage stability of mixed hyperalimentation solutions. *Am J Hosp Pharm.* 1973; 30:436–8.

191. Aro R (Senior Clinical Research Associate, Fujisawa USA): Personal communication, February 22, 1994.

192. Rodriguez Penin I, Yanez Gonzalez A, Camba Rodriguez A, et al. Estabilidad de la mezcla morfina-midazolam en un dispositivo de infusion continua. *Farm Hosp.* 1991; 15:407–9.

193. Nahata MC, Zingarelli JR, Durrell DE. Stability of caffeine injection in intravenous admixtures and parenteral nutrition solutions. *DICP.* 1989; 23:466–7.

194. Hull RL. Use of trace elements in intravenous hyperalimentation solutions. *Am J Hosp Pharm.* 1974; 31:759–61.

195. Johnson C, Cloyd J. Parenteral hyperalimentation. *Drug Intell Clin Pharm.* 1975; 9:493–9.

196. Hankins DA, Riella MC, Scribner BH, et al. Whole blood trace element concentrations during total parenteral nutrition. *Surgery.* 1976; 79:674–7.

197. Hamann MA. Trace element requirements in hyperalimentation. *Am J Hosp Pharm.* 1974; 31:1035.

198. Hull RL. Trace element requirements in hyperalimentation. *Am J Hosp Pharm.* 1974; 31:1038.

199. Heird WC, Winters RW. Total intravenous alimentation in pediatric patients. *South Med J.* 1975; 68:1173–6.

200. Baker JA, Kirkman H, Woodley C, et al. Computer-assisted pediatric hyperalimentation. *Am J Hosp Pharm.* 1974; 31:752–8.

201. Parish R. Hyperalimentation procedures. *Am J Hosp Pharm.* 1974; 31:1160.

202. Pomerance HH, Rader RE. Crystal formation: a new complication of total parenteral nutrition. *Pediatrics.* 1973; 52:864–6.

203. Bohart RD, Ogawa G. An observation on the stability of cis-dichlorodiammineplatinum (II): a caution regarding its administration. *Cancer Treat Rep.* 1979; 63:2117–8.

204. Prestayko AW, Cadiz M. Incompatibility of aluminum-containing iv administration equipment with cis-dichlorodiammineplatinum (II) administration. *Cancer Treat Rep.* 1979; 63:2118–9.

205. Shils ME. Minerals in total parenteral nutrition. *Drug Intell Clin Pharm.* 1972; 6:385–93.

206. Flack HL, Gans JA, Serlick SE, et al. The current status of parenteral hyperalimentation. *Am J Hosp Pharm.* 1971; 28:326–35.

207. McRae MP, King JC. Compatibility of antineoplastic, antibiotic, and corticosteroid drugs in intravenous admixtures. *Am J Hosp Pharm.* 1976; 33:1010–3.

208. Warren E, Synder RJ, Thompson CO, et al. Stability of ampicillin in intravenous solutions. *Mayo Clin Proc.* 1972; 47:34–5.

209. Raffanti EF, King JC. Effect of pH on the stability of sodium ampicillin solutions. *Am J Hosp Pharm.* 1974; 31:745–51.

210. Savello DR, Shangraw RF. Stability of sodium ampicillin solutions in the frozen and liquid states. *Am J Hosp Pharm.* 1971; 28:754–9.

211. Jacobs J, Nathan I, Superstine E, et al. Ampicillin and carbenicillin stability in commonly used infusion solutions. *Drug Intell Clin Pharm.* 1970; 4:204–8.

212. Hiranaka P, Frazier AG. Stability of ampicillin in aqueous solutions. *Am J Hosp Pharm.* 1972; 29:321–2.

213. Stratton M, Sandmann BJ. Stability studies of ampicillin sodium in intravenous fluids using optical activity. *Bull Parenter Drug Assoc.* 1975; 29:286–95.

214. Pincock RE, Kiovsky TE. Kinetics of reactions in frozen solutions. *J Chem Educ.* 1966; 43:358–60.

215. Hou JP, Poole JW. Kinetics and mechanism of degradation of ampicillin in solution. *J Pharm Sci.* 1969; 58:447–54.

216. Shils ME, Wright WL, Turnbull A, et al. Long-term parenteral nutrition through an external arteriovenous shunt. *N Engl J Med.* 1970; 283:341–4.

217. Zia H, Tehrani M. Kinetics of carbenicillin degradation in aqueous solutions. *Can J Pharm Sci.* 1974; 9:112–7.

218. Riff LJ, Jackson GG. Laboratory and clinical conditions for gentamicin inactivation by carbenicillin. *Arch Intern Med.* 1972; 130:887–91.

219. McLaughlin JE, Reeves DS. Clinical and laboratory evidence for inactivation of gentamicin by carbenicillin. *Lancet.* 1971; 1:261–4.

220. Klastersky J. Carbenicillin plus gentamicin. *Lancet.* 1971; 1:653–4.

221. Levison ME, Kaye D. Carbenicillin plus gentamicin. *Lancet.* 1971; 2:45–6.

222. Eykyn S, Phillips I. Gentamicin plus carbenicillin. *Lancet.* 1971; 1:545–6.

223. Riff L, Jackson GG. Gentamicin plus carbenicillin. *Lancet.* 1971; 1:592.

224. Zost ED, Yanchick VA. Stability of gentamicin in combination with carbenicillin. *Am J Hosp Pharm.* 1972; 29:388–90.

225. Jacoby GA. Carbenicillin and gentamicin. *N Engl J Med.* 1971; 284:1096–8.

226. Kleinberg ML (Professional Services, Immunex, Seattle, WA): Personal communication; 1993 Jun 14.

227. Baldini JT (Professional Services, Schering Laboratories, Kenilworth, NJ): Personal communication; 1972 Feb 11.

228. Koup JR, Gerbracht L. Combined use of heparin and gentamicin in peritoneal dialysis solutions. *Drug Intell Clin Pharm.* 1975; 9:388.

229. Reeves DS, Bywater MJ, Wise R, et al. Availability of three antibiotics after intramuscular injection into thigh and buttock. *Lancet.* 1974; 2:1421–2.

230. Jackson GG. Gentamicin. *Practitioner.* 1967; 198:855–66.

231. Preskey D, Kayes JB. Stability of sulfadiazine sodium as used in admixture with intravenous infusion fluids. *J Clin Pharm.* 1976; 1:39–48.

232. Physicians' desk reference. 49th ed. Oradell, NJ: Medical Economics Company; 1995.

233. Larsen SS, Jensen VG. Studies on stability of drugs in frozen systems. II. The stabilities of hexobarbital sodium and phenobarbital sodium in frozen aqueous solutions. *Dan Tidsskr Farm.* 1970; 44:21–31.

234. NCI investigational drugs pharmaceutical data. Bethesda, MD: National Cancer Institute; 1988, 1990, 1994.

235. Halpern NA, Colucci RD, Alicea M, et al. The compatibility of nicardipine hydrochloride injection with various ICU medications during simulated Y-site injection. *Int J Clin Pharmacol Ther Toxicol.* 1989; 27:250–4.

236. Anon. Kidney toxicity—main source of methotrexate complications. *J Am Med Assoc.* 1975; 223:1036–7.

237. Baker MBC Hospital Products Division, Abbott Laboratories, Abbott Park, Illinois: Personal Communication; 2003 Aug 27.

238. Hoeprich PD, Huston AC. Stability of four antifungal antimicrobics in vitro. *J Infect Dis.* 1978; 137:87–93.

239. Selam JL, Lord P, van Antwerp WP, et al. Heparin addition to insulin in implantable pumps to prevent catheter obstruction. *Diabetes Care.* 1989; 12:38–9.

240. Wang DP. Stability of procaine in aqueous systems. *Analyst.* 1983; 108:851–6.

241. Lapidas B. Cautions regarding the preparation of high-dose methotrexate infusions. *Am J Hosp Pharm.* 1976; 33:760.

242. Pelsor FR. Cautions regarding the preparation of high-dose methotrexate infusions. *Am J Hosp Pharm.* 1976; 33:760.

243. Pritchard J. Stability of heparin solutions. *J Pharm Pharmacol.* 1964; 16:487–9.

244. Turco SJ. I.V. drug incompatibilities—heparin sodium USP. *Am J IV Ther.* 1976; 3:16–9.

245. Kakkar VV, Corrigan TP. Prevention of fatal postoperative pulmonary embolism by low doses of heparin: an international multicentre trial. *Lancet.* 1975; 2:45–51.

246. Sherry S. Low-dose heparin prophylaxis for postoperative venous thromboembolism. *N Engl J Med.* 1975; 293:300–2.

247. Gallus AS, Hirsch J, O'Brien SE, et al. Prevention of venous thrombosis with small, subcutaneous doses of heparin. *JAMA.* 1976; 235:1980–2.

248. Hopefl AW. Low-dose heparin for the prevention of venous thromboembolism. *Hosp Pharm.* 1976; 11:223.

249. Wessler S. Heparin as an antithrombotic agent. Low-dose prophylaxis. *JAMA.* 1976; 236:389–91.

250. Erdi A, Kakkar VV, Thomas DP, et al. Effect of low-dose subcutaneous heparin on whole-blood viscosity. *Lancet.* 1976; 2:342–4.

251. Hadgraft JW. Adding drugs to intravenous infusions. *Lancet.* 1970; 2:1254.

252. Stock SL, Warner N. Heparin in acid solutions. *Br Med J.* 1971; 3:307.

253. Chessells JM, Braithwaite TA. Dextrose and sorbitol as diluents for continuous intravenous heparin infusion. *Br Med J.* 1972; 2:81–2.

254. Mitchell JF, Barger RC. Heparin stability in 5% dextrose and 0.9% sodium chloride. *Am J Hosp Pharm.* 1976; 33:540–2.

255. Thomas RB, Salter FJ. Heparin locks: their advantages and disadvantages. *Hosp Formul.* 1975; 10:536–8.

256. Deeb EN, DiMattia PE. The key question: how much heparin in the lock?. *Am J IV Ther.* 1976; 3:22–6.

257. DeFina E. How we use heparin locks. *Am J IV Ther.* 33 (Dec-Jan) 1976; 3:27.

258. Hanson RL, Grant AM. Heparin-lock maintenance with ten units of sodium heparin in one milliliter of normal saline solution. *Surg Gynecol Obstet.* 1976; 142:373–6.

259. Rebagay T, DeLuca PP. Residues in antibiotic preparations, ii: effect of pH on the nature and level of particulate matter in sodium cephalothin intravenous solutions. *Am J Hosp Pharm.* 1976; 33:443–8.

260. Albano D (Manager Drug Information, Wyeth-Ayerst). Personal Communication; 1994 Jan 5.

261. Hopefl AW. Room temperature stability of drug products. *Am J Hosp Pharm.* 1975; 32:1084.

262. Barger RC. Room temperature stability of drug products. *Am J Hosp Pharm.* 1975; 32:1089.

263. Rosenbloom AL. Advances in commercial insulin preparations. *Am J Dis Child.* 1974; 128:631–3.

264. Rosenberg JM, Simon WA, Sangkachand P, et al. Mixing insulin preparations. *Hosp Pharm.* 1976; 11:186.

265. Shainfeld FJ. Errors in insulin doses due to the design of insulin syringes. *Pediatrics.* 1975; 56:302–3.

266. Weisenfeld S, Podolsky S, Goldsmith L, et al. Adsorption of insulin to infusion bottles and tubing. *Diabetes.* 1968; 17:766–71.

267. Petty C, Cunningham NL. Insulin adsorption by glass infusion bottles, polyvinylchloride infusion containers, and intravenous tubing. *Anesthesiology.* 1974; 40:400–4.

268. Kraegen EW, Lazarus L, Meler H, et al. Carrier solutions for low-level intravenous insulin infusion. *Br Med J.* 1975; 3:464–6.

269. Semple P, Ratcliffe JG. Carrier solutions for low-level intravenous insulin infusion. *Br Med J.* 1975; 4:228–9.

270. Hays DP, Mehl B. I.V. drug incompatibilities—insulin. *Am J IV Ther.* 1976; 3:30–2.

271. Owen JA. The insulin revolution. *Hosp Formul.* 1976; 11:343.

272. Galloway JA (Medical Research Division, Eli Lilly and Company, Indianapolis, IN): Personal communication; 1967 Aug 29.

273. Rubin J, Humphries J, Smith G, et al. Antibiotic activity in peritoneal dialysate. *Am J Kidney Dis.* 1983; 3:205–8.

274. De Vroe C, De Muynck C, Remon JP, et al. The availability of diltiazem: a study on the sorption by intravenous delivery systems and on the stability of the drug. *J Pharm Pharmacol.* 1989; 41:273–5.

275. Kochevar M, Fry LK. Insulin and dead space volume. *Drug Intell Clin Pharm.* 1974; 8:33–4.

276. Bornstein M, Thomas PN, Coleman DL, et al. Stability of parenteral solutions of cefazolin sodium. *Am J Hosp Pharm.* 1974; 31:296–98.

277. Carone SM, Bornstein M, Coleman DL, et al. Stability of frozen solutions of cefazolin sodium. *Am J Hosp Pharm.* 1976; 33:639–41.

278. Royston DA (Consumer Technical Services, Eli Lilly and Company, Indianapolis, IN): Personal communication; 1976 Feb 19.

279. Brudney N, Eustace BT. Some formulations and compatibility problems with dimenhydrinate (Gravol). *Can Pharm J.* 1963; 96:470–1.

280. Acred P, Brown DM, Knudsen ET, et al. New semi-synthetic penicillin active against pseudomonas pyocyanea. *Nature (London).* 1967; 215:25–30.

281. Schwartz MA, Buckwalter FH. Pharmaceutics of penicillin. *J Pharm Sci.* 1962; 51:1119–28.

282. Thur MP (Parenteral Products, Travenol Laboratories, Deerfield, IL): Personal communication; 1976 Sep 20.

283. Ziemba LJ (Medical Information, ICI Pharmaceuticals Group, Wilmington, DE): Personal communication; 1990 Mar 15.

284. Yamana T, Tsuji A. Comparative stability of cephalosporins in aqueous solution: kinetics and mechanisms of degradation. *J Pharm Sci.* 1976; 65:1563–74.

285. Kleinman LM, Davignon JP, Cradock JC, et al. Investigational drug information. *Drug Intell Clin Pharm.* 1976; 10:48–9.

286. Chang SY, Evans TL. The stability of melphalan in the presence of chloride ion. *J Pharm Pharmacol.* 1979; 31:853–4.

287. Mitenko PA, Ogilvie RI. Rational intravenous doses of theophylline. *N Engl J Med.* 1973; 289:600–3.

288. Simons FER, Pierson WE. Current status of the use of intravenously administered aminophylline. *South Med J.* 1975; 68: 802–4.

289. Weinberger MW, Matthay RA, Ginchansky EJ, et al. Intravenous aminophylline dosage. Use of serum theophylline measurement for guidance. *JAMA.* 1976; 235:2110–3.

290. Nedich RL. Vitamin A absorption from plastic IV bags. *JAMA.* 1973; 224:1531–2.

291. Kaplan MA, Coppola WP, Nunning BC, et al. Pharmaceutical properties and stability of amikacin, part i. *Curr Ther Res Clin Exp.* 1976; 20:352–8.

292. Nunning BC, Granatek AP. Physical compatibility and chemical stability of amikacin sulfate in large-volume parenteral solutions, part ii. *Curr Ther Res Clin Exp.* 1976; 20:359–68.

293. Nunning BC, Granatek AP. Physical compatibility and chemical stability of amikacin sulfate in combination with antibiotics in large-volume parenteral solutions, part iii. *Curr Ther Res Clin Exp.* 1976; 20:369–416.

294. Nunning BC, Granatek AP. Physical compatibility and chemical stability of amikacin sulfate in combination with non-antibiotic drugs in large-volume parenteral solutions, part iv. *Curr Ther Res Clin Exp.* 1976; 20:417–91.

295. Koup JR, Gerbracht L. Reduction in heparin activity by gentamicin. *Drug Intell Clin Pharm.* 1975; 9:568.

296. McKinley JD (M.D. Anderson Hospital and Tumor Institute, Houston, TX): Personal communication; 1976 Aug 23.

297. Weiner B, McNeely DJ, Kluge RM, et al. Stability of gentamicin sulfate following unit dose repackaging. *Am J Hosp Pharm.* 1976; 33:1254–9.

298. Dinel BA, Ayotte DL, Behme RJ, et al. Comparative stability of antibiotic admixtures in minibags and minibottles. *Drug Intell Clin Pharm.* 1977; 11:226–39.

299. Dinel BA, Ayotte DL, Behme RJ, et al. Stability of antibiotic admixtures frozen in minibags. *Drug Intell Clin Pharm.* 1977; 11:542–8.

300. Lynn B. Pharmaceutics of the semi-synthetic penicillins. *Chem Drug.* 1967; 187:157–60.

301. Stanaszek WF, Pan IH. Analysis of hydroxyzine hydrochloride, meperidine hydrochloride and atropine sulfate in glass and plastic syringes. *Am J Hosp Pharm.* 1978; 35:1084–7.

302. Fraser GL. Incompatibility of magnesium sulfate and hydrocortisone sodium succinate. *Am J Hosp Pharm.* 1978; 35:783.

303. Kresel JJ, McDermott JS, Huffer LM, et al. Stability of carbenicillin and oxacillin frozen in syringes. *Am J Hosp Pharm.* 1978; 35:310–2.

304. Manning RE. Predicted expiration times for penicillin G in combination with multivitamin injections. *Am J Hosp Pharm.* 1976; 33:870.

305. Cloyd JC, Bosch DE. Concentration-time profile of phenytoin after admixture with small volumes of intravenous fluids. *Am J Hosp Pharm.* 1978; 35:45–8.

306. Bauman JL, Siepler JK. Phenytoin crystallization in intravenous fluids. *Drug Intell Clin Pharm.* 1977; 11:646–9.

307. Ashwin J, Lynn B. Ampicillin stability in saline or dextrose infusions. *Pharm J.* 1975; 214:487–9.

308. O'Brien MJ, Portnoff JB. Cefoxitin sodium compatibility with intravenous infusions and additives. *Am J Hosp Pharm.* 1979; 36:33–8.

309. Stevens JS. Incompatibility of diphenhydramine hydrochloride (Benadryl) with meglumine iodipamide (Cholografin). *Radiology.* 1975; 117:224–5.

310. Petrick RJ, Wolleben JE. Stability of frozen solutions of doxycycline hyclate for injection. *Am J Hosp Pharm.* 1978; 35: 1386–7.

311. Melberg SG, Havelund S, Villumsen J, et al. Insulin compatibility with polymer materials used in external pump infusion systems. *Diabet Med.* 1988; 5:243–7.

312. Gardella LA, Kesler H, Amann A, et al. Intropin (dopamine hydrochloride) intravenous admixture compatibility, part 3: stability with miscellaneous additives. *Am J Hosp Pharm.* 1978; 35:581–4.

313. Schuetz DH, King JC. Compatibility and stability of electrolytes, vitamins and antibiotics in combination with 8% amino acids solution. *Am J Hosp Pharm.* 1978; 35:33–44.

314. El-Nakeeb MA, Souccar N. Inactivation of various antibiotics by some vitamins. *Can J Pharm Sci.* 1976; 11:85–9.

315. Dixon FW, Weshalek J. Physical compatibility of nine drugs in various intavenous solutions. *Am J Hosp Pharm.* 1972; 29: 822–3.

316. Earhart RH. Instability of cis-dichlorodiammineplatinum in dextrose solution. *Cancer Treat Rep.* 1978; 62:1105–6.

317. Greene RF, Chatterji DC, Hiranaka PK, et al. Stability of cisplatin in aqueous solution. *Am J Hosp Pharm.* 1979; 36: 38–43.

318. Morrison RA, Oseekey KB. 5-Fluorouracil and methotrexate sodium: an admixture incompatibility?. *Am J Hosp Pharm.* 1978; 35:15.

319. King JC. 5-Fluorouracil and methotrexate sodium: an admixture incompatibility?. *Am J Hosp Pharm.* 1978; 35:18.

320. Rusmin S, Welton S, DeLuca P, et al. Effect of inline filtration on the potency of drugs administered intravenously. *Am J Hosp Pharm.* 1977; 34:1071–4.

321. Morris ME. Compatibility and stability of diazepam injection following dilution with intravenous fluids. *Am J Hosp Pharm.* 1978; 35:669–72.

322. Allen LV, Levinson RS. Compatibility of various admixtures with secondary additives at Y-injection sites of intravenous administration sets. *Am J Hosp Pharm.* 1977; 34:939–43.

323. Arnold TR, Eder J. Compatibility of primary-piggyback solution combinations. *Am J Hosp Pharm.* 1978; 35:249–50.

324. Jansen JR. Volume control sets and incompatibilities. *Am J Hosp Pharm.* 1975; 32:1225.

325. Aisenstein A, Kahn S. Study of the stability of some frozen antibiotics. *Hosp Pharm.* 1969; 4:17–21.

326. Parker WA. Physical compatibilities of preanesthetic medications. *Can J Hosp Pharm.* 1976; 29:91–2.

327. Cradock JC, Kleinman LM. Evaluation of some pharmaceutical aspects of intrathecal methotrexate sodium, cytarabine and hydrocortisone sodium succinate. *Am J Hosp Pharm.* 1978; 35: 402–6.

328. Sarubbi FA, Wilson B, Lee M, et al. Nosocomial meningitis and bacteremia due to contaminated amphotericin B. *JAMA.* 1978; 239:416–8.

329. The Upjohn Company. Solu-Medrol IV admixture, dilution, and compatibility information. 1978 Aug.

330. Parker WA, Morris ME. Incompatibility of diazepam injection in plastic intravenous bags. *Am J Hosp Pharm.* 1979; 36: 505–7.

331. Ingallinera T, Kapadia AJ, Hagman D, et al. Compatibility of glycopyrrolate injection with commonly used infusion solutions and additives. *Am J Hosp Pharm.* 1979; 36:508–10.

332. Bateman NE, Graham MD. Solubility of an ephedrine-phenobarbitone complex in water. *Australas J Pharm.* 1967; 48: S68–9.

333. Chang CH, Ashford WR, Ives DAJ, et al. Stability of oxytocin in various infusion solutions. *Can J Hosp Pharm.* 1972; 25: 152.

334. Lynn B. Administration of carbenicillin and ticarcillin—pharmaceutical aspects. *Eur J Cancer.* 1973; 9:425–33.

335. Block ER, Bennett JE. Stability of amphotericin B in infusion bottles. *Antimicrob Agents Chemother.* 1973; 4:648–9.

336. Gupta VD, Stewart KR. Quantitation of carbenicillin disodium, cefazolin sodium, cephalothin sodium, nafcillin sodium, and ticarcillin disodium by high-pressure liquid chromatography. *J Pharm Sci.* 1980; 69:1264–7.

337. Anon. Label changes on albumin—a reminder. *FDA Drug Bull.* 1978; 8:32.

338. Knoppert DC, Freeman D, Webb D. Stability of ceftizoxime in 5 percent dextrose and 0.9 percent sodium chloride. *Can J Hosp Pharm.* 1993; 46:13–6.

339. Koup JR, Schentag JJ, Vance JW, et al. System for clinical pharmacokinetic monitoring of theophylline therapy. *Am J Hosp Pharm.* 1976; 33:949–56.

340. Jusko WJ, Koup JR, Vance JW, et al. Intravenous theophylline therapy: nomogram guidelines. *Ann Intern Med.* 1977; 86: 400–4.

341. Travenol Laboratories. Product information on Travasol. Deerfield, IL; 1994 Jan.

342. McGaw Laboratories. Product information on FreAmine III. Irvine, CA; 1991 Sep.

343. Odne MAL, Lee SC. Rationale for adding trace elements to total parenteral nutrient solutions—a brief review. *Am J Hosp Pharm.* 1978; 35:1057–9.

344. Jeejeebhoy KN, Langer B, Tsallas G, et al. Total parenteral nutrition at home: studies in patients surviving 4 months to 5 years. *Gastroenterology.* 1976; (Dec):943–53.

345. Hull RL, Cassidy D. Trace element deficiencies during total parenteral nutrition. *Drug Intell Clin Pharm.* 1977; 11: 536–41.

346. Shils ME. More on trace elements in total parenteral nutrition solutions. *Am J Hosp Pharm.* 1975; 32:141–2.

347. Okada A, Takagi Y, Itakura T, et al. Skin lesions during intravenous hyperalimentation: zinc deficiency. *Surgery.* 1976; 80: 629–35.

348. Matoi JR, Jeffreys LP. Formulation of a trace element solution for long-term parenteral nutrition. *Am J Hosp Pharm.* 1978; 35: 165–8.

349. Athanikar N, Boyer B, Deamer R, et al. Visual compatibility of 30 additives with a parenteral nutrient solution. *Am J Hosp Pharm.* 1979; 36:511–3.

350. Finlayson JS. The birth and demise of "salt-poor" albumin. *Am J Hosp Pharm.* 1978; 35:898–900.

351. Winsnes M, Jeppsson R. Diazepam adsorption to infusion sets and plastic syringes. *Acta Anaesthesiol Scand.* 1981; 25:93–6.

352. Bonner DP, Mechlinski W, Schaffner CP. Stability studies with amphotericin B and amphotericin B methyl ester. *J Antibiot.* 1975; 28:132–5.

353. Shadomy S, Brummer DL. Light sensitivity of prepared solutions of amphotericin B. *Am Rev Resp Dis.* 1973; 107:303–4.

354. Fields BT Jr, Bates JH, Abernathy RS. Effect of rapid intravenous infusion on serum concentrations of amphotericin B. *Appl Microbiol.* 1971; 22:615–7.

355. Janknegt R, van den Berg T, de Jong M, et al. Compatibility study with midazolam. *Ziekenhuisfarmacie.* 1986; 2:45–8.

356. Arbuthnot R, Dullea A. Controlling thrombophlebitis from amphotericin B. *Am J Hosp Pharm.* 1978; 35:129.

357. Rosch JM, Pazin G. Mannitol and amphotericin B. *JAMA.* 1977; 237:27.

358. Moore DE, Sithipitaks V. Photolytic degradation of frusemide. *J Pharm Pharmacol.* 1983; 35:489–93.

359. Roberts JR. Cutaneous and subcutaneous complications of calcium infusions. *JACEP.* 1977; 6:16–20.

360. Smith Kline & French Laboratories. Product information on Tagamet. Philadelphia, PA; 1978 Oct.

361. Winters RE, Chow AW, Hecht RH, et al. Combined use of gentamicin and carbenicillin. *Ann Intern Med.* 1971; 75: 925–7.

362. Waitz JA, Drube CG, Moss EL, et al. Biological aspects of the interaction between gentamicin and carbenicillin. *J Antibiot.* 1972; 25:219–25.

363. Ervin FR, Bullock WE. Inactivation of gentamicin by penicillins in patients with renal failure. *Antimicrob Agents Chemother.* 1976; 9:1004–11.

364. Peterson CD, Kaatz BL. Ticarcillin and carbenicillin. *Drug Intell Clin Pharm.* 1977; 11:482–6.

365. Davies M, Morgan JR. Interactions of carbenicillin and ticarcillin with gentamicin. *Antimicrob Agents Chemother.* 1975; 7: 431–4.

366. Weibert R, Keane W, Shapiro F. Carbenicillin inactivation of aminoglycosides in patients with severe renal failure. *Trans Am Soc Artif Int Organs.* 1976; 22:439–43.

367. Weibert RT, Keane WF. Carbenicillin-gentamicin interaction in acute renal failure. *Am J Hosp Pharm.* 1977; 34:1137–9.

368. Bodey GP, Feld R. β-Lactam antibiotics alone or in combination with gentamicin for therapy of gram-negative bacillary infections in neutropenic patients. *Am J Med Sci.* 1976; 271: 179–86.

369. Schimpff S, Satterlee W, Young UM, et al. Empiric therapy with carbenicillin and gentamicin for febrile patients with cancer and granulocytopenia. *N Engl J Med.* 1971; 284:1061–5.

370. Hendeles L. Are carbenicillin and gentamicin synergists or antagonists? *Hosp Pharm.* 1972; (Sep)7:297–8.

371. Kole-James A. Electrolyte content of common intravenous solutions and antibiotics. *Hosp Pharm.* 1977; 12:394.

372. Donnelly RF, Tirona RG. Stability of citrated caffeine injectable solution in glass vials. *Am J Hosp Pharm.* 1994; 51:512–4.

373. Turco SJ, Hasan I. Comparison of features of Kefzol and Ancef. *Hosp Pharm.* 1976; 11:482.

374. Vukovich RA, Sugerman AA. Effect of 2% procaine hydrochloride solution on the bioavailability of cephradine after intramuscular injection. *Curr Ther Res Clin Exp.* 1975; 18: 711–9.

375. Stennett DJ, Simonson W. Effect of membrane filtration on 10–mg/mL cefazolin admixtures. *Am J Hosp Pharm.* 1979; 36: 657–60.

376. Klink PR, Frable RA, Bornstein M. Stability of mandol in parenteral fluids, frozen solutions and admixtures containing other drugs. Presented at 13th annual ASHP midyear clinical meeting. San Antonio, TX: 1978 Dec.

377. Henney JE, Von Hoff DD, Rozencweig M, et al. Thrombophlebitic potential of intravenous cytotoxic agents. *Drug Intell Clin Pharm.* 1977; 11:266–7.

378. Sillers BR. Irritant properties of diazepam. *Br Dent J.* 1968; 124:295.

379. Roche Products Ltd. Irritant properties of diazepam—reply. *Br Dent J.* 1968; 124:295.

380. Friedenberg W, Barker JD Jr. Intravenous diazepam administration. *JAMA.* 1973; 224:901–2.

381. Jusko WJ, Gretch M, Gassett R. Precipitation of diazepam from intravenous preparationsi. *JAMA.* 1973; 225:176.

382. Kortilla K, Sothman A. Polyethylene glycol as a solvent for diazepam: bioavailability and clinical effects after intramuscular administration, comparison of oral, intramuscular and rectal administration, and precipitation from intravenous solutions. *Acta Pharmacol Toxicol (Copenh).* 1976; 39:104–17.

383. Hillestad L, Hansen T, Melsome H, et al. Diazepam metabolism in normal man I. Serum concentrations and clinical effects after intravenous, intramuscular and oral administration. *Clin Pharmacol Ther.* 1974; 16:479–84.

384. Assaf RA, Dundee JW, Gamble JA. The influence of the route of administration on the clinical action of diazepam. *Anaesthesia.* 1975; 30:152–8.

385. Baxter MT, McKenzie DD. Dilution of diazepam in intravenous fluids. *Am J Hosp Pharm.* 1977; 34:124.

386. Thong YH, Abramson DC. Continuous infusion of diazepam in infants with severe recurrent convulsions. *Med Ann DC.* 1974; 43:63–5.

387. Khalid MS, Schultz H. Treatment and management of emergency status epilepticus. *Epilepsia.* 1976; 17:73–6.

388. Gibberd FB. Diseases of the central nervous system—epilepsy. *Br Med J.* 1975; 4:270–2.

389. Kawathekar P, Anusuya SR, Sriniwas P, et al. Diazepam (Calmpose) in eclampsia: a preliminary report of 16 cases. *Curr Ther Res Clin Exp.* 1973; 15:845–55.

390. Baskett TF, Bradford CR. Active management of severe preeclampsia. *Can Med Assoc J.* 1973; 109:1209–11.

391. Prensky AL, Raff MC, Moore MJ, et al. Intravenous diazepam in the treatment of prolonged seizure activity. *N Engl J Med.* 1967; 276:779–84.

392. Tehrani JB, Cavanaugh A. Diazepam infusion in the treatment of tetanus. *Drug Intell Clin Pharm.* 1977; 11:491.

393. McLean WN. Safety of diazepam infusion questioned. *Drug Intell Clin Pharm.* 1977; 11:690.

394. Trissel LA, Kleinman LM, Davignon JP, et al. Investigational drug information—daunorubicin hydrochloride and streptozotocin. *Drug Intell Clin Pharm.* 1978; 12:404–6.

395. Elsberry VA, Grangeia JM, Giorgianni SJ, et al. The lipid phase in TPN. *Am J IV Ther.* 1977; 4:22–8.

396. Belin RP, Bivins BA, Jona JZ, et al. Fat overload with a 10% soybean oil emulsion. *Arch Surg.* 1976; 111:1391–3.

397. McNiff BL. Clinical use of 10% soybean oil emulsion. *Am J Hosp Pharm.* 1977; 34:1080–6.

398. Roche Laboratories, Nutley, NJ: Personal communication.

399. McGaw Laboratories. McGaw compatibility studies: a preliminary report. Irvine, CA; 1978.

400. Bundgaard H, Norgaard T, Nielsen NM. Photodegradation and hydrolysis of furosemide and furosemide esters in aqueous solutions. *Int J Pharm.* 1988; 42:217–24.

401. Kresel JJ, Smith AL. Stability of gentamicin in plastic syringes. *Am J Hosp Pharm.* 1977; 34:570.

402. McNeely DJ, Weiner B, Stewart RB, et al. Stability of gentamicin in plastic syringes. *Am J Hosp Pharm.* 1977; 34:570.

403. Chrai SS, Ambrosio TJ. Gentamicin sulfate injection repackaging in syringes. *Am J Hosp Pharm.* 1977; 34:920.

404. Davis SM (Medical Information Manager, Astra Zeneca, Wilmington, Delaware): Personal communication, August 21, 2003.

405. Sohn C, Cupit GC. Concentration of heparin in heparin-locks. *Drug Intell Clin Pharm.* 1978; 12:112.

406. Okuno T, Nelson CA. Anticoagulant activity of heparin in intravenous fluids. *J Clin Pathol.* 1975; 28:494–7.

407. Joy RT, Hyneck ML, Berardi RR, et al. Effect of pH on the stability of heparin in 5% dextrose solutions. *Am J Hosp Pharm.* 1979; 36:618–21.

408. Brown J, Stead K. Anti-human lymphocyte globulin-heparin precipitate. *Drug Intell Clin Pharm.* 1976; 10:654.

409. Raab WP, Windisch J. Antagonism of neomycin by heparin. Further observations on the anaphylactoid activity of neomycin. *Arzneimittelforschung.* 1973; 23:1326–8.

410. Stella VJ. A case for prodrugs: Fosphenytoin. *Adv Drug Del Rev.* 1996; 19:311–30.

411. Dupuis LL, Wong B. Stability of propafenone hydrochloride in i.v. solutions. *Am J Health-Syst Pharm.* 1997; 54:1293–5.

412. Dupuis LL, Trope A, Giesbrecht E, et al. Compatibility and stability of propafenone hydrochloride with five critical-care medications. *Can J Hosp Pharm.* 1998; 51:55–7.

413. Storvick WO, Henry HJ. Effect of storage temperature on stability of commercial insulin preparations. *Diabetes.* 1968; 17: 499–502.

414. Jackson RL, Storvick WO, Hollinden CS, et al. Neutral regular insulin. *Diabetes.* 1972; 21:235–45.

415. Page MM, Alberti KGMM, Greenwood R, et al. Treatment of diabetic coma with continuous low-dose infusion of insulin. *Br Med J.* 1974; 2:687–90.

416. Kidson W, Casey J, Kraegen E, et al. Treatment of severe diabetes mellitus by insulin infusion. *Br Med J.* 1974; 2:691–94.

417. Semple PF, White C. Continuous intravenous infusion of small doses of insulin in treatment of diabetic ketoacidosis. *Br Med J.* 1974; 2:694–8.

418. Campbell LV, Lazarus L, Casey JH, et al. Routine use of low-dose intravenous insulin infusion in severe hyperglycaemia. *Med J Aust.* 1976; 2:519–22.

419. Martin MM, Martin ALA. Continuous low-dose infusion of insulin in the treatment of diabetic ketoacidosis in children. *J Pediatr.* 1976; 89:560-4.

420. Drop SLS, Duval-Arnould BJM, Gober AE, et al. Low-dose intravenous insulin infusion versus subcutaneous insulin injection: A controlled comparative study of diabetic ketoacidosis. *Pediatrics.* 1977; 59:733–8.

421. Fisher JN, Shahshahani MN. Diabetic ketoacidosis: low-dose insulin therapy by various routes. *N Engl J Med*. 1977; 297: 238–41.

422. Goldberg NJ, Levin SR. Insulin adsorption to an inline membrane filter. *N Engl J Med*. 1978; 298:1480.

423. Kristofferson J, Skobba TJ. Adsorption of insulin to infusion equipment. *Nor Farm Tidsskr*. 1977; 85:220–4.

424. Hirsch JI, Fratkin MJ, Wood JH, et al. Clinical significance of insulin adsorption by polyvinyl chloride infusion systems. *Am J Hosp Pharm*. 1977; 34:583–8.

425. Weber SS, Wood WA. Availability of insulin from parenteral nutrient solutions. *Am J Hosp Pharm*. 1977; 34:353–7.

426. Whalen FJ, LeCain WK. Availability of insulin from continuous low-dose insulin infusions. *Am J Hosp Pharm*. 1979; 36: 330–7.

427. Clarke BF, Campbell IW, Fraser DM, et al. Direct addition of small doses of insulin to intravenous infusion in severe uncontrolled diabetes. *Br Med J*. 1977; 2:1395–6.

428. Peterson L, Caldwell J. Insulin adsorbance to polyvinyl chloride surfaces with implications for constant-infusion therapy. *Diabetes*. 1976; 25:72–4.

429. Sadeghi A, Mehrbanpour J, Behmard S, et al. A trial of total dose infusion iron therapy as an outpatient procedure in rural Iranian villages (a three month follow-up). *Curr Ther Res Clin Exp*. 1976; 19:595–602.

430. Leach JK, Strickland RD, Millis DL, et al. Biological activity of dilute isoproterenol solution stored for long periods in plastic bags. *Am J Hosp Pharm*. 1977; 34:709–12.

431. Browning ML. IM MgSO$_4$ ampuls for IV use. *Hosp Pharm*. 1976; 11:325.

432. Epperson E, Nedich RL. Mannitol crystallization in plastic containers. *Am J Hosp Pharm*. 1978; 35:1337.

433. Chatterji DC, Gallelli JF. Thermal and photolytic decomposition of methotrexate in aqueous solutions. *J Pharm Sci*. 1978; 67:526–31.

434. Muller HJ, Berg J. Stabilitatsstudie zu tramadolhydrochlorid im PVC-infusionbeutel. *Krankenhauspharmazie*. 1997; 18:75–9.

435. Duttera MJ, Gallelli JF, Kleinman LM, et al. Intrathecal methotrexate. *Lancet*. 1972; 2:540.

436. Hartshorn EA. Oxidation of methyldopate hydrochloride in alkaline media. *Am J Hosp Pharm*. 1975; 32:244.

437. Parker EA. Oxidation of methyldopate hydrochloride in alkaline media. *Am J Hosp Pharm*. 1975; 32:244.

438. Hartline JV, Zachman RD. Vitamin A delivery in total parenteral nutrition solution. *Pediatrics*. 1976; 58:448–51.

439. Sina A, Youssef MK, Kassem AA, et al. Stability of oxytetracycline in solutions and injections. *Can J Pharm Sci*. 1974; 9: 44–9.

440. Colding H, Anderson GE. Stability of antibiotics and amino acids in two synthetic L-amino acid solutions commonly used for total parenteral nutrition in children. *Antimicrob Agents Chemother*. 1978; 13:555–8.

441. Schneider E (Knoll AG, Milan, Italy): Personal communication; 2000 Feb 25.

442. Perrier D, Rapp R, Young B, et al. Maintenance of therapeutic phenytoin plasma levels via intramuscular administration. *Ann Intern Med*. 1976; 85:318–21.

443. Sellers EM, Kalant H. Alcohol intoxication and withdrawal. *N Engl J Med*. 1976; 294:757–62.

444. Nahata MC. Formulation of caffeine injection for i.v. administration. *Am J Hosp Pharm*. 1987; 44:1308, 1312.

445. Anon. Intravenous phenytoin. *N Engl J Med*. 1976; 295:1078.

446. Anon. Intravenous phenytoin. *N Engl J Med*. 1976; 295:1078.

447. Frank JT. Author's response. *Drug Intell Clin Pharm*. 1973; 7: 419.

448. Woo E, Greenblatt DJ. Choosing the right phenytoin dosage. *Drug Ther*. 1977; 7:131–9.

449. Bighley LD, Wille J. Mixing of additives in glass and plastic intravenous fluid containers. *Am J Hosp Pharm*. 1974; 31: 736–9.

450. Schondelmeyer S, Gatlin L. Intravenous phenytoin (concluded). *N Engl J Med*. 1977; 296:111.

451. Bauman JL, Siepler JK. Intravenous phenytoin (concluded). *N Engl J Med*. 1977; 296:111.

452. Sistare F, Greene R. Phenytoin crystallization in intravenous fluids. *Drug Intell Clin Pharm*. 1978; 12:120.

453. Biberdorf RI, Spurbeck GH. Phenytoin in IV fluids: results endorsed. *Drug Intell Clin Pharm*. 1978; 12:300–1.

454. Williams RHP. Potassium overdosage: a potential hazard of non-rigid parenteral fluid containers. *Br Med J*. 1973; 1: 714–5.

455. Woodside W, King JA. Addition of potassium to non-rigid plastic intravenous infusion containers: a potential hazard. *J Hosp Pharm*. 1973; 31:192–4.

456. Lankton JW, Siler JN. Hyperkalemia after administration of potassium from nonrigid parenteral-fluid containers. *Anesthesiology*. 1973; 39:660–1.

457. Vrabel RB, Amerson AB. Reconstitution of sodium nitroprusside. *Am J Hosp Pharm*. 1975; 32:140–1.

458. Challen RG. Stability of sodium nitroprusside solutions. *Australas J Pharm*. 1967; 48:S110.

459. Martin T, Patel JA. Determination of sodium nitroprusside in aqueous solution. *Am J Hosp Pharm*. 1969; 26:51–3.

460. Frank MJ, Johnson JB. Spectrophotometric determination of sodium nitroprusside and its photodegradation products. *J Pharm Sci*. 1976; 65:44–8.

461. Ammar HO. Stability of injection solutions of vitamin B$_1$. *Pharmazie*. 1976; 31:373–4.

462. Anon. Correction: sodium in ticarcillin and carbenicillin. *Med Lett Drugs Ther*. 1977; 19:28.

463. Yamaji A, Yasuko F, Okuda H, et al. Photodegradation of vitamin K^1 and vitamin K^2 injections in preservation and in intravenous admixtures. *J Nippon Hosp Pharm Assoc Sci Ed*. 1978; 4:7–11.

464. Kobayashi NH, King JC. Compatibility of common additives in protein hydrolysate/dextrose solutions. *Am J Hosp Pharm*. 1977; 34:589–94.

465. Humphreys A, Marty JJ, Gooey SL, et al. Stability of methotrexate in an intravenous fluid. *Aust J Hosp Pharm*. 1978; 8: 66–7.

466. Clayton SK. Stability of intravenous additive preparations; studies on hydralazine as an additive. *J Clin Pharm*. 1978; 2: 247-56.

467. Anon. Mixing chlorpromazine and morphine. *Br Med J*. 1974; 3:681.

468. Crapper JB. Mixing chlorpromazine and morphine. *Br Med J*. 1975; 1:33.

469. Baird GM, Willoughby MLN. Photodegradation of dacarbazine. *Lancet*. 1978; 2:681.

470. Georget S, Vigneron J, Blaise N, et al. Stability of refrigerated and frozen solutions of tropisetron in either polyvinylchloride or polyolefin infusion bags. *J Clin Pharm Ther*. 1997; 22: 257–60.

471. Bergman HD. Cefamandole. *Drug Intell Clin Pharm*. 1979; 13: 144–9.

472. Indelicato JM, Wilham WL. Conversion of cefamandole nafate to cefamandole sodium. *J Pharm Sci*. 1976; 65:1175–8.

473. Palmer MA, Fraterrigo CC. Production of carbon dioxide gas after reconstitution of cefamandole nafate. *Am J Hosp Pharm*. 1979; 36:596–7.

474. Klink PR, McKeechan CW. Production of carbon dioxide gas after reconstitution of cefamandole nafate. *Am J Hosp Pharm*. 1979; 36:597.

475. Bornstein M, Klink PR, Farrell BT, et al. Stability of frozen solutions of cefamandole nafate. *Am J Hosp Pharm,*. 1980; 37: 98-101.

476. Buckles J, Walters V. Stability of amitriptyline hydrochloride in aqueous solution. *J Clin Pharm*. 1976; 1:107–12.

477. Enever RP, Po ALW, Millard BJ, et al. Decomposition of amitriptyline hydrochloride in aqueous solution: identification of decomposition products. *J Pharm Sci*. 1975; 64:1497–9.

478. Enever RP, Po ALW. Factors influencing decomposition rate of amitriptyline hydrochloride in aqueous solution. *J Pharm Sci*. 1977; 66:1087–9.

479. Holman BL, Dewanjee MK. Potential pH incompatibility of pharmacological and isotopic adjuncts to arteriography. *Radiology*. 1974; 110:722–3.

480. Kawilarang CRT, Georghiou K. The effect of additives on the physical properties of a phospholipid-stabilized soybean oil emulsion. *J Clin Hosp Pharm*. 1980; 5:151–60.

481. Bristol Laboratories. Stadol Q&A. Syracuse, NY; 1978 Nov:7.

482. Jacobs RS. Calcitonin-Salmon. *Drug Intell Clin Pharm*. 1975; 9:557–9.

483. Nahata MC, Zingarelli J, Durrell DE. Stability of caffeine citrate injection in intravenous admixtures and parenteral nutrition solutions. *J Clin Pharm Ther*. 1989; 14:53–5.

484. Davignon JP, Yang KW, Wood HB, et al. Formulation of three nitrosoureas for intravenous use. *Cancer Chemother Rep 3*. 1973; 4(3):7–11.

485. Buckles J, Walters V. Stability of imipramine hydrochloride solutions. *J Clin Pharm*. 1976; 1:113–8.

486. Andreu A, Garcia B, Pastor C, et al. Estudio de la estabilidad *in vitro* de la ranitidine i.v. en una solucion de nutricion parenteral total conteniendo lipidos. *Nutr Hosp*. 1988; 3:50–5.

487. Smith JL, Canham JE, Wells PA. Effect of phototherapy light, sodium bisulfite, and pH on vitamin stability in total parenteral nutrition admixtures. *J Parenter Enteral Nutr*. 1988; 12: 394–402.

488. Lauper RD. Leucovorin calcium administration and preparation. *Am J Hosp Pharm*. 1978; 35:377.

489. Tavoloni N, Guarino AM. Photolytic degradation of adriamycin. *J Pharm Pharmacol*. 1980; 32:860–2.

490. Black CD, Popovich NG. Stability of intravenous fat emulsions. *Arch Surg*. 1980; 115:891.

491. Bacon L. A review of two safety factors in the use of paraldehyde. *J R Coll Gen Pract*. 1980; 30:622–4.

492. Horton JK, Stevens MFG. Search for drug interactions between the antitumor agent DTIC and other cytotoxic agents. *J Pharm Pharmacol*. 1979; 31(Suppl):64P.

493. Zaccardelli DS, Krcmarik CS, Wolk R, et al. Stability of imipenem and cilastatin sodium in total parenteral nutrient solution. *JPEN J Parenter Enteral Nutr*. 1990; 14:306–309.

494. Kuehnle C, Moore TD. Sodium chloride residue provides potential for drug incompatibilities. *Am J Hosp Pharm*. 1979; 36: 881.

495. Trissel LA, Kleinman LM, Cradock JC, et al. Investigational drug information—ifosfamide and semustine. *Drug Intell Clin Pharm*. 1979; 13:340–3.

496. Horton JK, Stevens MFG. A new light on the photo-decomposition of the antitumour drug DTIC. *J Pharm Pharmacol*. 1981; 33:808–11.

497. Earp CM, Barriere SL. The lack of inactivation of tobramycin by cefazolin, cefamandole, and moxalactam in vitro. *Drug Intell Clin Pharm*. 1985; 19:677–9.

498. Elliott TSJ, Eley A, Cowlishaw A. Stability of tobramycin in combination with selected new beta-lactam antibiotics. *J Antimicrob Chemother*. 1986; 17:680–1.

499. Gu L, Chiang HS, Becker A. Kinetics and mechanisms of the autoxidation of ketorolac tromethamine in aqueous solution. *Int J Pharm*. 1988; 41:95–104.

500. Brown AF, Harvey DA, Hoddinott DJ. Freeze thaw stability of ceftazidime. *Br J Parenter Ther*. 1985; 6:43–5.

501. Grimble GK, Hunjan MK, Payne-James JJ, et al. Zantac and TPN. *Br J Intensive Care*. 1991; 32:7.

502. Vieth R, Ledermann SE, Kooh SW, et al. Losses of calcitrol to peritoneal dialysis bags and tubing. *Peritoneal Dial Int*. 1989; 9:277–80.

503. McNiff BL, McNiff EF. Potency and stability of extemporaneous nitroglycerin infusions. *Am J Hosp Pharm*. 1979; 36: 173–7.

504. Giamarellou H, Mavroudis K, Petrikkos G, et al. In vitro and in vivo interactions of recent cephalosporins with gentamicin and amikacin. *Chemioterapia*. 1984; 3:183–7.

505. Milano G, Etienne MC, Cassuto-Viguier E, et al. Long-term stability of 5-fluorouracil and folinic acid admixtures. *Eur J Cancer*. 1993; 29A:129–32.

506. Sturek JK, Sokolski TD, Winsley WT, et al. Stability of nitroglycerin injection determined by gas chromatography. *Am J Hosp Pharm*. 1978; 35:537–41.

507. Fung HL. Potency and stability of extemporaneously prepared nitroglycerin intravenous solutions (editorial). *Am J Hosp Pharm*. 1978; 35:528–9.

508. Grouthamel WG, Dorsch B, Shangraw R. Loss of nitroglycerin from plastic intravenous bags. *N Engl J Med*. 1978; 299:262.

509. Cossum PA, Galbraith AJ, Roberts MS, et al. Loss of nitroglycerin from intravenous infusion sets. *Lancet*. 1978; 2: 349–50.

510. Boylan JC, Robison RL. Stability of nitroglycerin solutions in Viaflex plastic containers. *Am J Hosp Pharm*. 1978; 35:1031.

511. Ludwig DJ, Ueda CT. Apparent stability of nitroglycerin in dextrose 5% in water. *Am J Hosp Pharm*. 1978; 35:541–4.

512. Brillaud AR. Interaction of platinol (cisplatin) and the metal aluminum. Syracuse, NY: Bristol Laboratories; 1979 Jul.

513. Baxter Healthcare, Clintec Nutrition Division, Product information on Intralipid 10% and 20%. Deerfield IL; 2007 Apr.

514. Reference number not in use.

515. Sewell DL, Golper TA. Stability of antimicrobial agents in peritoneal dialysate. *Antimicrob Agents Chemother.* 1982; 21:528–9.

516. El-Mallakh R. Incompatibilities with cimetidine hydrochloride injection. *Am J Hosp Pharm.* 1979; 36:1024.

517. Cutie MR. Letters. *Hosp Formul.* 1980; 15:502–3.

518. Tung EC, Gurwich EL, Sula JA, et al. Stability of five antibiotics in plastic intravenous solution containers of dextrose and sodium chloride. *Drug Intell Clin Pharm.* 1980; 14:848–50.

519. Benvenuto JA, Anderson RW, Kerkof K, et al. Stability and compatibility of antitumor agents in glass and plastic containers. *Am J Hosp Pharm.* 1981; 38:1914–8.

520. Jhunjhunwala VP, Bhalla HL. Compatibility of mephentermine sulfate with hydrocortisone sodium succinate or aminophylline in 5% dextrose injection. *Am J Hosp Pharm.* 1981; 38:1922–4.

521. Jhunjhunwala VP, Bhalla HL. Compatibility of aminophylline with hydrocortisone sodium succinate or dexamethasone sodium phosphate in 5% dextrose injection. *Am J Hosp Pharm.* 1981; 38:900–1.

522. Lee YC, Malick AW, Amann AH, et al. Bretylium tosylate intravenous admixture compatibility. II. Dopamine, lidocaine, procainamide and nitroglycerin. *Am J Hosp Pharm.* 1981; 38:183–7.

523. Colvin M, Hartner J. Stability of carmustine in the presence of sodium bicarbonate. *Am J Hosp Pharm.* 1980; 37:677–8.

524. Dorr RT. Incompatibilities with parenteral anticancer drugs. *Am J IV Ther.* 45, 46, 52 (Feb-Mar) 1979; 6:42.

525. Das Gupta V, Stewart KR. Stability of cefamandole nafate and cefoxitin sodium solutions. *Am J Hosp Pharm.* 1981; 38:875–9.

526. Poochikian GK, Cradock JC. Stability of anthracycline antitumor agents in four infusion fluids. *Am J Hosp Pharm.* 1981; 38:483–6.

527. Newton DW, Fung EYY. Stability of five catecholamines and terbutaline sulfate in 5% dextrose injection in the absence and presence of aminophylline. *Am J Hosp Pharm.* 1981; 38:1314–9.

528. Neil JM. A rational approach to intravenous additives. *Proc Guild.* 1979; 7:3–33.

529. Otterman GE, Samuelson DW. Incompatibility between carbenicillin injection and promethazine injection. *Am J Hosp Pharm.* 1979; 36:1156.

530. Marshall TR, Ling IT, Follis G, et al. Pharmacological incompatibility of contrast media with various drugs and agents. *Radiology.* 1965; 84:536–9.

531. Monder C. Stability of corticosteroids in aqueous solutions. *Endocrinology.* 1968; 82:318–26.

532. Kleinberg ML, Stauffer GL, Prior RB, et al. Stability of antibiotics frozen and stored in disposable hypodermic syringes. *Am J Hosp Pharm.* 1980; 37:1087–8.

533. Butler LD, Munson JM. Effect of inline filtration on the potency of low-dose drugs. *Am J Hosp Pharm.* 1980; 37:935–41.

534. Allen LV, Stiles ML. Compatibility of various admixtures with secondary additives at Y-injection sites of intravenous administration sets. Part 2. *Am J Hosp Pharm.* 1981; 38:380–1.

535. Kleinberg, ML, Stauffer GL, et al. Stability of five liquid drug products after unit dose repackaging. *Am J Hosp Pharm.* 1980; 37:680–2.

536. Kowaluk EA, Roberts MS, Blackburn HD, et al. Interactions between drugs and polyvinyl chloride infusion bags. *Am J Hosp Pharm.* 1981; 38:1308–14.

537. Zatz L, Sethia P. Stability of refrigerated aminophylline in 5% dextrose in water: a 96–hour study. *Hosp Pharm.* 1981; 16:548.

538. Scott KR, Bell AF. Drug interactions I: Folic acid and calcium gluconate. *J Pharm Sci.* 1980; 69:234.

539. Jurgens RW, DeLuca PP. Compatibility of amphotericin B with certain large-volume parenterals. *Am J Hosp Pharm.* 1981; 38:377–8.

540. Gotz VP, Mar DD. Compatibility of amphotericin B with drugs used to reduce adverse reactions. *Am J Hosp Pharm.* 1981; 38:378–9.

541. Lee YC, Baaske DM, Amann AH, et al. Bretylium tosylate intravenous admixture compatibility. I. Stability in common large-volume parenteral solutions. *Am J Hosp Pharm.* 1980; 37:803–8.

542. Yuhas EM, Lofton FT, Baldinus JG, et al. Cimetidine hydrochloride compatibility with preoperative medications. *Am J Hosp Pharm.* 1981; 38:1173–4.

543. Smith FM, Nuessle NO. Stability of lidocaine hydrochloride in 5% dextrose injection in plastic bags. *Am J Hosp Pharm.* 1981; 38:1745–7.

544. Finch ME. Sodium thiopental in 5% dextrose in lactated Ringer's precipitate. *Hosp Pharm.* 1979; 14:559–60.

545. Kirschenbaum HL, Lesko LJ, Mendes RW, et al. Stability of procainamide in 0.9% sodium chloride or dextrose 5% in water. *Am J Hosp Pharm.* 1979; 36:1464–5.

546. Baaske DM, Malick AW. Stability of procainamide hydrochloride in dextrose solutions. *Am J Hosp Pharm.* 1980; 37:1050–2.

547. Jeglum EL, Winter E. Nafcillin sodium incompatibility with acidic solutions. *Am J Hosp Pharm.* 1981; 38:462.

548. Cutie MR, Lordi NG. Compatibility of verapamil hydrochloride injection in commonly used large-volume parenterals. *Am J Hosp Pharm.* 1980; 37:675–6.

549. Rosenberg HA, Dougherty JT, Mayron D, et al. Cimetidine hydrochloride compatibility I: Chemical aspects and room temperature stability in intravenous infusion fluids. *Am J Hosp Pharm.* 1980; 37:390–3.

550. Yuhas EM, Lofton FT, Mayron D, et al. Cimetidine hydrochloride compatibility II: Room temperature stability in intravenous infusion fluids. *Am J Hosp Pharm.* 1981; 38:879–81.

551. Yuhas EM, Lofton FT, Rosenberg HA, et al. Cimetidine hydrochloride compatibility III: Room temperature stability in drug admixtures. *Am J Hosp Pharm.* 1981; 38:1919–22.

552. Dahlin PA, Paredes SM. Visual compatibility of dobutamine with seven parenteral drug products. *Am J Hosp Pharm.* 1980; 37:460.

553. Lesko LJ, Marion A, Ericson J, et al. Stability of trimethoprim-sulfamethoxazole injection in two infusion fluids. *Am J Hosp Pharm.* 1981; 38:1004–6.

554. Holmes CJ, Ausman RK, Walter CW, et al. Activity of antibiotic admixtures subjected to different freeze-thaw treatments. *Drug Intell Clin Pharm.* 1980; 14:353–7.

555. Holmes CJ, Ausman RK, Kundsin RB, et al. Effect of freezing and microwave thawing on the stability of six antibiotic admixtures in plastic bags. *Am J Hosp Pharm.* 1982; 39:104–8.

556. Boddapati S, Yang K. Physiochemical properties of aminophylline-dextrose injection admixtures. *Am J Hosp Pharm.* 1982; 39:108–12.

557. Canton EM, Baluch WM. Effect of freezing on particle formation in three antibiotic injections. *Am J Hosp Pharm.* 1982; 39: 124–5.

558. Chaudry IA, Bruey KP, Hurlburt LE, et al. Compatibility of netilmicin sulfate injection with commonly used intravenous injections and additives. *Am J Hosp Pharm.* 1981; 38:1737–42.

559. Cutie MR. Effects of cold and freezing temperatures on pharmaceutical dosage forms. *US Pharmacist.* 1979; 4:38–40.

560. Gove L, Walls ADF. Mixing parenteral nutrition products. *Pharm J.* 1979; 223:587.

561. Lauder AD. Mixing parenteral nutrition products. *Pharm J.* 1979; 223:587.

562. Hardin TC, Clibon U. Stability of 5-fluorouracil in a crystalline amino acid solution. *Am J IV Ther Clin Nutr.* 1982; 9:39–40.

563. Yamaji A, Fujii Y, Kurata Y, et al. Stability of pyridoxine hydrochloride in infusion solution under practical circumstances in wards. *Yakuzaigaku.* 1980; 40:143–50.

564. Dony J, Devleeschouwer MJ. Etude de la degradation photochimique de macrolides en presence de riboflavine. *J Pharm Belg.* 1976; 31:479–84.

565. Parker WA, Shearer CA. Metoclopramide compatibility. *Can J Hosp Pharm.* 1979; 32:38.

566. Parker WA. Compatibility of perphenazine and butorphanol admixtures. *Can J Hosp Pharm.* 1980; 33:152.

567. Stiles ML, Allen LV. Retention of drugs during inline filtration of parenteral solutions. *Infusion.* 1979; 3:67–9.

568. Somani P, Leathem WD, Barlow AL. Safflower oil emulsion: single and multiple infusions with or without added heparin in normal human volunteers. *JPEN J Parenter Enteral Nutr.* 1980; 4:307–11.

569. Rubin M, Bilik R, Gruenewald Z, et al. Use of 5-micron filter in administering 'all-in-one' mixtures for total parenteral nutrition. *Clin Nutr.* 1985; 4:163–8.

570. Moore RA, Feldman S, Treuting J, et al. Cimetidine and parenteral nutrition. *JPEN J Parenter Enteral Nutr.* 1981; 5:61–3.

571. Das Gupta V, Stewart KR. Stability of haloperidol in 5% dextrose injection. *Am J Hosp Pharm.* 1982; 39:292–4.

572. Cutie MR, Waranis R. Compatibility of hydromorphone hydrochloride in large-volume parenterals. *Am J Hosp Pharm.* 1982; 39:307–8.

573. Mirtallo JM, Caryer K, Schneider PJ, et al. Growth of bacteria and fungi in parenteral nutrition solutions containing albumin. *Am J Hosp Pharm.* 1981; 38:1907–10.

574. Holt HA, Broughall JM, McCarthy MM, et al. Interactions between aminoglycoside antibiotics and carbenicillin or ticarcillin. *Infection.* 1976; 4:107–9.

575. Pickering LK, Gearhart P. Effect of time and concentration upon interaction between gentamicin, tobramycin, netilmicin, or amikacin and carbenicillin or ticarcillin. *Antimicrob Agents Chemother.* 1979; 15:592–6.

576. Pieper JA, Vidal RA. Animal model distinguishing in vitro from in vivo carbenicillin-aminoglycoside interactions. *Antimicrob Agents Chemother.* 1980; 18:604–9.

577. Sturgeon RJ, Athanikar NK, Henry RS, et al. Titratable acidities of crystalline amino acid admixtures. *Am J Hosp Pharm.* 1980; 37:388–90.

578. Ausman RK, Kerkhof K, Holmes CJ, et al. Frozen storage and microwave thawing of parenteral nutrition solutions in plastic containers. *Drug Intell Clin Pharm.* 1981; 15:440–3.

579. Tortorici MP, Fearing D, Inman M, et al. Photoreaction involving essential amino acid injection. *Am J Hosp Pharm.* 1978; 35: 1030.

580. West KR, Sansom LN, Cosh DG, et al. Some aspects of the stability of parenteral nutrition solutions. *Pharm Acta Helv.* 1976; 51(1):19–22.

581. Jurgens RW, Henry RS. Amino acid stability in a mixed parenteral nutrition solution. *Am J Hosp Pharm.* 1981; 38:1358–9.

582. Mirtallo JM, Rogers KR, Johnson JA, et al. Stability of amino acids and the availability of acid in total parenteral nutrition solutions containing hydrochloric acid. *Am J Hosp Pharm.* 1981; 38:1729–31.

583. Rusho WJ, Standish R. A comparison of crystalline amino acid solutions for total parenteral nutrition. *Hosp Formul.* 1981; 16: 29–33.

584. Anon. Guidelines for essential trace element preparations for parenteral use. A statement by an expert panel. AMA Department of Foods and Nutrition. *JAMA..* 1979; 241:2051–54.

585. Freund H, Atamian S, Fischer JE. Chromium deficiency during total parenteral nutrition. *JAMA.* 1979; 241:496–8.

586. Heller RM, Kirchner SG, O'Neill JA, et al. Skeletal changes of copper deficiency in infants receiving prolonged total parenteral nutrition. *J Pediatr.* 1978; 92:947–9.

587. Moran DM, Russo J. Zinc deficiency dermatitis accompanying parenteral nutrition supplemented with trace elements. *Clin Pharm.* 1982; 1:169–76.

588. Askari A, Long CL, Blakemore WS. Zinc, copper, and parenteral nutrition in cancer. A review. *JPEN J Parenter Enteral Nutr.* 1980; 4:561–71.

589. Wolman SL, Anderson GH, Marliss EB, et al. Zinc in total parenteral nutrition: requirements and metabolic effects. *Gastroenterology.* 1979; 76:458–67.

590. Fliss DM, Lamy PP. Trace elements and total parenteral nutrition. *Hosp Formul.* 1979; 14:698–717.

591. Schneider PJ. Total parenteral nutrition: Part II: What goes into parenteral nutrition solutions?. *J Postgrad Pharm (Hosp Ed).* 1979; 1:18–27.

592. Isaacs JW, Millikan WJ, Stackhouse J, et al. Parenteral nutrition of adults with a 900 milliosmolar solution via peripheral veins. *Am J Clin Nutr.* 1977; 30:552–9.

593. Romankiewicz JA, McManus J, Gotz VP, et al. Medications not to be refrigerated. *Am J Hosp Pharm.* 1979; 36:1541–5.

594. Swerling R. Dilution of oral and intravenous aminophylline preparations. *Am J Hosp Pharm.* 1981; 38:1359–60.

595. Alcorn BT, Barnes SG. Pharmacy-initiated intravenous infusion guidelines. *Hosp Pharm.* 1982; 17:60–76.

596. Bowtle WJ, Heasman MJ, Prince AP, et al. Compatibility of the cephalosporin, cefamandole nafate, with injections. *Int J Pharm.* 1980; 4:263–5.

597. Anon. I.V. dosage guidelines for theophylline products. *FDA Drug Bull.* 1980; 10:4–5.

598. Tipple M, Shadomy S. Availability of active amphotericin B after filtration through membrane filters. *Am Rev Resp Dis.* 1977; 115:879–81.

599. Maddux MS, Barriere SL. A review of complications of amphotericin B therapy: recommendations for prevention and management. *Drug Intell Clin Pharm.* 1980; 14:177–81.

600. Lufter CH, Ball WD. Activity of amphotericin B after filtration. *Drug Intell Clin Pharm.* 1980; 14:719.

601. Kuchinskas EJ, Levy GN. Comparative stabilities of ampicillin and hetacillin in aqueous solutions. *J Pharm Sci.* 1972; 61:727–9.

602. Schwartz MA, Hayton WL. Relative stability of hetacillin and ampicillin in solution. *J Pharm Sci.* 1972; 61:906–9.

603. Bundgaard H. Polymerization of penicillins: kinetics and mechanism of di- and polymerization of ampicillin in aqueous solution. *Acta Pharm Suec.* 1976; 13:9–26.

604. Stjernstrom G, Olson OT, Nyqvist H, et al. Studies on the stability and compatibility of drugs in infusion fluids 6. Factors affecting the stability of ampicillin. *Acta Pharm Suec.* 1978; 15:33–50.

605. Johnson CA, Porter WA. Compatibility of azathioprine sodium with intravenous fluids. *Am J Hosp Pharm.* 1981; 38:871–5.

606. Kowaluk EA, Roberts MS. Interactions between drugs and intravenous delivery systems. *Am J Hosp Pharm.* 1982; 39:460–7.

607. Bryan CK, Darby MH. Bretylium tosylate: a review. *Am J Hosp Pharm.* 1979; 36:1189–92.

608. Henry RS, Jurgens RW, Sturgeon R, et al. Compatibility of calcium chloride and calcium gluconate with sodium phosphate in a mixed TPN solution. *Am J Hosp Pharm.* 1980; 37:673–4.

609. Eggert LD, Rusho WJ, MacKay MW, et al. Calcium and phosphorus compatibility in parenteral nutrition solutions for neonates. *Am J Hosp Pharm.* 1982; 39:49–53.

610. Robinson LA, Wright BT. Central venous catheter occlusion caused by body-heat-mediated calcium phosphate precipitation. *Am J Hosp Pharm.* 1982; 39:120–1.

611. Tuttle CB. Guidelines for phenytoin infusions. *Can J Hosp Pharm.* 1984; 37:137–9.

612. Stewart P, Lourwood D. Guidelines for the administration of a phenytoin loading dose via IVPB. *Hosp Pharm.* 1986; 21:1003–4.

613. Goldschmied S. An evaluation of the stability and safety of phenytoin infusion. *NY State J Pharm.* 1987; 7:45–7.

614. Kradjan WA, Burger R. In vivo inactivation of gentamicin by carbenicillin and ticarcillin. *Arch Intern Med.* 1980; 140:1668–70.

615. Young LS, Decker G. Inactivation of gentamicin by carbenicillin in the urinary tract. *Chemotherapy.* 1974; 20:212–20.

616. Henderson JL, Polk RE. In vitro inactivation of gentamicin, tobramycin, and netilmicin by carbenicillin, azlocillin, or mezlocillin. *Am J Hosp Pharm.* 1981; 38:1167–70.

617. Flournoy DJ. Inactivation of netilmicin by carbenicillin. *Infection.* 1978; 6:241.

618. Russo ME. Penicillin-aminoglycoside inactivation: another possible mechanism of interaction. *Am J Hosp Pharm.* 1980; 37:702–4.

619. Laskar PA, Ayres JW. Degradation of carmustine in aqueous media. *J Pharm Sci.* 1977; 66:1073–6.

620. Cardi V, Willcox GS. Reconstituting cefamandole and protecting from light. *Am J Hosp Pharm.* 1980; 37:334.

621. Kaiser GV, Gorman M. Cefamandole—a review of chemistry and microbiology. *J Infect Dis.* 1978; 137:S10–S16.

622. Wold JS, Joost RR, Black HR, et al. Hydrolysis of cefamandole nafate to cefamandole in vivo. *J Infect Dis.* 1978; 137:S17–S24.

623. Palmer MA, Fraterrigo CC. Clarification of "explosive-like" reaction occurring when reconstituted cefamandole nafate was stored in syringes. *Am J Hosp Pharm.* 1979; 36:1025.

624. Fites AL. Reconstituting cefamandole and protecting from light. *Am J Hosp Pharm.* 1980; 37:334.

625. Foster TS, Shrewsbury RP, Coonrod JD. Bioavailability and pain study of cefamandole nafate. *J Clin Pharmacol.* 1980; 20:526–33.

626. Indelicato JM, Stewart BA. Formylation of glucose by cefamandole nafate at alkaline pH. *J Pharm Sci.* 1980; 69:1183–8.

627. Tomecko GW, Kleinberg ML, Latiolais CL, et al. Stability of cefazolin sodium admixtures in plastic bags after thawing by microwave radiation. *Am J Hosp Pharm.* 1980; 37:211–5.

628. Janousek JP, Minisci MP. An evaluation of cefazolin sodium injection in an IV piggyback bottle. *Infusion.* 1978; 2:67–73.

629. Stiles ML. Effect of microwave radiation on the stability of frozen cefoxitin sodium solution in plastic bags. *Am J Hosp Pharm.* 1981; 38:1743–5.

630. Oberholtzer ER, Brenner GS. Cefoxitin sodium: solution and solid state chemical stability studies. *J Pharm Sci.* 1979; 68:863–6.

631. Bray RJ, Davies PA. The stability of preservative-free morphine in plastic syringes. *Anaesthesia.* 1986; 41:294–5.

632. Walker SE, Paton TW, Fabian TM, et al. Stability and sterility of cimetidine admixtures frozen in minibags. *Am J Hosp Pharm.* 1981; 38:881–3.

633. Cohen MR. Error 148—More on cisplatin storage. *Hosp Pharm.* 1980; 15:158–9.

634. LeRoy AF. Some quantitative data on cis-dichlorodiammineplatinum (II) species in solution. *Cancer Treat Rep.* 1979; 63:231–3.

635. Hincal AA, Long DF. Cis-platin stability in aqueous parenteral vehicles. *J Parenter Drug Assoc.* 1979; 33:107–16.

636. Mariani EP, Southard BJ, Woolever JT, et al. Physical compatibility and chemical stability of cisplatin in various diluents and in large-volume parenteral solutions. In: Cisplatin current status and new developments. New York, NY: Academic Press; 1980:305–16.

637. Repta AJ, Long DF. cis-Dichlorodiammineplatinum (II) stability in aqueous vehicles. *Cancer Treat Rep.* 1979; 63:229–30.

638. Gamble JA, Dundee JW, Assaf RA. Plasma diazepam levels after single dose oral and intramuscular administration. *Anaesthesia.* 1975; 30:164–9.

639. Langdon DE, Harlan JR, Bailey RL. Thrombophlebitis with diazepam used intravenously. *JAMA.* 1973; 223:184–5.

640. Dam M, Christiansen J. Diazepam: intravenous infusion in the treatment of status epilepticus. *Acta Neurol Scand.* 1976; 54:278–80.

641. Huber JW, Raymond GG. Additional conclusions on diazepam injectable precipitate: GC-MS confirmation. *Clin Toxicol.* 1979; 14:439–44.

642. Raymond G, Huber JW. Identification of injectable Valium precipitate. *Drug Intell Clin Pharm*. 1979; 13:612.

643. Newton DW, Driscoll DF, Goudreau JL, et al. Solubility characteristics of diazepam in aqueous admixture solutions: theory and practice. *Am J Hosp Pharm*. 1981; 38:179–82.

644. Mason NA, Cline S, Hyneck ML, et al. Factors affecting diazepam infusion: solubility, administration-set composition, and flow rate. *Am J Hosp Pharm*. 1981; 38:1449–54.

645. MacKichan J, Duffner PK. Adsorption of diazepam to plastic tubing. *N Engl J Med*. 1979; 301:332–3.

646. Parker WA, MacCara ME. Compatibility of diazepam with intravenous fluid containers and administration sets. *Am J Hosp Pharm*. 1980; 37:496–500.

647. Cloyd JC, Vezeau C. Availability of diazepam from plastic containers. *Am J Hosp Pharm*. 1980; 37:492–6.

648. Cloyd JC. Diluting diazepam injection. *Am J Hosp Pharm*. 1981; 38:32.

649. Dasta JF, Brier K. Loss of diazepam to drug delivery systems. *Am J Hosp Pharm*. 1980; 37:1176.

650. Boatman JA, Johnson JB. A four-stage approach to new-drug development. *Pharm Tech*. 1981; 5:46–56.

651. Martin CM. Chemical incompatibility of Renografin 76 and protamine sulfate. *Am Heart J*. 1976; 91:675–7.

652. Hoffman DM, Grossano DD, Damin L, et al. Stability of refrigerated and frozen solutions of doxorubicin hydrochloride. *Am J Hosp Pharm*. 1979; 36:1536–8.

653. Gardiner WA. Possible incompatibility of doxorubicin hydrochloride with aluminum. *Am J Hosp Pharm*. 1981; 38:1276.

654. Pfaller MA, Granich GG, Valdes R, et al. Comparative study of the ability of four aminoglycoside assay techniques to detect the inactivation of aminoglycosides by beta-lactam antibiotics. *Diagn Microbiol Infect Dis*. 1984; 2:93–100.

655. Hospira Inc. Product information on Liposyn III 10%, 20%, and 30%. Lake Forest, IL; 2005 Aug/Sep.

656. Black CD, Popovich NG. Study of intravenous emulsion compatibility: effects of dextrose, amino acids and selected electrolytes. *Drug Intell Clin Pharm*. 1981; 15:184–93.

657. Black CD, Popovich NG. Comment on intravenous emulsion compatibility. *Drug Intell Clin Pharm*. 1981; 15:908–9.

658. Pelham LD. Rational use of intravenous fat emulsions. *Am J Hosp Pharm*. 1981; 38:198–208.

659. Soussol C. Long-term parenteral nutrition: an artificial gut. *Int Surg*. 1976; 61:266–70.

660. Wretlind A. Current status of intralipid and other fat emulsions. In: Fat emulsion in parenteral nutrition. Chicago, IL: American Medical Association; 1975:109–19.

661. Higbee KC, Lamy PP. Use of Intralipid in neonates and infants. *Hosp Formul*. (Feb) 1980; 15:117–9, 122, 127.

662. Kleinberg ML, Stauffer GL. Effect of microwave radiation on redissolving precipitated matter in fluorouracil injection. *Am J Hosp Pharm*. 1980; 37:678–9.

663. Driessen O, deVos D. Adsorption of fluorouracil on glass surfaces. *J Pharm Sci*. 1978; 67:1494–5.

664. Ghanekar AG, Das Gupta V. Stability of furosemide in aqueous systems. *J Pharm Sci*. 1978; 67:808–11.

665. McLaughlin JE, Reeves DS. Gentamicin plus carbenicillin. *Lancet*. 1971; 1:864–5.

666. Young LS, Decker G. Inactivation of gentamicin by carbenicillin in the urinary tract. *Chemotherapy*. 1974; 20:212–20.

667. Murillo J, Standiford HC, Schimpff SC, et al. Gentamicin and ticarcillin serum levels. *JAMA*. 1979; 241:2401–3.

668. Storey P, Hill HH, St. Louis RH, et al. Subcutaneous infusions for control of cancer symptoms. *J Pain Symptom Manag*. 1990; 5:33–41.

669. Edwards ND, Fletcher A, Cole JR, et al. Combined infusions of morphine and ketamine for postoperative pain in elderly patients. *Anaesthesia*. 1993; 48:124–7.

670. Dormarunno CG (Associate Medical Information Scientist, Medical and Drug Information, Pharmacia Corp., Kalamazoo, MI): Personal communication; 2002 Mar 21.

671. Liles S (Department of Pharmacy, Christ Hospital, Cincinnati, OH): Personal communication; 2002 Feb 20.

672. Hayes DM, Reilly RM. The pharmaceutical stability of deferoxamine mesylate. *Can J Hosp Pharm*. 1994; 47:9–14.

673. Downie G, McRae N. Leaching of plasticizers by fat emulsion from polyvinyl chloride. *Br J Parenter Ther*. 1985; 6:142–4.

674. Anderson W, Harthill JE, Couper IA, et al. Heparin stability in dextrose solutions [proceedings]. *J Pharm Pharmacol*. 1977; 29:31P.

675. Bowie HM, Haylor V. Stability of heparin in sodium chloride solution. *J Clin Pharm*. 1978; 3:211–4.

676. Tunbridge LJ, Lloyd JV, Penhall RK, et al. Stability of diluted heparin sodium stored in plastic syringes. *Am J Hosp Pharm*. 1981; 38:1001–4.

677. Deeb EN, DiMattia PE. Standardization of heparin-lock maintenance solution. *N Engl J Med*. 1976; 294:448.

678. Holford NHG, Vozeh S, Coates P, et al. More on heparin lock. *N Engl J Med*. 1977; 296:1300–1.

679. Lynch CL, Linder GE. Frequently asked questions about insulin. *Hosp Pharm*. 1980; 15:213–4.

680. Graham DT, Pomeroy AR. Effects of freezing on commercial insulin suspensions. *Int J Pharm*. 1978; 1:315–22.

681. Hill JB. Adsorption of insulin to glass. *Proc Soc Exp Biol Med*. 1959; 102:75–7.

682. Hill JB. The adsorption of I^{131}-insulin to glass. *Endocrinology*. 1959; 65:515–7.

683. Wiseman R, Baltz BE. Prevention of insulin-I^{131} adsorption to glass. *Endocrinology*. 1961; 68:354–6.

684. Sonksen PH, Ellis JP, Lowy C, et al. Quantitative evaluation of the relative efficiency of gelatine and albumin in preventing insulin adsorption to glass. *Diabetologia*. 1965; 1:208–10.

685. Suess V, Froesch ER. Zur therapie des coma diabeticum: quantitative bedeutung des insulinuerlusts am infusionsbesteck. *Schweizer Med Wochanschr*. 1975; 105:1315–8.

686. Okamoto H, Kikuchi T. Adsorption of insulin to infusion bottles and plastic intravenous tubing. *Yakuzaigaku*. 1979; 39:107–11.

687. Wingert TD, Levin SR. Insulin adsorption to an air-eliminating inline filter. *Am J Hosp Pharm*. 1981; 38:382–3.

688. Hirsch JI, Wood JH. Insulin adsorption to polyolefin infusion bottles and polyvinyl chloride administration sets. *Am J Hosp Pharm*. 1981; 38:995–7.

689. Kerchner J, Cocaluca DM. Effect of whole blood on insulin adsorption onto intravenous infusion systems. *Am J Hosp Pharm*. 1980; 37:1323–5.

690. Galloway JA, Bressler R. Insulin treatment in diabetes. *Med Clin N Am*. 1978; 62:663–80.

691. Anon. Letter: Carrier solutions for low-level intravenous insulin infusion. *Br Med J*. 1976; 1:151–2.

692. Wan KK, Tsallas G. Dilute iron dextran formulation for addition to parenteral nutrient solutions. *Am J Hosp Pharm*. 1980; 37: 206–10.

693. Bornstein M, Lo AY, Thomas PN, et al. Moxalactam disodium compatibility with intramuscular and intravenous diluents. *Am J Hosp Pharm*. 1982; 39:1495–8.

694. Kleinberg ML, Latiolais CJ. Use of a microwave oven to redissolve crystallized mannitol injection (25%) in ampuls. *Hosp Pharm*. 1979; 14:391–2.

695. Hanson GG. Microwave oven explosion. *Hosp Pharm*. 1979; 14:612.

696. Kleinberg ML, Latiolais CJ. Microwave oven explosion. *Hosp Pharm*. 1979; 14:612.

697. Kana MJ. Microwave oven explosion. *Hosp Pharm*. 1980; 15: 104.

698. Post RE, Stephen SP. A warming cabinet for storing mannitol ampuls. *Hosp Pharm*. 1975; 10:102–3.

699. Scott KR, Bell AF, Thomas AJ. Warming kettle for storing mannitol injection. *Am J Hosp Pharm*. 1980; 37:16.

700. Herring P. Keeping mannitol in solution. *Hosp Pharm*. 1980; 15:530–1.

701. Church JJ. Continuous narcotic infusions for relief of postoperative pain. *Br Med J*. 1979; 1:977–9.

702. Townsend RJ, Puchala AH. Stability of methylprednisolone sodium succinate in small volumes of 5% dextrose and 0.9% sodium chloride injections. *Am J Hosp Pharm*. 1981; 38: 1319–22.

703. Knutsen CV, Epps DR, McCormick DC, et al. Total nutrient admixture guidelines. *Drug Intell Clin Pharm*. 1984; 18: 253–4.

704. Riggle MA, Brandt RB. Decomposition of TPN solutions. *J Pediatr*. 1982; 100:670.

705. Freund HR, Rimon B, Muggia-Sullam M, et al. The "All in one" system for TPN causes increased rates of catheter blockade. *J Parenter Enteral Nutr*. 1986; 10:543.

706. Cohen MR. Hazard warning—Flagyl IV (metronidazole hydrochloride) product reconstitution. *Hosp Pharm*. 1981; 16:398.

707. Little GB, Boylan JC. I.V. Flagyl reacts with aluminum. *Hosp Pharm*. 1981; 16:627.

708. Carmichael RR, Mahoney CD. Solubility and stability of phenytoin sodium when mixed with intravenous solutions. *Am J Hosp Pharm*. 1980; 37:95–8.

709. Salem RB, Yost RL, Torosian G, et al. Investigation of the crystallization of phenytoin in normal saline. *Drug Intell Clin Pharm*. 1980; 14:605–8.

710. Pfeifle CE, Adler DS. Phenytoin sodium solubility in three intravenous solutions. *Am J Hosp Pharm*. 1981; 38:358–2.

711. Reference number not in use.

712. Gupta VD, Stewart KR. Stability of cefuroxime sodium in some aqueous buffered solutions and intravenous admixtures. *J Clin Hosp Pharm*. 1986; 11:47–54.

713. Newton DW, Kluza RB. Prediction of phenytoin solubility in intravenous admixtures: physicochemical theory. *Am J Hosp Pharm*. 1980; 37:1647–51.

714. Cohen MR. Make sure your nurses mix drug additions to infusing I.V. solutions. *Hosp Pharm*. 1981; 16:164.

715. Schuna A, Nappi J, Kolstad J. Potassium pooling in non-rigid parenteral fluid containers. *J Parenter Drug Assoc*. 1979; 33: 184–6.

716. McCloskey WW, Jeffrey LP. Rational ordering of phosphate supplements. *Hosp Pharm*. 1979; 14:486–7.

717. Herman JJ. Phosphate: its valence and methods of quantification in parenteral solutions. *Drug Intell Clin Pharm*. 1979; 13: 579–85.

718. Benderev K. Hypophosphatemia and phosphorus supplementation. *Hosp Pharm*. 1980; 15:611–3.

719. Swerling R. Use and preparation of cardioplegic solutions in cardiac surgery. *Hosp Pharm*. 1980; 15:497–503.

720. Loucas SP, Mehl B, Maager P, et al. Stability of procaine HCl in a buffered cardioplegia formulation. *Am J Hosp Pharm*. 1981; 38:1924–8.

721. Amann AH, Baaske DM. Plastic i.v. container for nitroglycerin. *Am J Hosp Pharm*. 1980; 37:618.

722. Cacace LG, Harralson A, Clougherty T. Stability of NTG. *Am Heart J*. 1979; 97:817–8.

723. Yuen PH, Denman SL, Sokoloski TD, et al. Loss of nitroglycerin from aqueous solution into plastic intravenous delivery systems. *J Pharm Sci*. 1979; 68:1163–6.

724. Baaske DM, Amann AH, Wagenknecht DM, et al. Nitroglycerin compatibility with intravenous fluid filters, containers, and administration sets. *Am J Hosp Pharm*. 1980; 37:201–5.

725. Roberts MS, Cossum PA, Galbraith AJ, et al. Availability of nitroglycerin from parenteral solutions. *J Pharm Pharmacol*. 1980; 32:237–44.

726. Christiansen H, Skobba TJ, Andersen R, et al. Nitroglycerin infusion—factors influencing the concentration of nitroglycerin available to the patient. *J Clin Hosp Pharm*. 1980; 5:209–15.

727. Sokoloski TD, Wu CC. Rapid adsorptive loss of nitroglycerin from aqueous solution to plastic. *Int J Pharm*. 1980; 6:63–76.

728. Baaske DM, Amann AH, Karnatz NN, et al. Administration set for use with intravenous nitroglycerin. *Am J Hosp Pharm*. 1982; 39:121–2.

729. Little LA, Hatheway GJ. Problems with administration devices for commercially available nitroglycerin injection. *Am J Hosp Pharm*. 1982; 39:400.

730. Schad RF, Jennings R. Problems with administration devices for commercially available nitroglycerin injection. *Am J Hosp Pharm*. 1982; 39:400.

731. Turco SJ. Problems with administration devices for commercially available nitroglycerin injection. *Am J Hosp Pharm*. 1982; 39:977.

732. Vesey CJ, Batistoni GA. Determination and stability of sodium nitroprusside in aqueous solutions (determination and stability of SNP). *J Clin Pharm*. 1977; 2:105–7.

733. Milewski B, Jones D. Photodecomposition. *Hosp Pharm*. 1981; 16:178.

734. Nolly RJ, Stach PE, Latiolais CJ, et al. Stability of thiamine hydrochloride repackaged in disposable syringes. *Am J Hosp Pharm*. 1982; 39:471–4.

735. Polk RE, Kline BJ. Mail order tobramycin serum levels: low values caused by ticarcillin. *Am J Hosp Pharm*. 1980; 37:920.

736. Seitz DJ, Archambault JR, Kresel JJ, et al. Stability of tobramycin sulfate in plastic syringes. *Am J Hosp Pharm*. 1980; 37: 1614–5.

737. Levison ME, Knight R. In vitro evaluation of tobramycin, a new aminoglycoside antibiotic. *Antimicrob Agents Chemother.* 1972; 1:381–4.

738. Svensson LA. Stressed oxidative degradation of terbutaline in aqueous solution. *Acta Pharm Suec.* 1972; 9:141–6.

739. Cutie MR. Compatibility of verapamil with other additives. *Am J Hosp Pharm.* 1981; 38:231.

740. Lederle Laboratories. Hospital formulary monograph—Pipracil. Wayne, NJ; 1981 Nov.

741. Chan KK, Giannini DD, Staroscik JA, et al. 5-Azacytidine hydrolysis kinetics measured by high-pressure liquid chromatography and ¹³C-NMR spectroscopy. *J Pharm Sci.* 1979; 68: 807–12.

742. Rubin M, Bilik R, Aserin A, et al. Catheter obstruction: analysis of filter content of total nutrient admixture. *J Parenter Enteral Nutr.* 1989; 13:641–3.

743. Flora KP, Smith SL. Application of a simple high-performance liquid chromatographic method for the determination of melphalan in the presence of its hydrolysis products. *J Chromatogr.* 1979; 177:91–7.

744. Palmer AJ, Sewell GJ, Rowland CG. Qualitative studies on α-interferon-2b in prolonged continuous infusion regimes using gradient elution high-performance liquid chromatography. *J Clin Pharm Ther.* 1988; 13:225–31.

745. Morris ME, Parker WA. Compatibility of chlordiazepoxide HCl injection following dilution. *Can J Pharm Sci.* 1981; 16:43–5.

746. Cummings DS, Park MK. Compatibility of propranolol hydrochloride injection with intravenous infusion fluids in plastic containers. *Am J Hosp Pharm.* 1982; 39:1685–7.

747. Deans KW, Lang JR. Stability of trimethoprim-sulfamethoxazole injection in five infusion fluids. *Am J Hosp Pharm.* 1982; 39:1681–4.

748. Munson JW, Kubiak EJ. Cytosine arabinoside stability in intravenous admixtures with sodium bicarbonate and in plastic syringes. *Drug Intell Clin Pharm.* 1982; 16:765–7.

749. Kirschenbaum HL, Aronoff W, Perentesis GP, et al. Stability of dobutamine hydrochloride in selected large-volume parenterals. *Am J Hosp Pharm.* 1982; 39:1923–5.

750. Ray JB, Newton DW, Nye MT, et al. Droperidol stability in intravenous admixtures. *Am J Hosp Pharm.* 1983; 40:94–7.

751. Das Gupta V, Stewart KR. Stability of cefotaxime sodium and moxalactam disodium in 5% dextrose and 0.9% sodium chloride injections. *Am J IV Ther Clin Nutr.* 27–9 (Jan) 1983; 10:20.

752. Jett S, Eng SS. Prochlorperazine edisylate incompatibility. *Am J Hosp Pharm.* 1983; 40:210.

753. Porter WR, Johnson CA, Cohon MS, et al. Compatibility and stability of clindamycin phosphate with intravenous fluids. *Am J Hosp Pharm.* 1983; 40:91–4.

754. Hittel WP, Iafrate RP, Karnes HT, et al. Stability of pentobarbital sodium in 5% dextrose injection and 0.9% sodium chloride injection. *Am J Hosp Pharm.* 1983; 40:294–6.

755. Niemiec PW, Vanderveen TW, Hohenwarter MW, et al. Stability of aminophylline injection in three parenteral nutrition solutions. *Am J Hosp Pharm.* 1983; 40:428–32.

756. Perentesis GP, Piltz GW, Kirschenbaum HL, et al. Stability and visual compatibility of bretylium tosylate with selected large-volume parenterals and additives. *Am J Hosp Pharm.* 1983; 40: 1010–2.

757. Yuen PC, Taddei CR, Wyka BE, et al. Compatibility and stability of labetalol hydrochloride in commonly used intravenous solutions. *Am J Hosp Pharm.* 1983; 40:1007–9.

758. Pyter RA, Hsu LCC. Stability of methylprednisolone sodium succinate in 5% dextrose and 0.9% sodium chloride injection. *Am J Hosp Pharm.* 1983; 40:1329–33.

759. Gannon PM, Sesin GP. Stability of cytarabine following repackaging in plastic syringes and glass containers. *Am J IV Ther Clin Nutr.* 1983; 10:11–6.

760. Sesin GP, Millette LA. Stability study of 5-fluorouracil following repackaging in plastic disposable syringes and multidose vials. *Am J IV Ther Clin Nutr.* 29–30 (Sep) 1982; 9:23–5.

761. Parker WA. Compatibility of perphenazine and butorphanol admixtures. *Can J Hosp Pharm.* 1981; 34:38.

762. Jump WG, Plaza VM. Compatibility of nalbuphine hydrochloride with other preoperative medications. *Am J Hosp Pharm.* 1982; 39:841–3.

763. Dorr RT, Peng YM, Alberts DS. Bleomycin compatibility with selected intravenous medications. *J Med.* 1982; 13(1–:2):121–30.

764. Cutie MR. Compatibility of verapamil hydrochloride injection with commonly used additives. *Am J Hosp Pharm.* 1983; 40: 1205–7.

765. Shively CD, Redford A. Flagyl I.V., drug-drug physical compatibility. *Am J IV Ther Clin Nutr.* 1981; 8:9–16.

766. Souney PF, Steele L. Effect of vitamin B complex and ascorbic acid on the antimicrobial activity of cefazolin sodium. *Am J Hosp Pharm.* 1982; 39:840–1.

767. Keller JH, Ensminger WD. Stability of cancer chemotherapeutic agents in a totally implanted drug delivery system. *Am J Hosp Pharm.* 1982; 39:1321–3.

768. Rodanelli R, Comelli M, Pascale W, et al. Clinical pharmacology of some antibiotics: problems relating to their intravenous use in hospitals. *Farmaco Ed Prat.* 1982; 37:185–8.

769. Kowaluk EA, Roberts MS. Drug loss in polyolefin infusion systems. *Am J Hosp Pharm.* 1983; 40:118–9.

770. Illum L, Bundgaard H. Sorption of drugs by plastic infusion bags. *Int J Pharm.* 1982; 10:339–51.

771. Pfizer Laboratories. Vistaril IM, table of physical compatibilities. New York, NY; 1979 Jul.

772. Abbott Laboratories. Package insert on Neut. North Chicago, IL; 1988 Oct.

773. Jhunjhuowala VP, Bhalla HL. Sodium ampicillin: its stability in some large volume parenteral solutions. *Indian J Hosp Pharm.* 1981; 8:55–7.

774. Scheiner JM, Araujo MM. Thiamine destruction by sodium bisulfite in infusion solutions. *Am J Hosp Pharm.* 1981; 38: 1911–3.

775. Kirschenbaum HL, Aronoff W, Perentesis GP, et al. Stability and compatibility of lidocaine hydrochloride with selected large-volume parenterals and drug additives. *Am J Hosp Pharm.* 1982; 39:1013–5.

776. Lackner TE, Baldus D, Butler CD, et al. Lidocaine stability in cardioplegic solution stored in glass bottles and polyvinyl chloride bags. *Am J Hosp Pharm.* 1983; 40:97–101.

777. Russell WJ, Meyer-Witting M. The stability of atracurium in clinical practice. *Anaesth Intens Care.* 1990; 18:550–2.

778. Shank WA, Coupal JJ. Stability of digoxin in common large-volume injections. *Am J Hosp Pharm.* 1982; 39:844–6.

779. Solomon DA, Nasinnyk KK. Compatibility of haloperidol lactate and heparin sodium. *Am J Hosp Pharm.* 1982; 39:843–4.

780. Elliott GT, McKenzie MW, Curry SH, et al. Stability of cimetidine hydrochloride in admixtures after microwave thawing. *Am J Hosp Pharm.* 1983; 40:1002–6.

781. Tsallas G, Allen LC. Stability of cimetidine hydrochloride in parenteral nutrition solutions. *Am J Hosp Pharm.* 1982; 39:484–5.

782. Roberts MS, Cossum PA, Kowaluk EA, et al. Plastic syringes and intravenous infusions. *Med J Aust.* 1981; 2:580–1.

783. Das Gupta V, Stewart KR. Effect of tobramycin on the stability of carbenicillin disodium. *Am J Hosp Pharm.* 1983; 40:1013–6.

784. Simmons A, Allwood MC. Sorption to plastic syringes of drugs administered by syringe pump. *J Clin Hosp Pharm.* 1981; 6:71–3.

785. Nicholas E, Hess G. Degradation of penicillin, ticarcillin and carbenicillin resulting from storage of unit doses. *N Engl J Med.* 1982; 306:547–8.

786. Carpenter JP, Gomez EA. Administration of lorazepam injection through intravenous tubing. *Am J Hosp Pharm.* 1981; 38:1514–6.

787. Newton DW, Narducci WA, Leet WA, et al. Lorazepam solubility in and sorption from intravenous admixture solutions. *Am J Hosp Pharm.* 1983; 40:424–7.

788. Frable RA, Klink PR, Engel GL, et al. Stability of cefamandole nafate injection with parenteral solutions and additives. *Am J Hosp Pharm.* 1982; 39:622–7.

789. Kirschenbaum HL, Aronoff W, Piltz GW, et al. Compatibility and stability of dobutamine hydrochloride with large-volume parenterals and selected additives. *Am J Hosp Pharm.* 1983; 40:1690–1.

790. Bosch EH, van Doorne H, Brouwers JRBJ, et al. Vermindering van het sufentanilgehalte bij de bereiding en tijdens het gebruik van een epidurale toedieningsvorm. Een orienterend onderzoek. *Ziekenhuisfarmacie.* 1993; 9:97–101.

791. Cairns CJ. Incompatibility of amiodarone. *Pharm J.* 1986; 236:68.

792. Roney JV (Scientific Services, Hoechst-Roussel Pharmaceuticals, Somerville, NJ): Personal communication; 1983 Dec 4.

793. Berge SM, Henderson NL. Kinetics and mechanism of degradation of cefotaxime sodium in aqueous solution. *J Pharm Sci.* 1983; 72:59–63.

794. Smith FM, Nuessle NO. Stability of diazepam injection repackaged in glass unit-dose syringes. *Am J Hosp Pharm.* 1982; 39:1687–90.

795. Cossum PA, Roberts MS. Availability of isosorbide dinitrate, diazepam and chlormethiazole from I.V. delivery systems. *Eur J Clin Pharmacol.* 1981; 19:181–5.

796. Smith A, Bird G. Compatibility of diazepam with infusion fluids and their containers. *J Clin Hosp Pharm.* 1982; 7:181–6.

797. Yliruusi JK, Sothmann AG, Laine RH, et al. Sorptive loss of diazepam and nitroglycerin from solutions to three types of containers. *Am J Hosp Pharm.* 1982; 39:1018–21.

798. Kuhlman J, Abshagen U. Cleavage of glycosidic bonds of digoxin and derivatives as function of pH and time. *Naunyn Schmiedebergs Arch Pharmacol.* 1973; 276:149–56.

799. Gault MH, Charles JD, Sugden DL, et al. Hydrolysis of digoxin by acid. *J Pharm Pharmacol.* 1977; 29:27–32.

800. Sternson LA, Shaffer RD. Kinetics of digoxin stability in aqueous solution. *J Pharm Sci.* 1978; 67:327–30.

801. Khalil SA, El-Masry S. Instability of digoxin in acid medium using a nonisotopic method. *J Pharm Sci.* 1978; 67:1358–60.

802. Fagerman KE, Dean RE. Daily digoxin administration in parenteral nutrition solution. *Am J Hosp Pharm.* 1981; 38:1955.

803. Patterson MJ, Tjokrosetio R. Stability of adrenaline injection BP following resterilization. *Aust J Hosp Pharm.* 1981; 11:21–2.

804. Nazeravich DR, Otlen NHH. Effect of inline filtration on delivery of gentamicin at a slow infusion rate. *Am J Hosp Pharm.* 1983; 40:1961–4.

805. Zell M, Paone RP. Stability of insulin in plastic syringes. *Am J Hosp Pharm.* 1983; 40:637–8.

806. Benvenuto JA. Errors in oncolytic agent stability study. *Am J Hosp Pharm.* 1983; 40:1628.

807. Bisaillon S, Sarrazin R. Compatibility of several antibiotics or hydrocortisone when added to metronidazole solution for intravenous infusion. *J Parenter Sci Technol.* 1983; 37:129–132.

808. Gove L. Antibiotic interactions. *Pharm J.* 1983; 231:233.

809. Ennis CE, Merritt RJ, Neff DN. In vitro study of in line filtration of medications commonly administered to pediatric cancer patients. *JPEN J Parenter Enteral Nutr.* 1983; 7:156–8.

810. Buxton PC, Conduit SM. Stability of parentrovite in infusion fluids. *Br J IV Ther.* 1983; 4:5.

811. Das Gupta V, Stewart KR. Stability of dobutamine hydrochloride and verapamil hydrochloride in 0.9% sodium chloride and 5% dextrose injections. *Am J Hosp Pharm.* 1984; 41:686–9.

812. Hasegawa GR, Eder JF. Visual compatibility of dobutamine hydrochloride with other injectable drugs. *Am J Hosp Pharm.* 1984; 41:949–51.

813. Souney PF, Colucci RD, Mariani G, et al. Compatibility of magnesium sulfate solutions with various antibiotics during simulated Y-site injection. *Am J Hosp Pharm.* 1984; 41:323–4.

814. Lundergan FS, Lombardi TP, Neilan GE, et al. Stability of tobramycin sulfate mixed with oxacillin sodium and nafcillin sodium in human serum. *Am J Hosp Pharm.* 1984; 41:144–5.

815. Parker WA. Physical compatibility update of preoperative medications. *Hosp Pharm.* 1984; 19:475–8.

816. Hale DC, Jenkins R. In-vitro inactivation of aminoglycoside antibiotics by piperacillin and carbenicillin. *Am J Clin Pathol.* 1980; 74:316–9.

817. Rank DM, Packer AM. In vitro inactivation of tobramycin by penicillins. *Am J Hosp Pharm.* 1984; 41:1187–8.

818. Karlsen J, Thonnesen HH, Olsen IR, et al. Stability of cytotoxic intravenous solutions subjected to freeze-thaw treatment. *Nor Pharm Acta.* 1983; 45:61–7.

819. Cheung YW, Vishnuvajjala BR. Stability of cytarabine, methotrexate sodium, and hydrocortisone sodium succinate admixtures. *Am J Hosp Pharm.* 1984; 41:1802–6.

820. Bundgaard H, Larsen C. Influence of carbohydrates and polyhydric alcohols on the stability of cephalosporins in aqueous solution. *Int J Pharm.* 1983; 16:319–25.

821. Hamilton G. Adverse reactions to intravenous pyelography contrast agents. *Can Med Assoc J.* 1983; 129:405–6.

822. Miller B, Pesko L. Effect of freezing on particulate matter concentrations in five antibiotic solutions. *Am J IV Ther Clin Nutr.* 1984; 11:19–22.

823. Wagman GH, Bailey JV. Binding of aminoglycoside antibiotics to filtration materials. *Antimicrob Agents Chemother*. 1975; 7: 316–319.

824. Tindula RJ, Ambrose PJ. Aminoglycoside inactivation by penicillins and cephalosporins and its impact on drug-level monitoring. *Drug Intell Clin Pharm*. 1983; 17:906–8.

825. Gillies IR. Physical stability of Intralipid following drug addition. *Aust J Hosp Pharm*. 1980; 10:118–20.

826. Hardin TC, Clibon U, Page CP, et al. Compatibility of 5-fluorouracil and total parenteral nutrition solutions. *JPEN J Parenter Enteral Nutr*. 1982; 6:163–5.

827. Gaj E, Sesin GP. Evaluation of growth of five microorganisms in doxorubicin and floxuridine media. *Pharm Manufacturing*. 1984; 1:52–3.

828. Gaj E, Griffin RE. Evaluation of growth of six microorganisms in fluorouracil, bacteriostatic sodium chloride 0.9% and sodium chloride 0.9% media. *Hosp Pharm*. 1983; 18:348–9.

829. Turco SJ. Drug adsorption to membrane filters. *Am J IV Ther Clin Nutr*. 1982; 9:6.

830. Robinson WA, Krebs LU. The "real stuff" for intrathecal injection during leukaemia therapy. *Lancet*. 1982; 1:283.

831. Frear RS. Cefoperazone-aminoglycoside incompatibility. *Am J Hosp Pharm*. 1983; 40:564.

832. O'Bey KA, Jim LK, Gee JP, et al. Temperature dependence of the stability of tobramycin mixed with penicillins in human serum. *Am J Hosp Pharm*. 1982; 39:1005–8.

833. Bhatia J, Mims LC. Effect of phototherapy on amino acid solutions containing multivitamins. *J Pediatr*. 1980; 96:284–6.

834. Koshiro A, Fujita T. Interaction of penicillins with the components of plasma expanders. *Drug Intell Clin Pharm*. 1983; 17: 351–6.

835. Szucsova S, Slana M. Stability of infusion mixtures of 5% glucose solution with injection solutions. *Farm Obzor*. 1983; 52: 209–13.

836. Gillis J, Jones G, Pencharz P. Delivery of vitamins A, D, and E in total parenteral nutrition solutions. *JPEN J Parenter Enteral Nutr*. 1983; 7:11–4.

837. Farago S. Compatibility of antibiotics and other drugs in total parenteral nutrition solutions. *Can J Hosp Pharm*. 1983; 36: 43–51.

838. Gaj E, Sesin GP. Compatibility of doxorubicin hydrochloride and vinblastine sulfate—stability of a solution stored in Cormed reservoir bags or Monoject plastic syringes. *Am J IV Ther Clin Nutr*. 13–14, 19–20 (May) 1984; 11:8–9.

839. Bar-Or D, Kulig K, Marx JA, et al. Precipitation of verapamil. *Ann Intern Med*. 1982; 97:619.

840. Tucker R, Gentile JF. Precipitation of verapamil with nafcillin. *Am J Hosp Pharm*. 1984; 41:2588.

841. Hasegawa GR, Eder JF. Dobutamine-heparin mixture inadvisable. *Am J Hosp Pharm*. 1984; 41:2588.

842. Chen MF, Boyce HW, Triplett L. Stability of the B vitamins in mixed parenteral nutrition solution. *JPEN J Parenter Enteral Nutr*. 1983; 7:462–4.

843. Bowman BB, Nguyen P. Stability of thiamin in parenteral nutrition solutions. *JPEN J Parenter Enteral Nutr*. 1983; 7: 567–8.

844. Newton DW. Physicochemical determinants of incompatibility and instability in injectable drug solutions and admixtures. *Am J Hosp Pharm*. 1978; 35:1213–22.

845. Newton DW. Physicochemical determinants of incompatibility and instability of drugs for injection and infusion. In: Trissel LA. Handbook on injectable drugs. 3rd ed. Bethesda, MD: American Society of Hospital Pharmacists; 1983:XI-XXI.

846. Raymond G, Day P. Sodium content of commonly administered intravenous drugs. *Hosp Pharm*. 1982; 17:560–1.

847. Rich DS. Recent information about inactivation of aminoglycosides by carbenicillin and ticarcillin: clinical implications. *Hosp Pharm*. 1983; 18:41–3.

848. Lawrence RI, Flukes WK, Rust VJ, et al. Total parenteral nutrition using a combined nutrient solution. *Aust J Hosp Pharm*. 1981; 11:540–2.

849. Davis SS, Galloway M. Total parenteral nutrition. *Pharm J*. 1983; 6 (Jan 1 &: 8):230.

850. Travenol Laboratories. 3-in-1 admixture guide from Travenol. 1983 Nov.

851. Chan JC, Malekzadeh M, Hurley H. pH and titratable acidity of amino acid mixtures used in hyperalimentation. *JAMA*. 1972; 220:1119–20.

852. Kirk B, Sprake JM. Stability of aminophylline. *Br J IV Ther*. (Nov) 1982; 3:4, 6, 8.

853. Vogenberg FR, Souney PF. Stability guidelines for routinely refrigerated drug products. *Am J Hosp Pharm*. 1983; 40: 101–2.

854. Niemiec PW, Vanderveen TW. Compatibility considerations in parenteral nutrient solutions. *Am J Hosp Pharm*. 1984; 41: 893–911.

855. Irving JD, Reynolds PV. Disposable syringe danger. *Lancet*. 1966; 1:362.

856. Salter F (Bristol-Myers Squibb, Princeton, NJ): Personal communication; 1991 Feb 27.

857. Hopefl AW. Clinical use of intravenous acyclovir. *Drug Intell Clin Pharm*. 1983; 17:623–8.

858. Larsen C, Bundgaard H. Polymerization of penicillins VI. Timecourse of formation of antigenic di- and polymerization products in aqueous ampicillin sodium solutions. *Arch Pharm Chemi Sci Ed*. 1977; 5:201–9.

859. Carthy BJ, Hill GT. Some aspects of the analysis and stability of atracurium besylate. *Anal Proc*. 1983; 20:177–9.

860. D'Arcy PF. Comment on handling of anticancer drugs. *Drug Intell Clin Pharm*. 1984; 18:417.

861. Adams J, Wilson JP. Instability of bleomycin in plastic containers. *Am J Hosp Pharm*. 1982; 39:1636.

862. Levin VA, Zackheim HS. Stability of carmustine for topical application. *Arch Dermatol*. 1982; 118:450–1.

863. Chan KK, Zackheim HS. Stability of nitrosourea solutions. *Arch Dermatol*. 1973; 107:298.

864. Teil SM, Arwood LL. Stability of gentamicin and cefamandole in serum. *Am J Hosp Pharm*. 1982; 39:485–6.

865. Portnoff JB, Henley MW. Development of sodium cefoxitin as a dosage form. *J Parenter Sci Technol*. 1983; 37:180–5.

866. Vaughan LM, Poon CY. Stability of ceftazidime and vancomycin alone and in combination in heparinized and nonheparinized peritoneal dialysis solution. *Ann Pharmacother*. 1994; 28:572–6.

867. Muller RH, Heinemann S. Fat emulsions for parenteral nutrition. IV. Lipofundin MCT/LCT regimens for total parenteral nutrition (TPN) with high electrolyte load. *Int J Pharm*. 1994; 107:121–32.

868. Sorkin EM, Darvey DC. Review of cimetidine drug interactions. *Drug Intell Clin Pharm.* 1983; 17:110–20.

869. Raymond G, Day P. Multiple sources of sodium in injectable drugs. *Drug Intell Clin Pharm.* 1982; 16:703.

870. Eshaque M, McKay MJ. D-Mannitol platinum complexes. *Wadley Med Bull.* 1977; 7:338–48.

871. Ferguson DE. Degradation of clindamycin in frozen admixtures. *Am J Hosp Pharm.* 1982; 39:1156.

872. Ausman RK, Holmes CJ, Kundsin RB, et al. Degradation of clindamycin in frozen admixtures. *Am J Hosp Pharm.* 1982; 39:1156.

873. Cairns CJ, Robertson J. Incompatibility of ceftazidime and vancomycin. *Pharm J.* 1987; 238:577.

874. Sandoz. Sandimmune—pharmacy fact sheet. East Hanover, NJ; 1983 Nov.

875. Senholzi CS, Kerus MP. Crystal formation after reconstituting cefazolin sodium with 0.9% sodium chloride injection. *Am J Hosp Pharm.* 1985; 42:129–30.

876. Thompson DF, Allen LV, Desai SR, et al. Compatibility of furosemide with aminoglycoside admixtures. *Am J Hosp Pharm.* 1985; 42:116–9.

877. Geary TG, Akood MA, Jensen JB. Characteristics of chloroquine binding to glass and plastic. *Am J Trop Med Hyg.* 1983; 32:19–23.

878. Yayon A, Ginsburg A. A method for the measurement of chloroquin uptake in erythrocytes. *Anal Biochem.* 1980; 107:332–6.

879. D'Arcy PF. Drug interactions with medical plastics. *Drug Intell Clin Pharm.* 1983; 17:726–31.

880. Kowaluk EA, Roberts MS. Factors affecting the availability of diazepam stored in plastic bags and administered through intravenous sets. *Am J Hosp Pharm.* 1983; 40:417–23.

881. Kasahara K, Ruiz-Torres A. Einwirkung der verdauungssafe auf die bestandigkeit des digoxin-und digitoxin-molekuls. *Klin Wochenschr.* 1969; 47:1109–11.

882. Berman W, Whitman V, Marks KH, et al. Inadvertent overadministration of digoxin to low-birth-weight infants. *J Pediatr.* 1978; 92:1024–5.

883. Berman W, Dubynsky O, Whitman V, et al. Digoxin therapy in low-birth-weight infants with patent ductus arteriosus. *J Pediatr.* 1978; 93:652–5.

884. Hajratwala BR. Stability of prostaglandins. *Aust J Pharm Sci.* 1975; NS5(Jun):39–41.

885. Roseman TJ, Sims B. Stability of prostaglandins. *Am J Hosp Pharm.* 1973; 30:236–9.

886. Gupta VD, Stewart KR. Stability of cefsulodin in aqueous buffered solutions and some intravenous admixtures. *J Clin Hosp Pharm.* 1984; 9:21–7.

887. Williamson MJ, Luce JK. Doxorubicin hydrochloride-aluminum interaction. *Am J Hosp Pharm.* 1983; 40:214.

888. Chin TH (Professional Services, Miles Inc., West Haven, CT): Personal communication; 1993 Dec 3.

889. Hausrani PK, Davis SS. Preparation and properties of sterile intravenous emulsions. *J Parenter Sci Technol.* 1983; 37:145–50.

890. Gray MS, Singleton WS. Creaming of phosphatide stabilized fat emulsions by electrolyte solutions. *J Pharm Sci.* 1967; 56:1429–31.

891. Knutsen C, Miller P. Compatibility, stability, and effect of mixing 10% fat emulsion in TPN solutions. *JPEN J Parenter Enteral Nutr.* 1981; 5:579.

892. Burnham WR, Hansrani PK, Knott CE, et al. Stability of a fat emulsion based intravenous feeding mixture. *Int J Pharm.* 1983; 13:9–22.

893. Hardin TC. Complex parenteral nutrition solutions: II. Addition of fat emulsions. *Nutr Supp Serv.* 1983; 3:50–51.

894. Quebbeman EJ, Hamid AAR, Hoffman NE, et al. Stability of fluorouracil in plastic containers used for continuous infusion at home. *Am J Hosp Pharm.* 1984; 41:1153–6.

895. Barker A, Hebron BS, Beck PR, et al. Folic acid and total parenteral nutrition. *JPEN J Parenter Enteral Nutr.* 1984; 8:3–8.

896. Louie N, Stennett DJ. Stability of folic acid in 25% dextrose, 3.5% amino acids, and multivitamin solution. *JPEN J Parenter Enteral Nutr.* 1984; 8:421–6.

897. Koshiro A, Oie S, Harima Y, et al. Compatibility of gentamicin sulfate injection in parenteral solutions. *Jap J Hosp Pharm.* 1982; 7:377–80.

898. Godefroid RJ. Intravenous gentamicin dilution requirements. *Am J Hosp Pharm.* 1982; 39:1457.

899. Godefroid RJ. Comment on IV guidelines. *Drug Intell Clin Pharm.* 1984; 18:925.

900. Matthews H. Heparin anticoagulant activity in intravenous fluids utilising a chromagenic substrate assay method. *Aust J Hosp Pharm.* 1982; 12:S17–S22.

901. Turco SJ. Heparin locks. *Am J IV Ther Clin Nutr.* 1983; 10:9.

902. Swerling R: Normal saline or dilute heparin for heparin lock flush? *Infusion.* 1982; 6:123-124.

903. Epperson EL. Efficacy of 0.9% sodium chloride injection with and without heparin for maintaining indwelling intermittent injection sites. *Clin Pharm.* 1984; 3:626–9.

904. Kanke M, Eubanks JL. Binding of selected drugs to a "treated" inline filter. *Am J Hosp Pharm.* 1983; 40:1323–8.

905. Anderson W, Harthill JE. Anticoagulant activity of heparins in dextrose solutions. *J Pharm Pharmacol.* 1982; 34:90–6.

906. Enderlin G. Discoloration of hydralazine injection. *Am J Hosp Pharm.* 1984; 41:634.

907. Pingel M, Volund A. Stability of insulin preparations. *Diabetes.* 1972; 21:805–13.

908. Weber SS, Wood WA. Insulin adsorption controversy. *Drug Intell Clin Pharm.* 1976; 10:232–3.

909. Schildt B, Ahlgren T, Berghem L, et al. Adsorption of insulin by infusion materials. *Acta Anaesthesiol Scand.* 1978; 22:556–62.

910. Mitrano FP, Newton DW. Factors affecting insulin adherence to type I glass bottles. *Am J Hosp Pharm.* 1982; 39:1491–5.

911. Twardowski ZJ, Nolph KD, McGary TJ, et al. Insulin binding to plastic bags: a methodologic study. *Am J Hosp Pharm.* 1983; 40:575–9.

912. Twardowski ZJ, Nolph KD, McGary TJ, et al. Nature of insulin binding to plastic bags. *Am J Hosp Pharm.* 1983; 40:579–82.

913. Twardowski ZJ, Nolph KD, McGary TJ, et al. Influence of temperature and time on insulin adsorption to plastic bags. *Am J Hosp Pharm.* 1983; 40:583–6.

914. Sato S, Ebert CD. Prevention of insulin self-association and surface adsorption. *J Pharm Sci.* 1983; 72:228–32.

915. Phillips NC, Lauper RD. Review of etoposide. *Clin Pharm.* 1983; 2:112–9.

916. McCollam PL, Garrison TJ. Etoposide: A new chemotherapeutic agent. *Am J IV Ther Clin Nutr.* 27–28 (Mar) 1984; 11:24.

917. Stroup JW, Mighton-Eryou LM. Expiry date guidelines for a centralized IV admixture service. *Can J Hosp Pharm.* 1986; 39: 57–9.

918. Bishop BG. Adsorption of iron-dextran on membrane filters. *NZ Pharm.* 1981; 1:49.

919. Reed MD, Bertino JS. Use of intravenous iron dextran injection in children receiving total parenteral nutrition. *Am J Dis Child.* 1981; 135:829–31.

920. Halpin TC. Use of intravenous iron dextran in sick patients receiving TPN. *Nutr Supp Serv.* 1982; 2:19–20.

921. Shimada A. Adverse reactions to total-dose infusion of iron dextran. *Clin Pharm.* 1982; 1:248–9.

922. Thompson DF, Shimanek M. Stability of sterility study with magnesium sulfate admixtures. *Infusion.* 86 (May-June) 1983; 7:83.

923. Ausman RK, Crevar GE, Hagedorn H, et al. Studies in the pharmacodynamics of mechlorethamine and AB100. *J Am Med Assoc.* 1961; 178:143–6.

924. A.H. Robins Pharmaceutical Division. Compatibility chart for reglan injectable 5 mg/mL. Richmond, VA; 1983 Oct.

925. Bonati M, Gaspari F, D'Aranno V, et al. Physicochemical and analytical characteristics of amiodarone. *J Pharm Sci.* 1984; 73: 829–31.

926. Feroz RM, Puppala S, Chaudhry MA, et al. Compatibility of M.V.C. 9+3 (multivitamin concentrate for infusion) in different large volume parenteral solutions. LyphoMed, Inc., 1984.

927. Alam AS. Identification of labetalol precipitate. *Am J Hosp Pharm.* 1984; 41:74.

928. Wagenknecht DM, Baaske DM, Alam AS, et al. Stability of nitroglycerin solutions in polyolefin and glass containers. *Am J Hosp Pharm.* 1984; 41:1807–11.

929. Klamerus KJ, Ueda CT. Stability of nitroglycerin in intravenous admixtures. *Am J Hosp Pharm.* 1984; 41:303–5.

930. Scheife AH, Grisafe JA. Stability of intravenous nitroglycerin solutions. *J Pharm Sci.* 1982; 71:55–9.

931. Ingram JK, Miller JD. Plastic absorption adsorption of nitroglycerin solution. *Anesthesiology.* 1979; 51:S132.

932. Mathot F, Bonnard J, Hans P, et al. Les perfusions de nitroglycerine: Etude de l'absorption par differents materiaux plastiques. *J Pharm Belg.* 1980; 35:389–93.

933. Sokoloski TD, Wu CC. Nitroglycerin stability: effects on bioavailability, assay and biological dissolution. *J Clin Hosp Pharm.* 1981; 6:227–32.

934. Cawello VW, Bonn R. Bioverfugbarkeitseinflusse durch die wahl des infusionsmaterials bei der therapie mit nitroglycerin. *Arzneimittelforschung.* 1983; 33:595–7.

935. Rock CM, Gull J. Reducing IV-nitroglycerin loss to an intravenous administration set by preliminary preparation. *Am J IV Ther Clin Nutr.* 40–42 (Oct) 1982; 9:36.

936. Nix DE, Tharpe WN. Effects of presaturation on nitroglycerin delivery by polyvinyl chloride infusion sets. *Am J Hosp Pharm.* 1984; 41:1835–7.

937. Jacobi J, Dasta JF, Reilley TE, et al. Loss of nitroglycerin to pulmonary artery delivery systems. *Am J Hosp Pharm.* 1983; 40:1980–2.

938. Jacobi J, Dasta JF, Wu LS, et al. Loss of nitroglycerin to central venous pressure catheter. *Drug Intell Clin Pharm.* 1982; 16: 331–2.

939. Dasta JF, Jacobi J, Sokolowski TD, et al. Loss of nitroglycerin to cardiopulmonary bypass apparatus. *Crit Care Med.* 1983; 11: 50–2.

940. Dasta JF, Jacobi J, Sokoloski TD, et al. Extraction of nitroglycerin by a membrane oxygenator. *J Extra-Corp Tech.* 1983; 15: 101–3.

941. St. Peter JV, Cochran TG. Nitroglycerin loss from intravenous solutions administered with a volumetric infusion pump. *Am J Hosp Pharm.* 1982; 39:1328–30.

942. Hola ET. Loss of nitroglycerin during microinfusion. *Am J Hosp Pharm.* 1984; 41:142–4.

943. Yacobi A, Amann AH. Pharmaceutical considerations of nitroglycerin. *Drug Intell Clin Pharm.* 1983; 17:255–63.

944. Malick AW, Amann AH, Baaske DM, et al. Loss of nitroglycerin from solutions to intravenous plastic containers: a theoretical treatment. *J Pharm Sci.* 1981; 70:798–800.

945. Amann AH, Baaske DM. Loss of nitroglycerin from intravenous administration sets during infusion: a theoretical treatment. *J Pharm Sci.* 1982; 71:473–4.

946. Neftel KA, Walti M, Spengler H, et al. Effect of storage of penicillin G solutions on sensitization to penicillin G after intravenous administration. *Lancet.* 1982; 1:986–8.

947. Salem RB, Wilder BJ, Yost RL, et al. Rapid infusion of phenytoin sodium loading doses. *Am J Hosp Pharm.* 1981; 38: 354–7.

948. Gannaway WL, Wilding DC, Siepler JK, et al. Clinical use of intravenous phenytoin sodium infusions. *Clin Pharm.* 1983; 2: 135–8.

949. Boike SC, Rybak MJ, Tintinalli JE, et al. Evaluation of a method for intravenous phenytoin infusion. *Clin Pharm.* 1983; 2: 444–6.

950. Earnest MP, Marx JA, Drury LR. Complications of intravenous phenytoin for acute treatment of seizures. *JAMA.* 1983; 249: 762–5.

951. Giacona N, Bauman JL. Crystallization of three phenytoin preparations in intravenous solutions. *Am J Hosp Pharm.* 1982; 39: 630–4.

952. Lau A, Lee M, Flascha S, et al. Effect of piperacillin on tobramycin pharmacokinetics in patients with normal renal function. *Antimicrob Agents Chemother.* 1983; 24:533–7.

953. Autian J, Dhorda CN. Evaluation of disposable plastic syringes as to physical incompatibilities with parenteral products. *Am J Hosp Pharm.* 1959; 16:176–9.

954. Addy DP, Alesbury P. Paraldehyde and plastic syringes. *Br Med J.* 1978; 2:1434.

955. Fenton-May V, Lee F. Paraldehyde and plastic syringes. *Br Med J.* 1978; 2:1166.

956. Evans RJ. Effect of paraldehyde on disposable syringes and needles. *Lancet.* 1961; 2:1451.

957. Johnson CE, Vigoreaux JA. Compatibility of paraldehyde with plastic syringes and needle hubs. *Am J Hosp Pharm.* 1984; 41: 306–8.

958. Mahony C, Brown JE, Starget WW, et al. In vitro stability of sodium nitroprusside solutions for intravenous administration. *J Pharm Sci.* 1984; 73:838–9.

959. Fricker MP, Swerling R. Sodium nitroprusside reconstitution and administration. *Infusion*. 1981; 5:56.

960. Boehm JJ, Dutton DM. Shelf life of unrefrigerated succinylcholine chloride injection. *Am J Hosp Pharm*. 1984; 41:300–2.

961. Roach M. IV tetracycline. *Pharm J*. 1978; 220:143.

962. Chow MS, Qwintiliani R, Nightingale CH. In vivo inactivation of tobramycin by ticarcillin. A case report. *JAMA*. 1982; 247:658–9.

963. Baumgartner TG, Russell WL. Intravenous trimethoprim-sulfamethoxazole administration alert. *Am J IV Ther Clin Nutr*. 1983; 10:14–5.

964. Hiskey CF, Bullock E. Spectrophotometric study of aqueous solutions of warfarin sodium. *J Pharm Sci*. 1962; 51:43–6.

965. Nahata MC. Stability of ceftriaxone sodium in intravenous solutions. *Am J Hosp Pharm*. 1983; 40:2193–4.

966. Smith BR. Effect of storage temperature and time on stability of cefmenoxime, ceftriaxone, and cefotetan in 5% dextrose injection. *Am J Hosp Pharm*. 1983; 40:1024–5.

967. Vishnuvajjala BR, Cradock JC. Compatibility of plastic infusion devices with diluted *N*-methylformamide and *N,N*-dimethylacetamide. *Am J Hosp Pharm*. 1984; 41:1160–3.

968. Godefroid RJ. Vindesine: A new antineoplastic drug. *Cancer Chemother Update*. 1984; 2:4–7.

969. Cheung YW, Vishnuvajjala BR, Morris NL, et al. Stability of azacitidine in infusion fluids. *Am J Hosp Pharm*. 1984; 41:1156–9.

970. Bosanquet AG. Stability of melphalan solutions during preparation and storage. *J Pharm Sci*. 1985; 74:348–51.

971. Tabibi SE, Cradock JC. Stability of melphalan in infusion fluids. *Am J Hosp Pharm*. 1984; 41:1380–2.

972. Teresi M, Allison J. Interaction between vancomycin and ticarcillin. *Am J Hosp Pharm*. 1985; 42:2420.

973. Jorgensen JH, Crawford SA. Selective inactivation of aminoglycosides by newer beta-lactam antibiotics. *Curr Ther Res Clin Exp*. 1982; 32:25–35.

974. Bhatia J, Stegink LD, Ziegler EE. Riboflavin enhances photo-oxidation of amino acids under simulated clinical conditions. *JPEN J Parenter Enteral Nutr*. 1983; 7:277–9.

975. Smith G, Hasson K. Effects of ascorbic acid and disodium edetate on the stability of isoprenaline hydrochloride injection. *J Clin Hosp Pharm*. 1984; 9:209–15.

976. Hutchinson SM. Heparin and aminoglycosides instability. *Drug Intell Clin Pharm*. 1986; 20:886.

977. Johnston-Early A, McKenzie MA, Krasnow SH, et al. Drug trapping in intravenous infusion side arms. *JAMA*. 1984; 252:2392.

978. Parker WA. Physical compatibility of ranitidine HCl with pre-operative injectable medications. *Can J Hosp Pharm*. 1985; 38:160–1.

979. Das Gupta V, Stewart KR. Chemical stabilities of cefamandole nafate and metronidazole when mixed together for intravenous infusion. *J Clin Hosp Pharm*. 1985; 10:379–83.

980. Cohen MH, Johnston-Early A, Hood MA, et al. Drug precipitation within iv tubing: a potential hazard of chemotherapy administration. *Cancer Treat Rep*. 1985; 69:1325–6.

981. Marble DA, Bosso JA. Compatibility of clindamycin phosphate with amikacin sulfate at room temperature and with gentamicin sulfate and tobramycin sulfate under frozen conditions. *Drug Intell Clin Pharm*. 1986; 20:960–3.

982. Gove LF, Gordon NH, Miller J, et al. Pre-filled syringes for self-administration of epidural opiates. *Pharm J*. 1985; 234:378–9.

983. Bosso JA, Townsend RJ. Stability of clindamycin phosphate and ceftizoxime sodium, cefoxitin sodium, cefamandole nafate, or cefazolin sodium in two intravenous solutions. *Am J Hosp Pharm*. 1985; 42:2211–4.

984. Nahata MC, Durrell DE. Stability of tobramycin sulfate in admixtures with calcium gluconate. *Am J Hosp Pharm*. 1985; 42:1987–8.

985. Baker DE, Yost GS, Craig VL, et al. Compatibility of heparin sodium and morphine sulfate. *Am J Hosp Pharm*. 1985; 42:1352–5.

986. Carlson GH, Matzke GR. Particle formation of third-generation cephalosporin injections. *Am J Hosp Pharm*. 1985; 42:1578–9.

987. Nieves-Cordero AL, Luciw HM. Compatibility of narcotic analgesic solutions with various antibiotics during simulated Y-site injection. *Am J Hosp Pharm*. 1985; 42:1108–9.

988. Ogawa GS, Young R. Dispensing-pin problems. *Am J Hosp Pharm*. 1985; 42:1042.

989. Conklin CA, Kerege JF. Stability of an analgesic-sedative combination in glass and plastic single-dose syringes. *Am J Hosp Pharm*. 1985; 42:339–42.

990. Thompson M, Smith M, Gragg R, et al. Stability of nitroglycerin and dobutamine in 5% dextrose and 0.9% sodium chloride injection. *Am J Hosp Pharm*. 1985; 42:361–2.

991. Rhodes RS, Rhodes PJ. Stability of meperidine hydrochloride, promethazine hydrochloride, and atropine sulfate in plastic syringes. *Am J Hosp Pharm*. 1985; 42:112–5.

992. Kiel D, Connolly BJ. Visual compatibility of amrinone lactate with various i.v. secondary additives. *Parenterals*. (May-June) 1985; 3:1, 5–6.

993. Das Gupta V, Stewart KR. Chemical stabilities of hydrocortisone sodium succinate and several antibiotics when mixed with metronidazole injection for intravenous infusion. *J Parenter Sci Technol*. 1985; 39:145–8.

994. Foley PT, Bosso JA, Bair JN, et al. Compatibility of clindamycin phosphate with cefotaxime sodium or netilmicin sulfate in small-volume admixtures. *Am J Hosp Pharm*. 1985; 42:839–43.

995. Mansur JM, Abramowitz PW, Lerner SA, et al. Stability and cost analysis of clindamycin-gentamicin admixtures given every eight hours. *Am J Hosp Pharm*. 1985; 42:332–5.

996. Quock JR, Sakai RI. Stability of cytarabine in a parenteral nutrient solution. *Am J Hosp Pharm*. 1985; 42:592–4.

997. Walker SE, Bayliff CD. Stability of ranitidine hydrochloride in total parenteral nutrient solution. *Am J Hosp Pharm*. 1985; 42:590–2.

998. Baptista RJ, Palumbo JD, Tahan SR, et al. Stability of cimetidine hydrochloride in a total nutrient admixture. *Am J Hosp Pharm*. 1985; 42:2208–10.

999. Das Gupta V, Stewart KR. pH-Dependent effect of magnesium sulfate on the stability of penicillin G potassium solution. *Am J Hosp Pharm*. 1985; 42:598–602.

1000. Macias JM, Martin WJ. Stability of morphine sulfate and meperidine hydrochloride in a parenteral nutrient formulation. *Am J Hosp Pharm*. 1985; 42:1087–94.

1001. James MJ, Riley CM. Stability of intravenous admixtures of aztreonam and ampicillin. *Am J Hosp Pharm.* 1985; 42:1095–110.

1002. James MJ, Riley CM. Stability of intravenous admixtures of aztreonam and clindamycin phosphate. *Am J Hosp Pharm.* 1985; 42:1984–6.

1003. Thompson DF, Thompson GD. Effect of inline filtration on pediatric doses of gentamicin and tobramycin. *Infusion.* 1984; 8:31–2.

1004. Alexander SR, Arena R. Predicting calcium phosphate precipitation in premature infant parenteral nutrition solutions. *Hosp Pharm.* 1985; 20:656–8.

1005. Spruill WJ, McCall CY. In vitro inactivation of tobramycin by cephalosporins. *Am J Hosp Pharm.* 1985; 42:2506–9.

1006. Stevenson JG, Patriarca C. Incompatibility of morphine sulfate and prochlorperazine edisylate in syringes. *Am J Hosp Pharm.* 1985; 42:2651.

1007. Beijnen JH, Rosing H, deVries PA, et al. Stability of anthracycline antitumor agents in infusion fluids. *J Parenter Sci Technol.* 1985; 39:220–2.

1008. Baptista RJ, Lawrence RW. Compatibility of total nutrient admixtures and secondary antibiotic infusions. *Am J Hosp Pharm.* 1985; 42:362–3.

1009. Baptista RJ, Dumas GJ, Bistrian BR, et al. Compatibility of total nutrient admixtures and secondary cardiovascular medications. *Am J Hosp Pharm.* 1985; 42:777–8.

1010. Bullock L, Parks RB, Lampasona V, et al. Stability of ranitidine hydrochloride and amino acids in parenteral nutrient solutions. *Am J Hosp Pharm.* 1985; 42:2683–7.

1011. Henann NE, Jacks TT. Compatibility and availability of sodium bicarbonate in total parenteral nutrient solutions. *Am J Hosp Pharm.* 1985; 42:2718–20.

1012. Watson D. Piggyback compatibility of antibiotics with pediatric parenteral nutrition solutions. *JPEN J Parenter Enteral Nutr.* 1985; 9:220–4.

1013. Turner SA. Stability and clinical use of intravenous admixtures containing lipid emulsion. *Pharm J.* 1985; 234:799–800.

1014. El Eini D, Knott CE. Stability of iv lipid emulsions. *Pharm J.* 1985; 235:170.

1015. Hobbiss JH. Stability of iv lipid emulsions. *Pharm J.* 1985; 235:170.

1016. Allwood MC. Drop size of infusions containing fat emulsion. *Br J Parenter Ther.* 1984; 5:113–4.

1017. Iliano L, Delanghe M, van Den Baviere H, et al. Effect of electrolytes in the presence of some trace elements on the stability of all-in-one emulsion mixtures for total parenteral nutrition. *J Clin Hosp Pharm.* 1984; 9:87–93.

1018. Whateley TL, Steele G, Urwin J, et al. Particle size stability of Intralipid and mixed total parenteral nutrition mixtures. *J Clin Hosp Pharm.* 1984; 9:113–26.

1019. Harrie KR, Jacob M, McCormick D, et al. Comparison of total nutrient admixture stability using two intravenous fat emulsions, Soyacal and Intralipid 20%. *JPEN J Parenter Enteral Nutr.* 1986; 10:381–7.

1020. Riley CM, James MJ. Stability of intravenous admixtures containing aztreonam and cefazolin. *Am J Hosp Pharm.* 1986; 43:925–7.

1021. Kuhn RJ, Nahata MC. Stability of netilmicin sulfate in admixtures with calcium gluconate and aminophylline. *Am J Hosp Pharm.* 1986; 43:1241–2.

1022. Johnson CE, Cohen IA, Craft DA, et al. Compatibility of aminophylline and methylprednisolone sodium succinate intravenous admixtures. *Am J Hosp Pharm.* 1986; 43:1482–5.

1023. Bell RG, Lipford LC, Massanari MJ, et al. Stability of intravenous admixtures of aztreonam and cefoxitin, gentamicin, metronidazole, or tobramycin. *Am J Hosp Pharm.* 1986; 43:1444–53.

1024. Fitzgerald KA, MacKay MW. Calcium and phosphate solubility in neonatal parenteral nutrient solutions containing TrophAmine. *Am J Hosp Pharm.* 1986; 43:88–93.

1025. Sayeed FA, Johnson HW, Sukumaran KB, et al. Stability of Liposyn II fat emulsion in total nutrient admixtures. *Am J Hosp Pharm.* 1986; 43:1230–5.

1026. Marble DA, Bosso JA. Stability of clindamycin phosphate with aztreonam, ceftazidime sodium, ceftriaxone sodium, or piperacillin sodium in two intravenous solutions. *Am J Hosp Pharm.* 1986; 43:1732–6.

1027. Lee MG. Sorption of four drugs to polyvinyl chloride and polybutadiene intravenous administration sets. *Am J Hosp Pharm.* 1986; 43:1945–50.

1028. Riley CM, Lipford LC. Interaction of aztreonam with nafcillin in intravenous admixtures. *Am J Hosp Pharm.* 1986; 43:2221–4.

1029. Walker PC, Kaufmann RE. Compatibility of cefazolin and gentamicin in peritoneal dialysis solutions. *Drug Intell Clin Pharm.* 1986; 20:697–700.

1030. Beijnen JH, Neef C, Menwissen OJAT, et al. Stability of intravenous admixtures of doxorubicin and vincristine. *Am J Hosp Pharm.* 1986; 43:3022–7.

1031. Campbell S, Nolan PE, Bliss M, et al. Stability of amiodarone hydrochloride in admixtures with other injectable drugs. *Am J Hosp Pharm.* 1986; 43:917–21.

1032. Hasegawa GR, Eder JF. Visual compatibility of amiodarone hydrochloride injection with other injectable drugs. *Am J Hosp Pharm.* 1984; 41:1379–80.

1033. Allwood MC. Sorption of drugs to intravenous delivery systems. *Pharm Int.* 1983; 4:83–5.

1034. Khue NV, Jung L. Study of the retention of child-dose drugs on cellulose ester membranes during inline intravenous filtration. *S-T-P-Pharma.* 1985; 1:201–7.

1035. Das Gupta V, Shah KA. Stability of ampicillin sodium and penicillin G potassium solutions using high-pressure liquid chromatography. *Can J Pharm Sci.* 1981; 16:61–5.

1036. Janknegt R, Neil MJLE. De verenigbaarheid van antimicrobiele middelen in infusievloeistoffen. *Pharm Weekbl.* 1985; 120:638–40.

1037. Bouma J, Beijnen JH, Bult A, et al. Anthracycline antitumor agents, a review of physicochemical, analytical and stability properties. *Pharm Weekbl [Sci].* 1986; 8:109–33.

1038. Howard L, Chu R, Feman S, et al. Vitamin A deficiency from long-term parenteral nutrition. *Ann Intern Med.* 1980; 93:576–7.

1039. Shenai JP, Stahlman MT. Vitamin A delivery from parenteral alimentation solution. *J Pediatr.* 1981; 99:661–3.

1040. Kishi H, Yamaji A, Kataoka K, et al. Vitamin A and E requirements during total parenteral nutrition. *JPEN J Parenter Enteral Nutr.* 1981; 5:420–3.

1041. Knight P, Heer D, Abdenour G. CaxP and Ca/P in the parenteral feeding of preterm infants. *JPEN J Parenter Enteral Nutr.* 1983; 7:110–4.

1042. Poole RK, Rupp CA, Kerner JA Jr. Calcium and phosphorus in neonatal parenteral nutrition solutions. *JPEN J Parenter Enteral Nutr.* 1983; 7:358–60.

1043. Ritschel WA, Alcorn GJ, Streng WH, et al. Cimetidine-theophylline complex formation. *Methods Find Exp Clin Pharmacol.* 1983; 5:55–8.

1044. Glew RH, Pavuk RA. Stability of vancomycin and aminoglycoside antibiotics in peritoneal dialysis concentrate. *Nephron.* 1981; 28:241–3.

1045. Kamen BA, Gunther N, Sowinsky N, et al. Analysis of antibiotic stability in a parenteral nutrition solution. *Pediatr Infect Dis.* 1985; 4:387–9.

1046. Baumgartner TG, Sitren HS, Hall J, et al. Stability of urokinase in parenteral nutrition solutions. *Nutr Supp Serv.* 1985; 5: 41–3.

1047. Allwood MC. Influence of light on vitamin A degradation during administration. *Clin Nutr.* 1982; 1:63–70.

1048. Allwood MC, Plane JH. Degradation of vitamin A exposed to ultraviolet radiation. *Int J Pharm.* 1984; 19:207–13.

1049. Riggle MA, Brandt RB. Decrease of available vitamin A in parenteral nutrition solutions. *JPEN J Parenter Enteral Nutr.* 1986; 10:388–92.

1050. McKenna MC, Bieri JC. Loss of vitamin A from total parenteral nutrition (TPN) solutions. *Fed Proc.* 1980; 39:561.

1051. Bryant CA, Neufeld NJ. Differences in vitamin A content of enteral feeding solutions following exposure to a polyvinyl chloride enteral feeding system. *JPEN J Parenter Enteral Nutr.* 1982; 6:403–5.

1052. Riff LJ, Thomason JL. Comparative aminoglycoside inactivation by beta-lactam antibiotics—effect of cephalosporin and six penicillins on five aminoglycosides. *J Antibiot (Tokyo).* 1982; 35:850–7.

1053. Schutz VH, Schroder F. Heparin-natrium kompatibilitat bei gleichzeitiger applikation anderer pharmaka. *Krankenhauspharmazie.* 1985; 6:7–11.

1054. Wermeling DP, Rapp RP, DeLuca PP, et al. Osmolality of small-volume intravenous admixtures. *Am J Hosp Pharm.* 1985; 42:1739–44.

1055. Johnston SJ. Stability of tryptophan in total parenteral nutrient solutions. *Am J Hosp Pharm.* 1986; 43:1424.

1056. Allwood MC. Factors influencing the stability of ascorbic acid in total parenteral nutrition infusions. *J Clin Hosp Pharm.* 1984; 9:75–85.

1057. Parr MD, Bertch KE. Amino acid stability and microbial growth in total parenteral nutrient solutions. *Am J Hosp Pharm.* 1985; 42:2688–91.

1058. Nordfjeld K, Rasmussen M. Storage of mixtures for total parenteral nutrition: long-term stability of a total parenteral nutrition mixture. *J Clin Hosp Pharm.* 1983; 8:265–74.

1059. Nordfjeld K, Pedersen JL, Rasmussen M, et al. Storage of mixtures for total parenteral nutrition III. Stability of vitamins in TPN mixtures. *J Clin Hosp Pharm.* 1984; 9:293–301.

1060. Das Gupta V. Stability of vitamins in total parenteral nutrient solutions. *Am J Hosp Pharm.* 1986; 43:2132.

1061. Allwood MC. Stability of vitamins in total parenteral nutrient solutions. *Am J Hosp Pharm.* 1986; 43:2138.

1062. Louie N. Stability of vitamins in total parenteral nutrient solutions. *Am J Hosp Pharm.* 1986; 43:2138.

1063. Shine B, Farwell JA. Stability and compatibility in parenteral nutrition solutions. *Br J Parenter Ther.* 44–46, 50 (Mar) 1984; 5:4.

1064. Pamperl H, Kleinberger G. Stability of intravenous fat emulsions. *Arch Surg.* 1982; 117:859–860.

1065. Hardy G, Cotter R, Dawe R. The stability and comparative clearance of TPN mixtures with lipid. In: Johnson ID, ed. Advances in Clinical Nutrition: Selected Proceedings of the 2nd International Symposium. Lancaster, England: MTP Press; 1983:241–60.

1066. Hardy G, Klim RA. Stability studies of parenteral nutrition mixtures with lipids. *JPEN J Parenter Enteral Nutr.* 1981; 5: 569.

1067. Jeppsson RI, Sjoberg B. Compatibility of parenteral nutrition solutions when mixed in a plastic bag. *Clin Nutr.* 1984; 2: 149–58.

1068. Parry VA, Harrie KR. Effect of various nutrient ratios on the emulsion stability of total nutrient admixtures. *Am J Hosp Pharm.* 1986; 43:3017–22.

1069. Bettner FS, Stennett DJ. Effects of pH, temperature, concentration, and time on particle counts in lipid-containing total parenteral nutrition admixtures. *JPEN J Parenter Enteral Nutr.* 1986; 10:375–80.

1070. Schneider PJ. Three-in-one TPN formulations. *Infusion.* (May-June) 1984; 8:94–5, 101.

1071. Ernst JA, Williams JM, Glick MR, et al. Osmolality of substances used in the intensive care nursery. *Pediatrics.* 1983; 72: 347–52.

1072. Connors KA, Amidon GL, Stella VJ. Chemical stability of pharmaceuticals: a handbook for pharmacists. New York: John Wiley & Sons; 1986.

1073. Bosanquet AG. Stability of solutions of antineoplastic agents during preparation and storage for in vitro assays II. Assay methods, adriamycin and the other antitumor antibiotics. *Cancer Chemother Pharmacol.* 1986; 17:1–10.

1074. Grant AM (Medical Affairs, Abbott Laboratories, Abbott Park, IL): Personal communication; 1987 Mar 23.

1075. Bornstein M, Templeton RJ. Crystal formation after reconstituting cefazolin sodium with 0.9% sodium chloride injection. *Am J Hosp Pharm.* 1985; 42:2436.

1076. White JR, Campbell RK. Guide to mixing insulins. *Hosp Pharm.* 1991; 26:1046–48.

1077. Das Gupta V. Stability of cefotaxime sodium as determined by high-performance liquid chromatography. *J Pharm Sci.* 1984; 73:565–7.

1078. Carlson GH, Matzke GR. Particle formation of ceftizoxime sodium injections. *Am J Hosp Pharm.* 1985; 42:2651–2.

1079. Swenson E, Gooch WM. Visual compatibility of ceftizoxime sodium in four electrolyte injections. *Am J Hosp Pharm.* 1986; 43:2242–4.

1080. Barbero JR, Marino EL. Accelerated stability studies on Rocephin by high-efficiency liquid chromatography. *Int J Pharm.* 1984; 19:199–206.

1081. Smith RC. Overfill in cefuroxime sodium vials. *Am J Hosp Pharm.* 1985; 42:1045–6.

1082. Smith RC. No more overfill in cefuroxime sodium vials. *Am J Hosp Pharm.* 1986; 43:2154.

1083. DeVane CL, Wailand LA. Stability of chlorpromazine in five milliliter vials. *Can J Hosp Pharm.* 1984; 37:9.

1084. Mu-Chow KJ, Baptista RJ. Cost-effectiveness of parenteral nutrient solutions containing cimetidine hydrochloride. *Am J Hosp Pharm.* 1984; 41:1321.

1085. Parasrampuria J, Das Gupta V. Stability of acetazolamide sodium in 5% dextrose or 0.9% sodium chloride injection. *Am J Hosp Pharm.* 1987; 44:358–60.

1086. Zuber DE. Compatibility of morphine sulfate injections and prochlorperazine edisylate injections. *Am J Hosp Pharm.* 1987; 44:67.

1087. Cheung YW, Cradock JC, Vishnuvajjala BR, et al. Stability of cisplatin, iproplatin, carboplatin, and tetraplatin in commonly used intravenous infusion solutions. *Am J Hosp Pharm.* 1987; 44:124–30.

1088. LaFollette JM, Arbus MH. Stability of cisplatin admixtures in polyvinyl chloride bags. *Am J Hosp Pharm.* 1985; 42:2652.

1089. Hussain AA, Haddadin M. Reaction of cis-platinum with sodium bisulfite. *J Pharm Sci.* 1980; 69:364.

1090. Kirk B, Melia CD, Wilson JV, et al. Chemical stability of cyclophosphamide injection. *Br J Parenter Ther.* 1984; 5:90–7.

1091. Ptachcinski RJ, Logue LW, Burckart GJ, et al. Stability and availability of cyclosporine in 5% dextrose injection or 0.9% sodium chloride injection. *Am J Hosp Pharm.* 1986; 43:94–7.

1092. Venkataramanan R, Burckart GJ, Ptachcinski RJ, et al. Leaching of diethylhexyl phthalate from polyvinyl chloride bags into intravenous cyclosporine solution. *Am J Hosp Pharm.* 1986; 43:2800–2.

1093. Stevens MF, Peatey L. Photodegradation of solutions of the antitumour drug DTIC [proceedings]. *J Pharm Pharmacol.* 1978; 30(Suppl):47P.

1094. Williams BA, Tritton TR. Photoinactivation of anthracyclines. *Photochem Photobiol.* 1981; 34:131–4.

1095. Maloney TJ. Dilution of diazepam injection prior to intravenous administration. *Aust J Hosp Pharm.* 1983; 13:79.

1096. Hancock BG, Black CD. Effect of polyethylene-lined administration set on the availability of diazepam injection. *Am J Hosp Pharm.* 1985; 42:335–9.

1097. Yliruusi JK, Uotila JA. Effect of tubing length on adsorption of diazepam to polyvinyl chloride administration sets. *Am J Hosp Pharm.* 1986; 43:2789–94.

1098. Yliruusi JK, Uotila JA. Effect of flow rate and type of i.v. container on adsorption of diazepam to i.v. administration systems. *Am J Hosp Pharm.* 1986; 43:2795–9.

1099. Bell HE, Bertino JS. Constant diazepam infusion in the treatment of continuous seizure activity. *Drug Intell Clin Pharm.* 1984; 18:965–70.

1100. Dandurand KR, Stennett DJ. Stability of dopamine hydrochloride exposed to blue-light phototherapy. *Am J Hosp Pharm.* 1985; 42:595–7.

1101. Pluta PL, Morgan PK. Stability of erythromycin in intravenous admixtures. *Am J Hosp Pharm.* 1986; 43:2732.

1102. Deitel M, Faksa M, Kaminsky VM, et al. Growth of microorganisms in soybean oil emulsion and clinical implications. *Int Surg.* 1979; 64:27–32.

1103. Keammerer D, Mayhall CG, Hall GO, et al. Microbial growth patterns in intravenous fat emulsions. *Am J Hosp Pharm.* 1983; 40:1650–3.

1104. Kim CH, Lewis DE. Bacterial and fungal growth in intravenous fat emulsions. *Am J Hosp Pharm.* 1983; 40:2159–61.

1105. Allwood MC. Release of DEHP plasticizer into fat emulsion from iv administration sets. *Pharm J.* 1985; 235:600.

1106. Driscoll DF, Baptista RJ, Bistrian BR, et al. Practical considerations regarding the use of total nutrient admixtures. *Am J Hosp Pharm.* 1986; 43:416–9.

1107. Morgan DE, Bergdale S. Effect of syringe-pump position on infusion of fat emulsion with a primary solution. *Am J Hosp Pharm.* 1985; 42:1110–1.

1108. Neil JM, Fell AF. Evaluation of the stability of frusemide in intravenous infusions by reversed-phase high-performance liquid chromatography. *Int J Pharm.* 1984; 22:105–26.

1109. Dean T, Ridley P. Use of 0.9% sodium chloride injection without heparin for maintaining indwelling intermittent injection sites. *Clin Pharm.* 1985; 4:488.

1110. Chantelau EA, Berger M. Pollution of insulin with silicone oil, a hazard of disposable plastic syringes. *Lancet.* 1985; 1:1459.

1111. Furberg H, Jensen AK. Effect of pretreatment with 0.9% sodium chloride or insulin solutions on the delivery of insulin from an infusion system. *Am J Hosp Pharm.* 1986; 43:2209–13.

1112. Kane M, Jay M. Binding of insulin to a continuous ambulatory peritoneal dialysis system. *Am J Hosp Pharm.* 1986; 43:81–8.

1113. Hutchinson KG. Assessment of gelling in insulin solutions for infusion pumps. *J Pharm Pharmacol.* 1985; 37:528–31.

1114. Kamerman B. Dissolving mannitol crystals. *Hosp Pharm.* 1985; 20:360.

1115. Cano SB, Glogiewicz FL. Storage requirements for metronidazole injection. *Am J Hosp Pharm.* 1986; 43:2983.

1116. Schell KH, Copland JR. Metronidazole hydrochloride-aluminum interaction. *Am J Hosp Pharm.* 1985; 42:1040.

1117. Struthers BJ, Parr RJ. Clarifying the metronidazole hydrochloride-aluminum interaction. *Am J Hosp Pharm.* 1985; 42:2660.

1118. Quebbeman EJ, Hoffman NE, Ausman RK, et al. Stability of mitomycin admixtures. *Am J Hosp Pharm.* 1985; 42:1750–4.

1119. Edwards D, Selkirk AB. Determination of the stability of mitomycin C by high-performance liquid chromatography. *Int J Pharm.* 1979; 4:21–6.

1120. Young JB, Pratt CM, Farmer JA, et al. Specialized delivery systems for intravenous nitroglycerin. Are they necessary?. *Am J Med.* 1984; 76:27–37.

1121. Nix DE, Tharpe WN. Intravenous nitroglycerin delivery: dynamics and cost considerations. *Hosp Pharm.* 1985; 20:230–2.

1122. Schaber DE, Uden DL. Nitroglycerin adsorption to a combination polyvinyl chloride, polyethylene intravenous administration set. *Drug Intell Clin Pharm.* 1985; 19:572–5.

1123. Mendel S, Green JA. Comment: Nitroglycerin iv tubing adsorption. *Drug Intell Clin Pharm.* 1985; 19:946–7.

1124. Tarr BD, Campbell RK. Stability and sterility of biosynthetic human insulin stored in plastic insulin syringes for 28 days. *Am J Hosp Pharm.* 1991; 48:2631–4.

1125. Rayani S, Fakhreddin J. Stability of penicillin G sodium in 5% dextrose in water minibags after freezing. *Can J Hosp Pharm.* 1985; 38:162–3.

1126. Das Gupta V, Davis DD. Stability of piperacillin sodium in dextrose 5% and sodium chloride 0.9% injections. *Am J IV Ther Clin Nutr.* (Feb) 1984; 11:14–5, 18–19.

1127. Deardorff DL, Schmidt CN. Mixing additives by squeezing plastic bags. *Am J Hosp Pharm.* 1985; 42:533–4.

1128. Synave R, Vergote A. Stability of procaine hydrochloride in a cardioplegic solution containing bicarbonate. *J Clin Hosp Pharm.* 1985; 10:385–8.

1129. Raymond G, DeGennaro M. Effect of Neut on the pH of some commercially available intravenous solutions. *Infusion.* 1985; 9:144–6.

1130. Sewell GJ, Forbes DR. Stability of sodium nitroprusside infusion during the administration by motorized syringe-pump. *J Clin Hosp Pharm.* 1985; 10:351–60.

1131. Baaske DM, Smith MD, Karnatz N, et al. High-performance liquid chromatographic determination of sodium nitroprusside. *J Chromatogr.* 1981; 212:339–46.

1132. Elenbaas JK, Lander RD. Effect of inline filtration on tobramycin delivery. *Drug Intell Clin Pharm.* 1985; 19:122–5.

1133. Mehta J, Searcy CJ. Stability of terbutaline sulfate admixtures stored in polyvinyl chloride bags. *Am J Hosp Pharm.* 1986; 43: 1760–2.

1134. Das Gupta V, Stewart KR. Stability of vancomycin hydrochloride in 5% dextrose and 0.9% sodium chloride injections. *Am J Hosp Pharm.* 1986; 43:1729–31.

1135. Hazlet TK, Tankersley DL. Possible incompatibilities with immune globulin for i.v. use. *Am J Hosp Pharm.* 1993; 50: 654, 659–60.

1136. Richardson BL, Woodford JD, Andrews GD. Pharmacy of ceftazidime. *J Antimicrob Chemother.* 1981; 8:233–6.

1137. Cox ME, Roesner M. Production of carbon dioxide gas after reconstitution of ceftazidime. *Am J Hosp Pharm.* 1986; 43: 1422.

1138. Fites AL. Production of carbon dioxide gas after reconstitution of ceftazidime. *Am J Hosp Pharm.* 1986; 43:1422–3.

1139. Marwaha RK, Johnson BF. Simple stability-indicating assay for histamine solutions. *Am J Hosp Pharm.* 1985; 42:1568–71.

1140. Marwaha RK, Johnson BF. Long-term stability study of histamine in sterile bronchoprovocation solutions. *Am J Hosp Pharm.* 1986; 43:380–3.

1141. Bigley FP, Forsyth RJ. Compatibility of imipenem–cilastatin sodium with commonly used intravenous solutions. *Am J Hosp Pharm.* 1986; 43:2803–9.

1142. De NC, Alam AS. Stability of pentamidine isethionate in 5% dextrose and 0.9% sodium chloride injections. *Am J Hosp Pharm.* 1986; 43:1486–8.

1143. Lampasona V, Mullins RE. Stability of ranitidine admixtures frozen and refrigerated in minibags. *Am J Hosp Pharm.* 1986; 43:921–5.

1144. Gralla RJ, Tyson LB, Kris MG, et al. Management of chemotherapy-induced nausea and vomiting. *Med Clinics N Am.* 1987; 71:289–301.

1145. Forman JK, Souney PF. Visual compatibility of midazolam hydrochloride with common preoperative injectable medications. *Am J Hosp Pharm.* 1987; 44:2298–9.

1146. Thompson DF, Thompson GD. Visual compatibility of esmolol hydrochloride and furosemide in 5% dextrose or 0.9% sodium chloride injections. *Am J Hosp Pharm.* 1987; 44:2740.

1147. Ahmed I, Day P. Stability of cefazolin sodium in various artificial tear solutions and aqueous vehicles. *Am J Hosp Pharm.* 1987; 44:2287–90.

1148. McSherry TJ. Incompatibility between chlorpromazine and metacresol. *Am J Hosp Pharm.* 1987; 44:1574.

1149. Tebbett IR, Melrose E. Stability of promazine as an intravenous infusion. *Pharm J.* 1986; 237:172.

1150. Johnson CE, Cohen IA, Michelini TJ, et al. Compatibility of premixed theophylline and methylprednisolone sodium succinate intravenous admixtures. *Am J Hosp Pharm.* 1987; 44: 1620–4.

1151. Marti E, Cervera P. Compatibility of ranitidine hydrochloride with other injectable pharmaceuticals in common use. *Rev Assoc Esp Farm Hosp.* 1985; 9:169–72.

1152. Navarro JN, Aznar MT, Ruiz MD, et al. Stability of 5-fluorouracil in large volume intravenous solutions. *Rev Assoc Esp Farm Hosp.* 1985; 9:69–72.

1153. Biondi L, Nairn JG. Stability of 5-fluorouracil and flucytosine in parenteral solutions. *Can J Hosp Pharm.* 1986; 39:60–3.

1154. Parr MD, Barton SD, Haver VM, et al. Cyclosporine binding to components in medication administration sets. *Drug Intell Clin Pharm.* 1988; 22:173–4.

1155. Gasca M, Fanikos J. Visual compatibility of perphenazine with various antimicrobials during simulated Y-site injection. *Am J Hosp Pharm.* 1987; 44:574–5.

1156. Nolte MS, Poon V, Grodsky GM, et al. Reduced solubility of short-acting soluble insulins when mixed with longer-acting insulins. *Diabetes.* 1983; 32:1177–81.

1157. Forman JK, Lachs JR. Visual compatibility of acyclovir sodium with commonly used intravenous drugs during simulated Y-site injection. *Am J Hosp Pharm.* 1987; 44:1408–9.

1158. Nelson RW, Young R. Visual incompatibility of dacarbazine and heparin. *Am J Hosp Pharm.* 1987; 44:2028.

1159. Zbrozek AS, Marble DA, Bosso JA, et al. Compatibility and stability of clindamycin phosphate-aminoglycoside combinations within polypropylene syringes. *Drug Intell Clin Pharm.* 1987; 21:806–10.

1160. Perry M, Khalidi N. Stability of penicillins in total parenteral nutrient solution. *Am J Hosp Pharm.* 1987; 44:1625–8.

1161. Tu YH, Allen LV. Stability of papaverine hydrochloride and phentolamine mesylate in injectable mixtures. *Am J Hosp Pharm.* 1987; 44:2524–7.

1162. Seargeant LE, Kobrinsky NL, Sus CJ, et al. In vitro stability and compatibility of daunorubicin, cytarabine, and etoposide. *Cancer Treat Rep.* 1987; 71:1189–92.

1163. Baumgartner TG, Knudsen AK, Dunn AJ, et al. Norepinephrine stability in saline solutions. *Hosp Pharm.* (Jan) 1988; 23: 44, 49, 59.

1164. Marble DA, Bosso JA. Compatibility of clindamycin phosphate with aztreonam in polypropylene syringes and with cefoperazone sodium, cefonicid sodium, and cefuroxime sodium in partial-fill glass bottles. *Drug Intell Clin Pharm.* 1988; 22:54–7.

1165. Welty TE, Cloyd JC. Delivery of paraldehyde in 5% dextrose and 0.9% sodium chloride injections through polyvinyl chloride i.v. sets and burettes. *Am J Hosp Pharm.* 1988; 45:131–5.

1166. Thompson DF, Stiles ML, Allen LV, et al. Compatibility of verapamil hydrochloride with penicillin admixtures during simulated Y-site injection. *Am J Hosp Pharm.* 1988; 45:142–5.

1167. Pesko LJ, Arend KA, Hagman DE, et al. Physical compatibility and stability of metoclopramide injection. *Parenterals.* (Dec-Jan) 1988; 5:1–3, 6–8.

1168. Karnatz NN, Wong J, Kesler H, et al. Compatibility of esmolol hydrochloride with morphine sulfate and fentanyl citrate during simulated Y-site administration. *Am J Hosp Pharm.* 1988; 45: 368–71.

1169. Colucci RD, Cobuzzi LE. Visual compatibility of esmolol hydrochloride and various injectable drugs during simulated Y-site injection. *Am J Hosp Pharm.* 1988; 45:630–2.

1170. Schilling CG. Compatibility of drugs with a heparin-containing neonatal total parenteral nutrient solution. *Am J Hosp Pharm.* 1988; 45:313–4.

1171. Colucci RD, Cobuzzi LE. Visual compatibility of labetalol hydrochloride injection with various injectable drugs during simulated Y-site injection. *Am J Hosp Pharm.* 1988; 45:1357–8.

1172. Johnson CE, Lloyd CW, Aviles AI, et al. Compatibility of premixed theophylline and verapamil intravenous admixtures. *Am J Hosp Pharm.* 1988; 45:609–12.

1173. Askerud L, Finholt P. Intravenous infusion of theophylline in 5% dextrose solution—formulation and stability. *Medd Nor Farm Selsk.* 1981; 43:17–24.

1174. Morgan GJ, McClellan JD. Stability of a heparin urokinase mixture. *Br J Parenter Ther.* 1987; 8:89.

1175. Garren KW, Repta AJ. Incompatibility of cisplatin and Reglan injectable. *Int J Pharm.* 1985; 24:91–9.

1176. Sanburg AL, Lyndon RC. Effects of freezing, long-term storage and microwave thawing on the stability of three antibiotics reconstituted in minibags. *Aust J Hosp Pharm.* 1987; 17:31–4.

1177. Murase S, Ochiai K, Aoki M, et al. Study on compatibility of dopram with other drugs. *Jap J Hosp Pharm.* 1987; 13: 244–60.

1178. Borst DL, Sesin GP. Stability of selected beta-lactam antibiotics stored in plastic syringes. *NITA.* 1987; 10:368–72.

1179. Roberts DE, Cross MD, Thomas PH, et al. Azlocillin-aminoglycoside combinations in CAPD fluid. *Br J Pharm Pract.* 1987; 9:98–9.

1180. Robinson DC, Cookson TL. Concentration guidelines for parenteral antibiotics in fluid-restricted patients. *Drug Intell Clin Pharm.* 1987; 21:985–9.

1181. Sterchele JA. Update on stability guidelines for routinely refrigerated drug products. *Am J Hosp Pharm.* 1987; 44:2698.

1182. Dahl JM, Roche VF. Visual compatibility of cibenzoline succinate with commonly used acute care medications. *Am J Hosp Pharm.* 1987; 44:1123–5.

1183. Cano SM, Montoro JB, Pastor C, et al. Stability of ranitidine hydrochloride in total nutrient admixtures. *Am J Hosp Pharm.* 1988; 45:1100–2.

1184. Jimenez MD. Visual compatibility of nalbuphine hydrochloride and promethazine hydrochloride. *Am J Hosp Pharm.* 1988; 45: 1278.

1185. Pereira-Rosario R, Utamura T. Interaction of heparin sodium and dopamine hydrochloride in admixtures studied by microcalorimetry. *Am J Hosp Pharm.* 1988; 45:1350–2.

1186. Baptista RJ, Mitrano FP. Stability and compatibility of cimetidine hydrochloride and aminophylline in dextrose 5% in water injection. *Drug Intell Clin Pharm.* 1988; 22:592–3.

1187. Holmes CJ, Kubey WY. Viability of microorganisms in fluorouracil and cisplatin small-volume injections. *Am J Hosp Pharm.* 1988; 45:1089–91.

1188. Jay GT, Fanikos J. Visual compatibility of famotidine with commonly used critical-care medications during simulated Y-site injection. *Am J Hosp Pharm.* 1988; 45:1556–7.

1189. Tucker DR, Sieradzan R. Visual compatibility of ciprofloxacin lactate with five broad-spectrum antimicrobial agents during simulated Y-site injection. *Am J Hosp Pharm.* 1988; 45: 1910–1.

1190. Marquardt ED. Visual compatibility of hydroxyzine hydrochloride with various antineoplastic agents. *Am J Hosp Pharm.* 1988; 45:2127.

1191. Riley CM. Stability of milrinone and digoxin, furosemide, procainamide hydrochloride, propranolol hydrochloride, quinidine gluconate, or verapamil hydrochloride in 5% dextrose injection. *Am J Hosp Pharm.* 1988; 45:2079–91.

1192. Awang DV, Graham KC. Microwave thawing of frozen drug solutions. *Am J Hosp Pharm.* 1987; 44:2256.

1193. Bashaw ED, Amantea MA, Minor JR, et al. Visual compatibility of zidovudine with other injectable drugs during simulated Y-site administration. *Am J Hosp Pharm.* 1988; 45:2532–3.

1194. Souney PF, Fanikos J. Compatibility of cyclophosphamide solution with antibiotics during simulated Y-site injection. *Parenterals.* (Aug-Sep) 1988; 6:1, 2, 8.

1195. Beijnen JH, Vendrig DEMM. Stability of Vinca alkaloid anticancer drugs in three commonly used infusion fluids. *J Parenter Sci Technol.* 1989; 43:84–7.

1196. Fong PA, Ward J. Visual compatibility of intravenous famotidine with selected drugs. *Am J Hosp Pharm.* 1989; 46:125–6.

1197. Karnatz NN, Wong J, Baaske DM, et al. Stability of esmolol hydrochloride and sodium nitroprusside in intravenous admixtures. *Am J Hosp Pharm.* 1989; 46:101–4.

1198. Johnson CE, Lloyd CW, Mesaros JL, et al. Compatibility of aminophylline and verapamil in intravenous admixtures. *Am J Hosp Pharm.* 1989; 46:97–100.

1199. Parti R, Wolf W. Caveats with respect to storage of cisplatin and fluorouracil admixtures. *Am J Hosp Pharm.* 1989; 46:259.

1200. Johnson EG, Janosik JE. Manufacturer's recommendations for handling spilled antineoplastic agents. *Am J Hosp Pharm.* 1989; 46:318–9.

1201. Jarosinski PF, Kennedy PF. Stability of concentrated trimethoprim-sulfamethoxazole admixtures. *Am J Hosp Pharm.* 1989; 46:732–7.

1202. Bosanquet AG. Stability of solutions of antineoplastic agents during preparation and storage for in vitro assays III. Antimetabolites, tubulin-binding agents, platinum drugs, amsacrine, L-asparaginase, interferons, steroids and other miscellaneous antitumor agents. *Cancer Chemother Pharmacol.* 1989; 23: 197–207.

1203. Beijnen JH, Underberg WJM. Degradation of mitomycin C in acidic solution. *Int J Pharm.* 1985; 24:219–29.

1204. Beijnen JH, den Hartigh J. Quantitative aspects of the degradation of mitomycin C in alkaline solution. *J Pharm Biomed Anal.* 1985; 3:59–69.

1205. Beijnen JH, Rosing H. Stability of mitomycins in infusion fluids. *Arch Pharm Chemi Sci Ed.* 1985; 13:58–66.

1206. Janssen MJH, Crommelin DJA, Storm G, et al. Doxorubicin decomposition on storage. Effect of pH, type of buffer and liposome encapsulation. *Int J Pharm.* 1985; 23:1–11.

1207. Beijnen JH, van der Houwen OAGJ, Voskuilen MCH, et al. Aspects of the degradation kinetics of daunorubicin in aqueous solution. In: Beijnen JH, ed. Chemical stability of mitomycin and anthracycline antineoplastic drugs. Utrecht, The Netherlands: Drukkerij Elkinkwijk BV; 1986:245–60.

1208. Beijnen JH, van der Houwen OAGJ. Aspects of the degradation kinetics of doxorubicin in aqueous solution. *Int J Pharm.* 1986; 32:123–31.

1209. Fritz BL, Lockhart HE. Chemical stability of selected pharmaceuticals repackaged in glass and plastic. *Pharm Tech.* (Nov) 1988; 12:44, 46, 48, 50–2.

1210. Venkataraman PS, Brissie EO. Stability of calcium and phosphorus in neonatal parenteral nutrition solutions. *J Pediatr Gastroenterol Nutr.* 1983; 2:640–3.

1211. Fitzgerald KA, MacKay MW. Calcium and phosphate solubility in neonatal parenteral nutrient solutions containing Aminosyn PF. *Am J Hosp Pharm.* 1987; 44:1396–1400.

1212. Mikrut BA. Calcium and phosphate solubility in neonatal parenteral nutrient solutions containing Aminosyn PF or TrophAmine. *Am J Hosp Pharm.* 1987; 44:2702–4.

1213. Lenz GT, Mikrut BA. Calcium and phosphate solubility in neonatal parenteral nutrient solutions containing Aminosyn-PF or TrophAmine. *Am J Hosp Pharm.* 1988; 45:2367–71.

1214. Raupp P, von Kries R, Schmidt E, et al. Incompatibility between fat emulsion and calcium plus heparin in parenteral nutrition of premature babies. *Lancet.* 1988; 1:700.

1215. Waller DJ, Smith SR. Use of infusion devices with total nutrient admixtures. *Am J Hosp Pharm.* 1987; 44:1570.

1216. Gilbert M, Gallagher SC, Eads M, et al. Microbial growth patterns in a total parenteral nutrition formulation containing lipid emulsion. *JPEN J Parenter Enteral Nutr.* 1986; 10:494–7.

1217. Barat AC, Harrie K, Jacob M, et al. Effect of amino acid solutions on total nutrient admixture stability. *JPEN J Parenter Enteral Nutr.* 1987; 11:384–8.

1218. Cripps AL. Stability studies on total parenteral nutrition mixtures containing fat emulsions. *Br J Pharm Pract.* 1984; 6: 187–95.

1219. Davis SS, Galloway M. Studies on fat emulsions in combined nutrition solutions. *J Clin Hosp Pharm.* 1986; 11:33–45.

1220. Ang SD, Canham JE, Daly JM. Parenteral infusion with an admixture of amino acids, dextrose, and fat emulsion solution: compatibility and clinical safety. *JPEN J Parenter Enteral Nutr.* 1987; 11:23–7.

1221. du Plessis J, Van Wyk CJ. The stability of parenteral fat emulsions in nutrition admixtures. *J Clin Pharm Ther.* 1987; 12: 307–18.

1222. Sayeed FA, Tripp MG, Sukumaran KB, et al. Stability of total nutrient admixtures using various intravenous fat emulsions. *Am J Hosp Pharm.* 1987; 44:2271–80.

1223. Sayeed FA, Tripp MG, Sukumaran KB, et al. Stability of various total nutrient admixture formulations using Liposyn II and Aminosyn II. *Am J Hosp Pharm.* 1987; 44:2280–6.

1224. McGee CD, Mascarenhas MG, Ostro MJ, et al. Selenium and vitamin E stability in parenteral solutions. *JPEN J Parenter Enteral Nutr.* 1985; 9:568–70.

1225. Dahl GB, Jeppsson RI. Vitamin stability in a TPN mixture stored in an EVA plastic bag. *J Clin Hosp Pharm.* 1986; 11: 271–9.

1226. Shenkin A, Fraser WD, McLelland AJ, et al. Maintenance of vitamin and trace element status in intravenous nutrition using a complete nutritive mixture. *JPEN J Parenter Enteral Nutr.* 1987; 11:238–42.

1227. Yamaoka K, Nakajima Y, Okinaga S, et al. Variation by combination of hyperalimentation with fat emulsion. *Jap J Hosp Pharm.* 1987; 13:211–5.

1228. Sewell DL, Golper TA, Brown SD, et al. Stability of single and combination antimicrobial agents in various peritoneal dialysates in the presence of insulin and heparin. *Am J Kidney Dis.* 1983; 3:209–12.

1229. Nance KS, Matzke GR. Stability of gentamicin and tobramycin in concentrate solutions for automated peritoneal dialysis. *Am J Nephrol.* 1984; 4:240–3.

1230. Das Gupta V, Parasrampuria J. Quantitation of acetazolamide in pharmaceutical dosage forms using high-performance liquid chromatography. *Drug Dev Ind Pharm.* 1987; 13:147–57.

1231. Boak LR. Aminophylline stability. *Can J Hosp Pharm.* 1987; 40:155.

1232. Moore BR, Tindula R. Incompatibility between amphotericin B and evacuated i.v. containers. *Am J Hosp Pharm.* 1987; 44: 1312.

1233. Bretschneider H. Osmolalities of commercially supplied drugs often used in anesthesia. *Anaesth Analg.* 1987; 66:361–2.

1234. Odgers C. Drug/nutrient interactions and incompatibilities complicating TPN. *N.Z. Pharm.* 1986; 6:64–8.

1235. Kedzierewicz F, Finance C, Nicolas A, et al. Etude comparative de la stabilite de solutions de carbenicilline en fonction de la temperature. Interet du cycle congelation-decongelation au four a micro-ondes. *Pharm Acta Helv.* 1987; 62:109–15.

1236. Arbus MH. Room temperature stability guidelines for carmustine. *Am J Hosp Pharm.* 1988; 45:531.

1237. Frederiksson K, Lundgren P. Stability of carmustine—kinetics and compatibility during administration. *Acta Pharm Suec.* 1986; 23:115–24.

1238. Sewell GJ, Riley CM. The stability of carboplatin in ambulatory continuous infusion regimes. *J Clin Pharm Ther.* 1987; 12: 427–32.

1239. Ross MB. Additional stability guidelines for routinely refrigerated drug products. *Am J Hosp Pharm.* 1988; 45:1498–9.

1240. Goodell JA, Harry DJ, Low JR. More on production of a carbon dioxide gas after reconstitution of ceftazidime. *Am J Hosp Pharm.* 1987; 44:510.

1241. Savello DR. More on production of carbon dioxide gas after reconstitution of ceftazidime. *Am J Hosp Pharm.* 1987; 44: 512.

1242. Rovers JP, Menielly G, Souney PF, et al. The use of stability-indicating assays to determine the in vitro compatibility and stability of metronidazole/gentamicin admixtures. *Can J Hosp Pharm.* 1989; 42:143–6.

1243. Walker SE, Dranitsaris G. Stability of reconstituted ceftriaxone in dextrose and saline solutions. *Can J Hosp Pharm.* 1987; 40: 161–6.

1244. Martinez-Pancheco R, Vila-Jato JL. Effect of different factors on stability of ceftriaxone in solution. *Farmaco Ed Prat.* 1987; 42:131–7.

1245. Kedzierewicz F, Finance C, Nicolas A, et al. Stability of parenteral ceftriaxone disodium solutions in frozen and liquid states: effect of freezing and microwave thawing. *J Pharm Sci.* 1989; 78:73–7.

1246. Kristjansson F, Sternson LA. An investigation on possible oligomer formation in pharmaceutical formulations of cisplatin. *Int J Pharm.* 1988; 41:67–74.

1247. Anon. High-dose Maxolon mixes with cisplatin. *Pharm J.* 1985; 234:593.

1248. Kirk B. The evaluation of a light-protective giving set. The photosensitivity of intravenous dacarbazine solutions. *Br J Parenter Ther.* (May-June) 1987; 8:78, 81–2, 85–6.

1249. Bosanquet AG. Stability of solutions of antineoplastic agents during preparation and storage for in vitro assays. General considerations, the nitrosoureas and alkylating agents. *Cancer Chemother Pharmacol.* 1985; 14:83–95.

1250. Beijnen JH, Potman RP, van Ooijen RD, et al. Structure elucidation and characterization of daunorubicin degradation products. *Int J Pharm.* 1987; 34:247–57.

1251. Haronikova K, Pikulikova Z, Kral L, et al. Sorption of diazepam on the surface of the plastic infusion unit, part 2. *Farm Obz.* 1986; 55:485–94.

1252. Mathot F, Bonnard J, Paris P, et al. Influence des materiaux de perfusion sur les solutions de diazepam. *J Pharm Belg.* 1982; 37:153–6.

1253. Murphy A, Maltby S. Dissolution time, on reconstitution, of a new parenteral formulation of doxorubicin (Doxorubicin Rapid Dissolution). *Int J Pharm.* 1987; 38:257–9.

1254. Baumann TJ, Smythe MA, Kaufmann K, et al. Dissolution times of Adriamycin and Adriamycin RDF. *Am J Hosp Pharm.* 1988; 45:1667.

1255. Vogelzang NJ, Ruane M. Phase I trial of an implanted battery-powered, programmable drug delivery system for continuous doxorubicin administration. *J Clin Oncol.* 1985; 3:407–14.

1256. Keusters L, Stolk LML, Umans R, et al. Stability of solutions of doxorubicin and epirubicin in plastic minibags for intravesical use after storage at −20 °C and thawing by microwave radiation. *Pharm Weekbl [Sci].* 1986; 8:194–7.

1257. Williamson M, Luce JK. Microwave thawing of doxorubicin hydrochloride admixtures not recommended. *Am J Hosp Pharm.* 1987; 44:505.

1258. Adams S, Fernandez F. Intravenous use of haloperidol. *Hosp Pharm.* 1987; 22:306–7.

1259. Thoma K, Struve M. Untersuchungen zur photo- und thermostabilitat von adrenalin-losungen. *Pharm Acta Helv.* 1986; 61:2–9.

1260. David LM. Phlebitis with intravenous erythromycin. *Am J Hosp Pharm.* 1987; 44:732.

1261. Schwinghammer TL, Reilly M. Cracking of ABS plastic devices used to infuse undiluted etoposide injection. *Am J Hosp Pharm.* 1988; 45:1277.

1262. Beijnen JH, Holthuis JJM, Kerkdijk HG, et al. Degradation kinetics of etoposide in aqueous solution. *Int J Pharm.* 1988; 41:169–78.

1263. Brown DH, Simkover RA. Maximum hang times for i.v. fat emulsions. *Am J Hosp Pharm.* 1987; 44:282.

1264. Allwood MC. The release of phthalate ester plasticizer from intravenous administration sets into fat emulsion. *Int J Pharm.* 1986; 29:233–6.

1265. Nahata MC, Hipple TF. Stability of gentamicin diluted in 0.9% sodium chloride injection in glass syringes. *Hosp Pharm.* 1987; 22:1131–2.

1266. Dunn DL, Lenihan SF. The case for the saline flush. *Am J Nurs.* 1987; 87:7989.

1267. Shearer J. Normal saline flush versus dilute heparin flush. A study of peripheral intermittent I.V. devices. *NITA.* 1987; 10:425–7.

1268. Hamilton RA, Plis JM, Clay C, et al. Heparin sodium versus 0.9% sodium chloride injection for maintaining patency of indwelling intermittent infusion devices. *Clin Pharm.* 1988; 7:439–43.

1269. Lombardi TP, Gundersen B, Zammett LO, et al. Efficacy of 0.9% sodium chloride injection with or without heparin sodium for maintaining patency of intravenous catheters in children. *Clin Pharm.* 1988; 7:832–6.

1270. Cyganski JM, Donahue JM. The case for the heparin flush. *Am J Nurs.* 1987; 87:796–7.

1271. Bullock LS, Fitzgerald JF, Glick MR. Stability of famotidine in minibags refrigerated and/or frozen. *DICP.* 1989; 23:132–5.

1272. Swanson DJ, DeAngelis C, Smith IL, et al. Degradation kinetics of imipenem in normal saline and human serum. *Antimicrob Agents Chemother.* 1986; 29:936–7.

1273. Smith GB, Schoenewaldt EF. Stability of N-formimidoylthienamycin in aqueous solution. *J Pharm Sci.* 1981; 70:272–6.

1274. McElnay JC, Elliott DS. Binding of human insulin to burette administration sets. *Int J Pharm.* 1987; 36:199–203.

1275. Adams PS, Haines-Nutt RF. Stability of insulin mixtures in disposable plastic insulin syringes. *J Pharm Pharmacol.* 1987; 39:158–63.

1276. Mozzi G, Conegliani B, Lomi R, et al. Stabilita del calcio folinato in soluzioni acquose in funzione del pH e delta temperatura. *Boll Chim Farm.* 1986; 125:424–8.

1277. Powell MF. Stability of lidocaine in aqueous solution: effect of temperature, pH, buffer, and metal ions on amide hydrolysis. *Pharm Res.* 1987; 4:42–5.

1278. Das Gupta V, Stewart KR. Chemical stabilities of lignocaine hydrochloride and phenylephrine hydrochloride in aqueous solution. *J Clin Hosp Pharm.* 1986; 11:449–52.

1279. Kirk B. Stability of reconstituted mustine injection BP during storage. *Br J Parenter Ther.* (July-Aug) 1986; 7:86–7, 90–2.

1280. Wright MP, Newton JM. Stability of methotrexate injection in prefilled, plastic disposable syringes. *Int J Pharm.* 1988; 45:237–44.

1281. Dyvik O, Grislingaas AL, Tonnesen HH, et al. Methotrexate in infusion solutions—a stability test for the hospital pharmacy. *J Clin Hosp Pharm.* 1986; 11:343–8.

1282. Cabeza Barrera J, Bautista Paloma J, Garcia de Pesquera F, et al. Disminucion de la adsorcion de insulina a los envases de nutricion parenteral. *Rev Assoc Esp Farm Hosp.* 1988; 12:251–4.

1283. Beijnen JH, Fokkens RH, Rosing H, et al. Degradation of mitomycin C in acid phosphate and acetate buffer solutions. *Int J Pharm.* 1986; 32:111–21.

1284. Beijnen JH, Lingeman H, Van Munster HA, et al. Mitomycin antitumor agents: a review of their physico-chemical and analytical properties and stability. *J Pharm Biomed Anal.* 1986; 4:275–95.

1285. Stolk LML, Fruijtier A. Stability after freezing and thawing of solutions of mitomycin C in plastic minibags for intravesical use. *Pharm Weekbl [Sci]*. 1986; 8:286–8.

1286. Depiero D, Rekhi GS, Souney PF, et al. Stability of morphine sulfate solutions frozen in polyvinyl chloride intravenous bags. *Pharm Pract News*. (Oct) 1987; 14:1, 39–40.

1287. Hung CT, Young M. Stability of morphine solutions in plastic syringes determined by reversed-phase ion-pair liquid chromatography. *J Pharm Sci*. 1988; 77:719–23.

1288. Visor GC, Lin LH, Jackson SE, et al. Stability of ganciclovir sodium (DHPG sodium) in 5% dextrose or 0.9% sodium chloride injections. *Am J Hosp Pharm*. 1986; 43:2810–2.

1289. Behme RJ, Brooke D, Kensler TT, et al. Incompatibility of ifosfamide with benzyl-alcohol-preserved bacteriostatic water for injection. *Am J Hosp Pharm*. 1988; 45:627–8.

1290. Rowland CG, Bradford E, Adams P, et al. Infusion of ifosfamide plus mesna. *Lancet*. 1984; 2:468.

1291. Bristol-Myers Oncology Division. Product information on Mesnex (Mesna). Evansville, IN; 1989 Jun.

1292. Dorr RT. Mesnex dosing and administration guide. Evansville, IN: Bristol-Myers Company; 1989.

1293. Lederle Laboratories, American Cyanamid Company. Product information on Novantrone. Pearl River, NY; 1988.

1294. Nahata MC, Hipple TF. Stability of phenobarbital sodium diluted in 0.9% sodium chloride injection. *Am J Hosp Pharm*. 1986; 43:384–5.

1295. Dela Cruz FG, Kanter MZ, Fischer JH, et al. Efficacy of individualized phenytoin sodium loading doses administered by intravenous infusion. *Clin Pharm*. 1988; 7:219–24.

1296. Davidson SW, Lyall D. Sodium nitroprusside stability in light-protective administration sets. *Pharm J*. 1987; 239:599–601.

1297. Saunders A. Stability and light sensitivity of sodium nitroprusside infusions. *Aust J Hosp Pharm*. 1986; 16:55–6.

1298. Glascock JC, DiPiro JT, Cadwallader DE, et al. Stability of terbutaline sulfate repackaged in disposable plastic syringes. *Am J Hosp Pharm*. 1987; 44:2291–3.

1299. Raymond GG. Stability of terbutaline sulfate injection stored in plastic tuberculin syringes. *Drug Intell Clin Pharm*. 1988; 22:303–5.

1300. Das Gupta V, Gardner SN, Jalowsky CM, et al. Chemical stability of thiopental sodium injection in disposable plastic syringes. *J Clin Pharm Ther*. 1987; 12:339–42.

1301. Nahata MC, Miller MA. Stability of vancomycin hydrochloride in various concentrations of dextrose injection. *Am J Hosp Pharm*. 1987; 44:802–4.

1302. Greenberg RN, Saeed AMK, Kennedy DJ, et al. Instability of vancomycin in Infusaid drug pump model 100. *Antimicrob Agents Chemother*. 1987; 31:610–1.

1303. Tucker R, Gentile JF. Precipitation of verapamil in an intravenous line. *Ann Intern Med*. 1984; 101:880.

1304. Patel SD, Yalkowsky SH. Development of an intravenous formulation for the antiviral drug 9–(beta-D-arabinofuranosyl)-adenine. *J Parenter Sci Technol*. 1987; 41:15–20.

1305. Stolk LML, Huisman W, Nordemann HD, et al. Formulation of a stable vidarabine infusion fluid. *Pharm Weekbl [Sci]*. 1983; 5:57–60.

1306. Black J, Buechter DD. Stability of vinblastine sulfate when exposed to light. *Drug Intell Clin Pharm*. 1988; 22:634–6.

1307. Vendrig DEMM, Smeets BPGH, Beijnen JH, et al. Degradation kinetics of vinblastine sulphate in aqueous solutions. *Int J Pharm*. 1988; 43:131–8.

1308. Cartwight-Shamoon JM, McElnay JC. Examination of sorption and photodegradation of amsacrine during storage in intravenous burette administration sets. *Int J Pharm*. 1988; 42:41–6.

1309. Milano G, Etienne MC, Cassuto-Viguier E, et al. Long-term stability of 5-fluorouracil and folinic acid admixtures. *Eur J Cancer*. 1992; 29A:129–32.

1310. Kraynak MA. Pharmaceutical aspects of docetaxel. *Am J Health-Syst Pharm*. 1997; 54:S7–S10.

1311. Leigh PH, Buddle GC. Pentamidine infusion stability. *Br J Pharm Pract*. 1988; 10:22–3.

1312. Roos PJ, Glerum JH, Meilink JW. Stability of morphine hydrochloride in a portable pump reservoir. *Pharm Weekbl Sci*. 1992; 14:23–6.

1313. Wohlford JG, Fowler MD. Visual compatibility of hetastarch with injectable critical-care drugs. *Am J Hosp Pharm*. 1989; 46:995–6.

1314. Wohlford JG. Clarification of visual compatibility of hetastarch and ranitidine hydrochloride. *Am J Hosp Pharm*. 1989; 46:1772.

1315. Wohlford JG, Wright JC. More information on the visual compatibility of hetastarch with injectable critical-care drugs. *Am J Hosp Pharm*. 1990; 47:297–8.

1316. Dasta JF, Hale KN, Stauffer GL, et al. Comparison of visual and turbidimetric methods for determining short-term compatibility of intravenous critical-care drugs. *Am J Hosp Pharm*. 1988; 45:2361–6.

1317. Smith JA, Morris A, Duafala ME, et al. Stability of floxuridine and leucovorin calcium admixtures for intraperitoneal administration. *Am J Hosp Pharm*. 1989; 46:985–9.

1318. Perrin JH, Pereira-Rosario R. The interaction of dobutamine hydrochloride and heparin sodium in parenteral fluids. *Drug Dev Indust Pharm*. 1988; 14:1617–22.

1319. Lesko AB, Sesin GP. Ceftizoxime stability in iv solutions. *DICP, Ann Pharmacother*. 617–618 (July-Aug) 1989; 23:615.

1320. Mitrano FP, Baptista RJ. Stability of cimetidine HCl and copper sulfate in a TPN solution. *DICP, Ann Pharmacother*. 1989; 23:429–30.

1321. Schilling CG, Watson DM, McCoy HG, et al. Stability and delivery of vancomycin hydrochloride when admixed in a total parenteral nutrition solution. *JPEN J Parenter Enteral Nutr*. 1989; 13:63–4.

1322. Strong DK, Ho W. Visual compatibility of vancomycin and heparin in peritoneal dialysis solutions. *Am J Hosp Pharm*. 1989; 46:1832–3.

1323. Chilvers MR, Lysne JM. Visual compatibility of ranitidine hydrochloride with commonly used critical-care medications. *Am J Hosp Pharm*. 1989; 46:2057–8.

1324. Bullock L, Clark JH, Fitzgerald JF, et al. The stability of amikacin, gentamicin, and tobramycin in total nutrient admixtures. *JPEN J Parenter Enteral Nutr*. 1989; 13:505–9.

1325. Nahata MC. Stability of vancomycin hydrochloride in total parenteral nutrient solutions. *Am J Hosp Pharm*. 1989; 46:2055–7.

1326. Fox AS, Boyer KM. Antibiotic stability in a pediatric parenteral alimentation solution. *J Pediatr*. 1988; 112:813–7.

1327. Raymond GG, Reed MT, Teagarden JR, et al. Stability of procainamide hydrochloride in neutralized 5% dextrose injection. *Am J Hosp Pharm*. 1988; 45:2513–7.

1328. Zbrozek AS, Marble DA. Compatibility and stability of cefazolin sodium, clindamycin phosphate, and gentamicin sulfate in two intravenous solutions. *Drug Intell Clin Pharm*. 1988; 22: 873–5.

1329. Stewart CF, Hampton EM. Stability of cisplatin and etoposide in intravenous admixtures. *Am J Hosp Pharm*. 1989; 46: 1400–4.

1330. Shea BF, Ptachcinski RJ, O'Neill S, et al. Stability of cyclosporine in 5% dextrose injection. *Am J Hosp Pharm*. 1989; 46: 2053–5.

1331. Bullock L, Fitzgerald JF, Glick MR, et al. Stability of famotidine 20 and 40 mg/L and amino acids in total parenteral nutrient solutions. *Am J Hosp Pharm*. 1989; 46:2321–5.

1332. Bullock L, Fitzgerald JF. Stability of famotidine 20 and 50 mg/L in total nutrient admixtures. *Am J Hosp Pharm*. 1989; 46: 2326–9.

1333. Montoro JB, Pou L, Salvador P, et al. Stability of famotidine 20 and 40 mg/L in total nutrient admixtures. *Am J Hosp Pharm*. 1989; 46:2329–32.

1334. DiStefano JE, Mitrano FP, Baptista RJ, et al. Long-term stability of famotidine 20 mg/L in a total parenteral nutrient solution. *Am J Hosp Pharm*. 1989; 46:2333–5.

1335. Lor E, Takagi J. Visual compatibility of foscarnet with other injectable drugs. *Am J Hosp Pharm*. 1990; 47:157–9.

1336. Scott SM. Incompatibility of cefoperazone and promethazine. *Am J Hosp Pharm*. 1990; 47:519.

1337. Savitsky ME. Visual compatibility of neuromuscular blocking agents with various injectable drugs during simulated Y-site injection. *Am J Hosp Pharm*. 1990; 47:820–1.

1338. Smythe MA, Patel MA. Visual compatibility of narcotic analgesics with selected intravenous admixtures. *Am J Hosp Pharm*. 1990; 47:819–20.

1339. Stewart CF, Fleming RA. Compatibility of cisplatin and fluorouracil in 0.9% sodium chloride injection. *Am J Hosp Pharm*. 1990; 47:1373–7.

1340. Lee CY, Mauro VF. Visual and spectrophotometric determination of compatibility of alteplase and streptokinase with other injectable drugs. *Am J Hosp Pharm*. 1990; 47:606–8.

1341. Gupta VD, Bethea C. Chemical stabilities of cefoperazone sodium and ceftazidime in 5% dextrose and 0.9% sodium chloride injections. *J Clin Pharm Ther*. 1988; 13:199–205.

1342. Gupta VD, Parasrampuria J. Chemical stabilities of famotidine and ranitidine hydrochloride in intravenous admixtures. *J Clin Pharm Ther*. 1988; 13:329–34.

1343. Gupta VD, Pramar Y. Stability of acyclovir sodium in dextrose and sodium chloride injections. *J Clin Pharm Ther*. 1989; 14: 451–6.

1344. Underberg WJM, Koomen JM. Stability of famotidine in commonly used nutritional infusion fluids. *J Parenter Sci Technol*. 1988; 42:94–7.

1345. Messerschmidt W. Pharmazeutische kompatibilitat von ceftazidim und metronidazol. *Pharm Ztg*. 1990; 135:36–8.

1346. Messerschmidt W. Kompatibilitat von ciprofloxacin und metronidazol in mischinfusionen. *Pharm Ztg*. 1988; 133:26.

1347. Murdoch JM, Garner ST. Calcium gluconate compatibility. *Pharm J*. 1989; 242:634.

1348. Stoberski P, Zakrzewski Z. Bandanie stabilnosci furosemidu i soli sodowej hemibursztynianu hydrokortyzonu metoda RP-HPLC w wybranych plynach infuzyjnych. *Farm Pol*. 1988; 44: 398–401.

1349. Veechio M, Walker SE, Iazzetta J, et al. The stability of morphine intravenous infusion solutions. *Can J Hosp Pharm*. 1988; 41:5–9.

1350. Walker SE, Kirby K. Stability of ranitidine hydrochloride admixtures refrigerated in polyvinyl chloride minibags. *Can J Hosp Pharm*. 1988; 41:105–8.

1351. Gupta VD, Parasrampuria J, Bethea C, et al. Stability of clindamycin phosphate in dextrose and saline solutions. *Can J Hosp Pharm*. 1989; 42:109–12.

1352. Walker SE, Iazzetta J, Lau DWC, et al. Famotidine stability in total parenteral nutrient solutions. *Can J Hosp Pharm*. 1989; 42: 97–103.

1353. Walker SE, Dranitsaris G. Ceftazidime stability in normal saline and dextrose 5% in water. *Can J Hosp Pharm*. 1988; 41: 65–71.

1354. Walker SE, Birkhans B. Stability of intravenous vancomycin. *Can J Hosp Pharm*. 1988; 41:233–8.

1355. Halpern NA, Colucci RD, Alicea M, et al. Visual compatibility of enalaprilat with commonly used critical care medications during simulated Y-site injection. *Int J Clin Pharmacol Ther Toxicol*. 1989; 27:294–7.

1356. Allen LV Jr, Stiles ML. Stability of fentanyl citrate in 0.9% sodium chloride solution in portable infusion pumps. *Am J Hosp Pharm*. 1990; 47:1572–4.

1357. Kowalski SR, Gourlay GK. Stability of fentanyl citrate in glass and plastic containers and in a patient-controlled delivery system. *Am J Hosp Pharm*. 1990; 47:1584–7.

1358. Schaaf LJ, Robinson DH, Vogel GJ, et al. Stability of esmolol hydrochloride in the presence of aminophylline, bretylium tosylate, heparin sodium, and procainamide hydrochloride. *Am J Hosp Pharm*. 1990; 47:1567–71.

1359. Rosenberg LS, Hostetler CK, Wagenknecht DM, et al. An accurate prediction of the pH change due to degradation: correction for a "produced" secondary buffering system. *Pharm Res*. 1988; 5:514–7.

1360. Williams MF, Hak LJ. In vitro evaluation of the stability of ranitidine hydrochloride in total parenteral nutrient mixtures. *Am J Hosp Pharm*. 1990; 47:1574–9.

1361. Galante LJ, Stewart JT, Warren FW, et al. Stability of ranitidine hydrochloride with eight medications in intravenous admixtures. *Am J Hosp Pharm*. 1990; 47:1606–10.

1362. Galante LJ, Stewart JT, Warren FW, et al. Stability of ranitidine hydrochloride at dilute concentration in intravenous infusion fluids at room temperature. *Am J Hosp Pharm*. 1990; 47: 1580–4.

1363. Marquardt ED. Visual compatibility of tolazoline hydrochloride with various medications during simulated Y-site injection. *Am J Hosp Pharm*. 1990; 47:1802–3.

1364. Chandler SW, Folstad J. Aztreonam-vancomycin incompatibility. *Am J Hosp Pharm*. 1990; 47:1970.

1365. Trissel LA, Tramonte SM. Visual compatibility of ondansetron hydrochloride with other selected drugs during simulated Y-site injection. *Am J Hosp Pharm*. 1991; 48:988–92.

1366. Leak RE, Woodford JD. Pharmaceutical development of ondansetron injection. *Eur J Cancer Clin Oncol.* 1989; 25(Suppl 1):S67–S69.

1367. Mackinnon JW, Collin DT. The chemistry of ondansetron. *Eur J Cancer Clin Oncol.* 1989; 25(Suppl 1):S61.

1368. Adria Laboratories. Idamycin—hospital formulary product information form. Columbus, OH; 1990 Oct 19.

1369. Allwood M, Stanley A, Wright P. The cytotoxics handbook. 3rd ed. Oxford, England: Radcliffe Medical Press; 1997.

1370. Garinot O, Vitzling C, Mottu R, et al. Sandostatine: compatibility of sandostatine 100 mcg/mL and 500 mcg/mL infusions with various plastic syringes and infusion apparatus. Basle, Switzerland: Sandoz Pharmaceutical Research Center; 1988 Sep.

1371. Sandoz Laboratories. Sandostatin—compatibility between octreotide in the infusion and the giving set/container. Basle, Switzerland; 1986 Apr 3.

1372. Sandoz Laboratories. Sandostatin—stability in physiological salt solutions. Basle, Switzerland; 1986 Mar 26.

1373. Marchiarullo M. Stability of octreotide in various infusion supplies. East Hanover, NJ: Sandoz Pharmaceuticals Corporation; 1990 Mar 20.

1374. Beijnen JH, Beijnen-Bandhoe AU, Dubbelman AC, et al. Chemical and physical stability of etoposide and teniposide in commonly used infusion fluids. *J Parenter Sci Technol.* 1991; 45: 108–12.

1375. Santiero ML, Sagraves R. Osmolality of small-volume i.v. admixtures for pediatric patients. *Am J Hosp Pharm.* 1990; 47: 1359–64.

1376. Messerschmidt W. Kompatibilitat von cefuroxim mit metronidazole. *Krankenhauspharmazie.* 1987; 8:45–7.

1377. Rosen GH. Potential incompatibility of insulin and octreotide in total parenteral nutrient solutions. *Am J Hosp Pharm.* 1989; 46:1128.

1378. McElnay JC, Elliott DS, Cartwright-Shamoon J, et al. Stability of methotrexate and vinblastine in burette administration sets. *Int J Pharm.* 1988; 47:239–47.

1379. Williams DA. Stability and compatibility of admixtures of antineoplastic drugs. In: Lokich JJ, ed. Cancer chemotherapy by infusion. 2nd ed. Chicago, IL: Precept Press; 1990:52–73.

1380. Baaske DM, DeMay JF, Latona CA, et al. Stability of nicardipine hydrochloride in intravenous solutions. *Am J Health-Syst Pharm.* 1996; 53:1701–5.

1381. Trissel LA, Chandler SW. Visual compatibility of amsacrine with selected drugs during simulated Y-site injection. *Am J Hosp Pharm.* 1990; 47:2525–8.

1382. Townsend RS. In vitro inactivation of gentamicin by ampicillin. *Am J Hosp Pharm.* 1989; 46:2250–1.

1383. Vaughn LM, Small C. Incompatibility of iron dextran and a total nutrient admixture. *Am J Hosp Pharm.* 1990; 47:1745–6.

1384. Cutie MR. Verapamil precipitation. *Ann Intern Med.* 1983; 98: 672.

1385. Garner SS, Wiest DB. Compatibility of drugs separated by a fluid barrier in a retrograde intravenous infusion system. *Am J Hosp Pharm.* 1990; 47:604–6.

1386. Lokich J, Anderson N, Bern M, et al. Combined floxuridine and cisplatin in a 14–day infusion. *Cancer.* 1988; 62:2309–12.

1387. Anderson N, Lokich J, Bern M, et al. A phase I clinical trial of combined fluoropyrimidines with leucovorin in a 14–day infusion. *Cancer.* 1989; 63:233–7.

1388. Lokich J, Anderson N, Bern M, et al. Etoposide admixed with cisplatin. *Cancer.* 1989; 63:818–21.

1389. Lokich J, Bern M, Anderson N, et al. Cyclophosphamide, methotrexate, and 5-fluorouracil in a three-drug admixture. *Cancer.* 1989; 63:822–4.

1390. Anderson N, Lokich J, Bern M, et al. Combined 5-fluorouracil and floxuridine administered as a 14–day infusion. *Cancer.* 1989; 63:825–7.

1391. Stiles ML, Tu YH. Stability of cefazolin sodium, cefoxitin sodium, ceftazidime, and penicillin G sodium in portable pump reservoirs. *Am J Hosp Pharm.* 1989; 46:1408–12.

1392. Martens HJ, De Goede PN. Sorption of various drugs in polyvinyl chloride, glass, and polyethylene-lined infusion containers. *Am J Hosp Pharm.* 1990; 47:369–73.

1393. Baltz JK, Kennedy P, Minor JR, et al. Visual compatibility of foscarnet with other injectable drugs during simulated Y-site administration. *Am J Hosp Pharm.* 1990; 47:2075–7.

1394. Walker SE, Coons C, Matte D, et al. Hydromorphone and morphine stability in portable infusion pump casettes and minibags. *Can J Hosp Pharm.* 1988; 41:177–82.

1395. Smythe M, Malouf E. Visual compatibility of insulin with secondary intravenous drugs in admixtures. *Am J Hosp Pharm.* 1991; 48:125–6.

1396. Tu YH, Stiles ML. Stability of fentanyl citrate and bupivacaine hydrochloride in portable pump reservoirs. *Am J Hosp Pharm.* 1990; 47:2037–40.

1397. Pugh CB, Pabis DJ. Visual compatibility of morphine sulfate and meperidine hydrochloride with other injectable drugs during simulated Y-site injection. *Am J Hosp Pharm.* 1991; 48: 123–5.

1398. Pritts D, Hancock D. Incompatibility of ceftriaxone with vancomycin. *Am J Hosp Pharm.* 1991; 48:77.

1399. DeMuynck C, De Vroe C, Remon JP, et al. Binding of drugs to end-line filters: a study of four commonly administered drugs in intensive care units. *J Clin Pharm Ther.* 1988; 13:335–40.

1400. Aki H, Sawai N, Yamamoto K, et al. Structural confirmation of ampicillin polymers formed in aqueous solution. *Pharm Res.* 1991; 8:119–22.

1401. Bonhomme L, Postaire E, Touratier S, et al. Chemical stability of lignocaine (lidocaine) and adrenaline (epinephrine) in pH-adjusted parenteral solutions. *J Clin Pharm Ther.* 1988; 13: 257–61.

1402. Lee DKT, Lee A. Compatibility of cefoperazone sodium and furosemide in 5% dextrose injection. *Am J Hosp Pharm.* 1991; 48:108–10.

1403. Lee DKT, Wang DP. Compatibility of cefoperazone sodium and cimetidine hydrochloride in 5% dextrose injection. *Am J Hosp Pharm.* 1991; 48:111–3.

1404. Kirkpatrick AE, Holcome BJ. Effect of retrograde aminophylline administration on calcium and phosphate solubility in neonatal total parenteral nutrient solutions. *Am J Hosp Pharm.* 1989; 46:2496–500.

1405. Seay R, Bostrom B. Apparent compatibility of methotrexate and vancomycin. *Am J Hosp Pharm.* 1990; 47:2656.

1406. Johnson OL, Washington C, Davis SS, et al. The destabilization of parenteral feeding emulsions by heparin. *Int J Pharm.* 1989; 53:237–40.

1407. Lor E, Sheybani T. Visual compatibility of fluconazole with commonly used injectable drugs during simulated Y-site administration. *Am J Hosp Pharm.* 1991; 48:744–6.

1408. Tol A, Quik RFP. Adsorption of human and porcine insulins to intravenous administration sets. *Pharm Weekbl [Sci].* 1988; 10:213–6.

1409. Thompson DF, Allen LV Jr. Visual compatibility of enalaprilat with selected intravenous medications during simulated Y-site injection. *Am J Hosp Pharm.* 1990; 47:2530–1.

1410. Wilson TD, Forde MD. Stability of milrinone and epinephrine, atropine sulfate, lidocaine hydrochloride, or morphine sulfate injection. *Am J Hosp Pharm.* 1990; 47:2504–7.

1411. Lam NP, Kennedy PE, Jarosinski PF, et al. Stability of zidovudine in 5% dextrose injection and 0.9% sodium chloride injection. *Am J Hosp Pharm.* 1991; 48:280–2.

1412. Horrow JC, Digregorio GJ, Barbieri EJ, et al. Intravenous infusions of nitroprusside, dobutamine, and nitroglycerin are compatible. *Crit Care Med.* 1990; 18:858–61.

1413. Halstead DC, Guzzo J, Giardina JA, et al. In vitro bactericidal activities of gentamicin, cefazolin, and imipenem in peritoneal dialysis fluids. *Antimicrob Agents Chemother.* 1989; 33:1553–6.

1414. Drake JM, Myre SA, Staneck JL, et al. Antimicrobial activity of vancomycin, gentamicin, and tobramycin in peritoneal dialysis solution. *Am J Hosp Pharm.* 1990; 47:1604–6.

1415. Pavlik EJ, van Nagell JR, Hanson MB, et al. Sensitivity to anticancer agents in vitro: standardizing the cytotoxic response and characterizing the sensitivities of a reference cell line. *Gynecol Oncol.* 1982; 14:243–61.

1416. Pavlik EJ, Kenady DE, van Nagell JR, et al. Properties of anticancer agents relevant to in vitro determinations of human tumor cell sensitivity. *Cancer Chemother Pharmacol.* 1983; 11:8–15.

1417. Gora ML, Seth S, Visconti JA, et al. Stability of dobutamine hydrochloride in peritoneal dialysis solutions. *Am J Hosp Pharm.* 1991; 48:1234–7.

1418. Strom JG Jr, Miller SW. Stability and compatibility of methylprednisolone sodium succinate and cimetidine hydrochloride in 5% dextrose injection. *Am J Hosp Pharm.* 1991; 48:1237–41.

1419. Riley CM, Junkin P. Stability of amrinone and digoxin, procainamide hydrochloride, propranolol hydrochloride, sodium bicarbonate, potassium chloride, or verapamil hydrochloride in intravenous admixtures. *Am J Hosp Pharm.* 1991; 48:1245–52.

1420. Pennell AT, Allington DR. Effect of ceftazidime, cefotaxime, and cefoperazone on serum tobramycin concentrations. *Am J Hosp Pharm.* 1991; 48:520–2.

1421. Collins JL, Lutz RJ. In vitro study of simultaneous infusion of incompatible drugs in multilumen catheters. *Heart Lung.* 1991; 20:271–7.

1422. Gupta VD. Complexation of procainamide with dextrose. *J Pharm Sci.* 1982; 71:994–6.

1423. Gupta VD. Complexation of procainamide with hydroxide-containing compounds. *J Pharm Sci.* 1983; 72:205–7.

1424. Parasrampuria J, Gupta VD. Preformulation studies of acetazolamide: effect of pH, two buffer species, ionic strength, and temperature on its stability. *J Pharm Sci.* 1989; 78:855–7.

1425. Frazin BS. Maximal dilution of activase. *Am J Hosp Pharm.* 1990; 47:1016.

1426. Tripp MG. Automated 3–in-1 admixture compounding: a comparative study of simultaneous versus sequential pumping of core substrates on admixture stability. *Hosp Pharm.* 1990; 25:1090–3.

1427. Knowles JB, Cusson G, Smith M, et al. Pulmonary deposition of calcium phosphate crystals as a complication of home total parenteral nutrition. *JPEN J Parenter Enteral Nutr.* 1989; 13:209–13.

1428. Knight PJ, Buchanan S. Calcium and phosphate requirements of preterm infants who require prolonged hyperalimentation. *J Am Med Assoc.* 1980; 243:1244–6.

1429. Stennett DJ, Gerwick WH, Egging PK, et al. Precipitate analysis from an indwelling total parenteral nutrition catheter. *JPEN J Parenter Enteral Nutr.* 1988; 12:88–92.

1430. Mazur HI, Stennett DJ, Egging PK. Extraction of diethylhexylphthalate from total nutrient solution-containing polyvinyl chloride bags. *JPEN J Parenter Enteral Nutr.* 1989; 13:59–62.

1431. Smith JL, Canham JE, Kirkland WD, et al. Effect of Intralipid, amino acids, container, temperature, and duration of storage on vitamin stability in total parenteral nutrition admixtures. *JPEN J Parenter Enteral Nutr.* 1988; 12:478–83.

1432. Tripp MG, Menon SK. Stability of total nutrient admixtures in a dual-chamber flexible container. *Am J Hosp Pharm.* 1990; 47:2496–503.

1433. Dalton-Bunnow MF, Halvacks FJ. Update on room-temperature stability of drug products labeled for refrigerated storage. *Am J Hosp Pharm.* 1990; 47:2522–4.

1434. Kintzel PE, Kennedy PE. Stability of amphotericin B in 5% dextrose injection at concentrations used for administration through a central venous line. *Am J Hosp Pharm.* 1991; 48:283–5.

1435. Rice JK. Visual compatibility of amphotericin B and flush solutions. *Am J Hosp Pharm.* 1989; 46:2461.

1436. Trissel LA, Bready BB, Kwan JW, et al. The visual compatibility of sargramostim with selected chemotherapeutic drugs, anti-infectives, and other drugs during simulated Y-site injection. *Am J Hosp Pharm.* 1992; 49:402–6.

1437. Pilla TJ, Beshany SE. Incompatibility of hexabrix and papaverine. *Am J Roentgenol.* 1986; 146:1300–1.

1438. Irving HD, Burbridge BE. Incompatibility of contrast agents with intravascular medications. *Radiology.* 1989; 173:91–2.

1439. Trissel LA, Parks NPT. Visual compatibility of fludarabine phosphate with antineoplastic drugs, anti-infectives, and other selected drugs during simulated Y-site injection. *Am J Hosp Pharm.* 1991; 48:2186–9.

1440. Tidy PJ, Sewell GJ, Jeffries TM. Microwave freeze-thaw studies on azlocillin infusion. *Pharm J.* 1988; 241:R22–R23.

1441. Koberda M, Zieske PA, Raghavan NV, et al. Stability of bleomycin sulfate reconstituted in 5% dextrose injection or 0.9% sodium chloride injection stored in glass vials or polyvinyl chloride containers. *Am J Hosp Pharm.* 1990; 47:2528–9.

1442. Datapharm Publications Ltd. ABPI compendium of data sheets and summaries of product characteristics 1999/2000. London, England; 1999.

1443. Weir SJ, Szucs Myers VA, Bengston KD, et al. Sorption of amiodarone to polyvinyl chloride infusion bags and administration sets. *Am J Hosp Pharm.* 1985; 42:2679–83.

1444. Benedict MK, Roche VF, Banakar UV, et al. Visual compatibility of amiodarone hydrochloride with various antimicrobial agents during simulated Y-site injection. *Am J Hosp Pharm.* 1988; 45:1117–8.

1445. Capps PA, Robertson AL. Influence of amiodarone injection on delivery rate of intravenous fluids. *Pharm J.* 1985; 234:14–5.

1446. Tsuei SE, Nation RL. Sorption of chlormethiazole by intravenous infusion giving sets. *Eur J Clin Pharmacol.* 1980; 18: 333–8.

1447. Lingam S, Bertwistle H, Elliston HM, et al. Problems with intravenous chlormethiazole (Heminevrin) in status epilepticus. *Br Med J.* 1980; 280:155–6.

1448. Beaumont IM. Stability study of aqueous solutions of diamorphine and morphine using HPLC. *Pharm J.* 1982; 229:39–41.

1449. Kleinberg ML, Duafala ME, Nacov C, et al. Stability of heroin hydrochloride in infusion devices and containers for intravenous administration. *Am J Hosp Pharm.* 1990; 47:377–81.

1450. Jones VA, Hanks GW. New portable infusion pump for prolonged subcutaneous administration of opiod analgesics in patients with advanced cancer. *BMJ.* 1986; 292:1496.

1451. Jones VA, Hoskin PJ, Omar OA, et al. Diamorphine stability in aqueous solution for subcutaneous infusion. *Abs Br Soc Pharmacol Meet.* 1986; 66(Dec).

1452. Omar OA, Hoskin PJ, Johnston A, et al. Diamorphine stability in aqueous solution for subcutaneous infusion. *J Pharm Pharmacol.* 1989; 41:275–7.

1453. Al-Razzak LA, Benedetti AE, Waugh WN, et al. Chemical stability of pentostatin (NSC-218321), a cytotoxic and immunosuppressive agent. *Pharm Res.* 1990; 7:452–60.

1454. Allwood MC. Diamorphine mixed with antiemetic drugs in plastic syringes. *Br J Pharm Prac.* 1984; 6:88–90.

1455. Regnard C, Pashley S. Anti-emetic/diamorphine mixture compatibility in infusion pumps. *Br J Pharm Pract.* 1986; 8: 218–20.

1456. Collins AJ, Abathell JA, Holmes SG, et al. Stability of diamorphine hydrochloride with haloperidol in prefilled syringes for continuous subcutaneous administration. *J Pharm Pharmacol.* 1986; 38(S):51P.

1457. Page J, Hudson SA. Diamorphine hydrochloride compatibility with saline. *Pharm J.* 1982; 228:238–9.

1458. Kirk B, Hain WR. Diamorphine injection BP incompatibility. *Pharm J.* 1985; 235:171.

1459. Jones V, Murphy A. Solubility of diamorphine. *Pharm J.* 1985; 235:426.

1460. Wood MJ, Irwin WJ, Scott DK. Stability of doxorubicin, daunorubicin and epirubicin in plastic syringes and minibags. *J Clin Pharm Ther.* 1990; 15:279–89.

1461. Targett PL, Keefe PA. Stability of two concentrations of morphine tartrate in 10 mL polypropylene syringes. *Aust J Hosp Pharm.* 1997; 27:452–4.

1462. Keusters L, Stolk LML, Umans R, et al. Stability of solutions of doxorubicin and epirubicin in plastic minibags for intravesical use after storage at −20 °C and thawing by microwave radiation. *Pharm Weekbl [Sci].* 1986; 8:194–7.

1463. Wood MJ, Irwin WJ. Photodegradation of doxorubicin, daunorubicin, and epirubicin measured by high-performance liquid chromatography. *J Clin Pharm Ther.* 1990; 35:291–300.

1464. Lee MG, Fenton-May V. Absorption of isosorbide dinitrate by PVC infusion bags and administration sets. *J Clin Hosp Pharm.* 1981; 6:209–11.

1465. DeMuynck C, Remon JP. The sorption of isosorbide dinitrate to intravenous delivery systems. *J Pharm Pharmacol.* 1988; 40: 601–4.

1466. Struhar M, Mandak M, Heinrich J, et al. Sorption of isosorbide dinitrate on infusion sets. *Farm Obz.* 1989; 58:443–6.

1467. Allwood MC. Sorption of parenteral nitrates during administration with a syringe pump and extension set. *Int J Pharm.* 1987; 39:183–6.

1468. Wilson TD, Forde MD, Crain AVR, et al. Stability of milrinone in 0.45% sodium chloride, 0.9% sodium chloride, or 5% dextrose injections. *Am J Hosp Pharm.* 1986; 43:2218–20.

1469. Cook B, Hill SA. The stability of amoxycillin sodium in intravenous infusion fluids. *J Clin Hosp Pharm.* 1982; 7:245–50.

1470. Concannon J, Lovitt H, Ramage M, et al. Stability of aqueous solutions of amoxicillin sodium in the frozen and liquid states. *Am J Hosp Pharm.* 1986; 43:3027–30.

1471. McDonald C, Sunderland VB, Lau H, et al. The stability of amoxicillin sodium in normal saline and glucose (5%) solutions in the liquid and frozen states. *J Clin Pharm Ther.* 1989; 14: 45–52.

1472. McDonald C, Sunderland VB, Marshall CA, et al. Freezing rates of 50–mL infusion bags and some implications for drug stability as shown with amoxycillin. *Aust J Hosp Pharm.* 1989; 19: 194–7.

1473. Janknegt R, Schrouff GGM, Hooymans PM, et al. Quinolones and penicillins incompatibility. *DICP, Ann Pharmacother.* 1989; 23:91–2.

1474. Ashwin J, Lynn B. Stability and administration of intravenous Augmentin. *Pharm J.* 1987; 238:116–8.

1475. Lynn B. The stability and administration of intravenous penicillins. *Br J IV Ther.* 1981; 2:22–39.

1476. Landersjo L, Kallstrand G. Studies on the stability and compatibility of drugs in infusion fluids III. Factors affecting the stability of cloxacillin. *Acta Pharm Suec.* 1974; 11:563–80.

1477. Bundgaard H, Ilver K. Kinetics of degradation of cloxacillin sodium in aqueous solution. *Dansk Tidsskr Farm.* 1970; 44: 365–80.

1478. Brown AF, Harvey DA, Hoddinott DJ, et al. Freeze-thaw stability of antibiotics used in an IV additive service. *Br J Parenter Ther.* 1986; 7:42–4.

1479. Beatson C, Taylor A. A physical compatibility study of frusemide and flucloxacillin injections. *Br J Pharm Pract.* 1987; 9: 223–6.

1480. Nahata MC, Ahalt PA. Stability of cefazolin sodium in peritoneal dialysis solutions. *Am J Hosp Pharm.* 1991; 48:291–2.

1481. Paap CM, Nahata MC. Stability of cefotaxime in two peritoneal dialysis solutions. *Am J Hosp Pharm.* 1990; 47:147–50.

1482. Mehta AC, McCarty M. The chemical stability of cephradine injection solutions. *Intensive Ther Clin Monit.* 1988; 9:195–6.

1483. Lyall D, Blythe J. Ciprofloxacin lactate infusion. *Pharm J.* 1987; 238:290.

1484. Veljkovic VB, Lazic ML. Stability of bottled dextran solutions with respect to insoluble particle formations: a review. *Pharmazie*. 1989; 44:305–10.

1485. Veljkovic VB, Lazic ML. Mechanism of insoluble particle formation in bottled dextran solutions. *Pharmazie*. 1988; 43: 840–2.

1486. Shea BF, Souney PF. Stability of famotidine frozen in polypropylene syringes. *Am J Hosp Pharm*. 1990; 47:2073–4.

1487. Bullock LS, Fitzgerald JF. Stability of intravenous famotidine stored in polyvinyl-chloride syringes. *DICP, Ann Pharmacother*. 1989; 23:588–90.

1488. Thomas SMB. Stability of Intralipid in a parenteral nutrition solution. *Aust J Hosp Pharm*. 1987; 17:115–7.

1489. Stiles ML, Allen LV Jr. Stability of fluorouracil administered through four portable infusion pumps. *Am J Hosp Pharm*. 1989; 46:2036–40.

1490. Tu YH, Stiles ML, Allen LV Jr, et al. Stability study of gentamicin sulfate administered via Pharmacia Deltec CADD-VT pump. *Hosp Pharm*. 1990; 25:843–5.

1491. Parkinson R, Wilson JV, Ross M, et al. Stability of low-dosage heparin in pre-filled syringes. *Br J Pharm Pract*. 1989; 11:34.

1492. Menzies AR, Benoliel DM. The effects of autoclaving on the physical properties and biological activity of parenteral heparin preparations. *J Pharm Pharmacol*. 1989; 41:512–6.

1493. Farmitalia Carlo Erba. Stability of 4–demethoxydaunorubicin hydrochloride reconstituted solutions with water for injections, sodium chloride, dextrose, and sodium chloride with dextrose injections. Milan, Italy; 1986 Jun.

1494. Radford JA, Margison JM, Swindell R, et al. The stability of ifosfamide in aqueous solution and its suitability for continuous 7–day infusion by ambulatory pump. *Cancer Chemother Pharmacol*. 1990; 26:144–6.

1495. Shaw IC, Rose JWP. Infusion of ifosfamide plus mesna. *Lancet*. 1984; 1:1353–4.

1496. Bristol-Myers Oncology. Product information on IFEX (ifosfamide). Evansville, IN; 1990 Feb.

1497. Doglietto GB, Bellantone R, Bossola M, et al. Insulin adsorption to three-liter ethylen vinyl acetate bags during 24–hour infusion. *JPEN J Parenter Enteral Nutr*. 1989; 13:539–41.

1498. Donnelly RF. Immune globulin solubility in 5% dextrose injection. *Am J Hosp Pharm*. 1990; 47:1976.

1499. Prouix SM. Reconstitution of intravenous immunoglobulins. *Hosp Pharm*. 1987; 22:1133–4.

1500. Denson DD, Crews JC, Grummich KW, et al. Stability of methadone hydrochloride in 0.9% sodium chloride injection in single-dose plastic containers. *Am J Hosp Pharm*. 1991; 48: 515–7.

1501. Anderson BD, Taphouse V. Initial rate studies of hydrolysis and acyl migration in methylprednisolone 21–hemisuccinate and 17–hemisuccinate. *J Pharm Sci*. 1981; 70:181–6.

1502. Bogardus JB, Kaplan MA. Precipitation of teniposide during infusion. *Am J Hosp Pharm*. 1990; 47:518.

1503. Beijnen JH, van Gijn R. Chemical stability of the antitumor drug mitomycin C in solutions for intravesical installation. *J Parenter Sci Technol*. 1990; 44:332–5.

1504. Duafala ME, Kleinberg ML, Nacov C, et al. Stability of morphine sulfate in infusion devices and containers for intravenous administration. *Am J Hosp Pharm*. 1990; 47:143–6.

1505. Walker SE, Iazetta J. Stability of sulfite free high potency morphine sulfate solutions in portable infusion pump casettes. *Can J Hosp Pharm*. (Oct) 1989; 42:195–200, 218–9.

1506. Altman L, Hopkins RJ, Ahmed S, et al. Stability of morphine sulfate in Cormed III (Kalex) intravenous bags. *Am J Hosp Pharm*. 1990; 47:2040–2.

1507. Stiles ML, Tu YH. Stability of morphine sulfate in portable pump reservoirs during storage and simulated administration. *Am J Hosp Pharm*. 1989; 46:1404–7.

1508. Cante B, Monsarrat B, Lazorthes Y, et al. The stability of morphine in isobaric and hyperbaric solutions in a drug delivery system. *J Pharm Pharmacol*. 1988; 40:644–5.

1509. Martens HJ. Stabilitat wasserloslicher vitamine in verschiedenen infusionsbenteln. *Krankenhauspharmazie*. 1989; 10: 359–61.

1510. Tracy TS, Bowman L. Nitroglycerin delivery through a polyethylene-lined intravenous administration set. *Am J Hosp Pharm*. 1989; 46:2031–5.

1511. Loucas SP, Maager P, Mehl B, et al. Effect of vehicle ionic strength on sorption on nitroglycerin to a polyvinyl chloride administration set. *Am J Hosp Pharm*. 1990; 47:1559–62.

1512. DeRudder D, Remon JP. The sorption of nitroglycerin by infusion sets. *J Pharm Pharmacol*. 1987; 39:556–8.

1513. Jarosinski PF, Hirschfield S. Precipitation of ondansetron in alkaline solutions. *N Engl J Med*. 1991; 325:1315–6.

1514. Markowsky SJ, Kohls PR, Ehresman D, et al. Compatibility and pH variability of four injectable phenytoin sodium products. *Am J Hosp Pharm*. 1991; 48:510–4.

1515. Stolshek BS (Professional Services, Glaxo Inc.): Personal communication; 1990 Aug 27.

1516. Stewart JT, Warren FW, Johnson SM, et al. Stability of ranitidine in intravenous admixtures stored frozen, refrigerated, and at room temperature. *Am J Hosp Pharm*. 1990; 47:2043–6.

1517. Thibault L. Streptokinase flocculation in evacuated glass bottles. *Am J Hosp Pharm*. 1985; 42:278.

1518. Lerebours E, Ducable G, Francheschi A, et al. Catheter obstruction during prolonged parenteral alimentation. Are lipids responsible? *Clin Nutr*. 1985; 4:135–8.

1519. Den Hartigh J, Brandenburg HCR. Stability of azacitidine in lactated Ringer's injection frozen in polypropylene syringes. *Am J Hosp Pharm*. 1989; 46:2500–5.

1520. Waugh WN, Trissel LA. Stability, compatibility, and plasticizer extraction of taxol (NSC-125973) injection diluted in infusion solutions and stored in various containers. *Am J Hosp Pharm*. 1991; 48:1520–4.

1521. Strong DK, Morris LA. Precipitation of teniposide during infusion. *Am J Hosp Pharm*. 1990; 47:512.

1522. Outman WR, Mitrano FP. Visual compatibility of ganciclovir sodium and total parenteral nutrient solution during simulated Y-site injection. *Am J Hosp Pharm*. 1991; 48:1538–9.

1523. Outman WR, Monolakis J. Visual compatibility of haloperidol lactate with 0.9% sodium chloride injection or injectable critical-care drugs during simulated Y-site injection. *Am J Hosp Pharm*. 1991; 48:1539–41.

1524. Neels JT. Compatibility of hydromorphone hydrochloride and tetracaine hydrochloride. *Am J Hosp Pharm*. 1991; 48: 1682–83.

1525. Turowski RC, Durthaler JM. Visual compatibility of idarubicin hydrochloride with selected drugs during simulated Y-site injection. *Am J Hosp Pharm.* 1991; 48:2181–4.

1526. Woloschuk DMM, Wermeling JR. Stability and compatibility of fluorouracil and mannitol during simulated Y-site administration. *Am J Hosp Pharm.* 1991; 48:2158–60.

1527. Ishisaka DY, van Fleet J. Visual compatibility of indomethacin sodium trihydrate with drugs given to neonates by continuous infusion. *Am J Hosp Pharm.* 1991; 48:2442–3.

1528. Trissel LA, Bready BB. Turbidimetric assessment of the compatibility of taxol with selected other drugs during simulated Y-site injection. *Am J Hosp Pharm.* 1992; 49:1716–9.

1529. DiStefano JE, Outman WR. Additional data on visual compatibility of foscarnet sodium with morphine sulfate. *Am J Hosp Pharm.* 1992; 49:1672.

1530. Zanetti LA. Visual compatibility of diltiazem with commonly used injectable drugs during simulated Y-site administration. *Am J Hosp Pharm.* 1992; 49:1911.

1531. Martin KM. (Product Information Services, Lederle Laboratories, Pearl River, NY): Personal communication; 1992 Jan 14.

1532. Walker SE, DeAngelis C. Stability and compatibility of combinations of hydromorphone and a second drug. *Can J Hosp Pharm.* 1991; 44:289–95.

1533. Raineri DL, Cwik MJ, Rodvold KA, et al. Stability of nizatidine in commonly used intravenous fluids and containers. *Am J Hosp Pharm.* 1988; 45:1523–9.

1534. Hatton J, Holstad SG, Rosenbloom AD, et al. Stability of nizatidine in total nutrient admixtures. *Am J Hosp Pharm.* 1991; 48:1507–10.

1535. Wade CS, Lampasona V, Mullins RE, et al. Stability of ceftazidime and amino acids in parenteral nutrient solutions. *Am J Hosp Pharm.* 1991; 48:1515–9.

1536. Patel JP, Tran LT, Sinai WJ, et al. Activity of urokinase diluted in 0.9% sodium chloride injection or 5% dextrose injection and stored in glass or plastic syringes. *Am J Hosp Pharm.* 1991; 48:1511–4.

1537. Kintzel PE, Kennedy PE. Stability of amphotericin B in 5% dextrose injection at 25 °C. *Am J Hosp Pharm.* 1991; 48:1681.

1538. Stiles ML, Allen LV. Stability of doxorubicin hydrochloride in portable pump reservoirs. *Am J Hosp Pharm.* 1991; 48:1976–7.

1539. Sarkar MA, Rogers E, Reinhard M, et al. Stability of clindamycin phosphate, ranitidine hydrochloride, and piperacillin sodium in polyolefin containers. *Am J Hosp Pharm.* 1991; 48:2184–6.

1540. Ritchie DJ, Holstad SG, Westrich TJ, et al. Activity of octreotide acetate in a total nutrient admixture. *Am J Hosp Pharm.* 1991; 48:2172–5.

1541. Goodwin SD, Nix DE, Heyd A, et al. Compatibility of ciprofloxacin injection with selected drugs and solutions. *Am J Hosp Pharm.* 1991; 48:2166–71.

1542. Walker SE, DeAngelis C, Iazzetta J, et al. Compatibility of dexamethasone sodium phosphate with hydromorphone hydrochloride or diphenhydramine hydrochloride. *Am J Hosp Pharm.* 1991; 48:2161–6.

1543. Harkness BJ, Williams D, Stewart MC, et al. Change needed for i.v. rifampin preparation instructions. *Am J Hosp Pharm.* 1991; 48:2127–8.

1544. Wiest DB, Maish WA, Garner SS, et al. Stability of amphotericin B in four concentrations of dextrose injection. *Am J Hosp Pharm.* 1991; 48:2430–3.

1545. Silvestri AP, Mitrano FP, Baptista RJ, et al. Stability and compatibility of ganciclovir sodium in 5% dextrose injection over 35 days. *Am J Hosp Pharm.* 1991; 48:2641–3.

1546. Mitrano FP, Outman WR, Baptista RJ, et al. Chemical and visual stability of amphotericin B in 5% dextrose injection stored at 4 °C for 35 days. *Am J Hosp Pharm.* 1991; 48:2635–7.

1547. Rivers TE, McBride HA. Stability of cefotaxime sodium and metronidazole in an i.v. admixture at 8 °C. *Am J Hosp Pharm.* 1991; 48:2638–40.

1548. Rochard EB, Barthes DMC. Stability of fluorouracil, cytarabine, or doxorubicin hydrochloride in ethylene vinyl acetate portable infusion-pump reservoirs. *Am J Hosp Pharm.* 1992; 49:619–23.

1549. Letourneau M, Milot L. Visual compatibility of magnesium sulfate with narcotic analgesics. *Am J Hosp Pharm.* 1992; 49:838–9.

1550. Thompson DF, Heflin NR. Incompatibility of injectable indomethacin with gentamicin sulfate or tobramycin sulfate. *Am J Hosp Pharm.* 1992; 49:836.

1551. Munoz M, Girona V, Pujol M, et al. Stability of ifosfamide in 0.9% sodium chloride solution or water for injection in a portable i.v. pump cassette. *Am J Hosp Pharm.* 1992; 49:1137–9.

1552. Anderson PM, Rogosheske JR, Ramsay NKC, et al. Biological activity of recombinant interleukin-2 in intravenous admixtures containing antibiotic, morphine sulfate, or total parenteral nutrient solution. *Am J Hosp Pharm.* 1992; 49:608–12.

1553. Stiles ML, Allen LV. Stability of ondansetron hydrochloride in portable infusion-pump reservoirs. *Am J Hosp Pharm.* 1992; 49:1471–3.

1554. Couch P, Jacobson P. Stability of fluconazole and amino acids in parenteral nutrient solutions. *Am J Hosp Pharm.* 1992; 49:1459-62.

1555. McDonald C, Faridah. Solubilities of trimethoprim and sulfamethoxazole at various pH values and crystallization of trimethoprim from infusion fluids. *J Parenter Sci Technol.* 1991; 45:147–51.

1556. Trissel LA, Martinez JF. Turbidimetric assessment of the compatibility of taxol with 42 drugs during simulated Y-site injection. *Am J Hosp Pharm.* 1993; 50:300–4.

1557. Trissel LA, Martinez JF. Melphalan physical compatibility with selected drugs during simulated Y-site administration. *Am J Hosp Pharm.* 1993; 50:2359–63.

1558. Trissel LA, Martinez JF. Visual, turbidimetric, and particle-content assessment of compatibility of vinorelbine tartrate with selected drugs during simulated Y-site injection. *Am J Hosp Pharm.* 1994; 51:495–9.

1559. Pearson SD, Trissel LA. Stability and compatibility of minocycline hydrochloride and rifampin in intravenous solutions at various temperatures. *Am J Hosp Pharm.* 1993; 50:698–702.

1560. Graham CL, Dukes GE, Kao CF, et al. Stability of ondansetron in large-volume parenteral solutions. *Ann Pharmacother.* 1992; 26:768–71.

1561. Halasi S, Nairn JG. Stability of hydralazine hydrochloride in parenteral solutions. *Can J Hosp Pharm.* 1990; 43:237–41.

1562. Speaker TJ, Turco SJ, Nardone DA, et al. A study of the interaction of selected drugs and plastic syringes. *J Parenter Sci Technol.* 1991; 45:212–7.

1563. Reference number not in use.

1564. Adams PS, Haines-Nutt RF, Bradford E, et al. Pharmaceutical aspects of home infusion therapy for cancer patients. *Pharm J.* 1987; 238:476–8.

1565. Barnes AR. Chemical stabilities of cefuroxime sodium and metronidazole in an admixture for intravenous infusion. *J Clin Pharm Ther.* 1990; 15:187-96.

1566. Weir PJ, Ireland DS. Chemical stability of cytarabine and vinblastine injections. *Br J Pharm Pract.* (Feb) 1990; 12: 53, 54, 60.

1567. Vincke BJ, Verstraeten AE, El Eini DID, et al. Extended stability of 5-fluorouracil and methotrexate solutions in PVC containers. *Int J Pharm.* 1989; 54:181–9.

1568. Stevens RF, Wilkins KM. Use of cytotoxic drugs with an end-line filter—a study of four drugs commonly administered to paediatric patients. *J Clin Pharm Ther.* 1989; 14:475–9.

1569. Garner ST, Murdoch JM. Dopamine dilutions. *Pharm J.* 1990; 244:218.

1570. Schroder F, Schutz H. Kompatibilitat von heparin und gentamicin sulfat. *Pharm Ztg.* 1989; 134:24–6.

1571. Adams PS, Haines-Nutt RF. The stability of aminophylline intravenous infusion solutions. *Proc Guild.* 1988; 25:41–4.

1572. Schaaf LJ, Tremel LC, Wulf BG, et al. Compatibility of enalaprilat with dobutamine, dopamine, heparin, nitroglycerin, potassium chloride, and nitroprusside. *J Clin Pharm Ther.* 1990; 15:371–6.

1573. Kern JW, Lee KJ, Martinoff JT, et al. The in vivo availability of gentamicin when admixed with total nutrient solutions: a comparative study. *JPEN J Parenter Enteral Nutr.* 1990; 14: 523–6.

1574. Montoro JB, Galard R, Catalan R, et al. Stability of somatostatin in total parenteral nutrition. *Pharm Weekbl [Sci].* 1990; 12: 240–2.

1575. Sauer H. Aufbewahrung von zytostatika-losungen. *Krankenhauspharmazie.* 1990; 11:373–5.

1576. Shea BF, Souney PF. Stability of famotidine in a 3–in-1 total nutrient admixture. *DICP.* 1990; 24:232–5.

1577. De Vroe C, De Muynck C, Remon JP, et al. A study on the stability of three antineoplastic drugs and on their sorption by i.v. delivery systems and end-line filters. *Int J Pharm.* 1990; 65: 49–56.

1578. Raymond GG, Davis RL. Physical compatibility and chemical stability of amphotericin B in combination with magnesium sulfate in 5% dextrose injection. *DICP.* 1991; 25:123–6.

1579. Pramar Y, Gupta VD, Gardner SN, et al. Stabilities of dobutamine, dopamine, nitroglycerin, and sodium nitroprusside in disposable plastic syringes. *J Clin Pharm Ther.* 1991; 16:203–7.

1580. Stewart JT, Warren FW, Johnson SM, et al. Stability of ceftazidime in plastic syringes and glass vials under various storage conditions. *Am J Hosp Pharm.* 1992; 49:2765–8.

1581. Stiles ML, Allen LV Jr. Stability of ceftazidime (with arginine) and cefuroxime sodium in infusion-pump reservoirs. *Am J Hosp Pharm.* 1992; 49:2761–4.

1582. Kaufman MB, Scavone JM. Stability of undiluted trimethoprim-sulfamethoxazole for injection in plastic syringes. *Am J Hosp Pharm.* 1992; 49:2782–3.

1583. Nahata MC, Morosco RS. Stability of morphine sulfate in bacteriostatic 0.9% sodium chloride injection stored in glass vials at two temperatures. *Am J Hosp Pharm.* 1992; 49:2785–6.

1584. Nahata MC, Morosco RS. Stability of ceftazidime (with arginine) stored in plastic syringes at three temperatures. *Am J Hosp Pharm.* 1992; 49:2954–6.

1585. Mawhinney WM, Adair CG, Gorman SP, et al. Stability of ciprofloxacin in peritoneal dialysis solutions. *Am J Hosp Pharm.* 1992; 49:2956–9.

1586. Nahata MC, Morosco RS. Stability of aminophylline in bacteriostatic water for injection stored in plastic syringes at two temperatures. *Am J Hosp Pharm.* 1992; 49:2962–3.

1587. Allwood MC. The influence of buffering on the stability of erythromycin injection in small-volume infusions. *Int J Pharm.* 1992; 80:R7–R9.

1588. Toki N. Glass adsorption of highly purified urokinase. *Thromb Haemost.* 1980; 43:67.

1589. Zimmerman R, Schoffel G. Urokinase therapy: dose reduction by administration in plastic material. *Thromb Haemost.* 1981; 45:296.

1590. Walker SE, Iazzetta J. Compatibility and stability of pentobarbital infusions. *Anesthesiology.* 1981; 55:487–9.

1591. Walker SE, Iazzetta J. Cefotetan stability in normal saline and five percent dextrose in water. *Can J Hosp Pharm.* (1) 1992; 45:9–13, 37.

1592. Nahata MC. Stability of ceftriaxone sodium in peritoneal dialysis solutions. *DICP.* 1991; 25:741–2.

1593. Walker SE, Lau DWC, DeAngelis C, et al. Mitoxantrone stability in syringes and glass vials and evaluation of chemical contamination. *Can J Hosp Pharm.* 1991; 44:143–51.

1594. Walker S, Lau D, DeAngelis C, et al. Doxorubicin stability in syringes and glass vials and evaluation of chemical contamination. *Can J Hosp Pharm.* 1991; 44:71–78.

1595. Peterson GM, Khoo BHC, Galloway JG, et al. A preliminary study of the stability of midazolam in polypropylene syringes. *Aust J Hosp Pharm.* 1991; 21:115–8.

1596. Lecompte D, Bousselet M, Gayrard D, et al. Stability study of reconstituted and diluted solutions of calcium folinate. *Pharm Ind.* 1991; 53:90–4.

1597. Allwood MC. The stability of erythromycin injection in small-volume infusions. *Int J Pharm.* 1990; 62:R1–R3.

1598. Gupta VD, Pramar Y, Odom C, et al. Chemical stability of cefotetan disodium in 5% dextrose and 0.9% sodium chloride injections. *J Clin Pharm Ther.* 1990; 15:109–14.

1599. Poggi GL. Compatibility of morphine tartrate admixtures in polypropylene syringes. *Aust J Hosp Pharm.* 1991; 21:316.

1600. McLaughlin JP, Simpson C. The stability of reconstituted aztreonam. *Br J Pharm Pract.* (Oct) 1990; 12:328, 330, 334.

1601. Biejnen JH, van Gijn R, Horenblas S, et al. Chemical stability of suramin in commonly used infusion fluids. *DICP.* 1990; 24: 1056–8.

1602. Patel JP. Urokinase: stability studies in solution and lyophilized formulations. *Drug Dev Ind Pharm.* 1990; 16:2613–26.

1603. Driver AG, Worden JP Jr. Intravenous streptomycin. *DICP.* 1990; 24:826–8.

1604. Bosso JA. Clindamycin stability. *DICP.* 1990; 24:1008–9.

1605. Theuer H, Scherbel G, Distler F, et al. Cisplatin-injektionslosung. *Krankenhauspharmazie.* 1990; 11:288–91.

1606. Bluhm DP, Summers RS, Lowes MMJ, et al. Influence of container on vitamin A stability in TPN admixtures. *Int J Pharm.* 1991; 68:281–3.

1607. Bluhm DP, Summers RS, Lowes MMJ, et al. Lipid emulsion content and vitamin A stability in TPN admixtures. *Int J Pharm.* 1991; 68:277–80.

1608. Beijnen J, Koks CHW. Visual compatibility of ondansetron and dexamethasone. *DICP.* 1991; 25:869.

1609. Lawson WA, Longmore RB, McDonald C, et al. Stability of hyoscine in mixtures with morphine for continuous subcutaneous administration. *Aust J Hosp Pharm.* 1991; 21:395–6.

1610. Allwood MC. The stability of four catecholamines in 5% glucose infusions. *J Clin Pharm Ther.* 1991; 16:337–40.

1611. Van Asten P, Glerum JH, Spaanderman ER, et al. Compatibility of bupivacaine and iohexol in two mixtures for paediatric regional anaesthesia. *Pharm Weekbl [Sci].* 1991; 13:254–6.

1612. Sewell GJ, Palmer AJ. The chemical and physical stability of three intravenous infusions subjected to frozen storage and microwave thawing. *Int J Pharm.* 1991; 72:57–63.

1613. Janknegt R, Stratermans T, Cilissen J, et al. Ofloxacin intravenous—compatibility with other antibacterial agents. *Pharm Weekbl [Sci].* 1991; 13:207–9.

1614. Dunham B, Marcuard S, Khazanie PG, et al. The solubility of calcium and phosphorus in neonatal total parenteral nutrition solutions. *JPEN J Parenter Enteral Nutr.* 1991; 15:608–11.

1615. Delaney RA, Mikkelsen SL. Effects of heat treatment on selected plasma therapeutic drug concentrations. *Ann Pharmacother.* 1992; 26:338–40.

1616. McLeod HL, McGuire TR. Stability of cyclosporine in dextrose 5%, NaCl 0.9%, dextrose/amino acid solution, and lipid emulsion. *Ann Pharmacother.* 1992; 26:172–5.

1617. Andreu A, Cardona D, Pastor C, et al. Intravenous aminophylline: in vitro stability in fat-containing TPN. *Ann Pharmacother.* 1992; 26:127–8.

1618. Matsuura G. Visual compatibility of sargramostim (GM-CSF) during simulated Y-site administration with selected agents. *Hosp Pharm.* (Mar) 1992; 27:200, 202, 209.

1619. De Muynck C, Colardyn F. Influence of intravenous administration set composition on the sorption of isosorbide dinitrate. *J Pharm Pharmacol.* 1991; 43:601–4.

1620. Bullock L, Fitzgerald JF, Walter WV. Emulsion stability in total nutrient admixtures containing a pediatric amino acid formulation. *JPEN J Parenter Enteral Nutr.* 1992; 16:64–8.

1621. Olbrich A. Weichmacher als problematische bestandteile von mischinfusionen. *Krankenhauspharmazie.* 1991; 12:192–4.

1622. Cano SM, Montoro JB, Pastor C, et al. Stability of cimetidine in total parenteral nutrition. *J Clin Nutr Gastroenter.* 1987; 2: 40–3.

1623. Loeppky C, Tarka E. Compatibility of cephalosporins and aminoglycosides in peritoneal dialysis fluid. *Perit Dial Bull.* 1983; 3:128–9.

1624. Bhatt-Mehta V, Rosen DA, King RS, et al. Stability of midazolam hydrochloride in parenteral nutrient solutions. *Am J Hosp Pharm.* 1993; 50:285–8.

1625. Jacobson PA, Maksym CJ, Landvay A, et al. Compatibility of cyclosporine with fat emulsion. *Am J Hosp Pharm.* 1993; 50: 687–90.

1626. Johnson CE, Jacobson PA, Pillen HA, et al. Stability and compatibility of fluconazole and aminophylline in intravenous admixtures. *Am J Hosp Pharm.* 1993; 50:703–6.

1627. Allen LV Jr, Stiles ML, Wang DP, et al. Stability of bupivacaine hydrochloride, epinephrine hydrochloride, and fentanyl citrate in portable infusion-pump reservoirs. *Am J Hosp Pharm.* 1993; 50:714–5.

1628. Percy LA, Rho JP. Visual compatibility of ciprofloxacin with selected components of total parenteral nutrient solutions during simulated Y-site injection. *Am J Hosp Pharm.* 1993; 50: 715–6.

1629. Nieforth KA, Shea BF, Souney PF, et al. Stability of cyclosporine with magnesium sulfate in 5% dextrose injection. *Am J Hosp Pharm.* 1993; 50:470–2.

1630. Min DI, Brown T. Visual compatibility of tacrolimus with commonly used drugs during simulated Y-site injection. *Am J Hosp Pharm.* 1992; 49:2964–6.

1631. Dine T, Luyckx M, Cazin JC, et al. Stability and compatibility studies of vinblastine, vincristine, vindesine and vinorelbine with PVC infusion bags. *Int J Pharm.* 1991; 77:279–85.

1632. Inagaki K, Gill MA, Okamoto MP, et al. Stability of ranitidine hydrochloride with aztreonam, ceftazidime, or piperacillin sodium during simulated Y-site administration. *Am J Hosp Pharm.* 1992; 49:2769–72.

1633. Mitra AK, Narurkar MM. Kinetics of azathioprine degradation in aqueous solution. *Int J Pharm.* 1986; 35:165–71.

1634. Snyder RL. Filter clogging caused by albumin in i.v. nutrient solution. *Am J Hosp Pharm.* 1993; 50:63–4.

1635. Feldman F, Bergman G. Filter clogging caused by albumin in i.v. nutrient solution. *Am J Hosp Pharm.* 1993; 50:64.

1636. Bornstein M, Kao SH, Mercorelli M, et al. Stability of an ofloxacin injection in various infusion fluids. *Am J Hosp Pharm.* 1992; 49:2756–60.

1637. Heni J. Rekonstituierte ganciclovirlosung. *Krankenhauspharmazie.* 1991; 12:342–4.

1638. Theuer H, Scherbel G. Stabilitatsuntersuchungen von fentanylcitrat i.v.. *Krankenhauspharmazie.* 1991; 12:233–45.

1639. Burger DM, Brandjes DP, Koks CH, et al. Heparine in het heparineslot? *Pharm Weekbl.* 1991; 126:624–7.

1640. Witmer DR. Heparin lock flush solution versus 0.9% sodium chloride injection for maintaining patency. *Am J Hosp Pharm.* 1993; 50:241.

1641. Weber DR. Is heparin really necessary in the lock and, if so, how much? *DICP.* 1991; 25:399–407.

1642. Bosso JA, Prince RA. Stability of ondansetron hydrochloride in injectable solutions at −20, 5, and 25 °C. *Am J Hosp Pharm.* 1992; 49:2223–5.

1643. Parasrampuria J, Li LC, Stelmach AH, et al. Stability of ganciclovir sodium in 5% dextrose injection and in 0.9% sodium chloride injection over 35 days. *Am J Hosp Pharm.* 1992; 49: 116–8.

1644. Guo-jie JL. Compatibility of bumetanide injection and dextrose injection. *Yaoxue Tongbao.* 1989; 24:86–7.

1645. Buck GW, Wolfe KR. Interaction of sodium ascorbate with stainless steel particulate-filter needles. *Am J Hosp Pharm.* 1991; 48:1191.

1646. Floy BJ, Royko CG. Compatibility of ketorolac tromethamine injection with common infusion fluids and administration sets. *Am J Hosp Pharm.* 1990; 47:1097–100.

1647. Zieske PA, Koberda M, Hines JL, et al. Characterization of cisplatin degradation as affected by pH and light. *Am J Hosp Pharm.* 1991; 48:1500–6.

1648. Tu YH, Knox NL, Biringer JM, et al. Compatibility of iron dextran with total nutrient admixtures. *Am J Hosp Pharm.* 1992; 49:2233–5.

1649. Rivers TE, McBride HA, Trang JM. Stability of cefazolin sodium and metronidazole at 8 °C for use as an i.v. admixture. *J Parenter Sci Technol.* 1993; 47:135–7.

1650. Helbock HJ, Motchnik PA. Toxic hydroperoxides in intravenous lipid emulsions used in preterm infants. *Pediatrics.* 1993; 91:83–7.

1651. Washington C, Sizer T. Stability of TPN mixtures compounded from Lipofundin S and Aminoplex amino-acid solutions: comparison of laser diffraction and Coulter counter droplet size analysis. *Int J Pharm.* 1992; 83:227–31.

1652. Mason NA, Johnson CE. Stability of ceftazidime and tobramycin sulfate in peritoneal dialysis solution. *Am J Hosp Pharm.* 1992; 49:1139–42.

1653. Brawley V, Bhatia J. Hydrogen peroxide generation in a model paediatric parenteral amino acid solution. *Clin Sci.* 1993; 85: 709–12.

1654. Mawhinney WM, Adair CG, Gorman SP, et al. Stability of vancomycin hydrochloride in peritoneal dialysis solution. *Am J Hosp Pharm.* 1992; 49:137–9.

1655. Cervenka P, DeJong DJ, Butler BL, et al. Visual compatibility of injectable ciprofloxacin lactate with selected injectable drugs during simulated Y-site administration. *Hosp Pharm.* (Nov) 1992; 27:957–8, 961–2.

1656. Garrelts JC, LaRocca J, Ast D, et al. Comparison of heparin and 0.9% sodium chloride injection in the maintenance of indwelling intermittent i.v. devices. *Clin Pharm.* 1989; 8:34–9.

1657. Lewis JS. Justification for use of 1.2 micron end-line filters on total nutrient admixtures. *Hosp Pharm.* 1993; 28:656–8.

1658. Benvenuto JA, Adams SC, Vyas HM, et al. Pharmaceutical issues in infusion chemotherapy stability and compatibility. In: Lokich JJ, ed. Cancer chemotherapy by infusion. Chicago, IL: Precept Press; 1987:100–13.

1659. Briceland LL, Fudin J. Evaluation of microbial growth in select inoculated antineoplastic solutions. *Hosp Pharm.* 1990; 25: 338–40.

1660. Neels JT. Compatibility of bupivacaine hydrochloride with hydromorphone hydrochloride or morphine sulfate. *Am J Hosp Pharm.* 1992; 49:2149.

1661. Hauser AR, Trissel LA. Ondansetron compatible with sodium acetate. *J Clin Oncol.* 1993; 11:197.

1662. Pecosky DA, Parasrampuria J, Li LC, et al. Stability and sorption of calcitriol in plastic tuberculin syringes. *Am J Hosp Pharm.* 1992; 49:1463–6.

1663. Gregory R, Edwards S. Demonstration of insulin transformation products in insulin vials by high-performance liquid chromatography. *Diabetes Care.* 1991; 14:42–8.

1664. Seres DS. Insulin adsorption to parenteral infusion systems: case report and review of the literature. *Nutr Clin Pract.* 1990; 5: 111–7.

1665. Lazorova L, Haronikova K. Studium sorpcie inzulinu v priebehu infuznej terapie. *Farm Obz.* 1990; 59:157–64.

1666. Stolk LML, Chandi LS. Stabiliteit van fluorouracil (0,55 mg) in polypropyleen spuiten bij −20 °C. *Ziekenhuisfarmacie.* 1991; 7:12–3.

1667. de Vogel EM, Hendrikx MMP, van Dellen RT, et al. Adsorptie van sufentanil aan bacteriefilters. *Ziekenhuisfarmacie.* 1991; 7: 65–70.

1668. Hehenberger H. Fettemulsionen kompatibilitat wahrend der bypass-infusion. *Krankenhauspharmazie.* 1989; 10:513–8.

1669. Carstens G. Calcium-folinat uberlegungen zur stabilitat und zum einsatz verschiedener zubereitungen. *Krankenhauspharmazie.* 1989; 10:478–82.

1670. Washington C. The stability of intravenous fat emulsions in total parenteral nutrition mixtures. *Int J Pharm.* 1990; 66: 1–21.

1671. Allwood MC, Brown PW. The effect of buffering on the stability of reconstituted benzylpenicillin injection. *Int J Pharm Pract.* 1992; 1:242–4.

1672. Allwood MC. The stability of diamorphine alone and in combination with anti-emetics in plastic syringes. *Palliative Med.* 1991; 5:330–3.

1673. Lober CA, Dollard PA. Visual compatibility of gallium nitrate with selected drugs during simulated Y-site injection. *Am J Hosp Pharm.* 1993; 50:1208–10.

1674. Jahns BE, Bakst CM. Extension of expiration time for lorazepam injection at room temperature. *Am J Hosp Pharm.* 1993; 50:1134.

1675. Trissel LA, Martinez JF. Idarubicin hydrochloride turbidity versus incompatibility. *Am J Hosp Pharm.* 1993; 50:1134.

1676. Hunt-Fugate AK, Hennessey CK. Stability of fluconazole injectable solutions. *Am J Hosp Pharm.* 1993; 50:1186–7.

1677. Inagaki K, Takagi J, Lor E, et al. Stability of fluconazole in commonly used intravenous antibiotic solutions. *Am J Hosp Pharm.* 1993; 50:1206–8.

1678. Liao E, Fox JL. Inline filtration of ondansetron hydrochloride during simulated i.v. administration. *Am J Hosp Pharm.* 1993; 50:906.

1679. Belliveau PP, Shea BF. Stability of metoprolol tartrate in 5% dextrose injection or 0.9% sodium chloride injection. *Am J Hosp Pharm.* 1993; 50:950–2.

1680. Ringwood MA. Stability of cefepime for injection for IM or IV use following constitution/dilution. Syracuse, NY: Bristol-Myers Company; 1990 Aug 16.

1681. Ringwood MA, Vance VH. Cefepime IM, IV, and compatibility studies for U.S. registrational filing. Syracuse, NY: Bristol-Myers Company; 1992 May 13.

1682. Vance VH. Stability of cefepime admixed with vancomycin, metronidazole, ampicillin, clindamycin, tobramycin, netilmicin, TPN solution, and PD solution. Syracuse, NY: Bristol-Myers Company; 1992 Oct 14.

1683. Pearson SD, Trissel LA. Leaching of diethylhexyl phthalate from polyvinyl chloride containers by selected drugs and formulation components. *Am J Hosp Pharm.* 1993; 50:1405–9.

1684. Trissel LA, Pearson SD. Storage of lorazepam in three injectable solutions in polyvinyl chloride and polyolefin bags. *Am J Hosp Pharm.* 1994; 51:368–72.

1685. Reference number not in use.

1686. Trissel LA, Martinez JF. Compatibility of allopurinol sodium with selected drugs during simulated Y-site administration. *Am J Hosp Pharm.* 1994; 51:1792–9.

1687. Trissel LA, Martinez JF. Compatibility of filgrastim with selected drugs during simulated Y-site administration. *Am J Hosp Pharm.* 1994; 51:1907–13.

1688. Trissel LA, Martinez JF. Compatibility of piperacillin sodium plus tazobactam sodium with selected drugs during simulated Y-site injection. *Am J Hosp Pharm.* 1994; 51:672–8.

1689. Reference number not in use.

1690. Trissel LA, Xu Q, Martinez JF, et al. Compatibility and stability of ondansetron hydrochloride with morphine sulfate and hydromorphone hydrochloride in 0.9% sodium chloride injection at various temperatures. *Am J Hosp Pharm.* 1994; 51:2138–42.

1691. Belliveau PP, Nightingale CH. Stability of aztreonam and ampicillin/sulbactam in 0.9% saline for injection. *Am J Hosp Pharm.* 1994; 51:901–4.

1692. Fisher DM, Canfell C. Stability of atracurium administered by infusion. *Anesthesiology.* 1984; 61:347–8.

1693. Harper NJ, Pollard BJ, Edwards D, et al. Stability of atracurium in dilute solutions. *Br J Anaesth.* 1988; 60:344P–345P.

1694. Talton MA (Drug Information, Burroughs Wellcome Company, Research Triangle Park, NC): Personal communication; 1993 Jun 11.

1695. Perrone RK, Kaplan MA. Extent of cisplatin formation in carboplatin admixtures. *Am J Hosp Pharm.* 1989; 46:258–9.

1696. Northcott M, Allsopp MA, Powell H, et al. The stability of carboplatin, diamorphine, 5–fluorouracil and mitozantrone infusions in an ambulatory pump under storage and prolonged "in-use" conditions. *J Clin Pharm Ther.* 1991; 16:123–9.

1697. Ahmed ST, Parkinson R. The stability of drugs in pre-filled syringes: flucloxacillin, ampicillin, cefuroxime, cefotaxime, and ceftazidime. *Hosp Pharm Pract.* 1992; 2:285–9.

1698. Faouzi MA, Dine T, Luyckx M, et al. Stability and compatibility studies of pefloxacin, ofloxacin and ciprofloxacin with PVC infusion bags. *Int J Pharm.* 1993; 89:125–31.

1699. Stiles ML, Allen LV Jr. Gas production of three brands of ceftazidime. *Am J Hosp Pharm.* 1991; 48:1727–9.

1700. Dine T, Cazin JC, Gressier B, et al. Stability and compatibility of four anthracyclines: doxorubicin, epirubicin, daunorubicin, and pirarubicin with PVC infusion bags. *Pharm Weekbl [Sci].* 1992; 14:365–9.

1701. Trissel LA, Martinez JF. Sargramostim incompatibility. *Hosp Pharm.* 1992; 27:929.

1702. Trissel LA. Alternative interpretation for data. *Am J Hosp Pharm.* 1992; 49:570.

1703. Knapp AJ, Mauro VF. Incompatibility of ketorolac tromethamine with selected postoperative drugs. *Am J Hosp Pharm.* 1992; 49:2960–2.

1704. Reference number not in use.

1705. Cohon MS (Clinical Development and Medical Affairs, The Upjohn Company, Kalamazoo, MI): Personal communication; 1993 Dec 6.

1706. Chandler SW, Trissel LA, Weinstein SM. Combined administration of opioids with selected drugs to manage pain and other cancer symptoms: initial safety screening for compatibility. *J Pain Symptom Manage.* 1996; 12:168–71.

1707. Nation RL, Hackett LP. Uptake of clonazepam by plastic intravenous infusion bags and administration sets. *Am J Hosp Pharm.* 1983; 40:1692–3.

1708. Hooymans PM, Janknegt R. Comparison of clonazepam sorption to polyvinyl chloride-coated and polyethylene-coated tubings. *Pharm Weekbl [Sci].* 1990; 12:188–9.

1709. McLaughlin JP, Simpson C. The stability of reconstituted diethanolamine fusidate in a 5% dextrose infusion. *Hosp Pharm Pract.* 1992; 2:59–62.

1710. Olsen KM, Gurley BJ, Davis GA, et al. Stability of flumazenil with selected drugs in 5% dextrose injection. *Am J Hosp Pharm.* 1993; 50:1907–12.

1711. Reference number not in use.

1712. Larson PO, Ragi G, Swandby M, et al. Stability of buffered lidocaine and epinephrine used for local anesthesia. *J Dermatol Surg Oncol.* 1991; 17:411–4.

1713. Stewart JH, Cole GW. Neutralized lidocaine with epinephrine for local anesthesia. *J Dermatol Surg Oncol.* 1989; 15:1081–3.

1714. Nahata MC, Morosco RS. Stability of cimetidine hydrochloride and of clindamycin phosphate in water for injection stored in glass vials at two temperatures. *Am J Hosp Pharm.* 1993; 50:2559–61.

1715. Zeisler J, Alagna C. Incompatibility of labetalol hydrochloride and furosemide. *Am J Hosp Pharm.* 1993; 50:2521–2.

1716. Pfeifer RW, Hale KN. Precipitation of paclitaxel during infusion by pump. *Am J Hosp Pharm.* 1993; 50:2518.

1717. Hagan RL, Jacobs LF, Pimsler M, et al. Stability of midazolam hydrochloride in 5% dextrose injection or 0.9% sodium chloride injection over 30 days. *Am J Hosp Pharm.* 1993; 50:2379–81.

1718. Jones JW, Davis AT. Stability of bupivacaine hydrochloride in polypropylene syringes. *Am J Hosp Pharm.* 1993; 50:2364–5.

1719. Vogt C, Skipper PM. Compatibility of magnesium sulfate and morphine sulfate in 0.9% sodium chloride injection. *Am J Hosp Pharm.* 1993; 50:2311.

1720. Bailey LC, Tang KT. Stability of ceftriaxone sodium in infusion-pump syringes. *Am J Hosp Pharm.* 1993; 50:2092–4.

1721. Szof C, Walker PC. Incompatibility of cefotaxime sodium and vancomycin sulfate during Y-site administration. *Am J Hosp Pharm.* 1993; 50:2054.

1722. Jhee SS, Jeong EW, Chin A, et al. Stability of ondansetron hydrochloride stored in a disposable, elastomeric infusion device at 4 °C. *Am J Hosp Pharm.* 1993; 50:1918–20.

1723. Bartfield JM, Homer PJ, Ford DT, et al. Buffered lidocaine as a local anesthetic: an investigation of shelf life. *Ann Emerg Med.* 1992; 21:16–9.

1724. Peterfreund RA, Datta S. pH adjustment of local anesthetic solutions with sodium bicarbonate: laboratory evaluation of alkalinization and precipitation. *Reg Anesth.* 1989; 14:265–70.

1725. Trissel LA, Martinez JF. Screening teniposide for Y-site physical incompatibilities. *Hosp Pharm.* 1994; 29:1012–4.

1726. Woods K, Steinman W, Bruns L, et al. Stability of foscarnet sodium in 0.9% sodium chloride injection. *Am J Hosp Pharm.* 1994; 51:88–90.

1727. Parrish MA, Bailey LC. Stability of ceftriaxone sodium and aminophylline or theophylline in intravenous admixtures. *Am J Hosp Pharm.* 1994; 51:92–4.

1728. Lee MD, Hess MM, Boucher BA, et al. Stability of amphotericin B in 5% dextrose injection stored at 4 or 25 °C for 120 hours. *Am J Hosp Pharm.* 1994; 51:394–6.

1729. Reference number not in use.

1730. Pompilio FM, Fox JL, Inagaki K, et al. Stability of ranitidine hydrochloride with ondansetron hydrochloride or fluconazole during simulated Y-site administration. *Am J Hosp Pharm.* 1994; 51:391–4.

1731. Wolff DJ, Kline SS. Stability of amikacin, gentamicin, or tobramycin in 10% dextrose injection. *Am J Hosp Pharm.* 1994; 51:518–9.

1732. Bosso JA, Prince RA. Compatibility of ondansetron hydrochloride with fluconazole, ceftazidime, aztreonam, and cefazolin sodium under simulated Y-site conditions. *Am J Hosp Pharm.* 1994; 51:389–91.

1733. Stiles ML, Allen LV Jr, Prince SJ, et al. Stability of dexamethasone sodium phosphate, diphenhydramine hydrochloride, lorazepam, and metoclopramide hydrochloride in portable infusion-pump reservoirs. *Am J Hosp Pharm.* 1994; 51:514–7.

1734. Messerschmidt W. Kompatibilitat von ofloxacin mit ampicillin. *Krankenhauspharmazie.* 1994; 15:337–40.

1735. Messerschmidt W. Kompatibilitat von cefotaxim mit ofloxacin. *Pharmazie.* 1991; 136:42–4.

1736. Reference number not in use.

1737. Messerschmidt W. Kompatibilitat von cefotiam mit metronidazol. *Krankenhauspharmazie.* 1986; 7:263–5.

1738. Messerschmidt W. Pharmazeutische kompatibilitat der kombination cefotiam und ampicillin. *Krankenhauspharmazie.* 1992; 13:98–100.

1739. Cronquist SE, Daniels M. Precipitation of paclitaxel during infusion by pump. *Am J Hosp Pharm.* 1993; 50:2521.

1740. Fraser GL, Riker RR. Visual compatibility of haloperidol lactate with injectable solutions. *Am J Hosp Pharm.* 1994; 51:905–6.

1741. Burm JP, Jhee SS, Chin A, et al. Stability of paclitaxel with ondansetron hydrochloride or ranitidine hydrochloride during simulated Y-site administration. *Am J Hosp Pharm.* 1994; 51:1201–4.

1742. Mulye NV, Turco SJ. Stability of ganciclovir sodium in an infusion-pump syringe. *Am J Hosp Pharm.* 1994; 51:1348–9.

1743. Bonhomme L, Benhamou D, Comoy E, et al. Stability of adrenaline pH-adjusted solutions of local anaesthetics. *J Pharm Biomed Anal.* 1991; 9:497–9.

1744. Johnson CE, Jacobson PA. Stability of ganciclovir sodium and amino acids in parenteral nutrient solutions. *Am J Hosp Pharm.* 1994; 51:503–8.

1745. Abubakar AA, Mustapha A. An in vitro chemical interaction between promethazine hydrochloride and chloroquine phosphate. *Int J Pharm.* 1993; 7:14–9.

1746. Xu Q, Trissel LA. Stability of paclitaxel in 5% dextrose injection or 0.9% sodium chloride injection at 4, 22, or 32 °C. *Am J Hosp Pharm.* 1994; 51:3058-60.

1747. Kearney AS, Patel K. Preformulation studies to aid in the development of a ready-to-use injectable solution of the antitumor agent, topotecan. *Int J Pharm.* 1996; 127:229–37.

1748. Cilissen J, Hooymans PM. Indicatie van de stabiliteit van een mengsel van piperacilline en flucloxacilline in een reservoir voor een draagbare infusiepomp. *Ziekenhuisfarmacie.* 1994; 10: 10–1.

1749. Banerjee PS, Ghosh LK. Studies on the effects of some additives on the stability of injectable formulations of diazepam. *Indian Drugs.* 1992; 29:361–4.

1750. Lorillon P, Corbel JC, Mordelet MF, et al. Photosensibilite du 5-fluoro-uracile et du methotrexate dans des perfuseurs translucides ou opaques. *J Pharm Clin.* 1992; 11:285–95.

1751. Brouwers JRBJ, van Doorne H, Meevis RF, et al. Stability of sufentanil citrate and sufentanil citrate/bupivacaine mixture in portable infusion pump reservoirs. *Eur Hosp Pharm.* 1995; 1: 12–4.

1752. Chung KC, Moon YSK, Chin A, et al. Compatibility of ondansetron hydrochloride and piperacillin sodium-tazobactam sodium during simulated Y-site administration. *Am J Health-Syst Pharm.* 1995; 52:1554–6.

1753. Erickson SH, Ulici D. Incompatibility of cefotetan disodium and promethazine hydrochloride. *Am J Health-Syst Pharm.* 1995; 52:1347.

1754. Belliveau PP, Nightingale CH. Stability of cefotaxime sodium and metronidazole in 0.9% sodium chloride injection or in ready-to-use metronidazole bags. *Am J Health-Syst Pharm.* 1995; 52:1561–3.

1755. Roos PJ, Glerum JH. Stability of sufentanil citrate in a portable pump reservoir, a glass container and a polyethylene container. *Pharm Weekbl [Sci].* 1992; 14:196–200.

1756. Roos PJ, Glerum JH, Schroeders MJ. Effect of glucose 5% solution and bupivacaine hydrochloride on absorption of sufentanil citrate in a portable pump reservoir during storage and simulated infusion by an epidural catheter. *Pharm World Sci.* 1993; 15:269–75.

1757. Benaji B, Dine T, Luyckx M, et al. Stability and compatibility of cisplatin and carboplatin with PVC infusion bags. *J Clin Pharm Ther.* 1994; 19:95–100.

1758. Trissel LA, Martinez JF. Compatibility of aztreonam with selected drugs during simulated Y-site administration. *Am J Health-Syst Pharm.* 1995; 52:1086–90.

1759. Choi JS, Burm JP, Jhee SS, et al. Stability of piperacillin sodium-tazobactam sodium and ranitidine hydrochloride in 0.9% sodium chloride injection during simulated Y-site administration. *Am J Hosp Pharm.* 1994; 51:2273–6.

1760. Ishisaka DY. Visual compatibility of fluconazole with drugs given by continuous infusion. *Am J Hosp Pharm.* 1994; 51: 2290.

1761. Fawcett JP, Woods DJ, Munasiri B, et al. Compatibility of cyclizine lactate and haloperidol lactate. *Am J Hosp Pharm.* 1994; 51:2292.

1762. Hassan E, Leslie J. Stability of labetalol hydrochloride with selected critical care drugs during simulated Y-site injection. *Am J Hosp Pharm.* 1994; 51:2143–5.

1763. Wang DP, Chang LC, Wong CY, et al. Stability of cefazolin sodium-famotidine admixture. *Am J Hosp Pharm.* 1994; 51: 2205.

1764. Singh RF, Corelli RL. Sterility of unit dose syringes of filgrastim and sargramostim. *Am J Hosp Pharm.* 1994; 51:2811–2.

1765. Kleinberg ML. Sterility of repackaged filgrastim and sargramostim. *Am J Health-Syst Pharm.* 1995; 52:1101.

1766. Kirkham JC, Rutherford ET, Cunningham GN, et al. Stability of ondansetron hydrochloride in a total parenteral nutrient admixture. *Am J Health-Syst Pharm.* 1995; 52:1557–8.

1767. Gilbar PJ, Groves CF. Visual compatibility of total parenteral nutrition solution (Synthamin 17 premix) with selected drugs during simulated Y-site injection. *Aust J Hosp Pharm.* 1994; 24:167–70.

1768. Moon YSK, Chung KC, Chin A, et al. Stability of piperacillin sodium-tazobactam sodium in polypropylene syringes and polyvinyl chloride minibags. *Am J Health-Syst Pharm.* 1995; 52: 999–1001.

1769. Lumpkin MM, Burlington DB. Safety alert: hazards of precipitation associated with parenteral nutrition. *Am J Hosp Pharm.* 1994; 51:1427–8.

1770. Hasegawa GR. Caring about stability and compatibility. *Am J Hosp Pharm.* 1994; 51:1533–4.

1771. Trissel LA. Compounding our problems. *Am J Hosp Pharm.* 1994; 51:1534.

1772. Mirtallo JM. The complexity of mixing calcium and phosphate. *Am J Hosp Pharm.* 1994; 51:1535–6.

1773. Koorenhof MJC, Timmer JG. Stability of total parenteral nutrition supplied as "all-in-one" for children with chemotherapy-linked hyperhydration. *Pharm Weekbl [Sci].* 1992; 14:50–4.

1774. Picard C, Brazier M, Hary L, et al. Stabilite de quatre solutions de penicillines dans des poches et tubulures de perfusion en PVC plastifie. *J Pharm Clin.* 1992; 11:302–5.

1775. Szucsova S, Sykora J. Stablita injekcneho pripravku celaskon v infuznych zmesiach. *Farm Obzor.* 1992; 61:109–12.

1776. Walker SE, Iazzetta J, De Angelis C, et al. Stability and compatibility of combinations of hydromorphone and dimenhydrinate, lorazepam or prochlorperazine. *Can J Hosp Pharm.*. 1993; 46:61–5.

1777. Maswoswe JJ, Okpara AU. An old nemesis: calcium and phosphate interaction in TPN admixtures. *Hosp Pharm.* (July) 1995; 30:579–80, 582–6.

1778. Deardorff DL, Schmidt CN, Wiley RA. Effect of preparation techniques on mixing of additives in intravenous fluids in nonrigid containers. *Hosp Pharm.* (Apr) 1993; 28: 306, 309–10, 312–3.

1779. Stiles ML, Allen LV Jr. Stability of various antibiotics kept in an insulated pouch during administration via portable infusion pump. *Am J Health-Syst Pharm.* 1995; 52:70–4.

1780. Wang DP, Chang LC, Lee DKT, et al. Stability of fluorouracil-metoclopramide hydrochloride admixture. *Am J Health-Syst Pharm.* 1995; 52:98–9.

1781. Jackson CW, Cunningham K. Compatibility of haloperidol lactate with benztropine mesylate. *Am J Hosp Pharm.* 1994; 51: 2962–3.

1782. Mirtallo JM. Should the use of total nutrient admixtures be limited? *Am J Hosp Pharm.* 1994; 51(22):2831–4.

1783. Driscoll DF, Newton DW. Precipitation of calcium phosphate from parenteral nutrient fluids. *Am J Hosp Pharm.* 1994; 51: 2834–6.

1784. Gibler B, Kim MS. Visual compatibility of neuroleptics with anticholinergics or antihistamines in polyethylene syringes. *Am J Hosp Pharm.* 1994; 51:2709–10.

1785. Huang E, Anderson RP. Compatibility of hydromorphone hydrochloride with haloperidol lactate and ketorolac tromethamine. *Am J Hosp Pharm.* 1994; 51:2963.

1786. Mendenhall A, Hoyt DB. Incompatibility of ketorolac tromethamine with haloperidol lactate and thiethylperazine maleate. *Am J Hosp Pharm.* 1994; 51:2964.

1787. Harraki B, Guiraud P, Rochat MH, et al. Influence of copper, iron, and zinc on the physicochemical properties of parenteral admixture. *J Parenter Sci Technol.* 1993; 47:199–204.

1788. Aujoulat P, Coze C, Braguer D, et al. Compatibilite physicochimique du methotrexate avec les medicaments co-administres dans les protocols de chimiotherapie. *J Pharm Clin.* 1993; 12: 31–5.

1789. Johnson CE, Bhatt-Mehta V, Mancari SC, et al. Stability of midazolam hydrochloride and morphine sulfate during simulated intravenous coadministration. *Am J Hosp Pharm.* 1994; 51:2812–3.

1790. Burm JP, Choi JS, Jhee SS, et al. Stability of paclitaxel and fluconazole during simulated Y-site administration. *Am J Hosp Pharm.* 1994; 51:2704–6.

1791. Grassby PF, Roberts DE. Stability of epidural opiate solutions in 0.9 per cent sodium chloride infusion bags. *Int J Pharm Pract.* 1995; 3:174–7.

1792. Allwood MC, Brown PW. Stability of injections containing diamorphine and midazolam in plastic syringes. *Int J Pharm Pract.* 1994; 3:57–9.

1793. Kershaw BP, Monnier HL, Mason JH. Visual compatibility of premixed theophylline or heparin with selected drugs for i.v. administration. *Am J Hosp Pharm.* 1362–3 (July) 1993; 50: 1360.

1794. Trissel LA. Were the bubbles evolved or entrained? *Am J Health-Syst Pharm.* 1995; 52(7):757.

1795. Francomb MM, Ford JL. Adsorption of vincristine, doxorubicin and mitoxantrone to in-line intravenous filters. *Int J Pharm.* 1994; 103:87–92.

1796. Salomies HEM, Heinonen RM. Sorptive loss of diazepam, nitroglycerin and warfarin sodium to polypropylene-lined infusion bags (Softbags). *Int J Pharm.* 1994; 110:197–201.

1797. Haginaka J, Nakagawa T. Stability of clavulanic acid in aqueous solutions. *Chem Pharm Bull.* 1981; 29:3334–41.

1798. Bianchi C, Airaudo CB. Sorption studies of dipotassium clorazepate salt (Tranxene) and midazolam hydrochloride (Hypnovel) in polyvinyl chloride and glass infusion containers. *J Clin Pharm Ther.* 1992; 17:223–7.

1799. Sautou V, Chopineau J, Gremeau I, et al. Compatibility with medical plastics and stability of continuously and simultaneously infused isosorbide dinitrate and heparin. *Int J Pharm.* 1994; 107:111–19.

1800. Mitchell CL (Leo Pharmaceuticals, Buckinghamshire, United Kingdom): Personal communication; 1998 Sep 11.

1801. Hadzija BW, Lubarsky DA. Compatibility of etomidate, thiopental sodium, and propofol injections with drugs commonly administered during induction of anesthesia. *Am J Health-Syst Pharm.* 1995; 52:997–9.

1802. Stewart JT, Warren FW. Stability of ranitidine hydrochloride and seven medications. *Am J Hosp Pharm.* 1994; 51:1802–7.

1803. Palmquist KL, Quattrocchi FP. Compatibility of furosemide with 20% mannitol. *Am J Health-Syst Pharm.* 1995; 52:648.

1804. Trissel LA, Martinez JF. Compatibility of granisetron hydrochloride with selected alkaline drugs. *Am J Health-Syst Pharm.* 1995; 52:208.

1805. Bhatt-Mehta V, Paglia RE. Stability of propofol with parenteral nutrient solutions during simulated Y-site injection. *Am J Health-Syst Pharm.* 1995; 52:192–6.

1806. Hagan RL, Carr-Lopez SM. Stability of nafcillin sodium in the presence of lidocaine hydrochloride. *Am J Health-Syst Pharm.* 1995; 52:521–3.

1807. Gayed AA, Keshary PR. Visual compatibility of diltiazem injection with various diluents and medications during simulated Y-site injection. *Am J Health-Syst Pharm.* 1995; 52:516–20.

1808. Trissel LA. Amphotericin B does not mix with fat emulsion. *Am J Health-Syst Pharm.* 1995; 52:1463–4.

1809. Kirsch R, Goldstein R, Tarloff J, et al. An emulsion formulation of amphotericin B improves the therapeutic index when treating systemic murine candidiasis. *J Infect Dis.* 1988; 158:1065–70.

1810. Chavenet PY, Garry I, Charlier N, et al. Trial of glucose versus fat emulsion in preparation of amphotericin for use in HIV infected patients with candidiasis. *BMJ.* 1992; 305:921–5.

1811. Caillot D, Casanova O, Solary E, et al. Efficacy and tolerance of an amphotericin B lipid (Intralipid) emulsion in the treatment of candidaemia in neutropenic patients. *J Antimicrob Chemother.* 1993; 31:161–9.

1812. Fleming RA, Olsen DJ, Savage PD, et al. Stability of ondansetron hydrochloride and cyclophosphamide in injectable solutions. *Am J Health-Syst Pharm.* 1995; 52:514–6.

1813. Driscoll DF. Total nutrient admixtures: theory and practice. *Nutr Clin Pract.* 1995; 10:114–9.

1814. Driscoll DF, Bhargava HN, Li L, et al. Physicochemical stability of total nutrient admixtures. *Am J Health-Syst Pharm.* 1995; 52: 623–34.

1815. Pettei MJ, Israel D, Levine J. Serum vitamin K concentration in pediatric patients receiving total parenteral nutritionion. *JPEN J Parenter Enteral Nutr.* 1993; 17:465–7.

1816. Trissel LA, Martinez JF. Incompatibility of fluorouracil with leucovorin calcium or levoleucovorin calcium. *Am J Health-Syst Pharm.* 1995; 52:710–5.

1817. Montoya Garcia-Reol C, Sevilla Azzati E, Negro Vega E, et al. Estudio de la estabilidad de la mezcla fluorouracilo/folinato calcico en fluidos intravenosos. *Farm Hosp.* 1993; 17:99–103.

1818. Ward GH, Yalkowsky SH. Studies in phlebitis VI: dilution-induced precipitation of amiodarone HCl. *J Parenter Sci Technol.* 1993; 47:161–5.

1819. Ward GH, Yalkowsky SH. Studies in phlebitis IV: injection rate and amiodarone-induced phlebitis. *J Parenter Sci Technol.* 1993; 47:40–3.

1820. Allwood MC, Brown PW. Stability of ampicillin infusions in unbuffered and buffered saline. *Int J Pharm.* 1993; 97: 219–22.

1821. Lauper RD (Professional Services, Cetus Oncology Corporation, Emeryville, CA): Personal communication; 1993 Dec 20.

1822. Allen LV. Plasminogen activator. *US Pharmacist.* 1992; 17: 64–5, 70–1.

1823. Rochard E, Barthes D. Stability and compatibility of carboplatin with three portable infusion pump reservoirs. *Int J Pharm.* 1994; 101:257–62.

1824. Bailey LC, Cappel KM. Stability of ceftriaxone sodium in injectable solutions stored frozen in syringes. *Am J Hosp Pharm.* 1994; 51:2159–61.

1825. Mazzo DJ, Nguyen-Huu JJ, Pagniez S, et al. Compatibility of docetaxel and paclitaxel in intravenous solutions with polyvinyl chloride infusion materials. *Am J Health-Syst Pharm.* 1997; 54: 566–9.

1826. Kane MP, Bailie GR, Moon DG, et al. Stability of ciprofloxacin injection in peritoneal dialysis solutions. *Am J Hosp Pharm.* 1994; 51:373–7.

1827. Rochard E, Barthes D. Stability of cisplatin in ethylene vinyl-acetate portable infusion-pump reservoirs. *J Clin Pharm Ther.* 1992; 17:315–8.

1828. Pujol Cubells M, Prat Aixela J, Girona Brumos V, et al. Stability of cisplatin in sodium chloride 0.9% intravenous solution related to the container's material. *Pharm World Sci.* 1993; 15: 34–6.

1829. Islam MS, Asker AF. Photostabilization of dacarbazine with reduced glutathione. *J Pharm Sci Technol.* 1994; 48:38–40.

1830. Wiest DB, Garner SS. Stability of esmolol hydrochloride in 5% dextrose injection. *Am J Health-Syst Pharm.* 1995; 52:716–8.

1831. Baaske DM, Dykstra SD, Wagenknecht DM, et al. Stability of esmolol hydrochloride in intravenous solutions. *Am J Hosp Pharm.* 1994; 51:2693–6.

1832. Woloschuk DMM, Nazeravich DR. Etoposide precipitation. *Can J Hosp Pharm.* 1992; 45:136.

1833. Barthes DMC, Rochard EB, Pouliquen IJ, et al. Stability and compatibility of etoposide in 0.9% sodium chloride injection in three containers. *Am J Hosp Pharm.* 1994; 51:2706–9.

1834. Mathew M, Gupta VD. Stability of foscarnet sodium in 5% dextrose and 0.9% sodium chloride injections. *J Clin Pharm Ther.* 1994; 19:35–6.

1835. Stolk LM, Hendrikse H. Autoclave and long-term sterility of foscarnet sodium admixtures. *Am J Health-Syst Pharm.* 1995; 52:103.

1836. Phaypradith S, Vigneron J, Perrin A, et al. Stabilite des solutions diluees de ganciclovir sodique (Cymevan) en seringues polypropylene et en poches PVC pour perfusions. *J Pharm Belg.* 1992; 47:494–8.

1837. Chung KC, Chin A. Stability of granisetron hydrochloride in a disposable elastomeric infusion device. *Am J Health-Syst Pharm.* 1995; 52:1541–3.

1838. Flahive E (Medical Information, Ortho-McNeil, Raritan, NJ): Personal communication; 1995 Apr 6.

1839. Anon. ASHP therapeutic position statement on the institutional use of 0.9% sodium chloride injection to maintain patency of peripheral indwelling intermittent infusion devices. *Am J Hosp Pharm.* 1994; 51:1572–4.

1840. Nahata MC, Morosco RS. Stability of lorazepam diluted in bacteriostatic water for injection at two temperatures. *J Clin Pharm Ther.* 1993; 18:69–71.

1841. Pinguet F, Martel P, Rouanet P, et al. Effect of sodium chloride concentration and temperature on melphalan stability during storage and use. *Am J Hosp Pharm.* 1994; 51:2701–4.

1842. Chin A, Ramakrishnan RR, Yoshimura NN, et al. Paclitaxel stability and compatibility in polyolefin containers. *Ann Pharmacother.* 1994; 28:35–6.

1843. Trissel LA, Xu Q, Kwan J, et al. Compatibility of paclitaxel injection vehicle with intravenous administration and extension sets. *Am J Hosp Pharm.* 1994; 51:2804–10.

1844. McLaughlin JP, Simpson C, Taylor RA. When is flucloxacillin stable? *Hosp Pharm Pract.* 1993; 553–6.

1845. Trissel LA, Martinez JF. Compatibility of amifostine with selected drugs during simulated Y-site administration. *Am J Health-Syst Pharm.* 1995; 52:2208–12.

1846. Henry DW, Marshall JL, Nazzaro D, et al. Stability of cisplatin and ondansetron hydrochloride in admixtures for continuous infusion. *Am J Health-Syst Pharm.* 1995; 52:2570–3.

1847. Mantong ML, Marquardt ED. Visual compatibility of midazolam hydrochloride with selected drugs during simulated Y-site injection. *Am J Health-Syst Pharm.* 1995; 52:2567–8.

1848. Trissel LA, Xu QA. Compatibility and stability of aztreonam and vancomycin hydrochloride. *Am J Health-Syst Pharm.* 1995; 52:2560–4.

1849. Rivers TE, Webster AA. Stability of ceftizoxime sodium, ceftriaxone sodium, and ceftazidime with metronidazole in ready-to-use metronidazole bags. *Am J Health-Syst Pharm.* 1995; 52:2568–70.

1850. Wulf H, Gleim M. The stability of mixtures of morphine hydrochloride, bupivacaine hydrochloride, and clonidine hydrochloride in portable pump reservoirs for the management of chronic pain syndromes. *J Pain Symptom Manage.* 1994; 9:308–11.

1851. Korth-Bradley JM, Ludwig S. Incompatibility of amiodarone hydrochloride and sodium bicarbonate injections. *Am J Health-Syst Pharm.* 1995; 52:2340.

1852. Bhatt-Mehta V, Johnson CE, Leininger N, et al. Stability of fentanyl citrate and midazolam hydrochloride during simulated intravenous coadministration. *Am J Health-Syst Pharm.* 1995; 52:511–3.

1853. Matuschka PR, Smith WR. Compatibility of mannitol and sodium bicarbonate in injectable fluids. *Am J Health-Syst Pharm.* 1995; 52:320–1.

1854. Ku YM, Min DI, Kumar V, et al. Compatibility of tacrolimus injection with cimetidine hydrochloride injection in 0.9% sodium chloride injection. *Am J Health-Syst Pharm.* 1995; 52:2024–5.

1855. Swart EL, Mooren RAG. Compatibility of midazolam hydrochloride and lorazepam with selected drugs during simulated Y-site administration. *Am J Health-Syst Pharm.* 1995; 52:2020–2.

1856. Lam XM, Ward CA. Stability and activity of alteplase with injectable drugs commonly used in cardiac therapy. *Am J Health-Syst Pharm.* 1995; 52:1904–9.

1857. Alex S, Gupta SL, Minor JR, et al. Compatibility and activity of aldesleukin (recombinant interleukin-2) in presence of selected drugs during simulated Y-site administration: evaluation of three methods. *Am J Health-Syst Pharm.* 1995; 52:2423–6.

1858. Mancano MA, Boullata JI, Gelone SP, et al. Availability of lorazepam after simulated administration from glass and polyvinyl chloride containers. *Am J Health-Syst Pharm.* 1995; 52:2213–6.

1859. McMullin ST, Burns Schaif RA. Stability of midazolam hydrochloride in polyvinyl chloride bags under fluorescent light. *Am J Health-Syst Pharm.* 1995; 52:2018–20.

1860. Bednar DA, Klutman NE, Henry DW, et al. Stability of ceftazidime (with arginine) in an elastomeric infusion device. *Am J Health-Syst Pharm.* 1995; 52:1912–4.

1861. Trissel LA, Martinez JF. Compatibility of thiotepa (lyophilized) with selected drugs during simulated Y-site administration. *Am J Health-Syst Pharm.* 1996; 53:1041–5.

1862. Xu QA, Trissel LA. Compatibility of ondansetron hydrochloride with meperidine hydrochloride for combined administration. *Ann Pharmacother.* 1995; 29:1106–9.

1863. Bleasel MD, Peterson GM. Stability of midazolam in sodium chloride infusion packs. *Aust J Hosp Pharm.* 1993; 23:260–2.

1864. Taormina D, Abdallah HY, Venkataramanan R, et al. Stability and sorption of FK 506 in 5% dextrose injection and 0.9% sodium chloride injection in glass, polyvinyl chloride, and polyolefin containers. *Am J Hosp Pharm.* 1992; 49:119–22.

1865. Stiles ML, Allen LV Jr. Stability of ranitidine hydrochloride during simulated home-care use. *Am J Hosp Pharm.* 1994; 51:1706–7.

1866. Dorr RT, Likkil JD. Stability of mitomycin C in different infusion fluids: compatibility with heparin and glucocorticoids. *J Oncol Pharm Pract.* 1995; 1:19–24.

1867. Benaji B, Dine T, Goudaliez F, et al. Compatibility study of methotrexate with PVC bags after repackaging into two types of infusion admixtures. *Int J Pharm.* 1994; 105:83–7.

1868. Sanchez Alcaraz A, Quintana Vergara B. Estabilidad del midazolam en soluciones intravenosas gran volumen. *Farm Hosp.* 1992; 16:393–8.

1869. Trissel LA. Concentration-dependent precipitation of sodium bicarbonate with ciprofloxacin lactate. *Am J Health-Syst Pharm.* 1996; 53:84–5.

1870. Christen C, Johnson CE. Stability of bupivacaine hydrochloride and hydromorphone hydrochloride during simulated epidural coadministration. *Am J Health-Syst Pharm.* 1996; 53:170–3.

1871. Mewborn AL, Kessler JM. Compatibility and activity of enoxaparin sodium in 0.9% sodium chloride injection for 48 hours. *Am J Health-Syst Pharm.* 1996; 53:167–9.

1872. Ericsson O, Hallmen AC. Amphotericin B incompatible with lipid emulsion. *Ann Pharmacother.* 1996; 30:298.

1873. Hoey LL, Vance-Bryan K, Clarens DM, et al. Lorazepam stability in parenteral solutions for continuous intravenous administration. *Ann Pharmacother.* 1996; 30:343–6.

1874. Nyhammar EK, Johansson SG. Stability of doxorubicin hydrochloride and vincristine sulfate in two portable infusion-pump reservoirs. *Am J Health-Syst Pharm.* 1996; 53:1171–3.

1875. Chin A, Moon YSK, Chung KC, et al. Stability of granisetron hydrochloride with dexamethasone sodium phosphate for 14 days. *Am J Health-Syst Pharm.* 1996; 53:1174–6.

1876. Stewart JT, Warren FW, King DT, et al. Stability of ondansetron hydrochloride and five antineoplastic medications. *Am J Health-Syst Pharm.* 1996; 53:1297–300.

1877. Yamashita SK, Walker SE, Choudhury T, et al. Compatibility of selected critical care drugs during simulated Y-site administration. *Am J Health-Syst Pharm.* 1996; 53:1048–51.

1878. Ohls RK, Christensen RD. Stability of human recombinant epoetin alfa in commonly used neonatal intravenous solutions. *Ann Pharmacother.* 1996; 30:466–8.

1879. Nahata MC, Edmonds JJ. Stability of metronidazole and ceftizoxime sodium in ready-to-use metronidazole bags stored at 4 and 25°C. *Am J Health-Syst Pharm.* 1996; 53:1046–8.

1880. Lewis JD, El-Gendy A. Cephalosporin-pentamidine isethionate incompatibilities. *Am J Health-Syst Pharm.* 1996; 53:1461–2.

1881. Tanque N, Ueda H, Moriyama Y, et al. Compatibility of irinotecan hydrochloride injection with other injections. *Jpn J Hosp Pharm.* 1996; 22:457–65.

1882. Hagan RL, Mallett MS. Stability of ondansetron hydrochloride and dexamethasone sodium phosphate in infusion bags and syringes for 32 days. *Am J Health-Syst Pharm.* 1996; 53:1431–5.

1883. Mayron D, Gennaro AR. Stability and compatibility of grani-setron hydrochloride in i.v. solutions and oral liquids and during simulated Y-site injection with selected drugs. *Am J Health-Syst Pharm.* 1996; 53:294–304.

1884. Pinguet F, Rouanet P, Martel P, et al. Compatibility and stability of granisetron, dexamethasone, and methylprednisolone in injectable solutions. *J Pharm Sci.* 1995; 84:267–8.

1885. Lindsay CA, Dang K, Adams JM, et al. Stability and activity of intravenous immunoglobulin with neonatal dextrose and total parenteral nutrient solutions. *Ann Pharmacother.* 1994; 28:1014–7.

1886. Ukhun IA. Compatibility of haloperidol and diphenhydramine in a hypodermic syringe. *Ann Pharmacother.* 1995; 29:1168–9.

1887. Melonakos TK. Ciprofloxacin-ampicillin sulbactam incompatibility. *Ann Pharmacother.* 1996; 30:87.

1888. Digel S. Cefamandolnafat und metronidazol. *Krankenhauspharmazie.* 1995; 16:9–12.

1889. Heni J, Strehl E. Kompatibilitat von cefotiam. *Krankenhauspharmazie.* 1994; 15:187–92.

1890. Tham A (Medical Affairs, Chiron Therapeutics, Emeryville, CA): Personal communication; 1999 Nov 1.

1891. Mathew M, Gupta VD. Stability of ciprofloxacin in 5% dextrose and normal saline injections. *J Clin Pharm Ther.* 1994; 19:261–2.

1892. Pramar YV, Moniz D. Chemical stability and adsorption of succinylcholine chloride injections in disposable plastic syringes. *J Clin Pharm Ther.* 1994; 19:195–8.

1893. Wood MJ, Lund R. Stability of vancomycin in plastic syringes measured by high-performance liquid chromatography. *J Clin Pharm Ther.* 1995; 20:319–25.

1894. Strong ML, Schaaf LJ, Pankaskie MC, et al. Shelf-lives and factors affecting the stability of morphine sulphate and meperidine (pethidine) hydrochloride in plastic syringes for use in patient-controlled analgesic devices. *J Clin Pharm Ther.* 1994; 19:361–9.

1895. Giordano F, Bettinetti G, Cursano R, et al. A physicochemical approach to the investigation of the stability of trimethoprim-sulfamethoxazole (co-trimoxazole) mixtures for injectables. *J Pharm Sci.* 1995; 84:1254–8.

1896. Sianipar A, Parkin JE. Chemical incompatibility between procainamide hydrochloride and glucose following intravenous admixture. *J Pharm Pharmacol.* 1994; 46:951–5.

1897. Lau DWC, Law S, Walker SE, et al. Dexamethasone phosphate stability and contamination of solutions stored in syringes. *PDA J Pharm Sci Technol.* 1996; 50:261–7.

1898. Ambados F. Incompatibility between aminophylline and elemental zinc injections. *Aust J Hosp Pharm.* 1996; 26:370–1.

1899. Ambados F. Compatibility of morphine and ketamine for subcutaneous infusion. *Aust J Hosp Pharm.* 1995; 25:352.

1900. Boldu SP, Cubells MP, Brumos VG, et al. Stability study of azlocillin sodium in glass bottles and PVC bags containing intravenous admixtures. *Boll Chim Farm.* 1995; 134:467–71.

1901. LeBelle MJ, Savard C. Compatibility of morphine and midazolam or haloperidol in parenteral admixtures. *Can J Hosp Pharm.* 1995; 48:155–60.

1902. Donnelly RF, Yen M. Epinephrine stability in plastic syringes and glass vials. *Can J Hosp Pharm.* 1996; 49:62–5.

1903. Sadjak A, Wintersteiger R. Compatibility of morphine, baclofen, floxuridine and fluorouracil in an implantable medication pump. *Arzneim Forsch.* 1995; 45:93–8.

1904. Donnelly RF, Farncombe M. Compatibility of morphine or hydromorphone with salbutamol in a syringe. *Can J Hosp Pharm.* 1994; 47:252.

1905. Corbo DC, Suddith RL, Sharma B, et al. Stability, potency, and preservative effectiveness of epoetin alfa after addition of a bacteriostatic diluent. *Am J Hosp Pharm.* 1992; 49:1455–8.

1906. Lane G, Waite N. Erythropoietin stability. *Can J Hosp Pharm.* 1994; 47:182.

1907. Walker SE, Lau DWC. Compatibility and stability of hyaluronidase and hydromorphone. *Can J Hosp Pharm.* 1992; 45:187–92.

1908. Sastre Gervas I, Ferrandiz Gosalbez JR. Estabilidad fisica y quimica del sulfate magnesico combinado con heparina sodica en solucion salina al 0,9 por 100. *Farm Hosp.* 1995; 19:38–40.

1909. Halkiewicz A, Barteczko I. Interakcje fizykochemiczne izotonicznego roztworu teofiliny do wlewu dozylnego z niektorymi lekami do wstrzykiwan. *Farm Polska.* 1993; 49:11–5.

1910. Gila Azanedo JA, Mengual Sendra A, Fernandez Barral C, et al. Estudio de la estabilidad de una solucion de clorhidrato de morfina mas anestesicos locales en solucion salina 0,9 por 100 sin conservantes para uso epidural. *Farm Hosp.* 1994; 18:261–4.

1911. Sitaram BR, Tsui M, Rawicki HB, et al. Stability and compatibility of baclofen and morphine admixtures for use in an implantable infusion pump. *Int J Pharm.* 1995; 118:181–9.

1912. Allwood MC, Martin HJ. Long-term stability of cimetidine in total parenteral nutrition. *J Clin Pharm Ther.* 1996; 21:19–21.

1913. Jacolot A, Arnaud P, Lecompte D, et al. Stability and compatibility of 2.5 mg/mL methotrexate solution in plastic syringes over 7 days. *Int J Pharm.* 1996; 128:283–6.

1914. Wright A, Hecker J. Long term stability of heparin in dextrose-saline intravenous fluids. *Int J Pharm Pract.* 1995; 3:253–5.

1915. Kawano K, Matsunaga A, Terada K, et al. Loss of diltiazem hydrochloride in solutions in polyvinyl chloride containers or intravenous administration set—hydrolysis and sorption. *Jpn J Hosp Pharm.* 1994; 20:537–41.

1916. Reference number not in use.

1917. Kawano K, Takamatsu S, Yamashita J, et al. Effect of pH on the sorption of in-solution diazepam into the ethylene-vinylacetate copolymer membrane. *Jpn J Hosp Pharm.* 1994; 20:404–9.

1918. Picard C, Brazier M, Bou P, et al. Stabilite de quatre solutions de penicillines dans les poches de perfusion multicouches. *J Pharm Clin.* 1994; 13:45–9.

1919. Theuer H, Scherbel G, Balzulat S, et al. Herstellung und stabilitatuntersuchungen von carboplatin i.v. *Krankenhauspharmazie.* 1994; 15:120–30.

1920. Strehl E, Heni J. Amoxicillin, clavulansaure und metronidazol in kombination. *Krankenhauspharmazie.* 1994; 15:592–5.

1921. Hatton J, Luer M, Hirsch J, et al. Histamine receptor antagonists and lipid stability in total nutrient admixtures. *JPEN J Parenter Enteral Nutr.* 1994; 18:308–12.

1922. Ku YM, Min DI, Kumar V, et al. Stability of tacrolimus injection in total parenteral nutrition solution. *J Pharm Technol.* 1996; 12:58–61.

1923. Martinelli E, Muhlebach S. Kunststoffumbeutel als lichtschutz fur infusionen. *Krankenhauspharmazie*. 1995; 16:286–9.

1924. Teraoka K, Minakuchi K, Tsuchiya K, et al. Compatibility of ciprofloxacin infusion with other injections. *Jpn J Hosp Pharm*. 1995; 21:541–50.

1925. Asahara K, Goda Y, Shimomura Y, et al. Stability of thiamine in intravenous hyperalimentation containing multivitamin. *Jpn J Hosp Pharm*. 1995; 21:15–21.

1926. Namika Y, Fujiwara A, Kihara N, et al. Factors affecting tautomeric phenomenon of a novel potent immunosuppressant (FK506) on the design for injectable formulation. *Drug Dev Ind Pharm*. 1995; 21:809–22.

1927. Antipas AS, Vander Velde D. Factors affecting the deamidation of vancomycin in aqueous solutions. *Int J Pharm*. 1994; 109: 261–9.

1928. King AD, Stewart JT. Stability of cefmetazole-doxycycline mixtures in sodium chloride and dextrose injections. *J Clin Pharm Ther*. 1994; 19:317–25.

1929. Hughes IE, Smith JA. The stability of noradrenaline in physiologic saline solutions. *J Pharm Pharmacol*. 1978; 30:124–6.

1930. Anon. Infections linked to lax handling of propofol. *Am J Health-Syst Pharm*. 1995; 52:2061.

1931. Ordovas Baines JP, Ronchera Oms CL, Jimenez Torres NV, et al. Mezclas iv binarias de metronidazol y aminoglycosidos. *Revista AEFH*. 1988; 12:119–23.

1932. Nitescu P, Hultman E, Appelgren L, et al. Bacteriology, drug stability and exchange of percutaneous delivery systems and antibacterial filters in long-term intrathecal infusion of opioid drugs and bupivacaine in "refractory" pain. *Clin J Pain*. 1992; 8:324–37.

1933. Yao JD, Arkin CF, Karchmer AW. Vancomycin stability in heparin and total parenteral nutrition solutions: novel approach to therapy of central venous catheter-related infections. *JPEN J Parenter Enteral Nutr*. 1992; 16:268–74.

1934. Jim LK. Physical and chemical compatibility of intravenous ciprofloxacin with other drugs. *Ann Pharmacother*. 1993; 27: 704–7.

1935. Paesen J, Khan K, Roets E, et al. Study of the stability of erythromycin in neutral and alkaline solutions by liquid chromatography on poly(styrene-divinylbenzene). *Int J Pharm*. 1994; 113: 215–22.

1936. Keyi X, Gagnon N, Bisson C, et al. Stability of famotidine in polyvinyl chloride minibags and polypropylene syringes and compatibility of famotidine with selected drugs. *Ann Pharmacother*. 1993; 27:422–6.

1937. Pleasants RA, Vaughan LM, Williams DM, et al. Compatibility of ceftazidime and aminophylline admixtures for different methods of intravenous infusion. *Ann Pharmacother*. 1992; 26: 1221–6.

1938. Nahata MC, Morosco RS. Stability of diluted methylprednisolone sodium succinate injection at two temperatures. *Am J Hosp Pharm*. 1994; 51:2157–9.

1939. Nixon AR, O'Hare MCB. The stability of morphine sulphate and metoclopramide hydrochloride in various delivery presentations. *Pharm J*. 1995; 254:153–5.

1940. Lugo RA, Nahata MC. Stability of diluted dexamethasone sodium phosphate injection at two temperatures. *Ann Pharmacother*. 1994; 28:1018–9.

1941. Hanff PAJM, Van den Biggelaar JPFA. Stabiliteitsonderzoek van nitroglycerine-oplossingen voor parenteraal gebruik. *Ziekenhuisfarmacie*. 1994; 10:134–8.

1942. Forte FJ, Caravone D, Coyne MJ, et al. Albumin dilution as a cause of hemolysis during plasmapheresis. *Am J Health-Syst Pharm*. 1995; 52:207.

1943. Little G (Drug Information, Wyeth-Ayerst Laboratories, Philadelphia, PA): Personal communication; 1996 Mar 25.

1944. Andersin R, Tammilehto S. Photochemical decomposition of midazolam, part iv: study of pH-dependent stability by high-performance liquid chromatography. *Int J Pharm*. 1995; 123: 229–35.

1945. Boullata JI, Gelone SP, Mancano MA, et al. Precipitation of lorazepam infusion. *Ann Pharmacother*. 1996; 30:1037–8.

1946. Taylor RB, Richards RME, Low AS, et al. Chemical stability of polymyxin B in aqueous solution. *Int J Pharm*. 1994; 102: 201–6.

1947. Neuzil J, Darlow BA, Inder TE, et al. Oxidation of parenteral lipid emulsion by ambient and phototherapy lights: potential toxicity of routine parenteral feeding. *J Pediatr*. 1995; 126: 785–90.

1948. Katakam M, Banga AK. Aggregation of insulin and its prevention by carbohydrate excipients. *PDA J Pharm Sci Technol*. 1995; 49:160–5.

1949. Woloschuk DM. Drug precipitation and peristaltic pumps. *Am J Hosp Pharm*. 1994; 51:1473.

1950. Hehenberger H. Prednisolon-21–hemisuccinat-natrium. *Krankenhauspharmazie*. 1986; 7:128–32.

1951. Driscoll DF, Bacon M, Provost PS, et al. Automated compounders for parenteral nutrition admixtures. *JPEN J Parenter Enteral Nutr*. 1994; 18:385–6.

1952. Mehta AC, Kay EA. Admixtures' storage is extended. *Pharm Pract*. 1996; 6:113–4.

1953. Faouzi MA, Dine T, Luyckx M, et al. Stability and compatibility studies of cephaloridine, cefuroxime and ceftazidime with PVC infusion bags. *Pharmazie*. 1994; 49:425–9.

1954. Williams DA, Lokich J. A review of the stability and compatibility of antineoplastic drugs for multiple-drug infusions. *Cancer Chemother Pharmacol*. 1992; 31:171–81.

1955. Chevrier R, Sautou V, Pinon V, et al. Stability and compatibility of a mixture of the anti-cancer drugs etoposide, cytarabine and daunorubicine for infusion. *Pharm Acta Helv*. 1995; 70: 141–8.

1956. Christie JM, Jones CW. Chemical compatibility of regional anesthetic drug combinations. *Ann Pharmacother*. 1992; 26: 1078–80.

1957. Abdel-Moety EM, Al-Rashood KA, Rauf A, et al. Photostability-indicating HPLC method for determination of trifluoperazine in bulk form and pharmaceutical formulations. *J Pharm Biomed Anal*. 1996; 14:1639–44.

1958. Poochikian GK, Cradock JC. Heroin: stability and formulation approaches. *Int J Pharm*. 1983; 13:219–26.

1959. Kamitomo V, Olson K. Using normal saline to lock peripheral intravenous catheters in ambulatory cancer patients. *J Intraven Nurs*. 1996; 19:75–8.

1960. Burnakis TG. Insulin syringes: more than a one-shot deal. *Hosp Pharm*. 1996; 31:410.

1961. Sautou-Miranda V, Gremeau I, Chamard I, et al. Stability of dopamine hydrochloride and of dobutamine hydrochloride in plastic syringes and administration sets. *Am J Health-Syst Pharm.* 1996; 53:186.

1962. Murthey SS, Brittain HG. Stability of revex, nalmefene hydrochloride injection, in injectable solutions. *J Pharm Biomed Anal.* 1996; 15:221–6.

1963. Yuan LC, Samuels GJ. Stability of cidofovir in 0.9% sodium chloride injection and in 5% dextrose injection. *Am J Health-Syst Pharm.* 1996; 53:1939–43.

1964. Leader WG. Incompatibility between ceftriaxone sodium and labetalol hydrochloride. *Am J Health-Syst Pharm.* 1996; 53: 2639.

1965. Nahata MC, Morosco RS. Stability of ranitidine hydrochloride in water for injection in glass vials and plastic syringes. *Am J Health-Syst Pharm.* 1996; 53:1588–90.

1966. Lee DKT, Wong CY, Wang DP. Stability of cefazolin sodium and meperidine hydrochloride. *Am J Health-Syst Pharm.* 1996; 53(13):1608, 1610.

1967. Stiles ML, Allen LV Jr. Stability of deferoxamine mesylate, floxuridine, fluorouracil, hydromorphone hydrochloride, lorazepam, and midazolam hydrochloride in polypropylene infusion-pump syringes. *Am J Health-Syst Pharm.* 1996; 53: 1583–8.

1968. Quercia RA, Zhang J, Fan C, et al. Stability of granisetron hydrochloride in polypropylene syringes. *Am J Health-Syst Pharm.* 1996; 53:2744–6.

1969. Trissel LA, Martinez JF. Screening cladribine for Y-site physical compatibility with selected drugs. *Hosp Pharm.* 1996; 31: 1425–8.

1970. Allen LV Jr, Stiles ML, Prince SJ, et al. Stability of 14 drugs in the latex reservoir of an elastomeric infusion device. *Am J Health-Syst Pharm.* 1996; 53:2740–3.

1971. Benjamin BE. Ciprofloxacin and sodium phosphates not compatible during actual Y-site injection. *Am J Health-Syst Pharm.* 1996; 53:1850–1.

1972. Trissel LA. Everything in a compatibility study is important. *Am J Health-Syst Pharm.* 1996; 53:2990.

1973. Matuschka PR, Hill LJ. More on the compatibility of mannitol and sodium bicarbonate in injectable fluids. *Am J Health-Syst Pharm.* 1996; 53:2639.

1974. Veltri M, Lee CKK. Compatibility of neonatal parenteral nutrient solutions with selected intravenous drugs. *Am J Health-Syst Pharm.* 1996; 53:2611–3.

1975. Ritter H, Trissel LA, Anderson RW, et al. Electronic balance as quality assurance for cytotoxic drug admixtures. *Am J Health-Syst Pharm.* 1996; 53:2318–20.

1976. Zhang Y, Xu QA, Trissel LA, et al. Physical and chemical stability of methotrexate sodium, cytarabine, and hydrocortisone sodium succinate in Elliott's B solution. *Hosp Pharm.* 1996; 31: 965–70.

1977. Xu QA, Trissel LA. Stability and compatibility of fluorouracil with morphine sulfate and hydromorphone hydrochloride. *Ann Pharmacother.* 1996; 30:756–61.

1978. Kohut J III, Trissel LA. Don't ignore the details of drug-compatibility reports. *Am J Health-Syst Pharm.* 1996; 53:2339.

1979. Grillo JA, Barie PS. Precipitation of lorazepam during infusion by volumetric pump. *Am J Health-Syst Pharm.* 1996; 53:1850.

1980. Volles DF. More on usability of lorazepam admixtures for continuous infusion. *Am J Health-Syst Pharm.* 1996; 53:2753–4.

1981. Boullata JI, Gelone SP. More on usability of lorazepam admixtures for continuous infusion. *Am J Health-Syst Pharm.* 1996; 53:2754.

1982. Strozyk WR, Williamson R. Incompatibility of amiodarone hydrochloride and evacuated glass bottles. *Am J Health-Syst Pharm.* 1996; 53:184.

1983. Baud-Camus F, Crauste-Manciet S, Klein E, et al. Stability of fluorouracil in polypropylene syringes and ethylene vinyl acetate infusion-pump reservoirs. *Am J Health-Syst Pharm.* 1996; 53:1457.

1984. Chernin EL, Stewart JT. Stability of thiopental sodium and propofol in polypropylene syringes at 23 and 4 °C. *Am J Health-Syst Pharm.* 1996; 53:1576–9.

1985. Prankerd RJ, Jones RD. Physicochemical compatibility of propofol with thiopental sodium. *Am J Health-Syst Pharm.* 1996; 53:2606–10.

1986. Williams NA, Bornstein M. Stability of levofloxacin in intravenous solutions in polyvinyl chloride bags. *Am J Health-Syst Pharm.* 1996; 53:2309–13.

1987. Cleary JD. Amphotericin B formulated in a lipid emulsion. *Ann Pharmacother.* 1996; 30:409–12.

1988. Lopez RM, Ayestaran A, Pou L, et al. Stability of amphotericin B in an extemporaneously prepared i.v. fat emulsion. *Am J Health-Syst Pharm.* 1996; 53:2724–7.

1989. Manduru M, Fariello A, White RL, et al. Stability of ceftazidime sodium and teicoplanin sodium in a peritoneal dialysis solution. *Am J Health-Syst Pharm.* 1996; 53:2731–4.

1990. Plumridge RJ, Rieck AM, Annus TP, et al. Stability of ceftriaxone sodium in polypropylene syringes at −20, 4, and 20 °C. *Am J Health-Syst Pharm.* 1996; 53:2320–3.

1991. Plumridge RJ, Rieck AM, Annus TP, et al. Stability of ceftriaxone sodium reconstituted with lidocaine hydrochloride and stored in polypropylene syringes. *Am J Health-Syst Pharm.* 1996; 53:2323–5.

1992. Henderson F. 21–Day compatibility of hydromorphone hydrochloride and promethazine hydrochloride in a casette. *Am J Health-Syst Pharm.* 1996; 53:2338–9.

1993. Lima HA, Lennon J, Sesterhenn K, et al. Stability of dextrose and sodium chloride in injectable solutions stored in an elastomeric infusion device. *Am J Health-Syst Pharm.* 1996; 53: 794–5.

1994. Patel PR. Compatibility of meropenem with commonly used injectable drugs. *Am J Health-Syst Pharm.* 1996; 53:2853–5.

1995. Lougheed WD, Albisser AM, Martindale HM, et al. Physical stability of insulin formulations. *Diabetes.* 1983; 32:424–32.

1996. Gupta VD. Quantitation of papaverine hydrochloride in a discoloured injection. *Drug Stability.* 1996; 1:132–4.

1997. Akimoto K, Kawai A, Ohya K, et al. Photodegradation reactions of CPT-11, a derivative of camptothecin, part i: chemical structure of main degradation products in aqueous solution. *Drug Stability.* 1996; 1:118–22.

1998. Akimoto K, Kawai A. Photodegradation reactions of CPT-11, a derivative of camptothecin, part ii: photodegradation behaviour of CPT-11 in aqueous solution. *Drug Stability.* 1996; 1: 141–6.

1999. O'Connell C, Sabra K. Stability of reconstituted ceftriaxone solution in polypropylene syringes. *Eur Hosp Pharm.* 1996; 2: 47–8.

2000. Trissel LA, Gilbert DL. Compatibility of granisetron hydrochloride with selected drugs during simulated Y-site administration. *Am J Health-Syst Pharm.* 1997; 54:56–60.

2001. Zhang Y, Trissel LA, Martinez JF, et al. Stability of metoclopramide hydrochloride in plastic syringes. *Am J Health-Syst Pharm.* 1996; 53:1300–2.

2002. Kaijser GP, Aalbers T, Beijnen JH, et al. Chemical stability of cyclophosphamide, trofosfamide, and 2– and 3–dechloroethyl-fosfamide in aqueous solutions. *J Oncol Pharm Pract.* 1996; 2: 15–21.

2003. Nelson TJ, Graves SM. 0.9% Sodium chloride injection with and without heparin for maintaining peripheral indwelling intermittent-infusion devices in infants. *Am J Health-Syst Pharm.* 1998; 55:570–3.

2004. Martel P, Petit I, Pinguet F, et al. Long-term stability of 5-fluorouracil stored in PVC bags and in ambulatory pump reservoirs. *J Pharm Biomed Anal.* 1996; 14:395–9.

2005. Darbar D, Dell'Orto S, Wilkinson GR, et al. Loss of quinidine gluconate injection in a polyvinyl chloride infusion system. *Am J Health-Syst Pharm.* 1996; 53:655–8.

2006. Erkkila DM (Professional Services, Immunex Corporation): Personal communication; 1996 Mar 6.

2007. Xu QA, Trissel LA, Zhang Y, et al. Stability of thiotepa (lyophilized) in 5% dextrose injection at 4 and 23 °C. *Am J Health-Syst Pharm.* 1996; 53:2728–30.

2008. van Doorne H, Bernaards J. Ceftazidime degradation rates for predicting stability in a portable infusion-pump reservoir. *Am J Health-Syst Pharm.* 1996; 53:1302–5.

2009. Celesk RA (Medical Services, Bayer Pharmaceutical Division): Personal communication; 1996 May 7.

2010. Grandison D (Worldwide Medical Affairs, Du Pont Pharma): Personal communication; 1995 Dec 4.

2011. Martinez JF, Trissel LA. Compatibility of warfarin sodium with selected drugs and large-volume parenteral solutions. *Int J Pharm Compound.* 1997; 1:356–8.

2012. Williams DA. Zwitterions and pH-dependent solubility. *Am J Health-Syst Pharm.* 1996; 53:1732.

2013. Ariano RE, Kassum DA, Meatherhill RC, et al. Lack of in vitro inactivation of tobramycin by imipenem/cilastatin. *Ann Pharmacother.* 1992; 26:1075–7.

2014. Jenke DR. Drug binding by reservoirs in elastomeric devices. *Pharm Res.* 1994; 11:984–9.

2015. McCollom RA, Lange B, Bryson SM, et al. Polyvinylchloride containers do not influence the hemodynamic response to intravenous nitroglycerin. *Can J Hosp Pharm.* 1993; 46:165–70.

2016. Altavela JL, Haas CE, Nowak DR, et al. Clinical response to intravenous nitroglycerin infused through polyethylene or polyvinyl chloride tubing. *Am J Hosp Pharm.* 1994; 51:490–94.

2017. McCullough JM, Sprentall-Nankervis E, Potcova CA, et al. Recovery and biological activity of filgrastim after injection through silicone rubber catheters. *Am J Health-Syst Pharm.* 1995; 52:186–8.

2018. Park TW, Le-Bui LPK, Chung KC, et al. Stability of piperacillin sodium-tazobactam sodium in peritoneal dialysis solutions. *Am J Health-Syst Pharm.* 1995; 52:2022–4.

2019. Young D, Fadiran EO, Chang KT, et al. Stability of ticarcillin disodium in polypropylene syringes. *Am J Health-Syst Pharm.* 1995; 52:890.

2020. Stiles ML, Allen LV Jr, Resztak KE, et al. Stability of octreotide acetate in polypropylene syringes. *Am J Hosp Pharm.* 1993; 50: 2356–8.

2021. Ripley RG, Ritchie DJ. Stability of octreotide acetate in polypropylene syringes at 5 and −20 °C. *Am J Health-Syst Pharm.* 1995; 52:1910–1.

2022. Schepart BS, Burns BA, Evans S, et al. Long-term stability of interferon alfa-2b diluted to 2 million units/mL. *Am J Health-Syst Pharm.* 1995; 52:2128–30.

2023. Ikeda S, Frank PA, Schweiss JF, et al. In vitro cyanide release from sodium nitroprusside in various intravenous solutions. *Anesth Analg.* 1988; 67:360–2.

2024. Webster LK, Crinis NA, Davis JR, et al. Conversion of etoposide phosphate to etoposide under ambulatory infusion conditions. *J Oncol Pharm Pract.* 1995; 1:33–6.

2025. Hensrud DD, Burritt MF, Hall LG. Stability of heparin anticoagulant activity over time in parenteral nutrition solutions. *JPEN J Parenter Enteral Nutr.* 1996; 20:219–21.

2026. Gutcher GR, Lax AA. Vitamin A losses to plastic intravenous infusion devices and an improved method of delivery. *Am J Clin Nutr.* 1984; 40:8–13.

2027. Greene HL, Phillips BL, Franck L, et al. Persistently low blood retinol levels during and after parenteral feeding of very low birth weight infants: examination of losses into intravenous administration sets and a method of prevention by addition to a lipid emulsion. *Pediatrics.* 1987; 79:894–900.

2028. Henton DH, Merrott RJ. Vitamin A sorption to polyvinyl and polyolefin intravenous tubing. *JPEN J Parenter Enteral Nutr.* 1990; 14:79–81.

2029. Washington C, Ferguson JA. Computational prediction of the stability of lipid emulsions in total nutrient admixtures. *J Pharm Sci.* 1993; 82:808–12.

2030. Li LC, Sampogna TP. A factorial design study on the physical stability of 3–in-1 admixtures. *J Pharm Pharmacol.* 1993; 45: 985–7.

2031. Foresta K. Use of total nutrient admixtures should not be limited. *Am J Health-Syst Pharm.* 1995; 52:893.

2032. Driscoll DF. Use of total nutrient admixtures should not be limited. *Am J Health-Syst Pharm.* 1995; 52:893–4.

2033. Mirtallo JM. Use of total nutrient admixtures should not be limited. *Am J Health-Syst Pharm.* 1995; 52:894–5.

2034. Trissel LA. Use of total nutrient admixtures should not be limited. *Am J Health-Syst Pharm.* 1995; 52:895.

2035. Driscoll DF. Debate on total nutrient admixtures continues. *Am J Health-Syst Pharm.* 1995; 52:1921–2.

2036. Trissel LA. Debate on total nutrient admixtures continues. *Am J Health-Syst Pharm.* 1995; 52:1921–2.

2037. Hill SE, Heldman LS, Goo ED, et al. Fatal microvascular pulmonary emboli from precipitation of a total nutrient admixture solution. *JPEN J Parenter Enteral Nutr.* 1996; 20:81–7.

2038. MacKay MW, Fitzgerald KA, Jackson D. The solubility of calcium and phosphate in two specialty amino acid solutions. *JPEN J Parenter Enteral Nutr.* 1996; 20:63–6.

2039. Shatsky F, McFeely EJ. A table for estimating calcium and phosphorus compatibility in parenteral nutrition formulas that contain Trophamine plus cysteine. *Hosp Pharm.* 1995; 30: 690–2.

2040. Grassby PF, Hutchings L. Factors affecting the physical and chemical stability of morphine sulphate solutions stored in syringes. *Int J Pharm Pract*. 1993; 2:39–43.

2041. Ritter H, Trissel LA, Anderson RW, et al. Electronic balance as quality assurance for cytotoxic drug admixtures. *Am J Health-Syst Pharm*. 1996; 53:2318–20.

2042. Roos PJ, Glerum JH, Meilink JW, et al. Effect of pH on absorption of sufentanil citrate in a portable pump reservoir during storage and administration under simulated epidural conditions. *Pharm World Sci*. 1993; 15:139–44.

2043. Reference number not in use.

2044. Allen LV Jr, Stiles ML, Prince SJ, et al. Stability of cefpirome sulfate in the presence of commonly used intensive care drugs during simulated Y-site injection. *Am J Health-Syst Pharm*. 1995; 52:2427–33.

2045. Bureau A, Lahet JJ, D'Athis P, et al. Compatibilite PVC-psychotropes au cours d'une perfusion. *J Pharm Clin*. 1995; 14: 26–30.

2046. Streng WH, Brake NW. Dextrose adduct formation in aqueous teicoplanin solutions. *Pharm Res*. 1989; 6:1032–8.

2047. Hixt U. L-Alanyl-L-glutamine dipeptide for parenteral nutrition. *Eur Hosp Pharm*. 1996; 2:72–6.

2048. Tivnann H, Gaines-Gas R, Thorpe R, et al. An evaluation of the stability of granulocyte colony stimulating factor on the short-term storage and delivery from an elastomeric infusion system. *J Oncol Pharm Pract*. 1996; 2:107–12.

2049. Billion-Rey F, Guillaumont M, Frederich A, et al. Stability of fat-soluble vitamins A (retinol palmitate), E (tocopherol acetate), and K1 (phylloquinone) in total parenteral nutrition at home. *JPEN J Parenter Enteral Nutr*. 1993; 17:56–60.

2050. Dahl GB, Svensson L, Kinnander NJ, et al. Stability of vitamins in soybean oil fat emulsion under conditions simulating intravenous feeding of neonates and children. *JPEN J Parenter Enteral Nutr*. 1994; 18:234–9.

2051. Henry DW, Lacerte JA, Klutman NE, et al. Irreversibility of procainamide-dextrose complex in plasma in vitro. *Am J Hosp Pharm*. 1991; 48:2426–9.

2052. Martin M, Bepko R. Paclitaxel diluent and the case of the slippery spike. *Am J Hosp Pharm*. 1994; 51:3078.

2053. Faouzi MA, Dine T, Luyckx M, et al. Leaching of diethylhexyl phthalate from PVC bags into intravenous teniposide solution. *Int J Pharm*. 1994; 105:89–93.

2054. Haas CE, Nowak DR. Effect of using a standard polyvinyl chloride intravenous infusion set on patient response to nitroglycerin. *Am J Hosp Pharm*. 1992; 49:1135–7.

2055. Driver PS, Jarvi EJ. Stability of nitroglycerin as nitroglycerin concentrate for injection stored in plastic syringes. *Am J Hosp Pharm*. 1993; 50:2561–3.

2056. Casto DT. Stability of ondansetron stored in polypropylene syringes. *Ann Pharmacother*. 1994; 28:712–4.

2057. Bailey LC, Tang KT. Effect of syringe filter and i.v. administration set on delivery of propofol emulsion. *Am J Hosp Pharm*. 1991; 48:2627–30.

2058. Johnson CE, Christen C, Perez MM, et al. Compatibility of bupivacaine hydrochloride and morphine sulfate. *Am J Health-Syst Pharm*. 1997; 54:61–4.

2059. Ambados F. Compatibility of ketamine hydrochloride and meperidine hydrochloride. *Am J Health-Syst Pharm*. 1997; 54: 205.

2060. Hall PD, Yui D, Lyons S, et al. Compatibility of filgrastim with selected antimicrobial drugs during simulated Y-site administration. *Am J Health-Syst Pharm*. 1997; 54:185–9.

2061. Fausel CA, Newton DW, Driscoll DF, et al. Effect of fat emulsion and supersaturation on calcium phosphate solubility in parenteral nutrient admixtures. *Int J Pharm Compound*. 1997; 1: 54–9.

2062. Chiu MF, Schwartz ML. Visual compatibility of injectable drugs used in the intensive care unit. *Am J Health-Syst Pharm*. 1997; 54:64–5.

2063. Najari Z, Rusho WJ. Compatibility of commonly used bone marrow transplant drugs during Y-site delivery. *Am J Health-Syst Pharm*. 1997; 54:181–4.

2064. Xu QA, Trissel LA. Rapid loss of fentanyl citrate admixed with fluorouracil in polyvinyl chloride containers. *Ann Pharmacother*. 1997; 31:297–302.

2065. Gilbert DL Jr, Trissel LA. Compatibility of ciprofloxacin lactate with sodium bicarbonate during simulated Y-site administration. *Am J Health-Syst Pharm*. 1997; 54:1193–5.

2066. Trissel LA, Gilbert DL. Compatibility of propofol injectable emulsion with selected drugs during simulated Y-site administration. *Am J Health-Syst Pharm*. 1997; 54:1287–92.

2067. Asker AF, Ferdous AJ. Photodegradation of furosemide solutions. *PDA J Pharm Sci Technol*. 1996; 50:158–62.

2068. Anon. Compatibility of meropenem with commonly used injectable drugs. *Am J Health-Syst Pharm*. 1998; 55:735.

2069. Schobelock MJ (Medical Affairs Department, Roxane Laboratories, Inc.): Personal communication; 1997 Nov 4.

2070. Barnes AR, Nash S. Stability of bupivacaine hydrochloride and diamorphine hydrochloride in an epidural infusion. *Pharm World Sci*. 1995; 17:87–92.

2071. Grassby PF, Hutchings L. Drug combinations in syringe drivers: the compatibility and stability of diamorphine with cyclizine and haloperidol. *Palliat Med*. 1997; 11:217–24.

2072. Cohen MR. Volume limitations for IV drug infusions when sterile water for injection is used as a diluent. *Hosp Pharm*. 1998; 33:274–7.

2073. Pierce LR, Gaines A, Varricchio F, et al. Hemolysis and renal failure associated with use of sterile water for injection to dilute 25% human albumin solution. *Am J Health-Syst Pharm*. 1998; 55(10):1057, 1062, 1070.

2074. Trissel LA, Martinez JF. Compatibility of cisatracurium besylate with selected drugs during simulated Y-site administration. *Am J Health-Syst Pharm*. 1997; 54:1735–41.

2075. Trissel LA, Gilbert DL, Martinez JF, et al. Compatibility of remifentanil hydrochloride with selected drugs during simulated Y-site administration. *Am J Health-Syst Pharm*. 1997; 54: 2192–6.

2076. Ennis RD, Dahl TC. Stability of cidofovir in 0.9% sodium chloride injection for five days. *Am J Health-Syst Pharm*. 1997; 54(19):2204–6.

2077. Murray KM, Erkkila D, Gombotz WR, et al. Stability of thiotepa (lyophilized) in 0.9% sodium chloride injection. *Am J Health-Syst Pharm*. 1997; 54:2588–91.

2078. Bahal SM, Lee TJ, McGinnes M, et al. Visual compatibility of warfarin sodium injection with selected medications and solutions. *Am J Health-Syst Pharm*. 1997; 54:2599–600.

2079. Nolan PE, Hoyer GL, LeDoux JH, et al. Stability of ranitidine hydrochloride and human insulin in 0.9% sodium chloride injection. *Am J Health-Syst Pharm*. 1997; 54:1304–6.

2080. Stiles ML, Allen LV. Stability of nafcillin sodium, oxacillin sodium, penicillin G potassium, penicillin G sodium, and tobramycin sulfate in polyvinyl chloride drug reservoirs. *Am J Health-Syst Pharm*. 1997; 54:1068–70.

2081. Pujol M, Munoz M, Prat J, et al. Stability study of epirubicin in NaCl 0.9% injection. *Ann Pharmacother*. 1997; 31:992–5.

2082. Walker SE, DeAngelis C. Stability and compatibility of combinations of hydromorphone and a second drug. *Can J Hosp Pharm*. 1991; 44:289–95.

2083. Fischer JH, Cwik MJ, Luer MS, et al. Stability of fosphenytoin sodium with intravenous solutions in glass bottles, polyvinyl chloride bags, and polypropylene syringes. *Ann Pharmacother*. 1997; 31:553–9.

2084. Evrard B, Ceccato A, Gaspard O, et al. Stability of ondansetron hydrochloride and dexamethasone sodium phosphate in 0.9% sodium chloride injection and in 5% dextrose injection. *Am J Health-Syst Pharm*. 1997; 54:1065–8.

2085. Peddicord TE, Olsen KM, ZumBrunnen TL, et al. Stability of high-concentration dopamine hydrochloride, norepinephrine bitartrate, epinephrine hydrochloride, and nitroglycerin in 5% dextrose injection. *Am J Health-Syst Pharm*. 1997; 54:1417–9.

2086. Walker SE, Meinders A. Stability and compatibility of reconstituted sterile hydromorphone with midazolam. *Can J Hosp Pharm*. 1996; 49:290–8.

2087. Trissel LA, Gilbert DL. Compatibility of doxorubicin hydrochloride liposome injection with selected other drugs during simulated Y-site administration. *Am J Health-Syst Pharm*. 1997; 54:2708–13.

2088. Pramar YV, Loucas VA. Stability of midazolam hydrochloride in syringes and i.v. fluids. *Am J Health-Syst Pharm*. 1997; 54: 913–5.

2089. Patel PR, Cook SE. Stability of meropenem in intravenous solutions. *Am J Health-Syst Pharm*. 1997; 54:412–21.

2090. Cornish LA, Montgomery PA. Stability of bumetanide in 5% dextrose injection. *Am J Health-Syst Pharm*. 1997; 54:422–3.

2091. Bailey LC, Orosz ST. Stability of ceftriaxone sodium and metronidazole hydrochloride. *Am J Health-Syst Pharm*. 1997; 54: 424–7.

2092. Stewart JT, Warren FW, King DT, et al. Stability of ondansetron hydrochloride, doxorubicin hydrochloride, and dacarbazine or vincristine sulfate in elastomeric portable infusion devices and polyvinyl chloride bags. *Am J Health-Syst Pharm*. 1997; 54: 915–20.

2093. Owens D, Fleming RA, Restino MS, et al. Stability of amphotericin B 0.05 and 0.5 mg/mL in 20% fat emulsion. *Am J Health-Syst Pharm*. 1997; 54:683–6.

2094. Zhang Y, Xu QA, Trissel LA, et al. Compatibility and stability of paclitaxel combined with cisplatin and with carboplatin in infusion solutions. *Ann Pharmcother*. 1997; 31:1465–70.

2095. Gupta VD, Maswoswe J. Stability of ketorolac tromethamine in 5% dextrose injection and 0.9% sodium chloride injections. *Int J Pharm Compound*. 1997; 1:206–7.

2096. Zhang YP, Trissel LA. Stability of aminocaproic acid injection admixtures in 5% dextrose injection and 0.9% sodium chloride injection. *Int J Pharm Compound*. 1997; 1:132–4.

2097. Allen LV, Stiles ML. Stability of vancomycin hydrochloride in medication cassette reservoirs. *Int J Pharm Compound*. 1997; 1:123–4.

2098. Zhang YP, Trissel LA, Martinez JF, et al. Stability of acyclovir sodium 1, 7, and 10 mg/mL in 5% dextrose injection and 0.9% sodium chloride injection. *Am J Health-Syst Pharm*. 1998; 55: 574–7.

2099. Amador FD, Azzati ES. Stability of carboplatin in polyvinyl chloride bags. *Am J Health-Syst Pharm*. 1998; 55:602.

2100. Gupta VD, Maswoswe J. Stability of cefmetazole sodium in 5% dextrose injection and 0.9% sodium chloride injection. *Int J Pharm Compound*. 1997; 1:208–9.

2101. Gupta VD, Maswoswe J. Stability of ceftriaxone sodium when mixed with metronidazole injection. *Int J Pharm Compound*. 1997; 1:280–1.

2102. Gupta VD, Maswoswe J. Stability of cefepime hydrochloride in 5% dextrose injection and 0.9% sodium chloride injection. *Int J Pharm Compound*. 1997; 1:435–6.

2103. Mayhew SL, Quick MW. Compatibility of iron dextran with neonatal parenteral nutrient solutions. *Am J Health-Syst Pharm*. 1997; 54:570–1.

2104. Moshfeghi M, Ciuffo JD. Visual compatibility of fentanyl citrate with parenteral nutrient solutions. *Am J Health-Syst Pharm*. 1998; 55:1194.

2105. Gupta VD, Maswoswe J. Stability of indomethacin in 0.9% sodium chloride injection. *Int J Pharm Compound*. 1998; 2: 170–1.

2106. Wong F, Gill MA. Stability of milrinone lactate 200 mcg/mL in 5% dextrose injection and 0.9% sodium chloride injection. *Int J Pharm Compound*. 1998; 2:168–9.

2107. Nguyen D, Gill MA. Stability of milrinone lactate in 5% dextrose injection and 0.9% sodium chloride injection at concentrations of 400, 600, and 800 mcg/mL. *Int J Pharm Compound*. 1998; 2:246–8.

2108. Montgomery PA, Cornish LA, Johnson CE, et al. Stability of torsemide in 5% dextrose injection. *Am J Health-Syst Pharm*. 1998; 55:1042–3.

2109. Trissel LA, Gilbert DL, Martinez JF, et al. Compatibility of parenteral nutrient solutions with selected drugs during simulated Y-site administration. *Am J Health-Syst Pharm*. 1997; 54: 1295–1300.

2110. Pramar YV. Chemical stability of amiodarone hydrochloride in intravenous fluids. *Int J Pharm Compound*. 1997; 1:347–8.

2111. Wang DP, Wang MT, Wong CY, et al. Compatibility of vancomycin hydrochloride and famotidine in 5% dextrose injection. *Int J Pharm Compound*. 1997; 1:354–5.

2112. Bhatt-Mehta V, Hirata S. Physical compatibility and chemical stability of atracurium besylate and midazolam hydrochloride during intravenous coinfusion. *Int J Pharm Compound*. 1998; 2:79–82.

2113. Stendal TL, Klem W, Tonnesen HH, et al. Drug stability and pyridine generation in ceftazidime injection stored in an elastomeric infusion device. *Am J Health-Syst Pharm*. 1998; 55: 683–5.

2114. Ketkar VA, Kolling WM, Nardviriyakul N, et al. Stability of undiluted and diluted adenosine at three temperatures in syringes and bags. *Am J Health-Syst Pharm*. 1998; 55:466–0.

2115. Naud C, Marti B, Fernandez C, et al. Stability of adenosine 6 mcg/mL in 0.9% sodium chloride solution. *Am J Health-Syst Pharm.* 1998; 55:1161–4.

2116. Xu QA, Zhang YP, Trissel LA, et al. Stability of cisatracurium besylate in vials, syringes, and infusion admixtures. *Am J Health-Syst Pharm.* 1998; 55:1037–41.

2117. Trissel LA, Gilbert DL. Incompatibility and compatibility of amphotericin B cholsteryl sulfate complex with selected other drugs during simulated Y-site administration. *Hosp Pharm.* 1998; 33:284–92.

2118. Allwood MC, Martin J. How does storage affect propofol? The stability of propofol in plastic syringes. *Pharm Pract.* 1997; 7: 15–6.

2119. Harris MC, Como JA. Heparin flush solutions: how much is enough? *South J Health-Syst Pharm.* 1997; 2:10–4.

2120. Meyer BA, Little CJ, Thorp JA, et al. Heparin versus normal saline as a peripheral line flush in maintenance of intermittent intravenous lines in obstetric patients. *Obstet Gynecol.* 1995; 85:433–6.

2121. Danek GD, Noris EM. Pediatric i.v. catheters: efficacy of saline flush. *Pediatr Nurs.* 1992; 18:111–3.

2122. Hook ML, Reuling J, Luettgen ML, et al. Comparison of the patency of arterial lines maintained with heparinized and non-heparinized infusions. The Cardiovascular Intensive Care Unit Nursing Research Committee of St. Luke's Hospital. *Heart Lung.* 1987; 16:693–9.

2123. Kulkarni M, Elsner C, Ouellet D, et al. Heparinized saline versus normal saline in maintaining patency of the radial artery catheter. *Can J Surg.* 1994; 37:37–42.

2124. Clifton GD, Branson P, Kelly HJ, et al. Comparison of normal saline and heparin solutions for maintenance of arterial catheter patency. *Heart Lung.* 1991; 20:115–8.

2125. Butt W, Shann F, McDonnell G, et al. Effect of heparin concentration and infusion rate on the patency of arterial catheters. *Crit Care Med.* 1987; 15:230–2.

2126. Smith S, Dawson S, Hennessey R, et al. Maintenance of the patency of indwelling central venous catheters: is heparin necessary? *Am J Pediatr Hematol Oncol.* 1991; 13(2):141–3.

2127. O'Neill TJ, Tierney LM Jr, Proulx RJ. Heparin lock-induced alterations in the activated partial thromboplastin time. *JAMA.* 1974; 227:1297–8.

2128. Passannante A, Macik BG. Case report: the heparin flush syndrome: a cause of iatrogenic hemorrhage. *Am J Med Sci.* 1988; 296:71–3.

2129. Heeger PS, Backstrom JT. Heparin flushes and thrombocytopenia. *Ann Intern Med.* 1986; 105:143.

2130. Laster J, Cikrit D, Walker N, et al. The heparin-induced thrombocytopenia syndrome: an update. *Surgery.* 1987; 102: 763–70.

2131. Rizzoni WE, Miller K, Rick M, et al. Heparin-induced thrombocytopenia and thromboembolism in the postoperative period. *Surgery.* 1988; 103:470–6.

2132. Doty JR, Alving BM, McDonnell DE, et al. Heparin-associated thrombocytopenia in the neurosurgical patient. *Neurosurgery.* 1986; 19:69–72.

2133. Mehta AC, Kay EA. Storage time can be extended. *Pharm Pract.* (June) 1997; 7:305, 306, 308.

2134. Brittain HG, Lafferty L, Bousserski P, et al. Stability of Revex, nalmefene hydrochloride injection. *PDA J Pharm Sci Technol.* 1996; 50:35–9.

2135. McKinnon BT. FDA Safety Alert: hazards of precipitation associated with parenteral nutrition. *Nutr Clin Pract.* 1996; 11: 59–65.

2136. Seidner DL, Speerhas R. Can octreotide be added to parenteral nutrition? Point-counterpoint. *Nutr Clin Pract.* 1998; 13:84–8.

2137. Dodds HM, Craik DJ. Photodegradation of irinotecan (CPT-11) in aqueous solutions: identification of fluorescent products and influence of solution composition. *J Pharm Sci.* 1997; 86: 1410–6.

2138. Gremeau I, Sautou-miranda V, Picq F, et al. Influence de la nature de la membrane sur le passage du nitrate d'isosorbide et de son metabolite actif au cours d'une dialyse. *J Pharm Clin.* 1997; 16:19–23.

2139. Graham AE, Speicher E. Analysis of gentamicin sulfate and a study of its degradation in dextrose solution. *J Pharm Biomed Anal.* 1997; 15:537–43.

2140. Craig SB, Bhatt UH. Stability and compatibility of topotecan hydrochloride for injection with common infusion solutions and containers. *J Pharm Biomed Anal.* 1997; 16:199–205.

2141. Pramar YV, Loucas VA. Chemical stability and adsorption of atracurium besylate injections in disposable plastic syringes. *J Clin Pharm Ther.* 1996; 21:173–5.

2142. Galanti LM, Hecq JD, Vanbeckbergen D, et al. Long-term stability of cefuroxime and cefazolin sodium in intravenous infusions. *J Clin Pharm Ther.* 1996; 21:185–9.

2143. Kawano K, Takamatsu S, Mochizuku C, et al. Loss of isosorbide dinitrate or nitroglycerin solution content in practice injection or precision continuous drip infusion. *Jpn J Hosp Pharm.* 1996; 22:167–72.

2144. Yoshida H, Takaba D, Uchida Y, et al. Research for the crystal material produced in the continuous infusion line of midazloam (Dormicium) and butorphanol (Stadol). *Jpn J Hosp Pharm.* 1997; 23:531–8.

2145. Mawhinney WM, Adair CG, Gorman SP, et al. Long-term stability of teicoplanin in dialysis fluid: implications for the home-treatment of CAPD peritonitis. *Int J Pharm Pract.* 1991; 1: 90–3.

2146. Allwood MC, Martin H. The extraction of diethylhexylphthalate (DEHP) from polyvinyl chloride components of intravenous infusion containers and administration sets by paclitaxel injection. *Int J Pharm.* 1996; 127:65–71.

2147. Valiere C, Arnaud P, Caroff E, et al. Stability and compatibility study of a carboplatin solution in syringes for continuous ambulatory infusion. *Int J Pharm.* 1996; 138:125–8.

2148. Khalfi F, Dine T, Gressier B, et al. Compatibility and stability of vancomycin hydrochloride with PVC infusion material in various conditions using stability-indicating high-performance liquid chromatographic assay. *Int J Pharm.* 1996; 139:243–7.

2149. Hourcade F, Sautou-Miranda V, Normand B, et al. Compatibility of granisetron towards glass and plastics and its stability under various storage conditions. *Int J Pharm.* 1997; 154: 95–102.

2150. Rabouan-Guyon SM, Guet AF, Courtois PY, et al. Stability study of cefepime in different infusion solutions. *Int J Pharm.* 1997; 154:185–90.

2151. Anon. How I survived a direct injection of potassium chloride. *Hosp Pharm.* 1997; 32:298–300.

2152. Kramer I. Stability of meropenem in elastomeric portable infusion devices. *Eur Hosp Pharm.* 1997; 3:168–71.

2153. Uges DRA, Ruige M. Vancomycin adsorption to teflon tubing. *Eur Hosp Pharm.* 1996; 2:38.

2154. Daouphars M, Vigneron J, Perrin A, et al. Stability of cladribine in either polyethylene containers or polyvinyl chloride bags. *Europ Hosp Pharm.* 1997; 3:154–6.

2155. Girona V, Prat J, Pujol M, et al. Stability of vinblastine sulphate in 0.9% sodium chloride in polypropylene syringes. *Boll Chim Farm.* 1996; 135:413–4.

2156. Smith BA, Hilmi SC, McDonald C, et al. The stability of foscarnet in the presence of potassium. *Aust J Hosp Pharm.* 1996; 26:560–1.

2157. Jaffe GJ, Green GDJ. Stability of recombinant tissue plasminogen activator. *Am J Ophthal.* 1989; 108:90–1.

2158. Ward C, Weck S. Dilution and storage of recombinant tissue plasminogen activator (Activase) in balanced salt solutions. *Am J Ophthal.* 1990; 109:98–9.

2159. Grewing R, Mester U, Low M. Clinical experience with tissue plasminogen activator stored at -20 °C. *Ophthalmic Surg.* 1992; 23:780–1.

2160. Kramer I. Viability of microorganisms in novel antineoplastic and antiviral drug solutions. *J Oncol Pharm Pract.* 1998; 4: 32–7.

2161. Schneider JJ, Wilson KM. A study of the osmolality and pH of subcutaneous drug infusion solutions. *Aust J Hosp Pharm.* 1997; 27:29–31.

2162. Vermeire A, Remon JP. The solubility of morphine and the stability of concentrated morphine solutions in glass, polypropylene syringes and PVC containers. *Int J Pharm.* 1997; 146: 213–23.

2163. Kearney MCJ, Allwood MC, Martin H, et al. The influence of amino acid source on the stability of ascorbic acid in TPN mixtures. *Nutrition.* 1998; 14:173–8.

2164. Casasin Edo T, Roca Massa M. Sistema de distribucion de medicamentos utilizados en anestesia mediante jeringas precargadas. Estudio de estabilidad. *Farm Hosp.* 1996; 20:55–9.

2165. Malcomson C, Zilka S, Saum J, et al. Investigations into the compatibility of teicoplanin with heparin. *Eur J Parenter Sci.* 1997; 2:51–5.

2166. Walker SE, Walshaw PR. Imipenem stability and staining of teeth. *Can J Hosp Pharm.* 1997; 50:61–7.

2167. Gilbar P, McAllan Z. Ticarcillin-potassium clavulanate and vancomycin incompatibility. *Aust J Hosp Pharm.* 1997; 27:470.

2168. Burm JP. Stability of ondansetron and fluconazole in 5% dextrose injection and normal saline during Y-site administration. *Arch Pharm Res.* 1997; 20:171–5.

2169. Truelle-Hugon B, Tourrette G, Couineaux B, et al. Etude de stabilite du chlorhydrate de morphine Lavoisier dans differents systemes actifs pour perfusion apres reconstitution dans divers solvents. *Ann Pharm Fr.* 1997; 55:216–23.

2170. Sitaram BR, Tsui M, Rawicki HB, et al. Stability and compatibility of intrathecal admixtures containing baclofen and high concentrations of morphine. *Int J Pharm.* 1997; 153:13–24.

2171. Trinkle R. Compatibility of hydromorphone and prochlorperazine, and irritation due to subcutaneous prochlorperazine infusion. *Ann Pharmacother.* 1997; 31:789–90.

2172. Guchelar HJ, Hartog ME. De stabiliteit van clonazepaminjectievloeistof. *Ziekenhuisfarmacie.* 1997; 13:21–3.

2173. Leboucher G, Charpiat B. Incompatibilite physico-chimique entre l'omeprazole et la vancomycine. *Pharm Hosp Fr.* 1997; 121: 124.

2174. Taylor A. Review of clarithromycin mixtures. *Pharm Pract.* (Oct) 1997; 7:473, 474, 476.

2175. Farhang-Asnafi S, Callaert S, Barre J, et al. Influence du solvant de dilution sur la stabilite de la nouvelle forme de 5-fluorouracile en perfusion. *J Pharm Clin.* 1997; 16:45–8.

2176. Oustric-Mendes AC, Huart B, Le Hoang MD, et al. Study protocol: stability of morphine injected without preservative, delivered with a disposable infusion device. *J Clin Pharm Ther.* 1997; 22:283–90.

2177. Schoffski P, Freund M, Wunder R, et al. Safety and toxicity of amphotericin B in glucose 5% or Intralipid 20% in neutropenic patients with pneumonia or fever of unknown origin: randomised study. *BMJ.* 1998; 317:379–84.

2178. Heinemann V, Kahny B, Jehn U, et al. Serum pharmacology of amphotericin B applied in lipid emulsions. *Antimicrob Agents Chemother.* 1997; 41:728–32.

2179. Gupta VD, Maswoswe J. Stability of mitomycin aqueous solution when stored in tuberculin syringes. *Int J Pharm Compound.* 1997; 1:282–3.

2180. Targett PL, Keefe PA. Compatibility and stability of drug adjuvants and morphine tartrate in 10 mL polypropylene syringes. *Aust J Hosp Pharm.* 1997; 27:207–12.

2181. Goren MP, Lyman BA. The stability of mesna in beverages and syrup for oral administration. *Cancer Chemother Pharmacol.* 1991; 28:298–301.

2182. Xu QA, Trissel LA. Compatibility of paclitaxel in 5% glucose and 0.9% sodium chloride injections with EVA minibags. *Aust J Hosp Pharm.* 1998; 28:156–9.

2183. Xu QA, Zhang YP, Trissel LA, et al. Stability of busulfan injection admixtures in 5% dextrose injection and 0.9% sodium chloride injection. *J Oncol Pharm Pract.* 1996; 2:101–5.

2184. Sarver JG, Pryka R, Alexander KS, et al. Stability of magnesium sulfate in 0.9% sodium chloride and lactated Ringer's solutions. *Int J Pharm Compound.* 1998; 2:385–8.

2185. Jobet-Hermelin I, Mallvais ML, Jacquot C, et al. Proposition d'une concentration limite acceptable du plastifiant librere par le poly(chlorure de vinyle) dans les solutions injectables aqueuses. *J Pharm Clin.* 1996; 15:132–6.

2186. Jacobson PA, West NJ, Spadoni V, et al. Sterility of filgrastim (G-CSF) in syringes. *Ann Pharmacother.* 1996; 30:1238–42.

2187. Trissel LA, Spadoni VT. Comment: filgrastim sterility in syringes. *Ann Pharmacother.* 1997; 31:500–1.

2188. Appenheimer MM, Schepart BS, Poleon GP, et al. Stability of albumin-free interferon alfa-2b for 42 days. *Am J Health-Syst Pharm.* 1998; 55:1602–5.

2189. Trissel LA, Gilbert DL. Concentration dependency of vancomycin hydrochloride compatibility with beta-lactam antibiotics during simulated Y-site administration. *Hosp Pharm.* 1998; 33: 1515–22.

2190. McLaughlin JP, Simpson C. How stable is acyclovir in PVC bags? The stability of reconstituted acyclovir sodium in a 0.9% w/v sodium chloride infusion when stored at room temperature. *Pharm Pract.* 1995; 5:53–8.

2191. Mehta AC, Kay EA. How stable is alfentanil? Stability of alfentanil hydrochloride in 5% dextrose stored in syringes. *Pharm Pract.* 1995; 5:303–4.

2192. McLaughlin JP, Simpson C. How stable are Zinacef & Metrovex? The stability of cefuroxime sodium and metronidazole infusion when stored in a refrigerator. *Pharm Pract.* 1995; 5: 100–6.

2193. Bonferoni MC, Mellerio G, Giunchedi P, et al. Photostability evaluation of nicardipine HCl solutions. *Int J Pharm.* 1992; 80: 109–17.

2194. Erdman SH, McElwee CL, Kramer JM, et al. Central line occlusion with three-in-one nutrition admixtures administered at home. *JPEN J Parenter Enteral Nutr.* 1994; 18:177–81.

2195. Allwood MC, Martin H. Factors influencing the stability of ranitidine in TPN mixtures. *Clin Nutr.* 1995; 14:171–6.

2196. Hoie EB, Narducci WA. Laser particle analysis of calcium phosphate precipitate in neonatal TPN admixtures. *J Ped Pharm Pract.* 1996; 1:163–7.

2197. Ambados F, Brealey J. Incompatibilities with trace elements during TPN solution admixture. *Aust J Hosp Pharm.* 1998; 28: 112–4.

2198. Xu QA, Trissel LA. Compatibility of paclitaxel injection diluent with two reduced-phthalate administration sets for the Acclaim pump. *Int J Pharm Compound.* 1998; 2:382–4.

2199. Stewart JT, Warren FW, King DT, et al. Stability of ondansetron hydrochloride and 12 medications in plastic syringes. *Am J Health-Syst Pharm.* 1998; 55:2630–4.

2200. Donnelly RF, Bushfield TL. Chemical stability of meperidine hydrochloride in polypropylene syringes. *Int J Pharm Compound.* 1998; 2:463–5.

2201. Jappinen AL, Kokki H, Rasi AS, et al. Stability of sufentanil in a syringe pump under simulated epidural infusion. *Int J Pharm Compound.* 1998; 2:466–8.

2202. Wilson KM, Schneider JJ. Stability of midazolam and fentanyl in infusion solutions. *J Pain Symptom Manage.* 1998; 16: 52–8.

2203. Gupta VD, Pramar Y. Stability of lorazepam in 5% dextrose injection. *Int J Pharm Compound.* 1998; 2:322–4.

2204. Heide PE. Precipitation of amphotericin B from i.v. fat emulsion. *Am J Health-Syst Pharm.* 1997; 54:1449.

2205. Heide PE, Hehenberger H. Tensiometrische und konduktometrische stabilitatuntersuchungen von amphotericin B in fettmulsionen. *Oesterreichische Krankenhaus Pharmazie.* 1996; 10: 36–43.

2206. To TP, Garrett MK. Stability of flucloxacillin in a hospital in the home program. *Aust J Hosp Pharm.* 1998; 28:289–90.

2207. Levanda M. Noticeable difference in admixtures prepared from lorazepam 2 and 4 mg/mL. *Am J Health-Syst Pharm.* 1998; 55: 2305.

2208. Share MJ, Harrison RD, Folstad J, et al. Stability of lorazepam 1 and 2 mg/mL in glass bottles and polypropylene syringes. *Am J Health-Syst Pharm.* 1998; 55:2013–5.

2209. Inagaki K, Kambara M, Mizuno M, et al. Compatibility and stability of ranitidine hydrochloride with six cephalosporins during simulated Y-site administration. *Int J Pharm Compound.* 1998; 2:318–21.

2210. Ray LR, Chen DA. Stability of somatropin stored in plastic syringes for 28 days. *Am J Health-Syst Pharm.* 1998; 55: 1508–11.

2211. Patel K, Craig SB, McBride MG, et al. Microbial inhibitory properties and stability of topotecan hydrochloride injection. *Am J Health-Syst Pharm.* 1998; 55:1584–7.

2212. English BA, Riggs RM, Webster AA, et al. Y-site stability of fosphenytoin and sodium phenobarbital. *Int J Pharm Compound.* 1999; 3:64–6.

2213. Lieu CL, Chin A. Five-day stability of vinorelbine in 5% dextrose injection and in 0.9% sodium chloride injection at room temperature. *Int J Pharm Compound.* 1999; 3:67–8.

2214. Akkerman SR, Zhang H, Mullins RE, et al. Stability of milrinone lactate in the presence of 29 critical care drugs and 4 i.v. solutions. *Am J Health-Syst Pharm.* 1999; 56:63–8.

2215. Trissel LA, Gilbert DL, Martinez JF, et al. Compatibility of medications with 3–in–1 parenteral nutrition admixtures. *JPEN J Parenter Enteral Nutr.* 1999; 23:67–74.

2216. Johnson CE, vandenBussche HL, Chio CC, et al. Stability of tacrolimus with morphine sulfate, hydromorphone hydrochloride, and ceftazidime during simulated intravenous coadministration. *Am J Health-Syst Pharm.* 1999; 56:164–9.

2217. Stamatakis MK, Leader WG. Stability of high-dose vancomycin and ceftazidime in peritoneal dialysis solutions. *Am J Health-Syst Pharm.* 1999; 56:246–8.

2218. Trissel LA, Martinez JF. Compatibility of etoposide phosphate with selected drugs during simulated Y-site injection. *J Am Pharm Assoc.* 1999; 39:141–5.

2219. Zhang Y, Trissel LA. Physical and chemical stability of etoposide phosphate solutions. *J Am Pharm Assoc.* 1999; 39: 146–50.

2220. Stewart JT, Warren FW. Stability of cefepime hydrochloride injection in polypropylene syringes at -20 °C, 4 °C, and 22–24 °C. *Am J Health Syst Pharm.* 1999; 56:457–9.

2221. Stewart JT, Maddox FC. Stability of cefepime hydrochloride in polypropylene syringes. *Am J Health-Syst Pharm.* 1999; 56: 1134.

2222. Burkiewicz JS. Incompatibility of ceftriaxone sodium with lactated Ringer's injection. *Am J Health-Syst Pharm.* 1999; 56: 384.

2223. Riggs RM, English BA, Webster AA, et al. Fosphenytoin Y-site stability studies with lorazepam and midazolam hydrochloride. *Int J Pharm Compound.* 1999; 3:235–8.

2224. Trissel LA, Gilbert DL. Compatibility of docetaxel with selected drugs during simulated Y-site administration. *Int J Pharm Compound.* 1999; 3:241–4.

2225. Johnson CE, Truong NM. Stability and compatibility of tacrolimus and fluconazole in 0.9% sodium chloride. *J Am Pharm Assoc.* 1999; 39:505–8.

2226. Trissel LA, Martinez JF. Compatibility of gemcitabine hydrochloride with 107 selected drugs during simulated Y-site injection. *J Am Pharm Assoc.* 1999; 39:514–8.

2227. Xu Q, Zhang Y. Physical and chemical stability of gemcitabine hydrochloride solutions. *J Am Pharm Assoc.* 1999; 39:509–13.

2228. Walker SE, Gray S. Stability of reconstituted indomethacin sodium trihydrate in original vials and polypropylene syringes. *Am J Health-Syst Pharm.* 1998; 55:154–8.

2229. Schlatter J, Saulnier JL. Inline filtration of ranitidine hydrochloride solutions. *Am J Health-Syst Pharm.* 1998; 55:840.

2230. Zhang Y, Trissel LA. Paclitaxel compatibility with a triple-lumen polyurethane central catheter. *Hosp Pharm.* 1998; 33: 547–51.

2231. Xu QA, Trissel LA. Paclitaxel compatibility with the IV Express filter unit. *Int J Pharm Compound.* 1998; 2:243–5.

2232. Xu QA, Trissel LA. Paclitaxel compatibility with a TOTM-plasticized PVC administration set. *Hosp Pharm.* 1997; 32:1635–8.

2233. Saltsman CL, Tom CM, Mitchell A, et al. Compatibility of levofloxacin with 34 medications during simulated Y-site administration. *Am J Health-Syst Pharm.* 1999; 56:1458–9.

2234. Trissel LA, Gilbert DL. Compatibility screening of gatifloxacin during simulated Y-site administration with other drugs. *Hosp Pharm.* 1999; 34:1409–16.

2235. Voytilla KL, Rusho WJ. Compatibility of alatrofloxacin mesylate with commonly used drugs during Y-site delivery. *Am J Health-Syst Pharm.* 2000; 57:1437–9.

2236. Johnson CE, Truong NM. Stability and compatibility of tacrolimus and fluconazole in 0.9% sodium chloride. *J Am Pharm Assoc.* 1999; 39:505–8.

2237. Xu QA, Trissel LA. Stability of amphotericin B cholesteryl sulfate complex after reconstitution and admixture. *Hosp Pharm.* 1998; 33:1203–7.

2238. Balthasar JP. Concentration-dependent incompatibility of vinorelbine tartrate and heparin sodium. *Am J Health-Syst Pharm.* 1999; 56:1891.

2239. Wolfe JL, Thoma LA, Du C, et al. Compatibility and stability of vincristine sulfate, doxorubicin hydrochloride, and etoposide in 0.9% sodium chloride injection. *Am J Health-Syst Pharm.* 1999; 56:985–9.

2240. Peek BT, Webster KD. Stability and compatibility of promethazine hydrochloride and dihydroergotamine mesylate in combination. *Am J Health-Syst Pharm.* 1999; 56:1835–8.

2241. Webster AA, English BA, McGuire JM, et al. Stability of dobutamine hydrochloride 4 mg/mL in 5% dextrose injection at 5 and 23 (C. *Int J Pharmaceut Compound.* 1999; 3:412–4.

2242. Thiesen J, Kramer I. Physico-chemical stability of docetaxel premix solution and docetaxel infusion solutions in PVC bags and polyolefine containers. *Pharm World Sci.* 1999; 21:137–41.

2243. Kramer I, Thiesen J. Stability of topotecan infusion solutions in polyvinylchloride bags and elastomeric portable infusion devices. *J Oncol Pharm Pract.* 1999; 5:75–82.

2244. Hecq JD, Evrard JM, Gillet P, et al. Etude de stabilite visuelle du chlorydrate de chlorpromazine, du chlorure de potassium, de la furosemide et de l'heparine sodique en perfusion continue. *Pharmakon.* 1998; 116:145–8.

2245. Mayron D, Gennaro AR. Stability and compatibility of topotecan hydrochloride with selected drugs. *Am J Health-Syst Pharm.* 1999; 56:875–81.

2246. Harvey SC, Toussaint CP, Coe SE, et al. Stability of meperidine in an implantable infusion pump using capillary gas chromatography-mass spectrometry and a deuterated internal standard. *J Pharm Biomed Anal.* 1999; 21:577–83.

2247. Trissel LA, Xu QA. Compatibility and stability of paclitaxel combined with doxorubicin hydrochloride in infusion solutions. *Ann Pharmacother.* 1998; 32:1013–6.

2248. Reference number not in use.

2249. Bergquist PA, Zimmerman J, Kenney RR, et al. Stability of tirofiban hydrochloride in three commonly used i.v. solutions and polyvinyl chloride administration sets. *Am J Health-Syst Pharm.* 1999; 56:1627–9.

2250. Bergquist PA, Hunke WA, Reed RA, et al. Compatibility of tirofiban HCl with dopamine HCl, famotidine, sodium heparin, lidocaine HCl and potassium chloride during simulated Y-site administration. *J Clin Pharm Ther.* 1999; 24:125–32.

2251. McLaughlin JP, Simpson C. How stable is ganciclovir? *Pharm Pract.* 1998; 8:329–30, 332.

2252. Galanti LM, Hecq JD, Vanbeckbergen D, et al. Long-term stability of vancomycin hydrochloride in intravenous infusions. *J Clin Pharm Ther.* 1997; 22:353–6.

2253. Hor MMS, Chan SY, Yow KL, et al. Stability of admixtures of pethidine and metoclopramide in aqueous solution, 5% dextrose and 0.9% sodium chloride. *J Clin Pharm Ther.* 1997; 22:339–45.

2254. Hor MM, Chan SY, Yow KL, et al. Stability of morphine sulphate in saline under simulated patient administration conditions. *J Clin Pharm Ther.* 1997; 22:405–10.

2255. Mittner A, Vincze Z. Stability of cyclophosphamide containing infusions. *Pharmazie.* 1999; 54:224–5.

2256. Mittner A, Vincze Z. Stability of vinblastine sulphate containing infusions. *Pharmazie.* 1999; 54:625–6.

2257. Schrijvers D, Tai-Apin C, De Smet MC, et al. Determination of compatibility and stability of drugs used in palliative care. *J Clin Pharm Ther.* 1998; 23:311–4.

2258. Kopelent-Frank H, Schimper A. HPTLC-based stability assay for the determination of amiodarone in intravenous admixtures. *Pharmazie.* 1999; 54:542–4.

2259. Inagaki K, Miyamoto Y, Kurata N, et al. Stability of ranitidine hydrochloride with cefazolin sodium, cefbuperazone sodium, cefoxitin sodium, and cephalothin sodium during simulated Y-site administration. *Int J Pharmaceut Compound.* 2000; 4:150–3.

2260. Roy JJ, Hildgen P. Stability of morphine-ketamine mixtures in 0.9% sodium chloride injection packaged in syringes, plastic bags and Medication Cassette reservoirs. *Int J Pharmaceut Compound.* 2000; 4:225–8.

2261. Grant EM, Zhong MK, Ambrose PG, et al. Stability of meropenem in a portable infusion device in a cold pouch. *Am J Health-Syst Pharm.* 2000; 57:992–5.

2262. Xu QA, Trissel LA. Compatibility and stability of linezolid injection admixed with three cephalosporin antibiotics. *J Am Pharm Assoc.* 2000; 40:509–14.

2263. Zhang Y, Xu QA, Trissel LA, et al. Compatibility and stability of linezolid injection admixed with aztreonam or piperacillin sodium. *J Am Pharm Assoc.* 2000; 40:520–4.

2264. Trissel LA, Williams KY. Compatibility screening of linezolid injection during simulated Y-site administration with other drugs and infusion solutions. *J Am Pharm Assoc.* 2000; 40:515–9.

2265. Zhang Y, Xu QA, Trissel LA, et al. Physical compatibility of calcium acetate and potassium phosphates in parenteral nutrition solutions containing Aminosyn II. *Int J Pharmaceut Compound.* 1999; 3:415–20.

2266. Ambados F, Brealey J. Precipitation of potassium sulphate during TPN solution admixture. *Aust J Hosp Pharm.* 1998; 28:444.

2267. Ambados F. Destabilization of fat emulsion in total nutrient admixtures by concentrated albumin 20% infusion. *Aust J Hosp Pharm.* 1999; 29:210–2.

2268. Peterson GM, Miller KA, Galloway JG, et al. Compatibility and stability of fentanyl admixtures in polypropylene syringes. *J Clin Pharm Ther*. 1998; 23(1):67–72.

2269. Picard C, Hary L, Bou P, et al. Stability of three aminoglycoside solutions in PVC and multilayer infusion bags. *Pharmazie*. 1999; 54:854–6.

2270. Shella C. How to shake insulin. *Hosp Pharm*. 1999; 34:518.

2271. Bjorkman S, Roth B. Chemical compatibility of mitoxantrone and etoposide (VP-16). *Acta Pharm Nord*. 1991; 3:251.

2272. Charland SL, Davis DD. Activity of enoxaparin sodium in tuberculin syringes for 10 days. *Am J Health-Syst Pharm*. 1998; 55:1296–8.

2273. Couldry R, Sanborn M, Klutman NE, et al. Continuous infusion of ceftazidime with an elastomeric infusion device. *Am J Health-Syst Pharm*. 1998; 55:145–9.

2274. Tanoue N, Kishita S, Shiotsu K, et al. Compatibility of irinotecan hydrochloride injection with other injections. *Jpn J Hosp Pharm*. 1998; 24:420–8.

2275. Stiles ML, Allen LV Jr. Stability of two concentrations of heparin sodium prefilled in CADD-Micro pump syringes. *Int J Pharmaceut Compound*. 1997; 1:433–4.

2276. Nii LJ, Chin A, Cao TM, et al. Stability of sumatriptan succinate in polypropylene syringes. *Am J Health-Syst Pharm*. 1999; 56: 983–5.

2277. Proot P, Van Schepdael A, Raymakers AA, et al. Stability of adenosine in infusion. *J Pharm Biomed Anal*. 1998; 17:415–8.

2278. Biellmann-Berlaud V, Willemin JC. Stabilite de la vancomycine en poches de polyolefine ou polychlorure de vinyle et en flacons de verre. *J Pharm Clin*. 1998; 17(3):145–8.

2279. Mayer JLR, Pascale VJ, Clyne LP, et al. Stability of low-dose vancomycin hydrochloride in heparin sodium 100 IU/mL. *J Pharm Tech*. 1999; 15:13–7.

2280. Demange C, Vailleau JL, Wacquier S, et al. Etude de photosensibilite et fixation de la chlorpromazine sur le chlorure de polyvinyle pour administration en perfusion intraveineuse. *J Pharm Clin*. 1998; 17:77–82.

2281. Saito H, Tanida N, Inukai K, et al. Stability of iphosphamide and mesna in mixed infusion solutions. *Jpn J Hosp Pharm*. 1998; 24:96–99.

2282. Silvers KM, Darlow BA, Winterbourn CC. Pharmacologic levels of heparin do not destabilize neonatal parenteral nutrition. *JPEN J Parenter Enteral Nutr*. 1998; 22:311–4.

2283. Williamson JC, Volles DF, Lynch PLM, et al. Stability of cefepime in peritoneal dialysis solution. *Ann Pharmacother*. 1999; 33:906–9.

2284. Kramer I, Maas B. Compatibility of amsacrine (Amsidyl) concentrate for infusion with polypropylene syringes. *Pharmazie*. 1999; 54:538–41.

2285. Farina A, Porra R, Cotichini V, et al. Stability of reconstituted solutions of ceftazidime for injections: an HPLC and CE approach. *J Pharm Biomed Anal*. 1999; 20:521–30.

2286. Yokoyama H, Aoyama T, Matsuyama T, et al. The cause of polyurethane catheter cracking during constant infusion of etoposide (VP-16) injection. *Yakugaku Zasshi*. 1998; 118:581–8.

2287. Torres-Bondia FI, Carmona-Ibanez G, Guevara-Serrano J, et al. Estabilidad del valproate sodico en fluidos intravenosos. *Farm Hosp*. 1999; 23:320–2.

2288. Priston MJ, Sewell GJ. Stability of three cytotoxic drug infusions in the Graseby 9000 ambulatory infusion pump. *J Oncol Pharm Pract*. 1998; 4:143–9.

2289. Zeidler C, Dettmering D, Schrammel W, et al. Compatibility of various drugs used in intensive care medicine in polyethylene, PVC, and glass infusion containers. *Europ Hosp Pharm*. 1999; 5:106–10.

2290. Reference number not in use.

2291. Shay DK, Fann LM. Respiratory distress and sudden death associated with receipt of a peripheral parenteral nutrition admixture. *Infect Control Hosp Epidemiol*. 1997; 18:814–7.

2292. Zhan X, Yin G. Improved stability of 25% vitamin C parenteral formulation. *Int J Pharm*. 1998; 173:43–9.

2293. Mittner A, Vincze Z. Stability of cisplatin containing infusions. *Pharmazie*. 1998; 53:490–2.

2294. Carleton BC, Primmett DR, Levine M, et al. Sterility of unit-dosing filgrastim (G-CSF). *J Ped Pharm Pract*. 1999; 4: 68–74.

2295. Oliva A, Santovena A, Llabres M, et al. Stability study of human albumin pharmaceutical preparations. *J Pharm Pharmacol*. 1999; 51:385–92.

2296. Stephens D, Bares D, Robinson D, et al. Determination of amylose/particulate relationship in hydroxyethylstarch. *PDA J Pharm Sci Technol*. 1999; 53:181–5.

2297. Parsons TJ, Upton RN, Martinez AM, et al. No loss of undiluted propofol by sorption into administration systems. *Pharm Pharmacol Commun*. 1999; 5:377–81.

2298. Brigas F, Sautou-Miranda V, Normand B, et al. Compatibility of tropisetron with glass and plastics. Stability under different storage conditions. *J Pharm Pharmacol*. 1998; 50(4):407–11.

2299. Tse CST, Abdullah, R. Dissolving phenytoin precipitate in central venous access device. *Ann Intern Med*. 1998; 128:1049.

2300. Akinwande KI, Keehn DM. Dissolution of phenytoin precipitate with sodium bicarbonate in an occluded central venous access device. *Ann Pharmacother*. 1995; 29:707–9.

2301. Fuloria M, Friedberg MA, DuRant RH, et al. Effect of flow rate and insulin priming on the recovery of insulin from microbore infusion tubing. *Pediatrics*. 1998; 102:1401–6.

2302. Muller HJ, Frank C. Stabilitatstudie zu pentoxifyllin im PVC-infusionsbeutel. *Krankenhauspharmazie*. 1998; 19:469–72.

2303. Stahlmann SA, Frey OR. Stabilitatstudie zu fosfomycin-dinatrium (Fosfocin p.i. 5,0) in applikationfertigen perfusorspritzen. *Krankenhauspharmazie*. 1998; 19:553–7.

2304. Muller HJ, Frank C. Stabilitatstudie zu alizaprid im PVC-infusionsbeutel. *Krankenhauspharmazie*. 1999; 20:55–8.

2305. Sattler A, Jage J. Physico-chemical stability of infusion solutions for epidural administration containing fentanyl and bupivacaine or lidocaine. *Pharmazie*. 1998; 53:386–91.

2306. Laborie S, Lavoie JC, Pineault M, et al. Protecting solutions of parenteral nutrition from peroxidation. *JPEN J Parenter Enteral Nutr*. 1999; 23(2):104–8.

2307. Wakiya Y, Saiki A, Kondou N, et al. Stability of vitamins in the TPN mixture at a clinical site. *Jpn J Hosp Pharm*. 1999; 25: 40–7.

2308. Pertkkiewicz M, Knyt A, Majewska K, et al. Badania stabilnosci mieszanin odzywczych z aminomel 10%E i aminomel 12,5%E oraz emulsja tluszczowa ivelip 10% i 20%. *Farm Polska*. 1999; 55(16):756–63.

2309. Brawley V, Bhatia J. Effect of sodium metabisulfite on hydrogen peroxide production in light-exposed pediatric parenteral amino acid solutions. *Am J Health-Syst Pharm*. 1998; 55: 1288–92.

2310. Brawley V, Bhatia J. Hydrogen peroxide generation in a model paediatric parenteral amino acid solution. *Clin Sci*. 1993; 85: 709–12.

2311. Driscoll DF, Lawrence KR, Lewis K, et al. Particle size distribution of propofol injection from ampules and vials: the benefits of filtration. *Int J Pharmaceut Compound*. 1997; 1:118–20.

2312. Malesker MA, Malone PM, Cingle CM, et al. Extravasation of i.v. promethazine. *Am J Health-Syst Pharm*. 1999; 56:1742–3.

2313. Boersma HH, Groothuijsen HJG, Stolk LML, et al. Goed loudbaar onder normale omstandigheden. *Pharmaceut Weekblad*. 1999; 134:1444–8.

2314. Reference number not in use.

2315. Khalfi F, Dine T, Gressier B, et al. Compatibility of cefpirome and cephalothin with PVC bags during simulated infusion and storage. *Pharmazie*. 1998; 53:112–6.

2316. Laborie S, Lavoie JC, Pineault M, et al. Contribution of multivitamins, air, and light in the generation of peroxides in adult and neonatal parenteral nutrition solutions. *Ann Pharmacother*. 2000; 34:440–5.

2317. Laborie S, Lavoie JC. Paradoxical role of ascorbic acid and riboflavin in solutions of total parenteral nutrition: implication in photoinduced peroxide generation. *Pediat Res*. 1998; 43: 601–6.

2318. Rhoney DH, Coplin WM. Urokinase activity after freezing: implications for thrombolysis in intraventricular hemorrhage. *Am J Health-Syst Pharm*. 1999; 56:2047–51.

2319. Hrubisko M, McGown AT, Prendiville JA, et al. Suitability of cisplatin solutions for 14–day continuous infusion by ambulatory pump. *Cancer Chemother Pharmacol*. 1992; 29:252–5.

2320. Dine T, Khalfi F, Gressier B, et al. Stability study of fotemustine in PVC infusion bags and sets under various conditions using a stability-indicating high-performance liquid chromatographic assay. *J Pharm Biomed Anal*. 1998; 18:373–81.

2321. Hadfield JA, McGown AT, Dawson MJ, et al. The suitability of carboplatin solutions for 14–day continuous infusion by ambulatory pump: an HPLC-dynamic FAB study. *J Pharm Biomed Anal*. 1993; 11:723–7.

2322. Frey OR, Maier L. Polyethylene vials of calcium gluconate reduce aluminum contamination of TPN. *Ann Pharmacother*. 2000; 34:811–12.

2323. Louie S, Chin A. Activity of dalteparin sodium in polypropylene syringes. *Am J Health-Syst Pharm*. 2000; 57:760–2.

2324. Stewart JT, Maddox FC. Stability of cefepime hydrochloride injection and metronidazole in polyvinyl chloride bags at 4 °C and 22 °C-24 °C. *Hosp Pharm*. 2000; 35:1057–64.

2325. Ling J, Gupta VD. Stability of nafcillin sodium after reconstitution in 0.9% sodium chloride injection and storage in polypropylene syringes for pediatric use. *Int J Pharmaceut Compound*. 2000; 4:480–1.

2326. Gupta VD. Stability of levothyroxine sodium injection in polypropylene syringes. *Int J Pharmaceut Compound*. 2000; 4: 482–3.

2327. Davis SN, Vermeulen L, Banton J, et al. Activity and dosage of alteplase dilution for clearing occlusions of venous-access devices. *Am J Health-Syst Pharm*. 2000; 57:1039–45.

2328. Generali J, Cada DJ. Alteplase (t-PA) bolus: occluded catheters. *Hosp Pharm*. 2001; 36:93–103.

2329. Phelps KC, Verzino KC. Alternatives to urokinase for the management of central venous catheter occlusion. *Hosp Pharm*. 2001; 36:265–74.

2330. Haire WD, Herbst SL. Use of alteplase (t-PA) for the management of thrombotic catheter dysfunction: guidelines from a consensus conference of the National Association of Vascular Access Networks (NAVAN). *Nutr Clin Pract*. 2000; 15:265–75.

2331. Gupta VD, Ling J. Stability of hydrocortisone sodium succinate after reconstitution in 0.9% sodium chloride injection and storage in polypropylene syringes for pediatric use. *Int J Pharmaceut Compound*. 2000; 4:396–7.

2332. Xu QA, Trissel LA, Zhang Y, et al. Compatibility and stability of linezolid injection admixed with gentamicin sulfate and tobramycin sulfate. *Int J Pharmaceut Compound*. 2000; 4: 476–9.

2333. Trissel LA, Zhang Y. Incompatibility of erythromycin lactobionate and sulfamethoxazole/trimethoprim with linezolid injection. *Hosp Pharm*. 2000; 35:1192–6.

2334. Zhang Y, Xu QA, Trissel LA, et al. Compatibility of linezolid injection admixed with three quinolone antibiotics. *Ann Pharmacother*. 2000; 34:996–1001.

2335. Xu QA, Zhang Y, Trissel LA, et al. Adequacy of a new chlorhexidine-bearing polyurethane central catheter for administration of 82 selected parenteral drugs. *Ann Pharmacother*. 2000; 34:1109–16.

2336. Trissel LA. Drug compatibility differences with propofol injectable emulsion products. *Crit Care Med*. 2001; 29:466–8.

2337. Favier M, De Cazanove F, Coste A, et al. Stability of carmustine in polyvinyl chloride bags and polyethylene-lined trilayer plastic containers. *Am J Health-Syst Pharm*. 2001; 58(3):238–41.

2338. Zhang Y, Trissel LA. Compatibility of linezolid injection with intravenous administration sets. *J Am Pharm Assoc*. 2001; 41: 285–6.

2339. Trissel LA, Williams KY. Compatibility screening of Hextend during simulated Y-site administration with other drugs. *Int J Pharmaceut Compound*. 2001; 5:69–73.

2340. Gupta VD. Chemical stability of methylprednisolone sodium succinate after reconstitution in 0.9% sodium chloride injection and storage in polypropylene syringes. *Int J Pharmaceut Compound*. 2001; 5:148–50.

2341. Ling J, Gupta VD. Stability of cefepime hydrochloride after reconstitution in 0.9% sodium chloride injection and storage in polypropylene syringes for pediatric use. *Int J Pharmaceut Compound*. 2001; 5:151–2.

2342. Sterling J. Intralipids and tubing changes. *Hosp Pharm*. 2001; 36:258–9.

2343. Yuan P, Grimes GJ, Shankman SE, et al. Compatibility and stability of vincristine sulfate, doxorubicin hydrochloride, and etoposide phosphate in 0.9% sodium chloride injection. *Am J Health-Syst Pharm*. 2001; 58:594–8.

2344. Baker MT. Yellowing of metabisulfite-containing propofol emulsion. *Am J Health-Syst Pharm*. 2001; 58:1042.

2345. Gupta VD, Ling J. Stability of piperacillin sodium after reconstitution in 0.9% sodium chloride injection and storage in polypropylene syringes for pediatric use. *Int J Pharmaceut Compound*. 2001; 5:230–1.

2346. Bethune K, Allwood M, Grainger C, et al. Use of filters during the preparation and administration of parenteral nutrition: position paper and guidelines prepared by a British Pharmaceutical Nutrition Group Working Party. *Nutrition.* 2001; 17:403–8.

2347. Gellis C, Sautou-Miranda V, Arvouet A, et al. Stability of methylprednisolone sodium succinate in pediatric parenteral nutrition mixtures. *Am J Health-Syst Pharm.* 2001; 58:1139–42.

2348. Redhead HM, Jones CB. Pharmaceutical and antimicrobial differences between propofol emulsion products. *Am J Health-Syst Pharm.* 2000; 57:1174.

2349. Mirejovsky D, Ghosh M. Pharmaceutical and antimicrobial differences between propofol emulsion products. *Am J Health-Syst Pharm.* 2000; 57:1176–7.

2350. Trissel LA, Zhang Y. The stability of diluted vincristine sulfate used as a deterrent to inadvertent intrathecal injection. *Hosp Pharm.* 2001; 36:740–5.

2351. Thoma LA, Johnson-Singh A, Wood GC, et al. Physical compatibility of 10% alcohol in 5% dextrose injection with selected drugs during simulated Y-site administration. *Am J Health-Syst Pharm.* 2000; 57:2286–7.

2352. Chalmers JR, Bobek MB, Militello MA. Visual compatibility of amiodarone hydrochloride injection with various intravenous drugs. *Am J Health-Syst Pharm.* 2001; 58:504–6.

2353. Gupta VD, Bailey RE. Stability of alatrofloxacin mesylate in 5% dextrose injection and 0.45% sodium-chloride injection. *Int J Pharmaceut Compound.* 2000; 4:66–8.

2354. Gupta VD. Stability of levothyroxine sodium injection in polypropylene syringes, *Int J Pharmaceut Compound.* 2000; 4:482–3.

2355. Garabito MJ, Jimenez L, Bautista FJ, et al. Stability of tirofiban hydrochloride in 0.9% sodium chloride injection for 30 days. *Am J Health-Syst Pharm.* 2001; 58:1850–1.

2356. Bergquist PA, Manas D, Hunke WA, et al. Stability and compatibility of tirofiban hydrochloride during simulated Y-site administration with other drugs. *Am J Health-Syst Pharm.* 2001; 58:1218–23.

2357. Seto W, Trope A, Carfrae L, et al. Visual compatibility of sodium nitroprusside with other injectable medications given to pediatric patients. *Am J Health-Syst Pharm.* 2001; 58:1422–6.

2358. Zhang Y, Trissel LA. Stability of piperacillin and ticarcillin in AutoDose infusion system bags. *Ann Pharmacother.* 2001; 35:1360–3.

2359. Godwin DA, Kim NH, Zuniga R. Stability of baclofen and clonidine hydrochloride admixture for intrathecal administration. *Hosp Pharm.* 2001; 36:950–4.

2360. Quay I, Tan E. Compatibility and stability of potassium chloride and magnesium sulfate in 0.9% sodium chloride injection and 5% dextrose injection solutions. *Int J Pharmaceut Compound.* 2001; 5:323–4.

2361. Vega E, Sola N. Quantitative analysis of metronidazole in intravenous admixture with ciprofloxacin by first derivative spectrophotometry. *J Pharm Biomed Anal.* 2001; 25:523–30.

2362. Inagaki K, Miyamoto Y, Kurata N, et al. Stability of ranitidine hydrochloride with cefazolin sodium, cefbuperazone sodium, cefoxitin sodium and cephalothin sodium during simulated Y-site administration. *Int J Pharmaceut Compound.* 2000; 4:150–3.

2363. Trissel LA, Xu QA, Zhang Y, et al. Stability of ciprofloxacin and vancomycin hydrochloride in AutoDose infusion system bags. *Hosp Pharm.* 2001; 36:1170–3.

2364. Galanti LM, Hecq JD, Jeuniau P, et al. Assessment of the stability of teicoplanin in intravenous infusions. *Int J Pharmaceut Compound.* 2001; 5:397–400.

2365. Storms ML, Stewart JT, Warren FW. Stability of ephedrine sulfate at ambient temperature and 4 °C in polypropylene syringes. *Int J Pharmaceut Compound.* 2001; 5:394–6.

2366. Faouzi MA, Khalfi F, Dine T, et al. Stability, compatibility and plasticizer extraction of quinine injection added to infusion solutions and stored in polyvinyl chloride (PVC) containers. *J Pharmaceut Biomed Anal.* 1999; 21:923–30.

2367. della Cuno FSR, Mella M, Magistrali G, et al. Stability and compatibility of methylprednisolone acetate and ropivacaine hydrochloride in polypropylene syringes for epidural administration, *Am J Health-Syst Pharm.* 2001; 58:1753–6.

2368. Voytilla KL, Tyler LS, Rusho WJ. Visual compatibility of azithromycin with 24 commonly used drugs during simulated Y-site delivery. *Am J Health-Syst Pharm.* 2002; 59:853–5.

2369. Trissel LA, Zhang Y, Baker MB. Stability of fenoldopam mesylate in two infusion solutions. *Am J Health-Syst Pharm.* 2002; 59:846–8.

2370. Xu QA, Trissel LA, Saenz CA, et al. Stability of three cephalosporin antibiotics in AutoDose infusion system bags, *J Am Pharm Assoc.* 2002; 42:428–31.

2371. Gupta VD. Stability of cefotaxime sodium after reconstitution in 0.9% sodium chloride injection and storage in polypropylene syringes for pediatric use. *Int J Pharmaceut Compound.* 2002; 6:234–6.

2372. Walker SE, Dufour A, Iazzetta J. Concentration and solution dependent stability of cloxacillin intravenous solutions. *Can J Hosp Pharm.* 1998; 51:13–9.

2373. Trissel LA, Saenz CA. Compatibility screening of bivalirudin during simulated Y-site administration with other drugs. *Int J Pharmaceut Compound.* 2002; 6:311–4.

2374. Baroletti S, Hartman C, Churchill W. Visual compatibility of abciximab with selected drugs. *Am J Health-Syst Pharm.* 2002; 59:466–7.

2375. Li WY, Koda RT. Stability of irinotecan hydrochloride in aqueous solutions. *Am J Health-Syst Pharm.* 2002; 59:539–44.

2376. Trissel LA, Xu QA, Pham L. Physical and chemical stability of morphine sulfate 5 mg/mL and 50 mg/mL packaged in plastic syringes. *Int J Pharmaceut Compound.* 2002; 6:62–5.

2377. Trissel LA, Xu QA, Pham L. Physical and chemical stability of hydromorphone hydrochloride 1.5 mg/mL and 80 mg/mL packaged in plastic syringes. *Int J Pharmaceut Compound.* 2002; 6:74–6.

2378. Trissel LA, Xu QA, Pham L. Physical and chemical stability of low and high concentrations of morphine sulfate with bupivacaine hydrochloride packaged in plastic syringes. *Int J Pharmaceut Compound.* 2002; 6:70–3.

2379. Xu QA, Trissel LA, Saenz CA, et al. Stability of gentamicin sulfate and tobramycin sulfate in AutoDose infusion system bags. *Int J Pharmaceut Compound.* 2002; 6:152–4.

2380. Xu QA, Trissel LA, Pham L. Physical and chemical stability of low and high concentrations of morphine sulfate with clonidine hydrochloride packaged in plastic syringes. *Int J Pharmaceut Compound.* 2002; 6:66–9.

2381. Veltri MA, Conner KG. Physical compatibility of milrinone lactate injection with intravenous drugs commonly used in the pediatric intensive care unit. *Am J Health-Syst Pharm*. 2002; 59: 452–4.

2382. Elwell RJ, Spencer AP, Barnes JF, et al. Stability of furosemide in human albumin solution. *Ann Pharmacother*. 2002; 36: 423–6.

2383. Trissel LA, Saenz CA, Ingram DS, et al. Compatibility screening of Precedex during simulated Y-site administration with other drugs. *Int J Pharmaceut Compound*. 2002; 6:230–3.

2384. Zhang Y, Trissel LA. Stability of ampicillin sodium, nafcillin sodium, and oxacillin sodium in AutoDose infusion system bags. *Int J Pharmaceut Compound*. 2002; 6:226–9.

2385. Stewart JT, Storms ML, Warren FW. Stability of tubocurarine chloride injection at ambient temperature and 4 °C in polypropylene syringes. *Int J Pharmaceut Compound*. 2002; 6: 308–10.

2386. El Aatmani M, Poujol S, Astre C, et al. Stability of dacarbazine in amber glass vials and polyvinyl chloride bags. *Am J Health-Syst Pharm*. 2002; 59:1351–6.

2387. Jappinen A, Kokki H, Naaranlahti T. pH stability of injectable fentanyl, bupivacaine, or clonidine solution or a ternary mixture in 0.9% sodium chloride in two types of propylene syringes. *Int J Pharmaceut Compound*. 2002; 6:471–4.

2388. Wu CC, Wand DP, Wong CY, et al. Stability of cefazolin in heparinized and nonheparinized peritoneal dialysis solutions. *Am J Health-Syst Pharm*. 2002; 59:1537–8.

2389. Donnelly RF. Chemical stability of furosemide in minibags and polypropylene syringes. *Int J Pharmaceut Compound*. 2002; 6: 468–70.

2390. Schlesser V, Hecq JD, Vanbeckbergen D, et al. Effect of freezing, long-term storage, and microwave thawing of the stability of cefepime in 5% dextrose infusion in polyvinyl chloride bags. *Int J Pharmaceut Compound*. 2002; 6:391–4.

2391. Hartman CA, Baroletti SA, Churchill WW, et al. Visual compatibility of argatroban with selected drugs. *Am J Health-Syst Pharm*. 2002; 59:1784–5.

2392. Gupta VD. Chemical stability of dexamethasone sodium phosphate after reconstitution in 0.9% sodium chloride injection and storage in polypropylene syringes. *Int J Pharmaceut Compound*. 2002; 6:395–7.

2393. Trissel LA, Zhang Y. Stability of methylprednisolone sodium succinate in AutoDose infusion system bags. *J Am Pharm Assoc*. 2002; 42:868–70.

2394. Certain E, Beteta F, Goudou-Sinha C, et al. Stability of mycophenolate mofetil in 5% dextrose injection in polyvinyl chloride infusion bags. *Am J Health-Syst Pharm*. 2002; 59:2434–9.

2395. Beijnen JH, van Gijn R. Chemical stability of the cardioprotective agent ICRF-187 in infusion fluids. *J Parenter Sci Technol*. 1993; 47:166–71.

2396. Fatou A, Denis P, Conrath G, et al. Campto 20 mg/mL concentrate for infusion, stability during infusion, stability of the diluted parenteral solution prepared ahead of time in glass bottles and PVC bags.

2397. Bobineau V, Nguyen-Huu JJ. CPT-11 (RP 64174A) 20 mg/mL solution for injection, study of the stability of infusion solutions reconstituted in glass bottles or PVC infusion bags after 24 hours' storage at room temperature.

2398. Stolk LML, Chandi LS. Stabiliteit van cladribine in natriumchloride-oplossing 0,9% voor infusie, *Ziekenhuisfarmacie*. 1994; 10:138–9.

2399. Tiefenbacher EM, Haen E, Przybilla B, et al. Photodegradation of some quinolones used as antimicrobial therapeutics. *J Pharm Sci*. 1994; 83:463–7.

2400. Calis KA, Cullinane AM, Horne MK. Bioactivity of cryopreserved alteplase solutions. *Am J Health-Syst Pharm*. 1999; 56: 2056–7.

2401. Kaijser GP, Beijnen JH, Bult A, et al. A systematic study on the chemical stability of ifosfamide. *J Pharmaceut Biomed Anal*. 1991; 9:1061–7.

2402. Lau DWC, Walker SE, Fremes SE, et al. Adenosine stability in cardioplegic solutions. *Can J Hosp Pharm*. 1995; 48:167–71.

2403. Muller HJ, Berg J. Stabilitatstude zu apomorphine-hydrochlorid im PVC-infusionsbeutel, *Krankenhauspharmazie*. 1997; 18:468–73.

2404. Andrisano V, Gotti R, Leoni A, et al. Photodegradation studies on atenolol by liquid chromatography. *J Pharmaceut Biomed Anal*. 1999; 21:851–7.

2405. Blaise N, Vigeron J, Perrin A, et al. Stability of refrigerated and frozen solutions of ondansetron hydrochloride. *Eur J Hosp Pharm*. 1994; 4:12–3.

2406. Lougheed WD, Woulfe-Flanagan H, Clement JR, et al. Insulin aggregation in artificial delivery systems. *Diabetologia*. 1980; 19:1–9.

2407. Meyer G, Henneman PL. Buffered lidocaine. *Ann Emerg Med*. 1991; 20:218–9.

2408. Murakami CS, Odland PB, Ross BK. Buffered local anesthetics and epinephrine degradation. *J Dermatol Surg Oncol*. 1994; 20: 192–5.

2409. Hinshaw KD, Fiscella R, Sugar J. Preparation of pH-adjusted local anesthetics. *Ophthalmol Surg*. 1995; 26:194–9.

2410. Avelar MA, Walker SE. Stability and compatibility of reconstituted hydromorphone with potassium chloride or heparin. *Can J Hosp Pharm*. 1996; 49:140–5.

2411. Crowther J, Hrazdil J, Jolly DT, et al. Growth of microorganisms in propofol, thiopental, and a 1:1 mixture of propofol and thiopental. *Anesth Analg*. 1996; 82:475–8.

2412. El-Yazigi A, Wahab Fam, Afrane B. Stability study and content uniformity of prochlorperazine in pharmaceutical preparations by liquid chromatography. *J Chromatog A*. 1995; 690:71–6.

2413. Ekmore RL, Contois ME, Kelly K, et al. Stability and compatibility of admixtures of intravenous ciprofloxacin and selected drugs. *Clin Ther*. 1996; 18:246–55.

2414. Luo D, Dong H, Tang XZ, et al. Stability of amphotericin B in 50 g/L dextrose injection. *Chin Pharm J*. 1998; 33:220–2.

2415. Sewell GJ, Allsopp M, Collinson MP, et al. Stability studies on admixtures of 5-fluorouracil with carboplatin and 5-fluorouracil with heparin for administration in continuous infusion regimens. *J Clin Pharm Ther*. 1994; 19:127–33.

2416. Lugo RA, MacKay M, Rucho WJ. Stability of lorazepam 0.2 mg/L, 0.5 mg/mL, and 1 mg/mL in polypropylene syringes. *J Pediatr Pharmacol Ther*. 2001; 6:122–9.

2417. Zhao L, Yalkowsky SH. Stabilization of epitifibitide by cosolvents. *Int J Pharm*. 2001; 218:43–56.

2418. Gupta VD, Ling J. Stability of piperacillin sodium after reconstitution in 0.9% sodium chloride injection and storage in polypropylene syringes for pediatric use. *Int J Pharmaceut Compound*. 2001; 5: 230–1.

2419. Thiesen J, Kramer I. Physicochemical stability of irinotecan injection concentrate and diluted infusion solutions in PVC bags. *J Oncol Pharm Pract.* 2000; 6:115–21.

2420. Beitz C, Einberger C, Wehling M. Stabilitat und Kompatibilitat von Zytostatika-Zubereitungen mit Infusionslosungsbehaltern aus Polyethylene. *Krankenhauspharmazie.* 1999; 20:121–5.

2421. Favetta P, Allombert C, Breysse C, et al. Fortum stability in different disposable infusion devices by pyridine assay. *J Pharmaceut Biomed Anal.* 2002; 27:873–9.

2422. Orwa JA, Govaerts C, Gevers K, et al. Study of the stability of polymyxins B_1, E_1, and E_2 in aqueous solution using liquid chromatography and mass spectrometry. *J Pharmaceut Biomed Anal.* 2002; 29:203–12.

2423. Mayer MI, Weickum RJ, Solimando DA, et al. Stability of cisplatin, doxorubicin, and mitomycin combined with Iversol for chemoembolization. *Ann Pharmacother.* 2001; 35:1548–51.

2424. Loff S, Kabs F, Witt K, et al. Polyvinylchloride infusion lines expose infants to large amounts of toxic plasticizers. *J Ped Surg.* 2000; 35:1775–81.

2425. Storms ML, Stewart JT, Warren FW. Stability of neostigmine methylsulfate injection at ambient temperature and 4 °C in polypropylene syringes. *Int J Pharmaceut Compound.* 2002; 6:475–7.

2426. Ulsaker G, Teien G. Degradation of methylprednisolone sodium succinate in a diluent-containing vial. *Am J Health-Syst Pharm.* 2002; 59:2456–7.

2427. Johnson TJ, Voss G. Continuous infusion of undiluted lorazepam injection. *Am J Health-Syst Pharm.* 2002; 59:78–9.

2428. Storms ML, Stewart JT, Warren FW. Stability of lidocaine hydrochloride injection at ambient temperature and 4 °C in polypropylene syringes. *Int J Pharmaceut Compound.* 2002; 6:388–90.

2429. Gupta VD. Stability of pentobarbital sodium after reconstitution in 0.9% sodium chloride injection and repackaged in glass and polypropylene syringes. *Int J Pharmaceut Compound.* 2001; 6:482–4.

2430. Beitz C, Bertsch T, Hannak D, et al. Compatibility of plastics with cytotoxic drug solutions – comparison of polyethylene with other container materials. *Int J Pharm.* 1999; 185:113–21.

2431. Gupta VD: Stability of ketamine hydrochloride injection after reconstitution in water for injection and storage in 1–mL tuberculin polypropylene syringes for pediatric use. *Int J Pharmaceut Compound.* 2002; 6:316–7.

2432. Andrisano V, Hrelia P, Gotti R, et al. Photostability and phototoxicity studies on diltiazem. *J Pharmaceut Biomed Anal.* 2001; 25:589–97.

2433. Svedberg KO, McKenzie EJ, Larrivee-Elkins C. Compatibility of ropivacaine with morphine, sufentanil, fentanyl, or clonidine. *J Clin Pharm Ther.* 2002; 27:39–45.

2434. Servais H, Tulkens PM. Stability and compatibility of ceftazidime administered by continuous infusion to intensive care patients. *Antimicrob Agents Chemother.* 2001; 45:2643–7.

2435. Parti R, Mankarious S. Stability assessment of lyophilized intravenous immunoglobulin after reconstitution in glass containers and poly(vinyl chloride) bags. *Biotechnol Appl Biochem.* 1997; 23:13–8.

2436. Jappinen A, Kokki H, Naaranlahti TJ, et al. Stability of buprenorphine, haloperidol and glycopyrrolate mixture in a 0.9% sodium chloride solution. *Pharm World Sci.* 1999; 21:272–4.

2437. Jappinen A, Kokki H, Naaranlahti TJ, et al. Chemical stability of a mixture of fentanyl citrate, bupivacaine hydrochloride and clonidine hydrochloride in 0.9% sodium chloride injection stored in syringes and medication cassettes. *Pharm World Sci Suppl.* 1996; A11:119–21.

2438. Storms ML, Stewart JT, Warren FW. Stability of succinylcholine chloride injection at ambient temperature and 4 °C in polypropylene syringes. *Int J Pharmaceut Compound.* 2003; 7:68–70.

2439. Storms ML, Stewart JT, Warren FW. Stability of glycopyrrolate injection at ambient temperature and 4 °C in polypropylene syringes. *Int J Pharmaceut Compound.* 2003; 7:65–7.

2440. Mitchell AL, Gailey RA. Compatibility of caffeine citrate with other medications commonly used in a neonatal intensive care unit. *J Pediatr Pharm Pract.* 1999; 4:239–42.

2441. Wang DP, Lee DKT, Wang CN. Stability of sodium cefazolin and tenoxicam in 5% dextrose. *Chin Pharmaceut J.* 2001; 53:185–9.

2442. Shi A, Walker SE, Law S. Stability of ketorolac tromethamine in IV solutions and waste reduction. *Can J Hosp Pharm.* 2000; 53:263–9.

2443. Yano R, Nakamura T, Aono H, et al. The amount of the loss of cyclosporine A dose correlated with the amount of leaching di (2-ethylhexyl) phthalate from polyvinyl chloride infusion tube. *Yakugaku Zasshi.* 2001; 121:139–44.

2444. Micard S, Rieutord A, Prognon P, et al. Stability and sterility of meglumine gadoterate injection repackaged in plastic syringes. *Int J Pharm.* 2001; 212:93–9.

2445. Han H, Davis SS, Washington C. Physical properties and stability of two emulsion formulations of propofol. *Int J Pharm.* 2001; 215:207–20.

2446. Deitcher SR, Fesen MR, Kiproff PM, et al. Safety and efficacy of alteplase for restoring function in occluded central venous catheters: results of the cardiovascular thrombolytic to open occluded lines trial. *J Clin Oncol.* 2002; 20:317–24.

2447. Demore D, Vigeron J, Perrin A, et al. Leaching of diethylhexyl phthalate from polyvinyl chloride bags into intravenous etoposide solution. *J Clin Pharm Ther.* 2002; 27:139–42.

2448. Sakazume S, Sasahara K, Kawada T, et al. The adsorption of recombinant factor VIII (Kogenate) to infusion sets and inline filters. *Jpn J Pharm Health Care Sci.* 2001; 27:143–7.

2449. Little G (Director, Drug Information, Wyeth-Ayerst Pharmaceuticals, Philadelphia, PA): Personal communication; 1999 Mar 5.

2450. Hecq JD, Lebrun J, Vanbeckbergen D, et al. Effect of freezing, long-term storage, and microwave thawing on the stability of ketorolac tromethamine and tramadol hydrochloride in 5% dextrose infusion.

2451. Nguyen-Huu JJ, Bousquet O, Bobee JM. Compatibility of taxotere infusion solution with intravenous administration/extension sets, Rhone Poulenc Rorer, 2002.

2452. Suzuki M, Takamatsu S, Muramatsu E, et al. Loss of tacrolimus solution content and leaching of di-2-ethylhexyl phthalate in practice injection of precision continuous drip infusion. *Jpn J Hosp Pharm.* 2000; 26:7–12.

2453. He Y, Yu YC. Study on the stability of tetracaine hydrochloride injection. *Chin Pharm J.* 2001; 36:33–5.

2454. Chikuma T, Shinoda T, Taguchi K, et al. Stability of morphine hydrochloride in a total parenteral nutrient solution. *Jpn J Hosp Pharm.* 2000; 26:316–21.

2455. Farhang-Asnafi S, Barre J, Callaert S, et al. Compatibilite et stabilite du mélange bupivacaine-sufentanil en poche. *J Pharm Clin.* 2000; 19:248–51.

2456. Smith D. Akorn Laboratories. Arsenic trioxide injection, 1 mg/mL, 2001.

2457. Smith D. Akorn Laboratories. Arsenic trioxide injection, 1 mg/mL, 2000.

2458. Ball PA. Particulate contamination in parenteral nutrition solutions: still a cause for concern? *Nutrition.* 2001; 17:926–9.

2459. Allwood MC, Martin HJ. The photodegradation of vitamin A and E in parenteral nutrition mixtures during infusion. *Clin Nutr.* 2000; 19:339–42.

2460. Sforzini A, Bersani G, Stancari A, et al. Analysis of all-in-one parenteral nutrition admixtures by liquid chromatography and laser diffraction: study of stability. *J Pharmaceut Biomed Anal.* 2001; 24:1099–1109.

2461. Gibbons E, Allwood MC, Neal T, et al. Degradation of dehydroascorbic acid in parenteral nutrition mixtures. *J Pharmaceut Biomed Anal.* 2001; 25:605–11.

2462. Proot P, de Pourcq L, Raymakes AA. Stability of ascorbic acid in a standard total parenteral nutrition mixture. *Clin Nutr.* 1994; 13:273–9.

2463. Allwood MC, Brown PW, Ghedini C, et al. The stability of ascorbic acid in TPN mixtures stored in a multilayer bag. *Clin Nutr.* 1992; 11:284–8.

2464. Hak EB, Storm MC, Helms RA. Chromium and zinc contamination of parenteral nutrient solution components commonly used in infants and children. *Am J Health-Syst Pharm.* 1998; 55:150–4.

2465. Mehta RC, Head LF, Hazrati AM, et al. Fat emulsion particle-size distribution in total nutrient admixtures. *Am J Hosp Pharm.* 1992; 49:2749–55.

2466. Song YH, Burgess DJ, Herson VC, et al. Solubility of calcium acetate (CaAce) and sodium phosphate (NaP) in pediatric parenteral nutrition (PN) solution. *J Parenter Enteral Nutr.* 2000; 24:S22.

2467. Trissel LA, Saenz CA, Ogundele AB, et al. Compatibility of fenoldopam mesylate with other drugs during simulated Y-site administration. *Am J Health-Syst Pharm.* 2003; 60:80–5.

2468. Levadoux E, Sautou V, Bazin JE, et al. Medical plastics: compatibility of alfentanil and propofol alone or mixed. Stability of the alfentanil-propofol mixture. *Int J Pharm.* 1996; 127: 255–9.

2469. Trissel LA, Xu Q, Zhang Y, et al. Use of cysteine hydrochloride injection to increase the solubility of calcium and phosphates in FreAmine III-containing parenteral nutrition solutions. *Int J Pharmaceut Compound.* 2003; 7:71–3.

2470. Bell MS, Nolt DH. Visual compatibility of doxapram hydrochloride with drugs commonly administered via a Y-site in the intensive care nursery. *Am J Health-Syst Pharm.* 2003; 60: 193–4.

2471. Trissel LA, Xu QA. Stability of Imipenem–cilastatin sodium in AutoDose infusion system bags. *Hosp Pharm.* 2003; 38: 130–4.

2472. Naughton CA, Duppong LM, Forbes KD, et al. Stability of multidose, preserved formulation epoetin alfa in syringes for three and six weeks. *Am J Health-Syst Pharm.* 2003; 60:464–8.

2473. Xu QA, Trissel LA. Stability of clindamycin phosphate in AutoDose infusion system bags, *Int J Pharmaceut Compound.* 2003; 7:149–51.

2474. Gupta VD. Chemical stability of cefazolin sodium after reconstituting in 0.9% sodium chloride injection and storage in polypropylene syringes for pediatric use. *Int J Pharmaceut Compound.* 2003; 7:152–4.

2475. Zhang Y, Trissel LA. Stability of amikacin sulfate in AutoDose infusion system bags. *Int J Pharmaceut Compound.* 2003; 7: 230–2.

2476. Phares KR, Weiser WE, Miller SP, et al. Stability and preservative effectiveness of treprostinil sodium after dilution in common intravenous diluents. *Am J Health-Syst Pharm.* 2003; 60: 916–22.

2477. Hildebrand KR, Elsberry DD, Hassenbusch SJ. Stability and compatibility of morphine-clonidine admixtures in an implantable infusion system. *J Pain Symp Manage.* 2003; 25:464–71.

2478. Feddema S, Rusho WJ, Tyler LS, et al. Physical compatibility of vasopressin with medications commonly used in cardiac arrest. *Am J Health-Syst Pharm.* 2003; 60:1271–2.

2479. Trissel LA, Xu QA. Stability of cefepime hydrochloride in AutoDose infusion system bags. *Ann Pharmacother.* 2003; 37: 804–7.

2480. Lin YF, Wu CC, Lin SH, et al. Stability of cefazolin sodium in icodextrin-containing peritoneal dialysis solution. *Am J Health-Syst Pharm.* 2002; 59:2362–3.

2481. Cohen M (President, Institute for Safe Medication Practices, Huntingdon Valley, PA): Personal communication; 2003 Sep 5.

2482. Greenberg L. Errors and near misses linked to i.v. administration of sterile water for injection. *Pharm Pract News.* 2003; 30: 24.

2483. Roberts S, Sewell GJ. Stability and compatibility of 5-fluorouracil infusions in Braun Easypump. *J Oncol Pharm Pract.* 2003; 9:109–12.

2484. Laposata M, Johnson SM. Assessment of the stability of dalteparin sodium in prepared syringes for up to thirty days: an in vitro study. *Clin Ther.* 2003; 25:219–25.

2485. Gupta VD. Chemical stability of cefuroxime sodium after reconstitution in 0.9% sodium chloride injection and storage in polypropylene syringes for pediatric use. *Int J Pharmaceut Compound.* 2003; 7:310–2.

2486. Menard C, Bourguignon C, Schlatter J, et al. Stability of cyclophosphamide and mesna admixtures in polyethylene infusion bags. *Ann Pharmacother.* 2003; 37:1789–92.

2487. McQuade MS, Van Nostrand V, Schariter J, et al. Stability and compatibility of reconstituted ertapenem with commonly used i.v. infusion and coinfusion solutions. *Am J Health-Syst Pharm.* 2004; 61:38–45.

2488. Trissel LA, Saenz CA. Physical compatibility of antithymocyte globulin (rabbit) with heparin sodium and hydrocortisone sodium succinate. *Am J Health-Syst Pharm.* 2003; 60:1650–2.

2489. Musami P, Stewart JT, Taylor EW. Stability of zidovudine and dobutamine hydrochloride injections in 0.9% sodium chloride and 5% dextrose injections stored at ambient temperature (23 ± 2 °C) and 4 °C in 50-mL polyvinyl chloride bags up to 24 hours. *Int J Pharmaceut Compound.* 2004; 8:73–6.

2490. Masaki Y, Tanaka M, Nishikawa T. Physicochemical compatibility of propofol-lidocaine mixture. *Anesth Analg.* 2003; 97: 1646–51.

2491. Anderson PL, Miller S, Bushman LR. Stability of zidovudine with oxytocin in a simulated Y-site injection. *Am J Heath-Syst Pharm.* 2004; 61:394–96.

2492. Walker SE, Varrin S, Yannicelli D, et al. Stability of meropenem in saline and dextrose solutions and compatibility with potassium chloride. *Can J Hosp Pharm.* 1998; 51:156–68.

2493. Berlage V, Hecq JD, Vanbeckbergen D, et al. Long term stability of procaine hydrochloride cardioplegic infusion in P.V.C. bags at 4 °C. *Pharmakon.* 2003; 35:3–8.

2494. Kannan S. Incompatibility of prochlorperazine and ketoprofen. *Anaesthesia.* 2001; 56:920.

2495. Smith RPR, Jones M. Precipitation in Manchester:ketorolac/cyclizine. *Anaesthesia.* 2001; 56:494–5.

2496. Akhtar MJ, Khan MA, Ahmad I. Identification of photoproducts of folic acid and its degradation pathways in aqueous solution. *J Pharmaceut Biomed Anal.* 2003; 31:579–88.

2497. Tsui BCH, Cave D. Discoloration of parenteral ondansetron. *Anesth Analg.* 2003; 96:1239.

2498. Hartmann M, Knoth H, Kohler W. Stability of fentanyl/ropivacaine preparations for epidural application. *Pharmazie.* 2003; 58:434–5.

2499. Dager WE, Gosselin RC, King JH, et al. Anti-Xa stability of diluted enoxaparin for use in pediatrics. *Ann Pharmacother.* 2004; 38:569–73.

2500. Manley HJ, McClaran ML, Bedenbaugh A, et al. Linezolid stability in peritoneal dialysis solutions. *Perit Dial Int.* 2002; 22: 419–22.

2501. Semba CP, Weck S, Patapoff T. Alteplase: stability and bioactivity after dilution in normal saline solution. *J Vasc Interv Radiol.* 2003; 14:99–102.

2502. Faouzi MA, Dine T, Luyckx M, et al. Stability and compatibility studies of cephamandole nafate with PVC infusion bags. *J Pharmaceut Biomed Anal.* 1994; 12:99–104.

2503. Diduk N, Perez KG, de la Munoz L, et al. Estabilidad de ciclosporina inyectable (50 mg/ml). *Rev Mexicana Ciencias Farm.* 2000; 31:19–22.

2504. Bruch HR, Esser M. Catheter occlusion by calcium carbonate during simultaneous infusion of 5-FU and calcium folinate. *Onkologie.* 2003; 26:469–72.

2505. Vehabovic M, Hadzovic S, Stambolic F, et al. Stability of ranitidine in injectable solutions. *Int J Pharm.* 2003; 256: 109–15.

2506. Brodner G, Ermert T, Van Aken H, et al. Stability of sufentanil-ropivacaine mixture in glass and PVC reservoir. *Europ J Anesthesiol.* 2002; 19:295–7.

2507. Lettner A, Zollner P. Visuelle documentation der stabilitat der intravenosen losungen von omeprazole (Losec) und pantoprazole (Pantoloc). *Wien Med Wechenschr.* 2002; 152:568–78.

2508. Bosso JA, Taylor AJ, White RL, et al. Compatibility of two concentrations of recombinant human interleukin-1 receptor antagonist with selected antimicromial agents. *J Infect Dis Pharmacother.* 1995; 1:45–54.

2509. Nahata MC, Morosco RS, Sabados BK, et al. Stability and compatibility of anakinra with ceftriaxone sodium injection in 0.9% sodium chloride or 5% dextrose injection. *J Clin Pharm Ther.* 1997; 22:167–9.

2510. Nahata MC, Morosco RS, Sabados BK, et al. Stability and compatibility of anakinra and clindamycin phosphate injections in 0.9% sodium chloride injection. *J App Ther Res.* 1998; 2: 87–9.

2511. Nahata MC, Morosco RS, Sabados BK, et al. Stability and compatibility of anakinra with cimetidine hydrochloride or famotidine in 0.9% sodium chloride injection. *J Clin Pharm Ther.* 1995; 20:97–9.

2512. Nahata MC, Morosco RS, Sabados BK, et al. Stability and compatibility of anakinra with lorazepam injection in 0.9% sodium chloride injection. *J App Ther.* 1996; 1:191–2.

2513. Baririan N, Chanteux H, Viaene E, et al. Stability and compatibility study of cefepime in comparison with ceftazidime for potential administration by continuous infusion under conditions pertinent to ambulatory treatment of cystic fibrosis patients and to administration in intensive care units. *J Antimicrob Chemother.* 2003; 51:651–8.

2514. Sprauten PF, Beringer PM, Louie SG, et al. Stability and antibacterial activity of cefepime during continuous infusion. *Antimicrob Agents Chemother.* 2003; 47:1991–4.

2515. Vercaigne LM, Sitar DS, Penner SB, et al. Antibiotic-heparin lock: in vitro antibiotic stability combined with heparin in a central venous catheter. *Pharmacother.* 2000; 20:394–9.

2516. Vercaigne LM, Zhanel GG. Antibiotic-heparin lock: in vitro confirmation of antibacterial activity. *Can J Hosp Pharm.* 2000; 53:193–8.

2517. Sanchez del Aguila MJ, Jones MF, Vohra A. Premixed solutions of diamorphine in ropivacaine for epidural anaesthesia: a study on their long-term stability. *Br J Anaesthes.* 2003; 90:179–82.

2518. Ranchere JY, Latour JF, Fuhrman C, et al. Amphotericin B Intralipid formulation: stability and particle size. *J Antimicrob Chemother.* 1996; 37:1165–9.

2519. Hatem A, Marton S, Csoka G, et al. Preformulation studies of atenolol in oral liquid dosage form. I. Effect of pH and temperature. *Acta Pharmaceut Hung.* 1996; 66:177–80.

2520. Wiernikowski JT, Crowther M, Clase CM, et al. Stability and sterility of recombinant tissue plasminogen activator at −30 °C. *Lancet.* 2000; 355:2221.

2521. Barcia E, Reyes R, Luz Azuara M, et al. Compatibility of haloperidol and hyoscine-N-butyl bromide in mixtures for subcutaneous infusion to cancer patients in palliative care. *Support Care Cancer.* 2003; 11:107–13.

2522. Dix J, Weber RJ, Frye RF, et al. Stability of atropine sulfate prepared for mass chemical terrorism. *J Toxicol.* 2003; 41:771–5.

2523. Musami P, Stewart JT, Taylor EW. Stability of zidovudine and ranitidine in 0.9% sodium chloride and 5% dextrose injections stored at ambient temperature (23 ± 2 °C) and 4 °C in 50-mL polyvinylchloride bags up to 24 hours. *Int J Pharmaceut Compound.* 2004; 8:236–9.

2524. Gupta VD. Chemical stability of phenylephrine hydrochloride after reconstitution in 0.9% sodium chloride injection for infusion. *Int J Pharmaceut Compound.* 2004; 8:153–5.

2525. Norenburg JP, Achusim LE, Steel TH, et al. Stability of lorazepam in 0.9% sodium chloride in polyolefin bags. *Am J Health-Syst Pharm.* 2004; 61:1039–41.

2526. Lebrun J, Hecq JD, Vanbeckbergen D, et al. Effect of freezing, long-term storage and microwave thawing on the stability of tramadol in 5% dextrose infusion in polyvinyl chloride bags. *Int J Pharmaceut Compound.* 2004; 8:156–9.

2527. Sharley NA, Burgess NG. Stability and compatibility of alfentanil hydrochloride and morphine sulfate in polypropylene syringes. *J Pharm Pract Res*. 2003; 33:279–81.

2528. Xu QA, Trissel LA, Pham L. Physical and chemical stability of treprostinil sodium injection packaged in plastic syringe pump reservoirs. *Int J Pharmaceut Compound*. 2004; 8:228–30.

2529. Trissel LA, Saenz CA, Williams KY, et al. Incompatibilities of lansoprazole injection with other drugs during simulated Y-site coadministration. *Int J Pharmaceut Compound*. 2002; 5: 314–9.

2530. Braeden JU, Stendal TL, Fagernaes CB. Stability of dopamine hydrochloride 0.5 mg/mL in polypropylene syringes. *J Clin Pharm Ther*. 2003; 28:471–4.

2531. Good PD, Schneider JJ, Ravenscroft PJ. The compatibility and stability of midazolam and dexamethasone in infusion solutions. *J Pain Sympt Manag*. 2004; 27:471–5.

2532. Jaruratanasirikul S, Sriwiriyajan S. Stability of meropenem in normal saline solution after storage at room temperature. *Southeast Asian J Trop Med Pub Health*. 2003; 34:627–9.

2533. Xu QA, Trissel LA. Stability of palonosetron hydrochloride with paclitaxel and docetaxel during simulated Y-site administration. *Am J Health-Syst Pharm*. 2004; 61:1596–8.

2534. Sewell GJ, Rigsby-Jones AE, Priston MJ. Stability of intravesical epirubicin infusion: a sequential temperature study. *J Clin Pharm Ther*. 2003; 28:349–53.

2535. Trissel LA, Xu QA. Physical and chemical stability of palonosetron HCl in 4 infusion solutions. *Ann Pharmacother*. 2004; 38:1608–11.

2536. Curtis JM, Edwards DJ. Stability of trimethoprim in admixtures of trimethoprim-sulfamethoxazole prepared in polyvinyl chloride bags and glass bottles. *Can J Hosp Pharm*. 2002; 55: 207–11.

2537. La Forgia SP, Sharley NA, Burgess NG, et al. Stability and compatibility of morphine, midazolam, and bupivacaine combinations for intravenous infusion. *J Pharm Pract Res*. 2002; 32:65–8.

2538. Stecher AL, Morgantetti de Deus P, Polikarpov I, et al. Stability of L-asparaginase: an enzyme used in leukemia treatment. *Pharm Acta Helv*. 1999; 74:1–9.

2539. Arsene M, Favetta P, Favier B, et al. Comparison of ceftazidime degradation in glass bottles and plastic bags under various conditions. *J Clin Pharm Ther*. 2002; 27:205–9.

2540. Bennett J, Gross J, Nichols F, et al. The chemical and physical stability of a 1:1 mixture of propofol and methohexital. *Anesth Prog*. 2001; 48:61–5.

2541. Lepage R, Walker SE, Godin J. Stability and compatibility of etoposide in normal saline. *Can J Hosp Pharm*. 2000; 53: 338–44.

2542. Mayer JLR, Pascale VJ, Clyne LP, et al. Stability of low-dose vancomycin hydrochloride in heparin sodium 100 IU/mL. *J Pharm Tech*. 1999; 15:13–7.

2543. Park JW, Park ES, Chi SC, et al. The effect of lidocaine on the globule size distribution of propofol emulsions. *Anesth Analg*. 2003; 97:769–71.

2544. Vincentelli J, Braguer D, Guillet P, et al. Formulation of a flush solution of heparin, vancomycin, and colistin for implantation access systems in oncology. *J Oncol Pharm Pract*. 1997; 3: 18–23.

2545. Westphal M, Hohage H, Buerkle H, et al. Adsorption of sufentanil to epidural filters and catheters. *Europ J Anesthes*. 2003; 20:124–6.

2546. Hamilton MA, Stang L, Etches WS, et al. Stability of low molecular weight heparins stored in plastic syringes. *Thromb Res*. 2003; 112:1127–9.

2547. Vella-Brincat JWA, Begg EJ, Gallagher K, et al. Stability of benzylpenicillin during continuous home intravenous therapy. *J Antimicrob Chemother*. 2004; 53:675–7.

2548. Gill MA, Kislik AZ, Goree L, et al. Stability of advanced life support drugs in the field. *Am J Health-Syst Pharm*. 2004; 61: 597–602.

2549. Boitquin L, Hecq JD, Evrard JM, et al. Long-term stability of sufentanil citrate with levobupivacaine hydrochloride in 0.9% sodium chloride infusion PVC bags at 4 °C. *J Pain Symptom Manage*. 2004; 28:4–6.

2550. Jappinen A, Turpeinen M, Kokki H, et al. Stability of sufentanil and levobupivacaine solutions and a mixture in a 0.9% sodium chloride infusion stored in polypropylene syringes. *Europ J Pharm Sci*. 2003; 19:31–6.

2551. Gupta VD. Chemical stability of terbutaline sulfate injection after diluting with 0.9% sodium chloride injection when stored at room temperature in polyvinyl chloride bags. *Int J Pharmaceut Compound*. 2004; 8:404–6.

2552. Trissel LA, Zhang Y. Compatibility and stability of Aloxi (palonosetron hydrochloride) admixed with dexamethasone sodium phosphate. *Int J Pharmaceut Compound*. 2004; 8:398–403.

2553. Lai JJ, Brodeur SK. Physical and chemical compatibility of daptomycin with nine medications. *Ann Pharmacother*. 2004; 38: 1612–6.

2554. Smith DL, Bauer SM, Nicolau DP. Stability of meropenem in polyvinyl chloride bags and an elastomeric infusion device. *Am J Health-Syst Pharm*. 2004; 61:1682–5.

2555. Gong Y, Tian X, Xu Q. Compatibility of bumetanide injection combined with four kinds of injection. *China Pharm*. 2003; 6: 550–1.

2556. Ling J, Gupta VD. Stability of ethacrynate sodium after reconstitution in 0.9% sodium chloride injection and storage in polypropylene syringes for pediatric use. *Int J Pharmaceut Compound*. 2001; 5:73–5.

2557. Wang DP, Chiou HJ, Lee DKT. Compatibility and stability of ceftazidime sodium and tenoxicam in 5% dextrose injection. *Am J Health-Syst Pharm*. 2004; 61:1924–7.

2558. Ling J, Gupta VD. Stability of acyclovir sodium after reconstitution in 0.9% sodium chloride injection and storage in polypropylene syringes for pediatric use. *Int J Pharmaceut Compound*. 2001; 5:75–7.

2559. Xu XW, Du XL, Li DK, et al. Study on the sorption of fifteen injectable drugs in three different kinds of intravenous solution containers. *Chin Pharm J*. 2004; 39:205–7.

2560. Murata A, Okamoto Y, Sasa Y, et al. Effect of light and sodium bisulfite on the stability of thiamine in TPN fluids and integrated dose in period values. *Jpn J Pharm Health Care Sci*. 2004; 30: 266–70.

2561. Dedrick SC, Ramirez-Rico J. Potency and stability of frozen urokinase solutions in syringes. *Am J Health-Syst Pharm*. 2004; 61:1586–9.

2562. Valenzuela TD, Criss EA, Hammargen WM, et al. Thermal stability of prehospital medications. *Ann Emerg Med*. 1989; 18: 173–6.

2563. Ambados F, Brealey J. Compatibility of ketamine hydrochloride and fentanyl citrate in polypropylene syringes. *Am J Health-Syst Pharm*. 2004; 61:1438, 1445.

2564. Trissel LA, Saenz CA, Ogundele AB, et al. Physical compatibility of pemetrexed disodium with other drugs during simulated Y-site administration. *Am J Health-Syst Pharm*. 2004; 61: 2289–93.

2565. Alvarez JC, de Mazancourt P, Chartier-Kastler E, et al. Drug stability testing to support clinical feasibility investigations for intrathecal baclofen-clonidine admixture. *J Pain Sympt Manage*. 2004; 28:268–72.

2566. Trissel LA, Saenz CA, Ingram DS, et al. Compatibility screening of oxaliplatin during simulated Y-site administration with other drugs. *J Oncol Pharm Pract*. 2002; 8:33–7.

2567. White CM, Quercia R. Stability of extemporaneously prepared sterile testosterone solution in 0.9% sodium chloride solution large-volume parenterals in plastic bags. *Int J Pharmaceut*. 1999; 3:156–7.

2568. Kuti JL, Nightingale CH, Knauft RF, et al. Pharmacokinetic properties and stability of continuous-infusion meropenem in adults with cystic fibrosis. *Clin Ther*. 2004; 26:493–501.

2569. Ferreira E, Forest JM, Hildgen P. Compatibilite du dimenhydrinate injectable pour l'administration en Y. *Pharmactuel*. 2004; 37:17–20.

2570. Fubara JO, Notari RE. Influence of pH, temperature and buffers on cefepime degradation kinetics and stability predictions in aqueous solutions. *J Pharm Sci*. 1998; 87:1572–6.

2571. Brustugun J, Kristensen S, Hjorth Tonnesen H. Photostability of epinephrine—the influence of bisulfite and degradation products. *Pharmazie*. 2004; 59:457–63.

2572. Honisko ME, Fink JM, Militello MA, et al. Compatibility of argatroban with selected cardiovascular agents. *Am J Health-Syst Pharm*. 2004; 61:2415–8.

2573. Dooley DP, Tyler JR, Wortham WG, et al. Prolonged stability of antimicrobial activity in peritoneal dialysis solutions. *Perit Dial Int*. 2003; 23:58–62.

2574. Pere H, Chasse V, Forest JM, et al. Compatibilite du pantoprazole lors d'administration en Y. *Pharmactuel*. 2004; 37: 193–6.

2575. Baker MT, Gregerson MS, Martin SM, et al. Free radical and drug oxidation products in an intensive care unit sedative: propofol with sulfite. *Crit Care Med*. 2003; 31:787–92.

2576. Zaloga GP, Marik P. Sulfite-induced propofol oxidation: a cause for radical concern. *Crit Care Med*. 2003; 31:981–3.

2577. Lasak M. (Medical Information, Fujisawa): Personal communication. 2003; Sep 19.

2578. Boitquin LP, Hecq JD, Vanbeckbergen D, et al. Stability of sufentanil citrate with levobupivacaine hydrochloride in NaCl 0.9% infusion after microwave freeze-thaw treatment. *Ann Pharmacother*. 2004; 38:1836–9.

2579. Trissel LA, Zhang Y. Physical and chemical stability of palonosetron HCl with cisplatin, carboplatin, and oxaliplatin during simulated Y-site administration. *J Oncol Pharm Pract*. 2004; 10:191–5.

2580. Sprandal KA, Styrczula DE, Deyo K, et al. Stability and compatibility of levofloxacin and metronidazole during simulated and actual Y-site administration. *Am J Health-Syst Pharm*. 2005; 62:88–92.

2581. Trissel LA, Zhang Y. Palonosetron HCl compatibility and stability with doxorubicin HCl and epirubicin HCl during simulated Y-site administration. *Ann Pharmacother*. 2005; 39: 280–3.

2582. Lim SCB, Roberts MJ, Paech MJ, et al. Stability of insulin aspart in normal saline infusion. *J Pharm Pract Res*. 2004; 34: 11–3.

2583. Hildebrand KR, Elsberry DD, Deer TR. Stability, compatibility, and safety of intrathecal bupivacaine administered chronically via an implantable delivery system. *Clin J Pain*. 2001; 17: 239–44.

2584. Hildebrand KR, Elsberry DE, Anderson VC. Stability and compatibility of hydromorphone hydrochloride in an implantable infusion system. *J Pain Sympt Manag*. 2001; 22:1042–7.

2585. Classen AM, Wmbish GH, Kupiec TC. Stability of admixture containing morphine sulfate, bupivacaine hydrochloride, and clonidine hydrochloride in an implantable infusion system. *J Pain Sympt Manag*. 2004; 28:603–10.

2586. Gupta VD. Chemical stability of metoclopramide hydrochloride injection diluted with 0.9% sodium chloride injection in polypropylene syringes at room temperature. *Int J Pharmaceut Compound*. 2005; 9:72–4.

2587. Bourdeaux D, Sautou-Miranda V, Bagel-Boithias S, et al. Analysis by liquid chromatography and infrared spectrometry of di(2-ethylhexyl)phthalate released by multilayer infusion tubing. *J Pharmaceut Biomed Anal*. 2004; 35:57–64.

2588. Kambia K, Dine T, Gressier B, et al. Evaluation of childhood exposure to di(2-ethylhexyl)phthalate from perfusion kits during long-term parenteral nutrition. *Int J Pharm*. 2003; 262: 83–91.

2589. Driscoll DF, Dunbar JG, Marmarou A. Fat-globule size in a propofol emulsion containing sodium metabisulfite. *Am J Health-Syst Pharm*. 2004; 61:1276–80.

2590. Turnbull K, Bielech M, Walker SE, et al. Stability of oxycodone hydrochloride for injection in dextrose and saline solutions. *Can J Hosp Pharm*. 2002; 55:272–7.

2591. Rigge DC, Jones MF. Shelf lives of aseptically prepared medicines—stability of netilmicin injection in polypropylene syringes. *J Pharmaceut Biomed Anal*. 2004; 35:1251–6.

2592. Hecq JD, Boitquin LP, Vanbeckbergen D, et al. Effect of freezing and microwave thawing on the stability of cefuroxime in 5% dextrose infusion polyolefin bags at 4 °C. *Ann Pharmacother*. 2005; 39:1244–8.

2593. Rudich Z, Peng P, Dunn E, et al. Stability of clonidine in clonidine-hydromorphone mixture from implanted intrathecal infusion pumps in chronic pain patients. *J Pain Sympt Manag*. 2004; 28:599–602.

2594. Oh J, Gwak H, Moon H, et al. Stability of roxatidine acetate in parenteral nutrient solutions containing different amino acid formulations. *Am J Health-Syst Pharm*. 2005; 62:289–91.

2595. Noppawinyoowong C, Srisangchun J, Pongjanyakul T, et al. Chemical stability of frozen ganciclovir intravitreal injections. *Thai J Hosp Pharm*. 2003; 13:213–8.

2596. Kim YH, Heinze TM, Beger R, et al. A kinetic study on the degradation of erythromycin A in aqueous solution. *Int J Pharm*. 2004; 271:63–76.

2597. Ambados F. Incompatibility between calcium and sulfate ions in solutions for injection. *J Pharm Pract Res*. 2002; 32:307–9.

2598. Tang WM, Xue PH. Stability of ceftriaxone sodium injections. *Pharm Care Res*. 2002; 2:171–3.

2599. Torne GR, Luque AA, Pozo JF, et al. Estudio de la adsorcion de insulina en las bolsas de nutricion parenteral: influencia del tiempo de administracion y la temperatura. *J Clin Pharm*. 2003; 5:565–9.

2600. Gardiner PR. Compatibility of an injectable oxycodone formulation with typical diluents, syringes, tubings, infusion bags and drugs for potential co-administration. *Hosp Pharmacist*. 2003; 10:358–61.

2601. Sugiura M, Nakajima K, Yamada Y, et al. Adsorption of rhG-CSF (filgrastim) to extension tube. *Jpn J Pharm Health Care Sci*. 2003; 29:173–7.

2602. Priano RM, Hocht C, Oyola E, et al. Estabilidad de prostaglandina E1 fraccionada en jeringas de polipropileno. *Farm Hosp*. 2003; 27:304–7.

2603. Walker SE, Fau-Lun C, Wyllie A, et al. Physical compatibility of pantoprazole with selected medications during simulated Y-site administration. *Can J Hosp Pharm*. 2004; 57:90–7.

2604. Voges M, Faict D, Lechien G, et al. Stability of drug additives in peritoneal dialysis solutions in a new container. *Perit Dial Int*. 2004; 24:590–5.

2605. Bagel-Boithias S, Sautou-Miranda V, Bourseaux D, et al. Leaching of diethyl hexyl phthalate from multilayer tubing into etoposide infusion solutions. *Am J Health-Syst Pharm*. 2005; 62:182–8.

2606. Uebel RA, Wium CA, Schmidt AC. Stability evaluation of a prostaglandin E1 saline solution packed in insulin syringes. *Int J Impotence Res*. 2001; 13:16–7.

2607. Hennere G, Havard L, Bonan B, et al. Stability of cidofovir in extemporaneously prepared syringes. *Am J Health-Syst Pharm*. 2005; 62:506–9.

2608. Trissel LA, Xu QA. Physical and chemical stability of palonosetron hydrochloride with lorazepam and midazolam hydrochloride during simulated Y-site administration. *Int J Pharmaceut Compound*. 2005; 9:235–7.

2609. Trissel LA, Xu QA. Physical and chemical stability of palonosetron hydrochloride with topotecan hydrochloride and irinotecan hydrochloride during simulated Y-site administration. *Int J Pharmaceut Compound*. 2005; 9:238–41.

2610. Volonte MG, Valora PD, Cingolani A, et al. Stability of ibuprofen in injection solutions. *Am J Health-Syst Pharm*. 2005; 62:630–3.

2611. Phares KR, Wade M, Weiser WE, et al. Improved stability of treprostinil sodium with proper vial puncture technique and adapter use. *J Pharm Technol*. 2004; 20:270–5.

2612. He Y, Yu YC. Study on the stability of tetracaine hydrochloride injection. *Chin Pharm J*. 2001; 36:33–5.

2613. Priston MJ, Hughes JM, Santillo M, et al. Stability of epidural analgesic admixture containing epinephrine, fentanyl, and bupivacaine. *Anaesthesia*. 2004; 59:979–83.

2614. Hecq JD, Berlage V, Vanbeckbergen D, et al. Effects of freezing, long-term storage, and microwave thawing on the stability of piperacillin plus tazobactam in 5% dextrose for infusion. *Can J Hosp Pharm*. 2004; 57:276–82.

2615. Mann HJ, Demon SL, Boelk DA, et al. Physical and chemical compatibility of drotrecogin alfa (activated) with 34 drugs during simulated Y-site administration. *Am J Health-Syst Pharm*. 2004; 61:2664–71.

2616. Elwell RJ, Volino LR, Frye RF. Stability of cefepime in icodextrin peritoneal dialysis solution. *Ann Pharmacother*. 2004; 38:2041–4.

2617. Trissel LA, Ogundele AB. Compatibility of anidulafungin with other drugs during simulated Y-site administration. *Am J Health-Syst Pharm*. 2005; 62:834–7.

2618. Dupertuis YM, Morch A, Fathi M, et al. Physical characteristics of total parenteral nutrition bags significantly affect the stability of vitamins C and B1: A controlled prospective study. *J Parenter Enter Nutr*. 2002; 261:310–6.

2619. Driscoll DF, Nehne J, Peters H, et al. Physicochemical stability of intravenous lipid emulsions as all-in-one admixtures intended for the very young. *Clin Nutr*. 2003; 2:489–95.

2620. McNearney T, Bajaj C, Boyars M, et al. Total parenteral nutrition associated crystalline precipitates resulting in pulmonary artery occlusions and alveolar granulomas. *Digestive Dis Sci*. 2003; 48:1352–4.

2621. Lee MD, Yoon J, Kim S, et al. Stability of total nutrient admixtures in reference to ambient temperatures. *Nutrition*. 2003; 48:1352–4.

2622. Parikh MJ, Dumas G, Silvestri A, et al. Physical compatibility of neonatal total parenteral nutrient admixtures containing organic calcium and inorganic phosphate salts. *Am J Health-Syst Pharm*. 2005; 62:1177–83.

2623. Levi F, Metzger G, Massari C, et al. Oxaliplatin pharmacokinetics and chronopharmacological aspects. *Clin Pharmacokinet*. 2000; 38:1–21.

2624. Hoppe-Tichy T, Wenzel S, Gehring AK, et al. Stability of voriconazole concentrate and voriconazole in infusion bags. *Pharmazie*. 2005; 60:77–8.

2625. Nakamura L (Medical Information Department, Scios Inc., Fremont, CA). Personal communication; 2007 Jan 12.

2626. Steiner ME. Stability and sterility of dolasetron mesylate in syringes stored at room temperature. *Am J Health-Syst Pharm*. 2005; 62:896, 898–9.

2627. Trissel LA, Zhang Y. Physical and chemical stability of palonosetron hydrochloride with fluorouracil and with gemcitabine hydrochloride during simulated Y-site administration. *Int J Pharmaceut Compound*. 2005; 9:320–2.

2628. Lee G, Sabra K. Stability of morphine sulphate in ANAPA Plus ambulatory infusion device and PEGA infusion sets. *Europ J Hosp Pharm Sci*. 2006; 12:76–80.

2629. Chin A, Liu S, Ting-Chan J, et al. Extended stability of ascorbic acid in 5% dextrose injection and 0.9% sodium chloride injection. *Am J Health-Syst Pharm*. 2005; 62:1073–4.

2630. Patel K, Hursting MJ. Compatibility of argatroban with abciximab, eptifibatide, or tirofiban during simulated Y-site administration. *Am J Health-Syst Pharm*. 2005; 62:1381–4.

2631. Wazny L, Walker S, Moist L. Visual compatibility of gentamicin sulfate and 4% sodium citrate solutions. *Am J Health-Syst Pharm*. 2005; 62:1548, 1550.

2632. Barcia E, Martin A, Azuara ML, et al. Tramadol and hyoscine N-butyl bromide combined in infusion solutions: compatibility and stability. *Support Care Cancer*. 2007; 15:57–62.

2633. Laville I, Mercier L, Cachaty E, et al. Shelf-lives of morphine and pethidine solutions stored in patient-controlled analgesia devices: physico-chemical and microbiological stability study. *Pathol Biol (Paris)*. 2005; 53:210–6.

2634. Barcia E, Reyes R, Azuara ML, et al. Stability and compatibility of binary mixtures of morphine hydrochloride with hyoscine-n-butyl bromide. *Support Care Cancer*. 2005; 13:239–45.

2635. Fink JM, Capozzi DL, Shermock KM, et al. Alteplase for central catheter clearance: 1 mg/mL versus 2 mg/mL. *Ann Pharmacother*. 2004; 38:351–2.

2636. Lian MH, Shao MH, Yuan H, et al. Study on the stability of levofloxacin lactate for injection. *Chin J Antibiotics*. 2004; 29: 346–8.

2637. de Lemos M. Vinorelbine and venous irritation: optimal parenteral administration. *J Oncol Pharm Pract*. 2005; 11:79–81.

2638. DeFillippis MR, Bell MA, Heyob JA, et al. In vitro stability of insulin lispro in continuous subcutaneous insulin infusion. *Diabetes Tech Ther*. 2006; 8:358–68.

2639. Paul M, Razzouq N, Tixier G, et al. Stability of prostaglandin e_1 (pge_1) in aqueous solutions. *Europ J Hosp Pharm Sci*. 2005; 11:31–6.

2640. Xu QA, Trissel LA. Compatibility of palonosetron with cyclophosphamide and with ifosfamide during simulated Y-site administration. *Am J Health-Syst Pharm*. 2005; 62:1998–2000.

2641. Barker B, Feddema S, Rusho WJ, et al. Visual compatibility of vasopressin with other injectable drugs. *Am J Health-Syst Pharm*. 2005; 62:1969, 1975–6.

2642. Veggeland T. Visual compatibility of clonidine with selected drugs. *Am J Health-Syst Pharm*. 2005; 62:1968–9.

2643. Bougouin C, Thelcide C, Crespin-Maillard F, et al. Compatibility of ondansetron hydrochloride and methylprednisolone sodium succinate in multilayer polyolefin containers. *Am J Health-Syst Pharm*. 2005; 62:2001–5.

2644. Gupta VD. Chemical stability of hydralazine hydrochloride after reconstitution in 0.9% sodium chloride injection or 5% dextrose injection for infusion. *Int J Pharmaceut Compound*. 2005; 9: 399–401.

2645. Hecq JD, Boitquin LP, Venbeckbergen DF, et al. Effect of freezing, long-term storage, and microwave thawing on the stability of ketorolac tromethamine. *Ann Pharmacother*. 2005; 39: 1654–8.

2646. Onat D, Stathopoulos J, Rose A, et al. Reliability of nesiritide infusion via non-primed tubing and heparin-coated catheters. *Ann Pharmacother*. 2005; 39:1617–20.

2647. Voges M, Divino-Filho JC, Faict D, et al. Compatibility of insulin over 24 hours in standard and bicarbonate-based peritoneal dialysis solutions contained in bags made of different materials. *Perit Dial Int*. 2006; 26:498–502.

2648. Donnelly RF. Chemical stability of fentanyl in polypropylene syringes and polyvinyl chloride bags. *Int J Pharmaceut Compound*. 2005; 9:482–3.

2649. Lewis B, Jarvi E, Cady P. Atropine and ephedrine adsorption to syringe plastic. *AANA J*. 1994; 64:257–60.

2650. Nornoo AO, Elwell RJ. Stability of vancomycin in icodextrin peritoneal dialysis solution. *Ann Pharmacother*. 2006; 40: 1950–4.

2651. Velpandian T, Saluja V, Kumar Ravi A, et al. Evaluation of the stability of extemporaneously prepared ophthalmic formulation of mitomycin C. *J Ocular Pharmacol Ther*. 2005; 21:217–22.

2652. Abanmy NO, Zaghloul IY, Radwan MA. Compatibility of tramadol hydrochloride injection with selected drugs and solutions. *Am J Health-Syst Pharm*. 2005; 62:1299–302.

2653. Lee DKT, Wand DP, Harsono R, et al. Compatibility of fentanyl citrate, ketamine hydrochloride, and droperidol in 0.9% sodium chloride injection stored in polyvinyl chloride bags. *Am J Health-Syst Pharm*. 2005; 62:1190–2.

2654. Rigge DC, Jones MF. Shelf lives of aseptically prepared medicines—stability of hydrocortisone sodium succinate in PVC and non-PVC bags and in polypropylene syringes. *J Pharm Biomed Anal*. 2005; 38:322–6.

2655. Robinson RF, Morosco RS, Smith CV, et al. Stability of cefazolin sodium in four heparinized and non-heparinized dialysate solutions at 38 °C. *Perit Dial Int*. 2006; 26:593–7.

2656. Johnson CE. Stability of pantoprazole in 0.9% sodium chloride injection in polypropylene syringes. *Am J Health-Syst Pharm*. 2005; 62:2410–2.

2657. Swart EL, van Reij EML, Lee WC, et al. Visual compatibility of atosiban acetate with four drugs. *Am J Health-Syst Pharm*. 2005; 62:2459, 2463.

2658. Thalhammer F, Maier-Salamon A, Jager W. Examination of stability and compatibility of flucloxacillin (Floxapen) and ceftazidime (Fortum) in two infusion media: relevance for clinical practice. *Wien Med Wochenschr*. 2005; 155:337–43.

2659. Han J, Washington C. Partition of antimicrobial additives in an intravenous emulsion and their effect on emulsion physical stability. *Int J Pharm*. 2005; 288:263–71.

2660. Trissel LA, Xu QA, Baker M. Drug compatibility with new polyolefin infusion solution containers. *Am J Health-Syst Pharm*. 2006; 63:2379–82.

2661. Rodenbach MP, Hecq JD, Vanbeckbergen D, et al. Stability of cefuroxime infusion: the brand-name drug versus a generic product. *Europ J Hosp Pharm Sci*. 2006; 12:32–4.

2662. Cadrobbi J, Hecq JD, Lebrun C, et al. Long-term stability of voriconazole 4 mg/mL in dextrose 5% polyvinyl chloride bags at 4°C. *Europ J Hosp Pharm Sci*. 2006; 12:57–9.

2663. Andre P, Cisternino S, Chiadmi F, et al. Stability of bortezomib 1-mg/mL solution in plastic syringe and glass vial. *Ann Pharmacother*. 2005; 39:1462–6.

2664. Chan V. Influence of temperature and drug concentration on nafcillin precipitation. *Am J Health-Syst Pharm*. 2005; 62: 1347–8.

2665. Nguyen-Xuan T, Griffiths W, Kern C, et al. Stability of morphine sulfate in polypropylene infusion bags for use in patient-controlled analgesia pumps for postoperative pain management. *Int J Pharmaceut Compound*. 2006; 10:69–73.

2666. Wang DP. Stability of tetracaine in aqueous systems. *J Taiwan Pharm Assoc*. 1983; 35:132–41.

2667. Rigge DC, Jones MF. Shelf lives of aseptically prepared medicines—stability of piperacillin/tazobactam in PVC and non-PVC bags. *J Pharm Biomed Anal*. 2005; 39:339–43.

2668. Weck S, Cheung S, Hiraoka-Sutow M, et al. Alteplase as a catheter locking solution: in vitro evaluation of biochemical stability and antimicrobial properties. *J Vasc Interven Radiol*. 2005; 16:379–83.

2669. Pourroy B, Botta C, Solas C, et al. Seventy-two-hour stability of Taxol in 5% dextrose or 0.9% sodium chloride in Viaflo, Freeflex, Ecoflac, and Macoflex N non-PVC bags. *J Clin Pharm Ther*. 2005; 30:455–8.

2670. Ariz Ozdemir F, Anilanmert B, Pekin M. Spectrophotometric investigation of the chemical compatibility of the anticancer drugs irinotecan-HCl and epirubicin-HCl in the same infusion solution. *Cancer Chemother Pharmacol.* 2005; 56:529–34.

2671. Trissel LA, Zhang Y, Douglass K, et al. Extended stability of oxytocin in common infusion solutions. *Int J Pharmaceut Compound.* 2006; 10:156–8.

2672. Negro S, Martin A, Azuara ML, et al. Stability of tramadol and haloperidol for continuous subcutaneous infusion at home. *J Pain Symptom Manage.* 2005; 30:192–9.

2673. Sautou-Miranda V, Brigas F, Vanheerswynghels S, et al. Compatibility of paclitaxel in 5% glucose solution with ECOFLAC low-density polyethylene containers—stability under different storage conditions. *Int J Pharm.* 1999; 178:77–82.

2674. Trittler R. Stability of intravenous admixtures of doxorubicin and vincristine confirmed by LC-MS. *Europ J Hosp Pharm Sci.* 2006; 12:10–2.

2675. Chan J, Walker SE, Law S. Stability of dolasetron mesylate in 0.9% sodium chloride and 5% dextrose in water. *Can J Hosp Pharm.* 2003; 56:87–92.

2676. Zhang Y, Trissel LA. Physical and chemical stability of pemetrexed solutions in plastic syringes. *Ann Pharmacother.* 2005; 39:2026–8.

2677. Watson DG, Lin M, Morton A, et al. Compatibility and stability of dexamethasone sodium phosphate and ketamine hydrochloride subcutaneous infusions in polypropylene syringes. *J Pain Symptom Manage.* 2005; 30:80–6.

2678. Lee G, Sabra K, Doyle L, et al. Stability of morphine sulphate in P.C.A.s. *Europ J Hosp Pharm Sci.* 2003; 8:1–9.

2679. Theou N, Havard L, Maestroni ML, et al. Leaching of di(2-ethylhexyl)phthalate from polyvinyl chloride medical devices: recommendations for taxanes infusion. *Europ J Hosp Pharm Sci.* 2005; 11:55–61.

2680. Hartman CA, Faria CE, Mago K. Visual compatibility of bivalirudin with selected drugs. *Am J Health-Syst Pharm.* 2004; 61:1774, 1776.

2681. Trissel LA, Zhang Y, Xu QA. Physical and chemical stability of palonosetron hydrochloride with dacarbazine and with methylprednisolone sodium succinate during simulated Y-site administration. *Int J Pharmaceut Compound.* 2006; 10:234–6.

2682. Rodenbach MP, Hecq JD, Vanbeckbergen ED, et al. Effect of freezing, long-term storage and microwave thawing on the stability of vancomycin hydrochloride in 5% dextrose infusions. *Europ J Hosp Pharm Sci.* 2005; 11:111–3.

2683. Trusley C, Kupiec TC, Trissel LA. Compatibility of micafungin injection with other drugs during simulated Y-site co-administration. *Int J Pharmaceut Compound.* 2006; 10:230–3.

2684. Robinson JL, Tawfik G, Saxinger L, et al. Stability of heparin and physical compatibility of heparin/antibiotic solutions in concentrations appropriate for antibiotic lock therapy. *J Antimicrob Chemother.* 2005; 56:951–3.

2685. Corvino TF, Nahata MC, Angelos MG, et al. Availability, stability, and sterility of pralidoxime for mass casualty use. *Ann Emerg Med.* 2006; 47:272–7.

2686. Robinson RF, Morosco R. Stability of ciprofloxacin in four heparinized and nonheparinized dialysate solutions at 38°C. *ASHP Midyear Clinical Meeting Poster.* Dec 2005; 40:P442E.

2687. Faria CE, Fiumara K, Patel N, et al. Visual compatibility of furosemide with phenylephrine and vasopressin. *Am J Health-Syst Pharm.* 2006; 63:906, 908.

2688. Boothby LA, Madabushi R, Kumar V, et al. Extended stability of oxytocin in Ringer's lactate solution at 4° and 25°C. *Hosp Pharm.* 2006; 41:437–41.

2689. Zhang Y, Trissel LA. Physical and chemical stability of pemetrexed in infusion solutions. *Ann Pharmacother.* 2006; 40:1082–5.

2690. Driscoll DF. Lipid injectable emulsions: pharmacopeial and safety issues. *Pharm Res.* 2006; 23:1959–69.

2691. Anacardio R, Bartolini S, Gentile MM, et al. HPLC investigated physicochemical compatibility between artrosilene injectable solution and other pharmaceutical products frequently used for combined therapy into elastomeric Baxter LV5 infusion device. *Inter J Immunopath Pharmacol.* 2005; 18:791–8.

2692. Gupta VD. Chemical stability of pyridoxine hydrochloride 100-mg/mL injection, preservative free. *Int J Pharmaceut Compound.* 2006; 10:318–9.

2693. Zhang Y, Trissel LA. Physical instability of frozen pemetrexed solutions in PVC bags. *Ann Pharmacother.* 2006; 40:1289–92.

2694. Sahraoui L, Chiadmi F, Schlatter J, et al. Stability of voriconazole injection in 0.9% sodium chloride and 5% dextrose injection. *Am J Health-Syst Pharm.* 2006; 63:1423–6.

2695. Hamada C, Hayashi K, Shou I, et al. Pharmacokinetics of calcitriol and maxacalcitol administered into peritoneal dialysate bags in peritoneal dialysis patients. *Perit Dial Int.* 2005; 25:570–5.

2696. Carpenter JF, McNulty MA, Dusci LJ, et al. Stability of omeprazole sodium and pantoprazole sodium diluted for intravenous infusion. *J Pharm Technol.* 2006; 22:95–8.

2697. Mendez ASL, Dalomo J, Steppe M, et al. Stability and degradation kinetics of meropenem in powder for injection and reconstituted samples. *J Pharm Biomed Anal.* 2006; 41:1363–6.

2698. Kumarvel V, Gandhimani P, Cundill G. Frozen succinylcholine chloride. *Anaesthesia.* 2006; 61:202.

2699. Stone J, Fawcett W. A case of frozen succinylcholine chloride encountered during emergency Cesarean delivery. *Anesth Analg.* 2002; 95:1465.

2700. Negro S, Reyes R, Azuara ML, et al. Morphine, haloperidol and hyoscine N-butyl bromide combined in s.c. infusion solutions: compatibility and stability evaluation in terminal oncology patients. *Int J Pharm.* 2006; 307:278–84.

2701. Negro S, Azuara ML, Sanchez Y, et al. Physical compatibility and in vivo evaluation of drug mixtures for subcutaneous infusion to cancer patients in palliative care. *Support Care Cancer.* 2002; 10:65–70.

2702. Shields D, Montenegro R, Ragusa M. Chemical stability of admixtures combining ziconotide with morphine or hydromorphone during simulated intrathecal administration. *Neuromodulation.* 2005; 4:257–63.

2703. Shields D, Montenegro R. The chemical stability of admixtures combining ziconotide and clonidine during simulated intrathecal administration. *7th Congress International Modulation Society Poster.* Jun 2005.

2704. Shields D, Montenegro R, Aclan J. The chemical stability of admixtures combining ziconotide and bupivacaine hydrochloride during simulated intrathecal administration. *7th Congress International Modulation Society Poster.* Jun 2005.

2705. Huang L. Effect of pH and temperature on the stability of 1% tetracaine hydrochloride injection. *Yaoxue Tongbao.* 1982; 17: 208–9.

2706. Kambia NK, Luyckx M, Dine T, et al. Stability and compatibility of paracetamol injection admixed with ketoprofen. *Europ J Hosp Pharm Sci.* 2006; 12:81–4.

2707. Hecq JD, Boitquin L, Lebrun C, et al. Freeze thaw treatment of ketorolac tromethamine in 5% dextrose infusion polyolefin bags: effect of drug concentration and microwave power on the long-term stability at 4°C. *Europ J Hosp Pharm Sci.* 2006; 12: 72–5.

2708. Donyai P, Sewell GJ. Physical and chemical stability of paclitaxel infusions in different container types. *J Oncol Pharm Pract.* 2006; 12:211–2.

2709. Fielding H, Kyaterekera N, Skellern GG, et al. The compatibility and stability of octreotide acetate in the presence of diamorphine hydrochloride in polypropylene syringes. *Palliative Med.* 2000; 14:205–7.

2710. Vranken JH, van Kan HJ, van der Vegt MH. Stability and compatibility of a meperidine-clonidine mixture in portable pump reservoirs for the management of cancer pain syndromes. *J Pain Symptom Manage.* 2006; 32:297–9.

2711. Negro S, Rendon AL, Azuara ML, et al. Compatibility and stability of furosemide and dexamethasone combined in infusion solutions. *Arnzneim-Forsch.* 2006; 56:714–20.

2712. Fernandez-Varon E, Marin P, Espuny A, et al. Stability of moxifloxacin injection in peritoneal dialysis solution bags (Dianeal PD1 1.36% and Dianeal PD1 3.86%). *J Clin Pharm Ther.* 2006; 31:641–3.

2713. Shields D, Aclan J, Szatkowski A, et al. The chemical stability of an admixture containing 25 mcg/mL ziconotide and 20 mg/mL morphine sulfate during simulated intrathecal administration. *N Amer Neuromodulation Soc Poster.* 2006.

2714. Ludwig S, Vencl-Joncic M, Gandhi P, et al. Simulated Y-site compatibility testing of various diluents and drug products with tigecycline, a first-in-class intravenous glycylcycline. *ASHP Summer Meeting Poster.* 2006; P62E.

2715. Carroll JA. Stability of flucloxacillin in elastomeric infusion devices. *J Pharm Pract Res.* 2005; 35:90–2.

2716. Trusley C, Ben M, Kupiec TC, et al. Physical and chemical stability of palonosetron with metoclopramide and promethazine during simulated Y-site administration. *Int J Pharmaceut Compound.* 2007; 11:82–5.

2717. Chapalain-Pargrade S, Laville I, Paci A, et al. Microbiological and physicochemical stability of fentanyl and sufentanil solutions for patient-controlled delivery systems. *J Pain Symptom Manage.* 2006; 32:90–7.

2718. Dalle M, Sautou-Miranda V, Balayssac D, et al. Can solutions of docetaxel be conditioned in PVC bags?. *J Pharm Clin.* 2006; 25:147–52.

2719. Kovalick LJ, Pikalov AA, Ni N, et al. Short-term physical compatibility of intramuscular aripiprazole with intramuscular lorazepam. *Am J Health-Syst Pharm.* 2008; 65:2007–8.

2720. Trissel LA, Trusley C, Ben M, et al. Physical and chemical stability of palonosetron hydrochloride with five opiate agonists during simulated Y-site administration. *Am J Health-Syst Pharm.* 2007; 64:1209–13.

2721. Driscoll DF, Sivestri AP, Nehne J, et al. Physicochemical stability of highly concentrated total nutrient admixtures for fluid-restricted patients. *Am J Health-Syst Pharm.* 2006; 63:79–85.

2722. Pietroski N (Associate Director, Medical Services, Merck & Co., North Wales, PA). Personal communication; 2007 Jun 15.

2723. Pietroski N (Associate Director, Medical Services, Merck & Co., North Wales, PA). Personal communication; 2007 Jun 29.

2724. Hecq JD, Evrard JM, Vanbeckbergen DF, et al. Effect of freezing, long term storage and microwave thawing on the stability of ceftriaxone sodium in 5% dextrose infusion polyolefin bags at 2–8 °C. *Europ J Hosp Pharm Sci.* 2006; 12:52–6.

2725. Sudekum MJ (Manager, Clinical Pharmacy Services, Botsford Hospital, Farmington Hills, MI): Personal communication; 2007 Jun 6.

2726. Nolin TD, Lambert DA, Owens RC Jr. Stability of cefepime and metronidazole prepared for simplified administration as a single product. *Diag Microbiol Infect Dis.* 2006; 56:179–84.

2727. Serrurier C, Chenot ED, Vigneron J, et al. Assessment of injectable drugs' administration in two intensive care units and determination of potential physico-chemical incompatibilities. *Europ J Hosp Pharm Sci.* 2006; 12:96–9.

2728. Kraft MD, Johnson CE, Chung C, et al. Stability of metoprolol tartrate injection 1 mg/mL undiluted and 0.5 mg/mL in 0.9% sodium chloride injection and 5% dextrose injection. *Am J Health-Syst Pharm.* 2008; 65:636–8.

2729. Kattige A. Long-term physical and chemical stability of a generic paclitaxel infusion under simulated storage and clinical-use conditions. *Europ J Hosp Pharm Sci.* 2006; 12:129–34.

2730. Griffiths W, Favet J, Ing H, et al. Chemical stability and microbiological potency of intravenous vancomycin hydrochloride in polypropylene syringes for use in the neonatal intensive care unit. *Europ J Hosp Pharm Sci.* 2006; 12:135–9.

2731. Anon. Rocephin (ceftriaxone sodium) for injection (posted 07/05/2007). FDA MedWatch 2007. http://www.fda.gov/Safety/MedWatch/SafetyInformation/SafetyAlertsforHuman-MedicalProducts/ucm152863.htm.

2732. Vanneaux V, Proust V, Cheron M, et al. A physical and chemical stability study of amphotericin B lipid complexes (Abelcet) after dilution in dextrose 5%. *Europ J Hosp Pharm Sci.* 2007; 13:10–3.

2733. Rondelot G, Serrurier C, Vigneron J, et al. Stability of pemetrexed 25 mg/mL in a glass vial and 5 mg/mL in a PVC container after storage for one month at 2–8 °C. *Europ J Hosp Pharm Sci.* 2007; 13:14–6.

2734. Anon. Colistimethate (marketed as Coly-Mycin M and generic products) (posted 6/28/2007). FDA MedWatch 2007. http://www.fda.gov/Safety/MedWatch/SafetyInformation/Safety-AlertsforHumanMedicalProducts/ucm152109.htm.

2735. Johnson CE, Cober MP. Stability of vecuronium in sterile water for injection stored in polypropylene syringes for 21 days. *Am J Health-Syst Pharm.* 2007; 64:2356–8.

2736. Johnson CE. Stability of a 12.5 mg/mL dolasetron injection in a 12-mL polypropylene syringe. *ASHP Midyear Clinical Meeting Poster.* Dec 2006.

2737. Kiser TH, Oldland AR, Fish DN. Stability of phenylephrine hydrochloride injection in polypropylene syringes. *Am J Health-Syst Pharm.* 2007; 64:1092–5.

2738. Cochran BG, Sowinski KM, Fausel C, et al. Physical compatibility and chemical stability of mycophenolate mofetil during simulated Y-site administration with commonly coadministered drugs. *Am J Health-Syst Pharm.* 2007; 64:1410–4.

2739. Karstens A, Kramer I. Chemical and physical stability of diluted busulfan infusion solutions. *Europ J Hosp Pharm Sci.* 2007; 13: 40–7.

2740. Karstens A, Kramer I. Viability of micro-organisms in novel anticancer drug solutions. *Europ J Hosp Pharm Sci.* 2007; 13: 27–32.

2741. Ponton JL, Munoz C, Rey M, et al. The stability of (lyophilized) gemcitabine in 0.9% sodium chloride injection. *Europ J Hosp Pharm.* 2002; 1:23–5.

2742. Adnet F, Le Moyec L, Smith CE, et al. Stability of succinylcholine solutions stored at room temperature studied by nuclear magnetic resonance spectroscopy. *Emerg Med J.* 2007; 24: 168–9.

2743. Brammer MK, Chan P, Heatherly K, et al. Compatibility of doripenem with other drugs during simulated Y-site administration. *Am J Health-Syst Pharm.* 2008; 65:1261–5.

2744. Andre P, Cisternino S, Roy AL, et al. Stability of oxaliplatin in infusion bags containing 5% dextrose injection. *Am J Health-Syst Pharm.* 2007; 64:1950–4.

2745. Cohen V, Jellinek SP, Teperikdis L, et al. Room-temperature storage of medications labeled for refrigeration. *Am J Health-Syst Pharm.* 2007; 64:1711–5.

2746. Dice JE. Physical compatibility of alprostadil with commonly used IV solutions and medications in the neonatal intensive care unit. *J Pediatr Pharmacol Ther.* 2006; 11:233–6.

2747. Negro S, Salama A, Sanchez Y, et al. Compatibility and stability of tramadol and dexamethasone in solution and its use in terminally ill patients. *J Clin Pharm Ther.* 2007; 32:441–4.

2748. Parti R, Schoppmann A, Lee H, et al. Stability of lyophilized and reconstituted plasma/albumin-free recombinant human factor VIII (ADVATE rAHF-PFM). *Haemophilia.* 2005; 11: 492–6.

2749. Ben M, Trusley C, Kupiec TC, et al. Palonosetron hydrochloride compatibility and stability with three β-lactam antibiotics during simulated Y-site administration. *Int J Pharmaceut Compound.* 2007; 11:520–4.

2750. Girbau J, Jane S. Diltiazem-HCl 1 mg/mL prediluted in normal saline and dextrose 5%: compounding with the Gri-Fill 3.0 system and stability study up to 90 days in Gri-Bag. November 2007.

2751. Shields D, Montenegro R, Aclan J. Chemical stability of an admixture combining ziconotide and bupivacaine during simulated intrathecal administration. *Neuromodulation.* 2007; 10: S1–5.

2752. Shields D, Montenegro R. Chemical stability of ziconotide-clonidine hydrochloride admixtures with and without morphine sulfate during simulated intrathecal administration. *Neuromodulation.* 2007; 10:S6–11.

2753. Shields D, Montenegro R, Aclan J. Chemical stability of admixtures combining ziconotide with baclofen during simulated intrathecal administration. *Neuromodulation.* 2007; 10: S12–17.

2754. Reference number not in use.

2755. Dura JV, Hinkle GH. Stability of a mixture of technetium Tc 99m sulfur colloid and lidocaine hydrochloride. *Am J Health-Syst Pharm.* 2007; 64:2477–9.

2756. Cober MP, Johnson CE. Stability of 70% alcohol solutions in polypropylene syringes for use in ethanol-lock therapy. *Am J Health-Syst Pharm.* 2007; 64:2480–2.

2757. Psathas PA. Stability of doripenem for injection (500 mg) in representative infusion fluids and containers. *ASHP Summer Meeting Poster.* 2007; 64(Jun):P57e.

2758. Chan P, Healtherly K, Kupiec TC, et al. Compatibility of caspofungin acetate injection with other drugs during simulated Y-site coadministration. *Int J Pharmaceut Compound.* 2008; 12: 276–8.

2759. Kaiser JD, Vigneron J, Zenier H, et al. Chemical and physical stability of dexrazoxane, diluted with Ringer's lactate solution, in polyvinyl and polyethylene containers. *Europ J Hosp Pharm Sci.* 2007; 13:55–9.

2760. Kupiec TC, Aloumanis V, Ben M, et al. Physical and chemical stability of esomeprazole sodium solutions. *Ann Pharmacother.* 2008; 42:1247–51.

2761. Walker SE. Stability of docetaxel solution after dilution in ethanol and storage in vials and after dilution in normal saline and storage in bags. *Can J Hosp Pharm.* 2007; 60:231–7.

2762. Chan P, Bishop A, Kupiec TC, et al. Compatibility of ceftobiprole medocaril with selected drugs during simulated Y-site administration. *Am J Health-Syst Pharm.* 2008; 65:1545–51.

2763. Roy JJ, Boismenu D, Mamer OA, et al. Room temperature stability of injectable succinylcholine dichloride. *Int J Pharmaceut Compound.* 2008; 12:83–5.

2764. Trusley C, Ben M, Kupiec TC, et al. Compatibility and stability of palonosetron hydrochloride with four neuromuscular blocking agents during simulated Y-site administration. *Int J Pharmaceut Compound.* 2008; 12:156–60.

2765. Kupiec TC, Ben M, Trusley C, et al. Compatibility and stability of palonosetron hydrochloride with gentamicin, metronidazole, or vancomycin during simulated Y-site administration. *Int J Pharmaceut Compound.* 2008; 12:170–3.

2766. Condie CK, Tyler LS, Barker B, et al. Visual compatibility of caspofungin acetate with commonly used drugs during simulated Y-site delivery. *Am J Health-Syst Pharm.* 2008; 65: 454–7.

2767. Brousseau P, Nickerson J, Dobson G. Dexamethasone and ondansetron incompatibility in polypropylene syringes. *Can J Anesth.* 2007; 54:953–4.

2768. Walker SE, Milliken D, Law S. Stability of bortezomib reconstituted with 0.9% sodium chloride at 4 °C and room temperature (23 °C). *Can J Hosp Pharm.* 2008; 61:14–20.

2769. Chandler C, Gryniewicz CM, Pringle T, et al. Insulin temperature and stability under simulated transit conditions. *Am J Health-Syst Pharm.* 2008; 65:953–63.

2770. Walker SE, Law S. Physical [visual] Y-site compatibility of Voluven with 38 other intravenous medications. *CSHP Annual Meeting Poster.* Aug 2007.

2771. Kupiec TC, Trusley C, Ben M, et al. Physical and chemical stability of palonosetron hydrochloride with five common parenteral drugs during simulated Y-site administration. *Am J Health-Syst Pharm.* 2008; 65:1735–9.

2772. Shields DE, Aclan J, Szatkowski A. Chemical stability of admixtures combining ziconotide with fentanyl or sufentanil during simulated intrathecal administration. *Int J Pharmaceut Compound*. 2008; 12:463–6.

2773. Ben M, Trusley C, Kupiec TC, et al. Physical and chemical stability of palonosetron hydrochloride with glycopyrrolate and neostigmine during simulated Y-site administration. *Int J Pharmaceut Compound*. 2008; 12:368–72.

2774. Goldenberg NA, Jacobson L, Hathaway H, et al. Anti-Xa stability of diluted dalteparin for pediatric use. *Ann Pharmacother*. 2008; 42:511–5.

2775. Ben M, Kupiec TC, Trusley C, et al. Compatibility and stability of palonosetron hydrochloride with lactated Ringer's, hetastarch in lactated electrolyte, and mannitol injections during simulated Y-site administration. *Int J Pharmaceut Compound*. 2008; 12:460–2.

2776. Tremblay M, Lessard MR, Trepanier CA, et al. Stability of norepinephrine infusions prepared in dextrose and normal saline solutions. *Can J Anesth*. 2008; 55:163–7.

2777. Kaestner S, Sewell G. A sequential temperature cycling study for the investigation of carboplatin infusion stability to facilitate "dose-banding". *J Oncol Pharm Pract*. 2007; 13:119-26.

2778. Newton DW, Driscoll DF. Chemistry and safety of phosphates injections. *Am J Health-Syst Pharm*. 2008; 65:1761–6.

2779. Stucki MC, Fleury-Souverain S, Sautter AM, et al. Development of ready-to-use ketamine hydrochloride syringes for safe use in post-operative pain. *Europ J Hosp Pharm Sci*. 2008; 14:14–8.

2780. Shields DE, Aclan J, Szatkowski A. Chemical stability of admixtures containing ziconotide 25 mcg/mL and morphine sulfate 10 mg/mL or 20 mg/mL during simulated intrathecal administration. *Int J Pharmaceut Compound*. 2008; 12:553–7.

2781. Donnelly RF, Corman C. Physical compatibility and chemical stability of a concentrated solution of atropine sulfate (2 mg/mL) for use as an antidote in nerve agent casualties. *Int J Pharmaceut Compound*. 2008; 12:550–2.

2782. Junker A, Roy S, Desroches MC, et al. Stability of oxaliplatin solution. *Ann Pharmacother*. 2009; 43:390–1.

2783. Taiwo T (Medical Communications, Hospira, Inc., Lake Forest, IL). Personal communication; 2009 Feb 23.

2784. Anon. Information for healthcare professionals ceftriaxone (marketed as Rocephin and generics). FDA Update 4/14/2009. http://www.fda.gov/Drugs/DrugSafety/PostmarketDrugSafety-InformationforPatientsandProviders/DrugSafety-InformationforHeathcareProfessionals/ucm084263.htm.

2785. Martinez JN, Alminana MA, Sales OD. Establidad en suero fisiologico del busulfan intravenoso en un envase de poliolefinas. *Farm Hosp*. 2008; 32:344–8.

2786. Schmid R, Koren G, Klein J, et al. The stability of a ketamine-morphine solution. *Anesth Analg*. 2002; 94:898–900.

2787. Lau MH, Hackman C, Morgan DJ. Compatibility of ketamine and morphine injections. *Pain*. 1998; 75:389–90.

2788. Trissel LA, Trusley C, Kupiec TC, et al. Compatibility and stability of palonosetron hydrochloride and propofol during simulated Y-site administration. *Int J Pharmaceut Compound*. 2009; 13:78–80.

2789. Valverde Molina E, Gonzalez Muniz V, Gomez-Maldonado J, et al. Stability of pantoprazole in parenteral nutrition units. *Farm Hosp*. 2008; 32:290–2.

2790. Donnelly RF, Willman E, Andolfatto G. Stability of ketamine-propofol mixtures for procedural sedation and analgesia in the emergency department. *Can J Hosp Pharm*. 2008; 61:426–30.

2791. McCluskey SV, Graner KK, Kemp J, et al. Stability of fentanyl 5 μg/mL diluted with 0.9% sodium chloride injection and stored in polypropylene syringes. *Am J Health-Syst Pharm*. 2009; 66:860–3.

2792. Aloumanis V, Ben M, Kupiec TC, et al. Drug compatibility with a new generation of VISIV polyolefin infusion solution containers. *Int J Pharmaceut Compound*. 2009; 13:162–5.

2793. Xu M, WArren FW, Bartlett MG. Stability of low-concentration ceftazidime in 0.9% sodium chloride injection and balanced salt solutions in plastic syringes under various storage conditions. *Int J Pharmaceut Compound*. 2009; 13:166–9.

2794. Canann D, Tyler LS, Barker B, et al. Visual compatibility of i.v. medications routinely used in bone marrow transplant recipients. *Am J Health-Syst Pharm*. 2009; 66:727–9.

2795. Newland AM, Mauro VF, Alexander KS. Physical compatibility of metoprolol tartrate injection with selected cardiovascular agents. *Am J Health-Syst Pharm*. 2009; 66:986–7.

2796. Vazquez R, Le Hoang MD, Martin J, et al. Simultaneous quantification of water-soluble and fat-soluble vitamins in parenteral nutrition admixtures by HPLC-UV-MS/MS. *Eur J Hosp Pharm Sci*. 2009; 15:28–35.

2797. Donnelly RF. Physical compatibility and chemical stability of ketamine-morphine mixtures in polypropylene syringes. *Can J Hosp Pharm*. 2009; 62:28–33.

2798. Walker S, Iazzetta J, Law S. Extended stability of pantoprazole for injection in 0.9% sodium chloride or 5% dextrose at 4 °C and 23 °C. *Can J Hosp Pharm*. 2009; 62:135–41.

2799. Ensom MYY, Decarie D, Leung K, et al. Stability of hydromorphone-ketamine solutions in glass bottles, plastic syringes, and IV bags for pediatric use. *Can J Hosp Pharm*. 2009; 62:112–8.

2800. Pourroy B, Bausset EM, Boulamery A, et al. Incompatibility of imipenem-cilastatin and amoxicillin. *Am J Health-Syst Pharm*. 2009; 66:1253–4.

2801. Psathas P, Gilmor TP, Schaufelberger DE, et al. Stability of high and low concentrations of doripenem (500 mg) for injection in representative infusion fluids and containers. *ASHP Summer Meeting Poster*. Jun 2009.

2802. Gole DJ, Ilias J, Vermeersch H, et al. Stability of ceftobiprole for injection (500 mg) in representative infusion fluids and containers. *ASHP Summer Meeting Poster*. Jun 2009.

2803. Newton DW, Driscoll DF. Calcium and phosphate compatibility: revisited again. *Am J Health-Syst Pharm*. 2008; 65:73–80.

2804. Eroles AA, Bafalluy IM, Arnaiz JAS. Stability of docetaxel diluted to 0.3 to 0.9 mg/mL with 0.9% sodium chloride injection and stored in polyolefin or glass containers. *Am J Health-Syst Pharm*. 2009; 66:1565–8.

2805. Eiden C, Philibert L, Bekhtari K, et al. Physicochemical stability of oxaliplatin in 5% dextrose injection in polyvinyl chloride, polyethylene, and polypropylene infusion bags. *Am J Health-Syst Pharm*. 2009; 66:1929–33.

2806. Donnelly RF. Stability of aseptically prepared tazocin solutions in polyvinyl chloride bags. *Can J Hosp Pharm*. 2009; 62:226–31.

2807. Galanti L, Lebitassy MP, Hecq JD, et al. Long-term stability of 5-fluorouracil in 0.9% sodium chloride after freezing, microwave thawing, and refrigeration. *Can J Hosp Pharm*. 2009; 62: 34–8.

2808. Crandon JL, Sutherland C, Nicolau DP. Enhanced room temperature (RT) stability of doripenem (DOR) within two infusion devices. *Infectious Disease Society of America Meeting Poster*. Oct 2009.

2809. Crandon JL, Sutherland C, Nicolau DP. Stability of doripenem in polyvinyl chloride bags and elastomeric pumps. *Am J Health-Syst Pharm*. 2010; 67:1539–44.

2810. Almoazen H, Bhattacharjee H, Samsa AC, et al. Stability of mesna in ReadyMed infusion devices. *Ann Pharmacother*. 2010; 44:224–5.

2811. Athanapoulos A, Hecq JD, Vanbeckbergen D, et al. Long-term stability of tramadol chlorhydrate and metoclopramide hydrochloride in dextrose 5% polyolefin bag at 4 °C. *J Oncol Pharm Pract*. 2009; 15:195–200.

2812. Ikesue H, Vermuelen LC, Hoke R, et al. Stability of cetuximab and panitumumab in glass vials and polyvinyl chloride bags. *Am J Health-Syst Pharm*. 2010; 67:223–6.

2813. Walker SE, Law S, Garland J, et al. Stability of norepinephrine solutions in normal saline and 5% dextrose in water. *Can J Hosp Pharm*. 2010; 63:113–8.

2814. Moriyama B, Henning SA, Jin H, et al. Physical compatibility of magnesium sulfate and sodium bicarbonate in a pharmacy-compounded hemofiltration solution. *Am J Health-Syst Pharm*. 2010; 67:562–5.

2815. Pascuet E, Donnelly RF, Garceau D, et al. Buffered lidocaine hydrochloride solution with and without epinephrine: stability in polypropylene syringes. *Can J Hosp Pharm*. 2009; 62: 375–80.

2816. He J, Figueroa DA, Tze-Peng L, et al. Stability of polymyxin B sulfate diluted in 0.9% sodium chloride injection and stored at 4 or 25 °C. *Am J Health-Syst Pharm*. 67:1191–4.

2817. Wear J, McPherson TB, Kolling WM. Stability of sodium bicarbonate solutions in polyolefin bags. *Am J Health-Syst Pharm*. 2010; 67:1026–9.

2818. Khondkar D, Chopra P, McArter JP, et al. Chemcial stability of hydromorphone hydrochloride in patient-controlled analgesia injector. *Int J Pharmaceut Compound*. 2010; 14:160–4.

2819. Walker SE, Iazetta J, Law S, et al. Stability of commonly used antibiotic solutions in an elastomeric infusion device. *Can J Hosp Pharm*. 2010; 63:212–4.

2820. Baker DS, Waldrop B, Arnold J. Compatibility and stability of cefotaxime, vancomycin, and ciprofloxacin in antibiotic solutions containing heparin. *Int J Pharmaceut Compound*. 2010; 14:346–9.

2821. Kumar A, Mann HJ. Visual compatibility of oritavancin diphosphate with selected coadministered drugs during simulated Y-site administration. *Am J Health-Syst Pharm*. 2010; 67: 1640–4.

2822. Rolin C, Jecq JD, Vanbeckbergen DF, et al. Stability of ondansetron and dexamethasone infusion upon refrigeration. *Ann Pharmacother*. 2011; 45:130–1.

2823. Strong DK, Decarie D, Ensom MHH. Stability of levothyroxine in sodium chloride for IV administration. *Can J Hosp Pharm*. 2010; 63:437–43.

2824. Cote D, Lok CE, Battistella M, et al. Stability of trisodium citrate and gentamicin solution for catheter locks after storage in plastic syringes at room temperature. *Can J Hosp Pharm*. 2010; 63:304–11.

2825. Schutz L, Elder E, Jones K, et al. Stability of sodium nitroprusside and sodium thiosulfate 1:10 intravenous admixture. *Hosp Pharm*. 2010; 45:779–84.

2826. Singh BN, Dedhiya MG, DiNunzio J, et al. Compatibility of ceftaroline fosamil for injection with selected drugs during simulated Y-site administration. *Am J Health-Syst Pharm*. 2011; 68:2163-9.

2827. Amri A, Ben Achour A, Chachaty E, et al. Microbiology and physicochemical stability of oxycodone hydrochloride solutions for patient-controlled delivery systems. *J Pain Symptom Manage*. 2010; 40:87–94.

2828. Tsiouris M, Ulmer M, Yurcho JF, et al. Stability and compatibility of reconstituted caspofungin in select elastomeric infusion devices. *Int J Pharmaceut Compound*. 2010; 14:436–9.

2829. Tennant D (Senior Medical Information Specialist, Hospira, Inc., Lake Forest, IL): Personal communication; 2011 Mar 22.

2830. Housman ST, Tessier PR, Nicolau DP, et al. Physical compatibility of telavancin with select intravenous drugs during simulated Y-site administration. *Am J Health-Syst Pharm*. in press.

INDEX

Nonproprietary drug names appear in **bold** type and trade names in regular type.